Online Supplements

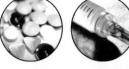

O9-AIC-255

- 500 NCLEX Review Questions
- Nursing Care Plans
- Audio Glossary
- Category Catchers
- Medication Errors Checklists
- IV Therapy Checklists

- Calculators
- Frequently Asked Questions
- Content Updates
- Supplemental Resources
- Answers to Case Studies and Critical Thinking Activities

Animations*

- Acute Myocardial Infarction
- Adenosine Infusion, Cardiac Effects
- Agonists/Antagonists
- Aldosterone Regulation Mechanism
- Amiodarone Treatment for Ventricular Tachycardia
- Amiodarone, Antidarrhythmic Drug; Treatment of Ventricular Fibrillation
- Antibiotics
- Antivirals
- Atropine
- Atropine Therapy for Sinus Bradycardia
- Autonomic Neurotransmitters
- Beta Blockers
- Calcium Channel Blockers
- Cancer Treatment: Chemotherapy
- Cholesterol-Lowering Medications
- Corticosteroids
- Diltiazem Injection, Cardiac Effects
- Distribution: Fat- vs. Water-Soluble Drugs
- Diuretics
- Dopamine Release
- Drug Movement through the Body
- Epinephrine

- Epinephrine and CPR
- Furosemide
- Half-Life of Intravenously Administered Ampicillin
- Heparin for Acute Coronary Syndrome
- Heparin for Atrial Fibrillation
- Impact of Surface Area
- Infusion
- Insulin Function
- Intravenous Antibiotic Therapy
- IV Fluid Administration
- Mix-O-Vials
- Mixing Two Medications in One Pre-Filled Cartridge and the Second Medication Is Available in a Vial
- Mixing Two Medications in One Syringe from One Vial and One Ampule
- Mixing Two Medications in One Syringe from Two Vials
- Normal Electrophysiology
- NSAID Treatment for Vasculitis
- Opiate Intoxication
- Overview of Pharmacokinetics: Oral Administration

- Palpitations
- Passive Diffusion
- Passive Transport
- Patient Noncompliance
- Pharmacokinetic Profiles: Normal, Renal Failure, and Hemodialysis
- Procedure for Drawing up Medication from an Ampule
- Procedure for Withdrawing Medication from a Vial
- Procedure to Insert a Pre-Filled Cartridge with Needle into the Carpuject Syringe
- Receptor Interaction
- Renin-Angiotensin in Control of Blood Pressure
- Thrombolytic Drugs; Clot Dissolving Drugs
- Thyroid Release
- Type 1 Diabetes
- Type 2 Diabetes
- Vaccination

*Selected pharmacology animations prepared by Ed Tessier, PharmD, MPH, BCPS.

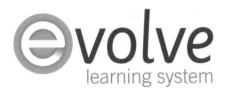

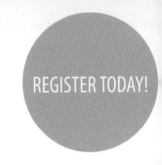

To access your Student Resources, visit:

http://evolve.elsevier.com/Lilley

Evolve Student Learning Resources for Lilley: Pharmacology and the Nursing Process, sixth edition, offers the following features:

- ## Prepare for Class, Clinical, or Lab
  Animations, Nursing Care Plans, Audio Glossary, Category Catchers (handouts with need-to-know information about various drug categories), Medication Errors Checklists, IV Therapies Checklists, Calculators, Frequently Asked Questions, Content Updates

- ## Prepare for Exams
  Review Questions for the NCLEX® Examination—500 questions with rationales help you review and apply content and prepare for the NCLEX® Examination!

- ## Additional Resources
  Supplemental Resources, Answers to Case Studies and Critical Thinking Activities, Appendixes

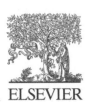

ELSEVIER

Pharmacology
and the NURSING
PROCESS

edition **6**

Pharmacology
and the NURSING
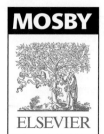 ## PROCESS

With Study Skills content by

Diane Savoca
Coordinator of Student Transition
St. Louis Community College at Florissant Valley
St. Louis, Missouri

With special thanks to

Richard E. Lake, BS, MS, MLA
For his contribution to the first edition Study Skills content

Linda Lane Lilley, RN, PhD
University Professor and Associate Professor Emeritus
School of Nursing
Old Dominion University
Virginia Beach, Virginia

Shelly Rainforth Collins, PharmD
Coordinator of Clinical Pharmacy Services
Chesapeake Regional Medical Center
Chesapeake, Virginia
President
Drug Information Consultants
Chesapeake, Virginia

Scott Harrington, PharmD
Independent Drug Information Consultant
Tucson, Arizona

Julie S. Snyder, MSN, RN-BC
Adjunct Faculty
School of Nursing
Old Dominion University
Norfolk, Virginia

MOSBY

ELSEVIER

3251 Riverport Lane
St. Louis, MO 63043

PHARMACOLOGY AND THE NURSING PROCESS, SIXTH EDITION   ISBN: 978-0-323-05544-4

Notice

Knowledge and best practice in this field are constantly changing. As new research and experience broaden our knowledge, changes in practice, treatment and drug therapy may become necessary or appropriate. Readers are advised to check the most current information provided (i) on procedures featured or (ii) by the manufacturer of each product to be administered, to verify the recommended dose or formula, the method and duration of administration, and contraindications. It is the responsibility of the practitioner, relying on their own experience and knowledge of the patient, to make diagnoses, to determine dosages and the best treatment for each individual patient, and to take all appropriate safety precautions. To the fullest extent of the law, neither the Publisher nor the [Editors/Authors] [delete as appropriate] assumes any liability for any injury and/or damage to persons or property arising out of or related to any use of the material contained in this book.

The Publisher

Previous editions copyrighted 2007, 2005, 2001, 1999, and 1996

Library of Congress Cataloging-in-Publication Data
Pharmacology and the nursing process / Linda Lane Lilley . . . [et al.] ; with study skills content by Diane Savoca. -- 6th ed.
        p. ; cm.
   Rev. ed. of: Pharmacology and the nursing process / Linda Lane Lilley, Scott Harrington, Julie S. Snyder. 5th ed. c2007
   Includes bibliographical references and index.
   ISBN 978-0-323-05544-4 (pbk. : alk. paper) 1. Pharmacology. 2. Nursing. I. Lilley, Linda Lane. II. Savoca, Diane. III. Lilley, Linda Lane. Pharmacology and the nursing process.
   [DNLM: 1. Pharmacology--Nurses' Instruction.   2. Drug Therapy--Nurses' Instruction.
3. Pharmaceutical Preparations--administration & dosage--Nurses' Instruction.   QV 4 P5363 2011]
   RM301.L466 2011
   615'.1--dc22

                                2009047493

Acquisitions Editor: Kristin Geen
Developmental Editor: Jamie Horn
Editorial Assistant: Jennifer Palada
Publishing Services Manager: Jeff Patterson
Senior Project Manager: Clay Broeker
Design Direction: Teresa McBryan

Printed in Canada

Last digit is the print number: 9   8   7   6   5   4   3   2   1

About the Authors

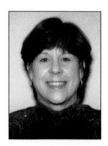

Linda Lane Lilley, RN, PhD

Linda Lilley received her diploma from Norfolk General School of Nursing, her BSN from the University of Virginia, her Master of Science (Nursing) from Old Dominion University, and her PhD in Nursing from George Mason University. As an Associate Professor Emeritus and University Professor at Old Dominion University, her teaching experience in nursing education spans over 25 years, including almost 20 years at Old Dominion University. Linda's teaching expertise includes drug therapy and the nursing process, adult nursing, physical assessment, fundamentals in nursing, oncology nursing, nursing theory, and trends in health care. The awarding of the University's most prestigious title of University Professor reflects her teaching excellence as a tenured faculty member. She has also been a two-time university nominee for the State Council of Higher Education in Virginia award for excellence in teaching, service, and scholarship. While at Old Dominion University, Linda mentored and taught undergraduate and graduate students as well as registered nurses returning for their BSN. She continues to serve as a member on dissertation committees with the College of Health Sciences. Since retirement in 2005, Linda has continued to be active in nursing, with membership and involvement in the American Nurses Association, Virginia Nurses Association, Sigma Theta Tau International, Phi Kappa Phi, and other professional organizations. Linda's research interests include the identification of factors affecting recruitment and retention of minority students in baccalaureate schools of nursing. Dr. Lilley's professional service varies, having served as a consultant with school nurses in the city of Virginia Beach, a member on the City of Virginia Beach's Health Advisory Board, and currently a member of the City of Virginia Beach's Community Health Advisory Board. Linda also served as an appointed member on the national advisory panel on medication errors prevention with the U.S. Pharmacopeia in Rockville, Maryland. She continues to educate nursing students and professional nurses about drug therapy and the nursing process. She also speaks to various groups about safe medication use in the elderly, humor and healing, and grief and loss.

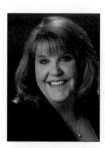

Shelly Rainforth Collins, PharmD

Shelly Rainforth Collins received her Doctor of Pharmacy degree from the University of Nebraska, College of Pharmacy in 1985, with High Distinction. She then completed a clinical pharmacy residency at Memorial Medical Center of Long Beach in Long Beach California. She worked as a pediatric clinical pharmacist, neonatal specialist, at Memorial Medical Center before moving to Mobile, Alabama. She was the Assistant Director of Clinical Pharmacy Services at Mobile Infirmary Medical Center. She currently serves as the Coordinator of Clinical Pharmacy Services at Chesapeake Regional Medical Center in Chesapeake, Virginia. Her practice focuses on developing and implementing clinical pharmacy services as well as medication safety and Joint Commission medication management standards and national patient safety goals. She also works as staff pharmacist at Chesapeake Regional Medical Center. She is president

of Drug Information Consultants, a business offering consultation and expert witness review for attorneys on medical malpractice cases. Shelly was awarded the Clinical Pharmacist of the Year Award in 2007 from the Virginia Society of Healthsystem Pharmacists. She led a multidisciplinary team that won the Clinical Achievement of the Year Award from George Mason University School of Public Health in 2007 for promoting safety with narcotics in patients with sleep apnea. This program has also received national recognition. She was awarded the Service Excellence Award from Chesapeake Regional Medical Center. Shelly's professional affiliations include the American Society of Healthsystem Pharmacists and the Virginia Society of Healthsystem Pharmacists.

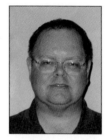

Scott Harrington, PharmD

Scott Harrington received his Associate of Science in Pharmacy Technology with High Honors from Pima Community College, Tucson, Arizona, in 1991. He then worked as both an outpatient and inpatient pharmacy technician while completing his Doctor of Pharmacy degree at the University of Arizona College of Pharmacy, which he received in 1997. He then completed two postdoctoral residency training programs. The first was a specialty residency in Pharmacocybernetics at Creighton University in Omaha, Nebraska, which he completed in 1998. The second was an additional specialty residency in Drug Information and Pharmaceutical Informatics at the University of California—San Francisco Medical Center and First DataBank in San Bruno, California, which he completed in 1999. Since that time he has worked in a variety of settings, including outpatient retail pharmacy where he also compounded customized prescriptions. He has since worked in hospital pharmacy and has served as a proofreader and content reviewer for Elsevier since 1999. He is now Director of Pharmacy for Northern Cochise Community Hospital in Willcox, Arizona, and most recently a staff pharmacist for Walgreens Pharmacy. Scott also regularly offers public education regarding medication use in mental illness during public outreach support groups at the office of the National Alliance for the Mentally Ill of Southern Arizona in Tucson. Scott's professional affiliations include the American Society of Health-System Pharmacy, the American Society for Consultant Pharmacists, the American Pharmacists Association, the Society for Technical Communicators, the American Medical Informatics Association, and the American College of Clinical Pharmacy. Scott is also a member of American MENSA.

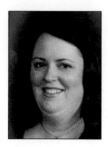

Julie S. Snyder, MSN, RN-BC

Julie Snyder received her diploma from Norfolk General Hospital School of Nursing and her BSN and MSN from Old Dominion University. After working in medical-surgical nursing for over 10 years, she began working in nursing staff development and community education. After 8 years, she transferred to teaching in a school of nursing, and since then she has taught fundamentals of nursing, pharmacology, physical assessment, gerontologic nursing, and adult medical-surgical nursing. She has been certified by the ANCC in Nursing Continuing Education and Staff Development and currently holds ANCC certification in Medical-Surgical Nursing. She is a member of Sigma Theta Tau International and was inducted into Phi Kappi Phi as Outstanding Alumni for Old Dominion University. She has worked for Elsevier as a reviewer and ancillary writer since 1997. Julie's professional service has included serving on the Virginia Nurses' Association Continuing Education Committee, serving as Educational Development Committee chair for the Epsilon Chi chapter of Sigma Theta Tau, serving as an item writer for the ANCC, working with a regional hospital educators' group, and serving as a consultant on various projects for local hospital education departments.

Contributors and Reviewers

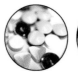

CONTRIBUTORS

Tom Lynch, PharmD, BCPS
Associate Professor
Department of Family and Community Medicine
Eastern Virginia Medical School
Norfolk, Virginia
Chapter 32

Timothy McGuire, PharmD, BCOP, FCCP
Associate Professor
University of Nebraska College of Pharmacy
Omaha, Nebraska
Chapters 47 and 48

Stephanie C. Butkus, MSN, RN, CPNP, CLC
Assistant Professor, Division of Nursing
Kettering College of Medical Arts
Kettering, Ohio
NCLEX Review Questions, Category Catchers, Medication Errors Checklists, and IV Therapy Checklists on the Evolve website

REVIEWERS

JoAnn Acierno, MSN, RN
Assistant Professor
Baccalaureate Nursing
Clarkson College
Omaha, Nebraska

Jan Belden, MSN, APRN, BC
Pain and Palliative Medicine Nurse Practitioner
Advanced Practice Nursing
Loma Linda University Medical Center
Loma Linda, California

Billie E. Blake, RN, BSN, MSN, EdD
Professor of Nursing
Nursing Education
St. John's River Community College
Palatka, Florida

Jacqueline L. Rosenjack Burchum, DNSc, APRN, BC, FNP
Assistant Professor
College of Nursing
University of Tennessee Health Science Center
Memphis, Tennessee

Teresa Burckhalter, MSN, RN, BC
Nursing Faculty
Technical College of the Lowcountry
Beaufort, South Carolina

Daniel Burfeind, RN, DNC
Nurse Educator
Amerisource Bergen ICS
Cookstown, New Jersey

Cynthia Carnes, PharmD, PhD
Associate Professor of Pharmacy and Biophysics
College of Pharmacy
Ohio State University
Columbus, Ohio

Sally Gaines, MSN, RN
Nursing Instructor
West Texas A&M University
Canyon, Texas

Susie M. Huyer, RN, MSN, CHPN
Administrator
Heartland Hospice
Fairfax, Virginia
Online Nursing Faculty
University of Phoenix
Phoenix, Arizona

Julie Kendall, MSN, RNC, WHNP, LCCE
Professor, Associate Degree Nursing
North Harris College
Houston, Texas

Ujjaini Khanderia, MS, PharmD
Clinical Associate Professor of Pharmacy
University of Michigan
Ann Arbor, Michigan

Catherine Lein, MS, APRN, BC
Assistant Professor/Nurse Practitioner
College of Nursing
Michigan State University
East Lansing, Michigan

Tom Lynch, PharmD, BCPS
Associate Professor
Department of Family and Community Medicine
Eastern Virginia Medical School
Norfolk, Virginia

Mary E. Malone, RN, BSN, BTh, MA, MSN
Professor of Nursing
Jefferson Community and Technical College
Louisville, Kentucky

Joan C. Martin, RN, MN, BSN
Assistant Professor of Nursing, Coordinator of the RN B(s)N Program
Department of Nursing
University of Central Missouri
Warrensburg, Missouri

Tina Mitchell Martin, RN, PhD
Associate Professor, School of Nursing
Associate Professor, Department of Neurology
University of Mississippi Medical Center
Jackson, Mississippi

Dottie Mathers, MSN, RN
Associate Professor of Nursing
Pennsylvania College of Technology
Williamsport, Pennsylvania

Dorothy Upson McCabe, RN, MS, MEd
Director, Divisions of Nursing and Health and Safety
Massachusetts Nurses Association
Canton, Massachusetts

Timothy McGuire, PharmD, BCOP, FCCP
Associate Professor
University of Nebraska College of Pharmacy
Omaha, Nebraska

Tara McMillan-Queen, RN, BSN, MN, ANP, GNP
Nursing Faculty
Mercy School of Nursing
Charlotte, North Carolina

Joy L. Meier, PharmD, PA
Pharmacoeconomics Pharmacist and Data Mart Manager
Department of Veterans Affairs
Northern California Health Care System
Martinez, California
Adjunct Associate Professor
Samuel Merritt College Physician Assistant Program
Oakland, California

Patricia Ann Montano, MS, RN, CPHQ, PhD (c)
Instructor of Nursing
New York Institute of Technology
Old Westbury, New York

Mariann M. Montgomery, RN, MSN
Assistant Professor of Nursing
School of Nursing
Kent State University Tuscarawas
New Philadelphia, Ohio

Diane Muckenhirn, MSN, RN, CNP
Hutchinson Medical Center
Hutchinson, Minnesota

Marianne Murray, BSN, RN-C
Faculty Member
Department of Professional Nursing
Baptist School of Health Professions
San Antonio, Texas

LaDonna Northington, DNS, RN
Associate Professor of Nursing
University of Mississippi
Jackson, Mississippi

Dan Ostrowski, RPh, MS
Infectious Disease Pharmacist
Chesapeake General Hospital
Chesapeake, Virginia

Randolph E. Regal, BS, PharmD
Clinical Pharmacist/Clinical Assistant Professor
Adult Internal Medicine
University of Michigan Hospital/College
   of Pharmacy
Ann Arbor, Michigan

Nancy C. Robbins, CFNP, CDE
Family Nurse Practitioner
Virginia Beach Family Practice
Sentara Healthcare
Virginia Beach, Virginia

Susan A. Sandstrom, MSN, RN, BC, CNE
Associate Professor in Nursing
College of Saint Mary
Omaha, Nebraska

Anna Sanford, RN, ANP, MSN
Associate Professor
Northern Michigan University
Marquette, Michigan

Stephen M. Setter, PharmD, DVM, CDE, CGP, FASCP
Associate Professor of Pharmacotherapy
Washington State University
Spokane, Washington

Virginia Shaw, MSN, RN
Assistant Professor
University of Texas Health
Science Center at San Antonio School of Nursing
San Antonio, Texas

Robert F. Shaw, PharmD, MPH
Clinical Pharmacy Specialist/Assistant Professor
University of Iowa College of Pharmacy/Iowa
   City VA Medical Center
Iowa City, Iowa

Brenda K. Shelton, MS, RN, CCRN, AOCN
Clinical Nurse Specialist
Sidney Kimmel Comprehensive Cancer Center
   at Johns Hopkins
Johns Hopkins Hospital
Baltimore, Maryland

Jennifer J. G. Steffensmeier, PharmD
Inpatient Clincial Pharmacy Specialist/Assistant
   Professor
University of Iowan College of Pharmacy
Iowa City, Iowa

Mavis M. TeSlaa, MSN, BSN, CRRN
Assistant Professor
Allen College
Waterloo, Iowa

Lindsay Vogel, MSN, RN
Assistant Professor
Allen College
Waterloo, Iowa

Valerie Warner, MS, RN
Professor of Nursing
College of Southern Idaho
Twin Falls, Idaho

Linda Wilson, RN, PhD, CPAN, CAPA, BC, CNE
Assistant Professor
College of Nursing and Health Professions
Drexel University
Philadelphia, Pennsylvania

Preface

Now in its sixth edition, *Pharmacology and the Nursing Process* provides the most current and clinically relevant information in an appealing, understandable, and practical format. The accessible size, readable writing style, and full-color design are ideal for today's busy nursing student. This text takes a unique approach to the study of pharmacology by presenting study skills content that will help students understand and learn the particularly demanding subject of pharmacology. Each part begins with a Study Skills Tips section, which features a discussion of researched and proven study skills and applies the discussion to the content in that part. Students are encouraged to use research-based study skills to enhance their study of pharmacology and nursing.

MARKET RESEARCH

This text incorporates many suggestions from focus group participants composed of nursing instructors from 2-, 3-, and 4-year degree programs in Chicago, Philadelphia, and Los Angeles. The focus groups assessed changes that have occurred in the teaching of pharmacology and determined what was needed to better teach pharmacology to nursing students. Based on faculty descriptions of their courses and students, these general recommendations were made:
- Accommodate the reading styles and abilities of the growing number of nontraditional nursing students.
- Increase the use of tables, boxes, illustrations, graphics, and other visually oriented approaches.
- Use color to increase interest and highlight important drug interactions and processes.

We have taken a truly collaborative approach with this text. The concerns raised by faculty members in market research have been addressed, as have additional improvements suggested by faculty members who served as reviewers or consultants, either formally or informally, throughout the manuscript's development and by the authors and editors of this text.

ORGANIZATION

This book includes 58 chapters presented in 10 parts and organized by body system. The 10 concepts chapters in Part 1 lay a solid foundation for the subsequent drug units and address the following topics:
- Study skills tips applied to learning pharmacology
- The nursing process and drug therapy
- Pharmacologic principles
- Life span considerations related to pharmacology
- Cultural, legal, and, ethical considerations
- Gene therapy and pharmacogenomics
- Preventing and responding to medication errors
- Patient education and drug therapy
- Over-the-counter drugs and herbal and dietary supplements

- Substance abuse
- Photo atlas of drug administration techniques, including over 100 illustrations and photographs

Parts 2 through 10 present pharmacology and nursing management in a traditional body systems/drug function framework. This approach facilitates learning by grouping functionally related drugs and drug groups. It provides an effective means to integrate the content into medical-surgical or adult health nursing courses or for teaching pharmacology in a separate course.

The 48 drug chapters in these parts constitute the main portion of the book. Drugs are presented in a consistent format with an emphasis on drug groups and key similarities and differences among the drugs in each group. Each chapter is subdivided into two discussions, beginning with a brief review of anatomy and physiology and pathophysiology of disease processes and a complete discussion of pharmacology, followed by a comprehensive yet succinct discussion of the nursing process. Pharmacology is presented for each drug group in a consistent format:
- Mechanism of Action and Drug Effects
- Indications
- Contraindications
- Adverse Effects (often including Toxicity and Management of Overdose)
- Interactions
- Dosages

Drug group discussions are followed by Drug Profiles, or brief narrative capsules of individual drugs in the class or group, including Pharmacokinetics tables for each drug. Key drugs, or prototypical drugs within a class, are identified with the ♦ symbol for easy identification. These individual drug profiles are followed by a Nursing Process discussion relating to the entire drug group. The nursing content is covered in the following functional nursing process format:
- Assessment
- Nursing Diagnoses
- Planning (including Goals and Outcome Criteria)
- Implementation
- Evaluation

At the end of each nursing process section is a Patient Teaching Tips box that summarizes key points for nursing students and/or nurses to include in the education of patients about their medications, with attention to how the drugs work, possible interactions, adverse effects, and other information related to the safe and effective use of the drug(s). The role of the nurse as patient educator and advocate continues to grow in importance in professional practice; thus there is emphasis of this key content in each chapter in this edition.

Additionally, each part begins with a Study Skills Tips section that presents a study skills topic and relates it to the unit being discussed. Topics include time management, note taking, studying, test taking, and others. This unique approach to teaching pharmacology is intended to aid students who find pharmacology difficult and to provide a tool that may prove beneficial throughout their nursing school careers. Coverage of this study skills content is limited to the beginning of each part so that instructors who choose not to require their students to read this material can easily eliminate it. However, this arrangement of content may be beneficial to faculty members who teach pharmacology through an integrated approach because it helps the student identify key content and concepts. This arrangement also facilitates location of content for either required or optional reading.

NEW TO THIS EDITION

Most importantly, the pharmacology and nursing content has been thoroughly revised to reflect the latest drug information and research. This includes:

- Critical Thinking Activities: Best Action questions that require critical thinking about how the nurse needs to prioritize
- NCLEX Examination Review Questions at the end of each chapter now include Alternate Item formats
- Expanded Case Studies, with one case study now provided for every chapter
- Expanded Pharmacokinetic Bridge to the Nursing Process sections that transition from the pharmacology content into the nursing process content by applying key pharmacokinetic information to nursing practice
- New "Anatomy, Physiology, and Disease Overview" and "Pharmacology Overview" headings introduce diseases and drug classes

FEATURES

This book includes several qualities that help set it apart from the rest, including:

- A focus on the role of prioritization in nursing care
- A strong focus on drug classes to help students acquire a better knowledge of how various drugs work in the body, allowing them to apply this knowledge to individual drugs
- Ease of readability throughout the text to make this difficult content more understandable

This book includes various pedagogic features that prepare the student for important content covered in each chapter and encourage review and reinforcement of that content. Chapter opener pedagogy includes the following:

- Learning Objectives
- e-Learning Activities boxes listing related content and exercises on the Evolve website
- Summary boxes listing the Drug Profiles in the chapter with page number references
- Glossaries of key terms with definitions and page number references (glossary terms are bolded in the narrative to emphasize this essential terminology)

The following features appear at the end of each chapter:

- Patient Teaching Tips related to drug therapy
- Points to Remember boxes summarizing key points
- NCLEX Examination Review Questions, with answers provided upside-down at the bottom of the section for quick and easy review
- Critical Thinking Activities, with answers provided on the Evolve website

Special features that appear throughout the text include the following:

- Cultural Implications boxes
- Herbal Therapies and Dietary Supplements boxes
- Legal and Ethical Principles boxes
- Life Span Considerations boxes for The Pediatric Patient and also The Elderly Patient
- Case Studies, with answers provided on the Evolve website, as well as in the Instructor's Manual
- Dosages tables listing generic and trade names, pharmacologic class, usual dosage ranges, and indications for the drugs
- Evidence-Based Practice boxes
- Laboratory Values Related to Drug Therapy boxes
- Preventing Medication Errors boxes

For a more comprehensive listing of the special features, please see the last page and inside back cover of the book.

Additional special features in this book include the following:

- A tear-out IV Compatibilities Chart that provides students with a portable reference on incompatible drugs administered intravenously
- A Bibliography listing references for more information

COLOR

The first edition of this book was the first full-color pharmacology text for nursing students. Faculty members suggested that color be used in both a functionally and visually appealing manner to more fully engage students in this typically demanding yet important content. Full color is used throughout to do the following:

- Highlight important content
- Illustrate how drugs work in the body in numerous anatomic and drug process color figures
- Improve the visual appearance of the content to make it more engaging and appealing to today's more visually sophisticated reader

We believe that the use of color in these ways significantly improves students' involvement and understanding of pharmacology.

SUPPLEMENTAL RESOURCES

A comprehensive ancillary package is available to students and instructors using *Pharmacology and the Nursing Process*. The following supplemental resources have been thoroughly revised for this edition and can significantly assist teaching and learning of pharmacology:

Study Guide

The carefully prepared student workbook includes the following:

- Student Study Tips that reinforce the study skills explained in the text and provide a "how to" guide to applying test-taking strategies
- Worksheets for each chapter with NCLEX-style multiple-choice questions (now with more application-based and alternate-item questions!), critical thinking and application questions, case studies, and other activities
- In-depth case studies followed by related critical thinking questions
- An increased focus on prioritization to help students identify the most important nursing diagnoses and interventions

- A special, updated Overview of Dosage Calculations with helpful tips for calculating doses, sample drug labels, practice problems, and a quiz
- Answers to all questions provided in the back of the book to enable self-study

Evolve Website

Located at http://evolve.elsevier.com/Lilley, the Evolve website for this book includes the following:

For students:

- 500 NCLEX Examination review questions
- 55 state-of-the-art animations (25 NEW!)
- An audio glossary that provides pronunciations for key terms in the book
- Printable Nursing Care Plans related to drug therapy and the nursing process
- Category Catcher handouts with the need-to-know information about each drug category
- Printable IV therapy and medication errors checklists that provide this crucial content in an on-the-go format
- Various calculators
- Frequently Asked Questions
- Content updates
- A variety of supplemental resources, including information on diagnostic drugs; a list of common formulas, weights, and equivalents; and more
- Answers to critical thinking activities and case studies from the book

For instructors:

- Course Management System
- Instructor's Manual that features overview summaries, key terms, learning objectives, chapter outlines, teaching strategies, critical thinking activities, additional resources listing, case studies, quizzes, and answer key
- ExamView Test Bank that features over 700 (100 NEW!) NCLEX-format test questions (including alternate item questions) with text page references, rationales, and answers coded for NCLEX Client Need category, nursing process, and cognitive level; the ExamView program allows instructors to create new tests; edit, add, and delete test questions; sort questions by NCLEX category, cognitive level, and nursing process step; and administer and grade online tests
- Image Collection with approximately 220 full-color images from the book for instructors to use in lectures
- PowerPoint Lecture Slides containing more than 2100 customizable text slides for instructors to use in lectures; the presentations include applicable illustrations from the Image Collection
- Audience Response Questions for i-Clicker and Other Systems (200 questions)
- Teaching Tips
- Access to all student resources listed above

Pharmacology Online

Pharmacology Online for *Pharmacology and the Nursing Process*, sixth edition (ISBN: 978-0-323-06889-5), is a dynamic, unit-by-unit online course resource that includes interactive self-study modules, a collection of interactive learning resources, and a media-rich library of supplemental resources:

- *Self-Study Modules* go beyond the basic principles of pharmacology, with animations and NCLEX examination-style questions to help you assess your understanding of pharmacology concepts.
- *Interactive Case Studies* immerse you in true-to-life scenarios that require you to make important choices in patient care and patient teaching.
- *"Roadside Assistance"* video clips use humor and analogy in a uniquely fun and engaging way to teach key concepts.
- Also includes Interactive Learning Activities, Flashcards, Practice Quizzes for the NCLEX Examination, and much more!

Evolve Select ebook ⊜ebooks

Spend less time searching and more time learning with electronic access to *Pharmacology and the Nursing Process*, sixth edition. With easy access from a computer or any internet browser, students can search across all of their Elsevier e-textbooks, paste important text and images from multiple sources into a custom document, make notes, highlights, and more. Please contact your Elsevier sales representative for more information, or visit http://evolve.elsevier.com/ebooks.

▌Acknowledgments

This book truly has been a collaborative effort. We wish to thank the instructors who provided input on an ongoing basis throughout the development of the previous editions. In addition, we would like to thank the following people: Rick Brady, Dottie Mathers, Chuck Dresner, Judith Myers, Ted Huff, Donald O'Connor, Linda Wendling, Ken Turnbough, Greg McVicar, Anthony Saranita, and Susan Orf. We thank Carolyn Duke and the Saint Louis University School of Nursing for their assistance and cooperation. Thanks also to Chesapeake Regional Medical Center for assistance with the fourth edition photo shoot.

We thank Kristin Geen and Jamie Horn for their contributions and support throughout the fourth, fifth, and sixth editions. We are also grateful to Jeff Patterson and Clay Broeker for very capably guiding the project through to publication and to Teresa McBryan for her effective design. Diane Savoca lent her study skills expertise and has updated the unique and appropriate feature for students, and for her collaboration we are most grateful. Finally, we thank Joe Albanese for his contributions to the first edition, Bob Aucker for his contributions to the first three editions of the book, and Scott Harrington for contributions through the latest edition.

Linda thanks her husband Les and daughter Karen for their constant support and encouragement. Long hours and time spent researching and writing has preempted time with family, but they have been there through all six editions. Linda wishes to dedicate this book to Les and Karen as they are her inspiration and constant support for all professional endeavors and personal accomplishments. The memory of Linda's parents, John and Thelma Lane, who passed away during the fourth edition, and in-laws, J.C. and Mary Anne Lilley, who passed away during the fifth and sixth editions, have continued to provide inspiration and a sense of pride in all her work. Students and graduates of Old Dominion

University School of Nursing have been eager to provide feedback and support, beginning with the class of 1990 and continuing through the class of 2005. Without their participation, the book would not have been so user-friendly and helpful to students beginning the study of drug therapy and subsequently applying this knowledge to nursing practice. Linda attributes her successes and accomplishments to a strong sense of purpose, faith, family and appreciation for the light-hearted side of life. To Jibby Baucom, Linda offers many thanks because without her recommendation to Mosby, Inc., the book would never have been developed. Robin Carter, Kristin Geen, and Jamie Horn have been constant resources and more than just editors with Elsevier; they have been sources of strength and encouragement. Their excellent work ethic, positivity, and calming natures will be forever appreciated. The fifth and six editions have also involved Clay Broeker, who has been a tremendous resource with editorial issues; his contributions to this edition have been strong and forward-thinking. Elsevier has shared some of its best employees with Linda beginning with day one of the first edition; for that, Linda is most thankful.

Shelly would like to thank Linda Lilley, Julie Snyder, Jamie Horn, and Kristin Geen for the opportunity to be part of this wonderful project .It is truly an honor to be associated with all of you and with this awesome book. I never envisioned my career would take me down the path as an author, but the experience has proven to be more than rewarding, albeit a little overwhelming at times. An extra special thanks to Julie Snyder, for recognizing my potential and for the numerous late night words of encouragement. Shelly would like to thank her parents, Charles and Rogene Rainforth of Hastings, Nebraska. You have always been there with unconditional love and support, and for that I am forever grateful. You have taught me so many things, most importantly the importance of the work ethic. Although we may be separated by distance, we are always close at heart. Shelly would also like to thank the talented pharmacy staff at Chesapeake Regional Medical Center. Thanks for the curbside consults. I am proud to not only call you my colleagues, but also my friends. Shelly would also like to thank the pharmacists at Long Beach Memorial Medical Center, for the knowledge you imparted during my residency training. I think I finally have captured the elusive "clinical experience." Last but certainly not least, Shelly would like to thank her daughter, Kristin, the best daughter anyone could wish for. Thanks for putting up with microwave dinners and understanding when mom had to "work." Thanks for sharing my passion for the finer things in life; you give me the motivation to keep working! Life may not always be easy, but with hard work and perseverance you can achieve anything. You have a very bright future, and I love watching the amazing woman you are becoming. I am very proud of you! Finally, I dedicate my portion of this edition to my nephew Chris Rainforth, an up-and-coming pharmacy student at Creighton University in Omaha, Nebraska. Even though you chose the "other school," I hope the profession is as rewarding and challenging for you as it has been for me.

Scott extends his thanks to his fellow staff members at Northern Cochise Community Hospital. Thank you for all of your consultations and questions that continuously help make me a better pharmacist. Thanks to both hospital staff and citizens of Willcox and Tucson, Arizona, as well as family and friends, who have been kind enough to show interest in this project and ask me how it was coming along. Your interest and enthusiasm helped me down the long road to completion. Thank you also to the staff and volunteers of the National Alliance for the Mentally Ill of Southern Arizona (NAMISA), where I continue to grow and learn through volunteer work, for your continued support and encouragement for this and other endeavors and for allowing me to be a part of your team as well. Very special thanks to my dear friend Gerry Bovell, who allowed me to work on this project for many months at his home and congratulated me as I finished each chapter. Both he and my other friend Ed Thorpe also sometimes brought me food. Thanks to both of them for their support and encouragement. Lastly, I offer heartfelt thanks to my mother and father Bonnie and John Harrington who granted me this life to begin with. My mother has an amazing heart and my father has an amazing mind. I believe that I was fortunate enough to inherit some of the best of both.

Julie thanks her husband, Jonathan, her daughter Emily, and her parents, Willis and Jean Simmons, for their unfailing support and encouragement. They were all patient despite the long hours working on revisions. Thanks also to those who participated in the fourth edition photo shoot. The pharmacists at Chesapeake Regional Medical Center have always been great resources. It has been a pleasure to work with Shelly Rainforth Collins on this new edition; thank you for all your hard work! Thanks also to Kristin Geen, Jamie Horn, and others at Elsevier for keeping the project organized and on track, as well as for providing all the support needed for such a project. Deep appreciation goes to Dr. Linda L. Lilley for her encouragement and mentoring over the years. Thanks also to each student who has provided feedback and comments on the text and study aids. Lastly, the support and encouragement of family and friends is vital to projects like this, so thanks and gratitude to all.

Finally, to those who teach, although your work may seem to go unnoticed or unappreciated, your impact will always be remembered in the accomplishments of your students. Your inspiration and motivation shape the future.

We always welcome comments from instructors and students who use this book so that we may continue to make improvements and be responsive to your needs in future editions. Please send any comments you may have in care of the publisher.

Contents

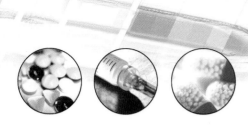

PART 1

Pharmacology Basics

STUDY SKILLS TIPS

Introduction to Study Skills Concepts　•　PURR　•　Pharmacology Basics

---

INTRODUCTION TO STUDY SKILLS CONCEPTS

What to study? When to study? How much to study? How to study? In the best of worlds, every student would have all the skills necessary to be effective in all academic areas. Unfortunately, many students do not know how to study effectively or have developed techniques that work well in some circumstances but not in others. The purpose of this Study Skills Tips is to introduce you to the steps to follow in learning text and maintaining focus on the appropriate material. This section also offers some specific examples for selected chapters in Part 1 to help you apply the study techniques and strategies discussed here.

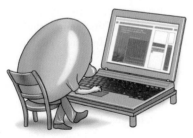

Extensive discussion of study skills, including how to manage time, take lecture notes, master the text, prepare for and take examinations, establish effective study groups, and develop vocabulary are presented in the Study Guide that accompanies this text. These tools are important to any student, but for students in challenging technical areas such as nursing and pharmacology, they become even more valuable. The techniques described here and in the Study Guide will not necessarily make learning easy, but they will help you achieve your goals as a student.

PURR

PURR is a handy mnemonic device representing a four-step process that will lead to mastery of material. These steps are as follows:
- Prepare
- Understand
- Rehearse
- Review

The PURR approach has positive and negative aspects. The negative is that it requires you to go through every chapter four times. The good news is that you will not actually *read* the chapter four times. You will only *go through* it four times. Only one of those times consists of a slow, careful, intensive reading. The other trips through the chapter are much quicker. The first time you go through the chapter it should take only 5 or 10 minutes. Each time you go through the chapter, you are processing the information in distinctly different ways. The PURR approach will enhance your learning, and if you use it from the first assignment on, you will find that it takes you less time than you were spending before you adopted the PURR approach to learn what you need.

Prepare

Reading the text, like any complex process, is not something to dive into without thought and planning. *Pharmacology and the Nursing Process* is organized to help you learn the material, but you have to take advantage of what the authors have done for you to facilitate this. Preparing to read means setting goals and objectives for your own learning, but the tools you need to help you do this are already in place. Look at the opening pages of any chapter in the text and you will see a standard structure.

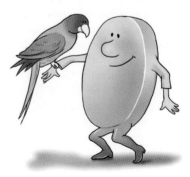

Every chapter begins with a **title.** Learn to use the title as the first step in preparing to learn. Chapter 4 is entitled "Cultural, Legal, and Ethical Considerations." This instantly identifies what the chapter is about. Do not start reading immediately; instead think about the title for a few seconds. Are there any unfamiliar terms? If your answer is "No," great. If it is "Yes," then you already have some focus for your reading, because you know you will need to learn the unfamiliar terms and their meanings.

The next feature of every chapter is the **objectives.** You need objectives for learning, and the authors have anticipated this. Read the objectives actively. Do not just look at the words; think about the objectives. Ask yourself the following questions: What do I already know about this material? How do these objectives relate to earlier assignments? How do they relate to objectives the instructor has given? The chapter objectives identify things you should be able to do after you have read the material. Do not wait until you have read the chapter to start trying to respond. *Prepare* means getting the brain engaged from the beginning. Studying the chapter objectives establishes a direction and purpose for your reading. This will enable you to maintain concentration and focus while you read.

Another feature in the opening pages of each chapter is the **glossary.** This is one of the most valuable tools the authors have provided. They know that there are many terms to learn and are giving you a head start on learning them. Spend a few minutes with the glossary. Notice the terms that are also used in the chapter objectives and are bolded in the text. Go back and look at the objectives and think about what you have learned from the glossary. As you study the glossary, look for shared root words, prefixes, or suffixes. If words share such common word elements, these words also have a shared meaning. Learning the meaning of common word elements can simplify the whole process of learning vocabulary. Perhaps you remember in elementary school being told to "look for the little words in the big word." This is essentially the same technique—one that worked then and one that will work now.

Now make a quick pass through the chapter or the assigned pages from the chapter. Focus on the text conventions, which are described later in this chapter. Look for anything that stands out in the chapter, such as boldfaced text, boxed material, and tables. This provides a quick overview of the chapter, which will make the next steps in the PURR process much more effective and efficient.

The **chapter headings** show the major points to be covered. Study them and notice the major headings (topics) and the subordinate headings (subtopics). They essentially provide a picture of the chapter, and using this picture is a fundamental step in preparing to read. As you read through the chapter headings, turn the topics and subtopics into a series of questions that you want to be able to answer when you finish reading. Think about the objectives and how these headings relate to them. Finally, in the headings devoted to specific classes of drugs, notice that there are elements that are common to every class. The last two headings are always "Implementation" and "Evaluation." This tells you that these are two common elements that you will be expected to know at the end of every chapter. The minutes you spend *preparing* will pay off in a big way when you start to read.

Preparing makes the whole approach to learning an active one. It may not make the chapters the most exciting reading you will ever do, but it will help you accomplish your personal learning objectives as well as those set by the authors.

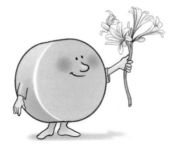

On-the-Run Action

Preparing is great to do during "found" time. It should not take more than 5 or 10 minutes. Time between classes, time spent waiting for the coffee water to boil, or any other small block of time that usually just slips away can be used to accomplish this step.

Understand

Now read the assignment. Go to your desk, the library, or wherever you have chosen for serious study. Reading the assignment is where all your preparation pays off. If you did the *Prepare* step earlier in the day, it is not a bad idea to spend a minute or two going through the chapter features again to get your focus. As you read the assignment, remember the chapter objectives and notice the chapter headings in the body of the chapter. As you read, rephrase the chapter headings as questions to help keep you focused on the task at hand. Because this is the first time you are really focusing on the concepts and the details, this is not the time to do any text notations. Read and, as you read, think. Terms from the glossary are repeated, and their meanings are often expanded and clarified in the body of the text. Pay attention to these terms as you read. Think about what they mean and how you would define them to someone else. Read for meaning. Read to *understand*. Do not read just to get to the end of the assignment. That is a passive action. Ask yourself questions. Analyze, respond, and react as you read.

Often, reading assignments are too long to be read with complete understanding in one session. If you find that your concentration is flagging or you do not remember anything you read on the previous page, it is time to take a break. All too often students have only one objective—to finish the assignment. You might be able to force yourself to continue reading, but you will not learn much. Mark your place and take a 5- or 10-minute break. Take a walk, read the daily comic strips, get a soda or a cup of coffee, and then go back to reading. When you come back to the assignment, spend the first 3 or 4 minutes reviewing. Look back at the previous chapter heading and think about what you were reading before the break. The chapter can be broken down into many small reading sessions, but it is critical that you not lose sight of the chapter as a whole. Spending these minutes in review may seem like time that could be better spent continuing with the reading, but this fast review will save time in the long run.

There is no quick way to read a chapter. You will not find an "on-the-run action" for this step because it cannot be done this way. However, if you do the *Prepare* step first, you will be surprised at how much more easily you get the reading done and how much more learning you have achieved in the process.

Rehearse

Rehearsing is the third step. It starts the process of consolidating your learning and establishing a basis for long-term memory. Rehearsal accomplishes two things. First, it helps you find out what you understand from the reading. Knowing what you know is really important. Second, it identifies what you do not understand, and this may be an even more

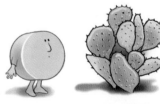

important ben... K... ...ot know before it comes

...*nderstand* steps comes
...should begin with the
...text to the beginning of
...begin to quiz yourself
...ur questions pertaining
...em to your satisfaction.
...both literal (asking for
...pter) and interpretive
...nd relationships). An
...apter 4 title might be,
...*l*, and *ethical?*" This
...you can satisfactorily
...g and answering ques-
...ning from short-term
...ery important to help
...ology contained in the
...sary to ask questions
...nd the relationships
...the chapter. An ex-
...the Chapter 4 title
...*al, legal,* and *ethical*
...etimes you will find
...the authors have an-
...the direct answer to
...formulate your own
...f information from
...ential for the chap-
...move on to the chapter objectives. Use the same process
here. Rephrase the objectives as questions and try to answer
them. Remember that the object of rehearsal is to reinforce what
you have learned and to identify areas where you need to spend
additional time (review).

Go to the glossary. Cover the definitions and try to define each
term in your own words. Another method is to cover the term and,
on the basis of the definition, name the term. Do not just memorize the definition, because you may find the information presented differently on an examination, and you will then be unable
to respond.

Now proceed to the chapter or assigned pages. The chapter
headings are the main tools for rehearsal. Apply the same question-
and-answer technique used for the title and objectives to test what
you may already know about the chapter content. Turn the headings into questions and answer them. Look at the text for boldfaced
and italicized items, lists, and other text conventions. These too can
become the basis for questions. The tables and diagrams should
also be used for this purpose. Keep in mind the importance of asking both literal and interpretive questions. Some of the questions
you ask yourself should also tie different topic headings together.
Ask yourself how topic A relates to topic B.

As you proceed through the chapter, do not worry if you cannot answer the questions you ask. As stated earlier, one of the
goals of the rehearsal process is to identify what you need to
spend more time on. If you can give no response to a particular
question, put a mark in the margin of the pertinent place in the

text to remind yourself to come back and spend more time on this
material, but move on at this point. Rehearsal should be a relatively quick procedure. Once you become accustomed to using
the PURR method, it should take no more than 15 or 20 minutes
to rehearse 15 pages after completing the *Prepare* and *Understand* steps.

As you reach the end of
the chapter, skim the *Implementation* and *Evaluation*
sections. Make sure that the
relationship between these
sections and the information
in the rest of the chapter is
clear. If you have questions
or concerns, note them in the
margins and ask your instruc-
tor to clarify these points. Although the objective is to master the
chapter content as an independent learner, sometimes it is essential to ask questions of the instructor to facilitate the process.

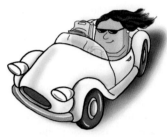

When to Rehearse

Ideally rehearsal should take place almost immediately after
you finish reading the material. Take a 10- to 15-minute break,
and then start the process. The longer the gap between reading
and rehearsal, the more you will forget and the longer it will
take to rehearse. If you are breaking down a reading assignment
into smaller segments, do the rehearsal for each segment before
you begin reading the new material. This helps maintain the
sense of continuity in the chapter. This seems like a lot of work
to do in a study session, but with practice it will go quickly and
you will be pleasantly surprised at the quality and quantity of
your learning.

Review

Review is the fourth and final step in the PURR process, and it is
an essential step. No matter how well you have learned material
in the preceding steps, forgetting will always occur. Reviewing is
the only way to store what you have learned in long-term memory. The good news is that, using the PURR approach, the review
can be done for small segments of material and can be accomplished relatively quickly.

How to Review

The basic review process is essentially the same as the rehearsal
process, with some limited rereading as the only difference.
When you cannot immediately answer a question, read the pertinent material again. *This does not mean you should read the entire chapter again.* Often the answer to the question will pop into
your mind after you have read only a few lines. When this happens, stop reading and go back to responding to your question.
The idea is to reread only as much material as is necessary to
make the answer clear. One or two words or one or two sentences
may trigger personal recall, but it may also take two or three
paragraphs for this to happen.

How Often to Review

How many times should you review material in this way? This
actually depends on many factors, such as the difficulty of the
material, the length of the assignment, and your personal back-

ground. Only you can determine how often you need to review, but there are some guidelines that will help you decide this for yourself.

First, consider the difficulty of the material. If it is very complex, contains many new terms and difficult concepts, and seems difficult to grasp, then you should review very frequently. On the other hand, if the material is straightforward and you are able to relate it well to what you have already learned, then less frequent reviews will serve to keep the material in your memory.

Second, consider how well the review went. If you had difficulty answering many questions to your satisfaction or had to do a lot of rereading, you should schedule another review soon (a day or two later at most).

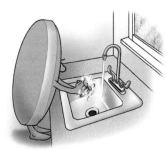

The success of each review session should be used to help you determine when to schedule another session. The review step is a means of monitoring the success of the learning process. If reviews go well, limited rereading is necessary, and you are able to give clear answers to your questions, then you can wait several days (4 or 5) before reviewing this material again. A mediocre review, more extensive rereading, and poor answers indicate that you should let only 2 or 3 days go by before reviewing the material again. If the review goes very poorly, you should plan to review the material again the next day. It is up to you to judge the success of each review and to decide how often you need to review. The nice thing about PURR is that it enables you to monitor your success and to regulate the learning process easily.

Techniques for Rehearsal and Review

Both rehearsal and review foster active learning, which helps you maintain interest in the material and strengthens your memory. For these benefits to occur, it is essential that the review and rehearsal processes be done orally. Talking to yourself is one way to accomplish this, but working with a study group is another and sometimes more interesting way to rehearse and review. Strategies for establishing and maintaining effective study groups can be found in the Study Guide that accompanies this text. You can find a short overview in the introduction to Part 3 of this text. Study groups are not for everyone. The key is to do what works for you. If studying alone produces the results you want, then continue. If not, you may want to try a study group.

When you ask questions and give your answers out loud, this forces you to think about the material. It helps you organize it and translate it into your own words. The object is not to memorize everything you have read but to understand and be able to explain it. Eventually you will need to answer questions on an examination. Framing questions as a part of the learning process is a way to anticipate examination questions. The more questions you ask yourself during study time, the more likely some of the questions on the examination will be ones you have asked yourself. When you work with a study group you have

several brains anticipating test questions. Further, by doing the rehearsal and review orally, you will find it easier to recall the answers during the examination, because this oral model requires more than just remembering seeing the material; you will actually be able to hear the rehearsed answers in your mind. As stated earlier, another advantage of performing the rehearsal and review processes orally is that it helps to identify what needs further study. When your oral answer is fragmentary, contains many "uhs," and is really disorganized, then you know that you need to devote more time to learning the given term, fact, or concept.

The PURR system may seem like a lot of work at first. The idea of going through a chapter four times understandably seems daunting. Add to this the need for several review sessions, and the first reaction is likely to be, "This won't work" or "I don't have the time to do this." Don't take that attitude. This system does work. It cultivates interest, aids concentration, fosters mastery of the material, and ensures long-term memory for the material, which is important not just for doing well on examinations but also for doing well as a nurse, when the safe care of patients at stake. The PURR system will work if you use it. It may take 3 or 4 weeks to get comfortable with the system, but if you keep at it, pretty soon it will become a good habit. After a while you will not be able to imagine studying in any other way.

Like all study systems, the PURR method is a model. As you use it, you may discover ways of changing it that work better for you. That is okay. Do not hesitate to make adjustments that better suit your learning style and strategies. Just remember as you start out that *Preparation, Understanding, Rehearsal,* and *Review* are solid learning principles and cannot be ignored.

Study skills tips are included on the pages at the beginning of each part of the book. These hints are directly applied to the content found within the chapters of the following unit.

PHARMACOLOGY BASICS

Prepare

As you begin to work with individual chapters, consider how the first step in the PURR system can be used to help you set a purpose and become an active learner.

Chapter 1 Objectives

Consider Objective 1 of Chapter 1: "List the five phases of the nursing process." Now turn the objective into a question: What are the five phases of the nursing process? Now move to Objective 2 and make it a question: What are the components of the assessment process for patients receiving medications, including collection and analysis of subjective and objective data? You might recognize that this question relates to Objective 1 because assessment is one phase of the nursing process. By putting Objective 2 into a question format you will begin to expand the focus of the first objective, and you will begin to concentrate on active learning with a clear purpose.

When you begin to read Chapter 1 you will discover that the five phases of the nursing process are repeated as topic headings, and you have the Objective 2 question on which to focus your reading. Begin now to develop the habit of applying this strategy to the objectives in every chapter assigned before you begin to read. Remember to look at the chapter headings at this point as well. It is amazing how much can be learned by using the text structures provided.

Vocabulary Development

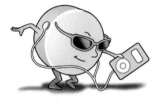

Turn to Chapter 2. Objective 1 makes an important point: "Define the common terms used in pharmacology." Success depends heavily on knowledge of the "language." The objective makes it clear that this chapter contains a number of terms that the author views as important to be mastered. This is only Chapter 2, and now is the time to begin to apply yourself to mastering the language of this content. Look at the glossary. There are six terms that share the common element *pharmaco*. Although each of these six words has a different meaning, the words have something in common. *Pharmaco* is an example of a group word. No matter what prefixes, group words, and/or suffixes are added to it, a part of the meaning of any word containing *pharmaco* will be "drug" or "medicine." Look up a word containing *pharmaco* in any dictionary and you will find that its definition pertains to "drug" or "medicine" in some way. Although you probably already knew that, it is always beneficial to start working on a new technique with something that is familiar. Look at four of the words that begin with *pharmaco*, and consider the rest of the word:

dynamics   genetics   gnosy   kinetics

What does each of these word parts mean? The meaning of *pharmacodynamics* is simply the combination of the meanings of *pharmaco* and *dynamics*. The definition, according to the glossary, begins "the study of the biochemical and physiologic inter-

actions of drugs." You could simply memorize this definition, which would seem to accomplish Objective 1. However, memorization does not always equal understanding. Try another approach. What does *dynamics* mean? Think about the word and relate it to your own experience and background. It appears to deal with movement or action. If you look it up in the dictionary, all the meanings given seem to relate in some fashion to the idea of motion and/or action. A simplistic definition of *pharmacodynamics* would be "drugs in action." Certainly this is not a technical or medical definition, but it contributes a great deal to an understanding of the definition provided in the glossary. This is the object of learning vocabulary. Do not memorize words without understanding. Apply a little thought and relate the term and definition in a way that makes the meaning personal for you. When you do that, you will find that you understand the glossary definition better, and your ability to retain the meaning will be significantly improved. This means that the test item asking you to select the definition for *pharmacodynamics* from a list of similar definitions will be much easier to answer, because you will remember action and movement and look for the choice that best represents that concept.

Apply this same strategy to the word part *genetics*. You already know what genetics means. Now you must determine how to connect that to the meaning in the text. After you have the definitions for *gnosy* and *kinetics,* you can apply the same procedure. When you have done this with all four word parts, you will discover that you will not need to spend a great amount of time trying to memorize esoteric definitions. You will have personalized the meanings. These meanings will stay with you much more readily than those learned by rote memorization. By the way, do you know what *biochemical* and *physiologic* mean? These terms are used in the glossary definition of *pharmacodynamics*. You need to know what they mean to fully understand *pharmacodynamics*.

The Nursing Process and Drug Therapy

OBJECTIVES

When you reach the end of this chapter, you should be able to do the following:

1 List the five phases of the nursing process.

2 Identify the components of the assessment process for patients receiving medications, including collection and analysis of subjective and objective data.

3 Discuss the process of formulating nursing diagnoses for patients receiving medications.

4 Identify goals and outcome criteria for patients receiving medications.

5 Discuss the evaluation process as it relates to the administration of medications and as reflected by goals and outcome criteria.

6 Develop a nursing care plan that is based on the nursing process as it relates to medication administration.

7 Briefly discuss the "Six Rights" associated with safe medication administration.

8 Discuss the professional responsibility and standards of practice for the professional nurse as related to the medication administration process.

9 Discuss the additional rights associated with safe medication administration.

e-Learning Activities

http://evolve.elsevier.com/Lilley

NCLEX Review Questions • Animations • Nursing Care Plans • Audio Glossary • Category Catchers • Medication Errors Checklists • IV Therapy Checklists • Calculators • Frequently Asked Questions • Content Updates • Supplemental Resources • Answers to Case Studies and Critical Thinking Activities

Glossary

Compliance Implementation or fulfillment of a prescriber's or care-giver's prescribed course of treatment or therapeutic plan by a patient. Also called *adherence.* (p. 8)

Goals Statements that are time specific and describe generally what is to be accomplished to address a specific nursing diagnosis. (p. 6)

Medication error Any preventable adverse drug event involving inappropriate medication use by a patient or health care professional; it may or may not cause the patient harm. (p. 14)

Noncompliance An informed decision on the part of the patient not to adhere to or follow a therapeutic plan or suggestion. Also called *nonadherence.* (p. 9)

Nursing process An organizational framework for the practice of nursing. It encompasses all steps taken by the nurse in caring for a patient: assessment, nursing diagnoses, planning (with goals and outcome criteria), implementation of the plan (with patient teaching), and evaluation. (p. 6)

Outcome criteria Descriptions of specific patient behaviors or responses that demonstrate meeting of or achievement of goals related to each nursing diagnosis. These statements, like goals, should be verifiable, framed in behavioral terms, measurable, and time specific. Outcome criteria are considered to be specific, whereas goals are broad. (p. 6)

Prescriber Any health care professional licensed by the appropriate regulatory board to prescribe medications. (p. 8)

• • •

OVERVIEW OF THE NURSING PROCESS

The **nursing process** is a well-established, research-supported framework for professional nursing practice. It is a flexible, adaptable, and adjustable five-step process consisting of assessment, nursing diagnoses, planning (including establishment of **goals** and **outcome criteria**), implementation (including patient education), and evaluation. As such, the nursing process ensures the delivery of thorough, individualized, and quality nursing care to patients, regardless of age, gender, medical diagnosis, or setting. Through use of the nursing process combined with knowledge and skills, the professional nurse will be able to develop effective solutions to meet patient's needs. The nursing process is usually discussed in nursing courses and/or textbooks that deal with the fundamentals of nursing practice, nursing theory, physical assessment, adult or pediatric nursing, and other nursing specialty areas. However, because of the importance of the nursing process in the care of patients, the process in all of its five phases is described in each chapter as it relates to specific drug groups or classifications.

Critical thinking is a major part of the nursing process and involves the use of the mind and thought processes to gather information and then develop conclusions, make decisions, draw inferences, and reflect upon all aspects of patient care. The elements of the nursing process address the physical, emotional, spiritual, sexual, financial, cultural, and cognitive aspects of a patient. Attention to these many aspects allows a more holistic approach to patient care. For example, a cardiologist may focus on cardiac functioning and pathology, a physical therapist on movement, and a chaplain on the spiritual aspects of patient care. However, it is the professional nurse who thinks critically about, processes, and incorporates all of these aspects and points of information about the patient and then uses this information to develop and coordinate patient care. Therefore, the nursing process remains a central process and framework for nursing care.

Box 1-1 provides a sample nursing care plan related to drug therapy and the nursing process. Other more specific nursing care plans are available online at *http://evolve.elsevier.com/Lilley*.

ASSESSMENT

During the initial assessment phase of the nursing process, data are collected, reviewed, and analyzed. Performing a comprehensive assessment allows the nurse to formulate a nursing diagnosis related to the patient's needs—for the purposes of this textbook, specifically needs related to drug administration. Information about the patient may come from a variety of sources, including the patient; the patient's family, caregiver, or significant other; and the patient's chart. Methods of data collection include interviewing, direct and indirect questioning, observation, medical

---

BOX 1-1   Sample Nursing Care Plan Related to Drug Therapy and the Nursing Process

This sample presents information useful for developing a nursing process–focused care plan for patients receiving medications. Brief listings and discussions of what should be contained in each phase of the nursing process are included. This sample may be used as a template for formatting nursing care plans in a variety of patient care situations. Only one nursing diagnosis is presented with each care plan at *http://evolve.elsevier.com/Lilley*.

Assessment
Objective Data
Objective data include information available through the senses, such as what is seen, felt, heard, and smelled. Among the sources of data are the chart, laboratory test results, reports of diagnostic procedures, health history, physical assessment, and examination findings. Examples of specific data are age, height, weight, allergies, medication profile, and health history.

Subjective Data
Subjective data include all spoken information shared by the patient, such as complaints, problems, or stated needs (e.g., patient complains of "dizziness, headache, vomiting, and feeling hot for 10 days").

Nursing Diagnoses
Once the assessment phase has been completed the nurse analyzes objective and subjective data about the patient and the drug and formulates nursing diagnoses. The following is an example of a nursing diagnosis statement: "Deficient knowledge related to lack of experience with medication regimen and second-grade reading level as an adult as evidenced by inability to perform a return demonstration and inability to state adverse effects to report to the prescriber." This statement of the nursing diagnosis can be broken down into three parts, as follows:
- Part 1—"Deficient knowledge." This is the statement of the human response of the patient to illness, injury, medications, or significant change. This can be an actual response, an increased risk, or an opportunity to improve the patient's health status. The nursing diagnosis related to knowledge may be identified as either a deficiency or the patient's readiness for enhancement (of knowledge).
- Part 2—"Related to lack of experience with medication regimen and second-grade reading level as an adult." This portion of the statement identifies factors related to the response; it often includes multiple factors with some degree of connection between them. The nursing diagnosis statement does not necessarily claim that there is a cause-and-effect link between these factors and the response, only that there is a connection.

- Part 3—"As evidenced by inability to perform a return demonstration and inability to state adverse effects to report to the prescriber." This statement lists clues, cues, evidence, and/or data that support the nurse's claim that the nursing diagnosis is accurate.

Nursing diagnoses are prioritized in order of criticality based on patient needs or problems. The ABCs of care (airway, breathing, and circulation) are often used as a basis for prioritization. Prioritizing always begins with the most important, significant, or critical need of the patient. Nursing diagnoses that involve actual responses are always ranked above nursing diagnoses that involve only risks.

Planning: Goals and Outcome Criteria
The planning phase includes the identification of goals and outcome criteria, provides time frames, and is patient oriented. Goals are objective, realistic, and measurable patient-centered statements with time frames and are broad, whereas outcome criteria are more specific descriptions of patient goals. See the Antihypertensive Drug Therapy nursing care plan available at *http://evolve.elsevier.com/Lilley* for examples of goal and outcome criteria statements.

Implementation
In the implementation phase, the nurse intervenes on behalf of the patient to address specific patient problems and needs. This is done through independent nursing actions; collaborative activities such as physical therapy, occupational therapy, and music therapy; and implementation of medical orders. Family, significant others, and caregivers assist in carrying out this phase of the nursing care plan. Specific interventions that relate to particular drugs (e.g., giving a particular cardiac drug only after monitoring the patient's pulse and blood pressure), nonpharmacologic interventions that enhance the therapeutic effects of medications, and patient education are major components of the implementation phase. See previous text discussion of the nursing process for more information on nursing interventions.

Evaluation
Evaluation is the part of the nursing process that includes monitoring whether patient goals and outcome criteria related to the nursing diagnoses are met. Monitoring includes observing for therapeutic effects of drug treatment as well as for adverse effects and toxicity. Many indicators are used to monitor these aspects of drug therapy as well as the results of appropriately related nonpharmacologic interventions. If the goals and outcome criteria are met, the nursing care plan may or may not be revised to include new nursing diagnoses; such changes are made only if appropriate. If goals and outcome criteria are not met, revisions are made to the entire nursing care plan with further evaluation.

records review, head-to-toe physical examination, and a nursing assessment. Data are categorized into objective and subjective data. Objective data may be defined as any information gathered through the senses or that which is seen, heard, felt, or smelled. Objective data may also be obtained from a nursing physical assessment; nursing history; past and present medical history; results of laboratory tests, diagnostic studies or procedures; measurement of vital signs, weight, and height; and medication profile. A medication profile should include, but not be limited to, the following information: (1) any and all drug use, (2) use of home or folk remedies and herbal and/or homeopathic treatments, plant or animal extracts, and dietary supplements, (3) intake of alcohol, tobacco, and caffeine, (4) current or past history of illegal drug use, (5) use of over-the-counter (OTC) medications (e.g., aspirin, acetaminophen, vitamins, laxatives, cold preparations, sinus medications, antacids, acid reducers, antidiarrheals, minerals, elements), (6) use of hormonal drugs (e.g., testosterone, estrogens, progestins, oral contraceptives), (7) past and present health history and associated drug regimen(s), (8) family history and racial, ethnic, and/or cultural attributes with attention to specific or different responses to medications as well as any unusual individual responses, and (9) growth and developmental stage (e.g., Erikson's developmental tasks) and issues related to the patient's age and medication regimen. A holistic nursing assessment includes gathering of data about the whole individual, including physical/emotional realms, religious preference, health beliefs, sociocultural characteristics, race, ethnicity, lifestyle, stressors, socioeconomic status, educational level, motor skills, cognitive ability, support systems, lifestyle, and use of any alternative and complementary therapies. Subjective data include information shared through the spoken word by any reliable source, such as the patient, spouse, family member, significant other, and/or caregiver.

Assessment about the specific drug is also important and involves the collection of specific information about prescribed, OTC, and herbal/complementary/alternative therapeutic drug use, with attention to the drug's action; signs and symptoms of allergic reaction; adverse effects; dosage and routes of administration; contraindications; drug incompatibilities; drug-drug, drug-food, and drug–laboratory test interactions; and toxicities and available antidotes. Nursing pharmacology textbooks provide a more nursing-specific knowledge base regarding drug therapy as related to the nursing process. Use of current references or those dated within the last 3 years is highly recommended. Some examples of authoritative sources include the *Physicians' Desk Reference, Mosby's Drug Consult,* drug manufacturers' inserts, drug handbooks, and/or licensed pharmacists. Reliable online resources include, but are not limited to, the following: U.S. Pharmacopeia (USP) *(http://www.usp.org)*, U.S. Food and Drug Administration *(http://www.fda.gov)*, and *http://www.WebMD.com.* Other online resources are cited throughout this textbook and at *http://evolve.elsevier.com/Lilley.*

Additional data about the patient and a given drug may be gathered by asking these simple questions: (1) What is the patient's oral intake? Tolerance of fluids? Swallowing ability for pills, tablets, capsules, and liquids? If there is difficulty swallowing, what is the degree of difficulty and are there solutions to the problem, such as use of thickening agents with fluids or use of other dosage forms? (2) What are laboratory tests and other diag-

CASE STUDY

The Nursing Process and Pharmacology

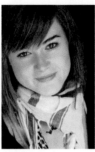
© Jose AS Reyes

Dollie, a 27-year-old social worker, is visiting the clinic today for a physical examination. She states that she and her husband want to "start a family," but she has not had a physical for several years. She was told when she was 22 years of age that she had "anemia" and was given iron tablets, but Dollie states that she has not taken them for years. She said she "felt better" and did not think she needed them. She denies any use of tobacco and illegal drugs; she states that she may have a drink with dinner once or twice a month. She uses tea tree oil on her face twice a day to reduce acne breakouts. She denies using any other drugs.

1. What other questions should be asked during this assessment phase?
2. Dollie is told, after laboratory work is performed, that she is slightly anemic and should resume taking iron supplements as well as folic acid. She is willing to try again and says that she is "all about doing what's right to stay healthy and become a mother." What nursing diagnoses would be appropriate at this time?
3. Dollie is given a prescription that reads as follows: "Ferrous sulfate 325 mg, PO for anemia." When she goes to the pharmacy, the pharmacist tells her that the prescription is incomplete. What is missing? What should be done?
4. After 4 weeks, her latest laboratory results indicate that she still has anemia. However, Dollie states, "I feel so much better that I'm planning to stop taking the iron tablets. I hate to take medicine." How should the nurse handle this?

For answers, see *http://evolve.elsevier.com/Lilley.*

nostic tests related to organ functioning and drug therapy? What do renal studies (e.g., blood urea nitrogen level, serum creatinine level) show? What are the results of hepatic function tests (e.g., total protein level, serum levels of bilirubin, alkaline phosphatase, creatinine phosphokinase, other liver enzymes)? What are the patient's white and red blood cell counts? Hemoglobin and hematocrit levels? (3) Current as well as past health status and presence of illness? What are the patient's experiences with use of any drug regimen? (4) What has been the patient's relationship with health care professionals and/or experiences with previous therapeutic regimens? (5) What are current and past values for blood pressure, pulse rate, temperature, and respiratory rate? (6) What medications is the patient currently taking and how is the patient taking and tolerating them? Are there issues of **compliance** (also called *adherence*)? Any use of folk medicines or folk remedies? (7) What is the patient's understanding of the medication? Are there any age-related concerns? If patients are not reliable historians, family members, significant others, and/or caregivers may provide answers to these questions.

Once assessment of the patient and the drug has been completed, the specific prescription or medication order from any **prescriber** must be checked for the following six elements: (1) patient's name, (2) date the drug order was written, (3) name of drug(s), (4) drug dosage amount and frequency, (5) route of administration, and (6) prescriber's signature.

It is also important during assessment to consider the traditional, nontraditional, expanded, and collaborative roles of the nurse. Physicians and dentists are no longer the only practitioners legally able to prescribe and write medication orders. Nurse practitioners and physician assistants have gained the professional privilege of legally prescribing medications. Nurses should always be aware of these legal regulations and be familiar with the specific state nurse practice acts and standards of care.

Analysis of Data

Once data about the patient and drug have been collected and reviewed, the nurse must critically analyze and synthesize the information. All information should be verified and documented appropriately, and it is at this point that the sum of the information about the patient and drug are used in the development of nursing diagnoses.

NURSING DIAGNOSES

Nursing diagnoses are developed by professional nurses and are used as a means of communicating and sharing information about the patient and the patient experience. Nursing diagnoses are the result of critical thinking, creativity, and accurate collection of data regarding the patient as well as the drug. Nursing diagnoses related to drug therapy will most likely grow out of data associated with the following: deficient knowledge; risk for injury; **noncompliance;** and various disturbances, deficits, excesses, impairments in bodily functions, and/or other problems or concerns as related to drug therapy. The development and classification of nursing diagnoses has been carried out by the North American Nursing Diagnosis Association (NANDA). NANDA is the formal organization recognized by professional nursing groups (e.g., the American Nurses Association [ANA]). NANDA is considered to be the major contributor to the development of nursing knowledge and the leading authority (on nursing diagnoses). The purpose of NANDA is to increase the visibility of nursing's contribution to the care of patients and to further develop, refine, and classify the information and phenomena related to nurses and professional nursing practice. In 2000, a classification system was adopted with a taxonomy including 13 domains divided into 106 classes and over 150 nursing diagnoses. Using this system, the nurse was able to choose a nursing diagnosis from the NANDA list and individualize the nursing care plan. The 2009-2011 revised NANDA nursing diagnoses are still characterized with domains and classes but also with many changes, including several new, revised and retired nursing diagnoses. See Box 1-2 for more information about NANDA and current changes/revisions in the writing of nursing diagnoses.

Formulation of nursing diagnoses is usually a three-step process with nursing diagnoses stated as follows: Part One of the statement is the human response of the patient to illness, injury, or significant change. This response can be an actual problem, an increased risk of developing a problem, or an opportunity or intent to improve the patient's health. Part Two of the nursing diagnosis statement identifies the factor(s) related to the response, with more than one factor often named. The nursing diagnosis statement does not necessarily claim a cause-and-effect link between these factors and the response;

BOX 1-2 A Brief Look at NANDA and the Nursing Process

The North American Nursing Diagnosis Association (NANDA) fulfills the following roles: (1) increases the visibility of nursing's contribution to patient care, (2) develops, refines, and classifies information and phenomena related to professional nursing practice, (3) provides a working organization for the development of evidence-based nursing diagnoses, and (4) supports for the improvement of quality nursing care through evidence-based practice and access to a global network of professional nurses. In 1987, NANDA and the American Nurses Association endorsed a framework for establishing nursing diagnoses and in 1990 *Nursing Diagnoses* became the official journal of NANDA. In 2001 and 2003, NANDA modified and updated the listing of nursing diagnoses but nursing diagnoses continued to be submitted for consideration by the Ad Hoc Research Committee of NANDA. This period resulted in changes such as replacement of the phrase *potential for* with *risk for.* The terms *impaired, deficient, ineffective, decreased, increased,* and *imbalanced* replaced the outdated terms *altered* and *alteration,* although the outdated terms may still be in use. In 2007-2008, there were 188 nursing diagnoses (up from 172) with changes to defining characteristics and related or risk factors. There were also some 15 newly approved nursing diagnoses. More significant changes occurred with the 2009-2011 version of NANDA's *Nursing Diagnoses: Definitions and Classifications,* with 21 new, 9 revised, and 6 retired nursing diagnoses. A companion website for more information about nursing diagnoses, their statement, and their domains and classes may be found at *www.blackwellpublishing.com/nursingdiagnoses.*

---

it indicates only that there is a connection between them. Part Three of the nursing diagnosis statement contains a listing of clues, cues, evidence, or other data that support the nurse's claim that this diagnosis is accurate. Tips for writing nursing diagnoses include the following: (1) Start with a statement of a human response. (2) Connect the first part of the statement or the human response with the second part, the cause, using the phrase "related to." (3) Be sure that the first two parts are not restatements of one another. (4) When appropriate, include several factors in the second part of the statement, such as associated factors. (5) Select a cause for the second part of the statement that can be changed by nursing interventions. (6) Avoid negative wording or language. (7) Finally, list clues or cues that led to the nursing diagnosis in the third part of the statement, which may also include more defining characteristics (e.g., "as evidenced by"). A listing of NANDA-approved nursing diagnoses (2009-2011) related to drug therapy is provided in Box 1-3. These nursing diagnoses, as well as all other phases of the nursing process, will be presented in the chapters that follow because the nursing process provides the framework of practice for all professional nurses and is also used to organize the nursing sections of this text.

PLANNING

After data are collected and nursing diagnoses are formulated, the planning phase begins; this includes identification of goals and outcome criteria. The major purposes of the planning phase are to prioritize the nursing diagnoses and specify goals and outcome criteria, including the time frame for their achievement.

BOX 1-3   Current NANDA-Approved Nursing Diagnoses Most Relevant to Drug Therapy

Activity intolerance
Acute pain
Airway clearance, ineffective
Allergy response, latex (and risk for)
Aspiration, risk for
Body image, disturbed
Body temperature, risk for imbalanced
Bowel incontinence
Breathing pattern, ineffective
Cardiac output, decreased
Comfort, readiness for enhanced
Communication (impaired verbal or readiness for enhanced)
Confusion (acute, chronic, or risk for acute)
Constipation (perceived or risk for)
Diarrhea
Falls, risk for
Fatigue
Fluid volume (deficient, excess, risk for deficient, and risk for imbalanced)
Gas exchange, impaired
Health maintenance, ineffective
Health-seeking behaviors
Home maintenance, impaired
Immunization status, readiness for enhanced
Incontinence (functional urinary, overflow urinary, reflex urinary, stress urinary, urge urinary, risk for urge urinary)
Infection, risk for
Injury, risk for
Insomnia
Knowledge (deficient, readiness for enhanced)

Lifestyle, sedentary
Liver function, risk for impaired
Memory, impaired
Mobility (impaired bed, impaired physical, impaired wheelchair)
Nausea
Noncompliance
Nutrition, imbalanced (less than body requirements, more than body requirements)
Oral mucous membrane, impaired
Pain (acute, chronic)
Peripheral neurovascular dysfunction, risk for
Poisoning, risk for
Self-care deficit (bathing/hygiene, dressing/grooming, feeding, toileting)
Self-esteem (chronic low, situational low, risk for situational low)
Sensory perception, disturbed
Sexual dysfunction
Sleep deprivation
Stress overload
Suicide, risk for
Surgical recovery, delayed
Swallowing, impaired
Therapeutic regimen management (ineffective, ineffective family, readiness for enhanced)
Tissue integrity, impaired
Tissue perfusion, ineffective
Urinary elimination (impaired, readiness for enhanced)
Urinary retention
Ventilation, impaired spontaneous
Walking, impaired

NANDA, North American Nursing Diagnosis Association.
From *Nursing diagnoses: definitions and classification 2009-2011.* Copyright 2009, 2007, 2005, 2003, 2001, 1998, 1996, 1994 by NANDA International. Used by arrangement with Wiley-Blackwell Publishing, a company of John Wiley & Sons, Inc.

The planning phase provides time to obtain special equipment for interventions, review the possible procedures or techniques to be used, and gather information for oneself (the nurse) or for the patient. This step leads to the provision of safe care if professional judgment is combined with the acquisition of knowledge about the patient and the medications to be given.

Goals and Outcome Criteria

Goals are objective, measurable, and realistic, with an established time period for achievement of the outcomes, which are specifically stated in the outcome criteria. Patient goals reflect expected and measurable changes in behavior through nursing care and are developed in collaboration with the patient. Patient goals developed in the planning phase of the nursing process are behavior based and may be categorized into physiologic, psychologic, spiritual, sexual, cognitive, motor, and/or other domains.

Outcome criteria are concrete descriptions of patient goals. As such, they should be patient focused, succinct, and well thought out. Outcome criteria should include expectations for behavior indicating something that can be changed and with a specific time frame or deadline. The ultimate aim of these criteria is the safe and effective administration of medications. These criteria should reflect each nursing diagnosis and guide the implementation phase of the nursing process. Formulation of outcome criteria begins with the analysis of the judgments made about patient data and subsequent nursing diagnoses and ends with the devel-

opment of a nursing care plan. Outcome criteria provide a standard for measuring movement toward goals. With regard to medication administration, these outcomes may address special storage and handling techniques, administration procedures, equipment needed, drug interactions, adverse effects, and contraindications. In this textbook, specific time frames are *not* provided in each chapter's nursing process section because in every situation patient care is individualized. Nursing care plans showing application of the nursing process as related to drug therapy may be found at *http://evolve.elsevier.com/Lilley*.

IMPLEMENTATION

Implementation is guided by the preceding phases of the nursing process (i.e., assessment, nursing diagnoses, and planning). Implementation requires constant communication and collaboration with the patient and with members of the health care team involved in the patient's care, as well as with any family members, significant others, or other caregivers. Implementation consists of initiation and completion of specific actions by the nurse as defined by nursing diagnoses, goals, and outcome criteria. Implementation of nursing actions may be independent, collaborative, or dependent upon a prescriber's order. Statements of interventions should include frequency, specific instructions, and any other pertinent information. With medication administration, the nurse needs to know and understand all of the information about the patient and about each medication prescribed (see assessment questions). In years past, nurses adhered to the "Five Rights" of medication administration: right drug, right dose, right time, right route, and right patient. However, support now exists for referring to "Six Rights" of medication administration with the addition of "right documentation." The Six Rights are discussed in detail in the following section. These "rights" of medication administration have been identified as basic standards of care as related to drug therapy. However, even the implementation of the Six Rights does not reflect the complexity of the role of the professional nurse because they focus more on the individual/patient than on the system as a whole or the entire medication administration process beginning with the prescriber's order. Viewed from an individual/patient focus, there are additional rights (or entitlements) that should also be considered when administering medications. These include the right to:

- Patient safety, ensured by use of the correct procedures, equipment, and techniques of medication administration and documentation
- Individualized, holistic, accurate, and complete patient education
- Double-checking and constant analysis of the system (i.e., the process of drug administration including all personnel involved, such as the prescriber, the nurse, the nursing unit, and the pharmacy department, as well as patient education)
- Proper drug storage
- Accurate calculation and preparation of the dose of medication and proper use of all types of medication delivery systems
- Careful checking of the transcription of medication orders
- Accurate use of the various routes of administration and awareness of the specific implications of their use
- Close consideration of special situations (e.g., patient difficulty in swallowing, use of a nasogastric tube, unconsciousness of the patient, advanced patient age)
- Implementation of all appropriate measures to prevent and report medication errors

Six Rights of Medication Administration
Right Drug

The "right drug" begins with the registered nurse's valid license to practice. Some states allow licensed practical nurses to administer medications; they should also hold a current license. The registered nurse should check all medication orders and/or prescriptions. To ensure that the correct drug is given, the nurse must check the specific medication order against the medication label or profile three times before giving the medication. The nurse should conduct the first check of the right drug/drug name while preparing the medication for administration. At this time, the nurse should also consider whether the drug is appropriate for the patient and, if doubt exists or an error is deemed possible, the prescriber should be contacted immediately. It would also be appropriate at this time to note the drug's indication and be aware that a drug may have multiple indications. In this textbook a particular drug is discussed in the chapter that deals with its main indication, but the drug may also be cross-referenced in other chapters if it has multiple uses.

All medication orders or prescriptions should be signed by the prescriber involved in the patient's care. If a verbal order is given, the prescriber should sign the order within 24 hours or as per facility protocol. Verbal and/or telephone orders are often used in emergencies and time-sensitive patient care situations. To be sure that the right drug is given, information about the patient and drug (see previous discussion of the assessment phase) must be obtained to make certain that all variables and data have been considered. Information about prescribed drugs should come from authoritative sources (see earlier discussion). Reliance on the knowledge of peers should be avoided and is unsafe nursing practice. The professional nurse should be familiar with the generic (nonproprietary) drug name as well as the trade name (proprietary name that is registered by a specific drug manufacturer); however, use of the drug's generic name is now preferred in clinical practice to reduce the risk of medication errors. A single drug often has numerous trade names and drugs in different classes may have similarly spelled names, which leads to possible medication errors. Therefore, when it comes to the "right drug" phase of the medication administration process, generic names should be used to ensure safe nursing care and help avoid a medication error. (See Chapter 2 for more information on the naming of drugs).

Should the nurse have any questions at any time in the medication administration process, the prescriber should be contacted to clarify the order. The nurse should never assume anything when it comes to drug administration, and as previously emphasized in this chapter, the nurse should check to confirm the right drug, right dose, right patient, right route, and right time at least three times before giving the medication.

Right Dose

Whenever a medication is ordered, a dosage is identified from the prescriber's order. The nurse must always check the dose and confirm that it is appropriate for the patient's age and size, and also check the prescribed dose against the available drug stocks and against the normal dosage range. Any mathematical calculations should always be rechecked, and careful attention should be paid to decimal points, the misplacement of which could lead to a tenfold or even greater overdose. Leading zeros, or zeros placed before a decimal point, are allowed, but trailing zeros, or zeros following the decimal point, should *not* be used. For example, 0.2 mg is allowed, but 2.0 mg is not acceptable, because it could easily be mistaken for 20 mg, especially with unclear penmanship. Patient variables (e.g., vital signs, age, gender, weight, height) should be noted because of the need for dosage adjustments in response to specific parameters. Pediatric and elderly patients are more sensitive to medications than younger and middle-aged adult patients; thus, there is a need for extra caution with drug dosage amounts for these patients.

Right Time

Each health care agency or institution has a policy regarding routine medication administration times; therefore, the nurse must always check this policy. However, when giving a medication at the prescribed time, the nurse may be confronted with a conflict between the timing suggested by the prescriber and specific pharmacokinetic or pharmacodynamic drug properties, concurrent drug therapy, dietary influences, laboratory and/or diag-

---

EVIDENCE-BASED PRACTICE

Reducing Hospital Stays for Patients Discharged to Nursing Homes: An Evolving Program

This study looked at the need to reduce hospital lengths of stay for patients who are difficult to place in nursing homes. The efficient movement of patients between hospitals and nursing homes continues to be a significant challenge. Various approaches have been used in the United States and Canada to try to maintain continuity of care between acute health care providers and providers of long-term care, including hospital-based case management programs, diagnosis-specific initiatives, and the development of units providing specialized acute care for the elderly. The number of hospital patient-days used by elderly patients aged 65 years and older with extended stays continues to increase, with few options to provide appropriate post-discharge care. This study also looked at several initiatives for reducing hospital lengths of stay.

■ Type of Evidence

This study was conducted in Syracuse, New York, with a population of over 440,000 and with 16.5% being 65 years and older. The area was served by four general acute care facilities as well as a teaching hospital with an affiliated medical school. During 2007, these facilities generated over 74,000 total discharges to the Syracuse area, which was served by 12 skilled nursing facilities or some 2900 beds. Evaluation of the implementation of difficult-to-place and subacute programs in Syracuse was done, with further analysis on the changes in hospital utilization for discharges to nursing homes during 2006 and 2007 and on use of subacute programs. Evaluation of the impact of the programs was also done because a reduction in level of services for discharges to nursing homes was one of the objectives within the initiatives of the study. Further evidence included gathering data about patients receiving care in the appropriate setting as well as improvement in the efficiency of patient turnover.

■ Results of the Study

Data collected for hospital discharges to nursing homes showed that mean stays declined by a statistically significant 2.2 days while discharges increased significantly during the program's initial years of 2002-2004. Data analysis suggested that level of services reduction for discharges to nursing home became more difficult in more recent years. Additional data about the impact of the difficult-to-place patient and subacute programs were provided by an analysis of utilization involving extended stays (stays of 10 days or greater) or twice the mean level for medical-surgical patients. This long-stay population has provided major

obstacles to utilization efficiency of the health care system in Syracuse. For adult medicine, long-stay discharges declined statistically significantly, as did the number of discharges for adult surgical patients (excluding the years 2005-2007). These reductions were addressed through the difficult-to-place and subacute programs. The data analysis proved that while the number of patients difficult to place from hospitals to nursing homes increased significantly (2002-2005), their rate of admissions declined. Both numbers and rates of difficult-to-place admissions to nursing homes also increased significantly between 2005 and 2007. The initiatives identified in this research are important to mention in that they were developed in an attempt to reduce the length of stays. One initiative was the identification of specific medications/dosages used with patients in the hospital and nursing home that increased hospital stays, including newer antibiotics, antivirals or combination therapy. Other medication issues identified in this study included the costs of certain medications. Hospitals provided a certain level of reimbursement to nursing homes for patients requiring special medications in the subacute programs. It then became more difficult to move additional patients into nursing homes because the unplaced patients required very expensive medications that the nursing homes couldn't afford; therefore, an enhanced medication program was created to provide incentives and increase interest for earlier discharge to the nursing home. Other initiatives dealt with electronic distribution of patient data and use of uniform definitions of these patient populations among different hospitals.

■ Link of Evidence to Nursing Practice

This study showed that progress can be achieved in reducing stays for hospital patients who are discharged to nursing homes. The process of achieving these reductions has evolved over time because of the complexity of the issues involved; however, the Syracuse experience does not suggest that the challenges are likely to end in the near future. The study did indicate that creative solutions and initiatives are possible if the problem is approached in a thoughtful, systematic manner, much like the nursing process. The findings also suggest that the initiatives, solutions, and interventions should be developed with purpose and over time with constant evaluation and monitoring of the results of each intervention, also like the nursing process. More creative initiatives and interventions will be needed to decrease hospital lengths of stay for this patient population, especially as the challenges posed by ever-changing demographics confront the reality of limited resources.

Data from Lagoe RJ et al: Reducing hospital stays for patients discharged to nursing homes: an evolving program, *Topics in Advanced Practice Nursing eJournal,* 8(2):1-5, 2008. Available at *http://www.medscape.com/viewarticle/572831.*

PREVENTING MEDICATION ERRORS

Right Dose?

The nurse is reviewing the orders for a newly admitted patient. One order reads: "Tylenol, 2 tablets PO, every 4 hours as needed for pain or fever."

The pharmacist calls to clarify this order, saying, "The dose is not clear." What does the pharmacist mean by this? The order says "2 tablets." Isn't that the dose?

NO! If you look up Tylenol (acetaminophen) in a drug resource book, you will see that Tylenol tablets are available in strengths of both 325 mg and 500 mg. The order is missing the "right dose" and needs to be clarified. Never assume the dose of a medication order!

nostic testing, and specific patient variables. For example, the prescribed right time for administration of antihypertensive drugs may be four times a day, but for an active, professional 42-year-old male patient working 14 hours a day, taking a medication four times daily may not be feasible, and this regimen may lead to noncompliance and subsequent complications. The nurse should contact the prescriber and inquire about another drug with a different dosing frequency (e.g., once or twice daily).

For routine medication orders, the medications must be given no more than ½ hour before or after the actual time specified in the prescriber's order (i.e., if a medication is ordered to be given at 0900 every morning, it may be given anytime between 0830 and 0930); the exception is medications designated to be given stat (immediately), which must be administered within ½ hour of the time the order is written. The nurse should always check the hospital or facility policy and procedure for any other specific information concerning the "½ hour before or after" rule. For medication orders with the annotation "prn" (*pro re nata,* or "as required"), the medication should be given at special times and under certain circumstances. For example, an analgesic is ordered every 4 to 6 hours *prn* for pain; after one dose of the medication, the patient complains of pain. After assessment, intervention with another dose of analgesic would occur, but only 4 to 6 hours after the previous dose. In addition, because of the increasing incidence of medication errors related to the use of abbreviations, many prescribers are using the wording "as required" or "as needed" instead of the abbreviation "prn." Military time is used when medication and other orders are written into a patient's chart (Table 1-1).

Nursing judgment may lead to some variations in timing, but the nurse should be sure to document any change and the rationale for the change. If medications are ordered to be given once every day, twice daily, three times daily, or even four times daily, the times of administration may be changed if it is not harmful to the patient or if the medication or the patient's condition does not require adherence to an exact schedule, but only if the change is approved by the prescriber. For example, suppose that an antacid is ordered to be given three times daily at 0900, 1300, and 1700, but the nurse has misread the order and gives the first dose at 1100. Depending on the hospital or facility policy, the medication, and the patient's condition, such an occurrence may not be considered an error, because the dosing may be changed once the prescriber is contacted, so that the drug is given at 1100, 1500, and 1900 without harm to the patient and without incident to the nurse. If this were an antihypertensive medication, the patient's condition and well-being could be greatly compromised by one missed or late dose. Thus, falling behind in dosing times is not to be taken lightly or ignored. The effect of a change in the dosing or timing of medication should never be underestimated, because one missed dose of certain medications can be life threatening.

Other factors must be considered in determining the right time, such as multiple-drug therapy, drug-drug or drug-food compatibility, scheduling of diagnostic studies, bioavailability of the drug (e.g., the need for consistent timing of doses around the clock to maintain blood levels), drug actions, and any biorhythm effects such as occur with steroids. It is also critical to patient safety to *avoid* using abbreviations for *any* component of a drug order (i.e., dose, time, route). The nurse should spell out *all* terms (e.g., "three times daily" instead of "tid"). The nurse must always be careful to write out all words and abbreviations, because the possibility of miscommunication or misinterpretation poses a risk to the patient.

Right Route

As previously stated, the nurse must know the particulars about each medication before administering it to ensure that the right drug, dose, and route are being used. A complete medication order includes the route of administration. If a medication order does not include the route, the nurse must ask the prescriber to clarify it. The nurse must never *assume* the route of administration.

TABLE 1-1 Conversion of Standard Time to Military Time

Standard Time	Military Time
1 AM	0100
2 AM	0200
3 AM	0300
4 AM	0400
5 AM	0500
6 AM	0600
7 AM	0700
8 AM	0800
9 AM	0900
10 AM	1000
11 AM	1100
12 PM (noon)	1200
1 PM	1300
2 PM	1400
3 PM	1500
4 PM	1600
5 PM	1700
6 PM	1800
7 PM	1900
8 PM	2000
9 PM	2100
10 PM	2200
11 PM	2300
12 AM (midnight)	2400

Right Patient

Checking the patient's identity before giving each medication dose is critical to the patient's safety. The nurse should ask the patient to state his or her name and check the patient's identification band to confirm the patient's name, identification number, age, and allergies. With pediatric patients, the parents and/or legal guardians are often the ones who identify the patient for the purpose of administration of prescribed medications. With newborns and in labor and delivery situations, the mother and baby have identification bracelets with matching numbers, which should be checked before giving medications. With elderly patients or patients with altered sensorium or level of consciousness, asking the patient his or her name or having the patient state his or her name is neither realistic nor safe. Therefore, checking the identification band against the medication profile, medication order, or other treatment or service orders is crucial to avoid errors. In 2008 the Joint Commission released National Patient Safety Goals for patient care. These goals emphasize the use of two identifiers when providing care, treatment, or services to patients. To meet these goals, the Joint Commission recommends that the patient be identified "reliably" and also that the service or treatment (e.g., medication administration) be matched to that individual. The Joint Commission's statement of National Patient Safety Goals indicates that the two identifiers may be in the same location, such as on a wristband. In fact, it is patient-specific information that is the identifier. Acceptable identifiers include the patient's name, an assigned identification number, a telephone number, or other patient-specific identifier. Armbands are commonly used in the acute care setting and may serve as one identifier, with the other one being date of birth, social security number, or home address.

Right Documentation

Documentation of information related to administration of medications is crucial to patient safety. Recording patient observations and nursing actions has always been an important ethical responsibility, but now it is becoming a major medical-legal consideration as well. Because of its significance in professional nursing practice, correct documentation is becoming known as the "sixth right" of medication administration. The patient's chart should *always* have the following information: date and time of medication administration, name of medication, dose, route, and site of administration. Documentation of drug action may also be made in the regularly scheduled assessments for changes in symptoms the patient is experiencing, adverse effects, toxicity, and any other drug-related physical and/or psychologic symptoms. Improvement in the patient's condition, symptoms, or disease process should be recorded, as well as no change or lack of improvement. Not only should these observations be documented promptly but they should also be reported in keeping with the nurse's critical thinking and judgment. Any teaching, as well as an assessment of the degree of understanding exhibited by the patient, should also be documented. Other information that should be documented includes the following: (1) if a drug is *not* administered and why with actions taken by the nurse, (2) refusal of a medication with information about the reason for refusal, if possible; if a medication is refused and the cause of refusal identified, the nursing care plan should be revised and further actions implemented, (3) actual time of drug administration, and (4) data regarding clinical observations and treatment of the patient if a medication error has occurred. If there is a medication error, documentation of completion of an incident report should not be included in the nurse's notes. However, an incident report should be completed with the entire event, surrounding circumstances, therapeutic response, adverse effects, and notification of the prescriber described in detail.

Medication Errors

When the Six Rights (and other rights) of drug administration are discussed, medication errors must be considered. Medication errors are a major problem for all of health care, regardless of the setting. The National Coordinating Council for Medication Error Reporting and Prevention defines a **medication error** as any *preventable* event that may cause or lead to inappropriate medication use or patient harm while the medication is in the control of the health care professional, patient, or consumer. Such events may be related to professional practice, health care products, procedures, or systems, including prescribing; order communication; product labeling, packaging, and nomenclature; compounding; dispensing; distribution; administration; education; monitoring; and use (*http://www. nccmerp.org/aboutMedErrors.html*). Both patient-related and system-related factors must always be considered when the medication administration process and the prevention of medication errors are being examined. For further discussion of medication errors and their prevention, see Chapter 6.

LEGAL AND ETHICAL PRINCIPLES

Charting Don'ts

- Don't record staffing problems (don't mention them in a patient's chart but instead talk with the nurse manager).
- Don't record a peer's conflicts, such as charting possible disputes between a patient and a nurse.
- Don't mention the term "incident report" in charting. These reports are confidential and filed separately. Chart only the facts of the medication error or incident.
- Don't use the following terms: "by mistake," "by accident," "accidentally," "unintentional," or "miscalculated."
- Don't chart anything but actual facts.
- Don't chart casual conversations with peers, prescribers, or other members of the health care team.
- Don't use abbreviations as a general rule. Some agencies or facilities may still keep a list of approved abbreviations, but overall their use is discouraged.
- Don't use negative language because it may come back to haunt you!

Modified from Institute for Safe Medication Practices: ISMP medication safety alert, Huntingdon Valley, Penn, February 20, 2003, The Institute; and Injury-Board.com: Medication and prescription errors, available at *http://www.injury-board.com*.

EVALUATION

Evaluation occurs after the nursing care plan has been implemented. It is systematic, ongoing, and a dynamic phase of the nursing process as related to drug therapy. It includes monitoring the fulfillment of goals and outcome criteria, as well as monitoring the patient's therapeutic response to the drug and its adverse effects and toxic effects. Documentation is also a very important component of evaluation and consists of clear, concise, abbreviation-free charting that records information related to goals and outcome criteria as well as information related to any aspect of the medication administration process, including therapeutic effects versus adverse effects or toxic effects of medications (see the Legal and Ethical Principles box).

Evaluation also includes monitoring the implementation of standards of care. Several standards are in place to help in the evaluation of outcomes of care, such as those established by state nurse practice acts and by the Joint Commission. Guidelines for nursing services policies and procedures are established by the Joint Commission. There are even specific standards regarding medication administration to protect both the patient and the nurse. The ANA *Code of Ethics* and Patient Rights statement are also used in establishing and evaluating standards of care.

In summary, the nursing process is an ongoing and constantly evolving process (see Box 1-1). The nursing process, as it relates to drug therapy, involves the way in which a nurse gathers, analyzes, organizes, provides, and acts upon data about the patient within the context of prudent nursing care and standards of care. The nurse's ability to make astute assessments, formulate sound nursing diagnoses, establish goals and outcome criteria, correctly administer drugs, and continually evaluate patients' responses to drugs increases with additional experience and knowledge.

POINTS TO REMEMBER

- The nursing process is an ongoing, constantly changing and evolving framework for professional nursing practice. It may be applied to all facets of nursing care, including medication administration.
- The phases of the nursing process include assessment; development of nursing diagnoses; planning, with establishment of goals and outcome criteria; implementation, including patient education; and evaluation.
- Nursing diagnoses are formulated based on objective and subjective data and help to drive the nursing care plan by suggesting specific goals and outcomes. Nursing diagnoses have been developed through a formal process conducted by NANDA and are constantly updated and revised. Safe, therapeutic, and effective medication administration is a major responsibility of professional nurses as they apply the nursing process to the care of their patients.
- Nurses are responsible for safe and prudent decision making in the nursing care of their patients, including the provision of drug therapy; in accomplishing this task, they attend to the Six Rights and adhere to legal and ethical standards related to medication administration and documentation. There are additional rights related to drug administration. These rights deserve worthy consideration before initiation of the medication administration process. Observance of all these rights enhances patient safety and helps avoid medication errors.

NCLEX EXAMINATION REVIEW QUESTIONS

1 An 86-year-old patient is being discharged to home on digitalis therapy and has very little information regarding the medication. Which statement best reflects a realistic goal or outcome of patient teaching activities?
  a The patient and patient's daughter will state the correct dosing and administration of the drug.
  b The nurse will provide teaching about the drug's adverse effects.
  c The patient will state all the symptoms of digitalis toxicity.
  d The patient will call the prescriber if adverse effects occur.

2 A patient has a new prescription for a blood pressure medication that may cause him to feel dizzy during the first few days of therapy. The best nursing diagnosis for this situation is
  a activity intolerance.
  b risk for injury.
  c disturbed body image.
  d self-care deficit.

3 A patient's chart includes an order that reads as follows: "Lanoxin 250 mcg once daily at 0900." Which action by the nurse is correct?
  a The nurse should give the drug via the transdermal route.
  b The nurse should give the drug orally.
  c The nurse should give the drug intravenously.
  d The nurse should contact the prescriber to clarify the dosage route.

4 The nurse is compiling a drug history for a patient. The most helpful question the nurse can ask is
  a "Do you depend on sleeping pills to get to sleep?"
  b "Do you have a family history of heart disease?"
  c "When you take your pain medicine, does it relieve the pain?"
  d "What childhood diseases did you have?"

5 A 77-year-old man who has been diagnosed with an upper respiratory tract infection tells the nurse that he is allergic to penicillin. Which is the most appropriate response by the nurse?
  a "That's to be expected—lots of people are allergic to penicillin."
  b "This allergy is not of major concern because the drug is given so commonly."
  c "What type of reaction did you have when you took penicillin?"
  d "Drug allergies don't usually occur in older individuals because they have built up resistance."

6 The nurse is preparing a care plan for a patient who has been newly diagnosed with type 2 diabetes mellitus. Put into correct order the steps of the nursing process, with 1 being the first step and 5 being the last step.
  a Implementation
  b Planning
  c Assessment
  d Evaluation
  e Nursing diagnoses

1. a, 2. b, 3. d, 4. c, 5. c, 6. a = 4, b = 3, c = 1, d = 5, e = 2.

CRITICAL THINKING ACTIVITIES: BEST ACTION

1 What are the crucial responsibilities of the nurse when implementing drug therapy?

2 When medications were administered during the night shift, a patient refused to take his 0200 dose of an antibiotic, claiming that he had just taken it. What is the best action by the nurse to maintain patient safety?

3 During a busy shift, the nurse notes that the chart of a newly admitted patient has a few orders for various medications and diagnostic tests, taken by telephone by another nurse. The nurse is on the way to the patient's room to do an assessment when the unit secretary tells the nurse that one of the orders reads as follows: "Lasix, 20 mg, stat." What should the nurse do first? How does the nurse go about giving this drug? Explain the best action to take in this situation.

For answers, see the *http://evolve.elsevier.com/Lilley.*

Pharmacologic Principles

OBJECTIVES

When you reach the end of this chapter, you should be able to do the following:

1 Define the common terms used in pharmacology (see the listing of terms in the glossary).

2 Understand the role of general concepts such as pharmaceutics, pharmacokinetics, and pharmacodynamics and their application in drug therapy and the nursing process.

3 Demonstrate an understanding of the various drug dosage forms as related to drug therapy and the nursing process.

4 Discuss the relevance of the four aspects of pharmacokinetics (absorption, distribution, metabolism, excretion) to professional nursing practice as related to drug therapy for a variety of patients and in a variety of health care settings.

5 Discuss the use of natural drug sources in the development of new drugs.

6 Develop a nursing care plan that takes into account general pharmacological principles, specifically pharmacokinetic principles, as they relate to the nursing process.

e-Learning Activities

http://evolve.elsevier.com/Lilley

NCLEX Review Questions • Animations • Nursing Care Plans • Audio Glossary • Category Catchers • Medication Errors Checklists • IV Therapy Checklists • Calculators • Frequently Asked Questions • Content Updates • Supplemental Resources • Answers to Case Studies and Critical Thinking Activities

Glossary

Additive effects Drug interactions in which the effect of a combination of two or more drugs with similar actions is equivalent to the sum of the individual effects of the same drugs given alone. For example, 1 + 1 = 2 (compare with *synergistic effects*). (p. 31)

Adverse drug event Any undesirable occurrence related to administering or failing to administer a prescribed medication. (p. 32)

Adverse drug reaction Any unexpected, unintended, undesired, or excessive response to a medication given at therapeutic dosages (as opposed to overdose). (p. 32)

Adverse effects A general term for any undesirable effects that are a direct response to one or more drugs. (p. 30)

Agonist A drug that binds to and stimulates the activity of one or more receptors in the body. (p. 29)

Allergic reaction An immunologic hypersensitivity reaction resulting from the unusual sensitivity of a patient to a particular medication; a type of adverse drug event. (p. 32)

Antagonist A drug that binds to and inhibits the activity of one or more receptors in the body. Antagonists are also called *inhibitors*. (p. 29)

Antagonistic effects Drug interactions in which the effect of a combination of two or more drugs is less than the sum of the individual effects of the same drugs given alone (1 + 1 = less than 2); it is usually caused by an antagonizing (blocking or reducing) effect of one drug on another. (p. 31)

Bioavailability A measure of the extent of drug absorption for a given drug and route (from 0% to 100%). (p. 20)

Biotransformation One or more biochemical reactions involving a parent drug. Biotransformation occurs mainly in the liver and produces a *metabolite* that is either inactive or active. Also known as *metabolism*. (p. 25)

Blood-brain barrier The barrier system that restricts the passage of various chemicals and microscopic entities (e.g., bacteria, viruses) between the bloodstream and the central nervous system. It still allows for the passage of essential substances such as oxygen. (p. 25)

Chemical name The name that describes the chemical composition and molecular structure of a drug. (p. 18)

Contraindication Any condition, especially one related to a disease state or other patient characteristic, including current or recent drug therapy, that renders a particular form of treatment improper or undesirable. (p. 29)

Cytochrome P-450 The general name for a large class of enzymes that play a significant role in drug metabolism. (p. 25)

Dependence A state in which there is a compulsive or chronic need, as for a drug. (p. 30)

Dissolution The process by which solid forms of drugs disintegrate in the gastrointestinal tract and become soluble before being absorbed into the circulation. (p. 19)

Drug Any chemical that affects the physiologic processes of a living organism. (p. 17)

Drug actions The cellular processes involved in the interaction between a drug and body cells (e.g., the action of a drug on a receptor protein); also called *mechanism of action*. (p. 18)

Drug effects The physiologic reactions of the body to a drug. They can be therapeutic or toxic and describe how the function of the body is affected as a whole by the drug. The terms *onset, peak,* and *duration* are used to describe drug effects (most often referring to therapeutic effects). (p. 26)

Drug-induced teratogenesis The development of congenital anomalies or defects in the developing fetus caused by the toxic effects of drugs. (p. 33)

Drug interaction Alteration in the pharmacologic activity of a given drug caused by the presence of one or more additional drugs; it is usually related to effects on the enzymes required for metabolism of the involved drugs. (p. 30)

Duration of action The length of time the concentration of a drug in the blood or tissues is sufficient to elicit a response. (p. 27)

Enzymes Protein molecules that catalyze one or more of a variety of biochemical reactions, including those related to the body's own physiologic processes as well as those related to drug metabolism. (p. 28)

First-pass effect The initial metabolism in the liver of a drug absorbed from the gastrointestinal tract before the drug reaches systemic circulation through the bloodstream. (p. 20)

Generic name The name given to a drug by the United States Adopted Names Council. Also called the *nonproprietary name*. The generic name is much shorter and simpler than the chemical name and is not protected by trademark. (p. 18)

Half-life In pharmacokinetics, the time required for half of an administered dose of drug to be eliminated by the body, or the time it takes for the blood level of a drug to be reduced by 50% (also called *elimination half-life*). (p. 26)

Idiosyncratic reaction An abnormal and unexpected response to a medication, other than an allergic reaction, that is peculiar to an individual patient. (p. 32)

Incompatibility The characteristic that causes two parenteral drugs or solutions to undergo a reaction when mixed or given together that results in the chemical deterioration of at least one of the drugs. (p. 31)

Intraarticular Within a joint (e.g., intraarticular injection). (p. 21)

Intrathecal Within a sheath (e.g., the *theca* of the spinal cord, as in an intrathecal injection into the subarachnoid space). (p. 21)

Medication error Any preventable adverse drug event involving inappropriate medication use by a patient or health care professional; it may or may not cause patient harm. (p. 32)

Medication use process The prescribing, dispensing, and administering of medications, and the monitoring of their effects. (p. 32)

Metabolite(s) A chemical form of a drug that is the product of one or more biochemical (metabolic) reactions involving the *parent drug* (see later). Active metabolites are those that have pharmacologic activity of their own, even if the parent drug is inactive (see *prodrug*). Inactive metabolites lack pharmacologic activity and are simply drug waste products awaiting excretion from the body (e.g., via the urinary, gastrointestinal, or respiratory tract). (p. 25)

Onset of action The time required for a drug to elicit a therapeutic response after dosing. (p. 27)

Parent drug The chemical form of a drug that is administered before it is metabolized by the body's biochemical reactions into its active or inactive metabolites (see *metabolite*). A parent drug that is not pharmacologically active itself is called a *prodrug*. A prodrug is then metabolized to pharmacologically active metabolites. (p. 20)

Peak effect The time required for a drug to reach its maximum therapeutic response in the body. (p. 27)

Peak level The maximum concentration of a drug in the body after administration, usually measured in a blood sample for therapeutic drug monitoring. (p. 27)

Pharmaceutics The science of preparing and dispensing drugs, including dosage form design. (p. 18)

Pharmacodynamics The study of the biochemical and physiologic interactions of drugs at their sites of activity. It examines the physicochemical properties of drugs and their pharmacologic interactions with body receptors. (p. 18)

Pharmacogenetics The study of the influence of genetic factors on drug response, including the nature of genetic aberrations that result in the absence, overabundance, or insufficiency of drug-metabolizing enzymes (also called *pharmacogenomics;* see Chapter 5). (p. 32)

Pharmacognosy The study of drugs that are obtained from natural plant and animal sources. (p. 19)

Pharmacokinetics The rate of drug distribution among various body compartments after a drug has entered the body. It includes the phases of absorption, distribution, metabolism, and excretion of drugs. (p. 18)

Pharmacology The broadest term for the study or science of drugs. (p. 17)

Pharmacotherapeutics The treatment of pathologic conditions through the use of drugs. (p. 18)

Prodrug An inactive drug dosage form that is converted to an active metabolite by various biochemical reactions once it is inside the body. (p. 25)

Receptor A molecular structure within or on the outer surface of a cell. Receptors bind specific substances (e.g., drug molecules), and one or more corresponding cellular effects *(drug actions)* occurs as a result of this drug-receptor interaction. (p. 28)

Steady state The physiologic state in which the amount of drug removed via elimination is equal to the amount of drug absorbed with each dose. (p. 26)

Substrates Substances (e.g., drugs or natural biochemicals in the body) on which an *enzyme* acts. (p. 25)

Synergistic effects Drug interactions in which the effect of a combination of two or more drugs with similar actions is greater than the sum of the individual effects of the same drugs given alone. For example, 1 + 1 is greater than 2 (compare with *additive effects*). (p. 31)

Therapeutic drug monitoring The process of measuring drug peak and trough levels to gauge the level of a patient's drug exposure and allow adjustment of dosages with the goals of maximizing therapeutic effects and minimizing toxicity. (p. 27)

Therapeutic effect The desired or intended effect of a particular medication. (p. 28)

Therapeutic index The ratio between the toxic and therapeutic concentrations of a drug. (p. 30)

Tolerance Reduced response to a drug after prolonged use. (p. 30)

Toxic The quality of being poisonous (i.e., injurious to health or dangerous to life). (p. 19)

Toxicity The condition of producing adverse bodily effects due to poisonous qualities. (p. 27)

Toxicology The study of poisons, including toxic drug effects, and applicable treatments. (p. 19)

Trade name The commercial name given to a drug product by its manufacturer; also called the *proprietary name*. (p. 18)

Trough level The lowest concentration of drug reached in the body after it falls from its peak level, usually measured in a blood sample for therapeutic drug monitoring. (p. 27)

• • •

OVERVIEW

Any chemical that affects the physiologic processes of a living organism can broadly be defined as a **drug.** The study or science of drugs is known as **pharmacology.** Pharmacology encompasses a variety of topics, including the following:

- Absorption
- Biochemical effects
- Biotransformation (metabolism)
- Distribution
- Drug history
- Drug origin
- Excretion
- Mechanisms of action
- Physical and chemical properties
- Physical effects
- Drug receptor mechanisms
- Therapeutic (beneficial) effects
- Toxic (harmful) effects

Pharmacology includes several subspecialty areas: pharmaceutics, pharmacokinetics, pharmacodynamics, pharmacogenetics, pharmacoeconomics, pharmacotherapeutics, pharmacognosy,

Chemical name (+/−)-2-(p-isobutylphenyl) propionic acid **Generic name** ibuprofen **Trade name** Motrin, others	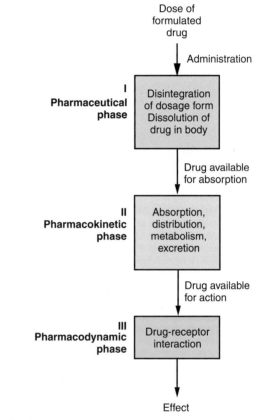

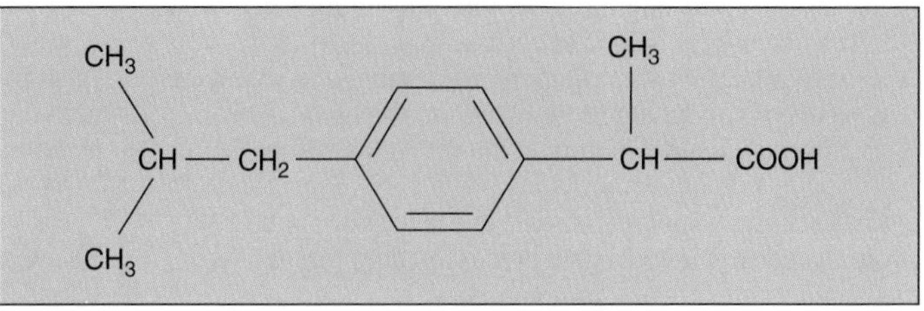

FIGURE 2-1   Chemical structure of the common analgesic ibuprofen and the chemical, generic, and trade names for the drug.

and toxicology. Knowledge of pharmacology enables the nurse to better understand how drugs affect humans. Without a sound understanding of basic pharmacologic principles, the nurse cannot fully appreciate the therapeutic benefits and potential toxicity of drugs.

Throughout the process of its development, a drug will acquire at least three different names. The **chemical name** describes the drug's chemical composition and molecular structure. The generic name, or nonproprietary name, is often much shorter and simpler than the chemical name. The **generic name** is used in most official drug compendiums to list drugs. The **trade name,** or proprietary name, is the drug's registered trademark, which indicates that its commercial use is restricted to the owner of the patent for the drug (Figure 2-1). The patent owner is usually the manufacturer of the drug. Trade names are generally created by the manufacturer with marketability in mind. For this reason, they are usually shorter and easier to pronounce and remember than generic drug names. The *patent life* of a newly discovered drug molecule is normally 17 years. This is the length of time from patent approval until patent expiration. Because the research processes for new drug development normally require about 10 years, a drug manufacturer generally has the remaining 7 years for sales profits before patent expiration. A significant amount of these profits serves to offset the multimillion-dollar costs for research and development of the drug.

After the patent for a given drug expires, other manufacturers may legally begin to manufacture *generic* drugs with the same active ingredient. At this point, the drug price usually falls substantially. Due to the high cost of drugs, many institutions have implemented programs in which one drug in a class of several drugs is chosen as the preferred agent, even though the drugs do not have the same active ingredients. Before one drug can be therapeutically substituted for another, the drugs must have been proven to have the same therapeutic effect in the body. This is called *therapeutic equivalence.*

Three basic areas of pharmacology—pharmaceutics, pharmacokinetics, and pharmacodynamics—describe the relationship between the dose of a drug given to a patient and the activity of that drug in treating the patient's disorder. **Pharmaceutics** includes the study of how various dosage forms influence the way in which the body metabolizes a drug and the way in which the drug affects the body. **Pharmacokinetics** is the study of what the body does to the drug molecules. Pharmacokinetics involves the processes of absorption, distribution, metabolism, and excretion. **Pharmacodynamics,** on the other hand, is the study of what the drug does to the body. Pharmacodynamics involves drug-receptor interactions. Figure 2-2 illustrates the three phases of

FIGURE 2-2   Phases of drug activity. (From McKenry LM, Tessier E, Hogan M: *Mosby's pharmacology in nursing,* ed 22, St Louis, 2006, Mosby.)

drug activity, starting with the pharmaceutical phase, proceeding to the pharmacokinetic phase, and finishing with the pharmacodynamic phase.

Pharmacotherapeutics (also called *therapeutics*) focuses on the clinical use of drugs to prevent and treat diseases. It defines the principles of **drug actions**—the cellular processes that change in response to the presence of drug molecules. Some drug mechanisms of action are more clearly understood than others. Drugs are categorized into pharmacologic classes according to their physiologic functions (e.g., beta-adrenergic blockers) and primary disease states treated (e.g., anticonvulsants, antiinfectives). The U.S. Food and Drug Administration (FDA) regulates the approval and clinical use of all drugs in the United States. The content of this book focuses almost exclusively on current FDA-approved indications for the different drugs discussed in each chapter and on drugs that are currently available in the United

States at the time of this writing. Only FDA-approved indications are permitted to be described in the manufacturer's written information, or *labeling*, for a given drug product. At times, prescribers may elect to prescribe drugs for non–FDA-approved indications. This is known as *off-label* prescribing and often requires seasoned clinical judgment on the part of the prescriber. Evolving over time in clinical practice, previously off-label indications often become FDA approved for a given drug.

The study of the adverse effects of drugs and other chemicals on living systems is known as **toxicology. Toxic** effects are often an extension of a drug's therapeutic action. Therefore, toxicology frequently involves overlapping principles of both pharmacotherapy and toxicology. The study of *natural* (vs. *synthetic*) drug sources (plants, animals, minerals) is called **pharmacognosy.** Pharmacoeconomics focuses on the economic aspects of drug therapy.

In summary, pharmacology is a very dynamic science incorporating several different disciplines. Traditionally, chemistry has been seen as the primary basis of pharmacology, but pharmacology also relies heavily on physiology and biology.

PHARMACEUTICS

Different drug dosage forms have different pharmaceutical properties. Dosage form design determines the rate at which drug **dissolution** (dissolving of solid dosage forms and their absorption, e.g., from gastrointestinal [GI] tract fluids) occurs. A drug to be ingested orally may be taken in either a solid form (tablet, capsule, or powder) or a liquid form (solution or suspension). Table 2-1 lists various oral drug preparations and the relative rate at which they are absorbed. Oral drugs that are liquids (e.g., elixirs, syrups) are already dissolved and are usually absorbed more quickly than solid dosage forms. Enteric-coated tablets, on the other hand, have a coating that prevents them from being broken down in the acidic pH environment of the stomach and therefore are not absorbed until they reach the higher (more alkaline) pH of the intestines. This pharmaceutical property results in slower dissolution and therefore slower absorption.

The size of the particles within a tablet or capsule can make different dosage forms of the same drug dissolve at different rates, become absorbed at different rates, and thus have different times to onset of action. A prime example is the difference between micronized glyburide and nonmicronized glyburide. Micronized glyburide reaches a maximum concentration peak faster than does the nonmicronized formulation. Dosage form design for injectable drugs tends to be more straightforward than that for oral dosage forms. However, some injections are carefully formulated to reduce drug toxicity (e.g., liposomal amphotericin B).

Combination dosage forms contain multiple drugs for simultaneous dosing of the patient. Examples of these combination forms include the cholesterol medication atorvastatin/amlodipine tablets (Caduet) and bacitracin/neomycin/polymyxin B/hydrocortisone ointment (generic). There are large numbers of such combination dosage forms; key examples are cited in the various chapters of this book, and the student may view additional examples on the Evolve website.

A variety of dosage forms exist to provide both accurate and convenient drug delivery systems (Table 2-2). These delivery systems are designed to achieve a desired therapeutic response

TABLE 2-1 Drug Absorption of Various Oral Preparations

Liquids, elixirs, and syrups	Fastest
Suspension solutions	
Powders	
Capsules	
Tablets	
Coated tablets	
Enteric-coated tablets	Slowest

TABLE 2-2 Dosage Forms

Route	Forms
Enteral	Tablets, capsules, pills, timed-release capsules, timed-release tablets, elixirs, suspensions, syrups, emulsions, solutions, lozenges or troches, rectal suppositories, sublingual or buccal tablets
Parenteral	Injectable forms, solutions, suspensions, emulsions, powders for reconstitution
Topical	Aerosols, ointments, creams, pastes, powders, solutions, foams, gels, transdermal patches, inhalers, rectal and vaginal suppositories

with minimal adverse effects. Many dosage forms have been developed to encourage patient adherence with the medication regimen. *Extended-release* tablets and capsules release drug molecules in the patient's GI tract over a prolonged period of time. This ultimately prolongs drug *absorption* as well as *duration of action*. This is the opposite of *immediate-release* dosage forms, which release all of the active ingredient immediately upon *dissolution* in the GI tract. Extended-release dosage forms are normally easily identified by various capital letter abbreviations attached to their names. Examples of this nomenclature are SR *(slow release* or *sustained release)*, SA *(sustained action)*, CR *(controlled release)*, XL *(extended length)*, and XT *(extended time)*. Convenience of administration correlates strongly with adherence to the medication regimen. Many of the extended-release oral dosage forms were designed with this in mind, because they often require fewer daily doses. Extended-release oral dosage forms should not be crushed, as this could cause accelerated release of drug from the dosage form and possible toxicity. Enteric-coated tablets also are usually not recommended for crushing. This causes disruption of the tablet coating designed to protect the stomach lining from the local effects of the drug and/or protect the drug from being prematurely disrupted by stomach acid. The ability to crush a tablet or open a capsule can facilitate drug administration when patients are unable or unwilling to swallow a tablet or capsule and also when medications need to be given through an enteral feeding tube. With capsules, powder or liquid contents can often be added to soft foods such as applesauce or pudding, or dissolved in a beverage. *Granules* contained in capsules are usually for extended drug release and normally should not be crushed or chewed by the patient. However, they can often be swallowed when sprinkled on one of the soft foods mentioned earlier. When in doubt about the appropriateness of crushing a tablet or opening a capsule prior to dosing, the nurse should consult a pharmacist, the product literature, or other suitable source.

An increasingly popular dosage form is drug products that dissolve in the mouth and are absorbed through the oral mucosa. These include *orally disintegrating tablets* as well as thin *wafers* that also dissolve in the mouth. Depending on the specific drug product, the dosage form may dissolve on the tongue, under the tongue, or in the buccal (cheek) pocket.

The specific characteristics of various dosage forms have a large impact on how and to what extent the drug is absorbed. If a drug is to work at a specific site in the body, either it must be applied directly at that site in an active form or it must have a way of getting to that site. Oral dosage forms rely on gastric and intestinal enzymes and pH environments to break the medication down into particles that are small enough to be absorbed into the circulation. Once absorbed through the mucosa of the stomach or intestines, the drug is then transported to the site of action by blood or lymph.

Many topically applied dosage forms work directly on the surface of the skin. Therefore, when the drug is applied, it is already in a form that allows it to act immediately. With other topical dosage forms, the skin acts as a barrier through which the drug must pass to get into the circulation; once there, the drug is then carried to its site of action (e.g., fentanyl transdermal patch for pain).

Dosage forms that are administered via injection are called *parenteral* forms. They must have certain characteristics to be safe and effective. The arteries and veins that carry drugs throughout the body can easily be damaged if the drug is too concentrated or corrosive. The pH of injections must be very similar to that of the blood for these drugs to be administered safely. Parenteral dosage forms that are injected intravenously are immediately placed into solution in the bloodstream and do not have to be dissolved in the body. Therefore, 100% absorption is assumed to occur immediately upon intravenous injection.

PHARMACOKINETICS

A drug's time to onset of action, time to peak effect, and duration of action are all characteristics defined by pharmacokinetics. Pharmacokinetics is the study of what happens to a drug from the time it is put into the body until the **parent drug** and all metabolites have left the body. Thus, drug absorption into, distribution and metabolism within, and excretion from the body represent the combined focus of pharmacokinetics.

Absorption

Absorption is the movement of a drug from its site of administration into the bloodstream for distribution to the tissues. A term used to express the extent of drug absorption is **bioavailability.** For example, a drug that is absorbed from the intestine must first pass through the liver before it reaches the systemic circulation. If a large proportion of a drug is chemically processed into inactive metabolites in the liver, then a much smaller amount of drug will pass into the circulation (i.e., will be bioavailable). Such a drug is said to have a high **first-pass effect** (e.g., oral nitrates). First-pass effect reduces the bioavailability of the drug to less than 100%. Many drugs administered by mouth have a bioavailability of less than 100%, whereas drugs administered by the

CASE STUDY

Pharmacokinetics

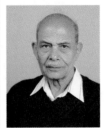
© Yellowcrest Media

Four patients with angina are receiving a form of nitroglycerin, as follows:

Mrs. A., age 88, takes 9 mg twice a day to prevent angina.

Mr. B., age 63, takes a form that delivers 0.2 mg/hr, also to prevent angina.

Mrs. C., age 58, takes 0.4 mg only if needed for chest pain.

Mr. D., age 62, is in the hospital with severe, unstable angina and is receiving 20 mcg/hr.

You may refer to the section on nitroglycerin in Chapter 24 or to a nursing drug handbook to answer the following questions.

1. State the route or form of nitroglycerin that each patient is receiving. In addition, specify the trade name(s) for each particular form.
2. For each patient, state the rationale for the route or form of drug that was chosen. Which forms have immediate action? Why would this be important?
3. Which form or forms are most affected by the first-pass effect? Explain.
4. What would happen if Mrs. A. chewed her nitroglycerin dose? If Mrs. C chewed her nitroglycerin dose?

For answers, see *http://evolve.elsevier.com/Lilley.*

intravenous route are 100% bioavailable, as noted earlier. If two medications have the same bioavailability and same concentration of active ingredient, they are said to be *bioequivalent* (e.g., a brand-name drug and the same generic drug).

Various factors affect the rate of drug absorption; specifics are discussed in the section on enteral drug delivery. How a drug is administered, or its *route of administration,* also affects the rate and extent of absorption of that drug. Although a number of dosage formulations are available for delivering medications to the body, they can all be categorized into three basic routes of administration: enteral (GI tract), parenteral, and topical.

Enteral Route

In enteral drug administration, the drug is absorbed into the systemic circulation through the mucosa of the stomach and/or small or large intestine. The rate of absorption can be altered by many factors. Normally, orally administered drugs are absorbed from the intestinal lumen into the blood system and transported to the liver. Once the drug is in the liver, hepatic enzyme systems metabolize it, and the remaining active ingredients are passed into the general circulation. Rectally administered drugs are often given for systemic effects (e.g., antinausea, analgesia, antipyretic effects), but they are also used to treat disease within the rectum or adjacent bowel (e.g., antiinflammatory ointment for hemorrhoids, corticosteroid enemas for colitis). In the latter case rectal administration can also be thought of as a *topical* route of drug administration.

Before orally administered drugs are passed into the portal circulation of the liver, they are absorbed in the small intestine, which has an enormous surface area. Many factors can alter the absorption of enterally administered drugs, including acid changes within the stomach, absorption changes in the intestines, and the presence or absence of food and fluid. Various factors that affect the acidity of the stomach include the time of day; the age of the patient; and the presence and types of medications (e.g., H_2 blockers or proton pump inhibitors [see Chapter 50]), foods, or beverages. Taking an enteric-coated medication (intended for *intestinal* dissolution and absorption) with a large amount food may result in dissolution of the enteric-coated dosage form by acidic stomach contents and reduced intestinal drug absorption. Anticholinergic drugs slow the GI *transit time* (or the time it takes for substances in the stomach to be dissolved for eventual transport to and absorption from the intestines). This may reduce the amount of drug absorption and therapeutic effect for acid-susceptible drugs that remain in the stomach for longer-than-ideal time periods. On the other hand, the presence of food may enhance the absorption of some fat-soluble drugs (depending on the fat content of the food) or drugs that are more easily broken down in an acidic environment.

Drug absorption may also be altered in patients who have had portions of the small intestine removed because of disease. This is known as *short bowel syndrome.* Similarly, bariatric weight loss surgery reduces the size of the stomach. As a result, medication absorption can be altered, because stomach contents are delivered to the intestines more rapidly than usual after such surgery. This is called *gastric dumping.* Examples of drugs to be taken on an empty stomach and those to be taken with food are provided in Box 2-1. The stomach and small intestine are highly vascularized. When blood flow to that area is decreased, absorption may also be decreased. Sepsis and exercise are examples of circumstances under which blood flow to the GI tract is often reduced. In both cases, blood tends to be routed to the heart and other vital organs. In the case of exercise, it is also routed to the skeletal muscles.

Sublingual and Buccal Routes Drugs administered by the *sublingual* route are absorbed into the highly vascularized tissue under the tongue—the oral mucosa. Sublingual nitroglycerin is an example. Sublingually administered drugs are absorbed rapidly because the area under the tongue has a large blood supply. These drugs bypass the liver and yet are systemically bioavailable. The same applies for drugs administered by the *buccal route* (the oral mucosa between the cheek and the gum). Through these routes, drugs such as nitroglycerin are absorbed rapidly into the bloodstream and delivered to their site of action (e.g., coronary arteries).

Parenteral Route

For most medications, the parenteral route is the fastest route by which a drug can be absorbed, followed by the enteral and topical routes. *Parenteral* is a general term meaning any route of administration other than the GI tract. It most commonly refers to injection. Intravenous injection delivers the drug directly into the circulation, where it is distributed with the blood throughout the body. Drugs given by intramuscular injection and subcutaneous injection are absorbed more slowly than those given intravenously. These drug formulations are usually absorbed over a period of several hours; however, some are specially formulated to be released over days, weeks, or months.

Drugs can be injected intradermally, subcutaneously, **intraarterially,** intramuscularly, **intrathecally,** intraarticularly, or intra-

---

BOX 2-1 Drugs to Be Taken on an Empty Stomach and Drugs to Be Taken with Food

Many medications are taken on an empty stomach with at least 6 oz of water. The nurse must give patients specific instructions regarding those medications that are not to be taken with food. Examples include alendronate sodium and risedronate sodium.

Medications that are generally taken with food include carbamazepine, iron and iron-containing products, hydralazine, lithium, propranolol, spironolactone, nonsteroidal antiinflammatory drugs, and theophylline.

Macrolides and oral opioids are often taken with food (even though they are specified to be taken with a full glass of water and on an empty stomach) to minimize the gastrointestinal irritation associated with these drugs. If doubt exists, a licensed pharmacist or a current authoritative drug resource should be consulted. An Internet source to use is *http://www.usp.org.*

---

venously. Medications given by the parenteral route also have the advantage of bypassing the first-pass effect of the liver. The parenteral route of administration offers an alternative route of delivery for those medications that cannot be given orally and there are fewer obstacles to absorption with parenteral administration. However, drugs that are administered by the parenteral route must still be absorbed into cells and tissues before they can exert their pharmacologic effect (see Table 2-3).

Subcutaneous, Intradermal, and Intramuscular Routes Injections into the fatty subcutaneous tissues under the dermal layer of skin are referred to as *subcutaneous* injections, whereas injections under the more superficial skin layers immediately underneath the epidermal layer of skin and into the dermal layer, are known as *intradermal* injections. Injections given into the muscle beneath the subcutaneous fatty tissue are referred to as *intramuscular* injections. Muscles have a greater blood supply than does the skin; therefore, drugs injected intramuscularly are typically absorbed faster than drugs injected subcutaneously. Absorption from either of these sites may be increased by applying heat to the injection site or by massaging the site. Both methods increase blood flow to the area, thereby enhancing absorption. In contrast, the presence of cold, hypotension, or poor peripheral blood flow compromises the circulation, reducing drug activity by reducing drug delivery to the tissues. Most intramuscularly injected drugs are absorbed over several hours. However, specially formulated long-acting intramuscular dosage forms known as *depot drugs* are designed for slow absorption and may be absorbed over a period of several days to a few months or longer. The intramuscular corticosteroid known as *methylprednisolone acetate* can provide antiinflammatory effects for several weeks. The intramuscular contraceptive medroxyprogesterone acetate normally prevents pregnancy for 3 months per dose.

Topical Route

The topical route of drug administration involves the application of medications to various body surfaces. Several different topical drug delivery systems exist. Topically administered drugs can be applied to the skin, eyes, ears, nose, lungs, rectum, or vagina. Topical application delivers a more uniform amount of drug over a longer period of time, but the effects of the drug are usually slower in their onset and more prolonged in their duration of ac-

TABLE **2-3** **Routes of Administration and Related Nursing Considerations**

Route	Advantages	Disadvantages	Nursing Considerations
Intravenous (IV)	Provides rapid onset (drug delivered immediately to bloodstream); allows more direct control of drug level in blood; gives option of larger fluid volume, therefore diluting irritating drugs; avoids first-pass metabolism	Higher cost; inconvenience (e.g., not self-administered); irreversibility of drug action in most cases and inability to retrieve medication; risk of fluid overload; greater likelihood of infection; possibility of embolism	Continuous IV infusions require frequent monitoring to be sure that the correct volume and amount are administered and that drug reaches safe, therapeutic blood levels. IV drugs and solutions should be checked for compatibilities. IV sites should be monitored for redness, swelling, heat, and drainage—all indicative of complications, such as thrombophlebitis. If intermittent IV infusions are used, clearing or flushing of the line with normal saline before and after is generally indicated to keep the IV site patent and minimize incompatibilities.
Intramuscular (IM); subcutaneous (subcut)	IM injections are good for poorly soluble drugs, which are often given in "depot" preparation form and are then absorbed over a prolonged period; onsets of action differ depending on route (e.g., IM injections often produce more rapid onset than subcut injections)	Discomfort of injection; inconvenience; bruising; slower onset of action compared to IV, although quicker than oral in most situations	Using landmarks to identify correct IM and subcut sites is always required and is recommended as a nursing standard of care. Ventral gluteal site is IM site of choice with use of 1½-inch (sometimes 1-inch in very thin or emaciated patients) and 21-25 gauge needle. Subcut injections are recommended to be given at 90-degree angle with proper size syringe and needle (½- to ⅝-inch needle); in emaciated or very thin patients, subcut angle should be 45 degrees. Selection of correct size of syringe and needle is key to safe administration by these routes and is based on thorough assessment of the patient as well as drug characteristics.
Oral	Usually easier, more convenient, and less expensive; safer than injection, dosing more likely to be reversible in cases of accidental ingestion (e.g., through induction of emesis, administration of activated charcoal)	Variable absorption; inactivation of some drugs by stomach acid and/or pH; problems with first-pass effect or presystemic metabolism; greater dependence of drug action on patient variables	Enteral routes include oral administration and involve a variety of dosage forms, e.g., liquids, solutions, tablets, and enteric-coated pills or tablets. Some medications should be taken with food and some should not be taken with food; oral forms should always be taken with at least 6-8 oz of fluid, such as water. Other factors to consider include other medicines being taken at the same time and concurrent use of dairy products or antacids. If oral forms are given via nasogastric tube or gastrostomy tube, tube should be assessed for placement in stomach and head should remain elevated; at least 30-60 mL of water or carbonated fluids should be used to flush tube prior to and after drug has been given to keep tube patent.
Sublingual, buccal (subtypes of oral, but more parenteral than enteral)	Absorbed more rapidly from oral mucosa and leads to more rapid onset of action; avoids breakdown of drug by stomach acid; avoids first-pass metabolism because gastric absorption is bypassed	Patients may swallow pill instead of keeping under tongue until dissolved; pills often smaller to handle	Drugs given via sublingual route should be placed under tongue; once dissolved, drug may then be swallowed. In buccal route, medication is placed between cheek and gum. Both of these dosage forms are relatively nonirritating; drug is usually without flavor and water soluble.
Rectal	Provides relatively rapid absorption; good alternative when oral route not feasible; useful for local or systemic drug delivery; usually leads to mixed first-pass and non–first-pass metabolism	Possible discomfort and embarrassment to patient; often higher cost than oral route	Absorption via this route is erratic and unpredictable, but it provides a safe alternative whenever nausea or vomiting prevents oral dosing of drugs. Patient should lie on left side for insertion of rectal dosage form. Suppositories are inserted using gloved hand or index finger and water-soluble lubricant. Drug should be administered exactly as ordered.
Topical	Delivers medication directly to affected area; decreases likelihood of systemic drug effects	Sometimes awkward to self-administer (e.g., eyedrops); can be messy; usually higher cost than oral route	Most dermatologic drugs are given via topical route in form of a solution, ointment, spray, or drops. Skin should be clean and free of debris; if measurement of ointment is necessary—such as with topical nitroglycerin—it should be done carefully and per instructions (e.g., apply 1 inch of ointment). Nurse should wear gloves to minimize cross contamination and prevent absorption of drug into his or her skin. If patient's skin is not intact, sterile technique is needed.

TABLE 2-3 Routes of Administration and Related Nursing Considerations—cont'd

Route	Advantages	Disadvantages	Nursing Considerations
Transdermal (subtype of topical)	Provides relatively constant rate of drug absorption; one patch can last 1-7 days, depending on drug; avoids first-pass metabolism	Rate of absorption can be affected by excessive perspiration and body temperature; patch may peel off; cost is higher; used patches must be disposed of safely	Transdermal drugs should be placed on alternating sites, on a clean and nonirritating area, and only after previously applied patch has been removed and area cleansed and dried. Transdermal drugs generally come in a single-dose, adhesive-backed drug application system.
Inhalational	Provides rapid absorption; drug delivered directly to lung tissues where most of these drugs exert their actions	Rate of absorption can be too rapid, increasing the risk of exaggerated drug effects; requires more patient education for self-administration; some patients may have difficulty with administration technique	Inhaled medications should be used exactly as prescribed and with clean equipment. Instructions should be given regarding the medications as well as the proper use, storage, and safe-keeping of inhalers, spacers, and nebulizers. Chapter 10 describes and shows how medications are inhaled.

PREVENTING MEDICATION ERRORS

Does IV = PO?

The physician writes an order for "Lasix 80 mg IV STAT" for a patient who is short of breath with pulmonary edema. When the nurse goes to give the drug, only the PO form is immediately available. Someone must go to the pharmacy to pick up the IV dose. Another nurse says, "Go ahead and give the pill. He needs it fast. It's all the same!" But is it?

Remember, the oral forms of medications must be processed through the gastrointestinal tract, absorbed through the small intestines, and undergo the first-pass effect in the liver before the drug can reach the intended site of action. However, IV forms are injected directly into the circulation and can act almost immediately because the first-pass effect is bypassed. The time until onset of action for the PO form is 30 to 60 minutes; for the IV form, this time is *5* minutes. This patient is in respiratory distress, and the immediate effect of the diuretic is desired. In addition, because of the first-pass effect, the available amount of orally administered drug that actually reaches the site of action would be less than the available amount of intravenously administered drug. Therefore, IV does NOT equal PO! Never change the route of administration of a medication; if questions come up, always check with the prescriber.

BOX 2-2 Drug Routes and First-Pass Effects

First-Pass Routes
Hepatic arterial
Oral
Portal venous
Rectal*

Non–First-Pass Routes
Aural (instilled into the ear)
Buccal
Inhaled
Intraarterial
Intramuscular
Intranasal
Intraocular
Intravaginal
Intravenous
Subcutaneous
Sublingual
Transdermal

*Leads to both first-pass and non–first-pass effects.

tion. This can be a problem if the patient begins to experience adverse effects from the drug and a considerable amount of drug has already been absorbed into the subcutaneous or mucosal tissues. All topical routes of drug administration also avoid first-pass effects of the liver, with the exception of rectal drug administration. Because the rectum is part of the GI tract, some drug will be absorbed into the capillaries that feed the portal vein to the liver. However, some drugs will also be absorbed locally into the perirectal tissues. Therefore, rectally administered drugs are said to have a mixed first-pass and non–first-pass absorption and metabolism. Box 2-2 lists the various drug routes and indicates whether they are associated with first-pass effects in the liver.

Ointments, gels, and creams are common types of topically administered drugs. Examples include sunscreens, antibiotics, and nitroglycerin ointment. The drawback to their use is that their systemic absorption is often erratic and unreliable. Generally, these medications are used for local effects, but some are used for systemic effects (e.g., nitroglycerin ointment for maintenance treatment of angina). Topically applied drugs can also be used in the treatment of various illnesses of the eyes, ears, and sinuses. Eye, ear, and nose drops are administered primarily for local effects, whereas nasal sprays may be used for both systemic and local effects (e.g., oxymetazoline for nasal sinus congestion, sumatriptan for migraine headaches). Vaginal medications may also be given for systemic effects (e.g., progestational hormone therapy with progesterone vaginal suppositories) but are more commonly used for local effects (e.g., treatment of vaginal yeast infection with miconazole [Monistat] vaginal cream).

Transdermal Route Transdermal drug delivery through adhesive patches is a more elaborate topical route of drug administration that is commonly used for systemic drug effects. Some examples of drugs administered by this route are fentanyl (for pain), nitroglycerin (for angina), nicotine (for smoking cessation), estrogen (for menopausal symptoms), and clonidine (for hypertension). Transdermal patches are usually designed to deliver a constant amount of drug per unit of time for a specified time period. For example, a nitroglycerin patch may deliver 0.1 or 0.2 mg/hr over 24 hours, whereas a fentanyl patch may deliver 25 to 100 mcg/hr over a 72-hour period. This route is suitable for patients who cannot tolerate orally administered medications and provides a practical and convenient method for drug delivery in other situations.

Inhaled Route Inhalation is another type of topical drug administration. Inhaled drugs are delivered to the lungs as micrometer-sized drug particles. This small drug size is necessary for the drug to be transported to the small air sacs within the lungs (alveoli). Once the small particles of drug are in the alveoli, drug absorption is fairly rapid. Many pulmonary and other types of diseases can be treated with such topically applied (inhaled) drugs. Examples of inhaled drugs are albuterol, which is used to treat bronchial constriction in individuals with asthma, and fluticasone, which is used for antiinflammatory purposes in patients with asthma and allergies.

Distribution

Distribution refers to the transport of a drug by the bloodstream to its site of action (Figure 2-3). The areas to which the drug is distributed first are those that are most extensively supplied with blood. Areas of rapid distribution include the heart, liver, kidneys, and brain. Areas of slower distribution include muscle, skin, and fat. Once a drug enters the bloodstream (circulation), it is distributed throughout the body. At this point it is also beginning to be eliminated by the organs that metabolize and excrete drugs—primarily the liver and the kidneys. Only drug molecules that are not bound to plasma proteins can freely distribute to ex-

travascular tissue (outside the blood vessels) to reach their site of action. If a drug is bound to plasma proteins, the drug-protein complex is generally too large to pass through the walls of blood capillaries into tissues (Figure 2-4). Albumin, the most common blood protein, carries the majority of protein-bound drug molecules. If a given drug binds to albumin as part of its chemical attributes, then there is only a limited amount of drug that is *not* bound. This unbound portion is pharmacologically active and is considered "free" drug, whereas "bound" drug is pharmacologically inactive. Certain conditions that cause low albumin levels, such as extensive burns, malnourished states, and negative nitrogen balance, result in a larger fraction of free (unbound and active) drug. This can raise the risk of drug toxicity.

When an individual is taking two medications that are highly protein bound, the medications may compete for binding sites on the albumin molecule. Because of this competition there is more free, unbound drug. This can lead to an unpredictable drug response called a *drug-drug interaction.* A drug-drug interaction occurs when the presence of one drug decreases or increases the actions of another drug that is administered concurrently (i.e., given at the same time).

A theoretical volume, called the *volume of distribution,* is sometimes used to describe the various areas in which drugs may be distributed. These areas, or *compartments,* may be the blood *(intravascular space),* total body water, body fat, or other body tissues and organs. Typically a drug that is highly water soluble (hydrophilic) will have a smaller volume of distribution and high blood concentrations. In contrast, fat-soluble drugs (lipophilic) have a larger volume of distribution and low blood concentrations. There are some sites in the body into which it may be very

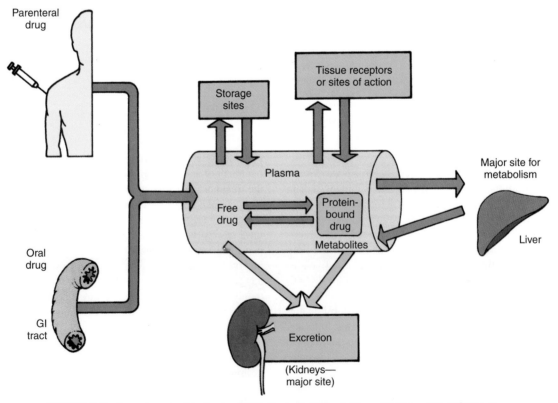

FIGURE 2-3   Drug transport in the body. *GI,* Gastrointestinal. (From McKenry LM, Salerno E: *Mosby's pharmacology in nursing,* ed 19, St Louis, 1995, Mosby.)

difficult to distribute a drug. These sites typically either have a poor blood supply (e.g., bone) or have physiologic barriers that make it difficult for drugs to pass through (e.g., the brain due to the **blood-brain barrier**).

Metabolism

Metabolism is also referred to as **biotransformation** because it involves the biochemical alteration of a drug into an inactive **metabolite,** a more soluble compound, a more potent active metabolite (as in the conversion of an inactive **prodrug** to its active form),

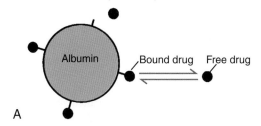

Reversible Binding of a Drug to Albumin

Albumin

Bound drug   Free drug

A

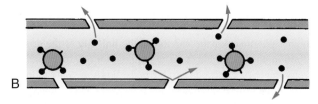

Retention of Protein-Bound Drug Within the Vasculature

B

FIGURE 2-4   Protein binding of drugs. **A,** Albumin is the most prevalent protein in plasma and the most important of the proteins to which drugs bind. **B,** Only unbound (free) drug molecules can leave the vascular system. Bound molecules are too large to fit through the pores in the capillary wall. (From Lehne RA: *Pharmacology for nursing care*, ed 7, St Louis, 2010, Saunders.)

or a less active metabolite. Metabolism is the next step after absorption and distribution. The organ most responsible for the metabolism of drugs is the liver. Other metabolic tissues include skeletal muscle, kidneys, lungs, plasma, and intestinal mucosa.

Hepatic metabolism involves the activity of a very large class of enzymes known as **cytochrome P-450** enzymes (or simply P-450 enzymes), also known as *microsomal* enzymes. These enzymes control a variety of reactions that aid in the metabolism of medications. They are largely targeted at lipid-soluble (*nonpolar* [no charge] drugs also known as *lipophilic* ["fat loving"]), which are typically very difficult to eliminate. These include the majority of medications. Those medications with water-soluble (polar or *hydrophilic* ["water loving"]) molecules may be more easily metabolized by simpler chemical reactions such as hydrolysis. Some of the chemical reactions by which the liver can metabolize drugs are listed in Table 2-4. Drug molecules that are the metabolic targets of specific enzymes are said to be **substrates** for those enzymes. Specific P-450 enzymes are identified by standardized number and letter designations. Some of the most common P-450 enzymes and their corresponding drug substrates are listed in Table 2-5. The P-450 system is one of the most important systems that influences drug-drug interactions. The list of drugs that are metabolized by the P-450 enzyme system is constantly changing as new drugs are introduced into the market. For further information, see websites such as *http://www.medicine. iupui.edu/flockhart/table.htm* and *http://www.nursinglink.com/ training/articles/320-clinically-significant-drug-interaction- with-the-cytochrome-p450-enzyme-system.*

The biotransformation capabilities of the liver can vary considerably from patient to patient. Various factors that can alter the biotransformation of a drug, including genetics, diseases, and the concurrent use of other medications, are listed in Table 2-6.

Many drugs can inhibit various drug-metabolizing enzymes and are called enzyme *inhibitors*. Decreased or delayed drug me-

---

TABLE 2-4 Mechanisms of Biotransformation

Type of Biotransformation	Mechanism	Result
Oxidation Reduction Hydrolysis	Chemical reactions	Increase polarity of chemical, making it more water soluble and more easily excreted. Often this results in a loss of pharmacologic activity.
Conjugation (e.g., glucuronidation, glycination, sulfation, methylation, alkylation)	Combination with another substance (e.g., glucuronide, glycine, sulfate, methyl groups, alkyl groups)	

TABLE 2-5 Common Liver Cytochrome P-450 Enzymes and Corresponding Drug Substrates

Enzyme	Common Drug Substrates
1A2	acetaminophen, caffeine, theophylline, warfarin
2C9	ibuprofen, phenytoin
2C19	diazepam, naproxen, omeprazole, propranolol
2D6	codeine, fluoxetine, hydrocodone, metoprolol, oxycodone, paroxetine, propoxyphene, risperidone, tricyclic antidepressants
2E1	acetaminophen, ethanol
3A4	acetaminophen, amiodarone, cyclosporine, diltiazem, ethinyl estradiol, indinavir, lidocaine, macrolides, progesterone, spironolactone, sulfamethoxazole, testosterone, verapamil

TABLE 2-6 Examples of Conditions and Drugs That Affect Drug Metabolism

Category	Example	Drug Metabolism	
		Increased	Decreased
Diseases	Cardiovascular dysfunction		X
	Renal insufficiency		X
Conditions	Starvation	X	
	Obstructive jaundice		X
	Genetic constitution		
	Fast acetylator	X	
	Slow acetylator		X
Drugs	Barbiturates	X	
	rifampin (P-450 inducer)	X	
	phenytoin (P-450 inducer)	X	
	ketoconazole (P-450 inhibitor)		X

tabolism results in the accumulation of the drug and prolongation of the effects of the drug, which can lead to drug toxicity. In contrast, stimulation of drug metabolism can cause diminishing pharmacologic effects. This often occurs with the repeated administration of some drugs that can stimulate the formation of new microsomal enzymes. Such drugs are said to be *enzyme inducers.*

Excretion

Excretion is the elimination of drugs from the body. Whether they are parent compounds or active or inactive metabolites, all drugs must eventually be removed from the body. The primary organ responsible for this elimination is the kidney. Two other organs that play an important role in the excretion of drugs are the liver and the bowel. Most drugs are metabolized in the liver by various mechanisms. Therefore, by the time most drugs reach the kidneys, they have undergone extensive biotransformation, and only a relatively small fraction of the original drug is excreted as the original compound. Other drugs may circumvent metabolism and reach the kidneys in their original form. Drugs that have been metabolized by the liver become more polar and water soluble. This makes their elimination by the kidneys much easier, because the urinary tract is water based. The kidneys themselves are also capable of metabolizing various drugs, although usually to a lesser extent than the liver.

The actual act of renal excretion is accomplished through *glomerular filtration, active tubular reabsorption,* and *active tubular secretion.* Free (unbound) water-soluble drugs and metabolites go through passive glomerular filtration. Many substances present in the nephrons go through active reabsorption and are taken back up into the systemic circulation and transported away from the kidney. This process is an attempt by the body to retain needed substances. Some substances may also be secreted into the nephron from the vasculature surrounding it. The processes of filtration, reabsorption, and secretion for urinary elimination are shown in Figure 2-5.

The excretion of drugs by the intestines is another common route of elimination. This process is referred to as *biliary excretion.* Drugs that are eliminated by this route are taken up by the liver, released into the bile, and eliminated in the feces. Once certain drugs, such as fat-soluble drugs, are in the bile, they may be reabsorbed into the bloodstream, returned to the liver, and again secreted into the bile. This process is called *enterohepatic recirculation.* Enterohepatically recirculated drugs persist in the body for much longer periods. Less common routes of elimination are the lungs and the sweat, salivary, and mammary glands.

Half-Life

Another pharmacokinetic variable is the **half-life** of the drug. By definition, the half-life is the time required for one half (50%) of a given drug to be removed from the body. It is a measure of the rate at which the drug is eliminated from the body. For instance, if the peak level of a particular drug is 100 mg/L and in 8 hours the measured drug level is 50 mg/L, then the estimated half-life of that drug is 8 hours. The concept of drug half-life viewed from several different perspectives is shown in Table 2-7.

After about five half-lives, most drugs are considered to be effectively removed from the body. At that time approximately 97% of the drug has been eliminated, and what little amount remains is usually too small to have either therapeutic or toxic effects.

The concept of half-life is clinically useful for determining when steady state will be reached in a patient taking a particular drug. With regard to blood levels, **steady state** of a drug refers to the physiologic state in which the amount of drug removed via elimination (e.g., renal clearance) is equal to the amount of drug absorbed with each dose. This physiologic plateau phenomenon typically occurs after four to five half-lives of administered drug. Therefore, if a drug has an extremely long half-life, it will take much longer for the drug to reach steady-state blood levels. Once steady-state blood levels have been reached, there are consistent levels of drug in the body that correlate with maximum therapeutic benefits.

Onset, Peak, and Duration

The pharmacokinetic terms *absorption, distribution, metabolism,* and *excretion* are all used to describe the movement of drugs through the body. Drug actions are the processes involved in the interaction between a drug and a cell (e.g., a drug's action on a receptor). In contrast, **drug effects** are the physiologic reactions of the body to the drug. The terms *onset, peak, duration,* and *trough* are used to describe drug effects. *Peak* and *trough* are also used to describe drug concentrations, which are usually measured from blood samples.

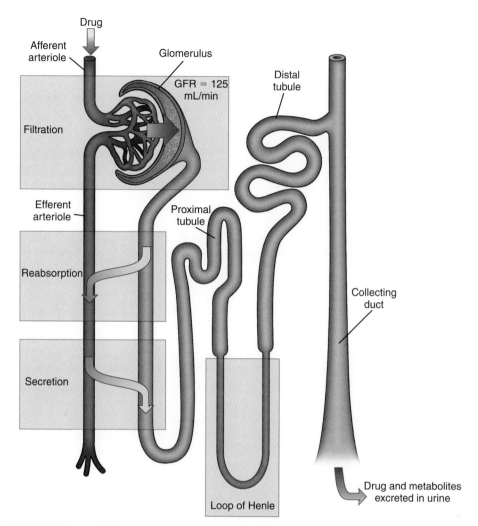

FIGURE 2-5   Renal drug excretion. The primary processes involved in drug excretion and the approximate location where these processes take place in the kidney are illustrated. *GFR,* Glomerular filtration rate.

TABLE 2-7 Example of Drug Half-Life Viewed from Different Perspectives

Metric	Changing Values					
Hours after peak concentration	0	8	16	24	32	40
Drug concentration (mg/L)	100 (peak)	50	25	12.5	6.25	3.125 (trough)
Number of half-lives	0	1	2	3	4	5
Percentage of drug removed	0	50	75	88	94	97

A drug's **onset of action** is the time required for the drug to elicit a therapeutic response. A drug's **peak effect** is the time required for a drug to reach its maximum therapeutic response. Physiologically, this corresponds to increasing drug concentrations at the site of action. The **duration of action** of a drug is the length of time that the drug concentration is sufficient (without more doses) to elicit a therapeutic response. These concepts are illustrated in Figure 2-6.

The length of time until the onset and peak of action and the duration of action often play an important part in determining the **peak level** (highest blood level) and **trough level** (lowest blood level) of a drug. If the peak blood level is too high, then drug toxicity may occur. The toxicity may be mild, such as intensification of the effects of the given drug (e.g., excessive sedation resulting from overdose of a drug with sedative properties). However, it can also be severe (e.g., damage to vital organs due to excessive drug exposure). If the trough blood level is too low, then the drug may not be at therapeutic levels. (A common example is antibiotic drug therapy with aminoglycoside antibiotics [see Chapter 39]). In **therapeutic drug monitoring,** *peak* (highest) and *trough* (lowest) values are measured to verify adequate drug exposure, maximize therapeutic effects, and minimize drug toxicity. This monitoring is often carried out by a clinical pharmacist working with other members of the health care team. The

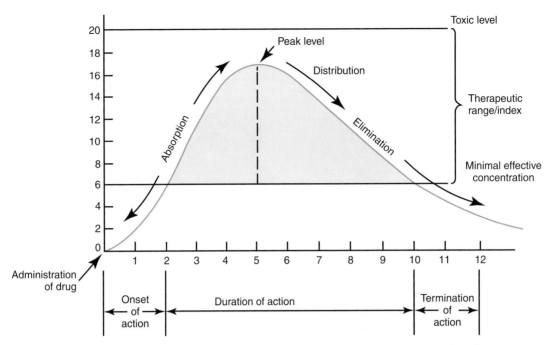

FIGURE 2-6   Characteristics of drug effect and relationship to the therapeutic window. (From McKenry LM, Tessier E, Hogan M: *Mosby's pharmacology in nursing,* ed 22, St Louis, 2006, Mosby.)

use of therapeutic drug monitoring will be described for specific drugs in various chapters when clinically relevant.

PHARMACODYNAMICS

Pharmacodynamics is concerned with the mechanisms of drug action in living tissues. Drug-induced alterations in normal physiologic functions are explained by the principles of pharmacodynamics. A positive change in a faulty physiologic system is called a **therapeutic effect** of a drug. Such an effect is the goal of drug therapy. Understanding the pharmacodynamic characteristics of a drug can aid in assessing the drug's therapeutic effect.

Mechanism of Action

Drugs can produce actions (therapeutic effects) in several ways. The effects of a particular drug depend on the characteristics of the cells or tissue targeted by the drug. Once the drug is at the site of action, it can modify (increase or decrease) the rate at which that cell or tissue functions, or it can modify the strength of function of that cell or tissue. A drug cannot, however, cause a cell or tissue to perform a function that is not part of its natural physiology.

Drugs can exert their actions in three basic ways: through *receptors, enzymes,* and *nonselective interactions.* These mechanisms are discussed in the following sections. It should also be noted that not all mechanisms of action have been identified for all drugs. Thus, a drug may be said to have an unknown or unclear mechanism of action, even though it has observable therapeutic effects in the body.

Receptor Interactions

A **receptor** can be defined as a reactive site on the surface or inside of a cell. If the mechanism of action of a drug involves a receptor interaction, then the molecular structure of the drug is

critical. Drug-receptor interaction is the selective joining of the drug molecule with a reactive site on the surface of a cell or tissue. Most commonly, this site is a protein structure within the cell membrane. Once a drug binds to and interacts with the receptor, a pharmacologic response is produced (Figure 2-7). The degree to which a drug attaches to and binds with a receptor is called its *affinity*. The drug with the best "fit" and strongest affinity for the receptor will elicit the greatest response from the cell or tissue. A drug becomes bound to the receptor through the formation of chemical bonds between the receptor on the cell and the active site on the drug molecule. Drugs that bind to receptors interact with receptors in different ways either to elicit or to block a physiologic response. Table 2-8 describes the different types of drug-receptor interaction.

Enzyme Interactions

Enzymes are the substances that catalyze nearly every biochemical reaction in a cell. Drugs can produce effects by interacting with these enzyme systems. For a drug to alter a physiologic response in this way, it may either inhibit (more common) or enhance (less common) the action of a specific enzyme. This process is called *selective interaction.* Drug-enzyme interaction occurs when the drug chemically binds to an enzyme molecule in such a way that it alters (inhibits or enhances) the enzyme's interaction with its normal target molecules in the body.

Nonselective Interactions

Drugs with nonspecific mechanisms of action do not interact with receptors or enzymes. Instead, their main targets are cell membranes and various cellular processes such as metabolic activities. These drugs can either physically interfere with or chemically alter cellular structures or processes. Some cancer drugs and antibiotics have this mechanism of action. By incorporating themselves into the normal metabolic process, they cause a defect in the final product or state. This defect may be an improperly formed cell wall that results in cell death through cell lysis or it may be the lack of a necessary energy substrate, which leads to cell starvation and death.

PHARMACOTHERAPEUTICS

Before drug therapy is initiated, an end point or expected outcome of therapy should be established. This desired therapeutic outcome should be patient specific, should be established in collaboration with the patient, and, if appropriate, should be determined with other members of the health care team. Outcomes should ideally be clearly defined and must be either measurable or observable by the patient or caregiver. A time line for these outcomes should also be specified. The progress being made should be monitored. Outcome goals should be realistic and prioritized so that drug therapy begins with interventions that are essential to the patient's well-being. Examples include curing a disease, eliminating or reducing a preexisting symptom, arresting or slowing a disease process, preventing a disease or other unwanted condition, or otherwise improving the quality of life. These goals and outcomes are not the same as nursing goals and outcomes. See Chapter 1 for a more specific discussion of the nursing process.

Patient therapy assessment is the process by which a practitioner integrates his or her knowledge of medical and drug-related facts with information about a specific patient's medical and social history. Items that should be considered in the assessment are drugs currently used (prescription, over the-counter, herbal, and illicit or street drugs), pregnancy and breast-feeding status, and concurrent illnesses that could contraindicate initia-

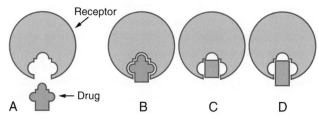

FIGURE 2-7 **A,** Drugs act by forming a chemical bond with specific receptor sites, similar to a key and lock. **B,** The better the "fit," the better the response. Drugs with complete attachment and response are called *agonists.* **C,** Drugs that attach but do not elicit a response are called *antagonists.* **D,** Drugs that attach, elicit some response, and also block other responses are called *partial agonists* or *agonist-antagonists.* (From Clayton BD, Stock YN: *Basic pharmacology for nurses,* ed 14, St Louis, 2007, Mosby.)

tion of a given medication. A **contraindication** for a medication is any patient condition, especially a disease state, that makes the use of the given medication dangerous for the patient. Careful attention to this assessment process helps to ensure an optimal therapeutic plan for the patient. The implementation of a treatment plan can involve several types and combinations of therapies. The type of therapy can be categorized as acute, maintenance, supplemental (or replacement), palliative, supportive, prophylactic, or empiric.

Acute Therapy

Acute therapy often involves more intensive drug treatment and is implemented in the acutely ill (those with rapid onset of illness) or even the critically ill. It is often needed to sustain life or treat disease. Examples are the administration of vasopressors to maintain blood pressure and cardiac output after open heart surgery, the use of volume expanders in a patient who is in shock, and intensive chemotherapy for a patient with newly diagnosed cancer.

Maintenance Therapy

Maintenance therapy typically does not eradicate problems the patient may have but does prevent progression of a disease or condition. It is used for the treatment of chronic illnesses such as hypertension. In the latter case, maintenance therapy maintains the patient's blood pressure within given limits, which prevents certain end-organ damage. Another example of maintenance therapy is the use of oral contraceptives for birth control.

Supplemental Therapy

Supplemental or replacement therapy supplies the body with a substance needed to maintain normal function. This substance may be needed either because it cannot be made by the body or because it is produced in insufficient quantity. Examples are the administration of insulin to diabetic patients and of iron to patients with iron-deficiency anemia.

Palliative Therapy

The goal of palliative therapy is to make the patient as comfortable as possible. It is typically used in the end stages of an illness when all attempts at curative therapy have failed. Examples are the use of high-dose opioid analgesics to relieve pain in the final stages of cancer and the use of oxygen in end-stage pulmonary disease.

Supportive Therapy

Supportive therapy maintains the integrity of body functions while the patient is recovering from illness or trauma. Examples are provision of fluids and electrolytes to prevent dehydration in a patient with influenza who is vomiting and has diarrhea, and

TABLE 2-8 Drug-Receptor Interactions

Drug Type	Action
Agonist	Drug binds to the receptor; there is a response.
Partial agonist (agonist-antagonist)	Drug binds to the receptor; the response is diminished compared with that elicited by an agonist.
Antagonist	Drug binds to the receptor; there is no response. Drug prevents binding of agonists.
Competitive antagonist	Drug competes with the agonist for binding to the receptor. If it binds, there is no response.
Noncompetitive antagonist	Drug combines with different parts of the receptor and inactivates it; agonist then has no effect.

administration of fluids, volume expanders, or blood products to a patient who has lost blood during surgery.

Prophylactic Therapy and Empiric Therapy

Prophylactic therapy is drug therapy provided to *prevent* illness or other undesirable outcome during *planned* events. A common example is the use of preoperative antibiotic therapy for surgical procedures. The antibiotic is given before the incision is made, so that the antibiotic can kill any potential pathogens. Another example is the administration of disease-specific vaccines to individuals traveling to geographic areas where a given disease is known to be endemic.

Empiric therapy is based on clinical probabilities. It involves drug administration when a certain pathologic condition has an uncertain but high likelihood of occurrence based on the patient's initial presenting symptoms. A common example is use of antibiotics active against the organism most commonly associated with a specific infection before the results of the culture and sensitivity reports are available.

Monitoring

Once the appropriate therapy has been implemented, the effectiveness of the therapy—that is, the clinical response of the patient to the treatment—must be evaluated. Evaluating the clinical response requires familiarity with both the drug's intended therapeutic action (beneficial effects) and its unintended possible **adverse effects** (predictable adverse drug reactions). Examples of monitoring are observing for the therapeutic effect of reduced blood pressure following administration of antihypertensive drugs and observing for the toxic effect of leukopenia after administering antineoplastic (cancer chemotherapy) drugs. Another example is performing a pain assessment after giving pain medication. It should be noted that this text generally highlights only the most common adverse effects of a given drug; however, the drug may have many other less commonly reported adverse effects. One must always keep in mind that patients may sometimes experience less common, and therefore less readily identifiable, adverse drug effects. The nurse should consult comprehensive references, pharmacists, or poison and drug information center staff whenever there is uncertainty regarding adverse effects that a patient may be experiencing.

All drugs are potentially toxic and can have cumulative effects. Recognizing these toxic effects and knowing their manifestations in the patient are integral components of the monitoring process. A drug accumulates when it is absorbed more quickly than it is eliminated or when it is administered before the previous dose has been metabolized or cleared from the body. Knowledge of the organs responsible for metabolizing and eliminating a drug, combined with knowledge of how a particular drug is metabolized and excreted, enables the nurse to anticipate problems and treat them appropriately if they occur.

Therapeutic Index

The ratio of a drug's toxic level to the level that provides therapeutic benefits is referred to as the drug's **therapeutic index.** The safety of a particular drug therapy is determined by this index. A low therapeutic index means that the difference between a therapeutically active dose and a toxic dose is small. A drug with a low

therapeutic index has a greater likelihood than other drugs of causing an adverse reaction, and therefore its use requires closer monitoring. Examples of such drugs are warfarin and digoxin. In contrast, a drug with a high therapeutic index, such as amoxicillin, is rarely associated with overdose events.

Drug Concentration

All drugs reach a certain concentration in the blood. Drug concentrations can be an important tool for evaluating the clinical response to drug therapy. Certain drug levels are associated with therapeutic responses, whereas other drug levels are associated with toxic effects. Toxic drug levels are typically seen when the body's normal mechanisms for metabolizing and excreting drugs are compromised. This commonly occurs when liver and kidney functions are impaired or when the liver or kidneys are immature (as in neonates). Dosage adjustments should be made in these patients to appropriately accommodate their impaired metabolism and excretion.

Patient's Condition

Another patient-specific factor to be considered when monitoring drug therapy is the patient's concurrent diseases or other medical conditions. A patient's response to a drug may vary greatly depending on physiologic and psychologic demands. Disease of any kind, infection, cardiovascular function, and GI function are just a few of the physiologic elements that can alter a patient's therapeutic response. Stress, depression, and anxiety can also be important psychologic factors affecting response.

Tolerance and Dependence

Drug therapy monitoring requires a knowledge of tolerance and dependence and an understanding of the difference between the two. **Tolerance** is a decreasing response to repeated drug doses. **Dependence** is a physiologic or psychologic need for a drug. *Physical dependence* is the physiologic need for a drug to avoid physical withdrawal symptoms (e.g., tachycardia in an opioid-addicted patient). *Psychologic dependence* is also known as *addiction* and is the obsessive desire for the euphoric effects of a drug. Addiction typically involves the recreational use of various drugs such as benzodiazepines, opioids, and amphetamines. See Chapter 9 for further discussion of dependence and addiction.

Interactions

Drugs may interact with other drugs, with foods, or with agents administered as part of laboratory tests. Knowledge of drug interactions is vital for the appropriate monitoring of drug therapy. The more drugs a patient receives, the more likely that a drug interaction will occur. This is especially true in older adults, who typically have an increased sensitivity to drug effects and are receiving several medications. In addition, over-the-counter medications and herbal therapies can interact significantly with prescribed medications. Food also can interact significantly with certain drugs. See Table 2-9 for the most common food-drug interactions.

Alteration of the action of one drug by another is referred to as **drug interaction.** A drug interaction can either increase or decrease the actions of one or both of the involved drugs. Drug interactions can be either beneficial or harmful. The more drugs a patient is taking, the greater the risk of drug interactions. Careful

TABLE 2-9 Common Food and Drug Interactions

Food	Drug (Category)	Result
Leafy green vegetables	warfarin (anticoagulant)	Decreased anticoagulant effect from warfarin
Dairy products	tetracycline, levofloxacin, ciprofloxacin, moxifloxacin (antibiotics)	Chemical binding of the drug leading to decreased effect and treatment failures
Grapefruit juice	amiodarone (antidysrhythmic) buspirone (antianxiety) carbamazepine (antiseizure) cyclosporine, tacrolimus (immunosuppressants) felodipine, nifedipine, nimodipine, nisoldipine (calcium channel blockers) simvastatin, atorvastatin (anticholesterol drugs)	Decreased metabolism of drugs and increased effects
Aged cheese, wine	Monoamine oxidase inhibitors	Hypertensive crisis

TABLE 2-10 Examples of Drug Interactions and Their Effects on Pharmacokinetics

Pharmacokinetic Phase	Drug Combination	Mechanism	Result
Absorption	Antacid with levofloxacin	Antacids bind to the levofloxacin preventing adequate absorption	Decreased effectiveness of levofloxacin, resulting from decreased blood levels (harmful)
Distribution	warfarin with amiodarone	Both drugs compete for protein-binding sites	Higher levels of free (unbound) warfarin and amiodarone, which increases actions of both drugs (harmful)
Metabolism	erythromycin with cyclosporine	Both drugs compete for the same hepatic enzymes	Decreased metabolism of cyclosporine, possibly resulting in toxic levels of cyclosporine (harmful)
Excretion	amoxicillin with probenecid	Inhibits the secretion of amoxicillin into the kidneys	Elevation and prolongation of plasma levels of amoxicillin (can be beneficial)

patient care combined with knowledge of all drugs being administered can decrease the likelihood of a harmful drug interaction.

Understanding the mechanisms of drug interactions can help prevent them from occurring. Concurrently administered drugs may interact with each other and alter the pharmacokinetics of one another during any of the four phases of pharmacokinetics: absorption, distribution, metabolism, or excretion. Table 2-10 provides examples of drug interaction during each of these phases. Most commonly, drug interactions occur when there is competition between two drugs for metabolizing enzymes, such as the cytochrome P-450 enzymes listed in Table 2-5. As a result, the speed of metabolism of one or both drugs may be enhanced or reduced. This change in metabolism of one or both drugs can lead to subtherapeutic or toxic drug actions. Because there are often hundreds of theoretically possible drug interactions among the several drugs a given patient might be receiving, this book focuses on those interactions that are more commonly reported.

Many terms are used to categorize drug interactions. When two drugs with similar actions are given together, they can have **additive effects** (1 + 1 = 2). Examples are the many combinations of analgesic products, such as antihistamine and opioid combinations (e.g., promethazine and codeine) for treatment of cold symptoms, and acetaminophen and opioid combinations (e.g., acetaminophen and oxycodone) for treatment of pain. Often drugs are used together for their additive effects so that smaller doses of each drug can be given.

Synergistic effects occur when two drugs administered together interact in such a way that their combined effects are greater than the sum of the effects for each drug given alone (1 + 1 = more than 2). The combination of hydrochlorothiazide with lisinopril for the treatment of hypertension is an example.

Drug effects that are the opposite of synergistic effects are known as **antagonistic effects.** Antagonistic effects are said to occur when the combination of two drugs results in drug effects that are less than the sum of the effects for each drug given separately (1 + 1 = less than 2). An example of this type of interaction occurs when the antibiotic ciprofloxacin is given simultaneously with antacids, vitamins, iron, or dairy products. These drugs reduce the absorption of ciprofloxacin and lead to decreased effectiveness of the antibiotic.

Incompatibility is a term most commonly used to describe parenteral drugs. Drug incompatibility occurs when two parenteral drugs or solutions are mixed together and the result is a chemical deterioration of one or both of the drugs or formation of a physical precipitate. The combination of two such drugs usually produces a precipitate, haziness, or color change in the solution. Before administering any intravenous medication, the nurse should always inspect the bag for precipitate. If the solution appears cloudy or visible flecks are seen, that bag should be discarded and not given to the patient. An example of incompatible drugs is the combination of parenteral furosemide and heparin.

Adverse Drug Events

The recognition of the potential hazards and actual detrimental effects of medication use is a topic that continues to receive much attention in the literature. This focus has contributed to an increasing body of knowledge regarding this topic as well as the development of new terminology. Health care institutions are under increasing pressure to develop effective strategies for preventing adverse effects of drugs.

Adverse drug event is a broad term for any undesirable occurrence involving medications. A similarly broad term also seen in the literature is *drug misadventure.* Patient outcomes associated with adverse drug events vary from no effects to mild discomfort to life-threatening complications, permanent disability, disfigurement, or death. Adverse drug events can be preventable (see discussion of medication errors later) or nonpreventable. Fortunately, many adverse drug events result in no measurable patient harm. The most common causes of adverse drug events *external* to the patient are errors by caregivers (both professional and nonprofessional) and malfunctioning of equipment (e.g., intravenous infusion pumps). An adverse drug event can also be *patient induced,* such as when a patient fails to take medication as prescribed or drinks alcoholic beverages that he or she was advised not to consume while taking a given medication. In these situations as well, the patient may experience no ill effects or may suffer varying degrees of harm. An impending adverse drug event that is noticed before it actually occurs should be considered a *potential* adverse drug event (and appropriate steps should be taken to avoid such a "near miss" in the future). A less common situation, but one still worth mentioning, is an *adverse drug withdrawal event.* This is an adverse outcome associated with discontinuation of drug therapy, such as hypertension caused by abruptly discontinuing blood pressure medication or return of infection caused by stopping antibiotic therapy too soon.

The two most common broad categories of adverse drug event are medication errors and adverse drug reactions. A **medication error** is a preventable situation in which there is a compromise in the "Six Rights" of medication use: *right patient, right drug, right time, right route, right dose,* and *right documentation.* Medication errors are more common than adverse drug reactions. Medication errors occur during the *prescribing, dispensing, administering,* or *monitoring* of drug therapy. These four phases are collectively known as the **medication use process.** Medication errors are discussed in more detail in Chapter 6.

An **adverse drug reaction** is any reaction to a drug that is unexpected and undesirable and occurs at therapeutic drug dosages. Adverse drug reactions may or may not be caused by medication errors. Adverse drug reactions may result in hospital admission, prolongation of hospital stay, change in drug therapy, initiation of supportive treatment, or complication of a patient's disease state. Adverse drug reactions are caused by processes inside the patient's body. They may or may not be preventable, depending on the situation. Mild adverse drug reactions (e.g., *drug adverse effects*—see later) usually do not require a change in the patient's drug therapy or other interventions. More severe adverse drug reactions, however, are likely to require changes to a patient's drug regimen. Severe adverse drug reactions can be permanently or significantly disabling, life threatening, or fatal. They may require or prolong hospitalization, lead to organ dam-

age (e.g., to the liver, kidneys, bone marrow, skin), cause congenital anomalies, or require specific interventions to prevent permanent impairment or tissue damage.

Adverse drug reactions that are specific to particular drug groups are discussed in the corresponding drug chapters in this book. Four general categories are discussed here: pharmacologic reaction, hypersensitivity (allergic) reaction, idiosyncratic reaction, and drug interaction.

A pharmacologic reaction is an extension of the drug's normal effects in the body. For example, a drug that is used to lower blood pressure in a patient with hypertension causes a pharmacologic adverse drug reaction when it lowers the blood pressure to the point at which the patient becomes unconscious. Pharmacologic reactions that result in adverse effects are predictable, well-known adverse drug reactions resulting in minor or no changes in patient management. They have predictable frequency and intensity, and their occurrence is related to the dose. They also usually resolve upon discontinuation of drug therapy.

An **allergic reaction** (also known as a *hypersensitivity reaction*) involves the patient's immune system. Immune system proteins known as *immunoglobulins* (see Chapters 45 and 46) recognize the drug molecule, its metabolite(s), or another ingredient in a drug formulation as a dangerous foreign substance. At this point, an *immune response* may occur in which immunoglobulin proteins bind to the drug substance in an attempt to neutralize the drug. Various chemical mediators, such as *histamine,* as well as *cytokines* and other inflammatory substances (e.g., *prostaglandins* [see Chapter 44]) usually are released during this process. This response can result in reactions ranging from mild reactions such as skin erythema or mild rash to severe, even life-threatening reactions such as constriction of bronchial airways and tachycardia.

It can be assumed throughout this book that use of any drug is contraindicated if the patient has a known allergy to that specific drug product. Allergy information may be reported by the patient as part of his or her history or may be observed by health care personnel during a patient encounter. In either case, every effort must be made to document as fully as possible the name of the drug product and the degree and details of the adverse reaction that occurred. For example: "Penicillin; skin rash, pruritus" or "Penicillin; skin rash, urticaria, and anaphylactic shock requiring emergency intervention."

In more extreme cases of disease or injury (e.g., cancer, snakebite), it may be deemed reasonable to administer a given drug *in spite of* a reported allergic or other adverse reaction. In such cases, the patient will likely be premedicated with additional medications (e.g., acetaminophen [Tylenol], diphenhydramine [Benadryl], prednisone) as an attempt to control any adverse reactions that may occur.

An **idiosyncratic reaction** is not the result of a known pharmacologic property of a drug or of a patient allergy but instead occurs unexpectedly in a particular patient. Such a reaction is a genetically determined abnormal response to normal dosages of a drug. Genetically inherited traits that result in the abnormal metabolism of drugs are distributed throughout the population. The study of such traits, which are solely revealed by drug administration, is called **pharmacogenetics** (see Chapter 5). Idiosyncratic drug reactions are usually caused by a deficiency or excess of drug-metabolizing enzymes. Many pharmacogenetic disorders exist. An example is glucose-6-phosphate dehydrogenase (G6PD) deficiency. This pharmacogenetic disease affects approximately 100 million people. People who lack proper levels of G6PD have idiosyncratic reactions to a wide range of drugs. There are more than 80 variations of the disease, and all produce some degree of drug-induced hemolysis. Drugs capable of inducing hemolysis in such patients are listed in Box 2-3.

The final type of adverse drug reaction is due to drug interaction. As described earlier, drug interaction occurs when the presence of two (or more) drugs in the body produces an unwanted effect. This unwanted effect can result when one drug either enhances or reduces the effects of another drug. Some drug interactions are intentional and beneficial (see Table 2-10). However, most clinically significant drug interactions are harmful. Drug interactions specific to particular drugs are discussed in detail in the chapters dealing with those drugs.

Other Drug Effects

Other drug-related effects that must be considered during drug therapy are teratogenic, mutagenic, and carcinogenic effects. These can result in devastating patient outcomes and can be prevented in many instances by appropriate monitoring.

Teratogenic effects of drugs or other chemicals result in structural defects in the fetus. Compounds that produce such effects are called *teratogens*. Prenatal development involves a delicate programmed sequence of interrelated embryologic events. Any significant disruption in this process of *embryogenesis* can have a teratogenic effect. Drugs that are capable of crossing the placenta can cause **drug-induced teratogenesis.** Drugs administered during pregnancy can produce different types of congenital anomalies. The period during which the fetus is most vulnerable to teratogenic effects begins with the third week of development and usually ends after the third month. Chapter 3 describes the FDA safety classification for drugs used by pregnant women.

Mutagenic effects are permanent changes in the genetic composition of living organisms and consist of alterations in chromosome structure, the number of chromosomes, or the genetic code of the deoxyribonucleic acid (DNA) molecule. Drugs capable of inducing mutations are called *mutagens*. Radiation, viruses, chemicals (e.g., industrial chemicals such as benzene), and drugs can all act as mutagenic agents in human beings. Drugs that affect genetic processes are active primarily during cell reproduction *(mitosis).*

Carcinogenic effects are the cancer-causing effects of drugs, other chemicals, radiation, and viruses. Agents that produce such effects are called *carcinogens*. Some exogenous causes of cancer are listed in Box 2-4.

PHARMACOGNOSY

The source of all early drugs was nature, and the study of these natural drug sources (plants and animals) is called *pharmacognosy*. Although many drugs in current use are synthetically derived, most were first isolated in nature. The four main sources for drugs are plants, animals, minerals, and laboratory synthesis. Plants provide many weak acids and weak bases *(alkaloids)* that are very useful and potent drugs. Alkaloids are more common, including atropine (belladonna plant), caffeine (coffee bean), and

---

BOX 2-3 Drugs to Avoid in Patients with Glucose-6-Phosphate Dehydrogenase Deficiency

aspirin
nitrofurantoin
primaquine
probenecid
sulfonamides

CULTURAL IMPLICATIONS

Glucose-6-Phosphate Dehydrogenase Deficiency

Glucose-6-phosphate dehydrogenase (G6PD) is an enzyme found in abundant amounts in the tissues of most individuals. It reduces the risk of hemolysis of red blood cells when they are exposed to oxidizing drugs such as aspirin. Approximately 13% of African American men and 20% of African American women carry the gene that results in G6PD deficiency. Approximately 14% of Sardinians and more than 50% of the Kurdish Jewish population also show G6PD deficiencies. When exposed to drugs such as sulfonamides, antimalarials, and aspirin, patients with this deficiency may suffer life-threatening hemolysis of the red blood cells, whereas individuals with adequate quantities of the enzyme have no problems in taking these drugs.

BOX 2-4 Exogenous Causes of Cancer

Dietary customs
Drug abuse
Carcinogenic drugs
Workplace chemicals
Radiation
Environmental pollution
Food-processing procedures
Food production procedures
Oncogenic viruses
Smoking

---

nicotine (tobacco leaf). Animals are the source of many hormone drugs. Conjugated estrogens are derived from the urine of pregnant mares, hence the drug trade name Premarin. *Equine* is the term used for any horse-derived drug. Insulin comes from two sources: pigs *(porcine)* and humans. Human insulin is now far more commonly used than animal insulins thanks to the use of recombinant DNA techniques. Heparin is another commonly used drug that is derived from pigs (porcine heparin). Some common mineral sources of currently used drugs are salicylic acid, aluminum hydroxide, and sodium chloride.

PHARMACOECONOMICS

Pharmacoeconomics is the study of the economic factors influencing the cost of drug therapy. One example is performing a *cost-benefit analysis* of one antibiotic versus another when competing drugs are considered for inclusion in a hospital formulary. Such studies typically examine treatment outcomes data (e.g.,

TABLE 2-11 Common Causes of Poisoning and Antidotes*

Substance	Antidote
acetaminophen	acetylcysteine
organophosphates (e.g., insecticides)	atropine
tricyclic antidepressants, quinidine	sodium bicarbonate
calcium channel blockers	intravenous calcium
iron salts	deferoxamine
digoxin and other cardiac glycosides	digoxin antibodies
ethylene glycol (e.g., automotive antifreeze solution), methanol	ethanol (same as alcohol used for drinking), given intravenously
benzodiazepines	flumazenil
beta-blockers	glucagon
opiates, opioid drugs	naloxone
carbon monoxide (by inhalation)	oxygen (at high concentration), known as *bariatric therapy*

*Note that these and other antidotes are discussed throughout this textbook where applicable.

how many patients recovered and how soon) in relation to the comparative total costs of treatment with the drugs in question.

TOXICOLOGY

The study of poisons and unwanted responses to both drugs and other chemicals is known as *toxicology*. Toxicology is the science of the adverse effects of chemicals on living organisms. Clinical toxicology deals specifically with the care of the poisoned patient. Poisoning can result from a variety of causes, ranging from prescription drug overdose to ingestion of household cleaning agents to snakebite. Poison control centers are health care institutions equipped with sufficient personnel and information resources to recommend appropriate treatment for the poisoned patient.

Effective treatment of the poisoned patient is based on a system of priorities, the first of which is to preserve the patient's vital functions by maintaining the airway, ventilation, and circulation. The second priority is to prevent absorption of the toxic substance and/or speed its elimination from the body using one or more of the variety of clinical methods available. Several common poisons and their specific antidotes are listed in Table 2-11.

CONCLUSION

A thorough understanding of the pharmacologic principles of pharmacokinetics, pharmacodynamics, pharmacotherapeutics, pharmacognosy, and toxicology is essential to the implementation of drug therapy in the nursing process and to safe, quality nursing practice. Medications may be very helpful in treating disease, but unless the nurse has an adequate, up-to-date knowledge base and clinical skills and engages in critical thinking and good decision making, any treatment may become harmful. Application of pharmacologic principles enables the nurse to provide safe and effective drug therapy while always acting on behalf of the patient and respecting the patient's rights. Nursing considerations associated with various routes of drug administration are summarized in Table 2-3.

POINTS TO REMEMBER

- The following definitions related to drug therapy are important to remember: pharmacology—the study or science of drugs; pharmacokinetics—the study of drug distribution among various body compartments after a drug has entered the body, including the phases of absorption, distribution, metabolism, and excretion; pharmaceutics—the science of dosage form design.
- The nurse's role in drug therapy and the nursing process as it relates to pharmacologic treatment is more than just the memorization of the names of drugs, their uses, and associated interventions. It involves a thorough comprehension of all aspects of pharmaceutics, pharmacokinetics, and pharmacodynamics and

the sound application of this drug knowledge to a variety of clinical situations. Refer to Chapter 1 for more detailed discussion of drug therapy as it relates to the nursing process.
- Drug actions are related to the pharmacologic, pharmaceutical, pharmacokinetic, and pharmacodynamic properties of a given medication, and each of these has a specific influence on the overall effects produced by the drug in a patient.
- Selection of the route of administration is based on patient variables and the specific characteristics of a drug.
- Nursing considerations vary depending on the drug as well as the route of administration.

NCLEX EXAMINATION REVIEW QUESTIONS

1 An elderly woman took a prescription medicine to help her to sleep; however, she felt restless all night and did not sleep at all. The nurse recognizes that this woman has experienced a(an)
   a allergic reaction.
   b idiosyncratic reaction.
   c mutagenic effect.
   d synergistic effect.

2 While caring for a patient with cirrhosis or hepatitis, the nurse knows that abnormalities in which phase of pharmacokinetics may occur?
   a Absorption
   b Distribution
   c Metabolism
   d Excretion

3 A patient who has advanced cancer is receiving opioid medications around the clock to "keep him comfortable" as he nears the end of his life. Which term best describes this type of therapy?
   a Palliative therapy
   b Maintenance therapy
   c Supportive therapy
   d Supplemental therapy

4 The nurse is giving medications to a patient in cardiogenic shock. The intravenous route is chosen instead of the intramuscular route. The nurse knows that the factor that most influences the decision about which route to use is the patient's

   a altered biliary function.
   b increased glomerular filtration.
   c reduced liver metabolism.
   d diminished circulation.

5 A patient has just received a prescription for an enteric-coated stool softener. When teaching the patient, the nurse should include which statement?
   a "Take the tablet with 2 to 3 oz of orange juice."
   b "Avoid taking all other medications with any enteric-coated tablet."
   c "Crush the tablet before swallowing if you have problems with swallowing."
   d "Be sure to swallow the tablet whole without chewing it."

6 Each statement describes a phase of pharmacokinetics. Put the statements in order, with 1 indicating the phase that occurs first and 4 indicating the phase that occurs last.
   a Enzymes in the liver transform the drug into an inactive metabolite.
   b Drug metabolites are secreted through passive glomerular filtration into the renal tubules.
   c A drug binds to the plasma protein albumin and circulates through the body.
   d A drug moves from the intestinal lumen into the mesenteric blood system.

1. b, 2. c, 3. a, 4. d, 5. d, 6. a = 3, b = 4, c = 2, d = 1.

CRITICAL THINKING ACTIVITIES: BEST ACTION

1 A patient tells the nurse during the assessment that he experiences some "strange" problem with drug metabolism that he was born with, so he is not to take certain medications. What type of disorder is this patient referring to, and what are the problems it can cause in the patient when specific medications are taken? What is the nurse's best action when a patient shares this information?

2 Mr. L. is admitted to the trauma unit with multisystem injuries from an automobile accident. He arrived at the unit with multiple abnormal findings, including shock from blood loss, de-

creased cardiac output, and urinary output of less than 30 mL/hr. Which route of administration would be the best choice for this patient? Explain your reasoning.

3 You are administering medications to a patient who had an enteral tube inserted 2 days earlier for continuous feedings. As you review the medication list, you note that one drug is an enteric-coated tablet given twice a day. What is the best action regarding giving this drug to this patient?

For answers, see *http://evolve.elsevier.com/Lilley.*

CHAPTER 3

Life Span Considerations

OBJECTIVES

When you reach the end of this chapter, you should be able to do the following:

1 Discuss the influences of the patient's age on the effects of drugs and drug responses.

2 Identify drug-related concerns during pregnancy and lactation and provide an explanation of the physiologic basis for these concerns.

3 Summarize the impact of age-related physiologic changes on the pharmacokinetic aspects of drug therapy.

4 Explain how these age-related changes in drug pharmacokinetics influence various drug effects and drug responses across the life span.

5 Provide several examples of how age affects the absorption, distribution, metabolism, and excretion of drugs.

6 Calculate a drug dose for a pediatric patient using the various formulas available.

7 Identify the importance of a body surface area nomogram for drug calculations in pediatric patients.

8 Develop a nursing care plan for drug therapy and the nursing process that takes into account life span considerations.

e-Learning Activities

http://evolve.elsevier.com/Lilley

NCLEX Review Questions • Animations • Nursing Care Plans • Audio Glossary • Category Catchers • Medication Errors Checklists • IV Therapy Checklists • Calculators • Frequently Asked Questions • Content Updates • Supplemental Resources • Answers to Case Studies and Critical Thinking Activities

Glossary

Active transport The active (energy-requiring) movement of a substance between different tissues via biomolecular pumping mechanisms contained within cell membranes. (p. 36)

Diffusion The passive movement of a substance (e.g., a drug) between different tissues from areas of higher concentration to areas of lower concentration. (Compare with *active transport*.) (p. 36)

Elderly Pertaining to a person who is 65 years of age or older. (NOTE: Some sources consider "elderly" to be 55 years of age or older.) (p. 40)

Neonate Pertaining to a person younger than 1 month of age; newborn infant. (p. 36)

Nomogram A graphic tool for estimating drug dosages using various body measurements. (p. 38)

Pediatric Pertaining to a person who is 12 years of age or younger. (p. 38)

Polypharmacy The use of many different drugs concurrently in treating a patient, who often has several health problems. (p. 41)

• • •

Most of the experience with drugs and pharmacology has been gained from the adult population. The great majority of drug studies and articles on drugs have focused on the population between the ages of 13 and 65 years. It has been estimated that 75% of currently approved drugs lack U.S. Food and Drug Adminis-

tration (FDA) approval for pediatric use and therefore lack specific dosage guidelines for **neonates** and children. Fortunately, many excellent pediatric drug dosage books are available. Most drugs are effective in younger and older patients, but drugs often behave very differently in these patients at the opposite ends of the age spectrum. It is therefore vitally important from the standpoint of safe and effective drug administration to understand what these differences are and how to adjust for them.

During the time from the beginning to the end of life, the human body changes in many ways. These changes have a dramatic effect on the four phases of pharmacokinetics—drug absorption, distribution, metabolism, and excretion. Newborn, pediatric, and elderly patients each have special needs, which are discussed in this chapter. Drug therapy at the two ends of the spectrum of life is more likely to result in adverse effects and toxicity. This is especially true if certain basic principles are not understood and followed. Fortunately, response to drug therapy changes in a predictable manner in younger and older patients. Knowing the effect that age has on the pharmacokinetic characteristics of drugs helps predict these changes.

DRUG THERAPY DURING PREGNANCY

A fetus is exposed to many of the same substances as the mother, including any drugs that she takes—prescription, nonprescription, or street drugs. Therefore, it is important to know and understand drug effects during gestational life. The first trimester of pregnancy is generally the period of greatest danger of drug-induced developmental defects.

Transfer of both drugs and nutrients to the fetus occurs primarily by **diffusion** across the placenta, although not all drugs cross the placenta. Recall from chemistry that diffusion is a passive process based on differences in concentration between different tissues, whereas **active transport** requires the expenditure of energy and often involves some sort of cell-surface protein

36

pump. The factors that contribute to the safety or potential harm of drug therapy during pregnancy can be broadly broken down into three areas: drug properties, fetal gestational age, and maternal factors.

Drug properties that impact drug transfer to the fetus include the drug's chemistry, dosage, and concurrently administered drugs. Examples of relevant chemical properties include molecular weight, protein binding, lipid solubility, and chemical structure. Important drug dosage variables include dose and duration of therapy.

Fetal gestational age is an important factor in determining the potential for harmful drug effects to the fetus. The fetus is at greatest risk for drug-induced developmental defects during the first trimester of pregnancy. During this period the fetus undergoes rapid cell proliferation, and the skeleton, muscles, limbs, and visceral organs are developing at their most rapid rate. Self-treatment of any minor illness should be strongly discouraged anytime during pregnancy, but especially during the first trimester. Gestational age is also important in determining when a drug can most easily cross the placenta to the fetus. During the last trimester the greatest percentage of maternally absorbed drug gets to the fetus.

Maternal factors can also play a role in determining drug effects on the fetus. Any change in the mother's physiology that could impact the pharmacokinetic characteristics of drugs can affect the amount of drug to which the fetus may be exposed. Maternal kidney and liver function play a major role in drug metabolism and excretion and are critical factors, especially if the drug crosses the placenta. Impairment in either kidney or liver function may result in higher drug levels than normal and/or prolonged drug exposure. Maternal genotype may also affect how and to what extent certain drugs are metabolized (pharmacogenetics), which in turn affects drug exposure of the fetus. The lack of certain enzyme systems may result in adverse drug effects to the fetus when the mother is exposed to a drug that is normally metabolized by the given enzyme.

Although exposure of the fetus to drugs is most detrimental during the first trimester, drug transfer to the fetus is more likely during the last trimester. This is the result of enhanced blood flow to the fetus, increased fetal surface area, and increased amount of free drug in the mother's circulation.

Although it is important to use drugs judiciously during pregnancy, there are certain situations that require their use. Without drug therapy, maternal conditions as such hypertension, epilepsy, diabetes, and infection could seriously endanger both the mother and the fetus, and the potential for harm far outweighs the risks of appropriate drug therapy.

The FDA classifies drugs according to their safety for use during pregnancy. This system of drug classification is based primarily on animal studies and limited human studies. This is due in part to ethical dilemmas surrounding the study of potential adverse effects on fetuses. We have learned from some unfortunate mistakes, such as the maternal use of thalidomide, which induces birth defects, and diethylstilbestrol (DES), which causes a high incidence of gynecologic malignancy in female offspring. Although some clinicians dispute its adequacy, the most widely used index of potential fetal risk of a given drug is the FDA's pregnancy safety category system. The five safety categories are described in Table 3-1. It should be noted that the FDA is in the process of changing the pregnancy categories, but the information is not yet published at the time of printing. The reader is referred to *http://evolve.elsevier.com/Lilley*.

DRUG THERAPY DURING BREAST-FEEDING

Breast-fed infants are also at risk for exposure to drugs consumed by the mother. A wide variety of drugs easily cross from the mother's circulation into the breast milk and subsequently to the breast-feeding infant. Drug properties similar to those discussed in the previous section influence the exposure of infants to drugs that are taken by breast-feeding mothers. The primary drug characteristics that increase the likelihood that a drug given to a breast-feeding mother will end up in the breast milk include fat solubility, low molecular weight, nonionization, and high concentration.

Fortunately, breast milk is not the primary route for maternal drug excretion. Drug levels in breast milk are usually lower than those in the maternal circulation. The actual amount of drug to which a breast-feeding infant is exposed depends largely on the volume of milk consumed. The ultimate decision as to whether a breast-feeding mother should take a particular drug depends on the risk/benefit ratio. The risks of transfer of maternal medication to the infant in relation to the benefits of continuing breast-feeding and the therapeutic benefits to the mother must be considered on a case-by-case basis.

CONSIDERATIONS FOR NEONATAL AND PEDIATRIC PATIENTS

In terms of age, a *child* is defined differently from a *neonate* or an *infant*. Therefore, the term *child* should be used only when referring to patients between 1 year and 12 years of age. The age ranges that correspond to the various terms applied to young patients are shown in Table 3-2. This classification is used throughout this book.

TABLE **3-1** Pregnancy Safety Categories

Category	Description
Category A	Studies indicate no risk to human fetus.
Category B	Studies indicate no risk to animal fetus; information for humans is not available.
Category C	Adverse effects reported in animal fetus; information for humans is not available.
Category D	Possible fetal risk in humans reported; however, consideration of potential benefit vs. risk may, in selected cases, warrant use of these drugs in pregnant women.
Category X	Fetal abnormalities reported and positive evidence of fetal risk in humans available from animal and/or human studies. These drugs should not be used in pregnant women.

TABLE 3-2 Classification of Young Patients

Age Range	Classification
Younger than 38 wk gestation	Premature or preterm infant
Younger than 1 mo	Neonate or newborn infant
1 mo up to 1 yr	Infant
1 yr up to 12 yr	Child

NOTE: The meaning of the term *pediatric* may vary with the individual drug and clinical situation. Often the maximum age for a pediatric patient may be identified as 16 years of age. Consult manufacturer's guidelines for specific dosing information.

Physiology and Pharmacokinetics

The anatomic and physiologic characteristics unique to **pediatric** patients account for most of the differences in the pharmacokinetic and pharmacodynamic behavior of drugs in this age group. The immaturity of organs is the physiologic factor most responsible for these differences. In both neonates and older pediatric patients, anatomic structures and physiologic systems and functions are still in the process of developing. The Life Span Considerations: The Pediatric Patient box on this page lists those physiologic factors that alter the pharmacokinetic properties of drugs in young patients.

Pharmacodynamics

Drug actions (or pharmacodynamics) are altered in young patients, and the maturity of various organs plays a role in how drugs act in the body. In young patients, certain drugs may be more toxic whereas others may be less toxic. The sensitivity of receptor sites may also vary with age; thus, higher or lower dosages may be required depending on the drug. In addition, rapidly developing tissues may be more sensitive to certain drugs, and therefore smaller dosages may be required. Because of this, certain drugs are contraindicated during the growth years. For instance, tetracycline may permanently discolor a young person's teeth; corticosteroids may suppress growth when given systemically (but not when delivered via asthma inhalers, for example); and quinolone antibiotics may damage cartilage.

Dosage Calculations for Pediatric Patients

Many drugs commonly used in adults have not been sufficiently investigated to ensure their safety and effectiveness in children. Most drugs administered in pediatric care are given on an empirical basis. In spite of this, there are numerous excellent pediatric dosage references. Because pediatric patients (especially premature infants and neonates) are small and have immature organs, they are very susceptible to many drug interactions, toxicity, and unusual drug responses and therefore require very different dosage calculations. Characteristics of pediatric patients that have a significant effect on dosage include the following:

- Skin is thinner and more permeable.
- Stomach lacks acid to kill bacteria.
- Lungs have weaker mucous barriers.
- Body temperature is less well regulated and dehydration occurs easily.
- Liver and kidneys are immature and therefore drug metabolism and excretion are impaired.

LIFE SPAN CONSIDERATIONS: The Pediatric Patient

Pharmacokinetic Changes in the Neonate and Pediatric Patient

Absorption
- Gastric pH is less acidic because acid-producing cells in the stomach are immature until approximately 1 to 2 years of age.
- Gastric emptying is slowed because of slow or irregular peristalsis.
- First-pass elimination by the liver is reduced because of the immaturity of the liver and reduced levels of microsomal enzymes.
- Intramuscular absorption is faster and irregular.

Distribution
- Total body water is 70% to 80% in full-term infants, 85% in premature newborns, and 64% in children 1 to 12 years of age.
- Fat content is lower in young patients because of greater total body water.
- Protein binding is decreased because of decreased production of protein by the immature liver.
- More drugs enter the brain because of an immature blood-brain barrier.

Metabolism
- Levels of microsomal enzymes are decreased because the immature liver has not yet started producing enough.
- Older children may have increased metabolism and require higher dosages once hepatic enzymes are produced.
- Many variables affect metabolism in premature infants, infants, and children, including the status of liver enzyme production, genetic differences, and substances to which the mother was exposed during pregnancy.

Excretion
- Glomerular filtration rate and tubular secretion and resorption are all decreased in young patients because of kidney immaturity.
- Perfusion to the kidneys may be decreased, which results in reduced renal function, concentrating ability, and excretion of drugs.

Many formulas for pediatric dosage calculation have been used throughout the years. Formulas involving age, weight, and body surface area (BSA) are most commonly employed as the basis for calculations. BSA-based formulas are the most accurate of these dosage formulas.

To use the BSA method, the nurse needs the following information:

- Drug order with drug name, dose, route, time, and frequency
- Information regarding available dosage forms
- Pediatric patient's height in centimeters (cm) and weight in kilograms (kg)
- BSA **nomogram** for children (e.g., West nomogram, shown in Figure 3-1)
- Recommended adult drug dosage

The West nomogram (see Figure 3-1) uses a child's height and weight to determine the child's BSA. This information is then inserted into the BSA formula to obtain a drug dosage for a specific pediatric patient. Consider the following examples:

$$\frac{\text{BSA of adult}}{\text{BSA of child}} \times \text{adult dose} = \text{estimated child's dose}$$

$$\text{BSA of child (m}^2) \times \frac{\text{manufacturer's recommended dose}}{\text{m}^2} = \text{estimated child's dose}$$

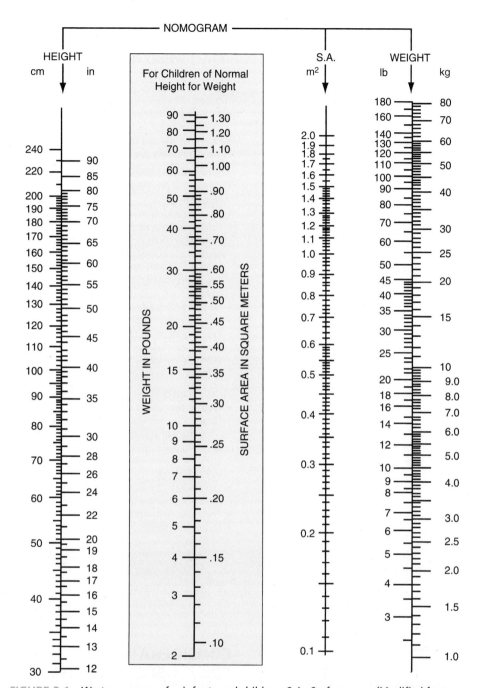

FIGURE 3-1   West nomogram for infants and children. *S.A.,* Surface area. (Modified from data by E. Boyd and C. D. West. In Kliegman RM et al: *Nelson textbook of pediatrics,* ed 18, Philadelphia, 2007, Saunders.)

Calculating the drug dosage according to the body weight is the most commonly used method today. Most drug references recommend dosages based on milligrams per kilogram of body weight. The following information is needed to calculate the pediatric dosage:

- Drug order (as discussed previously)
- Pediatric patient's weight in kilograms (1 kilogram = 2.2 pounds)
- Pediatric dosage as per manufacturer or drug formulary guidelines
- Information regarding available dosage forms

When using either of the previous methods, the nurse does the following:

- Determines the pediatric patient's weight in kilograms
- Uses a current drug reference to determine the usual dosage range per 24 hours in milligrams per kilogram
- Determines the dose parameters by multiplying the weight by the minimum and maximum daily doses of the drug (the safe range)
- Determines the total amount of the drug to administer per dose and per day

LIFE SPAN CONSIDERATIONS: The Pediatric Patient

Age-Related Considerations for Medication Administration from Infancy to Adolescence

General Interventions

- Always come prepared for the procedure (e.g., prepare for injections with needleless syringe and gather all needed equipment).
- Ask the parent and/or child (if age appropriate) if the parent should or should not remain for the procedure (for in-hospital administration).
- Assess for comfort methods that are appropriate before and after drug administration.

Infants

- While maintaining safe and secure positioning of the infant (e.g., with parent holding, rocking, cuddling, soothing), perform the procedure (e.g., injection) swiftly and safely.
- Allow self-comforting measures as age appropriate (e.g., use of pacifier, fingers in mouth, self-movement).

Toddlers

- Offer a brief, concrete explanation of the procedure but with realistic expectations of the child's actual understanding of the information. Parents, caregivers, or other legal guardians must be part of the process. Hold the child securely while administering the medication.
- Accept aggressive behavior as a healthy response, but only within reasonable limits.
- Provide comfort measures immediately after the procedure (e.g., touching, holding).
- Help the child understand the treatment and his or her feelings through puppet play or play with stuffed animals or hospital equipment such as empty, needleless syringes.
- Provide for healthy ways to release aggression such as age-appropriate supervised playtime.

Preschoolers

- Offer a brief, concrete explanation of the procedure at the patient's level and with the parent or caregiver present.
- Provide comfort measures after the procedure (e.g., touching, holding).

- Identify and accept aggressive responses and provide age-appropriate outlets.
- Make use of magical thinking (e.g., using ointments or "special medicines" to make discomfort go away).
- Note that the role of the parent in providing comfort and understanding is very important.

School-Aged Children

- Explain the procedure, allowing for some control over body and situation.
- Provide comfort measures.
- Explore feelings and concepts through the use of therapeutic play. Art may be used to help the patient express fears. Use of age-appropriate books and realistic hospital equipment may also be helpful.
- Set appropriate behavior limits (e.g., okay to cry or scream, but not to bite).
- Provide activities for releasing aggression and anger.
- Use the opportunity to teach about the relationship between receiving medication and body function and structure (e.g., what a seizure is and how medication helps prevent the seizure).
- Offer the complete picture (e.g., need to take medication, relax with deep breaths; medication will help prevent pain).

Adolescents

- Prepare the patient in advance for the procedure but without scare tactics.
- Allow for expression in a way that does not cause losing face, such as giving the adolescent time alone after the procedure (e.g., once a seizure is controlled) and giving the adolescent time to discuss his or her feelings.
- Explore with the adolescent any current concepts of self, hospitalization, and illness, and correct any misconceptions.
- Encourage self-expression, individuality, and self-care.
- Encourage participation in procedures as appropriate.

Modified from McKenry LM, Salerno E: *Mosby's pharmacology in nursing*, ed 22, St Louis, 2006, Mosby; Blaber M: Related to nursing intervention in pain. Newington's Children's Hospital manual for global pediatric nursing assessment (unpublished).

- Compares the drug dosage prescribed with the calculated safe range
- If the drug dosage raises any concerns or varies from the safe range, contacts the health care provider or prescriber immediately and does not give the drug!

A common source of medication error and potential toxicity is confusing pounds with kilograms. Unless otherwise noted, the child's weight should be given in kilograms, not pounds. Great care should be taken to ensure that the correct weight is reported to the prescriber. The nurse should never underestimate the importance of organ maturity, along with BSA, age, and weight, in calculating pediatric dosage. If all of these physical developmental factors are considered, the likelihood of safe and effective drug administration is increased. Emotional developmental considerations must also be a part of the decision-making process in drug therapy for pediatric patients (see Life Span Considerations: The Pediatric Patient box on this page).

CONSIDERATIONS FOR ELDERLY PATIENTS

The **elderly** patient has special needs because of the decline in organ function, which contributes to various pharmacokinetic changes. Therefore, drug therapy is much more likely to result in adverse effects and toxicity.

In this book, the word *elderly* is used instead of the word *geriatric;* however, these terms are synonymous. An elderly patient is defined as a person who is 65 years of age or older. This segment of the population is growing at a dramatic pace (see the Life Span Considerations: The Elderly Patient box on p. 42). At the beginning of the twentieth century, the elderly constituted a mere 4% of the total population. At that time more people died of infections than of chronic illnesses such as heart disease, cancer, and diabetes. As medical and health care technology has advanced, so has the ability to prolong life. This has resulted in a

LIFE SPAN CONSIDERATIONS: The Elderly Patient		
Percentage of Population over 65 Years of Age		
Year	Percentage over Age 65	
1900	4%	
2000	12%	
2020	20%	

growing population of older adults. Today patients over 65 years of age constitute 13% of the population. At any given time, the average elderly patient takes four or five prescription drugs as well as two OTC medications, which can increase the risk of drug interactions. Life expectancy is currently approximately 78.1 years, and it is estimated that by the year 2030, 20% of the population will be 65 years of age or older. These trends are expected to continue as new disease prevention and treatment methods are developed.

Issues in Clinical Drug Use in the Elderly

The growing elderly population consumes a larger proportion of all medications than other population groups, taking 30% of all prescription drugs and over 40% of OTC drugs. Commonly prescribed drugs for the elderly include antihypertensives, beta-blockers, diuretics, insulin, and potassium supplements. The most commonly used OTC drugs are analgesics, laxatives, and nonsteroidal antiinflammatory drugs (NSAIDs). Elderly patients, especially those of certain ethnicities, may use various folk remedies of unknown composition that are unfamiliar to their health care providers.

Not only do elderly patients consume a greater proportion of prescription and OTC medications, they commonly take multiple medications on a daily basis. About 1 in 3 elderly patients take more than 8 different drugs each day, with many taking 15 or more. More complicated medication regimens predispose elderly patients to self-medication errors, especially those with reduced visual acuity and manual dexterity. Such sensory and motor deficits can be particularly problematic when elderly patients split their own tablets. The practice of pill splitting occurs commonly for financial reasons, because lower- and higher-strength tablets often have similar costs. Furthermore, some insurance companies *require* tablet splitting for this reason. Other factors that may contribute to medication errors in the elderly include lack of adequate patient education and understanding of their drug regimens, and use of multiple prescribers and multiple pharmacies. One reason for patients' use of so many medications is the occurrence of more chronic diseases, which now have even more drug options for treatment. More than 80% of patients taking eight or more drugs have one or more chronic illness. In this age of medical specialization, patients may see several prescribers for their many illnesses. Because of this, it is very important for the patient to use only one pharmacy, so that monitoring for drug interactions and duplicate therapy can occur.

Elderly patients are hospitalized frequently due to adverse drug reactions. Complementary and alternative medicines such as herbal remedies and dietary supplements can interact with prescription drugs. The simultaneous use of multiple medications is called **polypharmacy.** As the number of medications a person takes increases, so does the risk of drug interaction. For example, the chance of a drug interaction is approximately 6% for a patient receiving two medications. This risk rises dramatically as the number of drugs the patient is taking increases. For a patient taking five medications, the chance of a drug interaction is 50%, and for those taking 10 or more medications, 100%.

Some drugs may be given specifically to counteract the adverse effects of other drugs (e.g., a potassium supplement to counteract the potassium loss caused by certain diuretic medications). This is one example of what is known as the *prescribing cascade.* This is where a provider prescribes a medication to treat the adverse effects of another medication. Sometimes it is difficult to distinguish adverse drug effects from disease symptoms. Although such prescribing is sometimes appropriate, it also increases the potential for even more adverse drug events (including drug interactions, hospitalization or prolonged hospital stays, hip fractures secondary to drug-induced falls, addiction risk, anorexia, confusion, urinary retention, and fatigue). Recognizing polypharmacy and taking steps to reduce it whenever possible by decreasing the number and/or dosages of drugs taken can significantly reduce the incidence of adverse outcomes. Appropriate drug doses for elderly patients may sometimes be one half to two thirds of the standard adult dose. As a general rule, dosing for the elderly should follow the admonition, "Start low and go slow," which means to start with the lowest possible dose (often less than an average adult dose) and increase the dose slowly, based on patient response.

Another important issue is *noncompliance* or *nonadherence* with prescribed medication regimens. Drug nonadherence is reported to occur in roughly 40% of elderly patients and is associated with increased rates of hospitalization. Some patients want to adhere to their medication regimen but truly cannot afford the medicine. Patients in this situation should be referred to a health care social worker or their prescriber. Many drug companies offer patient assistance for expensive medications.

Physiologic Changes

The physiologic changes associated with aging affect the action of many drugs. As the body ages, the functioning of several organ systems slowly declines. The collective physiologic changes associated with the aging process have a major effect on the disposition and action of drugs. Table 3-3 lists some of the body systems most affected by the aging process.

The sensitivity of the elderly patient to many drugs is altered as a result of physiologic changes; therefore, drug usage should be adjusted. For instance, with aging there is a general decrease in body weight. However, the drug dosages administered to elderly patients are often the same as those administered to younger adults. The criteria for drug dosages in older adults should include consideration of body weight and organ functioning, with emphasis on liver, renal, cardiovascular, and central nervous system function (similar to the criteria for pediatric dosages).

Changes in drug molecule receptors in the body can make a patient more or less sensitive to certain medications. For example, elderly patients commonly have increased sensitivity to central nervous system depressant medications (e.g., anxiolytics,

TABLE 3-3 Physiologic Changes in the Elderly Patient

System	Physiologic Change
Cardiovascular	↓ Cardiac output = ↓ absorption and distribution
	↓ Blood flow = ↓ absorption and distribution
Gastrointestinal	↑ pH (alkaline gastric secretions) = altered absorption
	↓ Peristalsis = delayed gastric emptying
Hepatic	↓ Enzyme production = ↓ metabolism
	↓ Blood flow = ↓ metabolism
Renal	↓ Blood flow = ↓ excretion
	↓ Function = ↓ excretion
	↓ Glomerular filtration rate = ↓ excretion

tricyclic antidepressants) because of reduced integrity of the blood-brain barrier.

It is important to monitor the results of laboratory tests that have been ordered for elderly patients. These values serve as a gauge of organ function. The most important organs from the standpoint of the breakdown and elimination of drugs are the liver and the kidneys. Kidney function is assessed by measuring serum *creatinine* and blood urea nitrogen levels. Creatinine is a byproduct of muscle metabolism. Because muscle mass declines with age, serum creatinine level may provide a misleading index of renal function. For example, a frail elderly female may have a reported serum creatinine value that is lower than normal, and this may lead one to falsely think that her renal function is above normal. In actuality, because this patient has no muscle mass, she cannot produce creatinine, so the value is low. But the seasoned clinician knows that renal function declines with age and that this value alone does not give an accurate estimate of renal function. The most accurate way to determine creatinine clearance is by collecting a patient's urine for 24 hours. This test is quite cumbersome, however, and is not used very often. Fortunately, several equations exist that allow pharmacists and prescribers to accurately assess renal function in the elderly. Frequency of testing for renal function is often dictated by the degree of renal dysfunction and the type of medications being prescribed or used.

Liver function is assessed by testing the blood for liver enzymes such as aspartate aminotransferase (AST) and alanine aminotransferase (ALT). These laboratory values can help in the assessment of an older patient's ability to metabolize and eliminate medications and can aid in anticipating the risk of toxicity and/or drug accumulation. Laboratory assessments should ideally be conducted at least annually for most elderly patients, both for preventive health monitoring and for screening for possible toxic effects of drug therapy. Such assessments may be indicated more frequently (e.g., every 1, 3, or 6 months) in those patients requiring higher-risk drug regimens.

Pharmacokinetics

The pharmacokinetic phases of absorption, distribution, metabolism, and excretion may be different in the older adult than in the younger adult. Awareness of these differences helps the nurse ensure appropriate administration of drugs and monitoring of elderly patients taking medications. The Life Span Consider-

LIFE SPAN CONSIDERATIONS: The Elderly Patient

Pharmacokinetic Changes

Absorption
- Gastric pH is less acidic because of a gradual reduction in the production of hydrochloric acid in the stomach.
- Gastric emptying is slowed because of a decline in smooth muscle tone and motor activity.
- Movement throughout the gastrointestinal (GI) tract is slower because of decreased muscle tone and motor activity.
- Blood flow to the GI tract is reduced by 40% to 50% because of decreased cardiac output and decreased perfusion.
- The absorptive surface area is decreased because the aging process blunts and flattens villi.

Distribution
- In adults 40 to 60 years of age, total body water is 55% in males and 47% in females; in those over 60 years of age, total body water is 52% in males and 46% in females.
- Fat content is increased because of decreased lean body mass.
- Protein (albumin) binding sites are reduced because of decreased production of proteins by the aging liver and reduced protein intake.

Metabolism
- The levels of microsomal enzymes are decreased because the capacity of the aging liver to produce them is reduced.
- Liver blood flow is reduced by approximately 1.5% per year after 25 years of age, which decreases hepatic metabolism.

Excretion
- Glomerular filtration rate is decreased by 40% to 50%, primarily because of decreased blood flow.
- The number of intact nephrons is decreased.

ations: The Elderly Patient box on this page lists the four pharmacokinetic phases and summarizes how they are altered by the aging process.

Absorption

Absorption in the older person can be altered by many mechanisms. Advancing age results in reduced absorption of both dietary nutrients and drugs. Several physiologic changes account for this, including a gradual reduction in the ability of the stomach to produce hydrochloric acid, which results in a decrease in gastric acidity and may alter the absorption of some drugs. In addition, the combination of decreased cardiac output and advancing atherosclerosis results in a general reduction in the flow of blood to major organs, including the stomach. By 65 years of age, there is an approximately 50% reduction in blood flow to the gastrointestinal (GI) tract. Absorption, whether of nutrient or drug, is dependent on good blood supply to the stomach and intestines. The absorptive surface area of an elderly person's GI tract is often reduced. Age-related changes reduce overall GI absorptive capabilities, including drug absorption.

GI motility is important for moving substances out of the stomach and also for moving them throughout the GI tract. Muscle tone and motor activity in the GI tract are reduced in older adults. This often results in constipation, for which older adults frequently take laxatives. This use of laxatives may accelerate GI motility enough to actually reduce the absorption of drugs.

Distribution

The distribution of medications throughout the body is different in older adults than it is in younger adults. There seems to be a gradual reduction in the total body water content with aging. Therefore, the concentrations of highly water-soluble *(hydrophilic)* drugs may be higher in elderly patients because they have less body water in which the drugs can be diluted. The composition of the body also changes with aging. The lean muscle mass decreases, which results in increased body fat. In both men and women there is an approximately 20% reduction in muscle mass between the ages of 25 and 65 years and a corresponding 20% increase in body fat. Fat-soluble or *lipophilic* drugs such as hypnotics and sedatives that are primarily distributed to the fatty tissues and may have prolonged drug actions and/or toxicity.

Elderly patients may have reduced protein concentrations, due in large part to reduced liver function. In addition, reduced dietary intake and/or poor GI protein absorption can cause nutritional deficiencies and reduced blood protein levels. Regardless of the cause, the result is a reduced number of protein-binding sites for highly protein-bound drugs. This results in higher levels of unbound drug in the blood. Remember that only drugs that are not bound to proteins are active. Therefore, the effects of highly protein-bound drugs may be enhanced if their dosages are not adjusted to accommodate any reduced serum albumin concentrations. Some highly protein-bound drugs include warfarin and phenytoin.

Metabolism

Metabolism declines with advancing age. The transformation of active drugs into inactive metabolites is primarily performed by the liver. The liver actually loses mass with age and slowly loses its ability to metabolize drugs effectively due to reduced production of microsomal *(cytochrome P-450)* enzymes. There is also a reduction in blood flow to the liver because of reduced cardiac output and atherosclerosis. A reduction in the hepatic blood flow of approximately 1.5% per year occurs after 25 years of age. All of these factors contribute to prolonging the half-life of many drugs (e.g., warfarin), which can potentially result in drug accumulation if serum drug levels are not closely monitored.

Excretion

Renal function declines in roughly two thirds of elderly patients. A reduction in the *glomerular filtration rate* of 40% to 50%, combined with a reduction in cardiac output leading to reduced renal perfusion, can result in delayed drug excretion and therefore drug accumulation. This is especially true for drugs with a low *therapeutic index* such as digoxin. Renal function should be monitored frequently as described earlier. Appropriate dose and interval adjustments may be determined based on the results of renal and liver function studies as well as the presence of therapeutic levels of the drug in the serum. If a decrease in renal and liver function is known, the dosage should be adjusted, so that drug accumulation and toxicity may be avoided or minimized.

Problematic Medications for the Elderly

Drugs in certain classes are more likely to cause problems in elderly patients because of many of the physiologic alterations and pharmacokinetic changes already discussed. Table 3-4 lists some of the more common medications that are problematic. Some of the drugs that should be avoided in the elderly have been identified by various professional organizations such as the American Nurses Association as well as by various other authoritative sources. Since the 1990s, a very effective tool, the

TABLE 3-4 Medications and Conditions Requiring Special Considerations in the Elderly Patient

Medication	Common Complications
Analgesics	
Opioids	Confusion, constipation, urinary retention, nausea, vomiting, respiratory depression, decreased level of consciousness, falls
Nonsteroidal antiinflammatory drugs (NSAIDs)	Edema, nausea, abdominal distress, gastric ulceration, bleeding, renal toxicity
Anticoagulants (heparin, warfarin)	Major and minor bleeding episodes, many drug interactions, dietary interactions
Anticholinergics	Blurred vision, dry mouth, constipation, confusion, urinary retention, tachycardia
Antidepressants	Sedation and strong anticholinergic adverse effects (see above)
Antihypertensives	Nausea, hypotension, diarrhea, bradycardia, heart failure, impotence
Cardiac glycosides (e.g., digoxin)	Visual disorders, nausea, diarrhea, dysrhythmias, hallucinations, decreased appetite, weight loss
Central nervous system (CNS) depressants (muscle relaxants, opioids)	Sedation, weakness, dry mouth, confusion, urinary retention, ataxia
Sedatives and hypnotics	Confusion, daytime sedation, ataxia, lethargy, forgetfulness, increased risk of falls
Thiazide diuretics	Electrolyte imbalance, rashes, fatigue, leg cramps, dehydration

Condition	Drugs Requiring Special Caution and Monitoring
Bladder flow obstruction	Anticholinergics, antihistamines, decongestants, antidepressants
Clotting disorders	NSAIDs, aspirin, antiplatelet drugs
Chronic constipation	Calcium channel blockers, tricyclic antidepressants, anticholinergics
Chronic obstructive pulmonary disease	Long-acting sedatives or hypnotics, narcotics, beta-blockers
Heart failure and hypertension	Sodium, decongestants, amphetamines, over-the-counter cold products
Insomnia	Decongestants, bronchodilators, monoamine oxidase inhibitors
Parkinson's disease	Antipsychotics, phenothiazines
Syncope, falls	Sedatives, hypnotics, opioids, CNS depressants, muscle relaxants, antidepressants, antihypertensives

Update on Application of the Beers Criteria for Evaluation of Drug Use in the Elderly

■ Review

The Beers criteria are basic guidelines for identifying drugs that are "potentially inappropriate medications" for the elderly. These criteria, originally developed in 1991 by a panel of experts led by Mark H. Beers, MD, are to be used to evaluate drug therapy in the elderly population for the purpose of predicting adverse drug reactions (ADRs). The panel updated its work in 1997 and 2002. The Beers criteria provide a listing of drugs and drug classes that should be avoided in the elderly, although this list is controversial. They also identify disease states that are contraindications for some drugs. In 2005, a research study was conducted to confirm the relationship between potentially inappropriate drug prescribing as defined by the Beers criteria and the occurrence of ADRs in elderly patients treated at outpatient clinics.

■ Type of Evidence

The research method used a prospective cohort study design in which over 500 elderly patients who were prescribed drugs on their first visit to an outpatient clinic were surveyed by telephone 1 week later. Statistical analysis focused on the possible relationship between ADRs and inappropriate drug prescribing for the elderly.

■ Results of Study

The 2005 study provided evidence that the Beers criteria can be used successfully to predict ADRs among elderly outpatients and to examine the possible impact of potentially inappropriate drug prescribing. Of the 500+ patients surveyed, 64 were prescribed potentially inappropriate drugs and 126 experienced ADRs. Statistical analysis confirmed an association between ADRs and potentially inappropriate drug prescribing. The results of this investigation have been extremely beneficial, because few studies have focused on drug-related problems experienced by the elderly. In 1999, the Centers for Medicare and Medicaid Services adapted the Beers criteria and incorporated them into nursing home regulatory guidelines—although such a use was not the intent of the original study panel.

■ Link of Evidence to Nursing Practice

This study showed a positive association between potentially inappropriate drug prescriptions as defined by the Beers criteria and ADRs. The study alerts prescribers to the possibility of ADRs in the elderly and raises concerns about certain medications. Health care providers should remain aware of and sensitive to these criteria as well as other factors contributing to negative outcomes of medication use in the elderly, including noncompliance. The Beers criteria attempt to fill a knowledge gap about the elderly, medication use, and related ADRs, but further research is needed using more well-developed research methods and analysis to strengthen evidence-based practice and decrease medication-related risks.

Data from Chang CM et al: Use of the Beers criteria to predict adverse drug reactions among first-visit elderly outpatients, *Pharmacotherapy* 25(6):831-838, 2005. Available at *http://www.medscape.com/viewarticle/507059*; Wick JY: The Beers criteria: red flags for elders, *Pharmacy Times,* p 56, June 2006. Available at *http://www.pharmacytimes.com/issues/articles/2006-06_3593.asp*.

Beers criteria, has been used to identify drugs that may be inappropriately prescribed, ineffective, or cause adverse drug reactions in elderly patients (see the Evidence-Based Practice box on this page). The Beers criteria are very useful and help determine risk-associated situations for the elderly and specific drugs that may be problematic.

NURSING PROCESS

Assessment

Before any medication is administered to a *pediatric* patient, a health history and medication history should be obtained with assistance from parents, caregivers, or legal guardian. The following should be included:
- Age
- Age-related concerns about organ functioning
- Age-related fears
- Allergies to drugs and food
- Baseline values for vital signs
- Head-to-toe physical assessment findings
- Height in feet/inches and centimeters
- Weight in kilograms and pounds
- Level of growth and development and related developmental tasks
- Medical and medication history (including adverse drug reactions); current medications and related dosage forms and routes and the patient's tolerance of the forms and/or routes

- State of anxiety of the patient and/or family members or caregiver
- Use of prescription and OTC medications in the home setting
- Usual method of medication administration, such as use of a calibrated spoon or needleless syringe
- Usual response to medications
- Motor and cognitive responses and their age appropriateness
- Resources available to the patient and family

In addition, the prescriber's orders should be checked and rechecked by the nurse, because there is no room for error when working with pediatric patients (or any patients). The medication dosage should be calculated and rechecked several times for accuracy. Calculations for dosages should take into account a variety of information and variables that may affect patient response and should use BSA formulas and body weight formulas (milligrams per kilogram). If any doubts exist regarding the calculation, time should always be taken to have the calculations rechecked. In addition to an assessment of the patient, an assessment of the drug should be performed, focusing specifically on information about the drug's purpose, dosage ranges, routes of administration, cautions, and contraindications. The saying that pediatric patients are just "small adults" is incorrect, because in pediatric patients every organ is anatomically and physiologically immature and not fully functioning. As pediatric patients grow older, their BSA and weight are still lower, so continual, extreme caution is needed when giving them medications. Immature organ and system development will influence pharmacokinetics and thus affect the way the pediatric patient responds to a drug.

Organ function may be determined through laboratory testing. The following studies may be ordered by the prescriber before beginning drug therapy as well as during and after drug therapy: hepatic and renal function studies, red and white blood cell counts, and measurement of hemoglobin and hematocrit levels and serum protein levels.

Assessment data to be gathered for the *elderly* patient may include the following:

- Age
- Allergies to drugs and food
- Dietary habits
- Sensory, visual, hearing, cognitive, and motor skill deficits
- Financial status and any limitations
- List of all health-related care providers, including physicians, dentists, optometrists and ophthalmologists, podiatrists, and alternative medicine health care practitioners such as osteopathic physicians, chiropractors, and nurse practitioners
- Past and present medical history
- Listing of medications, past and present, including prescription drugs, OTC medications, herbals, nutritional supplements, vitamins, and home remedies
- Existence of polypharmacy (the use of more than one medication)
- Self-medication practices
- Laboratory test results, especially those indicative of renal and liver function
- History of smoking and use of alcohol with notation of amount, frequency, and years of use
- Risk situations related to drug therapy identified by the Beers criteria (see the Evidence-Based Practice box on p. 44)

One way to collect data about the various medications or drugs being taken by the elderly is to obtain that information from the patient and/or caregiver using the brown-bag technique. This is an effective means of identifying various drugs the patient is taking, regardless of the patient's age, and should be used in conjunction with a complete review of the patient's medical history or record. The brown-bag technique requires the patient/caregiver to place all medications used in a bag and bring them to the health care provider. All medications should be brought in their original containers. A list of medications with generic names, dosages, routes of administration, and frequencies is then compiled. The list of medications should be compared with what is prescribed or with what the patient states he or she is actually taking. Medication reconciliation procedures are performed in health care facilities when assessing and tracking medications taken by the patient (see Chapter 6). In addition, the patient's insight into his or her medical problems is a very beneficial piece of information in developing a plan of care. It is also important for the nurse to realize that although elderly patients may be able to provide the required information themselves, many may be confused or poorly informed about their medications and/or health condition. In such cases, a more reliable historian, such as a significant other, family member, or caregiver, should be consulted. Elderly patients may also have sensory deficits that require the nurse to speak slowly, loudly, and clearly while facing the patient.

With the elderly patient—as with a patient of any age—the nurse should always assess support systems and the patient's ability to take medications safely. Whenever possible with the elderly, health care providers and prescribers should opt to use a nonpharmacologic approach to treatment first if appropriate. Other data the nurse should gather include information about acute or chronic illnesses, nutritional problems, cardiac problems, respiratory illnesses, and GI tract disorders. Laboratory tests related to life span considerations that should be performed include hemoglobin level and hematocrit, red and white blood cell counts, blood urea nitrogen level, serum and urine creatinine levels, urine specific gravity, serum electrolyte levels, and protein and serum albumin levels.

Nursing Diagnoses

- Risk for injury related to adverse effects of medications or to the method of drug administration
- Risk for injury related to idiosyncratic reactions to drugs due to age-related drug sensitivity
- Imbalanced nutrition, less than body requirements, related to age or drug therapy and possible drug adverse effects
- Deficient knowledge related to information about drugs and their adverse effects or about when to contact the prescriber

---

LIFE SPAN CONSIDERATIONS: The Elderly Patient

Alzheimer's Disease

- Alzheimer's disease was estimated to affect approximately 5.2 million Americans in 2008, of whom 5 million were people aged 65 or older and 200,000 were individuals under the age of 65 who have earlier-onset Alzheimer's disease. Alzheimer's disease is presently the sixth leading cause of death in adults in the United States. Unfortunately, every 71 seconds someone develops the disorder, and by midcentury, someone will develop Alzheimer's disease every 33 seconds. Approximately one in eight persons aged 65 and older has Alzheimer's disease. Ten million baby boomers will develop Alzheimer's disease in their lifetime.
- The disease process has a major impact on the patient's mental and physical abilities. Due to deterioration of mental status and chronic physical decline, these patients need assistance in performing the activities of daily living, including assistance with medication administration.
- The direct and indirect costs of Alzheimer's and other dementias to Medicare, Medicaid, and businesses amount to more than $148 billion each year.
- Caregivers and family members need to be informed of the short-term and long-term characteristics of the illness, and resources need to be provided in either a private care setting or through special needs units in assisted living settings or nursing homes.
- In 2007, 9.8 million family members, friends, and neighbors provided unpaid care for a person with Alzheimer's disease or another dementia.
- One in six women and one in ten men who live to be at least age 55 will develop Alzheimer's disease in their remaining lifetime.
- Family and other unpaid caregivers of people with Alzheimer's disease or another dementia are more likely than noncaregivers to have high levels of stress hormones, reduced immune function, and slow wound healing.

Data from Alzheimer's Association: 2008 Alzheimer's disease facts and figures, *Alzheimer's Dement* 4(2):110-133, 2008. Available at *http://www.alz.org/ national/documents/report_alzfactsfigures2008.pdf.*

Planning

Goals

- Patient states measures to minimize complications and adverse effects associated with the drugs taken during the therapeutic regimen.
- Patient states the importance of adhering to the prescribed drug therapy (or takes medication as prescribed with assistance).
- Patient contacts the prescriber when appropriate (such as when unusual effects occur) during drug therapy.

Outcome Criteria

- Patient (or parent, legal guardian, or caregiver) states the importance of taking the medication as prescribed (e.g., improved condition, decreased symptoms) for the duration of the recommended drug therapy.
- Patient (or parent, legal guardian, or caregiver) follows instructions specific to the administration of the medication ordered (e.g., special application of an ointment, proper administration of a liquid, correct dosage) for the duration of treatment.
- Patient (specifically the elderly patient) states why he or she is taking a specific medication and identifies what the drug looks like and when the drug is to be taken during the duration of drug treatment.
- Patient shows improvement in the condition being treated that is related to compliance with the medication regimen and successful medication therapy during the treatment period.
- Patient takes or receives medications safely and without injury to self over the duration of therapy.
- Patient (or parent, legal guardian, or caregiver) states specific situations in which the prescriber must be contacted (e.g., occurrence of fever, pain, vomiting, rash, or diarrhea; worsening of the condition being treated; bronchospasm; dyspnea; intolerable adverse effects; signs of major adverse effects).

Implementation

In general, it is always important to emphasize and practice the Six Rights of medication administration (see Chapter 1) and follow the prescriber's order and/or medication instructions. All drugs should be checked three times against the Six Rights and the prescriber's order before the drug is given to the patient. This usually applies for acute care and long-term care inpatient situations. For the *pediatric* patient, some specific nursing actions are as follows: (1) If necessary, mix medications in a substance or fluid other than essential foods such as milk, orange juice, or cereal, because the child may develop a dislike for the food in the future. Instead of such foods, find a liquid or food item that can be used to make the medications taste better, such as sherbet or another form or flavor of ice cream. This intervention should be used only if the patient is not able to swallow the dosage form. (2) Do not add drug(s) to fluid in a cup or bottle because the amount of drug consumed would then be impossible to calculate should the entire amount of fluid not be taken. (3) Always document special techniques of drug administration so that others involved in the care of the patient may benefit from and use the same techniques. For example, if having the child eat a frozen popsicle before giving an unpleasant-tasting pill, liquid, or tablet helps to get the medication administered, then share that information with others involved in the child's care. (4) Unless con-

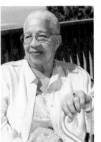
traindicated, add small amounts of water or fluids to elixirs so that the child may tolerate the medication. Remember, however, that it is essential that the child take the entire volume, so be very cautious with this practice and only use an amount of fluid mixture that you know the child can tolerate. (5) Avoid using the word *candy* in place of the word *drug* or *medication*. Medications should be called medicines and their dangers made known to children. No games should be played with this information. (6) Keep all medications out of the reach of children of all ages and be sure that parents and other family members understand this requirement and know to request child-protective lids or tops for medication containers. Childproof locks or closures should be used on cabinets holding medications. (7) Always ask about how the pediatric patient is used to taking medications (e.g., liquid vs. pill or tablet dosage forms) and whether there are any methods that the family or caregiver has found to be helpful in administering medications in general and in administering unpleasant-tasting drugs. See the Life Span Considerations: The Pediatric Patient box on p. 40 for further information regarding medication administration in patients from infancy through adolescence. For more information about dosage calculations for medication administration in pediatric patients, online sites providing examples and programs to help with pediatric drug dosage calculations including the following: *http://www.testandcalc.com* and *http://www.mapharm.com/dosage_calc.htm.*

Elderly patients should be encouraged to take medications as directed and not to discontinue them or double up on doses unless recommended or ordered to do so by their health care provider/prescriber. The nurse should ensure that the patient or caregiver understands treatment- and/or medication-related instructions and understands safety measures related to drug therapy, such as keeping all medications out of the reach of children. Written and oral instructions should be provided concerning the drug name, action, purpose, dosage, time of administration, route, adverse effects, safety of administration, storage, interactions, and any cautions about or contraindications to its use. Remember that simple is always best! Always try to find ways to simplify the patient's therapeutic regimen and be especially alert to polypharmacy. If a nurse advocate or a nurse practitioner with prescription privileges has the opportunity to review the patient's chart, he or she should take the time to simplify and write down the use or purpose of the drug, the best way to take the drug, and a list of adverse effects. Provide this information on paper in bold, large print. Among the specific interventions that have proven to be helpful in promoting medication safety in the elderly is the use of the Beers criteria (see the Evidence-Based Practice box on p. 44). These criteria provide a systematic way of identifying prescription medications that are potentially harmful to elderly patients. The prescriber and nurse must constantly remember that clinical judgment and knowledge base are important in making critical decisions about a patient's care and drug therapy. In addition, keeping abreast of evidence-based nursing practice, such as application of the Beers criteria, is important for the nurse to remain current in clinical nursing practice. Specific

guidelines for medication administration by various routes are presented in detail in the photo atlas in Chapter 10.

In summary, drug therapy across the life span must be well thought out, with full consideration to the patient's age, gender, cultural background, ethnicity, medical history, and medication profile. When all phases of the nursing process and the specific life span considerations discussed in this chapter are included, there is a better chance of decreasing adverse effects, reducing risks to the patient, and increasing drug safety.

Evaluation

In general, when the nurse is dealing with life span issues and drug therapy, the nurse's observation and monitoring for therapeutic effects as well as adverse effects is critical to safe and effective therapy. The nurse must know the patient's profile and history as well as information about the drug. The drug's purpose, specific use in the patient, simply stated actions, dose, frequency of dosing, adverse effects, cautions, and contraindications should be listed and kept available at all times. This information will allow more comprehensive monitoring of drug therapy, regardless of the age of the patient.

POINTS TO REMEMBER

- There are many age-related pharmacokinetic effects that lead to dramatic differences in drug absorption, distribution, metabolism, and excretion in the young and the elderly. At one end of the life span is the pediatric patient and at the other end is the elderly patient, both of whom are very sensitive to the effects of drugs.
- Most common dosage calculations use the milligrams per kilogram formula related to age; however, BSA is also used in drug calculations, and organ maturity is considered. It is important for the nurse to know that many elements besides the mathematical calculation itself contribute to safe dosage calculations. Safety should be the number one concern, with full consideration of the Six Rights of medication administration (see Chapter 1).

- The percentage of the population over the age of 65 years continues to grow; therefore, nurses will continue to come in contact with an increasing number of elderly patients. Polypharmacy raises many concerns for the elderly; thus, the patient should carry a current listing of all his or her medications at all times. If this is not appropriate, then the list should be kept by a caregiver or family member involved in the patient's nursing care.
- The nurse's responsibility is to act as a patient advocate as well as to be informed about growth and developmental principles and the effects of various drugs during the life span and in various phases of illness.

NCLEX EXAMINATION REVIEW QUESTIONS

1 The nurse is reviewing factors that influence pharmacokinetics in the neonatal patient. Which factor puts the neonatal patient at risk with regard to drug therapy?
  a Immature renal system
  b Hyperperistalsis in the GI tract
  c Irregular temperature regulation
  d Smaller circulatory capacity
2 The physiologic differences in the pediatric patient compared with the adult patient affect the amount of drug needed to produce a therapeutic effect. The nurse is aware that one of the main differences is that infants have
  a increased protein in circulation.
  b fat composition lower than 0.001%.
  c more muscular body composition.
  d water composition of approximately 75%.
3 While teaching a 76-year-old patient about the adverse effects of his medications, the nurse encourages him to keep a journal of the adverse effects he experiences. This intervention is impor-

tant for the elderly patient because of alterations in pharmacokinetics, such as
  a increased renal excretion of protein-bound drugs.
  b more alkaline gastric pH, resulting in more adverse effects.
  c decreased blood flow to the liver, resulting in altered metabolism.
  d less adipose tissue to store fat-soluble drugs.
4 When the nurse is reviewing a list of medications taken by an 88-year-old patient, the patient says, "I get dizzy when I stand up." She also states that she has nearly fainted "a time or two" in the afternoons. Her systolic blood pressure drops 15 points when she stands up. Which type of medication may be responsible for these effects?
  a NSAIDs
  b Cardiac glycosides
  c Anticoagulants
  d Antihypertensives

Continued

NCLEX EXAMINATION REVIEW QUESTIONS—cont'd

5 A pregnant patient who is at 32 weeks' gestation has a cold and calls the office to ask about taking an OTC medication that is rated as pregnancy category A. Which answer by the nurse is correct?
  a "This drug causes problems in the human fetus, so you should not take this medication."
  b "This drug may cause problems in the human fetus, but nothing has been proven in clinical trials. It is best not to take this medication."
  c "This drug has not caused problems in animals, but no testing has been done in humans. It is probably safe to take."
  d "Studies indicate that there is no risk to the human fetus, so it is okay to take this medication as directed, if you need it."

6 The nurse is preparing to administer an injection to a preschool-aged child. Which approaches are appropriate for this age group? (Select all that apply.)
  a Explain to the child in advance about the injection.
  b Provide a brief, concrete explanation about the injection.
  c Encourage participation in the procedure.
  d Make use of magical thinking.
  e Provide comfort measures after the injection.

1. a, 2. d, 3. c, 4. d, 5. d, 6. b, d, e.

CRITICAL THINKING ACTIVITIES: BEST ACTION

1 A mother calls the clinic to ask how to give a tablet to her 4-year-old son. He is refusing to swallow it and won't chew it because it "tastes icky." What is the best response by the nurse?

2 A woman in her third trimester of pregnancy is having a checkup and asks for aspirin for a headache. What is the nurse's best response?

3 A 22-year-old woman has brought her 16-month-old daughter to see the nurse practitioner because the toddler has symptoms of a sinus infection. After examining the toddler, the nurse practitioner writes a prescription for an antibiotic. The mother says, "Oh, I have tetracycline suspension at home that I took for an infection. Can't I just use that and save money?" What is the nurse's best answer?

For answers, see *http://evolve.elsevier.com/Lilley*.

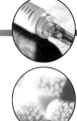

CHAPTER 4

Cultural, Legal, and Ethical Considerations

OBJECTIVES

When you reach the end of this chapter, you should be able to do the following:

1 Discuss the various cultural, genetic, and racial or ethnic factors that may influence an individual's response to medications.

2 Identify various cultural phenomena affecting health care and use of medications.

3 List the drugs that more commonly show variations in response due to cultural, racial, and ethnic factors.

4 Develop a nursing care plan that addresses the cultural care of patients in drug therapy and the nursing process.

5 Briefly discuss the important components of drug legislation at the state and federal levels.

6 Provide examples of how drug legislation impacts drug therapy and the nursing process.

7 Discuss the various categories of controlled substances and give specific drug examples in each category.

8 Identify the process involved in the development of new drugs, including the investigational new drug application, the phases of investigational drug studies, and the process for obtaining informed consent.

9 Discuss the nurse's role in the development of new and investigational drugs and the informed consent process.

10 Discuss the ethical aspects of drug administration as they relate to drug therapy and the nursing process.

11 Identify the ethical principles involved in making an ethical decision.

12 Develop a nursing care plan that addresses the legal and ethical care of patients with a specific focus on drug therapy and the nursing process.

e-Learning Activities

http://evolve.elsevier.com/Lilley

NCLEX Review Question • Animations • Nursing Care Plans • Audio Glossary • Category Catchers • Medication Errors Checklists • IV Therapy Checklists • Calculators • Frequently Asked Questions • Content Updates • Supplemental Resources • Answers to Case Studies and Critical Thinking Activities

Glossary

Bias Any systematic error in a measurement process. One common effort to avoid bias in research studies involves the use of blinded study designs (see later). (p. 54)

Black box warning A type of warning that appears in a drug's prescribing information, required by the U.S. Food and Drug Administration alerting prescribers of serious adverse events that have occurred with the given drug. (p. 55)

Blinded investigational drug study A research design in which the subjects are purposely unaware of whether the substance they are administered is the drug under study or a placebo. This method serves to eliminate bias on the part of research subjects in reporting their body's responses to investigational drugs. (p. 54)

Controlled substances Any drugs listed on one of the "schedules" of the Controlled Substance Act (also called *scheduled drugs*). (p. 52)

Double-blind investigational drug study A research design in which both the investigator(s) and the subjects are purposely unaware of whether the substance administered to a given subject is

the drug under study or a placebo. This method eliminates bias on the part of both the investigator and the subject. (p. 54)

Drug polymorphism Variation in response to a drug because of a patient's age, gender, size, and/or body composition. (p. 50)

Expedited drug approval Acceleration of the usual investigational new drug approval process by the U.S. Food and Drug Administration (FDA) and pharmaceutical companies, usually for drugs used to treat life-threatening diseases. (p. 53)

Health Insurance Portability and Accountability Act (HIPAA) An act that protects health insurance coverage for workers and their families when they change jobs. It also protects patient information. If confidentiality of a patient is breached, severe fines may be imposed. (p. 52)

Informed consent Written permission obtained from a patient consenting to the performance of a specific procedure (e.g., receiving an investigational drug), after the patient has been given information regarding the procedure deemed necessary for the patient to make a sound or "informed" decision. (p. 54)

Investigational new drug (IND) A drug not approved for marketing by the FDA but available for use in experiments to determine its safety and efficacy; also, the actual name of the category of application that the drug manufacturer submits to the FDA to obtain permission for human (clinical) studies following successful completion of animal (preclinical) studies. (p. 54)

Investigational new drug application The type of application that a drug manufacturer submits to the FDA following successful completion of required human research studies. (p. 54)

Legend drugs Another name for prescription drugs. (p. 52)

Narcotic A legal term established under the Harrison Antinarcotic Act of 1914. It originally applied to drugs that produced insensibility or stupor, especially the opioids (e.g., morphine, heroin). The term is currently used in clinical settings to refer to any medically adminis-tered controlled substance and in legal settings to refer to any illicit or "street" drug. (p. 52)

Orphan drugs A special category of drugs that have been identi-fied to help treat patients with rare diseases. (p. 52)

Over-the-counter drugs Drugs available to consumers without a prescription. Also called *nonprescription drugs*. (p. 52)

Placebo An inactive (inert) substance (e.g., saline, distilled water, starch, sugar), that is not a drug but is formulated to resemble a drug for research purposes. (p. 54)

• • •

CULTURAL CONSIDERATIONS

The United States is a very culturally diverse nation. Because the health care system emphasizes cure, prescribed drugs are often a major part of a patient's therapeutic regimen. The demographics of the United States continue to change. According to the 2008 population projections of the U.S. Census Bureau, minority groups—which now comprise roughly one third of the U.S. population—are expected to become the majority by 2042 and will represent 54% of the nation's population by 2050. That is, the combined population of all groups except non-Hispanic, single-race whites is projected to be approximately 235 million out of a total U.S. population of 439 million in 2050. The non-Hispanic, single-race white population is projected to be only slightly larger in 2050 (at about 203 million) than in 2008. It is predicted that nearly one in three U.S. residents will be Hispanic by 2050. The African American population is projected to in-crease from 41 million (about 14%) to about 66 million (or 15%) by 2050. The Asian population is projected to increase from 15 million to about 40 million, rising from a current 5.1% to 9.2% of the total. Of the remaining racial groups, American In-dians and Alaska Natives are projected to increase in number from 4.9 million to 8.6 million (or from 1.6% to 2% of the total population). The population of Native Hawaiians and other Pa-cific Islanders is expected to more than double, from 1.1 million to 2.6 million. The number of people who identify themselves as being of two or more races is projected to more than triple, from about 5 million to 16 million.

The field of *ethnopharmacology* provides an expanding body of knowledge for understanding the specific impact of cultural factors on patient drug response. It is hampered, however, by the lack of clarity in terms such as *race, ethnicity,* and *culture.* For example, although some researchers have used the term *Hispanic* to encompass geographic groups as diverse as Puerto Ricans, Mexicans, and Peruvians, other researchers have used it to denote a specific racial group. It is impossible to know a patient's geno-type by either physical appearance or health care history.

The nurse must be up to date in his or her basic knowledge of the nursing process and understanding of the art and science of professional nursing practice. Cultural assessment, along with other types of assessment, should be part of the assess-ment phase of the nursing process. Acknowledgment and ac-ceptance of the influences of a patient's cultural beliefs, values, and customs is necessary to promote optimal health and well-ness. Some relevant terms are defined in the Cultural Implica-tions box on this page.

CULTURAL IMPLICATIONS

Cultural Terms Related to Nursing Practice

Culture: An integrated system of beliefs, values, and customs that are associated with a particular group of people and are generally handed down from generation to generation.

Cultural competence: The ability to work with patients with proper consideration for the cultural context, which includes patients' belief systems and values regarding health, wellness, and illness. It also involves learning about different patients and their specific responses to treatment, including drug therapies.

Ethnicity: Ethnic affiliation based on shared culture or genetic heritage or both.

Ethnopharmacology: The study of the effect of ethnicity on drug responses, specifically drug absorption, metabolism, distribution, and excretion (i.e., pharmacokinetics; see Chapter 2) as well as the study of genetic variations to drugs (i.e., pharmacogenetics).

Race: Often defined as a class of individuals with a common lineage. In genetics, a race is considered to be a population having a somewhat different genetic composition or gene frequencies. Race is also used to refer to geographical origins of ancestry.

Influence of Ethnicity and Genetics on Drug Response

The concept of polymorphism is critical to an understanding of how the same drug may result in very different responses in differ-ent individuals. For example, why does a Chinese patient require lower dosages of an antianxiety drug than a white patient? Why does an African American patient respond differently to antihyper-tensives than a white patient? **Drug polymorphism** refers to the effect of a patient's age, gender, size, body composition, and other characteristics on the pharmacokinetics of specific drugs. Factors contributing to drug polymorphism may be loosely categorized into environmental factors (e.g., diet and nutritional status), cul-tural factors, and genetic (inherited) factors.

Medication response depends greatly on the level of the pa-tient's compliance with the therapy regimen. Yet compliance may vary depending on the patient's cultural beliefs, experiences with medications, personal expectations, family expectations, family influence, and level of education. Compliance is not the only is-sue, however. Prescribers must also be aware that some patients use alternative therapies, such as herbal and homeopathic reme-dies, that can inhibit or accelerate drug metabolism and therefore alter a drug's response.

Environmental and economic factors (such as diet) can con-tribute to drug response. For example, a diet high in fat has been documented to increase the absorption of the drug griseofulvin (an antifungal drug). Malnutrition with deficiencies in protein, vitamins, and minerals may modify the functioning of metabolic enzymes, which may alter the body's ability to absorb or elimi-nate a medication.

Historically, most clinical drug trials were conducted using white men, often college students, as research subjects. However, there are data that demonstrate the impact of genetic factors on drug *pharmacokinetics* and drug *pharmacodynamics* or drug re-sponse. Some individuals of European and African descent, for example, are known to be *slow acetylators*. This means that their bodies attach acetyl groups to drug molecules at a relatively slow rate, which results in elevated drug concentrations. This situation may warrant lower drug dosages. One classic example of a drug whose metabolism is affected by this characteristic is the antituberculosis drug isoniazid. In contrast, some patients of Japanese and Inuit descent are more rapid acetylators and metabolize drugs more quickly, which predisposes the patient to subtherapeutic drug concentrations and may require higher drug dosages.

Levels of the *cytochrome P-450* enzymes are also known to vary between ethnic groups. This has effects on the ability to metabolize psychotropic drugs. Most psychotropic drugs are metabolized in the liver in a two-phase process. Cytochrome P-450 enzymes often control phase I of the hepatic metabolism of both antidepressants and antipsychotic drugs. This can affect plasma drug levels, and therefore the intensity of drug response, at different doses. Groups of Asian patients have been shown to be "poor metabolizers" of these drugs and often require lower dosages to achieve desired therapeutic effects. In contrast, white patients are more likely to be classified as "ultrarapid metabolizers" and may require higher drug dosages.

Variations are also reported between ethnic groups in the occurrence of adverse effects. For example, African Americans are more likely to develop lethargy and dizziness than white patients taking lithium. For the treatment of hypertension, thiazide diuretics appear to be more effective in African Americans than in whites. Several additional examples of racial and ethnic differences in drug response are outlined in Table 4-1.

Individuals throughout the world share many common views and beliefs regarding health practices and medication use. However, specific cultural influences, beliefs, and practices related to medication administration do exist. Awareness of cultural differences is critical for the care of patients in the United States today because of the constantly changing U.S. demographics. As a result of these changes, nurses need to attend to and be concerned with each patient's cultural background to ensure safe and quality nursing care, including medication administration.

For example, some African Americans have health beliefs and practices that include an emphasis on proper diet and rest; the use of herbal teas, laxatives, and protective bracelets; and the use of folk medicine, prayer, and the "laying on of hands." Reliance on various home remedies can also be an important component of their health practices. Some Asian American patients, especially the Chinese, believe in the concepts of *yin* and *yang*. Yin and yang are opposing forces that lead to illness or health, depending on which force is dominant in the individual and whether the forces are balanced. Balance produces healthy states. Other common health practices of Asian Americans include use of acupuncture, herbal remedies, and heat. All such beliefs and practices need to be considered—especially when the patient values their use more highly than the use of medications. Many of these beliefs are strongly grounded in religion. The Asian and Pacific Islander racial-ethnic group also includes Thais, Vietnamese, Filipinos, Koreans, and Japanese, among others.

Some Native Americans believe in preserving harmony with nature or keeping a balance between the body and mind and the environment to maintain health. Ill spirits are seen as the cause of disease. The traditional healer for this culture is the medicine man, and treatments vary from massage and application of heat to acts of purification. Some individuals of Hispanic descent view health as a result of good luck and living right and illness as a result of bad luck or committing a bad deed. To restore health, these individuals seek a balance between the body and mind through the use of cold remedies or foods for "hot" illnesses (of blood or yellow bile) and hot remedies for "cold" illnesses (of phlegm or black bile). Hispanics may use a variety of religious rituals for healing (e.g., lighting of candles), which may also be practiced by adherents of other religions and/or belief systems. It is very important to remember that these beliefs vary from patient to patient; therefore, the nurse should always consult with the patient rather than assume that the patient holds certain beliefs because he or she belongs to one group or another.

Barriers to adequate health care for the culturally diverse U.S. patient population include language, poverty, access, pride, and beliefs regarding medical practices. Medications may have a different meaning to different cultures, as would any form of medical treatment. Therefore, before any medication is administered, a thorough cultural assessment should ideally be completed. This assessment should include questions regarding the following:

- Languages spoken, written, and understood; need for an interpreter
- Health beliefs and practices
- Past uses of medicine
- Use of herbal treatments, folk remedies, home remedies, or supplements

TABLE 4-1   Examples of Varying Drug Responses in Different Racial or Ethnic Groups

Racial or Ethnic Group	Drug Classification	Response
African Americans	Antihypertensive drugs	African Americans respond better to diuretics than to beta-blockers and angiotensin-converting enzyme inhibitors. African Americans respond less effectively to beta-blockers. African Americans respond best to calcium channel blockers, especially diltiazem. African Americans respond less effectively to single-drug therapy.
Asians and Hispanics	Antipsychotic and antianxiety drugs	Asians need lower dosages of certain drugs such as haloperidol. Asians and Hispanics respond better to lower dosages of antidepressants. Chinese require lower dosages of antipsychotics. Japanese require lower dosages of antimanic drugs.

NOTE: The comparison group for all responses is whites.

- Use of **over-the-counter drugs**
- Usual responses to illness
- Responsiveness to medical treatment
- Religious practices and beliefs (e.g., many Christian Scientists believe in taking no medications at all)
- Support from the patient's cultural community that may provide resources or assistance as needed, such as religious connections, leaders, family members, friends
- Dietary habits

U.S. DRUG AND RELATED LEGISLATION

Until the beginning of the twentieth century there were no federal rules and regulations in the United States to protect consumers from the dangers of medications. The various legislative interventions that have occurred have often been prompted by large-scale serious adverse drug reactions. One example is the sulfanilamide tragedy of 1937. Over 100 deaths occurred in the United States when people ingested a diethylene glycol solution of sulfanilamide that had been marketed as a therapeutic drug. Diethylene glycol is a component of automobile antifreeze solution, and the drug containing it was never tested for its toxicity. Another prominent example is the thalidomide tragedy that occurred in Europe between the 1940s and 1960s. Many pregnant women who took this sedative-hypnotic drug gave birth to seriously deformed infants.

A recent and significant piece of legislation is the **Health Insurance Portability and Accountability Act (HIPAA)** of 1996. HIPAA requires all health care providers, health and life insurance companies, public health authorities, employers, and schools to maintain patient privacy regarding protected health information. Protected health information includes any individually identifying information such as patients' health conditions, account numbers, prescription numbers, medications, and payment information. Such information can be oral and/or recorded in any paper or electronic form. The primary purpose of these types of federal legislation is to ensure the safety and efficacy of new drugs and, in the case of HIPAA, to protect patient confidentiality. Table 4-2 provides a timeline summary of major U.S. drug legislation.

NEW DRUG DEVELOPMENT

The research into and development of new drugs is an ongoing process. The pharmaceutical manufacturing industry is a multibillion-dollar industry, and pharmaceutical companies must continuously develop new and better drugs to maintain a competitive edge. The research required for the development of these new drugs may take several years. Hundreds of substances are isolated that never make it to market. Once a potentially beneficial drug has been identified, the pharmaceutical company must follow a very regulated, systematic process before the drug can be sold on the open market. This highly sophisticated process is regulated and carefully monitored by the Food and Drug Administration (FDA). The primary purpose of the FDA is to protect the patient and ensure drug effectiveness.

This U.S. system of drug research and development is one of the most stringent in the world. It was developed out of concern for patient safety and drug efficacy. To ensure that these two very important objectives are met with some degree of certainty requires much time, funding, and documentation. Many drugs are marketed and used in foreign countries long before they

---

TABLE 4-2 Summary of Major U.S. Drug and Related Legislation

Name of Legislation (Year)	Provisions/Comments
Federal Food and Drugs Act (FFDA, 1906)	Required drug manufacturers to list on the drug product label the presence of dangerous and possibly addicting substances; recognized the *U.S. Pharmacopeia* and *National Formulary* as printed references standards for drugs
Sherley Amendment (1912) to FFDA	Prohibited fraudulent claims for drug products
Harrison Narcotic Act (1914)	Established the legal term **narcotic** and regulated the manufacture and sale of habit-forming drugs
Federal Food, Drug, and Cosmetic Act (FFDCA, 1938; amendment to FFDA)	Required drug manufacturers to provide data proving drug safety with FDA review; established the investigational new drug application process (prompted by sulfanilamide elixir tragedy)
Durham-Humphrey Amendment (1951) to FFDCA	Established **legend drugs** or prescription drugs; drug labels must carry the legend, "Caution—Federal law prohibits dispensing without a prescription"
Kefauver-Harris Amendments (1962) to FFDCA	Required manufacturers to demonstrate both therapeutic efficacy *and* safety of new drugs (prompted by thalidomide tragedy)
Controlled Substance Act (1970)	Established "schedules" for **controlled substances** (Tables 4-3 and 4-4); promoted drug addiction education, research, and treatment
Orphan Drug Act (1983)	Enabled the FDA to promote research and marketing of **orphan drugs** used to treat rare diseases
Accelerated Drug Review Regulations (1991)	Enabled faster approval by the FDA of drugs to treat life-threatening illnesses (prompted by HIV/AIDS epidemic)
Health Insurance Portability and Accountability Act (1996)	More commonly known by its acronym, HIPAA, officially required health-related organizations as well as all schools to maintain privacy of protected health information
Medicare Prescription Drug Improvement and Modernization Act (2003)	More commonly known as *Medicare Part D;* provides seniors and disabled persons with an insurance benefit program for prescription drugs; the cost of medications is shared by the patient and the federal government

AIDS, Acquired immunodeficiency syndrome; *FDA,* Food and Drug Administration; *HIV,* human immunodeficiency virus.

TABLE 4-3 Controlled Substances: Schedule Categories

Schedule	Abuse Potential	Medical Use	Dependency Potential
C-I	High	None	Severe physical and psychologic
C-II	High	Accepted	Severe physical and psychologic
C-III	Less than C-II	Accepted	Moderate to low physical or high psychologic
C-IV	Less than C-III	Accepted	Limited physical or psychologic
C-V	Less than C-IV	Accepted	Limited physical or psychologic

TABLE 4-4 Controlled Substances: Categories, Dispensing Restrictions, and Examples

Schedule	Dispensing Restrictions	Examples
C-I	Only with approved protocol	Heroin, lysergic acid diethylamide (LSD), marijuana, mescaline, peyote, psilocybin, and methaqualone
C-II	Written prescription only* No prescription refills Container must have warning label	Codeine, cocaine, hydromorphone, meperidine, morphine, methadone, secobarbital, pentobarbital, oxycodone, amphetamine, methylphenidate, and others
C-III	Written or oral prescription that expires in 6 mo No more than five refills in 6-mo period Container must have warning label	Codeine with selected other medications (e.g., acetaminophen), hydrocodone, pentobarbital rectal suppositories, and dihydrocodeine combination products
C-IV	Written or oral prescription that expires in 6 mo No more than five refills in 6-mo period Container must have warning label	Phenobarbital, chloral hydrate, meprobamate, the benzodiazepines (e.g., diazepam, temazepam, lorazepam), dextropropoxyphene, pentazocine, and others
C-V	Written prescription or over the counter (varies with state law)	Medications generally for relief of coughs or diarrhea containing limited quantities of certain opioid controlled substances

*Legally permitted to be telephoned in for major emergencies only. If telephoned in, written prescription required within 72 hr.

receive approval for use in the United States. However, drug-related calamities are more likely to be avoided by this more stringent drug approval system. The thalidomide tragedy mentioned earlier, which resulted from the use of a drug that was marketed in Europe but not in the United States, is an illustrative example. A balance must be achieved between making new lifesaving therapies available and protecting consumers from potential drug-induced adverse effects. Historically, the FDA has had markedly less regulatory authority over vitamin, herbal, and homeopathic preparations because they are designated as dietary supplements rather than drugs. In 1994, Congress passed the Dietary Supplement Health and Education Act, which requires manufacturers of such products at least to ensure their safety (although not necessarily their efficacy) and prohibits them from making any unsubstantiated claims in the product labeling. For example, a product label may read "For depression" but cannot read "Known to cure depression." Reliable, objective information about these kinds of products is limited but is growing as more formal research studies are conducted. In 1998, Congress established the National Center for Complementary and Alternative Medicine as a new branch of the National Institutes of Health. The function of this center is to conduct rigorous scientific studies of alternative medical treatments and to publish the data from such studies. Consumer demand for and interest in these alternative medicine products continues to drive this process. Patients should be advised to exercise caution in using such products and to communicate regularly with their health care providers regarding their use.

U.S. Food and Drug Administration Drug Approval Process

The FDA is responsible for approving drugs for clinical safety and efficacy before they are brought to the market. There are stringent steps, each of which may take years, that must be approved before the drug can be approved. The FDA has attempted to make lifesaving investigational drug therapies clinically available sooner than usual by offering an **expedited drug approval** process, also known as "fast track" approval. AIDS was the first major public health crisis for which the FDA began granting expedited drug approval. This process allowed pharmaceutical manufacturers to shorten the approval process to allow prescribers to give medications that showed promise during early phase I and phase II clinical trials to qualified patients with AIDS. In such cases, when a trial continues to show favorable results, the overall process of drug approval is hastened as much as possible. The concept of expedited drug approval became controversial after the FDA-initiated manufacturer recall of the antiinflammatory drug rofecoxib (Vioxx) in 2004. This recall followed multiple case reports of severe cardiovascular events, including fatalities, associated with the use of this drug. Evidence then emerged suggesting that the FDA had granted approval for this drug without receiving the requisite safety data from its manufacturer. This example has reduced the number of drugs approved via the expedited approval process. More information and specific drugs approved under this fast-track process can be found at *http://www.fda.gov*.

The drug approval process is quite complex and prolonged. It normally begins with *preclinical* testing phases, which include *in vitro* studies (using tissue samples and cell cultures) and animal studies. *Clinical* (human) studies follow the preclinical phase. There are four clinical phases. The drug is put on the market after phase III is completed if an **investigational new drug application** submitted by the manufacturer is approved by the FDA. Phase IV consists of postmarketing studies. The collective goal of these phases is to provide information on the safety, toxicity, efficacy, potency, bioavailability, and purity of the new drug.

Preclinical Investigational Drug Studies

Current medical ethics still require that all new drugs undergo laboratory testing using both *in vitro* (cell or tissue) and animal studies before any testing in human subjects can be done. *In vitro* studies include testing of the response of various types of mammalian (including human) cells and tissues to different concentrations of the investigational drug. Various types of cells and tissues used for this purpose are collected from living or dead animal or human subjects (e.g., surgical or autopsy specimens). *In vitro* studies help researchers to determine early on if a substance might be too toxic for human patients. Many prospective new drugs are ruled out for human use during this preclinical phase of drug testing. However, a small percentage of the many drugs tested in this manner are referred on for further clinical testing in human subjects.

Four Clinical Phases of Investigational Drug Studies

Before any testing on humans begin, the subjects must sign an informed consent. **Informed consent** involves the careful explanation to the human test patient or *research subject* of the purpose of the study in which he or she is being asked to participate, the procedures to be used, the possible benefits, and the risks involved. This explanation is followed by written documentation in the form of a *consent form*. The informed consent document, or consent form, must be written in a language understood by the patient and must be dated and signed by the patient and at least one witness. Informed consent is always voluntary. By law, informed consent must be obtained more than a given number of days or hours before certain procedures are performed and must always be obtained when the patient is fully mentally competent. The informed consent process may be carried out by a nurse or other health care professional, depending on how a given study is arranged.

The principles of medical ethics dictate that participants in experimental drug studies be informed volunteers and not be uninformed or coerced to participate in any way. Therefore, informed consent must be obtained from all patients (or their legal guardians) before they can be enrolled in an **investigational new drug (IND)** study. Some patients may have unrealistic expectations of the IND's usefulness. Often they have the misconception that because an investigational drug is new it must automatically be better than existing forms of therapy. Other volunteers may be reluctant to enter the study because they think they will be treated as "guinea pigs." Whatever the circumstances of the study, the research subjects must be informed of all potential hazards as well as the possible benefits of the new therapy. It should be stressed to all patients that involvement in IND studies is voluntary and that any individual can either decline to participate or quit the study at any time without affecting the delivery of any previously agreed upon health care services.

Phase I

Phase I studies usually involve small numbers of healthy subjects rather than those who have the disease or ailment that the new drug is intended to treat. An exception might be a study involving a very toxic drug used to treat a life-threatening illness. In this case the only study subjects might be those who already have the illness and for whom other viable treatment options may not be available. The purpose of phase I studies is to determine the optimal dosage range and the pharmacokinetics of the drug (i.e., absorption, distribution, metabolism, and excretion) and to ascertain if further testing is needed. Blood tests, urinalyses, assessments of vital signs, and specific monitoring tests are also performed.

Phase II

Phase II studies involve small numbers of volunteers who have the disease or ailment that the drug is designed to diagnose or treat. Study participants are closely monitored to determine the drug's effectiveness and identify any adverse effects. This is also the phase during which therapeutic dosage ranges are refined. If no serious adverse effects occur, the study can progress to phase III.

Phase III

Phase III studies involve large numbers of patients who are followed by medical research centers and other types of health care facilities. The patients may be treated at the center itself or may be spread over a wider geographic area and be followed at a local inpatient or outpatient facility. The purpose of this larger sample size is to provide information about infrequent or rare adverse effects that may not yet have been observed during previous smaller studies. Information obtained during this clinical phase helps identify any risks associated with the new drug. To enhance objectivity, many studies are designed to incorporate a placebo. A **placebo** is an inert substance that is not a drug (e.g., normal saline). The rationale for administering a placebo to a portion of the research subjects is to separate out the real benefits of the investigational drug from the apparent benefits arising out of researcher or subject **bias** regarding expected or desired results of the drug therapy. A study incorporating a placebo is called a *placebo-controlled study.* If the study subject does not know whether the drug he or she is administered is a placebo or the investigational drug, but the investigator does know, the study is referred to as a **blinded investigational drug study.** In most studies neither the research staff nor the subjects being tested know which subjects are being given the real drug and which are receiving the placebo. This further enhances the objectivity of the study results and is known as a **double-blind investigational drug study** because both the researcher and the subject are "blinded" to the actual identity of the substance administered to a given subject. Both drug and placebo dosage forms given to patients often look identical except for a secret code that appears on the medication itself and/or its container. At the completion of the study, this code is revealed or broken to determine which study patients received the drug and which were given the placebo. The code can also be broken before study completion by the principle investigator in the event of a clinical emergency that requires a determination of what substance individual patients received.

The three objectives of phase III studies are to establish the drug's clinical effectiveness, safety, and dosage range. After phase III is completed, the FDA receives a report from the manufacturer, at which time the drug company submits a new drug application (NDA). The approval of the application paves the way for the pharmaceutical company to market the new drug exclusively until the patent for the drug molecule expires. This is normally 17 years after discovery of the molecule and includes the 10- to 12-year period generally required to complete drug research. Therefore, a new drug manufacturer typically has 5 to 7 years after drug marketing to recoup research costs, which are usually in the hundreds of millions of dollars for a single drug.

Phase IV

Phase IV studies are postmarketing studies voluntarily conducted by pharmaceutical companies to obtain further proof of the therapeutic and adverse effects of the new drug. Data from such studies are usually gathered for at least 2 years after the drug's release. Often these studies compare the safety and efficacy of the new drug with that of another drug in the same therapeutic category. An example would be a comparison of a new nonsteroidal antiinflammatory drug with ibuprofen in the treatment of osteoarthritis. Some medications make it through all phases of clinical trials without causing any problems among study patients. When they are used in the larger general population, however, severe adverse effects may appear for the first time. If a pattern of severe reactions to a newly marketed drug begins to emerge, the FDA may request that the manufacturer of the drug issue a **black box warning** or a voluntary recall. A black box warning indicates that serious adverse effects have been reported with the drug. The drug can still be prescribed, however the prescriber must be aware of the potential risk (see Table 4-2). In the rare occasion if the drug manufacturer refuses to recall the medication, and if the number and/or severity of reactions reaches a certain level, then the FDA may seek court action to condemn the product and allow it to be seized by legal authorities. Such an action, in effect, becomes an involuntary recall on behalf of the manufacturer. There are three designated classes of drug recall based on FDA response to postmarketing data for a given drug:

- **Class I:** The most serious type of recall—use of the drug product carries a reasonable probability of serious adverse health effects or death.
- **Class II:** Less severe—use of the drug product may result in temporary or medically reversible health effects, but the probability of lasting major adverse health effects is low.
- **Class III:** Least severe—use of the drug product is not likely to result in any significant health problems.

Notification by the FDA of a drug recall or drug warnings may take the form of press releases, website announcements *(http://www.fda.gov)*, or letters to health professionals. Such FDA news items provide the latest information when a drug has newly identified hazards. The FDA has a voluntary program called MedWatch, where professionals are encouraged to report any adverse events seen with newly approved drugs. Information can be found at *www.fda.gov/medwatch.* Drug information of this kind is continually evolving as new events are observed and reported by clinicians and patients. However, recommended actions also change with time, and so clinicians should use the most current information available along with sound clinical judgment.

CULTURAL, LEGAL, AND ETHICAL CONSIDERATIONS FOR NURSING PRACTICE

Cultural Issues

Nurses need to be knowledgeable about drugs that may elicit varied responses in culturally diverse patients or those from different racial-ethnic groups. Varied responses may include differences in therapeutic dosages and adverse effects, so that some patients may have therapeutic responses at lower dosages than are typically recommended. Much of this information was previously discussed in the first section of this chapter, but a few examples are worthy of consideration. For example, in Hispanic individuals taking traditional antipsychotics, symptoms may be managed effectively at lower dosages than the usual recommended dosage range. African American patients taking lithium may need to be monitored more closely for symptoms of drug toxicity, because serum drug levels may be higher than in white patients given the same dosage. Likewise, Japanese and Taiwanese patients may require lower dosages of lithium. Another aspect of cultural care as it relates to drug therapy is the recognition that patterns of communication may differ based on patients' race or ethnicity.

Critical to the cultural care of patients is an understanding of various health beliefs, because these beliefs may vary greatly and may influence how patients respond to drug therapy. Significant differences in values, beliefs, and attitudes may affect a patient's adherence to the drug regimen, for example, (1) different cultures attach different symbolic meanings to medications and various drug therapies, and (2) the use of herbal remedies and alternative and complementary therapies may be common practice among various racial-ethnic groups and these may interfere with prescribed medications.

Some general nursing considerations include the following: (1) Develop good interpersonal skills in communicating with patients from various cultures and ask questions with due consideration of their racial-ethnic backgrounds. (2) Focus on specific aspects of patients' drug therapy rather than asking questions that are too broad or general. (3) Be informed about different communication patterns across cultures; for example, Chinese patients are known to rarely complain, and Asian patients are likely to express their problems in behavioral or somatic terms rather than in emotional terms. (4) Always consider the patient's cultural beliefs, attitudes, and values when administering medications and in patient education. (5) Identify any potential conflicts between medications and cultural beliefs and work with the patient and the health care team to help achieve optimal patient outcomes. (6) Identify any herbal, complementary, or alternative therapies as well as home remedies or folk medicine practices being used. (7) Be alert to the patient's response to medications, because a change in drug therapy may be warranted should un-

---

BOX 4-1   **Cultural Assessment Tools and Related Web Links**

- Several cultural assessment tools have been developed over the last decade. Madeline Leininger's Sunrise Model focuses on seven major areas of cultural assessment, including educational, economic, familial and social, political, technologic, religious and philosophic, and cultural values, beliefs, and practices.
- Other comprehensive cultural assessment tools include those developed by Andrews and Bowls, 1999; Friedman, Bowden, and Jones, 2003; Giger and Davidhizar, 1999; and Purnell and Paulanka, 1998. Rani Srivastava's (2006), found in *The Healthcare Professional's Guide to Clinical Cultural Competence* (Healthcare Professional's Guides), contains further discussion on how populations are viewed by health care workers and not through the use of ethno-cultural/religious labels.

CULTURAL IMPLICATIONS

Common Practices of Selected Cultural Groups

Cultural Group	Common Practices
African	Practice folk medicine; employ "root workers" as healers
Asian	Believe in traditional medicine; use physicians and herbalists in their health care
Hispanic	View health as a result of good luck and living right, and illness as a result of doing a bad deed; use heat and cold as remedies
European	Hold traditional health beliefs; some still practice folk medicine
Native American	Believe in harmony with nature; view ill spirits as causing disease
Western	Show increased participation in health care; demand more explanation about diseases and treatment, as well as the prevention of diseases

---

usual effects or other untoward reactions occur. See Box 4-1 and the Cultural Implications box on p. 56 as well as Table 4-1 for more information.

Legislative and Legal Issues

State and federal legislation dictate the boundaries within which professional nurses practice. First is the development of *standards of care and practice,* including the definition of the scope and role of the professional nurse. Guidelines of professional nursing groups and institutional policies and procedures also help identify the legal boundaries of nursing practice. For example, nursing standards of care include legal guidelines for minimally safe and adequate nursing practice and are defined in each state's nurse practice acts of the state board of nursing. Nurse practice acts further define the scope of nursing practice, indicate expanded nursing roles, identify the educational requirements for nurses, and distinguish between nursing practice and medical practice. In addition, state boards of nursing also define specific nursing practices such as rules concerning the administration of intravenous therapy. State and federal hospital licensing laws, professional and specialty organization standards, and the

---

LEGAL AND ETHICAL PRINCIPLES

Ethical Terms Related to Nursing Practice

Autonomy: Self-determination and the ability to act on one's own; related nursing actions include promoting a patient's decision making, supporting informed consent, and assisting in decisions or making a decision when a patient is posing harm to himself or herself.

Beneficence: The ethical principle of doing or actively promoting good; related nursing actions include determining how the patient is best served.

Confidentiality: The duty to respect privileged information about a patient; related nursing actions include not talking about a patient in public or outside the context of the health care setting.

Justice: The ethical principle of being fair or equal in one's actions; related nursing actions include ensuring fairness in distributing resources for the care of patients and determining when to treat.

Nonmaleficence: The duty to do no harm to a patient; related nursing actions include avoiding doing any deliberate harm while rendering nursing care.

Veracity: The duty to tell the truth; related nursing actions include telling the truth with regard to placebos, investigational new drugs, and informed consent.

---

written policies and procedures of the employing institution also address professional nursing standards of care. There is also case law or common law consisting of prior court rulings that affect professional nursing practice.

The American Nurses Association (ANA) has developed standards for nursing practice, policy statements, and similar resolutions (last updated in 2001). The standards describe the scope, function, and role of the nurse and establish clinical practice standards. The Joint Commission requires that accredited hospitals fulfill certain standards with regard to nursing practice. One such requirement is that these institutions must have written policies and procedures. These policies are usually quite specific and are contained in policy and procedure manuals found on most nursing units. For example, a policy and procedure will outline the steps to take when changing a dressing or administering a medication. The nurse must know the policies and procedures of his or her employing institution, because if the nurse is involved in a lawsuit, this is one of the standards by which the nurse will be measured. Nursing specialty organizations also define standards of care for nurses who are certified in specialty areas, such as oncology, surgical care, or critical care. Standards of care help to determine whether a nurse is acting appropriately when performing professional duties. It is critical to safe nursing practice to remain up to date on the ever-changing obligations and standards of practice and care. Current nursing literature remains an authoritative resource for information on new standards of care.

The legal-ethical dimensions of professional nursing care are also addressed in the legislation passed to amplify the guidelines contained in HIPAA (1996). Under these federal regulations (see p. 52), the privacy of patient information is protected, and standards are included for the handling of electronic data about patients. HIPAA also defines the rights and privileges of patients in order to protect privacy without diminishing access to quality health care. The assurance of privacy—even prior to establishment of the HIPAA guidelines—was based on the principle of respect of an individual's right to determine when, to what extent, and under what circumstances private information can be shared or withheld from others, including family members. In addition, confidentiality must be preserved; that is, the individual identities of patients or research study participants should not be linked to information they provide and should not be publicly divulged. HIPAA addresses the issues of confidentiality and privacy by prohibiting prescribers, nurses, and other health care providers from sharing with others any patient health care information, including laboratory results, diagnoses, and prognoses, without the patient's consent. Conflicting obligations arise when a patient wants to keep information away from insurance companies, and matters remain complicated and challenging in the era of improving technology and computerization of medical records. Health care facilities continue to work diligently; however, to adhere to HIPAA guidelines and use special access codes to limit who can access information in computerized documents and charts.

In summary, federal and state legislation, standards of care, and nurse practice acts provide the legal framework for safe nursing practice, including drug therapy and medication administration. Further, as discussed in Chapter 1, the standard "Six Rights" of medication administration are yet another measure for ensuring safety and adherence to laws necessary for protecting the patient. Other patient rights were also discussed in Chapter 1 that should become a part of the standards of practice of every licensed, registered nurse and every student studying the art and science of nursing.

Ethical Issues

Ethical nursing practice is based on fundamental principles such as beneficence, autonomy, justice, veracity, and confidentiality. The American Nurses Association *Code of Ethics for Nurses* (Box 4-2) and the International Council of Nurses *ICN Code of Ethics for Nurses* (Box 4-3) should be familiar frameworks of practice for all nurses and serve as ethical guidelines for nursing care. Adherence to these ethical principles and codes of ethics ensures that the nurse is acting on behalf of the patient and with the patient's best interests at heart. As a professional, the nurse has the responsibility to provide safe nursing care to patients regardless of the setting, person, group, community, or family involved. Although it is not within the nurse's realm of ethical and professional responsibility to impose his or her own values or standards on the patient, it *is* within the nurse's realm to provide information and to assist the patient in making decisions regarding health care.

The nurse also has the right to refuse to participate in any treatment or aspect of a patient's care that violates the nurse's personal ethical principles. However, this should be done without deserting the patient, and in some facilities the nurse may be transferred to another patient care assignment only if the transfer is approved by the nurse manager or nurse supervisor. The nurse must always remember, however, that the *Code of Ethics* and professional responsibility and accountability require the nurse to provide nonjudgmental nursing care from the start of the patient's treatment until the time of the patient's discharge. If transferring to a different assignment is not an option because of institutional policy and because of the increase in the acuteness of patients' conditions and the high patient-to-nurse workload, the nurse must always act in the best interest of the patient while remaining an objective patient

---

BOX 4-2 American Nurses Association *Code of Ethics for Nurses*

The American Nurses Association (ANA) *Code of Ethics for Nurses* was revised in 1985, and further revisions were made by the ANA House of Delegates in 2001. The *Code of Ethics* continues to serve as an integral part of the foundation of professional nursing and is applicable to contemporary nursing practice. The *Code* draws on a broad knowledge base of ethical principles and theories, humanist perspectives, and ethics of care.

***Provisions of the* Code**

- The nurse, in all professional relationships, practices with compassion and respect for the inherent dignity, worth, and uniqueness of every individual, unrestricted by considerations of social or economic status, personal attributes, or the nature of health problems.
- The nurse's primary commitment is to the patient, whether an individual, family group, or community.
- The nurse promotes, advocates for, and strives to protect the health, safety, and rights of the patient.
- The nurse is responsible and accountable for individual nursing practice and determines the appropriate delegation of tasks consistent with the nurse's obligation to provide optimum patient care.
- The nurse owes the same duty to self as to others, including the responsibility to preserve integrity and safety, to maintain competence, and to continue personal and professional growth.
- The nurse participates in establishing, maintaining, and improving health care environments and conditions of employment conducive to the provision of quality health care and consistent with the values of the profession through individual and collective action.
- The nurse participates in the advancement of the profession through contributions to practice, education, administration, and knowledge development.
- The nurse collaborates with other health professionals and the public in promoting community, national, and international efforts to meet health needs.
- The profession of nursing, as represented by associations and their members, is responsible for articulating nursing values, for maintaining the integrity of the profession and its practice, and for shaping social policy.

Reprinted with permission from American Nurses Association: *Code of ethics for nurses with interpretive statements,* copyright 2001, Nursebooks.org, Silver Spring, MD.

---

advocate. It is always the nurse's responsibility to provide the highest quality nursing care and to practice within the professional standards of care. The ANA *Code of Ethics for Nurses,* the *ICN Code of Ethics for Nurses,* nurse practice acts, federal and state codes, ethical principles, and the previously mentioned legal principles and legislation are readily accessible and provide nurses with a sound, rational framework for professional nursing practice.

Another area of ethical consideration related to drug therapy and the nursing process is the use of placebos. A placebo is a drug dosage form (e.g., tablet or capsule) without any pharmacologic activity due to a lack of active ingredients. However, there may be reported therapeutic responses, and placebos have been found to be beneficial in certain patients, such as those being treated for anxiety. Placebos are also administered frequently in experimental studies of new drugs to evaluate and measure the pharmacologic effects of a new medicine compared with those of an inert placebo. Except in new drug studies, however, placebo use is often considered to be unethical and deceitful, possibly creating mistrust among the nurse, the prescriber, and the patient. In current clinical practice guidelines for pain management, the American Pain Society and the Agency for Health Care Policy and Research recommend the avoidance of placebos, because their use is believed to be deceitful and to violate a patient's rights to the highest quality care possible. Many health care agencies limit the use of placebos to research only to avoid the possible deceit and mistrust. Should an order be received for a placebo for a patient, it is within the legal purview of a professional nurse to inquire about the order and to ask why a placebo is being prescribed; the order should never be taken lightly. Should administration of the placebo be part of a research study or clinical trial, the informed consent process should be thorough and the patient should be informed of his or her right to (1) leave the study at any time without any pressure or coercion to stay, (2) leave the study without consequences to medical care, (3) receive full and complete information about the study, and (4) be aware of all alternative options and receive information on all treatments, including placebo therapy, being administered in the study.

NURSING PROCESS

Assessment

A thorough cultural assessment is needed for the provision of culturally competent nursing care. A variety of assessment tools and resources are available for the professional nurse to incorporate into nursing care and are provided in Box 4-1. However, various factors must be assessed, and these are listed below along with specific questions about the patient's physical, mental, and spiritual health.

Maintaining Health

- *For physical health:* Where are special foods and clothing items purchased? What types of health education are of the patient's culture? Where does the patient usually obtain information about health and illness? Folklore? Where are health services obtained? Who are health care providers (e.g., physicians, nurse practitioners, community services organizations, health departments, healers)?
- *For mental health:* What are examples of culturally specific activities for the mind and for maintaining mental health, as well as beliefs about stress reduction, rest, and relaxation?
- *For spiritual health:* What are resources for meeting spiritual needs?

Protecting Health

- *For physical health:* Where are special clothing and everyday essentials? What are examples of the patient's symbolic clothing, if any?
- *For mental health:* Who within the family and community teaches the roles in the patient's specific culture? Are there rules about avoiding certain persons or places? Are there special activities that must be performed?
- *For spiritual health:* Who teaches spiritual practices and where can special protective symbolic objects such as crystals or amulets be purchased? Are they expensive and how available are they for the patient when needed?

Restoring Health

- *For physical health:* Where are special remedies purchased? Can individuals produce or grow their own remedies, herbs, etc.? How often are traditional and nontraditional services obtained?
- *For mental health:* Who are the traditional and nontraditional resources for mental health? Are there culture-specific activities for coping with stress and illness?
- *For spiritual health:* How often and where are traditional and nontraditional spiritual leaders or healers accessed? (Modified from Spector RE: *Cultural care: guides to heritage assessment and health traditions,* ed 2, Upper Saddle River, NJ, 2000, Pearson/Prentice Hall, pp 24-25.)

Nursing Diagnoses

- Risk for injury related to interruption of daily activities and cultural patterns of health and wellness
- Risk for injury related to decreased sensorium and confusion caused by unfamiliar hospital environment
- Insomnia related to a lack of adherence to cultural practices for encouraging stress release and sleep induction
- Risk for injury related to reactions to drug therapy and impact of cultural, racial, and/or ethnic factors on pharmacokinetics (ethnopharmacology)
- Deficient knowledge related to lack of experience with and information about drug therapy

Planning

Goals

- Patient states the need for assistance while in the hospital or while health status is altered.
- Patient requests assistance in implementing cultural practices.
- Patient states specific needs related to performance of activities of daily living (ADLs), relaxation, healing, sleep, or rest.
- Patient states the importance of racial, ethnic, and cultural influences on nonpharmacologic and pharmacologic treatment regimens.

Outcome Criteria

- Patient experiences minimal or no difficulty in obtaining assistance with special needs and ADLs.
- Patient identifies specific cultural practices such as use of herbal teas and other herbal preparations, yin and yang balancing, aromatherapy, crystal therapy, and healing bracelets that will help with healing during illness.
- Patient is able to implement cultural practices as an integral part of a holistic nursing care plan and treatment regimen.

Implementation

There are numerous interventions for implementation of culturally competent nursing care, but one very important requirement is that the nurse maintain up-to-date knowledge about various cultures and related activities and practices of daily living, health beliefs, and emotional and spiritual health practices and beliefs. With regard to drug therapy, the nurse's knowledge about drugs that may elicit varied responses in specific racial and ethnic groups must remain current, and critical thinking must be used in applying the concepts of culturally competent care and ethnopharmacology to each patient care situation. One important factor is the impact of enzymes, specifically cytochrome P-450 enzymes, on certain phases of drug metabolism of (see previous discussion on p. 25). Specific examples of differences in certain cytochrome P-450 enzymes can be found on p. 51. Additional factors to consider during implementation are lifestyle and health belief systems. For example, with regard to adherence with the treatment regimen, Hispanics with hypertension have been found in some studies to be less likely than African Americans or whites to continue to take medication as prescribed, a finding that may reflect the patients' health belief systems. Other lifestyle decisions (e.g., use of tobacco or alcohol) may also affect responses to drugs and must be considered during drug administration. In addition, a patient's cultural background and associated socioeconomic status may create a situation that leads the patient to skip pills, split doses, and not obtain refills. This culture of poverty may be a causative factor in noncompliance and requires astute attention and individualized nursing actions.

Evaluation

The impact of cultural, legal, and ethical factors on the therapeutic effects of drug therapy should be evaluated for the duration of therapy. Evaluation should also include monitoring to ensure that goals and outcome criteria are met as well as observation for therapeutic effects versus adverse and toxic effects.

CASE STUDY

Clinical Drug Trial

© Andrew Gentry

A patient on the telemetry unit has had a serious heart condition for years and has been through every known protocol for treatment. The cardiac physician has admitted him to a telemetry unit for observation during a trial of a new investigational drug. The patient exclaims, "I have high hopes for this drug. I've read about it on the Internet and the reports are wonderful. I can't wait to get better!"

1. How should the nurse answer this statement?

The cardiac physician meets with the patient and the nurse to explain the medication and how the double-blind experimental drug study will work. The purpose of the medication and potential hazards of the therapy are described, as well as the laboratory tests that will be performed to measure the drug's effectiveness. The physician then asks the nurse to have the patient sign the consent form. When the nurse goes to get the patient's signature, the patient says, "I'll sign it, but I really didn't understand what that doctor told me about the placebo."

2. Should the nurse continue with getting the consent form signed? Explain.

3. The patient tells the nurse, "How can I make sure I have the real drug and not the fake drug? I really want to see if it will help my situation." How should the nurse respond?

4. After a week, the patient tells the nurse, "I don't see that this drug is helping me. In fact, I feel worse. But I'm afraid to tell the doctor that I want to stop the medicine. What do I do?" What is the nurse's best response?

For answers, see *http://evolve.elsevier.com/Lilley*.

POINTS TO REMEMBER

- A variety of culturally based assessment tools are available for use in patient care and drug therapy.
- Drug therapy and subsequent patient responses may be affected by racial and ethnic variations in levels of specific enzymes and metabolic pathways of drugs.
- Various pieces of federal legislation, as well as state law, state practice acts, and institutional policies, have been established to help ensure the safety and efficacy of drug therapy and the nursing process.
- HIPAA guidelines have increased awareness concerning patient confidentiality and privacy. It is important to understand this federal legislation as it relates to drug therapy and the nursing process.
- The Controlled Substance Act of 1970 provides nurses and other health care providers with information on drugs that cause little

Continued

POINTS TO REMEMBER—cont'd

to no dependence versus those associated with a high level of abuse and dependency.

- Informed consent should always be obtained as needed, and nurses must thoroughly understand their role and responsibilities as patient advocate in obtaining such consent.
- The nurse's role in the IND research process should be one of adhering to the study protocol while also acting as a patient advocate and honoring the patient's right to safe, quality nursing care.

- Adherence to legal guidelines, ethical principles, and the ANA *Code of Ethics for Nurses* ensures that the nurse's actions are based on a solid foundation.
- Placebo use remains controversial, and if a placebo is ordered the prescriber should be questioned about the specific cause for its use.

NCLEX EXAMINATION REVIEW QUESTIONS

1 A patient is undergoing major surgery and asks the nurse about a living will. He states, "I don't want anybody making decisions for me. And I don't want to prolong my life." The patient is demonstrating
   a autonomy.
   b beneficence.
   c justice.
   d veracity.

2 When caring for an elderly Chinese patient, the nurse recognizes that which of the following cultural issues may influence the care of this patient?
   a Radiographs are seen as a break in the soul's integrity.
   b Hospital diets are interpreted as being healing and healthful.
   c The use of heat may be an important practice for this patient.
   d Being hospitalized is a source of peace and socialization for this culture.

3 A patient is being counseled for possible participation in a clinical trial for a new medication. After the patient meets with the physician, the nurse is asked to obtain the patient's signature on the consent forms. The nurse knows that this "informed consent" indicates which of the following?
   a Once therapy has begun, the patient cannot withdraw from the clinical trial.
   b The patient has been informed of all potential hazards and benefits of the therapy.
   c The patient has received only the information that will help to make the clinical trial a success.
   d No matter what happens, the patient will not be able to sue the researchers for damages.

4 A new drug has been approved for use and the drug manufacturer has made it available for sale. During the first 6 months, the FDA receives reports of severe adverse effects that were not discovered during the testing and considers whether to withdraw the drug. This illustrates which phase of investigational drug studies?
   a Phase I
   b Phase II
   c Phase III
   d Phase IV

5 A patient of Japanese descent describes a family trait that manifests frequently: she says that members of her family often have "strong reactions" after taking certain medications, but her white friends have no problems with the same dosages of the same drugs. The nurse recognizes that, because of this trait, which statement applies?
   a She may need lower dosages of the medications prescribed.
   b She may need higher dosages of the medications prescribed.
   c She should not receive these medications because of potential problems with metabolism.
   d These situations vary greatly, and her accounts may not indicate a valid cause for concern.

6 When evaluating polymorphism and medication administration, the nurse considers which factors? (Select all that apply.)
   a Nutritional status
   b Drug route
   c Patient's ethnicity
   d Cultural beliefs
   e Patient's age

1.a, 2.c, 3.b, 4.d, 5.a, 6.a, c, d, e.

CRITICAL THINKING ACTIVITIES: BEST ACTION

1 During a busy shift, the nurse is called to the phone to speak to a family member of Mrs. H., who was admitted with pneumonia. The caller states, "I'm her grandson, and I want to know if that pneumonia she has is that very contagious bug that's going around hospitals. Is she going to die?" What guidelines should the nurse follow when giving a response?

2 The nurse is assessing a newly admitted 85-year-old woman. During the assessment, the nurse finds that the patient is wearing a copper ring around her left ankle. The ankle is swollen, with grade 3+ edema, and the copper ring is actually cutting into the skin. What is the best action for the nurse to take at this time?

3 Interview someone who is not in your racial or ethnic group about cultural practices and drug therapy, using the suggestions given on p. 55. Compare their practices with those of your family.

For answers, see *http://evolve.elsevier.com/Lilley*.

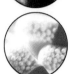

CHAPTER 5

Gene Therapy and Pharmacogenetics

OBJECTIVES

When you reach the end of this chapter, you should be able to do the following:

1 Understand the basic terms related to genetics and drug therapy.
2 Briefly discuss the major concepts of genetics as an evolving segment of health care, such as principles of genetic inheritance; deoxyribonucleic acid (DNA), ribonucleic acid (RNA), and their functioning; the relationship of DNA to protein synthesis; and the importance of amino acids.
3 Describe the basis of the Human Genome Project and its impact on the role of genetics in health care.
4 Discuss the different gene therapies currently available.
5 Differentiate between direct and indirect forms of gene therapy.
6 Identify the regulatory and ethical issues related to gene therapy as related to nursing and health care professionals.
7 Briefly discuss pharmacogenomics and pharmacogenetics.
8 Discuss the evolving role of professional nurses as related to gene therapy.

e-Learning Activities

http://evolve.elsevier.com/Lilley

NCLEX Review Questions • Animations • Nursing Care Plans • Audio Glossary • Category Catchers • Medication Errors Checklists • IV Therapy Checklists • Calculators • Frequently Asked Questions • Content Updates • Supplemental Resources • Answers to Case Studies and Critical Thinking Activities

Glossary

Acquired disease Any disease triggered by external factors and not *directly* caused by a person's genes (e.g., an infectious disease, noncongenital cardiovascular diseases). (p. 62)

Alleles The two or more alternative forms of a gene that can occupy a specific locus (location) on a chromosome (see *chromosomes*). (p. 62)

Chromatin A collective term for all of the chromosomal material within a given cell. (p. 63)

Chromosomes Structures in the nuclei of cells that contain linear threads of deoxyribonucleic acid (DNA), which transmits genetic information, and are associated with ribonucleic acid (RNA) molecules and synthesis of protein molecules. (p. 62)

Gene The biologic unit of *heredity;* a segment of a DNA molecule that contains all of the molecular information required for the synthesis of a biologic product such as an RNA molecule or an amino acid chain (protein molecule). (p. 62)

Gene therapy New therapeutic technologies that directly target human genes in the treatment or prevention of illness. (p. 64)

Genetic disease Any disorder caused directly by a genetic mechanism. (p. 62)

Genetic material DNA or RNA molecules or portions thereof. (p. 62)

Genetic polymorphisms (PMs) Allele variants that occur in the chromosomes of 1% or more of the general population (i.e., they occur too frequently to be caused by a random recurrent mutation). (p. 65)

Genetic predisposition The presence of certain factors in a person's genetic makeup, or *genome* (see below), that increase the individual's likelihood of eventually developing one or more diseases. (p. 62)

Genetics The study of the structure, function, and inheritance of genes. (p. 62)

Genome The complete set of genetic material of any organism. It may be contained in multiple chromosomes (groups of DNA or RNA molecules) in higher organisms; in a single chromosome, as in bacteria; or in a single DNA or RNA molecule, as in viruses. (p. 63)

Genomics The study of the structure and function of the genome, including DNA *sequencing, mapping,* and *expression,* and the way genes and their products work in both health and disease. (p. 63)

Genotype The particular alleles present at a given site (locus) on the chromosomes of an organism (e.g., human, animal, plant) that determine a specific genetic trait for that organism (compare *phenotype*). (p. 62)

Heredity The characteristics and qualities that are genetically passed from one generation to the next through reproduction. (p. 62)

Human Genome Project (HGP) A scientific project of the U.S. Department of Energy and National Institutes of Health to describe in detail the entire genome of a human being. (p. 63)

Inherited diseases Genetic diseases that result from defective alleles passed from parents to offspring. (p. 62)

Nucleic acids Molecules of DNA and RNA in the nucleus of every cell. DNA makes up the chromosomes and encodes the genes. (p. 62)

Personalized medicine The use of tools such as molecular and genetic characterizations of both disease processes and the patient for the customization of drug therapy. (p. 65)

Pharmacogenetics A general term for the study of the genetic basis for variations in the body's response to drugs, with a focus on variations related to a single gene. (p. 65)

Pharmacogenomics A branch of *pharmacogenetics* (see earlier) that involves the survey of the entire genome to detect multigenic (multiple-gene) determinants of drug response. (p. 65)

Phenotype The expression in the body of a genetic trait that results from a person's particular *genotype* (see earlier) for that trait. (p. 62)

Proteome The entire set of proteins produced from the information encoded in an organism's genome. (p. 63)

Proteomics The detailed study of the proteome, including all biologic actions of proteins. (p. 63)

Recombinant DNA (rDNA) DNA molecules that have been artificially synthesized or modified in a laboratory setting. (p. 64)

• • •

Genetic processes are a highly complex part of physiology and are far from completely understood by scientists. However, genetic research is one of the most active branches of science today, involving many types of health care professionals, including nurses. Expected outcomes of this research include an increasingly deeper knowledge of the genetic influences on disease, along with the development of gene-based therapies. The practice of nursing will also increasingly require an understanding of genetic concepts as well as genetically related health issues and therapeutic techniques. The goal of this chapter is to introduce some of the major concepts in this very complex and emerging branch of health science. In 1996, the *National Coalition for Health Professional Education in Genetics (NCHPEG)* was founded as a joint project of the American Medical Association, the American Nurses Association, and the National Human Genome Research Institute *(http://www.nchpeg.org)*. The purpose of NCHPEG is to promote the education of health professionals and the public regarding advances in applied genetics.

Since the 1960s, published clinical literature has described the role of nursing in genetics and genetic research. The Genetics Nursing Network was formed in 1984 and later became the International Society of Nurses in Genetics (ISONG). In 1997, the American Nurses Association designated genetics nursing as an official nursing specialty. In 2001, ISONG approved formation of the Genetic Nursing Credentialing Commission (GNCC), which has since certified the first genetic clinical nurses. The growing understanding of genetics is quickly creating demand for clinicians in all fields who can educate patients and provide clinical care that tailors health care services to each patient's inherent genetic constitution. This reality also calls for increasing the level of genetics education in nursing school curricula as well as continuing nursing education. Interestingly, the study of genetics has already become commonplace in secondary and even primary education.

BASIC PRINCIPLES OF GENETIC INHERITANCE

Nucleic acids are biochemical compounds consisting of two types of molecules: *deoxyribonucleic acid (DNA)* and *ribonucleic acid (RNA)*. DNA molecules make up the **genetic material** that is passed between all types of organisms during reproduction. In some

viruses (e.g., human immunodeficiency virus), it is actually RNA molecules that pass the virus's genetic material between generations; however, this is an exception to the norm. A chromosome is essentially a long strand of DNA that is contained in the nuclei of cells. DNA molecules, in turn, act as the template for the formation of RNA molecules, from which proteins are made. Humans normally have 23 pairs of **chromosomes** in each of their *somatic cells.* Somatic cells are all the cells in the body other than the *sex cells* (sperm cells or egg cells), which have only 23 single (unpaired) chromosomes. One pair of chromosomes in each cell are termed the *sex chromosomes,* which can be designated as either X or Y. The sex chromosomes are normally XX for females and XY for males. One member of each pair of chromosomes in somatic cells comes from the father's sperm and one from the mother's egg. **Alleles** are the alternative forms of a **gene** that can vary with regard to a specific genetic trait. Genetic traits can be desirable (e.g., lack of allergies) or undesirable (e.g., predisposition toward a specific disease). Each person has two alleles for every gene-coded trait: one allele from the mother, the other from the father. An allele may be dominant or recessive for a given genetic trait. The particular combination of alleles, or **genotype,** for a given trait normally determines whether or not a person manifests that trait, or the person's **phenotype.** Genetic traits that are passed on differently to male and female offspring are said to be *sex-linked traits* because they are carried on either the X or Y chromosome. For example, hemophilia genes are carried by females but manifest as a bleeding disorder only in males. Hemophilia is an example of an **inherited disease;** that is, a disease caused by passage of a genetic defect from parents to offspring. A more general term is **genetic disease,** which is any disease caused by a genetic mechanism. Note, however, that not all genetic diseases are inherited diseases, because chromosomal abnormalities *(aberrations)* can also occur spontaneously during embryonic development. In contrast, an **acquired disease** is any disease that develops in response to external factors and is not *directly* related to a person's genetic makeup. Genetics can play an indirect role in acquired disease, however. For example, atherosclerotic heart disease is often acquired in mid or later life. Many people have certain genes in their cells that increase the likelihood of this condition. This is known as a **genetic predisposition.** In some cases, as for this example, a person may be able to offset his or her genetic predisposition by lifestyle choices, such as consuming a healthy diet and exercising to avoid developing heart disease.

Current literature differentiates "old genetics," which focused on single-gene inherited diseases such as hemophilia, from the "new genetics." This new genetic perspective recognizes that common diseases, including Alzheimer's disease, cancer, and heart disease, are the product of complex relationships between genetic and environmental factors. These environmental factors, such as diet or toxic exposures, can initiate or worsen disease processes. New research into disease treatment is beginning to look at genetically tailored therapy.

DISCOVERY, STRUCTURE, AND FUNCTION OF DNA

Genetics is the study of the structure, function, and inheritance of genes, whereas **heredity** refers to the qualities that are genetically transferred from one generation to the next during reproduction. A major turning point in the current understanding of genetics came in 1953, when Drs. James Watson and Francis Crick first reported the chemical structures of human genetic material and named the primary biochemical compound *deoxyribonucleic acid.* They later received a Nobel Prize for their discovery.

It is now recognized that DNA is the primary molecule in the body that serves to transfer genes from parents to offspring. It exists in the nucleus of all body cells as strands in chromosomes, collectively called **chromatin.** As described in Chapter 40, DNA molecules contain four different organic bases, each of which has its own alphabetical designation: *adenine (A), guanine (G), thymine (T),* and *cytosine (C).* These bases are linked to a type of sugar molecule known as *deoxyribose.* In turn, these sugar molecules are linked to a "backbone" chain of phosphate molecules, which results in the classic *double-helix* structure of two side-by-side, spiral macromolecular chains. An important related biomolecule is RNA. RNA has a chemical structure similar to that of DNA, except that its sugar molecule is the compound *ribose* instead of deoxyribose and it contains the base *uracil (U)* in place of thymine. RNA more commonly occurs as a single-stranded molecule, although in some genetic processes it can also be double-stranded. In double-stranded nucleic acid structures, the base of each strand binds (via hydrogen bonds) to that of the other strand in the space between the two strands. This binding is based on complementary base pairings determined by the chemistry of the base molecules themselves. Specifically, adenine can only bind with guanine, whereas cytosine can only bind with thymine or uracil.

A *nucleotide* is the structural unit of DNA and consists of a single base and its attached sugar and phosphate molecules. A *nucleoside* is the base and attached sugar without the phosphate molecule. A relatively small sequence of nucleotides is called an *oligonucleotide* (the prefix *oligo-* means "a small number"). Certain new drug therapies involve several synthetic analogues of both nucleosides and nucleotides (see Chapters 40, 47, 48, and 49). A related field is targeted drug therapy. Targeted drug therapy currently focuses on modifying the function of immune system cells (*T cells* and *B cells*) and biochemical mediators of immune response *(cytokines).* However, it is expected to focus on modifying specific genes as well. Current examples of targeted drug therapy are presented in Chapters 45, 46, 47, and 48. One of these drugs, the ophthalmic antiviral drug fomivirsen, is an oligonucleotide with a chemical structure that is *opposite* (complementary) to that of a critical part of the messenger RNA (mRNA) of the cytomegalovirus. For this reason it is called an *antisense oligonucleotide,* and it is the first of this new class of drugs. Other types of antisense oligonucleotide drugs are anticipated in the near future as one type of gene therapy but are not yet available in the United States as of this writing. An organism's entire DNA structure is its **genome.** This word is a combination of the terms *gene* and *chromosome,* and it refers to all the genes in an organism taken together. **Genomics** is the relatively new science of determining the location *(mapping),* structure (DNA base *sequencing*), identification *(genotyping),* and expression *(phenotyping)* of individual genes along the entire genome, and determining their function in both health and disease processes.

Protein Synthesis

Protein molecules drive the functioning of all biochemical reactions in living organisms. Protein synthesis is the primary function of DNA in human cells. There is a direct relationship between DNA nucleotide sequence and corresponding amino acid sequences. This allows for precision in protein synthesis. Interestingly, it is estimated that only 2% to 3% of the human genome is involved in protein synthesis. Amino acid sequences control the *shape* of protein molecules, which ultimately affects their ability to function in the body. *Mutations,* undesired changes in DNA sequence, can ultimately affect the shape of protein molecules and impair or destroy their functioning.

In the cell nuclei, the double strands of DNA uncoil and separate, and a strand of mRNA forms on each separate DNA strand through complementary base pairing as described earlier. This process is called *transcription* of the DNA. These mRNA molecules then detach from their corresponding DNA strands, leave the cell nucleus, and enter the cytoplasm, where they are then "read," or *translated,* by the *ribosomes.* Ribosomes are composed of a second type of RNA, known as *ribosomal RNA (rRNA),* as well as several accessory proteins. Individual sequences of three bases at a time along the mRNA molecule serve to code for specific amino acid molecules. This translation process involves molecules of a third type of RNA, *transfer RNA* (tRNA). The tRNA molecules transport the corresponding amino acid molecules to the site of ribosomal translation along the mRNA strand in sequence according to the three-base codes along the mRNA strand. This in turn results in the creation of chains of multiple amino acids *(polypeptide chains),* which are known as protein molecules. The specificity of this *genetic code* is very important for proper protein synthesis, and the process is similar for all living organisms—plant and animal.

There are countless specific amino acid sequences (polypeptides) that result in the synthesis of many thousands of types of protein molecules. Proteins include hormones, enzymes, immunoglobulins, and numerous other biochemical molecules that regulate processes throughout the body. They are involved in both healthy (normal) physiologic processes and the pathophysiologic processes of many diseases. The biomedical literature continues to identify and describe many proteins that are part of disease processes. Manipulation of genetic material, as in *gene therapy* (see later), can theoretically modify the synthesis of these proteins and therefore aid in the treatment of disease. This emerging science continues to give rise to novel terminology. The entire set of proteins produced by a genome is now known as the **proteome. Proteomics** is the newest genetic science, taking the discovery process one step further than genomics. It is the study of the proteome, including protein expression, modification, localization, and function, as well as the protein-protein interactions that are part of biologic processes. This science is expected to provide new drug therapies in the future. Furthermore, most contemporary clinically approved drugs interact with body proteins such as cell membrane receptors, hormones, and enzymes.

Human Genome Project

In 1990, an unprecedented genetic research project began in the United States, the **Human Genome Project (HGP).** It was coordinated by the U.S. Department of Energy and the National Institutes of Health (NIH). The project was completed in 2003, two years ahead of schedule. The goals of this project were to identify the estimated 30,000 genes and 3 billion base pairs in the DNA of an entire human genome. Additional goals included developing new tools for genetic data analysis and storage, transferring newly developed technologies to the private sector, and addressing the inherent ethical, legal, and social issues involved in genetic research and clinical practice. However, the ultimate goal of this research is to develop improved prevention, treatment, and cures for disease. When the HGP began, there were 100 known human disease-related genes. By its completion there were 1400.

GENE THERAPY

Background

One result of the work of the HGP is the continued development of various types of **gene therapy.** This therapy involves the treatment or prevention of disease by transferring *exogenous* (foreign) genetic material (DNA or RNA) into the body of an individual. The main driving force of gene therapy research is the ongoing discovery of new details regarding cellular processes, including biochemical processes that occur at the molecular level. In addition, the increased understanding of *allelic variation* and its role in disease susceptibility can be used to guide attempts at preventive therapy based on a person's genotypic risk factors.

Although hundreds of gene therapy clinical trials have been approved by the U.S. Food and Drug Administration (FDA), no gene therapy to date has been approved for routine treatment of disease. The general goal of gene therapy is to transfer to the patient exogenous genes that will either provide a temporary substitute for, or initiate permanent changes in, the patient's own genetic functioning to treat a given disease. Originally projected to provide treatment primarily for inherited genetic diseases, gene therapy techniques are now being researched for treatment of acquired illnesses such as cancer, cardiovascular diseases, diabetes, infectious diseases, and substance abuse. In the more distant future *in utero* gene therapy may be used to prevent the development of serious diseases as part of prenatal care for the unborn infant.

Description

During gene therapy segments of DNA are usually injected into the patient's body in a process called *gene transfer.* These artificially produced DNA *splices* are also known as **recombinant DNA (rDNA)** and must usually be inserted into some kind of carrier or *vector* for the gene transfer process. Vectors currently being evaluated by researchers include spherical lipid compounds known as *liposomes,* free DNA splices known as *plasmids,* DNA *conjugates* in which DNA splices are linked (conjugated) to either protein or gold particles, and various types of viruses. Viruses are the most widely studied rDNA vectors thus far. One commonly used group of viruses are the *adenoviruses,* which include the human influenza (flu) viruses. If the desired rDNA segment can be inserted into the viral genome, the virus can then be injected into the patient to therapeutically infect human cells. If this planned infectious process is successful, the viral genome will be combined with the human host cell genome, and specific proteins will be produced to counter a disease process. Ideally, this would result in a permanent positive physiologic change in the host.

Limitations

Viruses used for gene transfer can also induce viral disease and can be immunogenic in the human host. The proteins produced by artificial methods can also be immunogenic. Even in the ab-

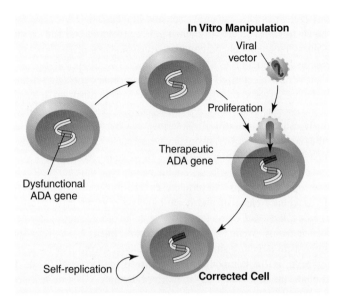

FIGURE 5-1 Gene therapy for adenosine deaminase (ADA) deficiency attempts to correct this immunodeficiency state. The viral vector containing the therapeutic gene is inserted into the patient's lymphocytes. These cells can then make the ADA enzyme. (From Lewis SM et al: *Medical-surgical nursing: assessment and management of clinical problems,* ed 7, St Louis, 2007, Mosby.)

sence of significant virus-induced disease, the positive effects (e.g., supplemented protein synthesis) may only be temporary, and therefore further treatments may be required. As a result, viruses must be carefully chosen and modified in an effort to optimize therapeutic effects while minimizing undesirable adverse effects. The determination of an ideal gene transfer method remains a major challenge for gene therapy researchers. Figure 5-1 provides a clinical example of the potential use of gene therapy.

Current Application

One indirect form of gene therapy is already well established. It involves the use of rDNA vectors in the laboratory to make recombinant forms of drugs, especially biologic drugs such as hormones, vaccines, antitoxins, and monoclonal antibodies (discussed in previous chapters). One of the most common examples is the use of the *Escherichia coli* bacterial genome to manufacture a recombinant form of human insulin. When the human insulin gene is inserted into the genome of the bacterial cells, the resulting culture artificially generates human insulin on a large scale. Although this insulin must be isolated and purified from its bacterial culture source, the majority of the world's medical insulin supply has been produced by this method for well over a decade.

Regulatory and Ethical Issues Regarding Gene Therapy

Gene therapy research is inherently complex, and this therapy can also carry great risks for its recipients. Thus, the issue of patient safety becomes significant. Research subjects who receive gene therapy often have a life-threatening illness, such as cancer, which may justify the risks involved. However, case reports of patient deaths in gene therapy trials have underscored these risks and raised the awareness of patient safety among researchers. In the 1980s the NIH Recombinant DNA Advisory Committee was assigned responsibility for oversight of gene therapy research in the United States. It reviews clinical trials involving human gene transfer and schedules public forums to discuss pertinent issues. The FDA must also review and approve all human clinical gene therapy trials, as it does for any type of drug therapy.

Any institution that conducts any type of research involving human subjects must have an *institutional review board,* whose purpose is to protect research subjects from unnecessary risks. Also required for institutions engaging in gene therapy research is an *institutional biosafety committee.* The role of this committee is to ensure compliance with the *NIH Guidelines for Research Involving Recombinant DNA Molecules.*

Another major ethical issue related to gene therapy techniques is that of *eugenics.* Eugenics is the intentional selection before birth of genotypes that are considered more desirable than others. For similar reasons, the prospect of being able to manipulate genes in human *germ cells* (sperm and eggs), even at a preembryonic stage, is also cited as a potential ethical hazard of gene therapy experimentation. Theoretically, even cosmetic modifications could be attempted by using such techniques as a part of routine family planning. Because of ethical concerns such as these, U.S. gene therapy research is limited to somatic cells only. Gene therapy in *germ-line* (reproductive) cells is currently illegal in the United States. This limitation remains despite arguments from those who believe that human germ-cell research could potentially yield cures for many serious chronic illnesses and disabilities, such as Parkinson's disease and spinal paralysis.

PHARMACOGENETICS AND PHARMACOGENOMICS

Pharmacogenetics is the most general term for the study of genetic variations in drug response and focuses on *single-gene* variations. A related science that pertains more directly to the HGP is **pharmacogenomics.** This is a newer branch of pharmacogenetics and involves working with the entire genome to determine multiple individual genetic factors that influence a person's response to specific medications. For example, a given patient may be more likely to benefit from, or suffer toxicity from, a certain type of drug therapy, depending on the presence or absence of specific alleles in his or her genome. Both of these disciplines, along with *proteomics,* described earlier, mark the most rapidly expanding areas of pharmacology and focus on how genes and proteins account for variations in drug responses among individuals or groups. The ultimate goal of these sciences is to predict patient drug response and proactively tailor drug selection and dosages for optimal treatment outcomes.

Individual differences in alleles that occur in at least 1% of a population are known as **genetic polymorphisms (PMs).** The word *polymorphism* literally means "many forms." Polymorphisms are considered to be too frequent to result from random genetic mutations. Polymorphisms that alter the amount or functioning of drug-metabolizing enzymes can alter the body's reactions to medications. Known examples include PMs that affect the metabolism of certain antimalarial drugs, the antituberculosis drug isoniazid, and the variety of drugs that are metabolized by the several subtypes of cytochrome (CYP) enzymes. They can also alter the functioning of *drug receptor* proteins, cell membrane *ion channels* and drug *transport proteins,* and intracellular *second messenger* proteins (which carry out drug actions after a drug molecule binds to a cell membrane receptor).

Differences in CYP enzymes are the best studied PM effects thus far. Depending on their existing genes for these enzymes, patients can be genetically classified as "poor" or "rapid" metabolizers of CYP-metabolized drugs such as warfarin, phenytoin, codeine, and quinidine. Dosages could then theoretically be adjusted accordingly, although this is not yet current widespread clinical practice. With warfarin and phenytoin, an ultrarapid metabolizer may need a higher dose of medication for the same effect, whereas a lower dose may be best for a poor metabolizer. With codeine, however, a counterintuitive dosing regimen may be better. A poor metabolizer may actually need a higher dose to get the same analgesic effect that occurs when codeine is metabolized to morphine in the body. In contrast, a rapid metabolizer may convert codeine to morphine too quickly, resulting in oversedation, and therefore, a lower dose may be sufficient. A similar situation is also likely to occur with quinidine. Because CYP enzymes are known to vary among racial and ethnic groups, the principle of "cultural safety" becomes one of the imperatives for routine gene-based drug dosing.

Studying both the genome of the patient and the presenting genetic features of the pathology (e.g., tumor cells, infectious organisms) before treatment could also allow for customized drug selection and dosing. Such analysis could permit the avoidance of drugs less likely to be effective as well as optimization of drug dosages to minimize the risk of adverse drug effects for a given patient. These applications of pharmacogenomics are examples of **personalized medicine.**

DNA Microarray Technology

Most drug dosage changes are still usually made on a trial-and-error basis by monitoring patient response. Researchers have already developed an analytical tool known as a *high-density microarray.* This technology applies methods used in computer chip manufacture to design tiny microchip plates that contain thousands of microscopic DNA samples. A patient's blood can then be screened for thousands of corresponding DNA sequences that bind from the patient's blood sample to the sequences on the chip. This allows determination of the presence or absence of various genes, such as those related to drug metabolism. For example, the long-recognized enzymes in the CYP system help metabolize from 25% to 30% of currently available drugs. Over 40 specific CYP genes have been identified thus far. In December 2004, the FDA approved the first DNA microchip for clinical use—the AmpliChip Microarray. It is used to screen blood samples for the individual's CYP enzyme profile. It is believed that within 5 years, all new drugs will have a target gene sequence in the public domain. Although this type of genotypic profiling is not yet practical for widespread use, it will eventually become a standard in clinical practice.

Table 5-1 lists several other examples of current clinical applications of pharmacogenomics.

TABLE 5-1 Clinical Applications of Pharmacogenomics

Genetic Technique	Application
Genotyping for the presence of CYP2D6 isoenzyme and for the CYP2D6 alleles determining whether patients are poor, intermediate, extensive, or ultrarapid metabolizers related to these enzymes (under study)	*Psychiatry* and *general medicine:* Helps guide prescribing of selected medications such as anticoagulants, immunosuppressants, antidepressants, antipsychotics, mood stabilizers, anticonvulsants, beta-blockers, and antidysrhythmics
Genotyping for the presence of the *p-glycoprotein* drug transport protein (under study)	*Cardiology, infectious diseases, oncology,* and other practice areas: Assists in drug selection and dosing for drugs such as digoxin, antiretrovirals, and antineoplastics
Genotyping for the presence of thiopurine methyltransferase enzyme	*Oncology:* Used to temper toxicity through more careful dosing of the cancer drug 6-mercaptopurine in pediatric leukemia patients
Genotyping for variations in beta-adrenergic receptors (under study)	*Pulmonology:* Determines which asthma patients are more or less responsive to beta-agonist therapy (e.g., albuterol) and which patients might benefit from other types of drug therapy
Genotyping for the presence of the Philadelphia chromosome	*Oncology:* Identifies those patients with chronic myelogenous leukemia who may be stronger candidates for therapy with the cancer drug imatinib (Gleevec)
Genotyping for the presence of the *HER2/neu* protooncogene	*Oncology:* Identifies a subset of breast cancer patients whose tumors express this gene, which indicates their suitability for treatment with the cancer drug trastuzumab (Herceptin)
Viral genotyping of hepatitis C viruses (under study)	*Infectious diseases:* Can determine whether a particular infection warrants 26 versus 48 weeks of drug therapy (thereby reducing both costs and adverse drug effects)
Genotyping for the presence of *factor V* gene mutation	*Women's health:* Identifies women with a 7 to 100 times greater risk of thrombosis with oral contraceptive use compared to women without the mutation
Muscle biopsy test for patients with a family history of *malignant hyperthermia*	*Surgery:* Assesses patients risk of this adverse effect known to occur with administration of various inhalation anesthetics and intraoperative paralyzing drugs
Genotyping for the presence of sodium channels associated with renin-angiotensin receptors and adrenal gland receptors	*Cardiology:* Allows refined antihypertensive drug selection
Race-based drug selection	*Cardiology:* Indicates use of the drug isosorbide dinitrate/hydralazine (BiDil) for treatment of hypertension in African American patients due ultimately to genotypic variations in this patient population

CYP2D6, Cytochrome P-450 enzyme subtype 2D6; *HER2/neu,* human epidermal growth factor receptor 2.

APPLICATION OF GENETIC PRINCIPLES RELATED TO DRUG THERAPY AND THE NURSING PROCESS

As noted previously, the recognition that genetic factors contribute, at some level, to most diseases continues to grow. Thus, nursing care delivery will routinely be affected by genetic influences on health, including the interaction of genetic and environmental (nongenetic) factors. In general, it is expected that in the next few years genetic research will move from the laboratory to clinical practice.

Nurses in general practice settings will not be expected to perform in-depth genetic testing or counseling. Nurses—or other health care providers—with specialty certification in the field of genetics will conduct genetic testing and counseling. However, all nurses will need to have a working knowledge of relevant genetic principles. In this era of the "new genetics" paradigm, nurses are fully aware of the fact that nearly all diseases have a genetic component. Conditions such as myocardial infarction, cancer, mental illness, diabetes, and Alzheimer's disease are now viewed in a different light because of the known complex interactions between a number of factors, including the influence of one or more genes and a variety of environmental exposures for patients.

There are several other applicable skills regarding genetics for nurses in general practice settings. Assessment is the first step of the nursing process, and during the assessment the nurse may uncover factors that may point to a risk for genetic disorders. During the initial assessment, the nurse obtains a patient's personal and family history. The family history should cover at least three generations and include the current and past health status of each family member. In addition, the nurse should assess for factors that may indicate a risk for genetic disorders. A few examples of such factors are a higher incidence of a particular disease or disorder in the patient's family than in the general population; diagnosis of a disease in family members at an unusually young age; diagnosis of a family member with an unusual form of cancer or with more than one type of cancer.

The nurse should ask about any unusual reactions to a drug—on the part of both the patient and family members. An unusual or other than expected reaction to a drug in family members may point to a difference in the patient's ability to metabolize certain drugs. As indicated earlier in this chapter (as well as in Chapter 2), genetic factors may alter a patient's metabolism of a particular drug, resulting in either increased or decreased drug action. Each and every time a medication is administered, the patient's response to that drug should be assessed. Any unusual medication responses in a patient may point to a need for further investigation. Once a genetic variation is known, drug therapy may be adjusted accordingly.

As DNA chip technology becomes more affordable and accessible, it will be possible for patients to know in advance their relative risks for different diseases in later life. Genotype testing to identify a patient's drug-metabolizing enzymes will help prescribers better predict a patient's response to drug therapy.

Teaching about genetic testing and counseling may be another responsibility of the nurse. Patients will have questions and concerns about genetic testing and other issues. Nurses in general practice are not experts in genetic issues. However, the nurse may help with suggestions about genetic counseling if appropriate. If genetic testing is ordered, the nurse may be a part of the testing process and will need to ensure that the informed decision-making and consent procedure has been carried out correctly.

Maintaining privacy and confidentiality is of utmost importance during genetic testing and counseling. The patient is the one who decides whether to include or exclude any family members from the discussion and from knowledge of the results of genetic testing. The patient should be reminded that he or she is not required to undergo the genetic test and that the patient has the right to disclose or withhold test results from anyone. Nurses must protect against improper disclosure of information to other family members, friends of the family, other health care providers, and insurance providers. Nurses share the responsibility with other health care providers to protect patients and their families against the misuse of the patients' genetic information.

Other responsibilities of the professional nurse may include development of clinical and social policy such as genetic nondiscrimination and prenatal testing policies, testing of genetic products for reliability, and tasks in genetic *informatics* to meet the challenge of sifting through a continually expanding body of knowledge.

SUMMARY

Increasing scientific understanding of genetic processes is expected to revolutionize modern health care in many ways. The artificial manipulation and transfer of genetic material, although not yet a standard treatment for disease, is the focus of over 300 current human clinical gene therapy trials. The spectrum of diseases that may eventually be treatable by gene therapy includes inherited diseases that are present from birth, disabilities such as paralysis from spinal cord injuries, life-threatening illnesses such as cancer, and even chronic illnesses acquired later in life for which a person may have a genetic predisposition. The science of pharmacogenomics has already identified some of the genetic nuances in how different individuals' bodies metabolize drugs to their benefit or harm. Continued study in this area is expected to result in proactive customization of drug therapy to promote therapeutic benefits while minimizing or eliminating toxic effects. Genetic procedures and therapeutic techniques will likely become an increasing part of nursing practice as well as of health care delivery in general. As the role and impact of genetics and genetically based drug therapy increase, so will their role in the nursing process.

CASE STUDY

Genetic Counseling

© Felix Mizioznikov

During the nurse's assessment of a newly admitted 38-year-old patient, the patient tells the nurse, "I'm allergic to codeine. Whenever I take it, it just knocks me out!" The patient tells the nurse that codeine does the same thing to all of her sisters.

1. Does the patient have an actual allergy to codeine? What else could be happening?

The next day, the patient's oncologist comes in and explains the results of a genetic test that was performed on an outpatient basis. The patient agrees to allow the nurse to sit in on the conversation. The physician tells the patient that she has a gene which indicates that she has a strong chance of developing breast cancer within the next 5 years. The oncologist recommends that she undergo a bilateral mastectomy soon to avoid the possibility of developing breast cancer and suggests that she share this information with her sisters and her daughter, who is 18 years old. After the physician leaves, the patient tells the nurse, "I don't know what to do. I haven't talked to one of my sisters for years and I just know she won't believe me. I also don't want to worry my daughter. She is so young and I'm sure she's too young to get cancer."

2. Should the nurse tell the patient's sister and daughter? Explain.

3. How should the nurse handle this situation?

For answers, see *http://evolve.elsevier.com/Lilley.*

POINTS TO REMEMBER

- Genetic processes are a highly complex facet of human physiology, and genetics is becoming an integral part of health care that holds much promise in the form of new treatments for alterations in health.
- The Human Genome Project (HGP), spearheaded by the U.S. Department of Energy and the NIH, described in detail the entire genome of a human individual.
- Basic genetic inheritance is carried by 23 pairs of chromosomes in each of the somatic cells; one pair of chromosomes in each cell

is the *sex chromosomes,* identified as XX for females and XY for males.
- Applicable skills for general nurses include taking thorough patient, family, and drug histories, recognizing situations that may warrant further investigation through genetic testing, identifying resources for patients, maintaining confidentiality and privacy, and ensuring that informed consent is obtained for genetic testing and counseling.

NCLEX EXAMINATION REVIEW QUESTIONS

1 Which is the most appropriate example of an indirect form of gene therapy?
a Stem cells
b Insulin
c Antigen substitution
d Platelet inhibitors

2 The general goal of gene therapy is to transfer exogenous genes to a patient to
a change the patient's own genetic functioning to treat a given disease.
b improve drug metabolism.
c prevent genetic disorders in the patient's future children.
d stimulate the growth of stem cells.

3 The NIH Recombinant DNA Advisory Committee has the responsibility for which of the following?
a Approving all forms of human clinical gene therapy
b Identifying all major risks to the human subjects in a specific research protocol
c Reviewing clinical trials involving human gene transfer and scheduling public forums
d Analyzing genomes and determining whether they appear mutagenic

4 The presence of certain factors in a person's genetic makeup that increase the likelihood of eventually developing one or more diseases is known as a
a genetic mutation.
b genetic polymorphism.
c genetic predisposition.
d genotype.

5 Which of the following is a commonly studied adenovirus?
a Hepatitis A and C virus
b Genovirum
c Human influenza virus
d Pallodium

6 General responsibilities of the nurse regarding genetics may include which of the following? (Select all that apply.)
a Assessing the patient's personal and family history
b Referring the patient to a genetic counselor or other genetics specialist
c Communicating the results of genetic tests to the patient and patient's family
d Maintaining privacy and confidentiality during the testing process
e Answering questions about genetic test results

1. b, 2. a, 3. c, 4. c, 5. c, 6. a, b, d.

CRITICAL THINKING ACTIVITIES: BEST ACTION

1 You are working on a medical-surgical unit as a newly graduated nurse. During an assessment, your patient states, "My doctor told me that I need to have genetic testing. I just don't understand. If they change my genes, then it will change the way I look!" What should you, as the nurse, do to best answer the patient's concerns?

2 An indirect form of gene therapy is already seen in contemporary health care practice. Explain this statement and provide examples.

3 Analyze the process for producing human insulin and suggest a few theoretical examples of how this same process could be used in other areas of health care.

For answers, see *http://evolve.elsevier.com/Lilley.*

CHAPTER 6

Medication Errors: Preventing and Responding

OBJECTIVES

When you reach the end of this chapter, you should be able to do the following:

1 Compare the following terms related to drug therapy in the context of professional nursing practice: *adverse drug event, adverse drug reaction, allergic reaction, idiosyncratic reaction, medical error,* and *medication error.*

2 Describe the most commonly encountered medication errors.

3 Develop a framework for professional nursing practice for prevention of medication errors.

4 Identify potential physical and emotional consequences of a medication error.

5 Discuss the impact of culture and age on the occurrence of medication errors.

6 Analyze the various ethical dilemmas related to professional nursing practice associated with medication errors.

7 Identify agencies concerned with prevention of and response to medication errors.

8 Discuss the possible consequences of medication errors for professional nurses and other members of the health care team.

e-Learning Activities

http://evolve.elsevier.com/Lilley

NCLEX Review Questions • Animations • Nursing Care Plans • Audio Glossary • Category Catchers • Medication Errors Checklists • IV Therapy Checklists • Calculators • Frequently Asked Questions • Content Updates • Supplemental Resources • Answers to Case Studies and Critical Thinking Activities

Glossary

Adverse drug event Any undesirable occurrence related to administration of or failure to administer a prescribed medication. (p. 69)

Adverse drug reactions Unexpected, unintended, undesired, or excessive responses to medications given at therapeutic dosages (as opposed to overdose); one type of adverse drug event. (p. 69)

Allergic reaction An immunologic hypersensitivity reaction resulting from an unusual sensitivity of a patient to a particular medication; a type of adverse drug event and a subtype of adverse drug reactions. (p. 70)

Idiosyncratic reaction Any abnormal and unexpected response to a medication, other than an allergic reaction, that is peculiar to an individual patient. (p. 70)

Medical error A broad term commonly used to refer to any error in any phase of clinical patient care that causes or has the potential to cause patient harm. (p. 69)

Medication errors Any preventable adverse drug events involving inappropriate medication use by a patient or health care professional; they may or may not cause the patient harm. (p. 69)

Medication reconciliation A procedure implemented by health care providers to maintain an accurate and up-to-date list of medications for all patients between all phases of health care delivery. (p. 75)

• • •

GENERAL IMPACT OF ERRORS ON PATIENTS

According to a landmark 1999 report of the Institute of Medicine (IOM), the number of patient deaths in U.S. hospitals ranged from 44,000 to 98,000 annually based on data from two large-scale studies. The IOM conducted a similar study in 2006 and found that medical errors harm at least 1.5 million people per year. Although **medical error** is often used as an umbrella term in the published literature, errors can occur during all phases of health care delivery and involve all categories of health professionals. Some of the more common types of error include misdiagnosis, patient misidentification, lack of patient monitoring, wrong-site surgery, and medication errors. Most studies have looked at medical errors occurring in hospitals; however, many serious medication errors occur in the home. Errors are occurring in homes more frequently because dangerous drugs once used only in hospitals are now being prescribed for outpatients. The majority of fatal errors at home involved the mixing of prescription drugs with alcohol or other drugs. Intangible losses resulting from such adverse outcomes include patient dissatisfaction with, and loss of trust in, the health care system. This, in turn, can lead to adverse health outcomes because patients are afraid to seek health services. This chapter focuses on the issues related to medication errors and ways to prevent and respond to these errors. Included is an overview of various institutional, educational, and sociologic factors that may contribute to such errors.

MEDICATION ERRORS

As mentioned in Chapter 2, **adverse drug event** is a general term that encompasses all types of clinical problems related to medication use. These include **medication errors** and **adverse drug**

reactions. The various subsets of adverse drug events and their interrelationships are illustrated in Figure 6-1. Adverse drug reactions are reactions that have been reported to occur with the use of the particular drug. Two types of adverse drug reactions are **allergic reaction** (often predictable) and **idiosyncratic reaction** (usually unpredictable). Medication errors are a common cause of adverse health care outcomes, which can range in severity from having no significant effect on the patient to directly causing patient disability or death. In the 2006 Institute of Medicine Study, it was estimated that some form of medication error resulted in patient harm to 1.5 million patients, including 400,000 in hospitals and up to 800,000 in long-term care settings per year. Estimates of preventable adverse drug events in outpatients were found to be approximately 530,000 per year.

It is important to consider all of the steps involved in the medication use system when discussing medication errors. Iden-

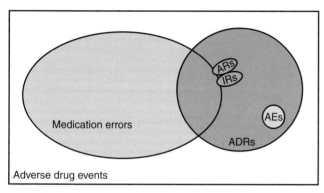

FIGURE 6-1 Diagram illustrating the various classes and subclasses of adverse drug events. *ADRs,* Adverse drug reactions; *AEs,* adverse (drug) effects; *ARs,* allergic reactions; *IRs,* idiosyncratic reactions.

tifying, responding to, and ultimately preventing medication errors requires an examination of the entire medication use process. Attention must be focused on all persons and all steps involved in the medication administration process, including the prescriber, the transcriber of the order from the chart, nurses, pharmacists, and any other ancillary staff involved. A system analysis approach takes the Six Rights one step further and examines the entire health care system, the health care professionals involved, and any other factor that has an impact on the error.

Some of the categories of drugs commonly involved in severe medication errors include central nervous system drugs, anticoagulants, and chemotherapeutic drugs. "High-alert" medications have been identified as those medications that, because of their potentially toxic nature, require special care when prescribing, dispensing, and/or administering. High-alert medications are not necessarily involved in more errors than other drugs; however, the potential for patient harm is higher with these medications. Some high-alert medications are listed in Box 6-1. Many medication errors result from the fact that there are an increasing number of drugs on the market which have similarities in spelling and/or pronunciation (i.e., look-alike or sound-alike names). Several acronyms have been created to refer to these drugs, including SALAD (sound-alike, look-alike drugs) and LASA (look alike, sound alike). Mixups between such drugs is most dangerous when two drugs from very different therapeutic classes have similar names. This can result in effects on the patient that are grossly different from those intended as part of the drug therapy. The Preventing Medication Errors box on p. 71 lists examples of commonly confused drug names. More information on high-alert medications and sound-alike, look-alike drugs can be found at the website of the Institute for Safe Medication Practice at *http://www.ismp.org.*

It is widely recognized that the majority of medication errors result from weaknesses in the systems within health care organizations rather than from individual shortcomings. Such weak-

---

BOX 6-1 Examples of High-Alert Medications

Drug Classes/Categories
- Adrenergic agonists, IV (e.g., epinephrine, phenylephrine, norepinephrine)
- Adrenergic antagonists, IV (e.g., propranolol, metoprolol, labetalol)
- Anesthetic agents, general, inhaled and IV (e.g., propofol, ketamine)
- Antidysrhythmics, IV (e.g., lidocaine, amiodarone)
- Antithrombotic agents (anticoagulants), including warfarin, low-molecular-weight heparin, IV unfractionated heparin, factor Xa inhibitors (e.g., fondaparinux), direct thrombin inhibitors (e.g., argatroban, lepirudin, bivalirudin), thrombolytics (e.g., alteplase, reteplase, tenecteplase), and glycoprotein IIb/IIIa inhibitors (e.g., eptifibatide)
- Cardioplegic solutions
- Chemotherapeutic agents, parenteral and oral
- Dextrose, hypertonic, 20% or greater
- Dialysis solutions, peritoneal and hemodialysis
- Epidural or intrathecal medications
- Hypoglycemics, oral
- Inotropic drugs, IV (e.g., digoxin, milrinone)
- Moderate sedation drugs, IV (e.g., midazolam)
- Moderate sedation agents, oral, for children (e.g., chloral hydrate)

- Narcotics/opiates, IV, transdermal, and oral (including liquid concentrates, immediate- and sustained-release formulations)
- Neuromuscular blocking agents (e.g., succinylcholine, rocuronium, vecuronium)
- Radiocontrast agents, IV
- Total parenteral nutrition solutions

Specific Drugs
- Insulin, subcutaneous and IV
- Magnesium sulfate injection
- Methotrexate, oral, nononcologic use
- Opium tincture
- Oxytocin, IV
- Nitroprusside sodium for injection
- Potassium chloride for injection concentrate
- Potassium phosphates injection
- Promethazine, IV
- Sodium chloride for injection, hypertonic (greater than 0.9% concentration)
- Sterile water for injection, inhalation, and irrigation (excluding pour bottles) in containers of 100 mL or more

From Institute for Safe Medication Practices: ISMP's list of high-alert medications, 2008, available at *http://www.ismp.org/Tools/highalertmedications.pdf.*

PREVENTING MEDICATION ERRORS

Institute for Safe Medication Practices: Examples of Look-Alike, Sound-Alike (LASA) Commonly Confused Drug Names

Names of Medications	Comments
Accupril vs. Aciphex	Antihypertensive vs. proton pump inhibitor (stomach acid blocker)
carboplatin vs. cisplatin	Two different antineoplastics
Celebrex vs. Celexa	Antiinflammatory drug vs. antidepressant drug
Darvon vs. Diovan	Analgesic vs. antihypertensive
Depakote vs. Depakote ER	Same drug; immediate-release vs. extended-release dosage forms
dopamine vs. dobutamine	Vasopressor drugs of markedly different strengths; dobutamine is also a strong inotropic affecting the heart
fentanyl vs. sufentanil	Both are injectable anesthetics but with a significant difference in potency and duration of action
glipizide vs. glyburide	Two different antidiabetic drugs
Humulin vs. Humalog	Short-acting vs. rapid-acting insulin
Lamictal vs. Lamisil	Anticonvulsant/mood stabilizer vs. antifungal
metronidazole vs. metformin	Antibiotic vs. antidiabetic
MiraLax vs. Mirapex	Laxative vs. antiparkinson drug
oxycodone vs. OxyContin	Immediate-release vs. long-acting oxycodone
Paxil vs. Plavix	Antidepressant vs. antiplatelet drug
Trazodone vs. tramadol	Antidepressant vs. analgesic

Additional examples can be found at *http://www.ismp.org/Tools/ confuseddrugnames.pdf.*

nesses include failure to create a "just culture" or nonpunitive work atmosphere for reporting errors, excessive workload with minimal time for staff preventive education, and lack of interdisciplinary communication and collaboration. All hospitals are required to analyze medication errors and implement ways to prevent them. Nurses must take the time to report errors, because without reporting, no changes can be made. When errors are reported, trends can be identified and processes can be changed to prevent the errors from occurring again.

PSYCHOSOCIAL ISSUES THAT CONTRIBUTE TO ERRORS

Organizational Issues

Medication errors can occur at any step in the medication process: procuring, prescribing, transcribing, dispensing, administering, and monitoring. One study noted that half of all preventable adverse drug events begin with an error at the medication ordering (prescribing) stage. Most prescribing errors can be caught by the pharmacist before order entry and by nurses prior to administration. The next most common point in the process at which medication errors occur is administration of the drug by the nurse; followed by dispensing errors and transcription errors. It is very important for nurses to have good relationships with pharmacists, because the two professions, working together, can

have a major impact in preventing medication errors. Hospital pharmacists are usually available 24/7 and should be called upon anytime a nurse has any question regarding drug therapy.

The Joint Commission, the major accreditation body for hospitals, began a patient public awareness campaign in 2006 called *Speak Up.* Its focus is on encouraging patients to take a more active role in their health care by "speaking up" and asking questions of all health care providers whenever they feel the need to do so. The value to patients is twofold: learning more about their illness and the care provided, and advocating for their own safety at each health care encounter. Specific topics on the campaign website (see the Bibliography) include asking questions about care in general, learning about living organ donation, preventing infections in the hospital, avoiding medication errors, participating in research studies, planning for follow-up care, avoiding errors in medical tests, and knowing about patients rights in general (see Box 6-3).

Effective use of technologies such as computerized prescriber order entry and bar coding of medication packages has been shown to reduce medication errors. In February 2004, the U.S. Food and Drug Administration (FDA) announced new regulations requiring bar codes for all prescription and over-the-counter medications. However, only a small percentage of U.S. hospitals have implemented bar-code scanning technology. This is largely due to prohibitive cost. Cost is a barrier to technologic improvements in general, because most hospital administrators are under continuous pressure to reduce expenses. The cost of implementing current technology, including automated drug dispensing cabinets with electronic charting and computerized order entry, may range from hundreds of thousands of dollars to over $20 million. Nonetheless, these various technologic advances have been shown to reduce medication errors. For example, computerized order entry eliminates handwriting and standardizes many prescribing functions, especially dosage specifications. Bar coding of medications has allowed the use of electronic devices by nurses for verification of correct medication at the patient's bedside. Computer programs are often used in the pharmacy to screen for potential drug interactions. Despite all the benefits technology has to offer, workload issues (i.e., nursing staff shortage), which may prevent adequate education in the use of the equipment, or difficulties in mastering the use of complex technology can prevent the technology from eliminating errors as it was designed to do. Self-medication by patients (e.g., patient-controlled analgesia) has been shown to reduce errors, provided patients have adequate cognitive ability and mental alertness.

Educational System Issues and Their Potential Impact on Medication Errors

All health professionals should feel free to double-check any necessary information before proceeding. This includes stopping and checking medication orders and being comfortable with one's immediate knowledge of the given drug *before* administering the drug. Authoritative sources for information about drugs include current drug reference guides such as *Mosby's Drug Consult, Physicians' Desk Reference, Drug Formulary,* and others written by legitimate experts. Even the most capable health care provider cannot know everything or have immediate recall of every fact ever read. This is especially true given the increasing complexity of health care practice. Patient safety begins in

BOX 6-2　Preventing Medication Errors

- As the first step to defend against errors, assess information about drug allergies, vital signs, and laboratory test results.
- Use two patient identifiers before giving medications.
- Never give medications that you have not drawn up or prepared yourself.
- Minimize the use of verbal and telephone orders. If used, be sure to repeat the order to confirm with the prescriber. Speak slowly and clearly and spell the drug name aloud.
- List the reason for use of each drug on the medication administration record and any educational materials.
- Avoid abbreviations, medical shorthand, and acronyms, because they can lead to confusion, miscommunication, and risk of error (see the Legal and Ethical Principles box).
- Never assume anything about any drug order or prescription, including route. If a medication order is questioned for any reason (e.g., dose, drug, indication), never assume that the prescriber is correct. Always be the patient's advocate and investigate the matter until all ambiguities are resolved.
- Do not try to decipher illegibly written orders; instead, contact the prescriber for clarification. Illegible orders fall below applicable standards for quality medical care and endanger patient safety. If in doubt about any part of an order, always check with the prescriber. Compare the medication order against what is on hand by checking for the RIGHT patient, dose, drug, time, and route.
- Never use trailing zeros (e.g., 1.0 mg) in writing and/or transcribing medication orders. Use of trailing zeros is associated with increased occurrence of overdose. For example, "1.0 mg warfarin sodium" could be misread as "10 mg warfarin," a tenfold dose increase. Instead, use "1 mg" or even "one mg."
- Failure to use leading zeros can also lead to overdose. For example, .25 mg digoxin could be misread as 25 mg digoxin, a dose that is 100 times the dose ordered. Instead, write "0.25 mg."
- Carefully read all labels for accuracy, expiration dates, dilution requirements, and warnings (e.g., black box warnings).
- Remain current with new techniques of administration and new equipment.
- Encourage the use of generic names to avoid medication errors due to many sound-alike trade names.

- Listen to and honor any concerns expressed by patients. Should the patient voice a concern about being allergic to a medication or state that a pill has already been taken or that the medication is not what the patient usually takes—STOP, listen, and investigate.
- Strive to maintain your own health to remain alert, and never be too busy to stop, learn, and inquire. In addition, engage in ongoing continuing education.
- Become a member of professional nursing organizations to network with other nursing students or professional nurses to advocate for improved working conditions and to stand up for the rights of nurses and patients.
- Know where to find the latest information on which dosage forms can or should not be crushed or opened (e.g., capsules) and educate patients accordingly.
- Safeguard any medications that the patient had on admission or transfer so that additional doses are not given or taken by mistake. In such situations, safeguarding is accomplished by compiling a current medication history and resolving any discrepancies rather than ignoring them.
- Always verify new medication administration records if they have been rewritten or reentered for any reason and follow policies and procedures about this action.
- Make sure the weight of the patient is always recorded before carrying out a medication order to help decrease dosage errors.
- Provide for mandatory recalculation of every drug dosage for high-risk drugs (e.g., highly toxic drugs) or high-risk patients (e.g., pediatric or elderly patients), because there is a narrow margin between therapeutic serum drug levels and toxic levels (e.g., for chemotherapeutic or digitalis drugs, or in the presence of altered liver or kidney function in a patient).
- Always suspect an error whenever an adult dosage form is dispensed for a pediatric patient.
- Seek translators when appropriate—never guess what patients are trying to say.
- Educate patients to take an active role in medication error prevention, both in the hospital setting and at home.
- Involve yourself politically in advocating for legislation that improves patient safety.

LEGAL AND ETHICAL PRINCIPLES

Use of Abbreviations

Medication errors often occur as a result of misinterpretation of abbreviations. Therefore, the National Coordinating Council for Medication Error Reporting and Prevention recommends that the following abbreviations be written out in full and the abbreviations avoided. The U.S. Pharmacopeia and Institute of Safe Medication Practices endorse the avoidance of abbreviations whenever possible. Most hospitals and nursing care units are adopting this significant change in documentation. NOTE: It is the philosophy of the authors of this textbook that abbreviations should be avoided whenever possible.

Abbreviation	Intended Meaning	Common Error
U	Units	Mistaken for a zero (0), a four (4), or cc.
mcg (μg)	Micrograms	Mistaken for mg (milligrams).
Q.D.	Latin abbreviation for "every day"	The period after the "Q" can be mistaken for an "I" so that a medication is given "QID" (four times daily) instead of once daily.
Q.O.D.	Latin abbreviation for "every other day"	Misinterpreted as "QD" (daily) or QID. If "O" is poorly written it may look like a period or "I."
D/C	Discharge or discontinue	Medications have been prematurely discontinued when D/C (intended to mean "discharge") was misinterpreted as "discontinue" because it was followed by a list of drugs. Use the word *Stop*.
HS	Half strength	Misinterpreted as the Latin abbreviation "HS" (hour of sleep).
cc	Cubic centimeters	Mistaken for "U" (units) when written poorly.
AU, AS, AD	Both ears, left ear, right ear	Misinterpreted as the Latin abbreviation "OU" (both eyes), "OS" (left eye), "OD" (right eye). Also, some people forget which is right or left or both, and which is eye or ear.

BOX 6-3 WHO Collaborating Centre for Patient Safety Solutions and Speak Up Initiatives about Medications and Health

On its website the World Health Organization (WHO) posts information regarding initiatives to promote patient safety in medication administration and other aspects of health care. As the WHO notes, no adverse event should ever occur anywhere in the world if the knowledge exists to prevent it from happening. Knowledge is of little use, however, if it is not applied in practice. The WHO Collaborating Centre for Patient Safety Solutions has developed patient safety initiatives that can serve as a guide in redesigning the patient care process to prevent the inevitable errors from ever reaching patients. Patient safety solutions are defined by the WHO as any system design feature or intervention that has demonstrated the ability to prevent or mitigate patient harm arising from the health care process. Information about the first group of patient safety solutions (2008/2009) approved by the WHO center is available at *http://www.ccforpatientsafety.org*. These patient safety concerns include avoiding confusion of medications with look-alike, sound-alike names; ensuring correct patient identification; enhancing communication during patient "hand-overs" between care units or care teams; ensuring performance of the correct procedure at the correct body site; maintaining control of concentrated electrolyte solutions; ensuring medication accuracy at transition points in care; avoiding catheter and tubing misconnections; and promoting single use of injection devices and improved hand hygiene to prevent health care–associated infections.

More information about patient safety and safety initiatives is also provided in a national campaign supported by the Joint Commission and the Centers for Medicare and Medicaid. These initiatives encourage patients to take a role in preventing health care errors by becoming more active, involved, and informed regarding all aspects of their health care. The *Speak Up* campaign features various brochures, posters, and buttons addressing a variety of patient safety issues and encourages the public to do the following: **S**peak up if you have any questions. **P**ay attention to your health care and make sure that any treatments or medications are appropriate and are ordered by the proper health care professionals. **E**ducate yourself about medical diagnoses and be informed. **A**sk a family member or friend you trust to be your advocate. **K**now the medications you take and the reason for taking them. **U**se a hospital, ambulatory or urgent care center, or other type of health care facility. **P**articipate in all decisions about your treatment, because you are the very center and heart of the health care team. The success of the Speak Up initiatives is well documented in the results of a 2005 survey of more than 600 accredited health care organizations, of which approximately 81% reported that campaigns like Speak Up bring more value to the accreditation process and 82% would like to see the Joint Commission sponsor more patient education programs in the future. Some 91% of these 600 organizations viewed the initiatives and program as excellent, very good, or good. For more information on the use of Speak Up and to look at the materials available, visit *http://www.jointcommission.org/GeneralPublic/Speak1Up/about_speakup.htm* or contact Joint Commission Resources at 877-223-6866 or the Joint Commission Resources web store at *http://store.jcrinc.com*. Other sources of information are listed at *http://www.ccforpatientsafety.org*.

---

the educational process with nursing students and faculty members. Adopting the philosophy that "no question is a stupid question" allows students to begin their careers with greater confidence and with a healthy habit of self-monitoring during health care delivery. In contrast, berating or otherwise penalizing a student for not immediately recalling a given fact, or for simply asking questions, instills fear and shame. It also discourages dialogue that would otherwise promote and enhance student learning and mastery of concepts. Commonly reported student nurse errors involve the following situations: unusual dosing times, medication administration record issues (unavailability of the record, failure to document resulting in administration of extra doses, failure to review the record before medicating patients), administration of discontinued or "held" medications, failure to monitor vital signs or laboratory results, administration of oral liquids as injections, preparation of medications for multiple patients at the same time, and dispensing of medications in different doses than those ordered (e.g., tablets that need to be broken in half). The World Health Organization has developed information about patient safety concerns, safety initiatives, and patient safety solutions (see Box 6-3).

Medication Errors and Related Sociologic Factors

It is well documented that effective communication among all members of the health care team contributes to improved patient care. However, a 2002 study published in the *American Journal of Nursing* identified disruptive physician behavior and lack of institutional response to it as significant factors affecting nurse job satisfaction and nursing staff retention. A more recent article in the March 2008 issue of *American Nurse Today* provided further discussion of the problem of disruptive behavior, reporting on a survey of nurses, physicians, and health care executives. Ninety-six percent of the nurses surveyed said they had witnessed or experienced disruptive behavior by a physician. Other literature shows that nurses are the primary victims of disruptive behavior and that this behavior may not only undermine patient care but also lead to staff dissatisfaction and turnover. In response to this increasing problem, the Joint Commission calls for the establishment of procedures for managing disruptive behavior by physicians and others who are granted clinical privileges. Disruptive behavior, as defined by the American Medical Association (AMA), is personal verbal or physical conduct that affects or potentially may affect patient care in a negative fashion. These behaviors are classified into four types by the AMA: (1) intimidation and violence, (2) inappropriate language or comments, (3) sexual harassment, and (4) inappropriate responses to patient needs or staff requests. Although all of these types are significant, the last type is most closely related to drug therapy because it includes behaviors such as showing disregard for policies and blaming others for adverse patient outcomes.

Fortunately, communication between prescribers and other members of the health care team has improved somewhat over the years with newer generations of prescribers. This is due in large part to more progressive approaches in medical education that emphasize a team orientation. Such approaches recognize the ever-increasing complexities of health care delivery and the reality that no one team member can know every fact and provide for all patient care needs.

PREVENTING, RESPONDING TO, REPORTING, AND DOCUMENTING MEDICATION ERRORS: A NURSING PERSPECTIVE

Preventing Medication Errors

As indicated earlier in this chapter, medication errors are considered to be any preventable event that could lead to inappropriate medication use or harm while that medication is in the control of the professional nurse, student nurse, health professional, prescriber, patient, or consumer. The major categories of medication error are defined by the 2005 National Coordinating Council for Medication Error Reporting and Prevention as (1) no error, although circumstances or events occurred that could have led to an error, (2) medication error that causes no harm, (3) medication error that causes harm, and (4) medication error that results in death. Medication errors may be prevented through a variety of strategies, including the following: (1) Multiple systems of checks and balances should be implemented to prevent medication errors. (2) Prescribers should write legible orders that contain correct information or orders should be written electronically if the technology is available. (3) Authoritative resources, such as pharmacists or current drug literature, should be consulted if there is any area of concern, beginning with the medication order and continuing throughout the entire medication administration process. (4) Nurses should always check the medication order three times before giving the drug and consult with authoritative resources (see earlier) if any questions or concerns exist. Faculty members should not be the student's research source regarding medications, and the safe practice of using appropriate resources should begin early in the educational process. (5) The "Six Rights" of medication administration should be used consistently, which has been shown to substantially reduce the likelihood of a medication error. See Box 6-2 for a more concise and detailed listing of ways to help prevent medication errors and the Life Span Considerations: The Pediatric Patient box on p. 74 for discussion of medication errors in pediatric patients and special considerations for this age group.

Responding to, Reporting, and Documenting Medication Errors

Responding to and reporting medication errors are part of the professional responsibilities for which the nurse is accountable. If a medication error does occur, it must be reported, regardless of whether the error was made by a nursing student or a professional nurse. Facility policies and procedures for reporting and documenting the error should be followed closely and cautiously. Once the patient has been assessed and urgent safety issues have been addressed, the error should be reported immediately to the appropriate prescriber and nursing management personnel, for example, the nurse manager or supervisor. If the patient cannot be left alone due to deterioration of the patient's condition or the need for close monitoring after the medication error, a fellow nurse or other qualified health care professional should remain with the patient and provide appropriate care while the prescriber is contacted. Follow-up procedures or tests may be ordered or an antidote prescribed. These orders should be implemented as indicated by the prescriber. Remember that the nurse's highest priority at all times during the medication administration process and during a medication error is the patient's physiologic status and safety.

LIFE SPAN CONSIDERATIONS: The Pediatric Patient

Medication Errors

Of all the ways a pediatric patient may be harmed during medical treatment, medication errors are the most common. As with elderly patients, when medication errors occur, there is a higher risk of death. The findings of several studies indicate that medication errors involving inpatient pediatric patients occur at a rate of 4.5 to 5.7 errors per 100 drugs used. The most common medication errors in pediatrics are dosing errors. Research has begun to identify some of the groups of pediatric patients who are at highest risk of medication errors. These include the following patients: (1) those younger than 2 years of age, (2) those in intensive care units (ICUs), specifically the neonatal ICU, (3) those in the emergency department between the hours of 4 AM and 8 AM or on the weekend and who are seriously ill, (4) those receiving intravenous and/or chemotherapeutic drugs, and (5) those whose weight not determined or recorded. Mathematical dosage calculations for pediatric patients are also problematic. In determination of the correct dosage once the drug has been ordered, the problems of most concern include the following: (1) inability of the nurse to understand/perform the correct calculation or dilution, (2) infrequent use of calculations, and (3) decimal point misplacement, with potential overdosing or underdosing.

The following are some of the actions that can be taken to prevent pediatric medication errors:

- Report all medication errors, because this information is part of the practice of professional nursing and helps in identifying causes of medication error.
- Know the drug thoroughly, including its on- and off-label uses, action, adverse effects, dosage ranges, routes of administration, high-alert drug status cautions (see Box 6-1), and contraindications (e.g., is it recommended for use in pediatric patients?).
- Confirm information about the patient each and every time a dose is given and check three times before giving the drug by comparing the drug order with the patient's medication profile and verifying for the right drug, right dose, right route, right time, and right patient.
- Double-check and verify information in handwritten orders that may be incomplete, unclear, or illegible.
- Avoid verbal telephone orders in general. When they are unavoidable, always repeat them back to the prescriber over the phone. Insist that the prescriber sign off any emergency in-person verbal orders before leaving the unit.
- Avoid distractions while giving medications.
- Communicate with everyone (e.g., parent, caregiver) involved in patient care.
- Make sure all orders are clear and understood with shift changes.
- Use authoritative resources such as drug handbooks, *Physicians' Desk Reference*, or information from the Food and Drug Administration website (*http://www.fda.gov*). For off-label use of drugs, see *http://www.fda.gov/cder/pediatric/labelchange.htm*.

When a medication error has occurred, the nurse should complete all appropriate forms—including an incident report—as per the facility's policies and procedures, and provide appropriate documentation. The medication error should be documented, however, by providing only factual information about the error. Documentation should always be accurate, thorough, and objective. The use of judgmental words such as *error* should be avoided in the documentation. Instead, the nurse should chart factual information such as the medication that was administered, the actual dose given, and other details regarding the order (e.g., wrong patient, wrong route, and/or wrong time). Any observed changes in the patient's physical and mental status should also be noted. In addition, the fact that the prescriber was notified and any follow-up actions or orders that were implemented should be documented. Patient monitoring should be ongoing.

Most facilities require additional documentation when a medication error occurs consisting of an incident report or unusual occurrence report. Facility policies and procedures or protocols should always be followed in completing an incident report. Documentation should include only factual information about the error as well as all corrective actions taken. Any additional sections of the form should be completed to help with the investigation of the incident. Because these forms are forwarded to the facility's risk management department, this complete and factual information may help prevent errors in the future. It should not be documented on the patient's chart that an incident report was filled out, and a copy of the incident report should not be kept. Incident reports are not to be placed in the patient's chart. The reporting of actual and suspected medication errors should offer the option of anonymity. This may help to foster improved error reporting and safe medication practices. Internal, facility-based systems of error tracking may generate data to help customize policy and procedure development. All institutional pharmacy departments are required to have an adverse drug event monitoring program.

Nurses as well as health care facilities may also be involved in external reporting of medication errors. There are nationwide confidential reporting programs that collect and disseminate safety information on a larger scale. One such program is the U.S. Pharmacopeia Medication Errors Reporting Program (USPMERP). The U.S. Pharmacopeia (USP) has created a nationwide database of medication errors and their causes, as well as potential errors. Any health care professional can report an error by contacting the USPMERP at 800-23-ERROR. Many important institutional changes have been made based on the data collected by this program. MedWatch is another useful error and adverse event reporting program provided by the FDA. Any member of the public can report problems with medications or medical devices via telephone or mail, or online at the FDA website. The Institute for Safe Medication Practices and the Joint Commission also provide useful information and reporting services to health care providers aimed at safety enhancement. See the Evolve website for specific addresses and points of contact for these and other helpful organizations.

Performing Medication Reconciliation

In 2005 the Institute for Healthcare Improvement *(http://www.ihi. org)* launched its 18-month 100,000 Lives Campaign. This was a safety campaign aimed at all health care facilities. Its goal was to prevent the approximately 100,000 reported avoidable deaths in these institutions. It was replaced by the Five Million Lives campaign of 2006 to 2008. The goal of this campaign was to prevent a projected 5 million cases of "medical harm" of any type during this period. One of the key strategies of both campaigns was the prevention of medication errors through medication reconciliation. **Medication reconciliation** is a process that seeks to prevent medication errors through the ongoing assessment and updating of information on patients' medications throughout the health care process and the timely communication of this information to both patients and their prescribers. Since 2006, implementation of this procedure has been required by both Medicare and the Joint Commission *(http://www.jointcommission.org)* for all health care facilities that receive Medicare reimbursement and/or Joint Commission accreditation. Driving implementation of this procedure is the fact that poorly communicated medical information is the cause of

---

CASE STUDY

Preventing Medication Errors

© Oliver Hoffmann

During your busy clinical day as a student nurse, the staff nurse assigned to your patient comes to you and says, "Would you like to give this injection? We have a 'now' order for Sandostatin (octreotide) 200 mcg subcutaneously. I've already drawn it up; 200 mcg equals 2 mL. It needs to be given as soon as possible, so I drew it up to save time." She hands you a syringe that has 2 mL of a clear fluid in it and the patient's medication administration record (MAR).

1. Should you give this medication "now," as ordered? Why or why not?

You decide to check the order that is handwritten on the MAR with the order written on the chart. The physician wrote, "Octreotide, 200 mcg now, subcutaneously, then 100 mcg every 8 hours as needed." Before you have a chance to find your instructor, the nurse returns and says, "Your instructor probably won't let you give the injection unless you can show the medication ampules. Here are the ampules I used to draw up the octreotide. Be quick—your patient needs it now!"

You take the order, the MAR, the two ampules, and the syringe to your instructor. Together you read the order, then check the ampules. Each ampule is marked "Sandostatin (octreotide) 500 mcg/mL."

2. If the nurse drew up 2 mL from those two ampules, how much octreotide is in the syringe? How does that amount compare with the amount on the order?

The nurse is astonished when you point out that the ampules read "500 mcg/mL." She goes into the automated medication dispenser and sees two identical boxes of Sandostatin next to each other in the refrigerated section. One box is labeled "100 mcg/mL" and the other box is labeled "500 mcg/mL." She then realizes that she chose an ampule of the wrong strength of drug and drew up an incorrect dose.

3. What would have happened if you had given the injection?

4. What should be done at this point? What contributed to this potential medication error, and how can it be prevented in the future?

For answers, see *http://evolve.elsevier.com/Lilley.*

---

up to 50% of hospital medication errors. Medication reconciliation is also one of the Joint Commission's 2009 National Patient Safety Goals (available at *http://www.jointcommission.org/PatientSafety/ NationalPatientSafetyGoals/*).

Unfortunately, implementation of the medication reconciliation process has been associated with unintended medication errors, primarily stemming from the fact that patients may not remember the exact dose or frequency of their medications. In 2009, The Joint Commission actually stopped scoring this goal and is in the process of reworking the requirements.

Medication reconciliation involves three steps (additional information can be found on either of the websites mentioned previously):

1. Verification—Collection of the patient's medication information with a focus on medications currently used (including prescription drugs as well as over-the-counter medications and supplements)
2. Clarification—Professional review of this information to ensure that medications and dosages are appropriate for the patient
3. Reconciliation—Further investigation of any discrepancies and documentation of relevant communications and changes in medication orders

To ensure ongoing accuracy of medication use, the steps listed should be repeated at each stage of health care delivery:

a. Admission

b. Status change (e.g., from critical to stable). It is the role of the provider to evaluate current medications and specify, in writing, which medications are to be continued or discontinued with any status change, transfer, or discharge.

c. Patient transfer within or between facilities or provider teams

d. Discharge (the latest medication list should be provided to the patient to take to his or her next health care provider or this information should be otherwise forwarded to the provider; applicable confidentiality guidelines should be followed)

Some applicable assessment and education tips regarding medication reconciliation are the following:

1. Ask the patient open-ended questions and gradually move to yes-no questions to help determine specific medication information. (Details are important, maybe even critical!)

2. Avoid the use of medical jargon unless it is clear that the patient understands and is comfortable with such language.

3. Prompt the patient to try to remember all applicable medications (e.g., patches, creams, eyedrops, inhalers, professional samples, injections, dietary supplements). If the patient provides a medication list, make a copy for the patient's chart as part of this process.

4. Clarify unclear information to the extent possible (e.g., by talking with the home caregiver or the outpatient pharmacist who fills the patient's prescriptions, if needed).

5. Record the foregoing information in the patient's chart as the first step in the medication reconciliation process.

6. Emphasize to the patient the importance of always maintaining a current and complete medication list and bringing it to each health care encounter (e.g., as a wallet card or other list). Many patients use their own computers for this. Also encourage patients to learn the names and current dosages of their medications.

OTHER ETHICAL ISSUES

Notification of Patients Regarding Errors

An article published in the *Journal of Clinical Outcomes Management* in 2001 recognized the obligation of institutions and health care providers to provide full disclosure to patients when errors have occurred in their care. The article not only emphasized the ethical basis for this practice but also addressed the legal implications and was a starting point for understanding the issue of notification of patients regarding medication errors. The point was made that patients who seek attorney services are often motivated primarily by a perceived imbalance in power between themselves and their health care providers and by fear of financial burden. Health care organizations can choose to proactively apologize and accept responsibility for obvious errors and even offer needed financial support (e.g., for travel expenses, temporary loss of wages). Research indicates that such actions help health care organizations to avoid litigation and potentially much larger financial settlements.

Possible Consequences of Medication Errors for Nurses

As mentioned earlier, the possible effects of medication errors on patients range from no significant effect to permanent disability and even death in the most extreme cases. However, medication errors may also affect health care professionals, including nurses and student nurses, in a number of ways. An error that involves significant patient harm or death may take an extreme emotional toll on the nurse involved in the error. Nurses may be named as defendants in malpractice litigation, with possibly serious financial consequences. Many nurses choose to carry personal malpractice insurance for this reason, although nurses working in institutional settings are usually covered by the institution's liability insurance policy. Nurses should obtain clear written documentation of any institutional coverage provided before deciding whether to carry individual malpractice insurance.

Administrative responses to medication errors vary from institution to institution and depend on the severity of the error. One possible response is a directive to the nurse involved to obtain continuing education or refresher training. Disciplinary action, including suspension or termination of employment, may also occur depending on the specific incident. However, many hospitals have implemented a non-punitive approach to medication errors. Nurses who have violated regulations of their state's nurse practice act may also be counseled or disciplined by their state nursing board, which may suspend or permanently revoke their nursing license. Student nurses, given their lack of clinical experience, should be especially careful to avoid medication errors, as well as errors in general. When in doubt about the correct course of action, students should consult with clinical instructors or more experienced staff nurses. Nonetheless, if a student nurse realizes that he or she has committed an error, the student should notify the responsible clinical instructor immediately. The patient may require additional monitoring or medication, and the prescriber may also need to be notified. Although such events are preferably avoided, they can ultimately be useful, though stressful, learning experiences for the student nurse. However, student nurses who commit sufficiently serious errors or display a pattern of errors can expect more severe disciplinary action. This may range from a requirement for extra clinical time or repeating of a clinical course to suspension or expulsion from the nursing school program (see the earlier section Educational System Issues and Their Potential Impact on Medication Errors).

SUMMARY

The increasing complexity of nursing practice also increases the risk for medication errors. Widely recognized and common causes of error include misunderstanding of abbreviations, illegibility of prescriber handwriting, miscommunication during verbal or telephone orders, and confusing drug nomenclature. The structure of various organizational, educational, and sociologic systems involved in health care delivery may also contribute directly or indirectly to the occurrence of medication errors. Understanding these influences can help the nurse take proactive steps to improve these systems. Such actions can range from fostering improved communication with other health care team members, including students, to advocating politically for safer conditions for both patients and staff. The first priority when an error does occur is to protect the patient from further harm whenever possible. All errors should serve as red flags that warrant further reflection, detailed analysis, and future preventive actions on the part of nurses, other health care professionals, and possibly even patients themselves.

POINTS TO REMEMBER

- To prevent medication errors from misinterpretation of the prescriber's orders, abbreviations should be avoided. Medication errors include giving a drug to the wrong patient, confusing sound-alike and look-alike drugs, administering the wrong drug or wrong dose, giving the drug by the wrong route, and giving the drug at the wrong time.
- Measures to help prevent medication errors include being prepared and knowledgeable and taking time to always triple-check for the right patient, drug, dosage, time, and route. It is also important for nurses always to be aware of the entire medication administration process and to take a systems analysis approach to medication errors and their prevention.
- Encourage patients to ask questions about their medications and to question any concern about the drug or any component of the medication administration process.

- Encourage patients to always carry drug allergy information on their persons and to keep a current list of medications in their wallets or purses and on their refrigerators. This list should include the drug's name, reason the drug is being used, usual dosage range and dosage prescribed, expected adverse effects and possible toxicity of the drug, and the prescriber's name and contact information.
- Medication errors should be reported. Assessment of patient status before, during, and after the medication error, as well as specific orders carried out in response to the error, are important to include in this documentation.

NCLEX EXAMINATION REVIEW QUESTIONS

1 The nurse keeps in mind that measures to reduce the risk of medication errors include:
   a When questioning a drug order, keep in mind that the prescriber is correct.
   b Be careful about questioning the drug order a board-certified physician has written for a patient.
   c Always double-check the many drugs with sound-alike and look-alike names because of the high risk of error.
   d If the drug route has not been specified, use the oral route.
2 During the medication administration process, it is important that the nurse remembers which guideline?
   a When in doubt about a drug, ask a colleague about it before giving the drug.
   b Ask what the patient knows about the drug before giving it.
   c When giving a new drug, be sure to read about it after giving it.
   d If a patient expresses a concern about a drug, stop, listen, and investigate the concerns.
3 If a student nurse realizes that he or she has made a drug error, the instructor should remind the student of which concept?
   a The student bears no legal responsibility when giving medications.
   b The major legal responsibility lies with the health care institution at which the student is placed for clinical experience.
   c The major legal responsibility for drug errors lies with the faculty members.

   d Once the student has committed a medication error, his or her responsibility is to the patient and to being honest and accountable.
4 The nurse is giving medications to a newly admitted patient who is to receive nothing by mouth (NPO status) and finds an order written as follows: "Digoxin, 250 mcg stat." Which action is appropriate?
   a Give the medication immediately (stat) by mouth because the patient has no intravenous (IV) access at this time.
   b Clarify the order with the prescribing physician before giving the drug.
   c Ask the charge nurse what route the physician meant to use.
   d Start an IV line, then give the medication IV so that it will work faster, because the patient's status is NPO at this time.
5 Which digoxin dose is written correctly?
   a Digoxin .25 mg
   b Digoxin .250 mg
   c Digoxin 0.250 mg
   d Digoxin 0.25 mg
6 The nurse is administering medications. Examples of high-alert medications include: (Select all that apply.)
   a Insulins
   b Cancer chemotherapy drugs
   c Opiates
   d Anticoagulants
   e Potassium chloride for injection

1. c, 2. d, 3. d, 4. b, 5. d, 6. a, b, c, d, e.

CRITICAL THINKING ACTIVITIES: BEST ACTION

1 The physician has ordered a stat IV vancomycin infusion, but when the bag comes up from the pharmacy, the nurse notices that the dose is incorrect. It takes 2 hours for the pharmacy to send up an IV bag with the correct dose. While checking the medication, the nurse notes that it is the right drug, right dose, and so on, yet it has been 2 hours since it was ordered stat. What, if anything, should the nurse do before giving this medication?
2 Just after the nurse administers an oral antihypertensive drug, the patient asks, "Wasn't that supposed to be a half-tablet? I

just took the whole tablet!" The nurse realizes that the patient was given twice the ordered amount. The order was for 25 mg, a half-tablet, and the entire 50-mg tablet was given. What should the nurse say to the patient at this time?
3 The nurse is reviewing orders on a newly admitted patient and reads this order: "Humalog insulin, 4 U qd." What problems, if any, should the nurse see in this order?

For answers, see *http://evolve.elsevier.com/Lilley.*

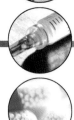

CHAPTER 7

Patient Education and Drug Therapy

OBJECTIVES

When you reach the end of this chapter, you should be able to do the following:

1 Discuss the importance of patient education in the safe and efficient administration of drugs (e.g., prescription drugs, over-the-counter drugs, herbal preparations, dietary supplements).

2 Summarize the various teaching and learning principles related patient education and drug therapy across the life span that are applicable in any health care setting.

3 Identify the impact of the various developmental phases (as described by Erikson) on patient education as it relates to drug therapy and the nursing process.

4 Develop a complete patient teaching plan as part of a comprehensive nursing care plan for drug therapy for the adult patient.

e-Learning Activities

http://evolve.elsevier.com/Lilley

NCLEX Review Questions • Animations • Nursing Care Plans • Audio Glossary • Category Catchers • Medication Errors Checklists • IV Therapy Checklists • Calculators • Frequently Asked Questions • Content Updates • Supplemental Resources • Answers to Case Studies and Critical Thinking Activities

Glossary

Affective domain The most intangible component of the learning process. Affective behavior is conduct that expresses feelings, needs, beliefs, values, and opinions. (p. 79)

Cognitive domain The domain involved in the learning and storage of basic knowledge. It is the thinking portion of the learning process and incorporates a person's previous experiences and perceptions. (p. 78)

Learning The acquisition of knowledge or skill. (p. 79)

Psychomotor domain The domain involved in the learning of a new procedure or skill; often called the *doing* domain. (p. 79)

Teaching A system of directed and deliberate actions intended to induce learning. (p. 79)

• • •

Given the constant change in today's health care climate and increased consumer awareness, the role of the nurse as an educator continues to increase and remains a significant part of patient care, both in and out of the hospital environment. Patient education is essential in any health care setting and is a critical component of safe and effective health care. Without patient education, the highest quality of care cannot be provided. Patient education is crucial for helping patients adapt to illness, prevent illness, maintain health and wellness, and provide self-care. Patient edu-

cation is a process—much like the nursing process in that it provides patients a framework of knowledge that assists them in learning healthy behaviors and assimilating these behaviors into their lifestyle.

For nurses, patient education may be one of the more satisfying aspects of patient care, because it is essential to improved health outcomes. In fact, in the current era of increasing acuteness of patient conditions and the need to decrease length of stays in hospitals, patient education and family teaching become even more essential to meet outcome criteria effectively and efficiently. Patient education has also been identified as a valued activity and one that brings professional satisfaction in professional nursing practice. In addition, patient education is a qualifier in professional and accreditation standards. Health teaching is not only included in the American Nurses Association document *Nursing: Scope and Standards of Practice* (2004) but is also one of the grading criteria used by The Joint Commission, which was formerly known as the Joint Commission on Accreditation for Healthcare Organizations (JCAHO, 2006).Contributing to the effectiveness of patient education is an understanding of and attention to the three domains of learning: the cognitive, affective, and psychomotor domains. One or a combination of these domains should be addressed in any patient educational session. The **cognitive domain** refers to the level at which basic knowledge is learned and stored. It is the thinking portion of the learning process and incorporates a person's previous experiences and perceptions. Previous experiences with health and wellness influence the learning of new materials, and prior knowledge and experience can serve as the foundation for adding new concepts. Thus, the learning process should begin with the identification of what experiences the person has had with the subject. The nurse should remember, however, that thinking involves more than the delivery of new information because a patient must build relationships between prior and new experiences to formulate new meanings. At a higher level in the thinking process, the new information is used to question something that is uncertain, to recognize when to seek additional information, and to make decisions during real-life situations.

The **affective domain** is the most intangible component of the learning process. Affective behavior is conduct that expresses feelings, needs, beliefs, values, and opinions. It is well known that individuals view events from different perspectives and often choose to internalize feelings rather than express them. Nurses must be willing to approach patients in a nonjudgmental fashion, listen to their concerns, recognize the nonverbal messages being given, and assess patient needs with an open mind. Should the nurse be successful in gaining the trust and confidence of patients and family members, it may have a powerful effect on their attitudes and thus on the learning process. The **psychomotor domain** involves the learning of a new procedure or skill and is often called the *doing* domain. Learning is generally accomplished by demonstration of the procedure or task using a step-by-step approach with return demonstrations by the learner to verify whether the procedure or skill has been mastered.

Using a teaching approach that engages these domains—whether one, two, or a combination of all—will certainly add to the quality and effectiveness of patient education sessions and subsequent learning.

The result of effective patient education is learning. **Learning** is defined as a change in behavior, and **teaching** as a sharing of knowledge. Although nurses may never be certain that patients will take medications as prescribed, they may carefully assess, plan, implement, and evaluate the teaching they provide to help maximize outcome criteria. Just like the nursing process, the medication administration process provides a systematic framework for professional nursing practice. The remainder of this chapter provides a brief look at patient education as related to the nursing process.

ASSESSMENT OF LEARNING NEEDS RELATED TO DRUG THERAPY

The patient education process is similar to the nursing process. A very important facet of the patient education process is a thorough assessment of learning needs to be completed before patients begin any form of drug therapy. This assessment, as related to patient education and drug therapy, should include gathering subjective and objective data about the following:

- Adaptation to any illnesses
- Barriers to learning (Box 7-1)
- Cognitive abilities
- Coping mechanisms
- Cultural background
- Developmental status for age group with attention to cognitive and mental processing abilities
- Education received including highest grade level completed and literacy level
- Emotional status
- Environment at home and work
- Folk medicine, home remedies, or use of alternative therapies (e.g., physical therapy, chiropractic, osteopathic medicine, meditation, yoga, aromatherapy)
- Family relationships
- Financial status

BOX 7-1 Strategies to Enhance Patient Education and Reduce Barriers to Learning

- Work with available educational resources in nursing and pharmacy to collect or order and distribute materials about drug therapy. Make sure that written materials are available to all individuals and are prepared on a reading level that is most representative of the geographical area, such as an eighth-grade reading level. Most acute care facilities and other health care facilities have electronic resources, so that printing educational materials is easy. Some examples of electronic or computerized programs are Micromedex and Lexi-PALS; these offer patient pamphlets that are in different languages and at appropriate reading levels.
- No English only! Be sure that written and verbal instructions are available in the language most commonly spoken, such as Spanish. Identify resources within the facility and in the community that can provide assistance with translation, such as nurses or other health care providers who are proficient in Spanish and other languages. Have the information available so that education is carried out in a timely and effective manner.
- Perform a cultural assessment that includes questions about level of education, learning experiences, past and present successes of therapies and medication regimens, language spoken, core beliefs, value system, meaning of health and illness, perceived cause of illness, family roles, social organization, and health practices or lack thereof.
- Make sure that written materials are available on the most commonly used medications and that all materials are updated annually to ensure that information is current.
- Have available information for patients on how they can prevent medication errors. The Institute for Safe Medication Practices offers informative pamphlets on the patient's role in preventing medica-

tion errors as well as web-based resources such as alerts for consumers with the proper citation.
- Work collaboratively in the health care setting, inpatient and outpatient, to develop a listing of medications that may be considered error prone, such as cardiac drugs, chemotherapeutic drugs, low molecular weight heparin, digoxin, metered-dose inhaled drugs, and acetaminophen. Lack of time for patient education is often a concern for nurses, but efforts should be undertaken to make materials available and to review these with patients and those involved in their care. Use all available resources, such as videotapes, verbal instructions, pictures, and other health care providers.
- For the adolescent, be sure to provide clear and simple directions for each medication, including clarification of information that may well be misinterpreted. For example, teenaged girls may have the false idea that oral contraceptives prevent them from contracting sexually transmitted diseases.
- Use readability tools in the development of patient education materials if you are involved in this process. Several tools are available, such as the SMOG (Simple Measure of Gobbledygook) readability measure and the Fry readability formula. It is important to know that evidenced-based measures such as these are available to help in the creation of written materials and verbal instructions for patients. Online resources include *http://www.utexas.edu/vp/ecs/communications/SMOG.pdf* and *http://www.idph.state.ai.us/health_literacy/common/pdf/tools/fry.pdf*.
- Never wait until discharge to teach patients. Include family or caregivers whenever possible, so that they become contributors to patient education and not barriers!

BOX 7-2 Erikson's Stages of Development

Infancy (birth to 1 year of age): Trust versus mistrust. Infant learns to trust himself or herself, others, and the environment; learns to love and be loved.

Toddlerhood (1 to 3 years of age): Autonomy versus shame and doubt. Toddler learns independence; learns to master the physical environment and maintain self-esteem.

Preschool age (3 to 6 years of age): Initiative versus guilt. Preschooler learns basic problem solving; develops conscience and sexual identity; initiates activities as well as imitates.

School age (6 to 12 years of age): Industry versus inferiority. School-aged child learns to do things well; develops a sense of self-worth.

Adolescence (12 to 18 years of age): Identity versus role confusion. Adolescent integrates many roles into self-identity through imitation of role models and peer pressure.

Young adulthood (18 to 45 years of age): Intimacy versus isolation. Young adult establishes deep and lasting relationships; learns to make commitment as a spouse, parent, and/or partner.

Middle adulthood (45 to 65 years of age): Generativity versus stagnation. Adult learns commitment to the community and world; is productive in career, family, and civic interests.

Older adulthood (over 65 years of age): Integrity versus despair. Older adult appreciates life role and status; deals with loss and prepares for death.

- Psychosocial growth and development level according to Erikson's stages (Box 7-2)
- Health beliefs, including beliefs about health, wellness, and/or illness
- Information the patient understands about past and present medical conditions, medical therapy, and medications
- Language(s) spoken
- Level of knowledge about any medications being taken
- Limitations (physical, psychologic, cognitive, and motor)
- Medications currently taken (including OTC drugs, prescription drugs, and herbal products)
- Misinformation about drug therapy
- Mobility and motor skills
- Motivation
- Nutritional status
- Past and present health behaviors
- Past and present experience with drug regimens and other forms of therapy, including levels of compliance
- Race and/or ethnicity
- Readiness to learn
- Religion or religious beliefs
- Self-care ability
- Sensory status
- Social support

During the assessment of learning needs, the nurse must be astutely aware of the patient's verbal and nonverbal communication. Often a patient will not tell the nurse how they truly feel. A seeming discrepancy is an indication that the patient's emotional or physical state may need to be further assessed in relation to their actual readiness and motivation for learning. Use of open-ended questions is encouraged, because they stimulate more discussion and greater clarification from the patient than closed-ended questions that require only a yes or no answer. Level of anxiety must also be assessed, because mild levels of anxiety have been identified as being motivating, whereas moderate to severe levels may be obstacles. In addition, if there are physical needs that are not being met, such as relief from pain, vomiting, or other physical distress, these needs become obstacles to learning. These physical issues should be managed appropriately before any patient teaching occurs.

NURSING DIAGNOSES RELATED TO LEARNING NEEDS AND DRUG THERAPY

Some of the most commonly used North American Nursing Diagnosis Association–approved nursing diagnoses related to patient education and drug therapy are the following (see Chapter 1 for a more complete listing):

- Deficient knowledge
- Ineffective health maintenance
- Ineffective self health management management
- Risk for injury
- Impaired memory
- Noncompliance

As an example of how nursing diagnoses related to patient education are derived, *deficient knowledge* refers to a situation in which the patient, caregiver, or significant other has a limited knowledge base or skills with regard to the medication or medication regimen. A nursing diagnosis of *deficient knowledge* develops out of objective and/or subjective data showing that there is limited, no understanding or misunderstanding of the medication and its action, indications, adverse reactions, toxic effects, drug-drug and/or drug-food interactions, cautions and contraindications. This diagnosis may also reflect decreased cognitive ability or impaired motor skill needed to perform self medication. *Deficient knowledge* differs from *noncompliance* in that the latter occurs when the patient does not take the medication as prescribed or at all—in other words, the patient does not comply with or adhere to the instructions given about the medication. Noncompliance (also called *nonadherence*) is usually a patient's choice. A nursing diagnosis of *noncompliance* is made when data collected from the patient show that the condition or symptoms for which the patient is taking the medication have recurred or were never resolved because the patient did not take the medication per the prescriber's orders or did not take the medication at all. Although noncompliance is usually a patient decision, other factors should always be assessed to determine the cause of the noncompliance (e.g., lack of ability of the parent, family, or caregiver to administer the medication; other physical, emotional, or socioeconomic factors).

PLANNING RELATED TO LEARNING NEEDS AND DRUG THERAPY

The planning phase of the teaching-learning process occurs as soon as a learning need has been assessed and then identified in the patient, family, or caregiver. With mutual understanding, the nurse and patient identify goals and outcome criteria that are associated with the identified nursing diagnosis and are able to relate them to the specific medication the patient is taking. The following is an example of a measurable goal with outcome criterion related to a nursing diagnosis of deficient knowledge for a patient who is self-administering an oral antidiabetic drug and has many questions about the medication therapy. *Sample goal:* The patient safely self-administers the prescribed oral antidiabetic drug within a given time frame. *Sample outcome criterion:* The patient remains without signs and symptoms of overmedication with an oral antidiabetic drug, such as hypoglycemia with tachycardia, palpitations, diaphoresis, hunger, and fatigue. When drug therapy goals and outcome criteria are developed, appropriate time frames for meeting outcome criteria should also be identified (see Chapter 1 for more information on the nursing process). In addition, goals and outcome criteria should be realistic, based on patient needs, stated in patient terms, and include behaviors that are measurable, such as *list, identify, demonstrate, self-administer, state, describe,* and *discuss.*

IMPLEMENTATION RELATED TO PATIENT EDUCATION AND DRUG THERAPY

After the nurse has completed the assessment phase, identified nursing diagnoses, and created a plan of care, the implementation phase of the teaching-learning process begins. This phase should include conveying specific information about the medication to the patient, family, or caregiver. Teaching-learning sessions should incorporate clear, simple, concise written instructions; oral instructions; and written pamphlets, pictures, videotapes, or any other learning aids that will help ensure patient learning. The nurse may have to conduct several brief teaching-learning sessions with multiple strategies, depending on the needs of the patient. Several changes related to the growth and aging of patients affect teaching-learning, and Table 7-1 lists educational strategies for accommodating these changes in a plan of care. The nurse may also need to identify aids to help the patient in the safe administration of medications at home, such as the use of

medication day or time calendars, pill reminder stickers, daily medication containers with alarms, weekly pill containers with separate compartments for different dosing times for each day for the week, and/or a method of documenting doses taken to avoid overdosage or omission of doses. Special issues arise when the patient speaks limited or no English. The nurse should communicate with the patient in the patient's native language if at all possible. If the nurse is not able to speak the patient's native language, a translator should be made available to prevent communication problems, minimize errors, and help boost the patient's level of trust and understanding of the nurse. In practice, this translator may be another nurse or health care professional, a nonprofessional member of the health care team, or a layperson, family member, adult friend, or religious leader or associate. The nurse should keep in mind that some of these individuals may not be competent in or comfortable with communicating technical clinical information, and other resources should be used if that is the case. As the United States experiences rapid growth in minority populations, our health care system will see a staggering increase in the percentage of non–English-speaking patients. According to the August 2008 projections of the U.S. Census Bureau, demographic changes will be significant, with minority groups—which currently comprise one third of the U.S. population—growing to become the majority by 2042 and projected to increase to 54% of the population by 2050. This growth in cultural diversity will continue to demand that nursing and related health care professions provide patient education materials in both English and Spanish. Publications provided for non–English-speaking patients may enable the nurse to convey a suf-

TABLE 7-1 Educational Strategies to Address Common Changes Related to Aging That May Influence Learning

Change Related to Aging	Educational Strategy
Cognitive and Memory Impairment	
Slowed cognitive functioning	Slow the pace of the presentation and attend to verbal and nonverbal patient cues to verify understanding.
Decreased short-term memory	Provide smaller amounts of information at one time. Repeat information frequently. Provide written instructions for home use.
Decreased ability to think abstractly	Use examples to illustrate information. Use a variety of methods, such as audiovisuals, props, videotapes, large-print materials, materials with vivid color, return demonstrations, and practice sessions.
Decreased ability to concentrate	Decrease external stimuli as much as possible.
Increased reaction time (slower to respond)	Always allow sufficient time and be patient. Allow more time for feedback.
Disturbed Sensory Perception	
Hearing Impairment	
Diminished hearing	Perform a baseline hearing assessment. Use tone- and volume-controlled teaching aids; use bright, large-print material to reinforce.
Decreased ability to distinguish sounds (e.g., differentiate words beginning with S, Z, T, D, F, and G)	Speak distinctly and slowly, and articulate carefully.
Decreased conduction of sound	Sit on the side of the patient's best ear.
Loss of ability to hear high-frequency sounds	Do not shout; speak in a normal voice but a lower voice pitch.
Partial to complete loss of hearing	Face the patient so that lip reading is possible. Use visual aids to reinforce verbal instruction. Reinforce teaching with easy-to-read materials. Decrease extraneous noise. Use community resources for the hearing impaired.
Visual Impairment	
Decreased visual acuity	Ensure that the patient's glasses are clean and in place and that the prescription is current.
Decreased ability to read fine detail	Use printed material with large print that is brightly and clearly colored.
Decreased ability to discriminate among blue, violet, and green; tendency for all colors to fade, with red fading the least	Use high-contrast materials, such as black on white. Avoid the use of blue, violet, and green in type or graphics; use red instead.
Thickening and yellowing of the lenses of the eyes, with decreased accommodation	Use nonglare lighting and avoid contrasts of light (e.g., darkened room with single light).
Decreased depth perception	Adjust teaching to allow for the use of touch to gauge depth.
Decreased peripheral vision	Keep all teaching materials within the patient's visual field.
Touch and Vibration Impairment	
Decreased sense of touch	Increase the time allowed for the teaching of psychomotor skills, the number of repetitions, and the number of return demonstrations.
Decreased sense of vibration	Teach the patient to palpate more prominent pulse sites (e.g., carotid and radial arteries).

Modified from Weinrich SP, Boyd M, Nussbaum J: Continuing education: adapting strategies to teach the elderly, *J Gerontol Nurs* 15(11):17-21, 1989; McKenry LM, Salerno E: *Mosby's pharmacology in nursing,* ed 22, St Louis, 2006, Mosby.
NOTE: These strategies may also be appropriate for younger patients.

CULTURAL IMPLICATIONS

Patient Education

The nurse must research various cultures to enhance an individualized approach to nursing care. For example, with Mexican American patients, aspects of nursing care must be approached in a sensitive manner with strong consideration for the family, communication needs, and religion. Approximately 90% of native Mexicans are Roman Catholic. To help meet the needs of these patients more effectively, the nurse should consider speaking with them about their desire for clergy visits while in the hospital. Family members are generally involved, and Mexican Americans often have large extended families; therefore, the nurse should take the time to include family members in the patient's care and when providing discharge instructions and medication instructions.

Modified from McKenry LM, Salerno E: *Mosby's pharmacology in nursing,* ed 22, St Louis, 2006, Mosby.

ficient amount of information in the patient's language to help effectively educate the patient and also allow the nurse to share materials with family members and caregivers for their use. Companies now also publish a variety of patient education materials for the discharge process in both English and Spanish.

Health care professionals who work in a geographic area where a variety of non-English languages are widely spoken should consider making an effort to learn one or more of these languages. Adult foreign language education is available in most U.S. cities, often at 2- and 4-year colleges or universities. Many classes are designed for working professionals and are scheduled at a variety of convenient times during the day and evening to accommodate demanding work schedules. Community colleges often offer quality courses that meet as little as 1 day or evening per week. Many employers will pay for job-related courses, and some courses may qualify for professional continuing education credits. Language courses provide a means of networking and

Patient Education and Anticoagulant Therapy

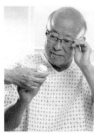

M.S., an 82-year-old retired librarian, has developed atrial fibrillation. As part of his medical therapy, he is started on the oral anticoagulant warfarin (Coumadin). His wife reports that he has some trouble hearing yet refuses to consider getting hearing aids. In addition, this is his first illness and his wife states that he has always "hated taking medications. He's read about herbs and folk healing and would rather try natural therapy." The nurse is planning education about oral anticoagulant ther-

© Supri Suharjoto

apy, and M.S. says that he'll "give it a try" for now, but he "knows nothing about this drug."

1. What should the nurse assess, including possible barriers to learning, before teaching?
2. Formulate an education-related nursing diagnosis for this patient based on the information given above. In addition, provide a goal and one example of an outcome criterion for the nursing diagnosis.
3. What education strategies should the nurse use, considering any age-related changes the patient may have?

For answers, see *http://evolve.elsevier.com/Lilley.*

Discharge Teaching

The safest practices for discharge teaching are the following:

- Always follow the health care facility's policy on discharge teaching with regard to how much information to impart to the patient.
- Do not assume that any patient has received adequate teaching before interacting with you.
- Always begin discharge teaching as soon as possible when the patient is ready.
- Minimize any distractions during the teaching session.
- Evaluate any teaching of the patient and/or significant others by having the individuals repeat the instructions you have given them.
- Contact the institution's social services department or the discharge planner if there are any concerns regarding the learning capacity of the patient.
- Document what you taught, who was present with the patient during the teaching, what specific written instructions were given, what the responses of the patient and significant other or caregiver were, and what your own nursing actions were, such as specific demonstrations or referrals to community resources.
- Document teaching-learning strategies used, such as videotapes and pamphlets.

Modified from U.S. Pharmacopeia Safe Medication Use Expert Committee Meeting, Rockville, Md, May 2003. Available at *http://www.usp.org.*

developing quality friendships with other highly motivated, empathic individuals both within and outside of the health care profession. A variety of self-study materials are also available.

Non–English-speaking patients tend to notice and appreciate their health professionals' efforts to speak their own language and will often help teach them new words or phrases, if there is enthusiasm and interest. This experience may lead to significantly greater rapport, put the patient at ease, and show respect for their culture or race/ethnicity. Obtaining and keeping available a foreign language dictionary may be helpful. Keeping notes about newly learned words, phrases, or sentences may be helpful, too. Even if the professional does not use the correct verb tenses, they may often communicate sufficiently with the patient for the purpose at hand. As one begins to learn a foreign language, a major challenge may be to speak with a patient over the phone. The important goal is to try to increase one's *listening* speed to match the *speaking* speed of the patient. With effort, this *can* be accomplished. If one can grasp even a few words of what the patient is saying, one may be able, with continued conversation with the patient, to determine and respond to the patient's needs. However, be aware that patients who are native English speakers may also have problems learning about their medications and treatment regimens because of learning deficits or difficulties, hearing and speech deficits, lack of education, or minimal previous exposure to treatment regimens and medication use.

The teaching of manual skills for specific medication administration is also part of the teaching-learning session. Sufficient time should be allowed for the patient to become familiar with any equipment and to perform several return demonstrations to the nurse or other health care provider. Teaching-learning needs will vary from patient to patient. Family members, significant others, or caregivers should also be included in this session or sessions for

reinforcement purposes. Audiovisual aids may be incorporated and based on findings from the learning needs and nursing assessment. Resources for information about medications include *USP Drug Information* volume II, *Advice for the Patient,* which is published annually (along with the *Health Care Professional* volume) by Thomson Micromedex; this information would be appropriate to share with the patient. This type of resource may be helpful to the patient when he or she seeks information about a medication (e.g., purpose, adverse effects, method of administration, drug interactions) and helpful to the nurse in developing a patient teaching plan. A safe, nonthreatening, nondistracting environment for learning should be created as well as being open and receptive to the patient's questions. The following strategies may help ensure an effective teaching-learning session:

- Begin the teaching-learning process upon the patient's admission to the health care setting (see Legal and Ethical Principles box).
- Individualize the teaching session to the patient.
- Provide positive rewards or reinforcement after accurate return demonstration of a procedure, technique, and/or skill during the teaching session.
- Complete a medication calendar that includes the names of the drugs to be taken along with the dosage and frequency. Allow the patient to see what the medications look like for future reference.
- Use audiovisual aids.
- Involve family members or significant others in the teaching session, as deemed appropriate.
- Keep the teaching on a level that is most meaningful to the given patient; general research on reading skills has shown that materials should be written at an eighth-grade reading level.

BOX 7-3 General Teaching and Learning Principles

- Make learning patient centered and individualized to each patient's needs, including his or her learning needs. This includes assessment of the patient's cultural beliefs, educational level, previous experience with medications, level of growth and development (to best select a teaching-learning strategy), age, gender, family support system, resources, ability to learn and way he or she learns best, and level of sophistication with regard to health care and own health care treatment.
- Assess the patient's motivation and readiness to learn.
- Assess the patient's ability to use and interpret label information on medication containers.
- Some studies have shown that as much as 20% of the U.S. population is functionally illiterate. Therefore, ensure that educational strategies and materials are at a level that the patient is able to understand, while taking care to not embarrass the patient.
- If a patient is illiterate, he or she still needs to be instructed on safe medication administration. Use pictures, demonstrations, and return demonstrations to emphasize instructions.
- Consider, assess, and appreciate language and ethnicity during patient teaching. Make every effort to educate non–English-speaking

patients in their native language. Ideally the patient should be instructed by a health professional familiar with the patient's clinical situation who also speaks the patient's native language. At the very least, provide the patient detailed written instructions in his or her native language.
- Assess the family support system for adequate patient teaching. Family living arrangements, financial status, resources, communication patterns, the roles of family members, and the power and authority of different family members should always be considered.
- Make the teaching-learning session simple, easy, fun, thorough, effective, and not monotonous. Make it applicable to daily life and schedule it at a time when the patient is ready to learn.
- Remember that learning occurs best with repetition and periods of demonstration and with the use of audiovisuals and other educational aids.
- Patient teaching should focus on the various processes in the cognitive, affective, and/or psychomotor domains (see earlier discussion).
- Consult online resources for help in obtaining the most up-to-date and accurate patient teaching materials and information.

Box 7-3 lists some general teaching and learning principles for the nurse to consider in providing patient education.

Upon completion of any teaching-learning process or patient education session, documentation should be completed and should include notes about the content provided, strategies used, and patient response to the teaching session, and an overall evaluation of learning. Because of the significance of patient education related to drug therapy and the nursing process, this textbook integrates patient education into each chapter in the implementation phase of the nursing process. In addition, a Patient Teaching Tips section is included at the end of most chapters.

EVALUATION OF PATIENT LEARNING RELATED TO DRUG THERAPY

Evaluation of patient learning is a critical component of safe and effective drug administration. To verify the success—or lack of success—of patient education, nurses should always ask specific questions related to patient outcomes and request that the patient repeat information or give a return demonstration of skills, if appropriate. The patient's behavior—such as adherence to the schedule for medication administration with few or no complications—is one key to determining whether or not teaching was successful and learning occurred. If a patient's behavior evidences noncompliance or an inadequate level of learning, a new plan of teaching should be developed, implemented, and evaluated.

SUMMARY

Patient education is a critical part of patient care, and patient education about medication administration, therapies, or regimens is no exception. From the time of initial contact with the patient throughout the time the nurse works with the patient, the patient is entitled to all information about medications prescribed

as well as other aspects of his or her care. Evaluation of patient learning and compliance with the medication regimen should be a continuous process, and the nurse should always be willing to listen to the patient about any aspect of the patient's drug therapy. Professional nurses are teachers and serve as patient advocates and thus have a responsibility to facilitate learning for patients and families. Accurate assessment of learning needs and readiness to learn always requires a look at the whole patient, including cultural values, health practices, and literacy issues. Every effort should be made to see that the patient receives effective learning to ensure successful outcomes with regard to drug therapy—and all parts of the patient's health care.

It is important to consult the resources mentioned earlier, as well as the U.S. Pharmacopeia (at *http://www.usp.org*) which serves as an advocate for patient safety and establishes standards for medications. This organization is a tremendous resource for the health care professional in obtaining information for the patient so that quality patient education can be provided. The U.S. Pharmacopeia values patient education as a means of enhancing patient safety as well as a means of decreasing medication errors in the hospital setting or at home. In addition, the Institute for Safe Medication Practices (at *http://www.ismp.org*) provides nurses with a wealth of information related to patient education, safety, and prevention of medication errors. As a nonprofit organization, this institute works closely with nurses, prescribers, regulatory agencies, and professional organizations to provide education about medication errors and their prevention, and is a premier resource in all matters pertaining to safe medication practices in health care organizations. In summary, it is professional nurses who usually have the most contact with patients and see patients in a variety of settings, and because of this nurses need to continue to be patient advocates and take the initiative to plan, design, create, and present educational materials for teaching about drug therapy.

PATIENT TEACHING TIPS

- Teaching needs to focus on either the cognitive, affective, or psychomotor domain or a combination of all three. The cognitive domain may involve recall for synthesis of facts, with the affective domain involving behaviors such as responding, valuing, and organizing. The psychomotor domain includes teaching someone how to perform a procedure.
- Realistic patient teaching goals and outcome criteria should be established with the involvement of the patient, caregiver, or significant other.

- Keep patient teaching on a level that is most meaningful to the individual. Most research indicates that reading materials should be written at an eighth-grade reading level but should be adjusted accordingly to patient assessment.
- Follow teaching and learning principles when developing and implementing patient education.

POINTS TO REMEMBER

- The effectiveness of patient education relies on an understanding of and attention to the cognitive, affective, and psychomotor domains of learning. After the nurse has completed the assessment phase, identified nursing diagnoses, and created a plan of care, the implementation phase of the teaching-learning process begins; reevaluation of the teaching plan should occur frequently and as needed. The growth in cultural diversity, in particular the increase in the Hispanic population, demands that nursing and related health care professions provide patient education materials in both English and Spanish.
- In educational sessions, patients need to receive information through as many senses as possible, such as verbally and visually

(as through pamphlets, videotapes, and diagrams), to maximize learning. Information should also be on the patient's reading level, in the patient's native language (if possible), and suitable for the patient's level of cognitive development (see Erikson's stages in Box 7-2).
- Teaching and learning principles should also be integrated into patient education plans. Evaluation of patient learning is a critical component of safe and effective drug administration.
- To verify the success—or lack of success—of patient education, nurses should always ask specific questions related to patient outcomes and request the patient repeat information or perform a return demonstration of skills, if appropriate.

NCLEX EXAMINATION REVIEW QUESTIONS

1 A 47-year-old patient with diabetes is being discharged to home and must take insulin injections twice a day. The nurse keeps in mind which concepts when considering patient teaching?
  a Teaching should begin at the time of diagnosis or admission and should be individualized to the patient's reading level.
  b The nurse can assume that because the patient is in his forties he will be able to read any written or printed documents provided.
  c The majority of the teaching can be done with pamphlets that the patient can share with family members.
  d A thorough and comprehensive teaching plan designed for an eleventh-grade reading level should be developed.
2 The nurse is developing a discharge plan regarding a patient's medication. The plan should
  a be developed right before the patient leaves the hospital.
  b be developed only after the patient is comfortable or after pain medications are administered.
  c include videotapes, demonstrations, and instructions written at least at the fifth-grade level.
  d be individualized and based on the patient's level of cognitive development.
3 The nurse is responsible for preoperative teaching for a patient who is mildly anxious about receiving opioids postoperatively. The nurse recognizes that this level of anxiety may
  a impede learning because anxiety is always a barrier to learning.
  b lead to major emotional unsteadiness.
  c result in learning by increasing the patient's willingness to learn.
  d reorganize the patient's thoughts and lead to inadequate potential for learning.

4 What action by the nurse is the best way to assess a patient's learning needs?
  a Quiz the patient daily on all medications
  b Begin with validation of the patient's present level of knowledge
  c Assess family members' knowledge of the prescribed medication even if they are not involved in the patient's care
  d Question other caregivers about their level of experience with the drug regimen and assume lack of interest if no answers are given
5 Which technique would be most appropriate to use when the nurse is teaching a patient with a potential language barrier?
  a Obtain an interpreter who can speak in the patient's native tongue for teaching sessions
  b Use detailed explanations, speaking slowly and clearly
  c Assume that the patient understands the information presented if the patient has no questions
  d Provide only written instructions
6 A nursing student is identifying situations that involve the psychomotor domain of learning as part of a class project. Which are examples of learning activities that involve the psychomotor domain? (Select all that apply.)
  a Teaching a patient how to self-administer eyedrops
  b Having a patient list the adverse effects of an antihypertensive drug
  c Discussing what foods to avoid while taking antilipemic drugs
  d Teaching a patient how to measure the pulse before taking a beta-blocker
  e Teaching a family member how to give an injection
  f Teaching a patient the rationale for checking a drug's blood level

CRITICAL THINKING ACTIVITIES: BEST ACTION

1 A 65-year-old woman with diabetes mellitus is to begin treatment with insulin injections. Using the guidelines and principles for patient education discussed in this chapter, develop a 10-minute teaching plan on the basics of subcutaneous self-administration of insulin.

2 A nurse has been trying to communicate with a patient who does not speak English, but so far none of the communication techniques has been successful. What are the best strategies the nurse can use to develop a plan of care that addresses the patient's need for medication information on the cardiac drug digoxin and also focuses on the potential for toxicity? (Note: You may need to look up the drug in the textbook if you are not familiar with it.)

3 A patient has had hip replacement surgery and will be going home in a few days. The surgeon has requested that the nurses teach the patient and a family member how to give subcutaneous injections of the low molecular weight heparin that will be prescribed for him after his discharge. When is the best time for the nurse to begin this patient education? Explain.

For answers, see *http://evolve.elsevier.com/Lilley.*

CHAPTER 8

Over-the-Counter Drugs and Herbal and Dietary Supplements

OBJECTIVES

When you reach the end of this chapter, you should be able to do the following:

1 Discuss the differences between prescription drugs, over-the-counter (OTC) drugs, herbals, and dietary supplements.

2 Briefly discuss the differences between the federal legislation governing the promotion and sale of prescription drugs and the legislation governing OTC drugs, herbals, and dietary supplements.

3 Describe the advantages and disadvantages of the use of OTC drugs, herbals, and dietary supplements.

4 Discuss the role of nonprescription drugs, specifically herbals and dietary supplements, in the integrative (often called *alternative* or *complementary*) approach to nursing and health care.

5 Discuss the potential dangers associated with the use of OTC drugs, herbals, and dietary supplements.

6 Develop a nursing care plan related to OTC, herbal, and dietary supplement drug therapy and the nursing process.

e-Learning Activities

http://evolve.elsevier.com/Lilley

NCLEX Review Questions • Animations • Nursing Care Plans • Audio Glossary • Category Catchers • Medication Errors Checklists • IV Therapy Checklists • Calculators • Frequently Asked Questions • Content Updates • Supplemental Resources • Answers to Case Studies and Critical Thinking Activities

Glossary

Alternative medicine Herbal medicine, chiropractic, acupuncture, reflexology, and any other therapies traditionally not emphasized in Western medical schools but popular with many patients. (p. 90)

Complementary medicine *Alternative medicine* when used simultaneously with, rather than instead of, standard Western medicine. (p. 90)

Conventional medicine The practice of medicine as taught in Western medical schools. (p. 90)

Dietary supplement A product taken by mouth that contains an ingredient intended to supplement the diet, including vitamins, minerals, herbs or other botanicals, amino acids, and substances such as enzymes, organ tissues, glandular preparations, metabolites, extracts, and concentrates. (p. 90)

Herbal medicine The practice of using herbs to heal. (p. 90)

Herbs Plant components including bark, roots, leaves, seeds, flowers, and fruit of trees, shrubs, and woody vines, and extracts of these plants and materials that are valued for their savory, aromatic, or medicinal qualities. (p. 90)

Iatrogenic effects Unintentional adverse effects that are caused by the actions of a prescriber or other health care professional or by a specific treatment. (p. 90)

Legend drugs Medications that are not legally available without a prescription from a prescriber (e.g., physician, nurse practitioner, physician assistant; also called *prescription drugs*). (p. 91)

Over-the-counter (OTC) drugs Medications that are legally available without a prescription. (p. 87)

Phytochemicals The pharmacologically active ingredients in herbal remedies. (p. 92)

• • •

OVER-THE-COUNTER DRUGS

Health care consumers are becoming increasingly involved in the diagnosis and treatment of common ailments. This has led to a great increase in the use of nonprescription or **over-the-counter (OTC) drugs.** More than 80 classes of OTC drugs are marketed to treat a variety of illnesses ranging from acne to cough and cold, pain relief, and weight control. There are currently more than 300,000 OTC products containing over 800 major active ingredients. OTC medications now account for about 60% of all medications used in the United States. Health care consumers use OTC drugs to treat or cure more than 400 different ailments. Over 700 medications that formerly required a prescription are now available OTC. Some 40% to 87% of people aged 65 or older living in the community use one OTC product regularly, and 5.7% take five or more OTC or dietary supplements daily.

For nurses to understand current OTC classification, it is helpful to have some knowledge of the U.S. Food and Drug Administration (FDA) approval process for OTC medications. In 1972 the FDA initiated an OTC Drug Review to ensure the safety and effectiveness of the OTC products available at that time as well as to establish appropriate labeling standards for these drugs. As a result of this review, approximately one third of the more than 500 OTC products then available were determined to be safe and effective for their intended uses and one third were found to be ineffective. A small number were considered to be unsafe, and the remainder required submission of

---

BOX 8-1 Criteria for Over-the-Counter Status

Indication for Use
- Consumer must be able to easily
  - Diagnose condition
  - Monitor effectiveness
- Benefits of correct usage must outweigh risks

Safety Profile
Drug should have
- Favorable adverse event profile
- Limited interaction with other drugs
- Low potential for abuse
- High therapeutic index*

Practicality for Over-the-Counter Use
Drug should be
- Easy to use
- Easy to monitor

*Ratio of toxic to therapeutic dosage.

BOX 8-2 Reclassified Over-the-Counter Products

Analgesics
ibuprofen (Advil, Motrin)
ketoprofen (Orudis KT)
naproxen sodium (Aleve, Naprosyn)

Histamine Blockers
H_1 Receptors
chlorpheniramine maleate (Chlor-Trimeton)
diphenhydramine hydrochloride (Benadryl)
loratadine (Claritin)
cetirizine (Zyrtec)

H_2 Receptors
cimetidine (Tagamet HB)
famotidine (Pepcid AC)
nizatidine (Axid AR)
ranitidine (Zantac)

Proton Pump Inhibitors
omeprazole (Prilosec-OTC)

Smoking Deterrents
nicotine polacrilex gum (Nicorette)
nicotine transdermal patches (Nicoderm) (other dosage forms available)

Topical Medications
clotrimazole (Lotrimin)
miconazole (Monistat)
minoxidil solution and hydrocortisone acetate 1% cream (Rogaine)

Weight Loss Products
orlistat (Allī)

---

additional data before their safety and effectiveness could be established. Products determined to be unsafe were removed from the market. Some established products that were found to be ineffective but not unsafe were "grandfathered" in and allowed to remain on the market. Many of these have gradually slipped into obscurity and are no longer sold. As of 2006, the FDA required new, stricter "drug facts" labeling for OTC products that includes information in the following categories: uses, directions for use, active ingredients, warnings, storage information, and inactive ingredients. According to a report of the Institute for Safe Medication Practices, one study found that parents gave children incorrect doses of OTC fever medications over 50% of the time. Use of OTC medications can be hazardous for patients with various chronic illnesses, including diabetes, enlarged prostate, hypertension, cardiovascular disease, and glaucoma. Patients are encouraged to read labels carefully and consult a qualified health professional when in doubt.

Another result of the OTC Drug Review was the reclassification from prescription to OTC status of more than 40 primary product ingredients. The FDA's Nonprescription Drugs Advisory Committee is responsible for the reclassification of prescription drug products to OTC status. A drug must meet the criteria listed in Box 8-1 to be considered for reclassification. The required information is obtained from clinical trial results and postmarketing safety surveillance data, which are submitted to the FDA by the manufacturer. Drug manufacturers often test consumers' ability to understand label instructions and even include consumers who should *not* use a given product due to their health conditions. Although this reclassification procedure has been criticized as overly time consuming, it is structured to ensure that products reclassified to OTC status are safe and effective when used by the average consumer.

OTC status has many advantages over prescription status. Patients can conveniently and effectively self-treat many minor ailments. Some professionals argue that allowing patients to self-treat minor illnesses enables prescribers to spend more time caring for patients with serious health problems. Others argue that it delays patients from seeking medical care until they are very ill.

The financial effect of this status change is enormous: by the year 2010, OTC sales in the United States will reach an estimated $22 billion. Manufacturers often benefit by prolonging market exclusivity without competition from generic products.

Reclassification of a prescription drug as an OTC drug may increase out-of-pocket costs for many patients because third-party health insurance payers usually do not cover OTC products. However, overall health care costs tend to decrease when products are reclassified as OTC due to a direct reduction in drug costs, elimination of prescriber office visits, and avoidance of pharmacy dispensing fees. A case in point is the reclassification of cough and cold products to OTC status. This reclassification resulted in annual consumer health care savings of approximately $1 billion. Some examples of drugs that have recently been reclassified as OTC products appear in Box 8-2.

The importance of patient education cannot be overstated. Many patients are inexperienced in the interpretation of medication labels, which results in misuse of the products (Figure 8-1). This lack of experience as well as possibly deficient knowledge about the medication may lead to adverse events or drug interactions with prescription medications or even other OTC medications. Small print on OTC package labels often complicates the situation, especially for elderly patients. Another problem associated with OTC drugs is that their use may postpone effective management of chronic disease states and may delay treatment of serious and/or life-threatening disorders. This is because the OTC medication may relieve symptoms without necessarily

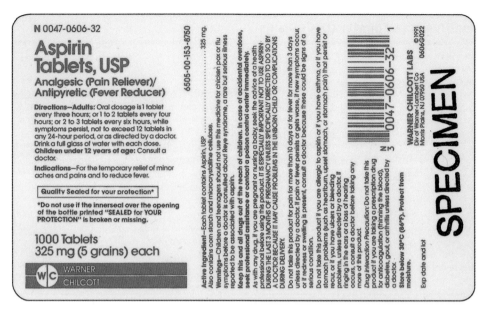

FIGURE 8-1   Example of an over-the-counter drug label.

addressing the cause of the disorder. This situation is often complicated when patients are afraid to visit a provider, are uninsured and have difficulty paying out of pocket for health care services, or simply want to avoid the inconvenience of visiting a provider and instead are hoping for a "quick fix" for themselves or their children.

OTC medications also have their own toxicity profiles. For example, cough and cold products usually include one or more of the following ingredients: nasal decongestants (for stuffy nose), expectorants (for loosening chest mucus), antihistamines (for sneezing and runny nose), and antitussives (for cough). In 2008, the FDA issued recommendations that OTC cough and cold products not be used in children under 2 years of age. This followed numerous case reports of symptoms such as oversedation, seizures, tachycardia, and even death in toddlers medicated with such products. There is also evidence that such medications are simply not efficacious in small children, and parents are advised to consult their pediatricians on the best ways to manage these illnesses. The FDA continues to evaluate the safety and efficacy of cough and cold products for children aged 2 to 11 years but has issued no guidelines to date. However, parents are advised to be mindful of how much medication they give to their children and to be careful not to give two products that contain the same active ingredient(s). Two other major current examples of OTC drug hazards include OTC products containing acetaminophen (e.g., Tylenol) and *nonsteroidal antiinflammatory drugs (NSAIDs)* such as ibuprofen (e.g., Advil, Motrin) and naproxen (e.g., Aleve). Hepatic toxicity is associated with excessive doses of acetaminophen. Acetaminophen doses should not exceed a total of 4 g/day, and some experts recommended not exceeding 3 g/day in elderly patients. A 2005 study showed that OTC acetaminophen use accounted for more than 40% of U.S. cases of acute liver failure. Gastrointestinal ulceration, myocardial infarction, and stroke are risks with NSAIDs. Patients may sometimes choose

excessive dosages of these and other OTC medications out of ignorance or simply in hopes of easing their symptoms. The FDA is currently considering mandatory new product labeling to enhance consumer awareness of these risks. Another interesting example of the potential hazards of OTC drug products is the nasal decongestant pseudoephedrine. Found in a variety of cough and cold products, this drug is also used to manufacture the widely abused street drug methamphetamine. For this reason, products containing pseudoephedrine must be sold from behind the pharmacy counter, and patients must sign a log book held by the pharmacist (see Chapter 9). OTC nasal sprays can cause rebound congestion and dependency.

Normally, OTC medications should be used only for short-term treatment of common minor illnesses. An appropriate medical evaluation should be sought for all chronic health conditions, even if the final decision is to prescribe OTC medications. Patient assessment should include questions regarding OTC drug use, including what conditions OTC medications are being used to treat. Such questions may help uncover more serious ongoing medical problems. Patients should be informed that OTC medications, including herbal products, are still medications. Because of this, their use may have associated risks depending on the specific OTC drugs used, concurrent prescription medications, and the patient's overall health status and disease states.

Health care professionals have an excellent opportunity to prevent common problems associated with the use of reclassified drugs. Up to 60% of patients consult a health care professional when selecting an OTC product. Patients should be provided with information about choice of an appropriate product, correct dosing, common adverse effects, and drug interactions with other medications.

For specific information on various OTC drugs, see the appropriate drug chapters later in this text. (Table 8-1 provides cross-references to these chapters.)

TABLE 8-1 Common Over-the-Counter (OTC) Drugs

Type of OTC Drug	Examples	Where Discussed in This Book
Acid-controlling drugs (H$_2$ blockers), antacids, and proton pump inhibitors	cimetidine (Tagamet HB), famotidine (Pepcid AC), nizatidine (Axid AR), ranitidine (Zantac); aluminum- and magnesium-containing products (Maalox, Mylanta); calcium-containing products (Tums), omeprazole (Prilosec-OTC)	Chapter 50: Acid-Controlling Drugs
Antifungal drugs (topical)	clotrimazole (Lotrimin), miconazole (Monistat)	Chapter 56: Dermatologic Drugs
Antihistamines and decongestants	brompheniramine (Dimetapp), cetirizine (Zyrtec) chlorpheniramine (Contac, Theraflu), diphenhydramine (Benadryl), guaifenesin (Robitussin), loratadine (Claritin), pseudoephedrine (Sudafed)	Chapter 36: Antihistamines, Decongestants, Antitussives, and Expectorants
Eyedrops	artificial tears (Moisture Eyes, Murine)	Chapter 57: Ophthalmic Drugs
Hair growth drugs (topical)	minoxidil (Rogaine)	Chapter 56: Dermatologic Drugs
Pain-relieving drugs		
Analgesics	acetaminophen (Tylenol)	Chapter 11: Analgesic Drugs
Nonsteroidal antiinflammatory drugs	aspirin, ibuprofen (Advil, Motrin), naproxen sodium (Aleve)	Chapter 44: Antiinflammatory and Antigout Drugs

HERBALS AND DIETARY SUPPLEMENTS

History

Dietary supplement is a broad term for orally administered alternative medicines and includes the category of herbal supplement. Basic definitions are provided here to ensure complete understanding and to prevent confusion in how these terms are used. Dietary supplements are products taken by mouth that contain ingredients intended to augment the diet and include vitamins, minerals, herbs or other botanicals, amino acids, and substances such as enzymes, organ tissues, glandular products, metabolites, extracts, and concentrates. Dietary supplements may be produced in many forms, such as tablets, capsules, softgels, gelcaps, liquids, and powders. These supplements may also be found in nutritional, breakfast, snack, or health food bars, drinks, and shakes. Labeling is required by law but must *not* represent the product to be a conventional food item.

Herbs come from nature and include the leaves, bark, berries, roots, gums, seeds, stems, and flowers of plants. They have been used for thousands of years to help maintain good health. Herbs have been an integral part of society because of their culinary and medicinal properties, and herbs have made numerous contributions to the commercial drug preparations that are currently manufactured. About 30% of all modern drugs are derived from plants (Table 8-2). In the early nineteenth century, scientific methods became more advanced and became the preferred means of healing. At this time, the practice of botanical healing was dismissed as quackery. **Herbal medicine** lost ground to new synthetic medicines as the development of patent medicines grew during the early part of the twentieth century. These new synthetically derived medicines were touted by scientists and physicians as more effective and reliable.

In the 1960s, concerns were expressed over the **iatrogenic effects** of **conventional medicine.** These concerns, along with a desire for more self-reliance, led to a renewed interest in "natural health," and as a result the use of herbal products increased. In

TABLE 8-2 Conventional Medicines Derived from Plants

Medicine*	Plant
atropine	*Atropa belladonna*
capsaicin	*Capsicum frutescens*
cocaine	*Erythroxylon coca*
codeine	*Papaver somniferum*
ipecac	*Cephaelis ipecacuanha*
quinine	*Cinchona officinalis*
scopolamine	*Datura fastuosa*
senna	*Cassia acutifolia*
paclitaxel	*Taxis brevifolia*
vincristine	*Catharanthus roseus*

*Includes both over-the-counter and prescription drugs.

1974 the World Health Organization encouraged developing countries to use traditional plant medicines. In 1978 the German equivalent of the FDA published a series of herbal recommendations known as the *Commission E monographs.* These monographs focus on herbs whose effectiveness for specific indications is supported by the research literature. Worldwide use of herbal medicines again became popular. Recognition of the rising use of herbal products and other nontraditional remedies, known as **alternative medicine,** led to the establishment of the Office of Alternative Medicine by the National Institutes of Health in 1992. This office was later renamed the National Center for Complementary and Alternative Medicine (NCCAM). **Complementary medicine** refers to the simultaneous use of both traditional and alternative medicine. This practice is also referred to as *integrative medicine.* NCCAM classifies complementary and alternative medicine into the following five categories: (1) alternative medical systems, (2) mind-body interventions, (3) biologically based therapies, (4) manipulative and body-based methods, and (5) energy therapies.

Many controversies remain about the safety and control of herbals and dietary supplements, although they continue to be used in the United States and abroad. Their uses and touted advantages are widely publicized. As a result, these products are sold in grocery stores, pharmacies, health food stores, and fitness gyms, and can even be ordered through television, radio, and the Internet. With greater use, their therapeutic effects have been acknowledged, and they are believed by some to be more beneficial than existing synthetic and natural prescription drugs. Adverse effects are considered to be minimal by the public as well as by the companies and businesses that sell these supplements. However a false sense of security has been created by their widespread use and the view of the public tends to be that if a product is "natural," then it is safe.

For many years, neither federal legislation nor the FDA provided any safeguards and monitoring of dietary supplements. Instead, manufacturers were responsible only for ensuring product safety and for not making unproven claims about their efficacy. In 1993, FDA Commissioner David Kessler threatened to remove dietary supplements from the market. The American public reacted with a massive letter-writing campaign to Congress, and the 103rd Congress responded by passing the Dietary Supplement and Health Education Act (DSHEA) of 1994. The DSHEA defined dietary supplements and provided a regulatory framework. In 2002, the U.S. Pharmacopeia, an independent organization that is the government's official standard-setting authority for dietary supplements, announced that it had begun to issue certification for hundreds of products that it had independently tested as part of its Dietary Supplement Verification Program. In June 2007, the FDA announced that all manufacturers of dietary supplements would be required to comply with current *good manufacturing practices* by 2010. Under these new requirements, manufacturers must provide data that demonstrate product identity, composition, quality, purity, and strength of active ingredients. They must also demonstrate that products are free from contaminants such as microbes, pesticides, and heavy metals (e.g., lead).

A major difference between **legend drugs** (prescription drugs) and dietary supplements is that the DSHEA requires no proof of efficacy or safety and sets no standards for quality control for products labeled as supplements. In contrast, the FDA has specific and stringent requirements for manufacturers of legend drugs. Manufacturers of supplements may claim an effect but cannot promise a specific cure on the product label. Unlike legend drugs, dietary supplements do not need approval from the FDA before they are marketed. A manufacturer does not have to provide the FDA with the evidence on which it relies to substantiate the safety or effectiveness of a product before or after it markets the product, except in the case of a new dietary ingredient. The FDA does post recent warnings on herbal products on its website *(http://www.fda.gov)*. In contrast, regulating agencies in Germany, France, the United Kingdom, and Canada require manufacturers to meet standards of herbal quality and safety.

Consumer Use of Dietary Supplements

Estimates of consumer use of dietary supplements indicate that they are used by 12% to 61% of adults. In a 2006 *Consumer Reports* paper it was reported that 40% of U.S. adults have used alternative medicine, and that one fourth of the 44 million people who use them experience adverse reactions. In general, consumers use dietary supplements therapeutically for the treatment of diseases and pathologic conditions, prophylactically for long-term prevention of disease, and proactively to preserve health and wellness and boost the immune system (e.g., reduce cardiovascular risk factors, increase liver and immune system functions, increase feelings of wellness). In addition, herbs and phytomedicinals may be used as adjunct therapy to support conventional pharmaceutical therapies. Such use is seen especially in societies in which phytotherapy, or the use of herbal medicines in clinical practice, is considerably more integrated with conventional medicine, such as in Germany.

Some herbal products may be used to treat minor conditions and illnesses (e.g., coughs, colds, stomach upset) in much the same way that conventional FDA-approved OTC nonprescription drugs are used. As the number of herbal products on the market increases, nurses will need to respond to patients' educational needs about these products.

Safety

Dietary supplements, and especially herbal medicines, are often perceived as being natural and therefore harmless; however, this is not the case. Many examples exist of allergic reactions, toxic reactions, and adverse effects caused by herbs. Some herbs have been shown to have possible mutagenic effects and to interact with drugs (see the Herbal Therapies and Dietary Supplements box for drug interactions with herbal and dietary supplements). It is estimated that 70% of patients using dietary supplements do not disclose this to their health care providers. In addition, one study identified a relatively low level of knowledge of these products and their risks, even among regular users. This demonstrates the need for health care providers to develop a clinical knowledge base regarding these products and know where to find key information as the need arises. Cases have also been reported in which whole plants or parts of plants have not been identified properly and thus are mislabeled. Because of underreporting, present knowledge may represent but a small fraction of potential safety concerns. Also, as mentioned previously, the FDA has limited oversight of how dietary supplements are prepared, whether herbal or not.

There are certainly fewer published scientific data regarding the relative safety of dietary supplements than regarding the safety of synthetic drugs. Two recent examples indicating some of the growing concerns about herbal remedies include the FDA warnings about possible liver toxicity with the use of kava and possible cardiovascular and stroke risks with the use of ephedra. Sale of ephedra was officially banned by the FDA in April 2004. Kava remains on the market despite a 2002 FDA consumer warning letter regarding the risk of liver toxicity. Health care providers should be on the alert for announcements about the safe and effective use of dietary supplements as well as reported adverse effects or problems. For some dietary supplements, the risk may be lower than that for conventional drugs. The discriminating and proper use of some dietary supplements is safe and may provide some therapeutic benefits, but the indiscriminate or excessive use of dietary supplements can be dangerous. The FDA has established MedWatch, which has a toll-free number (800-332-1088) consumers can call to report adverse effects of dietary supplements or of any drugs or medical devices.

HERBAL THERAPIES AND DIETARY SUPPLEMENTS

Selected Herbs and Dietary Supplements and Their Possible Drug Interactions

Herb or Dietary Supplement	Possible Drug Interaction
Chamomile	Increased risk for bleeding with anticoagulants
Cranberry	Decreased elimination of many drugs that are renally excreted
Echinacea	Possible interference with or counteraction to immunosuppressant drugs
Evening primrose	Possible interaction with antipsychotic drugs
Garlic	Possible interference with hypoglycemic therapy
Ginger root	At high dosages, possible interference with cardiac, antidiabetic, or anticoagulant drugs
Grapefruit	Decreases metabolism of drugs used for erectile dysfunction
	Decreases metabolism of estrogens, some psychotherapeutic drugs (sertraline)
	Increases risk of toxicity of immunosuppressants and some psychotherapeutic drugs (pimozide, escitalopram)
	Increases intensity and duration of effects of caffeine
Hawthorn	May lead to toxic levels of cardiac glycosides (e.g., digitalis)
Kava	May increase the effect of barbiturates and alcohol
Saw palmetto	May change the effects of hormones in oral contraceptive drugs, patches, or hormonal replacement therapies
St. John's wort	If other serotonergic drugs are also used (such as selective serotonin reuptake inhibitors [see Chapter 17]), may lead to serotonin syndrome
Valerian	Increases central nervous system depression if used with sedatives

Modified from Huang SM et al: Drug interactions with herbal products and grapefruit juice, *Clin Pharmacol Ther* 75(1):1-12, 2004; Wolinsky I, Williams L: *Nutrition in pharmacy practice,* Washington, DC, 2003, APHA Publications.

Level of Use

The FDA estimates that over 29,000 different dietary supplements are currently used in the United States, with approximately 1000 new products introduced annually. The many different herbs in these preparations contain a wide variety of active **phytochemicals** (plant compounds). A great deal of public interest in the use of dietary supplements remains. Estimates of the prevalence of dietary supplement use differ greatly, with various studies concluding that between 3% and 93% of the U.S. population, including nearly 16% of those taking prescription drugs, use these products. The wide disparity in these estimates is most likely due to the use of varying terminology (e.g., "herbs" vs. "dietary supplements") and differences in the wording of questions regarding length of use (e.g., "have you ever used" vs. "have you used in the last 12 months"). One recent estimate of the amount spent on dietary supplements was $17.8 billion annually in the United States. Although this figure is high, the use of botanical medicines is generally greater in other parts of the world (e.g., Europe) than in the United States.

Herbal medicine is based on the premise that plants contain natural substances that can promote health and alleviate illness. Some of the more common ailments and conditions treated with herbs are anxiety, arthritis, colds, constipation, cough, depression, fever, headache, infection, insomnia, intestinal disorders, premenstrual syndrome, menopausal symptoms, stress, ulcers, and weakness.

Herbal products constitute the largest growth area in retail pharmacy. Their use is increasing at a rate of 20% to 25% a year, which far exceeds the growth in the use of conventional drugs. Insurance plans and managed care organizations are beginning to offer reimbursement for alternative treatments. One managed care organization made the decision to cover herbal remedies based on a survey showing that 33% of its 1.5 million members had sought alternative treatments in the previous 2 years. Some

CULTURAL IMPLICATIONS

Drug Responses and Cultural Factors

Responses to drugs—including over-the-counter (OTC) drugs, herbals, and dietary supplements—may be affected by beliefs, values, and genetics as well as by culture, race, and ethnicity (see Chapter 4 for more discussion of cultural considerations). As one example of the impact of culture on drug response and use, if patients who are Japanese experience nausea, vomiting, or bowel changes as adverse effects of OTC drugs, herbals, and/or dietary supplements, these often are not mentioned. The reason is that this culture finds it unacceptable to complain about gastrointestinal symptoms, and so they may go unreported to the point of causing risk to the patient.

Herbal and alternative therapies may also be used more extensively in some cultures than in others. Wide acceptance of herbal use without major concern for the effects on other therapies may be very problematic because of the many interactions of conventional drugs with herbals and dietary supplements. For example, the Chinese herb ginseng may inhibit or accelerate the metabolism of a specific medication and significantly affect the drug's absorption or elimination.

One genetic factor that has an influence on drug response is acetylation polymorphism; that is, prescription drugs, OTC drugs, herbals, and dietary supplements may be metabolized in different ways that are genetically determined and vary with race or ethnicity. For example, populations of European or African descent contain approximately equal numbers of individuals showing rapid and slow acetylation (which affects drug metabolism), whereas Japanese and Inuit populations may contain more rapid acetylators. See Chapter 4 for a more in-depth discussion of these specific genetic attributes.

Modified from Munoz C, Hilgenberg C: Ethnopharmacology, *Am J Nurs* 105(8):40-49, 2005.

of the most commonly used herbal remedies are aloe, black cohosh, chamomile, echinacea, feverfew, garlic, ginger, ginkgo biloba, ginseng, goldenseal, hawthorn, St. John's wort, saw palmetto, and valerian. These products are covered in more detail in the Herbal Therapies and Dietary Supplements boxes that appear in the various drug chapters (see the inside back cover for a complete listing of these boxes with page numbers).

NURSING PROCESS

Assessment
Over-the-Counter Drugs

Nursing assessments are always important to perform but they are especially important in situations in which a patient is self-medicating. Reading level, cognitive level, motor abilities, previous use of *OTC drugs,* successes versus failures with drug therapies and self-medication, and caregiver support are just a few of the variables to be assessed, as deemed appropriate. Other assessment data should include allergies to any of the ingredients of the drug. A medication history should include a list of *all* medications and substances used by the patient, including OTC drugs, prescription drugs, herbal products, vitamins, and minerals, as well as any alcohol, tobacco, and caffeine use. Also needed is a past and present medical history, so that possible drug interactions, contraindications, and cautions may be identified. Patients should be screened carefully before recommendation of an OTC drug, because patients often assume that if a drug is sold OTC it is completely safe to take and without negative consequences. This is not true—OTC drugs can be just as lethal or problematic as prescription drugs if they are not taken properly or are taken in high dosages and without regard to directions (see earlier pharmacologic discussion in this chapter).

Assessment of the patient's knowledge about the components of self-medication, including the positive or negative consequences of the use of a given OTC drug, should be included. Assessment of the patient's (or caregiver's or family member's) level of knowledge and experience with OTC self-medication is critical to the patient's safety, as is assessment of attitudes toward and beliefs about their use, especially a too-casual attitude or a lack of respect for and concern about the use of OTC drugs. This is especially true if a casual attitude is combined with a lack of knowledge. Obviously this could result in overuse, overdosage, and potential complications. For more information on patient education, see Chapter 7.

Generally speaking, laboratory tests are not ordered before the use of OTC drugs, because they are self-administered and self-monitored. However, there are situations in which patients may be taking certain medications that react adversely with these drugs and laboratory testing may be needed. Some patient groups are also at higher risk for adverse reactions to OTC drugs (as to most drugs in general), including pediatric and elderly patients; patients with single and/or multiple acute and chronic illnesses; those who are frail or in poor health, debilitated, or nutritionally deficient; and those with suppressed immune systems. OTC drugs should also be used with caution or may be contraindicated in patients with a history of renal, hepatic, cardiac, or vascular dysfunction. More assessment information for OTC drugs, herbals, and dietary supplements is also provided in the various drug chapters when relevant (see Table 8-1). Drug interactions should be identified. The nurse should remember that consumer safety begins with education, and thus the best way for patients to help themselves is for them to learn how to assess each situation,

weigh all the factors, and find out all they can about the OTC drug they wish to take *before* taking it!

Herbal Products and Dietary Supplements

Many *herbal products* and *dietary supplements* are readily available in drug, health food, and grocery stores as well as in home gardens, kitchens, and medicine cabinets. As noted earlier, among the more commonly used herbals are aloe, black cohosh, chamomile, echinacea, feverfew, garlic, ginger, ginkgo biloba, ginseng, goldenseal, hawthorn, St. John's wort, saw palmetto, and valerian. Although patients generally self-administer these products and do not perform an assessment, the nurse in various settings may be able to assess the patient through a head-to-toe physical examination, medical and nursing history, and medication history. Assessment data and factors and variables to consider should be shared with the patient for the patient's safety. This sharing of assessment information allows the nurse or health care provider to be sure that the patient is taking the herbal product in as safe a manner as possible. Many herbals and dietary supplements may lead to a variety of adverse effects. For example, some may cause dermatitis when used topically, whereas some taken systemically may be associated with kidney disorders such as nephritis. Therefore, for example, patients with existing skin problems or kidney dysfunction should seek medical advice before using certain herbals. Other contraindications, cautions, and potential drug-drug and drug-food interactions should also be considered. See the Herbal Therapies and Dietary Supplements box on p. 92 for more information on drug interactions.

Nursing Diagnoses

Nursing diagnoses appropriate for the patient who is taking OTC drugs, herbals, and/or dietary supplements include the following (without related causes, because these are too numerous to include):

- Activity intolerance
- Acute/chronic pain
- Fatigue
- Health-seeking behaviors
- Impaired memory
- Impaired physical mobility
- Insomnia
- Risk for injury
- Impaired urinary retention

Planning
Goals

- Patient is able to increase activity and mobility as tolerated.
- Patient experiences pain relief or relief of the symptoms of the disease process or injury within the expected time period.
- Patient experiences increase in energy within the expected time frame.
- Patient seeks out healthy behaviors with questions about the drug, its action, therapeutic effects versus adverse effects, toxicity, cautions, contraindications, drug-drug or drug-food interactions, and appropriate dosage formulation administration.
- Patient experiences increased alertness and improved short-term and long-term memory with continued use of the drug.

- Patient experiences pain relief or relief of symptoms of the disease process, condition, injury, or problem (e.g., insomnia, urinary incontinence, lack of energy, nausea, fever, swelling, cold or flu symptoms) within the expected time period.
- Patient has minimal complaints and minimal adverse effects related to the use of the drug.
- Patient remains free from injury while taking the OTC drug, herbal, and/or dietary supplement.

Outcome Criteria

- Patient states that the actions of the OTC drug, herbal, or dietary supplement have been beneficial (e.g., relief of symptoms, increase activity, increase in energy, decreased insomnia) and have improved overall well-being and health status with minimal adverse effects or complications.
- Patient identifies factors that aggravate or alleviate symptoms for which the drug is being taken and incorporates this information into a self-directed plan.
- Patient describes nonpharmacologic approaches to the treatment of symptoms, such as the use of hot or cold packs, physical therapy, massage, relaxation therapy, biofeedback, imagery, and hypnosis.
- Patient states the importance of immediately reporting any severe adverse effects or complications associated with the use of an OTC drug, herbal, or dietary supplement to the health care provider as well as to the pharmacist and to contact poison control center if needed.
- Patient is able to self-administer these drugs using the appropriate dose, frequency and administration technique (e.g., transdermal patch, suppository, liquid, quick-dissolve tablet).

Implementation

With *OTC drugs, herbals,* and *dietary supplements,* an important strategy to enhance patient safety is patient education. Patients need to receive as much information as possible about the safe use of these products and to be informed that, even though these are not prescription drugs, they are *not* completely safe and are not without toxicity. Instructions should include information about safe use, frequency of dosing and dose, specifics of how to take the medication (e.g., with food or at bedtime), as well as strategies to prevent adverse effects, drug interactions, and toxicity. Another consideration is the dosage form, because a variety are available such as liquids, tablets, enteric-coated tablets, transdermal patches, gum, and quick-dissolve tablets or strips. For transdermal patches (e.g., for smoking cessation), it is important to emphasize proper use and application. The patient should be told that the FDA does not regulate these products unless there are sufficient data to support a recall. The companies that manufacture OTC drugs, herbals, and dietary supplements are not required to provide evidence of safety and effectiveness. As previously mentioned, many consumers believe that no risks exist if a medication is available OTC or is an herbal or a "natural" substance. See Box 8-1 for more information about the criteria for moving a drug from prescription to OTC status. The fact that a drug is an herbal or a dietary supplement does not mean that it can be safely administered to children, infants, pregnant or lactating women, or patients with certain health conditions that put them at risk.

ing women, or patients with certain health conditions that put them at risk.

Evaluation

Patients taking *OTC drugs, herbals,* or *dietary supplements* should carefully monitor themselves for unusual or adverse reactions and therapeutic responses to the medication to prevent overuse and overdosing. The range of therapeutic responses will vary, depending on the specific drug and the indication for which it is used. Therapeutic responses also vary depending on the drug's action; a few examples are the following: decreased pain; decreased stiffness and swelling in joints; decreased fever; increased activity or mobility, as in increased ease of carrying out activities of daily living; increased hair growth; increased ease in breathing; decrease in constipation, diarrhea, bowel irritability, or gastrointestinal reflux or hyperacidity; resolution of allergic symptoms; decreased vaginal itching and discharge; increased healing; increased sleep; decreased fatigue or improved energy. For more specific information about nursing diagnoses, planning with goals and outcome criteria, implementation, and evaluation related to various OTC drugs, herbals, and dietary supplements, see the appropriate chapters later in the book. (Table 8-1 provides cross-references to these chapters.)

CASE STUDY

Over-the-Counter Drugs and Herbal Products

© David Gilder

J.V., a 28-year-old graduate student, is at the student health clinic for a physical examination that is required before he goes on a research trip out of the country. As he completes the paperwork, he asks the nurse, "The form is asking about my medications. I don't have any prescribed medicines, but I take several herbal products and over-the-counter medicines. Do you need to know about these?"

1. How should the nurse answer J.V.?

On the form, J.V. lists the following items:

  1 baby aspirin each day to prevent blood clots
  Sleep-Well herbal product with valerian at night if needed
  Benadryl as needed for allergies, especially at night
  Stress-Away herbal product with ginseng as needed
  Generic ibuprofen, 3 or 4 tablets three times a day for muscle aches from working out
  Memory Boost herbal product with ginkgo every morning

2. Examine the products on J.V.'s list and state whether there are any concerns with interactions or adverse effects. You may need to refer to descriptions of the individual herbal products (see the inside back cover for a listing of the Herbal Therapies and Dietary Supplements boxes located throughout the text) or to the appropriate drug chapters for more information.

3. Upon further questioning, J.V. remembers that he has had problems with "acid stomach" for about a year and takes Prilosec-OTC for that as needed. What concerns, if any, are there about this?

For answers, see *http://evolve.elsevier.com/Lilley.*

PATIENT TEACHING TIPS

- Provide verbal and written information about how to choose an appropriate OTC drug or herbal or dietary supplement as well as information about correct dosing, common adverse effects, and possible interactions with other medications.
- Many patients believe that no risks exist if a medication is herbal and "natural" or if it is sold OTC, so provide adequate education about the drug or product as well as all the advantages and disadvantages of its use, because this is crucial to patient safety.
- Provide instructions on how to read OTC drug, herbal, and dietary supplement labels.
- Emphasize the importance of taking all OTC drugs, herbals, and dietary supplements with extreme caution, and being aware of all the possible interactions and/or concerns associated with the use of these products.
- Instruct the patient that all health care providers (e.g., nurses, dentists, osteopathic and chiropractic physicians) should be informed about the use of any OTC drugs, herbals, and dietary supplements (and, of course, any prescription drug use).

- Encourage journaling of any improvement of symptoms noted with the use of a specific OTC drug, herbal, and/or dietary supplement.
- Encourage the use of appropriate and authoritative resources for patient information, such as a registered pharmacist, literature provided from the drug company and pharmacist, and web-based information from reliable sites (e.g., *http://www.WebMD.com*).
- Instruct the patient that all medications, whether OTC drug, herbal, or dietary supplement, should be kept out of the reach of children and pets.
- Provide thorough instructions regarding the various dosage forms of OTC drugs, herbals, and dietary supplements. Provide specific instructions such as how to mix powders and how to properly use transdermal patches, inhalers, ointments, lotions, nose drops, ophthalmic drops, elixirs, suppositories, vaginal suppositories or creams, and all other dosage forms (see Chapter 9); also provide information about proper storage and cleansing of any equipment.

POINTS TO REMEMBER

- Consumers use herbal products therapeutically for the treatment of diseases and pathologic conditions, prophylactically for long-term prevention of disease, and proactively for the maintenance of health and wellness.
- The FDA has established the MedWatch program to track adverse events and/or problems related to drug therapy. The toll-free number for reporting adverse effects of prescription drugs, OTC drugs, herbals, and dietary supplements is 800-332-1088. Nurses may report adverse events anonymously and without consequence.

- Herbal products are not FDA-approved drugs, and therefore their labeling cannot be relied on to provide consumers and patients with adequate instructions for use or even information about warnings.
- The fact that a drug is an herbal product, dietary supplement, or OTC medication is no guarantee that it can be safely administered to children, infants, pregnant or lactating women, or patients with certain health conditions that may put them at risk.

NCLEX EXAMINATION REVIEW QUESTIONS

1 The nurse is reviewing dietary supplements and recalls that under the DSHEA, manufacturers of dietary supplements are required to
  a follow FDA standards for quality control.
  b prove efficacy and safety of dietary supplements.
  c list the ingredients of the dietary supplement on the label.
  d obtain FDA approval before the products are marketed.
2 When educating patients about the safe use of herbal products, the nurse remembers to include which concept?
  a Herbal and OTC products are approved by the FDA and under strict regulation.
  b Herbal products are tested for safety by the FDA and the U.S. Pharmacopeia.
  c No adverse effects are associated with these products because they are natural and may be purchased without a prescription.
  d Labeling is not reliable in providing proper instructions or warnings, and the products should be taken with caution.

3 When taking a patient's drug history, the nurse asks about use of OTC drugs. The patient responds by saying, "Oh, I frequently take aspirin for my headaches, but I didn't mention it because aspirin is nonprescription." What is the best response from the nurse?
  a "That's true, over-the-counter drugs are generally not harmful."
  b "Aspirin is one of the safest drugs out there."
  c "Although aspirin is over the counter, it's still important to know why you take it, how much you take, and how often."
  d "We need you to be honest about the drugs you are taking—are there any others that you haven't told us about?"
4 When making a home visit to a patient who was recently discharged from the hospital, the nurse notes that she has a small pack over her chest and that the pack has a strong odor. She also is drinking herbal tea. When asked about the pack and the tea, the patient says, "Oh, my grandmother never used medicines

Continued

from the doctor. She told me that this plaster and tea were all I would need to fix things." Which response by the nurse is most appropriate?

a "You really should listen to what the doctor told you if you want to get better."

b "What's in the plaster and the tea? When do you usually use them?"

c "These herbal remedies rarely work, but if you want to use them, then it is your choice."

d "It's fine if you want to use this home remedy, as long as you use it with your prescription medicines."

5 A patient tells the nurse that he has been using an herbal supplement that contains kava for several years to help him to relax in the evening. However, the nurse notes that he has a yellow tinge to his skin and sclera, and is concerned about liver toxicity. The nurse advises the patient to stop taking the kava and to see his

health care provider for an examination. What else, if anything, should the nurse do at this time?

a Report this incident to MedWatch.

b Notify the state's pharmaceutical board.

c Contact the supplement manufacturer.

d No other action is needed.

6 The nurse is reviewing the drug history of a patient, and during the interview the patient asks, "Why are some drugs over-the-counter and others are not?" The nurse keeps in mind that criteria for over-the-counter status include: (Select all that apply.)

a The condition must be diagnosed by a health care provider.

b The benefits of correct usage of the drug outweigh the risks.

c The drug has limited interaction with other drugs.

d The drug is easy to use.

e The drug company sells OTC drugs at lower prices.

1. c, 2. d, 3. c, 4. b, 5. a, 6. b, c, d.

1 The nurse is discussing over-the-counter drugs and herbal products with neighbors. One neighbor comments, "Oh, the over-the-counter drugs and herbals are safe. As long as you use the recommended amounts there won't be any bad side effects." What is the best response from the nurse?

2 The nurse is teaching a patient about pain control at home with OTC products. What are the most important points to include in this discussion?

3 A patient tells the clinic nurse that he has been taking a "blood thinner" for several months and wants to ask about taking ginkgo to prevent memory loss. He says his sister uses it and it "works wonders." He also says, "I think it would be safe because I can buy it at the grocery store. They wouldn't sell harmful drugs." What is the nurse's best response to this patient? (You may need to look up the drug warfarin and the herbal product elsewhere in the text.)

For answers, see *http://evolve.elsevier.com/Lilley.*

CHAPTER 9

Substance Abuse

OBJECTIVES

When you reach the end of this chapter, you should be able to do the following:

1 Discuss substance abuse and the significance of the problem in the United States.

2 Identify the drugs or chemicals that are most frequently abused.

3 Contrast the signs and symptoms of the most commonly abused drugs/chemicals.

4 Compare the treatments for drug withdrawal for the most commonly abused opioids (narcotics), central nervous system (CNS) depressants, amphetamines and other CNS stimulants, nicotine, and alcohol.

5 Describe alcohol abuse syndrome with a focus on signs and symptoms, mild to severe alcohol withdrawal symptoms, and associated treatment.

6 Describe other drug abuse syndromes, signs and symptoms, withdrawal symptoms, and treatment regimens.

7 Identify various assessment tools used in the nursing assessment of substance abuse.

8 Develop a nursing care plan encompassing all phases of the nursing process for a patient undergoing treatment for substance abuse and dependency.

---

e-Learning Activities

Glossary

Addiction Strong psychologic or physical dependence on a drug or other psychoactive substance. (p. 98)

Amphetamine A drug that stimulates the central nervous system. (p. 99)

Enuresis Urinary incontinence. (p. 100)

Habituation Development of tolerance to a substance following prolonged medical use but without psychologic or physical dependence (addiction). (p. 98)

Illicit drug use The use of a drug or substance in a way that it is not intended to be used or the use of a drug that is not legally approved for human administration. (p. 99)

Intoxication Stimulation, excitement, or stupefaction produced by a chemical substance. (p. 98)

Korsakoff's psychosis A syndrome of anterograde and retrograde amnesia with confabulation (making up of stories) associated with chronic alcohol abuse; it often occurs together with *Wernicke encephalopathy*. (p. 103)

Micturition Urination, the desire to urinate, or the frequency of urination. (p. 100)

Narcolepsy A sleep disorder characterized by sleeping during the day, disrupted nighttime sleep, cataplexy, sleep paralysis, and hypnagogic hallucinations. (p. 100)

Opioid analgesics Synthetic pain-relieving substances that were originally derived from the opium poppy. Naturally occurring opium derivatives are called *opiates*. (p. 98)

Physical dependence A condition characterized by physiologic reliance on a substance, usually indicated by tolerance to the effects of the substance and development of withdrawal symptoms when use of the substance is terminated. (p. 97)

Psychoactive properties Drug properties that affect mood, behavior, cognitive processes, and mental status. (p. 100)

Psychologic dependence A condition characterized by strong desires to obtain and use a substance. (p. 97)

Raves Increasingly popular all-night parties that typically involve dancing, drinking, and the use of various illicit drugs. (p. 100)

Roofies Pills that are classified as benzodiazepines. They have recently gained popularity as a recreational drug; chemically known as *flunitrazepam*. (p. 101)

Substance abuse The use of a mood- or behavior-altering substance in a maladaptive manner that often compromises health, safety, and social and occupational functioning, and causes legal problems. (p. 97)

Wernicke's encephalopathy A neurologic disorder characterized by apathy, drowsiness, ataxia, nystagmus, and ophthalmoplegia; it is caused by thiamine (vitamin B₁) deficiency secondary to chronic alcohol abuse. (p. 103)

Withdrawal A substance-specific mental disorder that follows the cessation or reduction in use of a psychoactive substance that has been taken regularly to induce a state of intoxication. (p. 98)

• • •

Anatomy, Physiology, and Disease Overview

Substance abuse affects people of all ages, sexes, and ethnic and socioeconomic groups. **Physical dependence** and **psychologic dependence** on a substance are chronic disorders with remissions and relapses, such as occur with any other chronic illness. Relapses should not be seen as failures but as indications to intensify treatment. Recognizing physical or psychologic dependence and understanding the basis and various guidelines for treatment are important skills for the individual caring for these patients. **Habituation** refers to situations in which a patient becomes accustomed to a certain drug (develops tolerance) and may have mild psychologic dependence on it but does not show compulsive dose escalation, drug-seeking behavior, or major withdrawal symptoms on drug discontinuation. This might occur, for example, in a postsurgical patient who receives opioid pain therapy regularly for only a few weeks.

In 2007, the Office of Applied Studies of the U.S. Substance Abuse and Mental Health Services Administration conducted a survey indicating that some 19.9 million Americans aged 12 or older were currently illicit drug users; that is, they reported using an illicit drug during the month prior to the survey interview. This number represents 8% of the population aged 12 years and older. Marijuana was identified as the most commonly used illicit drug, followed by psychotherapeutic drugs, pain relievers, tranquilizers, stimulants and sedatives used for non-medical purposes.

Nearly 50% of the adult patients seen in many family practice clinics have an alcohol or drug disorder. Some 25% to 40% of hospital admissions are related to substance abuse and its sequelae. Of outpatients seen in a general medicine practice, 10% to 16% are seeking treatment for problems related to substance abuse. Substance abuse is also strongly associated with many types of mental illness. Treatment of both disorders concurrently is often very difficult, in part because of the high risk of drug interactions with the abused substances (see Chapter 17). Assessment, intervention, prescription of medications, collaboration in implementing specific **addiction** treatment strategies, and monitoring of recovery are essential to the care of this patient population.

This chapter focuses on three major classes of commonly abused substances and two commonly abused individual drugs. A description of the category or the individual drug, possible effects, signs and symptoms of **intoxication** and **withdrawal,** peak period and duration of withdrawal symptoms, and drugs used to treat withdrawal are discussed. The list of substances of abuse in Box 9-1 is not all inclusive, but it contains some of the substances most commonly abused at this time.

The specific drugs used to treat withdrawal symptoms are discussed in the sections covering the major drug category or the individual drug whose withdrawal symptoms they are intended to treat. Pharmacologic therapies are indicated for patients with addictive disorders to prevent life-threatening withdrawal complications, such as seizures and delirium tremens, and to increase compliance with psychosocial forms of addiction treatment.

Pharmacology Overview

OPIOIDS

Opioid analgesics are synthetic versions of pain-relieving substances that were originally derived from the opium poppy plant. The natural plant compounds are called *opiates.* More than 20 different alkaloids are obtained from the unripe seed of the opium poppy plant, only a few of which are clinically useful, including morphine and codeine. The multitude of other opioid analgesics that are currently used in medical practice are synthetic or semisynthetic derivatives of these two drugs.

Diacetylmorphine (better known as *heroin*) and opium are also opioids. Heroin and opium are classified as Schedule I drugs

---

BOX 9-1   Commonly Abused Substances
Major Categories
Opioids
Stimulants
Depressants
Individual Drugs
Alcohol
Methamphetamine
Methylenedioxymethamphetamine (MDMA, Ecstasy)
Nicotine

---

and are not available in the United States for therapeutic use. Heroin is a potent analgesic whose use is allowed for medical pain control purposes in Europe, where governmental programs also exist to provide addicts with the drug to reduce crime. Heroin was banned in the United States in 1924 because of its high potential for abuse and the increasing number of heroin addicts. Heroin is one of the most commonly abused opioids. Some of the other commonly abused substances in the opioid category are codeine, hydrocodone, hydromorphone, meperidine, morphine, opium, oxycodone, and propoxyphene.

Currently heroin remains one of the top 10 most abused drugs in the United States and often is used in combination with the stimulant drug cocaine (discussed later in Stimulants). When heroin is injected (called *mainlining* or *skin popping*), sniffed (known as *snorting*), or smoked, it binds with opiate receptors found in many regions of the brain. The result is intense euphoria, often referred to as a *rush.* This rush lasts only briefly and is followed by a relaxed, contented state that persists for a couple of hours. In large doses, heroin, like other opioids, can reduce or stop respiration.

Mechanism of Action and Drug Effects

Opioids work by blocking receptors in the central nervous system (CNS). When these receptors are blocked, the perception of pain is blocked. There are three main receptor types to which opioids bind. These receptors and their physiologic effects when stimulated are discussed in Chapter 11. One of the reasons that opioids are abused is their ability to produce euphoria.

The drug effects of opioids are primarily centered in the CNS. However, these drugs also act outside the CNS, and many of their unwanted effects stem from these actions. In addition to analgesia, opioids produce drowsiness, euphoria, tranquility, and other alterations of mood. The mechanism by which opioids produce these latter effects is not entirely clear. The effects of opioids can be collectively referred to as *narcosis* or *stupor,* which involves reduced sensory response, especially to painful stimuli. For this reason, opioid analgesics are also referred to as *narcotics* (see Chapter 4), especially by law enforcement authorities.

Indications

The intended drug effects of opioids are to relieve pain, reduce cough, relieve diarrhea, and induce anesthesia. Many have a high potential for abuse and are therefore classified as Schedule II controlled substances (see Table 4-3). Relaxation and euphoria are the most common drug effects that lead to abuse and psychologic dependence. Sustained-release oxycodone (e.g.,

OxyContin) is one example of an opioid narcotic that is controversial because it is often overprescribed, misused, and grossly abused. Numerous deaths have been reported when sustained-release oxycodone was crushed and the entire 12-hour supply was released at one time.

Certain opioid drugs are themselves used to treat opioid dependence. Historically, methadone has been used most commonly for this purpose. Its long half-life of up to 12 to 24 hours allows patients to be dosed once daily at federally approved methadone maintenance clinics. In theory, the ultimate goal of such programs is to reduce the patient's dosage gradually so that eventually the patient can live permanently drug free. Unfortunately, relapse rates are often high in these programs. However, patients who remain on long-term opioid maintenance therapy in a medical setting still benefit by avoiding the hazards associated with obtaining and using illegal street drugs.

Contraindications

Contraindications to the therapeutic use of opioid medications include known drug allergy, pregnancy (high dosage or prolonged use is contraindicated), respiratory depression or severe asthma when resuscitative equipment is not available, and *paralytic ileus* (bowel paralysis).

Adverse Effects

The adverse effects of opioids can be broken down into two groups: CNS and non-CNS. The primary adverse effects of opioids are related to their actions in the CNS. The major CNS-related adverse effects are diuresis, miosis, convulsions, nausea, vomiting, and respiratory depression. Many of the non-CNS adverse effects are secondary to the release of histamine. This histamine release can cause vasodilation leading to hypotension; spasms of the colon leading to constipation; increased spasms of the ureter resulting in urinary retention; and dilation of cutaneous blood vessels leading to flushing of the skin of the face, neck, and upper thorax. The release of histamine is also thought to cause sweating, urticaria, and pruritus.

Management of Withdrawal, Toxicity, and Overdose

Box 9-2 lists the signs and symptoms of opioid drug withdrawal. The box also indicates the time when these symptoms are most likely to occur and their duration. See Chapter 11 for a detailed discussion of physical dependence and the management of acute intoxication, toxicity, and overdose. Withdrawal symptoms include nausea, dysphoria, muscle aches, lacrimation, rhinorrhea, pupillary dilation, piloerection (hair standing on end) or sweating, diarrhea, yawning, fever, and insomnia. The medications listed in Box 9-3 are intended to help decrease the desire for the abused opioid and reduce the severity of these withdrawal symptoms. The most serious adverse effect and the most common cause of death with opioids is respiratory depression.

Medications are sometimes used to prevent relapse use once an initial remission is achieved. These medications are useful only when concurrent counseling is provided and offer additional insurance against return to **illicit drug use.** For opioid abuse or dependence, naltrexone, an opioid antagonist, is administered (50 mg/day). Naltrexone works by blocking the opioid receptors so that use of opioid drugs does not produce euphoria. When euphoria is

---

> **BOX 9-2 Signs and Symptoms of Opioid Withdrawal**
>
> ***Peak Period***
> 1-3 days
>
> ***Duration***
> 5-7 days
>
> ***Signs***
> Drug seeking, mydriasis, piloerection, diaphoresis, rhinorrhea, lacrimation, vomiting, diarrhea, insomnia, elevated blood pressure and pulse rate
>
> ***Symptoms***
> Intense desire for drugs, muscle cramps, arthralgia, anxiety, nausea, malaise

---

> **BOX 9-3 Medications for Treatment of Opioid Withdrawal**
>
> ***Clonidine (Catapres) Substitution***
> Clonidine, 0.1 or 0.2 mg orally, is given every 4-6 hr as needed for signs and symptoms of withdrawal for 5-7 days. Days 2-4 are typically the most difficult days for the patient in detoxification. Check blood pressure before each dose, and do not give medication if patient is hypotensive.
>
> ***Methadone Substitution***
> Methadone test dose of 10 mg is given orally in liquid or as crushed tablet. Additional 10-20 mg doses are given for signs and symptoms of withdrawal every 4-6 hr for 24 hr after initial dose. Range for total daily dose is 15-30 mg. Repeat total first-day dose in two divided doses (stabilization dose) for 2-3 days, then reduce dosage by 5-10 mg/day until medication is completely withdrawn.

---

eliminated, the reinforcing effect of the drug is lost. The patient should be free from opioids for at least 1 week before beginning this medication, because naltrexone can produce withdrawal symptoms if given too soon. Naltrexone is also approved for use by alcohol-dependent patients. The same dose of naltrexone given to opioid-dependent patients, 50 mg/day, decreases craving for alcohol and reduces the likelihood of a full relapse if a slip occurs.

STIMULANTS

The abuse of stimulants is related to their ability to cause elevation of mood, reduction of fatigue, a sense of increased alertness, and invigorating aggressiveness. One stimulant drug that produces strong CNS stimulation and is commonly abused is **amphetamine.** Chemically, three classes of amphetamine exist: salts of racemic amphetamine, dextroamphetamine, and methamphetamine. These classes vary with respect to their potency and peripheral effects. Another stimulant drug of abuse is cocaine, which also produces strong CNS stimulation. Cocaine was originally classified as a narcotic, is considered a narcotic by the penal system and has been treated as a narcotic in terms of secured storage in health care facilities. However, unlike the opioid analgesics, cocaine does not normally induce a state of narcosis or stupor and is therefore more correctly categorized as a stimulant drug, which is its current classification. Other commonly abused substances in this category include methylphenidate, dextroamphetamine, and phenmetrazine.

There is currently widespread abuse of the CNS stimulant methamphetamine. Multiple slight chemical variants of methamphetamine exist. Table 9-1 lists commonly abused forms of amphetamine and cocaine and their street names.

These "designer drugs" have **psychoactive properties** along with their stimulant properties, which further enhances their abuse potential. Cocaine and amphetamine are two of the most commonly abused stimulants. Although these drugs have many therapeutic benefits, they are often abused and can lead to physical and psychologic dependence. Methamphetamine is a chemical class of amphetamine, but it has a much stronger effect on the CNS than the other two classes of amphetamine.

Methamphetamine is generally used in pill form orally or in powder form by snorting or injecting. It has 15 to 20 times the potency of amphetamine sulfate, the original drug in this class. Crystallized methamphetamine, known as *ice, crystal,* or *crystal meth,* is a smokable and more powerful form of the drug. Methamphetamine users who inject the drug and share needles are at risk for acquiring human immunodeficiency virus (HIV) infection and acquired immunodeficiency syndrome (AIDS), as well as hepatitis B and C. Marijuana and alcohol are commonly listed as additional drugs of abuse in those admitted for treatment of methamphetamine abuse. Most of the recorded methamphetamine-related deaths involved the use of methamphetamine in combination with at least one other drug, such as alcohol, heroin, or cocaine. The over-the-counter (OTC) decongestant pseudoephedrine is now commonly used to synthesize methamphetamine in secret drug laboratories, often in private homes. This practice has lead to dramatic increases in the abuse of this drug. In 2005, the Combat Methamphetamine Epidemic Act required restricted retail sales of all nonprescription drug products containing pseudoephedrine. Specific restrictions include allowing sales only from *behind* the pharmacy counter, requiring photo identification and electronic or paper record keeping of purchasers (which must remain on file for 2 years), and setting maximum allowable amount (in grams) of pseudoephedrine that can be sold per consumer per month.

Another synthetic amphetamine derivative is methylenedioxymethamphetamine (MDMA, "Ecstasy," or "E"), which is also usually prepared in secret home laboratories. This drug tends to have more calming effects than other amphetamine drugs. It is usually taken in pill form but can also be snorted or injected. Users often feel a strong sense of social bonding with and acceptance of other people, hence the nickname "love drug." The drug can also be very energizing, which makes it popular at **raves** (all-night dance parties). Originally synthesized by Merck Pharmaceuticals in 1914, it was studied by the U.S. Army as a "brainwashing" drug in the 1950s. Its popularity has grown widely since the Drug Enforcement Administration classified it as a Schedule I controlled substance in 1985.

Another illicit drug use problem is cocaine use. Cocaine is a white powder that is derived from the leaves of the South American coca plant. Cocaine is either snorted or injected intravenously. Cocaine tends to give a temporary illusion of limitless power and energy but afterward leaves the user feeling depressed, edgy, and craving more. Crack is a smokable form of cocaine that has been chemically altered. Cocaine and crack are highly addictive. The psychologic and physical dependence can erode physi-

TABLE 9-1 Various Forms of Amphetamine and Cocaine with Street Names

Chemical Name	Street Names
dimethoxymethylamphetamine	DOM, STP
methamphetamine (crystallized form)	Ice, crystal, glass
methamphetamine (powdered form)	Speed, meth, crank
methylenedioxyamphetamine	MDA, love drug
methylenedioxymethamphetamine	MDMA, Ecstasy
cocaine (powdered form)	Coke, dust, snow, flake, blow, girl
cocaine (crystallized form)	Crack, crack cocaine, freebase rocks, rock

cal and mental health and can become so strong that these drugs dominate all aspects of the addict's life.

Mechanism of Action and Drug Effects

Stimulants work by releasing *biogenic amines* from their storage sites in the nerve terminals. The primary biogenic amine released is norepinephrine. This release results in stimulation of the CNS. One effect of stimulant drugs is typically cardiovascular stimulation, which results in increased blood pressure and heart rate and possibly cardiac dysrhythmias. The effect on smooth muscle is seen primarily in the urinary bladder and results in contraction of the sphincter. This is helpful in treating **enuresis** (urinary incontinence) but results in painful and difficult **micturition** (voiding or urination) otherwise. Stimulants, particularly amphetamines, are very potent CNS stimulants. This CNS stimulation commonly results in wakefulness, alertness, and a decreased sense of fatigue; elevation of mood, with increased initiative, self-confidence, and ability to concentrate; often elation and euphoria; and an increase in motor and speech activity. Physical performance in athletes may be improved due to both enhanced alertness and reduction of fatigue. This quality leads to abuse of these drugs by many athletes, especially those under intense pressure to perform. However, these performance enhancement effects may reach a plateau and even result in a personal or professional crisis for an athlete who abuses these drugs on a long-term basis.

Indications

Many therapeutic uses for stimulants exist. Currently their most common use is in the treatment of attention deficit disorder or attention deficit hyperactivity disorder. Stimulants may be used to prevent or reverse fatigue and sleep, such as when they are used to treat **narcolepsy** (episodes of acute sleepiness). Another therapeutic effect of amphetamines is their ability to stimulate the respiratory center. Occasionally they are used after anesthesia to stimulate the respiratory center. Stimulants are also used to reduce food intake and treat obesity, however this therapeutic effect is limited because of rapid development of tolerance.

Contraindications

Contraindications to the therapeutic use of stimulant medications include drug allergy, diabetes, cardiovascular disorders, states of agitation, hypertension, known history of drug abuse, and Tourette syndrome.

Adverse Effects

The adverse effects of stimulants are commonly an extension of their therapeutic effects. The CNS-related adverse effects are restlessness, syncope (fainting), dizziness, tremor, hyperactive reflexes, talkativeness, tenseness, irritability, weakness, insomnia, fever, and sometimes euphoria. Confusion, aggression, increased libido, anxiety, delirium, paranoid hallucinations, panic states, and suicidal or homicidal tendencies occur, especially in mentally ill patients. Fatigue and depression usually follow the CNS stimulation. Cardiovascular effects are common and include headache, chilliness, pallor or flushing, palpitations, tachycardia, cardiac dysrhythmias, anginal pain, hypertension or hypotension, and circulatory collapse. Excessive sweating can also occur. Gastrointestinal (GI) effects include dry mouth, metallic taste, anorexia, nausea, vomiting, diarrhea, and abdominal cramps. A sometimes fatal hyperthermia can also occur, driven partly by excessive drug-induced muscular contractions.

Management of Withdrawal, Toxicity, and Overdose

Box 9-4 lists the signs and symptoms of withdrawal from stimulants. The box also indicates the peak period when these symptoms are most likely to occur and their duration. Death due to poisoning or toxic levels is usually a result of convulsions, coma, or cerebral hemorrhage and may occur during periods of intoxication or withdrawal.

DEPRESSANTS

Depressants are drugs that relieve anxiety, irritability, and tension when used as intended. They are also used to treat seizure disorders and induce anesthesia. The two main pharmacologic classes of depressant are benzodiazepines and barbiturates. Both of these drug classes are discussed further in Chapter 13. Benzodiazepines are relatively safe. They offer many advantages over older drugs used to relieve anxiety and insomnia. However, they are often intentionally and unintentionally misused. Ingestion of benzodiazepines together with alcohol can be lethal. Another depressant that is neither a benzodiazepine nor a barbiturate is marijuana. Derived from the cannabis plant, marijuana ("pot," "grass," "weed"), is the most commonly abused drug worldwide. Marijuana is generally smoked as a cigarette ("joint") or in a pipe ("bong") but can be mixed in food or tea.

A benzodiazepine that has recently gained popularity as a recreational drug is flunitrazepam. Flunitrazepam is not legally available for prescription in the United States, but it is legally sold in over 60 countries for treatment of insomnia. The drug, known as **roofies** among young people, creates a sleepy, relaxed, drunken feeling that lasts 2 to 8 hours. Roofies are commonly used in combination with alcohol and other drugs. They are sometimes taken to enhance a heroin high or to mellow or ease the experience of coming down from a cocaine or crack high. Used with alcohol, roofies produce disinhibition and amnesia.

Roofies have recently gained a reputation as a "date rape" drug. Girls and women around the country have reported being raped after being involuntarily sedated with roofies, which were often slipped into their drinks by their attackers. The drug has no taste or odor, so the victims do not realize what is happening. About 10 minutes after ingesting the drug, the woman may feel

BOX 9-4 Signs and Symptoms of Stimulant Withdrawal
Peak Period   1-3 days
Duration   5-7 days
Signs   Social withdrawal, psychomotor retardation, hypersomnia, hyperphagia
Symptoms   Depression, suicidal thoughts and behavior, paranoid delusions
Treatment   No specific pharmacologic treatments to reduce cravings or reverse acute toxicity and no known antidotes.

dizzy and disoriented, simultaneously too hot and too cold, and nauseous. She may experience difficulty speaking and moving and then pass out. Such a victim will have no memories of what happened while under the influence of the drug. Another popular date rape drug used in similar fashion is gamma-hydroxybutyric acid (GHB). GHB works by mimicking the natural inhibitory brain neurotransmitter gamma-aminobutyric acid (GABA). It is also known as "liquid Ecstasy." These drugs are also used simply for their depressant and hallucinogenic effects.

Mechanism of Action and Drug Effects

Benzodiazepines and barbiturates work by increasing the action of GABA. GABA is an amino acid in the brain that inhibits nerve transmission in the CNS. The alteration of GABA action in the CNS results in relief of anxiety, sedation, and muscle relaxation. The effects of depressants are primarily limited to the CNS. In addition to sedation, muscle relaxation, and reduced anxiety, their CNS effects include amnesia and unconsciousness. They have moderate effects outside the CNS, causing slight blood pressure decreases.

The active ingredients of the marijuana plant are known as cannabinoids, the most active of which is delta-9-trans-tetrahydrocannabinol, abbreviated *THC*. THC exerts its effects on the body by chemically binding to and stimulating two cannabinoid receptors in the CNS (CB1 and CB2). Smoking the drug leads to acute sensorial changes that start within 3 minutes, peak in 20 to 30 minutes, and last for 2 to 3 hours. Effects are longer when the drug is taken via the oral route. Specific effects include mild euphoria, memory lapses, dry mouth, enhanced appetite, motor awkwardness, and distorted sense of time and space. THC also stimulates sympathetic receptors and inhibits parasympathetic receptors in cardiac tissue, which leads to tachycardia. Other effects include hallucinations, anxiety, paranoia, and unsteady gait.

Indications

Many therapeutic uses of depressants exist. Benzodiazepines are more widely used and abused than barbiturates, and they are more commonly prescribed because they are felt by many to be safer than barbiturates. Benzodiazepines are used primarily to relieve anxiety, to induce sleep, to sedate, and to prevent seizures. Barbiturates are used as hypnotics, sedatives, and anticonvulsants and to induce anesthesia. Controversial medical uses for marijuana include treatment of chronic pain, reduction of nausea and vomiting associated with cancer treatment, and appetite stimulation in those with wasting syndromes, such as patients with cancer or AIDS. Dronabinol is a synthetic THC prescription capsule approved by the Food and Drug Administration (FDA) for the above indications (see Chapter 52 for further discussion of this drug). However, it is often not popular with those who claim that it is not as effective as inhaled marijuana.

Contraindications

Contraindications to the therapeutic use of depressant medications include known drug allergy, dyspnea or airway obstruction, narrow-angle glaucoma, and porphyria (a metabolic disorder).

Adverse Effects

The most common undesirable effect of benzodiazepines and barbiturates is an overexpression of their therapeutic effects. The CNS is the primary area of the body adversely affected by these drugs. Drowsiness, sedation, loss of coordination, dizziness, blurred vision, headaches, and paradoxical reactions (insomnia, increased excitability, hallucinations) are the primary CNS adverse effects. Occasional GI effects include nausea, vomiting, constipation, dry mouth, and abdominal cramping. Other possible adverse effects are pruritus and skin rash. Long-term use of marijuana may result in chronic respiratory symptoms (similar to those of tobacco abuse) and memory and attention deficit problems. A chronic depressive "amotivational" syndrome has also been observed, especially among younger users.

Management of Withdrawal, Toxicity, and Overdose

Box 9-5 lists the signs and symptoms of withdrawal from depressants. The box also indicates the peak periods when these symptoms are most likely to occur and their duration. Fatal poisoning is unusual with benzodiazepines when they are taken alone. When benzodiazepines are ingested with alcohol or barbiturates, however, the combination can be lethal. Death is typically due to respiratory arrest. Abrupt withdrawal of benzodiazepines when they have been taken for several months to years has resulted in autonomic withdrawal symptoms, seizures, delirium, rebound anxiety, myoclonus (involuntary muscle contractions), myalgia, and sleep disturbances.

Flumazenil is a benzodiazepine reversal agent. Flumazenil antagonizes the action of benzodiazepines on the CNS by directly competing with them for binding at the benzodiazepine receptor in the CNS and thus reversing sedation. The dosage regimen to be followed for the reversal of conscious sedation or general anesthesia induced by a benzodiazepine and the management of suspected benzodiazepine overdoses are summarized in Chapter 13 (Table 13-4).

Barbiturates and benzodiazepines are commonly implicated in suicides, especially in combination with alcohol. Generally speaking, depressants should not be regularly prescribed over a long period. Relatively safe hypnotic drugs such as the benzodiazepines are preferred whenever possible, especially in emotionally disturbed patients. Combinations of sedative-hypnotic drugs or in combination with alcohol should be avoided. Long-term use of hypnotic drugs leads to ineffective control of insomnia, de-

---

BOX 9-5 Signs, Symptoms, and Treatment of Depressant Withdrawal

Peak Period
2-4 days for short-acting drugs
4-7 days for long-acting drugs

Duration
4-7 days for short-acting drugs
7-12 days for long-acting drugs

Signs
Increased psychomotor activity; agitation; muscular weakness; hyperthermia; diaphoresis; delirium; convulsions; elevated blood pressure, pulse rate, and temperature; tremors of eyelids, tongue, and hands

Symptoms
Anxiety; depression; euphoria; incoherent thoughts; hostility; grandiosity; disorientation; tactile, auditory, and visual hallucinations; suicidal thoughts

Treatment of Benzodiazepine Withdrawal
A 7-10 day taper (10-14 day taper with long-acting benzodiazepines). Treat with diazepam (Valium) 10-20 mg orally qid on day 1, then taper until the dosage is 5-10 mg orally on last day. Avoid giving the drug "as needed." Adjustments in dosage according to the patient's clinical state may be indicated.

Treatment of Barbiturate Withdrawal
A 7-10 day taper or 10-14 day taper. Calculate barbiturate equivalence and give 50% of the original dosage (if actual dosage is known before detoxification); taper. Avoid giving the drug "as needed."

---

crease in rapid eye movement sleep, dependence, and drug withdrawal symptoms.

Effects of marijuana use are usually self-limiting and resolve within a few hours.

ALCOHOL

Alcoholic beverages have been used since the beginning of human civilization. Individuals of Arab descent introduced the technique of distillation to Europe in the Middle Ages. Alcohol has been called the "elixir of life" and has been touted as a remedy for practically all diseases, which led to the use of the term *whisky*, Gaelic for "water of life." Over time, it has been determined that the therapeutic value of alcohol is extremely limited, and long-term ingestion of excessive amounts is a major social and medical problem.

Mechanism of Action and Drug Effects

Alcohol, more accurately known as *ethanol* (abbreviated as *ETOH*), causes CNS depression by dissolving in lipid membranes in the CNS. The latest hypothesis is that ethanol causes a local disordering in the lipid matrix of the brain. This has been termed *membrane fluidization*. Some also believe that ethanol may augment GABA-mediated synaptic inhibition and fluxes of chloride. This enhancement of the action of GABA, an inhibitory neurotransmitter in the brain, causes CNS depression. The CNS is continuously depressed in the presence of ethanol. Moderate amounts of ethanol may stimulate or depress respirations. Effects of ethanol on the circulation are relatively minor. In moderate doses, ethanol causes vasodilation, especially of the cutaneous vessels, and produces warm, flushed skin. Ingestion of ethanol causes a feeling of warmth because it enhances cutaneous and gastric blood flow. Increased sweating may also occur. Heat is therefore lost more rapidly, and the internal body temperature consequently falls. The short-term (vs. long-term) ingestion of ethanol, even in intoxicating doses, probably produces little lasting change in hepatic function. Ethanol exerts a diuretic effect by virtue of its inhibition of antidiuretic hormone secretion and the resultant decrease in renal tubular reabsorption of water.

Indications

Few legitimate uses of ethanol and alcoholic beverages exist. Ethanol is an excellent solvent for many drugs and is commonly employed as a vehicle for medicinal mixtures. When applied topically to the skin, ethanol acts as a coolant. Ethanol sponges are therefore used to treat fever. Ethanol may also be used in liniments (oily medications used on the skin). Applied topically, ethanol is the most popular skin disinfectant. More commonly, however, the type of alcohol used on the skin is isopropyl alcohol, which is similar in structure to ethanol but is more toxic and is not drinkable.

Ethanol is still widely employed for its hypnotic and antipyretic effects in various cold and cough products. Systemic uses of ethanol are primarily limited to the treatment of methyl alcohol and ethylene glycol intoxication (e.g., from drinking automotive antifreeze solution). However, small amounts of ethanol preparations (such as red wine) have been shown to have cardiovascular benefits.

Adverse Effects

Long-term excessive ingestion of ethanol is directly associated with serious neurologic and mental disorders. These neurologic disorders can result in seizures. Nutritional and vitamin deficiencies, especially of the B vitamins, can occur and can lead to **Wernicke's encephalopathy, Korsakoff's psychosis,** polyneuritis, and nicotinic acid deficiency encephalopathy.

Moderate amounts of ethanol may stimulate or depress respirations. Large amounts produce dangerous or lethal depression of respiration. Although circulatory effects of ethanol are relatively minor, acute severe alcoholic intoxication may cause cardiovascular depression. Long-term excessive use of ethanol has largely irreversible effects on the heart, such as cardiomyopathy.

When consumed on a regular basis in large quantities, ethanol produces a constellation of dose-related negative effects such as alcoholic hepatitis or its progression to cirrhosis. Teratogenic effects can be devastating and are caused by the direct action of ethanol, which inhibits embryonic cellular proliferation early in gestation. This often results in a condition known as *fetal alcohol syndrome,* which is characterized by craniofacial abnormalities, CNS dysfunction, and both prenatal and postnatal growth retardation in the infant. Pregnant women should therefore be strongly advised not to consume alcohol during pregnancy, and appropriate treatment and counseling should be arranged for pregnant women addicted to alcohol or any other drug of abuse.

Management of Withdrawal, Toxicity, and Overdose

Box 9-6 lists the common signs and symptoms of ethanol withdrawal. Signs and symptoms may vary depending on the individual's usage pattern, his or her preferred type of ethanol, and

---

BOX 9-6   Signs, Symptoms, and Treatment of Ethanol Withdrawal

Mild Withdrawal
Signs and Symptoms
Systolic blood pressure higher than 150 mm Hg, diastolic blood pressure higher than 90 mm Hg, pulse rate higher than 110 beats/min, temperature above 100° F (37.7° C), tremors, insomnia, agitation

Moderate Withdrawal
Signs and Symptoms
Systolic blood pressure 150-200 mm Hg, diastolic blood pressure 90-140 mm Hg, pulse rate 110-140 beats/min, temperature 100°-101° F (37.7°-38.3° C), tremors, insomnia, agitation

Severe Withdrawal (Delirium Tremens)
Signs and Symptoms
Systolic blood pressure higher than 200 mm Hg, diastolic blood pressure higher than 140 mm Hg, pulse rate higher than 140 beats/min, temperature above 101° F (38.3° C), tremors, insomnia, agitation

Treatment
Benzodiazepines are the treatment of choice for ethanol withdrawal. The dosages are variable and differ from institution to institution. Lower dosages are used for mild symptoms and higher dosages are needed for severe withdrawal. The oral route is preferred; however, it is often necessary to use the intravenous route for patients experiencing severe withdrawal. Patients who are experiencing severe withdrawal often require monitoring in an intensive care unit for cardiac and respiratory function, fluid and nutrition replacement, vital signs, and mental status. Restraints are indicated for a patient who is confused or agitated to protect the patient from self and to protect others (delirium tremens can be a terrifying and life-threatening state). Thiamine administration, hydration, and magnesium replacement may be indicated depending on the severity of the withdrawal state.

TABLE 9-2   Disulfiram Adverse Effects: Acetaldehyde Syndrome

Body System Affected	Result
Cardiovascular	Vasodilation over the entire body, hypotension, orthostatic syncope, chest pain
Central nervous	Intense throbbing of the head and neck leading to a pulsating headache, sweating, marked uneasiness, weakness, vertigo, blurred vision, confusion
Gastrointestinal	Nausea, copious vomiting, thirst
Respiratory	Difficulty breathing

---

the presence of comorbidities. Ethanol withdrawal can be life threatening.

One pharmacologic option for the treatment of alcoholism is disulfiram. Disulfiram works by altering the metabolism of alcohol. It is not a cure for alcoholism, but it helps patients who have a sincere desire to stop drinking. The rationale for its use is that patients know that if they are to avoid the devastating experience of *acetaldehyde syndrome,* they cannot drink for at least 3 or 4 days after taking disulfiram. Table 9-2 outlines acetaldehyde syndrome. These adverse effects are obviously very uncomfortable and potentially dangerous for someone with any other major illnesses. For this reason, disulfiram is usually reserved as the treatment of last resort for "hard core" alcoholic patients for whom other treatment options (e.g., Alcoholics Anonymous, psychotherapy) have failed but who still hope to avoid continued alcohol abuse. When ethanol is ingested by an individual previously treated with disulfiram, the blood acetaldehyde concentration rises 5 to 10 times higher than in an untreated individual. Within about 5 to 10 minutes of alcohol ingestion, the individual's face feels hot, and soon afterward it is flushed and scarlet. After this, throbbing in the head and neck, nausea, copious vomiting, diaphoresis, dyspnea, hyperventilation, vertigo, blurred vision, and confusion occur. As little as 7 mL of alcohol will cause mild symptoms in a sensitive person. The effects last from 30 minutes to several hours. After the symptoms wear off, the patient is exhausted and may sleep for several hours. Most of the signs and symptoms observed after the ingestion of disulfiram plus alcohol are attributable to the resulting increase in the concentration of acetaldehyde in the body. There have even been a few published reports of localized disulfiram-alcohol skin reactions when alcohol preparations—even beer-containing shampoo—were placed on the skin. The usual dosage of disulfiram is 250 mg/day, or 125 mg/day in patients who experience adverse effects such as sedation, sexual dysfunction, and elevated liver enzyme levels.

A less noxious drug therapy option is the use of naltrexone, as mentioned previously in the section on opioids earlier in this chapter. The newest drug treatment indicated for alcoholism is acamprosate. Approved in 2004, it is used to maintain abstinence from alcohol in patients who are abstinent when starting the drug and who have additional psychosocial support. Its mechanism of action is not completely understood, but it may interact with *glutamate* and *GABA* receptors in the brain. The usual dosage is two 333-mg tablets taken three times daily.

NICOTINE

Nicotine was first isolated from the leaves of tobacco in 1828. The medical significance of nicotine grows out of its toxicity, presence in tobacco, and propensity for eliciting dependence in its users. The long-term effects of nicotine and the untoward effects of the long-term use of tobacco are considerable. Although many people smoke because they believe cigarettes calm their nerves, smoking releases epinephrine, a hormone that creates physiologic stress in the smoker rather than relaxation. The apparent calming effects may be related to the increased deep breathing associated with smoking. The use of tobacco is addictive. Most users develop tolerance for nicotine and need greater amounts to produce the desired effect. Smokers become physically and psychologically dependent and will suffer withdrawal symptoms. Smoking is particularly dangerous in adolescents because their bodies are still developing and changing. The 4000 chemicals, including 200 known poisons, present in cigarette smoke can adversely affect this maturation. Cigarettes are highly addictive. One third of young people who are "just experimenting" end up becoming addicted by the time they are 20 years of age.

Mechanism of Action and Drug Effects

Nicotine works by directly stimulating the autonomic ganglia of the nicotinic receptors. Its site of action is the ganglion itself rather than the preganglionic or postganglionic nerve fiber. The organs throughout the body that are innervated by nerves stimulated by nicotine actually contain nicotinic receptors. These receptors are so named because they were originally tested with nicotine to measure their responses. Nicotine can have multiple unpredictable and dramatic affects on the body because nicotinic receptors are found in several systems, including the adrenal glands, skeletal muscles, and CNS.

The major action of nicotine is transient stimulation, followed by more persistent depression of all autonomic ganglia. Small doses of nicotine stimulate the ganglion cells directly and facilitate the transmission of impulses. When larger doses of the drug are applied, the initial stimulation is followed quickly by a blockade of transmission.

Nicotine markedly stimulates the CNS, including respiratory stimulation. This stimulation of the CNS is followed by depression. Nicotine can have dramatic effects on the cardiovascular system as well, resulting in increases in heart rate and blood pressure. The GI system is generally stimulated by nicotine, which produces increased tone and activity in the bowel. This often leads to nausea and vomiting and occasionally to diarrhea.

Indications

The nicotine found in nature (i.e., tobacco plants) has no known therapeutic uses. It is medically significant because of its addictive and toxic properties. However, nicotine that is formulated into various drug products to reduce cravings and promote smoking cessation can be considered a therapeutic drug. It is available for this purpose as chewing gum, transdermal patches, and nasal spray.

Adverse Effects

Nicotine primarily affects the CNS. Large doses can produce tremors and even convulsions. Respiratory stimulation also commonly occurs. The initial stimulation of the CNS induced by nicotine is quickly followed by depression. Death can even result from respiratory failure, which is thought to be due to both central paralysis and peripheral blockade of respiratory muscles. The cardiovascular effects of nicotine are an increase in heart rate and blood pressure. The effects of nicotine on the GI system are largely due to parasympathetic stimulation, which results in increased tone and motor activity of the bowel. Nicotine induces vomiting by both central and peripheral actions. Centrally, nicotine's emetic effects are due to stimulation of the *chemoreceptor trigger zone* in the brain.

Management of Withdrawal, Toxicity, and Overdose

Smoking cessation is the primary cause for nicotine withdrawal, although discontinuation of any tobacco product can lead to this syndrome. An important and often overlooked problem in hospitalized patients is nicotine withdrawal, which manifests largely as cigarette craving. Irritability, restlessness, and a decrease in heart rate and blood pressure occur. Cardiac symptoms resolve over 3 to 4 weeks, but cigarette craving may persist for months or even years.

The nicotine transdermal system (patch) and nicotine polacrilex (gum) can be used to provide nicotine without the carcinogens in tobacco and are now available OTC. The patch system uses a stepwise reduction in subcutaneous delivery to gradually

TABLE 9-3 Nicotine Withdrawal Therapies

Drug	Dosage per Patch	Recommended Duration of Use
Transdermal Nicotine Systems		
Habitrol	7 mg/24 hr	2-4 wk
	14 mg/24 hr	2-4 wk
	21 mg/24 hr	4-8 wk
Nicoderm	7 mg/24 hr	2-4 wk
	14 mg/24 hr	2-4 wk
	21 mg/24 hr	4-8 wk
Nicotrol	5 mg/16 hr	2-4 wk
	10 mg/16 hr	2-4 wk
	15 mg/16 hr	4-12 wk
ProStep	11 mg/24 hr	2-4 wk
	22 mg/24 hr	4-8 wk
Nicotine Gum (Resin)	When the client has a strong urge to smoke, a stick of gum is chewed; use gradually reduced over a 2-3 mo period.	
Antidepressant		
bupropion (Zyban)	15-mg sustained-release tabs	15 mg on days 1-3, then 150 mg bid for 7-12 wk
Partial Nicotine Agonist		
varenicline (Chantix)	0.5 or 1 mg tabs	12-wk regimen, beginning with 0.5 mg orally bid, titrated to 1 mg daily by day 8.

decrease the nicotine dose, and patient treatment compliance seems higher than with the gum. Acute relief from withdrawal symptoms is most easily achieved with the use of the gum, because rapid chewing releases an immediate dose of nicotine. The dose is approximately half the dose the average smoker receives in one cigarette, however, and the onset of action is 30 minutes versus 10 minutes or less from smoking. These pharmacologic changes in delivery minimize the immediate reinforcement and self-reward effects that are prominent with the rapid nicotine delivery of cigarette smoking.

A sustained-release form of the antidepressant bupropion, called *Zyban,* has been approved as first-line therapy to aid in smoking cessation treatment. Sustained-release bupropion is an innovative treatment because it is the first nicotine-free prescription medicine to treat nicotine dependence. Table 9-3 lists the currently available drugs for nicotine withdrawal therapy.

A new medication for treatment was approved in 2006. Varenicline (Chantix) both activates and antagonizes the *alpha-4-beta-2* nicotinic receptors in the brain. This effect provides some stimulation to nicotine receptors, while also reducing the pleasurable effects of nicotine from smoking. This drug has demonstrated greater efficacy than bupropion mentioned earlier. The recommended 12-week treatment regimen begins with 0.5 mg orally twice daily, titrating up to 1 mg twice daily by day 8. An optional second 12-week regimen may be prescribed to help the patient maintain tobacco abstinence. The most common adverse effects are nausea, vomiting, headache, flatulence, insomnia, and taste disturbances. Drowsiness has also been reported, which prompted the FDA to recommend caution in driving and engaging in other potentially hazardous activities until the patient can determine how the drug affects his or her mental status. Although many highly addicted smokers are reporting significant success with varenicline, the FDA issued preliminary warnings in January 2008 regarding its use. Specifically, case reports have emerged of psychiatric symptoms including agitation, depression, and suicidality, as well as worsening of preexisting psychiatric illness, while using the drug. The FDA is recommending appropriate patient education and follow-up regarding these adverse effects. Varenicline is a pregnancy category C drug.

NURSING PROCESS

Assessment

The purpose of substance abuse assessment is to determine whether substance abuse exists, to evaluate the relationship between the abuse and other health concerns, and to begin the implementation of an effective health promotion and health restoration plan. Because of the prevalence of substance abuse and the role played by the professional nurse in a variety of settings, the nurse may be the first one to identify the risky behavior in a patient. Indications of abuse problems in patients may also present themselves during an abuser's hospitalization for an injury, illness, or surgery. Even when substance abuse is not suspected, however, a general nursing assessment and medication history should include questions about use of alcohol, nicotine, opioids, and so on (see pharmacology section of this chapter). All patients should be questioned about the use and misuse of substances, because addiction is found across the life span and therefore can be encountered in all clinical specialties. Additionally, abuse/misuse of substances/prescription medications may need to be assessed in family members because adolescents may be stealing their parents' prescription drugs.

The nurse's responsibilities relative to drug abuse and the nursing process must begin with the cultivation of excellent interpersonal communication skills. It is important for the nurse to acknowledge and address his or her individual beliefs about drug and alcohol use as well as any personal history of coping with addiction or dealing with addicted family members. This process will allow the nurse to anticipate his or her responses and behaviors toward this patient population and seek out resolution of these feelings. Acknowledging feelings and beliefs about this group of patients within a proper perspective and ethical framework will allow the nurse to resolve any personal animosity, judgmental attitudes, rejection, and/or enabling behaviors. Once detrimental behaviors and possible barriers to responsible and nonjudgmental care have been dealt with, the nurse can then focus on the patient and avoid being drawn into the manipulative and other negative behaviors of the abuser.

A thorough patient assessment and history must include specific questions about the substance(s) being used, the duration of abuse, related physical and mental health concerns, and withdrawal potential. In patients with suspected or confirmed substance abuse, honesty—on the part of the patient as well as the family or significant other—may be problematic when it comes to answering questions about drug use. Therefore, the nurse should use open-ended questions and maintain a nonjudgmental approach during the nursing process and in all contacts with the patient. A medication history should include information about all drugs being used, including prescription drugs, OTC drugs, herbals, dietary supplements, and illegal or "street" drugs. The names of these drugs, doses, and frequency and duration of use should be noted. The nurse must also be attentive to any clues the patient, family, or significant other may reveal, including behavioral and mood changes. A patient's reported use of multiple prescribed drugs as well as contact with multiple prescribers should raise a red flag as a possible sign of drug abuse. In addition, laboratory findings are important to assess, including results of renal and liver function studies and any drug screening studies. Results of HIV and hepatitis laboratory tests should also be assessed and monitored, once ordered. Baseline vital signs should also be measured and documented.

A number of assessment tools are available to nurses and health care professionals for use with patients suspected of drug or substance abuse, and their validity and reliability have been established. The goal of adequate screening for alcohol and other drug abuse or addiction is to identify patients who have or are at risk for developing alcohol or drug-related problems and to further engage them in discussion. This may help in further diagnosing and more accurately treating the patient's abuse problem. Laboratory tests are available to detect alcohol and other drugs in the blood and/or urine. These are used to identify more recent drug abuse rather than long-term use or dependence. However, there are other tests that are best used when assessing someone for confirmation of a diagnosis rather than screening. Some instruments available for screening alcohol and drug use in adults are the CAGE Alcoholism Screening Test Adapted to Include Drugs (CAGE-AID) and Substance Abuse Subtle Screening Inventory (SASSI). The Michigan Alcoholism Screening Test (MAST-G) is available for use in geriatric patients whereas the Problem Oriented Screening Instrument for Teenagers (POSIT) is available for use in adolescents. See Boxes 9-7 and 9-8 for examples of screening and detection tools and criteria for diagnosing substance abuse. If the findings of an assessment questionnaire are positive, the next step is for the nurse to explore the history of the patient's alcohol or drug use and problems. Further observation is needed to identify any physical, psychologic, and

---

> **BOX 9-7 CAGE Alcoholism Screening Test and CAGE Adapted to Include Drugs**
>
> ### CAGE
> The following questions are included in the **CAGE** questionnaire:
> **C** "Have you ever felt that you should **C**ut down on your drinking?"
> **A** "Have people **A**nnoyed you by criticizing your drinking?"
> **G** "Have you ever felt bad or **G**uilty about your drinking?"
> **E** "Have you ever had a drink, or an **E**ye-opener, first thing in the morning to steady your nerves or get rid of a hangover?"
> Two positive responses to these questions are considered a positive test result and indicate that further assessment is warranted.
>
> ### CAGE Adapted to Include Drugs (CAGE-AID)
> The following questions are included in the CAGE-AID questionnaire:
> 1. In the last 3 months, have you felt you should cut down or stop drinking *or using drugs?*
>   ☐ Yes
>   ☐ No
> 2. In the last 3 months, has anyone annoyed you or gotten on your nerves by telling you to cut down or stop drinking *or using drugs?*
>   ☐ Yes
>   ☐ No
> 3. In the last 3 months, have you felt guilty or bad about how much you drink *or use drugs?*
>   ☐ Yes
>   ☐ No
> 4. In the last 3 months, have you been waking up wanting to have an alcoholic drink *or use drugs?*
>   ☐ Yes
>   ☐ No
> Each affirmative response earns one point. One point indicates a possible problem. Two points indicates a probable problem.
>
> Modified from Ewing J: Detecting alcoholism: the CAGE questionnaire, *JAMA* 252:1905-1907, 1984; Dube C et al, editors: *Project ADEPT, curriculum for primary care physician training,* Vol. I: *Core modules,* Providence, RI, 1989, Brown University.

---

social signs of dependence and dysfunction. Maintaining communication with family members may also provide useful information. Should abuse be identified by a history-taking process, physical assessment, drug history profile, screening tests, or patient's confession of abuse, then confidentiality, privacy, and nonjudgmental behavior are key to ethical nursing practice. Although the substance abuse should be reported to the necessary health care professionals, the nurse must adhere to the American Nurses Association *Code of Ethics for Nurses* in making this report (see Chapter 4).

Assessment of *opioid* abuse includes, in addition to obtaining the assessment data mentioned earlier, determination of the route being used for drug delivery (e.g., oral vs. intravenous use). The use of intravenous drugs may give rise to health concerns such as HIV/AIDS or hepatitis. Respiratory assessment with attention to rate and rhythm are important because of the risk for respiratory depression with opioid overdose or overuse. Other more specific signs and symptoms have been described earlier in this chapter. Assessment for marijuana use includes appraisal of cognitive and motor function and assessment for the inability to carry out minor tasks. Hallucinogen abuse requires assessment for altered

BOX 9-8 Diagnosis of Dependence

The *Diagnostic and Statistical Manual of Mental Disorders* (American Psychiatric Association, 2000) identified criteria for the diagnosis of a dependence. The occurrence of at least *three* of the following symptoms within a 12-month period helps confirm a diagnosis of dependence:

- Tolerance or a marked need for increased amounts of the substance to achieve the desired effect
- Withdrawal symptoms
- Unsuccessful attempts to cut down or control use of the substance
- Abandonment or reduction of important social, occupational, or recreational activities due to substance use. The use continues regardless of recurrent physical/psychological problems.

Modified from Maurer FA: *Community/public health nursing practice: health for families and populations*, ed 3, Philadelphia, 2004, Saunders.

CASE STUDY

Substance Abuse and Adolescents

© Carme Balcells

You are having a discussion with a neighbor who has a 14-year-old son. The neighbor expresses concern about his son and substance abuse problems he has heard about.

1. The neighbor describes his son's friend, who was a bright and motivated student but has become sullen and withdrawn, and lacks the motivation he once had. In addition, he has a chronic cough but denies that he smokes cigarettes. This behavior change may indicate abuse of what substance? Are there any long-term effects?

2. The neighbor mentions "huffing," which his son told him has happened at several parties this year. The neighbor says, "Huffing is not harmful, right?" What should you tell him?

A few weeks later, the neighbor calls you because his son is extremely drowsy and unable to speak. The neighbor notes that his bottle of alprazolam (Xanax) is almost empty and worries that his son has taken an overdose.

3. What should you do first? What treatment would you expect his son to receive?

For answers, see *http://evolve.elsevier.com/Lilley.*

neurologic status, cognitive dysfunction, bizarre changes in mood and demeanor, feelings of paranoia or dysphoria, and a feeling of unreality. The nurse should also assess for and document flashbacks, irrational behavior, psychosis, combativeness, and violent tendencies.

Assessment of *CNS stimulant* abuse requires careful questioning about and observation for adverse effects, toxicity, and withdrawal signs and symptoms. Some of the more commonly abused CNS stimulants are amphetamines, dextroamphetamine, methamphetamine, butyl nitrite, designer drugs, and cocaine (see earlier discussion and Table 9-1). Signs and symptoms of CNS stimulant abuse have been previously discussed, such as changes in blood pressure and increased heart rate but a head-to-toe physical examination and assessment of any complaints or occurrence of vomiting, agitation, tremors, seizures, hyperactive reflexes, flushing, headache, high temperature, and mydriasis (pupil dilatation) should be documented. Vital signs and level of consciousness should be checked frequently. Any increased heart rate (tachycardia), irregular heart rhythm (dysrhythmia), increased motor and speech activity, and hyperthermia (which may be fatal) should be reported immediately to the health care provider.

The most dangerous substances in terms of withdrawal are *CNS depressants* such as barbiturates, benzodiazepines, and alcohol. Alcohol is considered to be a depressant and is discussed later in this chapter. Abuse of CNS depressants is manifested by a decrease in vital signs and mental functioning (see previous discussion); therefore, frequent monitoring of vital signs and neurologic status is needed for safe and prudent care. A comprehensive, thorough nursing history and medication profile must be obtained, as with any drug. Additional signs and symptoms of abuse are tremors and agitation with possible progression to hallucinations and sometimes death with continued abuse. Early withdrawal may be manifested by increased blood pressure and pulse rate and altered mental status. Because of the risk of respiratory and circulatory depression, the ABCs (*a*irway, *b*reathing, and *c*irculation) of care should always be performed. See the pharmacology section for more specific information. Marijuana, as a CNS depressant, may cause dizziness, disorientation, euphoria, and difficulty with speech and other motor activities. Chronic use/abuse has been previously discussed.

The signs and symptoms of ethanol (alcohol) withdrawal and toxicity are presented in Box 9-6. Assessment should also include gathering data about possible drug interactions, especially the use of other CNS depressants such as opioids, sedatives, and hypnotics. Blood alcohol levels are important to monitor, because the health issues and signs and symptoms that appear are directly related to the blood alcohol level. See *http://evolve. elsevier.com/Lilley* for further discussion of blood alcohol level, signs and symptoms of alcohol toxicity, and a brief discussion of the impact of long-term alcohol use on the brain, liver, GI tract, and nutritional status.

Abuse of *nicotine* (a CNS stimulant) is associated with adverse effects such as increase in heart rate and blood pressure. It can also result in vomiting and increased bowel tone and motor activity. Should the patient have a history of malnutrition, chronic lung disease, stroke, cancer, cardiac disease, or renal or liver dysfunction, relevant laboratory tests are generally ordered, and their results need to be examined by the nurse and those involved in the patient's care. Assessment should focus on vital signs, breath sounds, oxygen saturation levels, and monitoring for changes in neurologic functioning (e.g., level of consciousness, sensory/motor problems). Remember that smoking cessation and signs and symptoms of nicotine withdrawal (see pharmacology discussion) may happen abruptly in hospitalized patients. Being alert to any craving for nicotine associated with irritability, restlessness, and decrease in pulse rate and blood pressure, which will help in early identification of more serious problems.

Nursing Diagnoses

- Chronic low self-esteem related to the influence of substance abuse
- Deficient knowledge related to lack of information about abusive, addictive behaviors and their long-term management

- Ineffective health management of self related to substance abuse
- Risk for injury and falls related to substance abuse and/or abrupt withdrawal
- Risk for other-directed violence related to drug abuse or alcohol abuse

Planning

Goals

- Patient gains improved self-esteem during treatment for substance abuse.
- Patient remains without injury during treatment for substance abuse.
- Patient openly discusses their substance abuse problem and the benefit of a treatment regimen. Patient identifies any barriers to effective health maintenance and healthy self-image.
- Patient regains control of own behavior with assistance from the health care team and treatment modality.
- Patient identifies within a therapeutic environment the possibilities of violent behavior against self and others.

Outcome Criteria

- Patient exhibits improved body image and self-esteem through positive behaviors during treatment for abuse disorder.
- Patient exhibits participation and cooperation with a therapeutic regimen for abusive behaviors and related drug use.
- Patient undergoes safe withdrawal from the abused substance with stabilization of the aggravated and dysfunctional physical and emotional state caused by the substance abuse (see the specific drug and related signs and symptoms) and without injury to self or others.
- Patient receives appropriate referrals and humane treatment for the substance abuse problem in a safe, nonthreatening, healthy environment.
- Patient has a decreased number of violent responses and identifies possible preventative measures to avoid future violent behaviors.
- Patient verbalizes increased positive feelings of healthy adaptation and coping skills.

Implementation

The nurse plays a vital role in the care of patients manifesting abuse behaviors, intoxication, and withdrawal. It is also the nurse who, through the nursing process, helps to meet the patient's basic needs after developing a therapeutic relationship and teaches the patient, family, and/or significant others about addiction and its effect on the entire family. Nursing strategies for meeting actual or potential health problems are implemented for nursing diagnoses generated from assessment data. Nurses working with substance abuse patients need their own sound knowledge base as well as special understanding and empathy. Participation in training, seminars, and education about the process of substance abuse and related lifestyles is encouraged to assist the nurse in understanding the patient and developing a comprehensive plan of care. In general, nursing interventions involve maximizing all of the therapeutic plans and minimizing those factors contributing to the abusive behaviors. Once a therapeutic rapport has been established and a patient-nurse-health care provider contract has been agreed upon, maximizing recovery is the plan.

LIFE SPAN CONSIDERATIONS: The Elderly Patient

Substance Abuse

Alcohol and substance abuse among the elderly is a hidden national epidemic. It is believed that about 10% of this country's population abuses alcohol, but surveys have revealed that as many as 17% of adults older than age 65 have an alcohol abuse problem. Abuse of other substances by older adults is also an overlooked and often ignored problem. Older drug abusers are often poor, frail, and hidden from health professionals and service providers. The stigma associated with these problems keeps them, as well as family members, from coming forward to report problems. Although the overall rate of substance abuse is lower in older adults than in younger people, substance abuse in the elderly is a significant and growing problem. Alcohol abuse in the elderly is complicated by the fact that many abusers in this age group also use prescription and over-the-counter (OTC) medications. OTC drugs may cause adverse effects even when taken alone, and serious consequences may result when OTC drugs are taken with alcohol. The main problems are seen when the combining of alcohol with a drug results in intensification of the drug's action (e.g., heightened hypotensive effects when an antihypertensive drug is taken with alcohol); this can lead to increased adverse effects with significant negative consequences (such as dizziness and possible syncope due to the greater drop in blood pressure, which can result in falls and injury). Some of the signals indicating an alcohol or alcohol and medication-related problem in the elderly include trouble with memory after having a drink or taking a medication; loss of coordination, unsteadiness in walking or frequent falls; changes in sleeping habits; unexplained bruises; and irritability, sadness, depression, and being unsure of oneself.

Data from New York Office of Alcoholism and Substance Abuse Services: Elderly alcohol and substance abuse, 2005, available at *http://www.oasas.state. ny.us/AdMed/FYI/FYIINDepth-Elderly.cfin*.

Interventions are based on the patient's specific physical and emotional problems and are carried out accordingly and in order of priority of basic needs. For example, if the patient is experiencing hallucinations either from the substance or from withdrawal, the nurse must manage the ABCs of care and monitor vital signs and neurologic and mental status while providing a calm, quiet, nonjudgmental, and nonthreatening environment. Seizures may occur, so safety precautions are needed, including the use of protective measures such as attention to the airway, padding of side rails, and implementation of other seizure precautions (consult facility policies and procedures). For more information related to life span considerations (for adolescent and elderly patients) see the boxes on page 000.

Substance withdrawal is treated with a multimodal approach that includes pharmacologic and nonpharmacologic interventions. The nurse has the responsibility to remain nonjudgmental while assisting in the patient's recovery and rehabilitation. Nurses need to remain current in their knowledge about the different substances being abused as well as the various treatment and rehabilitation protocols. Of all interventions, ensuring patient safety is of utmost importance, beginning with the basic ABCs of care (see earlier) and moving through the plan of care for the patient's withdrawal, recovery, and rehabilitation. Patient education remains an essential part of patient care to help the patient, family, and/or significant others understand the need for long-term lifestyle changes. Whether it is disulfiram (Antabuse) treat-

LIFE SPAN CONSIDERATIONS: The Pediatric Patient

Abuse of Over-the-Counter Drugs and Huffing Practices in Adolescents

Adolescent patients are exposed to very real drug hazards connected with some everyday products within the home. Two major problems involving hazardous drug use are seen this population. The first is the abuse of over-the-counter cold products, specifically *dextromethorphan*-containing products. Dextromethorphan is the most commonly used and most effective nonprescription cough suppressant and is an ingredient in several over-the-counter products, including Robitussin DM cough syrup and Mucinex DM tablets. Some adolescents have discovered that taking dextromethorphan in large amounts leads to a "high" that is accompanied by hallucinations. The hallucinations have been documented to be similar to those associated with the street drug phencyclidine (PCP) and the anesthetic ketamine (see Chapter 12). The incidence of abuse varies; however, in April, 2005, the Medical News Today reported that 1 in 11 teens has abused dextromethorphan-containing medications (17th annual study; Partnership for a Drug-Free America). In addition, it has been found that teens who abuse dextromethorphan may also abuse other drugs such as lysergic acid diethylamide (LSD), PCP, Ecstasy, and inhalants. The hazardous short- or long-term effects that may occur with these drugs include nausea, hot flashes, reduced mental status, dizziness, seizures, loss of coordination and balance, brain damage, and death. The second problem is that of "huffing" or the abuse of inhalants, including the following substances: (1) *volatile solvents*—nail polish and paint thinner, (2)

aerosols—deodorants and cooking sprays, (3) *gases*—butane cigarette lighter fluid and nitrous oxide (laughing gas), and (4) *nitrites*—cyclohexyl nitrite (found in room deodorizers) and amyl nitrite and butyl nitrite (sold on the street in small sealed containers). While some studies reported an increase in inhalant abuse by teens in the past 10 years, a new report based upon the National Survey on Drug Use and Health found that fewer adolescents are using inhalants such as glue and lighter fluid, but that the number of inhalant abusers in U.S. teens has not declined. The Associated Press (March, 2009) reported that the number of adolescents actually abusing inhalants, as compared to those just trying them, remained at a stable rate between 2002-2007. Inhalant use often results in a euphoric feeling, but brain damage and even death can occur with just one huff. While the rate may be "stable," there is still a tremendous need for continued prevention and treatment efforts. Education should begin early on in elementary school, so that children learn of the problem and the related damaging effects to the brain before actual exposure to the practice. Education and awareness are important to prevent abuse and abuse behaviors, and a child is never too young to learn about these types of dysfunctional and life-threatening behaviors. Parents, other family members and relatives, and caregivers should be actively involved in any educational sessions about this specific practice, as well as about other drugs that are abused, and related signs and symptoms.

Data from Werner, E: Fewer teens sniffing inhalants to get high, Associated Press, Washington, DC, March 16, 2009; Join Together: Inhalant use declines among U.S. teens, March 19, 2009, available at *http://www.jointogether.org/news/headlines/inthenews/2009/inhalant-use-declines-among.html*; Prescription for danger: A report on the troubling trend of prescription and over-the-counter drug abuse among the nation's teens, January 2008, available at *http://theantidrug.com/pdfs/prescription report.pdf* or visit *www.ondcp.gov*, January 2008; The Partnership for a Drug-Free America: Generation RX: National study reveals new category of substance abuse emerging: Teens abusing RX and OTC medications intentionally to get high, available at *http://www.drugfree.org/Portal/About/NewsReleases/Generation_Rx_Teens_ Abusing_Rx_and_OTC_Medications*.

ment for alcohol abuse or bupropion therapy for nicotine withdrawal, patients need careful instructions and information about their treatment regimen.

Substance abuse has a major impact on family members and significant others. The family will also be in need of treatment and therapeutic support. But it is the caring, empathic, supportive, and educative responses by the nurse that will convey acceptance to the patient and family and help in the overall process of recovery and rehabilitation. A nonjudgemental attitude, caring, empathy, and quality care should be the center of Patient Rights as well as the ANA Code of Ethics (see Chapter 4) regardless of the admitting diagnosis and/or the type of substance being abused. Lifelong treatment is often indicated; the need for support during the long-term process of recovery should be emphasized and support recommended from within the family unit and extending outward to the community. (See Box 9-9 for a listing of various organizations and resources.) Methods to encourage recovery and minimize relapse should be individualized for each patient and should draw on all available resources, whether private or public. Communication techniques must be reinforcing and firm, yet sensitive to the patient's values and beliefs. Family members must be an integral part of all treatment and must participate in all educational sessions.

Evaluation

Patient safety is of utmost importance at all times during patient care but especially when the patient is experiencing the signs and symptoms of withdrawal. Patients may go from mild withdrawal to severe withdrawal and enter into life-threatening situations within a period of a day or two, and therefore complete evaluation of the

---

BOX 9-9 Organizations and Agencies Concerned with Substance Abuse

Alcoholics Anonymous
American Council for Drug Education
American Society of Addiction Medicine
International Nurses Society on Addictions
National Center on Addiction and Substance Abuse at Columbia University
National Clearinghouse for Alcohol and Drug Information
National Council on Alcoholism and Drug Dependence
National Inhalant Prevention Coalition
National Institute on Alcohol Abuse and Alcoholism
National Institute on Drug Abuse
Partnership for a Drug-Free America
Substance Abuse and Mental Health Services Administration
U.S. Drug Enforcement Administration

---

patient and environment must be ongoing. Evaluation of the recovery and rehabilitation process is important as well, with monitoring of the therapeutic effects of the treatment regimen and monitoring for any ill effects from the physiologic and/or psychologic withdrawal of the substance. Part of this evaluation process also is appraisal of the support provided by others such as family members, as well as review of the availability of needed resources during and after hospitalization. In addition, any abnormality in vital signs, laboratory test results, mental status, or other parameters should be reported immediately. This ongoing evaluation should also examine the availability of emotional, social, cultural, spiritual, and financial support, and the nursing care plan should be revised as needed.

PATIENT TEACHING TIPS

- Ensure that relevant, nondiscriminatory, current, and accurate information—at various reading levels—is available to the patient, family, or significant others regarding the specific abuse disorder, signs and symptoms, withdrawal, and treatment regimens. Making an informed decision is best for everyone involved in the process of recovery and rehabilitation.
- Educate the patient, family, and/or significant other about available support groups and community resources.
- Be sure that the patient understands the importance of having—on their person at all times—a current list of all medications, including treatment regimens for the abuse disorder. Include information about the drug, its action, why it is used and how, adverse effects, cautions, drug-drug and drug-food interactions, cautions, contraindications, dosing, and consequences of any missed doses.
- Patients should be educated about their rights to ethical and empathic treatment, regardless of the reason for treatment. One online resource available is at *http://www.healthline.com/galecontent/center-for-substance-abuse-prevention*. This site provides written information, resources, and video clips about drug/chemical abuse.

POINTS TO REMEMBER

- Physical dependence is a condition characterized by physiologic reliance on a substance, usually indicated by tolerance to the effects of the substance and development of withdrawal symptoms when use of the substance is terminated.
- Psychologic dependence is a condition characterized by strong desires to obtain and use a substance.
- Habituation refers to situations in which a patient becomes accustomed to a certain drug (develops tolerance) and may have mild psychologic dependence on it but does not show compulsive dose escalation, drug-seeking behavior, or major withdrawal symptoms upon drug discontinuation.
- Acamprosate is used to maintain abstinence from alcohol in patients who are abstinent when starting the drug and who have additional psychosocial support. Its mechanism of action is not completely understood.
- A new medication for smoking cessation is varenicline, which has shown better efficacy than bupropion.
- Because abuse is prevalent across the life span, the nurse may encounter this health issue in a variety of settings.

- Drug withdrawal symptoms vary with the class of drug and may even be the opposite of the drug's action. Signs and symptoms of *opioid withdrawal* include seeking the drug from more than one prescriber, mydriasis (pupil dilatation), rhinorrhea, diaphoresis, piloerection (goose bumps), lacrimation, diarrhea, insomnia, and elevated blood pressure and pulse rate. Signs and symptoms of *CNS stimulant withdrawal* include social isolation or withdrawal, psychomotor retardation, and hypersomnia. Signs and symptoms of *CNS depressant withdrawal* include increased psychomotor activity; agitation; muscular weakness; hyperthermia; diaphoresis; delirium; convulsions; elevated blood pressure, pulse rate, and temperature; and eyelid tremors. *Ethanol withdrawal* produces varying degrees of signs and symptoms depending on the specific blood alcohol level. Delirium tremens are characterized by hypertensive crisis, tachycardia, and hyperthermia and may be life threatening.
- Evaluation of the recovery and rehabilitation process is important, including monitoring of the therapeutic effects of the treatment regimen and monitoring for any physiologic and/or psychologic ill-effects from the withdrawal of the abused substance.

NCLEX EXAMINATION REVIEW QUESTIONS

1 A patient is experiencing withdrawal from opioids. The nurse expects to see which assessment finding most commonly associated with acute opioid withdrawal?
   a Elevated blood pressure
   b Decreased pulse
   c Lethargy
   d Constipation

2 During treatment for withdrawal from opioids, the nurse expects which medication to be ordered?
   a amphetamine (Dexedrine)
   b clonidine (Catapres)
   c diazepam (Valium)
   d disulfiram (Antabuse)

3 The nurse is presenting a seminar on substance abuse. Which drug is the most commonly used illicit drug in the United States?
   a Crack cocaine
   b Heroin
   c Marijuana
   d Methamphetamine

4 A patient taking disulfiram as part of an alcohol treatment program accidentally takes a dose of cough syrup that contains a small percentage of alcohol. The nurse expects to see which symptom as a result of acetaldehyde syndrome?
   a Lethargy
   b Copious vomiting
   c Hypertension
   d No ill effect because of the small amount of alcohol in the cough syrup

5 The nurse is assessing a patient for possible substance abuse. Which assessment finding indicates possible use of amphetamines?
   a Lethargy and fatigue
   b Cardiovascular depression
   c Talkativeness and euphoria
   d Difficulty swallowing and constipation

NCLEX EXAMINATION REVIEW QUESTIONS—cont'd

6 A patient experiencing ethanol withdrawal is beginning to show manifestations of delirium tremens. The nurse will plan to implement which interventions for management of delirium tremens? (Select all that apply.)
  a Doses of oral chlordiazepoxide (Librium)
  b Doses of intravenous chlordiazepoxide (Librium)
  c Restraints if the patient becomes confused, agitated, or a threat to himself or others
  d Thiamine supplementation
  e Oral disulfiram (Antabuse) treatment
  f Monitoring in the intensive care unit

1. a, 2. b, 3. c, 4. b, 5. c, 6. b, c, d, f

CRITICAL THINKING ACTIVITIES: BEST ACTION

1 A friend has revealed to the nurse that she has used crack cocaine often in the past few months and states that even though she enjoys the sensations she can "stop at any time." What is the nurse's best action in this situation?

2 A patient is admitted to the hospital for major abdominal surgery, and the physician has ordered that a transdermal nicotine patch be used while the patient is hospitalized because the patient was a heavy smoker. While the patch is applied, the patient asks, "Why in the world would you want to give me nicotine when I'm trying to stop smoking?" What is the nurse's best response to this question?

3 A patient has been admitted to the labor and delivery department. She has a history of heavy use of alcohol and appears to be intoxicated. What are the potential effects of alcohol use on a fetus, and what would be some concerns during the first few months of the newborn's life?

For answers, see *http://evolve.elsevier.com/Lilley.*

CHAPTER 10

Photo Atlas of Drug Administration

PREPARING FOR DRUG ADMINISTRATION

NOTE: This photo atlas is designed to illustrate general aspects of drug administration. For detailed instructions, please refer to a nursing fundamentals or skills book.

When giving medications, remember safety measures and correct administration techniques to avoid errors and to ensure optimal drug actions. Keep in mind the basic "Six Rights":

1. Right drug
2. Right dose
3. Right time
4. Right route
5. Right patient
6. Right documentation

Refer to Chapter 1 for additional rights regarding drug administration. Other things to keep in mind when preparing to give medications are the following:

- Remember to perform hand hygiene before preparing or giving medications (Box 10-1)
- If you are unsure about a drug or dosage calculation, do not hesitate to double-check with a drug reference or with a pharmacist. **DO NOT** give a medication if you are unsure about it!
- Be punctual when giving drugs. Some medications must be given at regular intervals to maintain therapeutic blood levels.
- Figure 10-1 shows an example of a computer-controlled drug-dispensing system. To prevent errors, obtain the drugs for one patient at a time.
- Remember to check the drug at least three times before giving it. The nurse is responsible for checking medication labels against the transcribed medication order. In Figure 10-2, the nurse is checking the drug against the medication administration record after taking it out of the dispenser drawer. The drug should also be checked before opening it and again after opening it but before giving it to the patient. Some drugs (i.e., heparin and insulin) must be checked by two licensed nurses.
- Health care facilities have various means of checking the medication record when a new one is printed, so be sure that you are working from one that has been checked or verified before giving the medication. If the patient's medication record has a new drug order on it, the best rule of practice is to double-check that order against the patient's chart.
- Check the expiration date of all medications. Medications used past the expiration date may be less potent or even harmful.
- Make sure that drugs that are given together are compatible. For example, antacids and bile acid sequestrants (see Chapters 29 and 50) should not be given with other drugs, because they will interfere with drug absorption and action. Check with a pharmacist if unsure.

- Before administering any medication, check the patient's identification bracelet. The Joint Commission's standards require two patient identifiers. In some facilities, patient information is in a barcode system that is scanned. In addition, the patient's drug allergies should be assessed (Figure 10-3).
- Be sure to take the time to explain the purpose of each medication, its action, possible adverse effects, and any other pertinent information, especially drug-drug or drug-food interactions, to the patient and/or caregiver.
- Open the medication at the bedside into the patient's hand or into a medicine cup. Try not to touch the drugs with your hands. Leaving the drugs in their packaging until you get to the patient's room helps to avoid contamination and waste should the patient refuse the drug.
- Discard any medications that fall to the floor or become contaminated by other means.
- Stay with the patient while the patient takes the drugs. Do not leave the drugs on the bedside table or the meal tray for the patient to take later.
- Chart the medication on the medication record (see Figure 10-9 on p. 116) as soon as it is given and before going to the next patient. Be sure also to document therapeutic responses, adverse effects (if any), and other concerns in the nurse's

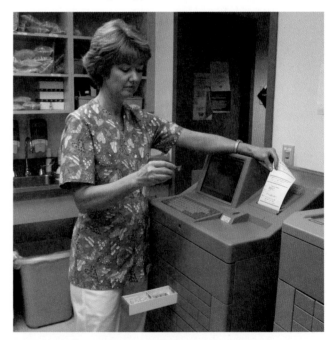

FIGURE 10-1 Using a computer-dispensing system to remove unit-dose medication.

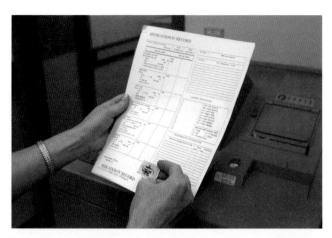

FIGURE 10-2   Checking the medication against the order on the medication administration record.

BOX 10-1 Standard Precautions

Always adhere to Standard Precautions, including the following:
- Wear clean gloves when exposed to, or when there is potential exposure to, blood, body fluids, secretions, excretions, and any items that may contain these substances. Always wash hands immediately when there is direct contact with these substances or any item contaminated with blood, body fluids, secretions, or excretions. Gloves should always be worn when giving injections and may be necessary during medication preparation. Be sure to assess the patient for latex allergies and use nonlatex gloves if indicated.
- Perform hand hygiene after removing gloves and between patient contacts. According to the Centers for Disease Control and Prevention, the preferred method of hand decontamination is with an alcohol-based hand rub, but washing with an antimicrobial soap and water is an alternative to the alcohol rub. When hands are visibly dirty, soap and water should be used to wash hands.
- Hand hygiene should be performed
  - Before direct contact with patients
  - After contact with blood, body fluids, excretions, mucous membranes, wound dressings, or nonintact skin

- After contact with a patient's skin (i.e., when taking a pulse or positioning a patient)
- After removing gloves
- Wear a mask, eye protective gear, and face shield during any procedure or patient care activity with the potential for splashing or spraying of blood, body fluids, secretions, or excretions. Use of a gown may also be indicated for these situations.
- When administering medications, once the exposure or procedure is completed and exposure is no longer a danger, remove soiled protective garments or gear and perform hand hygiene.
- Never remove, recap, cap, bend, or break any used needle or needle system. Be sure to discard any disposable syringes and needles in the appropriate puncture-resistant container.

For detailed information on Standard Precautions, see the guidelines posted on the Center for Disease Control and Prevention website at *http://www.cdc.gov/ncidod/dhqp/gl_isolation_standard.html.*

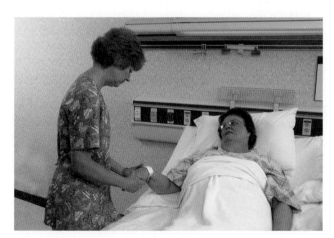

FIGURE 10-3   Always check the patient's identification, using two patient identifiers, and allergies before giving medications.

notes. Some facilities use manual documentation, and others use computer documentation.

- Return to evaluate the patient's response to the drug. Remember that the expected response time will vary according to the drug route. For example, responses to sublingual nitroglycerin or intravenous push medications should be evaluated within minutes, but it may take an hour or more for a response to be noted after an oral medication is given.
- See the Life Span Considerations: The Pediatric Patient box on p. 40 (Chapter 3) for age-related considerations for medication administration to infants and children.

ENTERAL DRUGS

Administering Oral Drugs

Always begin by performing hand hygiene and maintain Standard Precautions (see Box 10-1). When administering oral drugs, keep in mind the following points:

Oral Medications

- Administration of some oral medications (and medications by other routes) requires special assessments. For example, the apical pulse should be auscultated for 1 full minute before any digitalis preparation is given (Figure 10-4). Administration of other oral medications may require blood pressure monitoring. Be sure to document all parameters. In addition, do not forget to check the patient's identification and allergies before giving any oral medication (or medication by any other route).
- If the patient is experiencing difficulty swallowing (dysphagia), some types of tablets can be crushed with a clean mortar and pestle (or other device) (Figure 10-5) for easier administration. Crush one type of pill at a time, because if you mix together all of the medications before crushing (instead of crushing them one at a time) and then spill some, there is no way to tell which drug has been wasted. Also, if all are mixed together, you cannot check the Six Rights three times before giving the drug. Mix the crushed medication in a small amount of soft food, such as applesauce or pudding. Be sure that the pill-crushing device is clean before and after you use it. Refer to Chapter 2 for more information on medications that should not be crushed.
- **CAUTION:** Be sure to verify whether a medication can be crushed by consulting a drug reference book or a pharmacist. Some oral medications, such as capsules, enteric-coated tablets, and sustained-release or long-acting drugs, should *not* be crushed, broken, or chewed (Figure 10-6). These medications are formulated to protect the gastric lining from irritation or protect the drug from destruction by gastric acids, or are designed to break down gradually and slowly release the medication. If these drugs, designated with labels such as *sustained release* or *extended release,* are crushed or opened, then the intended action of the dosage form is destroyed. As a result, gastric irritation may occur, the drug may be inactivated by gastric acids, or the immediate availability of a drug that was supposed to be released slowly may cause *toxic* effects. Check with the prescriber to see if an alternate form of the drug is needed.
- Be sure to position the patient to a sitting or side-lying position to make it easier for the patient to swallow oral medica-

tions and to avoid the risk of aspiration (Figure 10-7). Always provide aspiration prevention measures as needed.

- Offer the patient a full glass of water; 4 to 6 oz of water or other fluid is recommended for the best dissolution and absorption of oral medications. *Age-related considerations:* Young patients and the elderly may not be able to drink a full glass of water but should take enough fluid to ensure that the medication reaches the stomach. If the patient prefers another fluid, be sure to check for interactions between the medication and the fluid of choice. If fluid restriction is ordered, be sure to follow the guidelines.
- If the patient requests, you may place the pill or capsule in his or her mouth with your gloved hand.
- Lozenges should not be chewed unless specifically instructed/ordered.
- Effervescent powders and tablets should be mixed with water and then given immediately after they are dissolved.
- Remain with the patient until all medication has been swallowed. If you are unsure whether a pill has been swallowed, ask the patient to open his or her mouth so that you can inspect to see if it is gone. Assist the patient to a comfortable position after the medication has been taken.
- Document the medication given on the medication record and monitor the patient for a therapeutic response as well as for adverse reactions.

Sublingual and Buccal Medications

The sublingual and buccal routes prevent destruction of the drugs in the gastrointestinal tract and allow for rapid absorption into the bloodstream through the oral mucous membranes. These routes are not often used. Be sure to provide instruction to the patient before giving these medications.

- Sublingual tablets should be placed under the tongue (Figure 10-8). Buccal tablets should be placed between the upper or lower molar teeth and the cheek.
- Be sure to wear gloves if you are placing the tablet into the patient's mouth. Adhere to Standard Precautions (see Box 10-1).
- Instruct the patient to allow the drug to dissolve completely before swallowing.
- Fluids should not be taken with these drug forms. Instruct the patient not to drink anything until the tablet has dissolved completely.
- Be sure to instruct the patient not to swallow the tablet.
- When using the buccal route, alternate sides with each dose to reduce risk of oral mucosa irritation.
- Document the medication given on the medication record (Figure 10-9) and monitor the patient for a therapeutic response as well as for adverse reactions.

Orally Disintegrating Medications

Orally disintegrating medications, either in tablet or medicated strip form, dissolve in the mouth without water within 60 seconds. These medications are placed *on* the tongue, not under the tongue, as in the sublingual route. The absorption through the oral mucosa is rapid with a faster onset of action than for drugs that are swallowed. The patient must be instructed to allow the medication to dissolve on the tongue and not to chew or swallow the medication.

- Be sure to wear gloves if you are placing the medication on the patient's tongue. Adhere to Standard Precautions (see Box 10-1).
- Make sure the patient has not eaten or had anything to drink for 5 minutes before and after taking these medications.
- Orally disintegrating medications are often packed in foil blister packs. Do not open the package until just before giving the medication. Carefully open *one* dose at a time. These medications are fragile and may break if they are pushed through the blister pack. Once a blister or foil pack is opened, the tablet must either be taken or discarded; it cannot be stored for another time.

- Orally disintegrating medications cannot be split, broken, or torn.
- Instruct the patient to hold the medication on the tongue to allow it to dissolve, instead of chewing or swallowing it. This should take about a minute. Warn the patient that there may be a sweet or even slightly bitter taste. Remind the patient not to drink water or to eat for 5 minutes after taking the medication.
- Document the medication given on the medication record (see Figure 10-9) and monitor the patient for a therapeutic response as well as for adverse reactions.

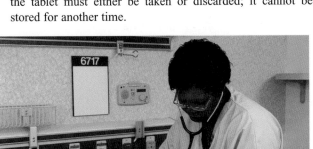
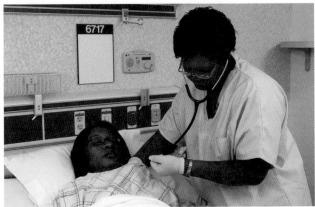

FIGURE 10-4   Some medications require special assessment before administration, such as taking an apical pulse.

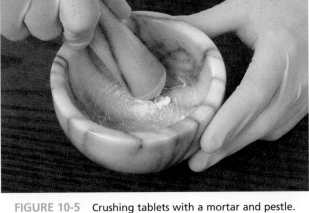

FIGURE 10-5   Crushing tablets with a mortar and pestle.

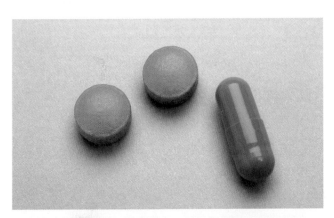

FIGURE 10-6   Enteric-coated tablets and long-acting medications should not be crushed.

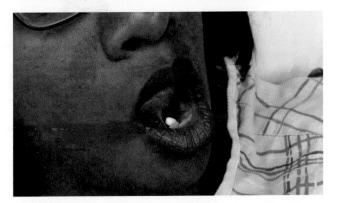

FIGURE 10-7   Giving oral medications.

FIGURE 10-8   Proper placement of a sublingual tablet.

MEDICATION ADMINISTRATION RECORD

Effective: 11/04/09 at 0600	11/04/09 0600-2400	11/05/09 0001-0559
ROUTINE ORDERS	*Time/Initials*	*Time/Initials*
lansoprazole (Prevacid) 15 mg 1 CAPSULE AC BREAKFAST DOSE = 1 CAP = 15 mg ORD#: 5	0730 *LLL*	
nitroglycerin 2% ointment 1 pkt NITRO-BID 2% OINT(unit dose) 1 packet Q 6 H TP 1 inch = 1 packet ORD#: 6	0900 *JSS* 1500 __ 2100 __	0300 __
enoxaparin (Lovenox) 30 mg 30 mg DAILY subcut DOSE = 30 mg = 0.3 mL (30 mg/0.3 mL premixed) DOCUMENT SITE ORD#: 7	0900 *JSS* Site: *RA*	
digoxin (Lanoxin) 0.125 mg ONE TABLET DAILY DOSE = 1 TAB = 0.125 MG CHECK & DOCUMENT APICAL PULSE ORD#: 8	0900 *JSS* AP = *90*	
PRN ORDERS		
acetaminophen 650 mg (Tylenol) 2 tablets Q 4 H prn PRN pain or headache DOSE = 650 mg = 2 TABLETS ORD #: 10		

ALLERGIES	INJECTION SITES
IVP DYE **PCN** **SULFA**	Abdomen LA = Left abdomen RA = Right abdomen LT = Left thigh RT = Right thigh LVG = Left ventrogluteal RVG = Right ventrogluteal LA = Left arm RA = Right arm O = Other (specify)

STAT and SINGLE DOSE MEDS

MED/DOSAGE/ROUTE	Date	Time	INITIALS
Lasix, 40 mg IV STAT	*11/04*	*1200*	*JSS*

INITIALS	MAR VERIFICATION/TIME
CTR	*Charles T. Ryan, RN/0500*

	SIGNATURE LOG
INITIALS	FULL SIGNATURE / TITLE
JSS	*Julie S. Snyder, RN*
LLL	*Linda L. Lilley, RN*

Patient Name: *Rue, Jeannie*

MR#: *06121958*   DOB: *05/25/40*

Admitting Dr: *Keadle, Ralph*   Room: *6717*

MAYFIELD GENERAL HOSPITAL

Virginia Shores, VA

PAGE 1 of 1

FIGURE 10-9   Example of a medication administration record.

Liquid Medications

- Liquid medications may come in a single-dose (unit-dose) package, may be poured into a medicine cup from a multi-dose bottle, or may be drawn up in an oral-dosing syringe (Figure 10-10).
- When pouring a liquid medication from a container, first shake the bottle gently to mix the contents if indicated. Remove the cap and place it on the counter, upside down. Hold the bottle with the label against the palm of your hand to keep any spilled medication from altering the label. Place the medication cup at eye level and fill to the proper level on the scale (Figure 10-11). Pour the liquid so that the base of the meniscus is even with the appropriate line measure on the medicine cup.
- If you overfill the medication cup, discard the excess in the sink. Do not pour it back into the multidose bottle. Before replacing the cap, wipe the rim of the bottle with a paper towel.
- Doses of medications that are less than 5 mL cannot be measured accurately in a calibrated medication cup. For small volumes, use a calibrated oral syringe. Do not use a hypodermic syringe or a syringe with a needle or syringe cap. If hypodermic syringes are used, the drug may be inadvertently given parenterally, or the syringe cap or needle, if not removed from the syringe, may become dislodged and accidentally aspirated by the patient when the syringe plunger is pressed.
- Document the medication given on the medication record (see Figure 10-9) and monitor the patient for a therapeutic response as well as for adverse reactions.

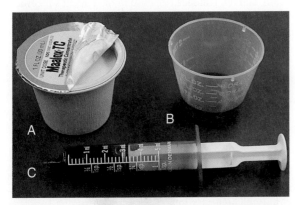

FIGURE 10-10   **A,** Liquid medication in a unit-dose package. **B,** Liquid measured into a medicine cup from a multidose container. **C,** Liquid medicine in an oral-dosing syringe.

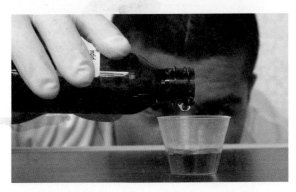

FIGURE 10-11   Measuring liquid medication.

Oral Medications for Infants and Children

- Liquids are usually ordered for infants and young children, because they cannot swallow pills or capsules.
- A plastic disposable oral-dosing syringe is recommended for measuring small doses of liquid medications. Use of an oral-dosing syringe prevents the inadvertent parenteral administration of a drug once it is drawn up into the syringe.
- Position the infant so that the head is slightly elevated to prevent aspiration. Not all infants will be cooperative, and many need to be partially restrained (Figure 10-12).
- Place the plastic dropper or syringe inside the infant's mouth, beside the tongue, and administer the liquid in small amounts while allowing the infant to swallow each time.
- An empty nipple may be used to administer the medication. Place the liquid inside the empty nipple and allow the infant to suck the nipple. Add a few milliliters of water to rinse any remaining medication into the infant's mouth, unless contraindicated.
- Take great care to prevent aspiration. A crying infant can easily aspirate medication. If the infant is crying, wait until the infant is calmer before trying again to give the medication.
- Do not add medication to a bottle of formula; the infant may refuse the feeding or may not drink all of it. Make sure that all of the oral medication has been taken, then return the infant to a safe, comfortable position.
- A child will reject oral medications that taste bitter. The drug may be mixed with a teaspoon of a sweet-tasting food such as jelly, applesauce, ice cream, or sherbet. Using honey in infants is *not* recommended because of the risk of botulism. Do not mix the medication in an essential food item, such as formula, milk, or orange juice, because the child may reject that food later. After the medication is taken, offer the child juice, a flavored frozen ice pop, or water.

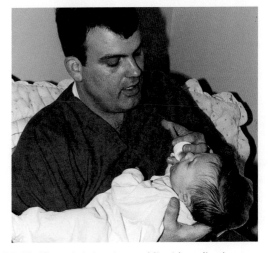

FIGURE 10-12   Administering oral liquid medication to an infant.

Administering Drugs Through a Nasogastric or Gastrostomy Tube

Always begin by performing hand hygiene and maintain Standard Precautions (see Box 10-1). Gloves should be worn. When administering drugs via these routes, keep in mind the following points:

- Before giving drugs via these routes, position the patient in a semi-Fowler's or Fowler's position and leave the head of the bed elevated for at least 30 minutes afterward to reduce the risk of aspiration (Figure 10-13).
- Assess whether fluid restriction or fluid overload is a concern. It will be necessary to give water along with the medications to flush the tubing.
- Check to see if the drug should be given on an empty or full stomach. In addition, some drugs are incompatible with enteral feedings. If the drug should be given on an empty stomach, or if incompatibility exists, the feeding may need to be stopped before and/or after giving the medication. Follow the guidelines for the specific drug if this is necessary. Examples of drugs that are not compatible with enteral feedings are phenytoin and carbidopa-levodopa. Whenever possible, give liquid forms of drugs to prevent clogging the tube.
- If tablets must be given, crush the tablets individually into a fine powder. Administer the drugs separately (Figure 10-14). Keeping the drugs separate allows for accurate identification if a dose is spilled. Be sure to check whether the medication should be crushed; enteric-coated and sustained-release tablets or capsules should not be crushed (see Chapter 2). Check with a pharmacist if you are unsure.

- Before administering the drugs, follow the institution's policy for verifying tube placement and checking gastric residual. Reinstill gastric residual per institutional policy, then clamp the tube.
- Dilute a crushed tablet or liquid medication in 15 to 30 mL of warm water. Some capsules may be opened and dissolved in 30 mL of warm water; check with a pharmacist.
- Remove the piston from an adaptable-tip syringe and attach it to the end of the tube. Unclamp the tube and pinch the tubing to close it again. Add 30 mL of warm water and release the pinched tubing. Allow the water to flow in by gravity to flush the tube, and then pinch the tubing closed again before all the water is gone to prevent excessive air from entering the stomach.
- Pour the diluted medication into the syringe and release the tubing to allow it to flow in by gravity. Flush between each drug with 10 mL of warm water (Figure 10-15). Be careful not to spill the medication mixture. Adjust fluid amounts if fluid restrictions are ordered, but sufficient fluid must be used to dilute the medications and to flush the tubing.
- If water or medication does not flow freely, you may apply gentle pressure with the plunger or bulb of the syringe. Do not try to force the medicine through the tubing.
- After the last drug dose, flush the tubing with 30 mL of warm water, then clamp the tube. Resume the tube feeding when appropriate.
- Have the patient remain in a high Fowler's or slightly elevated right-side-lying position to reduce the risk of aspiration.
- Document the medications given on the medication record, the amount of fluid given on the patient's intake and output record, and the patient's response in the patient's record.

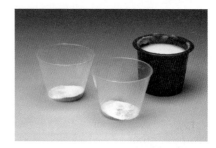

FIGURE 10-14 Medications given through gastric tubes should be administered separately. Dilute crushed pills in 15 to 30 mL of water before administration.

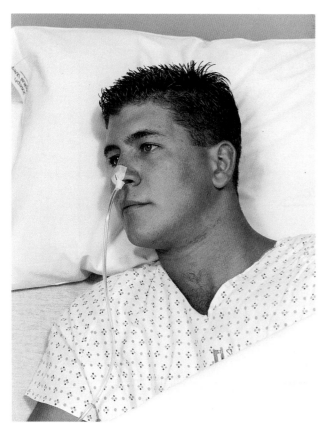

FIGURE 10-13 Elevate the head of the bed before administering medications through a nasogastric tube.

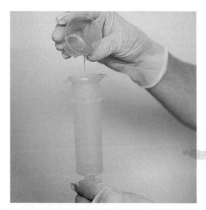

FIGURE 10-15 Pour liquid medication into the syringe, then unclamp the tubing and allow it to flow in by gravity.

Administering Rectal Drugs

Always begin by performing hand hygiene and maintain Standard Precautions (see Box 10-1). Gloves should be worn. When administering rectal drugs, keep in mind the following points:

- Assess the patient for the presence of active rectal bleeding or diarrhea, which generally are contraindications for the use of rectal suppositories.
- Suppositories should not be divided to provide a smaller dose. The active drug may not be evenly distributed within the suppository base.
- Position the patient on his or her left side, unless contraindicated. The uppermost leg should be flexed toward the waist (Sims' position). Provide privacy and drape.
- The suppository should not be inserted into stool. Gently palpate the rectal wall for the presence of feces. If possible, have the patient defecate. DO NOT palpate the patient's rectum if the patient has had rectal surgery.
- Remove the wrapping from the suppository and lubricate the rounded tip with water-soluble jelly (Figure 10-16).
- Insert the tip of the suppository into the rectum while having the patient take a deep breath and exhale through the mouth. With your gloved finger, quickly and gently insert the sup-

pository into the rectum, alongside the rectal wall, at least 1 inch beyond the internal sphincter (Figure 10-17).

- Have the patient remain lying on his or her left side for 15 to 20 minutes to allow absorption of the medication.
- *Age-related considerations:* With children it may be necessary to gently but firmly hold the buttocks in place for 5 to 10 minutes until the urge to expel the suppository has passed. Older adults with loss of sphincter control may not be able to retain the suppository.
- If the patient prefers to self-administer the suppository, the nurse should give specific instructions on the purpose and correct procedure. Be sure to tell the patient to remove the wrapper.
- Use the same procedure for medications administered by a retention enema, such as sodium polystyrene sulfonate (see Chapter 27). Drugs given by enemas are diluted in the smallest amount of solution possible. Retention enemas should be held for 30 minutes to 1 hour before expulsion, if possible.
- Document the medication on the medication record and monitor the patient for the therapeutic effects of the rectal medication.

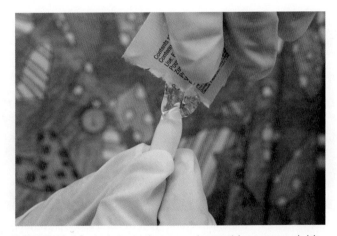

FIGURE 10-16   Lubricate the suppository with a water-soluble lubricant.

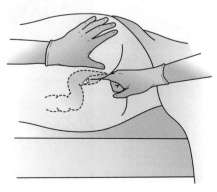

FIGURE 10-17   Inserting a rectal suppository.

PARENTERAL DRUGS

Preparing for Parenteral Drug Administration

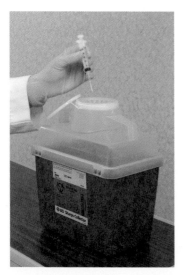

FIGURE 10-18 NEVER RECAP A USED NEEDLE! Always dispose of uncapped needles in the appropriate sharps container. Refer to Box 10-1 for Standard Precautions.

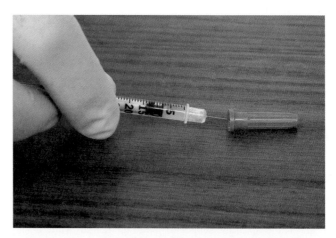

FIGURE 10-19 An UNUSED needle may need to be recapped before the medication is given to the patient. The "scoop method" is one way to recap an unused needle safely. Be sure not to touch the needle to the countertop or to the outside of the needle cap.

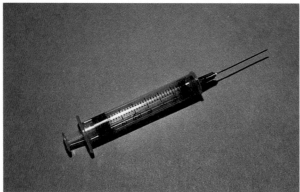

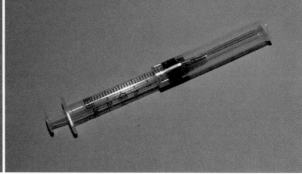

FIGURES 10-20 AND 10-21 There are several types of needlestick prevention syringes. This example (Figure 10-20) has a guard over the unused syringe. After the injection, the nurse pulls the guard up over the needle until it locks into place (Figure 10-21).

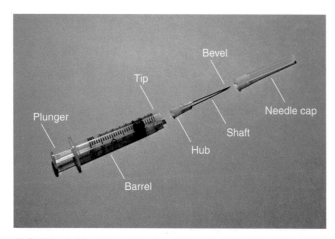

FIGURE 10-22 The parts of a syringe and hypodermic needle.

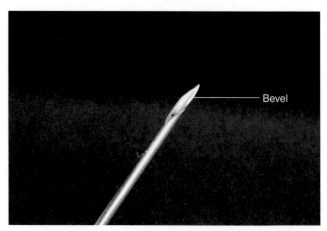

FIGURE 10-23 Close-up view of the bevel of a needle.

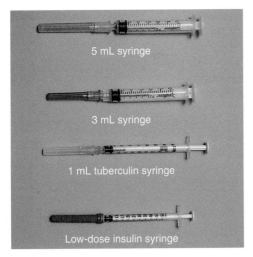

FIGURE 10-24   Be sure to choose the correct size and type of syringe for the drug ordered.

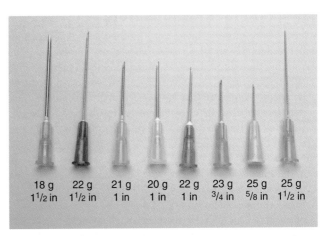

FIGURE 10-25   Needles come in various gauges and lengths. The larger the gauge number, the smaller the needle. Be sure to choose the correct needle—gauge and length—for the type of injection ordered.

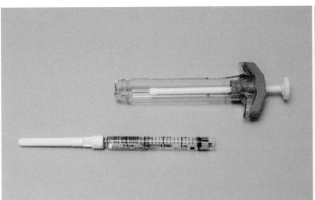

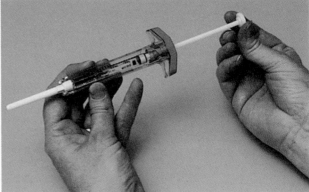

FIGURES 10-26 and 10-27   Some medications come in prefilled, sterile medication cartridges. Figures 10-26 and 10-27 show the Carpuject prefilled cartridge and syringe system. Follow the manufacturer's instructions for assembling prefilled syringes. After use, the syringe is disposed of in a sharps container; the cartridge is reusable. Some prefilled syringes come with an air bubble in the syringe; do not expel the bubble before administration.

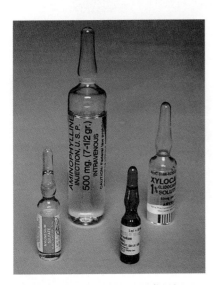

FIGURE 10-28   Ampules containing medications come in various sizes. The neck of the ampule must be broken carefully to withdraw the medication.

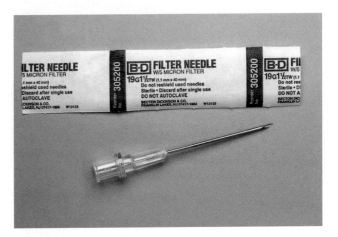

FIGURE 10-29   A filter needle should be used when withdrawing medication from an ampule. Filter needles help to remove tiny glass particles that may result from the ampule breakage. DO NOT USE A FILTER NEEDLE for injection into a patient! Some facilities may also require the use of a filter needle to withdraw medications from a vial.

Removing Medications from Ampules

Always begin by performing hand hygiene and maintain Standard Precautions (see Box 10-1). Gloves may be worn. When performing these procedures, keep in mind the following points:

- When removing medication from an ampule, use a sterile filter needle (Figure 10-29). These needles are designed to filter out glass particles that may be present inside the ampule after it is broken. The filter needle IS NOT intended for administration of the drug to the patient.
- Medication often rests in the top part of the ampule. Tap the top of the ampule lightly and quickly with your finger until all fluid moves to the bottom portion of the ampule (Figure 10-30).
- Place a small gauze pad or dry alcohol swab around the neck of the ampule to protect your hand. Snap the neck quickly and firmly and break the ampule *away* from your body (Figures 10-31 and 10-32).
- To draw up the medication, either set the open ampule on a flat surface or hold the ampule upside down. Insert the filter needle (attached to a syringe) into the center of the ampule opening. Do not allow the needle tip or shaft to touch the rim of the ampule (Figure 10-33).

- Gently pull back on the plunger to draw up the medication. Keep the needle tip below the fluid within the vial; tip the ampule to bring all of the fluid within reach of the needle.
- If air bubbles are aspirated, do not expel them into the ampule. Remove the needle from the ampule, hold the syringe with the needle pointing up, and tap the side of the syringe with your finger to cause the bubbles to rise toward the needle. Draw back slightly on the plunger and slowly push the plunger upward to eject the air. Do not eject fluid.
- Excess medication should be disposed of in a sink. Hold the syringe vertically with the needle tip up and slanted toward the sink. Slowly eject the excess fluid into the sink, then recheck the fluid level by holding the syringe vertically.
- Remove the filter needle and replace with the appropriate needle for administration. NEVER use a filter needle to administer medications to a patient!
- Dispose of the glass ampule pieces and the used filter needle in the appropriate sharps container.

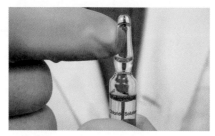

FIGURE 10-30   Tapping an ampule to move the fluid below the neck.

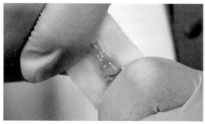 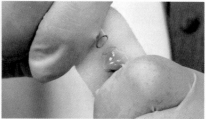

FIGURES 10-31 and 10-32   Breaking an ampule. Carefully break the neck of the ampule in a direction away from you.

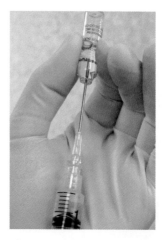

FIGURE 10-33   Using a filter needle to withdraw medication from an ampule.

Removing Medications from Vials

Always begin by performing hand hygiene and maintain Standard Precautions (see Box 10-1). Gloves may be worn. When performing these procedures, keep in mind the following points:

- Vials can contain either a single dose or multiple doses of medication. Follow the institution's policy for using opened multidose vials, such as vials of insulin. Multidose vials should be marked with the date and time of opening and the discard date (per facility policy). If you are unsure about the age of an opened vial of medication, discard it and obtain a new one.
- Check institutional policies regarding which type of needle to use to withdraw fluid from a vial. With the exception of insulin, which must be withdrawn using an insulin syringe, fluid may be withdrawn from a vial using a blunt fill needle or a filter needle. Using a blunt fill needle reduces the chance of injury with a sharp needle (Figure 10-34).
- If the vial is unused, remove the cap from the top of the vial.
- If the vial has been previously opened and used, wipe the top of the vial vigorously with an alcohol swab.
- Air must first be injected into a vial before fluid can be withdrawn. The amount of air injected into a vial should equal the amount of fluid that needs to be withdrawn.
- Determine the volume of fluid to be withdrawn from the vial. Pull back on the syringe's plunger to draw an amount of air into the syringe that is equivalent to the volume of medication to be removed from the vial. Insert the syringe into the vial, preferably using a needleless system. Figure 10-35 shows a needleless system for vial access. Inject the air into the vial.

- While holding onto the plunger, invert the vial and remove the desired amount of medication (Figure 10-36).
- Gently but firmly tap the syringe to remove air bubbles. Excess fluid, if present, should be discarded into a sink.
- Some vials are not compatible with needleless systems and therefore require a needle for fluid withdrawals (Figure 10-37). Use a blunt fill needle if available (see Figure 10-34).
- When an injection requires two medications from two different vials, begin by injecting air into the first vial (without touching the fluid in the first vial), then inject air into the second vial. Immediately remove the desired dose from the second vial. Change needles (if possible), then remove the exact prescribed dose of drug from the first vial. Take great care not to contaminate the drug in one vial with the drug from the other vial. Check with a pharmacist to make sure the two drugs are compatible for mixing in the same syringe.
- For injections, if a needle has been used to remove medication from a vial, always change the needle before administering the dose. Changing needles ensures that a clean and sharp needle is used for the injection. Medication that remains on the outside of the needle may cause irritation to the patient's tissues. In addition, the needle may become dull if used to puncture a rubber stopper. However, some syringes, such as insulin syringes, have needles that are fixed onto the syringe and cannot be removed.

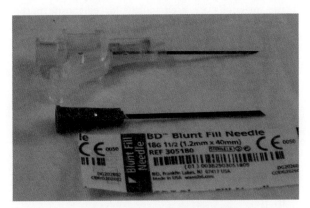

FIGURE 10-34 Comparison of the sharp tip of a needle for injection (*above*) with the blunt tip of a fill needle (*below*), which is used to remove fluid from a vial.

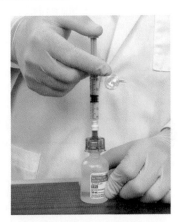

FIGURE 10-35 Insert air into a vial before withdrawing medication (needleless system shown).

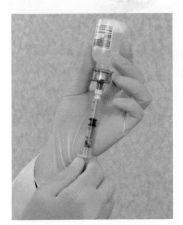

FIGURE 10-36 Withdrawing medication from a vial (needleless system shown).

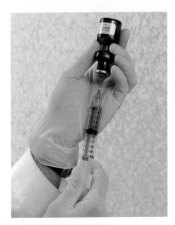

FIGURE 10-37 Using a needle and syringe to remove medication from a vial.

Injections Overview
Needle Insertion Angles for Intramuscular, Subcutaneous, and Intradermal Injections

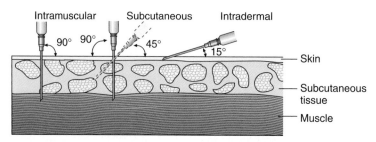

FIGURE 10-38   Comparison of angles of needle insertion for injections.

- For intramuscular (IM) injections, insert the needle at a 90-degree angle (Figure 10-38). Intramuscular injections deposit the drug deep into muscle tissue, where the drug is absorbed through blood vessels within the muscle. The rate of absorption of medication given by the intramuscular route is slower than that of medications given by the intravenous route but faster than that of medications given by the subcutaneous route. Intramuscular injections generally require a longer needle to reach the muscle tissue, but shorter needles may be needed for older patients, children, and adults who are malnourished. The site chosen will also determine the length of the needle needed. In general, aqueous medications can be given with a 22- to 27-gauge needle, but oil-based or more viscous medications are given with an 18- to 25-gauge needle. Average needle lengths for children range from ⅝ to 1 inch, and needles for adults range from 1 to 1½ inches. The nurse must choose the needle length based on the size of the muscle at the injection site, the age of the patient, and the type of medication used.
- For subcutaneous (subcut) injections, insert the needle at either a 45- or 90-degree angle. Subcutaneous injections deposit the drug into the loose connective tissue under the dermis. This tissue is not as well supplied with blood vessels as is the muscle tissue; as a result, drugs are absorbed more slowly than drugs given intramuscularly. In general, use a 25-gauge, ½- to ⅝-inch needle. A *90-degree angle* is used for an *average-sized* patient; a *45-degree angle* may be used for *thin, emaciated, and/or malnourished* patients and for children. To ensure correct needle length, grasp the skinfold with thumb and forefinger, and choose a needle that is approximately half the length of the skinfold from top to bottom.
- Intradermal (ID) injections are given into the outer layers of the dermis in very small amounts, usually 0.01 to 0.1 mL. These injections are used mostly for diagnostic purposes, such as testing for allergies or tuberculosis, and for local anesthesia. Very little of the drug is absorbed systemically. In general, choose a tuberculin or 1-mL syringe with a 25- or 27-gauge needle that is ⅜ to ⅝ inch long. The angle of injection is 5 to 15 degrees.
- For specific information about giving injections to children, see Box 10-2 on p. 130.

Air-Lock Technique

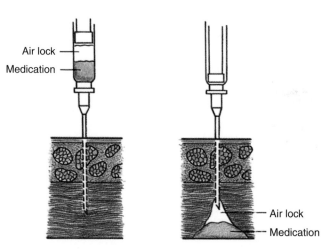

FIGURE 10-39   Air-lock technique for intramuscular injections.

- Some facilities recommend administering intramuscular injections using the air-lock technique (Figure 10-39). Check institutional policies.
- After withdrawing the desired amount of medication into the syringe, withdraw an additional 0.2 mL of air. Be sure to inject using a 90-degree angle. The small air bubble that follows the medication during the injection may help prevent the medication from leaking through the needle track into the subcutaneous tissues.

Intradermal Injections

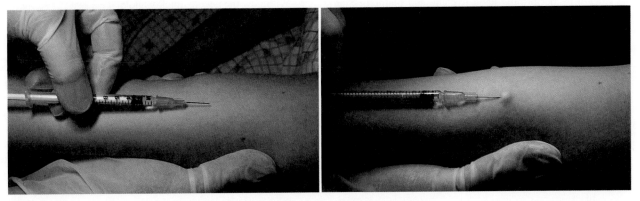

FIGURES 10-40 AND 10-41   Intradermal injection.

Always begin by performing hand hygiene and maintain Standard Precautions (see Box 10-1). Gloves should be worn. When giving an intradermal injection, keep in mind the following points:

- Be sure to choose an appropriate site for the injection. Avoid areas of bruising, rashes, inflammation, edema, or skin discoloration.
- Help the patient to a comfortable position. Extend and support the elbow and forearm on a flat surface.
- In general, three to four finger widths below the antecubital space and one hand width above the wrist are the preferred locations on the forearm. Areas on the back that are also suitable for subcutaneous injection may be used if the forearm is not appropriate for the intradermal injection.
- After cleansing the site with an alcohol swab and allowing it to dry, stretch the skin over the site with your nondominant hand.
- With the needle almost against the patient's skin, insert the needle, bevel UP, at a 5- to 15-degree angle until resistance is

felt, and then advance the needle through the epidermis, approximately 3 mm (Figures 10-40 and 10-41). The needle tip should still be visible under the skin.

- Do not aspirate. This area under the skin contains very few blood vessels.
- Slowly inject the medication. It is normal to feel resistance, and a bleb that resembles a mosquito bite (about 6 mm in diameter) should form at the site.
- Withdraw the needle slowly while gently applying a gauze pad at the site, but do not massage the site.
- Dispose of the syringe and needle in the appropriate container. DO NOT RECAP the needle. Perform hand hygiene after removing gloves.
- Provide instructions to the patient as needed for a follow-up visit for reading the skin testing, if applicable.
- Document in the medication record the date of the skin testing and the date that results should be read, if applicable.

Subcutaneous Injections

Always begin by performing hand hygiene and maintain Standard Precautions (see Box 10-1). Gloves should be worn. When giving a subcutaneous injection, keep in mind the following points:

- Be sure to choose an appropriate site for the injection. Avoid areas of bruising, rashes, inflammation, edema, or skin discoloration (Figure 10-42).
- Ensure that the needle size is correct. Grasp the skinfold between your thumb and forefinger and measure from top to bottom. The needle should be approximately half this length.
- Cleanse the site with an alcohol or antiseptic swab (Figure 10-43) and let the skin dry (occurs almost immediately).
- Tell the patient that he or she will feel a "stick" as you insert the needle.
- For an average-sized patient, pinch the skin with your non-dominant hand and inject the needle quickly at a 45- or 90-degree angle (Figure 10-44).
- For an obese patient, pinch the skin and inject the needle at a 90-degree angle. Be sure the needle is long enough to reach the base of the skinfold.
- *Age-related considerations:* For a child or thin patient, pinch the skin gently and be sure to use a 45-degree angle when injecting the needle.
- Injections given in the abdomen should be given at least 2 inches away from the umbilicus because of the surrounding vascular structure (Figure 10-45). In addition, the injection site should be 2 inches away from any incisions, stomas, or open wounds, if present.
- After the needle enters the skin, grasp the lower end of the syringe with your nondominant hand. Move your dominant hand to the end of the plunger—be careful not to move the syringe.
- Aspiration of medication to check for blood return is not necessary for subcutaneous injections, but some institutions may require it. Check institutional policy. Heparin injections and insulin injections are NOT aspirated before injection.

- With your dominant hand, slowly inject the medication.
- Withdraw the needle quickly and place a swab or sterile gauze pad over the site.
- Apply gentle pressure but do not massage the site. If necessary, apply a bandage to the site.
- Dispose of the syringe and needle in the appropriate container. DO NOT RECAP the needle. Perform hand hygiene after removing gloves.
- Document the medication given on the medication record and monitor the patient for a therapeutic response as well as for adverse reactions.
- For injections of heparin or other subcutaneous anticoagulants, follow the manufacturer's recommendations for injection technique as needed. Many manufacturers recommend the area of the abdomen known as the "love handles" for injection of anticoagulants. DO NOT ASPIRATE before injecting and DO NOT massage the site after injection. These actions may cause a hematoma at the injection site.

Insulin Syringes

- *Always use an insulin syringe to measure and administer insulin.* When giving small doses of insulin, use an insulin syringe that is calibrated for smaller doses. Figure 10-46 shows insulin syringes with two different calibrations. Notice that in the 100-unit syringe, each line represents 2 units; in the 50-unit syringe, each line represents 1 unit. NOTE: A unit of insulin is NOT equivalent to a milliliter of insulin!
- Figure 10-47 shows several examples of devices that can be used to help the patient self-administer insulin. These devices feature a multidose container of insulin and easy-to-read dials for choosing the correct dose. The needle is changed with each use.
- When two different types of insulin are drawn up into the same syringe, always draw up the clear insulin into the syringe first (Figure 10-48). See p. 123 for information about mixing two medications in one syringe.

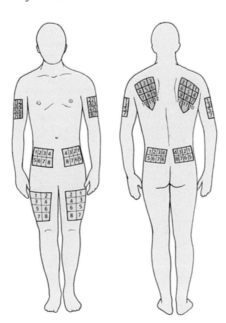

FIGURE 10-42 Potential sites for subcutaneous injections.

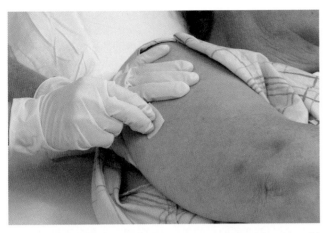

FIGURE 10-43 Before giving an injection, cleanse the skin with an alcohol or antiseptic swab.

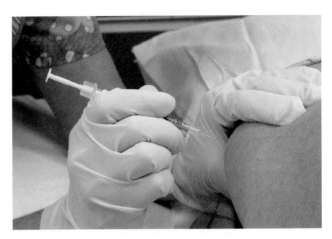

FIGURE 10-44 Giving a subcutaneous injection at a 90-degree angle.

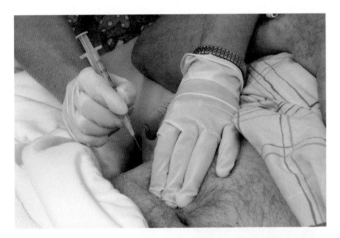

FIGURE 10-45 When giving a subcutaneous injection in the abdomen, be sure to choose a site at least 2 inches away from the umbilicus.

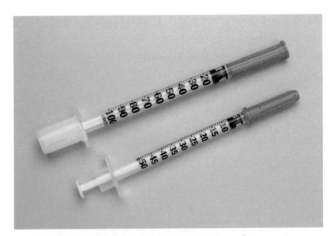

FIGURE 10-46 Insulin syringes are available in 100-unit and 50-unit calibrations.

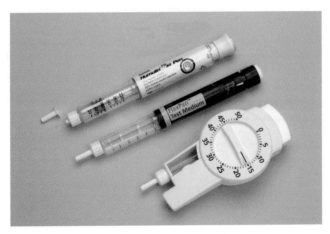

FIGURE 10-47 A variety of devices are available for insulin injections.

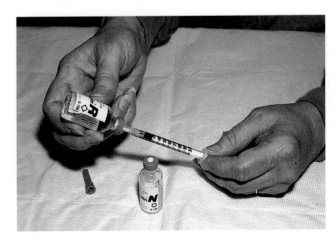

FIGURE 10-48 Mixing two types of insulin in the same syringe. NOTE: The clear insulin is always drawn up into the syringe first.

Intramuscular Injections

Always begin by performing hand hygiene and maintain Standard Precautions (see Box 10-1). Gloves should be worn. When giving an intramuscular injection, keep in mind the following points:

- Choose the appropriate site for the injection by assessing not only the size and integrity of the muscle but the amount and type of injection. Palpate potential sites for areas of hardness or tenderness and note the presence of bruising or infection.
- The dorsogluteal injection site is no longer recommended for injections because of the close proximity to the sciatic nerve and major blood vessels. Injury to the sciatic nerve from an injection may cause partial paralysis of the leg. The dorsogluteal site should not be used for intramuscular injections.
- Assist the patient to the proper position and ensure his or her comfort.
- Locate the proper site for the injection and cleanse the site with an alcohol swab. Keep the swab or a sterile gauze pad nearby and allow the alcohol to dry before injection.
- With your nondominant hand, pull the skin taut. Follow the instructions for the Z-track method (see later) if appropriate.
- Grasp the syringe with your dominant hand as if holding a dart and position the needle at a 90-degree angle to the skin.

Tell the patient that he or she will feel a "stick" as you insert the needle.

- Insert the needle quickly and firmly into the muscle. Grasp the lower end of the syringe with the nondominant hand while still holding the skin back, to stabilize the syringe. With the dominant hand, pull back on the plunger for 5 to 10 seconds to check for blood return.
- If no blood appears in the syringe, inject the medication slowly, at the rate of 1 mL every 10 seconds. After the drug is injected, wait 10 seconds, then withdraw the needle smoothly while releasing the skin.
- Apply gentle pressure at the site and watch for bleeding. Apply a bandage if necessary.
- If blood does appear in the syringe, remove the needle, dispose of the medication and syringe, and prepare a new syringe with the medication.
- Dispose of the syringe and needle in the appropriate container. DO NOT RECAP the needle. Perform hand hygiene after removing gloves.
- Document the medication given on the medication record and monitor the patient for a therapeutic response as well as for adverse reactions.

Z-Track Method

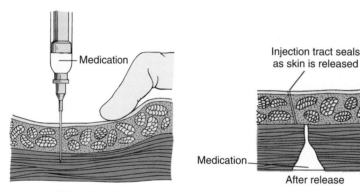

FIGURES 10-49 and 10-50   Z-track method for intramuscular injections.

- The Z-track method is used for injections of irritating substances such as iron dextran and hydroxyzine. The technique reduces pain, irritation, and staining at the injection site. Some facilities recommend this method for *all* intramuscular injections (Figures 10-49 and 10-50).
- After choosing and preparing the site for injection, use your nondominant hand to pull the skin laterally and hold it in this position while giving the injection. Insert the needle at a 90-degree angle, aspirate for 5 to 10 seconds to check for blood return, then inject the medication slowly. After injecting

the medication, wait 10 seconds before withdrawing the needle. Withdraw the needle slowly and smoothly, and maintain the 90-degree angle.
- Release the skin immediately after withdrawing the needle to seal off the injection site. This technique forms a Z-shaped track in the tissue that prevents the medication from leaking through the more sensitive subcutaneous tissue from the muscle site of injection. Apply gentle pressure to the site with a dry gauze pad.

Ventrogluteal Site

- The ventrogluteal site is the *preferred* site for adults and children. It is considered the safest of all sites because the muscle is deep and away from major blood vessels and nerves (Figure 10-51).
- The patient should be positioned on his or her side, with knees bent and upper leg slightly ahead of the bottom leg. If necessary, the patient may remain in a supine position.
- Palpate the greater trochanter at the head of the femur and the anterosuperior iliac spine. As illustrated in Figure 10-52, use the left hand to find landmarks when injecting into the patient's right ventrogluteal and use the right hand to find landmarks when injecting into the patient's left ventrogluteal site.

Place the palm of your hand over the greater trochanter and your index finger on the anterosuperior iliac spine. Point your thumb toward the patient's groin and fingers toward the patient's head. Spread the middle finger back along the iliac crest, toward the buttocks, as much as possible.

- The injection site is the center of the triangle formed by your middle and index fingers (see arrow in Figure 10-52).
- Before giving the injection you may need to switch hands so that you can use your dominant hand to give the injection (Figure 10-53).
- Follow the general instructions for giving an intramuscular injection.

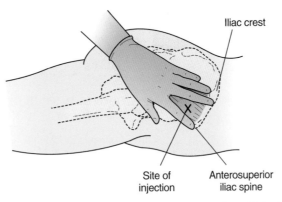

FIGURE 10-51   Finding landmarks for a ventrogluteal injection.

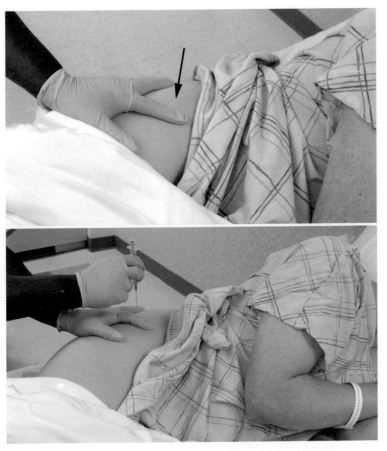

FIGURES 10-52 and 10-53   Ventrogluteal intramuscular injection.

Vastus Lateralis Site

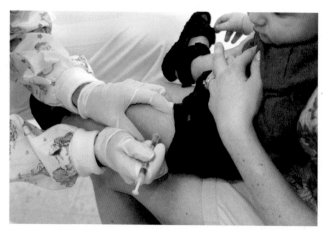

FIGURE 10-54   Vastus lateralis intramuscular injection in an infant.

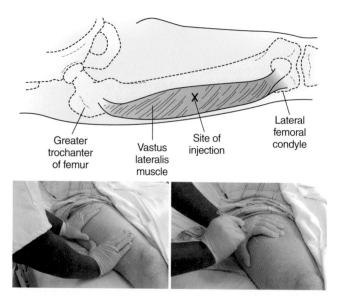

Greater trochanter of femur

Vastus lateralis muscle

Site of injection

Lateral femoral condyle

FIGURES 10-55, 10-56, AND 10-57   Vastus lateralis intramuscular injection.

- Generally the vastus lateralis muscle is well developed and not located near major nerves or blood vessels. It is the preferred site of injection of drugs such as immunizations for infants (Figure 10-54).

- The patient may be sitting or lying supine; if supine, have the patient bend the knee of the leg in which the injection will be given.

- To find the correct site of injection, place one hand above the knee and one hand below the greater trochanter of the femur. Locate the midline of the anterior thigh and the midline of the lateral side of the thigh. The injection site is located within the rectangular area (Figures 10-55, 10-56, and 10-57).

BOX 10-2 Pediatric Injections

Site selection is crucial for pediatric injections. Factors to consider are the age of the child, the size of the muscle at the injection site, the type of injection, the thickness of the solution, and the ease with which the child can be positioned properly. There is no universal agreement in the literature on the "best" intramuscular injection site for children. For infants, the preferred site is the vastus lateralis muscle. The ventrogluteal site may also be used in children of all ages. For immunizations in toddlers and older children, the deltoid muscle may be used *if* the muscle mass is well developed. Refer to facility policy.

Children are often extremely fearful of needles and injections. Even a child who appears calm may become upset and lose control during an injection procedure. For safety reasons, it is important to have another person available for positioning and holding the child.

Distraction techniques are helpful. Say to the child, "If you feel this you can ask me to take it out, please." Be quick and efficient when giving the injection.

Have a small, colorful bandage on hand to apply after the injection. If the child is old enough, have the child hold the bandage and apply it after the injection. If possible, offer a reward sticker after the injection.

After the injection, allow the child to express his or her feelings. For young children, encourage parents to offer comfort with holding and cuddling. Older children should be praised.

EMLA (lidocaine/prilocaine) cream or a vapocoolant spray, if available, may be used before the injection to reduce the pain from the needle insertion. However, because these agents do not absorb down into the muscle, the child may still experience pain when the medication enters the muscle. EMLA cream should be applied to the site at least 1 hour and up to 3 hours before the injection. Vapocoolant spray is applied to the site immediately before the injection. Another option is to apply a wrapped ice cube to the injection site for a minute before the injection.

From Hockenberry MJ et al: *Wong's nursing care of infants and children*, ed 8, St Louis, 2007, Mosby.

Deltoid Site

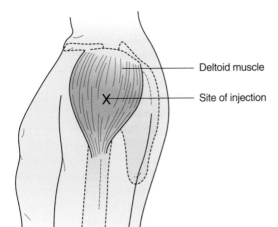

— Deltoid muscle

— Site of injection

FIGURES 10-58, 10-59, and 10-60   Deltoid intramuscular injection. The deltoid site is not considered a primary site for intramuscular injections but is used for immunizations for toddlers, older children, and adults. This site is not used for infants.

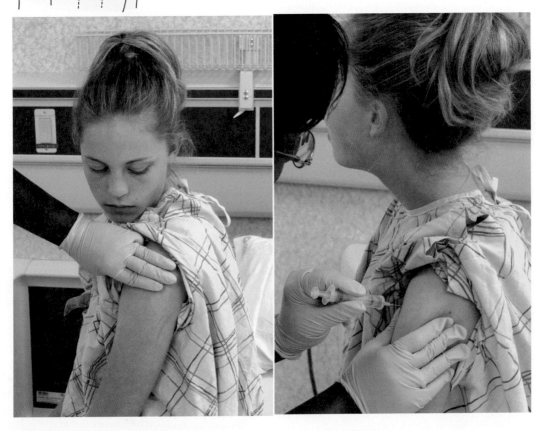

- Even though the deltoid site (Figure 10-58) is easily accessible, it is *not* the first choice for intramuscular injections because the muscle may not be well developed in some adults, and the site carries a risk for injury because the axillary nerve lies beneath the deltoid muscle. In addition, the brachial artery and radial, brachial, and ulnar nerves are also located in the upper arm. Always check medication administration policies, because some facilities do not permit the use of the deltoid site for intramuscular injections. The deltoid site should only be used for administration of immunizations to toddlers, older children, and adults (not infants) and only for small volumes of medication (0.5 to 1 mL).
- The patient may be sitting or lying down. Remove clothing to expose the upper arm and shoulder. Tight-fitting sleeves should not be rolled up. Have the patient relax his or her arm and slightly bend the elbow.
- Palpate the lower edge of the acromion process. This edge becomes the base of an imaginary triangle (Figure 10-59).
- Place three fingers below this edge of the acromion process. Find the point on the lateral arm in line with the axilla. The injection site will be in the center of this triangle, three finger widths (1 to 2 inches) below the acromion process.
- *Age-related considerations:* In children and smaller adults it may be necessary to bunch the underlying tissue together before giving the injection and/or use a shorter ($\frac{5}{8}$-inch) needle (Figure 10-60).
- To reduce patient anxiety, have the patient look away before giving the injection.

Preparing Intravenous Medications

Always begin by performing hand hygiene and maintain Standard Precautions (see Box 10-1). Gloves should be worn for most of these procedures. When administering intravenous (IV) drugs, keep in mind the following points:

- The intravenous route for medication administration provides for rapid onset and faster therapeutic drug levels in the blood than other routes. However, the intravenous route is also potentially more dangerous. Once an intravenous drug is given, it begins to act immediately and cannot be removed. The nurse must be aware of the drug's intended effects and possible side or adverse effects. In addition, hypersensitivity (allergic) reactions may occur quickly.
- Since the passage of the Needle Safety and Prevention Act of 2001, many institutions now use a needleless system for all infusion lines.
- Before giving an intravenous medication, assess the patient's drug allergies, assess the intravenous line for patency, and assess the site for signs of phlebitis or infiltration.
- When more than one intravenous medication is to be given, check with the pharmacy for compatibility if the medications are to be infused at the same time.
- Check the expiration date of both the medication and infusion bags.
- *Age-related considerations:* For children, infusion pumps *must* be used to prevent the risk of infusing the fluid and medication too fast.
- The Joint Commission requires that the pharmacy prepare intravenous solutions and intravenous piggyback (IVPB) admixtures under a special laminar airflow hood. Most IVPB medications come in vials that are added to the intravenous bag just before administration. On the rare occasion when you must dilute a drug for intravenous use, contact the pharmacist for instructions. Be sure to verify which type of fluid to use and the correct amount of solution for the dosage.
- It is important to choose the correct solution for diluting intravenous medications. For example, phenytoin must be infused with normal saline, not dextrose solutions (see Chapter 15). Check with the pharmacist if necessary.
- Most IVPB medications are provided as part of an "add-a-vial" system that allows the intravenous medication vial to be attached to a small-volume minibag for administration. Figure 10-61 shows two examples of IVPB medications attached to small-volume infusion bags.

- These IVPB medication setups allow for mixing of the drug and diluent immediately before the medication is given. Remember that if the seals are not broken and the medication is not mixed with the fluid in the infusion bag, then the medication stays in the vial! As a result, the patient does not receive the ordered drug dose; instead, the patient receives a small amount of plain intravenous fluid.
- One type of IVPB system that needs to be activated before administration is illustrated in Figure 10-62. To activate this type of IVPB system, snap the connection area between the intravenous infusion bag and the vial (Figure 10-63). Gently squeeze the fluid from the infusion bag into the vial and allow the medication to dissolve (Figure 10-64). After a few minutes, rotate the vial gently to ensure that all of the powder is dissolved. When the drug is fully dissolved, hold the IVPB apparatus by the vial and squeeze the bag; fluid will enter the bag from the vial. Make sure that all of the medication is returned to the IVPB bag.
- When hanging these IVPB medications, take care NOT to squeeze the bag. This may cause some of the fluid to leak back into the vial and alter the dose given.
- Always label the IVPB bag with the patient's name and room number, the name of the medication, the dose, the date and time mixed, your initials, and the date and time the medication was given.
- Some intravenous medications must be mixed using a needle and syringe. Again, in many facilities, this procedure will be performed in the pharmacy. Follow the facility policy. After checking the order and the compatibility of the drug and the intravenous fluid, wipe the port of the intravenous bag with an alcohol swab (Figure 10-65).
- Carefully insert the needle into the center of the port and inject the medication (Figures 10-66 and 10-67). Note how the medication remains in the lower part of the intravenous infusion bag. To infuse an even concentration of medication, gently shake the bag after injecting the drug (Figure 10-68).
- Always add medication to a *new* bag of intravenous fluid, not to a bag that has partially infused. The concentration of the medication may be too strong if it is added to a partially full bag.
- Always label the intravenous infusion bag when a drug has been added (Figure 10-69). Label as per institution policy and include the patient's name and room number, the name of the medication, the date and time mixed, your initials, and the date and time the infusion was started. In addition, label all intravenous infusion tubing per institution policy.

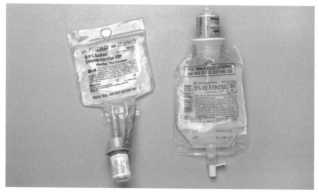

FIGURE 10-61 Two types of intravenous piggyback medication delivery systems. These intravenous systems must be activated before drug will be administered to the patient.

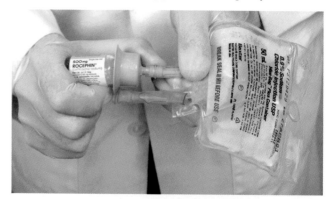

FIGURE 10-62 Activating an intravenous piggyback infusion bag (step 1).

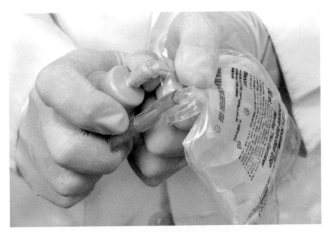

FIGURE 10-63   Activating an intravenous piggyback infusion bag (step 2).

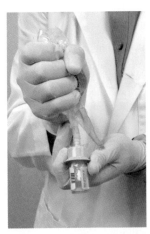

FIGURE 10-64   Activating an intravenous piggyback infusion bag (step 3).

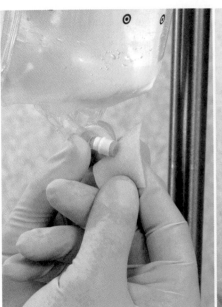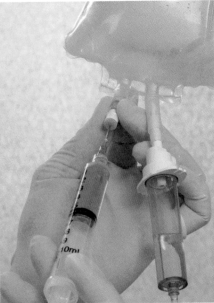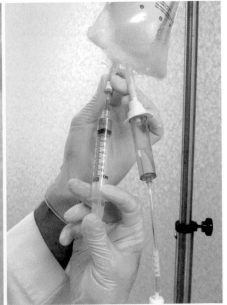

FIGURES 10-65, 10-66, AND 10-67   Adding a medication to an intravenous infusion bag with a needle and syringe.

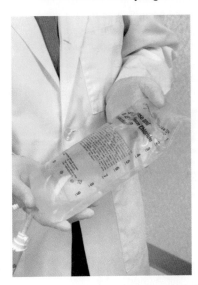

FIGURE 10-68   Mix the medication thoroughly before infusing.

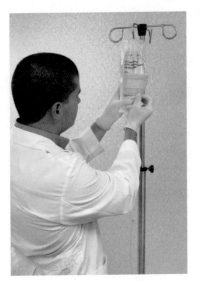

FIGURE 10-69   Label the intravenous infusion bag when medication has been added.

Infusions of Intravenous Piggyback Medications

Always begin by performing hand hygiene and maintain Standard Precautions (see Box 10-1). Gloves should be worn.

- If you are infusing the IVPB medication for the first time, you will need to attach the medication bag to the appropriate tubing and "prime" the tubing by allowing just enough fluid through the tubing to flush out the air. Take care not to waste too much of the medication when flushing the tubing.
- If you are adding IVPB medication to an infusion that already has tubing, then use the technique of "backpriming" to flush the tubing (Figure 10-70). Backpriming allows for the administration of multiple intravenous medications without multiple disconnections, and thus reduces the risk of contamination of the intravenous tubing system.
- Backpriming allows the removal of the old medication fluid that has remained in the IVPB tubing from the previous dose of intravenous medication. After ensuring that the medication in the primary infusion (if any) is compatible with the medication in the IVPB bag, close the roller clamp on the primary infusion if the intravenous fluid is infusing by gravity flow (not necessary if an infusion pump is used). Remove the empty IVPB container from the intravenous pole, lower it to below the level of the primary infusion bag, and open the clamp on the IVPB tubing. This will allow fluid to flow from the primary intravenous bag into the empty IVPB bag. Then, close the clamp on the IVPB tubing and squeeze the fluid that is in the drip chamber into the old IVPB bag to remove the old medication fluid. At this point you may add the new dose of intravenous medication to the IVPB tubing.
- Backpriming will not be possible if the primary intravenous infusion contains heparin, aminophylline, a vasopressor, or multivitamins. Check with a pharmacist if unsure about compatibility.
- Stopping intravenous infusions of medications such as vasopressors for an IVPB medication may affect a patient's blood pressure; stopping intravenous heparin may affect the patient's coagulation levels. Be sure to assess carefully before adding an IVPB medication to an existing infusion. A separate line may be necessary.
- Figure 10-71 shows an IVPB medication infusion (also known as the *secondary* infusion) with a primary gravity infusion. When the IVPB bag is hung higher than the primary intravenous infusion bag, the IVPB medication will infuse until empty, then the primary infusion will take over again.
- When beginning the infusion, attach the IVPB tubing to the upper port on the primary intravenous tubing. A back-check valve above this port prevents the medication from infusing up into the primary intravenous infusion bag.
- Fully open the clamp of the IVPB tubing and regulate the infusion rate with the roller clamp of the primary infusion tubing. Be sure to note the drip factor of the tubing and calculate the drops per minute to set the correct infusion rate for the IVPB medication.
- Monitor the patient during the infusion. Observe for hypersensitivity and for adverse reactions. In addition, observe the intravenous infusion site for infiltration. Have the patient report if pain or burning occurs.
- Monitor the rate of infusion during the IVPB medication administration. Changes in arm position may alter the infusion rate.

- When the infusion is complete, clamp the IVPB tubing and check the primary intravenous infusion rate. If necessary, adjust the clamp to the correct infusion rate.
- Figure 10-72 shows an IVPB medication infusion with a primary infusion that is going through an electronic infusion pump.
- When giving IVPB drugs through an intravenous infusion controlled by a pump, attach the IVPB tubing to the port on the primary intravenous tubing *above* the pump. Open the roller clamp of the IVPB medication tubing. Make sure that the IVPB bag is higher than the primary intravenous infusion bag.
- Following the manufacturer's directions, set the infusion pump to deliver the IVPB medication. Entering the volume of the IVPB bag and the desired time frame of the infusion (such as over a 60-minute period) will cause the pump to automatically calculate the flow rate for the IVPB medication. Start the IVPB infusion as instructed by the pump.
- Monitor the patient during the infusion, as described earlier.
- When the infusion is complete, the primary intravenous infusion will automatically resume.
- Be sure to document the medication given on the medication record and continue to monitor the patient for adverse reactions and therapeutic effects.
- When giving intravenous medications through a saline (heparin) lock, follow the facility's guidelines for the flushing protocol before and after the medication is administered.
- Figure 10-73 illustrates a volume-controlled administration set that can be used to administer intravenous medications. The chamber is attached to the infusion between the intravenous infusion bag and the intravenous tubing. Fill the chamber with the desired amount of fluid, then add the medication via the port above the chamber, as shown in the photo. Be sure to cleanse the port with an alcohol swab before inserting the needle in the port. The chamber should be labeled with the medication's name, dose, and time added and your initials. Infuse the drug at the prescribed rate.
- In patient-controlled analgesia (PCA) a specialized pump is used to allow patients to self-administer pain medications, usually opiates (Figure 10-74). These pumps allow the patient to self-administer only as much medication as needed to control the pain by pushing a button for intravenous bolus doses. Safety features of the pump prevent accidental overdoses. A patient receiving PCA pump infusions should be monitored closely for his or her response to the drug, excessive sedation, hypotension, and changes in mental and respiratory status. Follow the facility's guidelines for setup and use.

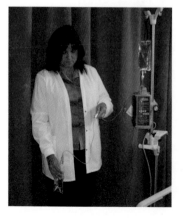

FIGURE 10-70 Flush the intravenous piggyback (secondary) tubing by using the backpriming method. Fluid is drained through the tubing into the old intravenous piggyback bag, which is then discarded. The new dose of medication is then attached to the primed tubing.

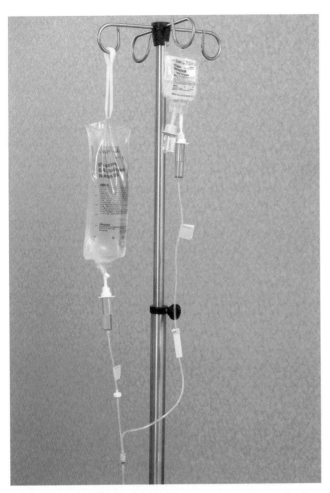

FIGURE 10-71   Infusing an intravenous piggyback medication with a primary gravity infusion. Note how the primary bag is lower than the IVPB.

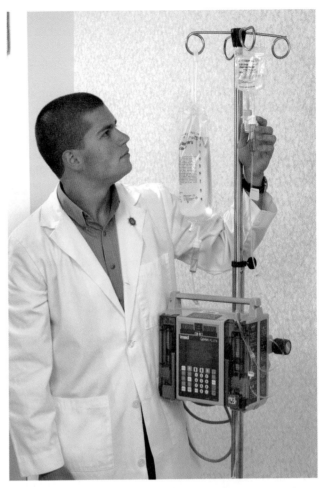

FIGURE 10-72   Infusing an intravenous piggyback medication with the primary infusion on an electronic infusion pump.

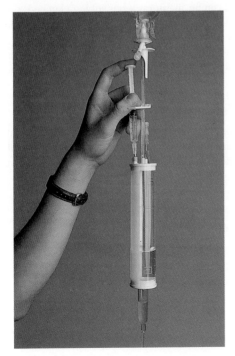

FIGURE 10-73   Adding a medication to a volume-controlled administration set.

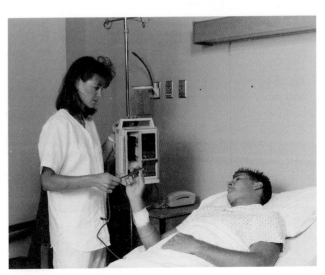

FIGURE 10-74   Instructing the patient on the use of a patient-controlled analgesia pump.

Intravenous Push Medications

Always begin by performing hand hygiene and maintain Standard Precautions (see Box 10-1).

When administering intravenous push (or bolus) medications, keep in mind the following points:

- Registered nurses are usually the only nursing staff members, besides a nurse anesthetist, allowed to give intravenous push medications. This may vary at different facilities.
- Intravenous push injections allow for rapid intravenous administration of a drug. The term *bolus* refers to a dose given all at once. Intravenous push injections may be given through an existing intravenous line, through an intravenous (saline or heparin) lock, or directly into a vein.
- Because the medication may have an immediate effect, monitor the patient closely for adverse reactions as well as for therapeutic effects.
- Follow the manufacturer's guidelines carefully when preparing an intravenous push medication. Some drugs require careful dilution. Consult a pharmacist if you are unsure about the dilution procedure. Improper dilution may increase the risk of phlebitis and other complications.
- Some drugs are *never* given by intravenous push. Examples include dopamine, potassium chloride, and antibiotics such as vancomycin.
- Small amounts of medication, less than 1 mL, need to be diluted in 5 to 10 mL of normal saline or another compatible fluid to ensure that the medication does not collect in a "dead space" of the tubing (such as the y-site port). Check the facility's policy.
- Most drugs given by intravenous push injection should be given over a period of 1 to 5 minutes to reduce local or systemic adverse effects. Always time the administration with your watch, because it is difficult to estimate the time accurately. Adenosine, however, must be given very rapidly, within 2 to 3 seconds, for optimal action. ALWAYS check packaging information for guidelines, because many errors and adverse effects have been associated with too-rapid intravenous drug administration.

Intravenous Push Medications Through an Intravenous Lock

- Obtain two syringes of 0.9% normal saline (NS). Most facilities provide prefilled 10 mL syringes. Prepare medication for injection. (Facilities may differ in the protocol for intravenous lock flushes—follow institutional policies.) If ordered, prepare a syringe with heparin flush solution.
- Follow the guidelines for a needleless system, if used.
- Cleanse the injection port of the intravenous lock with an antiseptic swab for 15 seconds after removing the cap, if present (Figure 10-75).

- Insert the syringe of NS into the injection port (Figure 10-76; needleless system shown). Open the clamp of the intravenous lock tubing, if present.
- Gently aspirate and observe for blood return. Absence of blood return does not mean that the intravenous line is occluded; further assessment may be required.
- Flush gently with saline while assessing for resistance. If resistance is felt, do not apply force. Stop and reassess the intravenous lock.
- Observe for signs of infiltration while injecting NS.
- Reclamp the tubing (if a clamp is present) and remove the NS syringe. Repeat cleansing of the port and attach the medication syringe. Open the clamp again.
- Inject the medication over the prescribed length of time. Measure time with a watch or clock (Figure 10-77).
- When the medication is infused, clamp the intravenous lock tubing (if a clamp is present) and remove the syringe.
- Repeat cleansing of the port; attach an NS syringe and inject the contents into the intravenous lock slowly. If a heparin flush is ordered, attach the syringe containing heparin flush solution and inject slowly (per the institution's protocol).

Intravenous Push Medications Through an Existing Infusion

- Prepare the medication for injection. Follow the guidelines for a needleless system, if used.
- Check compatibility of the intravenous medication with the existing intravenous solution.
- Choose the injection port that is closest to the patient.
- Remove the cap, if present, and cleanse the injection port with an antiseptic swab.
- Occlude the intravenous line by pinching the tubing just above the injection port (Figure 10-78). Attach the syringe to the injection port.
- Gently aspirate for blood return.
- While keeping the intravenous tubing clamped, slowly inject the medication according to administration guidelines. Be sure to time the injection with a watch or clock.
- After the injection, release the intravenous tubing, remove the syringe, and check the infusion rate of the intravenous fluid.

After Injection of Intravenous Push Medications

- Monitor the patient closely for adverse effects. Monitor the intravenous infusion site for signs of phlebitis and infiltration.
- Document medication given on the medication record and monitor for therapeutic effects.

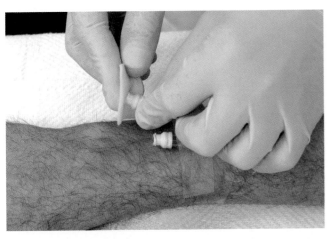

FIGURE 10-75   Cleanse the port for 15 seconds before attaching the syringe.

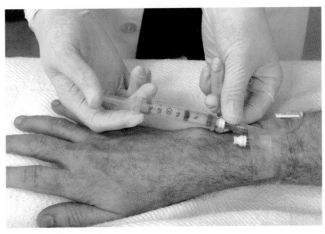

FIGURE 10-76   Attaching the syringe to the intravenous lock, using a needleless system.

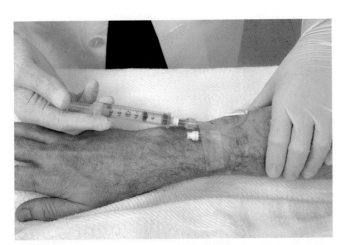

FIGURE 10-77   Slowly inject the intravenous push medication through the intravenous lock; use a watch to time the injection.

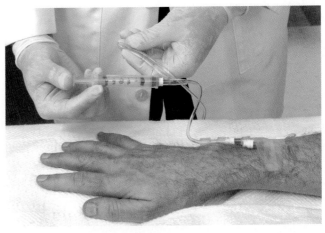

FIGURE 10-78   When giving an intravenous push medication through an intravenous line, pinch the tubing just above the injection port.

TOPICAL DRUGS

Administering Eye Medications

Always begin by performing hand hygiene and maintain Standard Precautions (see Box 10-1). Gloves should be worn. When administering eye preparations, keep in mind the following points:

- Assist the patient to a supine or sitting position. The patient's head should be tilted back slightly. Make sure the patient is not wearing contact lenses.
- Remove any secretions with a sterile gauze pad; be sure to wipe from the inner to outer canthus (Figure 10-79).
- Have the patient tilt his or her head slightly back and look up. With your nondominant hand, gently pull the lower lid open to expose the conjunctival sac.

Eyedrops

- With your dominant hand resting on the patient's forehead, hold the eye medication dropper 1 to 2 cm above the conjunctival sac. Do not touch the tip of the dropper to the eye or with your fingers (Figure 10-80).
- Drop the prescribed number of drops into the conjunctival sac. Never apply eyedrops to the cornea.
- If the drops land on the outer lid margins (if the patient moved or blinked), repeat the procedure.
- *Age-related considerations:* Infants often squeeze the eyes tightly shut to avoid eyedrops. To give drops to an uncooperative infant, restrain the head gently and place the drops at the corner near the nose where the eyelids meet. When the eye opens, the medication will flow into the eye.

Eye Ointment

- Gently squeeze the tube of medication to apply an even strip of medication (about 1 to 2 cm) along the border of the conjunctival sac. Start at the inner canthus and move toward the outer canthus (Figure 10-81).

After Instillation of Eye Medications

- Ask the patient to close the eye gently. Squeezing the eye shut may force the medication out of the conjunctival sac. A tissue may be used to blot liquid that runs out of the eye, but the patient should be instructed not to wipe the eye.
- You may apply gentle pressure to the patient's nasolacrimal duct for 30 to 60 seconds with a gloved finger wrapped in a tissue. This will help to reduce systemic absorption of the drug through the nasolacrimal duct and may also help to reduce the taste of the medication in the nasopharynx (Figure 10-82).
- If multiple eyedrops are due at the same time, then wait several minutes before administering the second medication. Check the instructions for the specific drug.
- Assist the patient to a comfortable position. Warn the patient that vision may be blurry for a few minutes.
- Document the medication given on the medication record and check the patient for a therapeutic response or adverse reactions.

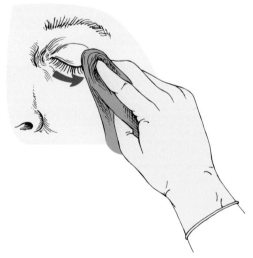

FIGURE 10-79   Cleanse the eye, washing from the inner to outer canthus, before giving eye medications.

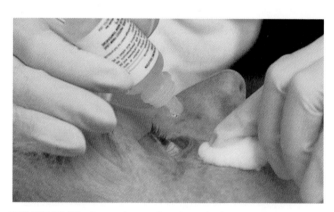

FIGURE 10-80   Insert the eyedrop into the lower conjunctival sac.

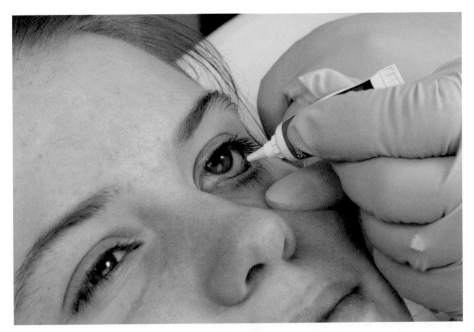

FIGURE 10-81   Applying eye ointment.

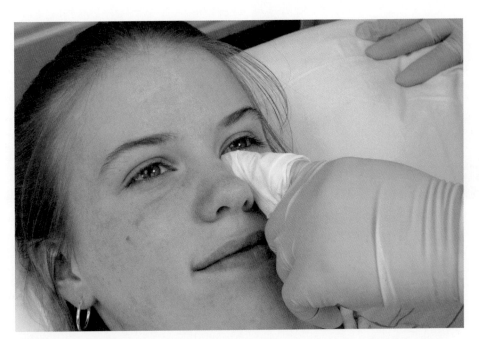

FIGURE 10-82   Applying gentle pressure against the nasolacrimal duct after giving eye medication.

Administering Eardrops

Always begin by performing hand hygiene and maintain Standard Precautions (see Box 10-1). Gloves may be worn. When administering ear preparations, keep in mind the following points:

- After explaining the procedure to the patient, assist the patient to a side-lying position with the affected ear facing up. If cerumen or drainage is noted in the outer ear canal, remove it carefully without pushing it back into the ear canal.
- Excessive amounts of cerumen should be removed before instillation of medication.
- If refrigerated, the ear medication should be warmed by taking it out of refrigeration for at least 30 minutes before administration. Instillation of cold eardrops can cause nausea, dizziness, and pain.
- *Age-related considerations:* For an adult or a child older than 3 years of age, pull the pinna up and back (Figure 10-83). For an infant or a child younger than 3 years of age, pull the pinna down and back (Figure 10-84).
- Administer the prescribed number of drops. Direct the drops along the sides of the ear canal rather than directly onto the eardrum.

- Instruct the patient to lie on his or her side for 5 to 10 minutes. Gently massaging the tragus of the ear with a finger will help to distribute the medication down the ear canal.
- If ordered, a loose cotton pledget can be gently inserted into the ear canal to prevent the medication from flowing out. The cotton should still be loose enough to allow any discharge to drain out of the ear canal. To prevent the dry cotton from absorbing the eardrops that were instilled, moisten the cotton with a small amount of medication before inserting the pledget. Insertion of cotton too deeply may result in increased pressure within the ear canal and on the eardrum. Remove the cotton after about 15 minutes.
- If medication is needed in the other ear, wait 5 to 10 minutes after instillation of the first eardrops before administering.
- Document the medication given on the medication record and observe the patient for a therapeutic response or adverse reactions.

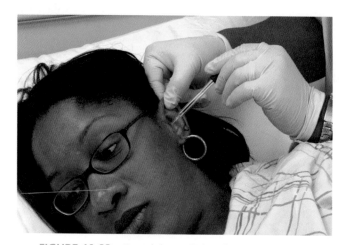

FIGURE 10-83   For adults, pull the pinna up and back.

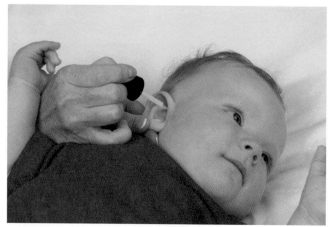

FIGURE 10-84   For infants and children younger than 3 years of age, pull the pinna down and back.

Administering Nasal Medications

Always begin by performing hand hygiene and maintain Standard Precautions (see Box 10-1). Patients may self-administer some of these drugs after proper instruction. Gloves should be worn. When administering nasal medications, keep in mind the following points:

- Before giving nasal medications, explain the procedure to the patient and tell him or her that temporary burning or stinging may occur. Instruct the patient that it is important to clear the nasal passages by blowing his or her nose, unless contraindicated (e.g., with increased intracranial pressure or nasal surgery), before administering the medication. Assess for deviated septum or a history of nasal fractures, because these may impede the patient's ability to inhale through the affected nostril.
- Figure 10-85 illustrates various delivery forms for nasal medications: sprays, drops, and dose-metered sprays.
- Assist the patient to a supine position. Support the patient's head as needed.
- If specific areas are targeted for the medication, position as follows:
  - For the posterior pharynx, position the head backward.
  - For the ethmoid or sphenoid sinuses, place the head gently over the top edge of the bed or place a pillow under the shoulders and tilt the head back.
  - For the frontal or maxillary sinuses, place the head back and turned toward the side that is to receive the medication.

Nasal Drops

- Hold the nose dropper approximately ½ inch above the nostril. Administer the prescribed number of drops toward the midline of the ethmoid bone (Figure 10-86).

- Repeat the procedure as ordered, instilling the indicated number of drops per nostril.
- Keep the patient in a supine position for 5 minutes.
- *Age-related considerations:* Infants are nose breathers, and the potential congestion caused by nasal medications may make it difficult for them to suck. If nose drops are ordered, administer them 20 to 30 minutes before a feeding.

Nasal Spray

- The patient should be sitting upright, with one nostril occluded. After gently shaking the nasal spray container, insert the tip into the nostril. Squeeze the spray bottle into the nostril while the patient inhales through the open nostril (Figure 10-87).
- Repeat the procedure as ordered, instilling the indicated number of sprays per nostril.
- Keep the patient in a supine position for 5 minutes.

After Administration of Nasal Medicines

- Offer the patient tissues for blotting any drainage, but instruct the patient to avoid blowing his or her nose for several minutes after instillation of the drops.
- Assist the patient to a comfortable position.
- Document the medication administration on the medication record and document drainage, if any. Monitor for adverse reactions and a therapeutic response.

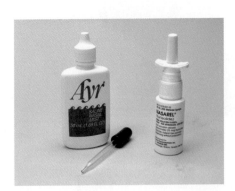

FIGURE 10-85 Nasal medications may come in various delivery forms.

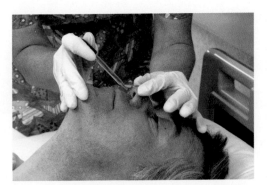

FIGURE 10-86 Administering nose drops.

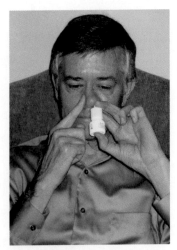

FIGURE 10-87 Before self-administering the nasal spray, the patient should occlude the other nostril.

Administering Inhaled Drugs

Always begin by performing hand hygiene and maintain Standard Precautions (see Box 10-1). Gloves may be worn. Patients with asthma should monitor their peak expiratory flow rates by using a peak flowmeter. A variety of inhalers are available (Figure 10-88). Be sure to check for specific instructions from the manufacturer as needed. Improper use will result in inadequate dosing. When administering inhaled preparations, keep in mind the following points.

Metered-Dose Inhalers

- Shake the metered-dose inhaler gently before using.
- Remove the cap; hold the inhaler upright and grasp with the thumb and first two fingers.
- Tilt the patient's head back slightly.
- If the inhaler is used without a spacer, do the following:
  1. Have the patient open his or her mouth; position the inhaler 1 to 2 inches away from the patient's mouth (Figure 10-89). For self-administration, some patients may measure this distance as 1 to 2 finger widths.
  2. Have the patient exhale, then press down once on the inhaler to release the medication; have the patient breathe in slowly and deeply for 5 seconds.
  3. Have the patient hold his or her breath for approximately 10 seconds, then exhale slowly through pursed lips.
- *Age-related considerations:* Spacers should be used with children and adults who have difficulty coordinating inhalations with activation of metered-dose inhalers (see Chapter 37). If the inhaler is used with a spacer, do the following:
  1. Attach the spacer to the mouthpiece of the inhaler after removing the inhaler cap (Figure 10-90).
  2. Place the mouthpiece of the spacer in the patient's mouth.
  3. Have the patient exhale.
  4. Press down on the inhaler to release the medication and have the patient inhale deeply and slowly through the spacer. The patient should breathe in and out slowly for 2 to 3 seconds, then hold his or her breath for 10 seconds (Figure 10-91).
- If a second puff of the same medication is ordered, wait 1 to 2 minutes between puffs.
- If a second type of inhaled medication is ordered, wait 2 to 5 minutes between medication inhalations or as prescribed.
- If both a bronchodilator and a corticosteroid inhaled medication are ordered, the bronchodilator should be administered first so that the passages will be more open for the second medication.
- The patient should be instructed to rinse his or her mouth after inhaling a corticosteroid medication to prevent the development of an oral fungal infection.
- Document the medication given on the medication record and monitor the patient for a therapeutic response as well as for adverse reactions.
- It is important to teach the patient how to calculate the number of doses in the inhaler and to keep track of uses. Simply shaking the inhaler to "estimate" whether it is empty is not accurate and may result in its being used when it is empty. The patient should be taught to count the number of puffs needed per day (doses) and divide this amount into the actual number of actuations (puffs) in the inhaler to estimate the number of days the inhaler will last. Then, a calendar can be marked a few days before this date with a note that it is time to obtain a refill. In addition, the date can be marked on the inhaler with a permanent marker. For example, an inhaler with 200 puffs, ordered to be used 4 times a day (2 puffs per dose, 8 puffs per day), would last for 25 days (200 divided by 8).
- Dry powder inhalers have varied instructions, and so the manufacturer's directions should be followed closely. Patients should be instructed to cover the mouthpiece completely with their mouths. Capsules that are intended for use with these inhalers should NEVER be taken orally. Some dry powder inhalers have convenient built-in dose counters.

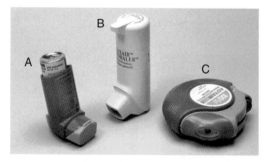

FIGURE 10-88   **A,** Metered-dose inhaler (MDI). **B,** Automated, or breath-activated, MDI. **C,** Dry powder inhaler that delivers powdered medication.

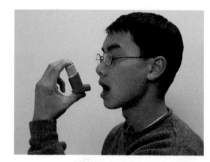

FIGURE 10-89   Using a metered-dose inhaler without a spacer.

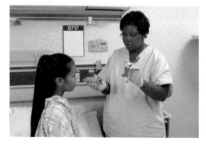

FIGURE 10-90   Instructing the patient on how to use a spacer device.

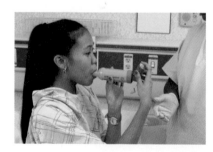

FIGURE 10-91   Using a spacer device with a metered-dose inhaler.

Small-Volume Nebulizers

- In some facilities, the air compressor is located in the wall unit of the room. In other facilities and at home, a small portable air compressor is used. Be sure to follow the manufacturer's recommendations for use.
- In some facilities, nebulizer treatments may be performed by a respiratory therapist. However, the nurse should closely monitor the patient before, during, and after the drug administration.
- Be sure to take the patient's baseline heart rate, especially if a beta-adrenergic drug is used. Some drugs may increase the heart rate.
- After gathering the equipment, add the prescribed medication to the nebulizer cup (Figure 10-92). Some medications will require a diluent; others are premixed with a diluent. Be sure to verify before adding a diluent.
- Have the patient hold the mouthpiece between his or her lips (Figure 10-93).
- *Age-related considerations:* A face mask should be used for a child or an adult who is too fatigued to hold the mouthpiece. Special adaptors are available if the patient has a tracheostomy.
- Before starting the nebulizer treatment, the patient should take a slow, deep breath, hold it briefly, then exhale slowly. Patients who are short of breath should be instructed to hold their breath every fourth or fifth breath.

- Turn on the small-volume nebulizer machine (or turn on the wall unit) and make sure that a sufficient mist is forming.
- Instruct the patient to repeat the breathing pattern mentioned previously during the treatment.
- Occasionally tap the nebulizer cup during the treatment and toward the end to move the fluid droplets back to the bottom of the cup.
- Monitor the patient throughout treatment to ensure that the nebulizer medication is properly administered.
- Monitor the patient's heart rate during and after the treatment.
- If inhaled steroids are given, instruct the patient to rinse his or her mouth afterward.
- After the procedure, clean and store the tubing per institutional policy.
- Document the medication given on the medication record and monitor the patient for a therapeutic response as well as for adverse reactions.
- If the patient will be using a nebulizer at home, instruct the patient to rinse the nebulizer parts after each use with warm, clear water and to air-dry. The parts should be washed daily with warm, soapy water and allowed to air-dry. Once a week, the nebulizer parts should be soaked in a solution of vinegar and water (four parts water and one part white vinegar) for 30 minutes; rinsed thoroughly with clear, warm water; and air-dried. Storing nebulizer parts that are still wet will encourage bacterial and mold growth.

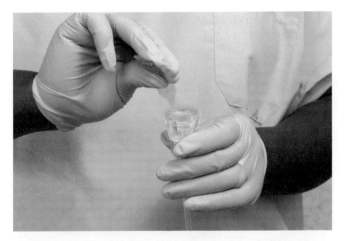

FIGURE 10-92   Adding medication to the nebulizer cup.

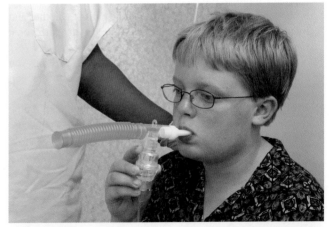

FIGURE 10-93   Administering a small-volume nebulizer treatment.

Administering Medications to the Skin

Always begin by performing hand hygiene and maintain Standard Precautions (see Box 10-1). Gloves should be worn. Avoid touching the preparations to your own skin. When administering skin preparations, keep in mind the following points.

Lotions, Creams, Ointments, and Powders

- Apply powder to clean, dry skin. Have the patient turn his or her head to the other side during application to avoid inhalation of powder particles.
- Apply lotion to clean, dry skin. Remove residual from previous applications with soap and water.
- Before administering any dose of a topical skin medication, ensure that the site is dry and free of irritation. Thoroughly remove previous applications using soap and water, if appropriate for the patient's condition, and dry the area thoroughly. Be sure to remove any debris, drainage, or pus if present.
- *Age-related considerations:* The skin of an older patient may be more fragile and easily bruised. Be sure to handle the skin gently when cleansing to prepare the site for medication and when applying medications.
- With lotion, cream, or gel, obtain the correct amount with your gloved hand (Figure 10-94). If the medication is in a jar, remove the dose with a sterile tongue depressor and apply to your gloved hand. Do not contaminate the medication in the jar.
- Apply the preparation with long, smooth, gentle strokes that follow the direction of hair growth (Figure 10-95). Avoid excessive pressure. Be especially careful with the skin of elderly persons, because age-related changes may result in increased capillary fragility and tendency to bruise.
- Some ointments and creams may soil the patient's clothes and linens. If ordered, cover the affected area with gauze or a transparent dressing.
- Nitroglycerin ointment in a tube is measured carefully on clean ruled application paper before it is applied to the skin (Figure 10-96). Unit-dose packages should not be measured. Do not massage nitroglycerin ointment into the skin. Apply the measured amount onto a clean, dry site and then secure the application paper with a transparent dressing or a strip of tape. Always remove the old medication before applying a new dose. Rotate application sites.

Transdermal Patches

- Be sure that the old patch is removed as ordered. Some patches may be removed before the next patch is due—check the order. Clear patches may be difficult to find, and patches may be overlooked in obese patients with skinfolds. Cleanse the site of the old patch thoroughly. Observe for signs of skin irritation at the old patch site. Rotate sites of application with each dose.
- Transdermal patches should be applied at the same time each day if ordered daily.
- The old patch can be pressed together, then wrapped in a glove as you remove the glove from your hand. Dispose in the proper container according to the facility's policy.
- Select a new site for application and ensure that it is clean and without powder or lotion. The site should be hairless and free from scratches or irritation. If it is necessary to remove hair, clip the hair instead of shaving to reduce irritation to the skin. Application sites may vary. Follow the drug manufacturer's specific instructions as to where the patch should be applied.
- Remove the backing from the new patch (Figure 10-97). Take care not to touch the medication side of the patch with your fingers.
- Place the patch on the skin site and press firmly (Figure 10-98). Press around the edges of the patch with one or two fingers to ensure that the patch is adequately secured to the skin. If an overlay is provided by the drug manufacturer, apply it over the patch.
- Instruct the patient not to cut transdermal patches. Cutting transdermal patches releases all of the medication at once and may result in a dangerous overdose.

After Administration of Topical Skin Preparations

- Chart the medication given on the medication record and monitor the patient for a therapeutic response as well as for any adverse reactions.
- Provide instruction on administration to the patient and/or caregiver.

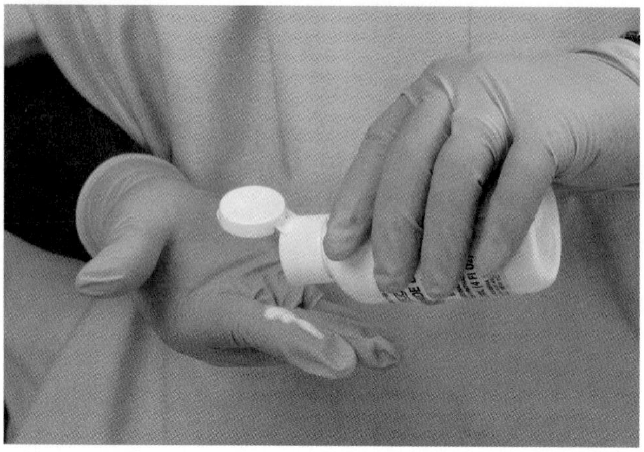

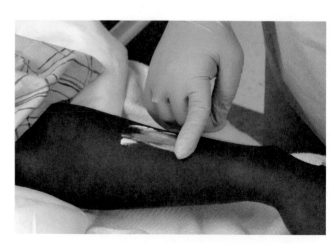

FIGURE 10-94 Use gloves to apply topical skin preparations.

FIGURE 10-95 Spread the lotion on the skin with long, smooth, gentle strokes.

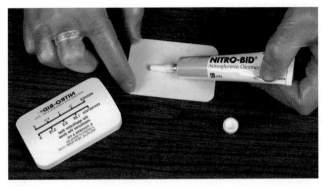

FIGURE 10-96   Measure nitroglycerin ointment carefully before application.

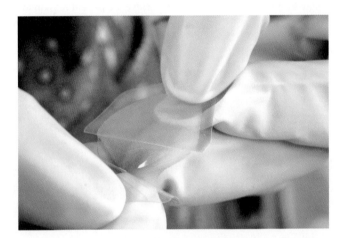

FIGURE 10-97   Opening a transdermal patch medication.

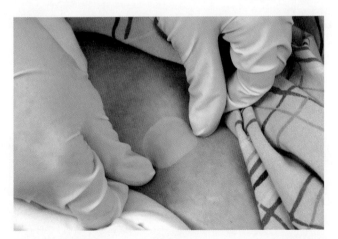

FIGURE 10-98   Ensure that the edges of the transdermal patch are secure after applying.

Administering Vaginal Medications

Always begin by performing hand hygiene and maintain Standard Precautions (see Box 10-1). Gloves should be worn. When administering vaginal preparations, keep in mind the following points:

- Vaginal suppositories are larger and more oval than rectal suppositories (Figure 10-99).
- Figure 10-100 shows examples of a vaginal suppository in an applicator and vaginal cream in an applicator.
- Before giving these medications explain the procedure to the patient and have her void the bladder.
- If possible, administer vaginal preparations at bedtime to allow the medications to remain in place as long as possible.
- Some patients may prefer to self-administer vaginal medications. Provide specific instructions if necessary.
- Position the patient in the lithotomy position and elevate the hips with a pillow, if tolerated. Be sure to drape the patient to provide privacy.

Creams, Foams, or Gels Applied with an Applicator

- Fit the applicator to the tube of the medication and then gently squeeze the tube to fill the applicator with the correct amount of medication.
- Lubricate the tip of the applicator with water-soluble lubricant.

- Use your nondominant hand to spread the labia and expose the vagina. Gently insert the applicator as far as possible into the vagina (Figure 10-101).
- Push the plunger to deposit the medication. Remove the applicator and wrap it in a paper towel for cleaning.

Suppositories or Vaginal Tablets

- For suppositories or vaginal tablets, remove the wrapping and lubricate the suppository with a water-soluble lubricant. Be sure that the suppository is at room temperature.
- Using the applicator provided, insert the suppository or tablet into the vagina, then push the plunger to deposit the suppository. Remove the applicator.
- If no applicator is available, use your dominant index finger to insert the suppository about 2 inches into the vagina (Figure 10-102).
- Have the patient remain in a supine position with hips elevated for 5 to 10 minutes to allow the suppository to melt and the medication to be absorbed.
- If the patient desires, apply a perineal pad.
- If the applicator is to be reused, wash with soap and water and store in a clean container for the next use.
- Document the medication given and the patient's response on the medication record. Monitor for a therapeutic response and adverse reactions.

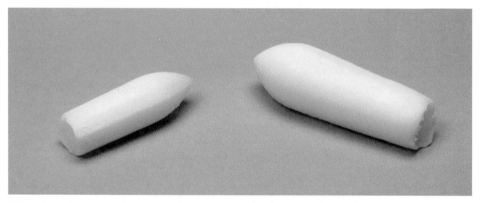

FIGURE 10-99   Vaginal suppositories *(right)* are larger and more oval than rectal suppositories *(left)*.

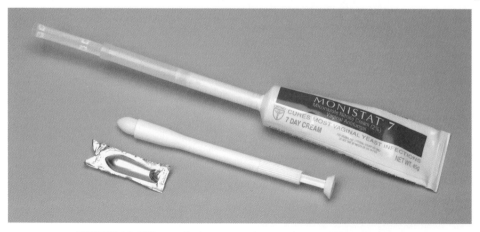

FIGURE 10-100   Vaginal cream and suppository, with applicators.

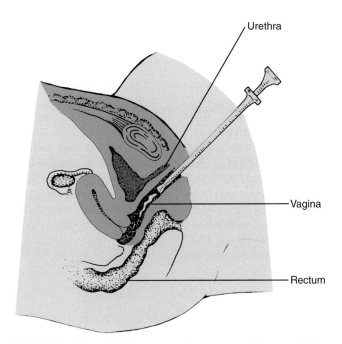

Urethra

Vagina

Rectum

FIGURE 10-101   Administering vaginal cream with an applicator.

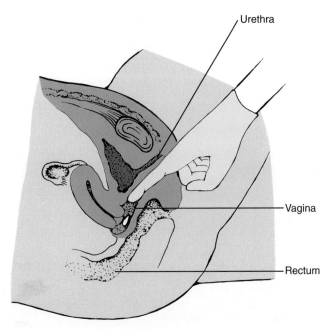

Urethra

Vagina

Rectum

FIGURE 10-102   Administering a vaginal suppository.

ILLUSTRATION CREDITS

Figures 10-1, 10-2, 10-3, 10-4, 10-5, 10-6, 10-7, 10-8, 10-11, 10-14, 10-16, 10-18, 10-19, 10-25, 10-29, 10-30, 10-31, 10-32, 10-33, 10-35, 10-36, 10-37, 10-43, 10-44, 10-45, 10-46, 10-47, 10-52, 10-53, 10-54, 10-56, 10-57, 10-59, 10-60, 10-61, 10-62, 10-63, 10-64, 10-65, 10-66, 10-67, 10-68, 10-69, 10-71, 10-72, 10-75, 10-76, 10-77, 10-78, 10-81, 10-82, 10-83, 10-84, 10-85, 10-86, 10-88, 10-90, 10-91, 10-92, 10-93, 10-94, 10-95, 10-97, 10-98, 10-99, 10-100, from Rick Brady, Riva, Md. Figures 10-10, 10-15, 10-39, 10-49, 10-80, 10-89, 10-101, 10-102, from Elkin MK, Perry AG, Potter PA: *Nursing interventions and clinical skills,* ed 3, St Louis, 2004, Mosby. Figure 10-12, courtesy Oscar H. Allison, Jr. In Clayton BD, Stock YN: *Basic pharmacology for nurses,* ed 14, St Louis, 2007, Mosby. Figure 10-17, modified from Perry AG, Potter PA: *Clinical nursing skills and techniques,* ed 6, St Louis, 2006, Mosby. Figures 10-20, 10-21, 10-22, 10-23, 10-40, 10-41, 10-48, courtesy Chuck Dresner. Figures 10-24, 10-26, 10-27, from Potter PA, Perry AG: *Basic nursing: theory and practice,* ed 3, St Louis, 1995, Mosby. Figure 10-28, from Potter PA, Perry AG: *Fundamentals of nursing,* ed 5, St Louis, 2001, Mosby. Figures 10-38, 10-79, 10-96, from Perry AG, Potter PA: *Clinical skills and techniques,* ed 6, St Louis, 2006, Mosby. Figure 10-42, from Potter PA, Perry AG: *Fundamentals of nursing: concepts, process, and practice,* ed 4, St Louis, 1997, Mosby. Figures 10-51, 10-55, 10-58, modified from Potter PA, Perry AG: *Fundamentals of nursing: concepts, process, and practice,* ed 3, St Louis, 1993, Mosby. Figure 10-73 from Potter PA, Perry AG: *Fundamentals of nursing,* ed 6, St Louis, 2005, Mosby.

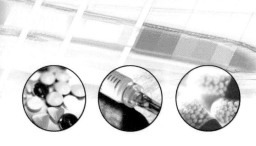

PART 2

Drugs Affecting the Central Nervous System

STUDY SKILLS TIPS

Vocabulary • Text Notation • Language Conventions

4.00021-9978-0-323-05544-4Introduction

VOCABULARY

In any subject matter, mastering the vocabulary is essential to mastering the content. But in a complex, technical subject such as nursing pharmacology, if the vocabulary is not mastered, understanding the content will be almost impossible. Each chapter in this text contains a glossary of unfamiliar terms at the beginning, and as an independent learner, you should spend some time and energy on the vocabulary contained in the glossary. Do not expect to completely understand and master the terms from the glossary alone. The terms are further defined and explained in the body of the chapter, and it is when you read the chapter that you should expect to fully master the vocabulary. However, the time you spend working on the glossary will pay off when you read the chapter.

Consider the terms *agonist* and *antagonist* in the Chapter 11 glossary. These terms share a common word part, which means the words are related in meaning. This is an important first step in mastering them. What does *agonist* mean? What is the similarity between *agonist* and *antagonist?* What is the essential difference between the two? Asking these questions as you start to work on Chapter 11 is a valuable technique for beginning to master the language of the content. Do not simply memorize the terms. Learn what they mean and link relationships between words with common elements. As you practice this technique it will become easier to retain the meaning.

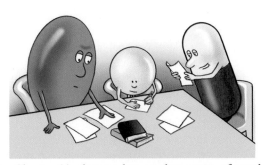

The Chapter 11 glossary has another group of words that should be viewed as a group that shares an important relationship. The first of these words is *pain.* The definition provided is clear and relatively easy to understand, but your focus should be not just on that single word, because there are 13 other words that relate to pain: *acute, breakthrough, cancer, central, chronic, deep, neuropathic, phantom, referred, somatic, superficial, vascular,* and *visceral.* Each of these words defines and categorizes pain in a very specific way. As you go about setting up vocabulary cards, look at the opening pages in this chapter. You will find considerable discussion of these terms, which is useful in helping you obtain the fullest understanding of these terms. Do not simply focus on a meaning of each term, but also ask what the similarities and/or differences are and how these words relate to one another.

TEXT NOTATION

The Study Skills Tips for Part One discussed a method for text underlining. If it is done carefully, this strategy is particularly useful for later review of text material. The object of text underlining is to pick out important terms, ideas, and key information so you can come back to it later for quick review. The three key elements in successful text notation are as follows:

1. Read the material once before attempting any underlining.

2. Be acutely aware of the author's language.

3. Be selective in underlining. The most common fault in underlining is to mark too much material.

The following are three paragraphs from Chapter 11 that have been underlined. The underlining should be viewed as an example of what can be done. Each reader will mark the text somewhat differently based on his or her background and experience. As you study this example, think not only about what has been underlined but also about why that material was chosen.

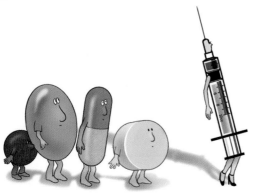

Pain is most commonly defined as an unpleasant sensory and emotional experience associated with either actual or potential tissue damage. It is a very personal and individual experience. Pain can be defined as whatever the patient says it is, and it exists whenever the patient says it does. Although the mechanisms of pain and the nature of pain pathways are becoming better understood, a patient's perception of pain is a complex process. Pain involves physical, psychologic, and even cultural factors. Because pain intensity cannot be precisely quantified, health care providers must cultivate relationships of mutual trust with their patients to provide optimal care.

There is no single approach to effective pain management. Instead, pain management should be tailored to each patient's needs and should consider the cause of the pain, if known; the existence of concurrent medical conditions; the characteristics of the pain; and the psychologic and cultural characteristics of the patient. It also requires ongoing reassessment of the pain and the effectiveness of treatment. The patient's emotional response to pain depends on his or her psychological experiences of pain, both current and prior. Pain results from the stimulation of sensory nerve fibers known as **nociceptors.** These receptors transmit pain signals from various body regions to the spinal cord and brain, which leads to the sensation of pain, or **nociception.**

The physical impulses that signal pain activate various nerve pathways from the periphery to the spinal cord and to the brain. The level of stimulus needed to produce a painful sensation is referred to as the **pain** threshold. Because this is technically a measure of the physiologic response of the nervous system, it is similar for most persons. However, variations in pain sensitivity may result from genetic factors.

LANGUAGE CONVENTIONS

Certain words and phrases are like signal lights at an intersection. They serve to tell the reader that something special, important, or noteworthy is happening. To the attentive, active reader these conventions contribute significantly to understanding what the author is trying to convey. Whether you are highlighting, underlining, writing margin notes, or studying the material using the PURR model, it is important that you become sensitive to these conventions.

The text following the topic heading *Anatomy, Physiology, and Disease Overview* in Chapter 11 contains several examples. The first sentence of the third paragraph contains the phrase *classified as.* Whenever an author says that something is being classified it means that there are at least two (and perhaps several more) elements of the term or idea that are being classified. This means that you should immediately ask a question about the reading, "What is being classified? How many classifications are there for this?" These questions will help you focus on what to learn and keep your attention firmly fixed on the process of learning.

As you read this chapter, or any other chapter, become aware of words and phrases like these that are intended to draw your attention to something the author especially wanted to emphasize. The more aware of language conventions you become, the easier it will be to become a selective reader. Selective readers do not try to remember everything they read, but they are able to select from the mass of information those concepts and/or terms that the writers tried to stress.

CHAPTER 11

Analgesic Drugs

OBJECTIVES

When you reach the end of this chapter, you should be able to do the following:

1 Define *acute pain* and *chronic pain.*

2 Contrast the signs, symptoms, and management of acute and chronic pain.

3 Describe pharmacologic and nonpharmacologic approaches for the management of acute and chronic pain.

4 Discuss the use of nonopioids, nonsteroidal antiinflammatory drugs, and opioids (opioid agonists, opioids with mixed actions, or opioid agonists-antagonists and antagonists) and miscellaneous drugs in the management of pain, including acute and chronic pain, cancer pain, and special pain situations.

5 Identify examples of drugs classified as nonopioids, nonsteroidal antiinflammatory drugs, opioid agonists, opioids with mixed actions, opioid antagonists, as well as any miscellaneous drugs.

6 Briefly describe the mechanism of action, indications, dosages, routes of administration, averse effects, toxicity, cautions, contraindications, and drug interactions of nonopioids, nonsteroidal antiinflammatory drugs (see Chapter 44), opioid agonists, opioids with mixed actions, antagonists, and miscellaneous drugs.

7 Contrast the pharmacologic and nonpharmacologic management of acute and chronic pain with the management of pain associated with cancer and pain experienced in terminal conditions.

8 Briefly describe special pain situations as well as specific standards of pain management as defined by the World Health Organization and the Joint Commission.

9 Develop a nursing care plan based on the nursing process related to the use of nonopioid and opioid drug therapy for patients in pain.

10 Identify various resources, agencies, and professional groups that are involved in establishing standards for the management of all types of pain and for promotion of a holistic approach to the care of patients with acute or chronic pain and those in special pain situations.

---

e-Learning Activities

http://evolve.elsevier.com/Lilley

NCLEX Review Questions • Animations • Nursing Care Plans • Audio Glossary • Category Catchers • Medication Errors Checklists • IV Therapy Checklists • Calculators • Frequently Asked Questions • Content Updates • Supplemental Resources • Answers to Case Studies and Critical Thinking Activities

Drug Profiles

* acetaminophen, p. 166
  codeine sulfate, p. 163
  fentanyl, p. 163
  lidocaine, p. 167
  meperidine hydrochloride, p. 164
  methadone hydrochloride, p. 164

* morphine sulfate, p. 161
* naloxone hydrochloride, p. 165
  naltrexone hydrochloride, p. 165
  oxycodone hydrochloride, p. 164
  tramadol hydrochloride, p. 166
  ziconotide, p. 167

  ◆ *Key drug.*

Glossary

Acute pain Pain that is sudden in onset, usually subsides when treated, and typically occurs over less than a 6-week period. (p. 153)

Addiction A primary, chronic, neurobiologic disease whose development is influenced by genetic, psychosocial, and environmental factors (same as *psychologic dependence*). (p. 156)

Adjuvant analgesic drugs Drugs that are added as a second drug for combined therapy with a primary drug and may have additive or independent analgesic properties, or both. (p. 152)

Agonist A substance that binds to a receptor and causes a response. (p. 158)

Agonists-antagonists Substances that bind to a receptor and cause a partial response that is not as strong as that caused by an agonist (also known as a *partial agonist*). (p. 158)

Analgesic ceiling effect What occurs when a given pain drug no longer effectively controls a patient's pain despite the administration of the highest safe dosages. (p. 158)

Analgesics Medications that relieve pain without causing loss of consciousness (sometimes referred to as *painkillers*). (p. 152)

Antagonist A drug that binds to a receptor and prevents (blocks) a response. (p. 158)

Breakthrough pain Pain that occurs between doses of pain medication. (p. 157)

Cancer pain Pain resulting from any of a variety of causes related to cancer and/or the metastasis of cancer. (p. 154)

Central pain Pain resulting from any disorder that causes central nervous system damage. (p. 154)

Chronic pain Persistent or recurring pain that is often difficult to treat. Includes any pain lasting longer than 3 to 6 months, pain lasting longer than 1 month after healing of an acute tissue injury, or pain that accompanies a nonhealing tissue injury. (p. 153)

Deep pain Pain that occurs in tissues below skin level; opposite of *superficial pain*. (p. 154)

151

Gate theory The most common and well-described theory of pain transmission and pain relief. It uses a gate model to explain how impulses from damaged tissues are sensed in the brain. (p. 154)

Narcotics A legal term established under the Harrison Narcotic Act of 1914. It originally applied to drugs that produce insensibility or stupor, especially the opioids (e.g., morphine, heroin). Currently used in clinical settings to refer to any medically used controlled substances and in legal settings to refer to any illicit or "street" drug. (NOTE: This term is falling out of use in favor of *opioid* and will not be used in this text.)

Neuropathic pain Pain that results from a disturbance of function or pathologic change in a nerve. (p. 154)

Nociception Processing of pain signals in the brain that gives rise to the feeling of pain. (p. 153)

Nociceptors A subclass of sensory nerves (A and C fibers) that transmit pain signals to the central nervous system from other body parts. (p. 153)

Nonopioid analgesics Analgesics that are not classified as opioids. (p. 153)

Nonsteroidal antiinflammatory drugs (NSAIDs) A large, chemically diverse group of drugs that are analgesics and also possess antiinflammatory and antipyretic activity but are not steroids. (p. 154)

Opioid analgesics Synthetic drugs that bind to opiate receptors to relieve pain but are not themselves derived from the opium plant. (p. 152)

Opioid naive Describes patients who are receiving opioid analgesics for the first time and who therefore are not accustomed to their effects. (p. 161)

Opioid tolerance A normal physiologic condition that results from long-term opioid use, in which larger doses of opioids are required to maintain the same level of analgesia and in which abrupt discontinuation of the drug results in withdrawal symptoms (same as *physical dependence*). (p. 156)

Opioid tolerant The opposite of opioid naive; describes patients who have been receiving opioid analgesics (legally or otherwise) for a period of time (1 week or longer) and who are therefore at greater risk of opioid withdrawal syndrome upon sudden discontinuation of opioid use. (p. 157)

Opioid withdrawal The signs and symptoms associated with abstinence from or withdrawal of an opioid analgesic when the body has become physically dependent on the substance. (p. 161)

Pain An unpleasant sensory and emotional experience associated with actual or potential tissue damage. (p. 152)

Pain threshold The level of a stimulus that results in the sensation of pain. (p. 153)

Pain tolerance The amount of pain a patient can endure without its interfering with normal function. (p. 153)

Partial agonist A drug that binds to a receptor and causes an activation response that is less than that caused by a full agonist (same as *antagonist-antagonist*). (p. 158)

Phantom pain Pain experienced in the area of a body part that has been surgically or traumatically removed. (p. 154)

Physical dependence A state of adaptation that is manifested by a drug class–specific withdrawal syndrome that can be produced by abrupt cessation, rapid dose reduction, decreasing blood level of the drug, and/or administration of an antagonist. The physical adaptation of the body to the presence of an opioid or other addictive substance. (p. 153)

Psychologic dependence A pattern of compulsive use of opioids or any other addictive substance characterized by a continuous craving for the substance and the need to use it for effects other than pain relief (also called *addiction*). (p. 156)

Referred pain Pain occurring in an area away from the organ of origin. (p. 154)

Somatic pain Pain that originates from skeletal muscles, ligaments, or joints. (p. 154)

Special pain situations The general term for pain control situations that are complex and whose treatment typically involves multiple medications, various health care personnel, and nonpharmacologic therapeutic modalities (e.g., massage, chiropractic care, surgery). (p. 175)

Superficial pain Pain that originates from the skin or mucous membranes; opposite of *deep pain*. (p. 154)

Synergistic effects Drug interactions in which the effect of a combination of two or more drugs with similar actions is greater than the sum of the individual effects of the same drugs given alone. For example, $1 + 1$ is greater than 2. (p. 157)

Tolerance The general term for a state of adaptation in which repetitive exposure to a given drug, over time, induces changes in drug receptors that reduce one or more of the drug's effects (same as *physical dependence*). (p. 153)

Vascular pain Pain that results from a pathology of the vascular or perivascular tissues. (p. 154)

Visceral pain Pain that originates from organs or smooth muscles. (p. 154)

World Health Organization An international body of health care professionals, including clinicians and epidemiologists among many others, that studies and responds to health needs and trends worldwide. (p. 158)

· · ·

Anatomy, Physiology, and Disease Overview

The management of pain is a very important aspect of nursing care in a variety of settings and across the life span. Pain is the most common reason that patients seek health care, resulting in some 70 million office visits annually in the United States. Surgical and diagnostic procedures often require pain management, as do several diseases including arthritis, diabetes, multiple sclerosis, cancer, and acquired immunodeficiency syndrome (AIDS). Pain leads to much suffering and is a tremendous economic burden in terms of lost workplace productivity, workers' compensation payments, and other related health care costs.

To provide quality patient care, nurses must be well informed about both pharmacologic and nonpharmacologic methods of pain management. This chapter focuses on pharmacologic methods of pain management. Nonpharmacologic methods of pain management are listed in Box 11-1.

Medications that relieve pain without causing loss of consciousness are classified as **analgesics.** They are also commonly referred to as *painkillers.* There are various classes of analgesics, determined by their chemical structures and mechanisms of action. This chapter focuses primarily on the **opioid analgesics,** which are normally used to manage moderate to severe pain. Often drugs from other chemical categories are added to the opioid regimen as **adjuvant analgesic drugs** (or adjuvants) and are described later.

Pain is most commonly defined as an unpleasant sensory and emotional experience associated with either actual or potential tissue damage. It is a very personal and individual experience. Pain can be defined as whatever the patient says it is, and it exists whenever the patient says it does. Although the mechanisms of pain and the nature of pain pathways are becoming better understood, a patient's perception of pain is a complex process. Pain involves physical, psychologic, and even

BOX 11-1 Nonpharmacologic Treatment Options for Pain

- Acupressure
- Acupuncture
- Art therapy
- Behavioral therapy
- Biofeedback
- Comfort measures
- Counseling
- Distraction
- Hot or cold packs
- Hypnosis
- Imagery
- Massage
- Meditation
- Music therapy
- Pet therapy
- Physical therapy
- Reduction of fear
- Relaxation
- Surgery
- Therapeutic baths
- Therapeutic communication
- Therapeutic touch
- Transcutaneous electric nerve stimulation
- Yoga

CULTURAL IMPLICATIONS

The Patient Experiencing Pain

- Each culture has its own beliefs, thoughts, and ways of approaching, defining, and managing pain. Attitudes, meanings and perceptions of pain vary with culture, race, and ethnicity
- African Americans believe in the power of healers who rely strongly on the religious faith of people and often use prayer and the laying on of hands for relief of pain.
- Hispanic Americans believe in prayer, the wearing of amulets, and the use of herbs and spices to maintain health and wellness. Specific herbs are used in teas and therapies, often including religious practices, massage, and cleansings.
- Some traditional methods of healing for the Chinese include acupuncture, herbal remedies, yin and yang balancing, and cold treatment. Moxibustion, in which cones or cylinders of pulverized wormwood are burned on or near the skin over specific meridian points, is another form of healing.
- Asian and Pacific Islander patients are often reluctant to express their pain because they believe that the pain is God's will or is punishment for past sins.
- For many Native Americans, treatments for pain include massage, the application of heat, sweat baths, herbal remedies, and being in harmony with nature.
- In Arab culture, patients are expected to express their pain openly and anticipate immediate relief, preferably through injections or intravenous drugs.
- Nurses should be aware of all cultural influences on health-related behaviors and on patients' attitudes toward medication therapy and thus, ultimately, on its effectiveness. A thorough assessment that includes questions about the patient's cultural background and practices is important to the effective and individualized delivery of nursing care.

cultural factors (see Cultural Implications box). Because pain intensity cannot be precisely quantified, health care providers must cultivate relationships of mutual trust with their patients to provide optimal care.

There is no single approach to effective pain management. Instead, pain management should be tailored to each patient's needs and should consider the cause of the pain, the existence of concurrent medical conditions; the characteristics of the pain; and the psychologic and cultural characteristics of the patient. It also requires ongoing reassessment of the pain and the effectiveness of treatment. The patient's emotional response to pain depends on his or her psychologic experiences of pain. Pain results from the stimulation of sensory nerve fibers known as **nociceptors.** These receptors transmit pain signals from various body regions to the spinal cord and brain, which leads to the sensation of pain, or **nociception** (Figure 11-1)**.**

The physical impulses that signal pain activate various nerve pathways from the periphery to the spinal cord and to the brain. The level of stimulus needed to produce a painful sensation is referred to as the **pain threshold.** Because this is technically a measure of the physiologic response of the nervous system, it is similar for most persons. However, variations in pain sensitivity may result from genetic factors.

There are three main receptors believed to be involved in pain. The mu receptors in the dorsal horn of the spinal cord appear to play a crucial role. Less important but still involved in pain sensations are the kappa and delta receptors. Pain receptors are located in both the central nervous system (CNS) and various body tissues. Pain perception—and, conversely, emotional well-being—is closely linked to the number of mu receptors. This number is controlled by a single gene, the mu opioid receptor gene. When the number of receptors is high, pain sensitivity is diminished. Conversely, when the receptors are reduced or missing altogether, relatively minor noxious stimuli may be perceived as painful.

The patient's emotional response to the pain is also molded by the patient's age, sex, culture, previous pain experience, and anxiety level. Whereas pain threshold is the physiologic element of pain, as described earlier, the psychologic element of pain is called **pain tolerance.** This is the amount of pain a patient can endure without its interfering with normal function. Because it is a subjective response, pain tolerance can vary from patient to patient and can be modulated by the patient's personality, attitude, environment, culture, and ethnic background. Pain tolerance can even vary within the same person depending on the circumstances involved. Table 11-1 lists the various conditions that can alter one's pain tolerance.

Pain can also be further classified in terms of its onset and duration as either acute or chronic. **Acute pain** is sudden and usually subsides when treated. One example of acute pain is postoperative pain. **Chronic pain** is persistent or recurring, lasting 3 to 6 months. It is often more difficult to treat, because changes occur in the nervous system that often require increasing drug dosages. This situation is known by the general term **tolerance** or **physical dependence** (see Chapter 9). Acute and chronic pain differ in their onset and duration, their associated diseases or conditions, and the way they are treated. Table 11-2 lists the different characteristics of acute and chronic pain and various diseases and conditions associated with each.

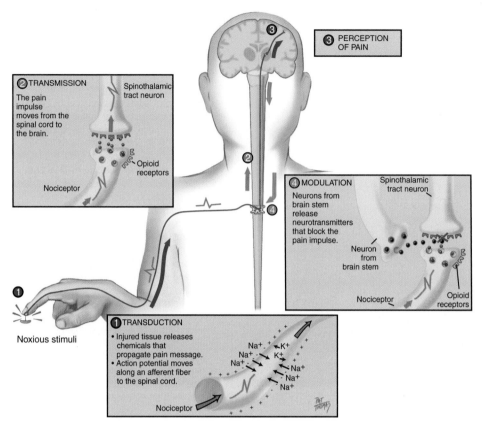

FIGURE 11-1 Illustration of the four processes of nociception. (From Jarvis C: *Physical examination and health assessment,* ed 5, Philadelphia, 2008, Saunders.)

TABLE 11-1 Conditions That Alter Pain Tolerance

Pain Threshold	Conditions
Lowered	Anger, anxiety, depression, discomfort, fear, isolation, chronic pain, sleeplessness, tiredness
Raised	Diversion, empathy, rest, sympathy, medications (analgesics, antianxiety drugs, antidepressants)

Pain can be further classified according to its source. The two most commonly mentioned sources of pain are somatic and visceral. **Somatic pain** originates from skeletal muscles, ligaments, and joints. **Visceral pain** originates from organs and smooth muscles. Sometimes pain is described as superficial. **Superficial pain** originates from the skin and mucous membranes, in contrast to **deep pain,** which occurs in tissues below skin level. Pain treatment may be more appropriately selected when the source of the pain is known. For example, visceral and superficial pain usually requires opioids for relief, whereas somatic pain (including bone pain) usually responds better to **nonopioid analgesics** such as **nonsteroidal antiinflammatory drugs (NSAIDs)** (see Chapter 44).

Pain may be further subclassified according to the diseases or other conditions that cause it. **Vascular pain** is believed to originate from pathology of the vascular or perivascular tissues and is thought to account for a large percentage of migraine headaches. **Referred pain** occurs when visceral nerve fibers or synapse at a level in the spinal cord close to fibers that supply specific subcutaneous tissues in the body. An example is the pain associated with cholecystitis, which is often referred to the back and scapular areas. **Neuropathic pain** usually results from damage to peripheral or CNS nerve fibers by disease or injury but may also be idiopathic (unexplained). **Phantom pain** occurs in the area of a body part that has been removed—surgically or traumatically—and is often described as burning, itching, tingling, or stabbing. It can also occur in paralyzed limbs following spinal cord injury. **Cancer pain** can be acute or chronic or both. It most often results from mechanical pressure of tumor mass against nerves, organs, or tissues. Other causes of cancer pain include hypoxia from blockage of blood supply to an organ, metastases, pathologic fractures, muscle spasms, and adverse effects of radiation, surgery, and chemotherapy. **Central pain** occurs with tumors, trauma, inflammation or disease (e.g., cancer, diabetes, stroke, multiple sclerosis) affecting CNS tissues.

Several theories attempt to explain pain transmission and pain relief. The most common and well described is the **gate theory.** This theory, proposed by Melzack and Wall in 1965, uses the analogy of a gate to describe how impulses from damaged tissues are sensed in the brain. First, the tissue injury causes the release of several substances from injured cells, such as bradykinin, histamine, potassium, prostaglandins, and serotonin. Some current pain medications work by altering the actions and levels of these substances (e.g., NSAIDs→prostaglandins; antidepressants→serotonin). The release of these pain-mediating chemicals initiates action potentials (electrical

TABLE **11-2** Acute Versus Chronic Pain

Type of Pain	Onset	Duration	Examples
Acute	Sudden (minutes to hours); usually sharp, localized; physiologic response (SNS: tachycardia, sweating, pallor, increased blood pressure)	Limited (has an end)	Myocardial infarction, appendicitis, dental procedures, kidney stones, surgical procedures
Chronic	Slow (days to months); long duration; dull, persistent aching	Persistent or recurring (endless)	Arthritis, cancer, lower back pain, peripheral neuropathy

SNS, Sympathetic nervous system.

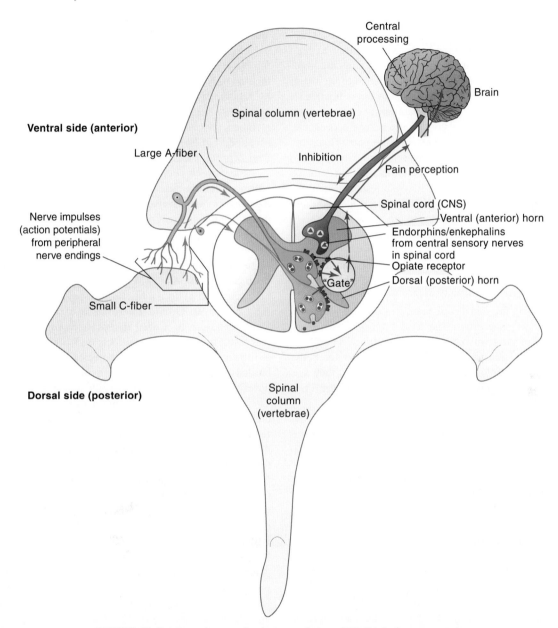

FIGURE 11-2   Gate theory of pain transmission. *CNS,* Central nervous system.

nerve impulses) at the distal end of sensory nerve fibers through pain receptors known as *nociceptors*. These nerve impulses are conducted along sensory nerve fibers and activate pain receptors in the *dorsal horn* of the spinal cord. It is here that the so-called gates are located. These gates regulate the flow of sensory nerve impulses. If impulses are stopped by a gate at this junction, no impulses are transmitted to the higher centers of the brain. Conversely, if the gates permit a sufficient number and intensity of action potentials to be conducted from the spinal cord to the cerebral cortex, the sensation of pain is then felt. This is known as *nociception.* Figure 11-2 depicts the gate theory of pain transmission.

TABLE 11-3 A and C Nerve Fibers

Type of Fiber	Myelin Sheath	Fiber Size	Conduction Speed	Type of Pain
A	Yes	Large	Fast	Sharp and well localized
C	No	Small	Slow	Dull and nonlocalized

Both the opening and the closing of this gate are influenced by the relative activation of the large-diameter A fibers and the small-diameter C fibers (Table 11-3). Closing of the gate seems to be affected by the activation of A fibers. This causes the inhibition of impulse transmission to the brain and avoidance of pain sensation. Opening of the gate is affected by the stimulation of the C fibers. This allows impulses to be transmitted to the brain and pain to be sensed. The gate is innervated by nerve fibers that originate in the brain and modulate the pain sensation by sending impulses to the gate in the spinal cord. These nerve fibers enable the brain to evaluate, identify, and localize the pain. Thus, the brain can control the gate, either keeping the gate closed or allowing it to open so that the brain is stimulated and pain is sensed. The cells that control the gate have a threshold. Impulses that reach these cells must rise above this threshold before an impulse is permitted to travel up to the brain.

The body is also equipped with certain endogenous neurotransmitters known as *enkephalins* and *endorphins.* These substances are produced within the body to fight pain and are considered the body's painkillers. Both are capable of bonding with opioid receptors and inhibiting the transmission of pain impulses by closing the spinal cord gates, in a manner similar to that of opioid analgesic drugs. The term *endorphin* is a condensed version of the term "endogenous morphine." These endogenous analgesic substances are released whenever the body experiences pain or prolonged exertion. For example, they are responsible for the phenomenon of "runner's high." Figure 11-1 depicts this entire process.

Another phenomenon of pain relief that may be explained by the gate theory is the fact that massaging a painful area often reduces the pain. When an area is rubbed or liniment is applied, large sensory A nerve fibers from peripheral receptors carry pain-modulating impulses to the spinal cord. Again, the A fibers tend to close the gate, which reduces pain sensation in the brain.

TREATMENT OF PAIN IN SPECIAL SITUATIONS

Estimates are that one of every three Americans experiences ongoing pain, and pain is poorly understood and often undertreated. In addition to enduring baseline chronic pain, patients with illnesses such as cancer, AIDS, and sickle cell anemia may also experience crisis periods of acute pain. Effective management of acute pain is often different from management of chronic pain in terms of medications and dosages used. Routes of drug administration may include oral, intravenous (IV), intramuscular (IM), subcutaneous (subcut), transdermal, and rectal. One intravenous route commonly used in the hospital setting is patient-controlled analgesia (PCA). In this situation, patients are able to self-medicate by pressing a switch on a PCA infusion pump. This has been shown to be very effective for many patients and even reduces the total opioid dose. Morphine and hydromorphone are commonly given by PCA. Potential hazards of PCA include well-meaning family members' pressing the dosing button rather than letting able patients do so on their own. For patients truly not able to self-medicate using the PCA pump, a different method of pain control should be used. Numerous deaths have occurred when well-meaning family members have administered too much of the opioid drug. This is called *PCA by proxy.* The Institute for Safe Medication Practices *(http://www.ismp.org)* advises against PCA by proxy.

Patients with complex pain syndromes often benefit from a holistic or multimodal clinical approach that involves pharmacologic and/or nonpharmacologic treatment. Effective drug therapy in such situations may include use of opioid and/or nonopioid drugs. The goals of pain management include reducing and controlling pain, and improving body function and quality of life.

In situations such as pain associated with malignancies, the main consideration in pain management is patient comfort and not prevention of drug **addiction** (or **psychologic dependence;** see Chapter 9). **Opioid tolerance** is a state of adaptation in which exposure to a drug induces changes in drug receptors that result in reduced drug effects over time. This can occur in as little as 1 week. Because of increasing pathology (e.g., tumor burden), patients usually require increasingly higher opioid doses and thus do become physically dependent on these drugs. These patients are therefore more likely to experience withdrawal symptoms (see Chapter 9) if opioid doses are abruptly reduced or discontinued. Although actual psychologic dependence or addiction in such patients is unusual, it is now believed to be more likely in patients who have a genetic predisposition for addiction. For long-term pain control situations such as these, oral, intravenous, subcutaneous, transdermal, and sometimes even rectal dosing routes are favored over multiple intramuscular injections, due to associated puncture trauma (bruising) and erratic drug absorption.

One controversial issue in pain management is the use of placebos, inert dosage forms that actually lack medication. Some prescribers feel that this practice may be helpful by taking advantage of the well-documented placebo effect. The placebo effect is a psychologic therapeutic effect that occurs even in the absence of actual medication. It is believed to arise from activation of patients' own endorphins. It is also attributed to the patient's belief that any "treatment" is effective, as well as the patient's high level of trust in the health care provider. Critics argue that the use of placebos is unethical, because it requires that the patient be deceived in the process. The use of placebos has fallen out of favor, and they are rarely used today (see Chapter 4 for further discussion).

The treatment of patients who are addicted to street opioids is of great concern to clinicians, who may be reluctant to prescribe opioid therapy for such patients. However, habitual street opioid users are also **opioid tolerant** and generally require high dosages. Longer-acting opioids such as methadone or extended-release oxycodone are usually better choices than shorter-acting immediate-release drug products for these patients. This is because the shorter-acting drugs are more likely to produce a psychologic "high" or euphoria, which only reinforces addictive tendencies. It should also be noted that genetic difference in cytochrome P-450 enzymes (see Chapters 2 and 5) can cause different patients, whether addicted or not, to respond more or less effectively to a given drug. For this reason, patients should not automatically be viewed with suspicion if they complain that a given drug does not work for them.

The label of "addict" can be used unfairly to justify refusal to prescribe pain medications, resulting in undertreatment of pain, even in patients who do not use street drugs. This is now generally regarded as inappropriate and inhumane clinical practice. In these situations, control of the patient's pain takes ethical and clinical priority over concerns regarding drug addiction. Nonetheless, prescribers must also contend with the reality of abuse of street and/or prescription drugs by patients without genuine pain conditions (see Chapter 9). Such patients often request excessive numbers of prescriptions and may also use multiple prescribers and/or pharmacies to get medication. At times, they may also forge prescriptions and/or use a telephone to call in prescriptions for non–Schedule II opioids such as hydrocodone/acetaminophen (Vicodin). Community pharmacists work collaboratively to detect such abuses and notify law enforcement authorities. Creating a phony prescription for a controlled substance is a felony under federal and state laws.

For patients receiving long-acting opioids, **breakthrough pain** often occur between doses of pain medications. This is because the analgesic effects wear off as the drug is metabolized and eliminated from the body. Treatment with prn (as needed) doses of immediate-release dosage forms (e.g., oxycodone IR), given between scheduled doses of extended-release dosage forms (e.g., oxycodone ER), is often helpful in these cases. It should be noted that chewing or crushing of any extended-release opioid drug can predispose the patient to oversedation, respiratory depression, and even death due to rapid drug absorption. If the patient is requiring larger doses for breakthrough pain, the dose of the scheduled extended-release opioid may need to be gradually titrated upward or a more potent drug started.

Drugs from other chemical categories are often added to the opioid regimen as adjuvant drugs. These assist the primary drugs in relieving pain. Such adjuvant drug therapy may include NSAIDs (see Chapter 44), antidepressants (see Chapter 17), anticonvulsants (see Chapter 15), and corticosteroids (see Chapter 33), all of which are discussed further in their corresponding chapters. This approach allows the use of smaller dosages of opioids. This reduces some of the adverse effects that are seen with higher dosages of opioids, such as respiratory depression, constipation, and urinary retention. It permits drugs with different mechanisms of action to produce **synergistic effects.** Antiemetics (see Chapter 52) and laxatives (see Chapter 51) may also be needed to prevent or relieve associated constipation, nausea, and vomiting (Box 11-2).

BOX 11-2 Potential Opioid Adverse Effects and Their Management

Constipation

Opioids decrease gastrointestinal (GI) tract peristalsis because of their central nervous system (CNS) depression, with subsequent constipation as an adverse effect. Stool becomes excessively dehydrated because it remains in the GI tract longer. **Preventative measures:** Constipation may be managed with increased intake of fluids, stool softeners such as docusate sodium, and use of mild cathartics such as senna. Less commonly used are bulk-forming laxatives such as psyllium, for which increased fluid intake is especially important to avoid fecal impactions or bowel obstructions.

Nausea and Vomiting

Opioids decrease GI tract peristalsis, and some also stimulate the vomiting center in the CNS, so nausea and vomiting are often experienced. **Preventative measures:** Nausea and vomiting may be managed with the use of antiemetics such as phenothiazines.

Sedation and Mental Clouding

Any change in mental status should always be evaluated to ensure that causes other than drug-related CNS depression are ruled out. **Preventative measures:** Persistent drug-related sedation may be managed with a decrease in the dosage of opioid or change in drug used. The prescriber may also order various CNS stimulants (see Chapter 14).

Respiratory Depression

Long-term opioid use is generally associated with tolerance to respiratory depression. **Preventative measures:** For severe respiratory depression, opioid antagonists may be used to improve respiratory status and, if they are titrated in small amounts, the respiratory depression may be reversed without analgesia reversal.

Subacute Overdose

Subacute overdose may be more common than acute respiratory depression and may progress slowly (over hours to days), with somnolence and respiratory depression. Before analgesic dosages are changed or reduced, advancing disease must be considered, especially in the dying patient. **Preventative measures:** Often, holding one or two doses of an opioid analgesic is enough to judge if the mental and respiratory depression are associated with the opioid. If there is improvement with this measure, the opioid dosage is often decreased by 25%.

Other Opioid Adverse Effects

Dry mouth, urinary retention, pruritus, myoclonus, dysphoria, euphoria, sleep disturbances, sexual dysfunction, and inappropriate secretion of antidiuretic hormone may occur but are less common than the aforementioned adverse effects. **Preventative measures:** Ongoing assessment is needed for each of the adverse effects so that appropriate measures may be implemented (e.g., sucking of sugar-free hard candy or use of artificial saliva drops or gum for dry mouth; use of diphenhydramine for pruritus).

One particularly common use of adjuvant drugs is in the treatment of neuropathic pain. Opioids often are not completely effective in such cases. Neuropathic pain usually results from some kind of nerve damage secondary to disease (e.g., diabetic neuropathy, postherpetic neuralgia secondary to shingles, trigeminal neuralgia, AIDS or injury, including nerve damage secondary to surgical procedures (e.g., postthoracotomy pain syndrome occurring after cardiothoracic surgery). Common symptoms include hypersensitivity or hyperalgesia to mild stimuli such as light touch or a pinprick, or the bed sheets on a person's feet. This is also known as *allodynia*. It can also manifest as hyperalgesia to uncomfortable stimuli, such as pressure from an inflated blood pressure cuff on a patient's limb. It may be described as heat, cold, numbness, tingling, burning, or electrical sensations. Examples of adjuvants commonly used in these cases are the antidepressant amitriptyline and the anticonvulsants gabapentin and pregabalin.

The three-step analgesic ladder defined by the **World Health Organization** (WHO) is often applied as the pain management standard for the use of nonopioid and opioid drugs in cancer pain. Examples of nonopioid analgesic drugs include NSAIDs (see Chapter 44) as well as acetaminophen and tramadol (see Drug Profiles). Step 1 is the use of nonopioids (with or without adjuvant medications) once the pain has been identified and assessed. If pain persists and/or increases, treatment moves to step 2, which is defined as the use of opioids with or without nonopioids and with or without adjuvants. Should pain persist or increase, management then rises to step 3, which is the use of opioids indicated for moderate to severe pain, administered with or without nonopioids or adjuvant medications. Many experts now question the effectiveness of Step 2, and the WHO is considering adjusting the ladder.

Pharmacology Overview

Opioids are classified as both mild **agonists** (codeine, hydrocodone, and propoxyphene) and strong agonists (morphine, hydromorphone, levorphanol, oxycodone, oxymorphone, meperidine, fentanyl, and methadone). Meperidine is not recommended for long-term use because of the accumulation of a neurotoxic metabolite, *normeperidine*. In fact, many hospitals have tried to prohibit the use of meperidine, due to its adverse CNS effects, including seizures. The opiate **agonists-antagonists** such as pentazocine and nalbuphine are associated with an **analgesic ceiling effect.** This means that the drug reaches a maximum analgesic effect, so that analgesia does not improve even with higher dosages (see Drug Profiles). Such drugs are useful only in patients who have not been previously exposed to opioids and can be administered for management of nonescalating moderate to severe pain. Finally, because of associated bruising and bleeding risks, as well as injection discomfort, there is now a strong trend away from intramuscular injections in favor of intravenous, oral, and transdermal routes of drug administration.

OPIOID DRUGS

The pain-relieving drugs currently known as *opioid analgesics* originated from the opium poppy plant. The word *opium* is a Greek word that means "juice." More than 20 different alkaloids are obtained from the unripe seed of the poppy. The properties of opium and its many alkaloids have been known for centuries. Opium-smoking immigrants brought opium to the United States, where unrestricted availability of opium prevailed until the early twentieth century.

Chemical Structure

Opioid analgesics are very strong pain relievers. They can be classified according to their chemical structure or their action at specific receptors. Of the 20 different natural alkaloids available

TABLE 11-4 Chemical Classification of Opioids

Chemical Category	Opioid Drugs
meperidine-like drugs	meperidine, fentanyl, remifentanil, sufentanil, alfentanil
methadone-like drugs	methadone, propoxyphene
morphine-like drugs	morphine, heroin, hydromorphone, oxymorphone, levorphanol, codeine, hydrocodone, oxycodone
Other	tramadol

TABLE 11-5 Opioid Receptors and Their Characteristics

Receptor Type	Prototypical Agonist	Effects of Opioid Stimulation
mu	morphine	Supraspinal analgesia, respiratory depression, euphoria, + + sedation
kappa	ketocyclazocine	Spinal analgesia, + + + + sedation, miosis
delta	Enkephalins	Analgesia

from the opium poppy plant, only three are clinically useful: morphine, codeine, and papaverine. Of these, only morphine and codeine are pain relievers; papaverine is a smooth muscle relaxant. Relatively simple synthetic chemical modifications of these opium alkaloids have produced the three different chemical classes of opioids: morphine-like drugs, meperidine-like drugs, and methadone-like drugs (Table 11-4).

Mechanism of Action and Drug Effects

Opioid analgesics can also be characterized according to their mechanism of action. They can be agonists, agonists-antagonists, or antagonists (nonanalgesic). An *agonist* binds to an opioid pain receptor in the brain and causes an analgesic response—the reduction of pain sensation. An *agonist-antagonist,* also called a **partial agonist** or a *mixed agonist,* binds to a pain receptor but causes a weaker pain response than a full agonist. Different drugs in this class exert their agonist and/or antagonist effects by binding in different degrees to kappa and mu opioid receptors. Although not normally used as first-line analgesics, they are sometimes useful in pain management in opioid-addicted patients as well as obstetrical patients (because they avoid oversedation of the mother and/or fetus). An **antagonist** binds to a pain receptor but does not reduce pain signals. It functions as a *competitive antagonist* because it competes with and reverses the effects of agonist and agonist-antagonist drugs at the receptor sites.

The actual receptors to which opioids bind to relieve pain are listed and their characteristics are summarized in Table 11-5. Although five types of opioid receptor have been identified to date: mu (μ), kappa (κ), sigma (σ), delta (δ), and epsilon (ϵ), the mu, kappa, and delta receptors are the most responsive to drug activity with the mu being the most important. Many of the characteristics of a particular opioid, such as its ability to sedate, its potency, and its ability to cause hallucinations, can be attributed to relative affinity for these various receptors.

BOX 11-3 Calculating Dosage Conversions Between Commonly Used Opioids

	Equianalgesic Doses			
	Oral Dose (mg)	Parenteral Dose (mg)	Oral-to-Parenteral Dose Ratio	Dosing Interval (hr)
Morphine	30	10	3:1	12 (continuous release) 4 (immediate release)
Hydromorphone	7.5	1.5	5:1	4 (immediate release)
Oxycodone	15	N/A	N/A	4 (immediate release)
Hydrocodone	30	N/A	N/A	N/A
Fentanyl	See fentanyl Drug Profile			

N/A, Not applicable.

Basic Conversion Equation

$$\frac{24\ \text{hour amount of current drug}}{X} = \frac{\text{EA dose of current drug}}{\text{EA dose of desired drug}}$$

Where X = amount of desired opioid in 24 hours and EA = equianalgesic dose obtained from table above

For example: A patient with colon cancer is currently taking oral oxycodone 80 mg every 12 hours and needs to be converted to intravenous morphine due to a bowel obstruction. What is the equivalent IV morphine dose?

Step 1: **Determine 24 hour amount of oxycodone taken by this patient:**
80 mg × 2 doses per 24 hours = 160 mg per 24 hours

Step 2: **Using the conversion table above, find the equianalgesic (EA) doses of oxycodone and parenteral morphine:**
15 mg oxycodone = 10 mg parenteral morphine

Step 3: **Use above equation and solve for X by cross multiplying.**

$$\frac{24\ \text{hr amount of oxycodone (160 mg)}}{X} = \frac{\text{EA of current oxycodone (15 mg)}}{\text{EA dose of parenteral morphine (10 mg)}}$$

Where X = amount of parenteral morphine in 24 hours (solve by cross multiplying)

$$160\ \text{mg} \times 10\ \text{mg} = 15\ \text{mg}\ X \qquad X = \frac{1600\ \text{mg}}{15\ \text{mg}}$$

$$X = 107\ \text{mg (approximately 100 mg of injectable morphine per 24 hours)}$$

An understanding of the relative potencies of various drugs becomes important in clinical settings. *Equianalgesia* refers to the ability to provide equivalent pain relief by calculating dosages of different drugs and/or routes of administration that provide comparable analgesia. Box 11-3 lists equianalgesic doses for several common opioids and shows how to calculate dosage conversions for patients. Because fentanyl is most commonly used transdermally, it is discussed separately in its drug profile.

Indications

The main use of opioids is to alleviate moderate to severe pain. The degree to which pain is relieved or unwanted adverse effects occur depends on the specific drug, the receptors to which it binds, and its chemical structure.

Strong opioid analgesics such as fentanyl, sufentanil, and alfentanil are commonly used in combination with anesthetics during surgery. These drugs are used not only to relieve pain but also to maintain a balanced state of anesthesia. The practice of using combinations of drugs to produce anesthesia is referred to as *balanced anesthesia* (see Chapter 12). Use of fentanyl injection for management of postoperative and procedural pain has become popular due to its rapid onset and short duration. Transdermal fentanyl comes in a patch formulation for use in long-term pain management and should not be used for postoperative or any other short-term pain control (see the Preventing Medication Errors box).

Strong opioids such as morphine, meperidine, hydromorphone, and oxycodone are often used to control postoperative and other types of pain. Because morphine and hydromorphone

PREVENTING MEDICATION ERRORS

Fentanyl Transdermal Patches

When giving fentanyl transdermal patches, the nurse needs to keep in mind several important points to avoid improper administration:

- These patches should be used only by patients who are considered opioid tolerant. To be considered opioid tolerant, a patient should have been taking, for a week or longer, morphine 60 mg daily, oral oxycodone 30 mg daily, or oral hydromorphone 8 mg daily (or an equianalgesic dose of another opioid). Giving fentanyl transdermal patches to non–opioid tolerant patients may result in severe respiratory depression. Thorough assessment is important.
- Patients should be taught that heat, such as from a heating pad, should never be applied over a fentanyl transdermal patch. The increased circulation that results from the application of heat may result in increased absorption of medication, causing an overdose.
- Patients should be taught to dispose of patches properly. Children have pulled used patches from the trash, which has resulted in death due to exposure to the drug. Used patches should be folded with sticky sides together and flushed down the toilet. Disposal practices may vary by area because of concerns for the water systems, but at this time flushing is still recommended for disposal because of concerns of the old patches either being stolen or touched by children or pets.

The Institute for Safe Medication Practices has described examples of fatal patient incidents resulting from failure to follow the above three points. It is essential for the patient's safety to read the product labeling and follow instructions precisely.

are available in injectable forms, they are often first-line analgesics in the immediate postoperative setting. There is a trend away from using meperidine due to its greater risk for toxicity (see its drug profile). All available oxycodone dosage forms are orally administered. The product OxyContin is a sustained-release form of oxycodone that is designed to last up to 12 hours. The "Contin" in the product name is a trademark of the original drug manufacturer, Purdue Frederick, and refers to the "continuous-release" nature of the drug formulation. Recall that a continuous- or extended-release dosage form of a drug means that it has a prolonged duration of action, most often 8 to 24 hours (see Chapter 2). Similarly, the drug product MS Contin is a long-acting or sustained-release form of morphine that is also designed to provide 8 to 12 hours of pain relief. The "MS" stands for morphine sulfate. Both drugs are also available generically.

In contrast to extended-release dosage forms, there are also immediate-release dosage forms of oxycodone and morphine in tablet, capsule, and liquid form. Meperidine is available only in immediate-release dosage forms, both oral and injectable. The analgesic effects of immediate-release oral dosage forms of all three drugs typically last for about 4 hours.

Opioids also suppress the medullary cough center, which results in cough suppression. The most commonly used opioid for this purpose is codeine. Hydrocodone is also used in many cough suppressants, either alone or in combination with other drugs. Sometimes the opioid-related cough suppressants have a depressant effect on the CNS and cause sedation. To avoid this problem, dextromethorphan, a nonopioid cough suppressant, is often given instead (see Chapters 9 and 36).

Constipation from decreased gastrointestinal (GI) tract motility is often an unwanted adverse effect of opioids related to their anticholinergic effects. It occurs because opioid drugs bind to intestinal opioid receptors. However, this effect is sometimes helpful in treating diarrhea. Some of the most common opioid-containing antidiarrheal preparations are camphorated opium tincture (paregoric) and diphenoxylate/atropine tablets.

Contraindications

Contraindications to the use of opioid analgesics include known drug allergy and severe asthma. It is not uncommon for patients to state they are allergic to codeine, when in the overwhelming majority of these patients, nausea was the "allergic" reaction. Many patients will claim to be allergic to morphine because it causes itching. Itching is a pharmacologic effect due to histamine release and not an allergic reaction. Thus, it is important for the nurse to determine the exact nature of a patient's stated allergy. Although these conditions are not absolute contraindications, extreme caution should be used in cases of respiratory insufficiency, especially when resuscitative equipment is not available; conditions involving elevated intracranial pressure (e.g., severe head injury); morbid obesity and/or sleep apnea; myasthenia gravis; paralytic ileus (bowel paralysis); and pregnancy, especially with long-term use or high dosages.

Adverse Effects

Many of the unwanted effects of opioid analgesics are related to their effects on parts of the body other than the CNS. Some of these unwanted effects can be explained by the respective drug's

TABLE 11-6 Opioid-Induced Adverse Effects by Body System

Body System	Adverse Effects
Cardiovascular	Hypotension, palpitations, flushing, bradycardia
Central nervous	Sedation, disorientation, euphoria, lightheadedness, dysphoria, lowered seizure threshold, tremors
Gastrointestinal	Nausea, vomiting, constipation, biliary tract spasm
Genitourinary	Urinary retention
Integumentary	Itching, rash, wheal formation
Respiratory	Respiratory depression and possible aggravation of asthma

For further information on transdermal fentanyl, visit *http://www.ismp.org/Newsletters/acutecare/articles/20050811.asp.*

selectivity for the receptors listed in Table 11-5. The various body systems that the opioids affect and their specific adverse effects are summarized in Table 11-6.

Opioids that have an affinity for mu receptors and have rapid onset of action produce marked euphoria. These are the opioids that are most likely to be abused and used recreationally. All opioid drugs have a strong abuse potential. They are common recreational drugs of abuse among the lay public and also among health care professionals, who often have relatively easy access. The person taking them to alter his or her mental status will soon become psychologically dependent (addicted; see Chapter 9).

In addition, opioids do cause some histamine release. It is thought that this histamine release is responsible for many of the drugs' unwanted adverse effects, such as itching or pruritus, rash, and hemodynamic changes. The histamine release causes peripheral arteries and veins to dilate, which leads to flushing and orthostatic hypotension. The amount of histamine release that an opioid analgesic causes is related to its chemical class. The naturally occurring opiates (e.g., morphine) elicit the most histamine release; the synthetic opioids (e.g., meperidine) elicit the least histamine release. (See Table 11-4 for a list of the various opioids and their respective chemical classes.)

The most serious adverse effect of opioid use is CNS depression, which may lead to respiratory depression. When death occurs from opioid overdose, it is almost always due to respiratory depression. When opioids are given, care should be taken to titrate the dose so that the patient's pain is controlled without respiratory function's being affected. Individual responses to opioids vary, and patients may occasionally experience respiratory compromise despite careful dose titration. Respiratory depression can be prevented in part by using drugs with very short duration of action and no active metabolites. Respiratory depression seems to be more common in patients with a preexisting condition causing respiratory compromise, such as asthma or chronic obstructive pulmonary disease. Respiratory depression is strongly related to the degree of sedation (see Toxicity and Management of Overdose later).

GI tract adverse effects are common in patients receiving opioids, due to stimulation of GI opioid receptors as noted previously. Nausea, vomiting, and constipation are the most common adverse effects associated with opioid analgesics. Opioids can

TABLE 11-7 Opioid Antagonists (Reversal Drugs)

Generic Name	Trade Name	Dosage	Adverse Effects
naloxone (IV)	Narcan	0.4-2 mg q2-3min (not more than 10 mg); IV infusion: 2 mg in 500 mL (titrate to response)	Raised or lowered blood pressure, dysrhythmias, pulmonary edema, withdrawal
naltrexone (PO)	ReVia	25-50 mg daily	Nervousness, headache, nausea, vomiting, pulmonary edema, withdrawal

IV, Intravenous; *PO,* oral.

irritate the GI tract, stimulating the chemoreceptor trigger zone in the CNS, which in turn may cause nausea and vomiting. Opioids slow peristalsis and increase absorption of water from intestinal contents. These two actions combine to produce constipation. This is more pronounced in hospitalized patients who are nonambulatory. Patients may require laxatives (Chapter 51) to help maintain normal bowel movements.

Urinary retention, or the inability to void, is another unwanted adverse effect of opioid analgesics, caused by increasing bladder tone. This is sometimes prevented by giving low dosages of an opioid agonist-antagonist or an opioid antagonist or a cholinergic agonist (see Chapter 20), such as bethanechol.

Severe hypersensitivity or anaphylactic reaction to opioid analgesics is rare. Many patients will experience GI discomforts or histamine-mediated reactions to opioids and call these "allergic reactions." However, true anaphylaxis is rare, even with intravenously administered opioids. Some patients may complain of flushing, itching, or wheal formation at the injection site, but this is usually local and histamine mediated, and not a true allergy. Box 11-2 provides additional information on opioid adverse effects and their management.

Toxicity and Management of Overdose

Opioid analgesics produce both beneficial and toxic effects. The opioid antagonists naloxone and naltrexone bind to and occupy all of the receptor sites (mu, kappa, delta). They are competitive antagonists with a strong affinity for these binding sites. Through such binding they can reverse the adverse effects induced by the opioid drug, such as respiratory depression. These drugs are used in the management of both opioid overdose and opioid addiction. The commonly used opioid antagonists (reversal drugs) are listed in Table 11-7.

When treating an opioid overdose or toxicity, the nurse must recognize the signs and symptoms of withdrawal. Some degree of physical dependence is expected in opioid-tolerant patients. The extent of opioid tolerance is most visible when an opioid drug is discontinued abruptly or when an opioid antagonist is administered. This usually leads to symptoms of **opioid withdrawal,** also known as *abstinence syndrome* (see Chapter 9). This can occur after as little as 2 weeks of opioid therapy in **opioid-naive** patients. Gradual dosage reduction after chronic opioid use, when possible, generally helps to minimize the risk and severity of withdrawal symptoms. Regardless of withdrawal symptoms, when a patient experiences severe respiratory depression, naloxone (an opioid antagonist) should be given.

Respiratory depression is the most serious adverse effect associated with opioids. Stimulation of the patient may be adequate to reverse mild hypoventilation. If this is unsuccessful, ventila-

tory assistance using a bag and mask or endotracheal intubation may be needed to support respiration. Administration of opioid antagonists (e.g., naloxone) may also be necessary to reverse severe respiratory depression. Careful titration of drug dose until the patient begins to breathe independently will prevent overreversal. The effects of naloxone are short lived and usually last about 1 hour. With long-acting opioids, respiratory depressant effects may reappear, and redosing of naloxone may be needed.

The timing of the onset of withdrawal symptoms is directly related to the half-life of the opioid analgesic being used. The withdrawal symptoms resulting from the discontinuance or reversal of therapy with short-acting opioids (codeine, hydrocodone, morphine, and hydromorphone) will appear within 6 to 12 hours and peak at 24 to 72 hours. The withdrawal symptoms associated with the long half-life drugs (methadone, levorphanol, and transdermal fentanyl) may not appear for 24 hours or longer after drug discontinuation and may be milder.

Interactions

Potential drug interactions with opioids are significant. Coadministration of opioids with alcohol, antihistamines, barbiturates, benzodiazepines, phenothiazine, and other CNS depressants can result in additive respiratory depressant effects. The combined use of opioids (such as meperidine) with monoamine oxidase inhibitors can result in respiratory depression, seizures, and hypotension.

Laboratory Test Interactions

Opioids can cause an abnormal increase in the serum levels of amylase, alanine aminotransferase, alkaline phosphatase, bilirubin, lipase, creatinine kinase, and lactate dehydrogenase. Other abnormal results include a decrease in urinary 17-ketosteroid levels and an increase in the urinary alkaloid and glucose concentrations.

Dosages

For the recommended initial dosages of selected analgesic drugs in opioid-naive patients, see the Dosages table on p. 162.

DRUG PROFILES

OPIOID AGONISTS
◆ morphine sulfate

Morphine, a naturally occurring alkaloid derived from the opium poppy, is the drug prototype for all opioid drugs. It is classified as a Schedule II controlled substance. This drug is indicated for severe pain and has a high abuse potential. It is available in oral, injectable, and rectal dosage forms. Extended-release forms include MS Contin, Kadian, and Avinza. Morphine also has a potentially toxic me-

DOSAGES

Selected Analgesic Drugs and Related Drugs

Drug (Pregnancy Category)	Pharmacologic Class	Usual Dosage Range	Indications/Uses
Opioids			
codeine sulfate (D)	Opiate analgesic; opium alkaloid	**Pediatric 2-5 yr** PO/subcut/IM: 2.5-5 mg q4-6h—do not exceed 30 mg/day	Cough relief
		Pediatric 6-11 yr 5-10 mg q4-6h	Cough relief
		Adult and pediatric older than 12 yr 10-20 mg q4-6h—do not exceed 120 mg/day	Cough relief
		Adult 15-60 mg tid-qid	Opioid analgesia
fentanyl citrate (Duragesic, Oralet, Actiq*) (D)	Opioid analgesic	All doses titrated to response, starting with lowest effective dose IV/IM doses available in 50 mcg/mL ampule or premixed infusion of varying strengths **Pediatric** IV/IM: 0.5-3 mcg/kg/dose	Procedural sedation or adjunct to general anesthesia
		Adult IV/IM: 20-100 mcg/dose titrated to response via continuous infusion Duragesic (transdermal patch): 12.5-200 mcg/hr q72h; Oralet, Actiq (buccal lozenges): begin with lowest dose (200 mcg) and titrate as needed Note that oral dosage forms are more commonly used in adults for safety due to high drug potency	Relief of moderate to severe acute pain; relief of chronic pain, including cancer pain
meperidine HCl (Demerol, Pethidine) (D)	Opioid analgesic	**Pediatric** PO/IM/subcut: 1-1.8 mg/kg q3-4h prn (max 100 mg/dose) IM/subcut: 0.5-1 mg/kg 30-90 min before anesthesia (max 600 mg/day)	Meperidine use should be restricted because of the unpredictable effects of neurometabolites at analgesic doses and risk for seizures
		Adult PO/IM/subcut: 50-150 mg q3-4h prn IM/subcut: 50-100 mg 30-90 min before anesthesia IV: 50-150 mg q3-4h	Obstetric analgesia, preoperative sedation
methadone HCl (Dolophine) (D)	Opioid analgesic	**Adult** PO/IM/IV/subcut: 2.5-10 mg q3-4h; 40 mg or more once daily	Opioid analgesia, relief of chronic pain, opioid detoxification, opioid addiction maintenance
morphine sulfate (MSIR, Roxanol, Kadian, Avinza, others) (D)	Opiate analgesic; opium alkaloid	**Pediatric** Subcut: 0.1-0.2 mg/kg dose—do not exceed a 15-mg single dose	Opioid analgesia
		Adult PO/IM/subcut: 5-30 mg q4h PR: 10-20 mg q4h IV: 2.5-20 mg q2-6h PCA pump, epidural: titrate to effect	Opioid analgesia
◆ morphine sulfate, continuous release (MS Contin, Oramorph) (D)	Opiate analgesic; opium alkaloid	**Adult only** PO: 15 mg q8h to 200 mg q 8-12h	Relief of moderate to severe pain
oxycodone, immediate release (OxyIR) (D)	Opioid, synthetic	**Pediatric** PO: 1.25-2.5 mg q6h prn	Relief of moderate to severe pain
		Adult PO: 5-20 mg q4-6h prn	Relief of moderate to severe pain
oxycodone, continuous release (OxyContin) (D) PO: 10-160 mg q8-12h	Opioid, synthetic Relief of moderate to severe pain	**Adult only**	

HCL, Hydrochloride; *IM,* intramuscular; *IV,* intravenous; *IR,* immediate release; *MS,* morphine sulfate; *MSIR,* morphine sulfate immediate release; *PCA,* patient-controlled analgesia; *PO,* oral; *PR,* rectal; *subcut,* subcutaneous.
*Actiq is not approved for use in patients under the age of 16.

DOSAGES

Selected Analgesic Drugs and Related Drugs—cont'd

Drug (Pregnancy Category)	Pharmacologic Class	Usual Dosage Range	Indications/Uses
Opioid Antagonists			
◆ naloxone HCl (Narcan)	Opioid antagonist	**Pediatric** IV 0.01 mg/kg IV followed by 0.1 mg/kg if needed; 0.0005-0.01 mg/kg IV—repeat at 2-3 min intervals	Treatment of opioid overdose, postoperative anesthesia reversal
		Adult IV 0.4-2 mg IV—repeat in 2-8 min if needed; 0.1-0.2 mg IV—repeat at 2-3 min intervals	Treatment of opioid overdose, postoperative anesthesia reversal
naltrexone HCl (Trexan)	Opioid antagonist	**Adult** PO: 50 mg q24h or 100 mg every other day	Maintenance of opioid-free state
Nonopioids			
◆ acetaminophen† (Tylenol, others) (B)	Nonopioid analgesic, antipyretic	**Pediatric** PO/PR: Variable doses by age from 40 to 480 mg q4-6h	Mild to moderate pain relief
		Adult PO/PR: 325-650 mg q4-6h; not to exceed 4 g/day In alcoholics, not to exceed 2 g/day	Relief of mild to moderate pain
tramadol (Ultram)	Nonopioid analgesic (with opioid-like activity)	**Adult** PO: 50-100 mg q4-6h; not to exceed 400 mg/day	Relief of moderate to moderately severe pain

†The maximum recommended daily dose of acetaminophen for a typical adult patient with *normal* liver function is 4000 mg/24 hr. For hepatically compromised patients, this dosage may be 2000 mg or even lower. If in doubt, check with a pharmacist or prescriber regarding a particular patient.

tabolite known as *morphine-6-glucuronide.* Accumulation of this metabolite is more likely to occur in patients with renal impairment. For this reason, other Schedule II opioids such as hydromorphone (Dilaudid), fentanyl (see fentanyl drug profile), and oxymorphone (Opana) may be safer analgesic choices for patients with renal insufficency. Drug profile information for hydromorphone is similar to that for morphine and meperidine. However, it is essential that all health care professionals realize that hydromorphone is about eight times more potent than morphine. One milligram of hydromorphone is equivalent to 8 mg of morphine. This difference in potency often is not taken into account when prescribing, and deaths have been reported when larger doses of hydromorphone are given. Morphine is available in oral, rectal, epidural, and injectable dosage forms, including PCA cartridges. Epidural dosage forms, usually physician administered, are injected onto the dura mater of the spinal cord. More recently, a liposomal epidural morphine product (DepoDur) has also become available. Liposomes are a lipid-based drug molecule vehicle that facilitates drug absorption through the lipid bilayer of cell membranes. Epidural analgesics have the potential for hazards arising from increased intracranial pressure, especially with multiple injections, and increased CNS depression when given with other CNS depressant drugs. Other CNS depressant drugs should not be given without orders from an anesthesiologist. For dosage information, see the table on p. 162.

PHARMACOKINETICS

Route	Onset of Action	Peak Plasma Concentration	Elimination Half-life	Duration of Action
IM	Rapid	30-60 min	1.7-4.5 hr	6-7 hr

codeine sulfate

Codeine sulfate is another natural opiate alkaloid (Schedule II) obtained from opium. It is similar to morphine in terms of its pharmacokinetic and pharmacodynamic properties. In fact, about 10% of a codeine dose is metabolized to morphine in the body. However, codeine is less effective as an analgesic and is the only agonist to possess a ceiling effect. Therefore it is more commonly used as an antitussive drug in an array of cough preparations. Codeine combined with acetaminophen (tablets or elixir) is classified as a Schedule III controlled substance and is commonly used for control of mild to moderate pain as well as cough. When codeine is not combined with other drugs, it classified as a Schedule II controlled substance, which implies a high abuse potential. Codeine causes GI tract upset, and, as noted earlier, many patients will say they are allergic to codeine, when in fact it just upsets their stomach. For dosage information, see the table on p. 162.

PHARMACOKINETICS

Route	Onset of Action	Peak Plasma Concentration	Elimination Half-life	Duration of Action
PO	15-30 min	34-45 min	2.5-4 hr	4-6 hr

fentanyl

Fentanyl is a synthetic opioid (Schedule II) used to treat moderate to severe pain. Like other opioids, it also has a high abuse potential. It is available in several dosage forms: parenteral injections (Sublimaze), transdermal patches (Duragesic), buccal lozenges (Fentora), and buccal lozenges on a stick or "lollipop" (Actiq). The buccal dosage forms are absorbed through the oral mucosa and are not "oral" dosage forms per se. They may be especially helpful in managing breakthrough and procedural pain. The injectable form is used most commonly in perioperative settings and in intensive care unit settings for sedation during mechanical ventilation. The oral and transdermal forms are used primarily for long-term control of both malignant and nonmalignant chronic pain. Fentanyl is a very potent analgesic. Fentanyl at a dose of 0.1 mg given intravenously is roughly equivalent to 10 mg of morphine given intravenously.

The transdermal delivery system (patch) has been shown to be highly effective in the treatment of various chronic pain syndromes such as cancer-induced pain, especially in patients who cannot take oral medications. This route should not be used in opioid-naive patients. Generally, fentanyl patches are best used for non-escalating pain because of the difficulty of titrating doses. To perform a conversion using the table in Box 11-3, first the daily (24-hour) opioid requirement of the patient should be determined. Second, if the opioid is not morphine, its dose should be converted to the equianalgesic dose of morphine using Box 11-3. Finally, the equipotent transdermal fentanyl dosage is calculated. These tables are conservative in their dosages for achieving pain relief, and supplemental short-acting opioid analgesics should be added as needed.

Nurses should also be aware that after the first patch is applied it will take 6 to 12 hours to reach steady-state pain control again, so that supplemental short-acting therapy is required. Most patients will experience adequate pain control for 72 hours with this method of fentanyl delivery. A new patch should be applied every 72 hours. It is important to remove the old patch when applying a new one. It should also be noted that it takes about 17 hours for the amount of fentanyl to reduce by 50% once the patch is removed.

In 2006, and again in 2007, the U.S. Food and Drug Administration (FDA) released safety warnings about the use of fentanyl patches. Fentanyl patches are intended for management of chronic or cancer pain in opioid-tolerant patients whose pain is not adequately controlled by other types of medications. These patches are not recommended for acute pain situations such as postoperative pain. Deaths have occurred from drug-induced respiratory arrest when these conditions have not been met. According to the FDA, patients who are considered opioid tolerant are those who have been taking at least 60 mg of oral morphine daily or at least 30 mg of oral oxycodone daily or at least 8 mg of oral hydromorphone daily or an equianalgesic dose of another opioid. Other hazards associated with the use of fentanyl patches are cutting the patch and exposing the patch to heat (e.g., via a heating pad or sauna), both of which accelerate the diffusion of the drug into the patient's body.

For dosage information, see the table on p. 162.

PHARMACOKINETICS

Route	Onset of Action	Peak Plasma Concentration	Elimination Half-life	Duration of Action
IV	Rapid	Minutes	1.5-6 hr	30-60 min
Transdermal	12-24 hr	48-72 hr	Delayed	13-40 hr
PO	5-15 min	20-30 min	5-15 hr	Unknown

meperidine hydrochloride

Meperidine hydrochloride (Demerol) is a synthetic opioid analgesic (Schedule II). Meperidine should be used with caution, if at all, in elderly patients and in patients who require long-term analgesia or who have kidney dysfunction. An active metabolite, normeperidine, can accumulate to toxic levels and lead to seizures. For this reason, meperidine is now used less commonly than before and is definitely not recommended for long-term pain treatment. However, it is still used for acute pain during postoperative periods, as well as in emergency department settings for acute migraine headaches. Meperidine is available in oral and injectable forms. For dosage information, see the table on p. 162.

PHARMACOKINETICS

Route	Onset of Action	Peak Plasma Concentration	Elimination Half-life	Duration of Action
IM	Rapid	30-60 min	3-5 hr	2-4 hr

methadone hydrochloride

Methadone hydrochloride (Dolophine) is a synthetic opioid analgesic (Schedule II). It is the opioid of choice for the detoxification treatment of opioid addicts in methadone maintenance programs. Use of agonist-antagonist opioids (e.g., pentazocine) in heroin-addicted patients or those in methadone maintenance programs can induce significant withdrawal symptoms. There has been renewed interest in the use of methadone for chronic (e.g., neuropathic) and cancer-related pain. The drug is readily absorbed through the GI tract with peak plasma concentrations at 4 hours for single dosing. Methadone is unique in that its half-life is longer than its duration of activity and it is bound into the tissues of the liver, kidneys and brain. With repeated doses, the drug accumulates in those tissues and is slowly released, thus allowing for 24 hour dosing. Methadone is eliminated through the liver, which makes it a safer choice than some other opioids for patients with renal impairment. Recent FDA reports have cited the prolonged half-life of the drug as a cause of unintentional overdoses and deaths. There is also concern that methadone may cause cardiac dysrhythmias. Methadone is available in oral and injectable forms. For dosage information, see the table on p. 162.

PHARMACOKINETICS

Route	Onset of Action	Peak Plasma Concentration	Elimination Half-life	Duration of Action
PO	30-60 min	1.5-2 hr	25 hr	22-48 hr

oxycodone hydrochloride

Oxycodone hydrochloride is an analgesic drug that is structurally related to morphine and has comparable analgesic activity (Schedule II). It is also commonly combined in tablets with acetaminophen (Percocet) and with aspirin (Percodan). Oxycodone is also available in immediate-release formulations (Oxy IR) and sustained-released formulations (OxyContin). A somewhat weaker but commonly used opioid is hydrocodone (Schedule III), which is available only in tablet form, most commonly in combination with acetaminophen (Vicodin) but also with aspirin and ibuprofen. It is available only for oral use. For dosage information, see the table on p. 162.

PHARMACOKINETICS (IMMEDIATE RELEASE)

Route	Onset of Action	Peak Plasma Concentration	Elimination Half-life	Duration of Action
PO	10-15 min	1 hr	2-3 hr	3-6 hr

OPIOID AGONISTS-ANTAGONISTS

Opioids with mixed actions are often called *agonists-antagonists* (Schedule IV). They bind to the mu receptor and can therefore compete with other substances for these sites. They either exert no action (i.e., they are competitive antagonists) or have only limited action (i.e., they are partial agonists). They are similar to the agonist opioid drugs in terms of their therapeutic indications; however, they have a lower risk of misuse and addiction. The antagonistic activity of this group can produce withdrawal symptoms in opioid-dependent patients. Their use is contraindicated in patients who have shown hypersensitivity reactions to the drugs.

Opioid agonist-antagonists have varying degrees of agonist and antagonist effects on the different opioid receptor subtypes. These drugs are normally used in situations requiring short-term pain control, such as after obstetric procedures. They are sometimes chosen for patients who have a history of opioid addiction. These medications can both help prevent overmedication and reduce posttreatment addictive cravings in these patients. These drugs are normally not strong enough for management of longer-term chronic pain (e.g., cancer pain, chronic lower back pain). They should also *not* be given concurrently with full opioid agonists, because they may both reduce analgesic effects and cause withdrawal symptoms in opioid-tolerant patients. Four opioid agonists-antagonists are currently available: buprenorphine (Buprenex), butorphanol (Stadol), nalbuphine (Nubain), and pentazocine (Talwin). They are available in various oral, injectable, and intranasal dosage forms as indicated in the dosage table. All except butorphanol are also available in combination with the opioid antagonist naloxone to enhance their opioid antagonistic effects, which are usually weaker than the agonistic effects of these drugs.

OPIOID ANTAGONISTS

Opioid antagonists produce their antagonistic activity by competing with opioids for CNS receptor sites.

◆ naloxone hydrochloride

Naloxone hydrochloride (Narcan) is a pure opioid antagonist because it possesses no agonistic morphine-like properties and works as a blocking drug for the opioid drugs. Accordingly, the drug does not produce analgesia or respiratory depression. Naloxone is the drug of choice for the complete or partial reversal of opioid-induced respiratory depression. It is also indicated in cases of suspected acute opioid overdose. Failure of the drug to significantly reverse the effects of the presumed opioid overdose indicates that the condition may not be related to opioid overdose. The primary adverse effect is opioid withdrawal syndrome, which can occur with abrupt overreversal in opioid-tolerant patients. Naloxone is available only in injectable dosage forms. Use of the drug is contraindicated in patients with a history of hypersensitivity to it. For dosage information, see the table on p. 162.

PHARMACOKINETICS

Route	Onset of Action	Peak Plasma Concentration	Elimination Half-life	Duration of Action
IV	Less than 2 min	Rapid	64 min	0.5-2 hr

naltrexone hydrochloride

Naltrexone hydrochloride (ReVia) is an opioid antagonist used as an adjunct for the maintenance of an opioid-free state in former opioid addicts. The FDA has identified it as a safe and effective adjunct to psychosocial treatments of alcoholism. It is also indicated for reversal of postoperative opioid-induced respiratory depression. Nausea and tachycardia are the most common adverse effects and are related to reversal of the opioid effect. Use of naltrexone hydrochloride is contraindicated in cases of known drug allergy and in patients with hepatitis or other severe liver dysfunction. It is available only for oral use. For dosage information, see the table on p. 162.

PHARMACOKINETICS

Route	Onset of Action	Peak Plasma Concentration	Elimination Half-life	Duration of Action
PO	Rapid	1 hr	4-13 hr	24-72 hr

NONOPIOID AND MISCELLANEOUS ANALGESICS

The most widely used nonopioid analgesic is acetaminophen. All drugs in the NSAID class, which includes aspirin, and the cyclooxygenase-2 (COX-2) inhibitors (e.g., Celebrex) are also nonopioid analgesics, and these drugs are discussed in greater detail in Chapter 44. These medications are commonly used for management of pain, especially pain associated with inflammatory conditions such as arthritis, because they have significant antiinflam-

matory effects in addition to their analgesic effects. Miscellaneous analgesics include tramadol and transdermal lidocaine. They are discussed in depth in their respective drug profiles.

Mechanism of Action and Drug Effects

The mechanism of action of acetaminophen is similar to that of the salicylates. It blocks peripheral pain impulses by inhibition of prostaglandin synthesis. Acetaminophen also lowers febrile body temperatures by acting on the hypothalamus, the structure in the brain that regulates body temperature. Heat is dissipated through resulting vasodilation and increased peripheral blood flow. In contrast to NSAIDs, acetaminophen lacks antiinflammatory effects. Although acetaminophen shares the analgesic and antipyretic effects of the salicylates and other NSAIDs, it does not have many of the unwanted effects of these drugs. For example, acetaminophen products are not usually associated with cardiovascular effects (e.g., edema) or platelet effects (e.g., bleeding) as do aspirin and other NSAIDs. They also do not cause the aspirin-related GI tract irritation or bleeding nor any of the aspirin-related acid-base changes.

Indications

Acetaminophen is indicated for the treatment of mild to moderate pain and fever. It is an appropriate substitute for aspirin because of its analgesic and antipyretic properties. Acetaminophen is a valuable alternative for those patients who cannot tolerate aspirin or for whom aspirin may be contraindicated.

Acetaminophen is also the antipyretic (antifever) drug of choice in children and adolescents with flu syndromes, because the use of aspirin in such populations is associated with a condition known as *Reye's syndrome.*

Contraindications

Contraindications to acetaminophen use include known drug allergy, severe liver disease, and the genetic disease known as *glucose-6-phosphate dehydrogenase deficiency.*

Adverse Effects

Acetaminophen is generally well tolerated and is therefore available over the counter (OTC) and in many combination prescription drugs. Possible adverse effects include rash, nausea, and vomiting. Much less common but more severe are the adverse effects of blood disorders or dyscrasias (e.g., anemias) and nephrotoxicities, and, of most concern, hepatotoxicity.

Toxicity and Management of Overdose

Many people do not realize that acetaminophen, despite its OTC status, is a potentially lethal drug when taken in overdose. Depressed patients (especially adolescents) may intentionally overdose on the drug as an attention-seeking gesture without realizing the grave danger involved.

The ingestion of large amounts of acetaminophen, as in acute overdose, or even chronic unintentional misuse can cause hepatic necrosis. Acute ingestion of acetaminophen doses of 150 mg/kg or more may result in hepatic toxicity. Acute hepatotoxicity can usually be reversed with acetylcysteine, where as long-term toxicity is more likely to be permanent.

The standard maximum daily dose of acetaminophen for healthy adults is 4000 mg. However, limitation to 2000 mg or less may be necessary for patients with risk factors such as advanced age (elderly) or liver dysfunction. Excessive dosing may also occur inadvertently with the use of combination drug products such as tablets that include a fixed ratio of an opioid drug plus acetaminophen (e.g., hydrocodone plus acetaminophen). Prescribers should be mindful of recommended daily dose limits when prescribing these medications.

The long-term ingestion of large doses of acetaminophen is more likely to result in severe hepatotoxicity, which may be irreversible. Because the reported or estimated quantity of drug ingested is often inaccurate and not a reliable guide to the therapeutic management of the overdose, serum acetaminophen concentration should be determined for this purpose no sooner than 4 hours after the ingestion. If a serum acetaminophen level cannot be determined, it should be assumed that the overdose is potentially toxic and treatment with acetylcysteine, the recommended antidote for acetaminophen toxicity, should be started. Acetylcysteine works by preventing the hepatotoxic metabolites of acetaminophen from forming. It is most effective when given within 10 hours of an overdose. Historically, the usual dosage regimen is a 140 mg/kg oral loading dose, followed by 70 mg/kg every 4 hours for 17 additional doses. This drug is notoriously bad tasting with an odor of rotten eggs, and vomiting of an oral dose is common. It is recommended that the dose be repeated if vomiting occurs within 1 hour of dosing. An intravenous dosage formulation of acetylcysteine (Acetadote) is also available. This is given in three intravenous doses of 150 mg/kg, 50 mg/kg, and 100 mg/kg over a 21-hour period.

Interactions

A variety of substances can interact with acetaminophen. Alcohol is potentially the most dangerous. Chronic heavy alcohol abusers may be at increased risk of liver toxicity from excessive acetaminophen use. For this reason, a maximum daily dose of 2000 mg is generally recommended for these persons. Health care professionals should alert patients with regular intake of moderate to large amounts of alcohol not to exceed recommended dosages of acetaminophen because of the risk of liver dysfunction and possible liver failure. Ideally, alcohol consumption should not exceed three drinks daily. Other hepatotoxic drugs should also be avoided. Other drugs that potentially can interact with acetaminophen include phenytoin, barbiturates, warfarin, isoniazid, rifampin, beta-blockers, and anticholinergic drugs, all of which are discussed in greater detail in later chapters.

DRUG PROFILES

◆ acetaminophen
Acetaminophen (Tylenol) is an effective and relatively safe nonopioid analgesic used for mild to moderate pain relief. It is contraindicated in patients with a hypersensitivity to it or intolerance to tartrazine (yellow dye no. 5), alcohol, sugar, or saccharin. Its use should be avoided in patients who are anemic or who have renal or hepatic disease. Acetaminophen is available in oral and rectal dosage forms. Repetitive acetaminophen dosing can also inhibit warfarin metabolism. Acetaminophen is also a component of several prescription combination drug products, including hydrocodone/acetaminophen (Vicodin) and oxycodone/acetaminophen (Percocet). Acetaminophen liquid is available in two different concentrations: infant drops contain 80 mg/0.8 mL, whereas ace-

taminophen liquid contains 160 mg/5 mL. It is very important for the nurse to specify which product is to be used. It is also important to discuss the amount needed in milligrams, not milliliters. For example, if a child is to receive 160 mg and the parent is told to give 5 mL, then if the parent uses the infant drops, that 5 mL would contain 500 mg versus 160 mg for the liquid. This difference could provide a fatal dose.

PHARMACOKINETICS

Route	Onset of Action	Peak Plasma Concentration	Elimination Half-life	Duration of Action
PO	10-30 min	0.5-2 hr	1-4 hr	3-4 hr

tramadol hydrochloride
Tramadol hydrochloride (Ultram) is categorized as a miscellaneous analgesic due to its unique properties. It is a centrally acting analgesic with a dual mechanism of action. It creates a weak bond to the mu opioid receptors and inhibits the reuptake of both norepinephrine and serotonin. Although it does have weak opioid receptor activity, tramadol is not currently classified as a controlled substance. Tramadol is indicated for the treatment of moderate to moderately severe pain. Tramadol is rapidly absorbed, and its absorption is unaffected by food. It is metabolized in the liver to an active metabolite and eliminated via renal excretion. Adverse effects are similar to those of opioids and include drowsiness, dizziness, headache, nausea, constipation, and respiratory depression. Seizures have been reported in patients taking tramadol and occur in patients taking both normal and excessive dosages. Patients who may be at risk are those receiving tricyclic antidepressants, selective serotonin reuptake inhibitor antidepressants (SSRIs), monoamine oxidase inhibitors, neuroleptics, or other drugs that reduce the seizure threshold. There is also an increased risk of developing serotonin syndrome when tramadol is taken concurrently with SSRIs (see Chapter 17).

Use of the drug is contraindicated in cases of known drug allergy, which may include allergy to opioids due to potential cross-reactivity. It is also contraindicated in cases of acute intoxication with alcohol, hypnotics, centrally acting analgesics, opioids, or psychotropic drugs. The drug is only available in oral dosage forms, including a newer combination with acetaminophen (Ultracet).

PHARMACOKINETICS

Route	Onset of Action	Peak Plasma Concentration	Elimination Half-life	Duration of Action
PO	30 min	2 hr	5-8 hr	6 hr

lidocaine, transdermal
Transdermal lidocaine is a topical anesthetic (see Chapter 12) and cardiac antidysrhythmic (see Chapter 23) that is formulated into a patch (Lidoderm), which is placed onto painful areas of the skin. It is indicated for the treatment of postherpetic neuralgia, a painful skin condition that remains after a skin outbreak of shingles. Shingles is caused by the herpes zoster virus, also known as the varicella-zoster virus, which causes chickenpox in children. Lidocaine patches provide local pain relief, and up to three patches may be placed on a large painful area. However, the patches should not be worn for longer than 12 hours a day to avoid potential systemic drug toxicity (e.g., cardiac dysrhythmias). Because they act topically, there are minimal systemic adverse effects. However, the skin at the site of treatment may develop redness or edema, and unusual skin sensations may occur. These reactions are usually mild and transient and resolve within a few minutes to hours. Patches should be applied only to intact skin with no blisters. They can be used either alone or as part of adjunctive treat-

ment with systemic therapies such as antidepressants (see Chapter 17), opioids, or anticonvulsants (see Chapter 15). Used patches should be disposed of securely because they may be dangerous to children or pets. Specific pharmacokinetic data are not listed due to the continuous nature of dosing. However, studies have demonstrated that a patch can provide varying degrees of pain relief for 4 to 12 hours.

ziconotide

The newly approved drug ziconotide (Prialt) is the first drug to be classified as an intrathecal analgesic. Intrathecal drugs are injected through the theca vertebralis membrane of the spinal cord into the subarachnoid space. Like epidural injections, intrathecal injections are normally physician administered. Ziconotide is a synthetic equivalent of a polypeptide protein found in certain sea snails. Its mechanism of action in humans is not yet fully defined. However, animal studies suggest that the drug works by binding to N-type calcium channels on nociceptive (pain) A and C nerve fibers in the spinal cord. This drug is indicated for severe, chronic pain that is refractory to other treatments. Because it is not an opiate, ziconotide does not cause opiate withdrawal symptoms and may be discontinued abruptly if needed. Adverse effects include severe psychotic symptoms and neurologic impairment, including reduced cognitive functioning, changes in mood and level of consciousness, and hallucinations. Drug interactions include increased sedation when taken with any other drug having sedative properties. The drug is contraindicated in cases of known drug allergy and in patients with preexisting psychoses, infection at the injection site, any uncontrolled bleeding, and any condition involving impairment of normal cerebral spinal fluid flow.

NURSING PROCESS

Pain may be acute or chronic and occurs in patients in all settings and across the life span, thus leading to much suffering. Patients experiencing pain pose many challenges to the nurse, prescribers, and other health care providers involved in their care. The challenge for the nurse is that pain is a complex and multifaceted problem that requires astute assessment skills with appropriate interventions based on the individual, the specific type of pain, and related diseases and/or health status.

Medical, health care, and nursing organizations and governing bodies have been involved in defining standards and outcomes of care related to assessment and management of pain. For example, the Joint Commission (see *http://www.joint commission.org*) and the Agency for Healthcare Research and Quality (see *http://www. ahrq.gov/whatsnew.asp#qt*) have developed such standards. In addition, the World Health Organization (see *http://www.who.int/en*) has developed standards related specifically to cancer pain. Professional nursing organizations, including the Oncology Nursing Society and the American Nurses Association, have also created standards of care related to pain assessment and management. Another organization, the American Pain Society, has published new opioid guidelines available at *http://www.jpain.org/article/PIIS1526590008008316/fulltext*.

Assessment

Adequate analgesia requires a holistic, comprehensive, and individualized patient assessment with specific attention to the type, intensity, and characteristics of the pain. Levels of comfort should also be assessed, with comfort defined as the extent of physical and psychologic ease that an individual experiences. A thorough health history, nursing assessment, and medication history should be obtained as soon as possible or upon the first encounter with the patient and should include questions about the following: (1) any allergies to nonopioids, opioids, partial or mixed agonists, and/or opioid antagonists (see previous pharmacologic discussion for examples of specific drugs); (2) any potential drug-drug and/or drug-food interactions; (3) presence of diseases or CNS depression; (4) any history of the use of alcohol, street drugs, or any illegal drug or substance and/or a history of substance abuse, with information about the substance, dose, and frequency of use; (5) the results of any laboratory tests ordered, such as levels of serum ALT, ALP, GGT, 5′-nucleotidase, and bilirubin (indicative of liver function), and/or levels of BUN and creatinine (reflective of renal function); abnormal liver or renal function may require that lower doses of the analgesic be used to prevent toxicity or overdosage; (6) the character and intensity of the pain, including onset, location, quality (stabbing/knifelike, throbbing, dull ache, sharp, diffuse, localized, or referred); actual rating of the pain using a pain assessment scale (see later); and any precipitating, aggravating, and/or relieving factors; (7) duration of the pain (acute vs. chronic); and (8) types of pharmacologic, nonpharmacologic, and/or adjunctive measures that have been implemented, with further explanation of the treatment's duration of use and overall effectiveness.

The assessment should also look at factors or variables that may impact an individual's pain experience, including physical factors (e.g., age, gender, pain threshold, overall state of health, disease processes or pathologies) as well as emotional, spiritual, and cultural variables (e.g., reaction to pain, pain tolerance, fear, anxiety, stressors, sleep patterns, societal influences, family roles, phase of growth and development, and religious, racial, and/or ethnic beliefs or practices). Age-appropriate assessment tools should be used to assess pain across the life span (see later discussion). For pediatric and elderly patients, nonverbal behavior or cues and information from family members or caregivers may be helpful in identifying pain levels. In an elderly individual, physical and cognitive impairments may affect reporting of pain; however, this does not mean that the elderly patient is not experiencing pain—the patient's reporting may just be altered. Chronic pain and pain associated with cancer are both complex and multifactorial problems requiring a holistic approach with attention to other patient complaints, such as a decrease in activities of daily living, insomnia, depression, social withdrawal, anxiety, personality changes, and quality of life issues.

A system-focused nursing assessment should also be carried out, with further collection of both subjective and objective data relating to the patient's neurologic status (e.g., level of orientation and alertness, level of sedation, sensory and motor abilities, reflexes), respiratory status (e.g., respiratory rate, rhythm, and depth; breath sounds), GI status (e.g., presence of bowel sounds; bowel patterns; complaints of constipation, diarrhea, nausea, vomiting, or abdominal discomfort), genitourinary status (e.g., urinary output; any burning or discomfort on urination; urinary retention), and cardiac status (e.g., pulse rate and rhythm, blood pressure, any problems with dizziness or syncope). Vital signs should be assessed and documented, including blood pressure,

---

LIFE SPAN CONSIDERATIONS: The Pediatric Patient

Opioid Use

- Assessment of the pediatric patient is challenging, and all types of behavior that may indicate pain, such as muscular rigidity, restlessness, screaming, fear of moving, and withdrawn behavior, must be carefully considered.
- Adequacy of pain management is more difficult to determine in children because of their inability to express themselves. Frequently the reason older pediatric patients do not verbalize their pain is their fear of treatment, such as injections. Compassionate and therapeutic communication skills, as well as the use of alternate routes of administration, as ordered, will help in these situations.
- The "ouch scale" is often used to determine the level of pain in children. This scale is used to obtain the child's rating of the intensity of pain from 0 to 5 by means of simple face diagrams, from a very happy face for level 0 (no pain) to a sad, tearful face for level 5 (severe pain). Assessment of pain is very important in pediatric patients because they are often undermedicated. The nurse should always thoroughly assess the pediatric patient and not underestimate the child's complaints and nonverbal behavior. Parents and caregivers play an important role in this assessment.
- The patient's baseline age, weight, and height are important to document, because drug calculations are often based on these variables. With the pediatric patient, *all* mathematical calculations should be checked and double-checked for accuracy to avoid excessive dosages; this is especially true for opioids.
- Analgesics should always be given before pain becomes severe, and oral dosage forms should be used first, if appropriate.
- If suppositories are used, the nurse must be careful to administer the exact dose and not to split, halve, or divide an adult dose into a child's dose. This may result in the administration of an unknown amount of medication and possible overdose.

- When subcutaneous, intramuscular, and intravenous medications are used, the principle of atraumatic care in the delivery of nursing care must be followed. One technique used to help ensure atraumatic care is the application of a mixture of local anesthetics or other prescribed substances to the injection site before the injection is given. EMLA (lidocaine/prilocaine) is a topical cream that anesthetizes the site of the injection; if ordered, it should be applied 1 to 2½ hours before the injection. Institutional policies and procedures should be consulted for further instructions regarding its use.
- Distraction and creative imagery may be used for older children such as toddlers or preschool-aged children.
- Pediatric patients should always be monitored very closely for any unusual behavior while receiving opioids.
- The following signs and symptoms of central nervous system changes should be reported to the prescriber immediately if they occur: dizziness, lightheadedness, drowsiness, hallucinations, changes in the level of consciousness, and sluggish pupil reaction. No further medication should be given until the nurse receives further orders from the prescriber.
- The nurse should always monitor and document vital signs before, during, and after the administration of opioid analgesics. Medication is usually withheld if respiration rate is less than 12 breaths/min or if there are any changes in the level of consciousness. Protocol should always be followed.
- Generally speaking, smaller doses of opioids, with very close and frequent monitoring, are indicated for the pediatric patient. Giving oral medications with meals or snacks may help to decrease gastrointestinal upset.

---

pulse rate, respirations, temperature, and level of pain (now considered as the fifth vital sign). It is important to pull from one's knowledge base and remember that during the acute pain response, stimulation of the sympathetic nervous system may result in elevated values for vital signs, with an increase in blood pressure (120/80 mm Hg or higher), pulse rate (100 beats/min or higher), and respiratory rate and depth (20 breaths/min or higher and shallow breathing).

A variety of pain assessment tools are available that may be used to gather information about the fifth vital sign. One very basic assessment tool is the Numeric Pain Intensity Scale (0 to 10 pain rating scale); patients are asked to rate their pain intensity by picking the number that most closely represents their level of pain. The Verbal Rating Scale, another pain assessment tool, uses verbal descriptors for pain, including words such as *mild, moderate, severe, aching, agonizing,* or *discomfort.* The FACES Pain Rating Scale is helpful in assessing pain in patients of all ages and educational levels because it relies on a series of faces ranging from happy to sad to sad with tears. The patient is asked to identify the face that best represents the pain he or she is experiencing at that moment. When the patient is in acute pain, when pain intensity is a primary focus for assessment, and/or when the need is to determine the efficacy of pain management intervention, the simple, one-dimensional scales (e.g., the Numeric Pain Intensity Scale) work best. The elderly, especially those with cognitive impairment, may need more time to respond to the assessment tool and may also require large-print versions of written tools. There are other assessment

tools that are multidimensional scales and are more beneficial in assessing patients who experience chronic rather than acute pain. One example is the Brief Pain Inventory assessment tool, which includes a body map so that the patient can identify on the figure the exact area where pain is felt. This tool also helps in obtaining information about the impact of pain on functioning. Pain should be assessed prior to, during, and after the pain intervention, as should pain level during activity and at rest. The following sections provide assessment information for specific drug classes.

Nonopioids

For patients receiving *nonopioid analgesics,* assessment should focus not only on general data as described earlier but also on the specific drug being given. For example, for patients taking acetaminophen, assessment should include determination of whether the patient has allergies, is pregnant, or is breast-feeding. There are no age-related precautions regarding acetaminophen use for children or the elderly; however, assessment should address contraindications, cautions, and drug interactions (see previous discussion). Once therapy has been initiated, there should be close monitoring for symptoms of chronic acetaminophen poisoning, as manifested by rapid, weak pulse, dyspnea, and cold and clammy extremities. Long-term daily use of acetaminophen may lead to increased risk of permanent liver damage, and thus the results of liver function studies should be monitored. Adults who ingest higher than recommended dosages may be at higher risk of liver dysfunction as well as other adverse effects such as loss of appe-

EVIDENCE-BASED PRACTICE

Strategies of Pain Assessment Used by Nurses on Surgical Units

■ Review
The purpose of this study was to identify various criteria that nurses use in the assessment of patients who are experiencing postoperative pain. In addition, the study looked at the kind of knowledge the nurses applied from their previous experiences in assessing these patients for pain.

■ Type of Evidence
Phenomenography, a qualitative research method, was used to analyze the data collected during interviews with 10 nurses as they performed pain assessments for 30 postsurgical patients. The study was carried out at a large urban New England hospital. It was anticipated that the number of years of nursing experience might be important in differentiating the types of criteria nurses used to assess pain. All patients had undergone surgery within the previous 24 hours and were experiencing pain. Patients were not using patient-controlled analgesia pump delivery systems and were not diagnosed with cancer. Patients did not have an altered level of consciousness. A series of five highly interactive, semistructured, audiotaped interviews were conducted with each nurse. Interviews focused on the nurse's perception of the patient's situation with consideration of how and on what basis the nurse judged the patient's pain.

■ Results of Study
Data from 30 clinical pain assessments performed by the 10 nurses identified multiple criteria used in each nurse's assessment of a patient. These same criteria were used as the framework from which the nurses developed and implemented variations in the assessment of pain. Nurses were found to draw on their past experiences in several ways

when working with patients: they learned how to focus on listening to patients, what to look for, and what to do for patients in pain. Both objective and subjective criteria were used by the nurses to assess pain. Objective criteria focused on the patient's appearance, whereas subjective criteria related more to what the patient said. This study was one of the first to empirically identify the criteria nurses use and the types of past knowledge they draw on when assessing patients for pain on a postoperative unit. Because it was a qualitative, descriptive study, the sample size was small; therefore, the strategies identified were by no means exhaustive or representative. Nevertheless, this study gave rise to true evidence-based practice, because the findings of this study prompted changes in pain assessment guidelines in this New England hospital, including adoption of a more subjective orientation and emphasis on the patient's self-report as one of the single most reliable indicators of the presence and intensity of pain.

■ Link of Evidence to Nursing Practice
The results of this study led to major policy changes regarding the criteria used in assessing patients' pain in a postoperative unit. However, questions that remain to be answered include the following: Does the strategy used for assessment influence the nurse's perception of the intensity of pain and the need for pain management? Does the assessment strategy used have an influence on pain management decisions? Quantification of the use of different pain assessment strategies in a large sample of nurses will allow the findings of this particular study to be extended to identify the strategies actually used in contemporary nursing practice and the resulting pain management techniques implemented by nurses.

Data from Kim HS et al: Strategies of pain assessment used by nurses on surgical units, *Pain Manag Nurs* 6(1):3-9, 2005.

---

tite, jaundice, nausea, and vomiting. Children are also at high risk of liver dysfunction if the recommended dosage ranges are exceeded. Use of the NSAIDs—such as ibuprofen, aspirin, and COX-2 inhibitors—requires assessment of renal and liver functioning as well as the gathering of information about GI disorders such as ulcers (see Chapter 44 for more information). With aspirin, age is important; this drug is not to be given to children and adolescent patients because of the risk of Reye's syndrome. Aspirin may also lead to bleeding and ulcers, so ruling out conditions that represent contraindications and cautions to its use before therapy begins is important to patient safety. With tramadol hydrochloride, assessment of age is again very important, because this drug should not be used by individuals 75 years of age or older.

A few miscellaneous nonopioid analgesics, including lidocaine transdermal and ziconotide, are newer options for managing different types of pain. For lidocaine transdermal patches, assessment should include information about the possible indications for this drug, for example, postherpetic neuralgia. When these patches are used, they must be kept away from children, and they should not be prescribed for very young, small, or debilitated patients, because such patients would be at higher risk for toxicity. Liver function should also be assessed. Ziconotide, given intrathecally, requires assessment for contraindications such as allergy to the drug, abnormal bleeding, infection at the site, and any problem involving the spinal fluid. See previous discussion for more information on contraindications, cautions, and drug interactions. Measurement of vital signs is also required.

▌ Opioids

When *opioid analgesics,* or any other CNS depressants, are prescribed, assessment should focus on vital signs; allergies; respiratory disorders; respiratory function (rate, rhythm, depth, and breath sounds); presence of head injury (which will mask signs and symptoms of increasing intracranial pressure); neurologic status, with attention to level of consciousness or alertness and the level of sedation; sensory and motor functioning; GI tract functioning (bowel sounds and bowel patterns); and genitourinary functioning (intake and output). In addition, opioids, except morphine, may cause spasms of the sphincter of Oddi in the gallbladder and are not recommended for those with biliary disease because they may lead to pain. If renal and liver function studies are ordered, results should be monitored, because the risk of toxicity increases with diminished function of these organs. An additional concern is any past or present history of neurologic disorders such as Alzheimer's disease, dementia, multiple sclerosis, muscular dystrophy, myasthenia gravis, or cerebrovascular accident or stroke, because the use of opioids may alter symptoms of the disease process, possibly masking symptoms or worsening the clinical presentation when no actual pathologic changes have occurred. In these situations, use of another analgesic or pain protocol may be indicated. Attention to age is also important, because both elderly and very young patients are more sensitive to opioids—as to many other medications. In fact, old or young age may be a contraindication to opioid use, depending on the specific drug. See the earlier pharmacology discussion regarding cautions, contraindications, and drug interactions.

Opioid Agonists-Antagonists

In patients taking *opioid agonists-antagonists,* such as buprenorphine hydrochloride, it is important to assess vital signs with attention to respiratory rate and breath sounds. The opioid agonists-antagonists still possess opioid agonist effects, and therefore the assessment information related to opioids is applicable to these drugs as well. It is also very important to remember during assessment that these drugs are still effective analgesics and still have CNS depressant effects but are subject to a ceiling effect (see earlier definition). Given the action of these drugs, the assessment should determine whether the patient is an abuser of opioids, because administering these agonists-antagonists with another opioid will lead to reversal of analgesia and possible opioid withdrawal. Age is another factor to assess, because these drugs are not recommended for use in patients 18 years or younger. See previous discussion for a listing of contraindications, cautions, and drug interactions.

Opioid Antagonists

The nurse must remember that the *opioid antagonists* are used mainly in reversing respiratory depression secondary to opioid overdosage. Naloxone may be used in patients of all ages, including neonates and children. Vital signs should be assessed and documented before, during, and after the use of the antagonist so that the therapeutic effects can be further assessed and documented and the need for further doses determined. In addition, the nurse must remember that the antagonist drug may not work with just one dosing and that repeated doses are generally needed to reverse the effects of the opioid. See the pharmacology section for information about contraindications, cautions, and drug interactions.

Nursing Diagnoses

- Acute pain related to specific disease processes or conditions and other pathologies leading to various levels and types of pain
- Chronic pain related to various disease processes, conditions, or syndromes causing pain
- Constipation related to the CNS depressant effects on the GI system
- Deficient knowledge related to lack of familiarity with opioids, their use, and their adverse effects
- Impaired gas exchange related to opioid-induced CNS effects and respiratory depression
- Risk for infection related to the adverse effect of urinary retention and subsequent urinary stasis from the use of opioids
- Risk for injury related to decreased sensorium or level of consciousness from use of either nonopioid or opioid analgesics
- Risk for injury related to possible overdosage and severe adverse reactions and/or drug interactions associated with the various classes of analgesics

Planning
Goals

- Patient states measures that will enhance the effectiveness of the analgesic regimen, such as taking medication as prescribed, using relaxation techniques, and practicing imagery.

- Patient identifies the rationale for use, therapeutic effects, and adverse effects associated with all types of analgesics.
- Patient states various measures to help minimize the occurrence of common adverse effects of nonopioids as well as opioids, such as forcing fluids (for constipation) and moving slowly and with assistance (to prevent injury).

Outcome Criteria

- Patient demonstrates increased comfort levels as seen by decreased use of analgesics, increased activity and performance of activities of daily living, decreased complaints of pain, and decreased levels of pain as rated on a scale of 1 to 10.
- Patient experiences minimal adverse effects and complications such as nausea, vomiting, and constipation associated with the use of analgesics, especially opioids.
- Patient uses nonpharmacologic measures such as relaxation therapy, distraction, and music therapy to help improve comfort and enhance any pharmacologic regimens.
- Patient manages adverse effects associated with analgesics, such as by using antiemetics, taking medication with meals, and implementing a bowel program.

Implementation

Once the cause of pain has been diagnosed or other assessment and data gathering have been completed, pain management should begin immediately and aggressively in conformity with the needs of each individual patient and each situation. Pain management is varied and multifaceted and should incorporate pharmacologic as well as nonpharmacologic approaches (see Box 11-1 and the Herbal Therapies and Dietary Supplements box). Pain management strategies should include consideration of the type of pain and pain rating as well as pain quality, duration, and precipitating factors, and interventions that help the pain. Some general principles of pain management are the following: (1) Individualize a plan of care based on the patient as a holistic and cultural being (see Cultural Implications box). (2) Manage mild pain with the use of nonopioid drugs such as acetaminophen, tramadol, and NSAIDs (see Chapter 44). (3) Manage moderate to severe pain with a stepped approach using opioids. Other analgesics or types of analgesics may be used in addition to other categories of medication (see pharmacology discussion). (4) Administer analgesics as ordered but before the pain gets out of control. (5) Always consider the use of nonpharmacologic comfort measures (see Box 11-1) such as homeopathic, folk, and herbal remedies; exercise; distraction; music or pet therapy; massage; and transcutaneous electrical stimulation. Although not always effective, these measures may prove beneficial for some patients. See Patient Teaching Tips for more information related to analgesics.

Nonopioids

Nonopioid analgesics should be given as ordered or as indicated for fever or pain. Acetaminophen should always be taken as prescribed and within the recommended dosage range over a 24-hour period because of the risk of liver damage and acute toxicity. If a patient is taking other OTC medications with acetaminophen, the patient should read the labels very carefully to identify the total amount of acetaminophen and any other drug-drug interactions. Patient education about the signs and symptoms of acetaminophen overdose should emphasize the follow-

HERBAL THERAPIES AND DIETARY SUPPLEMENTS

Feverfew *(Chrysanthemum parthenium)*

■ *Overview*

A member of the marigold family known for its antiinflammatory properties

■ *Common Uses*

Treatment of migraine headaches, menstrual cramps, inflammation, fever

■ *Adverse Effects*

Nausea, vomiting, constipation, diarrhea, altered taste sensations, muscle stiffness, joint pain

■ *Potential Drug Interactions*

Possible increase in bleeding with the use of aspirin and other nonsteroidal antiinflammatory drugs, dipyridamole, and warfarin

■ *Contraindications*

Contraindicated in those allergic to ragweed, chrysanthemums, and marigolds, as well as those about to undergo surgery

ing: bleeding, loss of energy, fever, sore throat, and easy bruising (due to hepatotoxicity). These should be reported immediately to the nurse and/or prescriber. The nurse should also instruct the patient to report a worsening of pain or changes in the nature of the pain.

Suppository dosage forms of acetaminophen—like suppository forms of other drugs—should be placed into a medicine cup of ice. Once the suppository is unwrapped, cold water should be run over it to moisten the suppository for easier insertion. The suppository is inserted into the rectum using a gloved finger and water-soluble lubricating gel, if necessary. Acetaminophen tablets may be crushed if needed. Adult patients who take more than 2.6 g in 24 hours are at risk for mild liver damage; those taking 10 g or more (e.g., deliberate overdoses) are at high risk for severe liver damage; and death is possible after ingestion of more than 15 g. Liver damage from acetaminophen may be minimized by timely dosing with acetylcysteine (see previous discussion). The patient should be warned about the foul taste and odor of acetylcysteine. Many patients say this drug smells and tastes like rotten eggs. Acetylcysteine is better tolerated if it is disguised by mixing with a drink such as cola or flavored water to increase its palatability. Use of a straw may help minimize contact with the mucous membranes of the mouth and is recommended. This antidote may be given through a nasogastric or orogastric tube, if necessary.

Tramadol may cause nausea and vomiting. Use of flat cola, ginger ale, or dry crackers may help to minimize this adverse effect. If dizziness, blurred vision, or drowsiness occur, the nurse should be sure to assist the patient with ambulation (as with the use of any analgesic that may lead to dizziness or lightheadedness) to minimize the risk of fall and injury. The patient should be educated about injury prevention, including the need to dangle the feet over the edge of the bed before full ambulation, change positions slowly, and use assistance. In addition, while the patient is taking tramadol—as well as any other analgesics, and especially opioids—the patient should avoid any tasks that require mental clarity and alertness. The patient should be encouraged to report any heart palpitations, seizures,

tremors, difficulty breathing, chest pain, and muscle weakness experienced while taking the medication.

▌ Opioids

When *opioids* (and other analgesics) are prescribed, the nurse should administer the drug as ordered after checking for the "Six Rights" of medication administration (see Chapter 1). After the prescriber's order has been double-checked, the medication profile and documentation should be examined to determine the last time the medication was given before another dose is administered. Patient's vital signs should be monitored at frequent intervals with special attention to respiratory changes. A respiratory rate of 10 breaths/min (some protocols still adhere to the parameter of 12 breaths/min) may indicate respiratory depression and should be reported to the prescriber. The drug dosage, frequency, and/or route may need to be changed or an antidote (opioid antagonist) given if respiratory depression occurs. Naloxone should always be available, especially with the use of intravenous and/or other parenteral dosage forms of opioids, such as PCA (see Chapter 10 and the discussion to follow), and/or epidural infusions. Naloxone is indicated to reverse CNS depression, specifically respiratory depression, but one must remember that this antidote also reverses analgesia. The patient's urinary output should also be monitored and should be at least 600 mL/24 hr. Bowel sounds should be monitored during therapy. Decreased peristalsis may indicate the need for a dietary change, such as increased fiber, or use of a stool softener or mild laxative (see Box 11-2). Pupil reactions should be assessed. Pinpoint pupils indicate an overdose.

Opioids or any analgesic should be given before the pain reaches its peak to help maximize the effectiveness of the opioid or other analgesic. Once the drug is administered, the nurse should return at the appropriate time (taking into consideration the times of onset and peak effect of the drug and the route) to assess the effectiveness of the drug and/or other interventions as well as observe for the presence of any adverse effects (see previous discussion of pain assessment tools). With regard to the route of administration, the recommendation is that oral dosage forms be used first, but only if ordered and if there is no nausea or vomiting. Taking the dose with food may help minimize GI upset. Should nausea or vomiting be problematic, an antiemetic may be ordered for administration before or with the dosing of medication. Crucial safety measures include keeping bed side rails up, turning bed alarms on (depending on the policies and procedures of the specific facility), and making sure the call bell is within the patient's reach. These measures will help to prevent falls or injury related to opioid use. Opioids and similar drugs lead to CNS depression with possible confusion, altered sensorium or alertness, hypotension, and altered motor functioning. Because of these drug effects, all patients are at risk for falls or injury, and the elderly are at higher risk (see the Life Span Considerations box on p. 172 and Box 11-2). Refer to Box 11-4 for more specific information concerning the handling of controlled substances and narcotics counts.

When managing pain with morphine and similar drugs, the nurse should withhold the dose and contact the prescriber if there is any decline in the patient's condition or if the vital signs are abnormal (see parameters mentioned earlier) and especially if the respiratory rate is less than 10 breaths/min. Intramuscular injections are rarely used because of the availability of other

---

LIFE SPAN CONSIDERATIONS: The Elderly Patient

Opioid Use

- The nurse should document the patient's weight and height before opioid therapy is begun. The patient should be monitored carefully for any changes in vital signs, level of consciousness, or respiratory rate, as well as any changes indicative of central nervous system depression, and any such changes should be documented.
- Many institutionalized or hospitalized elderly patients are very stoic about pain; elderly patients may also have altered presentations of common illnesses so that the pain experience manifests in a different way or may simply be unable to state how they feel in a clear manner. Each and every patient—regardless of age—has the right to a thorough pain assessment and adequate and appropriate pain management. It is a myth that aging increases one's pain threshold. The problem is that cognitive impairment and dementia are often major barriers to pain assessment. Nevertheless, many elderly patients are still reliable in their reporting of pain, even with moderate to severe cognitive impairment.
- Over time, the elderly may lose reliability in recalling and accurately reporting chronic pain. The elderly, especially those 75 years of age or older, are at higher risk for too much or too little pain management, and the nurse must remember that drugs have a higher peak and longer duration of action in these patients than in their younger counterparts.
- Smaller dosages of opioids are generally indicated for elderly patients because of their increased sensitivity to the central nervous system depressants and diminished renal and hepatic function. Paradoxical (opposite) reactions and/or unexpected reactions may also be more likely to occur in patients of this age group.
- In elderly male patients, benign prostatic hyperplasia or obstructive urinary diseases should be considered because of the urinary retention associated with the use of opioids. Urinary outflow can become further diminished in these patients and result in adverse reactions or complications. Dosage adjustments may need to be made by the prescriber.
- Polypharmacy is often a problem in older adults; therefore it is important for the nurse to have a complete list of all medications the patient is currently taking and to assess for drug interactions and treatment (drug) duplication.
- Frequent assessments of elderly patients are needed. The nurse should pay attention to level of consciousness, alertness, and cognitive ability while ensuring that the environment is safe by keeping a call bell or light at the bedside. Using bed alarms and/or raising side rails are indicated where appropriate.
- Decreased circulation causes variation in the absorption of intramuscular or intravenous dosage forms and often results in the slower absorption of parenteral forms of opioids.
- As stated by the American Geriatric Society on the Management of Pain, nonsteroidal antiinflammatory drugs should be used with caution because of their potential for renal and gastrointestinal toxicity. Acetaminophen is the drug of choice for relieving mild to moderate pain, but with cautious dosing because of hepatic and renal concerns. The oral route of administration is preferred for analgesia. The regimen should be as simple as possible to enhance compliance, and the nurse should be sure to note, report, and document any unusual reactions to the opioid drugs. Hypotension and respiratory depression may occur more frequently in elderly patients taking opioids; thus very careful vital sign monitoring is needed.

---

effective and convenient dosage forms, such as PCA pumps, transdermal patches, continuous subcutaneous infusions, and epidural infusions.

For transdermal patches (e.g., transdermal fentanyl), two systems are used. The oldest type of patch contains a reservoir system consisting of four layers beginning with the adhesive layer and ending with the protective backing. Between these two layers are the permeable rate-controlling membrane and the reservoir layer, which holds the drug in a gel or liquid form. The newer type of patch has a matrix system consisting of two layers: one layer containing the active drug with the releasing and adhesive mechanisms, and the protective impermeable backing layer. The advantages of the matrix system over the reservoir system are that the patch is slimmer and smaller, it is more comfortable, it is worn for up to 7 days (the older reservoir system patch is worn for up to 3 to 4 days), and it appears to result in more constant serum drug levels. In addition, the matrix system is alcohol free; the alcohol in the reservoir system often irritates the patient's skin. It is important for the nurse to know what type of delivery system is being used so that proper guidelines are followed to enhance the system's and drug's effectiveness.

Transdermal patches should be applied to a clean, nonhairy area. When the patch is changed, as ordered, the new patch should be placed on a new site, but only after the old patch has been removed and the old site cleansed of any residual medication. Rotation of sites helps to decrease irritation and enhance drug effects. Transdermal systems are beneficial for the delivery of many types of medications, especially analgesics, and have the benefits of allowing multiday therapy with a single application, avoiding first-pass metabolism, improving patient compliance, and minimizing frequent dosing. However, the patient should be watched carefully for the development of any type of contact dermatitis caused by the patch (the prescriber should be contacted immediately if this occurs) and should maintain his or her own pain journal when at home. Journal entries are a valid source of information for the nurse, other health care professionals, the patient, and family members to assess the patient's pain control and to monitor the effectiveness not only of transdermal analgesia but also any medication regimen.

With the intravenous administration of *opioid agonists* the nurse should always follow the manufacturer's guidelines and institutional policies regarding specific dilutional amounts and solutions as well as the time period for infusion. When PCA is used, the amounts and times of dosing should be noted in the appropriate records and tracked by appropriate personnel. The fact that a pump is being used, however, does not mean that it is 100% reliable or safe. To be sure that all is functioning properly, the nurse should monitor pain levels, response to medication, and vital signs just as frequently as—if not more frequently than—with other parenteral opioid administration. The nurse should follow dosage ranges for all opioid agonists and agonists-antagonists and pay special attention to the dosages of morphine and morphine-like drugs. For intravenous infusions, the nurse is responsible for monitoring the intravenous needle site and infusion rates and documenting any adverse effects or complications. Another point for the nurse to remember when administering opioids—as well as any other anal-

BOX 11-4 Controlled Substance/Opioid Counts— A Must Do!

Any medication that has the potential for abuse or is a controlled substance—often opioids—is handled differently from other medications. Opioids are delivered to a nursing unit by the pharmacy, and these and other controlled substances (see Chapter 4) are kept in a locked cabinet or in an automated dispensing system (see Chapter 10). At the beginning of each shift, two registered nurses must count all of the opioids and/or other controlled substances located in the locked cabinet and record the count on a controlled substance and/or opioid administration record. When opioids and other controlled substances are dispensed through an automated medication-dispensing system, such counting is unnecessary because these systems automatically count and record the nurse's electronic signature as each dose is dispensed. Any discrepancies found in the count of opioids or other controlled substances are investigated by registered nurses. If any opioids are unaccounted for, the nurse manager or supervisor should be contacted immediately. The nurse should adhere to the following guidelines when giving opioids and other controlled substances: (1) Check the opioid administration record for the number left in stock. (2) Compare this number with the actual supply available. (3) If the count is accurate, obtain the desired dose of drug. (4) If the count is incorrect, notify the nurse manager or supervisor and follow any institutional policy. (5) Record the count of the remaining supply. Once the dose is removed, the nurse may be required to record the patient's name, prescriber's name, patient's medical record number, dose of medication ordered, and the nurse's signature. (6) Administer the drug according to policy and procedures. If the controlled substance cannot be given to the patient because of patient refusal, medication contamination, changes in vital signs or status, or some other reason, the medication should be "wasted." However, wasting of controlled substances usually requires the signature of another nurse who witnesses the discarding or wasting of the medication and documentation on the appropriate form. Automated systems record this information within the computer system.

gesics—is that each medication has a different onset of action, peak, and duration of action, with the intravenous route producing the most rapid onset (e.g., within minutes) (see Table 11-8).

To reverse an opioid overdose or opioid-induced respiratory depression, an *opioid antagonist,* such as naloxone, must be administered. Naloxone is given intravenously in diluted form and administered slowly (such as over 15 seconds, or as ordered; see Table 11-7). However, packaging and manufacturer guidelines should also be followed. Emergency resuscitative equipment should be available in the event of respiratory or cardiac arrest.

Opioid Agonists-Antagonists

The nurse must remember when giving *agonists-antagonists* that they react very differently depending on whether they are given by themselves or with other drugs. When administered alone, they are effective analgesics because they bind with opiate receptors and produce an agonist effect (see discussion in pharmacology section). If given at the same time as other opioids, however, they lead to reversal of analgesia and acute withdrawal because of the blocking of opiate receptors. The nurse must also be very careful to check dosages and routes as well as to perform the interventions mentioned for opioid agonist drugs, including close assessment of vital signs, especially respiratory rate. Patient education should emphasize the need to report any dizziness, constipation, difficulty with urination, blurred vision, hallucinations, dyspnea or other changes in breathing, and tachycardia. The

drug's ability to reverse analgesia and the occurrence of withdrawal should be emphasized as well, and the patient should be given a list of drugs that should be avoided (other agonists).

Opioid Antagonists

Opioid antagonists should be given as ordered and should be readily available, especially when the patient is receiving PCA with an opioid, is opioid naive, or is receiving continuous doses of opioids. Several doses of these drugs are often required to ensure adequate opioid agonist reversal (see earlier discussion). Patients should report any nausea, vomiting, or palpitations.

• • •

The nurse should remain current on information of all forms of analgesics as well as protocols for pain management with focus on the specific drug(s) as well as differences in the treatment of mild to moderate pain, severe pain, and pain in special situations (e.g., cancer pain). The World Health Organization's three-step analgesic ladder provides a standard for pain management in cancer patients and should be reviewed as needed.

Dosing of medications for pain management is very important to the treatment regimen. As noted earlier, once a thorough assessment has been performed, it is best to treat the patient's pain before it becomes severe, which is the rationale for considering pain to be the fifth vital sign. When pain is present for more than 12 hours a day, analgesic doses should be individualized and are best administered around the clock rather than on an as-needed basis, but dosing should always be within the dosage guidelines for each drug used. Around-the-clock (or scheduled) dosing maintains steady-state levels of the medication and prevents drug troughs and escalation of pain. No given dosage of an analgesic will provide the same level of pain relief for every patient, and so titration upward or even downward should be carried out individually and should be implemented as long as the analgesic is needed. Aggressive titration may be necessary in difficult pain control cases and in cancer pain situations. Patients with severe pain, metastatic pain, or bone metastasis pain may need increasingly higher dosages of analgesic, so an opiate such as morphine should be titrated until the desired response is achieved or until adverse effects occur. A patient-rated pain level of less than 4 on a scale of 1 to 10 is considered to indicate effective pain relief.

If pain is not managed adequately by monotherapy, other drugs or adjuvants may need to be added to enhance analgesic efficacy. This includes the use of NSAIDs (for analgesic, antiinflammatory effects), acetaminophen (for analgesic effects), corticosteroids (for mood elevation and antiinflammatory, antiemetic, and appetite stimulation effects), anticonvulsants (for treatment of neuropathic pain), tricyclic antidepressants (for treatment of neuropathic pain and for their innate analgesic properties and opioid-potentiating effects), neuroleptics (for treatment of chronic pain syndromes), local anesthetics (for treatment of neuropathic pain), hydroxyzine (for mild antianxiety properties as well as sedating effects and antihistamine and mild antiemetic actions), or psychostimulants (for reduction of opioid-induced sedation when opioid dosage adjustment is not effective). See Table 11-9 for a listing of drugs that should *not* be used in patients experiencing cancer pain.

Dosage forms are also important, especially with chronic pain and cancer pain. Oral administration is always preferred but is not always tolerated by the patient and may not even be a viable option for pain control. If oral dosing is not appropriate, less in-

TABLE 11-8 Opioid Administration Guidelines

Opioid	Nursing Administration
buprenorphine and butorphanol	When giving IV, infuse over the recommended time (usually 3-5 min). Always assess respirations before, during and after use. Give IM as ordered.
codeine	Give PO doses with food to minimize GI tract upset; ceiling effects occur with oral codeine resulting in no increase in analgesia with increased dosage.
fentanyl	Administer parenteral doses as ordered and as per manufacturer guidelines in regard to mg/min to prevent CNS depression and possible cardiac or respiratory arrest. Transdermal patches come in a variety of dosages. Fentanyl lollipops are also available. Be sure to remove residual amounts of the old patch prior to application of a new patch. Dispose of patches properly to avoid inadvertent contact with children or pets.
hydromorphone	May be given subcut, rectally, IV, PO, or IM.
levorphanol	May be given PO, subcut, or IV; give IV forms over 5 min or as indicated by manufacturer guidelines; longer acting, lasting up to 6-8 hr.
meperidine	Given by a variety of routes: IV, IM, or PO; highly protein bound, so watch for interactions and toxicity. Monitor elderly patients for increased sensitivity.
morphine	Available in a variety of forms: subcut, IM, PO, IV, extended and immediate release; morphine sulfate (Duramorph) for epidural infusion. Always monitor respiratory rate.
nalbuphine	IV doses of 10 mg given undiluted over 5 min.
naloxone	Antagonist given for opioid overdose; 0.4 mg usually given IV over 15 sec or less. Reverses analgesia as well.
propoxyphene	PO dosing only; drug associated with high abuse potential.
oxycodone	Often mixed with acetaminophen or aspirin; PO and suppository dosage forms. Now available in both immediate and sustained-release tabs.
oxymorphone	Available in PO, IM, IV, subcut, and rectal suppository dosage forms.
pentazocine	Subcut, IV, and IM forms; mixed agonist-antagonist; IV dose of 5 mg to be given over 1 min.

CNS, Central nervous system; *GI,* gastrointestinal; *IM,* intramuscular(ly); *IV,* intravenous(ly); *PO,* oral(ly); *subcut,* subcutaneous(ly).

TABLE 11-9 Drugs *Not* Recommended for Treatment of Cancer Pain

Class	Drug	Reason for Not Recommending
Opioids with dosing around the clock	meperidine	Short (2-3 hr) duration of analgesia; administration may lead to CNS toxicity (tremor, confusion, or seizures)
Miscellaneous	Cannabinoids	Adverse effects of dysphoria, drowsiness, hypotension, and bradycardia, which preclude their routine use as analgesics; may be indicated for use in treating severe chemotherapy-induced nausea and vomiting
Opioid agonists-antagonists	pentazocine butorphanol nalbuphine	May precipitate withdrawal in opioid-dependent patients; analgesic ceiling effect; possible production of unpleasant psychologic adverse effects, including dysphoria, delusions, and hallucinations
	buprenorphine	Analgesic ceiling effect; can precipitate withdrawal if given with an opioid
Opioid antagonists	naloxone naltrexone	Reverses analgesia as well as CNS depressant effects, such as respiratory depression
Combination preparations	Brompton cocktails	No evidence of analgesic benefit over use of single opioid analgesic
	DPT* (meperidine, promethazine, and chlorpromazine)	Efficacy poor compared with that of other analgesics; associated with a higher incidence of adverse effects
Anxiolytics (as monotherapy) or sedatives-hypnotics (as monotherapy)	Benzodiazepines (e.g., alprazolam)	Analgesic properties not associated with these drugs except in some situations of neuropathic pain; common risk of sedation, which may put some patients at higher risk for neurologic complications
	Barbiturates Benzodiazepines	Analgesic properties not demonstrated; sedation is problematic and limits use

CNS, Central nervous system.
*DPT is the abbreviation for the trade names Demerol, Phenergan, and Thorazine.

vasive routes of administration include rectal and transdermal routes. Rectal dosage forms are safe, inexpensive, effective, and helpful if the patient is experiencing nausea or vomiting or altered mental status; however, this route would not be suitable for those with diarrhea, stomatitis, and/or low blood cell counts. Transdermal patches may provide up to 7 days of pain control but are not for rapid dose titration and are used only when stable analgesia has been previously achieved. Long-acting forms of morphine and fentanyl may be delivered via transdermal patches when a longer duration of action is needed. Intermittent injections or continuous infusions via the intravenous or subcutaneous route are often used for opioid delivery and may be administered at home in **special pain situations,** such as in hospice care or management of chronic cancer pain. Subcutaneous infusions are often used when there is no intravenous access. PCA pumps may be used to help deliver opioids intravenously, subcutaneously, or even intraspinally and can be managed in home health care or hospice care for the patient at home. Use of the intrathecal or epidural route requires special skill and expertise, and delivery of pain medications using these routes is available only from certain home health care agencies for at-home care. The main reason for long-term intraspinal opioid administration is intractable pain. Transnasal dosage forms are approved only for butorphanol, an agonist-antagonist drug, and this dosage form is generally not used or recommended. Regardless of the specific drug or dosage form used, a fast-acting rescue drug should always be ordered for patients with cancer pain and patients presenting other special challenges in pain management.

Summary

Regardless of the drug(s) used for the pain management regimen, the nurse must always remember that individualization of treatment is one of the most important considerations for effective and quality pain control. The nurse should also do or consider the following:

- At the initiation of pain therapy, conduct a review of all relevant histories, laboratory test values, and diagnostic study results in the patient's medical record. If there are underlying problems, the nurse should be sure to consider them but should not forget to treat the patient. The nurse should not let these problems overshadow the fact that there is a patient who is in pain.
- Always develop goals for pain management in conjunction with the patient, family members, significant others, and/or caregiver. These goals should include improving the level of comfort with increased levels of activities of daily living and ambulation.
- Collaborate with other members of the health care team to select a regimen that will be easy for the patient to follow while in the hospital and, if necessary, at home (e.g., for cancer patients and other patients with chronic pain).
- Be aware that most regimens for acute pain management include treatment with short-acting opioids plus the addition of other medications such as NSAIDs.
- Be familiar with equianalgesic doses of opioids, because lack of knowledge may lead to inadequate analgesia or overdose.
- Use an analgesic appropriate for the situation (e.g., short-acting opioids for severe pain secondary to a myocardial infarction, surgery, or kidney stones). For cancer pain, the regimen usually begins with short-acting opioids with eventual conversion to sustained-release formulations.
- Use preventative measures to manage adverse effects. In addition, a switch is made to another opioid as soon as possible if the patient finds that the medication is not controlling the pain adequately.
- Consider the option of analgesic adjuvants, especially in cases of chronic pain or cancer pain; these might include other prescribed drugs such as corticosteroids, antidepressants, anticonvulsants, and muscle relaxants. OTC drugs and herbals may be helpful.
- Be alert to patients with special needs, such as patients with breakthrough pain. Generally, the drug used to manage such pain is a short-acting form of the longer-acting opioid being

given (e.g., immediate-release morphine for breakthrough pain while sustained-release morphine is also used).
- Identify community resources that can assist the patient, family members, and/or significant others. These resources may include various web-based sites such as *http://www.WebMD.com*, *http://www.pain.com*, and *http://www.mayohealth.org*. Many other pain management sites may be found on the Internet by searching using the term *pain* or *pain clinic*.
- Because fall prevention is of utmost importance in patient care (after the ABCs of care are addressed), monitor the patient frequently after an analgesic is given. Frequent measurement of vital signs, inclusion of the patient in a frequent watch program, and/or use of bed alarms are encouraged.
- Restraints may cause many injuries; therefore, if restraints are necessary, follow the appropriate procedures, including specific institutional policies and rules. Assess, monitor, evaluate, and document the reason for the restraint; also document the patient's behavior, the type of restraint used, and the assessment of the patient after the placement of restraints. Use of restraints has been largely replaced with a bed watch system

---

CASE STUDY

Opioid Administration

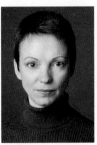
© Gpalmer

You are assigned to care for a patient who is in the terminal phases of breast cancer. As a home health care nurse, you have many responsibilities; however, you have not cared for many patients who are in the terminal phase of their illness. In fact, most of your patients are postoperative and have only required assessments, dressing changes, and wound care.

Ms. D. is 48 years of age and underwent bilateral mastectomy 4 years ago. She had lymph node involvement at the time of surgery, and recently metastasis to the bone has been diagnosed. She has been taking oxycodone (one 5-mg tab every 6 hours) at home but is not sleeping through the night and is now complaining of increasing pain to the point that her quality of life has decreased significantly. She wants to stay at home during the terminal phases of her illness but needs to have adequate and safe pain control. Her husband of 18 years is very supportive. They have no children. They are both college graduates and have medical insurance.

1. Ms. D.'s recent increase in pain has been attributed to bone metastasis in the area of the lumbar spine. At this time the oxycodone is not beneficial, and you as the home health care nurse need to advocate for Ms. D. to receive adequate pain relief. When discussing her pain medications with her physician, what type of medication would you expect to be ordered to relieve the bone pain, and what is the rationale for this medication? (Provide references from within this chapter to support the selection of the specific opioid drug.)
2. Ms. D.'s husband confides in you that he is worried that she will become addicted to the new medication. He is not sure he agrees with around-the-clock dosing. How do you address his concerns?
3. What should Mr. D. do if he feels that Ms. D. has had an overdose?

For answers, see *http://evolve.elsevier.com/Lilley*.

and the use of bed and/or wheelchair alarms. Instructions should be given to the patient, family members, and/or caregivers about the risk for falls and the need for safety measures. Restraints are not used in long-term care facilities.

Evaluation

Positive therapeutic outcomes of acetaminophen use are decreased symptoms, fever, and pain. Adverse reactions for which the nurse should monitor include anemias and the previously mentioned liver problems due to hepatotoxicity. In addition, abdominal pain and vomiting should be reported to the prescriber. During and after the administration of other *nonopioid analgesics* such as tramadol, *opioids,* and *mixed opioid agonists,* the nurse should monitor the patient for both therapeutic effects and adverse effects. Therapeutic effects include in-creased comfort levels as well as decreased complaints of pain and longer periods of comfort, with improvements in performance of activities of daily living, appetite, and sense of well-being. Adverse effects vary with each drug (see earlier discussions) but often consist of nausea, vomiting, constipation, dizziness, headache, blurred vision, decreased urinary output, drowsiness, lethargy, sedation, palpitations, bradycardia, bradypnea, dyspnea, and hypotension. Should vital signs change, the patient's condition decline, or pain continue, the prescriber should be contacted immediately and the patient closely monitored. Respiratory depression may be manifested by a respiratory rate of less than 10 breaths/min, dyspnea, diminished breath sounds, and/or shallow breathing. Evaluation should also include review of the effectiveness of multimodal and nonpharmacologic approaches to pain management.

PATIENT TEACHING TIPS

- Opioids should not be used with alcohol or with other CNS depressants, unless ordered, because of worsening of the depressant effects.
- A holistic approach to pain management may be appropriate, with the use of complementary modalities, including the following: biofeedback, imagery, relaxation, deep breathing, humor, pet therapy, music therapy, massage, use of hot or cold compresses, and use of herbal products.
- Dizziness, difficulty breathing, low blood pressure, excessive sleepiness (sedation), confusion, or loss of memory should be reported to the nurse, prescriber, or other health care providers.
- Opioids may result in constipation so forcing fluids (up to 3 L/day unless contraindicated), increasing fiber/bulk consumption, and exercising as tolerated is recommended. Stool softeners may also be necessary.
- Any nausea or vomiting should be reported. Antiemetic drugs may be prescribed.
- Any activities requiring mental clarity or alertness may need to be avoided if experiencing drowsiness or sedation. Ambulate with caution and/or assistance as needed.
- It is important for the patient to share any history of addiction with health care providers, but when such a patient experiences pain and is in need of opioid analgesia, the nurse must understand that the patient has a right to comfort. Any further issues with addiction may be managed during and after the use of opioids. Keeping an open mind regarding the use of resources, counseling, and other treatment options is important in dealing with addictive behaviors.
- If pain is problematic and not managed by monotherapy, then a combination of a variety of medications may be needed. Other drugs that may be used include antianxiety drugs, sedatives, hypnotics, or anticonvulsants.
- For the cancer patient or patient with special needs, the prescriber will monitor pain control and the need for other options for therapy or for dosing of drugs. For example, the use of transdermal patches, buccal tablets, and continuous infusions while the patient remains mobile or at home is often helpful in pain management. It is also important to understand that if morphine or morphine-like drugs are being used, the potential for addiction exists; however, in specific situations, the concern for quality of life and pain management is more important than the concern for addiction.
- Most hospitals have inpatient and outpatient resources such as pain clinics. The patient should seek out these options and remain active in his or her care for as long as possible.
- Tolerance does occur with opioid use, so if the level of pain increases while the patient remains on the prescribed dosage, the patient should contact the prescriber or other health care provider for assistance. The patient should never change dosages of or double-up on medication of any type unless prescribed.

POINTS TO REMEMBER

- Pain is individual and involves sensations and emotions that are unpleasant. It is influenced by age, culture, race, spirituality, and all other aspects of the person.
- Pain is associated with actual or potential tissue damage and may be exacerbated or alleviated depending on the treatment and type of pain.
- Types of analgesics include the following:
  - Nonopioids, including acetaminophen, aspirin, and NSAIDs
  - Opioids, which are natural or synthetic drugs that either contain or are derived from morphine (opiates) or have opiate-like effects or activities (opioids), and opioid agonist-antagonist drugs
- Pediatric dosages of morphine should be calculated very cautiously with close attention to the dose and kilograms of body weight. Cautious titration of dosage upward is usually the standard.
- Elderly patients may react differently than expected to analgesics, especially opioids and opioid agonists-antagonists.
- In treating the elderly, the nurse should remember that these patients experience pain the same as does the general population, but they may be reluctant to report pain and may metabolize opiates at a slower rate and thus are at increased risk for adverse effects such as sedation and respiratory depression. The best rule is to start with low dosages, reevaluate often, and go slowly during upward titration.

NCLEX EXAMINATION REVIEW QUESTIONS

1 For best results when treating severe pain associated with pathologic spinal fractures related to metastatic bone cancer, the nurse should remember that the best type of dosage schedule is to administer the pain medication
a as needed.
b around the clock.
c on schedule during waking hours only.
d around the clock, with additional doses as needed for breakthrough pain.

2 A patient is receiving an opioid via a PCA pump as part of his postoperative pain management program. During rounds, the nurse finds him unresponsive, with respirations of 8 breaths/min and blood pressure of 102/58 mm Hg. After stopping the opioid infusion, what should the nurse do next?
a Notify the charge nurse
b Administer oxygen
c Administer an opiate antagonist per standing orders
d Perform a thorough assessment, including mental status examination

3 A patient with bone pain caused by metastatic cancer will be receiving transdermal fentanyl patches. The patient asks the nurse what benefits these patches have. The nurse's best response includes which of the following features?
a More analgesia for longer time periods
b Less constipation and minimal dry mouth

c Less drowsiness than with oral opioids
d Lower dependency potential and no major adverse effects

4 The nurse suspects that a patient is showing signs of respiratory depression. Which drug could be the cause of this complication?
a naloxone (Narcan)
b hydromorphone (Dilaudid)
c acetaminophen (Tylenol)
d ziconotide (Prialt)

5 Several patients have standard orders for acetaminophen as needed for pain. When the nurse reviews their histories and assessments, the nurse discovers that one of the patients has a contraindication to acetaminophen therapy. Which patient is the one who should receive an alternate medication?
a A patient who has a fever of 103.4° F (39.7° C)
b A patient admitted with a deep vein thrombosis
c A patient admitted with severe hepatitis
d A patient who had abdominal surgery 1 week earlier

6 The nurse is administering an intravenous dose of morphine sulfate to a 48-year-old postoperative patient. The dose ordered is 3 mg every 3 hours as needed for pain. The medication is supplied in vials of 4 mg/mL. How much will be drawn into the syringe for this dose?

1. d, 2. c, 3. a, 4. b, 5. c, 6. 0.75 mL.

CRITICAL THINKING ACTIVITIES: BEST ACTION

1 The nurse is about to administer 5 mg of morphine sulfate intravenously to a patient with severe postoperative pain, as ordered. What is the most important assessment data that should be gathered before and after administering this drug? Explain your answer.
2 A patient complains that the drugs he is receiving for severe pain are not really helping. What would be the nurse's best response to this patient?

3 A young woman is brought by ambulance to the emergency department because she was found unconscious next to an empty bottle of acetaminophen. While the medical team assesses her, the nurse goes to question the family about the situation. What is the most important piece of information to know about this possible overdose?

For answers, see *http://evolve.elsevier.com/Lilley.*

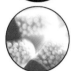

CHAPTER 12

General and Local Anesthetics

OBJECTIVES

When you reach the end of this chapter, you should be able to do the following:

1 Define *anesthesia*.

2 Describe the basic differences between general and local anesthesia.

3 List the most commonly used general and local anesthetics and associated risks.

4 Discuss the differences between depolarizing neuromuscular blocking drugs and nondepolarizing blocking drugs and their impact on the patient.

5 Compare the mechanisms of action, indications, adverse effects, routes of administration, cautions, contraindications, and drug interactions for general and local anesthesia as well as drugs used for moderate or conscious sedation.

6 Develop a nursing care plan for patients before anesthesia (preanesthesia), during anesthesia, and after anesthesia (postanesthesia) related to general anesthesia.

7 Develop a nursing care plan for patients undergoing local anesthesia and/or moderate or conscious sedation.

e-Learning Activities

http://evolve.elsevier.com/Lilley

NCLEX Review Questions • Animations • Nursing Care Plans • Audio Glossary • Category Catchers • Medication Errors Checklists • IV Therapy Checklists • Calculators • Frequently Asked Questions • Content Updates • Supplemental Resources • Answers to Case Studies and Critical Thinking Activities

Drug Profiles

isoflurane, p. 181
ketamine, p. 182
♦ lidocaine, p. 185
nitrous oxide, p. 182
pancuronium, p. 188

♦ propofol, p. 182
sevoflurane, p. 181
♦ succinylcholine, p. 188
♦ vecuronium, p. 189

♦ *Key drug.*

Glossary

Adjunct anesthetics Drugs used in combination with anesthetic drugs to control the adverse effects of anesthetics or to help maintain the anesthetic state in the patient. (See *balanced anesthesia*.) (p. 179)

Anesthesia The loss of the ability to feel pain resulting from the administration of an anesthetic drug or other medical intervention. (p. 178)

Anesthetics Drugs that depress the central nervous system (CNS) or peripheral nerves to produce diminution of consciousness, loss of responsiveness to sensory stimulation, or muscle relaxation. (p. 178)

Balanced anesthesia The practice of using combinations of different drug classes rather than a single drug to produce anesthesia. (p. 179)

General anesthesia A drug-induced state in which the CNS nerve impulses are altered to reduce pain and other sensations throughout the entire body. It normally involves complete loss of consciousness and depression of normal respiratory drive. (p. 178)

Local anesthesia A drug-induced state in which peripheral or spinal nerve impulses are altered to reduce or eliminate pain and other sensations in tissues innervated by these nerves. (p. 179)

Malignant hyperthermia A genetically linked major adverse reaction to general anesthesia characterized by a rapid rise in body temperature, as well as tachycardia, tachypnea, and sweating. (p. 180)

Moderate sedation A milder form of general anesthesia that causes partial or complete loss of consciousness but does not generally reduce normal respiratory drive. (p. 182)

Overton-Meyer theory A theory that describes the relationship between the lipid solubility of anesthetic drugs and their potency. (p. 179)

Spinal anesthesia Local anesthesia induced by injection of an anesthetic drug near the spinal cord to anesthetize nerves that are distal to the site of injection (also called *intraspinal anesthesia*). (p. 182)

• • •

Anatomy, Physiology, and Disease Overview

Anesthetics are drugs that reduce or eliminate pain by depressing nerve function in the central nervous system (CNS) and/or the peripheral nervous system (PNS). This state of reduced neurologic function is called **anesthesia.** Anesthesia is further classified as *general* or *local.* **General anesthesia** normally involves complete loss of consciousness, loss of body reflexes, elimination of pain and other sensations throughout the entire body, and skeletal and smooth muscle paralysis, including paralysis of respiratory muscles. This loss of normal respiratory function requires mechanical or manual ventilatory support to avoid brain damage and suffocation (death from respiratory arrest). **Local anesthesia** does not involve paralysis of respiratory function but does involve elimination of pain sensation in the tissues innervated by *anesthetized* nerves. Functions of the *autonomic nervous system*, which is a branch of the parasympathetic nervous system, may also be affected.

Pharmacology Overview
GENERAL ANESTHETICS

General anesthetics are drugs that induce general anesthesia and are most commonly used to induce anesthesia during surgical procedures. General anesthesia is achieved by the use of one or more drugs. Often a synergistic combination of drugs is used, which allows for smaller doses of each drug and better control of the patient's anesthetized state. Inhalational anesthetics are volatile liquids or gases that are vaporized or mixed with oxygen to induce anesthesia. For a historical perspective on general anesthesia, see Box 12-1.

Parenteral anesthetics (Table 12-1) are usually given intravenously and are used for induction and/or maintenance of general anesthesia, induction of amnesia, and as adjuncts to inhalation-type anesthetics (Table 12-2). The specific goal varies with the drug. Common intravenous anesthetic drugs include drugs classified solely as general anesthetics, such as etomidate and propofol.

In addition, there are also **adjunct anesthetics** or simply *adjuncts*. *Adjunct* is a general term for any drug or procedure that enhances clinical therapy for any condition when used simultaneously with another drug or procedure. Adjunct drugs can be thought of as "helper drugs" when their use complements the use of any other drug(s) and are used simultaneously with general anesthetics for anesthesia initiation (induction), sedation, reduction of anxiety, and amnesia. Adjuncts include neuromuscular blocking drugs (NMBDs; see Neuromuscular Blocking Drugs later in this chapter), sedative-hypnotics or anxiolytics (see Chapter 13) such as propofol (this chapter), benzodiazepines

(e.g., diazepam, midazolam), barbiturates (e.g., thiopental, methohexital; see Chapter 13), opioid analgesics (e.g., morphine, fentanyl, sufentanil; see Chapter 11), anticholinergics (e.g., atropine; see Chapter 21), and antiemetics (e.g., ondansetron, droperidol; see Chapter 52). Note that propofol can be used as a general anesthetic and/or sedative-hypnotic, depending on the dose (see Dosages table on p. 182). The simultaneous use of both general anesthetics and adjuncts is called **balanced anesthesia.** Common adjunctive anesthetic drugs are listed in Table 12-3.

Mechanism of Action and Drug Effects

Many theories have been proposed to explain the actual mechanism of action of general anesthetics. The drugs vary widely in their chemical structures, and their mechanism of action is not easily explained by a structure-receptor relationship. The concentrations of various anesthetics required to produce a given state of anesthesia also differ greatly. The **Overton-Meyer theory** has been used to explain some of the properties of anesthetic drugs since the early days of anesthesiology. In general terms, it proposes that, for all anesthetics, potency varies directly with lipid solubility. In other words, across a continuum of drug potency, fat-soluble drugs are stronger anesthetics than water-soluble drugs. Nerve cell membranes have a high lipid content, as does the *blood-brain barrier* (see Chapter 2). Lipid-soluble anesthetic drugs can therefore easily cross the blood-brain barrier to concentrate in nerve cell membranes.

The overall effect of general anesthetics is a progressive reduction of sensory and motor CNS functions. The degree and speed of this process varies with the anesthetics and adjuncts used along with their dosages and routes of administration. General anesthesia initially produces a loss of the senses of sight, touch, taste, smell, and hearing, along with loss of consciousness. Cardiac and pulmonary functions are usually the last to be inter-

---

BOX 12-1 General Anesthesia: A Historical Perspective

Until recently, general anesthesia was described as having several definitive stages. This was especially true with the use of many of the ether-based inhaled anesthetic drugs. Features of these distinctive stages were easily observable to the trained eye. They included specific physical and physiologic changes that progressed gradually and predictably with the depth of the patient's anesthetized state. Gradual changes in pupil size, progression from thoracic to diaphragmatic breathing, vital sign changes, and several other changes all characterized the various stages. Newer inhalational and intravenous general anesthetic drugs, however, often have a much more rapid onset of action and body distribution. As a result, the specific stages of anesthesia once observed with older drugs are no longer sufficiently well defined to be observable. Thus, the concept of stages of anesthesia is an outdated one in most modern surgical facilities. Registered nurses who pursue advanced training to become a certified registered nurse anesthetist often find this to be a rewarding and interesting area of nursing practice. Some nurses also find that this type of work offers greater flexibility in their work schedule than do other practice areas.

TABLE 12-1 Parenteral General Anesthetics

Generic Name	Trade Name
etomidate	Amidate
ketamine	Ketalar
methohexital	Brevital
propofol	Diprivan
thiamylal	Surital
thiopental	Pentothal

TABLE 12-2 Inhalational General Anesthetics

Generic Name	Trade Name
Inhaled Gas	
nitrous oxide (laughing gas)	
Inhaled Volatile Liquid	
desflurane	Suprane
enflurane	Ethrane
halothane	Fluothane
isoflurane	Forane
methoxyflurane	Penthrane
sevoflurane	Ultane

TABLE 12-3 Adjunctive Anesthetic Drugs

Drug	Pharmacologic Class	Usual Dosage Range	Indications/Uses
alfentanil (Alfenta)	Opioid analgesic	130-245 mcg/kg IV	Anesthesia induction
fentanyl (Sublimaze)		50-100 mcg/kg IV	
sufentanil (Sufenta)		8-30 mcg/kg IV	
diazepam (Valium)	Benzodiazepine	2-20 mg PO/IV/IM	Amnesia and anxiety reduction
midazolam (Versed)		0.05-0.35 mg/kg IV	
atropine	Anticholinergic	0.1-0.6 mg IV/IM/subcut	Drying up of excessive secretions
glycopyrrolate (Robinul)		0.0044 mg/kg IM	
scopolamine		0.3-0.6 mg subcut/IM	
meperidine (Demerol)	Opioid analgesic	50-100 mg IM/subcut	Pain prevention and pain relief
morphine		5-20 mg IM/subcut	
hydroxyzine (Atarax, Vistaril)	Antihistamine	25-100 mg IM	Amnesia and sedation
pentobarbital (Nembutal)	Sedative-hypnotic	150-200 mg IM	
promethazine (Phenergan)		25-50 mg IM	
secobarbital (Seconal)		100 mg PO	

IM, Intramuscularly; *IV,* intravenously; *PO,* orally; *subcut,* subcutaneously.

LIFE SPAN CONSIDERATIONS: The Elderly Patient

Anesthesia

- The elderly patient is affected more adversely by anesthesia than the young or middle-aged adult. With aging comes organ system deterioration. Declining liver function results in decreased metabolism of drugs, and a decline in renal functioning leads to decreased drug excretion. Either of these can lead to drug toxicity, unsafe levels, and/or overdose. If both of these organs are not functioning properly, the risk of drug toxicity or overdose is even greater. In addition, the elderly are more sensitive to the effects of drugs affecting the central nervous system.
- Presence of cardiac and respiratory diseases places the elderly patient at higher risk for cardiac dysrhythmias, hypotension, respiratory depression, atelectasis, and/or pneumonia during the postoperative or postanesthesia phase.
- The practice of polypharmacy is yet another concern in the elderly with regard to administration of any type of anesthetic. Because of the presence of various age-related diseases, the older patient is generally taking more than one medication. The more drugs a patient is taking, the higher the risk of adverse reactions and drug-drug interactions, including interactions with anesthetics.

---

rupted, because they are controlled by the *medulla* of the *brainstem,* the last area to be affected by general anesthetics. These are the classical "stages" of anesthesia. Again, mechanical ventilatory support is usually necessary. In more extensive surgical procedures, especially those involving the heart, pharmacologic cardiac support involving *adrenergic* drugs (see Chapter 18) and *inotropic* drugs (see Chapter 22) may also be required.

The reactions of various body systems to general anesthetics are further described in Table 12-4.

Indications

General anesthetics are used to produce unconsciousness as well as relaxation of skeletal and visceral smooth muscles for surgical procedures as well as in *electroconvulsive therapy* for severe depression (see Chapter 17).

Contraindications

Contraindications to the use of anesthetic drugs include known drug allergy and, depending on the drug type, may also include pregnancy, narrow-angle glaucoma, and known susceptibility to malignant hyperthermia (see Adverse Effects) from prior experience with anesthetics.

Adverse Effects

The adverse effects of general anesthetics are dose dependent and vary with the individual drug. The heart, peripheral circulation, liver, kidneys, and respiratory tract are the sites primarily affected. Myocardial depression is a common adverse effect. All of the halogenated anesthetics are capable of causing hepatotoxicity, and methoxyflurane can cause significant respiratory depression.

With the development and use of newer drugs, many of the unwanted adverse effects characteristic of the older drugs (such as hepatotoxicity and myocardial depression) are now a thing of the past. In addition, many of the bothersome adverse effects such as nausea, vomiting, and confusion have become less common since balanced anesthesia has become more widely used. It should also be noted that substance abuse (e.g., alcohol abuse; see Chapter 9) can predispose a patient to anesthetic-induced complications (e.g., liver toxicity). A positive determination of substance abuse during the anesthetist's history-taking interview may lead to dosage adjustments in one or more of the drugs used. A drug-abusing patient with a high tolerance for street drugs may require larger doses of anesthesia-related drugs (e.g., benzodiazepines, opioids) to achieve the desired sedative effects.

Malignant hyperthermia is an uncommon, but potentially fatal, genetically linked adverse metabolic reaction to general anesthesia. It is classically associated with the use of volatile inhalational anesthetics as well as the depolarizing NMBD succinylcholine (see Neuromuscular Blocking Drugs later in this chapter). Signs include rapid rise in body temperature, tachycardia, tachypnea, and muscular rigidity. Patients known to be statistically at greater risk for malignant hyperthermia include children, adolescents, and individuals with muscular and/or skeletal abnormalities such as hernias, strabismus, ptosis, scoliosis,

TABLE 12-4 Effects of Inhaled and Intravenous General Anesthetics

Organ/System	Reaction
Respiratory system	Depressed muscles and patterns of respiration; altered gas exchange and impaired oxygenation; depressed airway-protective mechanisms; airway irritation and possible laryngospasm
Cardiovascular system	Depressed myocardium; hypotension and tachycardia; bradycardia in response to vagal stimulation
Cerebrovascular system	Increased intracranial blood volume and increased intracranial pressure
Gastrointestinal system	Reduced hepatic blood flow and thus reduced hepatic clearance
Renal system	Decreased glomerular filtration
Skeletal muscles	Skeletal muscle relaxation
Cutaneous circulation	Vasodilation
Central nervous system (CNS)	CNS depression; blurred vision; nystagmus; progression of CNS depression to decreased alertness, sensorium, and decreased level of consciousness

---

LIFE SPAN CONSIDERATIONS: The Pediatric Patient

Anesthesia

- Premature infants, neonates, and pediatric patients are more adversely affected by anesthesia than the young or middle-aged adult patient. The reason for this difference in response is the increased sensitivity of the pediatric patient to anesthetics and related drugs because of immature functioning of the liver and kidneys, which leads to possible drug accumulation, toxicity, and subsequent complications. The central nervous system of pediatric patients is also more sensitive to the effects of anesthetics. Because of these risks of toxicity and complications with all forms of anesthesia, the nurse must take every precaution to ensure that the patient remains safe and free from harm.

- Cardiac and respiratory systems are not fully developed in the neonate, premature infant, and newborn, which makes this age group more susceptible to problems with the metabolism and excretion of drugs. Some of the more common problems include central nervous system depression with subsequent respiratory and cardiac depression, and development of atelectasis, pneumonia, and cardiac abnormalities.

- Neonates, in particular (see age group definitions and further discussion in Chapter 3), are at higher risk of upper airway obstruction during general anesthesia. During the anesthetic process, the risk of laryngospasm related to the intubation process may be increased for neonates because of the specific physical characteristics of the larynx and respiratory structures in this age group. Their higher metabolic rate and small airway diameter also put neonates at greater risk of experiencing complications during general anesthesia.

- Before any medications are given to the pediatric patient, a careful check and double-check of mathematical drug calculations should be performed. In addition to weight, body surface area and laboratory test results that may be indicative of organ dysfunction should always be taken into consideration in the actual drug calculation.

- Resuscitative equipment should be readily available on any neonatal or pediatric nursing care unit.

---

and muscular dystrophy. Malignant hyperthermia is treated with cardiorespiratory supportive care as needed to stabilize heart and lung function as well as with the skeletal muscle relaxant dantrolene (see Chapter 13). In fact, by law, all facilities that provide general anesthesia must maintain a certain amount of dantrolene on hand in case of malignant hyperthermia.

Toxicity and Management of Overdose

In large doses all anesthetics are potentially life threatening, with cardiac and respiratory arrest as the ultimate causes of death. However, these drugs are almost exclusively administered in a very controlled environment by personnel trained in advanced cardiac life support. These drugs are also very quickly metabolized. In addition, the medullary center, which governs the vital functions, is the last area of the brain to be affected by anesthetics and the first to regain function if it is lost. These factors combined make an anesthetic overdose rare and easily reversible.

Interactions

Some of the more common drugs that interact with general anesthetics are antihypertensives and beta-blockers, which have additive effects when combined with general anesthetics (i.e., increased hypotensive effects from antihypertensives, and increased myocardial depression with beta-blockers). No significant laboratory test interactions have been reported.

Dosages

For the recommended dosages of selected general anesthetic drugs, see the Dosages table on p. 182.

DRUG PROFILES

The dose of any anesthetic depends on the complexity of the surgical procedure to be performed and the physical characteristics of the patient. With regard to pharmacokinetics, all of the general anesthetics have a rapid onset of action along with rapid elimination upon discontinuation. Anesthesia is maintained intraoperatively by continuous administration of the drug.

isoflurane

Isoflurane (Forane) is a fluorinated ether that is a chemical isomer of the older fluorinated ether enflurane. It has a more rapid onset of action, causes less cardiovascular depression, and has little or no associated toxicity. This is in contrast to enflurane, which can cause seizures, and halothane, which is associated liver toxicity. Dosage information is given in the table on p. 182.

sevoflurane

Sevoflurane (Ultane) is the newest fluorinated ether and is now widely used. Its pharmacokinetics, with rapid onset and rapid elimination, make it especially useful in outpatient surgery settings. It is also nonirritating to the airway, which greatly facilitates induction of an unconscious state, especially in pediatric patients.

DOSAGES

Selected General Anesthetics

Drug	Pharmacologic Class	Usual Dosage Range	Indications/Uses
isoflurane (Forane)	Inhalation general anesthetic	0.1%-2% concentration with appropriate drugs	General anesthesia
ketamine (Ketalar)	Parenteral general anesthetic*	IV: 2 mg/kg bolus over 60 sec IV: 0.2-0.8 mg/kg bolus over 3 min	General anesthesia, moderate sedation
nitrous oxide (laughing gas)	Inorganic inhalation general anesthetic	20%-40% with oxygen (e.g., 70% with 30% oxygen)	Analgesia, anesthesia
◆ propofol (Diprivan)	Parenteral general anesthetic; sedative-hypnotic	IV: 100-150 mcg/kg/min IV: 25 mcg/kg/min	General anesthesia, moderate sedation

IV, Intravenous.
*Also available for subcutaneous, intramuscular, oral, rectal, topical, transdermal, and intranasal use for moderate sedation.

ketamine

Ketamine is a unique drug with multiple properties. Given intravenously, it can be used for both general anesthesia and moderate sedation. It is commonly used in the emergency department for setting broken bones. It can also provide moderate sedation when given intravenously and by several other routes, including subcutaneous, intramuscular, epidural, oral, intranasal, rectal, transdermal, and topical. It binds to receptors in both central and peripheral nervous systems, including opioid receptors. The most important receptors for the therapeutic activity of this drug, however, are the N-methyl-d-aspartate (NMDA) receptors located in the dorsal horn of the spinal cord. The drug is highly lipid soluble and penetrates the blood-brain barrier rapidly, which results in a rapid onset of action. It has a low incidence of reduction of cardiovascular, respiratory, and bowel function. Adverse effects can include disturbing *psychotomimetic* effects, including hallucinations. However, these are less likely to occur when benzodiazepines (see Chapter 13) are coadministered with the drug. Interacting drugs include NMBDs (prolonged paralysis) and halothane (reduced cardiac output and blood pressure). The drug is contraindicated in cases of known drug allergy. Selected dosage information appears in the Dosages table on p. 182.

nitrous oxide

Nitrous oxide, also known as *laughing gas,* is the only inhaled gas currently used as a general anesthetic. It is the weakest of the general anesthetic drugs and is used primarily for dental procedures or as a supplement to other, more potent anesthetics. Dosage information is given in the table on p. 182.

◆ propofol

Propofol (Diprivan) is a parenteral general anesthetic used for the induction and maintenance of general anesthesia and also for sedation for mechanical ventilation in intensive care unit (ICU) settings. In lower doses it can also be used as a sedative-hypnotic for *moderate sedation.* Some states allow nurses to administer propofol as part of a moderate sedation protocol. However, many state boards of nursing prohibit administration by nurses. Propofol also is typically well tolerated, producing few undesirable effects. Dosage information is provided in the Dosages table on p. 182.

DRUGS FOR MODERATE SEDATION

Moderate sedation, *conscious sedation,* and *procedural sedation* are synonymous terms for anesthesia that does not necessarily cause complete loss of consciousness and does not normally cause respiratory arrest. This technique uses combinations of several drugs that may be classified differently. For example, one or more benzodiazepines may be used with one or more opioids. Drugs may be given by intravenous, intramuscular, spinal, or oral routes. The net effect is a type of anesthesia that allows the patient to relax, have markedly reduced or no anxiety, yet still maintain his or her own open airway, as well as respond to verbal commands. Mild amnesia for the procedure is also a common effect. This is often desirable for helping patients not to remember painful medical procedures. All types of moderate sedation are associated with a more rapid recovery time than general anesthesia as well as a better safety profile because of lower cardiopulmonary risks. Persons who administer drugs for moderate sedation are required to have advanced cardiac life support training, and someone with the ability to intubate the patient must be present, in case the patient slips into a deeper state of sedation and is unable to maintain an open airway.

The oral route of drug administration is more commonly used in pediatric patients. This often involves administering an oral syrup form of midazolam with or without concurrent use of injected medications such as opiates. This technique can be especially helpful for pediatric patients who must undergo uncomfortable procedures such as wound suturing or diagnostic procedures requiring reduced movement such as *computed tomography* and *magnetic resonance imaging.* See Life Span Considerations: The Pediatric Patient box on p. 183 for other considerations.

LOCAL ANESTHETICS

Local anesthetics are the second major class of anesthetics. They reduce pain sensations at the level of peripheral nerves, although this can involve *intraspinal anesthesia* (see later). They are also called *regional anesthetics* because they render a specific portion of the body insensitive to pain. They do this by interfering with nerve transmission in specific areas of the body, blocking nerve conduction only in the area in which they are applied without causing loss of consciousness. They are most commonly used in clinical settings in which loss of consciousness is undesirable or unnecessary. These include childbirth and other situations in which **spinal anesthesia** is desired, dental procedures, suturing of skin lacerations, and diagnostic procedures (e.g., lumbar puncture, thoracentesis, biopsy).

LIFE SPAN CONSIDERATIONS: The Pediatric Patient

Moderate or Conscious Anesthesia

- The American Academy of Pediatrics recommends that moderate or conscious sedation (anesthesia) be used to reduce anxiety, pain, and fear in the pediatric patient. The use of moderate anesthesia in the pediatric patient allows a procedure to be performed restraint free in most situations while keeping the patient responsive.
- Pediatric dosing often conforms to the following guidelines:
  - Morphine—pediatric dosing may be at 0.05 to 0.1 mg/kg intravenously (IV) over a 2-minute period and is ideal for long procedures or cases in which pain is anticipated after the procedure.
  - Fentanyl—pediatric dosing may be at 0.5 to 1 mcg/kg with increments over 3 minutes to a maximum of three doses. Too rapid an IV injection may result in chest rigidity, which may need to be treated with muscle relaxants and possibly mechanical ventilation. Fentanyl is used often for short procedures.
  - Fentanyl citrate—oral transmucosal forms are dosed at 10 to 15 mcg/kg/hr and are used in monitored hospital settings. They are administered by having the patient suck on a stick (as with a lollipop).
  - Hydromorphone—pediatric dosing is at 0.015 to 0.02 mg/kg.
  - Meperidine—pediatric dosing is at 0.5 to 1 mg/kg over 2 minutes.

- Discharge status of the pediatric patient depends on the type of drugs and drug combinations used. Discharge after conscious or moderate sedation is based mainly on whether the following criteria are met:
  - Patient is alert and oriented compared with the baseline neurologic assessment.
  - Protective swallowing and gag reflexes are intact.
  - Vital signs are stable and consistent with baseline values for at least 30 minutes after the last dosing. Different health care facilities set different criteria that must be met and documented (blood pressure and pulse rate within normal limits or within 20 points of baseline, temperature lower than 101° F [38.3° C]).
  - Oxygen saturation is at least 95% on room air 30 minutes after the last dose.
  - Pain rating is at baseline levels or less.
  - Ambulation is at baseline level.
  - An adult is present to get the patient home and remain with the patient for at least two half-lives of the various drugs used for the anesthesia.
  - If a reversal drug was administered, there has been time for the drug to be excreted.

BOX 12-2 Types of Local Anesthesia

Central

Spinal or intraspinal anesthesia: Anesthetic drugs are injected into the area near the spinal cord within the vertebral column. Intraspinal anesthesia is commonly accomplished by one of two injection techniques: intrathecal and epidural.
- **Intrathecal anesthesia** involves injection of anesthetic into the subarachnoid space. Intrathecal anesthesia is commonly used for patients undergoing major abdominal or limb surgery for whom the risks of general anesthesia are too high or for patients who prefer this technique instead of complete loss of consciousness during their surgical procedure. More recently, intrathecal injection of anesthetics through implantable drug pumps is even being used on an outpatient basis in patients with severe chronic pain syndromes, such as those resulting from occupational injuries.
- **Epidural anesthesia** involves injection of anesthetic via a small catheter into the epidural space without puncturing the dura. Epidural anesthesia is commonly used to reduce maternal discomfort during labor and delivery and to manage postoperative acute pain after major abdominal or pelvic surgery. This route is becoming more popular for the administration of opioids for pain management.

Peripheral

- **Infiltration:** Small amounts of anesthetic solution are injected into the tissue that surrounds the operative site. This approach to anesthesia is commonly used for such procedures as wound suturing and dental surgery. Often drugs that cause constriction of local blood vessels (e.g., epinephrine, cocaine) are also administered to limit the site of action to the local area.
- **Nerve block:** Anesthetic solution is injected at the site where a nerve innervates a specific area such as a tissue. This allows large amounts of anesthetic drug to be delivered to a very specific area without affecting the whole body. This method is often reserved for more difficult-to-treat pain syndromes such as cancer pain and chronic orthopedic pain.
- **Topical anesthesia:** The anesthetic drug is applied directly onto the surface of the skin, eye, or any mucous membrane to relieve pain or prevent it from being sensed. It is commonly used for diagnostic eye examinations and skin suturing.

Most local anesthetics belong to one of two major groups of organic compounds, esters and amides, and are classified as either *parenteral* (injectable) or *topical* anesthetics. Parenteral anesthetics are most commonly given intravenously but may also be administered by various spinal injection techniques (Box 12-2). Topical anesthetics are applied directly to the skin and mucous membranes. They are available in the form of solutions, ointments, gels, creams, powders, suppositories, and ophthalmic drops. Their dosage strengths are listed in Table 12-5.

The injection of parenteral anesthetic drugs into the area near the spinal cord is known as spinal or intraspinal anesthesia. This type of anesthesia is generally used to block all peripheral nerves that branch out distal to the injection site. The result is elimination of pain and paralysis of the skeletal and smooth muscles of the corresponding innervated tissues. Some of the medications that may be used for spinal anesthesia include the opioids morphine, hydromorphone, fentanyl, and meperidine (see Chapter 11), and the local anesthetics lidocaine and bupivacaine. Because spinal anesthesia does not depress the CNS at a level that causes loss of consciousness, it can be thought of as a large-scale type of *local* rather than general anesthesia. Some of the common types of local anesthesia are described in Box 12-2. The paren-

TABLE 12-5 Topical Anesthetics

Drug	Route	Dose Strength
benzocaine (Dermoplast, Lanacane, Solarcaine)	Topical, aerosol, and spray	0.5%-20% ointment or cream
butamben (Butesin)	Topical	1% ointment
cocaine	Topical	4%-10% solution, jelly
dibucaine (Nupercainal)	Injection and topical	0.5%-1% solution, ointment, or cream
dibucaine	Topical	1% ointment
dyclonine (Dyclone, Sucrets)	Topical	0.5%-1% solution
ethyl chloride (Chloroethane)	Topical	Spray
lidocaine (Lidoderm)	Topical	5% patch
proparacaine (Alcaine, Ophthetic)	Ophthalmic	0.5% solution
pramoxine (Tronolane)	Topical	1% jelly, cream, or lotion
prilocaine/lidocaine (EMLA)	Topical	2.5% prilocaine and 2.5% lidocaine cream
tetracaine (Pontocaine)	Injection, topical, and ophthalmic	0.5%-2% solution, ointment, or cream

TABLE 12-6 Selected Parenteral Anesthetic Drugs*

Generic Name	Trade Name	Potency	Onset	Duration	Dose
lidocaine	Xylocaine	Moderate	Immediate	60-90 min	0.5%-4% injection
mepivacaine	Carbocaine	Moderate	Immediate	120-150 min	1%, 1.5%, 2%, 3% injection
procaine	Novocain	Lowest	2-5 min	30-60 min	1%, 2%, 10% injection
tetracaine	Pontocaine	Highest	5-10 min	90-120 min	0.2%, 0.3%, 1% injection

*Other common parenteral anesthetic drugs include bupivacaine (Marcaine, Sensorcaine), chloroprocaine (Nesacaine), etidocaine (Duranest), propoxycaine (Ravocaine), and ropivacaine (Naropin).

teral local anesthetic drugs and their pharmacokinetics are summarized in Table 12-6.

Local anesthesia of specific peripheral nerves is accomplished by *nerve block anesthesia* or *infiltration anesthesia*. The former involves relatively deep injections of drugs into locations adjacent to major nerve trunks or ganglia. It focuses on a relatively large body region but not necessarily as extensive as that affected by spinal anesthesia. In contrast, infiltration anesthesia involves multiple small injections (intradermal, subcutaneous, submucosal, or intramuscular) to produce a more limited or "local" anesthetic field. Finally, another subtype of local anesthesia involves *topical* application of a drug (e.g., lidocaine) onto the surface of the skin, mucous membranes, or eye.

Mechanism of Action and Drug Effects

Local anesthetics work by rendering a specific portion of the body insensitive to pain by interfering with nerve transmission in that area. Nerve conduction is blocked only in the area in which the anesthetic is applied, and there is no loss of consciousness. Local anesthetics block both the generation and conduction of impulses through all types of nerve fibers (sensory, motor, and autonomic) by blocking the movement of certain ions (sodium, potassium, and calcium) important to this process. They do this by making it more difficult for these ions to move in and out of the nerve fiber. For this reason, some of these drugs are also described as *membrane-stabilizing* because they alter the cell membrane of the nerve so that the free movement of ions is inhibited. The membrane-stabilizing effects occur first in the small fibers, then in the large fibers. In terms of paralysis, usually autonomic activity is affected first, then pain and other sensory functions are lost. Motor activity is the last to be lost. When the effects of the

local anesthetic wear off, recovery occurs in reverse order: motor activity returns first, then sensory functions, and finally autonomic activity.

Possible systemic effects of the administration of local anesthetics include effects on circulatory and respiratory function. The systemic adverse effects depend on where and how the drug is administered (e.g., injection at a certain level in the spinal cord or topical application of a drug that gains access to the circulation). Such adverse effects are somewhat unlikely unless large quantities of a drug are injected. Local anesthetics also produce *sympathetic blockade;* that is, they block the action of the two *neurotransmitters* of the sympathetic nervous system, *norepinephrine* and *epinephrine*. The cardiac effects of such a sympathetic blockade include a decrease in stroke volume, cardiac output, and peripheral resistance. The respiratory effects include reduced respiratory function and altered breathing patterns, but complete paralysis of respiratory function is unlikely because of the large amount of drug that would have to be absorbed. Some local anesthetics used for either infiltration or nerve block anesthesia are combined with vasoconstrictors such as epinephrine, phenylephrine, and norepinephrine to help confine the local anesthetic to the injected area and prevent systemic absorption.

Indications

Local anesthetics are used for surgical, dental, or diagnostic procedures, as well as for the treatment of various types of chronic pain. Spinal anesthesia is used to control pain during surgical procedures and childbirth. Nerve block anesthesia is used for surgical, dental, and diagnostic procedures and for the therapeutic management of chronic pain. Infiltration anesthesia is used for relatively minor surgical and dental procedures.

Contraindications

Contraindications for local anesthetics include known drug allergy. Only specially formulated dosage forms are intended for ophthalmic use (see Chapter 57).

Adverse Effects

The adverse effects of the local anesthetics are limited and of little clinical importance in most circumstances. The undesirable effects usually occur with high plasma concentrations of the drug, which result from inadvertent intravascular injection, an excessive dose or rate of injection, slow metabolic breakdown, or injection into a highly vascular tissue. One notable complication of spinal anesthesia is *spinal headache.* Spinal headache occurs in up to 70% of patients who either experience inadvertent dural puncture during epidural anesthesia or undergo intrathecal anesthesia. Spinal headache is most often self-limiting and is treated with bed rest and conventional analgesic medications. Oral or intravenous forms of the CNS stimulant caffeine (see Chapter 14) are also sometimes used. Severe cases of spinal headache may be treated by the anesthetist by injection of a small volume (roughly 15 mL) of venous sample of the patient's own blood into the patient's epidural space. The exact mechanism by which this *blood patch* provides relief is unknown, but it is effective in treating spinal headache in over 90% of cases.

True allergic reactions to local anesthetics are rare. However, allergic reactions can occur, ranging from skin rash, urticaria, and edema to anaphylactic shock. Such allergic reactions are generally limited to a particular chemical class of anesthetics called the *ester type.* Box 12-3 categorizes the local anesthetic drugs into the ester and amide chemical families. Different enzymes are responsible for the breakdown of these two groups of anesthetics in the body. Anesthetics belonging to the ester family are metabolized by cholinesterase in the plasma and liver. They are converted into a para-aminobenzoic acid (PABA) compound. This compound is mainly responsible for the allergic reactions. In contrast, the *amide type* of anesthetics is usually metabolized uneventfully to active and inactive metabolites in the liver by other enzymes. Often when an individual has an adverse reaction to one of the local anesthetics, using a drug from the alternate chemical class avoids this problem.

Toxicity and Management of Overdose

Local anesthetics have little opportunity to cause toxicity under most circumstances. However, systemic reactions are possible if sufficiently large quantities are absorbed into the systemic circulation. To prevent this from occurring, a *vasoconstrictor* such as epinephrine is often coadministered with the local anesthetic to maintain localized drug activity (e.g., lidocaine/epinephrine or bupivacaine/epinephrine). This property of epinephrine also serves to reduce local blood loss during minor surgical procedures. If for some reason significant amounts of the locally administered anesthetic are absorbed systemically, cardiovascular and respiratory function may be compromised. In extreme cases, such as inadvertent injection of drug into a major blood vessel, symptomatic and supportive cardiovascular and/or respiratory therapy may be required until the drug is metabolized and eliminated.

BOX 12-3 **Chemical Groups of Local Anesthetics**

Ester Type
benzocaine
chloroprocaine
cocaine
procaine
proparacaine
propoxycaine
tetracaine

Amide Type
bupivacaine
dibucaine
etidocaine
lidocaine
mepivacaine
prilocaine

Interactions

Few clinically significant drug interactions occur with the local anesthetics. When given with enflurane, halothane, or epinephrine, these drugs can lead to dysrhythmias.

Dosages

For the recommended dosages of lidocaine, see the Dosages table on p. 186.

DRUG PROFILES

Besides lidocaine, profiled here, local anesthetics include bupivacaine, chloroprocaine, etidocaine, mepivacaine, prilocaine, procaine, propoxycaine, ropivacaine, and tetracaine. As noted earlier, there are two major types of local anesthetics as determined by chemical structure: amides and esters. These designations refer to the type of linkage between the aromatic ring and the amino group of the chemical structures of the drug molecules. These structural components give these drugs their anesthetic properties.

◆ lidocaine

Lidocaine belongs to the amide class of local anesthetics. Some patients may report that they have allergic or anaphylactic reactions to the "caines," as they may refer to lidocaine and the other amide drugs. In these situations, it may be wise to try a local anesthetic of the ester type.

Lidocaine (Xylocaine) is one of the most commonly used local anesthetics. It is available in several strengths, both alone and in different concentrations with epinephrine, and is used for both infiltration and nerve block anesthesia. The vasoconstrictive properties of epinephrine reduce both blood loss and systemic drug absorption from minor surgical procedures. Lidocaine is also available in topical forms, including the unique product EMLA. This is a cream mixture of lidocaine and prilocaine that is applied to skin to ease the pain of needle punctures (e.g., starting an intravenous line). There is also a transdermal lidocaine patch for relief of *postherpetic neuralgia* (see Chapter 11). Parenteral lidocaine is also used to treat certain cardiac dysrhythmias (see Chapter 23). Contraindications include known drug allergy. Commonly recommended dosages are listed in the table on p. 186. Lidocaine is a pregnancy category B drug.

DOSAGES

Lidocaine

Drug	Pharmacologic Class	Usual Dosage Range	Indications/Uses
◆ lidocaine (Xylocaine)	Amide local anesthetic	0.5%, 1% solution: 5-300 mg	Percutaneous infiltration
		1% solution: 200-300 mg	Caudal obstetric analgesia, thoracic nerve block
		1% solution: 100 mg each side	Paracervical obstetric analgesia
		1% solution: 50-100 mg	Sympathetic lumbar nerve block
		1% solution: 30-50 mg	Paravertebral nerve block
		1% solution: 30 mg	Intercostal nerve block
		1% solution: 50 mg	Sympathetic cervical nerve block
		1.5% solution: 225-300 mg	Brachial nerve block, caudal surgical anesthesia
		2% solution: 20-100 mg	Dental procedures
		2% solution: 200-300 mg	Lumbar anesthesia

NEUROMUSCULAR BLOCKING DRUGS

Neuromuscular blocking drugs (NMBDs) prevent nerve transmission in skeletal and smooth muscles, leading to paralysis. They are often used as adjuncts with general anesthetics for surgical procedures. Neuromuscular blocking drugs also paralyze the skeletal muscles required for breathing: the *intercostal* muscles and the *diaphragm.* The patient is rendered unable to breathe on his or her own, and mechanical ventilation is required to prevent brain damage or death by suffocation. Deaths have been reported when an NMBD is accidentally mistaken for a different drug and given to a patient who is not mechanically ventilated. Most hospitals have taken extra precautions to keep NMBDs separated from other drugs, or at least marked with warning stickers. It is essential that the nurse ensure that the patient is ventilated before giving an NMBD and double-check that an NMBD is not inadvertently given. In the event of an error, the patient would experience a horrendous death, because the mind is alert but the patient cannot speak or move. (See Preventing Medication Errors box.)

Snakes and plants played a role in the identification of the chemical structure of substances that cause paralysis and the discovery of related receptor proteins in animals and humans. The beginning steps involved study of the irreversible nerve transmission inhibition caused by toxins in the venoms of krait snake species and the venoms of certain varieties of cobra. *Curare,* a general term for various South American arrow poisons, has a long and intriguing history. It has been used for centuries by natives of the Amazon River region and other parts of South America to kill wild animals for food. Animals shot with arrows soaked in this plant substance normally die from paralysis of respiratory muscles. Once the receptor sites of action of these venoms and toxins were identified, pharmacologic drugs were developed that mimic these substances by causing muscle paralysis. Curare can be considered the grandfather of modern NMBDs. Numerous curare-like drugs are now used in clinical practice. The first drug derived from curare to be used medicinally was d-tubocurarine, which was introduced into anesthesia practice in 1940; it has now been replaced by newer drugs such as pancuronium. Pancuronium has a pharmacodynamic profile similar to that of curare but produces fewer adverse effects.

PREVENTING MEDICATION ERRORS

Neuromuscular Blocking Drugs

Neuromuscular blocking drugs are considered high-alert drugs, because improper use may lead to severe injury or death. The Institute for Safe Medication Practices has reported several cases of patient death or injury as a result of medication errors involving neuromuscular blocking drugs. Because these drugs paralyze the respiratory muscles, incorrect administration without sufficient ventilator support has resulted in patient deaths. There have been medication errors due to "sound-alike" drug names as well (e.g., vancomycin and vecuronium). Most facilities have followed recommendations to restrict access to these drugs, provide warning labels and reminders, and increase staff awareness of the dangers of these drugs.

For more information, visit *http://www.ismp.org/Newsletters/acutecare/articles/20050922.asp.*

Mechanism of Action and Drug Effects

Neuromuscular blocking drugs (NMBDs) are classified into two groups based on mechanism of action: depolarizing and nondepolarizing. Depolarizing NMBDs work similarly to the neurotransmitter acetylcholine (ACh). They bind in place of ACh to cholinergic receptors at the motor endplates of muscle nerves or neuromuscular junctions. Thus they are competitive agonists (see Chapter 2). There are two phases of depolarizing block. During phase I (depolarizing phase) the muscles fasciculate (twitch). Eventually, after continued depolarization has occurred, muscles are no longer responsive to the ACh released; thus muscle tone cannot be maintained and the muscle becomes paralyzed. This is phase II, or the desensitizing phase. Depolarizing NMBDs include d-tubocurarine and succinylcholine (see later). The duration of action of succinylcholine after a single dose to facilitate intubation is only about 5 to 9 minutes because of the rapid breakdown of the drug by cholinesterase, the enzyme responsible for metabolizing succinylcholine.

Nondepolarizing NMBDs also bind to ACh receptors at the neuromuscular junction, but instead of mimicking ACh, they block its usual actions. Therefore, these drugs are *competitive antagonists* (see Chapter 2) of ACh. Consequently, the nerve cell membrane is not depolarized, the muscle fibers are not stimulated, and skeletal muscle contraction does not occur. Nondepolarizing NMBDs include vecuronium and pancuronium and are typically classified into three groups based on their duration of action: short-acting, intermediate-acting, and long-acting drugs.

The typical time course of NMBD-induced paralysis during a surgical procedure is as follows: The first sensation that is typically felt is muscle weakness. This is usually followed by a total flaccid paralysis. Small, rapidly moving muscles such as those of the fingers and eyes are generally the first to be paralyzed. The next are those of the limbs, neck, and trunk. Finally, the intercostal muscles and the diaphragm are paralyzed, which causes respiratory arrest. The patient can no longer breathe on his or her own. It must be noted that NMBDs, when used alone, do *not* cause sedation or relieve pain or anxiety. Therefore, the patient should also receive appropriate medications to manage pain and/or anxiety. Neuromuscular blocking drugs temporarily inactivate the body's natural drive to control respirations. Recovery of muscular activity after discontinuation of anesthesia usually occurs in the reverse order of the paralysis, and thus the diaphragm is ordinarily the first to regain function.

Indications

The main therapeutic use of NMBDs is for maintaining skeletal muscle paralysis to facilitate controlled ventilation during surgical procedures. Shorter-acting NMBDs are often used to facilitate intubation with an endotracheal tube. This is commonly done for a variety of diagnostic procedures such as laryngoscopy, bronchoscopy, and esophagoscopy. When used for this purpose, NMBDs are frequently combined with anxiolytics, analgesics, and anesthetics. Additional nonsurgical applications include reduction of laryngeal or general muscle spasms, reduction of spasticity from tetanus and neurologic diseases such as multiple sclerosis, and prevention of bone fractures during electroconvulsive therapy (see Chapter 17). These drugs are also used for the diagnosis of *myasthenia gravis,* a disease characterized by chronic muscular weakness.

Contraindications

Contraindications to NMBDs include known drug allergy and also may include previous history of malignant hyperthermia, penetrating eye injuries, and narrow-angle glaucoma.

Adverse Effects

The muscle paralysis induced by depolarizing NMBDs (e.g., succinylcholine) is sometimes preceded by muscle spasms, which may damage muscles. These muscle spasms are termed *muscle fasciculations* and are most pronounced in the muscle groups of the hands, feet, and face. Injury to muscle cells may cause postoperative muscle pain and release potassium into the circulation, resulting in hyperkalemia, which is usually self-limiting and reversible. Small doses of nondepolarizing NMBDs are sometimes administered with succinylcholine to minimize these muscle fasciculations. In spite of these disadvantages, however, succinylcholine is still popular due to its rapid onset of action, its depth of neuromuscular blockade, and its short duration of action. For these reasons, it is often preferred to nondepolarizing NMBDs for *rapid-sequence induction* of anesthesia (e.g., for emergency

TABLE 12-7 Effects of Ganglionic Blockade by Neuromuscular Blocking Drugs

Site	Part of Nervous System Blocked	Physiologic Effect
Arterioles	Sympathetic	Vasodilation and hypotension
Veins	Sympathetic	Dilation
Heart	Parasympathetic	Tachycardia
Gastrointestinal tract	Parasympathetic	Reduced tone and tract motility; constipation
Urinary bladder	Parasympathetic	Urinary retention
Salivary glands	Parasympathetic	Dry mouth

intubation). In addition, one general anesthetic drug that helps alleviate this common but undesirable effect is the newer inhalational drug sevoflurane.

The effects on the cardiovascular system vary depending on the NMBD used and the individual patient. Increases and decreases in blood pressure and heart rate have been seen. Some NMBDs cause a release of histamine, which can result in bronchospasm, hypotension, and excessive bronchial and salivary secretion. The gastrointestinal tract is seldom affected by NMBDs. When it is affected, decreased tone and motility typically result, which can lead to constipation or even ileus.

The key to limiting adverse effects with most NMBDs is to use only enough of the drug to block the neuromuscular receptors. If too much is used, the risk is increased that other ganglionic receptors will be affected. Blockade of these other ganglionic receptors leads to most of the undesirable effects of NMBDs. The effects of ganglionic blockade in various areas of the body are listed in Table 12-7.

Nondepolarizing NMBDs have relatively few adverse effects when used appropriately. Their cardiovascular effects include blockade of autonomic ganglia resulting in hypotension, blockade of muscarinic receptors resulting in tachycardia, and release of histamine resulting in hypotension. However, use of the depolarizing drug succinylcholine has been associated with hyperkalemia, dysrhythmias, fasciculations, muscle pain, myoglobinuria, and increased intraocular, intragastric, and intracranial pressure, as well as *malignant hyperthermia* described earlier.

Toxicity and Management of Overdose

The primary concern when NMBDs are overdosed is prolonged paralysis requiring prolonged mechanical ventilation (see the Preventing Medication Errors box). Cardiovascular collapse may also be seen and is thought to be the result of histamine release. Multiple medical conditions can predispose an individual to toxicity. These conditions increase the sensitivity of the individual to NMBDs and prolong their effects. These predisposing conditions are listed in Box 12-4. Some conditions make it more difficult for NMBDs to work, and therefore higher doses of NMBDs are required in these cases. Although these conditions do not necessarily lead to toxicity or overdose, they are worthy of mention and are listed in Box 12-5.

Anticholinesterase drugs such as neostigmine, pyridostigmine, and edrophonium are antidotes and are used to reverse

---

BOX 12-4 Conditions That Predispose Patients to Toxic Effects from Neuromuscular Blocking Drugs

Acidosis
Amyotrophic lateral sclerosis
Hypermagnesemia
Hypocalcemia
Hypokalemia
Hypothermia
Myasthenia gravis
Myasthenic syndrome
Neonatal status
Neurofibromatosis
Paraplegia
Poliomyelitis

BOX 12-5 Conditions That Oppose the Effects of Neuromuscular Blocking Drugs

Cirrhosis with ascites
Clostridial infections
Hemiplegia
Hypercalcemia
Hyperkalemia
Peripheral nerve transection
Peripheral neuropathies
Thermal burns

BOX 12-6 Drugs That Interact with Neuromuscular Blocking Drugs

Additive Effects
Aminoglycosides
Calcium channel blockers
clindamycin
cyclophosphamide
cyclosporine
dantrolene
furosemide
Inhalation anesthetics
Local anesthetics
magnesium
polymyxin
procainamide
quinidine

Opposing Effects
carbamazepine
Corticosteroids
phenytoin

---

muscle paralysis. They work by preventing the enzyme cholinesterase from breaking down ACh. This causes ACh to build up at the motor endplate, and it eventually displaces the nondepolarizing NMBD molecule, returning the nerve to its original state. The dysmetabolic syndrome known as *malignant hyperthermia* (see the earlier section General Anesthetics) can also occur with NMBDs, especially succinylcholine.

Interactions

Many drugs interact with NMBDs, which may lead to either synergistic or opposing effects. Aminoglycoside antibiotics, when given with an NMBD, can have additive effects. The tetracycline antibiotics can also produce neuromuscular blockade, possibly by chelation of calcium, and calcium channel blockers have also been shown to enhance neuromuscular blockade. Other notable drugs that interact with NMBDs are listed in Box 12-6.

Dosages

For the recommended dosages of selected NMBDs, see the Dosages table on page 189.

DRUG PROFILES

Neuromuscular blocking drugs are one of the most commonly used classes of drugs in the operating room. They are given primarily with general anesthetics to facilitate endotracheal intubation and to relax skeletal muscles during surgery. In addition to their use in the operating room, they are given in the ICU to paralyze mechanically ventilated patients. As noted earlier, the two basic types of NMBDs are depolarizing and nondepolarizing drugs. Nondepolarizing NMBDs are generally classified by their duration

of action. Box 12-7 lists examples of currently used nondepolarizing drugs.

DEPOLARIZING NEUROMUSCULAR BLOCKING DRUGS
◆ **succinylcholine**
Succinylcholine is the only currently available drug in the *depolarizing* subclass of NMBDs. Succinylcholine (Anectine) has a structure similar to that of the parasympathetic neurotransmitter ACh. It stimulates the same neurons as ACh and produces the same physiologic responses initially. Compared to ACh, however, succinylcholine is metabolized more slowly. Because of this slower metabolism, succinylcholine subjects the motor endplate to ongoing depolarizing stimulation. Repolarization cannot occur. As long as sufficient succinylcholine concentrations are present, the muscle loses its ability to contract, and flaccid muscle paralysis results. Because of its quick onset of action, succinylcholine is most commonly used to facilitate endotracheal intubation. It is seldom used over long periods because of its tendency to cause muscular fasciculations. It is contraindicated in patients with personal or familial history of malignant hyperthermia, skeletal muscle myopathies, and known hypersensitivity to the drug. It is available only in injectable form. Typical dosages are given in the table on p. 189.

PHARMACOKINETICS

Route	Onset of Action	Peak Plasma Concentration	Elimination Half-life	Duration of Action
IV	Rapid, less than 1 min	60 sec	Less than 1 min	4-6 min

NONDEPOLARIZING NEUROMUSCULAR BLOCKING DRUGS
Nondepolarizing NMBDs are commonly used to facilitate endotracheal intubation, reduce muscle contraction in an area that needs surgery, and facilitate a variety of diagnostic procedures. They are often combined with anxiolytics or anesthetics. They may also be used to induce respiratory arrest in patients on mechanical ventilation.

pancuronium
Pancuronium (Pavulon) is a long-acting nondepolarizing NMBD. It is used as an adjunct to general anesthesia to facilitate endotracheal intubation and to provide skeletal muscle relaxation during

DOSAGES

Selected Neuromuscular Blocking Drugs

Drug	Pharmacologic Class	Usual Dosage Range	Indications/Uses
pancuronium (Pavulon)	Nondepolarizing NMBD (long acting)	**Adults, children, and infants over 1 month** IV: 60-100 mcg/kg **Neonates up to 1 month** Because neonates are very sensitive to nondepolarizing NMBDs, give a test dose of 20 mcg/kg IV	Intubation
		Adult IV: 0.04-0.1 mg/kg Continuous infusion: 0.1 mg/kg/hr	Mechanical ventilation
◆ succinylcholine (Anectine, Quelicin, others)	Depolarizing NMBD (short acting)	**Pediatric** IV: 1-2 mg/kg IM: 3-4 mg/kg	Intubation
		Adult IV: 0.3-1.1 mg/kg IM: 3-4 mg/kg	Mechanical ventilation
◆ vecuronium (Norcuron)	Nondepolarizing NMBD (intermediate acting)	**Pediatric** IV: 0.08-0.1 mg/kg	Intubation
		Adult IV: 0.08-0.1 mg/kg Continuous infusion: 0.1 mg/kg/hr	Mechanical ventilation

IM, Intramuscular; *IV,* intravenous; *NMBD,* neuromuscular blocking drug.

BOX 12-7 Classification of Nondepolarizing Neuromuscular Blocking Drugs

Short-Acting Drug
mivacurium (Mivacron)

Intermediate-Acting Drugs
atracurium (Tracrium)
rocuronium (Zemuron)
vecuronium (Norcuron)

Long-Acting Drugs
doxacurium (Nuromax)
pancuronium (Pavulon)
tubocurarine (dTC)

---

surgery or mechanical ventilation. It is most commonly employed for long surgical procedures that require prolonged muscle paralysis. Use of pancuronium is contraindicated in cases of known drug allergy. It is available only in injectable form. Typical dosages are given in the table on p. 189.

PHARMACOKINETICS

Route	Onset of Action	Peak Plasma Concentration	Elimination Half-life	Duration of Action
IV	3-5 min	5 min	100 min	45-60 min

◆ vecuronium
Vecuronium (Norcuron) is an intermediate-acting nondepolarizing NMBD. It is used as an adjunct to general anesthesia to facilitate tracheal intubation and to provide skeletal muscle relaxation during surgery or mechanical ventilation, and is one of the most commonly used NMBDs. Long-term use in the ICU setting has resulted in prolonged paralysis and subsequent difficulty weaning from mechanical ventilation. This is believed to be due to an active metabolite, 3-desacetyl vecuronium, which tends to accumulate

with prolonged use. Use of vecuronium is contraindicated in cases of known drug allergy. It is available only in injectable form. Recommended dosages are given in the table on p. 189.

PHARMACOKINETICS

Route	Onset of Action	Peak Plasma Concentration	Elimination Half-life	Duration of Action
IV	2.5-3 min	3-5 min	65-76 min	25-40 min

PHARMACOKINETIC BRIDGE to Nursing Practice

With moderate (conscious or procedural) sedation or anesthesia, it is always important to understand the pharmacokinetic properties of the drug(s) used. For example, the intravenous form of diazepam has an immediate onset of action, peak effect time of 8 minutes, duration of action of 15 to 30 minutes, and half-life of 20 to 60 hours. Half-life is the time it takes for 50% of the drug to be excreted from the body. Therefore, if diazepam is used for sedation or anesthesia, the drug could be present in the body and cause effects for up to 60 hours. In the care of patients receiving drugs for anesthesia, whether for conscious or moderate sedation or general or local anesthesia, these drug profile properties help the nurse to predict the drug's onset of action, peak effect, and duration of action.

NURSING PROCESS

Assessment

Associated with each drug used for general and local anesthesia are some broad as well as very specific assessment parameters. First, for any form of anesthesia and during any of the phases of anesthesia, the major parameters to assess are airway, breathing and circulation (ABCs). The assessment should also include questions regarding allergies and use of prescription drugs, over-the-counter drugs, herbals, supplements, and social and/or illegal drugs. Another important area to assess is the patient's use of alcohol and nicotine. Excessive use of alcohol may alter the patient's response to general anesthesia, especially if there is liver impairment. Also, if the patient has a history of alcohol abuse, withdrawal symptoms may occur during the recovery from anesthesia and/or surgery. Respiratory assessment (e.g., respiratory rate, rhythm, and depth; breath sounds; oxygen saturation level) is needed, especially if the patient has a history of smoking or is currently a smoker. The patient's history of smoking is important because nicotine has a paralyzing effect on the cilia within the respiratory tract. Once they are malfunctioning, these cilia cannot perform their main function of keeping foreign bodies out of the lungs and allowing mucus and secretions to be coughed up with ease. Malfunctioning of the cilia can potentially lead to atelectasis or pneumonia. Other objective data include weight and height, because these parameters are often used in the dosing of anesthesia. Other studies that may be ordered by the anesthesiologist and/or surgeon include an electrocardiogram, chest radiograph, and tests of renal function (e.g., BUN level, creatinine level, urinalysis with specific gravity) and hepatic function (e.g., total protein and albumin levels; bilirubin level; ALP, AST, and ALT levels). Additional laboratory tests may include hgb, hct, WBC with differential, and tests that indicate clotting abilities, such as prothrombin time, partial thromboplastin time, and platelet count. Results of tests for serum electrolytes, specifically potassium, sodium, chloride, phosphorus, magnesium, and calcium, are also important to assess before anesthesia, because abnormalities may lead to further complications from the anesthesia. Results of a pregnancy test in females of childbearing age, if ordered, should also be assessed because of the possibility of teratogenic effects (adverse effects on the fetus) related to the anesthetic drug.

Neurologic assessment should include a thorough survey of the patient's mental status. Level of consciousness, alertness, and orientation to person, place, and time are important to determine and document prior to the anesthesia. Additional neurologic assessment should include motor assessments, with left-right and upper extremity versus lower extremity comparisons of strength, reflexes, grasp, and ability to move on command. Sensory assessment focuses the same anatomical areas, with comparisons of the response to various types of stimuli such as sharp, dull, soft, and cold versus warm. Swallowing ability and gag reflexes are also important to assess and document for baseline status and comparisons. When these motor, sensory, and cognitive parameters are within normal limits, there is proof of an intact neurologic system.

One very significant reaction to assess for in patients receiving general anesthesia is that of malignant hyperthermia. This is a rapid progression of hyperthermia that may be fatal if not promptly recognized and aggressively treated. The tendency is inherited, so questions about related signs and symptoms in the family's and patient's medical histories are important to document and report. A familial history of malignant hyperthermia would put the patient at risk. Signs and symptoms of malignant hyperthermia include a rapid rise in body temperature, tachycardia, tachypnea, muscle rigidity, cyanosis, irregular heartbeat, mottling of the skin, diaphoresis (profuse sweating), and an unstable blood pressure. If there is no documented problem with

CASE STUDY

Moderate (Conscious) Sedation

A 53-year-old woman is scheduled to have a colonoscopy this morning, and she is very anxious. The nurse anesthetist has explained the moderate (conscious) sedation that is planned, but the patient says after the anesthetist leaves the room, "I'm so afraid of feeling it during the test. Why don't they just put me to sleep?"

© Vgstudio

1. How does moderate sedation differ from general anesthesia?
2. What is the nurse's best answer to the patient's question?
3. What is important for the nurse to assess before this procedure is performed?

For answers, see *http://evolve.elsevier.Lilley.*

general anesthesia or if the patient is undergoing general anesthesia for the first time, it is important to perform an astute and careful examination of all medical and medication histories. With any type of anesthesia, it is often very slight changes in vital signs, other vital parameters, and laboratory test results that may provide nursing and other health care providers with a possible clue to the patient's reaction to anesthesia. Note that malignant hyperthermia occurs during the anesthesia process and in the surgical suite; nevertheless, close observation after anesthesia is still important and much needed. Intravenously administered anesthetic drugs are usually combined with adjuvant drugs (given at the same time) such as sedatives-hypnotics, antianxiety drugs, opioid and nonopioid analgesics, antiemetics, and anticholinergics. These drugs are used to decrease some of the undesirable aftereffects of inhaled anesthetics. If they are used, a complete assessment should be performed for each of the drugs, including obtaining a medical history and medication profile. Liver and kidney function studies are important in these patients as well, so that any risks of toxicity and complications can be anticipated.

For patients about to undergo anesthesia with *NMBDs*, a complete head-to-toe assessment should be performed with a thorough medical and medication history. Which specific drug is being used and whether it is depolarizing or nondepolarizing will guide nursing assessment, because of the action of NMBDs on the patient's neuromuscular functioning (see pharmacology discussion). All cautions, contraindications, and drug interactions must also be assessed. Another concern with the use of these drugs is that they are associated with an increase in intraocular pressure and intracranial pressure. Therefore, these anesthetic drugs should not be used or used with extreme caution (close monitoring of these pressures) in patients with glaucoma or closed head injuries. Patients receiving NMBDs should also receive a thorough respiratory assessment because of the effect of these drugs on the respiratory system. In particular, these drugs have a paralyzing effect on the muscles used for breathing and—for this very reason—are used to facilitate intubation for mechanical ventilation. Paralysis of respiratory muscles allows patient relaxation to the point where the patient will not fight against the breaths delivered by the ventilator. Also indicated with the use of NMBDs is careful assessment of serum electrolyte levels, specifically potassium and magnesium levels. Imbalances in these electrolytes may lead to increased action of the NMBD with exacerbation of the drug's actions and toxic effects. Allergic reactions to these drugs are most commonly characterized by rash, fever, respiratory distress, and pruritus. Drug interactions with herbal products are outlined in the Herbal Therapies and Dietary Supplements box. For more specific information on the differences between depolarizing and nondepolarizing NMBDs, see the pharmacology section of this chapter.

With the use of conscious or moderate sedation, as with any anesthesia technique, assessment for allergies, cautions, contraindications, and drug interactions is important. Because moderate sedation is commonly used across the life span, there should be close assessment of organ function and notation of diseases or conditions that could lead to excessive levels of the drug in the body, such as liver or kidney impairment. See Chapters 11 and 13 for more information about the assessment associated with the use of opioids and sedatives-hypnotics.

Use of spinal anesthesia requires thorough assessment with an emphasis on the ABCs, respiratory function, and vital signs, specifically blood pressure. Baseline respirations with attention to rate, rhythm, depth, and breath sounds are important to note, as are oxygen saturation levels obtained via pulse oximetry. Because of possible problems with vasodilatation from the spinal anesthetic, baseline blood pressure levels and pulse rate should also be documented. History of previous reactions to this form of anesthesia, allergies, and a listing of all medications should be recorded, and any abnormal reactions should be reported to the anesthesiologist and surgeon. Neurologic assessment with notation of sensory and motor intactness in the lower extremities, as well as documentation of any abnormalities, are important. The use of epidural anesthesia requires special attention to overall hemostasis through monitoring of vital signs and oxygen saturation levels. Baseline sensory and motor function in the extremities are important to assess, and an intact neurologic system should be documented (see nursing interventions for more detailed discussion). Spinal headaches may occur with either spinal anesthesia or epidural injections, and thus baseline assessment for the presence of headaches is important.

Local-topical anesthetics, such as lidocaine, used for either infiltration or nerve block anesthesia may be administered with or without a vasoconstrictor (e.g., epinephrine). The vasoconstrictors are used to help confine the local anesthetic to the injected area, prevent systemic absorption of the anesthetic, and reduce bleeding. If there is systemic absorption of the vasoconstrictor into the bloodstream, the patient's blood pressure could elevate to life-threatening levels, especially in patients who are at high risk (e.g., those with underlying arterial disease). Therefore, it is important to review the patient's medical history to assess for any preexisting illnesses, such as vascular disease, aneurysms, or hypertension, because these may be contraindications to the use of the vasoconstrictor with the anesthetic. In addition, with these local anesthetics, allergies to the drug as well as baseline vital signs should be assessed. Assessment for possible drug interactions should also occur, and prescription medications, herbal products, supplements, and over-the-counter medications should be noted. In summary, it is important with any type of anesthesia to assess the patient's level of homeostasis prior to actual administration of the drug. This assessment may include taking vital signs as well as checking the ABCs. Other parameters of interest may be oxygen saturation levels measured by pulse oximetry, cardiovascular and respiratory function and neurologic function.

Nursing Diagnoses

- Acute pain related to the adverse effect of spinal headache from epidural anesthesia
- Impaired gas exchange related to the general anesthetic's CNS depressant effect with altered respiratory rate and effort (decreased rate, decreased depth)
- Decreased cardiac output related to the systemic effects of anesthesia
- Risk for injury related to the impact of any form of anesthesia on the CNS (e.g., decreased sensorium)
- Deficient knowledge related to lack of information about anesthesia

Planning
Goals

- Patient states measures to help prevent adverse effect of spinal headache.
- Patient states the action and adverse effects of anesthesia, including decreased sensorium.
- Patient states the potential complications of anesthesia involving the respiratory and cardiac systems.
- Patient describes what to expect before, during, and after administration of anesthesia.
- Patient complies with postanesthesia care regimen to help with a healthy recovery.
- Patient follows instructions regarding preanesthesia and postanesthesia care.

Outcome Criteria

- Patient remains free of spinal headache after hydration with fluids and bed rest for 24 to 48 hours after epidural procedure.
- Patient experiences maximal effects of anesthesia with mini-

mal to no adverse effects such as respiratory and/or myocardial depression.

- Patient remains free of injury and/or falls during the preanesthesia period and throughout the postanesthesia period.
- Patient remains calm and experiences minimal anxiety as a result of adequate education.

Implementation

Regardless of the type of anesthesia used, one of the most important nursing considerations during the preanesthesia, intraanesthesia, and postanesthesia periods is close and frequent observation of all body systems. Specific attention begins with a focus on the ABCs of nursing care, vital signs, and oxygen saturation levels as measured by pulse oximetry. The observations from these interventions should be documented and the interventions repeated as needed, depending on the patient's status and in keeping with the standard of care for the type of anesthesia. Vital signs should be monitored frequently, and as needed, based on the patient's condition, including assessment of the fifth vital sign of pain (see discussion later in this section).

For patients undergoing general anesthesia, assessing the patient's temperature is especially important because of the risk of malignant hyperthermia, and close monitoring is required if malignant hyperthermia occurred during the anesthesia process. This sudden elevation in the patient's body temperature (e.g., higher than 104° F [40° C]) not only requires critical care during and immediately after anesthesia but also calls for close monitoring even during regular postoperative care (see earlier discussion). When intravenous, inhaled, or other forms of anesthesia are used, resuscitative equipment and medications, including opioid antidotes, are readily available in the surgical and postsurgical areas in case of cardiorespiratory distress or arrest. The anesthesiologist is the one who keeps control of the anesthetic drug, and he or she is well prepared for any emergency—as is the entire group of individuals in the surgical suite as well as in the postanesthesia recovery area. Continual monitoring of the status of breath sounds is an important intervention, because hypoventilation may be a complication of general and other forms of anesthesia. Oxygen is administered after a patient has received general and/or other forms of anesthesia to compensate for the respiratory depression that may have occurred during the anesthesia and surgical process. Because oxygen is a drug, a doctor's order is needed for its administration. Continuous monitoring of oxygen saturation levels is therefore an important intervention. In addition, hypotension and orthostatic hypotension are possible problems after anesthesia, so postural blood pressure measurements (supine and standing), in addition to regular blood pressure monitoring, may be needed. Additional nursing interventions may include monitoring of neurologic parameters such as reflexes, response to commands, level of consciousness or sedation, and pupil reaction to light. Monitoring for changes in sensation and movement in the extremities, distal pulses, temperature, and color should be part of the nursing care plan when nerve blocks and spinal anesthesia are used, because it is important to confirm that areas distal to the anesthetic site have remained intact.

Should the patient require pain management once the anesthesia has been terminated, the nurse must remember that the anesthetic and any adjuvant drugs used continue to have an effect on the patient until the period of the drugs' action has passed. There-

fore, administration of sedatives-hypnotics, opioids, nonopioids, and other CNS depressants for pain relief should be done cautiously and only with close monitoring of vital signs. If the patient has received some of these medications during postanesthesia, dosages of drugs used should be documented and then passed on during a report whenever the patient is transferred to another unit. Additional orders are usually provided by the physician/surgeon or anesthesiologist regarding doses of analgesics to administer once the patient has been transferred. If such orders have not been provided, however, and the patient is experiencing pain, the appropriate prescriber should be contacted. The concern here is that the patient will receive either too much or not enough analgesic.

Patients who receive *NMBDs* as part of an induction process for mechanical ventilation need to be monitored closely during and after initiation of mechanical ventilation. These patients are in intensive care or critical care units, and many protocols are provided regarding interventions after the intubation. These include measurement of vital signs and determination of neurologic status, including sensation and hand grasp strength. When mechanical ventilation is used, patients and family members need to be educated about the purpose of the paralysis (to prevent fighting against the ventilation provided by the machine) and informed that the patient can still hear the spoken word. Knowing what to expect is key to helping decrease fears and anxiety—for both the patient and those visiting the patient.

Patients undergoing moderate sedation as the method of anesthesia should receive patient education before and after the procedure. As noted earlier, recovery from this type of anesthesia is more rapid and the safety profile is better than that of general anesthesia, with its inherent cardiorespiratory risks. As with general anesthesia, however, the nurse should monitor the ABCs, vital signs, pulse oximetry oxygen saturation levels, and level of consciousness or sedation. See Box 12-8 for more information on conscious sedation.

With spinal anesthesia, nursing interventions should include constant monitoring for a return of sensation and motor activity below the anesthetic insertion site. Because of the risk that the anesthetic drug may move upward in the spinal cord and breathing may be affected, respiratory and breathing status should be continually monitored. In addition, because positioning is important to the movement of the anesthetic drug, the head of the bed should remain elevated. The nurse should remember, though, that this complication is usually identified and treated by the anesthesiologist, and patients will not return to their rooms on a nursing unit until all respiratory risks are identified and managed appropriately. Another major area of concern with spinal anesthesia is the risk for a sudden decrease in blood pressure. This drop in blood pressure is secondary to vasodilation caused by the anesthetic block to the sympathetic vasomotor nerves. Vital signs and oxygen saturation levels should return to normal before the patient is transferred out of postanesthesia care; however, these vital signs should continue to be monitored frequently after transfer. Another adverse reaction to intraspinal anesthesia is the occurrence of spinal headaches. These may occur with both intrathecal and epidural injections but are actually more frequent with the latter. Because intrathecal spinal needle designs have been technologically improved, the occurrence of spinal headaches administration is rare. Larger-bore needles are used to deliver epidural anesthetics, however, and these are more likely to

---

BOX 12-8 Moderate or Conscious Sedation: What to Expect and Questions to Ask

What questions should the patient or caregiver ask about the technique of moderate or conscious sedation?
- Who will be providing this type of anesthesia?
- Who will be monitoring me or my loved one?
- Will there be constant monitoring of blood pressure, pulse rate, respiratory rate, and temperature?
- Will there be emergency equipment in the room, in case of need?
- Are the personnel qualified to administer these drugs? To administer advanced cardiac life support?
- What do I need to know about care at home? Will I need help? Can I drive after having the procedure?

What are the adverse effects of moderate or conscious sedation?
- Brief periods of amnesia (loss of memory)
- Headache
- Hangover
- Nausea and vomiting

What should be expected immediately following the procedure?
- Frequent monitoring
- Written postoperative instructions and care
- If the patient is of driving age, no driving for at least 24 hours after undergoing moderate sedation
- A follow-up contact by phone to check on the patient

Who can administer the conscious sedation?
- Moderate or conscious sedation is safe when administered by qualified providers. Certified registered nurse anesthetists, anesthesiologists, other physicians, dentists, and oral surgeons are qualified to administer conscious sedation.

Which procedures generally require moderate sedation?
- Breast biopsy
- Vasectomy
- Minor foot surgery
- Minor bone fracture repair
- Plastic or reconstructive surgery
- Dental prosthetic or reconstructive surgery
- Endoscopy (such as diagnostic studies and treatment of stomach, colon, and bladder cancer)

What are the overall benefits of this type of anesthesia?
- It is a safe and effective option for patients undergoing minor surgeries or diagnostic procedures.
- It allows patients to recover quickly and resume normal activities in a relatively short period of time.

Data from American Association of Nurse Anesthetists: Conscious sedation: what patients should expect, 2005, available at *http://www.aana.com.*

BOX 12-9 Spinal Headaches: A Brief Look at a Terrible Pain!

Why do spinal headaches occur? As a result of penetration into and through the dura mater of the spinal cord (the covering of the spinal cord), a leakage of cerebrospinal fluid occurs from the insertion site. If enough of the spinal fluid leaks out, a spinal headache results. These headaches are more likely to be associated with epidural anesthesia than with intrathecal anesthesia because of the larger needles used with epidurals.

What are the symptoms of a spinal headache? Patients say that these headaches are worse than any other type! They are more severe when the patient is in an upright position and improve upon lying down. They may occur up to 5 days after the procedure and may be prevented with bed rest after the epidural procedure.

How are spinal headaches treated? Adequate hydration using intravenous fluids is often tried to help increase cerebral spinal fluid pressure. Another possible treatment is drinking a beverage high in caffeine, and strict bed rest for 24 to 48 hours is recommended. If the headaches are intolerable, however, the anesthesiologist may create a "blood patch" to help close up the leak. This requires insertion of a needle into the same space or very close to the area that was injected with the anesthesia. A small amount of blood is taken from the patient and injected into the epidural space, which closes the leak with a clot in the blood. A seal is formed and the headache relieved.

Data from Brenman EK (editor): Pain management: spinal headaches, 2007, available at *http://www.WebMD.com.*

give rise to spinal headache if they are inadvertently passed through the dura mater (the covering of the spinal cord). The patient should be kept hydrated and on bed rest as recommended by the anesthesiologist. See Box 12-9 for more information about these headaches and their treatment.

The use of epidural anesthesia (also called *regional anesthesia* in some textbooks) does not pose the same risk of respiratory complications, but monitoring is still needed to confirm overall homeostasis, such as measurement of vital signs and pulse oximetry to determine oxygen saturation levels. In addition, patients undergoing this form of anesthesia require monitoring for the return of motor function and tactile sensation. The patient should be checked frequently for the return of sensation bilaterally along the dermatome (area of the skin innervated by specific segments of the spinal cord); such monitoring is important to ensure patient safety as well as to maximize comfort. Touch sensation may be assessed through hand pressure or a gentle pinch of the skin. The nurse needs to know the level at which the epidural anesthesia was given to monitor properly for return of sensation. This monitoring process generally occurs in a postanesthesia care unit, and the patient is not returned to a regular nursing unit until all sensation and/or voluntary movement of the lower extremities is regained.

With regard to the use of *topical or local anesthetics* (e.g., lidocaine with or without epinephrine), solutions that are not clear and appear cloudy or discolored should not be used. Some anesthesiologists mix the solution with sodium bicarbonate to minimize local pain during infiltration, but this also causes a more rapid onset of action and a longer duration of sensory analgesia. If an anesthetic ointment or cream is used, the nurse should thoroughly cleanse and dry the area to be anesthetized before application of the drug. If a topical or local anesthetic is being used in the nose or throat, the nurse must remember that it may cause paralysis and/or numbness of the structures of the upper respiratory tract, which can lead to aspiration. If the patient receives a solution form of anesthetic, exact amounts of the drug should be used and at the exact dosing times or intervals. Local anesthetics are not to be swallowed unless the prescriber has so instructed. Should this occur, the nurse must closely observe the patient, check for the gag reflex, and expect to withhold food or drink until the patient's sensation and/or gag reflex has returned.

Once the patient has recovered from the anesthesia and procedure and is ready for discharge, patient teaching must be completed. Patient education should focus on what the patient's needs are and how these needs can be met at home. Home health care and/or rehabilitation services may be indicated, and arrangements should be made before the patient is discharged. If additional care or resources are needed at home, such as for a patient who lives alone, these arrangements should be completed in a timely fashion. Some examples of procedures for which help might be needed are wound care, dressing changes, surgical site care, drawing of blood for laboratory studies, and administration of various medications through the intravenous, intramuscular, or subcutaneous route. Some patients may also need assistance with taking oral medications at home. Pain management requires thorough and individualized patient teaching and also includes any necessary education for patients who will require home health care. See Chapter 11 for more information on analgesics. Simple instructions should be provided using age-appropriate teaching strategies (see Chapter 7). Sharing of information about community resources is also important, especially for those patients who need transportation, assistance with meals, housekeeping during recovery, and/or the services of additional health care providers (e.g., physical therapists, occupational therapists) in the home setting. Some of these community resources may be agencies that are supported by city or state social service programs. Meals on Wheels, senior citizen support groups, and church-sponsored groups are just a few examples of important resource groups. Many of these resources are free or have income-based fees. Additional suggestions regarding patient education are provided in Patient Teaching Tips.

Evaluation

The therapeutic effects of any general or local anesthetic include the following: loss of consciousness and reflexes during general anesthesia and loss of sensation to a particular area during local anesthesia (e.g., loss of sensation to the eye during corneal transplantation). The patient who has undergone general anesthesia should be constantly monitored for the occurrence of adverse effects of the anesthesia. These may include myocardial depression, convulsions, respiratory depression, allergic rhinitis, and decreased renal or liver function. Patients who have received a local anesthetic also need to be constantly monitored for the occurrence of adverse effects, including bradycardia, myocardial depression, hypotension, and dysrhythmias. In addition, as mentioned earlier in this chapter, significant overdoses of local anesthetic drugs or direct injection into a blood vessel may result in cardiovascular collapse or cardiac or respiratory depression. For those receiving spinal anesthesia, therapeutic effects include loss of sensation below the area of administration, and adverse effects includes hypotension, hypoventilation, urinary retention, the possibility of a prolonged period of decreased sensation or motor ability, and infection at the site. With epidural anesthesia, therapeutic effects are similar to those seen with intrathecal anesthesia; however, adverse effects include possible spinal headache (often severe) and/or loss of motor function or sensation below the area of administration. Moderate sedation provides the therapeutic effect of a decreased sensorium but without the complications of general anesthesia; however, there are CNS depressant effects associated with the drugs used.

PATIENT TEACHING TIPS

- Whenever general anesthesia is used, the prescriber's recommendations/orders about whether any medications should be discontinued or tapered before anesthetic administration should be emphasized.
- Make sure information about the anesthetic, route of administration, adverse effects, and special precautions is included in preprocedure and surgical educations.
- All fears and anxieties about anesthesia and related procedures/surgery should be discussed openly.
- Share with the patient and family instructions about the postanesthesia process and the need for close monitoring of vital signs, breath sounds, and neurologic intactness. Patients should expect frequent turning, coughing, and deep breathing to prevent atelectasis or pneumonia.
- Encourage patients to ambulate with assistance as needed and as ordered. Mobility helps increase circulation and improve ventilation to the alveoli of the lungs; consequently, circulation to the legs will be improved (which helps to prevent stasis of blood and possible blood clot formation in the leg veins). Assistance is needed to prevent falls or injury until recovery from the anesthetic.
- The patient should be encouraged to request pain medication, if needed, before pain becomes moderate to severe. The patient should be informed that, even though anesthesia has been administered, there may still be discomfort or pain from the procedure or surgery. The anesthesia will wear off, and adequate analgesia needed. The patient should be asked to rate his or her pain on a scale of 0 to 10, with 0 being no pain and 10 being the worst possible pain. See Chapter 11 for more information on assessment of pain and its management.
- The rationale for any other treatments or procedures related to the anesthesia (such as epidural catheter placement; delivery of oxygen; administration of a gas; use of various tubes, catheters, or intravenous lines) should be explained. Adequate patient education will help ease fears and anxieties and help in preventing adverse effects of complications.
- For a patient with diminished sensorium, the bed side rails should be up and a call button at the bedside. These actions are critical to patient safety. Note that bed alarms may be used instead of side rails. Everyone involved in the postanesthesia and postsurgical care (e.g., family members) should be educated about these safety measures.
- If appropriate, patients receiving NMBDs for mechanical ventilation should know that, although they may not be able to move due to the paralyzing effects of the drugs, they will still be able to hear. Being in this condition is extremely frightening, even with the most thorough patient education.
- With local anesthesia, the patient should understand the purpose and action of the local anesthetic as well as adverse effects.
- A patient receiving spinal anesthesia should be informed about the need for frequent assessments, measurement of vital signs, and system assessments during and after the procedure.

NCLEX EXAMINATION REVIEW QUESTIONS

1 A patient is in the hospital for removal of a lymph node from his arm under local anesthesia. The physician has requested "lidocaine *with* epinephrine." The nurse recognizes that the most important reason for adding epinephrine is that it
  a helps to calm the patient before the procedure.
  b minimizes the risk of an allergic reaction.
  c enhances the effect of the local lidocaine.
  d reduces bleeding in the surgical area.

2 The surgical nurse is reviewing operative cases scheduled for the day. Which of the following patients is more prone to complications from general anesthesia?
  a A 79-year-old female who is about to have her gallbladder removed
  b A 49-year-old male athlete who quit heavy smoking 12 years ago
  c A 30-year-old female who is in perfect health but has never had anesthesia
  d A 50-year-old female scheduled for outpatient laser surgery for vision correction

3 Which nursing diagnosis is possible for a patient who has been under general anesthesia for 3 to 4 hours during surgery?
  a Decreased urine output from use of vasopressors as anesthetics
  b Increased cardiac output related to the effects of general anesthesia
  c Risk for injury (fall) related to decreased sensorium for 2 to 4 days postoperatively
  d Decreased gaseous exchange due to the CNS depressant effect of general anesthesia

4 A patient is recovering from general anesthesia. What is the nurse's main concern during the immediate postoperative period?
  a Airway
  b Pupillary reflexes
  c Return of sensations
  d Level of consciousness

5 A patient is recovering from surgery during which he received an NMBD. As he wakes up during recovery, he looks as if he is panicking and yet is unable to speak. What is the best action by the nurse at this time?
  a Call the anesthesia department for reintubation because of an impaired airway
  b Reassure the patient that he is recovering and that the medication is still wearing off
  c Readminister the NMBD to help the patient calm down
  d Increase oxygen administration and monitor oxygenation

6 The nurse is administering an NMBD to a patient during a surgical procedure. Number the following phases of muscle paralysis in the order in which the patient will experience them. (Number 1 is the first step.)
  a Paralysis of intercostals and diaphragm muscles
  b Muscle weakness
  c Paralysis of muscles of the limbs, neck, and trunk
  d Paralysis of small rapidly moving muscles (fingers, eye)

1. d, 2. a, 3. d, 4. a, 5. b, 6. a = 4, b = 1, c = 3, d = 2.

CRITICAL THINKING ACTIVITIES: BEST ACTION

1 The nurse is monitoring a patient in the postanesthesia care unit. The patient had a colectomy with formation of a colostomy because of colon cancer. During this time, what is the primary focus of the nurse's assessment of the patient?

2 The nurse on the orthopedic surgery unit is monitoring the vital signs of a patient who had hip replacement surgery 2 hours earlier. At this time, the certified nursing assistant reports that the patient's temperature has changed from 98.9° F (37.2° C) to 104.8° F (40.4° C). Another nurse comments that the patient must be developing an infection from the hip replacement. What should the nurse do next?

3 The nurse is assessing a patient who is receiving mechanical ventilation because of respiratory problems. The patient's wife is visiting and asks the nurse, "He's awake but he can't move. Why is that?" What would be the nurse's best answer?

For answers, see *http://evolve.elsevier.Lilley.*

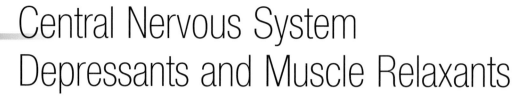

CHAPTER **13**

Central Nervous System Depressants and Muscle Relaxants

OBJECTIVES

When you reach the end of this chapter, you should be able to do the following:

1 Briefly describe the functions of the central nervous system.

2 Contrast the effects of central nervous system depressant drugs and central nervous system stimulant drugs (see Chapter 14) as relates to their basic actions.

3 Define the terms hypnotics, rapid eye movements, rapid eye movement sleep interference, rapid eye movement rebound, sedatives, sedatives-hypnotics, sleep, and therapeutic index.

4 Briefly discuss the problem of sleep disorders.

5 Identify the specific drugs within each of the following category of central nervous system depressant drugs: benzodiazepines, nonbenzodiazepines, muscle relaxants, and miscellaneous drugs.

6 Contrast the mechanism of action, indications, adverse effects, toxic effects, cautions, contraindications, dosage forms, routes of administration, and drug interactions of the following medications: benzodiazepines, nonbenzodiazepines, muscle relaxants, and miscellaneous drugs.

7 Discuss the nursing process as it relates to the nursing care of a patient receiving any central nervous system depressants and/or muscle relaxant.

8 Develop a thorough nursing care plan related to the use of pharmacologic and nonpharmacologic approaches to the treatment of sleep disorders.

e-Learning Activities

http://evolve.elsevier.com/Lilley

NCLEX Review Questions • Animations • Nursing Care Plans • Audio Glossary • Category Catchers • Medication Errors Checklists • IV Therapy Checklists • Calculators • Frequently Asked Questions • Content Updates • SupplementalResources • Answers to Case Studies and Critical Thinking Activities

Drug Profiles

◆ baclofen, p. 205
◆ cyclobenzaprine, p. 205
diazepam, p. 200
eszopiclone, p. 200
midazolam, p. 200
pentobarbital, p. 202

phenobarbital, p. 203
ramelteon, p. 201
◆ temazepam, p. 200
◆ zaleplon, p. 200
◆ zolpidem, p. 200

◆ *Key drug.*

Glossary

Barbiturates A class of drugs that are chemical derivatives of barbituric acid. They can induce sedation and sleep. (p. 201)
Benzodiazepines A chemical category of drugs most frequently prescribed as sedative-hypnotic and anxiolytic drugs. (p. 197)
Gamma-aminobutyric acid (GABA) An inhibitory neurotransmitter found in the brain. (p. 198)

Hypnotics Drugs that, when given at low to moderate dosages, calm or soothe the central nervous system (CNS) without inducing sleep but when given at high dosages do cause sleep. (p. 197)
Non–rapid eye movement (non-REM) sleep The largest portion of the sleep cycle. It characteristically has four stages and precedes REM sleep. Most of a normal sleep cycle consists of non-REM sleep. (p. 197)
Rapid eye movement (REM) sleep One of the stages of the sleep cycle. Some of the characteristics of REM sleep are rapid movement of the eyes, vivid dreams, and irregular breathing. (p. 197)
REM interference A drug-induced reduction of REM sleep time. (p. 197)
REM rebound Excessive REM sleep following discontinuation of a sleep-altering drug. (p. 197)
Sedatives Drugs that have an inhibitory effect on the CNS to the degree that they reduce nervousness, excitability, and irritability without causing sleep. (p. 197)
Sedatives-hypnotics Drugs that can act in the body either as sedatives or as hypnotics. (p. 197)
Sleep A transient, reversible, and periodic state of rest in which there is a decrease in physical activity and consciousness. (p. 197)
Sleep architecture The structure of the various elements involved in the sleep cycle, including normal and abnormal patterns of sleep. (p. 197)
Therapeutic index The ratio between the toxic and therapeutic concentrations of a drug. If the index is low, the difference between the therapeutic and toxic drug concentrations is small, and use of the drug is more hazardous. (p. 201)

• • •

196

Anatomy, Physiology, and Disease Overview

Drugs that have a calming effect or that depress the central nervous system (CNS) are referred to as *sedatives* and *hypnotics*. A drug is classified as either a sedative or a hypnotic drug depending on the degree to which it inhibits the transmission of nerve impulses to the CNS. **Sedatives** reduce nervousness, excitability, and irritability without causing sleep, but a sedative can become a hypnotic if it is given in large enough doses. **Hypnotics** cause sleep and have a much more potent effect on the CNS than do sedatives. Many drugs can act in the body as either a sedative or a hypnotic, depending on dose and patient responsiveness, and for this reason are called sedatives-hypnotics. **Sedatives-hypnotics** can be classified chemically into three main groups: barbiturates, benzodiazepines, and miscellaneous drugs.

PHYSIOLOGY OF SLEEP

Sleep is defined as a transient, reversible, and periodic state of rest in which there is a decrease in physical activity and consciousness. Normal sleep is cyclic and repetitive, and a person's responses to sensory stimuli are markedly reduced during sleep. During waking hours the body is bombarded with stimuli that provoke the senses of sight, hearing, touch, smell, and taste. These stimuli elicit voluntary and involuntary movements or functions. During sleep a person is no longer aware of the sensory stimuli within his or her immediate environment.

Sleep research involves study of the patterns of sleep, or what is sometimes referred to as **sleep architecture.** The architecture of sleep consists of two basic elements that occur cyclically: **rapid eye movement (REM) sleep** and **non–rapid eye movement (non-REM) sleep.** The normal cyclic progression of the stages of sleep is summarized in Table 13-1. Various sedative-hypnotic drugs affect different stages of the normal sleep pattern. If usage is prolonged, emotional and psychologic changes can occur. Prolonged sedative-hypnotic use may reduce the cumulative amount of REM sleep; this is known as **REM interference.** This can result in daytime fatigue, because REM sleep provides a certain component of the "restfulness" of sleep. On discontinuance of a sedative-hypnotic drug, **REM rebound** can occur in which the patient has an abnormally large amount of REM sleep, often leading to frequent and vivid dreams. Abuse of sedative-hypnotic drugs is common and is discussed in Chapter 9.

Pharmacology Overview

BENZODIAZEPINES AND MISCELLANEOUS HYPNOTIC DRUGS

Benzodiazepines used to be the most commonly prescribed sedative-hypnotic drugs; however, the nonbenzodiazepine drugs are now the most frequently used. The benzodiazepines show favorable adverse effect profiles, efficacy, and safety. Benzodiazepines are classified as either sedatives-hypnotics or anxiolytics depending on their primary usage. Anxiolytic drugs are used to reduce the intensity of feelings of anxiety. However, any of these drugs can function along a continuum as a sedative and/or hyp-

notic and/or anxiolytic depending on the dosage and patient sensitivity to drug action. The anxiolytic use of benzodiazepines is discussed further in Chapter 17. There are five benzodiazepines commonly used as sedative-hypnotic drugs. In addition, there are several miscellaneous drugs that are used primarily as hypnotics. They function much like benzodiazepines but are chemically distinct from them. All are listed in Table 13-2. One new hypnotic drug is ramelteon. It has a new mechanism of action and is profiled separately later in this chapter.

TABLE 13-1 Stages of Sleep

Stage	Characteristics	Average Percentage of Time in Stage (for Young Adult)
Non-REM Sleep		
1	Dozing or feelings of drifting off to sleep; person can be easily awakened; insomniacs have longer stage 1 periods than normal.	2%-5%
2	Relaxation, but person can easily be awakened; person has occasional REMs and also slight eye movements.	50%
3	Deep sleep; difficult to wake person; respiratory rates, pulse, and blood pressure may decrease.	5%
4	Very difficult to wake person; person may be very groggy if awakened; dreaming occurs, especially about daily events; sleepwalking or bedwetting may occur.	10%-15%
REM Sleep		
	REMs occur; vivid dreams occur; breathing may be irregular.	25%-33%

Modified from McKenry LM, Tessier E, Hogan MA: *Mosby's pharmacology in nursing,* ed 22, St Louis, 2006, Mosby.
REM, Rapid eye movement.

TABLE 13-2 Sedative-Hypnotic Benzodiazepines and Miscellaneous Drugs

Generic Name	Trade Name
Long Acting	
diazepam	Valium
estazolam	ProSom
eszopiclone*	Lunesta
flurazepam	Dalmane
lorazepam	Ativan
quazepam	Doral
Short Acting	
alprazolam	Xanax
midazolam	Versed
ramelteon*	Rozerem
temazepam	Restoril
triazolam	Halcion
zaleplon*	Sonata
zolpidem*	Ambien

*These drugs share many characteristics with the benzodiazepines but are classified as miscellaneous hypnotic drugs.

Mechanism of Action and Drug Effects

The sedative and hypnotic action of benzodiazepines is related to their ability to depress activity in the CNS. The specific areas they affect appear to be the hypothalamic, thalamic, and limbic systems of the brain. Although the mechanism of action is not certain, research suggests that there are specific receptors in the brain for benzodiazepines. These receptors are thought to be either **gamma-aminobutyric acid (GABA)** receptors or other adjacent receptors. GABA is the primary inhibitory neurotransmitter of the brain and serves to modulate CNS activity by inhibiting overstimulation. Like GABA itself, the depressant actions of benzodiazepines on the CNS appear to be related to their ability to inhibit stimulation of the brain. They have many favorable characteristics compared with the older drug class *barbiturates* (see the next section of this chapter). They do not suppress REM sleep to the same extent as do barbiturates. They also do not induce hepatic microsomal enzyme activity and are therefore safe to administer to patients who are taking medications metabolized by this enzyme system.

Indications

Benzodiazepines have a variety of therapeutic applications. They are commonly used for sedation, relief of agitation, treatment of depression, sleep induction, skeletal muscle relaxation (e.g., following injury), anxiety relief, and treatment of seizure disorders. They are often combined with anesthetics, analgesics, and neuromuscular blocking drugs in balanced anesthesia and also moderate sedation (see Chapter 12). They are used in this setting primarily for their amnesic properties to reduce memory of painful procedures. Finally, benzodiazepine receptors in the CNS are in the same area as those that play a role in alcohol addiction. Therefore, some benzodiazepines (e.g., diazepam) are used in the treatment and prevention of the symptoms of alcohol withdrawal (see Chapter 9). When these drugs are used to treat insomnia, it is generally recommended that they be used short term if clinically feasible to avoid dependency. However, many patients use

hypnotics on a long-term basis. Two newer products that have been approved by the U.S. Food and Drug Administration (FDA) for long-term use for insomnia include eszopiclone (Lunesta) and an extended-release form of zolpidem (Ambien CR). These two drugs are not benzodiazepines.

Contraindications

Contraindications to the use of benzodiazepines include known drug allergy, narrow-angle glaucoma, and pregnancy.

Adverse Effects

As a class, benzodiazepines have a relatively favorable adverse effect profile. The adverse effects associated with their use are usually mild and primarily involve the CNS. The more commonly reported undesirable effects are headache, drowsiness, paradoxical excitement or nervousness, dizziness or vertigo, cognitive impairment, and lethargy. Benzodiazepines can create a significant fall hazard in elderly patients, however, and their use should be avoided when possible in this patient population. To help prevent adverse effects, the lowest effective dosages are recommended for all patients, especially the elderly. Although these drugs have comparatively less intense effects on the normal sleep cycle, a "hangover" effect is sometimes reported (e.g., daytime sleepiness). Other less common adverse effects are palpitations, dry mouth, nausea, vomiting, hypokinesia, and occasional nightmares. Withdrawal symptoms such as rebound insomnia (i.e., greater insomnia than pretreatment) may occur with abrupt discontinuation.

Toxicity and Management of Overdose

An overdose of benzodiazepines may result in one or all of the following symptoms: somnolence, confusion, coma, and diminished reflexes. However, overdose of benzodiazepines alone rarely results in hypotension and respiratory depression. These effects are more commonly seen when benzodiazepines are taken with other CNS depressants such as alcohol or barbiturates. The same holds true for their lethal effects. In the absence of the concurrent ingestion of alcohol or other CNS depressants, benzodiazepine overdose rarely results in death.

The treatment of benzodiazepine intoxication is generally symptomatic and supportive. If ingestion is recent, decontamination of the gastrointestinal (GI) tract is indicated. Gastric lavage is generally the most effective means of gastric decontamination. Activated charcoal and a saline cathartic may be administered after gastric lavage to remove any remaining drug. Hemodialysis is not useful in the treatment of overdose. Flumazenil, a benzodiazepine antidote, can be used to acutely reverse the sedative effects of benzodiazepines, although this is normally done only in cases of excessive oral overdose or intravenous sedation. Flumazenil antagonizes the action of benzodiazepines on the CNS by directly competing with the benzodiazepine for binding at the receptors in the CNS. The dosage regimens to be followed for the reversal of conscious sedation or general anesthesia induced by benzodiazepines and the management of suspected overdose are summarized in Table 13-3.

Interactions

The potential drug interactions with the benzodiazepines are significant because of their intensity, particularly when they involve other CNS depressants (e.g., alcohol, opioids). These drugs may

TABLE 13-3 Flumazenil Treatment Regimen

Indication	Recommended Regimen	Duration
Reversal of moderate sedation or general anesthesia	Give 0.2 mg (2 mL) IV over 15 sec, then give 0.2 mg if consciousness does not occur; may be repeated at 60-sec intervals prn up to 4 additional times (maximum total dose, 1 mg)	1-4 hr
Management of suspected benzodiazepine overdose	Give 0.2 mg (2 mL) IV over 30 sec; wait 30 sec, then give 0.3 mg (3 mL) over 30 sec if consciousness does not occur; further doses of 0.5 mg (5 mL) can be given over 30 sec at intervals of 1 min up to a cumulative dose of 3 mg	1-4 hr

IMPORTANT NOTE: Flumazenil has a relatively short half-life and a duration of effect of 1-4 hr; therefore, if flumazenil is used to reverse the effects of a long-acting benzodiazepine, the dose of the reversal drug may wear off and the patient may become sedated again, requiring more flumazenil. *IV,* Intravenously.

TABLE 13-4 Benzodiazepines: Drug Interactions

Drug	Mechanism	Result
Cimetidine	Decreased benzodiazepine metabolism	Prolonged benzodiazepine action
CNS depressants	Additive effects	Increased CNS depression
MAOIs	Decreased metabolism	Increased benzodiazepine effects
Protease inhibitors	Decreased metabolism	Increased benzodiazepine effects

CNS, Central nervous system; *MAOIs,* monoamine oxidase inhibitors.

HERBAL THERAPIES AND DIETARY SUPPLEMENTS

Kava *(Piper methysticum)*

■ *Overview*

Kava consists of the dried rhizomes of *Piper methysticum.* The drug contains kava pyrones (kawain). Extended continuous intake can cause a temporary yellow discoloration of the skin, hair, and nails.

■ *Common Uses*

Relief of anxiety, stress, restlessness; promotion of sleep

■ *Adverse Effects*

Skin discoloration, possible accommodative disturbances and pupillary enlargement, scaly skin (with long-term use)

■ *Potential Drug Interactions*

Alcohol, barbiturates, psychoactive drugs

■ *Contraindications*

Contraindicated in patients with Parkinson's disease, liver disease, or alcoholism; in those operating heavy machinery; and in pregnant and breast-feeding women

HERBAL THERAPIES AND DIETARY SUPPLEMENTS

Valerian *(Valeriana officinalis)*

■ *Overview*

Valerian root, consisting of fresh underground plant parts, contains essential oil with monoterpenes and sesquiterpenes (valerianic acids).

■ *Common Uses*

Relief of anxiety, restlessness, sleep disorders

■ *Adverse Effects*

Central nervous system depression, hepatotoxicity, nausea, vomiting, anorexia, headache, restlessness, insomnia

■ *Potential Drug Interactions*

Central nervous system depressants, monamine oxidase inhibitors, phenytoin, warfarin; may have enhanced relative and adverse effects when taken with other drugs (including other herbal products) that have known sedative properties (including alcohol)

■ *Contraindications*

Contraindicated in patients with cardiac disease, liver disease, or those operating heavy machinery

result in further CNS depressant effects, including reduced blood pressure, respiratory rate, sedation, confusion, and diminished reflexes. This and other major drug interactions are listed in Table 13-4. Herbal remedies that interact with the benzodiazepines include kava and valerian, which may also lead to further CNS depression. Food-drug interactions include interactions with grapefruit and grapefruit juice, which alter drug absorption.

Dosages

Please see the Dosages table on p. 200.

DRUG PROFILES

Benzodiazepines and miscellaneous sedative-hypnotic drugs are all prescription-only drugs, and they are designated as Schedule IV controlled substances. Uses for benzodiazepines can vary, including treatment of insomnia, procedural sedation (see Chapter 12), muscle relaxation, anticonvulsant therapy (see Chapter 15), and anxiety relief (see Chapter 17). The miscellaneous drugs are normally used only for their hypnotic purposes to treat insomnia. Dosage information appears in the Dosages table for benzodiazepines and miscellaneous sedative-hypnotic drugs.

DOSAGES

Selected Benzodiazepine and Other Sedative-Hypnotic Drugs

Drug (Pregnancy Category) [Controlled Substance Schedule]	Onset and Duration	Usual Dosage Range	Indications/Uses
diazepam (Valium) (D) [IV]	Long acting	**Adult** PO/IV: 5-10 mg 1 hr before procedure PO: 5-10 mg	Moderate procedural sedation Muscle relaxation
midazolam (Versed) (D) [IV]	Short acting	**Adult** IV/IM: 2-5 mg just before procedure **Pediatric** PO: 1-5 mg 20-30 min before procedure	Moderate procedural sedation
◆ temazepam (Restoril) (D) [IV]	Short acting	**Adult** PO: 7.5-30 mg at bedtime	Sleep induction
◆ zaleplon (Sonata) [C] [IV]	Short acting	**Adult** PO: 5-10 mg at bedtime	Sleep induction
◆ zolpidem* (Ambien) (B) [IV]	Short acting	**Adult** PO: 5-10 mg at bedtime	Sleep induction
eszopiclone* (Lunesta) (C) [IV]	Long acting	**Adult** PO: 1-3 mg at bedtime	Sleep induction
ramelteon* (Rozerem) (C) [N/A]	Long acting	**Adult** PO: 8 mg at bedtime	Sleep induction

IM, Intramuscular; *IV,* intravenous; *N/A,* not applicable; *PO,* oral.
*Nonbenzodiazepine drugs.

BENZODIAZEPINES
diazepam
Diazepam (Valium) was the first clinically available benzodiazepine drug. It has varied uses, including treatment of anxiety (see Chapter 17), procedural sedation and anesthesia adjunct (see Chapter 12), anticonvulsant therapy (see Chapter 15), and skeletal muscle relaxation following orthopedic injury or surgery. It is available in oral, rectal, and injectable forms.

PHARMACOKINETICS

Route	Onset of Action	Peak Plasma Concentration	Elimination Half-life	Duration of Action
IV	Immediate	8 min	20-60 hr	15-30 min
PO	30 min	1-2 hr	20-60 hr	12-24 hr

midazolam
Midazolam (Versed) is most commonly used for procedural sedation. It is useful for this indication due to its ability to cause amnesia and anxiolysis (reduced anxiety) as well as sedation. This helps patients to feel less anxious about, and avoid remembering, uncomfortable medical procedures. The drug is normally given by injection in adults. However, a liquid oral dosage form is also available for children.
◆ temazepam
Temazepam (Restoril), a short-acting benzodiazepine, used to be one of the most commonly prescribed hypnotics. It is actually one of the metabolites of diazepam and normally induces sleep within 20 to 40 minutes. Temazepam has a long onset of action, so it is recommended that patients take it about 1 hour prior to going to bed. Although it is still an effective hypnotic, it has been replaced by the newer drugs.

PHARMACOKINETICS

Route	Onset of Action	Peak Plasma Concentration	Elimination Half-life	Duration of Action
PO	30-60 min	2-3 hr	9.5-12 hr	7-8 hr

NON-BENZODIAZEPINES
◆ zaleplon
Zaleplon (Sonata) is a short-acting nonbenzodiazepine hypnotic. A unique advantage of this drug stems from its very short half-life: patients whose sleep difficulties include early awakenings can dose themselves in the middle of the night as long as they take the drug at least 4 hours before they must arise.

PHARMACOKINETICS

Route	Onset of Action	Peak Plasma Concentration	Elimination Half-life	Duration of Action
PO	Rapid	1 hr	1 hr	6-8 hr

◆ zolpidem
Zolpidem (Ambien) is also a short-acting nonbenzodiazepine hypnotic. Its relatively short half-life and its lack of active metabolites contribute to a lower incidence of daytime sleepiness compared with benzodiazepine hypnotics. A newer dosage form, Ambien CR, is a longer-acting form with two separate drug reservoirs. One releases zolpidem faster than the other to induce hypnosis (sleep) more rapidly. The second reservoir also releases zolpidem but does so more slowly throughout the night to help maintain sleep. One special concern with this particular dosage form is the possibility of somnambulation or sleepwalking, which has been reported with its use. Nevertheless, Ambien CR is currently one of only two hypnotics to be FDA-approved for long-term use; the other is eszopiclone (Lunesta; see next profile).

PHARMACOKINETICS

Route	Onset of Action	Peak Plasma Concentration	Elimination Half-life	Duration of Action
PO	30 min	1.6 hr	1.4-4.5 hr	6-8 hr

eszopiclone
Eszopiclone (Lunesta) is one of the newest hypnotics and is a longer-acting nonbenzodiazepine drug. It was the first hypnotic to

be FDA-approved for long-term use. It is designed to provide a full 8 hours of sleep.

PHARMACOKINETICS

Route	Onset of Action	Peak Plasma Concentration	Elimination Half-life	Duration of Action
PO	30-60 min	1 hr	6 hr	8 hr

ramelteon

Ramelteon (Rozerem) is the newest prescription hypnotic. It is the first prescription hypnotic in 35 years with a new mechanism of action. This drug is structurally similar to the hormone melatonin, which is believed to regulate circadian rhythms (day-night sleep cycles) in the body. Recall from physiology that this hormone also controls skin color through its production of the dark pigment melanin in the skin. Over-the-counter dietary supplements containing melatonin have been available for several years. Ramelteon works as an agonist at the body's melatonin receptors in the CNS. Technically it is not a CNS depressant, but it is included here because of its use as a hypnotic. It is also not classified as a controlled substance because of its lack of observed dependency risk. It potentially has a shorter duration of action than other hypnotics and is therefore indicated primarily for patients who have difficulty with sleep *onset* rather than sleep maintenance. Its use is contraindicated in cases of severe liver dysfunction. It should also be avoided in patients receiving fluvoxamine (see Chapter 17), fluconazole, or ketoconazole (see Chapter 42), all of which can impede its metabolism. Rifampin (see Chapter 41) can reduce its absorption.

PHARMACOKINETICS

Route	Onset of Action	Peak Plasma Concentration	Elimination Half-life	Duration of Action
PO	30-60 min	45 min	1-2.5 hr	6-8 hr

BARBITURATES

Barbiturates were first introduced into clinical use in 1903 and were the standard drugs for treating insomnia and producing sedation. Chemically they are derivatives of barbituric acid. Although almost 50 different barbiturates are approved for clinical use in the United States, only a handful are in common clinical use today. This is due in part to the favorable safety profile and proven efficacy of the benzodiazepines. Barbiturates can produce many unwanted adverse effects. They are habit forming and have a low **therapeutic index** (i.e., there is only a narrow dosage range within which the drug is effective, and above that range it is rapidly toxic). Barbiturates can be classified into four groups based on their onset and duration of action. Table 13-5 lists the drugs in each category and summarizes their pharmacokinetic characteristics.

Mechanism of Action and Drug Effects

Barbiturates are CNS depressants that act primarily on the brainstem in an area called the reticular formation. Their sedative and hypnotic effects are dose related, and they act by reducing the nerve impulses traveling to the area of the brain called the *cerebral cortex.* Their ability to inhibit nerve impulse transmission is in part due to their ability to potentiate the action of the inhibitory neurotransmitter GABA, which is found in high concentrations in the CNS. Barbiturates also raise the seizure threshold.

TABLE 13-5 Sedative-Hypnotic Barbiturates

Generic Name	Trade Name
Ultrashort Acting	
methohexital	Brevital
thiopental	Pentothal
Short Acting	
pentobarbital	Nembutal
secobarbital	Seconal
Intermediate Acting	
butabarbital	Butisol
Long Acting	
phenobarbital	Solfoton, Luminal
mephobarbital	Mebaral

Indications

All barbiturates have the same sedative-hypnotic effects but differ in their potency, time to onset of action, and duration of action. They are used as hypnotics, sedatives, and anticonvulsants and also for anesthesia during surgical procedures. The various categories of barbiturates are used for the following therapeutic purposes:

Ultrashort acting: Anesthesia for short surgical procedures, anesthesia induction, control of convulsions, and reduction of intracranial pressure in neurosurgical patients

Short acting: Sedation/sleep induction and control of convulsive conditions

Intermediate acting: Sedation/sleep induction and control of convulsive conditions

Long acting: Sleep induction, epileptic seizure prophylaxis

Contraindications

Contraindications to barbiturate use include known drug allergy, pregnancy, significant respiratory difficulties, and severe kidney or liver disease. These drugs should be used with caution in elderly patients due to their sedative properties and increased fall risk.

Adverse Effects

Barbiturates as a class are notorious enzyme inducers. They stimulate the action of enzymes in the liver that are responsible for the metabolism or breakdown of many drugs. By stimulating the action of these enzymes, they cause many drugs to be metabolized more quickly, which usually shortens their duration of action. Other drugs that are enzyme inducers are warfarin, theophylline, and phenytoin.

The main adverse effects of barbiturates relate to the CNS and include drowsiness, lethargy, dizziness, hangover (prolongation of drowsiness, lethargy, and dizziness), and paradoxical restlessness or excitement. Their long-term effects on normal sleep architecture can be detrimental. Sleep research has shown that adequate rest is obtained from the sleep process only when there are proper amounts of REM sleep, which is sometimes referred to as *dreaming sleep.* Barbiturates deprive people of REM sleep, which can result in agitation and an inability to deal with normal daily stress. When the barbiturate is stopped and REM sleep once

TABLE 13-6 Barbiturates: Adverse Effects

Body System	Adverse Effects
Cardiovascular	Vasodilation and hypotension, especially if given too rapidly
Gastrointestinal	Nausea, vomiting, diarrhea, constipation
Hematologic	Agranulocytosis, thrombocytopenia, megaloblastic anemia
Nervous	Drowsiness; lethargy; vertigo; headache; mental depression; myalgic, neuralgic, or arthralgic pain
Respiratory	Respiratory depression, apnea, laryngospasm, bronchospasm, coughing
Other	Hypersensitivity reactions: urticaria, angioedema, rash, fever, serum sickness, Stevens-Johnson syndrome

again takes place, a rebound phenomenon can occur. As noted earlier, during this rebound the proportion of REM sleep is increased, the patient's dream time constitutes a larger percentage of total sleep, and the dreams are often nightmares. Common adverse effects of barbiturates are listed in Table 13-6. As is the case with most sedative drugs, barbiturates are also associated with an increased incidence of falls when used in the elderly. If they are recommended for older adults at all, the usual dose is reduced by half whenever possible.

Toxicity and Management of Overdose

Phenobarbital is also used to treat status epilepticus (prolonged uncontrolled seizures). In extreme cases, patients may be intentionally overdosed to the extent of causing therapeutic phenobarbital coma. Because of the inhibitory effects of barbiturates on nerve transmission in the brain (possibly GABA mediated), the uncontrollable seizures can be stopped until sufficient serum levels of anticonvulsant drugs are achieved. An overdose of barbiturates produces CNS depression ranging from sleep to profound coma and death. Respiratory depression progresses to Cheyne-Stokes respirations, hypoventilation, and cyanosis. Affected patients often have cold, clammy skin or are hypothermic, and later they can exhibit fever, areflexia, tachycardia, and hypotension. Pupils are usually slightly constricted but may be dilated in cases of severe drug toxicity.

Treatment of an overdose is mainly symptomatic and supportive. The mainstays of therapy are maintenance of an adequate airway, assisted ventilation, and oxygen administration if needed, along with fluid and pressor support as indicated. Barbiturates are highly metabolized by the liver, where they also induce enzyme activity. In an overdose, however, the amount of barbiturate may overwhelm the liver's ability to metabolize it. This is a situation in which administration of activated charcoal may be helpful. Activated charcoal adsorbs (binds to) drug molecules in the stomach. It also has the effect of drawing the drug from the circulation into the GI tract for elimination. Multiple-dose (every 4 hours) nasogastric administration of activated charcoal is a common regimen. Some of the barbiturates (phenobarbital and mephobarbital), because they are relatively acidic, can be eliminated more quickly by the kidneys when the urine is alkalized (pH is raised). This keeps the drug in the urine and prevents it

from being resorbed back into the circulation. Alkalization, along with forced diuresis using diuretics (e.g., furosemide [see Chapter 26]), can hasten elimination of the barbiturate.

Interactions

A major risk encountered in the coadministration of barbiturates with alcohol, antihistamines, benzodiazepines, opioids, and tranquilizers is additive CNS depression. Most of the drug-drug interactions involving barbiturates are secondary to the effects of barbiturates on the hepatic enzyme system. As mentioned previously, barbiturates increase the activity of hepatic microsomal or cytochrome P-450 enzymes (Chapter 2). This process is called enzyme induction. Induction of this enzyme system results in increased drug metabolism and breakdown. However, if two drugs are competing for the same enzyme system for metabolism, the result can be inhibited drug metabolism and possibly increased toxicity for the wide variety of drugs that are metabolized by these enzymes. Examples are the administration of monoamine oxidase inhibitors (MAOIs), anticoagulants, glucocorticoids, tricyclic antidepressants, quinidine, and oral contraceptives with barbiturates. Coadministration of MAOIs and barbiturates can result in prolonged barbiturate effects. Coadministration of anticoagulants with barbiturates can result in decreased anticoagulation response and possible clot formation. Coadministration of barbiturates with oral contraceptives can result in accelerated metabolism of the contraceptive drug and possible unintended pregnancy. Women taking both types of medication concurrently should be advised to consider an additional method of contraception as a backup.

Dosages

Barbiturates can act as either sedatives or hypnotics depending on the dosage. Selected barbiturates and their recommended sedative and hypnotic dosages are listed in the Selected Barbiturates.

DRUG PROFILES

Like benzodiazepines, barbiturates can also have varied uses, including preoperative sedation, anesthesia adjunct, and anticonvulsant therapy. All barbiturates are controlled substances but not all are on the same schedule, as illustrated in Table 13-7. Dosage information appears in the Dosages table for barbiturates.

pentobarbital

Pentobarbital (Nembutal) is a short-acting barbiturate. Formerly prescribed as a sedative-hypnotic for insomnia, pentobarbital is now principally used preoperatively to relieve anxiety and provide sedation. In addition, it is used occasionally to control status epilepticus or acute seizure episodes resulting from meningitis, poisons, eclampsia, alcohol withdrawal, tetanus, and chorea. Pentobarbital may also be used to treat withdrawal symptoms in patients who are physically dependent on barbiturates or nonbarbiturate hypnotics. It is available in oral, injectable, and rectal dosage forms.

PHARMACOKINETICS

Route	Onset of Action	Peak Plasma Concentration	Elimination Half-life	Duration of Action
PO	30-60 min	1-2 hr	20-45 min	3-4 hr

DOSAGES

Selected Barbiturates

Drug	Onset and Duration	Usual Dosage Range	Indications/Uses
pentobarbital (Nembutal)	Short acting	**Pediatric** IM/IV/PO/PR: 2-6 mg/kg/day (max 100 mg) depending on clinical purpose, age, and weight (suppositories should not be divided)	Anticonvulsant, preoperative sedative, sedative
		Adult IM: 150-200 mg PR: 120-200 mg at bedtime IV: 100 mg PO: 60-100 mg/day	Anticonvulsant, preoperative sedative, hypnotic
phenobarbital (Solfoton, Luminal)	Long acting	**Pediatric** PO: 6 mg/kg in 3 equally divided doses IM/IV: 1-3 mg/kg	Sedative Preoperative sedative
		Adult PO: 30-120 mg/day divided 100-320 mg at bedtime IM/IV: 100-200 mg 60-90 min before surgery	Sedative Hypnotic Preoperative sedative

IM, Intramuscularly; *IV*, intravenously; *PO*, orally; *PR*, rectally.

TABLE 13-7 Barbiturates: Controlled Substance Schedule

Schedule	Barbiturates
C-II	pentobarbital, secobarbital
C-III	butabarbital, thiopental
C-IV	mephobarbital, methohexital, phenobarbital

phenobarbital

Phenobarbital is the barbiturate most commonly prescribed, either alone or in combination with other drugs. It is considered the prototypical barbiturate and is classified as a long-acting drug. Phenobarbital is used for the prevention of generalized tonic-clonic seizures and fever-induced convulsions. In addition, it has been useful in the treatment of hyperbilirubinemia in neonates. It has also been used for the treatment of Gilbert syndrome. It is only rarely used today as a sedative-hypnotic drug. It is available in oral and injectable forms.

PHARMACOKINETICS

Route	Onset of Action	Peak Plasma Concentration	Elimination Half-life	Duration of Action
IV	5 min	30 min	50-120 hr	6-12 hr
PO	30 min	1-6 hr	50-120 hr	6-12 hr

OVER-THE-COUNTER HYPNOTICS

Nonprescription sleeping aids often contain antihistamines (see Chapter 36). These drugs also have a depressant effect on the CNS that should be recognized. The most common antihistamines contained in over-the-counter sleeping aids are doxylamine (Unisom) and diphenhydramine (Sominex). Analgesics (e.g., acetaminophen [see Chapter 11]) are sometimes added to offer some pain relief if pain, such as headache or backache, is a component of the sleep disturbance (e.g., acetaminophen/diphenhydramine [Extra Strength Tylenol PM]). As with other CNS depressants, concurrent use of alcohol can cause respiratory depression or arrest.

MUSCLE RELAXANTS

A variety of conditions such as trauma, inflammation, anxiety, and pain can be associated with acute muscle spasms. Although there is no completely satisfactory form of therapy available for relief of skeletal muscle spasticity, muscle relaxant drugs are capable of providing some relief. The muscle relaxants are a group of compounds that act predominantly within the CNS to relieve pain associated with skeletal muscle spasms. The majority of muscle relaxants are known as centrally acting skeletal muscle relaxants because their site of action is the CNS. Centrally acting skeletal muscle relaxants are similar in structures and action to other CNS depressants such as diazepam. It is believed that the muscle relaxant effects of these drugs are related to this CNS depressant activity. Only one of these compounds, dantrolene, acts directly on skeletal muscle. It belongs to a group of relaxants known as direct-acting skeletal muscle relaxants. It closely resembles GABA.

These drugs are most effective when they are used in conjunction with rest and physical therapy. When muscle relaxants are taken with alcohol, other CNS depressants, or opioid analgesics, enhanced CNS depressant effects are seen. In such cases, close monitoring and dosage reduction of one or both drugs should be considered.

Mechanism of Action and Drug Effects

The majority of the muscle relaxants work within the CNS. Their beneficial effects are believed to come from their sedative effects rather than from direct muscle relaxation. Dantrolene has direct effects on skeletal muscle. All others have no direct effects on muscles, nerve conduction, or muscle-nerve junctions. One of the more effective drugs in this class, baclofen, is a derivative of GABA. It is believed to work by depressing nerve transmission in the spinal cord. The other drugs in this class are not derivatives of GABA but act by enhancing GABA's central inhibitory effects at the level of the spinal cord. These drugs are generally less effective than baclofen. Dantrolene acts directly on the excitation-contraction coupling of muscle fibers and not at the level of the

DOSAGES

Selected Muscle Relaxants

Drug (Pregnancy Category)	Pharmacologic Class	Usual Dosage Range	Indications/Uses
◆ baclofen (Lioresal) (C)	Centrally acting	**Adult** PO: 5 mg three times daily (tid) for 3 days, then 10 mg tid for 3 days, then 20 mg tid, then titrated to response (max: 20 mg po qid) Intrathecal: 120-1500 mcg/day	Spasticity
◆ cyclobenzaprine (Flexeril) (B)	Centrally acting	**Adult** PO: 5-10 mg tid **Adults and adolescents 15 yrs and younger** The FDA-approved dosage has been reduced to 5 mg po 3 times daily based on clinical efficacy and safety data. In February 2003, cyclobenzaprine became available in 5- and 10-mg tablets to accomodate lower dosage recommendations. Dosage may be increased to 10 mg po 3 times daily if needed	Spasticity

PO, Orally.

CNS. It directly affects skeletal muscles by decreasing the response of the muscle to stimuli. It appears to exert its action by decreasing the amount of calcium released from storage sites in the sarcoplasmic reticula of muscle fibers.

Muscle relaxants have a depressant effect on the CNS. Their effects are the result of CNS depression in the brain primarily at the level of the brainstem, thalamus, and basal ganglia but also at the spinal cord. The effects of muscle relaxants are relaxation of striated muscles, mild weakness of skeletal muscles, decreased force of muscle contraction, and muscle stiffness. Other drug effects that may be experienced include generalized CNS depression manifested as sedation, somnolence, ataxia, and respiratory and cardiovascular depression.

Indications

Muscle relaxants are primarily used for the relief of painful musculoskeletal conditions such as muscle spasms, often following injuries. They are most effective when used in conjunction with physical therapy. They may also be used in the management of spasticity associated with severe chronic disorders such as multiple sclerosis and other types of cerebral lesions, cerebral palsy, and rheumatic disorders. Some relaxants are used to reduce choreiform movement in patients with Huntington's chorea, to reduce rigidity in patients with parkinsonian syndrome, or to relieve the pain associated with trigeminal neuralgia. Intravenous dantrolene is used for the management of the hypermetabolic skeletal muscle spasms that accompany the crisis condition known as malignant hyperthermia (see Chapter 12). Baclofen, has been shown to be effective in relieving hiccups.

Contraindications

The only usual contraindication to the use of muscle relaxants is known drug allergy, but contraindications for some drugs may also include severe renal impairment.

Adverse Effects

The primary adverse effects of muscle relaxants are an extension of their effects on the CNS and skeletal muscles. Euphoria, lightheadedness, dizziness, drowsiness, fatigue, and muscle weakness are often experienced early in treatment. These adverse effects are generally short lived, with patients growing tolerant to them over time. Less common adverse effects seen with the muscle relaxants include diarrhea, GI upset, headache, slurred speech, muscle stiffness, constipation, sexual difficulties in males, hypotension, tachycardia, and weight gain.

Toxicity and Management of Overdose

The toxicities and consequences of an overdose of muscle relaxants primarily involve the CNS. There is no specific antidote or reversal drug for muscle relaxant overdoses. They are best treated with conservative supportive measures. More aggressive therapies are generally needed when muscle relaxants are taken along with other CNS depressant drugs in an overdose. Gastric lavage and close observation of the patient are recommended. An adequate airway should be maintained, and means of artificial respiration should be readily available. Electrocardiographic monitoring should be instituted, and large quantities of intravenous fluids should be administered to avoid crystalluria.

Interactions

When muscle relaxants are administered along with other depressant drugs such as alcohol and benzodiazepines, caution should be used to avoid overdosage. Mental confusion, anxiety, tremors, and additive hypoglycemic activity have been reported with this combination as well. A dosage reduction and/or discontinuance of one or both drugs is recommended.

Dosages

For an overview of dosages for the more commonly used muscle relaxants, see the Dosages table on p. 204.

DRUG PROFILES

With the exception of dantrolene (Dantrium), muscle relaxants are classified as centrally acting drugs because of their site of action in the CNS. These include baclofen (Lioresal), carisoprodol (Soma), chlorzoxazone (Paraflex), cyclobenzaprine (Flexeril), metaxalone (Skelaxin), methocarbamol (Robaxin), and orphenadrine (Disipal), and tizanidine (Zanaflex). In contrast, dantrolene acts directly on skeletal muscle tissue. Use of all muscle relaxants is contraindicated in patients who have shown a hypersensitivity reaction to them or have compromised pulmonary function, active hepatic disease, or impaired myocardial function. Dosage information appears in the Dosages table for muscle relaxants.

◆ baclofen

Baclofen (Lioresal) is available in both oral and injectable dosage forms. The injectable form is for use with an implantable baclofen pump device. This method is sometimes used to treat chronic spastic muscular conditions. With this administration route, a test dose should be administered initially to test for a positive response. The injection is diluted before infusion. Both oral and injectable doses are titrated to desired response.

PHARMACOKINETICS

Route	Onset of Action	Peak Plasma Concentration	Elimination Half-life	Duration of Action
PO	0.5-1 hr	2-3 hr	2.5-4 hr	8 hr or longer

◆ cyclobenzaprine

Cyclobenzaprine (Flexeril) is available in a 5-mg and 10-mg dose. Cyclobenzaprine is a centrally acting muscle relaxant that is structurally and pharmacologically related to the tricyclic antidepressants. It is the most commonly used drug in this class to reduce spasms following musculoskeletal injuries. It is very common for patients to exhibit marked sedation from its use.

PHARMACOKINETICS

Route	Onset of Action	Peak Plasma Concentration	Elimination Half-life	Duration of Action
PO	1 hr	3-8 hr	8-37 hr	12-24 hr

NURSING PROCESS

Assessment

Before administering any *CNS depressant drug*, such as a benzodiazepine, nonbenzodiazepine, miscellaneous drug, muscle relaxant, or barbiturate, the nurse should perform an assessment focusing on some of the more common parameters and data, including the following: (1) in relation to sleep, any insomnia with attention to onset, duration, frequency, and pharmacologic as well as nonpharmacologic measures used; also, any documentation by the patient or family of sleep disorders, sleep patterns, difficulty in sleeping, or frequent awakenings as well as the time it takes to fall asleep and the energy level upon awakening; (2) vital signs with attention to blood pressure (both supine and standing measurements); pulse rate and rhythm; respiratory rate, rhythm, and depth, body temperature; and presence of pain, with notation of its onset, frequency, duration, and other characteristics (see Chapter 11); (3) results of a head-to-toe physical examination for baseline comparisons; (4) neurologic findings with a focus on any changes in mental status, memory, cognitive abilities, alertness, level of orientation (to person, place, and time) or level of sedation, mood changes, depression or other mental disorder, changes in sensations, anxiety, panic attacks, and other related neurologic findings; and (5) miscellaneous information such as medical history; allergies; use of alcohol and smoking history; caffeine intake; past and current medication profile, including use of any prescription drugs, over-the-counter drugs, and herbals; alternative or folk practices; any changes in health status, weight, nutrition, exercise, life stressors (including loss and grief), or lifestyle.

For patients taking *benzodiazepines* or *benzodiazepine-like drugs*, assessment should include, in addition to the aforementioned elements, the identification of disorders or conditions that represent cautions or contraindications to use of these drugs as well as drugs the patient is taking that might interact with benzodiazepines or benzodiazepine-like drugs (see earlier discussion). Close monitoring is needed in those who are anemic, are suicidal, or have a history of abusing drugs, alcohol, or other substances. Other significant cautions pertain to use of these drugs in the elderly and the very young because of their increased sensitivity to these drugs, as well as in pregnant or lactating women. The elderly and very young may require lower dosages due to potential ataxia and excessive sedation. In addition, before initiating drug therapy with the benzodiazepines and most other sedative-hypnotic drugs, including barbiturates, the prescriber may order blood studies such as CBC. Renal function studies (BUN or creatinine levels) and/or hepatic function studies (ALP level) may be ordered to rule out organ impairment and prevent potential toxicity or complications resulting from decreased excretion and/or metabolism. Potential drug interactions for benzodiazepines are presented Table 13-3. The nurse should pay particular attention to the use of other CNS depressants (e.g., opioids), because their concurrent use may lead to severe decreases in blood pressure, respiratory rate, reflexes, and level of consciousness.

With the *nonbenzodiazepines* such as zaleplon and zolpidem tartrate, assessment should include a head-to-toe physical assessment and thorough medication history with measurement of the vital signs and other parameters mentioned earlier. Allergies to these drugs and to aspirin should be assessed and documented. If the patient is allergic to aspirin, there is an associated risk of allergies to nonbenzodiazepines. Other considerations include the need for assessment of any confusion and lightheadedness, especially in the elderly because of their increased sensitivity to these drugs. Zaleplon and eszopiclone should not be used in those younger than 18 years of age, and extreme caution is necessary if there is a history of compromised respiratory status or drug, alcohol, or other substance abuse. Drug interactions include interactions with other CNS depressants (see previous discussion).

For *muscle relaxants*, drug allergies should be noted before use, and a complete head-to-toe assessment should be performed with focus on the neurologic system. In the elderly, there is increased risk of CNS toxicity with possible hallucinations, confusion, and excessive sedation. Assessment includes taking a thorough health and medication history and examining the complete patient profile with results of associated laboratory studies. See previous discussion about cautions, contraindications, and drug interactions.

The *miscellaneous* drug ramelteon is a newer medication that is used for insomnia but is not associated with CNS depression, does not carry the potential for abuse or dependence, and does not lead to withdrawal symptoms when treatment stops. Therefore, this drug can be used for patients who are likely to be abusers of CNS depressants. Assessment should include inquiry into sleep patterns and habits. Because this drug should not be used in patients with liver impairment, liver function studies are needed prior to beginning the medication. Respiratory assessment and assessment of other vital signs are needed as well. If the patient has a history of respiratory disorders such as chronic obstructive pulmonary disease or sleep apnea, or if the patient is a child, this medication would not be indicated.

Barbiturates are discussed further in Chapter 15 along with other antiepileptic drugs. However, a brief description is needed to emphasize the importance of conducting a thorough patient assessment as well as evaluating for cautions, contraindications, and drug interactions. These drugs should not be used by pregnant or lactating women because the drugs cross the placenta and are present in breast milk, posing the risk of respiratory depression in the fetus or neonate. It is important to note that withdrawal symptoms may appear in neonates born to women who have taken barbiturates during their last trimester of pregnancy. Barbiturates may also produce paradoxical excitement in children and confusion and mental depression in the elderly, so baseline neurologic assessment is needed. Assessment of renal and liver function is also important in those with compromised organ function and in the elderly to help avoid toxicity.

Nursing Diagnoses

- Impaired gas exchange related to the respiratory depression associated with CNS depressants
- Deficient knowledge related to inadequate information about the various CNS drugs
- Disturbed sleep patterns related to the drug's interference with REM sleep
- Risk for injury and falls related to drug-induced decreased sensorium
- Risk for injury related to possible drug overdose or adverse reactions related to drug-drug interactions (e.g., combined use of the drug with alcohol, tranquilizers, and/or analgesics)
- Risk for injury and addiction related to physical or psychologic dependency on CNS drugs

Planning

Goals

- Patient remains free of respiratory depression.
- Patient remains free of further sleep deprivation.
- Patient experiences little or no rebound insomnia.
- Patient remains free of self-injury and falls related to decreased sensorium.
- Patient complies with drug therapy and keeps follow-up appointments with the prescriber or other health care professional.
- Patient regains normal sleep patterns.
- Patient remains free of or experiences minimal adverse effects and toxic effects from sedative-hypnotic drugs, muscle relaxants, and other CNS depressants.
- Patient remains free of drug interaction effects.
- Patient experiences no problems with addiction.

Outcome Criteria

- Patient states the common adverse effects, toxic effects, and symptoms related to use of sedative-hypnotic drugs to be reported to the prescriber, such as drowsiness, confusion, and respiratory depression.
- Patient states ways to minimize self-injury and falls related to decreased sensorium, such as changing positions slowly.
- Patient states risk for REM interference from sedative-hypnotic drugs with associated sleep hangovers and uses nonpharmacologic measures as appropriate.

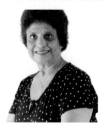

CASE STUDY

Drugs for Sleep

P.S., a 68-year-old retired secretary, comes to the office complaining of feeling "so tired" during the day. She has had trouble sleeping off and on for years, and a few weeks ago received a prescription for the benzodiazepine alprazolam (Xanax) to take "as needed for nerves." Upon closer questioning, the nurse discovers that P.S. has been using alprazolam almost every night for 3 weeks to help her get to sleep. She says, "I just could not fall asleep before! I am sleeping so well, but I'm so tired during the day. I don't understand how I can get such good sleep and still feel tired!"

1. Can you explain the reason for her tiredness?
2. P.S.'s nurse practitioner prescribes a period of decreasing doses of the alprazolam each evening, then every other evening, until the medication is stopped. Explain the rationale behind the tapering dosage schedule.
3. P.S. receives a prescription for ramelteon (Rozerem). How is this drug different from alprazolam?
4. What are nonpharmacologic measures that P.S. can try to improve her sleep?

For answers, see *http://evolve.elsevier.com/Lilley*.

- Patient states the common adverse effects related to use of muscle relaxants such as euphoria, dizziness, drowsiness, and fatigue.
- Patient minimizes adverse effects and toxic effects by taking medications as prescribed.
- Patient states the common drug interactions with alcohol and other medications (e.g., tranquilizers and analgesics) that may be life threatening.
- Patient states the importance of taking measures to minimize problems with addiction, such as taking medication only as needed.
- Patient, family, or significant other states the need to contact the prescriber about possible complications, such as respiratory depression.
- Patient demonstrates increased knowledge related to inadequate information about pharmacologic and nonpharmacologic treatment and regimen for sleeping disturbance.

Implementation

Patients taking *benzodiazepines* and other CNS depressants experience sedation and possible ataxia, thus the need for patient safety measures. Hospital or facility policies mandate the type of safety precautions to be taken, such as the use of side rails or bed alarms. Ambulation should occur with assistance when patients are sedated or are experiencing the adverse effects of these drugs. In addition, dependence may be a problem with the benzodiazepines, but not to the same degree as with the barbiturates. While taking these drugs, patients should avoid driving or participating in any activities that require mental alertness. These drugs should be taken on an empty stomach for faster onset of action; however, this often results in GI upset so, practically speaking, they should be taken with food, a light snack, or meals. Orally administered benzodiazepines have an onset of action of 30 minutes to 6 hours depending on the drug (see the pharmacokinetics information in the drug profiles), and the appropriate timing and intervals of dosing will be determined by these characteristics. For example, if a patient takes a benzodiazepine or other CNS drug to induce sleep and the drug's onset of action is 30 to 60 minutes, then the drug should be dosed 60 minutes prior to bedtime. In addition, it is crucial to patient compliance and safety to understand that drug tolerance may develop to many of these drugs, and so the patient may require larger dosages to produce the same therapeutic effect at some point. Interrupting therapy helps to decrease such tolerance.

Among the benzodiazepines, REM interference is less problematic with flurazepam, quazepam, and estazolam, primarily because they produce fewer active metabolites. In addition, patients should be informed that REM interference and rebound insomnia may occur with just a 3- to 4-week regimen of drug therapy. To minimize REM interference, benzodiazepines and other drugs should be used only when nonpharmacologic methods fail and should be used with caution in all patients with sleep disorders and for short periods of times. Zolpidem is also available in a sustained release product used for long-term management of sleep disorders. Gradual weaning-off periods are recommended for benzodiazepines and all CNS depressants. Hangover effects are also associated with many of the CNS depressants but occur less frequently with benzodiazepines and nonbenzodiazepines than with barbiturates.

Nonbenzodiazepines should be taken for the prescribed time and with attention to special instructions, such as the following: (1) Zaleplon should be taken as directed and immediately before bedtime due to its quick onset of action. Very heavy and/or high-fat meals should *not* be consumed within 2 hours of taking this drug because of interference with the drug's action. (2) Zolpidem should be taken at bedtime on an empty stomach with no crushing, chewing, or breaking of the oral dosage form. It is also important to emphasize that this drug may infrequently lead to temporary memory loss. To help avoid this adverse effect, it is recommended that the patient not take a dose of the drug unless he or she had a full night's sleep (e.g., at least 7 to 8 hours) the previous night (with or without the use of a sleep aid). As with any CNS depressant drug, tasks requiring mental alertness should be avoided until the patient's response to the drug is known. Tolerance and dependence are possible with prolonged use, and neither drug should be discontinued without gradual weaning.

Muscle relaxants have different indications than the barbiturates and benzodiazepines and are not used to treat insomnia. They are generally indicated for some forms of spasticity (see pharmacology discussion). However, when used they may lead to adverse effects and toxicities, so that frequent monitoring of airway, breathing, and circulation is needed. Early identification of toxicity is critical to provide prompt treatment and to prevent respiratory and other CNS depressant effects. Close monitoring of all vital parameters and level of consciousness or sedation is needed when these muscle relaxants are used, and the patient should ambulate only with assistance. Changing positions purposefully and slowly is recommended to prevent syncope or dizziness. The greatest risk for hypotension associated with these drugs is usually within 1 hour of dosing, so it is important for the patient to be more cautious about activity during this time.

The *miscellaneous* drug ramelteon is a newer product, and the nurse should emphasize that it should not be mixed with alcohol. Other important points are that the drug should be taken 30 minutes before bedtime and should *not* be taken along with or immediately after a high-fat meal.

Barbiturates are to be used with very close monitoring and extreme caution. Observation and documentation of the patient's level of consciousness or sedation; orientation to person, place, and time; respiratory rate; oxygen saturation; and other vital signs is needed. Oral doses should be taken with food or a light snack, and dosage forms should not be altered. A bed alarm system or side rails should be used and assistance with ambulation provided as needed or indicated prevent injury. Barbiturates also produce a hangover effect, and this residual drowsiness occurs upon awakening and results in impaired reaction times. The intermediate- and long-acting hypnotics are often the culprits in this adverse effect. Careful ambulation is needed, as are other safety measures discussed previously. Abrupt withdrawal of barbiturates after prolonged therapy may produce adverse effects ranging from nightmares, hallucinations, and delirium to seizures. In addition, while the patient is taking barbiturates it is important to monitor the patient's red blood cell count, hemoglobin level, and hematocrit because of the possible adverse effect of anemia. Long-term use of barbiturates also requires monitoring of therapeutic blood levels of the drug. For example, the level of phenobarbital should be 10 to 30 mcg/mL. Patients with serum levels above 40 mcg/mL may experience toxicity manifested by cold and clammy skin, respiratory rate of less than 10 breaths/min, and other signs of severe CNS depression.

Intravenous use of barbiturates, as with some with the benzodiazepines (e.g., diazepam), requires dilution of the drug with normal saline or other recommended solutions. Recommendations regarding rates of intravenous administration must be strictly followed for safe use. Most of the drugs should not be administered any faster than 1 mg/kg/min and a maximum amount per minute may be specified; the nurse should refer to an authoritative drug source or handbook or the manufacturer's insert before giving any of these drugs. Too rapid an infusion of a barbiturate may produce profound hypotension and marked respiratory depression. Should there be intravenous infiltration, the site may become swollen, erythematous, and tender. Tissue necrosis may occur with this infiltration, depending on the particular drug. There are antidote protocols for some of the intravenous barbiturates. For example, with phenobarbital intravenous infiltration, the solution should be discontinued, a 0.5% procaine solution injected into the affected area, and moist heat applied, as per institutional policy or procedure. Protocol for management of infiltration of an intravenous drug should always be checked before intervening, because in some situations the intravenous catheter may be left in place until antidotes are administered. Another area of concern with intravenous drugs is incompatibilities with other intravenously administered medications, and barbiturates have several. Some intravenous drugs with which barbiturates are incompatible are amphotericin B, hydrocortisone, and hydromorphone, and these drugs should be given only after the intravenous line has been adequately flushed with normal saline. With intramuscular injection, the solution should be given deep into a large muscle mass to prevent tissue sloughing; however, this route should be avoided and used only when absolutely necessary.

In summary, before giving any CNS depressant, it is always important to try nonpharmacologic measures to induce sleep. However, if medication therapy is indicated, preventing respiratory depression and other problems associated with CNS depression is of prime importance, as is maintaining patient safety and preventing injury. Documentation must be timely, clear, and concise and must reflect follow-up of the patient's response to the drug. It is also important for the nurse to document the dose, route, time of administration, and safety measures taken after each dose is given.

Evaluation

Some of the criteria by which to confirm a patient's therapeutic response to a *CNS depressant* include the following: an increased ability to sleep at night, fewer awakenings, shorter sleep induction time, few adverse effects such as hangover effects, and an improved sense of well-being because of improved sleep. Therapeutic effects related to *muscle relaxants* include decreased spasticity, reduction of choreiform movements in Huntington chorea, decreased rigidity in parkinsonian syndrome, and relief of pain from trigeminal neuralgia. The nurse must constantly watch for and document the occurrence of any of the adverse effects of benzodiazepines, barbiturates, and muscle relaxants. See the previous discussion of adverse effects for each type of drug. Toxic effects of the CNS depressants for which the nurse should evaluate range from severe CNS depression of all body systems to respiratory and circulatory collapse.

BOX 13-1 Sleep Diaries and Nonpharmacologic Treatment of Sleep Disorders

Information for a Sleep Diary
- What time do you usually go to bed and wake up?
- How long and how well do you sleep?
- When were you awake during the night and for how long?
- How easy was it to go to sleep?
- How easy was it to wake up in the morning?
- How much caffeine or alcohol do you consume?
- What time did you last eat or drink (if after dinner)?
- Did you have any bedtime snacks?
- What emotions or stressors are present?
- What medications do you take daily?
- Do you smoke? If so, how much and for how long?
- Do you consume alcohol? If so, how much and for how long?
- Do you take any over-the-counter drugs? If so, what drug and for what reason? How much and for how long?
- Do you take any herbals? If so, which ones? For what and for how long?

Nonpharmacologic Sleep Interventions
- Establish a set sleep pattern with a time to go to bed at night and a regular time to get up in the morning and stick to it. This will help to reset your internal clock.

- Sleep only as much as you need to feel refreshed and renewed. Too much sleep may lead to fragmented sleep patterns and shallow sleep.
- Keep bedroom temperatures moderate, if possible.
- Avoid caffeine-containing beverages and food within 6 hours of bedtime.
- Decrease exposure to loud noises.
- Avoid daytime napping.
- Avoid exercise late in the evening (i.e., not past 7 PM).
- Avoid alcohol in the evening. Rather than putting you to sleep, it actually results in fragmented sleep.
- Avoid tobacco at bedtime, because it disturbs sleep.
- Try to relax before bedtime with soft music, yoga, relaxation therapy, deep breathing, or light reading on a topic that is not intense or anxiety provoking.
- Drink a warm decaffeinated beverage, such as warm milk or chamomile tea, 30 minutes to 1 hour before bedtime.
- If you are still awake 20 minutes after going to bed, get up and engage in a relaxing activity (as noted previously) and go back to bed once you feel drowsy. Repeat as necessary.

PATIENT TEACHING TIPS

- Encourage individuals to keep a journal recording sleep habits, sleep patterns, and response to both drug and nondrug therapy (Box 13-1).
- Nonpharmacologic measures should be used first to enhance sleep. This is important, because the use of CNS depressants for treatment of sleep deficit or insomnia often leads to interference with the REM stage of sleep, hangover effects, and/or tolerance, as well as other adverse effects.
- Always check with the prescriber or pharmacist before taking any over-the-counter medications because of the many drug interactions with CNS depressants.
- These, and all medications, should be kept out of the reach of children.
- Emphasize that medications should be taken only as prescribed. The patient is usually told that if one dose does not work, the patient is not to double up on the dosage unless otherwise prescribed or directed.

- Educate about any time constraints related to driving, operation of heavy machinery or equipment, and participation in activities requiring mental alertness while the patient is taking these medications.
- These medications should not be abruptly discontinued or withdrawn, if possible, to avoid rebound insomnia.
- Sedative-hypnotic drugs (for sleep promotion) are not intended for long-term use because of their adverse effects, interference with REM sleep, and addictive properties.
- The patient should be made aware that hangover effects may occur with most of these drugs and that this is more problematic in the elderly or in patients with altered renal and hepatic function.
- The patient should be warned to avoid smoking when in bed or when lounging.

POINTS TO REMEMBER

- Nonpharmacologic measures to improve sleep should always be tried before resorting to treatment with medications.
- Nurses should understand the classification and pharmacokinetic properties of barbiturates. Short-acting barbiturates include pentobarbital sodium and secobarbital. Intermediate-acting barbiturates include amobarbital, aprobarbital, and butabarbital.
- The pharmacokinetics of each group of barbiturates lend specific characteristics to the drugs in that group. The nurse needs to understand how these drugs are absorbed orally and used parenterally, as well as their onset time, time until peak effect, and duration of action. In addition, the life-threatening potential of these drugs should never be minimized by the nurse or other health care providers administering the drugs, because too rapid an infusion may precipitate respiratory or cardiac arrest.

- Nursing interventions for barbiturates include careful consideration of parenteral administration. The nurse must have complete knowledge about incompatibilities with other drugs in solution as well as dilutional fluid incompatibilities.
- Most sedative-hypnotic drugs suppress REM sleep and should be used only for the recommended period of time. This time frame varies depending on the specific drug used.
- Muscle relaxants are often used for the treatment of muscle spasms, spasticity, and rigidity. They result in varying levels of decreased sensorium and CNS depression depending on the specific drug, dosage, and route of administration. Nurses need to understand that even though muscle relaxants are discussed in this chapter, they are not used as sedative-hypnotic drugs.

NCLEX EXAMINATION REVIEW QUESTIONS

1 A patient has been admitted to the emergency department because of an overdose of an oral benzodiazepine. He is very drowsy but still responsive. The nurse should prepare for which immediate intervention?
   a Hemodialysis to remove the medication
   b Administration of flumazenil
   c Administration of naloxone
   d Intubation and mechanical ventilation

2 An older adult has been given a benzodiazepine for sleep induction, but the night nurse noted that the patient was awake most of the night, watching television and reading in bed. This type of reaction is known as
   a an allergic reaction.
   b a teratogenic reaction.
   c a paradoxical reaction.
   d an idiopathic reaction.

3 The nurse is preparing to administer a medication for sleep. Which intervention applies to the administration of a nonbenzodiazepine, such as zolpidem?
   a These drugs need to be taken about 1 hour before bedtime.
   b Because of their rapid onset, they should be taken just before bedtime.
   c The patient should be cautioned about the high incidence of morning drowsiness that may occur after taking these drugs.
   d These drugs are less likely to interact with alcohol.

4 The nurse should monitor the patient who is taking a muscle relaxant for which adverse effect?
   a CNS depression
   b Hypertension
   c Peripheral edema
   d Blurred vision

5 A patient on a cardiac medical-surgical unit is complaining of having difficulty sleeping. Which action should the nurse take first to address this problem?
   a Administer a sedative-hypnotic drug if ordered
   b Offer tea made with the herbal preparation valerian
   c Encourage the patient to exercise by walking up and down the halls a few times if tolerated
   d Provide an environment that is restful and reduce loud noises

6 Which considerations are important for the nurse to remember when administering a benzodiazepine as a sedative-hypnotic drug? (Select all that apply.)
   a These drugs are intended for long-term management of insomnia.
   b The drugs can be administered safely with other CNS depressants for insomnia.
   c The dose should be given about an hour before the patient's bedtime.
   d The drug should be used as a first choice for treatment of sleeplessness.
   e The patient should be evaluated for the drowsiness that may occur the morning after a benzodiazepine is taken.

1. b, 2. c, 3. b, 4. a, 5. d, 6. c, e.

CRITICAL THINKING ACTIVITIES: BEST ACTION

1 A patient has a prescription for eszopiclone (Lunesta) because he has had trouble sleeping. The nurse is reviewing the use of this medication, and the patient says, "I've been drinking a glass of wine before bedtime to help me sleep. Can I still do that? This medication is not like Valium, right?" What is the nurse's best response?

2 During rounds on night shift, the nurse finds that a patient is lying in bed, wide-awake at 4 AM. The patient complains, "I can't sleep. I need my sleeping pill. Can I have it now?" The patient's

medication administration sheet has a prn (as needed) order for temazepam (Restoril). What is the nurse's best action at this time?

3 The nurse is talking to a patient about what adverse effects to expect when taking a muscle relaxant for injuries the patient received after an automobile accident. What is the most important adverse effect the nurse should discuss with the patient? Explain.

For answers, see *http://evolve.elsevier.com/Lilley.*

CHAPTER 14

Central Nervous System Stimulants and Related Drugs

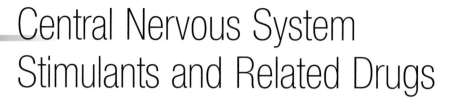

OBJECTIVES

When you reach the end of this chapter, you should be able to do the following:

1 Briefly review the anatomy, physiology and functions of the central nervous system with attention to stimulant effects on its function.

2 Review the glossary terms as they relate to the central nervous system and stimulant drugs.

3 Identify the various central nervous system stimulant drugs.

4 Discuss the mechanisms of action, indications, dosages, routes of administration, contraindications, cautions, drug interactions, adverse effects, and any related toxicity for the various central nervous system stimulants.

5 Develop a nursing care plan based on the nursing process for patients using central nervous system stimulant drugs.

e-Learning Activities

http://evolve.elsevier.com/Lilley

NCLEX Review Questions • Animations • Nursing Care Plans • Audio Glossary • Category Catchers • Medication Errors Checklists • IV Therapy Checklists • Calculators • Frequently Asked Questions • Content Updates • Supplemental Resources • Answers to Case Studies and Critical Thinking Activities

Drug Profiles

♦ amphetamines, p. 213
atomoxetine, p. 214
♦ caffeine, p. 219
doxapram, p. 220
♦ methylphenidate, p. 213
modafinil, p. 214

orlistat, p. 216
♦ phentermine, p. 216
♦ sibutramine, p. 216
sodium oxybate, p. 214
♦ sumatriptan, p. 217

♦ Key drug.

Glossary

Amphetamines The collective term for a class of stimulant drugs that includes the originally synthesized drug amphetamine sulfate and all of its drug derivatives. (p. 212)

Analeptics Central nervous system (CNS) stimulants that have generalized effects on the brainstem and spinal cord, which in turn produce an increase in responsiveness to external stimuli and stimulate respiration. (p. 219)

Anorexiants Drugs used to control or suppress appetite. (p. 215)

Attention deficit hyperactivity disorder (ADHD) A syndrome affecting children, adolescents, and adults characterized by difficulty in maintaining concentration on a given task and/or hyperactive behavior. The term *attention deficit disorder (ADD)* has been absorbed under this broader term. (p. 211)

Cataplexy A condition characterized by abrupt attacks of muscular weakness and hypotonia triggered by an emotional stimulus such as joy, laughter, anger, fear, or surprise. It is often associated with *narcolepsy*. (p. 211)

CNS stimulants Drugs that stimulate specific areas of the brain or spinal cord. (p. 210)

Ergot alkaloids Drugs that have been found to narrow or constrict blood vessels in the brain and provide relief of pain for certain migraine headaches. (p. 217)

Migraine A common type of recurring painful headache characterized by a pulsatile or throbbing quality, incapacitating pain, and photophobia. (p. 212)

Narcolepsy A syndrome characterized by sudden sleep attacks, *cataplexy*, sleep paralysis, and visual or auditory hallucinations at the onset of sleep. (p. 211)

Serotonin receptor agonists A new class of CNS stimulants used to treat migraine headaches; they work by stimulating 5-hydroxytryptamine 1 receptors in the brain and are sometimes referred to as *selective serotonin receptor agonists* or *triptans*. (p. 217)

Sympathomimetic drugs CNS stimulants such as noradrenergic drugs (and, to a lesser degree, dopaminergic drugs) whose actions resemble or mimic those of the sympathetic nervous system. (p. 211)

• • •

Anatomy, Physiology, and Disease Overview

Central nervous system (CNS) activity is regulated by a checks-and-balances system that consists of both excitatory and inhibitory neurotransmitters and their corresponding receptors in the brain and spinal cord tissues. CNS stimulation can result from either excessive stimulation of excitatory neurons or blockade of inhibitory neurons. **CNS stimulants** are a broad class of drugs that stimulate specific areas of the brain or spinal cord. Most

TABLE 14-1 Structurally Related CNS Stimulants

Chemical Category	CNS Stimulants and Related Drugs
Amphetamines and related stimulants	dextroamphetamine, methamphetamine, benzphetamine, methylphenidate, dexmethylphenidate, pemoline, mazindol
Serotonin agonists	almotriptan, eletriptan, frovatriptan, naratriptan, rizatriptan, sumatriptan, zolmitriptan
Sympathomimetics	phentermine, phendimetrazine
Xanthines	caffeine, theophylline, aminophylline
Miscellaneous	modafinil, sodium oxybate (CNS depressant), sibutramine (anorexiant), orlistat (lipase inhibitor), doxapram (analeptic)

CNS, Central nervous system.

TABLE 14-2 CNS Stimulants: Site of Action

Primary Site of Action	CNS Stimulants
Cerebrovascular system	Serotonin agonists
Cerebral cortex	Amphetamines, phenidates, mazindol, modafinil
Hypothalamic and limbic regions	Anorexiants
Medulla and brainstem	Analeptics

CNS, Central nervous system.

TABLE 14-3 CNS Stimulants and Related Drugs: Therapeutic Categories

Category	Drugs
Anti-ADHD	dextroamphetamine, methamphetamine, methylphenidate, atomoxetine (norepinephrine reuptake inhibitor)
Antinarcoleptic	dextroamphetamine, methamphetamine, methylphenidate, mazindol, modafinil, sodium oxybate (CNS depressant)
Anorexiant	methamphetamine, phentermine, phendimetrazine, diethylpropion, benzphetamine, sibutramine, orlistat (lipase inhibitor)
Antimigraine	almotriptan, eletriptan, frovatriptan, naratriptan, rizatriptan, sumatriptan, zolmitriptan (serotonin agonists); dihydroergotamine mesylate, ergotamine tartrate with caffeine (ergot alkaloids)
Analeptic	caffeine, doxapram, aminophylline, theophylline, modafinil (antinarcoleptic)

ADHD, Attention deficit hyperactivity disorder; *CNS*, central nervous system.

CNS stimulant drugs act by stimulating the excitatory neurons in the brain. These neurons contain receptors for excitatory neurotransmitters, including dopamine (dopaminergic drugs), norepinephrine (noradrenergic drugs), and serotonin (serotonergic drugs). Dopamine is a metabolic precursor of norepinephrine, which is also a neurotransmitter in the *sympathetic nervous system*. The actions of noradrenergic drugs often resemble or mimic the actions of the sympathetic nervous system. For this reason, noradrenergic drugs (and, to a lesser degree, dopaminergic drugs as well) are also called **sympathomimetic drugs.** Other sympathomimetic drugs are discussed further in Chapter 18.

There are three ways to classify CNS stimulant drugs. The first is on the basis of chemical structural similarities. Major chemical classes of CNS stimulants include amphetamines, serotonin agonists, sympathomimetics, and xanthines (Table 14-1). Second, these drugs can be classified according to their site of therapeutic action in the CNS (Table 14-2). Finally, they can be categorized according to five major therapeutic usage categories for CNS stimulant drugs (Table 14-3). These include anti–attention deficit, antinarcoleptic, anorexiant, antimigraine, and analeptic drugs. Anorexiants are drugs used to control obesity by suppression of appetite. Analeptics are drugs used by clinicians for specific CNS stimulation in certain clinical situations. Some therapeutic overlap exists among these drug categories.

ATTENTION DEFICIT HYPERACTIVITY DISORDER

Attention deficit hyperactivity disorder (ADHD), formerly known as *attention deficit disorder (ADD),* is the most common psychiatric disorder in children, affecting 3% to 10% of school-aged children. Boys are affected from two to nine times more often than girls, although the disorder may be underdiagnosed in girls. Primary symptoms of ADHD center around a developmentally inappropriate ability to maintain attention span and/or the presence of hyperactivity and impulsivity. The disorder may involve predominantly attention deficit, predominantly hyperactivity or impulsivity, or a combination of both. It usually begins before 7 years of age, sometimes earlier than age 4. It can officially be diagnosed when symptoms last at least 6 months and occur in at least two different settings (e.g., home and school), according to the *Diagnostic and Statistical Manual of Mental*

Disorders. Many children outgrow ADHD, but adult ADHD is also common. Drug therapy for both childhood and adult ADHD is essentially the same. Although there is some social controversy regarding possible overdiagnosis of, and overmedication for, this disorder, studies in twins indicate a degree of genetic predisposition and familial heritability. The disorder is commonly associated with other forms of mental illness, including depression, bipolar disorder, anxiety, and learning difficulties.

NARCOLEPSY

Narcolepsy is an incurable neurologic condition in which patients unexpectedly fall asleep in the middle of normal daily activities. These "sleep attacks" are reported to cause car accidents or near-misses in 70% or more of patients. Another major symptom of the disease is dysfunctional *rapid eye movement sleep* (see Chapter 13). **Cataplexy** is an associated symptom in at least 70% of narcolepsy cases. It involves sudden, acute skeletal muscle weakness. The condition is often associated with strong emotions (e.g., joy, anger), and commonly the knees buckle and the individual falls to the floor while still awake. Men and women are equally affected, with approximately 100,000 cases in the United States. Some genetic markers have been identified. Roughly half of patients with narcolepsy experience migraine headaches as well.

OBESITY

According to the National Institutes of Health and the Centers for Disease Control and Prevention, at least 30.5% of Americans are *obese* and nearly two thirds (64.5%) are *overweight.* This translates into more than 60 million obese adults, with a higher incidence of obesity among women and minorities. Obesity was formerly defined as being 20% or more above one's ideal body weight based on population statistics for height, body frame, and gender. More recent data are based on a measurement known as the body mass index (BMI), defined as weight in kilograms divided by height in meters squared (i.e., BMI = weight [kg] ÷ [height (m)]^2). *Overweight* is now defined as a BMI of 25 to 29.9, whereas *obesity* is now defined as a BMI of 30 or higher. At any given time, one third of women and one quarter of men are trying to lose weight. Moreover, the incidence of obesity in young people aged 6 to 19 years has more than tripled since 1980. Obesity increases the risk for hypertension, dyslipidemia, coronary artery disease, stroke, type 2 diabetes mellitus, gallbladder disease, gout, osteoarthritis, sleep apnea, and certain types of cancer, including breast and colon cancer. An estimated 70% of diabetes risk in the United States can be attributed to excess weight. Some 300,000 deaths each year are linked to obesity, which makes it the second leading cause of preventable deaths in the United States. The related health care costs alone are currently estimated at more than $90 billion. Yet many people who attempt weight loss do so for cosmetic reasons rather than health reasons. Obese people are often stigmatized, at times even by the health care professionals treating them.

MIGRAINE

A **migraine** is a common type of recurring headache, usually lasting from 4 to 72 hours. Typical features include a pulsatile quality with pain that worsens with each pulse. The pain is most commonly unilateral but may occur on both sides of the head. Associated symptoms include nausea, vomiting, *photophobia* (avoidance of light), and *phonophobia* (avoidance of sounds). In addition, a minority of migraines are accompanied by an *aura,* which is a predictive set of altered visual or other senses (formerly termed *classic migraine*). However, the majority of migraines are without an aura (formerly termed *common migraine*). Migraines affect about 12% of the U.S. population, with a reported incidence in females roughly three times that in males. These headaches can occur at any age, but migraines commonly begin after age 10 and peak between the mid-twenties and early forties. They often fade after age 50. Familial inheritance of migraine is also well recognized. Precipitating factors include stress, emotionality, hypoglycemia, menses, endogenous estrogen (including oral contraceptives), exercise, and intake of alcohol, caffeine, cocaine, nitroglycerin, aspartame, and the food additive monosodium glutamate (MSG). Interestingly, over 50% of patients with narcolepsy report nocturnal migraines. Historically, there have been several theories regarding the cause of migraines, including the "vascular hypothesis" and the "neurovascular hypothesis." The most recent evidence points to decreased serotonin levels. Thus, the majority of current investigations involve drugs that can increase the serotonin levels.

ANALEPTIC-RESPONSIVE RESPIRATORY DEPRESSION SYNDROMES

Analeptic drugs are now generally used much less frequently than they were in the earlier days of general anesthesia. This is because of advances in intensive respiratory care, including mechanical ventilation and improved anesthetic techniques, as well as the availability of newer medications with less toxicity. Nonetheless, there are several respiratory syndromes for which these medications are sometimes still used. *Neonatal apnea,* or periodic cessation of breathing in newborn babies, is a common condition seen in neonatal intensive care units. It occurs in about 25% of premature infants, whose pulmonary and CNS structures, including the *medullary* centers that control breathing, have not completed their gestational development due to preterm birth. Infants undergoing prolonged mechanical ventilation, especially at high pressures, often develop a chronic lung disease known as *bronchopulmonary dysplasia,* for which caffeine can also be helpful. *Postanesthetic respiratory depression* occurs when a patient's spontaneous respiratory drive does not resume adequately and in a timely manner after general anesthesia. Respiratory depression may also be secondary to abuse of some drugs. Hypercapnia, or elevated blood levels of carbon dioxide, is often associated with later stages of chronic obstructive pulmonary disease (COPD). Analeptic drugs such as theophylline, aminophylline, caffeine, and doxapram may be used to treat one or more of these conditions.

▮ Pharmacology Overview

DRUGS FOR ATTENTION DEFICIT HYPERACTIVITY DISORDER AND NARCOLEPSY

CNS stimulants are the first-line drugs of choice for both ADHD and narcolepsy. They are potent drugs with a strong potential for tolerance and psychologic dependence (addiction; see Chapter 9). They are classified as Schedule II drugs under the Controlled Substance Act. Although there has been some public controversy regarding their use, these drugs have led to a 65% to 75% improvement in symptoms in treated patients compared with a placebo. In general, CNS stimulants elevate mood, produce a sense of increased energy and alertness, decrease appetite, and enhance task performance impaired by fatigue or boredom. Two of the oldest known stimulants are cocaine and amphetamine, which are prototypical drugs for this class. Caffeine, contained in coffee and tea, is another plant-derived CNS stimulant.

Amphetamine sulfate was first synthesized in the late 1800s. It was subsequently used to treat narcolepsy and then to prolong the alertness of soldiers during World War II. Later derivatives of this drug, which are still used clinically, include its d-isomer dextroamphetamine sulfate, methamphetamine hydrochloride, benzphetamine and mixed amphetamine salts—salts of both amphetamine and dextroamphetamine. They are often collectively referred to simply as **amphetamines,** a term that includes amphetamine sulfate itself. Methylphenidate, a synthetic amphetamine derivative, was first introduced for the treatment of hyperactivity in children in 1958. Its d-isomer is the drug dexmethylphenidate. The phenidates are also Schedule II drugs. All of these amphetamine-related drugs are used to treat ADHD and/or narcolepsy. Nonamphetamine stimulants include pemoline and modafinil. In 2005, pemoline was taken off the market due to reports of liver failure associated with its use.

Atomoxetine is a nonstimulant drug that is also used to treat ADHD. Atomoxetine is a norepinephrine reuptake inhibitor. Because it is not an amphetamine, it is associated with a low incidence of insomnia and has low abuse potential. Another advantage is that phone-in refills are allowed for this drug (as opposed to Schedule CII drugs, which require a written prescription).

Mechanism of Action and Drug Effects

Amphetamines stimulate areas of the brain associated with mental alertness, such as the cerebral cortex and the thalamus. The pharmacologic actions of CNS stimulants are similar to the actions of the sympathetic nervous system in that the CNS and respiratory systems are the primary body systems affected. CNS effects include mood elevation or euphoria, increased mental alertness and capacity for work, decreased fatigue and drowsiness, and prolonged wakefulness. The respiratory effects most commonly seen are relaxation of bronchial smooth muscle, increased respiration, and dilation of pulmonary arteries.

The amphetamines and phenidates increase the effects of both norepinephrine and dopamine in CNS synapses by increasing their release and blocking their reuptake. As a result, both neurotransmitters are in contact with their receptors longer, which lengthens their duration of action. Modafinil is also classified as an analeptic. It promotes wakefulness like the amphetamines and phenidates. It lacks sympathomimetic properties, however, and appears to work primarily by reducing gamma-aminobutyric acid (GABA)–mediated neurotransmission in the brain. GABA is the principal inhibitory neurotransmitter in the brain. The nonstimulant drug, atomoxetine, is also being used to treat ADHD. It works in the CNS by selective inhibition of norepinephrine reuptake.

Indications

The various amphetamine derivatives, including methylphenidate, are currently used to treat both ADHD and narcolepsy. Dexmethylphenidate is currently indicated for ADHD alone. Amphetamine sulfate was also used to treat obesity in the early to mid twentieth century. However, the only amphetamines currently approved for this indication are benzphetamine and methamphetamine (see Anorexiants). The nonamphetamine stimulant modafinil is indicated for narcolepsy.

Specialists sometimes recommend periodic "drug holidays" (e.g., 1 day per week) without medication to mitigate the addictive tendencies of the stimulant drugs. School-aged children often do not take these drugs on weekends and school vacations.

Contraindications

Contraindications to the use of amphetamine and nonamphetamine stimulants include known drug allergy. These drugs can also exacerbate the following conditions: marked anxiety or agitation, Tourette syndrome and other tic disorders (hyperstimulation), and glaucoma (can increase intraocular pressure; see Chapter 57). The drugs should not be used in patients who have received therapy with any monoamine oxidase inhibitor (MAOI) in the preceding 14 days (see Chapter 17). Contraindications specific to atomoxetine include drug allergy, glaucoma, and recent MAOI use.

Adverse Effects

Both amphetamine and nonamphetamine stimulants have a wide range of adverse effects that most often arise when these drugs are administered at dosages higher than the therapeutic dosages. These drugs tend to "speed up" body systems. For example, effects on the cardiovascular system include increased heart rate and blood pressure. Other adverse effects include angina, anxiety, insomnia, headache, tremor, blurred vision, increased metabolic rate (beneficial in treatment of obesity), gastrointestinal (GI) distress, and dry mouth. Common adverse effects associated with atomoxetine include headache, abdominal pain, vomiting, anorexia, and cough.

Interactions

The drug interactions associated with these drugs vary greatly from class to class. Table 14-4 summarizes some of the more common interactions for all drug classes in this chapter.

Dosages

Dosages and other information for stimulant drugs are listed in the Dosages table on p. 218.

DRUG PROFILES

AMPHETAMINES AND RELATED STIMULANTS
As noted earlier, the principal drugs used to treat ADHD and narcolepsy are the amphetamine and nonamphetamine stimulants. Atomoxetine, a nonstimulant drug, is also used for ADHD.

◆ amphetamines
The various amphetamine salts are the prototypical CNS stimulants used to treat ADHD and narcolepsy. Amphetamine is available in prescription form only for oral use, both as single-component dextroamphetamine sulfate (Dexedrine) and as a mixture of dextroamphetamine sulfate, dextroamphetamine saccharate, amphetamine sulfate, and amphetamine aspartate (Adderall).

PHARMACOKINETICS (DEXTROAMPHETAMINE)

Route	Onset of Action	Peak Plasma Concentration	Elimination Half-life	Duration of Action
PO	30-60 min	90-120 min	7-14 hr	10 hr

◆ methylphenidate
Methylphenidate (Ritalin) was the first prescription drug indicated for ADHD and continues to be the most widely prescribed drug for the treatment of ADHD and is also used for narcolepsy. Extended-release dosage forms include Ritalin SR, Concerta, and Metadate CD. There is some controversy regarding drug therapy for ADHD. Some parents may also be understandably apprehensive regarding this type of drug therapy. However, with proper diagnosis of the disorder, proper dosing of the drug, and regular medical monitoring, many children can achieve significant improvement in school performance and social skills with this therapy. Psychosocial problems within a child's family

TABLE 14-4 CNS Stimulants: Common Drug Interactions

Drug	Interacting Drugs	Mechanism	Result
Amphetamine and Nonamphetamine Stimulants			
Amphetamines (various salts) Methylphenidate	Beta-blockers	Increased alpha-adrenergic effects	Hypertension, bradycardia, dysrhythmias, heart block
	CNS stimulants	Additive toxicities	Cardiovascular adverse effects, nervousness, insomnia, convulsions
	digoxin	Additive toxicity	Increased risk of dysrhythmias
	MAOIs	Increased release of catecholamines	Headaches, dysrhythmias, severe hypertension
	Tricyclic antidepressants	Additive toxicities	Cardiovascular adverse effects (dysrhythmias, tachycardia, hypertension)
Atomoxetine			
	Sympathomimetic drugs	Enhanced SNS effects	Cardiovascular adverse effects (dysrhythmias, tachycardia, hypertension)
	CYP2D6 inhibitors (MAOIs, paroxetine)	Reduced metabolism of atomoxetine	Enhanced atomoxetine toxicity
Anorexiants and Analeptics			
Phentermine Sibutramine	CNS stimulants	Additive toxicities	Nervousness, irritability, insomnia, dysrhythmias, seizures
	MAOIs	Increased release of catecholamines	Headaches, dysrhythmias, severe hypertension
	Quinolone antibiotics	Interference with metabolism	Reduced clearance of caffeine and prolongation of caffeine's effects
	Serotonergic drugs	Additive toxicity	Cardiovascular adverse effects, nervousness, insomnia, convulsions
Serotonin Agonists			
Sumatriptan and others	Ergot alkaloids, SSRIs, MAOIs	Additive toxicity	Cardiovascular adverse effects, nervousness, insomnia, convulsions
Ergot Alkaloids			
D.H.E.45, Caffergot	Protease inhibitors, azole antifungals, macrolide antibiotics	Increased ergot levels	Acute ergot toxicity; nausea, vomiting, hypotension or hypertension, seizures, coma, death; use with ergot alkaloids is contraindicated

CNS, Central nervous system; *CYP2D6,* cytochrome P-450 enzyme 2D6; *MAOIs,* monoamine oxidase inhibitors; *SNS,* sympathetic nervous system; *SSRIs,* selective serotonin reuptake inhibitors.

should be ruled out or addressed if they are contributing to the child's problems, regardless of whether the medication is prescribed.

PHARMACOKINETICS (IMMEDIATE RELEASE)

Route	Onset of Action	Peak Plasma Concentration	Elimination Half-life	Duration of Action
PO	30-60 min	1-3 hr	1-3 hr	4-6 hr

atomoxetine

Atomoxetine (Strattera) is the newest medication approved for treating ADHD in children older than 6 years of age and in adults. This medication is not a controlled substance because it lacks addictive properties, unlike amphetamines and phenidates. For this reason, it has rapidly gained popularity as a therapeutic option for treating ADHD and has been used to treat over 2 million patients to date. In September 2005, however, the FDA issued a warning describing cases of suicidal thinking and behavior in small numbers of adolescent patients receiving this medication, similar to its previous warnings regarding adolescent use of antidepressant medications (see Chapter 17). Atomoxetine currently remains on the market, but prescribers are advised to work with parents in providing prudent monitoring of any young patients taking this medication and to promptly reevaluate patients showing any behavioral symptoms of concern.

PHARMACOKINETICS

Route	Onset of Action	Peak Plasma Concentration	Elimination Half-life	Duration of Action
PO	60 min	1-2 hr	5-24 hr	24-120 hr

modafinil

Modafinil (Provigil) is indicated for improvement of wakefulness in patients with excessive daytime sleepiness associated with narcolepsy and also with *shift work sleep disorder*. It has less abuse potential than amphetamines and methylphenidate and is a Schedule IV drug.

PHARMACOKINETICS

Route	Onset of Action	Peak Plasma Concentration	Elimination Half-life	Duration of Action
PO	1-2 months*	2-4 hr	8-15 hr	Unknown

*Therapeutic effects.

MISCELLANEOUS NARCOLEPSY DRUGS
sodium oxybate

Sodium oxybate (Xyrem) is the sodium salt of gamma-hydroxybutyrate, one of the notorious "date rape" drugs. It is currently one of only two drugs approved by the FDA for the treatment of cata-

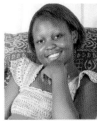
plexy. (The other is viloxazine [Catatrol], an antidepressant that blocks norepinephrine reuptake.) Cataplexy is a condition characterized by acute attacks of muscle weakness and is often associated with narcolepsy. Distribution of this drug is carefully controlled due to its abuse potential. Prescribers who wish to use this medication for this restricted population of patients must contact the Xyrem Success Program at 866-XYREM-88 (866-997-3688). Sodium oxybate is considered an orphan drug and is currently legally available only through such restricted dispensing programs. It is classified as a Schedule III controlled substance for this limited medical use and is technically a CNS depressant rather than a stimulant. This drug is contraindicated in cases of sleep apnea, substance abuse, or concurrent use of hypnotic drugs.

PHARMACOKINETICS

Route	Onset of Action	Peak Plasma Concentration	Elimination Half-life	Duration of Action
PO	30 min	30-75 min	30-60 min	1-5 hr

ANOREXIANTS

By definition, an *anorexiant* is any substance that suppresses appetite. Anorexiants are CNS stimulant drugs used to promote weight loss in obesity. These drugs include phentermine (Ionamin), benzphetamine (Didrex), methamphetamine (Desoxyn), phendimetrazine (Bontril), diethylpropion (Tenuate), and sibutramine (Meridia). Benzphetamine and methamphetamine are the only amphetamines currently approved for treating obesity. Orlistat (Xenical) is a related nonstimulant drug.

Mechanism of Action and Drug Effects

Anorexiants are CNS stimulants that are believed to work by suppressing appetite control centers in the brain. Some evidence suggests that they also increase the body's basal metabolic rate, including mobilization of adipose tissue stores and enhanced cellular glucose uptake, as well as reduce dietary fat absorption.

There are some minor differences between these drugs in terms of their individual actions. Phentermine, phendimetrazine, diethylpropion, methamphetamine, and benzphetamine resemble amphetamine sulfate in their chemical structures and CNS effects. These drugs are classified as both anorexiants and adrenergic (sympathomimetic) drugs. However, all appear to suppress appetite centers in the CNS through dopamine- and norepinephrine-mediated pathways. Sibutramine, the newest anorexiant, enhances dopamine, norepinephrine, and serotonin activity in the brain by inhibiting neuronal reuptake of these neurotransmitters. Its dopamine activity is weaker than its norepinephrine and serotonin activity. This kind of serotonergic activity is associated with enhanced feelings of satiety.

Another relatively new drug is orlistat, which differs from the others in that it is not a CNS stimulant per se but works by irreversibly inhibiting the enzyme lipase. This results in reduced absorption of dietary fat from the intestinal tract and increased fat elimination in the feces.

Indications

Anorexiants are used for the treatment of obesity. However, their effects are often minimal without accompanying behavioral modifications involving diet and exercise. They are most commonly used in higher-risk patients. These include obese patients with a BMI of 30 or higher, or in patients with a BMI of 27 who are also hypertensive or have high cholesterol or diabetes.

Contraindications

Contraindications to anorexiants include drug allergy, any severe cardiovascular disease, uncontrolled hypertension, hyperthyroidism, glaucoma, mental agitation, history of drug abuse, eating disorders (e.g., anorexia, bulimia), and use of monoamine oxidiase inhibitors (see Chapter 17) within the previous 14 days. In addition, sibutramine should not be used concurrently with other serotonergic drugs, including selective serotonin reuptake inhibitors, meperidine, lithium, or dihydroergotamine, due to risk of *serotonin syndrome* (see Chapter 17). Orlistat is contraindicated in cases of chronic malabsorption syndrome or cholestasis.

Adverse Effects

With the exception of diethylpropion, anorexiants may raise blood pressure and cause heart palpitations and even dysrhythmias at higher dosages. Ironically, at therapeutic dosages, they may actually reflexively slow the heart rate. Diethylpropion, however, has little cardiovascular activity. These drugs may also cause anxiety, agitation, dizziness, and headache. With sibutramine use, in addition to these effects, there have been case reports of mania, intestinal obstruction, cardiac arrest, and stroke, among several other serious consequences. However, it should be recognized that obese patients commonly have multiple risk fac-

An Applied Evidence-Based Review of the Diagnosis and Treatment of Obesity in Adults

■ Review

Because obesity is an epidemic in the United States and leads to substantial morbidity and mortality, a review was conducted to identify effective strategies for managing obesity and to provide a rationale for its diagnosis and treatment. This applied evidence-based review of research presents information about the diagnostic test characteristics of exact body mass index (BMI). The review provided support for the recommendations from the following scientific bodies that are known for their work on adult obesity: the National Heart, Lung, and Blood Institute; the World Health Organization; the Canadian Task Force on Preventative Health Care; and the U.S. Preventative Task Force. Data were obtained from pertinent studies identified using MEDLINE, the Database of Abstracts of Reviews of Effectiveness, and the Cochrane Database of Systematic Reviews.

■ Type of Evidence

This was an applied evidence-based review of methods for diagnosing and treating adults with obesity. Various data in the following areas were summarized: evidence of increased health risk associated with obesity, evidence that reducing weight decreases disease risk, and evidence that reducing weight increases disease risk (e.g., increased risk of hip fracture). The review was based on a compilation and synthesis of the data, focusing on the role of primary care health care providers in the diagnosis and treatment of adult obese patients.

■ Results of Study

The review focused on means of diagnosing obesity in adulthood that were based on BMI rather than the gender-height-age-specific tables previously used. BMI (weight in kilograms divided by the square of the height in meters) is easily calculated and is seen as a reliable measure of overweight and obesity in adults. Evidence on treatment modalities was also reviewed and presented. Data on the effectiveness of various interventions were reviewed. The weight loss interventions identified as being effective included diet, exercise, behavioral strategies, limited use of pharmacologic treatments in combination with strategies that change lifestyle, and surgery for selected morbidly obese patients. Because this chapter concerns central nervous system stimulants, it is relevant to mention that serotonin-norepinephrine reuptake inhibitors (e.g., sibutramine) and gastrointestinal lipase inhibitors (e.g., orlistat) were the specific drugs mentioned in this review. Surgical interventions discussed in the review were gastric bypass and gastroplasty.

■ Link of Evidence to Nursing Practice

This review emphasized the importance of using an applied evidence-based approach to investigate obesity management in adults. Diagnosis and treatment were the focus of the review, and excellent criteria were identified for the health care provider to use in everyday practice. Some of the key points relevant for clinicians to use when treating obese patients included the following: (1) Obesity should be managed as a chronic and relapsing disease. (2) BMI should be used as a tool to diagnose obesity and to guide decisions about treatment. (3) A reduction of 10% of total body weight (identified as a "modest" reduction) yields results in improving and preventing hypertension, diabetes, and hyperlipidemia. (4) Diet combined with exercise proved to be the most effective treatment method. (5) Patients should be counseled to set a goal of a 10% decrease in total body weight, to exercise for increasing energy expenditure. (6) Referral to a behavioral program to reinforce the health care provider's counseling should be considered. (7) Being an advocate for social policies that promote health, good nutrition, and increased physical activity is important.

This review summarized various therapies and lifestyle changes for treating obesity. The importance of viewing obesity management as a lifelong process and applying a "chronic disease care" model that incorporates collaborative approaches to care was emphasized. Effective methods of diagnosis and treatment of adult obesity were identified. Although the review concentrated on the actions of the primary care provider during the clinical encounter, this was identified as a reactive approach; a more proactive strategy on the part of health care providers is critical to successful therapy. Major changes must occur in the health care of adults and children (because habits start early!) to put in place the necessary social policies, good nutrition, and exercise habits that are needed to attack this problem. Nurses continue to play an important role in patient care and in the education of the community regarding all types of health care concerns, including the morbidity and mortality associated with obesity.

Data from Orzano JA, Scott JG: Diagnosis and treatment of obesity in adults: an applied evidence-based review, *J Am Board Fam Pract* 17(5):359-369, 2004. Available at *http://www.medscape.com/viewarticle/489073_print.*

tors for such adverse events even when this drug is not taken. The most common adverse effects of orlistat include headache, upper respiratory tract infection (mechanism uncertain), and GI distress, including fecal incontinence.

Interactions

See Table 14-4.

Amphetamine salts generally are no longer used for treatment of obesity because of their high abuse potential. The current major prescription anorexiants include phentermine and sibutramine. Several others have been mentioned earlier but are not as commonly prescribed. A newer nonstimulant drug also included here is the lipase inhibitor orlistat. All three of these medications offer generally improved safety and adverse effect profiles compared with the potent and highly addictive amphetamines.

◆ phentermine

Phentermine (Ionamin) is a sympathomimetic anorexiant that is structurally related to amphetamines but with much lower abuse potential. It is classified as a Schedule IV drug. This drug is not to be confused with several other drugs that were recalled by the FDA in the late 1990s (fenfluramine/dexfenfluramine [Phen-Fen]) and in 2000 (phenylpropanolamine) because of case reports of various adverse cardiovascular and/or pulmonary effects.

◆ sibutramine

Sibutramine (Meridia) is one of the newest anorexiants and is classified as a Schedule IV controlled substance. Sibutramine works by inhibiting the reuptake primarily of norepinephrine and serotonin (and, to a lesser extent, dopamine), which results in reduced appetite.

PHARMACOKINETICS

Route	Onset of Action	Peak Plasma Concentration	Elimination Half-life	Duration of Action
PO	8 wk*	6 mo	14-16 hr	12 mo

*Therapeutic effects.

orlistat

Orlistat (Xenical), one of the newer anorexiants, is unrelated to other drugs in its category. Allī is an over-the-counter (OTC) version released in 2007. As noted earlier, it works by binding to gastric and pancreatic enzymes called *lipases*. Blocking these enzymes reduces fat absorption by roughly 30%. Restricting dietary intake of fat to less than 30% of total calories can help reduce some of the GI adverse effects, which include oily spotting, flatulence, and fecal incontinence in 20% to 40% of patients. Decreases in serum concentrations of vitamins A, D, and E and beta carotene are seen as a result of the blocking of fat absorption. Supplementation with fat-soluble vitamins corrects this deficiency.

PHARMACOKINETICS

Route	Onset of Action	Peak Plasma Concentration	Elimination Half-life	Duration of Action
PO	3 mo*	6-8 hr	1-2 hr	Unknown

*Therapeutic effects.

ANTIMIGRAINE DRUGS

Serotonin receptor agonists, first introduced in the 1990s, have revolutionized the treatment of migraine headache. These drugs work by stimulating serotonin receptors in the brain. They include sumatriptan (Imitrex), almotriptan (Axert), eletriptan (Relpax), naratriptan (Amerge), rizatriptan (Maxalt), zolmitriptan (Zomig), and frovatriptan (Frova). Collectively, these drugs are referred to as *triptans*. Other pertinent drugs are described in other chapters. **Ergot alkaloids** are drugs that have been traditionally used as the mainstay of treatment of migraine headaches but have been replaced by the triptans. They are obtained from a fungus and cause vasoconstriction of dilated blood vessels in the brain and of the carotid arteries. They are contraindicated in patients with peripheral vascular disease, coronary artery disease, sepsis, impaired renal or hepatic function, and severe hypertension.

Mechanism of Action and Drug Effects

The chemical name for serotonin is 5-hydroxytryptamine, or 5-HT. Physiologists have further identified two 5-HT receptor subtypes on which these drugs have their greatest effect: 5-HT_{1B} and 5-HT_{1D}. Triptans stimulate these receptors in cerebral arteries, causing vasoconstriction and normally reducing or eliminating headache symptoms. They also reduce the production of inflammatory neuropeptides. This is known as *abortive* drug therapy because it treats a headache that has already started. Ergot alkaloids also narrow or constrict blood vessels in the brain. Although the cause of migraines is not fully understood, they are thought to be related to the blood vessels within the brain.

Indications

The triptan antimigraine drugs, also referred to as *selective serotonin receptor agonists (SSRAs)*, are indicated for abortive therapy of an acute migraine headache. Although they may be taken during aura symptoms in patients who have auras with their headaches,

these drugs are not indicated for *preventive* migraine therapy. Preventive therapy is indicated if migraine attacks occur one or more days per week. A variety of drugs are used for preventive therapy; most of them are discussed in more detail in other chapters. These include the ergot alkaloid dihydroergotamine mesylate (D.H.E. 45); nonsteroidal antiinflammatory drugs, including aspirin; acetaminophen; tricyclic antidepressants; MAOIs; beta-blockers; calcium channel blockers; anticonvulsants; antiemetics; sedatives; and the antihistamine cyproheptadine. Among the most commonly used products is a tablet or capsule containing fixed combinations of acetaminophen or aspirin plus the barbiturate butalbital (see Chapter 13) plus the analeptic caffeine, with or without codeine (Fioricet). In addition to potentiating the effects of the analgesics, caffeine can also enhance intestinal absorption of the ergot alkaloids and has a vasoconstricting effect, which can reduce cerebral blood flow to ease headache pain. Caffeine also has a diuretic effect, which may ultimately also reduce cerebral blood flow due to reduced vascular volume secondary to enhanced urinary output. In many cases, preventive drug therapy is sufficient for abortive therapy. When treatment is needed, triptans are the most commonly prescribed drug class.

Contraindications

Contraindications to triptans include drug allergy and the presence of serious cardiovascular disease, because of the vasoconstrictive potential of these medications. Contraindications to the use of ergot alkaloids include uncontrolled hypertension; cerebral, cardiac, or peripheral vascular disease; dysrhythmias; glaucoma; and coronary or ischemic heart disease.

Adverse Effects

Triptans have potential vasoconstrictor effects, including effects on the coronary circulation. Injectable dosage forms may cause local irritation at the site of injection. Other adverse effects include feelings of tingling, flushing (skin warmth and redness), and a congested feeling in the head or chest. Ergot alkaloids are associated with the adverse effects of nausea, vomiting, cold or clammy hands and feet, muscle pain, dizziness, numbness, a vague feeling of anxiety, a bitter or foul taste in the mouth or throat, and irritation of the nose (with the nasal spray dosage form).

Interactions

See Table 14-4.

DRUG PROFILES

SEROTONIN AGONISTS

The serotonin agonists are used to treat migraine headache. They can produce relief from moderate to severe migraines within 2 hours in 70% to 80% of patients. They work by stimulating 5-HT_1 receptors in the brain and are sometimes referred to as *SSRAs* or *triptans*. They are available in a variety of formulations, including oral tablets, sublingual tablets, subcutaneous self-injections, and nasal sprays. A common effect of migraines is nausea and vomiting. Orally administered medications are therefore not tolerated by some patients. Nonoral (including sublingual) forms are advantageous for this reason. They also often have a more rapid onset of action, producing relief in some patients in 10 to 15 minutes, compared with 1 to 2 hours for tablets. (See the Dosages table on p. 218.)

DOSAGES

Selected CNS Stimulants and Related Drugs

Drug (Pregnancy Category)	Pharmacologic Class	Usual Dosage Range	Indications/Uses
◆ amphetamine/dextroamphetamine (Adderall) (C)	CNS stimulant	**Pediatric 3-5 yr** PO: 2.5 mg/day, increased weekly until desired effect **Pediatric 6 yr and older and Adult** PO: 5 mg once or twice daily, increased weekly until desired effect to a daily max of 40 mg	ADHD, narcolepsy
atomoxetine (Strattera) (C)	Selective norepinephrine reuptake inhibitor	**Pediatric (less than 70 kg)** PO: 0.5-1.2 mg/kg/day divided once or twice daily **Adult (70 kg or more)** PO: 40-100 mg/day divided once or twice daily	ADHD
◆ caffeine (NoDoz Maximum Strength, Vivarin) (B)	Xanthine cerebral stimulant	**Adult** PO: 5-10 mg tid 0.5-1 hr before meals IM/IV: 500-1000 mg caffeine citrate or sodium benzoate **Premature infants** IV (caffeine citrate only): 20 mg/kg load followed by 5 mg/kg once daily	Need for mental alertness Respiratory depression (not commonly used in adults) Neonatal apnea, bronchopulmonary dysplasia
doxapram (Dopram) (B)	Respiratory stimulant (analeptic)	**Adult and pediatric older than 12 yr** 0.5-1 mg/kg IV as a single injection not to exceed 1.5 mg/kg, or infusion of 5 mg/min until desired effect, then reduced to 1-3 mg/min 1-2 mg IV given twice at 5-min intervals then repeated at 1-2 hr intervals prn Infusion of 1-2 mg/min for up to 2 hr	Postanesthetic respiratory depression Drug-induced respiratory depression COPD-associated hypercapnia
◆ methylphenidate, extended release (Concerta) (C)	CNS stimulant	**Pediatric and adult** 18-72 mg/day in a single dose	ADHD, narcolepsy
◆ methylphenidate (Ritalin) (C)	CNS stimulant	**Pediatric 6 yr and older** PO: 5 mg bid before breakfast and lunch and increased weekly until desired effect to max of 60 mg/day **Adult** PO: 20-60 mg/day divided bid-tid 30-45 min ac	ADHD, narcolepsy
◆ methylphenidate, extended release (Ritalin-SR) (C)	CNS stimulant	**Pediatric and adult** 20-60 mg/day in a single dose	ADHD, narcolepsy
modafinil (Provigil) (C)	CNS stimulant	**Adult** PO: 200 mg q AM; if second dose needed, give at noon	Narcolepsy
orlistat (Xenical, Allī) (B)	Lipase inhibitor	**Adult** PO: 120 mg tid with each meal containing fat	Obesity
◆ sibutramine (Meridia) (C)	CNS stimulant (anorexiant)	**Adult** PO: 10 mg/day, up to max of 15 mg/day	Obesity
sodium oxybate (Xyrem) (B)	CNS depressant	**Adult only** PO: 2.25 g qhs, repeat in 2.5-4 hr if needed	Cataplexy (associated with narcolepsy)
◆ sumatriptan (Imitrex) (C)	Serotonin agonist	**Adult** PO: 25, 50, or 100 mg, can repeat after 2 hr (max 200 mg/day) Subcut: 4-6 mg, can repeat in 1 hr (max 2 injections/day) Nasal spray: 5, 10, or 20 mg, can repeat after 2 hr (max 40 mg/day)	Acute migraine with or without aura

ADHD, Attention deficit hyperactivity disorder; *CNS*, central nervous system; *COPD*, chronic obstructive pulmonary disease; *IM*, Intramuscular; *IV*, intravenous; *PO*, oral; *subcut*, subcutaneous.

◆ **sumatriptan**

Sumatriptan (Imitrex) was the original prototype drug for this class. As noted earlier, there are now seven triptans. Slight pharmacokinetic differences exist between some of these products, but their effects are comparable overall.

PHARMACOKINETICS

Route	Onset of Action	Peak Plasma Concentration	Elimination Half-life	Duration of Action
PO	0.5-1 hr	2.5 hr	2.5 hr	4 hr

ERGOT ALKALOIDS

Ergot alkaloids, such as ergotamine, are still used in treatment and prevention of migraines but are rapidly being replaced by the triptans. Dihydroergotamine mesylate (D.H.E. 45) is available in injectable form and as a nasal spray (Migranal). Ergotamine tartrate with caffeine (Cafergot) is available in tablet form.

DRUGS FOR SPECIFIC RESPIRATORY DEPRESSION SYNDROMES: ANALEPTICS

Analeptics include doxapram (Dopram) and the methylxanthines aminophylline, theophylline, and caffeine. These drugs are sometimes used to treat neonatal and postoperative respiratory depression. Neonatal uses are more common. Postoperative respiratory depression is a less common problem than it was historically due to the design of newer anesthetic drugs with shorter durations of action.

Mechanism of Action and Drug Effects

Analeptics work by stimulating areas of the CNS that control respiration, mainly the medulla and spinal cord. Methylxanthine analeptics (caffeine, aminophylline, and theophylline) also inhibit the enzyme *phosphodiesterase.* This enzyme breaks down a substance called *cyclic adenosine monophosphate* (cAMP). When analeptics block this enzyme, cAMP accumulates. This results in relaxation of smooth muscle in the respiratory tract, dilation of pulmonary arterioles, and stimulation of the CNS in general. Aminophylline is a *prodrug* (a drug that is formulated for greater solubility to facilitate administration but must be metabolized to an active form); it is *hydrolyzed* to theophylline in the body. Theophylline, in turn, is metabolized to caffeine. Caffeine is inherently a stronger CNS stimulant; hence its popularity in coffee, tea, and soft drinks. As noted previously, it also helps to potentiate the effects of analgesics used for migraine therapy and has a diuretic effect. The stimulant effects of caffeine are attributed to its antagonism (blocking) of adenosine receptors in the brain. Adenosine is associated with sleep promotion. The mechanism of action of doxapram is similar to that of the methylxanthines, but it has a greater stimulant effect in the area of the brain that senses carbon dioxide content. When the carbon dioxide content of the blood is high, the respiratory center in the brain is stimulated to induce deeper and faster breathing in an attempt to exchange more carbon dioxide for inhaled oxygen.

Indications

Currently listed indications for analeptics include neonatal apnea, bronchopulmonary dysplasia, hypercapnia associated with COPD, postanesthetic respiratory depression, and respiratory depression secondary to drugs of abuse (e.g., opioids, alcohol, or barbiturates).

Postoperative respiratory depression is now more commonly treated with mechanical ventilation until the anesthetics wear off. In newborns, administration of caffeine is associated with less tachycardia, CNS stimulation, and feeding intolerance than administration of theophylline or aminophylline. The latter are also used to treat neonatal bradycardia as well as asthma in older children and adults.

Contraindications

Contraindications to the use of analeptics include drug allergy, peptic ulcer disease (especially for caffeine), and serious cardiovascular conditions. Concurrent use of other phosphodiesterase-inhibiting drugs such as sildenafil and similar drugs is also not recommended.

Doxapram use is contraindicated in newborns because of the benzyl alcohol contained in the injectable formulation of the drug. Its use is also contraindicated in patients with epilepsy or other convulsive disorders, those who have shown a hypersensitivity reaction to it, those showing evidence of head injury, those suffering from cardiovascular impairment or severe hypertension, and patients who have experienced a stroke.

Adverse Effects

At higher dosages, analeptics stimulate the vagal, vasomotor, and respiratory centers of the medulla in the brainstem, as well as skeletal muscles. Vagal effects include stimulation of gastric secretions, diarrhea, and reflex tachycardia. Vasomotor effects include flushing (warmth, redness) and sweating of the skin. Respiratory effects include elevated respiratory rate (which is normally desired). Skeletal muscle effects include muscular tension and tremors. Neurologic effects include reduced deep tendon reflexes.

Interactions

See Table 14-4.

DRUG PROFILES

Analeptic drugs include doxapram (Dopram), aminophylline, theophylline, and caffeine. The profiles for aminophylline and theophylline can be found in Chapter 37. The antinarcoleptic analeptic drug modafinil was discussed earlier in the narcolepsy section of this chapter. Dosage and other information appears in the table on p. 218.

◆ **caffeine**

Caffeine is a CNS stimulant that can be found in OTC drugs (e.g., NoDoz) and combination prescription drugs (e.g., Fioricet, Fiorinal). It is also contained in many beverages and foods. Just a few of the many foods and drugs that contain caffeine are listed in Table 14-5. Caffeine is contraindicated in patients with a known hypersensitivity to it and should be used with caution in patients who have a history of peptic ulcers or cardiac dysrhythmias or who have recently experienced a myocardial infarction. Caffeine is available in oral and injectable dosage forms.

PHARMACOKINETICS

Route	Onset of Action	Peak Plasma Concentration	Elimination Half-life	Duration of Action
PO	15-45 min	1 hr	3-4 hr	6 hr

There are two forms of intravenous caffeine, caffeine citrate and caffeine sodium benzoate. Caffeine citrate is recommended for neonatal apnea, including cases not responsive to other meth-

TABLE 14-5 Caffeine-Containing Beverages and Drugs

Medication or Beverage	Amount of Caffeine
Nonprescription Medications	
Analgesics	
Anacin	32 mg/tab
Excedrin, Excedrin Aspirin-Free, Excedrin Migraine	65 mg/tab
Stimulants	
NoDoz Maximum Strength	100 mg/tab
Vivarin	200 mg/tab
Prescription Medications (for Migraines)	
Fioricet, Fiorinal	40 mg/tab
Esgic	40 mg/tab
Cafergot	10 mg/suppository
Beverages	
Coffee (brewed, instant)	80-150 mg/5-oz cup
Coffee (decaffeinated)	2-4 mg/5-oz cup
Tea (brewed)	30-75 mg/5-oz cup
Soft drinks	35-60 mg/12-oz cup
Cocoa	5-40 mg/5-oz cup

ylxanthines such as theophylline. Caffeine sodium benzoate is used for respiratory depression in adults only, because it is associated with *gasping syndrome* in infants and may also displace bilirubin into the blood from albumin binding sites in the circulation. This, in turn, could cause or worsen hyperbilirubinemia, a common condition in high-risk infants.

doxapram

Doxapram (Dopram) is another analeptic that is commonly used in conjunction with supportive measures in cases of respiratory depression that involve anesthetics or drugs of abuse and in COPD-associated hypercapnia. Deep tendon reflexes, in addition to vital signs and heart rhythm, are monitored to prevent overdosage of this drug.

PHARMACOKINETICS

Route	Onset of Action	Peak Plasma Concentration	Elimination Half-life	Duration of Action
IV	Less than 30 sec	Less than 2 min	2-4 hr	5-12 min

NURSING PROCESS

Assessment

CNS stimulants are used for a variety of conditions and disorders. They have addictive potential, and so the following assessment data should be collected before their use, regardless of indication: (1) a thorough medical history with attention to preexisting diseases or conditions, especially those of the cardiovascular, cerebrovascular, neurologic, renal, and liver systems; (2) past and current history of addictive or substance abuse behaviors; (3) complete medication profile with a listing of prescription, OTC, and herbal drugs and any use of alcohol, nicotine, and/or social or illegal drugs; and (4) a complete nutritional and dietary history. All of these areas must be assessed because of the mechanism of action of CNS stimulants, which increases pulse rate and blood pressure,

and can lead to seizures, intracerebral bleeding, and toxicity (due to decreased metabolism and excretion). Stimulation of the respiratory system is actually desirable, and this action is beneficial in those patients suffering from CNS depression, such as postoperatively. Improvement of attention span is beneficial in those in need of the medication, but the possibility of adverse effects requires a thorough assessment to obtain baseline information. The anorexiant action may cause complications if the drugs are used or ordered inappropriately. When they are taken for appetite suppression, baseline height, weight, and dietary intake should be assessed and documented. Vital signs should always be measured, with specific attention to blood pressure and pulse rate.

To add to the thoroughness of the assessment, a complete nursing history should include inquiry about lifestyle, exercise, nutritional habits and patterns (a reduction in fat-soluble vitamins, history of any type of eating disorder), educational level, previous teaching and learning successes and failures, available support structures such as family and friends, self-esteem, stress levels, mental status and mental health problems (drugs may exacerbate psychosis), presence of diabetes (diabetic patients need closer monitoring and tighter glucose control), and information related to contraindications, cautions, and drug interactions (see Table 14-4).

With *drugs used for the management of attention deficit hyperactivity disorder*, very cautious and continuous assessment is required, including much of the information mentioned earlier. For the pediatric patient, assessment should include the baseline weight and height, growth and development patterns, vital signs, and complete blood counts. Adults should have baseline weight, height, vital signs, and complete blood counts. Usual sleep habits and patterns should be assessed and documented so that sleep disturbances may be anticipated and managed appropriately. Atypical behavior, loss in attention span, and history of social problems or problems in school are also important to assess and document before and during therapy for baseline comparison. For children with ADHD, parental support is important to the success of treatment, and so a home assessment may be needed. Attention to and documentation of daily dietary intake before drug therapy is important because of the risk of drug-related weight loss. It is also important that the pediatric patient not experience too rapid or too much weight loss; a thorough nutritional and dietary assessment is needed. Cardiac assessment is important because of the CNS stimulation. Blood pressure, pulse rate, heart sounds, and any history of chest pain or palpitations should be noted. Assessment should address possible contraindications, cautions, and drug interactions (see previous discussion), and findings should be documented along with notation of the patient's use of any prescription drugs, OTC drugs (e.g., nasal decongestants, which are also stimulants), and herbal preparations, specifically ginseng and caffeine (see Herbal Therapies and Dietary Supplements box).

The *serotonin agonists* commonly used in the treatment of migraines are not without adverse reactions, contraindications, cautions, and drug interactions (see previous discussion). Assessment should include a thorough cardiac history as well as measurement of blood pressure and pulse rate and rhythm. Should a patient have a history of hypertension, there is risk of further increases in blood pressure to dangerous levels with use of these drugs, and thus the need for careful assessment and documentation. In fact, generally these drugs are not prescribed for patients with migraines who also have coronary artery disease unless a

HERBAL THERAPIES AND DIETARY SUPPLEMENTS

Selected Herbal Compounds Used for Nervous System Stimulation*

Common Name(s)	Uses	Possible Drug Interactions (Avoid Concurrent Use)
Ginkgo biloba, ginkgo	To enhance mental alertness; to improve memory or dementia	Warfarin, aspirin
Ginseng	To enhance impaired mental function and concentration	Drugs for diabetes that lower blood sugar (e.g., insulin, oral hypoglycemic drugs), monoamine oxidase inhibitors
Guarana	To stimulate nervous system, suppress appetite	Adenosine, disulfiram, quinolones, oral contraceptives, beta-blockers, iron, lithium, phenylephrine (e.g., nasal spray), cimetidine, theophylline, tobacco

Data from Fetrow CW, Avila JR: *The complete guide to herbal remedies,* Springhouse, Pa, 2000, Springhouse.

*The information in this box does not imply author or publisher endorsement of these products. Although individual consumers often experience satisfying results with various herbal products, there is frequently little, if any, rigorously controlled research to demonstrate their efficacy at treating particular conditions. Patients should always be advised to communicate regularly with their health care practitioners about all medications used, including herbal remedies, to decrease the likelihood of possibly hazardous drug interactions.

Note also that sale of the herbal central nervous system stimulant known as *ephedra* or *ma huang* was officially banned by the Food and Drug Administration, effective April 2004, following its link to cases of myocardial infarction and stroke.

---

thorough cardiac evaluation has been performed. A careful assessment should be performed to identify other drugs the patient is taking that might lead to significant drug interactions, such as ergot alkaloids, selective serotonin receptor inhibitors, and MAOIs, because if serotonin agonists are taken within 2 weeks of the use of these drugs, there is high risk for an additive toxicity. Such toxicity would be manifested by nervousness, insomnia, cardiovascular complications, and convulsions.

Ergot alkaloids also have cautions, contraindications, and drug interactions (see previous discussion), which need to be assessed for and documented. A history of the migraines and their pattern, exacerbating factors, measures providing relief, and previous treatments should also be obtained. See *http://www. WebMD.com/migraines-headaches* for further discussion of migraine headaches.

An *analeptic* such as doxapram is used as a central respiratory stimulant; therefore, it is most likely be used in a hospital setting, specifically in intensive care units or postanesthesia units. The same concerns regarding contraindications, cautions, and drug interactions exist for this drug as for all CNS stimulants, and even closer attention must be paid to vital signs, especially heart rate and rhythm, and blood pressure. Any elevations in blood pressure and pulse rate may put the patient at a higher risk of complications. The same neurologic assessment data should be gathered as previously discussed because of associated risks of seizures. In addition, baseline reflexes (e.g., deep tendon reflexes) should also be assessed and documented.

Nursing Diagnoses

- Disturbed energy field, anxiety, and restlessness related to the adverse effects of CNS stimulants
- Decreased cardiac output related to the adverse effects of CNS stimulants (e.g., palpitations and tachycardia)
- Deficient knowledge related to lack of information and experience with a day-today or as-needed drug regimen
- Disturbed sleep patterns related to the action and adverse effects of CNS stimulants
- Imbalanced nutrition, more than body requirements, as manifested by the presence of obesity, related to poor nutritional habits

- Imbalanced nutrition, less than body requirements, related to adverse effects of CNS stimulants (e.g., amphetamines and anorexiants)
- Chronic pain related to the experience of or a history of migraine headaches
- Acute pain related to the adverse effects of CNS drugs (e.g., headache and dry mouth)
- Situational low self-esteem related to the impact of obesity and/or other nutritional disorders or to the impact of attention deficit hyperactivity disorder

Planning
Goals

- Patient appears less anxious or experiences no anxiety from the medication.
- Patient is free of cardiac symptoms and associated complications of drug therapy.
- Patient remains open to education about related drug and nondrug therapeutic regimens.
- Patient regains or maintains near normal body weight and BMI during therapy.
- Patient continues to undergo close to normal growth and development while taking medications.
- Patient experiences minimal sleep deprivation.
- Patient maintains positive self-esteem.
- Patient remains compliant with drug therapy and free from complications of treatment.

Outcome Criteria

- Patient communicates anxiety, anger, and feelings regarding self-image and self-esteem openly and as needed.
- Patient maintains appropriate weight loss without too rapid losses or gains throughout treatment while taking CNS stimulants (if a pediatric patient, normal growth and development patterns are continued with weight and height falling within normal limits on growth chart).
- Patient shows improved sensorium and level of consciousness with increased attention span and cognition.
- Patient experiences more restful sleep using nonpharmacologic measures.

- Patient's vital signs, especially blood pressure and pulse, remain within normal limits.
- Patient states symptoms (e.g., palpitations, chest pain) that should be reported to the prescriber immediately.
- Patient reports a decrease in headaches.
- Patient reports that medication is taken as ordered and consistently over the time of the therapeutic protocol.

Implementation

With *drugs used for the treatment of attention deficit hyperactivity disorder,* some pediatric patients may respond better to certain dosage forms such as immediate release. However, dosing should be individualized and based on the patient's needs at different times during the school day (e.g., a noon dose to help with music lessons later in the afternoon). Scheduling of these medications and close communication among the school, teachers, school nurse, and the family and patient is very important to successful treatment. It is also important to time the dosing of medications—but as ordered—for periods in which symptom control is most needed but without causing alterations in sleep patterns. Generally speaking, once-a-day dosing is used with extended-release or long-acting preparations. Adequate and proper dosing will be manifested by good control of behavior and improvement during school time. If extended-release dosage forms lead to acceptable outcomes for the pediatric patient, taking medications at school may not be necessary. Many times a stigma is associated with taking medications at school. This may be preventable with use of long-acting preparations or other scheduling. To help decrease the occurrence of insomnia, the last daily dose should be taken 4 to 6 hours before bedtime as ordered. During therapy, the patient will also be monitored for continued physical growth, with specific attention to weight and height. The prescriber may order medication-free times on weekends, holidays, and/or vacations; that is, the drug may be discontinued periodically so that the need for the medication can be reassessed and sensitivity increased.

Because *anorexiants* are generally used for a short period of time, it is very important to emphasize to the patient and all members of the patient's support system that a suitable diet, appropriate independent and/or supervised exercise program, and behavioral modifications are necessary to support a favorable result and to help the patient cease overeating and experience healthy weight loss. With a drug regimen, medications are usually taken first thing in the morning, as ordered, to minimize interference with sleep. These drugs should not be taken within 4 to 6 hours of sleep due to interference with sleep. If the patient has been taking these drugs for a prolonged period, there should be an interval of weaning before discontinuation to avoid withdrawal symptoms and to avoid any chance of a rebound increase in appetite. Weight should be assessed weekly or as ordered. The patient should be encouraged to keep a journal to record food intake as well as responses to the drug regimen, any adverse effects, socialization, exercise, and notes about how the patient is feeling day to day. Dry mouth may be managed with frequent mouth care and the use of sugar-free gum or hard candy. Sucking ice chips, as well as keeping a bottle of fresh water on hand at all times, may also be helpful. If headaches occur, acetaminophen will most likely be suggested. Caffeine in any form, including coffee, tea, sodas, and chocolate, should be avoided. Other products that may contain caffeine include some OTC analgesics; OTC compounds to treat menstrual

LEGAL AND ETHICAL PRINCIPLES

Handling of Prescription Drugs

It is important for the nurse to understand the following amendments to the federal laws that apply to the handling of all prescription drugs by the registered nurse. (NOTE: This is a summary and does not reflect the laws in their entirety.)

The registered nurse is prohibited from doing the following:
- Compounding or dispensing the designated drugs for legal distribution and administration.
- Distributing the drugs to any individuals who are not licensed or authorized by federal or state law to receive the drugs (e.g., those individuals outside the health care provider–patient relationship); the penalties for such actions are generally severe.
- Making, selling, keeping, or concealing any counterfeit drug equipment.
- Possessing any type of stimulant or depressant drug unless authorized to do so by a legal prescription (as a patient); any unauthorized possession is illegal.

It is important to adhere to these legal guidelines in the practice of drug administration to avoid legal penalties, including possible loss of license or other severe penalties.

symptoms; OTC products for cough, cold, flu, or congestion; and prescription drugs such as analgesics with ergotamine and caffeine, and butalbital with aspirin and caffeine (see following discussion). Supplementation with fat-soluble vitamins may be indicated with use of these drugs. It is also important to watch for tolerance to the anorexiant during the course of treatment. Other nursing considerations include emphasis on a holistic approach to treatment of obesity, including the possible use of hypnosis, biofeedback, and guided imagery, as ordered. Patients should be encouraged to keep follow-up visits with their prescribers and others involved in their care.

SSRAs come in a variety of dosage forms. Rizatriptan is available in oral tablets as well as in a disintegrating tablet or wafer that dissolves on the tongue. The latter dosage form leads to a more rapid absorption. Use of the nasal spray or self-injectable forms of the serotonin agonists is especially desirable in patients experiencing the nausea and vomiting that may occur with migraine headaches. Self-injectable forms and nasal sprays also have the benefit of an onset of action of 10 to 15 minutes compared with 1 to 2 hours for tablet forms. Administration of a test dose of the injectable and all other dosage forms is usually recommended. If the injectable form is prescribed, the patient should also receive instructions and demonstrations about the technique. See Patient Teaching Tips for more information.

Ergot alkaloids should be taken exactly as prescribed; for example, tablets should be taken with 6 to 8 oz of water or other fluid and work best when taken at the first sign of the migraine. This allows more successful treatment. With ergotamine tartrate and related drugs, the maximum dose is usually 6 tablets for a single headache and 10 tablets in any 7-day period. Dependence may occur with the ergots, and if they are withdrawn suddenly, rebound headaches may occur. The patient should report to the prescriber any headaches that are uncharacteristic or unusual, as well as any persistent headache, worsening of headaches, severe nausea, vomiting, dizziness, or restlessness. Any of the following should also be reported immediately to the prescriber: slow, fast, or irregular heartbeat; tingling, pain, or coldness in the fingers or toes; loss of feeling in the fingers or toes; muscle pain or weakness; severe stomach or abdominal pain; lower back pain; little or no urine. The patient should seek immediate medical attention if there is any chest pain, vision changes, confusion, or slurred speech. As mentioned previously, these medications should not be taken with triptans.

The *analeptic* doxapram may be administered intravenously (see the Dosages table on p. 218) but at different dosages depending on the purpose. Doxapram infusions should be given using an intravenous pump and with close monitoring. Because the patient's sensorium is generally diminished in this situation, placing the patient in the Sims' or semi-Fowler's position is necessary to prevent aspiration. The patient's airway, breathing, and circulation (ABCs of care) are of most importance. Should adverse effects occur (see the pharmacology discussion), the prescriber should be notified.

Evaluation

Therapeutic responses to *drugs for attention deficit hyperactivity disorder* include decreased hyperactivity, increased attention span and concentration, and improved behavior. Adverse effects range from loss of appetite to increased irritability, insomnia, palpitations, nausea, and headaches. Therapeutic effects of *anorexiants* include appetite control and weight loss for the treatment of obe-sity. Adverse effects of these drugs include dry mouth, headache, insomnia, constipation, tachycardia, cardiac irregularities, hypertension, changes in mental status or sensorium, changes in mood or affect, alteration of sleep patterns, and seizures (all due to excess CNS stimulation). Evaluating for any increased irritability and withdrawal symptoms (e.g., headache, nausea and vomiting) is also important. If the anorexiant affects fat metabolism, then there may be adverse effects such as flatulence with an oily discharge, spotting, and fecal urgency. The patient also needs to be closely evaluated for decreased levels of fat-soluble vitamins (A, D, E, and K), because their levels may be affected by the decreased absorption of fats. For *drugs used to treat narcolepsy,* therapeutic responses include a decrease in sleepiness and more wakefulness. Adverse effects for which to monitor include headache, nausea, nervousness, and anxiety. Therapeutic responses to the *serotonin agonists* include a decrease in the frequency, duration, and severity of migraine headaches with improved daily functioning and performance because of the reduction in headaches. Adverse effects for which to monitor include pain at the injection site (if a self-injectable form is used; such pain is temporary), flushing, chest tightness or pressure, weakness, sedation, dizziness, sweating, increase in blood pressure and pulse rate, and bad taste with the nasal spray formulation, which may precipitate nausea.

PATIENT TEACHING TIPS

General Information
- Serotonin agonists should be taken at the exact time and frequency ordered.
- Medications should be taken exactly as prescribed without skipping, omitting, or adding doses.
- Alcohol, OTC cold products, cough syrups that contain alcohol, nicotine, and caffeine should be avoided. All food items or beverages with caffeine should also be avoided.
- Keeping a journal of daily activities and response to drug therapy and any adverse effects is encouraged.
- Sudden withdrawal of medications should be avoided.

Drugs Used to Treat Attention Deficit Hyperactivity Disorder
- Medication should be taken on an empty stomach 30 to 45 minutes before eating for maximal effects.
- The importance of keeping all follow-up appointments is important to monitoring drug therapy.
- If the prescriber decides that the medication should be discontinued, a weaning process with careful supervision should be used.
- Extended-release or long-acting preparations should not be crushed, chewed, broken, or altered in any way and should be taken only as directed.
- Dosage should not be increased or decreased by the patient or family, because this may lead to drug-related complications. If there is any concern about the drug and its dosage amount or adverse effects, parents or caregivers should be encouraged to contact the prescriber.

Anorexiants
- The patient must be sure to follow all prescriber instructions regarding medications, diet, and exercise.
- Some of these medications may impair alertness and ability to think so patients should be cautious engaging in activities that may be adversely affected until these impairments are resolved.

- An unpleasant taste of the medicine and/or dry mouth may be minimized by the use of mouth rinses, ice chips, sugarless chewing gum, and/or hard candies.

Antimigraine Drugs
- Patients experiencing migraines should avoid foods containing tyramine, because they are known to trigger severe or migraine headaches. Tyramine-containing substances include beer, wine, aged cheese, food additives, preservatives, artificial sweeteners, chocolate, and caffeine (see Table 17-4).
- Before using a nasal spray form of an antimigraine drug, the patient should gently blow the nose to clear the nasal passages. With the head upright, the patient should close one nostril and insert the nozzle into the open nostril. While a breath is taken through the nose, the spray should be released. The nozzle should be removed, and the patient should gently breathe in through the nose and out through the mouth for 10 to 20 seconds. Some bad taste may be experienced.
- Until migraine is resolved, the patient should avoid doing things that require alertness and rapid skilled movements. It may be helpful to keep the room darkened and noise to a minimum. Should the headache not resolve and/or vomiting occur, the patient should contact the prescriber for further instructions to help avoid additional problems, such as dehydration.
- A journal should be kept of all headaches, precipitators, and relievers, and should rate each headache on a scale of 0 to 10, where 0 is no pain and 10 is the worst pain ever. The patient should be sure to record other symptoms such as photophobia, nausea, and vomiting, as well as their frequency and duration.
- When taking SSRAs, the patient should contact the prescriber immediately if he or she experiences palpitations, chest pain, and/or pain or weakness in the extremities.
- Injectable forms of sumatriptan should be given subcutaneously and as ordered. The patient should practice administering injections (without the medication) with the nurse at the prescriber's

Continued

PATIENT TEACHING TIPS—cont'd

office so that proper technique is used and comfort level achieved.

- Autoinjectors with prefilled syringes may be used. The syringe should be discarded in an appropriate container or receptacle after use and should be kept out of the reach of children.
- No more than two injections of sumatriptan should be administered during a 24-hour period and at least 1 hour should be allowed between injections.
- When using injectable sumatriptan, the patient should contact the prescriber or emergency services immediately if he or she experiences swelling around the eyes, pain or tightness in the chest or throat, wheezing, and/or heart throbbing.

- Treatment for migraine headaches can relieve the pain and symptoms of a migraine attack as well as prevent further migraine attacks. Some abortive therapies may offer rapid relief if drugs are given as ordered and before the headache worsens. Drugs may be given orally, sublingually, or by injection in the thigh. Abortive treatment medications include the triptans, such as sumatriptan. When a triptan does not work, an ergot alkaloid such as dihydroergotamine or ergotamine tartrate may be ordered. As mentioned in the pharmacology section, other drugs may also be used to try to prevent migraine headache, such as antiemetics, antidepressants, antiseizure medications, and beta-blockers.

POINTS TO REMEMBER

- CNS stimulants are drugs that stimulate the brain or spinal cord.
- The actions of these stimulants mimic those of the neurotransmitters of the sympathetic nervous system (e.g., norepinephrine, dopamine, and serotonin).
- Included in the family of CNS stimulants are amphetamines, analeptics, and anorexiants with therapeutic uses for attention deficit hyperactivity disorder, narcolepsy, and appetite control. Adverse effects associated with CNS stimulants include changes in mental status or sensorium, changes in mood or affect, tachycardia, loss of appetite, nausea, altered sleep patterns (e.g., insomnia), physical dependency, irritability, and seizures.
- Serotonin agonists may be administered as a subcutaneous injection, as a nasal spray, and as oral tablets. Any chest pain or tightness, tremors, vomiting, or worsening symptoms should be reported to the prescriber immediately.

- Anorexiants control or suppress appetite. They are used to stimulate the CNS and result in suppression of appetite control centers in the brain.
- Contraindications to the use of anorexiants, as well as other CNS stimulants, include hypersensitivity, seizure activity, convulsive disorders, and liver dysfunction.
- The SSRAs are a newer class of CNS stimulants and are used to treat migraine headaches. They should not be given to patients with coronary heart disease.
- Amphetamines elevate mood or produce euphoria, increase mental alertness and capacity for work, decrease fatigue and drowsiness, and prolong wakefulness.
- Journaling is helpful in evaluating the effects of all drugs used to treat attention deficit hyperactivity disorder, obesity, migraines, and narcolepsy.

NCLEX EXAMINATION REVIEW QUESTIONS

1 A patient with narcolepsy will begin treatment with a CNS stimulant. The nurse expects to see which adverse effect?
  a Bradycardia
  b Nervousness
  c Mental clouding
  d Drowsiness at night
2 A patient at a weight management clinic who was given a prescription for orlistat (Xenical) calls the clinic hotline complaining of a "terrible side effect." The nurse suspects that the patient is referring to
  a nausea.
  b sexual dysfunction.
  c urinary incontinence.
  d fecal incontinence.
3 The nurse is developing a plan of care for a patient receiving an anorexiant. Which nursing diagnosis is most appropriate?
  a Deficient fluid volume
  b Sleep deprivation
  c Impaired memory
  d Imbalanced nutrition, more than body requirements
4 A patient has a new prescription for sumatriptan (Imitrex). The nurse providing patient teaching on self-administration will include which information?
  a Correct technique for subcutaneous injections
  b Correct technique for intramuscular injections
  c Proper placement of the transdermal patch
  d The need to dissolve tablets under the tongue completely
5 The nurse is reviewing the history of a patient who will be starting the triptan sumatriptan (Imitrex) as part of treatment for migraine headaches. Which condition, if present, may be a contraindication to triptan therapy?
  a Cardiovascular disease
  b Chronic bronchitis
  c History of renal calculi
  d Diabetes mellitus type 2
6 The nurse is reviewing medication therapy with the parents of an adolescent with ADHD. Which statement is correct? (Select all that apply.)
  a "Be sure to have your child blow his nose before administering the nasal spray."
  b "This medication is used only when symptoms of ADHD are severe."
  c "The last dose should be taken 4 to 6 hours before bedtime to avoid interference with sleep."
  d "Be sure to contact the physician right away if you notice expression of suicidal thoughts."
  e "We will need to check your child's height and weight periodically to monitor physical growth."
  f "If adverse effects become severe, stop the medication for 3 to 4 days."

1. b, 2. d, 3. d, 4. a, 5. a, 6. c, d, e.

CRITICAL THINKING ACTIVITIES: BEST ACTION

1 The parents of a 10-year-old boy are concerned about the effects of the medication their son is taking for ADHD. They ask, "What should we be looking for when he starts this medicine?" What is the nurse's best response?
2 A patient calls the headache clinic because she is unhappy about her medication. She says, "I've been taking zolmitriptan (Zomig) to prevent headaches, but I am still having them." What is the nurse's best answer to this patient?
3 An obese patient is discussing options for appetite suppressant therapy and says, "I want to lose weight but I can't help myself—I'm hungry all the time! The doctor wants me to take a pill to stop my appetite, but I'm afraid there will be adverse effects." What is the nurse's best action at this time?

For answers, see *http://evolve.elsevier.com/Lilley.*

CHAPTER 15

Antiepileptic Drugs

OBJECTIVES

When you reach the end of this chapter, you should be able to do the following:

1 Briefly describe the pathophysiology of epilepsy.

2 Discuss the rationale for the use of the various classes of antiepileptic drugs (AEDs) administered for management of the different forms of epilepsy.

3 Identify the various drugs in each of the following drug classes: iminostilbenes, benzodiazepines, barbiturates, hydantoins, and miscellaneous drugs.

4 Identify the mechanisms of action, indications, cautions, contraindications, dosages, routes of administration, adverse effects, toxic effects, related therapeutic blood levels, and drug interactions for the drugs in each AED class.

5 Develop a nursing care plan, including patient education, based on the nursing process for patients receiving AEDs.

e-Learning Activities

Drug Profiles

♦ carbamazepine, p. 236
ethosuximide, p. 237
♦ gabapentin, p. 237
lamotrigine, p. 237
levetiracetam, p. 237
oxcarbazepine, p. 237
♦ phenobarbital and primidone, p. 233

♦ phenytoin and fosphenytoin, p. 235
pregabalin, p. 237
tiagabine, p. 238
topiramate, p. 238
♦ valproic acid, p. 236
zonisamide, p. 238

♦ *Key drug.*

Glossary

Anticonvulsants Substances or procedures that prevent or reduce the severity of *epileptic* or other *convulsive* seizures. (p. 228)

Antiepileptic drugs Substances that prevent or reduce the severity of epilepsy and different types of epileptic seizures, not just convulsive seizures. (p. 228)

Autoinduction A metabolic process in which a drug stimulates the production of enzymes that enhance its own metabolism over time, which leads to a reduction in therapeutic drug concentrations. (p. 237)

Convulsion A type of seizure involving excessive stimulation of neurons in the brain and characterized by the spasmodic contraction of voluntary muscles. (See also *seizure.*) (p. 226)

Electroencephalogram (EEG) A recording of the electrical activity that arises from spontaneous currents in nerve cells in the brain, derived from electrodes placed on the outer skull. (p. 227)

Epilepsy A general term for any of a group of neurologic disorders characterized by *recurrent* episodes of *convulsive seizures*, sensory disturbances, abnormal behavior, loss of consciousness, or any combination of these. (p. 227)

Primary epilepsy Epilepsy in which there is no identifiable cause. Also known as *idiopathic.* (p. 227)

Seizure Excessive stimulation of neurons in the brain leading to a sudden burst of abnormal neuron activity that results in temporary changes in brain function, primarily affecting sensory and motor activity. (p. 226)

Seizures, generalized onset Seizures originating simultaneously in both cerebral hemispheres. (p. 227)

Seizures, partial onset Seizures originating in a more localized region of the brain (also called *focal* seizures). (p. 227)

Status epilepticus A common seizure disorder characterized by generalized tonic-clonic convulsions that occur in succession. (p. 228)

Tonic-clonic seizures Seizures involving initial muscular contraction throughout the body (tonic phase), progressing to alternating contraction and relaxation (clonic phase). (p. 227)

• • •

Anatomy, Physiology, and Disease Overview

EPILEPSY

Epilepsy is a broad syndrome of central nervous system (CNS) dysfunction that can manifest in many ways, from momentary sensory disturbances to convulsive seizures. It is the most common chronic neurologic illness. It results from excessive electrical activity of neurons (nerve cells) located in the superficial area of the brain known as the *cerebral cortex* or *gray matter.* The terms *convulsion, seizure,* and *epilepsy* are often used interchangeably, but they do not have the same meaning. A **seizure** is a brief episode of abnormal electrical activity in the nerve cells of the brain, which may or may not lead to a convulsion. A **convulsion** is a more severe seizure characterized by involuntary spasmodic contractions of any or all voluntary muscles throughout the body, including skeletal, facial, and ocular muscles. Commonly reported symptoms include abnormal motor function, loss of consciousness, altered sensory awareness, and psychic changes. In contrast, **epilepsy** is a chronic, recurrent pattern of seizures. These excessive electrical discharges can often be detected by an **electroencephalogram (EEG),** which is commonly obtained to help diagnose epilepsy. Fluctuations in the brain's electrical potential are seen in the form of waves, which correlate well with different neurologic conditions and so are used as diagnostic indicators. In the case of epilepsy, they are used to identify specific seizure subtypes.

Because up to 50% of patients with epilepsy have normal EEGs, a careful history is also important for accurate diagnosis. Other applicable diagnostic tests include skull radiography, *computed tomography,* and *magnetic resonance imaging.* These procedures help to rule out structural causes of epilepsy, such as brain tumors. In particularly severe cases, patients may be observed in a hospital setting or sleep study laboratory. This allows for continuous EEG and video monitoring to identify detailed patterns of seizure activity and, it is hoped, to allow tailoring of an effective treatment.

Epilepsy occurs most commonly in children and the elderly. Epilepsy without an identifiable cause is known as **primary epilepsy** or *idiopathic* epilepsy. Primary epilepsy accounts for roughly 50% of cases. Evidence strongly indicates genetic predispositions, but these have yet to be clearly defined. Studies in the field of *pharmacogenetics* (see Chapter 5) are just beginning to attempt to clarify genetic factors that can help optimize antiepileptic drug therapy. In other cases, epilepsy has a distinct cause, such as trauma, infection, cerebrovascular disorder, or other illness. This type is known as *secondary* or *symptomatic* epilepsy. The chief causes of secondary epilepsy in children and infants are developmental defects, metabolic disease, and injury at birth. *Febrile seizures* occur in children aged 6 months to 5 years, and by definition are caused by fever. Children usually outgrow the tendency to have such seizures, and thus these seizures do not constitute a chronic illness. Antipyretic drugs (e.g., acetaminophen [see Chapter 11]) are normally adequate for acute treatment.

In adults, acquired brain disorder is the major cause of secondary epilepsy. Some examples include head injury, disease or infection of the brain and spinal cord, stroke, metabolic disorder, adverse drug reactions (e.g., meperidine [see Chapter 11], theophylline [see Chapter 37]), a primary or metastatic brain tumor, or other nonspecific neurologic diseases. Interestingly, the elderly have the highest incidence of new-onset epilepsy. Fortunately, seizures in the elderly are often well controlled with drug therapy.

Seizures are classified into different categories based on their presenting features. The International League Against Epilepsy *(http://www.ilae-epilepsy.org)* lists three major categories: *partial onset, generalized onset,* and *unclassified* seizures (Box 15-1). Furthermore, evidence provided by EEG and other diagnostic techniques mentioned previously indicates that different types of seizures originate from disruptions of normal brain electrical activity in different regions or *lobes* of the brain.

Generalized onset seizures, formerly called *grand mal* seizures, are characterized by neuronal activity that originates simultaneously in the gray matter of both hemispheres. There are

---

BOX 15-1 International League Against Epilepsy: Classification of Seizures

Partial Seizures
Description

Short alterations in consciousness, repetitive unusual movements (chewing or swallowing movements), psychologic changes, and confusion

Simple Seizures
- No impaired consciousness
- Motor symptoms (most commonly face, arm, or leg)
- Hallucinations of sight, hearing, or taste along with somatosensory changes (tingling)
- Autonomic nervous system responses
- Personality changes

Complex Seizures
- Impaired consciousness
- Memory impairment
- Behavioral effects
- Purposeless behaviors
- Aura, chewing and swallowing movements, unreal feelings, bizarre behavior
- Tonic, clonic, or tonic-clonic seizures

Generalized Seizures
Description

Most often seen in children and commonly characterized by temporary lapses in consciousness lasting a few seconds. Staring off into space, daydreaming, and inattentive look are common symptoms. Patients may exhibit rhythmic movements of their eyes, head, or hands but do not experience convulsions. Patients may have several attacks per day.
- Both cerebral hemispheres involved
- Tonic, clonic, myoclonic, atonic, or tonic-clonic seizures and infantile spasms possible
- Brief loss of consciousness for a few seconds with no confusion
- Head drop or falling-down symptoms

Unclassified Seizures
Description

Seizures that are not officially classified due to inadequate data, and seizures that do not fit into the above categories. These include neonatal seizures such as those manifested by rhythmic eye movements, chewing, and swimming movements.

---

several subtypes of generalized seizures. **Tonic-clonic seizures** begin with muscular contraction throughout the body (tonic phase) and progress to alternating contraction and relaxation (clonic phase). *Tonic* seizures involve spasms of the upper trunk with flexion of the arms. *Clonic* seizures are the same as tonic-clonic seizures but without the tonic phase. *Atonic* seizures, also known as *drop attacks,* involve sudden global muscle weakness and syncope. *Myoclonic seizures* are characterized by brief muscular jerks, but not as extreme as in other subtypes. Finally, *absence* seizures involve a brief loss of awareness that commonly occurs with repetitive spasmodic eye blinking for up to 30 seconds. This type occurs primarily in childhood and rarely after age 14 years.

Partial onset seizures originate in a localized or *focal* region (e.g., one lobe) of the brain. There are three types of partial onset seizures. The first type is known as *simple partial onset seizure,* formerly called *petit mal* seizure, and is characterized by brief loss of awareness (e.g., blank stare) but without loss of consciousness or spasmodic eye blinking as in absence seizures described previously. In the second type, *complex partial onset seizure,* the level of consciousness is reduced but is not completely lost. Partial onset seizures can progress to generalized tonic-clonic seizures in up to 40% of patients. This third type is known as a *secondary generalized tonic-clonic seizure.* The latter two types are also associated with postictal confusion, a term for the confused mental state that follows seizure activity.

Unclassified seizures are those that do not clearly fit into any of the other categories.

As noted, seizure episodes can sometimes start off as partial and then become generalized. If the partial component is not noticed, the patient may be misdiagnosed and receive suboptimal drug therapy. Another important seizure condition is **status epilepticus.** In status epilepticus, multiple seizures occur with no recovery between them. Hypotension, hypoxia, and cardiac dysrhythmias complicate the disorder, and brain damage and death quickly ensue if appropriate therapy is not started promptly. Febrile seizures can also sometimes progress to status epilepticus. In addition to the website of the International League Against Epilepsy mentioned earlier, other helpful websites include *http://www.epilepsyfoundation.org* and *http://www.epilepsy.com.*

Pharmacology Overview
ANTIEPILEPTIC DRUGS

Antiepileptic drugs are also called *anticonvulsants.* **Antiepileptic drugs** is a more appropriate term, because many of these medications are indicated for the management of all types of epilepsy, and not necessarily just convulsions. **Anticonvulsants,** on the other hand, are medications that are used to prevent the *convulsive* seizures typically associated with epilepsy.

The goal of antiepileptic drug therapy is to control or prevent seizures while maintaining a reasonable quality of life. Approximately 70% of patients can expect to become seizure free and most will take only one drug. The remaining 30% of cases are more complicated, and often multiple medications are required. Many antiepileptic drugs have adverse effects, and achieving seizure control while avoiding adverse effects is often a difficult balancing task. In most cases, the therapeutic goal is not to eliminate seizure activity but rather to maximally reduce the incidence of seizures while minimizing drug-induced toxicity. Many patients must take these drugs for their entire lives. Treatment may eventually be stopped in some, but others will experience repeated seizures if constant levels of antiepileptic drugs are not maintained in the blood. Abrupt discontinuation of these drugs can result in withdrawal seizures. In both children and adults, there is only a 40% chance of recurrence after the first partial or generalized seizure. Therefore, antiepileptic drug therapy is *not* recommended after a single isolated seizure event. However, antiepileptic drug therapy *is* recommended for patients who have had two or more seizures.

A number of antiepileptic drugs are available. Sometimes, a combination of drugs must be given to control the disorder. Nonetheless, most seizure disorders can be controlled. To optimize drug selection for each patient, neurologists consider the known efficacy of a given drug for a certain type of seizure, the adverse effects profile, the likelihood of drug interactions, the

---

LIFE SPAN CONSIDERATIONS: The Pediatric Patient

Antiepileptic Drugs

- Should a skin rash develop in a child or infant taking phenytoin, the drug should be discontinued immediately and the prescriber notified.
- Chewable dosage forms of antiepileptic drugs should not be used for once-a-day administration. Intramuscular injections of barbiturates or phenytoin should not be used in any patient.
- Family members, parents, significant others, or caregivers should be encouraged to keep a journal with a record of the signs and symptoms before, during, and after a seizure and before, during, and after the treatment with an antiepileptic drug.
- Wearing of a medical alert bracelet or necklace at all times with information about the diagnosis and medication therapy should be encouraged.
- Suspension dosage forms should always be shaken thoroughly before use. A graduated device or oral syringe should be used for more accurate dosing of this liquid.
- Pediatric patients are more sensitive to barbiturates and may respond to lower than expected dosages. They may also experience more profound central nervous system depressive effects related to the antiepileptic drug or show depression, confusion, or excitement (a paradoxical reaction).
- Any excessive sedation, confusion, lethargy, hypotension, bradypnea, tachycardia, and/or decreased movement in pediatric patients taking any antiepileptic drug should be reported to the prescriber immediately.
- Carbamazepine should be given with meals to reduce risk of gastrointestinal distress. All suspension forms should be shaken well before use.
- Oral forms of valproic acid should not be given with milk, because this may cause the drug to dissolve early and irritate the mucosa. The drug also should not be given with carbonated beverages.

---

cost, ease of use, and the availability of pediatric dosage forms. In addition, a number of these drugs are also used to treat other types of illnesses, including psychiatric disorders (see Chapter 17), migraine headaches (see Chapter 14), and neuropathic pain syndromes (see Chapter 11). Generally, single-drug therapy must fail before two-drug or multidrug therapy is attempted. Patients are normally started on a single antiepileptic drug and the dosage is slowly increased until the seizures are controlled or until clinical toxicity occurs. If the first antiepileptic drug is not effective, the drug should be tapered slowly while a second drug is introduced. Antiepileptic drugs should never be stopped abruptly unless a severe adverse effect occurs. It is sometimes difficult to control a patient's seizures using a single drug, but monotherapy is most likely to result in higher serum drug concentrations, fewer adverse effects, and better control.

Therapeutic drug monitoring (see Chapter 2) of serum drug concentrations provides a useful guideline in assessing the effectiveness of therapy. Maintaining serum drug levels within therapeutic ranges helps not only to control seizures but also to reduce adverse effects. Drugs that are routinely monitored in this way also have a low *therapeutic index* (see Chapter 2). There are established normal therapeutic ranges for many antiepileptic drugs, but these are useful only as guidelines (see Table 15-6). The serum concentrations of phenytoin, phenobarbital, carbamazepine, and primidone correlate better with seizure control and toxicity than do those of valproic acid, ethosuximide, and clonazepam. However,

TABLE 15-1 Currently Available Antiepileptic Drugs

Generic Name	Trade Name	Route
Traditional Antiepileptic Drugs		
Barbiturates		
phenobarbital	Solfoton	PO
	Luminal	IV
primidone	Mysoline	PO
Hydantoins		
phenytoin	Dilantin	PO, IV
fosphenytoin	Cerebyx	IV, IM
Iminostilbenes		
carbamazepine	Tegretol, Carbatrol	PO
oxcarbazepine	Trileptal	PO
Class Unspecified		
valproic acid	Depakene, Depakote	PO
	Depacon	IV
Miscellaneous Newer Antiepileptic Drugs		
gabapentin	Neurontin	PO
lamotrigine	Lamictal	PO
levetiracetam	Keppra	PO
pregabalin	Lyrica	PO
tiagabine	Gabitril	PO
topiramate	Topamax	PO
zonisamide	Zonegran	PO
lacosamide	Vimpat	PO, IV

IM, Intramuscular; *IV,* intravenous; *PO,* oral.

each patient should be monitored individually, and the dosages adjusted based on the individual case. In many patients, maintenance is successful at levels below or above the usual therapeutic range. The goal should be to slowly titrate to the lowest effective serum drug level that controls the seizure disorder. This reduces the risk for adverse drug effects and drug interactions. Successful control of a seizure disorder hinges on selection of the appropriate drug class and drug dosage, avoidance of drug toxicity, and patient compliance with the treatment regimen.

There are three classes of antiepileptic drugs traditionally used to manage seizure disorders—barbiturates, hydantoins, and iminostilbenes—plus valproic acid. Several newer drugs have also been marketed (Table 15-1). Newer drugs may have fewer adverse effects and drug interactions than the more traditional drugs. This may especially benefit elderly patients, who are more likely to be taking multiple medications and therefore are more prone to drug interactions. However, there is currently debate in the neurologic literature as to whether patients actually benefit more from newer than from older drugs.

Encouraging news was announced in December 2007 at the annual conference of the American Epilepsy Society. It is now believed that the majority of both pediatric and adult epilepsy patients who have been seizure free for 1 to 2 years while taking antiepileptic drugs can eventually stop taking them with medical supervision.

For many years only the name-brand form of phenytoin, Dilantin, was available. However, generic dosage forms have now also been available for several years, and both name-brand and generic phenytoin are commonly prescribed. Phenobarbital and valproic acid are used almost exclusively in the generic forms. The remainder of the newer antiepileptic drugs are still available in brand-name forms only, with the exception of gabapentin. All generic drug manufacturers are required to provide research data that demonstrate *bioequivalency* of their generic drugs to the corresponding original brand-name drugs. This means that the generic drug product must meet federal standards that include equality of absorption and distribution *(bioavailability)* as well as equal clinical efficacy compared with the brand-name drug. In spite of the existence of these standards, both the American Academy of Neurology and the American Epilepsy Society are both concerned that generic drug products may be less clinically efficacious than brand-name drug products. Of particular concern is the common requirement of health insurance companies that patients receive generic drugs when available. As of December 2007, the American Epilepsy society was helping to design a study that would demonstrate to the FDA the validity of these concerns regarding efficacy.

Mechanism of Action and Drug Effects

As with many classes of drugs, the exact mechanism of action of the antiepileptic drugs is not known with certainty. However, strong evidence indicates that they alter the movement of sodium, potassium, calcium, and magnesium ions. The changes in the movement of these ions induced by antiepileptics result in more stabilized and less excitable cell membranes.

The major pharmacologic effects of antiepileptics are threefold. First, they *increase the threshold* of activity in the area of the brain called the *motor cortex.* In other words, they make it more difficult for a nerve to be excited or they reduce the nerve's response to incoming electrical or chemical stimulation. Second, they act to *limit the spread* of a seizure discharge from its origin. They do this by suppressing the transmission of impulses from one nerve to the next. Third, they can *decrease the speed* of nerve impulse conduction within a given neuron. Less well understood are mechanisms of action that involve theoretical drug effects outside the neuron. For example, these drugs may indirectly affect seizure *foci* (locations) in the brain by altering the blood supply to these areas. Regardless of the mechanism, however, the overall effect is that antiepileptics stabilize neurons and keep them from becoming hyperexcited and generating excessive nerve impulses to adjacent neurons. Some work by enhancing the effects of the inhibitory neurotransmitter gamma-aminobutyric acid (GABA).

Indications

The major therapeutic use of antiepileptic drugs is the prevention or control of seizure activity. As evidenced by the wide range of seizure disorders listed in Box 15-1, epilepsy is a very diverse disorder. As a result, specific indications vary among drugs. The latest indications are noted, drug by drug, in Table 15-2, the Dosages table, and specific drug profiles. An accurate diagnosis is important, because some drugs may not be ideal for specific seizure types. For example, it is known that carbamazepine may worsen myoclonic or absence seizures. Other evidence supports the following generalizations: Phenobarbital, phenytoin, primidone, carbamazepine, and valproic acid are equally effective for partial onset seizures. Lamotrigine, topiramate, gabapentin, oxcarbazepine, zonisamide, levetiracetam, and tiagabine are all effective as *adjuncts* or adjunctive therapy for refractory partial

TABLE **15-2** Common Seizure Indications for Antiepileptic Drugs

	Partial	Secondary General	Generalized Tonic Clonic	Absence	Myoclonic
First Line	carbamazepine phenobarbital primidone phenytoin fosphenytoin	carbamazepine phenobarbital primidone phenytoin fosphenytoin	carbamazepine phenobarbital primidone phenytoin fosphenytoin valproic acid	valproic acid	valproic acid
Adjunct Drugs	clonazepam clorazepate oxcarbazepine gabapentin pregabalin lamotrigine levetiracetam tiagabine topiramate zonisamide	clonazepam oxcarbazepine gabapentin lamotrigine levetiracetam tiagabine topiramate zonisamide	clonazepam lamotrigine topiramate zonisamide	acetazolamide ethosuximide zonisamide	clonazepam zonisamide

TABLE **15-3** Antiepileptic Drugs Used to Treat Status Epilepticus

Drug	IV Dose (mg/kg)	Onset	Duration	Half-life	Adverse Effects
diazepam	0.15-0.25 (10 mg)*	3-10 min	Minutes	35 hr	Apnea, hypotension, somnolence
fosphenytoin	15-20 phenytoin equivalents	15-30 min	12-24 hr	10-60 hr	Comparable to those for phenytoin (see below)
lorazepam†	0.05-0.1	1-20 min	Hours	15 hr	Apnea, hypotension, somnolence
phenobarbital	20	10-30 min	4-10 hr	53-140 hr	Apnea, hypotension, somnolence
phenytoin	15-20	5-30 min	12-24 hr	10-60 hr	Cardiac dysrhythmias, hypotension

IV, Intravenous.
*Rectal products also available for emergency use for both adults and children of all ages.
†Off-label use (not a Food and Drug Administration–approved indication), but still sometimes used for this purpose.

TABLE **15-4** Adverse Effects of Selected Antiepileptic Drugs

Drug or Drug Class	Adverse Effects
First-Line Drugs	
Barbiturates: phenobarbital, primidone	Dizziness, drowsiness, lethargy, paradoxical restlessness, excitement, nausea
Hydantoins: phenytoin, fosphenytoin	Nystagmus, ataxia, dizziness, drowsiness, rash, gingival hyperplasia
Iminostilbenes: carbamazepine, oxcarbazepine	Nausea, headache, dizziness, drowsiness, unusual eye movements, visual changes, mental or mood changes, behavioral changes; rarely decrease in bone marrow function with aplastic anemia and agranulocytosis
Succinimides: ethosuximide	Nausea, abdominal pain, dizziness, drowsiness
valproic acid and derivatives, including valproate sodium and divalproex sodium	Dizziness, drowsiness, GI upset, weight gain, hair thinning, ankle edema, hepatotoxicity, pancreatitis
Adjunct Drugs	
gabapentin	Dizziness, drowsiness, nausea, ataxia, visual and speech changes, edema
pregabalin	Dizziness, drowsiness
lamotrigine	Dizziness, drowsiness, ataxia, headache, nausea, blurred or double vision and other visual changes
levetiracetam	Dizziness, drowsiness, hyperactivity, asthenia, unspecified infections, mood or behavior changes such as anxiety, hostility, agitation, or suicide
tiagabine	Dizziness, drowsiness, confusion, agitation, asthenia, GI upset
topiramate	Cognitive impairment, dizziness, drowsiness, GI upset, ataxia, headache
zonisamide	Dizziness, drowsiness, anorexia, ataxia, confusion, agitation, cognitive impairment

GI, Gastrointestinal.

onset seizures, that is, those that do not respond to the first-line drugs listed earlier. Specific antiepileptic drugs and the seizure disorders they are used to treat are listed in Table 15-2.

Antiepileptics are chiefly used for the long-term maintenance treatment of epilepsy. However, they are also useful for the acute treatment of convulsions and status epilepticus. In these cases the therapy is typically diazepam, which is considered by many to be the drug of choice. Other commonly used drugs are listed in Table 15-3.

Once status epilepticus is controlled, long-term drug therapy is begun with other drugs for the prevention of future seizures. Patients who undergo brain surgery or who have experienced severe head injuries may receive prophylactic antiepileptic therapy. These patients are at high risk for acquiring a seizure disorder, and often severe complications will arise if seizures are not controlled.

Contraindications

The only usual contraindication to antiepileptics is known drug allergy. Pregnancy is also a common contraindication, but the prescriber must consider the risks to mother and infant of untreated maternal epilepsy and the increased risks for seizure activity.

Adverse Effects

Antiepileptic drugs are plagued by many adverse effects, which often limit their usefulness. Drugs must be withdrawn from many patients because of some of these effects. The rate of birth defects in infants of epileptic mothers is somewhat higher than normal, regardless of whether the mother was receiving drug therapy. Epileptic women should ideally be monitored closely by both an obstetrician and a neurologist during pregnancy. Each antiepileptic drug is associated with its own diverse set of adverse effects. The various antiepileptic drugs and their most common adverse effects are listed in Table 15-4.

In December 2008, the U.S. Food and Drug Administration (FDA) required black box warnings on all antiepileptic drugs regarding the risk of suicidal thoughts and behavior. Patients being treated with antiepileptic drugs for any indication should be monitored for the emergence or worsening of depression, suicidal thoughts or behavior, or any unusual changes in mood or behavior. The FDA's action was based on a review of 199 clinical trials of 11 antiepileptic drugs which showed that patients receiving antiepileptic drugs had almost twice the risk of suicidal behavior compared with those receiving a placebo.

Interactions

Drug interactions that can occur with antiepileptic drugs are also numerous and are summarized in Table 15-5. The most clinically common interactions are those related to concurrent therapy with more than one antiepileptic drug. This is important, because many epileptic patients are treated with combination therapy.

Dosages

For certain antiepileptic drugs, the safe and toxic levels are very close together; that is, the therapeutic range is narrow. Table 15-6 lists the various drugs for which monitoring of therapeutic

TABLE 15-5 Selected Drug Interactions of Antiepileptic Drugs

AED Drug or Drug Class	Interacting Drug	Mechanism	Results
Barbiturates phenobarbital, primidone	carbamazepine	Altered CYP450 enzyme metabolism	Reduced levels of both drugs
	Hydantoins, valproic acid	Altered CYP450 enzyme metabolism	Increased barbiturate levels
	Succinimides	Altered CYP450 enzyme metabolism	Reduced barbiturate levels
	Beta-blockers, corticosteroids (e.g., prednisone), oral contraceptives, dihydropyridines (e.g., nifedipine), methadone, metronidazole, quinidine, theophylline	Altered CYP450 enzyme metabolism	Reduced effects of object drugs
	ethanol	Enhanced CNS depression	Can be fatal
Hydantoins phenytoin, ethotoin	allopurinol, amiodarone, benzodiazepines, azole antifungals, isoniazid, metronidazole, omeprazole, succinimide AEDs, sulfonamide antibiotics, valproic acid, SSRAs	Altered CYP450 enzyme metabolism	Reduced hydantoin clearance and increased effects
	aspirin, tricyclic antidepressants, valproic acid	Displacement of hydantoin molecule from plasma protein binding sites	Increased blood hydantoin levels and effects
	Barbiturates, carbamazepine	Altered CYP450 enzyme metabolism	Increased hydantoin clearance and reduced effects
	Antacids	Reduced GI absorption	Reduced hydantoin effects
	warfarin	Displacement of warfarin from plasma protein binding sites	Increased free warfarin levels and bleeding risk

AED, Antiepileptic drug; *CNS,* central nervous system; *CYP450,* cytochrome P-450; *GI,* gastrointestinal; *SSRAs,* selective serotonin receptor antagonists; *SSRIs,* selective serotonin reuptake inhibitors.

Continued

TABLE 15-5 Selected Drug Interactions of Antiepileptic Drugs—cont'd

AED Drug or Drug Class	Interacting Drug	Mechanism	Results
Iminostilbenes			
carbamazepine	Azole antifungals, diltiazem, isoniazid, loratadine, macrolides, niacin, protease inhibitor antiretrovirals, propoxyphene, SSRIs, valproic acid, verapamil	Altered CYP450 enzyme metabolism	Increased carbamazepine levels and toxicity risk
	cisplatin, barbiturates, hydantoins, rifampin, succinimides, theophylline	Altered CYP450 enzyme metabolism	Reduced carbamazepine levels and efficacy
	acetaminophen	Altered CYP450 enzyme metabolism	Increased hepatic metabolism of acetaminophen and toxicity risk and reduced efficacy
	Antipsychotics, antidepressants, benzodiazepines, cyclosporine, statins, lamotrigine, oxcarbazepine, tiagabine, topiramate, tramadol, thyroid hormones, oral contraceptives, zonisamide	Altered CYP450 enzyme metabolism	Reduced efficacy; patient response must be monitored
oxcarbazepine	Barbiturates, hydantoins	Altered CYP450 enzyme metabolism	Increased barbiturate and hydantoin levels and reduced oxcarbazepine levels
	valproic acid, verapamil	Altered CYP450 enzyme metabolism	Reduced oxcarbazepine levels
	lamotrigine	Altered CYP450 enzyme metabolism	Reduced lamotrigine levels
	Oral contraceptives	Altered CYP450 enzyme metabolism	Reduced oral contraceptive levels and increased likelihood of pregnancy
Valproic Acid and Derivatives			
valproic acid valproate sodium and divalproex sodium	aspirin	Displacement of valproic acid from plasma protein binding sites	Increased free valproic acid levels and toxicity risk
	cholestyramine	Reduced valproic acid absorption	Reduced valproic acid efficacy (give valproic acid 3 hr before cholestyramine)
	carbamazepine, ethosuximide, hydantoins, lamotrigine	Altered CYP450 enzyme metabolism	Reduced valproic acid efficacy; increased lamotrigine levels; increased or decreased ethosuximide and carbamazepine levels
	diazepam, warfarin	Displacement of diazepam, warfarin from plasma protein binding sites	Increased toxicity risk of diazepam, warfarin
	rifampin	Altered CYP450 enzyme metabolism	Reduced valproic acid efficacy
	Tricyclic antidepressants	Altered CYP450 enzyme metabolism	Increased toxicity risk of tricyclic antidepressants
	chloroquine (antimalarial)	Decreased levels of valproic acid	Loss of seizure control
Succinimides			
ethosuximide	Hydantoins, barbiturates, valproic acid	Altered CYP450 enzyme metabolism	Increased or reduced clearance of involved drugs
Miscellaneous AEDs			
gabapentin	Antacids	Reduced gabapentin absorption	Reduced gabapentin efficacy
	hydrocodone, morphine	Altered CYP450 enzyme metabolism	Increased gabapentin levels; reduced hydrocodone levels
pregabalin	None listed		
lamotrigine	acetaminophen, barbiturates, carbamazepine, hydantoins, oral contraceptives, oxcarbazepine, rifampin, succinimides	Altered CYP450 enzyme metabolism	Reduced lamotrigine levels and efficacy; may need dosage increase

TABLE **15-5** Selected Drug Interactions of Antiepileptic Drugs—cont'd

AED Drug or Drug Class	Interacting Drug	Mechanism	Results
Miscellaneous AEDs—cont'd			
lamotrigine—cont'd	valproic acid	Altered CYP450 enzyme metabolism	Increased lamotrigine levels and toxicity risk; may need dosage reduction
	topiramate	Altered CYP450 enzyme metabolism	Increased topiramate levels
levetiracetam	None listed		
tiagabine	Barbiturates, carbamazepine, hydantoins	Altered CYP450 enzyme metabolism	Increased tiagabine clearance and reduced efficacy
	Highly protein-bound drugs (e.g., warfarin)	Displacement of either drug from plasma protein binding sites	Increased or reduced free drug levels in blood with potential for toxicity or subtherapeutic efficacy
topiramate	carbamazepine, hydantoins, valproic acid	Altered CYP450 enzyme metabolism	Reduced topiramate and valproic acid levels
	hydrochlorothiazide, lamotrigine, metformin	Altered CYP450 enzyme metabolism	Increased topiramate and metformin levels
	Oral contraceptives	Altered CYP450 enzyme metabolism	Reduced oral contraceptive efficacy
	digoxin, lithium, risperidone	Altered CYP450 enzyme metabolism	Reduced efficacy of digoxin, lithium, risperidone
zonisamide	CYP450 enzyme inducers or inhibitors	Altered CYP450 enzyme metabolism	Increased or reduced clearance and effects

TABLE **15-6** Therapeutic Plasma Levels of Antiepileptic Drugs with a Narrow Therapeutic Range

Antiepileptic Drug	Therapeutic Plasma Level (mcg/mL)
carbamazepine	4-12
clonazepam	0.02-0.08
divalproex	50-100
ethosuximide	40-100
phenobarbital	15-40
phenytoin	10-20
primidone	5-12
valproic acid	50-100

plasma levels is required and their corresponding therapeutic values. For an overview of dosages, see the drug Dosages table on p. 234.

DRUG PROFILES

In most children and adults, epilepsy can be controlled with a first-line antiepileptic drug such as carbamazepine (Tegretol), phenobarbital (Luminal), phenytoin (Dilantin), or valproic acid (Depakene). For patients who do not respond to these first-line drugs, there are a number of second-line or *adjunct* antiepileptic drugs that are used occasionally, such ethosuximide (Zarontin), primidone (Mysoline), the benzodiazepines (see Chapter 13), diazepam (Valium), clonazepam (Klonopin), clorazepate (Tranxene), and the diuretic acetazolamide (Diamox [see Chapter 26]).

After valproic acid was introduced in 1978, no major new drugs for the treatment of epilepsy were introduced in the United States until the 1990s. Gabapentin (Neurontin), lamotrigine (Lamictal), and felbamate (Felbatol) all were approved during this decade. Although felbamate initially appeared to be a promising antiepileptic drug, there were several case reports of aplastic anemia and acute liver failure associated with its use. As a result, the FDA recommends that felbamate be given only to patients who have seizures that are refractory to treatment with all other medications and in whom risk-benefit considerations warrant its use. Weekly or biweekly complete blood counts and liver function tests are also recommended. Because of its rare clinical use, this drug is not discussed further in this book.

Antiepileptic drugs that have been approved more recently are levetiracetam (Keppra), topiramate (Topamax), zonisamide (Zonegran), tiagabine (Gabitril), and pregabalin (Lyrica). These drugs fall into the miscellaneous category of antiepileptics and have greatly expanded the options currently available to treat patients with seizure disorders. Common adverse effects and drug interactions are listed in the individual drug profiles and/or in Tables 15-3 and 15-4 if the list is extensive. Dosage information appears in the Dosages table on p. 234.

BARBITURATES
◆ phenobarbital and primidone
Originally, two of the most commonly used antiepileptic drugs were the barbiturates phenobarbital (Luminal) and primidone (Mysoline). Primidone is metabolized in the liver to phenobarbital and phenylethylmalonamide, both of which have anticonvulsant properties. Use of primidone can provide anticonvulsant activity with a lower serum level of phenobarbital than that attained when phenobarbital itself is administered. This can reduce the likelihood of sedation and fatigue associated with phenobarbital.

DOSAGES

Selected Antiepileptic Drugs

Drug (Pregnancy Category)	Pharmacologic Class	Usual Dosage Range	Seizure Indications
◆ carbamazepine (Tegretol, Tegretol XR) (D)	Iminostilbene	**Pediatric** PO: younger than 9 yr, 10-20 mg/kg/day PO: 6-12 yr, 200-1000 mg/day **Adult and pediatric older than 12 yr** PO: 400-1600 mg/day	Partial, secondary generalized, generalized tonic-clonic seizures
ethosuximide (Zarontin) (C)	Succinimide	**Pediatric** PO: 3-6 yr, 250 mg/day then adjust; older than 6 yr, 500 mg/day then adjust **Adult** PO: 500 mg/day then adjust	Absence seizures
◆ fosphenytoin (Cerebyx) (D)	Hydantoin	**Pediatric** IV: 10-20 PE*/kg loading dose; may begin maintenance dosing 8-12 hr later using pediatric phenytoin dosing guidelines (see below) **Adult** IV: 10-20 PE*/kg loading dose; maintenance dose 4-6 mg/kg/day	Partial, secondary generalized, generalized tonic-clonic seizures
◆ gabapentin (Neurontin) (C)	Miscellaneous	**Pediatric** PO: 10-15 mg/kg/day divided tid, then adjust **Adult** PO: over 18 yr, 900-1800 mg/day	Partial, secondary generalized seizures
lamotrigine (Lamictal) (C)	Miscellaneous	**Pediatric** PO: 2-12 yr, 5-15 mg/kg/day depending on other AEDs used **Adult** PO: 50-200 mg once daily or divided bid	Partial, secondary generalized, generalized tonic-clonic seizures; seizures associated with Lennox-Gastaut syndrome
levetiracetam (Keppra) (C)	Miscellaneous	**Pediatric** Per child neurologist **Adult** PO: 500 mg bid to 3000 mg/day	Partial, secondary generalized seizures
oxcarbazepine (Trileptal) (C)	Iminostilbene	**Pediatric** PO: 8-10 mg/kg/day divided bid; max 600 mg/day **Adult** 300-600 mg bid	Partial, secondary generalized seizures
◆ phenobarbital [oral], Luminal [injectable]) (D)	Barbiturate	**Pediatric** PO: 3-5 mg/kg/day **Adult** PO: 100-300 mg/day **Pediatric** IM/IV: 10-20 mg/kg load, may repeat 5 mg/kg every 15-30 min until seizure is controlled or total dose of 40 mg/kg **Adult** IM/IV: 200-800 mg followed by 120-240 mg dose every 20 min until seizure is controlled or a total dose of 1-2 g	Partial, secondary generalized, generalized tonic-clonic seizures, prophylaxis for febrile seizures, psychomotor seizures Partial, secondary generalized, generalized tonic-clonic Status epilepticus
◆ phenytoin (Dilantin) (D)	Hydantoin	**Pediatric** PO: 4-8 mg/kg/day IV: 15-20 mg/kg **Adult** PO: 300-600 mg/day IV: 15-20 mg/kg	Partial, secondary generalized, generalized tonic-clonic seizures Status epilepticus

AED, Antiepileptic drug; *IM,* intramuscular; *IV,* intravenous; *PE,* phenytoin equivalent; *PO,* oral.
*One PE = 1.5 mg fosphenytoin = 1 mg phenytoin. Therefore, 1.5 mg fosphenytoin should be given for each milligram of phenytoin desired.

DOSAGES

Selected Antiepileptic Drugs—cont'd

Drug (Pregnancy Category)	Pharmacologic Class	Usual Dosage Range	Seizure Indications
pregabalin (Lyrica) (C)	Miscellaneous	**Adult** PO: 150-600 mg/day divided into 2 or 3 doses	Partial seizures
◆ primidone (Mysoline) (D)	Barbiturate	**Pediatric** PO: younger than 8 yr, 125-250 mg/tid Dosage for pediatric younger than 8 yr is initially 50-125 mg at bedtime, slowly titrated up to 125-250 mg tid; older than 8 yr is initially 125-250 mg at bedtime, slowly titrated up to 250 mg; max 2 g/day	Partial, secondary generalized, generalized tonic-clonic seizures
		Adult and pediatric older than 8 yr 250 mg orally 4-6 times/day; max 2 g/day	Partial, secondary generalized, generalized tonic-clonic seizures
tiagabine (Gabitril) (C)	Miscellaneous	**Pediatric** PO: 12-18 yr, 4 mg daily to 32 mg divided bid-qid **Adult** 4 mg daily to 56 mg divided bid-qid	Partial, secondary generalized seizures
topiramate (Topamax) (C)	Miscellaneous	**Pediatric** PO: 1-9 mg/kg/day **Adult** PO: 25-1600 mg/day	Partial, secondary generalized, generalized tonic-clonic seizures
◆ valproic acid (Depacon, IV Depakote, Depakene oral) (D)	Miscellaneous	**Adult and pediatric** PO: 15-60 mg/kg/day divided bid-tid IV: 10-15 mg/kg/day as a 60-min infusion	Generalized tonic-clonic, absence, myoclonic seizures
zonisamide (Zonegran) (C)	Miscellaneous	**Pediatric** Over 16 yr, 100-400 mg/day **Adult** 100-400 mg/day	Partial, secondary generalized, generalized tonic-clonic, absence, myoclonic seizures

Phenobarbital is a Schedule IV controlled substance, whereas primidone is not controlled. Phenobarbital has been used since 1912, principally for controlling tonic-clonic and partial seizures. Phenobarbital is still one of the widely used drugs for the management of status epilepticus and is an effective prophylactic drug for the control of febrile seizures. Although phenobarbital is still frequently used to treat seizure emergencies the use of oral phenobarbital for seizure prevention is much less common. In developing third-world countries, however, oral phenobarbital is often the drug of choice for routine seizure prophylaxis because of its dramatically lower cost compared with the newer drugs. By far the most common adverse effect is sedation, but tolerance to this effect usually develops with continued therapy. Therapeutic effects are generally seen at serum drug levels of 15 to 40 mcg/mL. A major advantage of this drug is its long half-life, which allows once-a-day dosing. This can be a substantial advantage for patients who have a hard time remembering to take their medication or for those who have erratic schedules. Even if a patient takes his or her dose 12 or even 24 hours too late, therapeutic blood levels may still be maintained. In addition, phenobarbital is the most inexpensive antiepileptic drug, costing only pennies a day compared with several dollars a day for other drugs. Contraindications include known drug allergy, porphyria (a disorder of the synthesis of heme, a component of hemoglobin), liver or kidney impairment, and respiratory illness. Adverse effects include cardiovascular, CNS, gastrointestinal (GI), and dermatologic reactions (see Table 15-4). Phenobarbital interacts with many drugs because it is a major inducer of hepatic microsomal enzymes, including enzymes of the cytochrome P-450 system (see Chapter 2), which causes more rapid clearance of some drugs (see Table 15-5). Phenobarbital is available in oral and injectable forms, whereas primidone is available only for oral use.

PHARMACOKINETICS (phenobarbital)

Route	Onset of Action	Peak Plasma Concentration	Elimination Half-life	Duration of Action
PO	20-60 min	8-12 hr	50-120 hr	6-12 hr
IV	5 min	30 min	50-120 hr	6-12 hr

PHARMACOKINETICS (primidone)

Route	Onset of Action	Peak Plasma Concentration	Elimination Half-life	Duration of Action
PO	Unknown	3-4 hr	10-12 hr*	Unknown

*Longer for active metabolites, including phenobarbital.

HYDANTOINS
◆ phenytoin and fosphenytoin

Phenytoin (Dilantin) has been used as a first-line drug for many years. It is primarily indicated for the management of tonic-clonic and partial seizures. Contraindications include known drug allergy and heart conditions that involve bradycardia or blockage of electrocardiac function. Adverse effects and drug interactions both are numerous and are listed in Table 15-4 and 15-5, respectively. The most common adverse effects are lethargy, abnormal movements, mental confusion, and cognitive changes. *Gingival hyperplasia* (overgrowth of gum tissue) is also a well-known adverse effect of long-term oral phenytoin therapy. Scrupulous dental care can help prevent gingival hypertrophy. Long-term phenytoin therapy can cause gingival hyperplasia, acne, hirsutism, and hypertrophy of subcutaneous facial tissue resulting in an appearance known as *Dilantin facies.* Another long-term consequence of phenytoin therapy is osteoporosis. Vitamin D therapy may help to prevent this, particularly in women. Therapeutic drug levels are usually 10 to 20 mcg/mL. At toxic levels, phenytoin can cause nystagmus, ataxia, dysarthria, and encephalopathy. Phenytoin can interact with other medications for two main reasons. First, it is highly bound to plasma proteins and competes with other highly protein-bound medications for binding sites. Second, it induces hepatic microsomal enzymes, mainly cytochrome P-450 enzymes (see Chapter 2). This increases the metabolism of the majority of other drugs that are metabolized by these enzymes and reduces their blood levels.

Exaggerated phenytoin effects can be seen in patients with very low serum albumin concentrations. This most commonly occurs in patients who are malnourished or have chronic renal failure. In these patients, it may be necessary to maintain phenytoin levels well below 20 mcg/mL. With lower levels of albumin in the patient's body, more of the free, unbound, pharmacologically active phenytoin molecules will be present in the blood.

Phenytoin has many advantages from the standpoint of long-term therapy. It is usually well tolerated, highly effective, and relatively inexpensive. It can also be given intravenously if needed. Most often, however, phenytoin is taken orally. The long half-life of the drug allows for twice- or even once-daily dosing. This encourages patient adherence to drug therapy, which helps reduce seizure frequency.

Parenteral phenytoin is adjusted chemically to a pH of 12 for reasons of drug stability. It is very irritating to veins when injected and should be given by slow intravenous (IV) push (not exceeding 50 mg/min in adults) directly into a large vein through a large-gauge (20-gauge or larger) venous catheter. Each injection should be followed by an injection of a saline flush to avoid local venous irritation caused by the alkalinity of the solution. It is recommended that continuous IV infusion be avoided. Soft tissue irritation and inflammation can occur at the site of injection with or without extravasation. This can vary from slight tenderness to extensive necrosis and sloughing, and in rare instances can require amputation. Improper administration, including subcutaneous or perivascular injection, should be avoided to help prevent the possibility of such occurrences.

Fosphenytoin (Cerebyx) is an injectable prodrug of phenytoin that was developed in an attempt to overcome some of the chemical disadvantages of phenytoin sodium injection. Fosphenytoin is a water-soluble, phosphorylated phenytoin derivative that can be given intramuscularly or intravenously—by IV push or continuous infusion—without causing the burning on injection associated with phenytoin. Fosphenytoin is dosed in *phenytoin equivalents (PE)* as indicated in Table 15-7. Fosphenytoin should be given at a rate of 150 mg PE/min or less to avoid hypotension or cardiorespiratory depression. Should dysrhythmias or hypotension occur, the infusion should be discontinued. Fall prevention measures should be in place after infusion because of possible ataxia and dizziness, and vital signs should continue to be taken up to 2 hours after infusion. IV incompatibilities are numerous, so the nurse should always check available references and/or consult with a pharmacist before dosing.

TABLE 15-7 Comparison of Phenytoin Sodium and Fosphenytoin Sodium

	Phenytoin Sodium (Dilantin IV)	Fosphenytoin Sodium (Cerebyx IM/IV)
pH	12	8.6-9
Maximum infusion rate	50 mg/min	150 mg PE*/min
Admixtures	0.9% saline	0.9% saline or 5% dextrose

IM, Intramuscular; *IV,* intravenous; *PE,* phenytoin sodium equivalents.
*150 mg fosphenytoin sodium = 100 mg phenytoin sodium.

PHARMACOKINETICS (phenytoin)

Route	Onset of Action	Peak Plasma Concentration	Elimination Half-life	Duration of Action
PO	Unknown	12 hr	20-60 hr	Unknown
IV	Unknown	2-3 hr	20-60 hr	Unknown

UNSPECIFIED ANTIEPILEPTICS
◆ valproic acid

Valproic acid (Depakene) is used primarily in the treatment of generalized seizures (absence, myoclonic, and tonic-clonic). It is of an unspecified chemical class but is a longstanding antiepileptic drug. It has also been shown to be effective in controlling partial seizures. Contraindications include known drug allergy, liver impairment, and *urea cycle* disorders (genetic disorders of urea metabolism). Common adverse effects include drowsiness; nausea, vomiting, and other GI disturbances; tremor; weight gain; and transient hair loss (see Table 15-4). The most serious adverse effects are hepatotoxicity and pancreatitis. Valproic acid can interact with many medications (see Table 15-5). The main reasons for these interactions are protein binding and liver metabolism. It is highly bound to plasma proteins and competes with other highly protein-bound medications for binding sites. It also is highly metabolized by hepatic microsomal enzymes and competes for metabolism with other drugs. In contrast to phenobarbital and phenytoin, however, it is not a hepatic enzyme inducer. This drug is available in both oral and injectable forms. Valproic acid itself is chemically the simplest dosage form and is available as an oral liquid. Long-acting oral dosage forms are also available as a solid salt matrix, divalproex sodium (Depakote), which comes in delayed- and extended-release tablets as well as capsules with long-acting granules (Depakote Sprinkles) that can be opened and sprinkled into food. The injectable form is the salt valproate sodium (Depacon).

PHARMACOKINETICS

Route	Onset of Action	Peak Plasma Concentration	Elimination Half-life	Duration of Action
PO	15-30 min	1-4 hr	6-16 hr	4-6 hr
IV	Same	Same	Same	Same

IMINOSTILBENES
◆ carbamazepine

Carbamazepine (Tegretol) is the second most commonly prescribed antiepileptic drug in the United States, after phenytoin. It was marketed in the late 1960s for the treatment of epilepsy in adults after its efficacy and safety for the treatment of *trigeminal neuralgia* (a painful facial nerve condition) were proved. Approval was granted for its use in pediatric patients in 1976. It is chemically related to the *tricyclic* antidepressants (see Chapter 17) and is considered a first-line treatment for partial seizures and generalized tonic-clonic seizures. However, it may actually worsen myoclonic or absence seizures as noted previously. Therefore its use is contraindicated in both of these conditions as well as in cases of known drug allergy and bone marrow depression. Carbamazepine is associated with **autoinduction** of hepatic enzymes. Autoinduction is a process in which, over time, a drug stimulates the production of enzymes that enhance its own metabolism, which leads to lower than expected drug concentrations. With carbamazepine, this process usually occurs within the first 2 months after starting the drug. Adverse reactions and drug interactions are numerous; examples are given in Tables 15-4 and 15-5. Carbamazepine is available for oral use only.

PHARMACOKINETICS

Route	Onset of Action	Peak Plasma Concentration	Elimination Half-life	Duration of Action
PO	Slow	4-8 hr	25-65 hr	12-24 hr

oxcarbazepine

Oxcarbazepine (Trileptal) is a chemical analogue of carbamazepine. Its precise mechanism of action has not been identified, although it is known to block voltage-sensitive sodium channels, which aids in stabilizing excited neuronal membranes. It is indicated for partial seizures and secondarily generalized seizures. Contraindications include known drug allergy. Common adverse reactions include headache, dizziness, and nausea (see also Table 15-4). Unlike carbamazepine, this drug is not a hepatic enzyme inducer. As a result, it is associated with far fewer common drug interactions than is carbamazepine (see Table 15-5). Oxcarbazepine is available for oral use only.

PHARMACOKINETICS

Route	Onset of Action	Peak Plasma Concentration	Elimination Half-life	Duration of Action
PO	2-4 hr	2-3 days	2-9 hr	Unknown

SUCCINIMIDE
ethosuximide

Ethosuximide (Zarontin) is used in the treatment of uncomplicated absence seizures. It is not effective for secondary generalized tonic-clonic seizures. The only listed contraindication for either use is known allergy to succinimides. Adverse effects include GI and CNS effects (see Table 15-4). Drug interactions most commonly involve hepatic enzyme–inducing drugs (see Table 15-5). Succinimides are availably for oral use only.

PHARMACOKINETICS

Route	Onset of Action	Peak Plasma Concentration	Elimination Half-life	Duration of Action
PO	Unknown	4 hr	60 hr	Unknown

MISCELLANEOUS DRUGS
◆ gabapentin

Gabapentin (Neurontin) is a chemical analogue of *GABA*, a major neurotransmitter that inhibits brain activity. It is indicated as an adjunct drug for the treatment of partial seizures and for prophylaxis of partial seizures. Evidence also exists showing gabapentin to be effective as single-drug therapy for new-onset epilepsy. It is also commonly used to treat neuropathic pain. Contraindications include known drug allergy. Adverse effects include CNS and GI symptoms (see Table 15-4). Drug interactions include antacids and hydrocodone, which can reduce gabapentin levels, and cimetidine, morphine, naproxen, and oral contra-

ceptives, which can raise levels (see Table 15-5). The exact mechanism of action of gabapentin is unknown. Many believe that it works by increasing the synthesis and synaptic accumulation of GABA between neurons, hence, the drug name. Gabapentin is available for oral use only.

PHARMACOKINETICS

Route	Onset of Action	Peak Plasma Concentration	Elimination Half-life	Duration of Action
PO	Unknown	Unknown	5-7 hr	Unknown

pregabalin

Pregabalin (Lyrica), like gabapentin, is structurally related to the inhibitory neurotransmitter GABA. However, the drug binds not to GABA receptors but rather to the alpha$_2$-delta receptor sites, which affect calcium channels in CNS tissues. This is believed to be related to its mechanism of action, although the mechanism is still not fully understood. This drug is also a Schedule V controlled substance. The drug is indicated as adjunct therapy for partial seizures. However, it is most commonly used for *neuropathic pain* (see Chapter 11), and *postherpetic neuralgia* (see Chapter 40). Contraindications include known drug allergy. Adverse drug reactions are primarily CNS related (see Table 15-4). No clinically significant drug interactions are listed to date; however, as with all antiepileptic drugs, the potential for additive CNS depression exists when other sedating drugs are used. Pregabalin is available for oral use only.

PHARMACOKINETICS

Route	Onset of Action	Peak Plasma Concentration	Elimination Half-life	Duration of Action
PO	Unknown	1.5 hr	6 hr	Unknown

lamotrigine

Lamotrigine (Lamictal) is indicated for simple or complex partial seizures, for generalized seizures related to *Lennox-Gastaut syndrome* (an atypical form of absence epilepsy that may persist into adulthood), and, most recently, for primary generalized tonic-clonic seizures. It is also used for the treatment of bipolar disorder. It has no known contraindications other than drug allergy. Common adverse effects include relatively minor CNS and GI symptoms (see Table 15-4). However, one potentially serious adverse effect is a rash that can progress to the major dermatologic reaction known as *Stevens-Johnson syndrome*. This condition involves inflammation and sloughing of skin, potentially over the entire body, in a manner that resembles a third-degree burn. It is often reversible but can also be fatal. To avoid this condition, patients' doses are very slowly titrated over several weeks. Drug interactions chiefly involve other antiepileptic drugs as well as other CNS depressants, acetaminophen, and oral contraceptives (see Table 15-5). Lamotrigine is available for oral use only.

PHARMACOKINETICS

Route	Onset of Action	Peak Plasma Concentration	Elimination Half-life	Duration of Action
PO	Unknown	1.4-2.3 hr	24 hr	Unknown

levetiracetam

Levetiracetam (Keppra) is indicated as adjunct therapy for partial seizures with and without secondary generalization. It is contraindicated in cases of known drug allergy. Its mechanism of action is unknown. It is generally well tolerated, with the most common adverse effects being CNS related (see Table 15-4). No drug interactions are currently listed; however, like all antiepileptic drugs, the potential for excessive CNS depression exists when it is used in combination with other sedating drugs. Levetiracetam is available in both oral and injectable forms.

PHARMACOKINETICS

Route	Onset of Action	Peak Plasma Concentration	Elimination Half-life	Duration of Action
PO	Rapid	1 hr	6-8 hr	Unknown

tiagabine

Tiagabine (Gabitril) is indicated as adjunct therapy for partial seizures. Contraindications include known drug allergy. Its exact mechanism of action has not been identified, but the drug is known to have beneficial effects by inhibiting the reuptake of GABA from the neuronal synapses (spaces between neurons) in the brain. In February 2005, the FDA issued a special warning regarding the use of tiagabine for "off-label" (non–FDA-approved) indications. Although tiagabine is effective in controlling epileptic seizures, there have been several case reports of *paradoxical* seizures (opposite of what would intuitively be expected) in nonepileptic patients who are treated with the drug for other indications. Most of these cases involved patients being treated for psychiatric disorders such as bipolar disorder. Of even greater concern is the fact that in some of these cases the seizure episodes progressed to status epilepticus. For these reasons, prescribers are currently advised to avoid off-label use of this drug. Common adverse effects are CNS and GI symptoms (see Table 15-4). Drug interactions chiefly involve enzyme-inducing antiepileptic drugs (see Table 15-5). Tiagabine is available for oral use only.

PHARMACOKINETICS

Route	Onset of Action	Peak Plasma Concentration	Elimination Half-life	Duration of Action
PO	Rapid	45 min	7-9 hr	Unknown

topiramate

Topiramate (Topamax) is a structurally unique drug chemically related to fructose. It is indicated as adjunct therapy for partial and secondarily generalized seizures, for generalized tonic-clonic seizures, and for drop attacks in Lennox-Gastaut syndrome. Contraindications include known drug allergy. Its exact mechanism of action is unknown. Common adverse effects are primarily CNS related (see Table 15-4). However, angle-closure glaucoma can also occur, and the patient should be instructed to immediately report any visual changes. Common drug interactions involve chiefly other antiepileptic drugs but also drugs of various other classes, including antidiabetic drugs and oral contraceptives (see Table 15-5). Topiramate is available for oral use only.

PHARMACOKINETICS

Route	Onset of Action	Peak Plasma Concentration	Elimination Half-life	Duration of Action
PO	Unknown	2-4 hr	21 hr	Unknown

zonisamide

Zonisamide (Zonegran) is a sulfonamide derivative (see Chapter 38) indicated for a variety of seizure types, including partial and secondary generalized, primary generalized, absence, and myoclonic. It is contraindicated in patients with known drug allergy to the drug itself or to sulfa drugs (see Chapter 38). Common adverse effects include CNS and GI symptoms (see Table 15-4). Drugs with which it interacts include any inducers of cytochrome P-450 enzymes, which increase clearance of zonisamide, and la-

motrigine, which tends to reduce its clearance (see Table 15-5). Zonisamide is available for oral use only.

PHARMACOKINETICS

Route	Onset of Action	Peak Plasma Concentration	Elimination Half-life	Duration of Action
PO	Rapid	2-6 hr	63 hr	Unknown

NURSING PROCESS

Assessment

With use of any of the antiepileptic drugs, a thorough physical assessment should be performed and a comprehensive health and medication history obtained, so that any possible allergies, drug interactions, adverse reactions, cautions, and contraindications can be identified. The patient's medical history should be thoroughly reviewed, and any type of seizure disorder, precipitating events, and the duration, frequency, and intensity of the seizure activity should be noted. Information should be sought about any other problems or signs and symptoms occurring before, during, or after the seizure. The patient should be questioned about the occurrence of panic attacks because of the possible association between high levels of anxiety or stress and the precipitation of seizures in those at risk. The patient should also be assessed for signs and symptoms of autonomic nervous system responses associated with anxiety or stress such as cold, clammy hands, excessive sweating (diaphoresis), agitation, and trembling of the extremities. Additional assessment about other problems or symptoms is important because some antiepileptic medications may be indicated for other medical diagnoses, such as prevention of migraines or treatment of postherpetic neuropathy or neuropathic pain. A complete neurologic assessment with documentation of baseline CNS functioning is also important before administering antiepileptic drugs. This may include testing of the response of deep tendon reflexes, bilateral and upper and lower extremity sensory and motor testing, and questioning about the presence of any headaches, photosensitivity, occurrence of auras, or visual changes.

Laboratory test results to review before giving these drugs may include the results of red and white blood cell counts, clotting studies, and renal and/or liver function studies. Knowing baseline levels of these laboratory values is important to help identify any initial abnormalities as well as to provide a comparison value when assessing for possible adverse effects, cautions, contraindications, and interactions. Conditions other than epilepsy or seizure disorders may also cause loss of or alterations in consciousness and are worthy of consideration during assessment. These conditions include syncope, breath-holding practices, transient ischemic attacks, drug use, metabolic disorders, infections, head trauma, tumors, and psychogenic problems. Therefore, an attempt will most likely be made to rule out or eliminate many of these disorders or conditions during the diagnosing of epilepsy, so the nurse should be sure to analyze all the data available. An EEG may also be ordered to provide more information related to the diagnosis of epilepsy. Another diagnostic procedure, magnetic resonance imaging, may be performed for neuroimaging and further data gathering.

CASE STUDY

Medications for Seizures

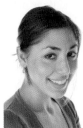
© ZanyZeus

Devin, a 21-year-old patient, has been brought to the emergency department in status epilepticus. Measures are taken to ensure her safety and prevent injury, and an intravenous (IV) line is started. The emergency department physician has ordered diazepam (Valium) 0.25 mg/kg IV push STAT.

1. Devin weighs 135 pounds How much medication will the nurse administer?

Soon after the IV diazepam is given, Devin's seizures stop, and she regains consciousness. She is admitted to a medical-surgical unit, and her mother goes to the room with her. The admitting orders call for an initial IV dose of phenytoin, followed by oral doses twice a day.

2. Why was the loading dose given intravenously?

3. After 2 days of observation, Devin is ready for discharge to her mother's home. Her phenytoin level is 16 mcg/mL. She is very concerned about how the phenytoin will affect her. What teaching regarding her self-care and the adverse effects of phenytoin should she receive?

4. After 4 months, the patient's mother calls to report that Devin has seemed "very sad lately" and has not wanted to join her friends for evenings out. "Devin just goes to work, then comes home and stays in her room." What should the nurse suggest?

For answers, see http://evolve.elsevier.com/Lilley.

The use of a *succinimide* such as ethosuximide requires assessment for the specific indication for this medication, that is, generalized absence seizures. In addition to performing a baseline neurologic assessment, the nurse should ask questions about any history of GI disorders or problems as well as questions about weight gain, dizziness, and fluid retention.

Miscellaneous drugs such as tiagabine, topiramate, and zonisamide are some of the more recently available antiepileptic drugs and have significant contraindications, cautions, and drug interactions, which have been discussed previously in the pharmacology section of this chapter and are summarized in Tables 15-3 and 15-4. In addition, vital signs and mental status should be assessed with attention to the patient's sensorium, level of alertness or consciousness, and any mental depression before, during, and after drug therapy and/or seizure activity. Document baseline problems with dizziness, drowsiness, confusion, and GI upset with tiagabine and topiramate.

If *barbiturates* have been ordered, careful assessment of not only the neurologic system but also vital signs is especially important because of the CNS depression associated with this class of drugs. All of the aforementioned general assessment data should also be obtained when barbiturates are prescribed. In addition, patients at high risk for excessive sedation should be identified. If the patient is in an acute care facility, the room should be assessed to ensure that safety measures are in place (e.g., side rails up or a bed alarm system in use depending on facility policy), noise level is controlled, and seizure precautions are available (oxygen, suctioning equipment, and airway devices nearby; padded side rails being used; and IV access obtained per facility policy). The age of the patient should also be assessed, because the very young and the elderly react with more sensitiv-

ity to these drugs with paradoxical reactions, irritability and hyperactivity (as compared to CNS depressant effects). Cautions, contraindications, and drug interactions have been previously discussed in the pharmacology section.

With *hydantoins* like phenytoin, the previously mentioned assessment procedure is appropriate. A skin assessment is also needed with documentation of intactness and the presence or absence of any rashes, because of the possibility of a measles-like rash. In addition, baseline dental hygiene habits and the status of the patient's gum and teeth are critical because of the adverse effects of gingival hyperplasia. As when any antiepileptic drugs are taken, assessment of baseline neurologic functioning is crucial and, for these drugs, should include the following: (1) a focus on vision with attention to any abnormalities, especially those related to eye movement; (2) baseline neuromuscular stability with attention to coordinated movements, gait, and reflexes; and (3) assessment of speech for clarity and ability to form and express words appropriately. In addition, when the phenytoins are taken, baseline liver function studies and complete blood counts are needed, and attention must be given to specific drug-related cautions, contraindications, and drug interactions.

Before administering carbamazepine, an *iminostilbene*, results of a complete blood count should be assessed, if ordered, and the findings documented for baseline comparisons because of the possible adverse effect of drug-related anemias (e.g., aplastic anemia). Baseline vision should be measured and any abnormalities noted because of the potential visual changes. Significant contraindications include conditions involving bone marrow suppression because it is a rare adverse effect.

Gabapentin requires a thorough neurologic assessment with attention to baseline energy levels, visual intactness, sensory and motor functioning, and any changes in speech. It is also important for the nurse to understand the rationale for gabapentin's use, so that appropriate education and instructions can be shared with the patient and family. For example, gabapentin may be used for seizure therapy, but it is also used to treat postherpetic neuralgia and neuropathic pain, and to prevent migraines. Thus, a plan of care with proper education would need to be developed from the appropriate assessment data. Pregabalin is similar to gabapentin and requires the same assessment.

Valproic acid should be given only after an assessment of the patient's medical history, medication profile, and neurologic system with information about seizure activity (see above). Assessment for drug allergies, cautions, contraindications, and drug interactions has been previously discussed but other assessment areas include baseline weight and liver studies as well as any history of pancreatitis.

Lamotrigine use requires a thorough neurologic assessment and documentation of baseline energy levels, vision acuity, and history of headaches for comparative purposes because of common adverse effects include headaches, vision changes, and drowsiness. Several newer *miscellaneous antiepileptic drugs* are available, such as levetiracetam, topiramate, zonisamide, tiagabine, and pregabalin. These miscellaneous drugs require the same thorough general assessment as with other antiepileptic drugs. A few additional points should be kept in mind. For example, in patients taking levetiracetam, the presence of any neuropsychiatric symptoms must be documented because of the potential for drug-related agitation, depression, anxiety, and other mood or behavioral changes. Although these adverse effects are rare, the assessment data must still be thorough. One interesting fact, as noted in the pharmacology section, is the lack of drug interactions with levetiracetam; however, because all antiepileptic drugs depress the CNS in some manner, assessment for the use of other CNS depressant drugs is important. In addition, liver and renal functioning should be assessed before therapy initiated. Topiramate is used not only for management of seizures but also for other indications as listed in the pharmacology section, such as cluster headaches and neuropathic pain. Therefore, assessment should also include a thorough review of the medical and medication history to understand the reason for the drug's use. Baseline energy levels should be documented, with complete blood counts as ordered.

Nursing Diagnoses

- Risk for injury related to decreased sensorium and CNS depression associated with the actions and adverse effects of antiepileptic drugs
- Deficient knowledge related to lack of familiarity and minimal experience with and lack of information concerning the use of antiepileptic drugs
- Noncompliance with the therapeutic regimen related to the patient's misuse of drugs or lack of understanding about the seizure disorder and its treatment
- Chronic low self-esteem related to diagnosis of a life-long disease and the adverse effects associated with antiepileptic drugs

Planning
Goals

- Patient experiences little to no adverse effects associated with the use of antiepileptic drugs.
- Patient remains without injury during drug therapy.
- Patient remains compliant with the therapy regimen, avoids adverse effects as much as possible, and experiences minimal problems with either overtreatment or undertreatment.
- Patient identifies the therapeutic effects of antiepileptic drugs.
- Patient remains without major harm to self during drug therapy.

Outcome Criteria

- Patient states the therapeutic drug effects (e.g., minimal to no seizure activity with minimal adverse effects of antiepileptic drugs such as sedation, confusion, ataxia, and drowsiness).
- Patient and/or family states the importance of taking the medication exactly as prescribed, such as at the same time every day, to help maximize therapeutic effectiveness.
- Patient states the dangers associated with sudden withdrawal of the medication, such as rebound seizure activity.
- Patient maintains a protective environment at home and at work to minimize self-injury.

Implementation

For patients taking all *antiepileptic* drugs, interventions are aimed at monitoring the patient while providing safety measures (see previous discussion) and securing the airway, breathing, and circulation. Airway maintenance is of critical importance for epileptic patients, because the tongue relaxes during seizure activity, falling backward and subsequently blocking the airway. The patient's airway may be maintained in the same way as during cardiopulmonary resuscitation using the chin lift or jaw thrust method. Rescue breathing should be provided if the patient is not breathing on his or her own at a rate of 1 breath every 5 seconds. If the patient is breathing, the airway is simply kept open through the proper positioning (as just described). In addition to performing these critical components of care, it is also important to maintain seizure precautions according to hospital policy. This may include making sure the patient is gently kept in bed or kept from falling, putting the side rails up, placing the patient in a side-lying position if needed, avoiding the use of tongue blades or other instruments to pry open the patient's mouth or clenched teeth, and ensuring quick access to oxygen and suctioning equipment at all times.

With antiepileptic drug administration, it is important to adhere closely to the drug dose and frequency of dosing, as ordered. Close monitoring of dosing is important to attain therapeutic blood levels. For example, if an antiepileptic drug is ordered to be administered every 6 hours, it is crucial to dose the drug so that it is given around the clock to maintain blood levels. Administering the antiepileptic drug at the same time every day is also important to maintain blood levels. See Patient Teaching Tips for more information.

With oral dosing of these drugs, it is recommended that the drug be taken with at least 6 to 8 oz of fluid, preferrably water, and with food, meals, or a snack to help decrease the risk of GI upset, a frequently encountered adverse effect. Juices, milk, and carbonated beverages are best avoided as the fluids of choice because of possible interactions with the drug. Oral suspensions should be shaken and the solution mixed thoroughly. Capsules should not be crushed, opened, or chewed—especially if extended- or long-release forms. The nurse should always check with an authoritative source if there are any doubts about the type of capsule, pill, or tablet or questions about recommended administration guidelines. Extended-release drugs are usually taken once a day, so the nurse should be cautious about their use, especially if more frequent dosing is ordered—always check and double-check! This is important to prevent too high or too low a serum level of the drug. If there are any questions about the medication order or the medication prescribed, the prescriber should be contacted immediately for clarification. *Topiramate* and *valproic acid* tablets and delayed or extended-release dosage forms should not be altered in any way. However, if the capsule is not delayed or extended-release, it can be opened and sprinkled in 1 teaspoon of soft food such as applesauce if needed.

The following interventions are specific to drugs and/or drug classes:

- *Carbamazepine:* This drug should *not* be given with grapefruit because this leads to increased toxicity of the antiepileptic drug. If the drug is to be replaced with another antiepileptic drug, a plan should be in place to decrease the dosages of the older drug before beginning low doses (at first) of the newer drug. Serum therapeutic levels are given in Table 15-6.
- *Hydantoins:* As a point of reference, 150 mg of fosphenytoin is the equivalent of 100 mg of phenytoin and the dose, concentration solution, and infusion rate of fosphenytoin is expressed as a

phenytoin equivalent (PE). Dilutional fluids include 5% dextrose in water (D5W) and 0.9% NaCl. Rates of infusion should follow manufacturer's guidelines and are usually 150 mg PE/min or less to avoid hypotension and cardiorespiratory depression. Should dysrhythmias or hypotension occur, the infusion should be discontinued, patient vital signs monitored, and the prescriber contacted immediately. Safety measures, such as assisting the patient with ambulation and having the patient move slowly and purposefully, should be implemented when this drug (or any other antiepileptic drug) is given because of the adverse effects of ataxia and dizziness. IV dose administration requires even more cautious use because of the rapid onset of action. CNS depression is always a concern; thus there is a need to frequently monitor the patient's vital signs. If existing IV lines are used that contain D5W or other solutions, the line should be flushed with normal saline before and after dosing to avoid precipitate formation. If infiltration of the IV site leads to subcutaneous tissue access, ischemia and sloughing may occur because of the high alkalinity of the drug. Hospital or facility policy as well as manufacturer's guidelines should be reviewed regarding the use of possible antidotes. If infiltration occurs, infusion of the solution should be discontinued but the needle should be left in place until all orders from the prescriber have been received. This practice allows any antidote medication to be administered through the IV catheter, if ordered. Oral dosage forms that are sustained or extended release should never be opened, punctured, chewed, or broken in pieces. Other regular forms of the drug may be crushed as needed. Gingival hyperplasia is an adverse effect and requires that the patient receive daily oral care as well as frequent dental visits. Complete blood counts are often monitored very closely within the first year of therapy (e.g., measured monthly for 1 year, then every 3 months).

- *Barbiturates* (e.g., phenobarbital): Abrupt withdrawal of these drugs, as well as of any antiepileptic drugs, should be avoided due to possible rebound seizure activity. Most of the oral dosage forms of this class of drugs should be taken with water, and elixirs should be mixed with fruit juice, milk, or water. If IV infusions are indicated, the dose should be safely calculated and an IV infusion pump used to administer the drug. Too rapid an infusion of IV dosage forms may lead to cardiovascular collapse and respiratory depression. In addition, vital signs and IV infusion rates should be monitored frequently and documented in the patient's chart. If any signs or symptoms of cardiovascular or respiratory depression are noted, the drug should be withheld and the prescriber contacted immediately; supportive care should be provided through maintenance of the airway, breathing, and circulation.
- *Gabapentin:* This is one of the antiepileptic drugs that can be taken without regard to meals. If discontinuation of the drug is indicated, dosage should be tapered over at least 1 week to avoid rebound seizures.
- *Lamotrigine:* Dosing regimen should be followed as ordered. See previous pharmacology discussion for more detailed in-

formation on dosage forms. The nurse should check for drug interactions and should be proactive and report any suicidal thoughts immediately.

- *Levetiracetam:* The most common adverse effects include sleepiness, weakness, dizziness, and infection. The prescriber should be contacted if any extreme adverse effects or any problems with moving, walking, or mood/behavioral changes occur. Any suicidal thoughts or psychotic symptoms should be reported. As with any antiepileptic drug, the patient should not drive, operate heavy machinery, or make major decisions when beginning therapy.
- *Oxcarbazepine:* This drug should be taken as prescribed and is usually given in two divided doses. Potential drug interactions should always be checked before administering (see previous discussion). The drug should be taken with food or snacks. Rash, tremors, abnormal walking or moving, or abdominal pain should be reported.
- *Pregabalin:* The daily dosage is usually given in two or three divided doses. Sudden or abrupt withdrawal is to be avoided. The patient should be monitored for any excessive dizziness, ocular or visual changes, or edema, and these should be reported immediately if they occur.
- *Tiagabine:* This drug should be taken with food, and any problems with generalized weakness, tremors, rash, or abdominal pain should be reported.
- *Valproic acid:* Oral dosage forms are not to be taken with carbonated beverages and should be taken with at least 4 to 6 oz of water. The drug should be given with fluids, food, or a snack to minimize any GI upset.

Evaluation

The occurrence of a therapeutic response to *antiepileptic drugs* does not mean that the patient has been cured of the seizures but only that seizure activity is decreased or absent. Any response to the medication should be documented in the nurse's notes. These classes of medications have other indications, such as management of chronic pain and migraines, and the existing problem or disorder should show improvement with minimal adverse effects. In addition, when monitoring and evaluating the effects of antiepileptic drugs, the nurse needs to constantly assess the patient for changes in mental status/level of consciousness, affect, eye problems or visual disorders, sore throat, and fever (blood dyscrasia is an adverse effect of the hydantoins). Measurements of serum levels of the specific antiepileptic drug are ordered at baseline or at the start of therapy and frequently thereafter to monitor the amount of drug in the blood and to determine if subsequent serum levels are subtherapeutic, therapeutic, or toxic. Subtherapeutic levels indicate that the dosage of the drug may need to be increased by the prescriber, and toxic levels require withholding or decreasing the dose—but only on the prescriber's order! Specific therapeutic blood levels are given in Table 15-6.

PATIENT TEACHING TIPS

- Educate about the sedating effects of drug therapy so that appropriate steps can be taken to ensure patient safety until a steady state is achieved (usually after four or five drug half-lives). The patient should not drive, operate heavy machinery, or make major decisions until steady state is achieved.
- The patient should report any suicidal thoughts or ideas immediately. Alcohol, caffeine intake, and smoking should be avoided.
- Antiepileptic drugs should never be abruptly discontinued as it may precipitate rebound seizure activity.
- The adverse effects that are most commonly associated with these drugs are drowsiness, GI upset, and CNS-depressing effects. The patient should be told that these effects often decrease after the drug has been taken for several weeks.
- The patient should be informed that a reoccurrence of seizure activity is usually due to a lack of compliance with the drug regimen.
- Some antiepileptic drugs may cause photosensitivity, so exposure to sunlight or tanning beds should be avoided. The patient should be instructed to use sunscreen and protective clothing.
- It should be emphasized to the patient that treatment of epilepsy is lifelong and that compliance with the treatment regimen is important for therapy to be effective. Community and other appropriate resources (e.g., national and local support groups) should be discussed with the patient.
- The patient should be told that any unusual reactions such as glandular swelling, fever, sore throat, tarry stools, back pain, hematuria, easy bruising, lethargy, or mouth ulcers should be reported to the prescriber immediately.
- Backup contraception is recommended for women of childbearing age who are taking topiramate.
- Important ways to improve *safety* in day to day activities while taking antiepileptic drugs should be discussed with the patient:

In the kitchen: Use an electric stove with no open flame, wear oven mitts, and cook only on rear burners. Cook in the microwave—it is the safest option. Have a plumber install a heat-control device on faucets to avoid burns. Carpet floors to help cushion any falls and use plastic dishes and containers instead of glass when possible. *In the bathroom:* Use heat-control devices on faucets. Carpet floors instead of using tile. Do not put a lock on the bathroom door so that help can be obtained, if needed. Bathe with only a few inches of water in the tub, and if seizure activity has not been fully controlled, bathe while someone else is present in the home. *During activities:* Always have someone along when engaging in sports and make sure the person is knowledgeable about management of airway and seizures. Bike riding with a helmet and swimming and water sports are okay if an accompanying adult is present who knows how to manage seizure activity and its consequences.
- Each state has different driving regulations for individuals with epilepsy, so the patient should be instructed to contact the department of motor vehicles of his or her state for further information. Many people with epilepsy work at steady jobs and have successful careers. Some are unable to work, but epilepsy should not prevent the individual from getting a job—such discrimination has been outlawed by the Americans with Disabilities Act of 1990 (Public Law 101-336).
- The patient should be encouraged to wear a medical alert bracelet or necklace and to keep a medical alert card on his or her person at all times.
- Keeping a daily diary or journal is important and is a helpful tool for the patient, prescriber, and/or caregivers. The date and time of any seizure should be recorded, and any details such as omitted drug doses, illnesses, and so on, should be documented.

POINTS TO REMEMBER

- *Epilepsy* is a disorder of the brain manifested as a chronic, recurrent pattern of seizures. A *seizure* is abnormal electrical activity in the brain.
- Seizures are classified as follows: partial onset seizures or those originating in a more localized region of the brain; status epilepticus, characterized by generalized tonic-clonic convulsions that occur repeatedly in succession; and tonic-clonic seizures involving initial muscular contraction throughout the body (tonic) and progressing alternating contraction and relaxation (clonic phase).
- Nurses must distinguish between the different types of seizure, with assessment and documentation of all symptoms, events, and problems that occur prior to, during and after any seizure activity. This information may aid in the diagnosis of the type of seizure the patient is experiencing.

- Noncompliance with the drug regimen is the most important factor leading to treatment failure.
- Therapeutic blood levels should be monitored at all times, and abrupt withdrawal of the antiepileptic drug must be avoided to prevent rebound seizure activity.
- IV infusions of antiepileptic drugs are very dangerous and should be managed cautiously, with adherence to hospital or facility policy and manufacturer's guidelines. Rapid infusions should always be avoided because of the risk for cardiac and/or respiratory arrest.
- Elderly may react with paradoxical reactions to antiepileptic drugs, with possible hyperactivity and irritability versus sedation.

NCLEX EXAMINATION REVIEW QUESTIONS

1 Which is the most appropriate nursing action for intravenous (IV) phenytoin (Dilantin)?
  a Give IV doses via rapid IV push
  b Administer in normal saline solutions
  c Administer in dextrose solutions
  d Ensure continuous infusion of the drug

2 The nurse is reviewing the drugs currently taken by a patient who will be starting drug therapy with carbamazepine. Which drug may raise a concern for interactions?
  a Digoxin (Lanoxin)
  b Acetaminophen (Tylenol)
  c Diazepam (Valium)
  d Warfarin (Coumadin)

3 Which response would the nurse expect to find in a patient with a phenytoin (Dilantin) level of 35 mcg/mL?
  a Ataxia
  b Hypertension
  c Seizures
  d No unusual response; this level is therapeutic.

4 A patient is taking pregabalin (Lyrica) but does not have a history of seizures. The nurse recognizes that this drug is also indicated for

  a postherpetic neuralgia.
  b viral infections.
  c Parkinson's disease.
  d depression.

5 The nurse is assessing a newly admitted patient who has a history of seizures. During the assessment, the patient has a generalized seizure that does not stop for several minutes. The nurse expects that which drug will be ordered for this condition?
  a Valproic acid (Depakote)
  b Neurontin (Gabapentin)
  c Carbamazepine (Tegretol)
  d Diazepam (Valium)

6 The nurse is administering an antiepileptic drug and will follow which guidelines? (Select all that apply.)
  a Monitor the patient for drowsiness.
  b Medications may be stopped if seizure activity disappears.
  c Give the medication at the same time every day.
  d Give the medication on an empty stomach.
  e Notify the prescriber if the patient is unable to take the medication.

1. b, 2. d, 3. a, 4. a, 5. d, 6. a, c, e.

CRITICAL THINKING ACTIVITIES: BEST ACTION

1 The nurse is about to administer the morning dose of phenobarbital to a patient with a history of seizures. Before the dose is given, the laboratory calls to report that the patient's phenobarbital blood level is 10 mcg/mL. What is the nurse's best action at this time?

2 The laboratory results indicate that the patient's phenytoin level is subtherapeutic, but the patient insists that he has not skipped any doses of medication. "I take it the same time every morn-

ing," he states emphatically. Upon further questioning, he mentions that he also takes an antacid in the morning because of heartburn. "Could that have any effect on my drug level?" he asks. What is the nurse's best response?

3 A patient is starting an antiepileptic drug and has many questions about it. The patient asks, "Will I be able to drive to work?" What is the nurse's best response?

For answers, see http:/evolve.elsevier.com/Lilley.

CHAPTER 16

Antiparkinsonian Drugs

OBJECTIVES

When you reach the end of this chapter, you should be able to do the following:

1 Briefly discuss the impact of acetylcholine and dopamine on the brain.
2 Describe the pathophysiology of Parkinson's disease.
3 Identify the different classes of medications used to manage Parkinson's disease, including first- and second-line drugs used in therapy.
4 Discuss the mechanisms of action, dosages, indications, routes of administration, contraindications, cautions, drug interactions, adverse effects, and toxic effects of antiparkinsonian drugs.
5 Develop a nursing care plan that includes all phases of the nursing process for patients taking antiparkinsonian drugs.

e-Learning Activities

Drug Profiles

amantadine, p. 250
apomorphine, p. 252
◆ benztropine mesylate, p. 253
bromocriptine, p. 251

◆ carbidopa-levodopa, p. 253
entacapone, p. 251
◆ ropinirole, p. 252
selegiline (and rasagiline), p. 247

◆ *Key drug.*

Glossary

Akinesia A reduction or absence of psychomotor activity that results in a masklike facial expression and impaired postural reflexes. A classic characteristic of Parkinson's disease. (p. 245)
Bradykinesia Slowness of movement; another classic symptom of Parkinson's disease. (p. 245)
Chorea A condition characterized by involuntary, purposeless, rapid motions such as flexing and extending the fingers, raising and lowering the shoulders, or grimacing. (p. 246)
Dyskinesia An impaired ability to execute voluntary movements. (p. 246)
Dystonia Impaired or distorted voluntary movement due to a disorder of muscle tone. (p. 246)
Exogenous A term describing any substance produced outside of the body that may be taken into the body (e.g., a medication, food, or environmental toxin). (p. 252)
On-off phenomenon A common experience of patients taking medication for Parkinson's disease in which they experience periods of greater symptomatic control ("on" time) alternating with periods of lesser symptomatic control ("off" time). (p. 246)
Parkinson's disease A slowly progressive, degenerative neurologic disorder characterized by resting tremor, pill-rolling of the fingers, masklike facies, shuffling gait, forward flexion of the trunk, loss of postural reflexes, and muscle rigidity and weakness. (p. 244)

Postural instability A decrease or change in motor and muscle movements that leads to unsteadiness and hesitation in movement and gait when the individual starts or stops walking; occurs in Parkinson's disease. (p. 245)
Presynaptic Drugs that exert their antiparkinsonian effects before the nerve synapse. (p. 250)
Rigidity Resistance of the muscles to passive movement; leads to the "cogwheel" rigidity seen in Parkinson's disease. (p. 245)
Tremor In Parkinson's disease, shakiness of the extremities seen mostly at rest. (p. 245)
Wearing off phenomenon A gradual worsening of Parkinsonian symptoms as a patient's medications begin to lose their effectiveness, despite maximal dosing with a variety of medications. (p. 246)

• • •

Anatomy, Physiology, and Disease Overview

PARKINSON'S DISEASE

Parkinson's disease is a chronic, progressive, degenerative disorder affecting the dopamine-producing neurons in the brain. Other chronic central nervous system (CNS) neuromuscular disorders are myasthenia gravis, dementia, and Alzheimer's disease. Parkinson's disease was initially recognized in 1817, at which time it was called *shaking palsy.* James Parkinson later described in more detail the symptoms of both the early and advanced stages of the disease. Not until the 1960s, however, was the underlying pathologic defect discovered. It was then first recognized that Parkinson's disease involved a dopamine deficit in the area of the cerebral cortex called the *substantia nigra,* which is contained within another brain structure known as the *basal ganglia.* Also relevant is the adjacent structure called the *globus pallidus.* All three structures are parts of the brain that are included in the *extrapyramidal system,* which is involved in motor function, including posture, muscle tone, and smooth muscle activity. In addition, the *thalamus* serves as a relay station for brain impulses, whereas the *cerebellum* also regulates muscle coordination (Figure 16-1).

Dopamine is an inhibitory neurotransmitter and *acetylcholine* is an excitatory neurotransmitter in this area of the brain. A cor-

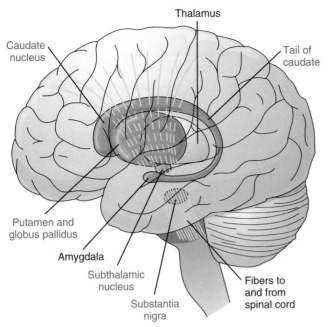

FIGURE 16-1   Basal ganglia and related structures of the brain. (From Copstead-Kirkhorn LC, Banasik JL: *Pathophysiology,* ed 4, St Louis, 2010, Saunders.)

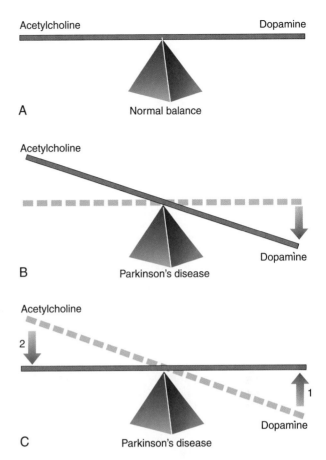

A, Normal balance of acetylcholine and dopamine in the CNS.
B, In Parkinson's disease, a decrease in dopamine results in an imbalance.
C, Drug therapy in Parkinson's disease is aimed at correcting the imbalance between acetylcholine and dopamine. This can be accomplished by:
   1. increasing the supply of dopamine
   2. blocking or lowering acetylcholine levels

FIGURE 16-2   The neurotransmitter abnormality in Parkinson's disease.

rect balance between these two neurotransmitters is needed for the proper regulation of posture, muscle tone, and voluntary movement. It is now recognized that Parkinson's disease results from an imbalance in these two neurotransmitters in the basal ganglia. This imbalance is caused by failure of the nerve terminals in the substantia nigra to produce dopamine. Dopamine acts in the basal ganglia to control movements. Destruction of the substantia nigra by Parkinson's disease leads to dopamine depletion. This dopamine deficiency often results in excessive, unopposed acetylcholine (cholinergic) activity due to the lack of a normal dopaminergic balancing effect. Figure 16-2 illustrates the difference in neurotransmitter concentrations in persons with normal balance and in patients with Parkinson's disease.

Some theorize that Parkinson's disease is the result of an earlier head injury or of excess iron in the substantia nigra, which undergoes oxidation and causes the generation of toxic free radicals. Another theory postulates that, because dopamine levels naturally decrease with age, Parkinson's disease represents a premature aging of the *nigrostriatal cells* of the substantia nigra resulting from environmental or intrinsic biochemical factors, or both. Evidence from animal studies suggests that environmental toxins, such as pesticides and metals, also contribute to the development of Parkinson's disease.

Parkinson's disease affects at least 1 million Americans. It is the second most common neurodegenerative disease after Alzheimer's disease. Some patients have both conditions. In most patients, the disease becomes apparent between 45 and 65 years of age, with a mean age of onset of 56 years. The number of patients with Parkinson's disease is expected to continue to increase as our elderly population grows. The disease occasionally occurs in younger people, especially after acute encephalitis or carbon monoxide or metallic poisoning. However, it is usually idiopathic (of no known cause). Overall, there is a 2% chance of developing the disease in one's lifetime. Men are affected more often than

women in a ratio of up to 3:2. In the past, family history did not appear to be a factor. However, evidence is now beginning to appear that supports the idea of genetic links, and up to 20% of patients have a family history of the disease.

There are no readily available laboratory tests that can detect or confirm Parkinson's disease. Results of computed tomography (CT), magnetic resonance imaging (MRI), cerebrospinal fluid analysis, and electroencephalography are usually normal and of little diagnostic value. Positron emission tomography (PET) may offer some additional information. CT, MRI, and PET may be useful tools for ruling out other possible diseases as causes of the symptoms, as well as for follow-up imaging after drug and surgical treatments. The diagnosis is usually made on the basis of the classic symptoms and physical findings. The classic symptoms of Parkinson's disease include **akinesia, bradykinesia, postural instability, rigidity,** and **tremors** (see Table 16-1).

Unfortunately, Parkinson's disease is a progressive condition. Over time, there is substantial reduction in the number of surviving dopaminergic terminals that can take up pharmacologically administered levodopa and convert it into dopamine. Rapid swings in the

TABLE 16-1 Classic Parkinsonian Symptoms

Symptom	Description
Akinesia	Reduction in or absence of psychomotor activity resulting in masklike facial expression and impaired postural reflexes (see postural instability)
Bradykinesia	Slowness of movement
Rigidity	"Cogwheel" rigidity, resistance to passive movement
Tremor	Pill rolling: tremor of the thumb against the forefinger, seen mostly at rest and less severe during voluntary activity; usually starts on one side then progresses to the other; is the presenting sign in 70% of cases
Postural instability	Unsteadiness that leads to danger of falling; hesitation in gait as patient starts or stops walking

TABLE 16-2 Currently Available Antiparkinsonian Drugs

Generic Name	Trade Name	Route
Dopamine Receptor Agonists		
Indirect Acting		
MAO-B Inhibitors		
selegiline	Eldepryl, Zelapar*	PO
rasagiline	Azilect	PO
Presynaptic Dopamine Release Enhancer		
amantadine	Symmetrel	PO
COMT Inhibitors		
tolcapone	Tasmar	PO
entacapone	Comtan	PO
Direct Acting		
Nondopamine Dopamine Receptor Agonists		
Ergot		
bromocriptine	Parlodel	PO
Nonergot		
pramipexole	Mirapex	PO
ropinirole	Requip	PO
apomorphine	Apokyn	Subcutaneous
Dopamine Replacement Drugs		
carbidopa*	Lodosyn	PO
carbidopa-levodopa	Sinemet, Parcopa**	PO
Anticholinergic Drugs (see Chapter 21)		
benztropine	Cogentin	PO, IV
trihexyphenidyl	Generic only (formerly Artane)	PO
Antihistamines (see Chapter 36)		
diphenhydramine	Benadryl	PO, IV

COMT, Catechol ortho-methyltransferase; *IV,* intravenous; *MAO-B,* monoamine oxidase type B; *PO,* oral.
*Not actually a dopamine replacement drug; used to reduce side effects associated with levodopa.
**Orally disintegrating tablet (see Chapter 2).

response to levodopa, called the **on-off phenomenon,** also occur. The result is worsening of the disease when too little dopamine is present, or dyskinesias when too much is present. In contrast, the **wearing-off phenomenon** occurs when anti–Parkinson's disease medications begin to lose their effectiveness, despite maximal dosing, as the disease progresses. **Dyskinesia** is the difficulty in performing voluntary movements that is commonly seen in the disease. The two dyskinesias most frequently associated with antiparkinsonian therapy are **chorea** (irregular, spasmodic, involuntary movements of the limbs or facial muscles) and **dystonia** (abnormal muscle tone leading to impaired or abnormal movements). Dystonia commonly involves the head, neck, and tongue and often occurs as an adverse effect of a medication. These motor complications make Parkinson's disease a prominent cause of disability. Dementia may also be a result of the disease whether or not the patient also has Alzheimer's disease. Other dyskinesias, such as hand tremor, can occur as an adverse effect of medications.

Symptoms of Parkinson's disease do not appear until approximately 80% of the dopamine store in the substantia nigra has been depleted. This means that by the time the disease is diagnosed, only approximately 20% of the patient's original nigral dopaminergic terminals are functioning normally.

Treatment of Parkinson's Disease

The first step in the treatment of Parkinson's disease is to provide a full explanation of the disease to the patient and his or her family members or significant others. Physical therapy, speech therapy, and occupational therapy are almost always needed when the patient is in the later stages of the disease.

Treatment of the disease normally centers around drug therapy. For especially severe cases, the surgical technique of *deep brain stimulation* may be used. This involves electrical stimulation of dopamine-deficient brain tissues in a way that helps to reduce Parkinson-associated dyskinesias. An electrical brain implant can be used for this purpose. Surgical treatments are for the more severe cases, and the patient must still respond well to levodopa drug therapy, discussed later in this chapter.

Pharmacology Overview

Because Parkinson's disease is thought to be due to imbalances of dopamine and acetylcholine, drug therapy is aimed at increasing the levels of dopamine and/or antagonizing the effects of acetylcholine to slow the progression of the disease. The drugs available for the treatment of Parkinson's disease are listed in Table 16-2.

Nerve terminals can take up substances, store them, and release them for use when needed. This forms the basis for antiparkinsonian drug therapy. As long as there are functioning nerve terminals that can take up dopamine, the symptoms of Parkinson's disease can be at least partially controlled. Parkinson's disease is essentially a deficiency of dopamine in the neurons in certain areas of the brain. Therefore, it seems logical that drug therapy focuses primarily on restoring and enhancing dopaminergic activity in these neurons. A variety of both indirect- and direct-acting drugs are available for this purpose. The indirect-acting drugs are often administered first in the disease process.

INDIRECT-ACTING DOPAMINERGIC DRUGS

MONOAMINE OXIDASE INHIBITORS

The enzyme *monoamine oxidase (MAO)* catalyzes the breakdown of *catecholamines* in the body, which include dopamine, norepinephrine, and epinephrine. There are two subclasses of MAO in the body: MAO-A and MAO-B. As early as 1965, nonselective monoamine oxidase inhibitors (MAOIs), which inhibit both MAO-A and MAO-B, were being used to improve the therapeutic effect of levodopa by preventing its metabolic breakdown. They were also among the first medications used to treat depression but have been widely replaced by newer drug categories (see Chapter 17). A major adverse effect of the nonselective MAOIs is that they interact with tyramine-containing foods (cheese, red wine, beer, and yogurt) because of their inhibitory activity against MAO-A. This has been called the *cheese effect,* and one hazardous result can be severe hypertension. Selegiline, an amphetamine derivative, is a selective MAO-B inhibitor, and is much less likely to elicit the classic cheese effect at dosages of 10 mg or less daily. It is approved for use in conjunction with levodopa therapy in the treatment of Parkinson's disease. There was earlier speculation by researchers that selegiline, as well as possibly vitamins E (tocopherol) and C (ascorbic acid), might have antiparkinsonian effects due to "neuroprotective" activity at the neuronal (nerve cell) level. The results of some animal studies suggested this as a possibility. However, no human or animal studies to date have conclusively demonstrated this to be the case for any of these three substances. Nonetheless, this theoretical neuroprotective effect is still debated in the literature.

Rasagiline is the newest antiparkinsonian drug and received FDA approval in 2008. Like selegiline, rasagiline is a selective MAO-B inhibitor. It is approved to be given once a day as monotherapy in the early stages of the disease, as well as in combination with other drugs in advanced cases. Drug interactions and adverse effects are similar to those of selegiline.

Mechanism of Action and Drug Effects

The MAO enzymes are widely distributed throughout the body. The areas where concentrations are high are the liver, kidney, stomach, intestinal wall, and brain. There are two subclasses of MAOs, A and B with most of MAO-B occurring in the CNS, primarily in the brain. Since the primary role of MAOs is the breakdown of catecholamines, such as dopamine, norepinephrine, and epinephrine, as well as serotonin, giving an MAO-B inhibitor such as selegiline causes an increase in the levels of dopaminergic stimulation in the CNS. This helps to counter the dopaminergic deficiency seen in Parkinson's disease. Administration of selegiline can also allow the dose of levodopa (discussed later in this chapter) to be reduced. Improvement in functional ability and decreased severity of symptoms are common after selegiline is added. However, only approximately 50% to 60% of patients show a positive response.

Indications

Selegiline is currently approved for use in combination with levodopa or carbidopa-levodopa. It is an adjunctive drug used when a patient's response to levodopa is fluctuating. Selegiline may also be somewhat beneficial as a prophylactic drug to delay reduction in a patient's response to levodopa. Several studies have shown that selegiline-treated patients required levodopa therapy approximately 1.8 times later than control patients. As Parkinson's disease progresses, it becomes more difficult to manage it with levodopa. Ultimately, levodopa no longer controls the disease, and the patient is seriously debilitated. This generally occurs between 5 and 10 years after the start of levodopa therapy.

Prophylactic selegiline use may delay the development of serious debilitating Parkinson's disease for 9 to 18 years. Since the average age of patients at the onset of Parkinson's disease is between 55 and 65 years, such a delay can prevent functional disability during the patient's life span.

Contraindications

Selegiline is contraindicated in cases of known drug allergy. Its concurrent use with the opioid analgesic meperidine (see Chapter 11) is also contraindicated due to well-documented drug interactions between MAOIs and meperidine (see section on interactions).

Adverse Effects

The most common adverse effects associated with selegiline use are mild and are listed in Table 16-3. At recommended dosages of 10 mg/day, the drug maintains its selective MAO-B inhibition. However, at dosages that exceed 10 mg/day, selegiline becomes a nonselective MAOI, which contributes to the development of the cheese effect described earlier.

Interactions

Selegiline interacts with relatively few drugs and the degree of interaction is dose dependent. Meperidine, when given with selegiline, has been associated with delirium, muscle rigidity, hyperpyrexia (high fever), and hyperirritability. Other reported reactions are rare and are listed in Table 16-3. Selegiline may safely be taken concurrently with catechol ortho-methyltransferase inhibitors (see later drug section).

Dosages

For the recommended dosage of selegiline, see the Dosages table on p. 248. Also see the Preventing Medication Errors box.

DRUG PROFILES

selegiline (and rasagiline)

Selegiline (Eldepryl) is a selective MAO-B inhibitor which is indicated for Parkinson's disease. It is used as an adjunctive drug along with levodopa to reduce the dosage of levodopa needed for symptom control. Adverse effects increased with doses greater than 10 mg when it loses its selectivity for MAO-B are listed in Table 16-3. Drug interactions are listed in Table 16-4. Selegiline was previously available only for oral use. However, there is now an orally disintegrating tablet for buccal use known as Zelapar, which can provide improved drug absorption. In addition, a new transdermal form of the drug known as Emsam has become available. Emsam is currently indicated only for major depressive disorder (see Chapter 17). Rasagiline (Azilect) is a newer selective MAO-B inhibitor comparable to selegiline. Its advantage is that it is approved as monotherapy for Parkinson's disease, whereas selegiline, as noted earlier, is normally used adjunctively with the dopamine replacement drug levodopa.

PHARMACOKINETICS

Route	Onset of Action	Peak Plasma Concentration	Elimination Half-life*	Duration of Action
PO	1 hr	0.5-2 hr	2 hr	1-3 days

*Selegiline has three active metabolites with long half-lives of 18 to 21 hr.

TABLE 16-3 Adverse Effects of Selected Antiparkinsonian Drugs

Drug or Drug Class	Adverse Effects
Indirect-Acting Dopamine Receptor Agonists	
MAO-B inhibitor: selegiline	Dizziness, dyskinesias, nausea, syncope
Presynaptic dopamine release enhancer: amantadine	Dizziness, insomnia, nausea
COMT inhibitors: entacapone, tolcapone	GI upset, dyskinesias, urine discoloration Tolcapone: liver failure
Direct-Acting Dopamine Receptor Agonists	
Ergot Derivative	
bromocriptine	Ataxia, confusion, dizziness, depression. drowsiness, GI upset, visual changes
Nonergot Drugs	
pramipexole, ropinirole	Leg edema, fatigue, syncope, dizziness, drowsiness, GI upset, viral infection (presumed unknown immunosuppressant effect)
apomorphine	Dyskinesias, dizziness, drowsiness, nausea, vomiting, hallucinations, leg edema
Dopamine Replacement Drugs	
levodopa, carbidopa	Heart palpitations, hypotension, urinary retention, depression, psychosis, dyskinesias, rhinorrhea

COMT, Catechol ortho-methyltransferase; *GI,* gastrointestinal; *MAO-B,* monoamine oxidase type B.

DOSAGES

Selected Antiparkinsonian Drugs

Drug (Pregnancy Category)	Pharmacologic Class	Usual Dosage Range	Indications
amantadine (Symmetrel) (C)	Indirect-acting dopamine agonist	**Adult** PO: 100-400 mg/day divided q12h	
apomorphine (Apokyn) (C)	Direct-acting dopamine agonist; nonergot	**Adult** Subcut: dose is 0.2 to 0.6 mL adjusted for "off" episodes	
◆ benztropine (Cogentin) (C)	Anticholinergic	**Adult** PO: 0.5-6 mg/day	
bromocriptine (Parlodel) (D)	Direct-acting dopamine agonist; ergot derivative	**Adult** PO: 2.5-90 mg/day	
carbidopa-levodopa (Sinemet, Sinemet CR, Parcopa) (C)	Direct-acting dopamine agonist/replacement	**Adult** PO: 10/100, 1 tab 3-8×/day; 25/100, 1 tab 3-6×/day; 25/250, 1 tab tid-qid CR: 1 tab bid; up to 2-8 tabs at 4- to 8-hr intervals PO (orally disintegrating tablet [Parcopa]): same as above	Parkinson's disease
entacapone (Comtan) (C)	Indirect-acting dopamine agonist	**Adult** PO: 200 mg with each dosage of levodopa, up to 8×/day	
◆ ropinirole (Requip) (C)	Direct-acting dopamine agonist; non–ergot derivative	**Adult** PO: 0.25 mg tid slowly titrating to max dose of 24 mg/day	
selegiline (Eldepryl, Zelapar) (C)	Indirect-acting dopamine agonist/selective MAOI	**Adult** PO: 5 mg bid with breakfast and lunch in combination with carbidopa-levodopa, or 10 mg qAM **Adult** PO (orally disintegrating tablet [Zelapar]): 1.25-2.5 mg once daily	

CR, Controlled release; *MAOI,* monoamine oxidase inhibitor; *PO,* oral; *subcut,* subcutaneous.

PREVENTING MEDICATION ERRORS

Look-Alike/Sound-Alike Drugs: Selegiline and Salagen

Be careful about look-alike/sound-alike drugs! Medication errors often occur when drug names are similar.

Selegiline is a monoamine oxidase inhibitor that is used to treat Parkinson's disease. Salagen, an oral form of pilocarpine hydrochloride, is prescribed for relief of dry mouth symptoms, also known as *xerosto-*

mia, in patients who have Sjögren's syndrome or who have received radiation therapy. To make it more confusing, both drugs are available in 5-mg tablets. Be sure to double-check the name and use of these drugs when receiving orders and instruct patients to check the drug names when getting these drugs filled at pharmacies.

For more information, visit *http://www.ismp.org/Newsletters/acutecare/articles/20050922_1.asp.*

TABLE 16-4 Selected Drug Interactions of Antiparkinsonian Drugs

Drug or Drug Class	Interacting Drug	Mechanism	Result
Indirect-Acting Dopamine Receptor Agonists			
MAO-B inhibitor:			
selegiline	meperidine and other opioids, tramadol; cyclobenzaprine, dextromethorphan, other MAOIs, serotonergic antidepressants, and sympathomimetic amines	Additive CNS stimulation	Serotonin syndrome
	carbamazepine, oxcarbazepine, oral contraceptives	Reduced selegiline clearance	Potential selegiline toxicity
	buspirone	Uncertain	Hypertension
Presynaptic dopamine release enhancer:			
amantadine	Anticholinergic drugs	Additive effects	Increased anticholinergic adverse effects
	Sulfonamide antibiotics, quinidine, thiazide diuretics, triamterene	Reduced amantadine clearance	Potential amantadine toxicity
COMT inhibitor:			
entacapone	MAOIs, catecholamines	Reduced catecholamine metabolism	Tachycardia, cardiac dysrhythmias, hypertension
	ampicillin, cholestyramine, erythromycin, rifampin	Reduced biliary clearance of entacapone	Increased catecholamine activity due to excessive COMT inhibition
Direct-Acting Dopamine Receptor Agonists			
Ergot Derivative			
bromocriptine	erythromycin	Cytochrome P-450 interactions	Increased bromocriptine effects with risk of toxicity
	Sympathomimetics	Additive effects	Hypertension, cardiac dysrhythmias
	Antihypertensives	Additive effects	Hypotension
Nonergot Drugs			
Ropinirole	acetaminophen, caffeine, warfarin, ciprofloxacin	Cytochrome P-450 interactions	Reduced ropinirole clearance with risk of toxicity
	Antipsychotics	Antidopaminergic activity	Reduced efficacy of ropinirole
apomorphine	Serotonin antiemetics	Uncertain	Profound hypotension
	Antihypertensives	Uncertain	Hypotension, falls
	Antipsychotics	Antidopaminergic activity	Reduced efficacy of apomorphine
	Any drugs that prolong QT interval on ECG	Uncertain	Cardiac dysrhythmias
Dopamine Replacement Drugs			
Levodopa, carbidopa	Antacids	Increased bioavailability of levodopa and/or carbidopa	Enhanced anti–Parkinson's disease effects
	metoclopramide	Increased bioavailability of levodopa and/or carbidopa; reduced efficacy of metoclopramide	Enhanced anti–Parkinson's disease effects; reduced gastric emptying and increased esophageal pressure
	Anticholinergics	Reduced levodopa absorption; additive effects	Reduced therapeutic effects; increased dyskinesias
	Benzodiazepines, hydantoins	Cytochrome P-450 interactions	Reduced anti–Parkinson's disease effects
	pyridoxine	Reversal of levodopa effects when levodopa used alone	Reduced therapeutic effects (can be avoided by using carbidopa-levodopa)
	Tricyclic antidepressants	Reduced levodopa absorption	Reduced therapeutic effects

CNS, Central nervous system; *COMT,* catechol ortho-methyltransferase; *ECG,* electrocardiogram; *MAO-B,* monoamine oxidase type B; *MAOI,* monoamine oxidase inhibitor.

PRESYNAPTIC DOPAMINE RELEASE ENHANCER

Only one drug is currently known to function as a **presynaptic** dopamine release enhancer. Amantadine (Symmetrel) was first recognized as an antiviral drug and was used for treating influenza virus infections. It is still used for this purpose (see Chapter 40) as well as for management of Parkinson's disease.

Mechanism of Action and Drug Effects

Amantadine appears to exert its antiparkinsonian effect by causing the release of dopamine and other catecholamines from their storage sites, or *vesicles*, in the presynaptic fibers of nerve cells within the basal ganglia that have not yet been destroyed by the disease process. Amantadine also blocks the reuptake of dopamine into the nerve fibers. This results in higher levels of dopamine in the synapses between nerves and improved dopamine neurotransmission between neurons. Because amantadine does not directly stimulate dopaminergic receptors, it is considered to be *indirect acting*. Amantadine also has some anticholinergic properties (see Chapter 21). This may further help by controlling symptoms of dyskinesia.

Indications

Amantadine is indicated for treatment of Parkinson's disease relatively early in the course of the disease, while there are still some intact neurons in the basal ganglia. It is usually effective for only 6 to 12 months, after which it often fails to relieve hypokinesia and rigidity. Once it becomes ineffective, a dopamine agonist such as bromocriptine is usually tried next (see later drug section). Amantadine is also indicated for influenza virus infection (see Chapter 40).

Contraindications

Amantadine is contraindicated in cases of known drug allergy.

Adverse Drug Effects

Common adverse effects associated with amantadine are relatively mild and include dizziness, insomnia, and nausea. Other effects are listed in Table 16-3.

Drug Interactions

Drugs that interact with amantadine include anticholinergic drugs and CNS stimulants. These and other interactions are described in Table 16-4.

Dosage

See Dosages table on p. 248.

DRUG PROFILE

amantadine

Amantadine (Symmetrel) is actually an antiviral drug that is used most often for influenza virus infection (see Chapter 40). It is also indicated for treatment of early Parkinson's disease, for which it helps to control symptoms of dyskinesia, including motor rigidity, by virtue of both its dopaminergic and anticholinergic effects. Common adverse reactions include dizziness, insomnia, and nausea (see Table 16-3). Interacting drugs include anticholinergics and

---

CNS stimulants (additive effects) (see Table 16-4). Amantadine is available only for oral use.

PHARMACOKINETICS

Route	Onset of Action	Peak Plasma Concentration	Elimination Half-life	Duration of Action
PO	48 hr	2-4 hr	11-15 hr	6-12 wk

CATECHOL ORTHO-METHYLTRANSFERASE INHIBITORS

The third category of indirect-acting dopaminergic drugs is the *catechol ortho-methyltransferase (COMT)* inhibitors. There are currently two drugs in this category: tolcapone (Tasmar) and entacapone (Comtan).

Mechanism of Action and Drug Effects

Tolcapone and entacapone, like amantadine, work presynaptically. Both drugs block COMT. COMT is the enzyme that catalyzes the breakdown of the body's catecholamines. Tolcapone differs slightly from entacapone in that it may act both centrally and peripherally. Entacapone cannot cross the blood-brain barrier and therefore can act only peripherally. The main positive effect of these drugs is that they prolong the duration of action of levodopa. This is especially true when levodopa is given with carbidopa (see section on dopamine replacement drugs later). This results in reduction of the *wearing off phenomenon*.

Indications

COMT inhibitors are indicated for the treatment of Parkinson's disease.

Contraindications

Both COMT inhibitors are contraindicated in cases of known drug allergy. Tolcapone is also contraindicated in cases of liver failure (see following section on adverse drug effects).

Adverse Effects

Commonly reported adverse effects with both COMT inhibitors include gastrointestinal (GI) upset, dyskinesias, and urine discoloration (see Table 16-3). Tolcapone has been associated with cases of severe liver failure. For this reason, the FDA announced in 1998 that this drug should be considered only in patients who do not respond to other Parkinson's disease drug therapy (see drug profile section).

Interactions

Neither tolcapone nor entacapone should be taken with nonselective MAOIs because of a dual cardiovascular risk of reduced catecholamine metabolism. However, the selective MAO-B inhibitor selegiline may be safely taken concurrently with COMT inhibitors. Similar hazards may occur when COMT inhibitors are given with catecholamines due to reduced catecholamine metabolism. These and other interactions are listed in Table 16-4.

Dosages

See the Dosages table on p. 248.

Inhibition of the enzyme in the body known as COMT is a new strategy for prolonging the duration of action of levodopa. Two compounds were developed for this purpose: tolcapone (Tasmar) and entacapone (Comtan). Both drugs are reversible inhibitors of COMT. The major difference between them is that tolcapone has a longer duration of action. Tolcapone has been associated with severe liver failure. It remains on the U.S. market but is used rarely. To date, no similar pattern of adverse outcomes has been shown with entacapone, which makes it a better first choice for COMT inhibitor therapy.

entacapone

Entacapone (Comtan) is a potent COMT inhibitor indicated for the adjunctive treatment of Parkinson's disease. Entacapone is normally taken with levodopa and should be effective from the first dose. A patient can feel the benefit of entacapone within a few days. Entacapone benefits patients who are experiencing wearing-off effects. Entacapone, when used with levodopa, can also reduce on-off effects. The levodopa dosage can often be reduced. Adverse reactions include GI upset, dyskinesias, and urine discoloration (see Table 16-3). Drug interactions (see Table 16-4) occur with nonselective MAOIs (see Chapter 17) and catecholamines (see Chapter 18). Entacapone is contraindicated in patients who have shown a hypersensitivity reaction to it and should be used with caution in patients with preexisting liver disease. Entacapone is available only for oral use. It is also now available in combination tablets that contain various doses of entacapone, carbidopa, and levodopa (Stalevo).

PHARMACOKINETICS

Route	Onset of Action	Peak Plasma Concentration	Elimination Half-life	Duration of Action
PO	1 hr	0.5-1.5 hr	1-3.5 hr	6 hr

DIRECT-ACTING DOPAMINE RECEPTOR AGONISTS

Direct-acting dopamine receptor agonists are a major class of drugs used to treat Parkinson's disease, especially in its later stages. These drugs include two subclasses: *nondopamine dopamine receptor agonists (NDDRAs)* and *dopamine replacement drugs*. NDDRAs are further subdivided into the ergot derivatives bromocriptine (Parlodel) and pergolide (Permax), and the nonergot drugs pramipexole (Mirapex), ropinirole (Requip), and apomorphine (Apokyn). The dopamine replacements drugs include levodopa (Larodopa), carbidopa (Lodosyn), and carbidopa-levodopa (Sinemet). Another NDDRA, rotigotine (Neupro), is a transdermal dosage form. However, it was recalled in April 2008 due to erratic crystallizations of drug within the skin patches with the potential for unpredictable patterns of drug absorption. Pergolide was taken off the U.S. market after severe adverse effects were reported.

NONDOPAMINE DOPAMINE RECEPTOR AGONISTS

Mechanism of Action and Drug Effects

All of the NDDRAs work by direct stimulation of presynaptic and/or postsynaptic dopamine receptors in the brain. They may be used in early or late stages of the disease. However, the dopa-

mine replacement drugs are often used as a last resort after other drug classes have failed or reached a wearing-off effect.

Chemically, bromocriptine is an ergot alkaloid similar to ergotamine (see Chapter 14) in its chemical structure. *Ergot* is the name of a pathologic fungal growth on plants such as the rye plant. The antiparkinsonian effects of bromocriptine are due to its ability to activate presynaptic dopamine receptors to stimulate the production of more dopamine. It chief site of activity is the D2 subclass of dopamine receptors. Pramipexole and ropinirole are two newer *nonergot* NDDRAs. Both are effective in early and late stages of Parkinson's disease.

Indications

Both ergot and nonergot NDDRAs are used to treat various stages of Parkinson's disease, either alone or in combination with other drugs. Bromocriptine also inhibits the production of the hormone *prolactin,* which stimulates normal lactation. For this reason, it is used to treat women with excessive or undesired breast milk production *(galactorrhea)* and is also used for treatment of prolactin-secreting tumors. Ropinirole is also used to treat a disorder known as *restless legs syndrome,* a nocturnal movement of the legs that disrupts sleep.

Contraindications

A contraindication to dopaminergic drugs is known drug allergy. These drugs also should not be used concurrently with catecholamines (see Chapter 18), due to the cardiovascular risks of excessive catecholamine activity. These drugs should not be taken until at least 14 days after the discontinuation of therapy with MAOIs (see Chapter 17), with the exception of selegiline and rasagiline, which are selective MAO-B inhibitors.

Adverse Effects

Many potential adverse effects are associated with the dopaminergic drugs. They are listed in Table 16-3.

Interactions

Interactions vary among drugs and are listed in Table 16-4.

Dosages

See the Dosages table on p. 248.

The traditional role of the NDDRAs bromocriptine, pramipexole, and ropinirole has been as adjuncts to levodopa for management of motor fluctuations only. These drugs differ from levodopa in that they do not replace dopamine itself but act by stimulation of dopaminergic receptors in the brain. The drugs have been evaluated as initial monotherapy and as combination therapy with low-dose levodopa in an attempt to either delay levodopa therapy or reduce the dosage of levodopa and its associated motor complications (see drug profile for levodopa). The newest antiparkinsonian drug, apomorphine (Apokyn), is an injectable drug used for refractory disease (see drug profile).

bromocriptine

Bromocriptine stimulates only the D2 receptors and antagonizes the D1 receptors. Eventually, carbidopa-levodopa is needed to control the patient's symptoms. Using amantadine until it fails and then using a nondopamine agonist until it also fails may postpone the need for levodopa therapy for up to 3 years. Bromocriptine may also be given with carbidopa-levodopa so that lower dosages of the levodopa are needed. This often results in prolonging the "on" periods and minimizing the "off" periods of the disease. Bromocriptine is indicated for Parkinson's disease as well as hyper-prolactinemia. Bromocriptine is contraindicated in cases of known drug allergy to any ergot alkaloids and also in patients with severe ischemic disease of any kind (e.g., peripheral vascular disease). This is because of the ability of bromocriptine to stimulate dopamine receptors in the peripheral tissues outside of the brain. This can result in vasoconstriction, which can worsen peripheral vascular disease. Adverse reactions include GI upset, dyskinesias, sleep disturbances, and others as listed in Table 16-3. Drug interactions occur with erythromycin, phenothiazines, and adrenergic drugs (see Table 16-4). Bromocriptine is available only for oral use.

PHARMACOKINETICS

Route	Onset of Action	Peak Plasma Concentration	Elimination Half-life	Duration of Action
PO	0.5-1.5 hr	1-3 hr	3-5 hr	4-8 hr

◆ ropinirole

Ropinirole (Requip) is a nonergot NDDRA. A similar drug is pramipexole (Mirapex). The nonergot drugs may have a better adverse effects profile (e.g., fewer dyskinesias) than bromocriptine. Ropinirole is also more specific than bromocriptine for the D2 subfamily of dopamine receptors (D2, D3, and D4). This in turn may result in more specific antiparkinsonian effects with fewer of the adverse effects associated with more generalized dopaminergic stimulation. Ropinirole can be effective in both early- and late-stage Parkinson's disease and appears to delay the need for levodopa therapy. Ropinirole is indicated for both monotherapy and adjunctive therapy with levodopa. It is also approved by the FDA for moderate to severe primary restless legs syndrome. The drug is contraindicated in patients with known drug allergy. Adverse effects include dizziness, GI upset, and somnolence (see Table 16-3). Drug interactions occur with any drug metabolized by cytochrome P-450 enzyme 1A2 (e.g., acetaminophen, caffeine, warfarin), theophylline, and digoxin (see Table 16-4). Ropinirole is available only for oral use.

PHARMACOKINETICS

Route	Onset of Action	Peak Plasma Concentration	Elimination Half-life	Duration of Action
PO	30 min	1-2 hr	3-5 hr	6-10 hr

apomorphine

Apomorphine (Apokyn) is a newer nonergot dopamine agonist introduced in 2004. It is given by subcutaneous injection only. The drug is indicated as adjunct drug therapy for both on-off and wearing-off episodes associated with advanced disease. It is contraindicated in cases of known drug allergy, allergy to the preservative metabisulfite or sulfa drugs, severe cardiovascular disease, and concurrent use of serotonin antiemetics (see Chapter 52). Adverse effects include severe nausea and vomiting, drowsiness, and hypotension (see Table 16-3). The dose is titrated to avoid hypotensive effects, and the drug should be prescribed in terms of *milliliters* and not milligrams to avoid potentially life-threatening overdose. Nausea and vomiting are to be expected and are treated with the antiemetic trimethobenzamide (see Chapter 52). Apomorphine interacts with 5-hydroxytryptamine 3 (serotonin)

antiemetics, which can also cause hypotension and syncope (see Table 16-4). Apomorphine is available only for injectable use.

PHARMACOKINETICS

Route	Onset of Action	Peak Plasma Concentration	Elimination Half-life	Duration of Action
PO	Unknown	10-60 min	30-60 min	Unknown

DOPAMINE REPLACEMENT DRUGS

The traditional cornerstone of therapy for Parkinson's disease has been with the drug levodopa, a biologic precursor of dopamine required by the brain for dopamine synthesis. However, levodopa cannot be used by itself in the brain and must be combined with another substance, carbidopa. The combination product carbidopa-levodopa provides **exogenous** sources of dopamine that directly replace the deficient neurotransmitter dopamine in the substantia nigra. These drugs are thus classified as *dopamine replacement* drugs and are drugs of choice in the later stages of Parkinson's disease.

Mechanism of Action and Drug Effects

Dopamine replacement drugs stimulate presynaptic dopamine receptors to increase brain levels of dopamine. Dopamine must be administered orally as levodopa, because exogenously administered dopamine cannot pass through the blood-brain barrier. Levodopa is the biologic precursor of dopamine and can penetrate into the CNS. However, levodopa is given in combination with carbidopa because very large oral doses of levodopa must be given to obtain adequate dopamine replacement in the brain, because much of the levodopa administered is broken down outside the CNS by the enzyme dopa decarboxylase. These large doses result in high peripheral levels of dopamine and lead to many unwanted adverse effects (see Table 16-3). These adverse effects include confusion, involuntary movements, GI distress, hypotension, and even cardiac dysrhythmias. These problems may be avoided when levodopa is given with carbidopa. Carbidopa is a peripheral decarboxylase inhibitor with little or no pharmacologic activity when given alone. When given in combination with levodopa, carbidopa inhibits the breakdown of levodopa in the periphery and thus allows smaller doses of levodopa to be used. Lesser amounts of levodopa result in fewer of the unwanted adverse effects.

Indications

Dopamine replacement drugs are used to directly restore dopaminergic activity in Parkinson's disease. Dopamine itself is also given by injection in critical care settings (see Chapter 18) as a pressor drug to raise blood pressure and enhance renal perfusion.

Contraindications

Levodopa and carbidopa are both contraindicated in cases of angle-closure glaucoma, because they can raise intraocular pressure. However, they may be used cautiously in patients with open-angle glaucoma (see Chapter 57). Neither drug should be used in patients with any undiagnosed skin condition, because both drugs can activate malignant melanoma.

Adverse Effects

Adverse effects of dopamine replacement drugs include cardiac dysrhythmias, hypotension, chorea, muscle cramps, and GI distress (see Table 16-3).

Interactions

Drugs that interact with levodopa and carbidopa include antacids, anticholinergics, MAOIs, and others, which are described in Table 16-4.

DRUG PROFILE

◆ carbidopa-levodopa

Carbidopa-levodopa (Sinemet), available orally, is one of the most commonly used drugs for Parkinson's disease. Carbidopa (Lodosyn) alone is not used as frequently. A variety of studies have shown that the controlled-release product Sinemet CR (or generic) increases on-time and decreases off-time. As with all sustained-release products, Sinemet CR should not be crushed. Drug interactions occur with antacids, tricyclic antidepressants, and other drugs (see Table 16-4).

PHARMACOKINETICS

Route	Onset of Action	Peak Plasma Concentration	Elimination Half-life	Duration of Action
PO	2-3 wk*	0.5-2 hr	1.5 hr	5 hr

*Therapeutic effect.

ANTICHOLINERGIC DRUGS

Anticholinergic drugs block the effects of the neurotransmitter acetylcholine at cholinergic receptors in the brain as well as in the rest of the body. They are discussed in greater detail in Chapter 21. Anticholinergics are used as adjunct drug therapy in Parkinson's disease due to their *antidyskinetic* properties. The purpose of their use is to reduce excessive cholinergic activity in the brain. Accumulation of acetylcholine in Parkinson's disease causes an overstimulation of the cholinergic excitatory pathways, which results in muscle tremors and muscle rigidity. One example of this is the *cogwheel rigidity* observed when an arm that is flexed toward the body is then extended at the elbow. The muscle tremors are usually worse when the patient is at rest and consist of a pill-rolling movement and bobbing of the head. Anticholinergic drugs help to alleviate these bothersome and often disabling symptoms. However, anticholinergics do little to relieve the *bradykinesia* (extremely slow movements) that are also associated with Parkinson's disease. Acetylcholine is also responsible for causing increased *s*alivation, *l*acrimation (tearing of the eyes), *u*rination, *d*iarrhea, increased *G*I motility, and possibly *e*mesis (vomiting). The acronym *SLUDGE* is often used to describe these cholinergic effects. The effects of anticholinergics are the opposite of the SLUDGE symptoms—such as *antisecretory* effects (dry mouth or decreased salivation), urinary retention, decreased GI motility (constipation), dilated pupils (*mydriasis*), and smooth muscle relaxation. Anticholinergic drugs readily cross the blood-brain barrier and therefore can get to the site of Parkinson's disease pathology in the brain, the substantia nigra.

The first drugs in this category to be used were the belladonna plant alkaloids and the synthetic drugs atropine and scopolamine.

However, the anticholinergic adverse effects of dry mouth, urinary retention, and blurred vision associated with these original anticholinergics can be excessive. Therefore, synthetic anticholinergics were developed that have better adverse effect profiles. The anticholinergics most commonly used include benztropine (Cogentin) and trihexyphenidyl (generic only; formerly Artane). Antihistamines (see Chapter 36) also have significant anticholinergic properties, they can also be used to manage cholinergic symptoms in Parkinson's disease. The most common choice is the drug diphenhydramine (Benadryl). Anticholinergics must be used cautiously in older adults because of significant potential adverse effects such as confusion, urinary retention, visual blurring, palpitations, and increased intraocular pressure.

DRUG PROFILE

◆ benztropine mesylate

Benztropine (Cogentin) is an anticholinergic drug used for Parkinson's disease and also for extrapyramidal symptoms from antipsychotic drugs (see Chapter 17). Benztropine should be used with caution in hot weather or during exercise because it may cause hyperthermia. Other adverse effects include tachycardia, confusion, disorientation, toxic psychosis, urinary retention, dry throat, constipation, nausea, and vomiting. Anticholinergic syndrome can occur when it is given with other drugs such as amantadine, phenothiazine, or tricyclic antidepressants that are associated with a high incidence of anticholinergic effects. Alcohol should be avoided. Benztropine is available as tablets and in injectable form. The normal dosage is 0.5 to 6 mg/day in one or two divided doses.

PHARMACOKINETICS

Route	Onset of Action	Peak Plasma Concentration	Elimination Half-life	Duration of Action
PO	1 hr	2-4 hr	4-8 hr	6-10 hr

NURSING PROCESS

Assessment

After patients are confronted with the diagnosis of Parkinson's disease, they soon experience the impact of the disease with every movement and activity of daily living. Not only will their lives never be the same, they will soon learn that their quality of life depends on drug therapy and nondrug measures. Before medications for Parkinson's disease are given, vital signs (e.g., blood pressure, pulse, respirations, temperature, pain) and ABCs (airway, breathing, and circulation) need to be assessed and documented. In addition, a complete nursing history must be obtained with a thorough physical, including compilation of a comprehensive medication profile. Because it may take several weeks to see a therapeutic response to medication regimens, a keen assessment and careful patient monitoring are even more critical to quality nursing care. A thorough assessment should include a health history, review of systems, determination of sensory and motor abilities, and head-to-toe examination. Other information to gather includes the following: (1) health history: complaint upon admission or the symptoms/event that led the patient to obtain medical treatment; past and current medical history with a focus on the presence or absence of head injury, seizures, diabetes, hypertension, heart disease, and/or cancer; family history of any neuromuscular or neurologic disorders, heart disease, diabetes, cancer, seizures, cerebrovascular accident (stroke), and/or Parkinson's disease; and (2) systems assessment, subjective and objective information in the following areas related the possible impact of Parkinson's disease:

- *Central nervous system*—The patient should be asked about any headaches, fatigue, weakness, paralysis, dizziness, and/or syncope. Any changes in walking or mobility, increase in rigidity or muscle movements, and/or changes in the ability to carry out activities of daily living should be noted. Also important are any changes in sensation in the extremities, changes in vision or hearing, loss of or changes in coordination, changes in gait and balance, and/or any changes in energy level. The assessment should also include questions about any changes in baseline levels of alertness; changes in memory (short term or long term); blackouts or seizures; numbness, tingling, or abnormal sensations in the extremities; changes in mood; changes in muscle movement or strength (e.g., any paralysis) or in voluntary versus involuntary motor control; and any muscle rigidity or tremors. Response to stimuli should be noted; the pupils should be examined with attention to size, shape, response to light, and symmetry in reactions; and deep tendon reflexes should be assessed with attention to strength bilaterally. The nurse should observe and document the patient's ability to walk and characterize the patient's gait as well as left-right and upper-lower extremity strength. The ability of the patient to feed self and carry out activities of daily living should be assessed.
- *Genitourinary and gastrointestinal systems*—The abdominal area should be assessed, with a general survey of the abdomen, auscultation of bowel sounds, and palpation for any distension. Baseline urinary and bowel patterns should be determined, and any changes in or loss of control of bladder or bowel functioning noted. Any changes in the ability to engage in toileting activities and need for assistance should be identified. The patient should be asked about any difficulty in swallowing (dysphagia) and any problems in feeding self or preparing meals. If such difficulties are identified, then the patient should be assessed for any subsequent nutritional excesses or deficits.
- *Skin*—The color, texture, turgor, and fragility of the skin should be assessed, and any breaks in the skin, bruises, lesions, masses, and/or swelling should be noted.
- *Oral and mucous membranes*—Color and moisture as well as the presence of any abnormal lesions should be documented.
- *Respiratory system*—Attention should be given to respiratory rate, rhythm, depth, effort, and breath sounds.
- *Psychologic and emotional status*—The patient should be assessed for any recent or past changes in mood, affect, or personality. Any other disease-related concerns such as depression, emotional ups and downs, increase in irritability, social withdrawal, or changes in sexual functioning or intimacy should also be noted.
- *Functional abilities*—Inquiry should be made about any changes in everyday function in the patient's personal and/or professional life. Any changes in daily task performance at the place of employment or need to take sick leave or sick days, as well as the patient's ability to exercise, drive, and/or shop for groceries and other necessities, should be noted.

> ### LIFE SPAN CONSIDERATIONS: The Elderly Patient
>
> #### Antiparkinsonian Drugs
>
> - Carbidopa-levodopa should be used cautiously and with close monitoring in elderly patients, especially those with a history of cardiac, renal, hepatic, endocrine, pulmonary, ulcer, or psychiatric disease.
> - Elderly patients taking carbidopa-levodopa are at an increased risk for experiencing adverse effects, especially confusion, loss of appetite, and orthostatic hypotension.
> - Carbidopa-levodopa is often started at a low dose because of the increased sensitivity of older patients to these medications and the need to save higher dosages for a later time during treatment.
> - Overheating is a problem in patients taking anticholinergics, and so elderly patients taking these drugs should avoid excessive exercise during warm weather and excessive heat exposure.
> - One of the main problems with the long-term use of carbidopa-levodopa is that its duration of effectiveness decreases over time; this is even more problematic in elderly patients. Catechol ortho-methyltransferase inhibitors hold much promise for elderly patients who are experiencing the wearing off phenomenon; they help turn "off" times into "on" times so that the drug begins to work throughout the entire day.

With *dopaminergic drugs,* such as amantadine, carbidopa-levodopa, and ropinirole, a patient assessment should include vital signs with supine and standing blood pressures, height, weight, medication and medical history, nursing history. This assessment should also include gathering information from family, caregivers, and/or significant others. Blood pressure is of significance because of drug-related postural hypotension. Contraindications, cautions, and drug interactions should be noted prior to administering these drugs (see previous pharmacology discussion). Motor skills, including abilities and deficiencies, should be assessed, and any akinesia, bradykinesia, postural instability, rigidity, tremors, staggering gait, or drooling should be specifically noted (see Glossary and Table 16-1). Assessment of urinary patterns is also important because of the possibility of drug-induced urinary retention. If BUN and creatinine measurements are ordered, the results should be examined, because these values are indicators of renal function. Alkaline phosphatase levels are indicators of liver function and should be assessed if this test is ordered. Dosage amounts of antiparkinsonian drugs may need to be altered if renal and liver dysfunction is present. For life span considerations, it is important to understand the gynecologic history of the patient and to know if the patient is pregnant and/or lactating. Some of the dopaminergics cross into the placenta and into breast milk and have unknown actions in the pediatric patient. Drug interactions related to these drugs are presented in Table 16-4. Apomorphine, a newer, *nonergot dopamine agonist drug,* should be given only after cautious assessment of drug allergies and drug interactions (see Table 16-4). It is important to note any cross allergies to sulfa drugs and sulfite preservatives. Other contraindications, cautions, and drug interactions have been previously discussed. A thorough baseline head-to-toe assessment with a focus on the cardiovascular, GI, genitourinary, and neurologic systems is important, as well.

When *anticholinergic drugs* are prescribed, the nurse should assess the patient carefully to determine gross level of organ functioning—especially in those systems most affected by Parkinson's disease, including the GI, genitourinary, visual, cardiac, and neurologic systems. Mental status should be assessed and agitation, confusion, or psychotic-like behavior identified; this is especially important in those 60 years of age or older, because this age group is at a higher risk for these problems, which could worsen with the use of anticholinergics. This age group is also at higher risk of toxicity and adverse effects because of declining organ function and an overall increased sensitivity to medications in general (see Chapter 3). Cautions, contraindications, and drug interactions have been previously discussed.

For the *dopamine agonists* that are also antiviral, (e.g., amantadine), the aforementioned baseline and general assessment information is also important. The patient's knowledge of the drug's use for Parkinson's disease (versus its use as an antiviral) and awareness that its onset of action will be delayed for several days or longer should also be confirmed. Continual assessment of the patient's status and improvement of disease-related symptoms is important, because a decline in this drug's effectiveness may occur within 3 to 6 months after initiation of therapy. If a dopamine agonist that is also a prolactin inhibitor is prescribed, the nurse must understand that this drug is also used for suppression of lactation and must assess for the appropriateness of its use. Elderly patients require additional CNS assessment because of the possible adverse effects related to that system (such as headache, lightheadedness, and visual or auditory changes). Also, if the patient is taking this medication long term, assessment for the following is crucial to patient safety: fainting (syncope), peptic ulcers, severe abdominal pain, and GI hemorrhage.

The antiparkinsonian drugs classified as *MAO-B inhibitors* (e.g., selegiline) require assessment of many of the same parameters described earlier. In addition, however, cardiac status is important to assess and document because of the possible adverse effects of cardiac irregularities and hypotension. Assessment of dosing is also important, because, as with other antiparkinsonian drugs, a low dose should be used initially with gradual increases over approximately a 3- to 4-week period. The lowest possible dose is recommended for initiation of therapy so that plenty of room exists for further increases in dosing as the disease progresses. These drugs also require careful neurologic assessment due to drug-related CNS depression (see Table 16-4).

For the *COMT inhibitors* (e.g., entacapone and tolcapone) assessment of baseline vital signs is also required, with a focus on standing and supine blood pressure because of the adverse effects of orthostatic hypotension and syncope. In fact, these adverse effects occur more frequently with the COMT inhibitors than with the other antiparkinsonian drugs, and thus increased caution and concern is needed. Assessment of dosing time is also important, because if these drugs are not given 1 hour before or 2 hours after meals, the bioavailability of the drug may be adversely effected. Serum transaminase levels should be assessed prior to and during drug therapy, and if the patient's ALT level is elevated to the upper range of normal or higher, the drug will most likely be discontinued by the prescriber because of the increased risk of hepatic failure. Elderly patients also experience a higher incidence of hallucinations

with these drugs than do other patients, and thus a thorough neurologic and mental status examination is needed.

Nursing Diagnoses

- Impaired physical mobility related to the disease process and adverse effects of the various antiparkinsonian medications
- Disturbed body image related to changes in appearance and mobility due to the disease process
- Urinary retention related to the pathophysiologic effects of the disease process on the bladder with incomplete emptying
- Constipation related to decreased GI peristalsis associated with the disease process
- Risk for injury related to the physical limitations and changes in mobility, gait, balance, and coordination produced by the disease process
- Imbalanced nutrition, less than body requirements, related to the disease process as well as adverse effects of drug therapy
- Deficient knowledge related to lack of exposure to and experience with a complex and long-term treatment regimen

Planning
Goals

- Patient remains free of self-injury.
- Patient states the purpose of the specific medications prescribed for the disease.
- Patient states the adverse effects and toxic effects of medications.
- Patient regains as normal as possible bowel and bladder elimination patterns.
- Patient maintains adequate nutritional status.
- Patient remains as independent as possible.
- Patient is less anxious and fearful.
- Patient regains a positive self-concept.
- Patient remains adherent with the therapy regimen.

Outcome Criteria

- Patient (and family and/or significant others) describes ways of preventing self-injury, such as the use of assistive devices.
- Patient states purposes, adverse effects, and toxic effects associated with the specific antiparkinsonian medications, such as emesis, nausea, instability, and palpitations.
- Patient states ways to prevent some of the adverse effects and toxic effects of antiparkinsonian medications, such as frequent mouth care and increased fluid intake.
- Patient discusses ways to minimize problems associated with drug-induced alterations in bowel and bladder elimination patterns through changes in diet and fluid intake.
- Patient discusses measures to ensure an adequate nutritional status with possible antiemetic therapy.
- Patient begins to perform activities of daily living more independently.
- Patient openly verbalizes fears, anxieties, and changes in self-image with members of the health care team and supportive staff.

Implementation

Nursing interventions associated with the various antiparkinsonian drugs will vary somewhat depending on the drug class, but close monitoring and comprehensive patient education are re-

CASE STUDY

Drugs for Parkinson's Disease

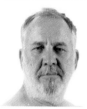
© Rohit Seth

Ben, a 62-year-old retired contractor, is undergoing surgery to repair an umbilical hernia. He has had Parkinson's disease for 5 years and is currently taking carbidopa-levodopa (Sinemet CR) and selegiline (Eldepryl). Other than the Parkinson's disease, he has no health problems. He has enjoyed fairly good control up until this week but is now experiencing more "bad times," as he calls them.

1. Patients who are taking long-term levodopa treatment often experience an "on-off" phenomenon in symptoms. Explain the physiology behind this phenomenon.
2. Explain the reason for giving selegiline along with the carbidopa-levodopa.
3. A nurse comments to you that the carbidopa-levodopa Ben is taking will probably be discontinued for the surgery to allow a "drug holiday" during the recovery. What is your reply?

Ben undergoes the surgery without any difficulties, and the following medication orders are noted on the chart:

> Continue previous orders for carbidopa-levodopa (Sinemet CR) 1 bid and selegiline (Eldepryl) 5 mg bid (taken with the Sinemet CR)
> Meperidine (Demerol) 10 mg IV every 4 hours as needed for pain
> Ondansetron (Zofran) 4 mg IV one time if needed for nausea
> Begin entacapone (Comtan) 200 mg bid with each dose of Sinemet

4. Are there any concerns regarding drug interactions? Explain.
5. What is the purpose of the entacapone?

IV, Intravenous.

---

quired for all these drugs. During the start of *dopaminergic drug* therapy, the patient should be assisted when walking because of the dizziness and possibly syncope caused by these drugs. Doses should be given several hours before bedtime to decrease the incidence of insomnia, a known adverse effect of these drugs. Oral doses should also be given with food to help minimize GI upset. Interaction of vitamin B$_6$ (pyridoxine) with levodopa was once a major concern because this vitamin was found to block the uptake of plain levodopa. However, a majority of patients taking a carbidopa-levodopa combination drug were found to have no problems with vitamin B$_6$. The National Parkinson's Disease Foundation (available at *http://www.pdf.org*) reports on its website that only patients who are very, very sensitive to the effects of any drug will have problems with vitamin B$_6$. If it is a problem, then the prescriber should be consulted for further instructions. In addition, amino acids from dietary protein may interfere with the uptake of levodopa in the brain. If the patient is taking carbidopa-levodopa, the patient should continue to eat high-protein foods (e.g., meat, fish, poultry, and dairy products) but use portion control (meat portion about the size of a deck of cards) and take the drug dose half an hour before a protein-containing meal. Timing is the issue, not the quantity of protein consumed over the course of the day. A nutritional consult may be beneficial to assist the patient in menu planning and teach the patient to divide the total quantity of protein among small frequent meals so that minimal amounts of protein are ingested throughout the day and are consumed at the proper time. Consumption of well-balanced meals is important, as is the forcing of fluids. The patient should aim to drink at least 3000 mL/day unless contraindicated. Drinking water is important, even if the patient is not thirsty or in need of hydration, to prevent and manage the adverse effect of constipation. Eating foods that are natural laxatives, such as prunes and vegetables and other foods high in fiber, should also be encouraged. If the adverse effect of dry mouth is problematic, taking fluids and sucking on hard candy or lozenges may be helpful. If nausea or vomiting occurs or problems with edema are persistent (the patient gains 2 pounds or more in 24 hours or 5 pounds or more in 1 week), the prescriber should be contacted immediately.

In the past, drug holidays were scheduled when the *dopamine agonists* were used. A drug holiday is a procedure in which all antiparkinsonian drugs the patient is taking are discontinued for a week or longer. Use of this procedure enabled some patients to resume taking the drug at a lower dosage and with fewer adverse effects, but these benefits lasted for only very short periods of time. This procedure is no longer recommended because it is a total shock to the patient's homeostasis and body, and it allows both the patient and family to witness how far the disease has actually progressed. Therefore, because of the extreme discomfort, especially for patients in the more advanced stages of the disease, it is almost never recommended except as deemed necessary by a neurologist with appropriate institutional support staff.

Patients taking *apomorphine* need to understand the method of and rationale for its use in the treatment of "off" episodes (times of difficulty moving, walking, and speaking that may occur as medication wears off or at random). Although apomorphine will not prevent "off" episodes, it will help improve symptoms when an "off" episode has already begun. Education must be complete and thorough on the use of this drug for its maximal therapeutic benefits to be realized. In addition to apomorphine, other medications will be ordered to minimize or prevent upset stomach and/or vomiting, and this therapy is important to initiate at the beginning of apomorphine treatment. The prescriber will give orders for when these other medications should be stopped. With apomorphine, the dosage should be gradually increased over a period of weeks. The prescriber should be contacted for further instructions should the drug be omitted, especially if longer than 1 week. This drug is given by subcutaneous injection and never intravenously. First doses of this drug are usually given in the prescriber's office, and instructions should be provided to the individual who will be responsible for giving the injections at home. The nurse should make sure that education is thorough and that the patient provides return demonstrations. The following points should be included: (1) Apomorphine solution comes in a glass cartridge to use with an injector pen. (2) Only new, sterile needles should be used and needles should be discarded in a puncture-resistant container and out of the reach of children. (3) Injections to be made into the subcutaneous areas of the stomach, upper outer area of the arm (middle third between the shoulder and elbow), or the upper leg (see Chapter 10 for injection sites) and at least 2 inches away from a wound, incision, umbilicus and never into area that is red, sore, bruised, oozing or abnormal. (4) Expiration dates of medications checked before administration. (5) Only clear solutions should be used. (6) The person giving the injection should make sure that the dose knob at the end of the injector pen is at the correct dose, which will show up in the pen's window, and should remember that the dose will be in milliliters (mL) and not in milligrams (mg); if there are any questions, the prescriber should be contacted. (7) If the drug solution accidentally gets onto the skin or into the eye area, the area should be flushed with cold water immediately. As with many other antiparkinsonian drugs, the patient should be alerted about the possibility of postural hypotension and given instructions to move and change positions slowly. Vomiting, constipation, diarrhea, weakness and changes in urinary patterns should be reported to the prescriber immediately.

With *anticholinergic drugs,* patients should take the medication as prescribed, after meals or at bedtime and not at the same time as with other medications. Patients should know that it may take a few days to several weeks for the drugs to show their therapeutic effectiveness (e.g., improvement in tremors). Because of the risk of stomach upset, these drugs should be taken with a snack, such as ginger ale and crackers. These medications are generally taken at night because of their sedating properties, and measures to help prevent and treat dry mouth are encouraged, such as increasing fluids and sucking on sugar-free hard candies. See Chapter 21 for further information about the use of these drugs, interventions and adverse effects to report. *Bromocriptine* should be taken as prescribed and should not be stopped abruptly. Because this drug may cause GI upset, it is best taken with a snack. Any severe dizziness, stomach upset, headache, vomiting, confusion, swelling of the feet or ankles, or irregular pulse rate should be reported immediately.

MAO-B inhibitors, such as selegiline, should be given as ordered. Selegiline is often given in upwardly titrated dosages while carbidopa-levodopa dose amounts are decreased. Oral disintegrating dosage forms should be placed on the tongue and not swallowed until the dosage form is melted. This dosage form should also be taken without liquids and given in the morning before breakfast. Foods and fluids should not be consumed for 5 minutes before or after the drug is taken. Postural hypotension may be a transient problem, and so the patient should move and change positions slowly and purposely. If dizziness is severe or if the patient experiences abdominal pain, hallucinations, or abnormal heart beats, the prescriber should be contacted for further instructions.

The newer *COMT inhibitors* have been shown to have greater efficacy in patients with advanced forms of Parkinson's disease. After treatment using the various dosage forms of levodopa or carbidopa-levodopa, a COMT inhibitor may then be added to the therapeutic regimen, and onset of therapeutic effects is rapid. These drugs should be administered as prescribed and may be taken without regard to meals or food. These and other antiparkinsonian drugs should never be discontinued abruptly and require a gradual weaning period to avoid worsening of Parkinson's disease or other dangerous effects. It should be emphasized to patients and caregivers that all appointments with the prescriber must be kept and all laboratory testing performed, as ordered. Patients should change positions slowly and purposely to avoid syncope due to orthostatic hypotension. Patients should be told that entacapone may turn their urine brownish orange but that this is not harmful. As with all medications, patients should keep a written list of prescription drugs, over-the-counter drugs, vitamins, minerals, and herbal therapies they are taking on their person at all times. This list of medications should be updated and taken each time the prescriber is visited and/or the patient is hospitalized so that health care providers are always aware of the medications taken on a regular basis. Patients should be educated to report the following to the prescriber: back pain, severe sweating, bruising, and orthostatic hypotension with feelings of dizziness or syncope (fainting) upon standing.

It is most important in the care of patients with Parkinson's disease to be aware of all other forms of therapies that may be beneficial, such as support groups, water aerobics, and occupational and physical therapy, to name a few. Some community resources that are available are community-wide recreation facilities, transportation services, and Meals on Wheels. Educational materials and emotional support resources should also be shared with family members, caregivers, and significant others because of the long-term and progressive nature of the disease. Contacting research institutes about new treatment protocols may be a viable option for patients and family members during the course of the disease. See Patient Teaching Tips for more specific information.

Evaluation

Monitoring the patient's response to any of the antiparkinsonian drugs is crucial to documenting treatment success or failure. Therapeutic responses to the antiparkinsonian drugs include an improved sense of well-being, improved mental status, increased appetite, ability to perform activities of daily living, improved concentration and ability to think more clearly, and a decrease in the intensity of parkinsonian symptoms (e.g., less tremor, shuffling of gait, and muscle rigidity, and fewer involuntary movements). In addition to monitoring for therapeutic responses, the nurse must also watch for the occurrence of adverse effects, such as confusion, anxiety, irritability, depression, paranoia, headache, weakness, lethargy, nausea, vomiting, anorexia, palpitations, postural hypotension, tachycardia, dry mouth, constipation, urinary retention, blurred vision, dark urine, difficulty swallowing, and nightmares. Patients should know to immediately report to their prescriber any of the following signs and symptoms indicating possible overdose: excessive twitching, drooling, or eye spasms. Therapeutic effects of *COMT inhibitors* (such as entacapone) may be noticed within a few days, whereas therapeutic effects of other antiparkinsonian drugs may take weeks to become manifest. Adverse effects for which to monitor with COMT inhibitors include those mentioned previously, but fewer dyskinesias are seen than with dopamine agonists.

PATIENT TEACHING TIPS

- All medications should be taken exactly as ordered. Around-the-clock dosing is usually prescribed to achieve steady blood levels, especially with the dopamine agonists.
- Alcohol, over-the-counter drugs, and herbals should be avoided unless approved by the prescriber.
- If experiencing postural hypotension, the patient should understand the rationale for changing positions slowly and the need to force fluids and wear compression stockings, unless contraindicated.
- Sustained-released drug forms should not be crushed, chewed, or altered in any way. The drug to be taken its whole form.
- Female patients of childbearing age who are using oral contraception should be told to use alternative methods of contraception.
- With dopamine agonists or anticholinergics, warn the patient about the adverse effect of dry mouth. Use of artificial saliva drops/ gum, frequent mouth care, forcing fluids, and sucking on sugarless gum or hard candy may be helpful.
- If an entacapone is used, the color of sweat and urine may darken, and the patient should be told that this adverse effect is harmless.
- Encourage patients to report any change in vision (e.g., blurring), decline in mental alertness, confusion, or lethargy experienced while taking any of the antiparkinsonian drugs. Any difficulty with urination, irregular pulse rate, or severe, uncontrolled movements of the arms, legs, mouth, or tongue should also be reported.
- Education about potential blood pressure problems should be emphasized. Such problems may occur as an adverse effect of drug therapy (e.g., postural hypotension) or may take the form of a hypertensive crisis if an MAOI is mistakenly taken with a drug containing levodopa. MAOIs should not be used with carbidopa-levodopa and related drugs; if such drugs are needed, a period of 2 weeks should pass between the time the MAOI is discontinued and the carbidopa-levodopa initiated.

- The patient and family must understand that dopaminergics are often titrated to the patient's response and that it may take 3 to 4 weeks for a therapeutic response to become evident.
- Some of the newer dopamine agonists, such as ropinirole, may result in "sleep attacks," which may occur without warning. The patient should be told how to handle these episodes, with an emphasis on safety measures.
- Fluids and dietary fiber should be increased to help prevent drug-related constipation.
- The patient should be told to take COMT inhibitors with food, meals, or a snack to minimize nausea and vomiting. Other instructions for COMT inhibitors include information about the adverse effects of dizziness and drowsiness (and nausea) that may occur in the beginning of therapy but that diminish as therapy continues. Mental clarity and motor skills may be decreased when therapy with these drugs is first begun, so the patient should be cautioned to avoid demanding mental or motor tasks or activities until these effects diminish.
- Any abnormal contractions of the head, neck, or trunk, as well as any syncope, falls, itching, and/or jaundice should be reported immediately to the prescriber.
- The patient should be educated about the goal of therapy, especially if entacapone is being used to help manage the wearing off phenomenon. The wearing off phenomenon is a waning of the effects of a dose of levodopa before the scheduled time of the next dose, resulting in diminished motor ability and the experience of more disease symptoms. If a COMT inhibitor is added to the carbidopa-levodopa, the wearing off phenomenon is minimized, and the therapeutic effects of the regimen are maximized. The patient can then expect that the "off" time will be eliminated and that the drugs will work through the whole day, which is the goal in the treatment of Parkinson's disease.

POINTS TO REMEMBER

- The neurotransmission-related abnormalities in Parkinson's disease include the chronic, progressive degeneration of dopamine-producing neurons in the brain. Patients with this disease also have elevated acetylcholine levels and lowered dopamine levels.
- Signs and symptoms of this disease process include bradykinesia (slow movements), muscle rigidity (cogwheel rigidity), tremor (pill rolling), postural instability, and dyskinesias (difficulty performing voluntary movements), two common ones of which are chorea (irregular, spasmodic, involuntary movements of the limbs or facial muscles) and dystonias (abnormal muscle tone in any tissue).

- Drug therapies for Parkinson's disease include dopamine agonists, MAOIs, anticholinergics, and COMT inhibitors.
- Patient considerations include providing individual and family support along with options for care of the family member with Parkinson's disease. The disease is long term and lifelong, as well as debilitating. A holistic approach in which all aspects of the patient and family are considered and respected is the key to quality nursing care.

NCLEX EXAMINATION REVIEW QUESTIONS

1 Which of the following should alert the nurse to a potential caution or contraindication regarding the use of a dopaminergic drug for treatment of mild Parkinson's disease?
a Diarrhea
b Tremors
c Angle-closure glaucoma
d Unstable gait

2 A patient is taking entacapone as part of the therapy for Parkinson's disease. Which intervention by the nurse is appropriate at this time?
a Notify the patient that this drug causes discoloration of the urine.
b Limit the patient's intake of tyramine-containing foods.
c Monitor results of liver studies because this drug can seriously affect liver function.
d Force fluids to prevent dehydration.

3 During a patient teaching session about antiparkinsonian drugs, the nurse will include which statement?
a The drug should be stopped when tremors and weakness are relieved.
b If a dose is missed, take two doses to avoid significant decreases in blood levels.
c Notify the physician if the urine turns brownish-orange in color.
d Change positions slowly to prevent falling due to postural hypotension.

4 A patient will be taking selegiline, 10 mg daily, in addition to dopamine replacement therapy for Parkinson's disease. The nurse will implement which precautions regarding selegiline?
a Teach the patient to avoid foods containing tyramine.
b Monitor for syncope or dizziness.
c Inform the patient that this drug may cause urine discoloration.
d Monitor for tachycardia and palpitations.

5 A patient with Parkinson's disease will start taking entacapone along with the carbidopa-levodopa therapy he has been taking for a few years. The nurse recognizes that the advantage of taking entacapone is that
a the entacapone can reduce on-off effects.
b the levodopa may be stopped in a few days.
c there is less GI upset with entacapone.
d it does not cause the cheese effect.

6 The nurse is assessing a patient who is going to begin therapy with apomorphine for Parkinson's disease. Which condition would be a concern if identified in the patient? (Select all that apply.)
a Severe cardiovascular disease
b Inability to swallow
c Advanced stage of Parkinson's disease
d Glaucoma
e Allergy to sulfa drugs

1. c, 2. a, 3. d, 4. b, 5. a, 6. a, e.

CRITICAL THINKING ACTIVITIES: BEST ACTION

1 A patient has been newly diagnosed with early-stage Parkinson's disease and will be starting therapy with amantadine. He asks the nurse, "How long will I have to take this medicine?" What would be the nurse's best answer?

2 The nurse is checking the orders for a patient who has Parkinson's disease. One order reads, "Apomorphine, 0.2 mg, subcutaneously, now." The nurse has discovered an error in the order. What is the error, and what is the nurse's best action? Explain.

3 The nurse is assessing a patient who is visiting the clinic for a 2-month follow-up appointment after starting selegiline, 10 mg daily. The patient is pleased with the improvement in his Parkinson's disease symptoms but states, "My wife looked up this drug and told me that I can't eat cheese or drink wine anymore. I hate that." What is the nurse's best action at this time?

For answers, see *http://evolve.elsevier.com/Lilley.*

CHAPTER 17

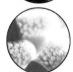

Psychotherapeutic Drugs

OBJECTIVES

When you reach the end of this chapter, you should be able to do the following:

1 Briefly discuss the various mental illnesses.

2 Identify the various psychotherapeutic drug classes, such as anxiolytic drugs, antidepressants, mood-stabilizing drugs, and antipsychotics.

3 Discuss the mechanisms of action, indications, therapeutic effects, adverse effects, toxic effects, drug interactions, contraindications, and cautions associated with the various psychotherapeutic drugs.

4 Develop a nursing care plan that includes all phases of the nursing process for patients taking psychotherapeutic drugs.

5 Develop patient education guidelines for patients receiving psychotherapeutic drugs.

e-Learning Activities

http://evolve.elsevier.com/Lilley

NCLEX Review Questions • Animations • Nursing Care Plans • Audio Glossary • Category Catchers • Medication Errors Checklists • IV Therapy Checklists • Calculators • Frequently Asked Questions • Content Updates • Supplemental Resources • Answers to Case Studies and Critical Thinking Activities

Drug Profiles

- ◆ alprazolam, p. 266
- ◆ amitriptyline, p. 270
- ◆ bupropion, p. 273
- buspirone, p. 266
- clozapine, p. 276
- ◆ diazepam, p. 266
- duloxetine, p. 274
- ◆ fluoxetine, p. 273

- haloperidol, p. 275
- ◆ lithium, p. 268
- ◆ lorazepam, p. 266
- ◆ mirtazapine, p. 273
- ◆ risperidone, p. 277
- selegiline transdermal patch, p. 271
- trazodone, p. 273

◆ *Key drug.*

Glossary

Affective disorders Emotional disorders that are characterized by changes in mood. (p. 262)

Agoraphobia Fear of leaving the familiar setting of home. (p. 262)

Akathisia Motor restlessness—a distressing experience of uncontrollable muscular movements that can occur as an adverse effect of many psychotropic medications. (p. 275)

Anxiety The unpleasant state of mind in which real or imagined dangers are anticipated and/or exaggerated. (p. 261)

Biogenic amine hypothesis A theory suggesting that depression and mania are due to alterations in the concentrations of neuronal and synaptic amines, primarily the catecholamines dopamine and norepinephrine, and the indolamines serotonin and histamine. (p. 268)

Bipolar disorder A major psychologic disorder characterized by episodes of *mania* or *hypomania*, cycling with depression; formerly called *manic-depressive illness*. (p. 262)

Depression An abnormal emotional state characterized by exaggerated feelings of sadness, melancholy, dejection, worthlessness, emptiness, and hopelessness that are inappropriate and out of proportion to reality. (p. 262)

Dopamine hypothesis A theory suggesting that dopamine dysregulation in certain parts of the brain is one of the primary contributing factors to the development of psychotic disorders (psychoses). (p. 262)

Dyskinesia The general term for abnormal and distressing involuntary movements. (p. 275)

Dysregulation hypothesis A theory that views depression and affective disorders as caused not simply by decreased or increased catecholamine and serotonin activity but by failure of the brain to *regulate* the levels of these neurotransmitters. (p. 269)

Dystonia A condition of acute muscle spasms that lead to dyskinesias. (p. 275)

Extrapyramidal symptoms The term for symptoms that arise adjacent to the *pyramidal* portions of the brain. Such symptoms include various motion disorders similar to those in Parkinson's disease and are an adverse effect associated with use of various antipsychotic drugs. (p. 275)

Gamma-aminobutyric acid An amino acid in the brain that functions to inhibit nerve transmission in the central nervous system. (p. 261)

Hypomania A less severe and less potentially hazardous form of mania. (p. 262)

Mania An acute illness characterized by an expansive emotional state, including extreme excitement, elation, hyperactivity, agitation, talkativeness, flight of ideas, reduced attention span, increased psychomotor activity, and sometimes violent, destructive, and self-destructive behavior. (p. 262)

Neuroleptic malignant syndrome An uncommon but serious adverse effect associated with the use of antipsychotic drugs and characterized by symptoms such as fever, cardiovascular instability, and myoglobinemia (presence in the blood of muscle breakdown proteins). (p. 275)

Neurotransmitters Endogenous chemicals in the body that serve to conduct nerve impulses between nerve cells (neurons). (p. 261)

Permissive hypothesis A theory postulating that reduced concentrations of serotonin (5-hydroxytriptamine) are the predisposing factors in individuals with affective disorders. (p. 268)

Psychosis (Plural: *psychoses*) A type of serious mental illness that can take several different forms and is associated with being truly out of touch with reality; that is, the individual is unable to distinguish imaginary from real circumstances and events. (p. 262)

Psychotherapeutics The treatment of emotional and mental disorders. (p. 261)

Psychotropic Capable of affecting mental processes; usually said of a medication. (p. 262)

Serotonin syndrome A collection of symptoms resulting from excessive activity of the neurotransmitter *serotonin* in the brain; may occur with the use of any psychotropic drug (e.g., antidepressants or buspirone) that enhances brain serotonin activity (see Box 17-1). (p. 272)

Stigma Widespread negative perceptions of and prejudice toward a specific group of people such as those with mental illness. (p. 261)

Tardive dyskinesia A serious drug adverse effect characterized by abnormal and distressing involuntary body movements and muscle tension that is associated with the use of antipsychotic medications. (p. 275)

• • •

Anatomy, Physiology, and Disease Overview

Most people experience normal emotions such as anxiety, depression, excitement, and grief. Sometimes such emotions are simply situational. They arise because of a specific event and subside with time. Treatment, if any, is often limited to psychotherapy, and possibly short-term drug therapy. However, when a person's emotions or behavior compromises his or her quality of life, ability to carry out normal activities of daily living, social functioning (interactions and relationships with others), or occupational functioning (employment, school, etc.) over a prolonged period (at least several months), longer-term pharmacotherapy in conjunction with psychotherapy is usually recommended.

The exact causes of mental disorders are not fully understood. Many theories have been advanced in an attempt to explain the causes and pathophysiology of mental dysfunction. In the *biochemical imbalance* theory, mental disorders are thought to arise as the result of abnormal levels of endogenous chemicals in the brain known as **neurotransmitters.** The conduction of messages between *neurons* (nerve cells) by neurotransmitters is called *neurotransmission.* This occurs in both the central nervous system (CNS) and the peripheral nervous system. However, the proposed mechanisms of both the pathology of and drug therapy for mental illness center around neurotransmission within the brain. There is strong evidence indicating that the brain levels of catecholamines (especially dopamine and norepinephrine; see Chapter 18) and indolamines (serotonin and histamine) play an important role in maintaining mental health. Other biochemical substances that seem necessary for the maintenance of normal mental function are the inhibitory neurotransmitter **gamma-aminobutyric acid;** the cholinergic neurotransmitter *acetylcholine* (see Chapter 20); and various inorganic ions such as sodium, potassium, and magnesium. Drugs used to treat anxiety, affective disorders, and psychoses work by blocking or stimulating the release of the endogenous neurotransmitters considered by these theories to play key roles in mental functioning.

The symptoms of the many different psychiatric disorders often overlap, which can make it difficult to accurately diagnose a disorder. Complicating this issue further is the inherent subjectivity of patients' experience of their symptoms. The *Diagnostic and Statistical Manual of Mental Disorders,* 4th edition, Text Revision (DSM-IV-TR) is a widely used reference published by the American Psychiatric Association. It presents demographic information and diagnostic criteria for recognized psychiatric disorders. Often a patient has ongoing symptoms that meet the criteria for several mental disorders. Such patients may be said to have a *spectrum disorder.* For example, research shows that more than half of chronically depressed adults also have a comorbid personality disorder, and one third have a comorbid anxiety disorder and/or a substance abuse disorder. The problem of comorbid substance abuse is especially troublesome. Usually, a patient must discontinue use of the abused substance(s) to have a chance at significant success in treating the concurrent psychiatric disorder. Unfortunately, this does not happen in the majority of patients.

Mentally ill people may be more susceptible to various physical health problems than the general population. For example, obesity is significantly more common in patients with mental disorders. These patients are therefore at greater risk for physical illnesses associated with obesity, including diabetes, hypertension, and heart disease. Because of the variety of economic, educational, and psychosocial issues that may preclude a mentally ill person from seeking psychiatric health care, many patients self-medicate with substances of abuse, including alcohol, tobacco, and illegal drugs. This generally compounds the problem of their baseline psychiatric illness.

Despite the development of newer, more effective treatments for mental illness, a longstanding societal **stigma** continues to be an obstacle for diagnosed patients. The National Alliance on Mental Illness (NAMI) is one major organization that works to reduce this stigma. NAMI seeks to promote consumer well-being and autonomy through public education, research funding, and legislative advocacy.

The treatment of mental disorders is called **psychotherapeutics.** Ideal mental health care usually involves many components, including a carefully detailed patient interview (to help ensure accurate and complete diagnosis) and carefully chosen and regularly monitored drug therapy, if indicated. Nonpharmacologic treatments include psychotherapy, support groups, social and family support systems, and often spiritual support systems. Other practices that promote mental health include physical exercise, good nutrition, and mental exercises such as meditation and visualization. In extreme cases, such as refractory depression, electroconvulsive therapy may be used (see the section on antidepressant drug therapy).

This chapter focuses on three common types of mental illness: anxiety, affective disorders, and psychoses.

Anxiety is the unpleasant state of mind chiefly characterized by a sense of dread and fear. It may be based on anticipated or past experiences, such as scheduled surgery or previous abuse. It may also stem from exaggerated responses to imaginary negative situations or to common everyday experiences that are only mildly disturbing to a mentally healthy person. Persistent anxiety is divided clinically into several distinct disorders, including the following:

- Obsessive-compulsive disorder
- Post-traumatic stress disorder
- Generalized anxiety disorder
- Panic disorder with or without agoraphobia
- Social phobia (also called *social anxiety disorder*)
- Simple phobia

Anxiety is a normal physiologic emotion; however, results of epidemiologic studies show that 2% to 6% of adults suffer from generalized anxiety disorder, 1% from panic disorder, 2% to 9% from posttraumatic stress disorder, and 4% to 5% from **agoraphobia** (the fear of leaving the familiar setting of home). Obsessive-compulsive disorder was previously thought to be rare but is now observed to be twice as common as schizophrenia or panic disorder in the general population. Anxiety may occur as a result of a wide range of medical illnesses (e.g., cardiovascular or pulmonary disease, hypothyroidism, hyperthyroidism, pheochromocytoma, and hypoglycemia).

Affective disorders, also called *mood disorders*, are characterized by changes in mood and range from **mania** (acutely pronounced emotions) to **depression** (acutely or chronically reduced emotions). Some patients may exhibit both mania and depression, experiencing periodic swings in emotions between these two extremes. This is referred to as **bipolar disorder. Hypomania** is a form of mania that is less severe and less potentially dangerous (to patient and others).

Bipolar disorder occurs in an estimated 2% to 3% of the population. Depression is currently reported to have prevalence rates ranging from 4.4% to 20%. Major depressive disorders are expected to become the second leading cause of disability by the year 2020. Common depressive symptoms include feelings of worthlessness, loss of interest in normally pleasurable activities, reduced energy level, reduced motivation and ability to meet routine responsibilities, drastic increase or decrease in appetite, insomnia or hypersomnia, and recurrent thoughts of death or suicide. In addition to being associated with drastic reductions in quality of life and occupational and social functioning, depression is also accompanied by the occurrence of major sleep disturbances in up to 80% of patients. Some sleep researchers report that a 1.5-hour loss of sleep on any given night may reduce alertness on the following day by 33%; therefore, insomnia associated with depression has far-reaching adverse effects on the patient. This decrease in the patient's level of alertness may be associated with accidents and even increased risk for suicide. Despite recent advances in pharmacotherapy for depression, it remains undertreated in many cases.

Psychosis is a severe mental disorder that often impairs mental function to the point of causing significant disability in performing the activities of daily living. A hallmark of psychosis is a loss of contact with reality. The primary psychotic disorders are schizophrenia and depressive and drug-induced psychoses. Schizophrenia may trigger hallucinations, delusions, and paranoia. It is estimated to affect 1% of the population. The **dopamine hypothesis** of psychotic illness grows out of the observation that psychotic patients often have excessive dopaminergic activity in the brain. Drug therapy is therefore aimed at reducing this activity. Note that this is in direct contrast to the treatment of Parkinson's disease (see Chapter 16), in which the therapeutic goal is to enhance brain dopaminergic activity.

Pharmacology Overview

Psychotropic drugs are among the most commonly prescribed drugs in the United States. Because of the inherent variability both in diagnoses and in the patient's description and reporting of symptoms of mental illness, the effects of these drugs are less easily quantified than are those of many other types of medications. For example, it is usually not known with certainty how long a given psychotropic drug works in the body (duration of action). Thus, the effectiveness of psychotropic drug therapy is often measured by verbal reports from patients regarding the level of improvement (if any) in their social and occupational functioning. Drug selection is often a trial-and-error process, which can be long and frustrating for both prescribers and patients. It is hoped that the emerging field of pharmacogenetics (see Chapter 5) will eventually allow more proactive and improved customization of psychotropic drug therapy. It is also common for the approved indications for a given drug to expand over time. This often occurs as more information is learned about the drug after its initial marketing.

A common problem with psychotropic drug therapy, as with other types of drug therapy, is nonadherence to the prescribed regimen. Many people do not want to accept a psychiatric diagnosis because of the associated stigma. As a result, they may remain in denial about the reality of their mental illness, including the need to take psychotropic medications. They may also have legitimate fears about adverse effects as well as fear of the unknown regarding their illness. Finally, they may dread the prospect of having to remain on medication to control their symptoms. Such patients can often be helped by support groups and other social supports. As they adjust to their diagnosis, it is hoped they will see enough benefits of treatment to strengthen their own role in maintaining their mental health.

ANXIOLYTIC DRUGS

Primary anxiolytic drugs include the benzodiazepine drug class and the miscellaneous drugs buspirone and meprobamate (Table 17-1) The benzodiazepines are commonly used as first-line drug therapy for both acute and chronic anxiety disorders. They are the focus of this section. Buspirone, and especially meprobamate, are much less commonly used. In addition there are other drug classes or single drugs that are effective. These include *selective serotonin reuptake inhibitors (SSRIs), tricyclic antidepressants (TCAs),* and *monoamine oxidase inhibitors (MAOIs)* (all discussed in the section on antidepressants), *antipsychotics* (see later section on antipsychotic drugs), and the antihistamine hydroxyzine (see Chapter 36).

Mechanism of Action and Drug Effects

All anxiolytic drugs decrease anxiety by reducing overactivity in the CNS. There are, however, differences among the various drug classes. Benzodiazepines seem to exert their effects by depressing activity in the areas of the brain called the brainstem and the limbic system. Benzodiazepines are believed to accomplish this by increasing the action of gamma-aminobutyric acid, which is an inhibitory neurotransmitter in the brain that inhibits nerve transmission in the CNS.

The drug buspirone is a miscellaneous anxiolytic in its own class and is described in further detail in its drug profile.

Indications

Benzodiazepines are the largest and most commonly prescribed anxiolytic drug class because they offer several advantages over the other drugs used to treat anxiety. Because of their wide range of therapeutic effects, anxiolytic drugs are sometimes used for certain other indications in addition to anxiety, such as ethanol withdrawal (see Chapter 9), insomnia and muscle spasms (see

TABLE 17-1 Currently Available Psychotherapeutic Drugs

Generic Name	Trade Name	Route	Generic Name	Trade Name	Route
Anxiolytics			**Newer Generation**		
Benzodiazepines			SSRIs		
alprazolam	Xanax	PO	citalopram	Celexa	PO
clorazepate	Tranxene T-Tab	PO	escitalopram	Lexapro	PO
chlordiazepoxide	Librium	PO, IM, IV	fluoxetine	Prozac	PO
clonazepam	Klonopin	PO	fluvoxamine	generic	PO
diazepam	Valium, Diastat	PO, PR, IM, IV	paroxetine	Paxil	PO
lorazepam	Ativan	PO, IM, IV	sertraline	Zoloft	PO
oxazepam	Serax	PO	SNRIs		
Miscellaneous			duloxetine	Cymbalta	PO
buspirone	BuSpar	PO	venlafaxine	Effexor	PO
meprobamate	Miltown	PO	Miscellaneous		
Antihistamines	See Chapter 36		bupropion	Wellbutrin	PO
Mood Stabilizers			nefazodone	generic	PO
lithium carbonate*	Lithobid		trazodone	generic	PO
lithium citrate*	Generic		*Antipsychotics*		
Antiepileptics	See Chapter 15		**Older Generation (Conventional)**		
Antidepressants			Phenothiazines		
Older Generation			chlorpromazine	Thorazine	PO, PR, IM, IV
Tricyclics			fluphenazine	generic	PO, IM
amitriptyline	Elavil	PO	perphenazine	generic	PO
amoxapine	Generic	PO	prochlorperazine	Compazine	PO, PR, IM, IV
clomipramine	Anafranil	PO	trifluoperazine	generic	PO
desipramine	Norpramin	PO	thioridazine	generic	PO
doxepin	Sinequan	PO	Thioxanthene		
imipramine	Tofranil	PO	thiothixene	Navane	PO
nortriptyline	Pamelor	PO	Phenylbutylpiperidines		
protriptyline	Vivactil	PO	haloperidol	Haldol	PO, IM
trimipramine	Surmontil	PO	pimozide	Orap	PO
Tetracyclics			Dihydroindolone		
maprotiline (older generation)	Generic	PO	molindone	Moban	PO
			Newer Generation (Atypical)		
mirtazapine (newer generation)	Remeron	PO	Dibenzodiazepines		
			clozapine	Clozaril	PO
MAOIs			loxapine	Loxitane	PO
isocarboxazid	Marplan	PO	olanzapine	Zyprexa	PO, IM
phenelzine	Nardil	PO	quetiapine	Seroquel	PO
tranylcypromine	Parnate	PO	Benzisoxazoles		
			paliperidone	Invega	PO
			risperidone	Risperdal	PO, IM
			ziprasidone	Geodon	PO, IM
			Quinolinone		
			aripiprazole	Abilify	PO, IM

IM, Intramuscular; *IV*, intravenous; *MAOIs*, monoamine oxidase inhibitors; *PO*, oral; *PR*, by rectum; *SNRIs*, serotonin-norepinephrine reuptake inhibitors; *SSRIs*, selective serotonin reuptake inhibitors.
*Also classified as an antipsychotic.

Chapter 13), and seizure disorders (see Chapter 15), and as adjuncts in anesthesia (see Chapter 12). They are also commonly used as adjunct therapy for depression because depressive and anxious symptoms often occur together.

Contraindications

Contraindications to benzodiazepines include known drug allergy; angle-closure glaucoma, due to their ability to cause mydriasis; and pregnancy, due to their sedative properties. A history of seizure is a relative contraindication.

Adverse Effects

The most common undesirable effect of the anxiolytic drugs is an overexpression of their therapeutic effects, in particular CNS depression. Benzodiazepines can also cause hypotension. Of particular note are *paradoxical* reactions (opposite of those that would normally be expected) to the benzodiazepines and antihistamines, including hyperactivity and aggressive behavior. Such reactions are relatively uncommon. They are more likely to occur in children and adolescents and in psychiatric patients. Also, rebound disinhibition can occur in elderly patients on discontinuation of these drugs. In rebound disinhibition, an elderly patient first experiences marked sedation for 1 to 2 hours, followed by marked agitation and confusion for several hours afterward. It should also be noted that all benzodiazepines are potentially habit-forming and addictive. Although they can provide significant symptom relief, they should be used judiciously and at the lowest effective doses needed for symptom control. (See Table 17-2 for more information on adverse effects.) Elderly patients tend to be more sensitive to the sedating effects of benzodiazepines; thus the elderly should be started at lower dosages.

Toxicity and Management of Overdose

When benzodiazepines are taken alone, an overdose is generally not life threatening. When they are combined with alcohol or other CNS depressants, the outcome is much more severe. An overdose of benzodiazepines may result in one or any combination of the following symptoms: somnolence, confusion, coma, and respiratory depression. The treatment of benzodiazepine intoxication is generally symptomatic and supportive. If ingestion is recent, decontamination of the gastrointestinal system is indicated. Flumazenil (Romazicon) is a benzodiazepine receptor blocker (antagonist) that is used to reverse the effects of benzodiazepines. It is commonly given to reverse benzodiazepine effects after procedures involving moderate sedation (see Chapter 12). The treatment regimen for the acute reversal of benzodiazepine effects is summarized in Chapter 13. Flumazenil should be used cautiously in known long-term benzodiazepine users, because it can cause an acute withdrawal syndrome, including seizures.

Interactions

Several notable drug interactions occur with the use of benzodiazepines. Alcohol and CNS depressants, when coadministered with benzodiazepines, can result in additive CNS depression and even death. This serious consequence is more likely to occur in patients with renal and/or hepatic compromise (e.g., the elderly). Cimetidine, disulfiram, MAOIs (see later section this chapter), and tobacco all can decrease the metabolism of benzodiazepines and result in increased CNS depression (Table 17-3).

TABLE 17-2 Adverse Effects of Selected Psychotropic Drugs by Class*

Drug or Drug Class	Adverse Effects
Anxiolytics	
Benzodiazepines	Amnesia, anorexia, ataxia, cognitive impairment, confusion, depression, dizziness, drowsiness, GI disturbance, euphoria, headache, vocal changes (e.g., slurred speech), visual changes
Miscellaneous	
buspirone	See drug profile
Antihistamines	See Chapter 36
Mood Stabilizers	
lithium salts	See drug profile
Antiepileptic drugs	See Chapter 15
Antidepressants	
Older Generation	
Tricyclics	Anorexia, dry mouth, blurred vision, mydriasis, constipation, gynecomastia, sexual dysfunction, altered libido, menstrual changes, altered blood glucose level, urinary retention, agitation, akathisia, anxiety, ataxia, cognitive impairment, dizziness, drowsiness, headache, hypomania, insomnia, skin rash, photosensitivity, mild GI disturbance, weight changes
MAOIs	See text for MAOIs in general, and drug profile for selegiline transdermal patch
Newer Generation	
Tetracyclics	
mirtazapine, maprotiline	See drug profile for mirtazapine; maprotiline, actually an older-generation drug, is rarely used
SSRIs	Anxiety, dizziness, drowsiness, headache, anorexia, mild GI disturbance, sexual dysfunction, asthenia (muscle weakness), tremor
SNRIs	See drug profile for duloxetine
Miscellaneous	
trazodone, bupropion	See drug profiles
Antipsychotics	
Older Generation (Conventional)	Akathisia, extrapyramidal symptoms, hypertension, neuroleptic malignant syndrome. confusion, headache, mild GI disturbance, dry mouth, amenorrhea, gynecomastia, visual disturbances, hyperpyrexia, edema, nasal congestion, asthma, tardive dyskinesia, skin rash, photosensitivity, weight gain, urinary retention
Newer Generation (Atypical)	Tachycardia, akathisia, agitation, asthenia, ataxia, seizures, dyskinesia, dizziness, drowsiness, headache, insomnia, dry mouth, dyspepsia, anxiety, increased appetite, weight gain

GI, Gastrointestinal; *MAOIs*, monoamine oxidase inhibitors; *SNRIs*, serotonin-norepinephrine reuptake inhibitors; *SSRIs*, selective serotonin reuptake inhibitors.
*See also drug profiles for drug-specific information.

TABLE 17-3 Drug Interactions of Selected Psychotropic Drugs by Class*

Drug Class	Interacting Drug(s)	Mechanism	Result
Anxiolytics Benzodiazepines	CNS depressants (e.g., alcohol, opioids)	Additive effects	Enhanced CNS depression (sedation, confusion, ataxia, etc.)
	Antacids	Reduced rate of absorption	Delayed drug effects
	cimetidine, oral contraceptives, disulfiram, SSRIs, isoniazid, azole antifungals, beta-blockers, opioids, probenecid, valproic acid	Impaired hepatic elimination of benzodiazepine	Enhanced benzodiazepine effects (e.g., CNS depression)
	rifampin	Enhanced benzodiazepine clearance	Reduced therapeutic effects
	theophylline	Antagonistic effects	Reduced sedative effects
	digoxin, phenytoin	Reduced clearance	Potential for digoxin toxicity and phenytoin toxicity
	levodopa	Enhanced levodopa clearance	Reduced therapeutic effects
Miscellaneous buspirone Antihistamines	See drug profile See Chapter 36		
Mood Stabilizers lithium salts Antiepileptic drugs	See drug profile See Chapter 15		
Antidepressants **Older-Generation** Tricyclics (TCAs)	carbamazepine, rifamycins	Enhanced TCA clearance	Reduced therapeutic effects
	carbamazepine	Reduced carbamazepine clearance	Potential for carbamazepine toxicity
	cimetidine, haloperidol, histamine H₂ antagonists, SSRIs, valproic acid	Reduced TCA clearance	Potential for TCA toxicity
	Anticholinergics	Additive anticholinergic effects	Potential for paralytic ileus
	clonidine	Reduced clonidine clearance	Potential for hypertensive crisis
	levodopa	Enhanced levodopa clearance	Reduced therapeutic effects; hypertensive crisis
	Quinolone antibiotics	Reduced quinolone clearance	Potential for life-threatening cardiac dysrhythmias
	Sympathomimetics	Enhanced sympathomimetic effects	Potential for cardiac dysrhythmias
MAOIs	See text for MAOIs in general, and drug profile for selegiline transdermal patch		
Newer-Generation Tetracyclics mirtazapine, maprotiline	See drug profile for mirtazapine; maprotiline, actually an older-generation drug, is rarely used		
SSRIs	MAOIs, linezolid, lithium, metoclopramide, sibutramine, sympathomimetics, tramadol	Additive effects	Potential for serotonin syndrome
	TCAs	Reduced TCA clearance	Potential TCA toxicity
	NSAIDs	Not listed	Increased risk of GI adverse effects
SNRIs duloxetine	See drug profiles		
Miscellaneous trazodone, bupropion	See drug profiles		
Antipsychotics **Older and Newer Generation**	alcohol, other CNS depressants	Additive drug effects	Enhanced CNS depression; dystonia with alcohol
	Antihypertensives	Enhanced antihypertensive effects	Potential for hypotension

CNS, Central nervous system; *CYP3A4*, cytochrome P-450 enzyme 3A4; *GI*, gastrointestinal; *MAOIs*, monoamine oxidase inhibitors; *NSAIDs*, nonsteroidal antiinflammatory drugs; *SNRIs*, serotonin-norepinephrine reuptake inhibitors; *SSRIs*, selective serotonin reuptake inhibitors.
*See also drug profiles for drug-specific information.

Continued

TABLE 17-3 Drug Interactions of Selected Psychotropic Drugs by Class*—cont'd

Drug Class	Interacting Drug(s)	Mechanism	Result
Antipsychotics—cont'd			
Older Generation (Conventional): Phenothiazines	Anticholinergics	Additive and antagonistic drug effects	Reduced phenothiazine efficacy; enhanced anticholinergic effects
	Beta-blockers	Additive drug effects	Potential toxicity of either drug
	Opioids	Additive drug effects	Excessive sedation, hypotension
	warfarin	Enhanced warfarin clearance	Increased bleeding potential
	phenytoin	Uncertain	Can increase or reduce phenytoin levels
	thiazide diuretics	Reduced diuretic clearance	Potential for hypotension
Newer Generation (Atypicals)*	CYP3A4 inhibitors (e.g., ketoconazole)	Reduced antipsychotic clearance	Potential for antipsychotic toxicity
	carbamazepine	Enhanced antipsychotic clearance	Reduced therapeutic effects

Dosages

For the recommended dosages of selected antianxiety drugs, see the Dosages table on p. 267.

DRUG PROFILES

BENZODIAZEPINES

Benzodiazepines are widely used anxiolytic drugs. Benzodiazepines are all classified as Schedule IV controlled substances. Dosage and indication information appears in the Dosages table on p. 267.

◆ alprazolam

Alprazolam (Xanax) is most commonly used as an anxiolytic. It is also indicated for the specific anxiety disorder known as *panic disorder.* Adverse effects include confusion, ataxia, headache, and others listed in Table 17-2. Interacting drugs include alcohol, antacids, oral contraceptives, and others listed in Table 17-3. Alprazolam is available only for oral use. Niravam, a new formulation of alprazolam, is an orally dissolving tablet that is indicated for the treatment of anxiety disorder, short-term relief of anxiety symptoms, treatment of anxiety associated with depression, and treatment of panic disorder with or without agoraphobia.

PHARMACOKINETICS

Route	Onset of Action	Peak Plasma Concentration	Elimination Half-life	Duration of Action
PO	30-60 min	1-2 hr	10-15 hr	6 hr

◆ diazepam

Diazepam (Valium) used to be one of the most commonly prescribed benzodiazepines; however, for treatment of anxiety it has generally been replaced by the shorter-acting benzodiazepines alprazolam and lorazepam. It is indicated for the relief of anxiety, management of alcohol withdrawal, reversal of status epilepticus, preoperative sedation, and as an adjunct for the relief of skeletal muscle spasms. Diazepam has active metabolites that can accumulate in patients with hepatic dysfunction, because it is metabolized primarily in the liver. This can result in additive, cumulative effects that may be manifested as prolonged sedation, respiratory depression, or coma. For this reason, it is probably best avoided in patients with major hepatic compromise. Adverse drug effects

include headache, confusion, slurred speech, and others listed in Table 17-2. Drugs with which it interacts include alcohol, antacids, oral contraceptives, ranitidine (reduces diazepam absorption), and others as shown in Table 17-3. Diazepam is available in oral, rectal, and injectable dosage forms.

PHARMACOKINETICS

Route	Onset of Action	Peak Plasma Concentration	Elimination Half-life	Duration of Action
PO	30-60 min	1-2 hr	20-80 hr	12-24 hr

◆ lorazepam

Lorazepam (Ativan) is an intermediate-acting benzodiazepine. Alprazolam is the shortest acting, whereas diazepam is the longest acting. Lorazepam is also available in an injectable form and may be given intramuscularly. It has excellent absorption and bioavailability when given by this route. The conversion between intramuscular and oral dosage forms is 1:1. Lorazepam can also be given by intravenous push, which is useful in the treatment of an acutely agitated patient. It is often administered as a continuous infusion to agitated patients who are undergoing mechanical ventilation. It is also commonly used to treat or prevent alcohol withdrawal (see Chapter 9). Indications, contraindications, and adverse effects are similar to those of alprazolam.

PHARMACOKINETICS

Route	Onset of Action	Peak Plasma Concentration	Elimination Half-life	Duration of Action
PO	30-60 min	2 hr	11-16 hr	8 hr

MISCELLANEOUS DRUG
buspirone

Buspirone (BuSpar) is an anxiolytic drug that is distinctly different both chemically and pharmacologically from the benzodiazepines. Its precise mechanism of action is unknown, but it appears to have agonist activity at a subset of both serotonin and dopamine receptors. It is indicated for treatment of anxiety and is always administered on a scheduled (not "as needed") basis. Its only reported contraindication is drug allergy. The advantages of buspirone over benzodiazepines include its lack of the sedative properties and dependency potential of the benzodiazepines. Adverse effects include paradoxical anxiety, dizziness, blurred vision, headache, and nausea. Potential drug interactions include a risk for serotonin

DOSAGES

Psychotropic Drugs

Drug (Pregnancy Category)	Pharmacologic Class	Usual Dosage Range*	Current FDA-Approved Indications/Uses
Anxiolytics			
◆ alprazolam (Xanax) (D)	Benzodiazepine	**Adult** PO: 0.25-2 mg tid; do not exceed 6 mg/day	Anxiety
◆ diazepam (Valium) (D)	Benzodiazepine	**Adult** PO: 2-10 mg 2-4×/day **Pediatric** PO: 1-2.5 mg 3-4×/day	Anxiety
		Adult IV/IM: 2-10 mg q1-4h, depending on situation **Pediatric** IV/IM: 0.25 mg/kg/dose; may repeat prn after 15-30 min	Preoperative sedation or anxiety, status epilepticus
Mood Stabilizers			
◆ lithium carbonate (D)	Inorganic salt	600-1800 mg/day divided bid-tid	Acute mania, prevention of mania
Antidepressants **Older Generation**			
◆ amitriptyline (generic only; formerly Elavil) (C)	Tricyclic	**Adult** PO: 10-300 mg/day divided	Depression (more commonly used for insomnia and neuropathic pain)
Newer Generation			
◆ bupropion (Wellbutrin, Zyban) (C)	Miscellaneous	PO: 200-300 mg/day, divided bid PO, SR: 150-400 mg/day	Depression (Wellbutrin), smoking cessation (Zyban)
duloxetine (Cymbalta) (C)	SNRI	PO: 20-40 mg/day; or 60 mg/day divided bid	Depression, GAD, diabetic peripheral neuropathy
◆ fluoxetine (Prozac) (C)	SSRI	PO: 10-20 mg daily; higher doses up to 80 mg/day divided bid	Depression, OCD, bulimia nervosa, panic disorder, premenstrual dysphoric disorder
◆ mirtazapine (Remeron) (C)	Tetracyclic	PO: 15-45 mg at bedtime	Depression, bipolar disorder
trazodone (Desyrel) (C)	Miscellaneous	PO: 25-600 mg/day, with larger doses divided	Depression (more commonly used for insomnia)
Antipsychotics **Older Generation**			
haloperidol (Haldol) (C)	Butyrophenone, phenylbutylpiperidine	**Adult** PO, IM: 0.5-5 mg bid-tid **Pediatric** PO: 25-50 mcg/kg/day IM (acute care only): 2-5 mg up to q1h prn	Schizophrenia, Tourette syndrome, severe refractory behavioral problems or hyperactivity
Newer Generation			
clozapine (Clozaril) (B)	Dibenzodiazepine	PO: 25-900 mg/day with larger doses divided tid	Schizophrenia; recurrent suicidal behavior in patients with schizophrenia or schizoaffective disorder
◆ risperidone (Risperdal) (C)	Benzisoxazole	PO: 1-8 mg/day in either one or two doses IM depot form (Risperdal Consta): 25-50 mg every 2 wk	Schizophrenia, mania, irritability associated with autism

FDA, Food and Drug Administration; *GAD*, generalized anxiety disorder; *IM*, intramuscular; *IV*, intravenous; *OCD*, obsessive-compulsive disorder; *PO*, oral; *SNRI*, serotonin norepinephrine reuptake inhibitor; *SSRI*, selective serotonin reuptake inhibitor.
*All dosages reflect usual adult dosage ranges. Pediatric dosages may be more variable and should be specified by a pediatric practitioner.

syndrome (see section on antidepressants in the chapter) when buspirone is used concurrently with any antidepressant with serotonergic activity. Patients receiving both types of medications together should be monitored carefully. It is recommended that MAOIs not be used concurrently with buspirone due to a risk of hypertension. A washout period of at least 14 days after discontinuation of MAOI therapy should be allowed before buspirone is started. Other drugs that interact with buspirone include *inhibitors* of the cytochrome P-450 enzyme system (see Chapter 2), specifically with CYP3A4 (e.g., ketoconazole, clarithromycin), which can reduce buspirone clearance; and *inducers* of these same enzymes, which can enhance buspirone clearance. In either case, the buspirone dosage may need to be adjusted. Buspirone is available only for oral use.

PHARMACOKINETICS

Route	Onset of Action	Peak Plasma Concentration	Elimination Half-life	Duration of Action
PO	2-3 wk	40-60 min	2-3 hr	Unknown

DRUGS USED TO TREAT AFFECTIVE DISORDERS

Several classes of drugs are used in the treatment of the affective disorders. The two main drug categories are mood-stabilizing drugs and antidepressant drugs.

MOOD-STABILIZING DRUGS

Drugs used to treat bipolar illness (cycles of mania, hypomania, and depression) are commonly referred to as *mood stabilizers.* Clinical evidence indicates that the catecholamines (dopamine and norepinephrine) play an important pathophysiologic role in the development of mania. Serotonin also appears to be involved. The original drugs still currently available that can effectively alleviate the symptoms of *acute* mania are the lithium salts lithium carbonate and lithium citrate. Lithium is also effective for the *maintenance* treatment of bipolar disorder. One possible explanation for its effectiveness is that it potentiates serotonergic neurotransmission. A variety of medications may be used in conjunction with lithium to regulate mood or achieve stability in manic or hypomanic patients including benzodiazepines (described earlier), antipsychotic drugs (see later) antiepileptic drugs (see Chapter 15), and dopamine receptor agonists (see Chapter 16). The antiepileptics valproic acid, lamotrigine, oxcarbazepine, and topiramate are commonly preferred to lithium because lithium has a narrow therapeutic range and requires blood level monitoring. These drugs are often effective in treating mania, hypomania, and, to a lesser degree, depressive symptoms. Other evidence has shown that the atypical antipsychotic drugs risperidone, olanzapine, quetiapine, and ziprasidone (see later) can also be effective in treating mania and hypomania.

DRUG PROFILE

◆ lithium
The antimanic effect of lithium is not fully understood. Research indicates that lithium ions alter sodium ion transport in nerve cells, which results in a shift in catecholamine metabolism. The therapeutic levels of lithium that are required are close to the toxic levels, but there is increasingly greater tolerance to these toxic levels during acute manic phases. For the management of acute mania, a lithium serum level of 1 to 1.5 mEq/L is usually required. Desirable long-term maintenance levels range between 0.6 and 1.2 mEq/L. Blood levels are best measured 8 to 12 hours after the last dose (roughly the midpoint of the drug half-life), because the half-life is usually between 18 and 24 hours. Both sodium and lithium are monovalent positive ions, and one can affect the other. Therefore, the patient's serum sodium levels should also be monitored. Keeping the sodium level in the normal range (135 to 145 mEq/L) helps to maintain therapeutic

lithium levels. Patients should be advised not to drastically change their sodium intake while taking lithium.

Lithium is indicated for the treatment of manic episodes in bipolar disorder as well as for maintenance therapy for prevention of such episodes. Contraindications to lithium therapy are relative and include dehydration, known sodium imbalance, and major renal or cardiovascular disease, because all of these conditions increase the risk of lithium toxicity. Renal dysfunction of any degree can increase lithium levels. Elderly patients are particularly prone to this effect, because renal function normally declines with advancing age. Adverse effects tend to correlate with serum levels. Levels exceeding 1.5 to 2.5 mEq/L begin to produce toxicity, including gastrointestinal discomfort, tremor, confusion, somnolence, seizures, and possibly death. The most serious adverse effect is cardiac dysrhythmia. Other effects include drowsiness, slurred speech, epilepsy-type seizures, choreoathetotic movements (involuntary wavelike movements of the extremities), ataxia (generalized disturbance of muscular coordination), and hypotension. Long-term treatment may cause hypothyroidism. Potentially interacting drugs include the thiazide diuretics, angiotensin-converting enzyme inhibitors, calcium channel blockers, and nonsteroidal antiinflammatory drugs, all of which can increase lithium toxicity. Lithium carbonate is available only for oral use.

PHARMACOKINETICS

Route	Onset of Action	Peak Plasma Concentration	Elimination Half-life	Duration of Action
PO	7-14 days*	0.5-2 hr	18-24 hr	2-24 hr

*Therapeutic benefit for maintenance control of mania.

ANTIDEPRESSANT DRUGS

Antidepressants are the pharmacologic treatment of choice for major depressive disorders. Not only are they very effective in treating depression, they are also useful in treating other disorders, such as *dysthymia* (chronic low-grade depression), schizophrenia (as an adjunctive drug), eating disorders, and personality disorders. Some of the antidepressant drugs are also commonly used in the treatment of various medical conditions, including migraine headaches, chronic pain syndromes, sleep disorders, premenstrual syndrome, and hot flashes associated with menopause. Both older- and newer-generation antidepressants are listed in Table 17-1.

Many of the drugs currently used to treat affective disorders increase the levels of monoamine neurotransmitter concentrations in the CNS. Monoamine neurotransmitters include serotonin (also known as *5-hydroxytryptamine,* or 5-HT), dopamine, and norepinephrine. This treatment is based on the belief that alterations in the levels of these neurotransmitters are responsible for causing depression. A widely held hypothesis advanced to explain depression in these terms is the **biogenic amine hypothesis.** Specifically, it postulates that depression results from a deficiency of neuronal and synaptic catecholamines (primarily norepinephrine) and mania from an excess of amines at the adrenergic receptor sites in the brain. This hypothesis is illustrated in Figure 17-1.

Another hypothesis regarding the cause of depression is the **permissive hypothesis,** which led to the creation of the class of drugs called the *selective serotonin reuptake inhibitors (SSRIs)* mentioned earlier. The permissive theory postulates that reduced concentrations of serotonin are the predisposing factor in patients with affective disorders. Depression results from decreases in both the serotonin and catecholamine levels, whereas mania results

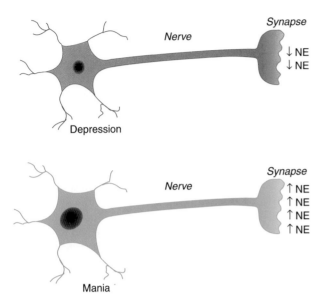

FIGURE 17-1   Biologic amine hypothesis. *NE,* Norepinephrine.

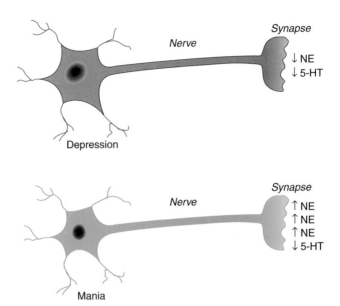

FIGURE 17-2   Permissive hypothesis. *NE,* Norepinephrine; *5-HT,* serotonin.

from increased catecholamine levels but decreased serotonin levels. The permissive hypothesis is illustrated in Figure 17-2.

A new leading theory attempting to explain the cause of affective disorders is the **dysregulation hypothesis.** It is essentially a reformulation of the biogenic amine hypothesis. This theory views depression and other affective disorders not simply in terms of decreased or increased catecholamine activity but as a failure of the regulation of these systems.

Recent research data indicate that early and aggressive antidepressant treatment increases the chances for full remission. The first 6 to 8 weeks of therapy constitute the acute phase. The primary goals during this time are to obtain a response to drug therapy and to improve the patient's symptoms. It is currently recommended that antidepressant drug therapy be maintained at the effective dose for an additional 8 to 14 months after remission of depressive symptoms. In choosing an antidepressant for a given patient, the patient's previous psychotropic drug response history (if any) should be considered. Information regarding any family history of depression with known drug responses may also be helpful. Therapeutic response is measured primarily by subjective patient feedback. In addition, a few measurement tools are available that attempt to quantify the patient's response to drug therapy, such as the Hamilton Rating Scale for Depression and the Symptom Checklist-90 anxiety factor scale. Anxiety and depression commonly occur together and reinforce each other. Similarly, there is much crossover in terms of symptom control between antidepressant and anxiolytic drugs. A therapeutic nonresponse to antidepressant drug therapy is defined as failure to respond to at least 6 weeks of therapy with adequate drug dosages. Twenty percent to 30% of patients who do not respond to the usual dosage of a given antidepressant drug will respond to higher dosages. Therefore, dosage optimization, which involves careful upward titration of medication dose for several weeks, is recommended before concluding that a given drug is ineffective in treating a particular patient. Research indicates that, in cases in which a switch to a different pharmacologic class of antidepressant is deemed appropriate, 40% to 60% of patients will re-

spond to the second drug class tried. Anxiolytic and antipsychotic drugs may also be used, either alone or as adjunct therapy.

The most severe cases of refractory depression may warrant an attempt at treatment with electroconvulsive therapy. Current electroconvulsive therapy techniques are greatly refined from the methods used in past decades, and treatment is generally carried out in a postanesthesia care unit setting under brief general anesthesia. Seizure activity is induced in the anesthetized patient via externally applied electric shocks to the brain.

It should be recognized that treatment failure in cases of depression may be due to a misdiagnosis or failure to treat comorbid mental illness (e.g., anxiety disorder, substance abuse) and/or comorbid nonpsychiatric illness (e.g., hypothyroidism). It may also be due to nonadherence to drug therapy. Careful choice of drug therapy to minimize adverse effects may improve patient compliance with treatment and therapeutic outcome. Another reason for treatment failure may be the discouragement associated with depression itself. This alone may cause patients to give up prematurely on their drug therapy, especially because antidepressants often take several weeks to reach their full effect. Effective psychotherapy and support groups can help encourage patients to be consistent with prescribed psychotropic drug therapy.

Newer-generation antidepressants are generally more commonly used to treat depression than are the older-generation drugs. In 2005, the U.S. Food and Drug Administration (FDA) issued special black box warnings regarding the use of all classes of antidepressants in both adult and pediatric patient populations. It should be kept in mind that most patients do not experience severe adverse effects from these medications, and many patients obtain significant relief. However, data from the FDA, including a meta-analysis combining data from 24 small studies of child and adolescent subjects, indicated a higher risk for suicide in patients receiving these medications (up to 4% of patients taking the drugs showed suicidal thoughts or behaviors compared with 2% receiving a placebo). Later in the same year, the agency expressed similar concerns regarding adult patients. As a result, current recommendations for all patients receiving antidepressants include regular monitoring for signs of worsening depressive symptoms, especially when the medication is started or the dosage is changed. Patients should be evaluated by their prescriber immediately if they report, or others observe, signs of worsening depression or other emotional instability.

TRICYCLIC ANTIDEPRESSANTS

One of the original first-generation antidepressants, TCAs have been largely superseded as first-line antidepressant drug therapy since the introduction of the SSRIs in the 1980s, beginning with fluoxetine (Prozac). Now TCAs are generally considered second-line drug therapy for patients for whom the newer drugs are ineffective or as adjunct therapy with newer drugs. TCAs are so named because of their characteristic three-ring chemical stricture.

Mechanism of Action and Drug Effects

TCAs are believed to work by correcting imbalance in the neurotransmitter concentrations of serotonin and norepinephrine at the nerve endings in the CNS (the biogenic amine hypothesis). This is accomplished by blocking the presynaptic reuptake of the neurotransmitters, which makes them available for transmission of nerve impulses to adjacent neurons in the brain. Some also believe that these drugs may help regulate malfunctioning neurons (the dysregulation hypothesis).

Indications

Originally used to treat depression currently, TCAs are most commonly used to treat neuropathic pain syndromes and insomnia. With the advent of the newer-generation antidepressant classes, their use as antidepressants is rare. Some of the TCAs have additional specific indications. For example, imipramine is used as an adjunct in the treatment of childhood enuresis (bedwetting), and clomipramine is useful in the treatment of obsessive-compulsive disorder.

Contraindications

Contraindications for TCAs include known drug allergy, use of MAOIs within the previous 14 days, and pregnancy. TCAs are also not recommended in patients with any acute or chronic cardiac problems or history of seizures, because both condition are associated with a greater likelihood of death upon TCA overdose.

Adverse Effects

The most common undesirable effects of TCAs are a result of their effects on various receptors, especially the muscarinic receptors (a type of cholinergic receptor) and, to a lesser degree, adrenergic, histaminergic, dopaminergic, and serotonergic receptors. Blockade of cholinergic receptors by TCAs results in many undesirable anticholinergic adverse effects, the most common being constipation and urinary retention. Adrenergic and dopaminergic receptor blockade can lead to disturbances in cardiac conduction and hypotension. Histaminergic blockade can cause sedation, and serotonergic blockade can alter the seizure threshold, and cause sexual dysfunction (see also Table 17-2).

Toxicity and Management of Overdose

Tricyclic antidepressant overdoses are notoriously lethal. It is estimated that 70% to 80% of patients who die of TCA overdose do so before reaching the hospital, especially if the drugs are taken with alcohol. The primary organ systems affected are the CNS and cardiovascular system, and death usually results from either seizures or dysrhythmias. It used to be taught that one should never give patients more than a 1-month supply of antidepressants because of the risk of suicide attempts. However, with the cost of drugs today, it is not uncommon to see a 3-month supply given with only one copay. This is a two-edged sword: the patient saves money, but now the depressed patient has more than enough drugs to cause death by overdose.

There is no specific antidote for TCA poisoning. Management efforts are aimed at reducing drug absorption by administering multiple doses of activated charcoal. Administration of sodium bicarbonate speeds up elimination of the TCA by alkalinizing the urine. CNS damage may also be minimized by the administration of diazepam, and cardiovascular events may be minimized by giving antidysrhythmics to control cardiac dysrhythmias. Other care includes basic life support in an intensive care setting to maintain vital organ functions. These interventions must continue until enough of the TCA is eliminated to permit restoration of normal organ function.

Interactions

Taking anticholinergics and phenothiazines with TCAs may result in increased anticholinergic effects. Combining CNS depressants with TCAs leads to additive CNS depressant effects. When MAOIs are taken with TCAs, the result may be increased therapeutic and toxic effects, including hyperpyretic crisis (excessive fever). TCAs can inhibit the metabolism of warfarin, which leads to increased anticoagulation effects (see Table 17-3.)

Dosages

For the recommended dosages of selected TCA drugs, see the Dosages table on p. 267.

DRUG PROFILE

TCAs are effective drugs in the treatment of various affective disorders, but they are also associated with serious adverse effects. Therefore, patients taking them need to be monitored closely. For this reason, all antidepressants are available only with a prescription, with the exception of some herbal products such as St. John's wort (see the Herbal Therapies and Dietary Supplements box on p. 271). Many drugs in this class are rated as pregnancy category D drugs, which makes their use by pregnant women relatively more hazardous than that of most of the newer drugs.

◆ amitriptyline

Amitriptyline (Elavil) is the oldest and most widely used of all the TCAs. Its original indication was depression, but it is now more commonly used to treat insomnia and neuropathic pain. Contraindications include known drug allergy and recent myocardial infarction. It has very potent anticholinergic properties, which can lead to many adverse effects such as dry mouth, constipation, blurred vision, urinary retention, and dysrhythmias (see also Table 17-2). Drugs with which it interacts include bupropion, haloperidol, MAOIs, and others listed in Table 17-3. Amitriptyline is available only for oral use.

PHARMACOKINETICS

Route	Onset of Action	Peak Plasma Concentration	Elimination Half-life	Duration of Action
PO	7-21 days	2-12 hr	10-50 hr	6-12 hr

HERBAL THERAPIES AND DIETARY SUPPLEMENTS

St. John's Wort (Hypericum perforatum)

■ *Overview*

St. John's wort herbal preparations consist of the dried above-ground parts of the plant species *Hypericum perforatum* gathered during flowering season. The herb is available over the counter in numerous oral dosage forms. St. John's wort is sometimes referred to as the *herbal Prozac*.

■ *Common Uses*

Depression, anxiety, sleep disorders, nervousness

■ *Adverse Effects*

Gastrointestinal upset, allergic reactions, fatigue, dizziness, confusion, dry mouth, possible photosensitization (especially in fair-skinned individuals)

■ *Potential Drug Interactions*

Monoamine oxidase inhibitors, selective serotonin reuptake inhibitors, cyclosporine, sympathomimetic amines, piroxicam, tetracycline, tyramine-containing foods, opioids, digoxin, estrogens, theophylline

■ *Contraindications*

Contraindicated in patients with bipolar depression, schizophrenia, Alzheimer's disease, and dementia

MONOAMINE OXIDASE INHIBITORS

MAOIs, along with TCAs, represent the first generation of antidepressant drug therapy. Although MAOIs are potent drugs, they are now rarely used. This is partly because newer, safer drugs are now available. A serious disadvantage to MAOI use is their potential to cause a hypertensive crisis when taken with a substance containing tyramine, which is found in many common foods and beverages (Table 17-4).

Currently four MAOI antidepressants are available. Isocarboxazid, phenelzine, and tranylcypromine are nonselective inhibitors of both MAO type A (MAO-A) and MAO type B (MAO-B). Selegiline is a selective MAO-B inhibitor, is actually a newer-generation antidepressant in that it comes in a new transdermal dosage form. It is profiled in detail in this section. An oral form of this drug is also used to treat Parkinson's disease (see Chapter 16). Because these drugs inhibit the MAO enzyme system in the CNS of patients experiencing depression, amines such as dopamine, serotonin, and norepinephrine are not broken down, and therefore higher levels of these substances occur. This, in turn, alleviates the symptoms of depression.

Most adverse effects of MAOIs stem from their interactions with food. A variety of over-the-counter drugs (especially for cough and cold) also can interact with MAOIs to cause adverse cardiovascular effects. For example, MAOIs may increase the CNS depressant effects of diphenhydramine and cetirizine. Patients taking MAOIs should always read labels and/or consult the pharmacist when using any such products. Dosage information for selected MAOIs appears in the Dosages table on p. 267.

Sympathomimetic drugs can also interact with the MAOIs, and together these drugs can cause a hypertensive crisis. MAOIs can markedly potentiate the effects of meperidine, and therefore their concurrent use is contraindicated. In addition, concurrent use of MAOIs with SSRIs carries the risk for serotonin syndrome. A washout period of 2 to 5 weeks between drugs is recommended.

TABLE 17-4 Food and Drink to Avoid When Taking Monoamine Oxidase Inhibitors

Food/Drink	Examples
High Tyramine Content—Not Permitted	
Aged mature cheeses	Cheddar, blue, Swiss
Smoked or pickled meats	Herring, sausage, corned beef, smoked fish or poultry, salami, pepperoni
Aged or fermented meats	Chicken or beef liver pâté, game fish or poultry
Yeast extracts	Brewer's yeast
Red wines	Chianti, burgundy, sherry, vermouth
Italian broad beans	Fava beans
Moderate Tyramine Content—Limited Amounts Allowed	
Meat extracts	Bouillon, consommé
Pasteurized light and pale beer	
Ripe avocado	
Low Tyramine Content—Permissible	
Distilled spirits	Vodka, gin, rye, scotch (in moderation)
Non-aged cheeses	American cheese, mozzarella, cottage cheese, cream cheese
Chocolate and caffeinated beverages	
Fruit	Figs, bananas, raisins, grapes, pineapple, oranges
Soy sauce	
Yogurt, sour cream	

Toxicity and Management of Overdose

Clinical symptoms of MAOI overdose generally do not appear until about 12 hours after ingestion. The primary signs and symptoms are cardiovascular and neurologic. The most serious cardiovascular effects are tachycardia and circulatory collapse, and the neurologic symptoms of major concern are seizures and coma. Hyperthermia and miosis are also generally present in overdose. Treatment is aimed at eliminating the ingested toxin and protecting the organs at greatest risk for damage—the brain and the heart. Recommended treatments are gastric lavage, urine acidification to a pH of 5, and hemodialysis. Treatment of hypertensive crisis resulting from consumption of tyramine-containing foods or beverages may require intravenous administration of hypotensive drugs along with careful monitoring in an intensive care setting.

DRUG PROFILE

selegiline transdermal patch

The selegiline transdermal patch (Emsam) is a new medication that is a selective MAO-B inhibitor. It is currently indicated strictly for major depression. The well-recognized drug-food interactions associated with MAOIs are listed in Table 17-4. The lowest strength of the selegiline transdermal patch (6 mg/24 hr) can be used without dietary restrictions. However, there are insufficient data to date to permit the same dietary freedom with the 9- and 12-mg patch strengths. Contraindications include known drug allergy. Adverse drug effects and drug interactions are the same as for the oral dosage form and can be found earlier in the discussion of MAOIs in general and in Chapter 16 for selegiline in particular. Patients should avoid exposing the patch to external sources of heat, such as a heating pad, electric blanket, sauna, or even prolonged direct sunlight. Standard pharmacokinetic parameters for the transdermal dosage form are not listed at this time.

PHARMACOKINETICS

Route	Onset of Action	Peak Plasma Concentration	Elimination Half-life	Duration of Action
Transdermal	Unknown	Unknown	Unknown	Unknown

NEWER-GENERATION ANTIDEPRESSANTS

Newer-generation antidepressants, called SSRIs are generally considered superior to TCAs and MAOIs in terms of their adverse effect profiles. They are associated with significantly fewer and less severe systemic adverse effects, especially anticholinergic and cardiovascular adverse effects. Because of this, they have largely replaced TCAs and MAOIs as first-line drug therapy for depression. Fluoxetine (Prozac) was the first SSRI available. Currently available newer-generation drugs are listed in Table 17-1. However, it does take approximately the same amount of time for them to reach maximum clinical effectiveness as it does for the TCAs and MAOIs, typically 4 to 6 weeks.

Mechanism of Action and Drug Effects

The inhibition of serotonin reuptake seems to be the primary clinically significant mechanism of action of the SSRIs, although the SSRIs may also have weak effects on norepinephrine and dopamine reuptake (see individual drug profiles). Patients should be educated that antidepressant drugs commonly must be taken for several weeks before full therapeutic effects are realized. This requires some patience and faithful dosing on the part of patients.

Indications

Although depression is their primary indication, classes of newer-generation antidepressants have shown benefit in treating a variety of other mental and physical disorders. Examples include bipolar disorder, obesity, eating disorders, obsessive-compulsive disorder, panic attacks or disorders, social anxiety disorder, posttraumatic stress disorder, premenstrual dysphoric disorder, the neurologic disorder myoclonus, and various substance abuse problems such as alcoholism. This list is expanding with continued research on these drugs.

Contraindications

Contraindications include known drug allergy, use of MAOIs in the previous 14 days, and therapy with certain antipsychotic drugs such as thioridazine or mesoridazine. In addition, a significant history of cardiac disease or seizure may be a contraindication due to the relatively uncommon, but reported, cardiac effects and alterations in seizure threshold (see later). Bupropion is also contraindicated in cases of eating disorder and seizure disorder because it can lower the seizure threshold.

Adverse Effects

The newer-generation drugs offer an advantage over TCAs and MAOIs in that their adverse effect profiles are generally much better. However, up to two thirds of all depressed patients may still discon-

---

> **BOX 17-1 Common Symptoms of Serotonin Syndrome**
>
> Common symptoms include delirium, agitation, tachycardia, sweating, myoclonus (muscle spasms), hyperreflexia, shivering, coarse tremors, and extensor plantar muscle (sole of foot) responses. In more severe cases, hyperthermia, seizures, rhabdomyolysis, renal failure, cardiac dysrhythmias, and disseminated intravascular coagulation may occur.

tinue therapy due to drug adverse effects. Some of the most common and bothersome adverse effects are insomnia (partly due to reduced rapid eye movement sleep), weight gain, and sexual dysfunction. Sexual dysfunction caused by the SSRIs is primarily related to inability to achieve orgasm. One potentially hazardous adverse effect of any drug or combination of drugs that have serotoninergic activity is known as **serotonin syndrome.** The symptoms of this condition are listed in Box 17-1. Fortunately, it is usually self-limiting on discontinuation of the causative drugs. (See also Table 17-2.)

Interactions

The newer-generation antidepressants are highly bound to albumin. When given with other drugs that are also highly protein bound (e.g., warfarin and phenytoin), they compete for binding sites on the surface of albumin. This results in a more free, unbound drug and therefore a more pronounced drug effect.

Some of the newer drugs may also inhibit cytochrome P-450 enzymes, though there is debate about this in the literature. The cytochrome P-450 system is an enzyme system in the liver that is responsible for the metabolism of several drugs (see Chapter 2). Inhibition of this enzyme system results in higher levels of these drugs with the potential for toxicity.

To prevent the potentially fatal pharmacodynamic interactions that can occur between the newer drugs and the MAOIs, a 2- to 5-week washout period is recommended between uses of these two classes of medications. Newer-generation antidepressants have a potentiating effect when given with opioid analgesics, in that the increased serotonin concentration at nerve endings appears to work synergistically with the opioid analgesic in relieving pain. (See also Table 17-3.)

Using the SSRIs with linezolid (Zyvox), an antibiotic used to treat resistant infections (see Chapter 39), can cause serotonin syndrome, and their combined use is contraindicated. This can be problematic, however, due to the long half-lives of some of the SSRIs, and abrupt discontinuation of the SSRIs can produce a withdrawal syndrome. The manufacturer of linezolid has gone on record stating that the SSRIs can be used with linezolid, but the patient should be monitored closely for signs of serotonin syndrome.

Dosages

For the recommended dosages of selected newer-generation antidepressants, see the Dosages table on p. 267.

DRUG PROFILES

The period from the 1980s to the present were decades of much development in psychotropic pharmacotherapy. Several new antidepressants alone were introduced during this period. Two of the first newer-generation antidepressants were trazodone (generic only; formerly Desyrel) and bupropion (Wellbutrin). Both are still commonly used. The SSRIs were also introduced. These include fluoxetine (Prozac), sertraline (Zoloft), paroxetine (Paxil), fluvoxamine (generic only; formerly Luvox), citalopram (Celexa), and escitalopram (Lexapro). The 1990s saw the introduction of still more antidepressants, including venlafaxine (Effexor), nefazodone (Serzone), and mirtazapine (Remeron), whereas two new drugs were introduced in the 2000s, including duloxetine (Cymbalta) and desvenlafaxine (Pristiq). Pristiq is just a different isomer of venlafaxine, of which the generic version will become available soon. All of these newer drugs have proved to be effective antidepressants. They also have generally better adverse effect profiles than first-generation antidepressants. They are now considered first-line drugs in the treatment of patients with depression, including patients with concurrent symptoms of anxiety and patients with depression with suicidal ideations.

trazodone

Trazodone (Desyrel) is unique in its chemical drug class of triazolopyridine. It was the first of the newer-generation antidepressants that could selectively inhibit serotonin reuptake but that negligibly affected norepinephrine reuptake. This is responsible for one advantage of trazodone over TCAs, namely, its minimal adverse effect on the cardiovascular system. Trazodone is indicated for the treatment of depression. However, it is also commonly used as a nonaddictive drug treatment for insomnia. Contraindications include known drug allergy. Adverse effects include strongly sedative qualities. These can be severe and can impair cognitive function in older adults. However, the sedating effect of trazodone is often advantageous in helping depressed patients, who commonly have comorbid anxiety and/or insomnia, obtain effective sleep. Trazodone also has been associated in rare cases with transient nonsexual *priapism*. This is a dangerously sustained penile erection that is reportedly the result of alpha-adrenergic blockade. Drugs with which trazodone interacts include azole antifungals, phenothiazines, and protease inhibitors, all of which can increase the risk of trazodone toxicity; carbamazepine, which can reduce trazodone levels, while carbamazepine levels are increased; CNS depressants (e.g., alcohol), whose effects can be potentiated by trazodone; digoxin and phenytoin, whose levels can be increased by trazodone; and warfarin, whose levels can be either increased or reduced. It is also recommended that trazodone be started gradually after a patient has recently stopped MAOI therapy. Trazodone is available only for oral use.

PHARMACOKINETICS

Route	Onset of Action	Peak Plasma Concentration	Elimination Half-life	Duration of Action
PO	1-2 wk	2-4 wk	6-9 hr	Several weeks

◆ fluoxetine

Fluoxetine (Prozac) was the first SSRI marketed for the treatment of depression. Since that time, it has become the top-prescribed antidepressant in the United States and one of the most commonly prescribed of all drugs. Although it was initially indicated for treatment of depression, the indications for fluoxetine have since expanded to include bulimia, obsessive-compulsive disorder, panic disorder, and premenstrual dysphoric disorder. Contraindications include known drug allergy and concurrent MAOI therapy. Adverse effects include anxiety, dizziness, drowsiness, insomnia, and others listed in Table 17-2. Interacting drugs include benzodiazepines (reduced benzodiazepine clearance); buspirone (reduced buspirone effects); antipsychotics (elevated antipsychotic levels); lithium (altered lithium levels); propafenone, ritonavir, trazodone,

and cyclosporine (elevated drug levels, serotonin syndrome with ritonavir); and others listed in Table 17-3. Fluoxetine is available only for oral use.

PHARMACOKINETICS

Route	Onset of Action	Peak Plasma Concentration	Elimination Half-life	Duration of Action
PO	1-4 wk	6-8 hr	1-3 days	2-4 wk

◆ bupropion

Bupropion (Wellbutrin) was originally approved by the FDA in 1985 but was withdrawn by the manufacturer because of its apparently high potential for inducing seizures in nondepressed patients being treated for bulimia. Subsequent investigations revealed that the overall estimated frequency of seizures was approximately 0.4%, and the drug was reintroduced in 1989. Bupropion is a unique antidepressant in terms of both its structure and mechanism of action. It has relatively weak, but measurable, effects on brain serotonin activity, but little to no effect on monoamine oxidase. Its strongest therapeutic activity appears to be primarily dopaminergic and noradrenergic.

Bupropion was originally indicated strictly for treatment of depression but is now also indicated as an aid in smoking cessation. It is sometimes added as an adjunct antidepressant for male patients experiencing sexual adverse effects secondary to SSRI therapy. Although the mechanism for it is unclear, the drug is often effective in this situation. A newer, sustained-release form of bupropion, Zyban, was approved for smoking cessation treatment. Sustained-release bupropion was an innovative new treatment because it was the first nicotine-free prescription medicine used to treat nicotine dependence. Its exact mechanism of action in treating nicotine dependence is unknown, but it is believed to be related to the drug's ability to modulate dopamine and norepinephrine levels in the brain. Both of these neurotransmitters are believed to play an important role in maintaining nicotine addiction. However, the newer smoking cessation drug varenicline (Chantix; see Chapter 9) is becoming more popular for this purpose.

Bupropion use is contraindicated in patients who have a known drug allergy, those with a seizure disorder (bupropion can lower the seizure threshold), those who currently have anorexia nervosa or bulimia or have had one of these disorders in the past, and those currently taking an MAOI. Common adverse effects include dizziness, confusion, tachycardia, agitation, tremor, and dry mouth. Drugs that interact with bupropion include amantadine, levodopa, nicotine replacement drugs, and ritonavir (increased risk of bupropion adverse effects), as well as drugs metabolized by the cytochrome P-450 enzyme system, specifically CYP2D6 (e.g., SSRIs, tricyclic antidepressants, antipsychotics, beta-blockers, antidysrhythmics), for all of which there is an increased risk of toxicity because bupropion inhibits this enzyme. Bupropion is available only for oral use.

PHARMACOKINETICS

Route	Onset of Action	Peak Plasma Concentration	Elimination Half-life	Duration of Action
PO	Up to 4 wk	3 hr	10-14 hr	Weeks to months

◆ mirtazapine

Mirtazapine (Remeron) is unique in that it promotes the presynaptic release in the brain of both serotonin and norepinephrine, due to its antagonist activity in the presynaptic alpha$_2$-adrenergic receptors, but does not inhibit the reuptake of either of these neurotransmitters. It is strongly associated with sedation in more than 50% of patients due to its histamine 1 (H$_1$) receptor activity and therefore is usually dosed once daily at bedtime. Furthermore, although clearance of the drug may be somewhat reduced in elderly patients, no dosage adjustment is currently recommended. Mirtazapine is indicated for treatment of depression, including that associated with bipolar disorder. It is also sometimes helpful (mechanism unknown) in reducing the sexual adverse effects in male patients receiving SSRI therapy. Mirtazapine is known to be an appetite stimulant and thus can be helpful in underweight depressed patients. Mirtazapine is contraindicated in cases of drug allergy and concurrent use of MAOIs. Adverse effects include drowsiness, abnormal dreams, dry mouth, constipation, increased appetite, and asthenia. Drug interactions include additive CNS depressant effects with alcohol and benzodiazepines. Mirtazapine is available only for oral use.

PHARMACOKINETICS

Route	Onset of Action	Peak Plasma Concentration	Elimination Half-life	Duration of Action
PO	1-3 wk	2 hr	20-40 hr	Unknown

duloxetine

Duloxetine (Cymbalta) is a relatively new antidepressant, introduced in 2004. Like venlafaxine, it is a serotonin-norepinephrine reuptake inhibitor. It is indicated for depression and generalized anxiety disorder. It is also indicated for pain resulting from diabetic peripheral neuropathy. This drug is contraindicated in cases of known drug allergy and concurrent MAOI use, and can worsen uncontrolled angle-closure glaucoma. Adverse effects include dizziness, drowsiness, headache, gastrointestinal upset, anorexia, and hepatotoxicity. Drugs with which duloxetine interacts include SSRIs and triptans (increased risk of serotonin syndrome), alcohol (increased risk of liver injury), and warfarin (increased bleeding risk). Duloxetine is available only for oral use.

PHARMACOKINETICS

Route	Onset of Action	Peak Plasma Concentration	Elimination Half-life	Duration of Action
PO	Unknown	6 hr	12 hr	Unknown

ANTIPSYCHOTIC DRUGS

Antipsychotic drugs are used to treat serious mental illnesses such as drug-induced psychoses, schizophrenia, and autism. Antipsychotics are also used to treat extreme mania (as an adjunct to lithium), bipolar disorder, certain movement disorders (e.g., Tourette syndrome), and certain other medical conditions (e.g., nausea, intractable hiccups). Antipsychotics have also been referred to as *tranquilizers* or *neuroleptics* because they produce a state of tranquility and act on abnormally functioning nerves. However, these are both older terms that are now less commonly used.

The phenothiazines are the largest chemical class of antipsychotic drugs, constituting about two thirds of all antipsychotics. They were also the original drugs in this category. Like many other drugs, phenothiazines were discovered by chance, in this case during research for new antihistamines. Chlorpromazine, isolated in 1951, was the first phenothiazine to be discovered in this way. The variety of currently available antipsychotics are listed in Table 17-1.

There are few overall differences between antipsychotics in terms of mechanism of action. Therefore, selection of an antipsychotic is based primarily on the patient's tolerance and the need

to minimize adverse effects. Of the currently available antipsychotic drugs, no single drug stands out for all patients as either more or less effective in the treatment of psychotic symptoms. It should also be stressed that antipsychotic drug therapy does not normally provide a cure for psychoses but is a way of chemically controlling the symptoms of the illness.

Antipsychotic drugs represent a significant advance in the treatment of mental illnesses, as borne out by the fact that the early treatment of mental illnesses (before the 1950s) consisted of such extreme measures as isolation, physical restraint, shock therapy, and even lobotomy.

More recently, a new class of antipsychotic medications has evolved. These newer-generation antipsychotics are referred to as *atypical* antipsychotics, as opposed to the older-generation drugs, which can also be thought of as *conventional* antipsychotics. Atypical antipsychotics differ from conventional drugs in that they tend to have better adverse effect profiles. The atypical antipsychotics still have adverse effects, but they are usually not as severe as those of the older-generation drugs.

Mechanism of Action and Drug Effects

One thing that all antipsychotics have in common is some degree of blockage of dopamine receptors in the brain, which decreases the dopamine concentration in the CNS. Specifically, the older phenothiazines block the receptors to which dopamine normally binds postsynaptically in certain areas of the CNS, such as the limbic system and the basal ganglia. These are the areas associated with emotions, cognitive function, and motor function. This receptor blocking produces a tranquilizing effect in psychotic patients. Both the therapeutic and toxic effects of these drugs are the direct result of the dopamine blockade in these areas. The newer atypical antipsychotic drugs block specific dopamine receptors called *dopamine 2 (D_2)* receptors, as well as specific serotonin receptors in the brain known as *serotonin 2 (5-HT_2)* receptors. These more refined mechanisms of action of the atypicals are responsible for their improved efficacy and safety profiles, compared with older drugs (see Adverse Effects).

All antipsychotics show some efficacy in improving the *positive* symptoms of schizophrenia, and, over time, these beneficial effects may even increase. So-called positive symptoms include hallucinations, delusions, and conceptual disorganization. Unfortunately, older-generation drugs are much less effective in managing negative symptoms. Negative symptoms are apathy, social withdrawal, blunted affect, poverty of speech, and catatonia. It is these negative symptoms that account for most of the social and vocational disability caused by schizophrenia. Fortunately, atypical antipsychotics have improved efficacy in treating both positive and negative symptoms.

Indications

Antipsychotic drugs are primarily indicated for psychotic illness, most commonly schizophrenia. As more has been learned about these drugs, especially the atypical antipsychotic drugs, their indications have expanded to include anxiety (see later) and mood disorders as well. It has already been noted that antipsychotics can also block serotonin receptors. This, in combination with their ability to block dopamine receptors in the *chemoreceptor trigger zone* in the brain and, more peripherally, to inhibit neurotransmission in the vagus nerve in the gastrointestinal tract,

TABLE 17-5 Antipsychotics: Receptor-Related Adverse Effects

Receptor	Adverse Effects	Drug Category
Alpha-adrenergic	Postural hypotension, lightheadedness, reflex tachycardia	Low-potency drugs
Dopamine	Extrapyramidal movement disorders, dystonia, parkinsonism, akathisia, tardive dyskinesia	High-potency drugs
Endocrine	Prolactin secretion (galactorrhea, gynecomastia), menstrual changes, sexual dysfunction	Low-potency drugs
Histamine	Sedation, drowsiness, hypotension, weight gain	Low-potency drugs
Muscarinic (cholinergic)	Blurred vision, worsening of angle-closure glaucoma, dry mouth, tachycardia, constipation, urinary retention, decreased sweating	Low-potency drugs

accounts for the ability of certain antipsychotics (e.g., prochlor-perazine) to function as antiemetics (see Chapter 52). Additional blocking of dopamine receptors in the brainstem *reticular system* also allows atypical drugs to have antianxiety effects.

Contraindications

Contraindications to the use of antipsychotic drugs include known drug allergy, comatose state, and, possibly, significant CNS depression, brain damage, liver or kidney disease, blood dyscrasias, or uncontrolled epilepsy.

Adverse Effects

The common adverse effects caused by blockade of the dopamine, muscarinic (cholinergic), histamine, and alpha-adrenergic receptors are listed in Table 17-5. Possible severe hematologic effects include agranulocytosis (lack of *granulocytes* in the blood) and hemolytic anemia. CNS effects include drowsiness, **neuroleptic malignant syndrome, extrapyramidal symptoms,** and **tardive dyskinesia.** Neuroleptic malignant syndrome is a potentially life-threatening adverse effect that may include high fever, unstable blood pressure, and myoglobinemia. Extrapyramidal symptoms are involuntary motor symptoms similar to those associated with Parkinson's disease (see Chapter 16). This drug-induced state is known as *pseudoparkinsonism* and is characterized by symptoms such as **akathisia** (distressing motor restlessness) and acute **dystonia** (painful muscle spasms). Two anticholinergic medications, benztropine (Cogentin) and trihexyphenidyl (Artane), are commonly used to treat these symptoms (see Chapter 16). *Tardive* is a word that means "late appearing." Tardive **dyskinesia** is characterized by involuntary contractions of oral and facial muscles (e. g., involuntary tongue thrusting) and choreoathetosis (wavelike movements of the extremities) and usually appears only after continuous long-term antipsychotic therapy. Theoretically these effects are possible with atypical antipsychotics as well as older drugs. However, evidence suggests that the incidence is lower with the newer drugs.

Cardiovascular effects, caused by alpha receptor blockade, include postural hypotension. In addition, electrocardiogram changes, notably prolonged QT interval, are associated to varying degrees with all classes of antipsychotic drugs. Baseline and periodic electrocardiograms, as well as measurement of serum potassium and magnesium levels, can help determine if a patient is at risk for such effects or diagnose newly acquired cardiac dysrhythmias. The older first-generation drugs such as the phenothiazines and haloperidol can also augment prolactin release, which can result in swelling of the breasts and milk secretion in women taking these drugs. Gynecomastia (breast tissue enlarge-

ment) can also be a distressing adverse effect in male patients. (See also Table 17-2.)

Interactions

Major drug interactions include the following. Antacids and *tannic acids* (also known as *tannins;* found in tea, grapes, wine, etc.) can reduce absorption of antipsychotics when taken with these drugs. Antihypertensives may have additive hypotensive effects and CNS depressants may have additive CNS depressant effects when taken with antipsychotics. Grapefruit juice can enhance the effects of clozapine (by reducing its metabolism) and nicotine can reduce its effects (by speeding its metabolism). (See also Table 17-3.)

Dosages

For the recommended dosages of selected antipsychotic drugs, see the Dosages table on p. 267.

DRUG PROFILES

The first-generation antipsychotic drugs are currently still available on the U.S. market (see Table 17-1). However, their use in common clinical practice has been replaced by the newer-generation or atypical antipsychotic drugs, which, as noted earlier, generally have better adverse effects profiles. All antipsychotics are prescription-only medications that are indicated for the treatment of various psychotic disorders. No single drug stands out as being either more or less effective in the treatment of the symptoms of psychosis. Some of the factors that should be considered before selecting an antipsychotic are the patient's history of response to a drug and the possible adverse effects profile. Patients should be started at a low dose with titration to the lowest effective dose to achieve a balance between symptom relief and adverse effects, if any. Dosage information for profiled drugs appears in the Dosages table on p. 267.

BUTYROPHENONE
haloperidol
Haloperidol (Haldol) is structurally different from the thioxanthenes and the phenothiazines but has similar antipsychotic properties. It is indicated primarily for the long-term treatment of psychosis. However, it has been largely replaced by the newer-generation antipsychotics because of its adverse effects (see later). Haloperidol is contraindicated in patients who have shown a hypersensitivity reaction to it, those in a comatose state, those taking large amounts of CNS depressants, and those with Parkinson's disease. It is a high-potency neuroleptic drug that has a favorable cardiovascular, anticholinergic, and sedative adverse effect profile, but it can cause extrapyramidal symptoms as well as tardive dyskinesia. Haloperidol

is available in three salt forms: base (for oral use), decanoate injection, and lactate injection. Haloperidol decanoate has an extremely long duration of action, which has historically made it useful in treating patients with schizophrenia who were nonadherent with their drug regimen. The lactate formulation is commonly given intravenously in acute situations. It is important to note that, although the manufacturer states that the drug should not be given intravenously, overwhelming clinical experience has shown the intravenous route to be safe and effective. Other adverse effects are listed in Table 17-2. Drugs with which haloperidol interacts include anticholinergics and rifamycins (can reduce haloperidol levels), azole antifungals and fluoxetine (can increase haloperidol levels), and lithium (case reports of CNS depression, encephalopathy, extrapyramidal symptoms, fever, and leukocytosis). Haloperidol is available in both oral and injectable forms.

PHARMACOKINETICS

Route	Onset of Action	Peak Plasma Concentration	Elimination Half-life	Duration of Action
PO	2 hr	2-6 hr	13-35 hr	8-12 hr
IM	Lactate: 20-30 min	Lactate: 30-45 min	13-35 hr	Lactate: 4-8 hr
	Decanoate: 3-9 days	Decanoate: unknown		Decanoate: 1 mo

ATYPICAL ANTIPSYCHOTICS

Between 1975 and 1990 not a single new antipsychotic drug was approved in the United States. In 1990, clozapine (Clozaril), the first of the atypical antipsychotics, was approved. Clozapine was followed by risperidone (Risperdal), olanzapine (Zyprexa), quetiapine (Seroquel), ziprasidone (Geodon), aripiprazole (Abilify), and (in 2006) paliperidone (Invega). The term *atypical antipsychotics* refers to the following advantageous properties of these drugs: reduced effect on prolactin levels compared with older drugs and improvement in the negative symptoms associated with schizophrenia. Although they are still fairly new compared with their first-generation counterparts, they also seem to show a lower risk for neuromuscular malignant syndrome, extrapyramidal adverse effects, and tardive dyskinesia. These new drugs—and several more in clinical trials—are revolutionizing the treatment of psychosis and schizophrenia. For these reasons, atypical antipsychotics are also referred to and recognized as *newer-generation antipsychotic drugs*. All six of the currently available atypical drugs have several pharmacologic properties in common. Antagonist activity at the D_2 receptor is believed to be the mechanism of their antimanic activity. Serotonergic (serotonin agonist) activity at various 5-HT receptor subtypes and alpha$_2$-adrenergic (agonist) activity are both associated with antidepressant activity. Alpha$_1$-adrenergic receptor antagonist activity is associated with orthostatic hypotension and H_1 receptor antagonist activity is associated with both sedative and appetite-stimulating effects. This latter activity accounts for the common adverse effect of weight gain that is associated to various degrees with antipsychotic drugs. This can cause or worsen obesity and even lead to diabetes. Clozapine and olanzapine are associated with the most weight gain, risperidone and quetiapine with less, and ziprasidone is considered weight neutral. Sedative effects may diminish over time and can actually be helpful for patients with insomnia. Although these drugs all have similar pharmacologic properties, they vary in the degree of affinity that each may have for the various types of receptors. These subtle pharmacologic differences, along with often unknown and unpredictable patient physiologic variation, help to explain why some patients respond better (or do not respond) to one medication versus another.

In April 2005, the FDA issued a special public health advisory concerning the use of atypical antipsychotic drugs in elderly patients for off-label (non–FDA-approved) uses. These medications are currently FDA approved for the treatment of schizophrenia and mania. In practice, however, they are also commonly used to control behavioral symptoms of agitation in elderly patients with dementia, including dementia related to Alzheimer's disease. The FDA data, including a meta-analysis combining the data of 17 smaller placebo-controlled studies found that elderly patients given atypical antipsychotics for this reason were up to 1.7 times more likely to die during treatment. The FDA announcement serves to remind prescribers that atypical antipsychotics are not officially indicated for dementia-related behavioral symptoms. The agency also recommends that patients so treated have their treatment plans reevaluated by their prescribers.

Dosage and indication information appears in the Dosages table on p. 267.

clozapine

Clozapine (Clozaril) was the first of the newer-generation or *atypical* antipsychotics. Compared to older-generation antipsychotic drugs, it more selectively blocks the dopaminergic receptors in the *mesolimbic* region of the brain. Older antipsychotic drugs block dopamine receptors in an area of the brain called the *neostriatum,* but blockade in this area is believed to give rise to extrapyramidal adverse effects. Because clozapine has very weak dopamine-blocking abilities in this area of the brain, it is associated with minor or no extrapyramidal symptoms. This often makes clozapine the drug of choice for treatment of psychotic disorders in patients who also have Parkinson's disease, because it will not worsen motor symptoms.

Clozapine has been extremely useful for the treatment of patients for whom therapy with other antipsychotic drugs has failed, especially those with schizophrenia. In particular, it is indicated for schizophrenic patients who have shown high risk for suicidal behavior. Adverse effects include the potential for agranulocytosis, a dangerous disorder of white blood cell (WBC) production that is drug induced. For this reason, patients beginning clozapine therapy require weekly monitoring of WBC counts for the first 6 months of therapy. The drug should be discontinued if the count falls below 3000/mm^3 and withheld until it rises above this value. It is also recommended that WBC counts be evaluated weekly for 4 weeks after discontinuation of the drug. Clozaril is available only through the Clozapine National Registry, with which the patient and prescriber must be registered. Other adverse effects are listed in Table 17-2. Clozapine is contraindicated in patients with known drug allergy; in those with myeloproliferative disorders, severe granulocytopenia, CNS depression, or angle-closure glaucoma; and in comatose patients. Interacting drugs include alcohol and other CNS depressants (increased CNS depression), antihypertensives (risk of hypotension), and others listed in Table 17-3. Clozapine is available only for oral use. Other atypical antipsychotics have features comparable to those of clozapine but do not require extensive WBC monitoring. Risperidone is described in the following profile as an example of these drugs. An orally disintegrating tablet form of clozapine, called FazaClo, is now available. This may improve compliance, because the tablet dissolves in the patient's mouth. The usual dosage is the same as that for regular tablets (see the Dosages table).

PHARMACOKINETICS

Route	Onset of Action	Peak Plasma Concentration	Elimination Half-life	Duration of Action
PO	1-6 hr	Weeks	6 hr	4-12 hr

◆ risperidone

Risperidone (Risperdal) is another atypical antipsychotic that was introduced a few years after clozapine. It is even more active than clozapine at the serotonin (5-HT$_{2A}$ and 5-HT$_{2C}$) receptors. It also has a high affinity for alpha$_1$- and alpha$_2$-adrenergic receptors and histamine H$_1$ receptors. This drug is indicated for schizophrenia, including negative symptoms, and causes minimal extrapyramidal adverse effects at therapeutic dosages of 1 to 6 mg/day.

Risperidone is contraindicated in cases of known drug allergy. Adverse effects include elevated prolactin levels, abnormal dreams, insomnia, dizziness, headache, and others listed in Table 17-2. Drugs interacting with risperidone include CNS depressants, antihypertensives, and others listed in Table 17-3. Risperidone is available for oral and injectable use. The long-acting injectable form is called Risperdal Consta, and one intramuscular injection lasts approximately 2 weeks. This is at least one option for helping patients maintain adherence with the prescribed drug regimen. Patients must continue to take oral risperidone for 3 weeks after the first injection of the Consta dosage form to ensure adequate blood levels from the injection.

PHARMACOKINETICS

Route	Onset of Action	Peak Plasma Concentration	Elimination Half-life	Duration of Action
PO	1-2 wk	Unknown	20-30 hr	7 days
IM	3 wk	Unknown	20-30 hr	2 wk

LIFE SPAN CONSIDERATIONS: The Elderly Patient

Psychotherapeutic Drugs

- Elderly patients show higher serum levels of psychotherapeutic drugs because they have age-related changes in drug distribution and metabolism, less serum albumin, decreased lean body mass, less water in tissues, and increased body fat. They also have decreased renal function. Because of these changes, elderly patients generally require lower dosages of antipsychotic and antidepressant drugs and are at greater risk for toxicity.
- Orthostatic hypotension, anticholinergic adverse effects, sedation, and extrapyramidal symptoms are more common in elderly patients taking psychotherapeutic drugs.
- Careful evaluation and documentation of baseline parameters, including neurologic findings, are important to the safe use of these drugs.
- Increased anxiety is often associated with the use of tricyclic antidepressants.
- Patients with a history of cardiac disease may be at a greater risk for experiencing dysrhythmias, tachycardia, stroke, myocardial infarction, or heart failure.
- Lithium is more toxic in elderly patients and lower dosages are often necessary. Close monitoring is important to its safe use in this age group. Central nervous system toxicity, lithium-induced goiter, and hypothyroidism are more common in elderly patients.

NURSING PROCESS

Assessment

Before any of the psychotherapeutic drugs is administered, a complete head-to-toe physical assessment and mental status examination should be completed and documented. The data obtained will serve as a comparative baseline for the patient during and after initiation of therapy. The patient's neurologic functioning should be thoroughly assessed, including level of consciousness, mental alertness, and level of motor and cognitive functioning. The Mini-Mental State Examination (MMSE) is one tool that may be used to assess cognitive status and help identify impairments often found in many mental illnesses. The MMSE is simple to use, is cost effective, and can be completed in about 20 minutes by the nurse or clinician. This tool is available in most nursing assessment, nursing fundamentals, and/or psychiatric or mental health nursing textbooks. Points are scored in the areas of patient level of orientation, attention and calculation ability, recall, and language skills. Other mental health assessment tools include the six-item Blessed Orientation-Memory-Concentration Test, clock drawing tasks and Functional Activities Questionnaire (for those with dementia), Alzheimer's Disease Assessment Scale, Mattis Dementia Rating Scale, Severe Impairment Battery, and Hamilton Rating Scale for Depression. In addition to performing examinations such as these, the nurse should note baseline levels of motor responses and reflexes, as well as the presence of any tremors and/or personality changes. The patient should also be assessed for the presence of cold clammy hands, sweating, and pallor, because these findings may indicate an altered autonomic nervous system response.

Constant assessment for any suicidal ideations or tendencies is important, with attention not only to overt cues and behaviors but also to covert thoughts and ideation. This is important because of the potential for suicide with psychotherapeutic drugs, with or without the concurrent use of other medications or alcohol. Suicide assessment tools are available and may be helpful in identifying an individual's risk for suicidal behaviors. One such tool, the Suicide Assessment Scale, has been found to be valid, reliable, and easy to use. The following are some questions that may be helpful: "What brings you to the doctor's office today?" "How has life been treating you?" "What are some of your worries or concerns?" "How would you describe your mood?" "Tell me about your thoughts." Should an assessment reveal any concerns and/or the patient acknowledge suicidal thoughts, the appropriate referral should be made for immediate assessment and/or treatment.

One must also remember that many of the patients who require psychotherapeutic drugs are so mentally distressed that their physical needs often go unmet. Their mental state leads to a complexity of other problems, such as insomnia, poor health status, and weight loss or gain. Each of these areas should be assessed (i.e., sleep, eating habits, physical history) so that a baseline is documented for comparative purposes. Drug allergies as well as any contraindications, cautions, and potential drug interactions should also be noted (see pharmacology discussion and Table 17-3). Blood pressure, pulse rate, and body temperature should be assessed and documented before, during, and after drug therapy. Postural blood pressures (i.e., blood pressure taken supine then standing) are particularly important to note because of the possible drug-related adverse effects of postural hypotension and dizziness. The more potent, older drugs, such as MAOIs or TCAs, may lead to a significant drop in blood pressure and warrant even more skillful assessment and close monitoring.

Results of any laboratory studies performed before and during the drug therapy should be reviewed. This is especially important

Psychotherapeutic Drugs

- Pediatric patients are more likely to experience adverse effects from psychotropic drugs, especially extrapyramidal effects.
- The incidence of Reye's syndrome and other adverse reactions is greater in pediatric patients who have had chickenpox, central nervous system infections, measles, acute illnesses, or dehydration and are taking psychotropic drugs.
- Lithium may lead to decreased bone density or bone formation in children; therefore, children receiving it should be closely monitored for signs and symptoms of lithium toxicity and bone disorders.
- Tricyclic antidepressants generally are not prescribed for patients younger than 12 years of age. However, some antidepressants are used in children with enuresis, attention deficit disorders, and major depressive disorders, and may be associated with adverse reactions such as electrocardiographic changes, nervousness, sleep disorder, fatigue, elevated blood pressure, and gastrointestinal upset.
- Pediatric patients are generally more sensitive to the effects of most drugs, and psychotherapeutic drugs are no exception. Nurses should be aware of the risk of toxicity, which can be fatal. Should confusion, lethargy, visual disturbances, insomnia, tremors, palpitations, constipation, or eye pain occur, the prescriber should be contacted immediately.

for patients who are receiving long-term drug therapy to prevent or identify any early complications or other possible adverse effects or toxicity. Laboratory studies may include, but are not limited to, tests to confirm therapeutic serum levels of the specific drug and, if appropriate, a complete blood cell count, erythrocyte sedimentation rate, serum electrolyte levels, glucose levels, BUN level, liver function studies, serum level of vitamin B_{12}, and thyroid studies. If the patient is experiencing forms of dementia, other types of testing may be needed, such as genetic studies, computed tomographic scanning, or magnetic resonance imaging.

With psychotherapeutic drug therapy, the nurse should assess the patient's mouth to make sure the patient has swallowed the entire oral dosage. This helps to prevent hoarding or cheeking of medications, a form of noncompliance that may lead to drug toxicity or overdose. If the assessment shows that this is a potential risk, the use of liquid dosage forms, when available, may minimize such problems. The assessment should also address appetite, sleeping patterns, addictive behaviors, elimination difficulties, hypersensitivity, and other symptoms, and the findings should be documented.

Antianxiety Drugs

Antianxiety drugs, specifically the benzodiazepines, are associated with many contraindications, cautions, and drug interactions (see pharmacology discussion).

When these drugs are used, the prescriber may order laboratory studies, such as complete blood cell counts, serum electrolyte levels, and liver and kidney function tests (see earlier discussion). Blood pressure readings are also very important to assess because of drug-related postural hypotension. The baseline neurologic examination should include assessment of alertness, orientation, and sensory and motor functioning. Any complaints of ataxia, headache, or other neurologic abnormalities should be

noted. A thorough medication profile should be compiled that includes all of the psychotherapeutic drugs taken, with documentation about other prescription drugs, over-the-counter drugs, vitamins, minerals, and herbal products the patient uses. Diazepam, although one of the more commonly prescribed benzodiazepines, is generally used for seizure disorders and preoperative sedation and requires assessment related to these uses (see Chapters 12 and 15). Specific concerns for pediatric and elderly patients are presented in the boxes on pp. 277 and 278. Elderly patients must be closely observed and assessed for oversedation and/or profound CNS depression during drug therapy. The elderly are often more sensitive to drugs and therefore more likely to experience adverse effects, and their safety should be a constant concern.

Eye problems may occur with the benzodiazepines, and thus baseline visual testing using a Snellen chart or an eye examination conducted by the appropriate health care provider (e.g., an ophthalmologist or optometrist) is needed. Allergic reactions to some of these medications, such as clonazepam, are characterized by a red, raised rash and should be noted. In addition, obese patients may experience toxicity in a shorter period of time than those who are not obese. This occurs because several antianxiety drugs are lipid soluble and have greater affinity for fatty tissues; therefore their half-life is increased in patients who are obese. Lorazepam should be given cautiously (under very close supervision) if the patient is suicidal because its use is associated with suicide attempts, and alprazolam should be administered only after very careful assessment of mental status, mood, sensorium, and sleep patterns as well as evaluation for anxiety or dizziness.

Some benzodiazepines are also associated with medication errors because of the existence of sound-alike or look-alike drugs. Assessing the drug order for the right drug is important because of the possibility of such an error and the negative consequences to the patient. Benzodiazepine drugs and the sound-alike medications with which they could be confused include the following: Klonopin (clonazepam) and clonidine; diazepam and Ditropan (oxybutynin); lorazepam and alprazolam; Versed (midazolam) and VePesid (etoposide) and Vistaril (hydroxyzine).

Buspirone is another antianxiety drug that is not a benzodiazepine. It is used because it has fewer adverse effects such as sedation and lack of dependency potential. However, it is associated with many drug interactions, cautions, and contraindications (see pharmacology discussion). General assessment of the neurologic system and a mental health assessment are also important to complete.

Antimanic Drugs

Before antimanic drugs such as lithium are administered, a thorough neurologic examination should be performed, and vital signs, especially blood pressure, should be assessed. Hydration status, dietary intake, skin tone, and presence of edema are also important to assess and document. Baseline levels of consciousness and alertness, gait and mobility levels, and overall motor functioning are also important to assess, because poor coordination, tremors, and weakness may be symptoms of toxic blood levels of antimanic drugs. Laboratory studies often ordered before and during drug therapy are serum sodium, albumin, and uric acid levels. A urinalysis, including urine specific gravity, may also be ordered. Serum levels of sodium are important to know because lithium toxicity is potentiated by the presence of hyponatremia and hypovolemia. In addition, serum lithium levels must be assessed once drug therapy is initiated and usually every 3 to 4 days, especially during the initial phase of therapy. In general, with lithium it is best to measure the levels 8 to 12 hours after the dose of drug (therapeutic levels are 0.6 to 1.2 mEq/L; toxic levels are above 1.5 mEq/L). It is also important to determine what other medications are being used for mood stabilization, such as antiepileptic drugs (see Chapter 15) and dopamine agonists (see Chapter 16). These drugs are often used as adjunctive therapies but must be fully understood prior to their use.

Antidepressants

There are many cautions, contraindications, and drug interactions for which to assess before giving antidepressants (see pharmacology discussion). Continuous assessment for any suicidal ideations or tendencies is important, because indicators of suicide risk may be covert as well as overt. Suicide should always be considered a potential risk when any psychotherapeutic medication, whether an antidepressant or other CNS-altering drug, is taken either alone or in combination with other drugs or alcohol.

The newer-generation antidepressants such as the SSRIs (e.g., fluoxetine) are associated with fewer and less severe adverse effects than the older antidepressants. Assessment of cardiac, neuromuscular systems and mental state would be important to document. These systems are important to assess because of the signs and symptoms of serotonin syndrome, such as agitation, tachycardia, tremors, sweating and muscle tremors. Contraindications, cautions, and drug interactions have been previously discussed and need to be thoroughly assessed for and documented.

Because the newer antidepressants are associated with fewer and less potent adverse effects, only very few MAOIs are used today in psychiatric mental health settings. Patients receiving these drugs who have a history of suicide attempts or suicidal ideations, or who have seizure disorders, hyperactivity, diabetes, or psychosis need to be closely monitored. Suicidal thoughts and suicide attempts are important to consider, because these drugs may be hoarded by the patient and then used to carry out suicide. These patients should be under the care of a health care professional (such as a psychiatrist, physician, or nurse practitioner) so that they may be closely monitored for destructive behaviors. MAOIs are also known for their potentiation of hypertensive

crisis when taken concurrently with SSRIs, meperidine, TCAs, and foods containing tyramine (see Table 17-4); thus blood pressure readings, including postural blood pressure measurements, must be monitored closely. Postural hypotension leads to a high risk of dizziness, fainting, and possible falls or injury. If the patient is hospitalized, supine/standing or sitting blood pressures should be monitored at least every 8 hours or more frequently, if needed. The nurse should wait 1 to 2 minutes after taking the supine blood pressure before measuring standing or sitting pressure and pulse rate. Laboratory tests that are often ordered for patients taking these drugs include complete blood counts and renal and liver function studies. In addition, it is crucial to understand that elderly patients should be given these drugs only if it is deemed absolutely necessary by the prescriber and only with careful monitoring. The extrapyramidal adverse effects (e.g., tremors) are often worse in the elderly and may result in inability to perform activities of daily living. This extrapyramidal reaction may lead to progressive deterioration of motor activities, and therefore a thorough baseline motor and neurologic assessment is needed. A hyperthermic crisis may occur if MAOIs are used with the antihypertensive drug, clonidine (thus the need for frequent temperature monitoring).

With second-generation antidepressants, cautious use in the elderly and cardiac patients is important. Bupropion may be preferred over other antidepressants because it has fewer anticholinergic, antiadrenergic, and cardiotoxic effects. However, patient age and the findings of an assessment of the patient's neurologic status, mental status, and cardiac systems should be documented before the drug is used. The onset of action of many of the second-generation antidepressants should be noted as well, because, as with bupropion, therapeutic effects may be delayed for up to 4 weeks. This information is also important for the safety of the patient, because of the need to closely watch the patient during this period for any suicidal tendencies or ideas. Availability of family support systems and other supportive resources for the patient should be assessed so that proper resources may be used, as needed. Because of the risk for seizures associated with second-generation antidepressants, patients with a history of seizures should be identified so that another medication may be used, if ordered. Third-generation antidepressants have several advantages over the older classes of antidepressants but still have contraindications, cautions, and drug interactions (see previous discussion). Concurrent use of third-generation antidepressants and any of the SSRI drugs carries the risk for serotonin syndrome and should be avoided. The patient should be assessed for serotonin syndrome (see Box 17-1).

Bupropion use is contraindicated in patients who have a known drug allergy, those with a seizure disorder (bupropion can lower the seizure threshold), those who currently have anorexia nervosa or bulimia or have had one of these disorders in the past, and those currently taking an MAOI. Common adverse effects include dizziness, confusion, tachycardia, agitation, tremor, and dry mouth.

▌ Antipsychotics

The use of antipsychotics requires careful assessment of all body systems, and assessment of cardiovascular, cerebrovascular, neurologic, gastrointestinal, genitourinary, renal, hepatic, and hematologic functioning is important to safe and efficacious drug therapy. The presence of significant disease in one or several organ systems may lead to a more adverse response to a drug and may even be dose limiting; thus, a careful and skillful assessment of the patient is needed before and during drug therapy. Weight gain may occur, and if the patient is experiencing deleterious health effects because of this, another drug may be ordered. Suicidal ideations, orthostatic changes in blood pressure, extrapyramidal symptoms, confusion, headache, gastrointestinal upset, abnormal muscle movements, rashes, photosensitivity, and dry

mouth may be associated with many of these drugs, so a thorough nursing history and mental status examination should be carried out and the findings documented before drug therapy is begun. The nurse should identify possible drug interactions with any prescription drugs, over-the-counter medications, and/or herbals the patient is taking should be identified, as well as any conditions that represent cautions or contraindications to use of the antipsychotic drug (see pharmacology discussion). The phenothiazine antipsychotics may still be prescribed in some situations but are mentioned here mainly for historical purposes. These antipsychotics are associated with significant extrapyramidal adverse effects (see earlier discussion) as well as with anticholinergic adverse effects such as dry mouth, urinary hesitancy, and constipation.

Haloperidol is similar to other high-potency antipsychotics, because its sedating effects are low but the incidence of extrapyramidal symptoms is high (see pharmacology discussion). Assessment of baseline motor, sensory, and neurologic functioning is therefore very important to patient safety. With some of the antipsychotic drugs, patients may experience adverse effects of tremors and muscle twitching from the drug's blockade of dopamine receptors (dopamine generally has an inhibitory effect on specific motor activity in the musculoskeletal system). These extrapyramidal movements are like those in parkinsonism (see Chapter 16) and may be very bothersome and uncomfortable. Therefore, it is important to document the patient's baseline motor and sensory functions and assess for underlying movement disturbances so that the best therapy can be selected.

Atypical antipsychotics such as clozapine and risperidone have many contraindications, cautions, and drug interactions (see previous pharmacology discussion). A thorough mental status examination should be performed and the findings documented before initiation of treatment with these and other antipsychotic drugs. An assessment of musculoskeletal functioning and monitoring for any extrapyramidal reaction is also important to patient safety. Liver and renal function studies, complete blood count, and urinalysis should be monitored before and during therapy. Blood pressure readings should be documented with close attention to postural readings. A drop of 20 mm Hg or more in the systolic blood pressure requires immediate attention and implementation of safety precautions. In addition, for the elderly patient, the prescriber may order reduced dosages to help prevent toxicity. These drugs are also associated with a high degree of sedation and should be used only when absolutely necessary and with extreme caution (close monitoring) in the elderly and other patients who are at risk for falls or have limited motor and sensory capabilities. Patients taking these drugs also require careful monitoring of heart sounds and observation for any abnormal heart rhythms.

Nursing Diagnoses

- Risk for injury related to the disease state and possible adverse effects of medications
- Impaired social interaction related to various inadequacies felt by the patient due to illness or isolation from others
- Imbalanced nutrition, less than body requirements, related to the consequences of illness and/or the medication used to treat it
- Sleep deprivation related to the mental illness and/or related drug therapy

- Situational low self-esteem related to the disease process and the adverse effects of medication, including sexual dysfunction
- Constipation related to treatment with psychotherapeutic drugs
- Urinary retention related treatment with psychotherapeutic drugs
- Deficient knowledge related to lack of information about the specific psychotherapeutic drugs and their adverse effects
- Sexual dysfunction related to treatment with psychotherapeutic drugs

Planning
Goals

- Patient does not sustain injury while taking medication.
- Patient experiences no further deterioration in thought processes.
- Patient exhibits improved nutritional status.
- Patient regains normal sleep patterns.
- Patient exhibits (overtly and internally) a more positive self-image.
- Patient remains free of any alterations in urinary elimination patterns.
- Patient remains free of altered bowel elimination patterns.
- Patient remains adherent with the therapy regimen.
- Patient is free of complications associated with the drug and with food-drug interactions.
- Patient is free of problems in sexual function.

Outcome Criteria

- Patient is free from falls, dizziness, and fainting attributable to drug adverse effects.
- Patient demonstrates improved or no deterioration in thought processes and is less hostile, withdrawn, and delusional once medication has reached a steady-state level.
- Patient demonstrates more open and appropriate behavior and communication with health care team and significant others.
- Patient shows healthy nutritional habits with appropriate weight gain and a diet that includes foods from the U.S. Department of Agriculture food pyramid *(http://www. mypyramid.gov).*
- Patient reports sleeping better and feeling more rested.
- Patient openly discusses feelings of poor self-image and self-concept with staff.
- Patient reports any problems with urinary retention and identifies measures to reduce its occurrence.
- Patient reports any difficulty with constipation if not manageable by fluids and dietary changes.
- Patient states the importance of taking medications exactly as prescribed at the same time every day and without omissions.
- Patient states the importance of keeping appointments with the prescriber or other health care providers to track improvement and monitor therapy.
- Patient states the common adverse effects of the medication being taken and those adverse effects that should be reported to the prescriber (e.g., confusion or changes in level of consciousness).
- Patient lists the medications and foods to be avoided while taking any psychotherapeutic medication.
- Patient reports any problems with sexual function.

Implementation

Regardless of the psychotherapeutic drug prescribed, several general nursing actions are important for safe administration. First and foremost is demonstration of a firm but patient attitude combined with therapeutic communication. Simple explanations about the drug, its action, and the length of time before therapeutic effects can be expected should be given after the patient's reading level and an effective means of teaching and learning have been established. A thorough psychosocial and holistic approach should always be adopted when caring for any patient with any illness. Vital signs should be monitored and the findings documented, especially during the initiation of therapy. Of great concern is administration of these medications to those who are elderly and to patients with a history of hypertension and cardiac disease. Generally speaking, all of the psychotherapeutic drugs should be taken exactly as prescribed and at the same time every day and without failure. If omission occurs, the prescriber should be contacted immediately. Abrupt withdrawal may have negative affects on the patient's physical and mental status. Help should be solicited from family members or others providing support so that there are options for assistance with drug administration. Adherence to the medication regimen is crucial to effective management, and all support systems and resources should be utilized to accomplish this.

Antianxiety Drugs

Specific nursing interventions related to the use of antianxiety drugs include frequent monitoring of vital signs with special attention to blood pressure and postural blood pressures; encouraging the use of elastic compression stockings and changing positions slowly to minimize dizziness and falls from orthostatic hypotension; creating a therapeutic environment for open communication—especially of all disturbing thoughts, including those of suicide; checking the patient's oral cavities for hoarding or "cheeking" of drugs; dispensing medications only as ordered to help minimize the risk for suicide attempts; using intravenous routes of administration only as prescribed and giving the drug over the recommended time with the proper diluent and at a rate indicated by the manufacturer and prescriber; and always administering intramuscular dosage forms in a large muscle mass and only as ordered or indicated (see Chapter 10 for more information on parenteral administration). See Patient Teaching Tips for more information.

Antimanic Drugs

Safe use of the antimanic drug lithium depends on adequate hydration and electrolyte status, because lithium may become toxic with dehydration and hyponatremia. See Patient Teaching Tips for more information.

Antidepressants

Antidepressants must be administered carefully and exactly as ordered. With antidepressants as well as other psychotherapeutic drugs, it is important to emphasize that it may take several weeks before therapeutic effects are evident. The nurse must make sure the patients understands this and continues to take the medication as prescribed—even if the patient feels his or her condition is not improving. Carefully monitoring the patient, being readily available, and providing supportive care during this time is critical to therapeutic effectiveness. The period before therapeutic effects are seen may be the time the patient is at highest risk for self-harm and/or suicide. Other nursing considerations include taking the drug(s) with food and at least 4 to 6 oz of fluid; assisting with ambulation and other activities if patient is weak, elderly or dizzy (from postural hypotension); and counseling patients about potential sexual dysfunction if appropriate and if an adverse effect of the drug. If sexual dysfunction occurs, information about various options should be shared (e.g., waiting to see if the adverse effect resolves, reducing the current dosage of the drug as ordered, taking a "drug holiday" if ordered by the prescriber). A drug holiday generally occurs in a hospital setting and the drug is removed but only under very close monitoring. See Patient Teaching Tips for more information.

Specific nursing interventions for MAOIs and TCAs include the education of adverse effects, drug and food interactions, keeping a list of all medications on their person and changing positions purposely and slowly. All health care providers should be informed that the patient is taking these drugs and weaning should occur when these drugs are to be discontinued. With TCAs, the patient should be told to report the following to their prescriber should they occur: blurred vision, excessive drowsiness, sleepiness, urinary retention, and constipation. It is also important to inform patients that with some of the second- and third-generation antidepressants, therapeutic effects may not be evident for up to 4 to 6 weeks and that tolerance to sedation will occur.

Antipsychotics

Patients need to be aware that these drugs should be taken exactly as prescribed to be effective. Different levels of paranoia or delusions may lead to suspicion and mistrust of the nurse and other members of the health care team, so maintaining a sufficient level of trust through consistency, empathy, and the establishment of therapeutic communication will be a key to compliance. Adherence/compliance is always a critical issue for patients with psychotic illnesses, because these patients are at higher risk for not taking medications and not keeping follow-up appointments. Nonadherence to the medical and treatment regimen is of major concern, because the serum levels of drugs such as haloperidol must be within a specified therapeutic range for the patient to feel better and be functional. If serum levels of haloperidol are less than 4 ng/mL, the patient may show symptoms of the mental disorder, whereas levels higher than 22 ng/mL may result in toxicity. Therefore, selection of an antipsychotic drug and its dosage, route of administration, risk for toxicity, and/or suicidal potential, as well as therapeutic communications and patient education, are all important factors for successful therapy. Because most antipsychotic drugs are quite potent, the nurse must be sure that oral dosage forms have actually been swallowed and have not been intentionally hidden in the side of the mouth ("cheeking") or under the tongue to be discarded at a later time or combined with other doses into an overdose that can have a potentially lethal outcome. Oral forms of the antipsychotics are generally well absorbed and will cause less gastrointestinal upset if taken with food or a full glass of water. Sucking on hard candy or gum may help to relieve dry mouth. With any of the dosage forms, perspiration may be increased; therefore, patients should be encouraged to avoid engaging in excessive activity or being exposed to heat or humidity. Excessive sweating can lead to dehydration and then drug toxicity.

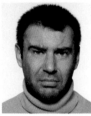
Haloperidol may not necessarily be the best drug to use because of the risk for undermedication or overmedication and troubling adverse effects (see Table 17-2). Therefore, other antipsychotics (e.g., clozapine and risperidone) may be preferred, as previously discussed. Clozapine and risperidone are therapeutically effective and carry a minimal risk of tardive dyskinesia and extrapyramidal symptoms. In addition, they usually lead to improvement in cognitive behavior. Clozapine should be taken as ordered and is usually given in divided doses; proper dosing is very important to therapeutic effectiveness. If any changes in blood counts (e.g., leukopenia) are noted or if abnormal cardiac functioning (e.g., tachycardia) is identified, the prescriber should be contacted immediately. In such a case, the medication may need to be discontinued, but only as ordered, and the patient monitored closely. Titration of doses of clozapine, either upward or downward, should also be done carefully with close monitoring of the patient for any exacerbation of the mental illness or suicidal tendencies.

Risperidone should be given as ordered and is administered by injection into a deep muscle mass. Hospital or facility policy and drug insert guidelines regarding the administration of this drug should be checked. Intramuscular injection dosage forms may be ordered along with oral doses of risperidone or possibly of another antipsychotic drug for several weeks, with maintenance doses of an intramuscular injection given every 2 to 4 weeks, as ordered. It is important to the integrity of tissue and muscle mass to always alternate intramuscular injection sites and to be sure that the site is not red, swollen, or irritated. Any changes must be documented and reported. Oral solution, tablets, and orally disintegrating tabs are other available dosage forms. Oral solutions should not be given with cola or tea, and the disintegrating tabs should be dissolved under the tongue before swallowing with or without liquid. The prescriber's orders for administering the drug should be followed. The daily amount is usually given in two divided doses, with dosage decreased in the elderly and in those with impaired renal or hepatic function. Any excess sedation, anxiety, extrapyramidal symptoms, tardive dyskinesia, or strokelike symptoms should be reported immediately. Measuring vital signs and monitoring for any postural hypotension is also important during treatment.

Once therapy with any of the antipsychotic drugs has been initiated, it is important for the nurse and other health care providers involved in the patient's care to monitor drug therapy closely, including measuring serum drug levels during follow-up visits. If the patient is suspected of being nonadherent and serum drug levels are subtherapeutic, the patient should be reevaluated by the prescriber for a possible change of drug or dosage form. The parenteral dosage forms usually come in a depot (longer-releasing) dosage formulation that releases the drug over 2 to 4 weeks, which leads to increased compliance and often a better therapeutic outcome.

Patient education (see Patient Teaching Tips) and patient adherence with the drug regimen are keys to successful treatment, regardless of the mental illness. Often it is the mental disorder itself that causes patient nonadherence. Keeping communication open with the patient, family, and/or caregiver is important to develop trust and a sense of empathy. Although patient education may have been thorough, it is always best to emphasize that the patient can call the prescriber, clinic, or hotline 24 hours a day. Phone numbers should be updated and shared frequently with the patient. Professional counseling with a mental health care provider (psychiatrist, nurse practitioner, or other licensed mental health professional) should be available as needed so that the patient's progress is consistently monitored. Group therapy and support groups are also available for the patient and significant others.

Evaluation

Both the therapeutic effects of psychotherapeutic medications and the patient's progress must be monitored before and during drug therapy. Mental alertness, cognition, affect, mood, ability to carry out activities of daily living, appetite, and sleep patterns are all areas that need to be closely monitored and documented. The patient must continue with other forms of therapy, in addition to drug therapy, with the goal of acquiring more effective coping skills. Other forms of treatment may include intense psychotherapy, relaxation therapy, stress reduction, and lifestyle changes. It is important to mention that blood levels of these drugs will be measured during follow-up visits to ensure that therapeutic levels are maintained. Such monitoring of serum drug levels helps identify both subtherapeutic and toxic levels.

The therapeutic effects of *antianxiety drugs* are evidenced by improved mental alertness, cognition, and mood; fewer anxiety and panic attacks; improved sleep patterns and appetite; more interest in self and others; less tension and irritability; and fewer feelings of fear, impending doom, and stress. Adverse effects to watch for in patients taking antianxiety drugs include hypotension, lethargy, fatigue, drowsiness, confusion, constipation, dry mouth, blood dyscrasias, lightheadedness, and insomnia. In general, adverse reactions to antidepressants consist of drowsiness, dry mouth, constipation, dizziness, postural hypotension, sedation, blood dyscrasias, and tremors. Overdose is evidenced by

irritability, agitation, CNS irritability, seizures, and then progression to CNS depression with respiratory or cardiac depression.

Therapeutic effects of lithium are decreased mania and stabilization of the patient's mood. Lithium is usually better tolerated by the patient during the manic phase. Therapeutic levels of lithium range from 0.6 to 1.2 mEq/L, and blood levels should be determined frequently, every few days initially and then at least every few months while the patient is taking the drug. The nurse should also monitor the patient's mood, affect, and emotional stability. Adverse reactions to lithium include dysrhythmias, hypotension, sedation, slurred speech, slowed motor abilities, and weight gain. Gastrointestinal symptoms such as diarrhea and vomiting, drowsiness, weakness, and unsteady gait are indicative of overdose. The prescriber should be consulted immediately if these occur.

When used as *antidepressants*, SSRIs may take up to 8 weeks to reach full therapeutic effect. A therapeutic response to these drugs includes improved depression or mental status, improved ability to carry out activities of daily living, less insomnia, and improved mood disorder with minimal adverse effects of weight gain, sedation, headache, insomnia, gastrointestinal complaints, dizziness, agitation, and sexual dysfunction. The patient should be monitored for symptoms of serotonin syndrome. Other therapeutic effects of these and other antidepressants are improved sleep patterns and nutrition, increased feelings of self-esteem, decreased feelings of hopelessness, and an increased interest in self and appearance. MAOIs and TCAs may also take up to 4 weeks to reach full therapeutic effectiveness. Adverse effects include sedation, dry mouth, constipation, postural hypotension, blurred vision, seizures, and tremors. Toxic reactions may be manifested by confusion or hypotension and possibly by respiratory or cardiac distress. Patients taking clozapine should exhibit improvement in their schizophrenic state. Evaluation for adverse effects should include monitoring of blood counts. It is important to remember that this drug is associated with minor or no extrapyramidal symptoms.

The therapeutic effects of haloperidol are similar to those of the other antipsychotic drugs, but the nurse should monitor the patient for adverse reactions that are specific to haloperidol. These include sedation; ticlike trembling movements of the hands, face, neck, and head; hypotension; and dry mouth. Overdose is manifested by severe sedation, hypotension, respiratory depression, and coma. It takes approximately 3 weeks for the therapeutic effects of haloperidol to appear, but it is still important for the nurse to monitor the patient for possible abnormal movements and trembling during this early period. Should these occur, the nurse should consult the prescriber immediately. The therapeutic effects of the antipsychotic drugs include improvement in mood and affect, and alleviation of the psychotic symptoms and episodes. Emotional instability, hallucinations, paranoia, delusions, garbled speech, and inability to cope should begin to abate once the patient has been taking the medication for several weeks. It is critical that the nurse carefully monitor the patient's potential to injure self or others during the delay between the start of therapy and symptomatic improvement.

PATIENT TEACHING TIPS

Antianxiety Drugs

- Patients should be encouraged to move around and change positions slowly, especially when rising from a sitting or reclining position, to avoid dizziness or fainting. Operating heavy machinery and driving should be avoided until the adverse effects of sedation or drowsiness have resolved.
- Educate about the development of tolerance to the sedating properties of benzodiazepines.
- Over-the-counter drugs or herbals should not be taken without seeking advice from the prescriber.
- Keep these and all psychotherapeutic drugs out of the reach of children. Alcohol and other CNS depressants should be avoided.
- A medical alert or other identification bracelet or necklace recording the patient's diagnosis should always be worn, and a list of the patient's drugs and allergies should be carried by the patient at all times. The drug list should be updated at least every 3 months.
- Medications should be taken exactly as ordered, and sudden withdrawal is to be avoided. If withdrawal of drug is needed, tapering/weaning of doses is needed.
- The prescriber should be contacted immediately if there is a lack of improvement or with an increase in fears, anxiety, or feelings of despair as well as excessive adverse effects.

Antimanic Drugs

- Lithium should be taken at the same time each day and specific instructions given on how to handle missed doses.
- The patient should be told that the adverse effects of lithium are usually transient but excessive tremors, increased thirst and urination, nausea, diarrhea, anorexia, muscle weakness, dizziness, syncope, and excessive sedation should be reported to the prescriber immediately.
- Encourage adequate hydration, with consumption of up to 8 to 10 glasses of water daily if not contraindicated.
- Follow-up visits with the prescriber are important so that serum drug levels and fluid and electrolyte status can be monitored to help decrease toxicity and maximize therapeutic effects.

Antidepressant Drugs

- Increased intake of dietary fiber and fluids to help minimize constipation should be encouraged. Fiber should be taken at least 2 hours before or after the dosing of medication to avoid interference with drug absorption.
- Measures to help with dry mouth include using saliva substitutes, chewing gum, and allowing hard candy to dissolve in the mouth. Sugar-free forms of candy and gum are available.
- Should sedation and drowsiness continue for longer than 2 to 3 weeks, the prescriber should be contacted immediately.
- Encourage the patient to openly discuss any concerns about the medication and adverse effects such as gastrointestinal upset, sexual dysfunction, or weight gain.
- Educate that discontinuation of SSRIs requires a tapering period of up to 1 to 2 months as ordered. Discontinuation syndrome

may occur without a tapering period; this includes symptoms of dizziness, diarrhea, movement disorders, insomnia, irritability, visual disturbance, lethargy, anorexia, and lowered mood.
- Provide a listing of drug-drug interactions, such as the strong interaction between SSRIs and MAOIs, St. John's wort (an herbal product), and tryptophan (a serotonin precursor found in foods). Such interactions may pose a risk for serotonin syndrome (see earlier discussion). Cold products and over-the-counter medications should always be approved by the prescriber.
- When the transdermal patch is used, the patient should be cautioned to avoid exposing the patch to external sources of heat, such as a heating pad, electric blanket, sauna, or even prolonged direct sunlight. The patch site should be rotated with each application; the patch should be placed on a nonhairy, healthy area, and any residue from the previous patch should be gently cleaned off before the new patch is applied.

Monoamine Oxidase Inhibitors and Tricyclic Antidepressants

- The prescriber should be contacted if any of the following signs and symptoms of overdosage or toxicity occur: increased pulse rate; seizure activity; changes in breathing, memory, or alertness; or restlessness.
- The patient should be made aware that therapeutic drug effects may be delayed for up to 4 weeks for MAOIs.
- If the patient is taking an MAOI, the patient should be cautioned to avoid over-the-counter cold and flu products. Foods or beverages high in tyramine should also be avoided (see Table 17-4). Combining these drugs with tyramine leads to serious elevations in blood pressure, heart palpitations or rapid heartbeat, neck stiffness, nausea and/or vomiting, and severe headache. Should these problems occur, the patient must seek out medical care immediately, because the drug interaction–related hypertensive crisis may lead to stroke.
- When the patient is taking a TCA, any blurred vision, excessive drowsiness or sleepiness, urinary retention, or constipation should be reported to the prescriber.
- Encourage wearing of a medical alert necklace or bracelet showing the diagnosis and a list of current drugs.

Haloperidol and Other Antipsychotics

- Hot baths, saunas, and hot climates should be avoided because of the risk of further drop in blood pressure, especially upon standing (postural hypotension). Injury to self may occur due to dizziness or fainting.
- Haloperidol and other antipsychotics should never be stopped abruptly because of the high risk of inducing a withdrawal psychosis.
- Sun exposure and tanning booths should be avoided. The patient should be encouraged to apply sunscreen liberally and wear sun-protective clothing or hats.
- Any sore throat, malaise, fever, or bleeding should be reported to the prescriber immediately.

POINTS TO REMEMBER

- Psychosis is a major emotional disorder that impairs mental function. A person experiencing psychosis cannot participate in everyday life and shows the hallmark symptom of loss of contact with reality.
- Affective disorders are emotional disorders characterized by changes in mood. They range from mania (abnormally elevated emotions) to depression (abnormally reduced emotions) and include anxiety, a normal emotion that may be a healthy reaction but becomes pathologic when it is life altering.
- Situational anxiety arises in response to specific life events, and nursing assessment is key to identifying patients at risk.

- Benzodiazepines remain the drugs of choice for treatment of anxiety. They are most often prescribed, are considered to be fairly safe, and interact with fewer other drugs than do other groups of psychotherapeutic medications.
- SSRIs are often prescribed because of their superiority to older antidepressants.
- Nursing considerations related to psychotherapeutic drugs include the need for skillful patient assessment with an emphasis on past and present medical history, physical examination, and a thorough medication history and profile. Medications should be taken exactly as prescribed.

NCLEX EXAMINATION REVIEW QUESTIONS

1 In caring for a patient experiencing alcohol withdrawal, the nurse knows that which medication or medication class is most likely to be ordered as treatment for this condition?
   a Lithium (Eskalith)
   b Benzodiazepines
   c Buspirone (BuSpar)
   d Antidepressants
2 Patient teaching for a patient receiving an MAOI would include instructions to the patient to avoid which food product?
   a Grapefruit juice
   b Milk
   c Shrimp
   d Swiss cheese
3 After a patient has been treated for depression for 4 weeks, the nurse calls the patient to schedule a follow-up visit. What concern should the nurse know to look for during the conversation with the patient?
   a Weakness
   b Hallucinations
   c Suicidal ideations
   d Difficulty with urination
4 The nurse is caring for a patient who has been taking clozapine (Clozaril) for 2 months. Which laboratory test(s) should be performed regularly while the patient is taking this medication?

   a Platelet count
   b WBC count
   c Liver function studies
   d Renal function studies
5 The nurse is giving medications to a patient. Which drug(s), when administered with lithium, increases the risk for lithium toxicity?
   a Thiazides
   b Levofloxacin
   c Calcium citrate
   d Beta-blockers
6 The nurse is teaching a patient about treatment with an SSRI antidepressant. Which teaching considerations are appropriate? (Select all that apply.)
   a The patient should be told which foods contain tyramine and instructed to avoid these foods.
   b The patient should be instructed to use caution when standing up from a sitting position.
   c The patient should be told that if sexual dysfunction occurs, the drug will be stopped.
   d This medication should not be stopped abruptly.
   e Drug levels may become toxic if dehydration occurs.
   f The patient should be told to check with the prescriber before taking any over-the-counter medications.

1. b, 2. d, 3. c, 4. b, 5. a, 6. b, d, f.

CRITICAL THINKING ACTIVITIES: BEST ACTION

1 A 22-year-old patient who has been taking lithium for 3 months has had severe vomiting and diarrhea from a gastrointestinal flu. The nurse assesses for what immediate concern?
2 A 68-year-old patient has been taking an SSRI antidepressant for 5 weeks. His wife calls and expresses concern because he has started to give away some of his keepsakes. What is the nurse's best action?

3 A patient has been admitted to the hospital because of a suspected overdose of a tricyclic antidepressant. What two problems are the nurse's priorities during this time?

For answers, see *http://evolve.elsevier.com/Lilley.*

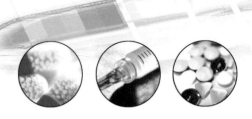

PART 3

Drugs Affecting the Autonomic Nervous System

STUDY SKILLS TIPS

PURR Application　•　Study Groups

PURR APPLICATION

Planning for the Part

The basic explanation provided for the PURR model in the Study Skills Tips for Part 1 demonstrates the application process as it relates to individual chapters. There is another application for the PURR model that can be very useful. This application encourages the learner to take a broader view of the assignment. In the case of this text, you have noticed that the chapters are grouped together into multiple chapter blocks called *parts*. Part organization is not some random process applied by the author to further complicate the subject. Part organization is a carefully considered process to put content together in a fashion that is logical and meaningful. Since the author has spent considerable time trying to link the chapters together in the most logical pattern, it is to your benefit as a student to learn to take advantage of the work already done for you.

Part Title

Begin the process of part planning by looking at the Part 3 title, "Drugs Affecting the Autonomic Nervous System." Then look at the part structure. There are four chapters contained in Part 3. All these chapters must be concerned with the autonomic nervous system. Even before you have read any chapter, you are beginning to look for the links that will establish a relationship—not only the links among the ideas in individual chapters but also the broader links that connect the four chapters in this part with each other and with the ideas that have come in earlier parts and will follow in later parts.

　　There is a clear example here of the way in which parts relate to one another. Look back at Part 2, "Drugs Affecting the Central Nervous System." Clearly that part deals with some aspect of the nervous system, as does this part. One learning objective you should establish for yourself is determining the relationship between these two parts. You must be able to define and explain

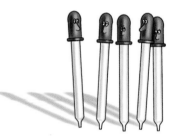

central nervous system and *autonomic nervous system*. However, just defining these terms and moving on limits the learning you can achieve. Ask yourself some additional questions that will help you establish a connection between these parts. What are the differences in functions of the central and the autonomic nervous systems? Are there pharmacologic drugs that have application in both the central and autonomic nervous systems? The principle is to keep stressing the links that must exist throughout all the parts and chapters you are studying. The normal study pattern that most students apply is one that focuses on the individual chapters, but it is essential to remain aware of the broader scope of chapter and part.

Part Chapters

After considering the part title and looking for relationships between the new part and the previous parts, the next step in applying the *Plan* step of PURR is to spend a few minutes studying the chapter titles and looking for the relationships that must exist. Part 3 has four chapters, and there is a clear pattern in these chapters. Chapters 18 and 19 both contain the term *adrenergic*. Clearly the two chapters are dealing with the same broad topic. However, Chapter 18 covers adrenergic drugs and Chapter 19 covers adrenergic-blocking drugs. Apply questioning strategies at this point. What does *adrenergic* mean? What is an *adrenergic drug?* These two questions are essential in mastering the content of Chapter 18 and should be questions that you ask yourself almost without thinking.

　　The next step is one that can greatly enhance your understanding when you start to read the material. This is a step that is easily overlooked. Notice that Chapter 18 deals with drugs and

Chapter 19 deals with blocking drugs. There must be a difference between a *drug* and a *blocking drug.* Focus now with a few questions that will keep you aware that the content in Chapter 18 has a direct relationship to the content in Chapter 19. What is the difference between a drug and a blocking drug? When is the pharmacologic application of a drug appropriate? Under what conditions should a blocking drug be chosen? Then ask a question to help maintain the focus on the concept of the entire part: What aspects of the autonomic nervous system are related to the adrenergic drugs and blocking drugs?

Once you begin to focus on the relationship of chapters within a part, certain things will begin to become apparent. Chapters 20 and 21 also cover drugs and blocking drugs. These two chapters develop the concept in relation to cholinergics rather than adrenergics. However, the same questions you used as a focus for Chapters 18 and 19 can be recycled in setting up the study of Chapters 20 and 21. Simply replace the term *adrenergic* with *cholinergic,* and you are ready to begin reading these two chapters with a clear personal learning objective.

Active Questioning

Active questioning is the key concept to master in working through the process of planning your learning for an entire part rather than for single chapters. The idea is to view the part as a whole rather than seeing only the content of individual chapters. The preceding discussion has provided a number of sample questions to help you begin the process. These questions should not be seen as the only questions you should ask, but rather as examples to help you develop a questioning process.

Keep in mind that you may or may not ask questions that are useful and appropriate when you are using only the chapter titles as the question stimulus. Some of the questions you devise will prove to be very useful when reading the chapter. On the other hand, some of the initial questions you generate may have little or no application as you read and understand the content of an individual chapter. Do not worry about the quality of your questions when planning at the part level. Questions can (and sometimes should) be revised or discarded when the details of the chapter become clearer. The important point is that you begin the part with some questions to help you focus your own reading and learning. Also, you will find that the more you apply active questioning as a part of your learning strategy, the better your questions will become.

STUDY GROUPS

A significant part of the PURR approach to learning is active questioning and rehearsing. When we engage others in this process, we have access to their ideas and understanding. We must also think through our own thoughts and make them clear to others. The best way to learn is to teach others.

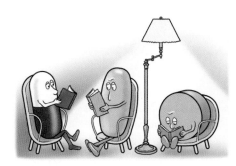

Study groups are particularly helpful when anticipating test questions. With several minds working, you increase your odds of being correct. In nursing, your textbook learning is of no value until you learn to apply the knowledge and skills you are learning. Study groups provide a discussion venue to stimulate thinking about the nursing process. The critical thinking activities at the end of each chapter can serve as a basis for small group discussions. Study group members can share lecture notes, which is of value if you need to be absent or if you have an instructor who talks too fast. Relating with a study group keeps you alert while you are studying. It is hard to fall asleep or daydream when you are in the middle of a discussion. There are many advantages to working with a study group; however, you must be careful when selecting the people to be in your group. Consider these four guidelines when establishing your study group:

1. Choose students who have **similar abilities and motivation** to yours. Socializing and gossiping can eat up valuable study time. Noncommitted and underprepared classmates can be a drain.

2. Look for students who have a **common time to meet.**

3. Select classmates who have learning styles **different** from yours. They might understand the reading material or lecture material better than you. They may be able to draw a diagram that will help your learning.

4. Find students that have **good communication skills;** that is, people who know how to listen, ask good questions, and explain concepts.

Study groups are not for everyone; however, they may be an alternative for you if you are having difficulty staying focused during your personal study time.

CHAPTER 18

Adrenergic Drugs

OBJECTIVES

When you reach the end of this chapter, you should be able to do the following:

1   Briefly describe the functions of the sympathetic nervous system and the specific effects of adrenergic stimulation.

2   List the various drugs classified as adrenergic agonists or sympathomimetics.

3   Discuss the mechanisms of action, therapeutic effects, indications, adverse and toxic effects, cautions, contraindications, drug interactions, and available antidotes to overdosage for the various adrenergic agonists or sympathomimetic drugs.

4   Develop a nursing care plan that includes all phases of the nursing process for patients taking adrenergic agonists.

e-Learning Activities

http://evolve.elsevier.com/Lilley

NCLEX Review Questions • Animations • Nursing Care Plans • Audio Glossary • Category Catchers • Medication Errors Checklists • IV Therapy Checklists • Calculators • Frequently Asked Questions • Content Updates • Supplemental Resources • Answers to Case Studies and Critical Thinking Activities

Drug Profiles

◆ dobutamine, p. 294   midodrine, p. 295
◆ dopamine, p. 294   ◆ norepinephrine, p. 295
◆ epinephrine, p. 294   phenylephrine, p. 295
  fenoldopam, p. 295

    ◆ *Key drug.*

Glossary

Adrenergic agonists Drugs that stimulate and mimic the actions of the sympathetic nervous system. Also called *sympathomimetics*. (p. 289)

Adrenergic receptors Receptor sites for the sympathetic neurotransmitters norepinephrine and epinephrine. (p. 289)

Alpha-adrenergic receptors A class of adrenergic receptors that are further subdivided into alpha$_1$- and alpha$_2$-adrenergic receptors, and are differentiated by their anatomic location in the tissues, muscles, and organs regulated by specific autonomic nerve fibers. (p. 289)

Autonomic functions Bodily functions that are involuntary and result from the physiologic activity of the autonomic nervous system. The functions often occur in pairs of opposing actions between the sympathetic and parasympathetic divisions of the autonomic nervous system. (p. 289)

Autonomic nervous system A branch of the peripheral nervous system that controls autonomic bodily functions. It consists of the sympathetic nervous system and the parasympathetic nervous system. (p. 289)

Beta-adrenergic receptors Receptors located on postsynaptic effector cells of tissues, muscles, and organs stimulated by specific autonomic nerve fibers. Beta$_1$-adrenergic receptors are located primarily in the heart, whereas Beta$_2$-adrenergic receptors are located in the smooth muscle fibers of the bronchioles, arterioles, and visceral organs. (p. 289)

Catecholamines Substances that can produce a sympathomimetic response. They are either endogenous catecholamines (such as epinephrine, norepinephrine, and dopamine) or synthetic catecholamine drugs (such as dobutamine). (p. 289)

Dopaminergic receptor A third type of adrenergic receptor (in addition to alpha-adrenergic and beta-adrenergic receptors) located in various tissues and organs and activated by the binding of the neurotransmitter dopamine, which can be either endogenous or a synthetic drug form. (p. 289)

Mydriasis Pupillary dilation, whether natural (physiologic) or drug induced. (p. 292)

Ophthalmics Drugs that are used in the eye (p. 292)

Positive chronotropic effect An increase in heart rate. (p. 292)

Positive dromotropic effect An increase in the conduction of cardiac electrical impulses through the atrioventricular node, which results in the transfer of nerve action potentials from the atria to the ventricles. This ultimately leads to a systolic heartbeat (ventricular contractions). (p. 292)

Positive inotropic effect An increase in the force of contraction of the heart muscle (myocardium). (p. 292)

Sympathomimetics Drugs used therapeutically that mimic the catecholamines epinephrine, norepinephrine, and dopamine. Also called *adrenergic agonists*. (p. 289)

Synaptic cleft The space either between two adjacent nerve cell membranes or between a nerve cell membrane and an effector organ cell membrane (also called *synapse*). (p. 290)

• • •

Anatomy and Physiology Overview

Adrenergic compounds include several exogenous (synthetic) and endogenous (produced in the body naturally) substances. They have a wide variety of therapeutic uses depending on their site of action and their effect on different types of adrenergic receptors. Adrenergics stimulate the sympathetic nervous system (SNS) and are also called **adrenergic agonists.** They are also known as **sympathomimetics,** because they mimic the effects of the SNS neurotransmitters norepinephrine, epinephrine, and dopamine. These three neurotransmitters are chemically classified as **catecholamines.** In considering the adrenergic class of medications, it is helpful to understand how the SNS operates in relation to the rest of the nervous system.

SYMPATHETIC NERVOUS SYSTEM

Figure 18-1 depicts the divisions of the nervous system and shows the relationship of the SNS to the entire nervous system. The SNS is the counterpart of the parasympathetic nervous system; together they make up the **autonomic nervous system.** They provide a checks-and-balances system for maintaining the normal homeostasis of the **autonomic functions** of the human body.

Throughout the body are receptor sites for the catecholamines norepinephrine and epinephrine. These are referred to as **adrenergic receptors,** and these are the sites at which adrenergic drugs bind and produce their effects. Adrenergic receptors are located in many anatomic sites. Many physiologic responses are produced when they are stimulated or blocked. Adrenergic receptors are further divided into **alpha-adrenergic receptors** and **beta-adrenergic receptors,** depending on the specific physiologic responses caused by their stimulation. Both types of adrenergic receptors have subtypes, designated 1 and 2, which provide a further means of checks and balances that control stimulation and blockade, vasoconstriction and vasodilation of blood vessels, and the increased and decreased production of various substances.

The alpha$_1$- and alpha$_2$-adrenergic receptors are differentiated by their location relative to nerves. The alpha$_1$-adrenergic receptors are located on postsynaptic effector cells (the tissue, muscle, or organ that the nerve stimulates). The alpha$_2$-adrenergic receptors are located on the presynaptic nerve terminals. They control the release of neurotransmitters. The predominant alpha-adrenergic agonist response is vasoconstriction and central nervous system (CNS) stimulation.

The beta-adrenergic receptors are all located on postsynaptic effector cells. The beta$_1$-adrenergic receptors are primarily located in the heart, whereas the beta$_2$-adrenergic receptors are located in the smooth muscle fibers of the bronchioles, arterioles, and visceral organs. A beta-adrenergic agonist response results in bronchial, gastrointestinal (GI), and uterine smooth muscle relaxation; glycogenolysis; and cardiac stimulation. Table 18-1 provides a more detailed listing of the adrenergic receptors and the responses elicited when they are stimulated by a neurotransmitter or a drug that acts like a neurotransmitter (Figure 18-2).

Another type of adrenergic receptor is the **dopaminergic receptor.** When stimulated by dopamine, these receptors cause the

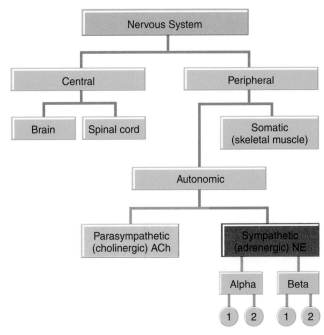

FIGURE 18-1   Sympathetic nervous system in relation to the entire nervous system. *ACh,* Acetylcholine; *NE,* norepinephrine.

TABLE 18-1   Adrenergic Receptor Responses to Stimulation

Location	Receptor	Response
Cardiovascular		
Blood vessels	Alpha$_1$	Vasoconstriction
	Beta$_2$	Vasodilation
Cardiac muscle	Beta$_1$	Increased contractility
Atrioventricular node	Beta$_1$	Increased heart rate
Sinoatrial node	Beta$_1$	Increased heart rate
Endocrine		
Liver	Alpha$_1$, beta$_2$	Glycogenolysis
Kidney	Beta$_1$	Increased renin secretion
Gastrointestinal		
Muscle	Alpha$_1$, beta$_2$	Decreased motility (relaxation of gastrointestinal smooth muscle)
Genitourinary		
Bladder sphincter	Alpha$_1$	Constriction
Penis	Alpha$_1$	Ejaculation
Uterus	Alpha$_1$	Contraction
	Beta$_2$	Relaxation
Respiratory		
Bronchial muscles	Beta$_2$	Dilation (relaxation of bronchial smooth muscles)
Ocular		
Pupillary muscles of the iris	Alpha$_1$	Mydriasis

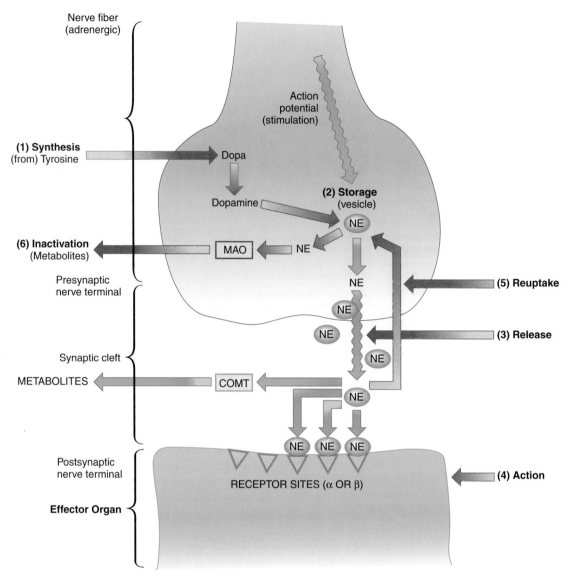

FIGURE 18-2 Mechanism by which stimulation of a nerve fiber results in a physiologic process; adrenergic drugs mimic this same process. *COMT,* Catechol ortho-methyltransferase; *MAO,* monoamine oxidase; *NE,* norepinephrine.

vessels of the renal, mesenteric, coronary, and cerebral arteries to dilate, which increases blood flow to these tissues. Dopamine is the only substance that can stimulate these receptors.

Catecholamine neurotransmitter molecules are produced by the SNS and are stored in vesicles or granules located in the ends of nerves. Here the transmitter waits until the nerve is stimulated, then the vesicles move to the walls of nerve endings and release their contents into the space between the nerve ending and the effector organ, known as the **synaptic cleft** or *synapse.* The released contents of the vesicles (catecholamines) then have the opportunity to bind to the receptor sites located all along the effector organ. Once the neurotransmitter binds to the receptors, the effector organ responds. Depending on the function of the particular organ, this response may involve smooth muscle contraction (e.g., skeletal muscles) or relaxation (e.g., GI and airway smooth muscles), an increased heart rate, the increased production of one or more substances (e.g., stress hormones), or constriction of a blood vessel. This process is halted by the action of

specific enzymes and by reuptake of the neurotransmitter molecules back into the nerve cell (neuron). Catecholamines are specifically metabolized by two enzymes, monoamine oxidase (MAO) and catechol ortho-methyltransferase (COMT). Each enzyme breaks down catecholamines but is responsible for doing it in a different area. MAO breaks down the catecholamines that are in the nerve ending, whereas COMT breaks down the catecholamines that are outside the nerve ending at the synaptic cleft (see Figure 18-2). Neurotransmitter molecules may also be actively taken back up into the presynaptic nerve fiber by the action of various protein pumps within the cell membrane, a phenomenon known as *active transport.* This restores the catecholamine to the vesicle and provides another means of maintaining an adequate supply of the substance for future sympathetic nerve impulses. This process is illustrated in Figure 18-2. The sympathetic branch of the autonomic nervous system is often described as having a "fight-or-flight" function, because it allows the body to respond in a self-protective manner to dangerous situations.

Pharmacology Overview

ADRENERGIC DRUGS

Drugs with effects that are similar to or mimic the effects of the SNS neurotransmitters norepinephrine, epinephrine, and dopamine are referred to as *adrenergics*. These neurotransmitters are known as *catecholamines*. Catecholamines produce a sympathomimetic response and are either endogenous substances such as epinephrine, norepinephrine, and dopamine or synthetic substances such as dobutamine and phenylephrine. These three endogenous catecholamines, (epinephrine, norepinephrine, and dopamine) are also available in synthetic drug form.

Catecholamine drugs that are used therapeutically produce the same result as endogenous catecholamines. When epinephrine, dobutamine, or any of the adrenergic drugs is given, it bathes the area between the nerve and the effector cell (i.e., the synaptic cleft). Once there, the drug has the opportunity to induce a response. This can be accomplished in one of three ways: by direct stimulation, by indirect stimulation, or by a combination of the two (mixed acting).

A direct-acting sympathomimetic binds directly to the receptor and causes a physiologic response (Figure 18-3). Epinephrine is an example of such a drug. An indirect-acting sympathomimetic is an adrenergic drug that, when given, causes the release of the catecholamine from the storage sites (vesicles) in the nerve endings; it then binds to the receptors and causes a physiologic response (Figure 18-4). Amphetamine and other related anorexiants are examples of such drugs. A mixed-acting sympathomimetic both directly stimulates the receptor by binding to it and indirectly stimulates the receptor by causing the release of the neurotransmitter stored in vesicles at the nerve endings (Figure 18-5). Ephedrine is an example of a mixed-acting adrenergic drug.

There are also noncatecholamine adrenergic drugs such as phenylephrine, metaproterenol, and albuterol. These are structurally dissimilar to the endogenous catecholamines and generally have a longer duration of action than either the endogenous or synthetic catecholamines. The noncatecholamine drugs show similar patterns of activity.

Catecholamines and noncatecholamines can act to varying degrees at different types of adrenergic receptors, depending on the amount of drug administered. Examples of catecholamines and the dose-specific selectivity of these drugs are given in Table 18-2. Although adrenergics work primarily peripherally at postganglionic receptors (the receptors that immediately innervate the effector organ, gland, muscle, and so on), they may also work more centrally in the nervous system at the preganglionic sympathetic nerve trunks. The ability to do so depends on the potency of the specific drug and the dose used.

Although adrenergic drugs are classified most technically by their specific receptor activities, they may also be categorized in terms of their clinical effects. For example, phenylephrine is both an alpha$_1$ agonist and a vasopressive drug (pressor), whereas albuterol is both an alpha$_2$ agonist and a bronchodilator. Both classifications are suitable for most clinical purposes. However, it may sometimes be necessary to carefully choose an adrenergic drug with greater selectivity for a particular receptor type to avoid undesired clinical effects. In such a situation, detailed knowledge of the type and degree of receptor selectivity of different drugs becomes important.

Mechanism of Action and Drug Effects

To fully understand the mechanism of action of adrenergics, one must have a working knowledge of normal adrenergic transmission, which takes place at the junction between the nerve (postganglionic sympathetic neuron) and the receptor site of the innervated organ or tissue (effector). The process of SNS stimulation

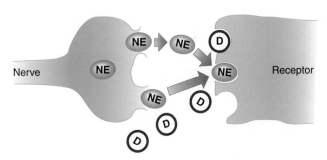

FIGURE 18-5 Mechanism of physiologic response to *mixed-acting* sympathomimetics. *D,* Drug; *NE,* norepinephrine.

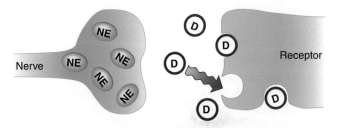

FIGURE 18-3 Mechanism of physiologic response to *direct-acting* sympathomimetics. *D,* Drug; *NE,* norepinephrine.

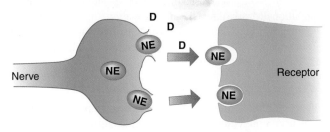

FIGURE 18-4 Mechanism of physiologic response to *indirect-acting* sympathomimetics. *D,* Drug; *NE,* norepinephrine.

TABLE 18-2 Catecholamines and Their Dose-Response Relationship

Drug	Dosage	Receptor
dobutamine (Dobutrex)	Maintenance: 2-15 mcg/kg/min High: 40 mcg/kg/min	Beta$_1$ >> beta B$_2$ > alpha$_1$
dopamine (Intropin)	Low: 0.5-2 mcg/kg/min	Dopaminergic
	Moderate: 2-4 or less than 10 mcg/kg/min	Beta$_1$
	High: 20-30 mcg/kg/min	Alpha$_1$
epinephrine (Adrenalin)	Low: 1-4 mcg/min	Beta$_1$ > beta$_2$ >> alpha$_1$
	High: 4-40 mcg/min	Alpha$_1$ ≥ beta$_1$

is illustrated in Figure 18-2 and was discussed earlier in this chapter. When adrenergic drugs stimulate alpha$_1$-adrenergic receptor sites located on smooth muscles, vasoconstriction most commonly occurs. The binding of adrenergic drugs to these alpha$_1$-adrenergic receptors on the smooth muscle of blood vessels causes smooth muscle contraction that results in vasoconstriction. However, such drug binding can also cause the relaxation of GI smooth muscle, contraction of the uterus and bladder, male ejaculation, and contraction of the pupillary muscles of the eye, which causes the pupils to dilate (see Table 18-1). Stimulation of alpha$_2$-adrenergic receptors, on the other hand, actually tends to reverse sympathetic activity but is not of great significance either physiologically or pharmacologically.

There are beta$_1$-adrenergic receptors on the myocardium and in the conduction system of the heart, including the sinoatrial node and the atrioventricular node. When these beta$_1$-adrenergic receptors are stimulated by an adrenergic drug, three things result: (1) an increase in the force of contraction **(positive inotropic effect)**, (2) an increase in heart rate **(positive chronotropic effect)**, and (3) an increase in the conduction of cardiac electrical nerve impulses through the atrioventricular node **(positive dromotropic effect)**. In addition, stimulation of beta$_1$ receptors in the kidney causes an increase in renin secretion. Activation of beta$_2$-adrenergic receptors produces relaxation of the bronchi (bronchodilation) and uterus, and also causes increased glycogenolysis (glucose release) from the liver (see Table 18-1).

Indications

Adrenergics, or sympathomimetics, are used in the treatment of a wide variety of illnesses and conditions. Their selectivity for either alpha- or beta-adrenergic receptors and their affinity for certain tissues or organs determine the settings in which they are most commonly used. Some adrenergics are used as adjuncts to dietary changes in the short-term treatment of obesity. These drugs are discussed in more detail in Chapter 14.

Respiratory Indications

Certain adrenergic drugs have an affinity for the adrenergic receptors located in the respiratory system and are classified as bronchodilators. They tend to preferentially stimulate the beta$_2$-adrenergic receptors and cause bronchodilation. Of the two subtypes of beta-adrenergic receptors, these drugs are attracted more to the beta$_2$-adrenergic receptors located on the bronchial, uterine, and vascular smooth muscles as opposed to the beta$_1$-adrenergic receptors located on the heart. The beta$_2$ agonists are helpful in treating conditions such as asthma and bronchitis. Some common bronchodilators that are classified as predominantly beta$_2$-selective adrenergic drugs include albuterol, ephedrine, epinephrine, formoterol, levalbuterol, metaproterenol, pirbuterol, salmeterol, and terbutaline. These drugs are discussed in more detail in Chapter 37.

Indications for Topical Nasal Decongestants

The intranasal application of certain adrenergics can cause the constriction of dilated arterioles and a reduction in nasal blood flow, which thus decreases congestion. These adrenergic drugs work by stimulating alpha$_1$-adrenergic receptors and have little or no effect on beta-adrenergic receptors. The nasal decongestants include epinephrine, ephedrine, naphazoline, oxymetazoline,

phenylephrine, and tetrahydrozoline. They are discussed in more detail in Chapter 36.

Ophthalmic Indications

Some adrenergics are applied to the surface of the eye. These drugs are called **ophthalmics,** and they work in much the same way as nasal decongestants except that they affect the vasculature of the eye. When administered, they stimulate alpha-adrenergic receptors located on small arterioles in the eye and temporarily relieve conjunctival congestion by causing arteriolar vasoconstriction. The ophthalmic adrenergics include epinephrine, naphazoline, phenylephrine, and tetrahydrozoline.

Adrenergics can also be used to reduce intraocular pressure and dilate the pupils **(mydriasis),** properties that make them useful in the treatment of open-angle glaucoma, as well as for diagnostic eye examinations. They produce these effects by stimulating alpha- or beta$_2$-adrenergic receptors, or both. The two adrenergics used for this purpose are epinephrine and dipivefrin. Ocular adrenergic drugs are discussed in more detail in Chapter 57.

Cardiovascular Indications

The final group of adrenergics is sometimes referred to as *vasoactive sympathomimetics, vasoconstrictive drugs* (also known as *vasopressive drugs, pressor drugs,* or *pressors*), *inotropes,* or *cardioselective sympathomimetics* because they are used to support the cardiovascular system during cardiac failure or shock. These drugs have a variety of effects on the various alpha- and beta-adrenergic receptors, and these effects can also be related to the specific dose of the adrenergic drug. Common vasoactive adrenergic drugs include dobutamine, dopamine, ephedrine, epinephrine, fenoldopam, midodrine, norepinephrine, and phenylephrine.

Contraindications

The only usual contraindications to the use of adrenergic drugs are known drug allergy and severe hypertension.

Adverse Effects

Some of the most common unwanted CNS effects of the alpha-adrenergic drugs are headache, restlessness, excitement, insomnia, and euphoria. Possible cardiovascular adverse effects of the alpha-adrenergic drugs include chest pain, vasoconstriction, hypertension, tachycardia, and palpitations or dysrhythmias. Effects on other body systems include anorexia (loss of appetite), dry mouth, nausea, vomiting, and, rarely, taste changes.

The beta-adrenergic drugs can adversely stimulate the CNS, causing mild tremors, headache, nervousness, and dizziness. These drugs can also have unwanted effects on the cardiovascular system, including increased heart rate (positive chronotropy), palpitations (dysrhythmias), and fluctuations in blood pressure. Other significant effects include sweating, nausea, vomiting, and muscle cramps. See the Life Span Considerations box on p. 293 for additional information.

Toxicity and Management of Overdose

The toxic effects of adrenergic drugs are mainly an extension of their common adverse effects (e.g., seizures from excessive CNS stimulation, hypotension or hypertension, dysrhythmias, palpitations, nervousness, dizziness, fatigue, malaise, insom-

---

LIFE SPAN CONSIDERATIONS: The Elderly Patient

Use of Beta-Adrenergic Agonists

- Several physiologic changes occur in the cardiovascular system of the older adult, including a decline in the efficiency and contractile ability of the heart muscle, decrease in cardiac output, and diminished stroke volume. In most cases, the older adult adjusts to these changes without too much difficulty, but if unusual demands are placed on the aging heart, problems and complications may arise. Examples of unusual demands include strenuous activities, excess stress, heat, and medication use. For instance, stress, heat, and use of beta-adrenergic agonists may lead to significant increases in blood pressure and pulse rate. The older adult may then react negatively with a diminished ability to compensate adequately for these changes.
- Baroreceptors do not work as effectively in the elderly patient. Reduced baroreceptor activity may lead to orthostatic hypotension even without the impact of certain medications and their associated mechanism of action and/or adverse effects.
- Because of the possible presence of concurrent medical conditions such as hypertension, peripheral vascular disease, cardiovascular disease, and/or cerebrovascular disease, the elderly patient must be monitored carefully before, during, and after administration of adrenergic drugs.
- An elderly patient should immediately report to the prescriber the occurrence of any chest pain, palpitations, blurred vision, headache, seizures, or hallucinations.
- Cautious use of over-the-counter drugs, herbals, supplements, and other medications is recommended. This caution is due to possible drug-drug interactions as well as the elderly person's increased sensitivity to many drugs and other chemicals.
- Vital signs, especially blood pressure and pulse rate, should be monitored frequently and as needed when the patient is taking any of the adrenergic drugs because of their cardiovascular and cerebrovascular effects.
- The elderly often have decreased motor and cognitive functioning. Therefore, use of additional equipment and certain facilitating aids as well as provision of special instructions are needed to help ensure proper dosing of medications.

---

nia, headache, tremor, dry mouth, and nausea). The two most life-threatening toxic effects involve the CNS and cardiovascular system. In the acute setting, seizures can be effectively managed with diazepam. Intracranial bleeding can also occur, often as the result of an extreme elevation in blood pressure. Such elevated blood pressure poses the risk of hemorrhage not only in the brain but elsewhere in the body as well. The best and most effective treatment in this situation is to lower the blood pressure using a rapid-acting sympatholytic drug (e.g., esmolol; see Chapter 19). This can directly reverse the adrenergic-induced state.

Many adrenergic drugs are either synthetic analogues of the naturally occurring neurotransmitters (norepinephrine, epinephrine, and dopamine) or the actual endogenous adrenergic compounds. The majority of these compounds have very short half-lives, and thus their effects are short lived. Therefore, when these drugs are taken in overdose or toxicity develops, reversing the adverse effects takes a relatively short time. Stopping the drug should quickly cause the toxic symptoms to subside. The recommended treatment for overdose is often to manage the symptoms and support the patient. If death occurs, it is usually the result of

either respiratory failure or cardiac arrest. The treatment of overdose should therefore be aimed at supporting the respiratory and cardiac systems.

Interactions

Numerous drug interactions can occur with adrenergic drugs. Although many of the interactions result only in a diminished adrenergic effect because of direct antagonism at and competition for receptor sites, some reactions can be life threatening. The following are some of the more serious drug-drug interactions involving adrenergic drugs: When alpha- and beta-adrenergic drugs are given with adrenergic antagonists (e.g., some classes of antihypertensive drugs), the drugs directly antagonize each other, which results in reduced therapeutic effects. Administration of adrenergics with anesthetic drugs can increase the risk of cardiac dysrhythmias. Tricyclic antidepressants, when given with adrenergics, can cause increased vasopressor effects, acute hypertensive crisis, and possibly respiratory depression. Administration of adrenergic drugs with MAO inhibitors may cause a possibly life-threatening hypertensive crisis (see Chapter 17). Antihistamines and thyroid preparations can also increase the effects of adrenergic drugs.

Laboratory Test Interactions

Alpha-adrenergic drugs can cause the serum levels of endogenous corticotropin (i.e., adrenocorticotropic hormone), corticosteroids, and glucose to be increased. Therefore, the results of laboratory tests for these substances should be interpreted with caution in patients receiving any of these medications.

Dosages

For the recommended dosages of various adrenergic drugs, see the Dosages table on p. 294.

DRUG PROFILES

Four frequently used therapeutic classes of adrenergic drugs are bronchodilators (see Chapter 37), ophthalmic drugs (see Chapter 57), nasal decongestants (see Chapter 36), and vasoactive drugs, which are emphasized in this chapter (see drug profiles) and in Chapter 24. It should be noted that receptor selectivity for the alpha$_1$, beta$_1$, and beta$_2$ receptor subtypes is *relative* (as opposed to *absolute*). Thus, there may be some overlap of drug effects between the different adrenergic classes of drugs, especially at higher dosages. In contrast, dopamine receptors are more specific for dopamine itself and/or specific dopaminergic drugs.

VASOACTIVE ADRENERGICS

Adrenergics that have primarily cardioselective effects are referred to as *vasoactive adrenergics*. They are used to support a failing heart or to treat shock. They may also be used to treat orthostatic hypotension. These drugs have a wide range of effects on alpha- and beta-adrenergic receptors, depending on the dosage. The vasoactive adrenergics are very potent, quick-acting, injectable drugs. Although dosage recommendations are given in the table on p. 294, all of these drugs are titrated to the desired physiologic response. All of the vasoactive adrenergics (with the exception of midodrine) are rapid in onset, and their effects very quickly cease when administration is stopped. Therefore, careful titration and monitoring of vital signs and electrocardiogram (ECG) are required.

DOSAGES

Selected Vasoactive Adrenergics

Drug	Pharmacologic Class	Usual Dosage Range	Indications
◆ dobutamine (Dobutrex)	Beta₁-adrenergic	**Pediatric** IV infusion: 2.5-15 mcg/kg/min **Adult** IV infusion: 2.5-40 mcg/kg/min	Cardiac decompensation
◆ dopamine (Intropin)	Beta₁-adrenergic	**Adult and pediatric** IV infusion: 1-50 mcg/kg/min	Shock syndrome, cardiopulmonary arrest
◆ epinephrine (Adrenalin)	Alpha- and beta-adrenergic	**Pediatric** Subcut: 10 mcg/kg repeated q15min ×2 then q4h prn **Adult** Subcut: 0.1-0.5 mg repeated q10-15min if required **Neonatal** IV: 10-30 mcg/kg q3-5min if required **Pediatric** IV: 10 mcg/kg q3-5min if required **Adult** IV: 0.5-1 mg q3-5min if required	Anaphylaxis, cardiopulmonary arrest
fenoldopam (Corlopam)	Dopamine 1 agonist	**Adult only** IV: 0.1-1.6 mcg/kg/min for up to 48 hr	Hypertensive emergency in hospital setting
midodrine (ProAmatine)	Alpha₁-adrenergic	**Adult only** PO: 10 mg tid (q3-4h when awake), max 40 mg/day	Orthostatic hypotension
◆ norepinephrine (Levophed)	Alpha- and beta-adrenergic	**Pediatric** IV infusion: 0.05-1 mcg/kg/min **Adult** IV infusion: 4-20 mcg/min	Hypotensive states
phenylephrine (Neo-Synephrine)	Alpha-adrenergic	**Pediatric** (for hypotension during spinal anesthesia) Subcut/IM: 0.1 mg/kg/dose **Adult** IV infusion: 10 mg/250 or 500 mL IV solution, start at 100-180 mcg/min and titrate down to 40-60 mcg/min IM/subcut: 2-5 mg IV: 0.1-0.5 mg	Hypotension, paroxysmal supraventricular tachycardia

IM, Intramuscular; *IV,* intravenous; *PO,* oral; *subcut,* subcutaneous.

◆ dobutamine

Dobutamine (Dobutrex) is a beta₁-selective vasoactive adrenergic drug that is structurally similar to the naturally occurring catecholamine dopamine. Through stimulation of the beta₁ receptors on heart muscle (myocardium), it increases cardiac output by increasing contractility (positive inotropy), which increases the stroke volume, especially in patients with heart failure. Dobutamine is available only as an intravenous drug and is given by continuous infusion. (See Dosages table.)

PHARMACOKINETICS

Route	Onset of Action	Peak Plasma Concentration	Elimination Half-life	Duration of Action
IV	Less than 2 min	Less than 10 min	2-5 min	Less than 10 min

◆ dopamine

Dopamine (Intropin) is a naturally occurring catecholamine neurotransmitter in the SNS. It has potent dopaminergic as well as beta₁- and alpha₁-adrenergic receptor activity, depending on the dosage. Dopamine, when used at low dosages, can dilate blood vessels in the brain, heart, kidneys, and mesentery, which increases blood flow to these areas (dopaminergic receptor activity). At higher infusion rates dopamine can improve cardiac contractility and output (beta₁-adrenergic receptor activity). Use of the drug is contraindicated in patients who have a catecholamine-secreting tumor of the adrenal gland known as a *pheochromocytoma*. The drug is available only as an intravenous injectable drug and is given by continuous infusion. (See Dosages table.)

PHARMACOKINETICS

Route	Onset of Action	Peak Plasma Concentration	Elimination Half-life	Duration of Action
PO	2-5 min	Rapid	Less than 2 min	10 min

◆ epinephrine

Epinephrine (Adrenalin) is an endogenous vasoactive catecholamine. It acts directly on both the alpha- and beta-adrenergic receptors of tissues innervated by the SNS. It is administered in emergency situations and is one of the primary vasoactive drugs used in many advanced cardiac life support protocols. The physiologic response it elicits is dose related. At low dosages it stimulates mostly beta$_1$-adrenergic receptors, increasing the force of contraction and heart rate. It is also used to treat acute asthma (see Chapter 37) and anaphylactic shock at these dosages because it has significant bronchodilatory effects via the beta$_2$-adrenergic receptors in the lungs. At high dosages (e.g., intravenous drip), it stimulates mostly alpha-adrenergic receptors, causing vasoconstriction, which elevates the blood pressure. (See Dosages table.)

PHARMACOKINETICS

Route	Onset of Action	Peak Plasma Concentration	Elimination Half-life	Duration of Action
Subcut	5-10 min	20 min	Variable	Unknown
IV	Less than 2 min	Rapid	Less than 5 min	5-30 min

fenoldopam

Fenoldopam (Corlopam) is a peripheral dopamine 1 (D$_1$) agonist indicated for parenteral use in lowering blood pressure. Fenoldopam produces its blood pressure–lowering effects by inducing arteriolar vasodilation mainly through stimulation of D$_1$ receptors. It appears to be as effective as sodium nitroprusside for short-term treatment of severe hypertension and may have beneficial effects on renal function because it increases renal blood flow. It is available as a 10-mg/mL injection. (See Dosages table.)

PHARMACOKINETICS

Route	Onset of Action	Peak Plasma Concentration	Elimination Half-life	Duration of Action
IV	5 min	20 min	More than 5 min	10 min

midodrine

Midodrine (ProAmatine) is a prodrug converted to its active form, desglymidodrine, in the liver. It is this active metabolite that is responsible for the primary pharmacologic action of midodrine, which is alpha$_1$-adrenergic receptor stimulation. This alpha$_1$ stimulation causes constriction of both arterioles and veins, resulting in peripheral vasoconstriction. Midodrine is primarily indicated for the treatment of symptomatic orthostatic hypotension. Midodrine is available as 2.5- and 5-mg tablets. (See Dosages table.)

PHARMACOKINETICS

Route	Onset of Action	Peak Plasma Concentration	Elimination Half-life	Duration of Action
PO	45-90 min	1 hr	More than 3-4 hr	6-8 hr

◆ norepinephrine

Norepinephrine (Levophed) acts predominantly by directly stimulating alpha-adrenergic receptors, which leads to vasoconstriction. It also has some direct-stimulating beta-adrenergic effects on the heart (beta$_1$-adrenergic receptors) but none on the lung (beta$_2$-adrenergic receptors). Norepinephrine is directly metabolized to dopamine and is used primarily in the treatment of hypotension and shock. It is given only by continuous infusion. (See Dosages table.)

PHARMACOKINETICS

Route	Onset of Action	Peak Plasma Concentration	Elimination Half-life	Duration of Action
PO	Rapid	1-2 min	Less than 5 min	1-2 min

phenylephrine

Phenylephrine (Neo-Synephrine) works almost exclusively on the alpha-adrenergic receptors. It is used primarily for short-term treatment to raise blood pressure in patients in shock, to control some dysrhythmias (supraventricular tachycardias), and to produce vasoconstriction in regional anesthesia. It is also administered topically as an ophthalmic drug (see Chapter 57) and as a nasal decongestant (see Chapter 36). (See Dosages table.)

PHARMACOKINETICS

Route	Onset of Action	Peak Plasma Concentration	Elimination Half-life	Duration of Action
IV	Rapid	Rapid	Less than 5 min	15-20 min

PREVENTING MEDICATION ERRORS

Neo-Synephrine and Norepinephrine

A common error that occurs is confusion between norepinephrine and the brand name for phenylephrine, which is Neo-Synephrine. It is not uncommon for both drugs to be ordered for patients, and because they sound alike, the wrong drug may be given. To avoid this confusion, many pharmacies list these drugs by their trade names as well: norepinephrine is called *Levophed* and phenylephrine is called *Neo-Synephrine*. See the Institute for Safe Medication Practices List of High-Alert Medications at *http://www.ismp.org/ Newsletters/acutecare/articles/20070809.pdf.*

NURSING PROCESS

Assessment

Adrenergic agonist drugs have a variety of effects depending on the receptors they stimulate. Stimulation of the alpha-adrenergic receptors results in vasoconstriction of blood vessels. Stimulation of beta$_1$-adrenergic receptors produces cardiac stimulation, and beta$_2$-adrenergic receptor stimulation results in bronchodilation. Because of these sympathomimetic properties, especially the cardiac effects, use of adrenergic agonists requires careful patient assessment and monitoring to maximize therapeutic effects and minimize possible adverse effects. This assessment should include taking a comprehensive health history with past and present medical history, performing a head-to-toe examination, and obtaining a medication history with a listing of drug allergies, medications routinely used or prescribed, and over-the-counter drugs and herbal products used. Other important assessment questions to pose because of the actions of adrenergic agonists and related uses, cautions, and contraindications include the following:

- Does the patient have any allergies to any medications, foods, topical products, environmental products, or other substance?
- Does the patient have asthma? If so, how frequent and severe are the acute episodes and what are factors that exacerbate the episodes and alleviate them? Are there any other signs and symptoms besides bronchospasms, wheezing, or dyspnea (shortness of breath)? What previous treatments for asthma have been tried? Any successes or failures?
- Does the patient have any history of transient ischemic attacks? Any history of cerebrovascular accident or stroke, hypertension, hypotension, cardiac irregularities, or other cardiovascular disease?

Assessment of renal and hepatic functioning is also important before initiation of treatment, especially in high-risk patients such as the elderly. With impaired functioning and altered metabolism and excretion, there is higher risk for adverse effects and toxicity (as with any drug). Assessment of cardiac functioning should include reviewing baseline heart rates, blood pressure, including postural blood pressures (discussed also in Chapter 17), and heart sounds, as well as asking questions about past and present cardiac disease states or symptoms. This should include inquiry about any occurrence of hypertension, bradycardia, tachycardia, myocardial infarction, or heart failure. A thorough cardiac assessment is needed because some of the adrenergic drugs can possibly put the patient at risk for worsening of preexisting cardiac disease states or symptoms.

Other baseline vital signs to be assessed and noted include temperature, respiratory rate, and breath sounds. Peripheral pulses, skin color, and capillary refill should also be assessed and documented. Specific to the use of midodrine is the assessment of postural blood pressures and pulse rates in supine, sitting, and standing positions before and during drug administration. In addition to measurement of postural blood pressures and pulse rates, the assessment should include inquiry about other significant symptoms such as dizziness, lightheadedness, and syncope. Assessment of the patient's symptoms and the patient's perception of either disease progression or a decrease in symptoms is very important for effective and successful treatment.

With other adrenergic drugs, such as those used for bronchodilating effects, there should be close assessment and documentation of the patient's respiratory rate, rhythm, and depth as well as the presence of normal and/or adventitious (abnormal) breath sounds. Asking questions about any complaints of difficulty in breathing and activity or exercise intolerance is also important. Pulse oximetry readings for oxygen saturation levels are also assessed and documented. Measurement of respiratory peak flow using a flow meter as well as measurement of the anterior-posterior diameter of the chest wall should also be included in the assessment, because a decrease in peak flow readings may indicate bronchospasms and an increase in anterior-posterior chest wall diameter is seen in chronic lung disorders such as emphysema. Prescribers may also order additional respiratory function studies such as measurement of arterial blood gas levels. Cautions or contraindications to drug use, life span considerations, and drug interactions should also be identified before use of any of the adrenergic agonist drugs (see previous pharmacology discussion). Elderly and very young patients may react with increased sensitivity to these drugs. In addition, some of these drugs are used only for acute episodes of asthma, whereas other drugs are used year-round as preventative drugs. For example, the drugs salmeterol (see Chapter 37) and formoterol are *not* used to treat acute asthmatic episodes, but albuterol is indicated for treatment of acute episodes.

Epinephrine and similar drugs are used for their cardiac, bronchial, antiallergic, ophthalmic, and vasopressor effects. Assessment should focus on vital signs, breath sounds, arterial blood gas levels, and ECG findings. Liver and renal function test results also need to be assessed and documented. In addition, each system related to the specific action of the drug (e.g., respiratory system for bronchodilation) must be assessed.

Overall, adrenergic drugs work in similar ways, but individual drugs may have some differences with regard to action, indications, and overall considerations. If the general class of drugs and the way in which they work is known, then the relevant assessment parameters, cautions, contraindications, drug interactions, and life span considerations are easy to determine. If the drug is a pure adrenergic agonist, the net effect is stimulation of alpha-adrenergic receptors with vasoconstriction of blood vessels and subsequent elevation of blood pressure and heart rate. The nurse would then know to expect specific actions from the drug as well as to anticipate certain adverse effects. The drug may be used for the therapeutic effect of increased blood pressure, but an unwanted adverse effect could then be a hypertensive crisis. If the drug is a beta-adrenergic agonist, it will stimulate both beta$_1$ and beta$_2$ receptors, which will lead to cardiac stimulation and bronchodilation. This beta$_1$ action can also result in too much stimulation with severe tachycardia and possibly chest pain if coronary artery disease is present. Thus, by knowing the actions of a given drug, the nurse may draw conclusions about, anticipate, and be very alert to the drug's therapeutic action, adverse effects, cautions, contraindications, drug interactions, and toxicity.

Nursing Diagnoses

- Decreased cardiac output related to cardiovascular adverse effects of adrenergic agonist drugs
- Ineffective cerebral and peripheral tissue perfusion related to intense vasoconstrictive actions of medications
- Acute pain related to adverse effects of tachycardia and palpitations
- Deficient knowledge of the therapeutic regimen, adverse effects, drug interactions, and precautions related to the use of adrenergic drugs
- Risk for injury related to possible adverse effects (nervousness, vertigo, hypertension, or tremors) or to potential drug interactions
- Disturbed sleep patterns related to CNS stimulation caused by adrenergic drugs
- Noncompliance with drug therapy related to lack of information about the importance of taking the medication as ordered

Planning

Goals

- Patient's symptoms improve because of the drug's therapeutic effects.
- Patient takes the drugs as ordered and follows directions explicitly.
- Patient remains adherent to the drug therapy regimen.
- Patient demonstrates adequate knowledge about the use of the specific medications.

Outcome Criteria

- Patient shows improvement in the disease process or condition for which the medication was given with subsequent decrease in the signs and symptoms of cardiac and/or respiratory problems.
- Patient states the importance of pharmacologic and nonpharmacologic treatment of the respiratory or other conditions that may be present, such as asthma.
- Patient states the importance of compliance with the drug regimen and adherence to the proper dosage of the medication to maximize therapeutic effects and minimize adverse effects.

- Patient experiences minimal adverse effects and complications, such as excessive CNS stimulation, insomnia, tachycardia, chest pain, and tremors.
- Patient states conditions and adverse effects associated with long-term at-home use that should be reported to the prescriber, such as chest pain, restlessness, and severe insomnia.
- Patient states the importance of scheduling and keeping follow-up appointments with the prescriber to monitor the effectiveness of drug therapy.

Implementation

There are several nursing interventions that may maximize the therapeutic effects of *adrenergic drugs* and minimize their adverse effects. The nurse should always check the package inserts for the types and amounts of dilutional solutions to use with parenteral dosage forms. For example, subcutaneous administration of the adrenergic agonist epinephrine to patients with asthma requires safe calculations and accurate dosing. A tuberculin syringe may be used for subcutaneous administration of epinephrine to help in accurate dosing for both adult and pediatric patients.

Use of epinephrine and some of the other pure alpha-adrenergics may not be indicated for shock-related symptoms, because these drugs lead to vasoconstriction of the renal vessels and subsequent renal damage or shutdown. Therefore, when a patient is in shock and requires medications, dopamine is generally the drug of choice (rather than epinephrine). Dopamine is used because in specific dosage ranges it helps treat a shock-related syndrome through its ability to produce vasoconstriction of peripheral blood vessels and increase blood pressure, but this is done without vasoconstriction of the renal vasculature. This lack of renal vasculature vasoconstriction helps improve perfusion through the kidneys and thus salvages the kidneys (while increasing blood pressure). With administration of dopamine and similar drugs, the intravenous site should be checked frequently for infiltration (e.g., every hour, as needed) to be sure that the site remains intact and that the drug is being infused at the proper rate. Infiltration of an intravenous solution containing an adrenergic drug may lead to tissue necrosis from excessive vasoconstriction around the intravenous site. Phentolamine is often used for the treatment of infiltration (see Chapter 19). Also, with intravenous infusions the nurse must use only clear solutions and a proper dilutional fluid, and must always administer the drug with an intravenous infusion pump with close monitoring of the cardiac system (e.g., vital signs, heart sounds, and/or ECG monitoring). All of these drugs should be given per the manufacturer's directions and suggested infusion rates to avoid precipitating dangerously high blood pressure and pulse rate, and subsequent complications.

When these drugs are given via an inhaler or nebulizer, patient instruction about correct use, storage, and care of equipment should be complete, thorough, and age appropriate. The patient also needs to know how to use a spacer correctly, because use of this device with the inhaler is often ordered. A spacer provides more effective delivery of inhaled doses of drug (see Chapter 10 and Patient Teaching Tips). When the adrenergics are dosed for bronchodilating effects, often two adrenergics are prescribed. This is because different medications are associated with different pharmacokinetics and actions. One inhaler may be for

use in *acute* situations and the other may be for *long-term* and/or *preventative* use. This type of treatment regimen requires that the patient receive thorough, simple, and complete instructions and explanations about the method of delivery as well as the drugs used. This will help to minimize overdosage and reduce the risk of severe adverse effects such as hypertension, severe tachycardia, tremors, and CNS overstimulation.

The nurse must emphasize in patient teaching that these medications are to be used only as prescribed with regard to amount, timing, and spacing of doses. Because of their synergistic effects, when these medications (especially asthmatics) are used in combination with other types of bronchodilators, the patient must be very clear about what to do before, during, and after the dose is delivered. If the patient is taking an inhaled dosage form, he or she may also be taking an oral or parenteral form of the same or a similar drug. The reason for the use of more than one drug of the same drug class and the use of more than one route of administration is to achieve combined therapeutic effects. Patient education requires extremely close attention with these regimens, because of the need to prevent exacerbation of adverse effects, minimize drug interactions, and prevent severe vascular and cardiovascular adverse effects. Patients should immediately report any complaints of chest pain, palpitations, blurred vision, headache, seizures, or hallucinations.

CASE STUDY

Dopamine Infusion

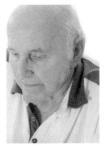
© Andi Berger

Mr. P., age 82 years, is receiving dopamine at a dose of 5 mcg/kg/min for heart failure. He has a history of hypothyroidism and takes a daily dose of thyroid replacement hormone. Yesterday, his vital signs were as follows:

Blood pressure, 150/88 mm Hg
Pulse rate, 92 beats/min
Respiration rate, 16 breaths/min

His heart rhythm showed sinus rhythm with rare ectopic beats. While at rest he had no shortness of breath but did experience some dyspnea when getting up to the bedside commode. He has edema in his lower legs rated as 2+ edema.

1. Explain how this dose of dopamine works to help treat Mr. P's heart failure.
2. What would you expect to happen if the dose were set to 1 mcg/kg/min? 20 mcg/kg/min?

This morning, you make rounds and find that Mr. P's vital signs are as follows:

Blood pressure, 170/94
Pulse rate, 120 beats/min
Respiration rate, 22 breaths/min

The heart monitor shows sinus tachycardia with two to three ectopic beats per minute. Mr. P. is complaining of palpitations and some shortness of breath at rest but says, "I've felt this before when I've had bad spells with my heart. I'm sure it will pass."

3. Do you think there is a concern at this time? Explain your reasoning and what should be done.

The physician decides to titrate the dopamine infusion to 3 mcg/kg/min, which you do immediately.

4. How quickly should you see a response from the patient to this decrease in dosage?

For answers, see *http://evolve.elsevier.com/Lilley.*

Infiltrating Intravenous Infusions

Nurses often encounter infiltrating intravenous (IV) infusions in the routine care of many of their patients. Every action taken is very important in meeting the standard of care for the patient and in ensuring that the nurse has acted as any prudent nurse would. The assessment and action of the nurse can be important for the patient, as in the case of *Macon-Bibb Hosp. Authority v. Ross* (335 S.E. 2d 633-GA).

Situation and Outcome

Ms. Ross was brought to the emergency department of the hospital with dyspnea, bradycardia, and a blood pressure (BP) of 250/150 mm Hg. She went into respiratory arrest at 2:55 PM; she was intubated with an endotracheal tube, and nitroprusside was administered IV to lower her BP. Because of the rapid drop in BP, an IV administration of dopamine was started at 3:28 PM in her right wrist to raise her BP. When her BP was stable at 4:30 PM, she was transferred to the cardiac care unit. At midnight, a nurse noted that the IV catheter site had a "bruise bluish in color." The next notation was at 11:00 AM the following day, in which it was recorded that the patient's right arm was swollen and painful with a large blistered area around the IV catheter site. The same notation was made at 4:00 PM. It was not until 6:50 PM that a note indicated that a physician was informed of the infiltration. As a result of the extravasation of dopamine, the patient's lower right arm was permanently scarred. On a jury verdict, the court entered judgment for the patient. The hospital appealed.

The court of appeals affirmed the judgment of the lower court. It was noted that, although an infiltration may result from an improper technique, it may also be due to the size of the needle, the status of the patient's veins, or specific intolerance to an IV catheter. However, according to the expert nurse's testimony, supported by suitable references, dopamine should be infused into a "large vein," such as a vein in the antecubital fossa, to minimize the risk for extravasation. In addition, a dopamine infusion should be monitored continuously for free flow. If extravasation of dopamine occurs, the recommended treatment of the site is infiltration with a saline solution of phentolamine (Regitine) within 12 hours.

The nurses were criticized for not being sufficiently knowledgeable regarding dopamine, which resulted in their failure to notify a physician of the patient's impaired tissue integrity.

From McKenry LM, Tessier E, Hogan M: *Mosby's pharmacology in nursing,* ed 22, St Louis, 2006, Mosby.

Patients with chronic lung disease who are receiving adrenergic drugs should also avoid anything that may exacerbate their respiratory condition (e.g., food or other allergens, cigarette smoking) and implement measures that may help diminish the risk of respiratory infection. These measures may include avoiding those who are ill with colds or flu, avoiding crowded areas, remaining well nourished and rested, and maintaining fluid intake of up to 3000 mL/day to ensure adequate hydration (unless contraindicated). Keeping a journal of symptoms and noting any improvement or worsening in the treated condition while taking the medications may be very helpful.

Salmeterol is not to be used for relief of acute symptoms, and education about its dosing is important. The dosage of salmeterol is usually two puffs twice daily 12 hours apart for maintenance effects. For prevention of exercise-induced asthma, it is recommended that patients take two puffs ½ to 1 hour before exercise and no additional doses for 12 hours. These orders and directions should always be rechecked. If another type of inhalant is used, such as a corticosteroid, the bronchodilator should be used first, with a 5-minute waiting period afterward before the second drug is taken. All equipment should be rinsed, and the patient should be encouraged to rinse the mouth thoroughly after the use of any inhalant form of medication. Further discussion of this medication is found in Chapter 37.

If ophthalmic forms of these drugs are used, the nurse must make sure that the medication has not expired and is also a clear solution. The eyedropper must not be allowed to touch the eye when the drug is applied to help prevent contamination of the remaining solution. With ophthalmic administration, drops and ointments should be applied into the conjunctival sac—not directly onto the eye itself.

Oral midodrine should be taken exactly as prescribed. This medication is usually ordered to be given with forcing of fluids before the patient gets out of bed in the morning. Doses of the drug are also often front loaded in their dosing schedule so that most of the doses occur in the morning when patients with orthostatic intolerance are usually more symptomatic. Patients should avoid taking this medication after 6 PM if at all possible to prevent insomnia and possible supine hypertension.

Evaluation

Therapeutic effects of *adrenergic drugs* include the following: For vasoactive drugs, therapeutic effects include improved cardiac output (with increased urinary output), return to normal vital signs (e.g., blood pressure of 120/80 mm Hg or higher or gradual increases in blood pressure as indicated, pulse rate greater than 60 but less than 120 beats/min), improved skin color (pallor to pink) and temperature (cool to warm) in the extremities, improved peripheral pulses, and increased level of consciousness. Therapeutic effects of drugs given for bronchial indications include a return to normal respiratory rate (more than 12 but fewer than 20 breaths/min), improved breath sounds throughout the lung field with fewer adventitious (abnormal) sounds, increased air exchange in all areas of the lungs, decreased to no coughing, less dyspnea, improved partial pressure of oxygen and pulse oximeter readings, and tolerance of slowly increasing levels of activity. If the drugs are used for nasal congestion, the patient should report less congestion and improved ability to breathe. Therapeutic effects of midodrine include improved level of functioning and improved performance of the activities of daily living, fewer episodes of postural intolerance (dizziness, lightheadedness, and syncopal episodes), and more energy.

Evaluation for the occurrence of adverse effects with adrenergic drugs includes monitoring for stimulation of the systems that are affected, such as the cardiac system and the CNS. Adverse effects such as cardiac irregularities, hypertension, and tachycardia may occur. The nurse should be sure to monitor for chest pain as well. With the use of nasal decongestants, adverse effects of rebound nasal congestion, rhinitis, and nasal mucosal ulcerations are possible. See previous discussion for additional information on adverse effects.

PATIENT TEACHING TIPS

- Medications should be taken as prescribed. Excessive dosing may cause CNS and cardiovascular stimulation with tremors, nervousness, tachycardia, and palpitations.
- Instructions for use of inhaled forms of medication, including nebulizers, inhalers, and metered-dose inhalers, should be clear and concise (see Chapter 10).
- The patient should be instructed to report any worsening of respiratory symptoms, dyspnea, distress, chest pain, and/or cardiac palpitations to the prescriber immediately.
- Over-the-counter medications and herbal supplements should be avoided unless the prescriber's approval is obtained.

- If adrenergic nasal decongestant sprays are used, the phenomenon of rebound nasal congestion may occur with overuse. Rebound can be prevented by taking the drug as prescribed and not overusing the drug. Should rebound nasal congestion occur, the patient should follow the instructions given by the prescriber or health care provider and use saline nasal spray for relief.
- Midodrine requires careful dosing, as ordered, and the patient should keep a journal to record adverse effects, improvements in symptoms, and any worsening of symptoms.

POINTS TO REMEMBER

- Catecholamines are substances that produce a sympathomimetic response (stimulate the SNS). The naturally occurring or endogenous catecholamines include epinephrine, norepinephrine, and dopamine. An example of an exogenous catecholamine is dobutamine.
- If the patient has a chronic respiratory disease, such as emphysema or chronic asthma or bronchitis, it is important for the patient to avoid contact with individuals who may have infections to help minimize situations that would exacerbate the original problem. Respiratory irritants should also be avoided.
- With nasal preparations, rebound nasal congestion or ulcerations of the nasal mucosa may occur if drugs are overused;

therefore, patients need to be educated to use these products only as directed.
- Midodrine use requires careful blood pressure monitoring, so patient education about supine blood pressure measurement and journaling of measured blood pressure values is very important to the effective use of the drug.
- Inhaled forms of beta$_2$ agonists are used for their bronchodilating action and must be taken only as prescribed, with caution to avoid any overuse of the drug. Overdosage of these drugs may lead to severe cardiovascular, CNS, and cerebrovascular adverse effects and stimulation.

NCLEX EXAMINATION REVIEW QUESTIONS

1 The nurse caring for a patient who is receiving beta$_1$ agonist drug therapy needs to be aware that these drugs cause
  a increased cardiac contractility.
  b decreased heart rate.
  c bronchoconstriction.
  d increased GI tract motility.
2 During a teaching session for a patient who is receiving inhaled salmeterol, the nurse emphasizes that the drug is indicated for
  a rescue treatment of acute bronchospasms.
  b prevention of bronchospasm.
  c reduction of airway inflammation.
  d long-term treatment of sinus congestion.
3 For a patient receiving a vasoactive drug such as intravenous dopamine, which action by the nurse is most appropriate?
  a Monitor the gravity drip infusion closely and adjust as needed
  b Assess the patient's cardiac function by checking the radial pulse
  c Assess the intravenous site hourly to rule out infiltration
  d Administer the drug by intravenous boluses according to the patient's blood pressure

4 A patient is receiving dobutamine for shock and is complaining of feeling more "skipping beats" than yesterday. The nurse's next action should be to
  a monitor for other signs of a therapeutic response to the drug.
  b titrate the drug to a higher dose to reduce the palpitations.
  c discontinue the dobutamine immediately.
  d assess the patient's vital signs and cardiac rhythm.
5 When a drug is characterized as having a negative chronotropic effect, the nurse knows to expect
  a improved sinoatrial nodal firing.
  b decreased heart rate.
  c decreased ectopic beats.
  d increased force of cardiac contractions.
6 The nurse is monitoring a patient who is receiving an infusion of a beta-adrenergic agonist. Which adverse effects may occur with this infusion? (Select all that apply.)
  a Mild tremors
  b Bradycardia
  c Tachycardia
  d Palpitations
  e Drowsiness
  f Nervousness

1. a, 2. b, 3. c, 4. d, 5. b, 6. a, c, d, f.

CRITICAL THINKING ACTIVITIES: BEST ACTION

1 While making initial morning rounds, the nurse checks the insertion site of a patient's dopamine infusion and finds the area swollen and cool to the touch. What should the nurse do first? Explain what actions will follow.

2 A patient with chronic emphysema is experiencing an episode of bronchoconstriction and wants to use his salmeterol inhaler. What is the nurse's best action?

3 A patient is experiencing a severe anaphylactic reaction after a dose of an antibiotic, and the emergency team is present. The nurse is expecting to give what drug first? Explain.

For answers, see *http://evolve.elsevier.com/Lilley*.

CHAPTER 19

Adrenergic-Blocking Drugs

OBJECTIVES

When you reach the end of this chapter, you should be able to do the following:

1 Briefly review the functions of the sympathetic nervous system and the specific effects of adrenergic blocking.

2 List the various drugs classified as adrenergic antagonists (blockers) or sympatholytics.

3 Discuss the mechanisms of action, therapeutic effects, indications, adverse and toxic effects, cautions, contraindications, drug interactions, dosages, routes of administration, and any antidotal management for the various alpha antagonists (blockers), beta nonselective blockers and the beta$_1$- and beta$_2$-blockers.

4 Develop a nursing care plan that includes all phases of the nursing process for patients taking adrenergic antagonists.

Drug Profiles

- ◆ atenolol, p. 306
- carvedilol, p. 306
- ◆ esmolol, p. 306
- labetalol, p. 306
- ◆ metoprolol, p. 307

- ◆ phentolamine, p. 304
- ◆ propranolol, p. 307
- sotalol, p. 308
- tamsulosin, p. 304

◆ *Key drug.*

Glossary

Agonists Drugs with a specific receptor affinity that mimic the body's natural chemicals (e.g., hormones, neurotransmitters). (p. 301)

Angina Paroxysmal (sudden) chest pain caused by myocardial ischemia. (p. 305)

Antagonists Drugs that bind to specific receptors and inhibit or block the response of the receptors. (p. 301)

Dysrhythmias Irregular heart rhythms; almost always called *arrhythmias* in clinical practice. (p. 305)

Extravasation The leaking of fluid from a blood vessel into the surrounding tissues, as in the case of an infiltrated intravenous infusion. (p. 303)

Intrinsic sympathomimetic activity The paradoxical action of some beta-blocking drugs (e.g., acebutolol) that mimics the action of the sympathetic nervous system. (p. 304)

Lipophilicity The chemical attraction of a substance (e.g., drug molecule) to lipid or fat molecules. (p. 305)

Pheochromocytoma A vascular adrenal gland tumor that is usually benign but secretes epinephrine and norepinephrine and thus often causes central nervous system stimulation and substantial blood pressure elevation. (p. 302)

Sympatholytics Drugs that inhibit the postganglionic functioning of the sympathetic nervous system. (p. 301)

• • •

Anatomy and Physiology Overview

The autonomic nervous system consists of the parasympathetic and sympathetic nervous systems. The class of drugs discussed in this chapter works primarily on the sympathetic nervous system (SNS). As discussed in Chapter 18, the adrenergic agonist drugs stimulate the SNS. Those drugs are called **agonists** because they bind to receptors and cause a response. The adrenergic blockers have the opposite effect and are therefore referred to as **antagonists.** They also bind to adrenergic receptors but in doing so inhibit or block stimulation by the SNS. They are also referred to as **sympatholytics** because they "lyse," or inhibit, SNS stimulation.

Throughout the body there are receptor sites for the endogenous sympathetic neurotransmitters norepinephrine and epinephrine. Such receptors are known as *adrenergic receptors,* and two basic types are found—alpha and beta. There are subtypes of both the alpha- and beta-adrenergic receptors, designated 1 and 2. The alpha$_1$- and alpha$_2$-adrenergic receptors are differentiated by their location on nerves. The alpha$_1$-adrenergic receptors are located on the tissue, muscle, or organ that the nerve is stimulating (postsynaptic effector cells). The alpha$_2$-adrenergic receptors are located on the actual nerves that stimulate the presynaptic effector cells. The alpha-$_2$ receptors are inhibitory. Thus, it is actually the stimulation or agonist activity at alpha-$_2$ receptors that causes the inhibitory effects of the SNS. Alpha$_2$–active drugs (i.e., clonidine) are discussed in Chapter 25 on antihypertensive drugs. The beta$_1$-

adrenergic receptors are located primarily in the heart. The beta$_2$-adrenergic receptors are located primarily on the smooth muscles of the bronchioles and blood vessels. It is at these various receptors that adrenergic blockers act, and they are classified by the type of adrenergic receptor they block—alpha or beta or, in a few cases, both. Hence, they are called *alpha-blockers, beta-blockers,* or *alpha/beta-blockers.*

Pharmacology Overview

ALPHA-BLOCKERS

Mechanism of Action and Drug Effects

The alpha-adrenergic–blocking drugs, or alpha-blockers, interrupt the stimulation of the SNS at the alpha$_1$-adrenergic receptors. More specifically, alpha-blockers work either by direct competition with the SNS neurotransmitter norepinephrine or by a noncompetitive process. Figure 19-1 illustrates these two mechanisms. The drugs have a greater affinity for the alpha-adrenergic receptor than does norepinephrine and can chemically displace norepinephrine molecules from the receptor. Adrenergic blockade at these receptors leads to effects such as vasodilation, reduced blood pressure, miosis (pupillary constriction), and reduced smooth muscle tone in organs like the bladder and prostate. Currently available alpha-blockers are listed in Table 19-1.

Indications

The alpha-blockers such as doxazosin, prazosin, and terazosin cause both arterial and venous dilation. This reduces peripheral vascular resistance and blood pressure, and these drugs are used to treat hypertension (see Chapter 25). The alpha-adrenergic receptors are also present in the prostate and bladder. By blocking stimulation of alpha$_1$ receptors, these drugs reduce smooth muscle contraction of the bladder neck and the prostatic portion of the urethra. For this reason, alpha-blockers are given to patients with benign prostatic hyperplasia (BPH) to decrease resistance to urinary outflow. This reduces urinary obstruction and relieves some of the effects of BPH. Tamsulosin and alfuzosin are used exclusively for treating BPH, whereas terazosin and doxazosin can be used for both hypertension and BPH.

Other alpha-blockers can inhibit excitatory responses to adrenergic stimulation. These drugs noncompetitively block alpha-adrenergic receptors on smooth muscle and various exocrine glands. Because of this action, these alpha-blockers are very useful in controlling or preventing hypertension in patients who have a **pheochromocytoma,** a tumor that forms on the adrenal gland on top of the kidney and secretes norepinephrine, thus causing SNS stimulation. The alpha-blockers are also useful in the treatment of patients who have any kind of increased endogenous alpha-adrenergic agonist activity, which results in vasoconstriction. Three conditions in which this occurs are Raynaud's disease, acrocyanosis, and frostbite. Phenoxybenzamine, in particular, is an

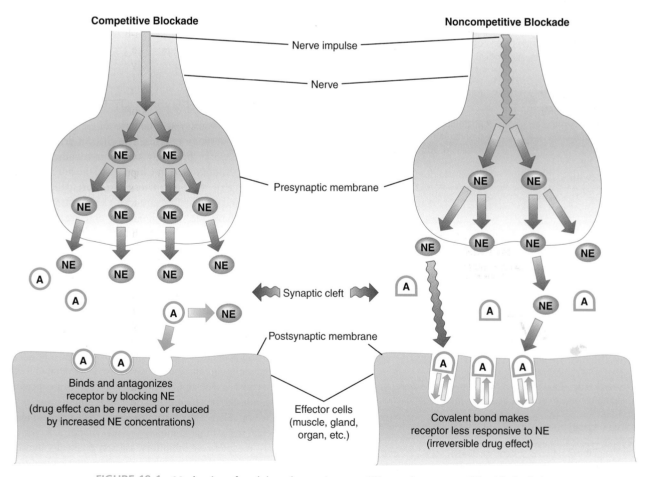

FIGURE 19-1   Mechanisms for alpha-adrenergic competitive and noncompetitive blockade by alpha-blockers. *A,* Alpha-blocker; *NE,* norepinephrine.

TABLE 19-1 Currently Available Adrenergic-Blocking Drugs

Generic Name	Trade Name	Route
Alpha₁-Blockers		
alfuzosin	Uroxatral	PO
doxazosin	Cardura	PO
phenoxybenzamine	Dibenzyline	PO
phentolamine	generic	IV, IM, IM/subcut/ intradermal (for extravasation wounds)
prazosin	Minipress	PO
terazosin	Hytrin	PO
tamsulosin	Flomax	PO
Beta-Blockers		
Nonselective		
carteolol	Cartrol	
carvedilol*	Coreg, Coreg CR	PO
labetalol*	Normodyne, Trandate	PO, IV
nadolol	Corgard	PO
penbutolol	Levatol	PO
pindolol	Visken	PO
propranolol*	Inderal	PO, IV
sotalol	Betapace	PO
timolol	Blocadren, Timoptic	PO, IV, ophthalmic
Cardioselective		
acebutolol	Sectral	PO
atenolol	Tenormin	PO, IV
betaxolol	Kerlone	PO
bisoprolol	Zebeta	PO
esmolol	Brevibloc	IV
metoprolol	Lopressor, Toprol-XL	PO, IV

IM, Intramuscular; *IV,* intravenous; *PO,* oral; *subcut,* subcutaneous.
*Has antagonist activity at alpha₁, beta₁, and beta₂ receptors.

TABLE 19-2 Alpha-Blockers: Adverse Effects

Body System	Adverse Effects
Cardiovascular	Palpitations, orthostatic hypotension, tachycardia, edema, dysrhythmias, chest pain
Central nervous	Dizziness, headache, drowsiness, anxiety, depression, vertigo, weakness, numbness, fatigue
Gastrointestinal	Nausea, vomiting, diarrhea, constipation, abdominal pain
Other	Incontinence, nosebleed, tinnitus, dry mouth, pharyngitis, rhinitis

TABLE 19-3 Alpha-Blockers: Common Drug Interactions

Interacting Drug	Mechanism	Result
Beta-blockers Calcium channel blockers Diuretics	Additive effects	Profound hypotension
Protein-bound drugs	Competition for plasma protein-binding sites	Effects of increased free drug levels in plasma

Adverse Effects

The primary adverse effects of alpha-blockers are those related to their effects on the vasculature. The primary adverse effects of the alpha-blockers are listed by body system in Table 19-2.

Toxicity and Management of Overdose

In an acute oral overdose, the patient's stomach should be emptied immediately by gastric lavage. After this, activated charcoal should be administered to bind to the drug and remove it from the stomach and the circulation. With overdoses of both oral and injectable forms, symptomatic and supportive measures should be instituted as needed. Blood pressure support with the administration of fluids, volume expanders, and vasopressor drugs and the administration of anticonvulsants such as diazepam for the control of seizures are examples of such measures.

Interactions

The most severe drug interactions with alpha-blockers are the ones that potentiate the effects of the alpha-blockers. The alpha-blockers are very highly protein bound and compete for binding sites with other drugs that are highly protein bound (see Chapter 2). Because of the limited sites for binding on proteins and the increased competition for these sites, more free alpha-blocker molecules circulate in the bloodstream. Only the drug that is not bound to protein is active. Thus more active drug results in a more pronounced drug effect. Some of the common drugs that interact with alpha-blockers and the results of these interactions are listed in Table 19-3.

Dosages

For the recommended dosages of alpha-blockers, see the Dosages table on p. 304.

alpha-blocker beneficial in the treatment of these syndromes, although its use is uncommon.

Still other alpha-blockers are effective at counteracting any excessive effects of injected catecholamines such as epinephrine and norepinephrine. They do this by causing peripheral vasodilation and reducing peripheral resistance by blocking catecholamine-stimulated vasoconstriction. Because of their potent vasodilating properties and their fast onset of action, they are also used to prevent skin necrosis and sloughing after the **extravasation** of vasopressors such as norepinephrine or epinephrine. When these drugs extravasate, or leak out of the blood vessel into the surrounding tissue, they cause vasoconstriction and ultimately tissue death, or necrosis. If the vasoconstriction is not reversed quickly, the entire limb can be lost. Phentolamine, in particular, can reverse this potent vasoconstriction and restore blood flow to the ischemic tissue.

Contraindications

Contraindications to the use of alpha-blocking drugs include known drug allergy and peripheral vascular disease and may include hepatic and renal disease, coronary artery disease, peptic ulcer, and sepsis.

DOSAGES

Selected Alpha-Adrenergic–Blocking Drugs

Drug (Pregnancy Category)	Pharmacologic Class	Usual Dosage Range	Indications
◆ phentolamine (Regitine) (C)	Alpha-blocker	**Adult** IM/IV: 5 mg; repeat if necessary	Hypertensive episodes with pheochromocytoma
		Adult 5-10 mg diluted in 10 mL NS injected into extravasation site	Alpha-adrenergic drug extravasation
		Pediatric 0.1-0.2 mg/kg into extravasation site	
tamsulosin (Flomax) (B)*	Alpha$_1$-blocker	**Adult** PO: 0.4 mg once daily; max dose 0.8 mg	Benign prostatic hyperplasia

IM, Intramuscular; *IV,* intravenous; *NS,* normal saline; *PO,* oral.
*Not indicated for use in women.

DRUG PROFILES

The alpha-blockers are commonly used to treat hypertension and/or benign prostatic hyperplasia. They include phentolamine, phenoxybenzamine, terazosin, alfuzosin, tamsulosin, and prazosin. Prazosin is discussed in Chapter 25 on antihypertensive drugs.

◆ phentolamine

Phentolamine (Regitine) is an alpha-blocker that reduces peripheral vascular resistance and is also used to treat hypertension. Like phenoxybenzamine, it is used to treat the high blood pressure caused by pheochromocytoma, but unlike phenoxybenzamine, phentolamine can also be used in the diagnosis of this catecholamine-secreting tumor. To help establish a diagnosis of pheochromocytoma, a single intravenous dose of phentolamine is given to the hypertensive patient who is suspected of having the tumor. If the blood pressure declines rapidly, it is highly likely that the patient has a pheochromocytoma. Phentolamine is available only as an injectable preparation. This confers some advantages, however, because it can be used to treat the extravasation of vasoconstricting intravenous drugs such as norepinephrine, epinephrine, and dopamine, which when given intravenously can leak out of the vein, especially if the intravenous tube is not correctly positioned. If such a drug is allowed to extravasate into the surrounding tissue, the result is intense vasoconstriction, decreased blood flow, necrosis, and potential loss of the limb. When phentolamine is injected subcutaneously in a circular fashion around the extravasation site, it causes alpha-adrenergic receptor blockade and vasodilation, which in turn increases blood flow to the ischemic tissue and thus prevents permanent damage. Its use is contraindicated in patients who have shown a hypersensitivity to it, those who have experienced a myocardial infarction (MI), and those with coronary artery disease. Adverse effects include tachycardia, dizziness, gastrointestinal upset, and others listed in Table 19-2. Drugs with which phentolamine interacts include alcohol (disulfiram-like reaction; see Chapter 9) and erectile dysfunction medications such as sildenafil (additive hypotensive effects; see Chapter 35). Epinephrine and ephedrine can counteract the desired effects of phentolamine. The recommended dosages are given in the table above.

PHARMACOKINETICS

Route	Onset of Action	Peak Plasma Concentration	Elimination Half-life	Duration of Action
IV	1 hr	4-6 hr	24 hr	3-4 days

tamsulosin

Tamsulosin (Flomax) is an alpha-blocker used primarily to treat BPH and is exclusively indicated for male patients. A similar drug with the same indication is alfuzosin. These drugs block alpha-adrenergic receptors on smooth muscle within the prostate and bladder. This results in relaxation of these smooth muscle fibers and improved urinary flow. Other similar drugs include terazosin and doxazosin, which can be used to treat both BPH and hypertension. Contraindications to tamsulosin include known drug allergy and concurrent use of erectile dysfunction drugs such as sildenafil. Adverse effects include headache, abnormal ejaculation, rhinitis, and others listed in Table 19-2. Interacting drugs include other alpha-blockers, calcium channel blockers and erectile dysfunction drugs (additive hypotensive effects); drugs that induce or inhibit hepatic enzymes may reduce or enhance, respectively, the effects of tamsulosin. Tamsulosin is available only for oral use.

PHARMACOKINETICS

Route	Onset of Action	Peak Plasma Concentration	Elimination Half-life	Duration of Action
PO	Unknown	4-7 hr	15 hr	unknown

BETA-BLOCKERS

Mechanism of Action and Drug Effects

The beta-adrenergic–blocking drugs (beta-blockers) block SNS stimulation of the beta-adrenergic receptors by competing with the endogenous catecholamines norepinephrine and epinephrine. The beta-blockers can be either selective or nonselective, depending on the type of beta-adrenergic receptors they antagonize. As mentioned earlier, beta$_1$-adrenergic receptors are located primarily in the heart. Beta-blockers selective for these receptors are sometimes called *cardioselective beta-blockers* or *beta$_1$-blocking drugs.* Other beta-blockers block both beta$_1$- and beta$_2$-adrenergic receptors, the latter of which are located primarily on the smooth muscles of the bronchioles and blood vessels. These beta-blockers are referred to as *nonselective beta-blockers.* In addition, beta-blockers can be further categorized according to whether or not they have **intrinsic sympathomimetic activity.** Drugs with intrinsic sympathomimetic activity (acebutolol, penbutolol, pindolol) not only block beta-adrenergic receptors but also partially stimulate them. This was initially believed to be an advantageous characteristic, but clinical experience has not borne this out. Two beta-blockers, carvedilol and labetalol, also have an alpha-receptor–blocking activity, especially at higher dosages. Table 19-1 lists the currently available beta-blockers.

Cardioselective beta$_1$-blockers block the beta$_1$ receptors on the surface of the heart. This reduces myocardial stimulation, which in turn reduces heart rate, slows conduction through the atrioventricular (AV) node, prolongs sinoatrial (SA) node recovery, and decreases myocardial oxygen demand by decreasing myocardial contractile force (contractility). Nonselective beta-blockers also have these cardiac effects, but they block beta$_2$ receptors on the smooth muscle of the bronchioles and blood vessels as well.

Smooth muscle also surrounds the airways in the lungs called *bronchioles.* When beta$_2$-receptors in the bronchioles are blocked, the smooth muscle contracts, causing these airways to narrow. This may lead to shortness of breath. In addition, the smooth muscle that surrounds blood vessels controls the size of the blood vessels and can cause dilation or constriction depending on whether the beta$_1$ or beta$_2$ receptors are stimulated. When beta$_2$ stimulation is blocked by a beta-blocker, the muscles are then stimulated by unopposed sympathetic activity at the beta$_1$ receptors, which causes them to contract. This in turn increases peripheral vascular resistance. Furthermore, catecholamines promote *glycogenolysis,* the production of glucose from glycogen, and mobilize glucose in response to hypoglycemia. Nonselective beta-blockers impair this process and also impede the secretion of insulin from the pancreas, which causes elevation of blood glucose level.

Finally, beta-blockers can cause the release of free fatty acids from adipose tissue. This may result in moderately elevated blood levels of triglycerides and reduced levels of the "good cholesterol" known as *high-density lipoprotein* (HDL).

Indications

Indications for beta-blockers include angina, MI, cardiac dysrhythmias, hypertension, and heart failure.

Beta-blockers are commonly used in the treatment of **angina,** or chest pain (see Chapter 24). These drugs work by decreasing the demand for myocardial energy and oxygen consumption, which helps shift the supply/demand ratio to the supply side and allows more oxygen to get to the heart muscle. This in turn helps relieve the pain in the heart muscle caused by the lack of oxygen.

Beta-blockers are also considered to be *cardioprotective* because they inhibit stimulation of the myocardium by circulating catecholamines. Catecholamines are released during myocardial muscle damage such as that caused by an MI, or heart attack. Unopposed stimulation by catecholamines would further increase the heart rate and the contractile force and thereby increase myocardial oxygen demand. When a beta-blocker drug occupies myocardial beta$_1$ receptors, circulating catecholamine molecules are prevented from binding to the receptors. Thus, the beta-blockers protect the heart from being stimulated by these catecholamines. Because of this characteristic, beta-blockers are commonly given to patients after they have experienced an MI to protect the heart.

As mentioned previously, beta-blockers also have a profound effect on the conduction system of the heart. The AV node normally receives impulse stimulation from the SA node and slows it down so that the ventricles have time to fill before they are

stimulated to contract. Conduction in the SA node, is slowed by beta-blockers, which results in a decreased heart rate. These drugs also slow conduction through the AV node. These effects of the beta-blockers on the conduction system of the heart make them useful drugs in the treatment of various types of irregular heart rhythms, called **dysrhythmias** (see Chapter 23).

The ability to reduce SNS stimulation of the heart, including reducing heart rate and the force of myocardial contraction (systole), renders beta-blockers useful in treating hypertension. Traditionally beta-blockers were thought to worsen heart failure. However, recent studies have shown benefit to the use of beta-blockers. Certain beta-blockers such as carvedilol and metoprolol have produced the best results to date. The form of heart failure that includes a diastolic dysfunction component responds especially favorably to beta-blockers.

Because of their **lipophilicity** (attraction to lipid or fat), some beta-blockers (e.g., propranolol) can easily gain entry into the central nervous system and are used to treat migraine headaches. In addition, the topical application of timolol to the eye has been very effective in treating ocular disorders such as glaucoma (see Chapter 57).

Contraindications

Contraindications to the use of beta-blockers include known drug allergies and may include uncompensated heart failure, cardiogenic shock, heart block or bradycardia, pregnancy, severe pulmonary disease, and Raynaud's disease.

Adverse Effects

The adverse effects of beta-blockers are primarily extensions of their pharmacologic activity. Most such effects are mild and diminish with time. Some of the most serious undesirable effects can be caused by acute withdrawal of the drug. For example, such sudden withdrawal may exacerbate the underlying angina the drug is being used to treat or it may precipitate an MI. Beta-blockers may delay the recovery from hypoglycemia in patients with type 1 diabetes patients (rarely in those with type 2). In addition, the nonselective beta-blockers can interfere with the normal responses to hypoglycemia, such as tremor, tachycardia, and nervousness, in essence masking the signs and symptoms of hypoglycemia. Adverse effects induced by beta-blockers are listed by body system in Table 19-4.

TABLE 19-4 Beta-Blockers: Common Adverse Effects

Body System	Adverse Effects
Cardiovascular	Atrioventricular block, bradycardia, heart failure, peripheral vascular insufficiency
Central nervous	Dizziness, fatigue, mental depression, lethargy, drowsiness, unusual dreams
Gastrointestinal	Nausea, vomiting, constipation, diarrhea, cramps, ischemic colitis
Hematologic	Agranulocytosis, thrombocytopenia
Metabolic	Hyperglycemia and/or hypoglycemia, hyperlipidemia
Other	Impotence, rash, alopecia, bronchospasms, wheezing, dry mouth

TABLE 19-5 Beta-Blockers: Drug Interactions

Interacting Drug	Mechanism	Result
Antacids (aluminum hydroxide type)	Decrease absorption	Decreased beta-blocker activity
Antimuscarinics, anticholinergics	Antagonism	Reduced beta-blocker effects
Digoxin	Additive effect	Enhanced bradycardic effects of digoxin
Diuretics and cardiovascular drugs	Additive effect	Additive hypotensive effects
Neuromuscular blocking drugs	Additive effect	Prolonged neuromuscular blockade
Oral hypoglycemic drugs, insulin	Additive hypoglycemic effects	Hypoglycemia
Mefloquine (antimalarial)	Unknown	Increased risk of cardiac dysrhythmias and cardiac arrest

Toxicity and Management of Overdose

After acute oral overdose of a beta-blocker, the stomach should be emptied immediately, either by induction of emesis or by gastric lavage. For overdoses of both oral and injectable dosage forms, treatment consists primarily of symptomatic and supportive care. Atropine may be given intravenously for the management of bradycardia. If the bradycardia still persists, placement of a transvenous cardiac pacemaker should be considered. For the treatment of severe hypotension, vasopressors should be titrated until the desired blood pressure and heart rate are achieved. Intravenously administered diazepam may be useful for the treatment of seizures. Most beta-blockers are dialyzable; therefore, hemodialysis may be useful in enhancing elimination in the event of severe overdose.

Interactions

Most of the drug interactions with beta-blockers result from either the additive effects of coadministered medications with similar mechanisms of action or the antagonistic effects of various drugs. Nonselective beta-blockers may mask the tachycardia from hypoglycemia caused by insulin and sulfonylureas, and the hypoglycemic effect of insulin and sulfonylureas may be enhanced (see Chapter 32). Some of the common drugs that interact with beta-blockers and the resulting effects are given in Table 19-5.

Dosages

For the recommended dosages of selected beta-blockers, see the Dosages table on p. 307.

DRUG PROFILES

Numerous beta-blockers currently available are listed in Table 19-1. Several beta-blockers are profiled in the following sections. Contraindications, adverse reactions, and drug interactions are comparable for these drugs and are listed in the previous text, Table 19-4, and Table 19-5, respectively.

◆ atenolol
Atenolol (Tenormin) is a cardioselective beta-blocker that is commonly used to prevent future heart attacks in patients who have had one. It is also used in the treatment of hypertension and angina. Atenolol is available for oral and injectable use. See the table on p. 307 for the recommended dosages.

PHARMACOKINETICS

Route	Onset of Action	Peak Plasma Concentration	Elimination Half-life	Duration of Action
IV	Immediate	Less than 5 min	6-7 hr	Less than 12 hr
PO	1 hr	2-4 hr	6-7 hr	24 hr

carvedilol
Carvedilol (Coreg) has many effects, including acting as a nonselective beta-blocker, an alpha$_1$-blocker, a calcium channel blocker, and possibly an antioxidant. It is used primarily in the treatment of heart failure but is also beneficial for hypertension and angina. It has been shown to slow the progression of heart failure and to decrease the frequency of hospitalization in patients with mild to moderate (class II or III) heart failure. Carvedilol is most commonly added to digoxin, furosemide, and angiotensin-converting enzyme inhibitors when used to treat heart failure. Carvedilol is available only for oral use. A controlled-release formulation, Coreg CR, was recently approved. The dosages are different from those for immediate-release Coreg, and the two cannot be interchanged. Recommended dosages are given in the table on p. 307.

PHARMACOKINETICS

Route	Onset of Action	Peak Plasma Concentration	Elimination Half-life	Duration of Action
PO	20-120 min	1-4 hr	6-8 hr	8-24 hr

◆ esmolol
Esmolol (Brevibloc) is a very potent short-acting beta$_1$-blocker. It is primarily used in acute situations to provide rapid temporary control of the ventricular rate in patients with supraventricular tachydysrhythmias. Because of its very short half-life, it is given only as an intravenous infusion and is titrated to achieve the serum levels that control the patient's symptoms. Recommended dosages are given in the table on p. 307.

PHARMACOKINETICS

Route	Onset of Action	Peak Plasma Concentration	Elimination Half-life	Duration of Action
IV	Immediate	6 min	9 min	15-20 min

labetalol
Labetalol (Normodyne) is unusual in that it can block both alpha- and beta-adrenergic receptors. It is used in the treatment of severe hypertension and hypertensive emergencies to quickly lower the blood pressure before permanent damage is done. Labetalol is available for oral and injectable use. The normal dosages are given in the table on p. 307.

DOSAGES

Selected Beta-Adrenergic–Blocking Drugs

Drug (Pregnancy Category)	Pharmacologic Class	Usual Dosage Range	Indications
◆ atenolol (Tenormin) (C)	Beta$_1$-blocker	**Adult** PO: 50-200 mg/day daily or divided bid, (max 200 mg/day) IV: 5 mg over 5 min; may repeat in 10 min	Hypertension, angina Acute myocardial infarction (MI)
carvedilol (Coreg) (C)	Alpha- and beta-blocker	**Adult** PO: 3.125 mg bid; may double dose every 2 wk to highest tolerated dose, max 50 mg/day (100 mg/day for patients with heart failure who weigh over 85 kg)	Heart failure, angina, hypertension
◆ esmolol (Brevibloc) (C)	Beta$_1$-blocker	**Adult** IV: Bolus of 500 mcg/kg over 1 min, followed by 4 min at 50 mcg/kg/min and evaluate IV: 80 mg bolus over 30 min followed by 150 mcg/kg/min infusion	Supraventricular tachydysrhythmias Intraoperative/postoperative hypertension
labetalol (Normodyne, Trandate) (C)	Alpha$_1$- and beta-blocker	**Adult** PO: 200-800 mg/day divided bid IV: 20 mg with additional doses of 40-80 mg at 10-min intervals until desired effect or a total dose of 300 mg is injected; maintenance infusion of 2 mg/min initially and titrated to response	Hypertension Severe hypertension
◆ metoprolol (Lopressor, Toprol XL) (C)	Beta$_1$-blocker	**Adult** PO: 100-450 mg/day divided bid-tid IV/PO: 3 bolus injections of 5 mg at 2-min intervals followed in 15 min by 50 mg PO q6h for 48 hr; thereafter 100 mg PO bid	Hypertension, late MI Early MI
◆ propranolol (Inderal) (C)	Beta-blocker	**Adult** PO: 80-320 mg/day divided bid-qid 120-640 mg/day divided bid-tid 10-30 mg tid-qid 180-240 mg divided tid-qid 20-40 mg tid-qid 120-320 mg/day divided 160-240 mg/day divided 30-60 mg/day divided for 3 days before surgery with an alpha-blocker also IV: 1 mg slow IV push, may repeat every 5 min up to 5 mg	Angina Hypertension Dysrhythmias Post-MI Hypertrophic subaortic stenosis Essential tremor Migraine Pheochromocytoma surgery Serious dysrhythmias
sotalol (Betapace) (B)	Beta-blocker	**Adult** PO: 160-320 mg/day divided	Life-threatening ventricular dysrhythmias

IV, Intravenous; *PO,* oral.

PHARMACOKINETICS

Route	Onset of Action	Peak Plasma Concentration	Elimination Half-life	Duration of Action
IV	2-5 min	5-15 min	2.5-8 hr	2-4 hr
PO	20-120 min	1-4 hr	2.5-8 hr	8-24 hr

◆ metoprolol

Metoprolol (Lopressor) is a beta$_1$-blocker that has become a favorite of cardiologists for use in patients after MI. Recent studies of metoprolol have shown increased survival in patients given the drug after they have experienced an MI. Metoprolol is available for oral and injectable use. Commonly recommended dosages are given in the table above.

PHARMACOKINETICS

Route	Onset of Action	Peak Plasma Concentration	Elimination Half-life	Duration of Action
IV	1 min	20 min	3-8 hr	5-8 hr
PO	1 hr	2-4 hr	3-8 hr	10-20 hr

◆ propranolol

Propranolol (Inderal) is the prototypical nonselective beta$_1$- and beta$_2$-blocking drug. It was one of the very first beta-blockers to be used. The lengthy experience with it has revealed many uses for it. In addition to the indications mentioned for metoprolol, propranolol has been used for the treatment of tachydysrhythmias associated with cardiac glycoside intoxication and for the treatment of hypertrophic subaortic stenosis, pheochromocytoma, thyrotoxicosis, migraine headache, essential tremor, and many other conditions. The same contraindications that apply to the cardioselective beta-blockers discussed earlier hold for propranolol as well. In addition, its use is contraindicated in patients with bronchial asthma. Propranolol is available for oral and injectable use. The recommended dosages are given in the table on p. 307.

PHARMACOKINETICS

Route	Onset of Action	Peak Plasma Concentration	Elimination Half-life	Duration of Action
IV	2 min	1-4 hr	3-5 hr	3-6 hr
PO	1-2 hr	1-4 hr	3-5 hr	6-12 hr

sotalol

Sotalol (Betapace) is a nonselective beta-blocker that has very potent antidysrhythmic properties. It is commonly used for the management of difficult-to-treat dysrhythmias. Often these dysrhythmias are life-threatening ventricular dysrhythmias such as sustained ventricular tachycardia. It has properties characteristic of both a class II and a class III antidysrhythmic drug (see Chapter 23). Because it is a nonselective beta-blocker, it causes some of the unwanted adverse effects typical of these drugs (e.g., hypotension). Sotalol is available only for oral use. Commonly recommended dosages are given in the table on p. 307.

PHARMACOKINETICS

Route	Onset of Action	Peak Plasma Concentration	Elimination Half-life	Duration of Action
PO	1-2 hr	2.5-4 hr	12 hr	8-16 hr

PREVENTING MEDICATION ERRORS

Look-Alike Drugs: Toprol-XL, Topamax, and Tegretol

Be careful about look-alike drugs! Medication errors often occur when drug names are similar. The Food and Drug Administration has reported errors in prescribing and dispensing involving a mix-up between Topamax (topiramate), which is indicated for the treatment of epilepsy and prophylaxis of migraines, and Toprol-XL (metoprolol succinate), which is used for the treatment of hypertension and heart failure as well as the long-term treatment of angina pectoris. Other errors have occurred when Toprol-XL and Tegretol (carbamazepine), a drug used for various types of seizures and trigeminal neuralgia, have been confused. Consider what would happen if a patient with a history of seizures receives a beta-blocker instead of the prescribed antiepileptic drug! These cases reinforce the importance of checking the drug name carefully (using both trade and generic names).

For more information, go to *http://www.fda.gov/medwatch/safety/2005/toprol_dhcp.pdf.*

NURSING PROCESS

Assessment

Adrenergic-blocking drugs, or sympatholytics, produce a variety of effects on the patient, depending on the type of receptor(s) blocked. Because of the impact of these drugs, primarily on the cardiac and respiratory systems, their use requires careful assessment to help minimize the adverse effects and maximize the therapeutic effects. Understanding the basic anatomy and physiology of adrenergic receptors and their subsequent actions if stimulated or blocked is also critical in carrying out assessment and other aspects of the nursing process and drug therapy. If an adrenergic-blocking drug is nonselective, it blocks both alpha and beta (beta$_1$ and beta$_2$) receptors. Alpha receptor blocking affects blood vessels, whereas beta$_1$ receptor blocking affects heart rate and beta$_2$ blocking affects bronchial smooth muscle. Therefore, a nonselective adrenergic blocker will have the following actions: (1) alpha-blocking leading to blockade of the sympathetic stimulation of blood vessels (i.e., vasoconstriction) and resulting in vasodilation and a subsequent decrease in blood pressure; (2) beta$_1$-blocking leading to blockade of the sympathetic effects on heart rate, contractility, and conduction with resulting bradycardia, negative inotropic effects (i.e., decrease in contractility), and a decrease in conduction; and (3) beta$_2$-blocking leading to blockade of the sympathetic effects on bronchial smooth muscle with the net effect of bronchoconstriction. However, if the drug is only an alpha-, beta$_1$-, or beta$_2$-blocker, the resulting effect will be related to the specific receptor being blocked (or combination of receptors, depending on the drug). An understanding of these basic physiologic concepts is necessary to critical thinking and decision making in the administration of these drugs.

To begin a thorough assessment, the nurse should gather information about the patient's allergies and past and present medical conditions. Conducting a system overview and taking a thorough medication history should also be part of this process. Questions about the following should be asked and findings documented: allergies to medications and/or foods; presence of chronic obstructive pulmonary disease (e.g., emphysema, asthma, chronic bronchitis), other respiratory diseases, hypertension or hypotension, cardiac disease, bradycardia, congestive heart failure, and/or cardiac dysrhythmias. This information is crucial to patient safety, because alpha-blockers may precipitate hypotension, and therefore patients with baseline low blood pressure readings may need frequent monitoring (blood pressure measurement) or may not tolerate the medication prescribed for them. Beta-blocking drugs may precipitate bradycardia, hypotension, heart block, heart failure, bronchoconstriction, and/or increased airway resistance. Therefore, any preexisting condition that might be worsened by the concurrent use of any of these medications may then represent a contraindication or caution. More specifically, with beta$_1$-blocking drugs, patients with preexisting bradycardia, decreased cardiac contractility, heart failure, and/or decreased conduction with heart block would not be able to take these drugs without significant negative consequences. As another example, patients with a history of asthma, emphysema, bronchitis, or any condition with increased airway resistance or bronchoconstriction cannot take beta$_2$-blocking drugs without experiencing major negative effects on their underlying disease condition. For a complete listing of drug interactions see Tables 19-3 and 19-5. Adverse effects are listed in Tables 19-2 and 19-4.

Nursing Diagnoses

- Ineffective airway clearance related to the adverse effect of bronchoconstriction caused by beta-adrenergic drugs as well as any underlying restrictive airway conditions
- Ineffective cerebral and peripheral tissue perfusion related to the adverse effects of the disease of hypertension and the adverse effects of the adrenergic-blocking drugs (hypotension)

- Disturbed sensory perception related to the central nervous system adverse effects of the adrenergic-blocking drugs
- Risk for injury related to possible adverse effects of the adrenergic-blocking drugs (e.g., postural hypotension, numbness and tingling of the fingers and toes)
- Imbalanced nutrition, less than body requirements, due to nausea and vomiting related to the adverse effects of the adrenergic blockers
- Deficient knowledge related to lack of information about the therapeutic regimen, drug adverse effects, drug interactions, and precautions to be taken during drug treatment

Planning

Goals

- Patient maintains or regains effective airway clearance and airway exchange.
- Patient maintains or regains adequate tissue perfusion.
- Patient's perception and central nervous system functioning remain intact.
- Patient is free of injury to self related to adverse effects of the medications.
- Patient takes medication exactly as prescribed and with minimal impact on nutrition.
- Patient experiences improvement in hypertension or relief of the symptoms for which the medication was prescribed.
- Patient remains adherent to the drug therapy regimen.
- Patient demonstrates adequate knowledge concerning the use of the specific medications, their adverse effects, and the appropriate dosing routine to be followed at home.

Outcome Criteria

- Patient states that respirations are performed with ease and in a regular rhythm, and without any bronchospasms or wheezing.
- Patient states that blood pressure readings are within the normal range and that adverse effects are minimal.
- Patient reports fewer symptoms of hypertension as well as more energy and clearer thinking without profound adverse effects.
- Patient is free of injury to self related to adverse effects of the medications.
- Patient states the importance of both the pharmacologic and nonpharmacologic treatment of hypertension or other indication for the drug therapy.
- Patient states reasons for adhering with the medication therapy regimen without risking nutritional status.
- Patient reports effective blood pressure lowering or other treatment with an adrenergic blocker without risks and complications such as syncope, dizziness, and hypotension.
- Patient demonstrates the correct method of self-measurement of blood pressure using a digital cuff device or community resources.
- Patient states the conditions that may occur of which the prescriber should be informed immediately, such as palpitations, chest pain, insomnia, and excessive agitation.
- Patient keeps all follow-up appointments with the prescriber to maintain safe therapy.
- Patient follows instructions to avoid sudden withdrawal of hypertensive drugs to prevent rebound hypertensive crises, and experiences minimal complications.

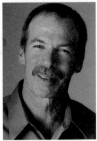
Implementation

Several nursing interventions may help maximize therapeutic effects of *adrenergic-blocking drugs* and minimize their adverse effects. Patients taking alpha-blockers should be encouraged to change positions slowly and with purpose to prevent or minimize postural hypotension with subsequent dizziness and/or syncope. Alpha-blockers and their indications in treatment of hypertensive disease and/or hypertensive crises are discussed further in Chapter 25. Use of the newer alpha-blocker tamsulosin in patients with BPH is quite common, and patients taking this drug should inform all health care providers—including dentists—that this is part of their medical regimen, especially before any type of surgery. In addition, anything leading to vasodilation should be avoided to prevent postural hypotension with resultant dizziness, lightheadedness, and syncope. This includes alcohol intake, excessive exercise, exposure to hot climates, and use of saunas, hot tubs, and heated showers or baths. See Patient Teaching Tips for more information.

When either an alpha- or beta-blocker drug is used, apical pulse should be counted for one full minute and both supine and standing blood pressures should be measured and documented. If the patient has any problems with dizziness, fainting, or lightheadedness, or if the systolic blood pressure is lower than 100 mm Hg systolic or the pulse rate is lower than 60 beats/min, the prescriber should be contacted immediately. Daily weight measurement is important to monitor the progress of therapy and check for the adverse effect of edema. A good rule of thumb is that if the patient shows an increase of 2 pounds or more over a 24-hour period or 5 pounds or more within 1 week, the prescriber should be contacted. The patient should keep a daily journal documenting not only daily weights but blood pressures, pulse rates, adverse effects, and overall feeling of wellness or lack thereof. Other symptoms to report to the prescriber are muscle weakness, shortness of breath, and collection of fluid in the lower extremities as manifested by difficulty in putting on shoes or socks and weight gain. Patients taking any of these medications must be weaned off the drug slowly, because an abrupt discontinuation could lead to rebound hypertension or chest pain. The nurse should remember basic anatomy and physiology, as mentioned previously, because this knowledge will help guide nursing actions related to these drugs. See Patient Teaching Tips for more specific information.

Evaluation

Therapeutic effects for which to monitor in patients receiving *adrenergic-blocking drugs* include, but are not limited to, a decrease in blood pressure, pulse rate, and palpitations (in patients with these specific problems before drug therapy); alleviation of the symptoms of the disorder for which the drug was indicated; a return to normal blood pressure and pulse with lowering of the blood pressure toward 120/80 mm Hg and the pulse toward 60 beats/min in patients with diagnosed hypertension; and a decrease in chest pain in patients with angina. Patients must also be monitored for the occurrence of the adverse effects associated with these medications, including bradycardia, depression, fatigue, and hypotension. See Tables 19-2 and 19-4 for other potential adverse effects.

PATIENT TEACHING TIPS

- Written and verbal information should be given to the patient about drug indications, actions, adverse effects, cautions, contraindications, and drug interactions. This information should be age specific and tailored to the specific learning needs of the patient.
- The need to wear a medical alert bracelet or necklace that identifies the specific medical diagnoses and provides access to a list of all medications, including prescription drugs, over-the-counter drugs, and herbals and supplements, should be emphasized to the patient. The patient should also carry this information in written form on his or her person at all times and update the information at least every few months or whenever there are major changes in the diagnosis and treatment regimen. The patient should also keep a card in his or her wallet or purse to record blood pressure readings by date and time. This information may then be shared with other health care professionals.
- Caution the patient to take medications exactly as prescribed and to never abruptly discontinue them due to risk of rebound hypertension. Should there be concern about omitted or skipped doses, the prescriber should be contacted immediately.
- Caffeine and other central nervous system stimulants should be avoided while taking adrenergic-blocking drugs to prevent further irritability of the cardiac and central nervous systems and subsequent negative effects on health status.
- Alcohol ingestion should be avoided because it causes vasodilation, which increases the risk of hypotension and postural blood pressure changes.
- Encourage the patient to contact the prescriber if they experience palpitations, chest pain, confusion, weight gain (2 pounds

or more in 24 hours or 5 pounds or more in 1 week), dyspnea, nausea, or vomiting. Other problems to report include swelling in the feet and ankles, shortness of breath, excessive fatigue, dizziness, and syncope.
- The alpha-blocker tamsulosin must be taken as directed and with cautious use by patients with blood pressure problems (e.g., hypotension). The drug should also be used with caution by the elderly and while driving or engaging in other activities requiring alertness, because the adverse effects of this drug include blurred vision, dizziness, and drowsiness.
- Possible drug interactions should be reviewed for any adrenergic-blocking drug (see pharmacology discussion).
- The patient should be cautioned to change positions slowly to avoid dizziness and/or syncope. Excessive exercise, exposure to hot climates, use of a sauna or tanning bed, and alcohol consumption exacerbate vasodilation from the adrenergic-blocking drugs and lead to a greater drop in blood pressure with even more risk of dizziness and syncope.
- Constipation may develop as an adverse effect, and the patient should be encouraged to prevent this by increasing the intake of fluids, roughage, and fiber.
- Urinary hesitancy related to the adverse effect of bladder distension may be manifested by extreme discomfort over the pubic symphysis area, and the patient should report this to the prescriber.
- The patient should be instructed to report immediately to the prescriber any confusion, depression, hallucinations, nightmares, palpitations, dizziness, or syncope.

POINTS TO REMEMBER

- Adrenergic-blocking drugs block the stimulation of the alpha-, beta$_1$-, and/or beta$_2$-adrenergic receptors, with the net result of blocking the effects of either norepinephrine or epinephrine on the receptors. This blocking action leads to a variety of physiologic responses depending on which receptors are blocked. Knowing how these receptors work allows the nurse to under-

stand and predict the expected therapeutic effects of the drugs as well as the expected adverse effects.
- With alpha-blockers the predominant response is vasodilation. This is due to blocking of the alpha-adrenergic effect of vasoconstriction, which results in blood vessel relaxation.

POINTS TO REMEMBER—cont'd

- Vasodilation of blood vessels with the alpha-blockers results in a drop in blood pressure and a reduction in urinary obstruction, which may lead to increased urinary flow rates. These are effects for which to monitor in patients taking alpha-blockers.
- Beta-blockers inhibit the stimulation of beta-adrenergic receptors by blocking the effects of the SNS neurotransmitters norepinephrine, epinephrine, and dopamine. Stimulation of beta$_1$ receptors leads to an increase in heart rate, conduction, and contractility. Stimulation of beta$_2$ receptors results in bronchial smooth muscle relaxation or bronchodilation. Blocking of beta$_1$ receptors results in a *decrease* in heart rate, conduction, and contractility. Blocking of beta$_2$ receptors leads to a *decrease* in bronchial smooth muscle relaxation, or bronchoconstriction.
- Beta-blockers are classified as either selective or nonselective. Selective beta-blockers are also called *cardioselective beta-blockers* and block only the beta-adrenergic receptors in the heart that are located on the postsynaptic effector cells (i.e., the cells that nerves stimulate). The beneficial effects of the cardioselective beta-block-

ers include decreased heart rate, reduced cardiac conduction, and decreased myocardial contractility with no bronchoconstriction. These drugs are a good choice for patients with hypertension who also have bronchospastic airway disease or other pulmonary disease.
- Nonselective beta-blockers block both beta$_1$- and beta$_2$-adrenergic receptors and affect the heart and bronchial smooth muscle. These drugs are used to treat patients with hypertension who do not have a problem with bronchospasm or pulmonary airway disease.
- Nursing considerations for patients taking alpha- and beta-blockers include teaching patients that they should weigh themselves daily, avoid sudden changes in position, and increase intake of fluids and fiber. Weight gain, dizziness, fainting, and/or a decrease in heart rate below 60 beats/min or a blood pressure of less than 100 mm Hg systolic or less than 80 mm Hg diastolic should be reported immediately.

NCLEX EXAMINATION REVIEW QUESTIONS

1 When a patient has experienced infiltration of a peripheral infusion of dopamine, the nurse knows that injecting the alpha-blocker phentolamine (Regitine) will result in local
  a vasoconstriction.
  b vasodilation.
  c analgesia.
  d hypotension.
2 When administering beta-blockers, the nurse knows that which guideline for administration and monitoring is correct?
  a The drug may be discontinued at any time.
  b Postural hypotension is not a problem with this drug.
  c Weaning off the medication is necessary to prevent rebound hypertension.
  d The patient should stop taking the medication at once if he or she gains 3 to 4 pounds in a week.
3 The nurse providing teaching for a patient who has a new prescription for beta$_1$-blockers will keep in mind that these drugs may result in which effect?
  a Tachycardia
  b Tachypnea
  c Bradycardia
  d Bradypnea

4 A patient who has recently had an MI has started therapy with a beta-blocker. The nurse explains that the main purpose of the beta-blocker for this patient is to
  a cause vasodilation of the coronary arteries.
  b prevent hypertension.
  c increase conduction through the SA node.
  d protect the heart from circulating catecholamines.
5 Before initiating therapy with a nonselective beta-blocker, the nurse should assess the patient for the presence of
  a hypertension.
  b liver disease.
  c pancreatitis.
  d asthma.
6 A patient is taking an alpha-blocker as treatment for benign prostatic hypertrophy. The nurse monitors for which potential drug effects? (Select all that apply.)
  a Orthostatic hypotension
  b Increased blood pressure
  c Increased urine flow
  d Headaches
  e Bradycardia

1. b, 2. c, 3. c, 4. d, 5. d, 6. a, c, d.

CRITICAL THINKING ACTIVITIES: BEST ACTION

1 A 46-year-old woman is now taking propranolol (Inderal) for the control of tachycardia and hypertension. What is the nurse's best response if the patient states, "Well, if it doesn't work after a month or two, I'll just quit taking it!"?
2 You are reviewing orders and find one for carvedilol (Coreg). When you go to the automated drug-dispensing machine to retrieve the drug, you find Coreg CR in the drawer. Should you give the drug? What is your best action at this time?

3 A 73-year-old man is given a new prescription for tamsulosin (Flomax) for treatment of BPH. He lives at home with his wife and uses a cane to help him walk because of the effects of a stroke he had 5 years ago. During the patient education session, what is the most important item the nurse should emphasize?

For answers, see *http://evolve.elsevier.com/Lilley.*

CHAPTER 20

Cholinergic Drugs

OBJECTIVES

When you reach the end of this chapter, you should be able to do the following:

1   Briefly review the functions of the autonomic nervous system and the impact of the parasympathetic division.
2   List the various drugs classified as cholinergic agonists or parasympathomimetics.
3   Discuss the mechanisms of action, therapeutic effects, indications, adverse and toxic effects, drug interactions, cautions, contraindications, dosages, routes of administration, and any antidotal management for the various cholinergic agonists or parasympathomimetics.
4   Develop a nursing care plan that includes all phases of the nursing process for patients taking cholinergic agonists.

e-Learning Activities

Drug Profiles

♦ bethanechol, p. 315
♦ donepezil, p. 315
♦ memantine, p. 316
♦ physostigmine, p. 316

♦ *Key drug.*

Glossary

Acetylcholine The neurotransmitter responsible for transmission of nerve impulses to effector cells in the parasympathetic nervous system. (p. 312)

Acetylcholinesterase The enzyme responsible for the breakdown of acetylcholine (also referred to simply as *cholinesterase*). (p. 313)

Alzheimer's disease A disease of the brain that is characterized by progressive mental deterioration manifested by confusion, disorientation, and loss of memory, ability to calculate, and visual-spatial orientation. (p. 314)

Cholinergic receptor A nerve receptors that is stimulated by acetylcholine. (p. 312)

Miosis The contraction of the pupil. (p. 314)

Muscarinic receptors Cholinergic receptors that are located postsynaptically in the *effector organs* such as smooth muscle, cardiac muscle, and glands supplied by parasympathetic fibers. (p. 312)

Nicotinic receptors Cholinergic receptors located in the *ganglia* (where presynaptic and postsynaptic nerve fibers meet) of both the parasympathetic nervous system and the sympathetic nervous system; so named because they can be stimulated by the alkaloid nicotine. (p. 312)

Parasympathomimetics Drugs that mimic the parasympathetic nervous system; also referred to as *cholinergic agonist drugs.* (p.312)

• • •

Anatomy and Physiology Overview

Cholinergics, cholinergic agonists, and *parasympathomimetics* are all terms that refer to the class of drugs which stimulate the parasympathetic nervous system. For a better understanding of how these drugs work, it is helpful to know how the parasympathetic nervous system operates in relation to the rest of the nervous system.

PARASYMPATHETIC NERVOUS SYSTEM

The parasympathetic nervous system is the branch of the autonomic nervous system with nerve functions generally opposite those of the sympathetic nervous system (Figure 20-1). The neurotransmitter responsible for the transmission of nerve impulses to effector cells in the parasympathetic nervous system is **acetylcholine.** A receptor that binds acetylcholine and mediates its actions is called a **cholinergic receptor.** There are two types of cholinergic receptors, as determined by their location and their action once stimulated. **Nicotinic receptors** are located in the ganglia of both the parasympathetic nervous system and sympathetic nervous system. They are called *nicotinic* because they can also be stimulated by the alkaloid nicotine that is found in the tobacco plant. The other type of cholinergic receptor is the **muscarinic receptors.** These receptors are located postsynaptically in the effector organs (i.e., smooth muscle, cardiac muscle, and glands) supplied by the parasympathetic fibers. They are called *muscarinic* because they are stimulated by the alkaloid muscarine, a substance isolated from mushrooms. Figure 20-2 shows how the nicotinic and muscarinic receptors are arranged in the parasympathetic nervous system.

Pharmacology Overview

CHOLINERGIC DRUGS

Cholinergic drugs, also known as cholinergic *agonists,* mimic the effects of acetylcholine and are therefore sometimes referred to as **parasympathomimetics.** These drugs can stimulate choliner-

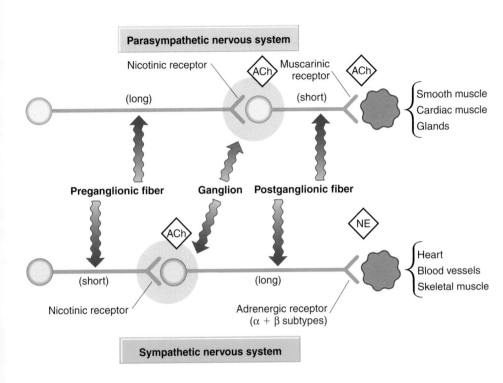

FIGURE 20-1 Parasympathetic and sympathetic nervous systems and their relationship to one another. *ACh,* Acetylcholine; *NE,* norepinephrine.

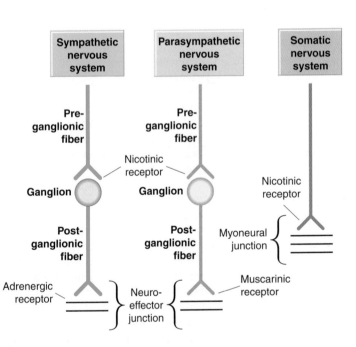

FIGURE 20-2 Sympathetic, parasympathetic, and somatic nervous systems. Note the location of the nicotinic and muscarinic receptors in the parasympathetic nervous system.

gic receptors either directly or indirectly. *Direct-acting* cholinergic agonists bind directly to cholinergic receptors and activate them. *Indirect-acting* cholinergic agonists stimulate postsynaptic nerve cell (neuronal) release of acetylcholine at the receptor site. This then allows acetylcholine to bind to and stimulate the receptor. Indirect-acting cholinergic drugs work by inhibiting the action of **acetylcholinesterase,** the enzyme responsible for breaking down acetylcholine. Acetylcholinesterase is also referred to simply as *cholinesterase.* The indirect-acting cholinergic drugs bind to cholinesterase in one of two ways: reversibly or irreversibly. *Reversible* cholinesterase inhibitors bind to cholinesterase

for a period of minutes to hours. *Irreversible* cholinesterase inhibitors bind to cholinesterase and form a permanent covalent bond. The body must then generate new enzymes to override the effects of the irreversible drugs. Box 20-1 lists the direct- and indirect-acting cholinergics.

Mechanism of Action and Drug Effects

When acetylcholine directly binds to its receptor, stimulation occurs. Once binding takes place on the membranes of an effector cell (cell of the target tissue or organ), the permeability of the cell changes, and calcium and sodium are permitted to flow into the

BOX 20-1 Cholinergic Drugs

Direct-Acting Drugs
bethanechol (Urecholine)
carbachol (Carboptic, others)
pilocarpine (Salagen, Pilocar [see Chapter 57], others)
succinylcholine (Anectine, Quelicin; see Chapter 12)

Indirect-Acting Drugs
ambenonium (Mytelase)
donepezil (Aricept)
echothiophate (Phospholine Iodide; see Chapter 57)
edrophonium (Tensilon, others)
galantamine (Razadyne)
neostigmine (Prostigmin)
physostigmine (Antilirium)
pyridostigmine (Mestinon)
rivastigmine (Exelon)
tacrine (Cognex)

TABLE 20-1 Cholinergic Agonists: Drug Effects

Body Tissue/Organ	Response to Stimulation	
	Muscarinic	Nicotinic
Bronchi (lung)	Increased secretion, constriction	None
Cardiovascular		
Blood vessels	Dilation	Constriction
Heart rate	Slowed	Increased
Blood pressure	Decreased	Increased
Eye	Pupil constriction, decreased accommodation	Pupil constriction, decreased accommodation
Gastrointestinal		
Tone	Increased	Increased
Motility	Increased	Increased
Sphincters	Relaxed	None
Genitourinary		
Tone	Increased	Increased
Motility	Increased	Increased
Sphincter	Relaxed	Relaxed
Glandular secretions	Increased intestinal, lacrimal, salivary, and sweat gland secretion	—
Skeletal muscle	—	Increased contraction

cell. This then depolarizes the cell membrane and stimulates the effector organ.

The effects of direct- and indirect-acting cholinergics are those that are generally seen when the parasympathetic nervous system is stimulated. There are many mnemonics to aid in remembering these effects. One is to think of the parasympathetic nervous system as the "rest and digest" system, in contrast to the "flight or fight" sympathetic nervous system.

Cholinergic drugs stimulate the intestine and bladder, which results in increased gastric secretions, gastrointestinal (GI) motility, and urinary frequency. They also stimulate constriction of the pupil, termed **miosis.** This helps decrease intraocular pressure. In addition, parasympathomimetic drugs cause increased salivation and sweating. Their cardiovascular effects include reduced heart rate and vasodilation. These drugs also cause the bronchi of the lungs to constrict and the airways to narrow.

Acetylcholine is needed for normal brain function. It is in short supply in patients with **Alzheimer's disease.** At recommended dosages, cholinergics primarily affect the muscarinic receptors, but at high dosages the nicotinic receptors can also be stimulated. The desired effects come from muscarinic receptor stimulation; many of the undesirable adverse effects are due to nicotinic receptor stimulation. The various effects of the cholinergic drugs are listed in Table 20-1 according to the receptors stimulated.

Indications

Some of the direct-acting drugs, such as carbachol, pilocarpine, and echothiophate, are used topically to reduce intraocular pressure in patients with glaucoma or in those undergoing ocular surgery (see Chapter 57). They are poorly absorbed orally because they have large quaternary amines in their chemical structure. This limits their use mostly to topical application. One exception is the direct-acting cholinergic drug bethanechol, which can be administered orally or by subcutaneous injection. It primarily affects the detrusor muscle of the urinary bladder and the smooth muscle of the GI tract. When given, it causes increased bladder and GI tract tone and motility, which thereby increases the movement of contents through these areas. It also causes the sphincters in the bladder and the GI tract to relax, which allows

them to empty. It is therefore used to treat atony of the bladder and GI tract. Atony sometimes occurs after a surgical procedure. Another direct-acting drug, cevimeline, is used to treat excessively dry mouth (xerostomia) resulting from a disorder known as *Sjögren's syndrome.* Oral pilocarpine can also be used for this purpose. Still another direct-acting cholinergic is the drug succinylcholine, which is used as a neuromuscular blocker in general anesthesia (see Chapter 12).

Indirect-acting drugs work by increasing acetylcholine concentrations at the receptor sites, which leads to stimulation of the effector cells. Indirect-acting drugs cause skeletal muscle contraction and are therefore used for the diagnosis and treatment of myasthenia gravis. Their ability to inhibit acetylcholinesterase also makes them useful for the reversal of neuromuscular blockade produced either by neuromuscular blocking drugs or by anticholinergic poisoning. For this reason, the indirect-acting drug physostigmine is considered the antidote for anticholinergic poisoning as well as poisoning by irreversible cholinesterase inhibitors such as the organophosphates and carbonates, common classes of insecticides.

In the treatment of Alzheimer's disease, cholinergic drugs increase concentrations of acetylcholine in the brain and thereby improve cholinergic function. The ability of the drugs to increase acetylcholine levels in the brain by inhibiting cholinesterase and preventing the degradation of endogenously released acetylcholine helps to enhance and maintain memory and learning capabilities. The last two decades have seen the introduction of four new medications that are specifically used to arrest or slow the progression of Alzheimer's disease. All are indirect-acting anticholinergic drugs, which means that they are inhibitors of the enzyme acetylcholinesterase. Although their therapeutic efficacy is often limited (it has been reported that only 15% to 30% of patients treated actually see benefits), these drugs can sometimes enhance a patient's mental status enough to cause a noticeable, if temporary, improvement in the quality of life for patients as well as caregivers and family members. The most commonly used of these medications at this time is donepezil. It should be kept in mind that patient response to these drugs, as with most other drug classes, is highly variable. For this reason, a failure to respond to maximally titrated dosages of one of these drugs should not necessarily rule out an attempt at therapy with another. Dosage information for all of these drugs appears in the Dosages table on p. 316.

Contraindications

Contraindications to the use of cholinergic drugs include known drug allergy, GI or genitourinary (GU) tract obstruction (which may require surgical correction), bradycardia, defects in cardiac impulse conduction, hyperthyroidism, epilepsy, hypotension, chronic obstructive pulmonary disease, and Parkinson's disease (see Chapter 16).

Adverse Effects

The primary adverse effects of cholinergic drugs are the consequence of overstimulation of the parasympathetic nervous system. They are extensions of the cholinergic reactions that affect many body functions. The major effects are listed by body system in Table 20-2.

Toxicity and Management of Overdose

There is little systemic absorption of the topically administered drugs and therefore little systemic toxicity. When administered locally in the eye, they can cause temporary ocular changes such as transient blurring and dimming of vision, which can be bothersome to the patient. Systemic toxicity with topically applied cholinergics is seen most commonly when longer-acting drugs are given repeatedly over a long period. This can result in overstimulation of the parasympathetic nervous system and all the attendant responses. Treatment is generally symptomatic and supportive, and the administration of a reversal drug (e.g., atropine) is rarely required.

The likelihood of toxicity is greater for cholinergics that are given orally or intravenously. The most severe consequence of an overdose of a cholinergic drug is a cholinergic crisis. The symptoms of such a reaction may include circulatory collapse, hypotension, bloody diarrhea, shock, and cardiac arrest. Early signs include abdominal cramps, salivation, flushing of the skin, nausea, and vomiting. Transient syncope, transient complete heart block, dyspnea, and orthostatic hypotension may also occur. These can be reversed promptly by the administration of atropine, a cholinergic antagonist. Severe cardiovascular reactions or bronchoconstriction may be alleviated by epinephrine, an adrenergic agonist. One way of remembering the effects of cholinergic poisoning is to use the acronym *SLUDGE*, which stands for salivation, lacrimation, urinary incontinence, diarrhea, GI cramps, and emesis.

Interactions

Anticholinergics (such as atropine), antihistamines, and sympathomimetics may antagonize cholinergic drugs and lead to a reduced response to them. Other cholinergic drugs may have additive effects.

TABLE 20-2 Cholinergic Agonists: Adverse Effects

Body System	Adverse Effects
Cardiovascular	Bradycardia, hypotension, conduction abnormalities (atrioventricular block and cardiac arrest)
Central nervous	Headache, dizziness, convulsions
Gastrointestinal	Abdominal cramps, increased secretions, nausea, vomiting
Respiratory	Increased bronchial secretions, bronchospasms
Other	Lacrimation, sweating, salivation, loss of ocular accommodation, miosis

Dosages

For the recommended dosages of the cholinergic drugs, see the Dosages table on p. 316.

DRUG PROFILES

◆ bethanechol

Bethanechol (Urecholine) is a direct-acting cholinergic agonist. It is used in the treatment of acute postoperative and postpartum nonobstructive urinary retention and for the management of urinary retention associated with neurogenic atony of the bladder. It has also been used to prevent and treat the adverse effects of other classes of drugs, such as bladder dysfunction induced by phenothiazine and tricyclic antidepressants (see Chapter 17). In addition, it is used in the treatment of postoperative GI atony and gastric retention, chronic refractory heartburn, and familial dysautonomia, as well as in diagnostic testing for infantile cystic fibrosis. Bethanechol injection is given only subcutaneously; intramuscular and intravenous use are contraindicated. Contraindications include known drug allergy, hyperthyroidism, peptic ulcer, active bronchial asthma, cardiac disease or coronary artery disease, epilepsy, and parkinsonism. The drug should also be avoided in patients with conditions in which the strength or integrity of the GI tract or bladder wall is questionable or with conditions in which increased muscular activity could prove harmful, such as known or suspected mechanical obstruction.

Adverse effects include hypotension, tachycardia, headache, seizure, GI upset, and asthmatic attacks. Drugs that interact with bethanechol include acetylcholinesterase inhibitors (i.e., indirect-acting cholinergics), which can enhance the adverse effects of bethanechol. Bethanechol is available in both oral and parenteral formulations. Commonly recommended dosages are given in the table on p. 316.

PHARMACOKINETICS

Route	Onset of Action	Peak Plasma Concentration	Elimination Half-life	Duration of Action
PO/injection	30-90 min	Less than 30 min	Unknown	1-6 hr

◆ donepezil

Donepezil (Aricept) is an indirect-acting anticholinesterase drug that works centrally in the brain to increase levels of acetylcholine by inhibiting acetylcholinesterase. It is used in the treatment of mild to moderate Alzheimer's disease. Similar drugs in this class include tacrine, galantamine, and rivastigmine. Rivastigmine is also approved for treating dementia associated with Parkinson's disease. Contraindications for donepezil include known drug allergy. Adverse effects are normally mild and resolve on their own. They can often be avoided by careful dose titration. They include GI upset, drowsiness, insomnia, and muscle cramps. Interacting drugs include

DOSAGES

Selected Cholinergic Agonist Drugs

Drug (Pregnancy Category)	Pharmacologic Class	Usual Dosage Range	Indications/Uses
◆ bethanechol (Urecholine) (C)	Direct-acting muscarinic	**Adult** PO: 10-50 mg tid-qid (usually start with 5-10 mg, repeating hourly until urination, max 50 mg/cycle)	Postoperative and postpartum functional urinary retention
◆ donepezil (Aricept) (C)	Anticholinesterase (indirect acting)	**Adult** PO: 5-10 mg/day as a single dose	Alzheimer's dementia
◆ memantine (Namenda) (B)	NMDA-receptor antagonist	**Adult only** PO: Initial dose is 5 mg/day; titrate by 5 mg/wk up to a target dose of 10 mg/bid (20 mg/day)	Alzheimer's dementia
◆ physostigmine (Antilirium) (C)	Anticholinesterase (indirect acting)	**Pediatric** IM/IV: 0.01-0.03 mg/kg repeated at 5-10 min intervals until desired effect or dose of 2 mg reached **Adult** IM/IV: 0.5-2 mg repeated q20min if needed	Myasthenia gravis, reversal of anticholinergic drug effects and TCA overdose

IM, Intramuscular; *IV,* intravenous; *NMDA,* N-methyl-ᴅ-aspartate; *PO,* oral; *TCA,* tricyclic antidepressant.

anticholinergics (counteract donepezil effects) and nonsteroidal antiinflammatory drugs (see Chapter 44); donepezil increases gastric secretions, increasing ulcer risk. Donepezil is available only for oral use. Recommended dosages are given in the table above.

PHARMACOKINETICS

Route	Onset of Action	Peak Plasma Concentration	Elimination Half-life	Duration of Action
PO	3 wk	3-4 hr	70 hr	2 wk

◆ memantine

In 2003, the Food and Drug Administration (FDA) approved a new medication for the treatment of Alzheimer's disease, memantine (Namenda). Memantine is not a cholinergic drug, per se, but is being included here in the discussion of drugs for Alzheimer's dementia. It is classified as an N-methyl-ᴅ-aspartate (NMDA) receptor antagonist due to its inhibitory activity at the NMDA receptors in the central nervous system. Stimulation of these receptors is believed to be part of the Alzheimer's disease process. Memantine blocks this stimulation and thereby helps to reduce or arrest the patient's degenerative cognitive symptoms. As with all other currently available medications for this debilitating illness, the effects of this drug are likely to be temporary but may still afford some improvement in quality of life and general functioning for some patients. Its only current contraindication is known drug allergy. Reported adverse effects are relatively uncommon but include hypotension, headache, GI upset, musculoskeletal pain, dyspnea, and fatigue. No clearly defined drug interactions are listed. Memantine is available only for oral use. The recommended dosage is given in the table above.

PHARMACOKINETICS

Route	Onset of Action	Peak Plasma Concentration	Elimination Half-life	Duration of Action
PO	Unknown	5 hr	70 hr	Unknown

◆ physostigmine

Physostigmine (Antilirium) is a synthetic quaternary ammonium compound that is very similar in structure to other drugs in this class, including edrophonium, pyridostigmine, neostigmine, and ambenonium. All are indirect-acting cholinergic drugs that work to increase acetylcholine by inhibiting acetylcholinesterase. Physostigmine has been shown to improve muscle strength and is therefore used to relieve the symptoms of myasthenia gravis. Neostigmine, pyridostigmine, and ambenonium are the standard drugs used for symptomatic treatment of myasthenia gravis. Edrophonium, another indirect-acting cholinergic drug, is commonly used to diagnose this disorder. Neostigmine and pyridostigmine are also useful for reversing the effects of nondepolarizing neuromuscular blocking drugs (see Chapter 12) after surgery. They are also used in the treatment of severe overdoses of tricyclic antidepressants because of the significant anticholinergic effects associated with the tricyclic antidepressants. Physostigmine, neostigmine, and pyridostigmine are also used as an antidote after toxic exposure to nondrug anticholinergic agents, including those used in chemical warfare. Contraindications to these drugs include known drug allergy, prior severe cholinergic reactions, asthma, gangrene, hyperthyroidism, cardiovascular disease, and mechanical obstruction of the GI or GU tracts. Adverse effects include GI upset and excessive salivation. Interacting drugs include anticholinergic drugs, which can counteract the therapeutic effects of physostigmine and other indirect-acting cholinergic drugs. Physostigmine is available only in injectable form. Recommended dosages are given in the table above.

PHARMACOKINETICS

Route	Onset of Action	Peak Plasma Concentration	Elimination Half-life	Duration of Action
IV/IM	Less than 5 min	5 min	15-40 min	30-60 min

CASE STUDY

Donepezil (Aricept) for Alzheimer's Disease

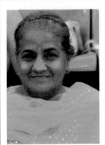
© Gina Smith

E. is a 72-year-old woman married to F., aged 73 years. F. has noticed that E. is becoming more forgetful but did not worry about it until she got lost while driving home from the grocery store. F. makes an appointment for E. to see their primary care physician, Dr. Smythe. After the examination, Dr. Smythe tells F., in private, that she thinks that E. is in the early stages of Alzheimer's disease but will order some tests to rule out other problems. F. then accompanies Dr. Smythe while she tells E. of the tentative diagnosis. Understandably, E. is upset to hear this news.

1. In her discussion with E. and her husband, Dr. Smythe mentioned a drug called donepezil (Aricept) that can be used in the early stages of Alzheimer's disease. It can be started after the other diagnostic tests are performed. After Dr. Smythe leaves the room, E. asks the nurse, "What will this drug do for me? Will it stop the Alzheimer's disease?" What should the nurse tell E.?

   Several diagnostic tests are performed, including a complete blood count, serum electrolyte levels, vitamin B_{12} levels, liver and thyroid function tests, and a magnetic resonance imaging scan to rule out other neurologic disease. Results of all tests are within normal limits. Dr. Smythe decides to prescribe donepezil, 5 mg, daily, for E..

2. After a week, F. calls the nurse to ask about giving E. an over-the-counter antihistamine for her allergies. "She always needs an allergy pill this time of year." He also says that she needs to take a pain pill for her mild arthritis but is not sure whether to use acetaminophen or ibuprofen. What should the nurse tell F.?

3. After 6 weeks, F. brings E. back to the doctor's office for a follow-up appointment. F. privately tells Dr. Smythe that he is "upset" because he has noticed very little improvement. E. tells Dr. Smythe that she feels "fine" and has not noticed any problems. What do you think will be Dr. Smythe's next order at this time? Is E.'s response to the donepezil typical? Explain.

For answers, see *http://evolve.elsevier.com/Lilley.*

HERBAL THERAPIES AND DIETARY SUPPLEMENTS

Ginkgo *(Ginkgo biloba)*

■ *Overview*
The dried leaf of the ginkgo plant contains flavonoids, terpenoids, and organic acids that help ginkgo preparations exert their positive effects as an antioxidant and inhibitor of platelet aggregation.

■ *Common Uses*
Organic brain syndrome, peripheral arterial occlusive disease, vertigo, tinnitus

■ *Adverse Effects*
Stomach or intestinal upset, headache, bleeding, allergic skin reaction

■ *Potential Drug Interactions*
Aspirin, nonsteroidal antiinflammatory drugs, warfarin, heparin, anticonvulsants, ticlopidine, clopidogrel, dipyridamole, tricyclic antidepressants

■ *Contraindications*
None

NURSING PROCESS

Assessment

Cholinergic drugs, or parasympathomimetics, produce a variety of effects stemming from their ability to stimulate the parasympathetic nervous system and mimic the action of acetylcholine. These effects include a decrease in heart rate, increase in GI and GU tone through increased contractility of the smooth muscle of the bowel and bladder, increase in the contractility and tone of bronchial smooth muscle, increased respiratory secretions, and miosis or pupillary constriction. Therefore, if the patient has any preexisting conditions such as heart block or the patient is taking other drugs mimicking the actions of the parasympathetic system, adverse effects or toxicity could be increased. Before cholinergic drugs are given, a thorough head-to-toe physical examination should be performed, and a nursing history and medication history (including prescription drugs, over-the-counter drugs, and herbals) should be obtained. Drug allergies and past and present medical conditions need to be documented as well. Cautions, contraindications, and drug interactions also need to be identified and documented if a cholinergic drug is given (see previous pharmacology discussion). Vitals signs need to be assessed and documented.

Before a drug for Alzheimer's disease, such as donepezil or memantine, is used, the patient should be assessed for allergies, cautions, contraindications, and drug interactions (see previous discussion). There should also be close assessment and documentation of the patient's neurologic status with attention to short- and long-term memory; level of alertness; motor, cognitive, and sensory functioning; any suicidal tendencies or thoughts; musculoskeletal intactness; and GI, GU, and cardiovascular functioning. Any abnormalities and/or complaints should be reported to the prescriber immediately. Presence or absence of family support systems should also be noted because of the chronic nature of this illness. Once the patient has begun taking medication, it is critical for the nurse to continue to assess the patient's response to the drug. Changes in symptoms within the first 6 weeks of therapy should especially be noted. Journaling may be helpful to the prescriber to assess any positive changes and any adverse effects and/or lack of improvement. Ginkgo may be used by some health care providers for organic brain syndrome (see the Herbal Therapies and Dietary Supplements box above).

Nursing Diagnoses

- Acute pain related to the adverse effect of abdominal cramping caused by the medication
- Deficient knowledge of the therapeutic regimen, adverse effects, drug interactions, and precautions for cholinergic drugs
- Risk for injury related to the possible adverse effects of cholinergic drugs, such as bradycardia and hypotension, with possible falls or syncope
- Decreased cardiac output related to drug-related cardiovascular adverse effects of dysrhythmias, hypotension, and bradycardia
- Disturbed sensory perception related to the adverse central nervous system effects of cholinergic drugs, such as somnolence

Planning

Goals

- Patient receives or takes medications as prescribed.
- Patient experiences relief of the symptoms for which the medication was prescribed.
- Patient remains adherent to the drug therapy regimen.
- Patient demonstrates adequate knowledge concerning the use of the specific medication, its adverse effects, and the appropriate dosing at home.
- Patient remains free of self-injury resulting from the adverse effects of the medication.

Outcome Criteria

- Patient states the importance of both the pharmacologic and nonpharmacologic treatment of the GI or GU tract disorder or glaucoma in achieving good health.
- Patient states reasons for adherence to the drug therapy and the risks associated with nonadherence as well as the complications associated with overuse of the medication, such as bronchospasm, increased abdominal cramping, and decreased pulse and blood pressure.
- Patient states conditions under which to contact the prescriber, such as the occurrence of wheezing, bradycardia, and/or increased abdominal pain.
- Patient states the importance of scheduling and keeping follow-up appointments with the prescriber related to the management of the disorder for which medication has been prescribed.

Implementation

Several nursing interventions may help to maximize the therapeutic effects of cholinergic drugs and minimize their adverse effects. If the patient has just undergone surgery and the cholinergic drugs are indicated, then ambulation and increased intake of fluids and fiber should be encouraged, unless contraindicated. Early ambulation helps to increase GI peristalsis and possibly prevent the need for drugs such as bethanechol. Bethanechol is used to treat decreased or absent peristalsis related to the surgery and/or anesthesia. However, these drugs should not be administered if a mechanical obstruction is suspected. Use of these drugs in such a situation could possibly result in bowel perforation. Subcutaneous injections of bethanechol should be administered as ordered (see Chapter 10), and sites rotated if injections are frequent. It is always preferable to use nonpharmacologic measures rather than pharmacologic regimens to treat the anticipated postoperative problems of decreased peristalsis and/or urinary retention (see above). For drugs used to treat myasthenia gravis, the oral medication should be given about 30 minutes before meals to allow for onset of action and therapeutic effects (e.g., decreased dysphagia or decreased difficulty swallowing). Atropine is the antidote to a cholinergic overdose; therefore, this medication should be readily available and given per the prescriber's order.

None of the drugs used for treatment of Alzheimer's disease provides a cure, but these drugs do improve function and cognition to some degree. It is crucial that the fact that the disease has no cure be discussed with empathy and compassion, because the di-

agnosis of Alzheimer's disease and/or dementia is shocking, at best. Those involved in the care of the patient need to be honest in sharing information with the patient, family, significant others, and caregivers. The nurse should always follow ethical standards of practice when working with patients and adhere to the American Nurses Association Code of Ethics. This code outlines behaviors required to maintain a high level of professionalism and specific actions that demonstrate respect for patient rights in any patient care situation. However, any sharing of information with the patient, family, significant others, and caregivers must be done with the approval of the prescriber, with good intent, in compliance with any research protocol, and/or with the goal of being a patient advocate. When beginning any of these medications, the patient will most likely need continued assistance and help with activities of daily living and ambulation (because the medication may increase dizziness and cause gait imbalances at the initiation of treatment). The patient, family members, and/or caregivers also need to understand the importance of taking the medication exactly as ordered. In addition, the patient and anyone involved in the patient's daily care should be instructed about how the medication should be taken, for example, taking the drug with food to decrease GI upset. The patient and family or caregiver should be encouraged to educate themselves about the use of the drug, its adverse effects, possible interactions, and potential for harm, and should be told the importance of *not* withdrawing the medication abruptly. The patient must be weaned off all drugs over a period of time designated by the prescriber, because of the potential for serious complications if weaning does not occur.

Most of the cholinergic agonists have dose-limiting adverse effects that include severe GI disturbances such as nausea and vomiting. Blood pressure readings and pulse rates should be taken and recorded before, during, and after initiation of drug therapy. Dizziness may occur with therapy and thus the need for assistance with ambulation and other ADLs. Ataxia, or unsteady gait, may also indicate the need for further assessment and intervention by the nurse and prescriber. Maintenance of a journal that records daily doses of drugs, ability of the patient to participate in activities of daily living, motor ability, gait, mental status, cognition, and any adverse effects will provide valuable information to any health care provider or caregiver involved in the patient's day-to-day care.

Dosages of these medications may be changed by the prescriber after about 6 weeks if no therapeutic response occurs. For patient safety, the patient's blood pressure, pulse rate, and electrocardiogram should be carefully monitored throughout therapy. The patient, family or caregiver should report any cardiac distress (e.g., chest discomfort or palpitations), GI bleeding, or blood in vomitus or stool. Dissolving forms of the medication donepezil should be placed on the tongue and allowed to dissolve before the patient drinks fluids or swallows.

In summary, because most of the cholinergic drugs are used to treat patients diagnosed with Alzheimer's disease, it is important that the patient's family and other support personnel be monitored closely and that their questions be answered and their needs met. Often family members, significant others, and other caregivers have many questions and short- and long-term concerns. Preplanning education addressing these concerns is an important part of a holistic approach to patient care and to the

EVIDENCE-BASED PRACTICE

Exercise and Improved Cognition

■ Review

As the average age of the population in the United States and elsewhere continues to increase, the number of people living with Alzheimer's disease is expected to rise from the current 26.6 million to more than 106 million by 2050. It has been estimated that if the onset of dementia could be delayed by about 12 months, there would be approximately 9.2 million fewer cases worldwide. Several clinical trials have examined the ability of pharmacologic therapies such as cholinesterase inhibitors (e.g., donepezil), vitamin E, and rofecoxib to prevent progression to dementia in those at risk for Alzheimer's disease, but outcomes have been largely negative. However, many observational studies have suggested that physical activity may reduce the risk for cognitive decline. Because the evidence supporting a preventative effect of exercise is sparse, a randomized trial was designed to determine whether a program of regular exercise could slow the rate of cognitive decline in older adults at risk. This study is one of the first to demonstrate that exercise improves cognitive functioning in older adults experiencing subjective and objective mild cognitive impairment.

■ Type of Evidence

This study was a randomized, controlled trial in which one group of patients participated in a 24-week home-based program of physical activity consisting mainly of walking, whereas a second control group received only education and the usual care. Study participants were individuals who reported memory problems but did not meet the criteria for dementia. A total of 170 participants were randomly assigned to the two study groups, but only 138 actually completed the 18-month assessment. Those participating in the exercise program increased their physical activity by the relatively modest amount of about 20 minutes per day. Cognitive function was measured over a period of 18 months using the Alzheimer's Disease Assessment Scale—Cognitive Subscale (ADAS-Cog).

■ Results of Study

In an intent-to-treat analysis, participants in the physical activity group showed an average improvement of 0.26 points in their ADAS-Cog scores at the end of the 6-month intervention, while those in the usual care group showed deterioration by an average of 1.04 points; thus,

the absolute improvement of the physical activity group over the usual care group was 1.3 points. The researchers noted that this result compares favorably with the reported improvement of 0.5 points associated with the use of donepezil. After the 6-month intervention period, patients in the physical activity group were encouraged to remain active, and a newsletter was sent out periodically to reinforce the goals of the program. No further intervention was offered. By 18 months, those in the physical activity group had improved by an average of 0.73 points in ADAS-Cog score, compared with an improvement of 0.04 points for those in the usual care group. Modest improvements were also seen in scores on some other tests, including word list delayed recall and Clinical Dementia Rating sum of boxes, but no significant changes were seen in scores on tests of word list total immediate recall, digit symbol coding, or verbal fluency. Beck Depression Inventory scores and scores on the Medical Outcomes 36-Item Short Form Health Survey physical and mental component summaries also improved in the physical activity group.

■ Link of Evidence to Nursing Practice

A very important achievement of this study is its demonstration of the potential benefit of the simple, nonpharmacologic intervention of exercise, which is almost universally available, in the prevention of cognitive decline. For these participants as well as many other patients with physical and/or mental disease, the benefits of exercise go beyond improvement in cognition and include a positive impact on depression, quality of life, and cardiovascular function, as well as a decrease in falls and disability. Although advances are being made in health and technology and people are living longer, there is a need to find alternative therapies as well as therapies that are nonpharmacologic and simple to implement to prevent and treat diseases such as Alzheimer's dementia and other catastrophic brain disorders. Nurses can educate patients and family members on the importance of habitual exercise as well as encourage the provision of consistent medical care, a suitable environment, adequate nutritional intake, and social interactions to help prevent mental and physical deterioration associated with certain disease states. These simple measures are easy to implement and may contribute significantly to the improvement of the individual's well-being in

Data from Jeffery S: Exercise may improve cognition in adults with memory impairment, *JAMA* 300:1027-1037, 1077-1079, 2008.

meeting of patient needs. Often the best place to begin in terms of education is to prepare answers to the following questions that are often posed: What should we expect for our loved one? What will happen to the person emotionally and physically? What treatments are available and what drugs are deemed safe? What are the common adverse effects of drug therapy and how can they be minimized? What about diet, fluids, and exercise for our loved one? Are there herbals or any supplements or over-the-counter drugs that would help with the disease or should they be avoided? What will we need to do for long-term care or other living situations for our loved one? What are the expected costs of our lived one's care now and in the future? What are the costs of drug therapy? Other costs? What kind of help can we all receive emotionally? What about emotional support for our loved one? How can this disease affect intimate relationships? What type of attorney should we seek out? What

about durable power of attorney and living wills? Other types of wills? Are these needed right away if we don't have these legal documents already? How do we all go on with our lives when our loved one is changing so drastically? Will life ever be normal again? What about research and clinical trials for treatment regimens? Should we pursue other treatments or do nothing new? What about drugs that are not yet FDA approved? How long will this process take? Just what can we expect over time?

Evaluation

The following are some therapeutic effects for which to monitor in patients receiving cholinergic drugs: In patients with myasthenia gravis, the signs and symptoms of the disease should be decreased but may not be completely alleviated. In patients experiencing a decrease in GI peristalsis postoperatively, there should be an increase in bowel sounds, the passage of flatus, and the occurrence of bowel movements that indicate increased peristalsis. In patients who have a hypotonic bladder with urinary retention, micturition (voiding) should occur within about 60 minutes of the administration of bethanechol. The nurse must also be alert to the occurrence of the adverse effects of these medications, including increased respiratory secretions, bronchospasms, nausea, vomiting, diarrhea, hypotension, bradycardia, and conduction abnormalities. For other adverse effects, see Table 20-2.

Therapeutic effects of the drugs used to manage Alzheimer's disease–related dementia or cognitive impairment include an improvement of the symptoms of the disease, but in most cases it takes up to 6 weeks for these effects to become apparent. Varying degrees of improvement in mood and a decrease in confusion usually occur. Adverse effects include nausea, vomiting, dizziness, and others (see individual drug profiles for specific information).

PATIENT TEACHING TIPS

- Medications should be taken exactly as ordered and with meals to minimize GI upset. Medications should never be increased except on the advice of the prescriber. Specific instructions should be given on what to do if a medication dose has been omitted.
- Intervals between doses of medication should be timed consistently to optimize therapeutic effects and minimize adverse effects and toxicity.
- Patients, family, significant others, and/or caregivers should be encouraged to call the prescriber or other health care provider if there is any increased muscle weakness, abdominal cramps, diarrhea, dizziness, ataxia, and/or difficulty breathing. Caregiver(s) should be provided with the appropriate phone numbers and contact information for 24/7 support.
- Community resources should be utilized and information about these resources made available to patients and their caregiver(s), family, and significant others. Such resources may include, but are not be limited to, Meals on Wheels; local, state, and national chapters of the Alzheimer's Association; adult day care and/or alternate care resources; special prescription services (e.g., Nationwide Prescription Assistance at the toll-free number 888-812-5152 or online at *http://www.FreeMedicine.com*); and respite care and/or home health care services.
- The signs and symptoms of improvement of myasthenia gravis, such as a decrease in or absence of ptosis (eyelid drooping) and diplopia (double vision), less difficulty swallowing and chewing, and an improvement in muscle weakness, should be emphasized.
- If the medication is being taken for myasthenia gravis, the patient should take it 30 minutes before meals so that the drug begins to work before the patient chews and swallows. This will help strengthen the muscles for chewing and eating.
- Sustained-released or extended-release dosage forms should be taken in their entirety and should not be crushed, chewed, or broken in any way.
- The patient should wear a medical alert bracelet or necklace or carry a medical alert card on his or her person at all times that gives the medical diagnoses and provides access to a list of medications and allergies, and any special requirements regarding emergency treatment.

POINTS TO REMEMBER

- *Cholinergics, cholinergic agonists,* and *parasympathomimetics* are all appropriate terms for the class of drugs that stimulate the parasympathetic nervous system, which is the branch of the autonomic nervous system that opposes the sympathetic nervous system.
- The primary neurotransmitter of the parasympathetic nervous system is acetylcholine, and there are two types of cholinergic receptors: nicotinic and muscarinic.
- Nursing considerations for the administration of cholinergic drugs include giving the drug as directed and monitoring the patient carefully for the occurrence of bradycardia, hypotension, headache, dizziness, respiratory depression, and bronchospasms. If these occur in a patient taking cholinergics, the prescriber must be contacted immediately.
- It may take up to 6 weeks for a therapeutic response to occur with some of the medications used with Alzheimer's disease.
- Patients taking cholinergics should always change positions slowly to avoid dizziness and fainting resulting from postural hypotension.

NCLEX EXAMINATION REVIEW QUESTIONS

1 A patient is taking the direct-acting cholinergic drug bethan-echol (Urecholine) before meals. After 3 days, he calls his health care provider's office and complains of occasional nausea and vomiting. The nurse should give which instruction?
   a "Continue to take it on an empty stomach to minimize GI upset."
   b "If this continues, you can skip a dose and try it again tomorrow."
   c "If these symptoms continue, take the doses in the evening."
   d "Take this medication with meals to reduce GI upset."
2 The family of a patient who has recently been diagnosed with Alzheimer's disease is asking about the new drug prescribed to treat this disease. The patient's wife says, "I'm so excited that there are drugs that can cure this disease! I can't wait for him to start treatment." Which reply from the nurse is appropriate?
   a "The sooner he starts the medicine, the sooner it can have this effect."
   b "These effects won't be seen for a few months."
   c "These drugs do not cure Alzheimer's disease. Let's talk about what the physician said to expect with this drug therapy."
   d "His response to this drug therapy will depend on how far along he is in the disease process."
3 The nurse is giving a dose of bethanechol (Urecholine) to a post-operative patient. The nurse is aware that contraindications to bethanechol include:
   a Bladder atony
   b Peptic ulcer

   c Urinary retention
   d Gastric retention
4 A patient took an accidental overdose of a cholinergic drug while at home. He comes to the emergency department with severe abdominal cramping and bloody diarrhea. The nurse expects that which drug will be used to treat this patient?
   a Atropine
   b Physostigmine
   c Lidocaine
   d Protamine sulfate
5 A patient with myasthenia gravis has received a prescription for pyridostigmine (Mestinon). The nurse should include which teaching point for this patient?
   a The drug is taken once in the mornings for maximum effect.
   b The drug should be taken 30 minutes before eating meals.
   c The drug should be taken 30 minutes after eating meals.
   d This drug can be given without regard to meals.
6 When giving intravenous cholinergic drugs, the nurse must watch for symptoms of a cholinergic crisis, such as: (Select all that apply.)
   a Peripheral tingling
   b Hypotension
   c Dry mouth
   d Syncope
   e Dyspnea
   f Tinnitus

1. d, 2. c, 3. b, 4. a, 5. b, 6. b, d, e.

CRITICAL THINKING ACTIVITIES: BEST ACTION

1 An elderly neighbor wants to take Ginkgo (Ginkgo biloba) because he is worried about "losing his mind." He asks you if this drug would help him. He has lived alone since being widowed last year and does not have any family members in the area. What is your best answer for this neighbor? Review the Herbal Therapies and Dietary Supplements box in this chapter and other sources, if desired.
2 A patient who has been newly diagnosed with myasthenia gravis has received a dose of physostigmine in the morning, just before

breakfast. She says, "Oh, I know this won't cure me, but I'm so glad that this drug makes me feel better. Will it last all day?" What is the nurse's best answer?
3 A patient is admitted to the emergency department after an industrial accident in which he was exposed to a large amount of organophosphate insecticide. The patient is having difficulty breathing. What is the nurse's priority of action at this time, and what antidote will be prepared?

For answers, see *http://evolve.elsevier.com/Lilley.*

CHAPTER 21

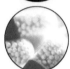

Cholinergic-Blocking Drugs

OBJECTIVES

When you reach the end of this chapter, you should be able to do the following:

1　Briefly review the functions of the sympathetic nervous system and the specific effects of blocking cholinergic receptors (parasympatholytic effects).

2　List the various drugs classified as cholinergic antagonists (blocking) or sympatholytics.

3　Discuss the mechanisms of action, therapeutic effects, indications, adverse and toxic effects, drug interactions, cautions, contraindications, dosages, routes of administration, and any antidotal management for the various cholinergic antagonists (blockers).

4　Develop a nursing care plan that includes all phases of the nursing process for patients taking cholinergic antagonists.

e-Learning Activities

http://evolve.elsevier.com/Lilley

NCLEX Review Questions • Animations • Nursing Care Plans • Audio Glossary • Category Catchers • Medication Errors Checklists • IV Therapy Checklists • Calculators • Frequently Asked Questions • Content Updates • Supplemental Resources • Answers to Case Studies and Critical Thinking Activities

Drug Profiles

♦ atropine, p. 326
♦ dicyclomine, p. 326
　glycopyrrolate, p. 326

　oxybutynin, p. 326
　scopolamine, p. 326
♦ tolterodine, p. 326

♦ *Key drug.*

Glossary

Cholinergic-blocking drugs Drugs that block the action of acetylcholine and substances similar to acetylcholine at receptor sites in the synapse. Such drugs block the action of the cholinergic nerves that transmit impulses through the release of acetylcholine at their synapse. (p. 322)

Mydriasis Dilation of the pupil of the eye caused by contraction of the dilator muscle of the iris. (p. 323)

Parasympatholytics Drugs that reduce the activity of the parasympathetic nervous system; also called *anticholinergics.* (p. 322)

• • •

Anatomy and Physiology Overview

PARASYMPATHETIC NERVOUS SYSTEM

The parasympathetic nervous system is the branch of the autonomic nervous system with nerve functions generally opposite those of the sympathetic nervous system. The neurotransmitter responsible for the transmission of nerve impulses to effector cells in the parasympathetic nervous system is *acetylcholine.* A receptor that binds acetylcholine and mediates its actions is called a *cholinergic receptor.* This chapter focuses on cholinergic-blocking drugs, which inhibit the effects of the parasympathetic nervous system.

Pharmacology Overview

CHOLINERGIC-BLOCKING DRUGS

Cholinergic blockers, anticholinergics, **parasympatholytics,** and *antimuscarinic drugs* are all terms that refer to the class of drugs that block or inhibit the actions of acetylcholine in the parasympathetic nervous system. These drugs were first discussed in Chapter 16 in relation to treatment of Parkinson's disease.

Cholinergic blockers have many important therapeutic uses and are one of the oldest groups of therapeutic drugs. Originally they were derived from various plant sources, but today these naturally occurring substances are only part of a larger group of cholinergic blockers that also include synthetic and semisynthetic drugs. Box 21-1 lists the currently available cholinergic blockers grouped according to their chemical class.

Mechanism of Action and Drug Effects

Cholinergic-blocking drugs block the action of the neurotransmitter acetylcholine at the muscarinic receptors in the parasympathetic nervous system. Acetylcholine released from a stimulated nerve fiber is then unable to bind to the receptor site and fails to produce a cholinergic effect. This is why the cholinergic blockers are also referred to as *anticholinergics.* Blocking the parasympathetic nerves allows the sympathetic (adrenergic) nervous system to dominate. Because of this, cholinergic blockers have many of the same effects as the adrenergics. Figure 21-1 illustrates the site of action of the cholinergic blockers in the parasympathetic nervous system.

Cholinergic blockers are largely *competitive antagonists.* They compete with acetylcholine for binding at the muscarinic receptors of the parasympathetic nervous system. Once they have bound to the receptor, they inhibit cholinergic nerve transmission. This generally occurs at the neuroeffector junction, or the point where the nerve ending reaches the effector organs such as smooth muscle, cardiac muscle, and glands. Cholinergic blockers have little effect at the nicotinic receptors, although at high doses they can have partial blocking effects.

The major sites of action of the anticholinergics are the heart, respiratory tract, gastrointestinal (GI) tract, urinary bladder, eye, and exocrine glands. In general the anticholinergics have effects opposite those of the cholinergics at these sites of action. The blockade of acetylcholine by these drugs causes the pupils to dilate and increases intraocular pressure. This occurs because the ciliary muscles and the sphincter muscle of the iris are innervated by cholinergic nerve fibers. Cholinergic blockers therefore keep the sphincter muscle of the iris from contracting. The result is dilation of the pupil (**mydriasis**) and paralysis of the ocular lens (cycloplegia). This can be detrimental to patients with glaucoma,

however, because it results in increased intraocular pressure (see Chapter 57).

In the GI tract, cholinergic blockers cause a decrease in GI motility, GI secretions, and salivation. In the cardiovascular system these drugs cause an increase in heart rate. In the genitourinary (GU) system, anticholinergics lead to decreased bladder contraction, which can result in urinary retention. In the skin they reduce sweating, and in the respiratory system they dry mucous membranes and cause bronchial dilation. These and other effects are listed by body system in Table 21-1. Many of these cholinergic-blocking drugs are available in a variety of forms, including intravenous, intramuscular, oral, and subcutaneous preparations.

Indications

At the level of the central nervous system, cholinergic blockers have the therapeutic effect of decreasing muscle rigidity and diminishing tremors. This is of benefit in the treatment of both Parkinson's disease (see Chapter 16) and drug-induced extrapyramidal reactions such as those associated with antiparkinsonian drugs. These conditions involve dysfunction of the extrapyramidal parts of the brain and include motor dysfunctions such as chorea, dystonia, and dyskinesia. The therapeutic cardiovascular effects of anticholinergics are related to their cholinergic-blocking actions on the heart's conduction system. At low dosages the anticholinergics may actually slow the heart rate through their effects on the cardiac center in the portion of the brain called the *medulla.* At high dosages, cholinergic blockers block the inhibitory vagal (i.e., parasympathetic or cholinergic) effects on the pacemaker cells of the sinoatrial and atrioventricular nodes, which leads to acceleration of the heart rate due to unopposed sympathetic activity. Atropine is used primarily in the management of cardiovascular disorders, such as in the diagnosis of sinus node dysfunction, the treatment of patients with symptomatic second-degree atrioventricular block, and provision of advanced life support in the treatment of sinus bradycardia that is accompanied by hemodynamic compromise. It also has ophthalmic uses (see Chapter 57).

When the cholinergic stimulation of the parasympathetic nervous system is blocked by cholinergic blockers, the sympathetic nervous system effects go unopposed. In the respiratory tract this results in decreased secretions from the nose, mouth, pharynx, and bronchi. It also causes relaxation of the smooth muscles in the bronchi and bronchioles, which results in decreased airway resistance and bronchodilation. Because of this, the cholinergic

---

BOX 21-1 Cholinergic Blockers Grouped According to Chemical Class

Natural Plant Alkaloids with Synthetic Drug Trade Names
atropine (Sal-Tropine)
belladonna (Belladonna Tincture)
hyoscyamine (Levsin)
scopolamine (Transderm-Scōp)

Synthetic and Semisynthetic Drugs
benztropine (Cogentin; Chapter 16)
biperiden (Akineton)
dicyclomine (Bentyl)
glycopyrrolate (Robinul)
homatropine (Isopto Homatropine; Chapter 57)
ipratropium (Atrovent; Chapter 37)
mepenzolate (Cantil)
methscopolamine (Pamine)
oxybutynin (Ditropan)
procyclidine (Kemadrin)
propantheline (Pro-Banthine)
solifenacin (VESIcare)
tolterodine (Detrol)
trihexyphenidyl (generic; Chapter 16)

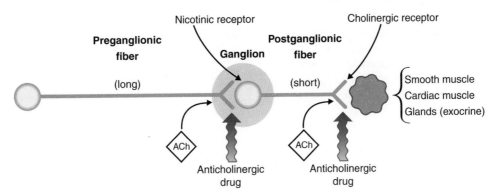

FIGURE 21-1 Site of action of cholinergic blockers in the parasympathetic nervous system. *ACh,* Acetylcholine.

TABLE 21-1 Cholinergic Blockers: Drug Effects

Body System	Cholinergic-Blocking Effects
Cardiovascular	Small doses: decrease heart rate Large doses: increase heart rate
Central nervous	Small doses: decrease muscle rigidity and tremors Large doses: cause drowsiness, disorientation, hallucinations
Eye	Dilate pupils (mydriasis), decrease accommodation by paralyzing ciliary muscles (cycloplegia)
Gastrointestinal	Relax smooth muscle tone of gastrointestinal tract, decrease intestinal and gastric secretions, decrease motility and peristalsis
Genitourinary	Relax detrusor muscle of bladder, increase constriction of internal sphincter; these two effects may result in urinary retention
Glandular	Decrease bronchial secretions, salivation, and sweating
Respiratory	Decrease bronchial secretions, dilate bronchial airways

TABLE 21-2 Cholinergic Blockers: Adverse Effects

Body System	Adverse Effects
Cardiovascular	Increased heart rate, dysrhythmias
Central nervous	Central nervous system excitation, restlessness, irritability, disorientation, hallucinations, delirium
Eye	Dilated pupils, decreased visual accommodation, increased intraocular pressure
Gastrointestinal	Decreased salivation, gastric secretions, and motility
Genitourinary	Urinary retention
Glandular	Decreased sweating
Respiratory	Decreased bronchial secretions

blockers have proved beneficial in treating exercise-induced bronchospasms, chronic bronchitis, asthma, and chronic obstructive pulmonary disease. They are also used preoperatively to reduce salivary secretions, which aids in intubation and other procedures (e.g., endoscopy) involving the oral cavity.

Gastric secretions and the smooth muscles responsible for producing gastric motility are both controlled by the parasympathetic nervous system, which is primarily under the control of muscarinic receptors. Cholinergic blockers antagonize these receptors, causing reduced secretions, relaxation of smooth muscle, and reduced GI motility and peristalsis. For these reasons cholinergic blockers are commonly used in the treatment of irritable bowel disease and GI hypersecretory states.

The effects that anticholinergics have on the bladder have made them useful in the treatment of such GU tract disorders as reflex neurogenic bladder and incontinence. They relax the detrusor muscles of the bladder and increase constriction of the internal sphincter. The ability of cholinergic blockers to decrease glandular secretions also makes them potentially useful drugs for reducing gastric and pancreatic secretions in patients with acute pancreatitis.

Contraindications

Contraindications to the use of anticholinergic drugs include known drug allergy, angle-closure glaucoma, acute asthma or other respiratory distress, myasthenia gravis, acute cardiovascular instability (some exceptions were listed previously), and GI or GU tract obstruction (e.g., benign prostatic hyperplasia) or other acute GI or GU illness.

Adverse Effects

Many body systems are affected adversely by cholinergic blockers because of the site of action of these drugs. The muscarinic receptors are located in a variety of tissues, organs, and glands throughout the body (see Chapter 20). Therefore, blockade of these receptors by the anticholinergics produces a wide range of effects, some desirable, as described in the previous section, and

some not so desirable, depending on the clinical situation. The various adverse effects of cholinergic blockers are listed by body system in Table 21-2.

Other factors contributing to the wide variety of possible adverse effects of cholinergic blockers are the relative affinity of the muscarinic receptors for specific drugs and the drug dosage. Certain patient populations are also more susceptible to the effects of these drugs. These groups include infants, older adults, fair-skinned children with Down syndrome, and children with spastic paralysis or brain damage.

Toxicity and Management of Overdose

The dosage of cholinergic blockers is particularly important, because there is a very small difference between therapeutic and toxic dosages. Drugs with this characteristic are commonly referred to as having a *low therapeutic index*. The treatment of cholinergic blocker overdose consists of symptomatic and supportive therapy. The patient should be hospitalized, and close, continuous monitoring, including continuous electrocardiographic monitoring, should be initiated. The stomach should be emptied by gastric lavage. Activated charcoal has also proven very effective in removing from the GI tract any drug that has not yet been absorbed.

Fluid therapy and other standard measures used for the treatment of shock should be instituted as needed. Delirium, hallucinations, coma, and cardiac dysrhythmias respond favorably to treatment with the cholinergic drug physostigmine. Its routine use as an antidote for cholinergic blocker overdose is controversial because it has the potential to produce severe adverse effects such as seizures and cardiac asystole, and it should therefore be reserved for the treatment of patients who show extreme delirium or agitation or who could inflict injury upon themselves.

Interactions

The drug interactions most commonly reported for the anticholinergics are additive anticholinergic effects when taken with amantadine, antihistamines, and tricyclic antidepressants; reduced antipsychotic effects of phenothiazines when taken with anticholinergic drugs; and increased effects of digoxin (see Chapter 22) when combined with anticholinergics.

Dosages

For the recommended dosages of selected cholinergic blockers, see the Dosages table on p. 325.

DOSAGES

Selected Cholinergic Antagonist (Anticholinergic) Drugs

Drug (Pregnancy Category)	Usual Dosage Range	Indications/Uses
◆ atropine (generic) (C)	**Pediatric** 0.01-0.02 mg/kg/dose preoperative and/or q4-6h	Preoperative control of secretions, therapeutic anticho- linergic effect
	0.02 mg/kg, max 0.5 mg	Treatment of bradycardia
	0.05 mg/kg initial dose, repeat q10-30min prn	Anticholinesterase effect for organophosphate or carbamate poisoning (e.g., insecticides)
	Adult IM: 1 mg	Hypotonic radiography
	IV: 0.5-1 mg (max of 3 mg)	Treatment of bradycardia, cardiopulmonary resuscitation
	IV: 1-3 mg/dose, repeat prn until signs of atropine intoxication appear (e.g., tachycardia)	Anticholinesterase effect for organophosphate or carbamate poisoning (e.g., insecticides)
◆ dicyclomine (Bentyl) (B)	**Pediatric** PO: 5-10 mg tid-qid	Treatment of irritable bowel syndrome
	Adult PO: 80-160 mg/day divided qid	
glycopyrrolate (Robinul) (B)	**Pediatric** PO: 40-100 mcg/kg/dose tid-qid	Control of secretions
	IM/IV: 4-10 mcg/kg/dose q3-4h, max 0.2 mg/dose or 0.8 mg/day	
	IV (intraoperative): 4 mcg/kg, max 0.1 mg; may repeat q2-3min prn	Intraoperative control of secretions
	Adult and pediatric 12 yr and older PO: 1-2 mg bid-tid	Treatment of peptic ulcer
	IM/IV: 0.1-0.2 mg tid-qid	
	IM: 4.4 mcg/kg 30-60 min preoperative	Preoperative control of secretions
	IV (intraoperative): 0.1 mg, may repeat q2-3min prn	Intraoperative control of secretions
	Adult and pediatric 0.2 mg for each 1 mg of neostigmine or 5 mg of pyridostigmine	Reversal of neuromuscular blockade
oxybutynin (Ditropan, Ditropan XL, Oxytrol [transdermal patch])	**Pediatric 1-5 yr** PO: 0.2 mg/kg/dose bid-qid	Antispasmodic for neurogenic bladder (e.g., following spinal cord injury), overactive bladder
	Adult and pediatric older than 5 yr PO: 5 mg bid-qid	
	Adult only PO ER tab: 5-30 mg/day in single or divided doses	
	Adult Transdermal patch: 1 patch (3.9 mg/day) applied twice weekly (every 3-4 days) (for overactive bladder)	
scopolamine (generic injection; Transderm-Scōp patch) (C)	**Pediatric** 6 mcg/kg/dose, max 0.3 mg/dose; may repeat q6-8h	Preoperative control of secretions
	Adult IM/IV/subcut: 0.3-0.65 mg	Preoperative control of secretions
	Transdermal patch: 1.5 mg patch behind ear every 3 days (delivers approx 1 mg scopolamine over 3 days); apply at least 4 hr before transportation	Motion sickness prevention
◆ tolterodine (Detrol, Detrol XL) (C)	**Adult only** PO: 1-2 mg bid	Treatment of overactive bladder
	PO ER cap: 2-4 mg qd	

ER, Extended release; *IM,* intramuscular; *IV,* intravenous; *PO,* oral; *subcut,* subcutaneous; *XL,* extended release.

▌ DRUG PROFILES

Among the oldest and best known naturally occurring cholinergic blockers are the belladonna alkaloids. It is the belladonna alkaloid contained in the anticholinergic drugs that is responsible for their therapeutic effects. Of these, atropine is the prototypical drug. It has been in use for hundreds of years and continues to be widely administered because of its effectiveness. Besides atropine, scopolamine and hyoscyamine are the other major naturally occurring drugs. These drugs come from a variety of plants in the potato family.

Many of the semisynthetic and synthetic cholinergic blockers are therapeutically useful drugs. These drugs are used in the treatment of a variety of illnesses and conditions ranging from irritable bowel syndrome to the symptoms of the common cold and are also administered preoperatively to dry up secretions. They are the synthetic counterparts of the plant-derived belladonna alkaloids and are generally more specific in binding predominantly with muscarinic receptors. They may also be associated with fewer adverse effects. Adverse effects and drug interactions are comparable for the different anticholinergic drugs and are detailed in Table 21-2 and previous text, respectively, unless otherwise noted.

◆ atropine

Atropine is a naturally occurring antimuscarinic. It may be prepared synthetically but is usually obtained by extraction from various members of the potato family. In general, atropine is more potent than scopolamine in its cholinergic-blocking effects on the heart and in its effects on the smooth muscles of the bronchi and intestines. Atropine is effective in the treatment of many of the conditions listed in the Indications section. It is also used preoperatively to reduce salivation and GI secretions, as is glycopyrrolate. Its use is contraindicated in patients with angle-closure glaucoma, adhesions between the iris and lens, certain types of asthma (not cholinergic associated), advanced hepatic and renal dysfunction, hiatal hernia associated with reflux esophagitis, intestinal atony, obstructive GI or GU conditions, and severe ulcerative colitis. It is available in injectable, oral, and ophthalmic forms (see Chapter 57). It is also combined with the opiate diphenoxylate to make Lomotil tablets, a common antidiarrheal preparation. The recommended dosages are given in the table on p. 325.

PHARMACOKINETICS

Route	Onset of Action	Peak Plasma Concentration	Elimination Half-life	Duration of Action
IV	Immediate	2-4 min	2.5 hr	4-6 hr

◆ dicyclomine

Dicyclomine (Bentyl) is a synthetic antispasmodic cholinergic blocker used primarily in the treatment of functional disturbances of GI motility such as irritable bowel syndrome. It has also been used alone and in combination with phenobarbital for the treatment of colic and enterocolitis in infants. Use of the drug is contraindicated in patients who have a known hypersensitivity to anticholinergics and in those with angle-closure glaucoma, GI tract obstruction, myasthenia gravis, paralytic ileus, GI atony, or toxic megacolon. It is available in injectable and oral form. The recommended dosages can be found in the table on p. 325.

PHARMACOKINETICS

Route	Onset of Action	Peak Plasma Concentration	Elimination Half-life	Duration of Action
PO	1-2 hr	60-90 min	9-10 hr	3-4 hr

glycopyrrolate

Glycopyrrolate (Robinul) is a synthetic antimuscarinic drug that blocks receptor sites in the autonomic nervous system which control the production of secretions and the concentration of free acids in the stomach. It is most commonly used preoperatively to reduce salivation and excessive secretions in the respiratory and GI tracts. Its use is contraindicated in patients who are hypersensitive to it and in those with angle-closure glaucoma, myasthenia gravis, GI or GU tract obstruction, tachycardia, myocardial ischemia, hepatic disease, ulcerative colitis, or toxic megacolon. It also should not be given to children younger than 3 years of age. Glycopyrrolate is available in injectable and oral form. The normal recommended dosages are given in the table on p. 325.

PHARMACOKINETICS

Route	Onset of Action	Peak Plasma Concentration	Elimination Half-life	Duration of Action
IV	1 min	10-15 min	Variable	4 hr
PO	Up to 45 min	1 hr	Variable	6 hr

oxybutynin

Oxybutynin (Ditropan) is a synthetic antimuscarinic drug used for treatment of overactive bladder. It is also used as an antispasmodic for neurogenic bladder associated with spinal cord injuries and congenital conditions such as spina bifida. Contraindications include drug allergy, urinary or gastric retention, and uncontrolled angle-closure glaucoma. Oxybutynin is available for oral use. A new transdermal patch (Oxytrol) is now also available and approved for treatment of overactive bladder. For recommended dosages see the table on p. 325.

PHARMACOKINETICS

Route	Onset of Action	Peak Plasma Concentration	Elimination Half-life	Duration of Action
PO	Unknown	1 hr	2-3 hr	Unknown

scopolamine

Scopolamine is another naturally occurring cholinergic blocker and one of the principal belladonna alkaloids. It appears to be the most potent antimuscarinic for the prevention of motion sickness. It seems to accomplish this by correcting the imbalance between acetylcholine and norepinephrine in the higher centers in the brain, particularly in the vomiting center, that is responsible for the symptoms of motion sickness. Ipratropium, a derivative of scopolamine, has potent therapeutic effects on the lungs and is discussed in Chapters 36 and 37. Scopolamine is available in several different delivery systems that make it very useful for various indications. For the prevention of motion sickness it is available in a convenient transdermal delivery system (Transderm-Scōp), a patch that can be applied just behind the ear 4 to 5 hours before travel. Transdermal scopolamine may cause drowsiness, dry mouth, and blurred vision. Using scopolamine with central nervous system depressants or alcohol may increase sedation. Scopolamine is also available in several parenteral formulations for injection by various routes: intravenous, intramuscular, and subcutaneous. Scopolamine is also available for ocular indications and in oral form. The contraindications that apply to atropine apply to scopolamine as well. The recommended dosages for various indications can be found in the table on p. 325.

PHARMACOKINETICS

Route	Onset of Action	Peak Plasma Concentration	Elimination Half-life	Duration of Action
IV	30-60 min	30-45 min	Variable	4 hr
Transdermal	4-5 hr	6 hr	Variable	72 hr

◆ tolterodine

Tolterodine (Detrol) is a relatively new muscarinic receptor blocker now being widely promoted for treatment of urinary frequency, urgency, and urge incontinence caused by bladder (detrusor) overactivity. Another, much older drug that is commonly used to treat these conditions is oxybutynin (profiled previously), which is one of the most commonly prescribed. Other drugs also used include propantheline, hyoscyamine, flavoxate, and the tricyclic antidepressant imipramine. The newest drug for this purpose is solifenacin. These drugs are less commonly used than tolterodine because of their antimuscarinic adverse effects, particularly dry mouth. Tolterodine appears to be associated with a much lower incidence of dry mouth, in part because of its pharmacologic specificity for the bladder as opposed to the salivary glands.

Tolterodine should not be used in patients with angle-closure glaucoma or urinary retention. Patients with markedly decreased hepatic function or poor metabolizers taking drugs that inhibit cytochrome P-450 enzyme 3A4, such as erythromycin or ketoconazole, should start with 1 mg twice a day instead of the normal recommended dose of 2 mg twice a day. Tolterodine is available only for oral use. Recommended dosages are given in the table on p. 325.

PHARMACOKINETICS

Route	Onset of Action	Peak Plasma Concentration	Elimination Half-life	Duration of Action
PO	1 hr	1-2 hr	2-4 hr	5 hr

NURSING PROCESS

Assessment

The drugs known as *parasympatholytics, cholinergic blockers, cholinergic antagonists,* or *anticholinergics* (an older term) produce a number of physiologic effects that result from the blocking of cholinergic receptors. These effects include smooth muscle relaxation, decreased glandular secretion, and mydriasis (pupil dilation). Knowing the way these drugs work and the related physiology will assist in the safe assessment and nursing care of patients taking these drugs. A thorough medical history; complete medication history with a listing of prescription drugs, over-the counter drugs, and herbals; as well as a thorough head-to-toe examination will help identify the presence of any contraindications, cautions, and/or potential drug interactions associated with the cholinergic blocking drugs (see pharmacology discussion). The assessment data will help in documenting baseline findings and providing information for evaluating drug effectiveness. Life span considerations for the very young or pediatric patient and the elderly include a need for close assessment and monitoring because of the increased susceptibility of these groups to the adverse effects of confusion, delirium, constipation, blurred vision, and tachycardia as well as their increased sensitivity to these drugs.

Assessment associated with atropine and other cholinergic blockers includes checking for allergies, glaucoma, certain eye conditions such as adhesions in the iris and lens of the eye, gastroesophageal reflux disease, poor intestinal motility, obstructions of the GI and GU systems, and severe ulcerative colitis. These conditions and others are exacerbated by the cholinergic blockers (see pharmacology discussion in this chapter and in Chapters 18 through 20) and would be considered contraindications. Dicyclomine, glycopyrrolate, and oxybutynin also have associated cautions, contraindications, and drug interactions that should be addressed in the assessment with appropriate documentation. A thorough assessment also includes noting any disorders of the bladder or GI tract. The transdermal dosage form of scopolamine should be applied only after the order has been reviewed and the skin assessed.

Nursing Diagnoses

- Ineffective tissue perfusion (cardiopulmonary) related to drug-induced tachycardia
- Risk for injury related to possible excessive central nervous system stimulation and adverse effects of tremors, confusion, and sedation
- Constipation related to adverse effects of cholinergic blocking drugs

- Impaired gas exchange related to adverse effects of thickened respiratory secretions
- Urinary retention related to loss of bladder tone from adverse effects of cholinergic-blocking drugs
- Risk for injury related to decreased sweating and loss of normal heat-regulating mechanisms (especially in elderly patients and in those who engage in excessive exercise or who are exposed to high environmental temperatures) and possible heat stroke due to the impact of the drug on the temperature-regulating mechanisms
- Risk for falls related to changes in vision caused by mydriasis (pupil dilation) and sedation
- Deficient knowledge related to lack of information about the therapeutic regimen, adverse effects, drug interactions, and precautions related to the use of cholinergic blocking drugs

Planning
Goals

- Patient self-administers medication as prescribed.
- Patient experiences relief of the symptoms for which the medication was prescribed.
- Patient remains adherent to the drug therapy regimen.

- Patient demonstrates adequate knowledge about the use of the specific medication, adverse effects, and appropriate dosing at home.
- Patient is free of injury to self resulting from adverse effects from the medication.

Outcome Criteria

- Patient states the rationale for the use of cholinergic blockers in preoperative preparation, such as decreasing the risk of complications associated with anesthesia.
- Patient states the importance of compliance with the medication regimen, such as avoiding complications of Parkinson's disease.
- Patient states the importance of taking the medication as prescribed and not suddenly withdrawing the medication because of the risk of increasing adverse effects.
- Patient states those conditions of which the prescriber should be notified immediately if they occur (e.g., palpitations, dysrhythmias, chest pain).
- Patient keeps follow-up appointments with the prescriber to avoid unnecessary adverse effects or complications of treatment or nonadherence to the drug regimen.

Implementation

A preventative focus for nursing care is important to the effective use of *cholinergic-blocking drugs*, especially with regard to patient teaching about how to decrease the need for these medications. There are several nursing interventions that may maximize the therapeutic effects of these drugs and minimize the adverse effects. Some important nursing interventions include giving the drug same time each day and per the prescriber's orders, and giving the medication with adequate fluid intake (6 to 8 glasses of water daily).

Because drugs such as atropine and glycopyrrolate are compatible with some of the commonly used opioids (e.g., meperidine and morphine), they may be used in combination with these drugs and mixed in the same syringe for parenteral dosing. Checking for the compatibility of drugs combined in the same syringe is important with any medication, and compatibility should always be double-checked for patient safety. If a cholinergic-blocking drug is given via the ophthalmic route, the nurse must always check the concentration of the drug and, once it is given, apply light pressure with a tissue to the inner canthus of the eye for approximately 15 to 30 seconds. This helps to minimize the possibility of systemic absorption of the drug.

Atropine may be combined with other cholinergic-blocking drugs (e.g., hyoscyamine) for treatment of lower urinary tract discomfort or to help decrease GI and GU hypermotility, but the drug should be given via the correct route and with proper dosing as prescribed. The anticholinergic adverse effect of dry mouth may be managed with frequent mouth care, oral rinses, forcing of fluids, and use of sugar-free gum or hard candy. Oxybutynin should be taken as directed (with fluids) either 1 hour before or 2 hours after meals, if tolerated. Tolterodine should be taken as directed and with food. Transdermal forms of these medications (e.g., scopolamine and oxybutynin) should be applied to the skin only after the previous dosage form has been removed and the area gently cleansed of residual medication. Transdermal patches may be applied to any dry, nonhairy, nonirritated area. Rotation of transdermal sites is recommended to decrease skin irritation.

CASE STUDY

Transdermal Scopolamine

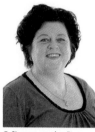

© Simone van den Berg

Jan, a 53-year-old schoolteacher, is going on a cruise to Alaska with her husband, Jake, for their thirtieth anniversary. She is very excited about the trip but is also worried because she gets "very seasick" whenever she is on a boat. She calls her doctor's office for a prescription for a medicine for motion sickness. Her physician prescribes transdermal scopolamine (Transderm-Scōp).

1. Before Jan picks up the prescription, the nurse assesses for contraindications to scopolamine. What are the contraindications to the use of the scopolamine patch?

The nurse provides patient education, and Jan indicates that she understands how to use the patch. On the first day of the cruise, she applies the patch 4 hours before they board the ship.

2. That evening, Jan and Jake go to dinner. Jan is feeling somewhat drowsy, but thirsty. The waiter asks if they would like to have champagne as part of the first-night-of-the-cruise celebration. How should Jan respond?

3. The next morning, while out on the deck, Jake and Jan are taking pictures of the bright, snow-covered shoreline views. Jake looks at Jan and exclaims, "Look at your eyes! Is that a side effect of that patch?" What has Jake noticed about Jan's blue eyes? What should Jan be doing because of what Jake has noticed?

4. Later that day, Jan tells Jake, "I'm feeling great! I don't think I need this patch. I'm going to take it off, but I'll save it for later in case I get nauseated." Is this a good idea? Explain.

For answers, see *http://evolve.elsevier.com/Lilley.*

Also associated with the cholinergic-blocking drugs are the adverse effects of constipation and inability to sweat or perspire. Because these may be significant to patients, education should be given about how to minimize these adverse effects. See Patient Teaching Tips for more information on these specific drugs.

Evaluation

Monitoring of goals and outcome criteria should be a starting place for effective evaluation of therapy with these medications. In particular, therapeutic effects of cholinergic-blocking drugs include the following: (1) improved ability to carry out the activities of daily living and fewer problems with tremors, salivation, and drooling in patients with Parkinson's disease; (2) decreased GI symptoms, such as hyperacidity, abdominal pain, nausea, and vomiting, and improved comfort; (3) decreased GU hypermotility with increased comfort and improved patterns of voiding with an increase in time between voidings; and (4) fewer bronchospasms with induction of anesthesia and fewer problems with thickened, viscous secretions in patients before, during, and after surgery. The nurse must also monitor the patient for the occurrence of adverse effects such as constipation, tachycardia, tremors, confusion, hallucinations, central nervous system depression (which occurs with large dosages of atropine), sedation, urinary retention, hot and dry skin, and fever. Toxic effects of these drugs include possible central nervous system depression with confusion and hallucinations. However, cardiovascular stimulation with severe tachycardia and palpitations may also occur at toxic levels of some of the cholinergic blockers.

PATIENT TEACHING TIPS

- Medications should be taken exactly as prescribed. Overdosage of anticholinergics may cause life-threatening problems, especially in the cardiovascular and central nervous systems.
- Anticholinergics may lead to dry mouth. Regular and thorough oral hygiene is required with brushing of teeth twice daily and dental flossing. Dry mouth may be minimized by forcing fluids, if not contraindicated, use of artificial saliva drops/gum or sucking on sugar-free hard candy, as needed. Regularly scheduled dental visits should be encouraged because of the risk of dental caries and gum disease with dry mouth. The use of water pick devices may stimulate gums and help prevent gum disease.
- Exercise should be done with caution and excessive sweating avoided because of drug-induced altered sweating. This may cause hyperthermia in the elderly or those with already altered sweating mechanisms. If there is sedation and/or blurred vision, the patient should avoid driving or engaging in activities that require quick decision making, alertness, or clear vision, such as operating heavy machinery, taking tests, and making important decisions. These adverse effects will decrease over time.
- Wearing dark or tinted glasses or sunglasses is encouraged because of the increased sensitivity to light associated with these medications.
- The patient should always consult the prescriber or other health care provider before taking any other medications, including prescription drugs, over-the-counter medications, herbals, and supplements.
- The elderly patient has existing age-related changes in body temperature–regulating mechanisms. With these medications, especially at high dosages, there is an increased risk of heat stroke or hyperthermia because of the drug's interference with the body's heat-regulating mechanisms. To prevent hyperthermia in the elderly, they should stay in shaded areas or inside in an air-conditioned or cooled environment when external temperatures are warm; remain well hydrated with cool fluids; wear protective clothing and hats; avoid saunas, hot tubs, excessive heat, and strenuous exercise in warm environments; and keep portable fans on hand and maintain adequate ventilation in heated environments to prevent overheating.
- All health care providers should be informed about the treatment regimen, and a list of the patient's drugs should be given to all involved in the care of a patient taking anticholinergics or cholinergic blockers. The prescriber should be contacted if there is any unresolved constipation, palpitations, alterations in gait or balance, excessive dizziness, or inability to void.
- Constipation may be managed by the increased dietary intake of fluids, bulk, and fiber and/or the use of over-the-counter fiber-containing supplements, such as psyllium products.

POINTS TO REMEMBER

- *Cholinergic blockers, parasympatholytics,* and *antimuscarinics* are all terms that refer to the drugs that block or inhibit the actions of acetylcholine in the parasympathetic nervous system.
- The use of these cholinergic blockers allows the sympathetic nervous system to dominate. These drugs are classified chemically as natural, semisynthetic, and synthetic cholinergic blockers. These drugs may be competitive antagonists (blockers) and compete with acetylcholine at the muscarinic receptors. In high dosages they result in partial blocking actions at nicotinic receptors.

NCLEX EXAMINATION REVIEW QUESTIONS

1 The nurse is providing education about anticholinergic drug therapy to an elderly patient. An important point to emphasize would be to
  a avoid exposure to high temperatures.
  b limit liquid intake to avoid fluid overload.
  c begin an exercise program to avoid adverse effects.
  d stop the medication if excessive mouth dryness occurs.
2 When giving anticholinergic drugs, the nurse keeps in mind that contraindications include:
  a Chronic bronchitis
  b Peptic ulcer disease
  c Irritable bowel syndrome
  d Benign prostatic hyperplasia
3 When assessing for adverse effects of anticholinergic drug therapy, the nurse would expect to find that the patient complains of which drug effect?
  a Diaphoresis
  b Dry mouth
  c Diarrhea
  d Urinary frequency
4 The nurse administering a cholinergic-blocking drug to a patient who is experiencing drug-induced extrapyramidal effects would assess for which therapeutic effect?
  a Decreased muscle rigidity and tremors
  b Increased heart rate
  c Decreased bronchial secretions
  d Decreased GI motility and peristalsis
5 During the assessment of a patient about to receive a cholinergic-blocking drug, the nurse should determine whether the patient is taking any drugs that may potentially interact with the anticholinergic, including:
  a Opioids, such as morphine sulfate
  b Antibiotics, such as penicillin
  c Tricyclic antidepressants, such as amitriptyline
  d Anticonvulsants, such as phenobarbital
6 A patient has been given a prescription for transdermal scopolamine patches for use during a vacation cruise. The nurse will include which instructions? (Select all that apply.)
  a "Apply the patch as soon as you board the ship."
  b "Apply the patch 3 to 4 hours before boarding the ship."
  c "The patch should be placed on a nonhairy area on your upper chest or upper arm."
  d "The patch should be placed on a nonhairy area just behind your ear."
  e "Change the patch every 3 days."
  f "Rotate the application sites."

1.a, 2.d, 3.b, 4.a, 5.c, 6.b, d, e, f.

CRITICAL THINKING ACTIVITIES: BEST ACTION

1 You are getting ready to administer atropine sulfate and an opioid, ordered as standard preoperative medications, to a 75-year-old woman who will be undergoing minor surgery. When you check her medical history, you see that she has a history of smoking and has angle-closure glaucoma. What is your best action at this time regarding administration of the preoperative medications? Explain.

2 In preparing a patient for emergency surgery, the order was to give 0.5 mg of atropine sulfate to the patient intravenously. The vial concentration is 1 mg/mL. In the haste of this emergency situation, 5 mL of the atropine solution is given. How much atropine did the patient receive? What should the nurse do next?

3 A patient who has a history of heart failure starts taking oxybutynin (Ditropan) for urge incontinence. One week later, she calls the office and tells the nurse, "I get so thirsty on this drug. I've been drinking lots of water, but it seems that I can't drink enough water to keep from getting thirsty!" What is the nurse's best response to this patient?

For answers, see *http://evolve.elsevier.com/Lilley.*

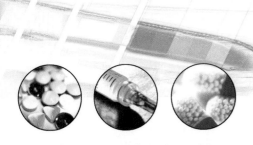

PART 4

Drugs Affecting the Cardiovascular and Renal Systems

STUDY SKILLS TIPS

Linking Learning   •   Text Notation

LINKING LEARNING

The Part Three Study Skills Tips stressed the importance of planning for the part as a whole. With that in mind, what is the focus of Part Four? The part title is Drugs Affecting the Cardiovascular and Renal Systems. What is the first question you think you should ask about this part? I would begin by asking, "What are the cardiovascular and renal systems?" This is a very obvious question and might seem to be so basic that it need not be asked, but the next eight chapters will all develop around this part title. Asking the obvious question is sometimes exactly the thing that should be done to get started.

Chapter Structure

Just as there is a structure to each part in the text, which is constant from one part to the next, there is also a structure in the chapters. This structure is a repeating model that was created by the authors in an attempt to organize the material and present it in the clearest way possible. The chapter structure is a valuable learning asset for those who make use of it.

Chapter Objectives

Each chapter begins with a set of objectives. These are established by the authors and serve to tell you what they expect you will know and be able to do when you have completed the chapter. It is sometimes tempting to ignore the objectives and get right on with the task of reading the chapter. Do not give in to that temptation. Read the objectives and spend some time thinking about what they reveal about the content of the chapter.

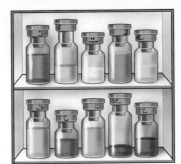

Example Based on Chapter 22 Objectives

Objective 1: Differentiate between the terms *inotropic, chronotropic,* and *dromotropic.*

What can you learn from this objective? First, there is the vocabulary. This objective makes it clear that you have some terms to learn. This means that you may want to have some blank note cards available to start setting up vocabulary cards for this chapter. In fact, you should write each of the terms in objective 1 on a separate card and be ready to complete the card as the terms are introduced and explained in the chapter.

The next thing that stands out in this first objective is that the three terms contain a common element: *-tropic.* This should bring active questioning into play. What does the suffix *-tropic* mean? Asking this question now is a way of noting that these three terms do have some common meaning. Also it serves to provide an immediate focus for personal learning when you begin to read the chapter.

Objective 2: Briefly discuss the pathophysiology of heart failure.

From this comes the potential for a new question relating to the first objective. What do *inotropic, chronotropic,* and *dromotropic* have to do with the heart? Just as it is essential to see the relationship between parts and chapters, it is also essential to see relationships within the chapters. These first two objectives should cause you to consider those relationships and make your own learning much more active.

Chapter Headings

The next chapter structure to consider in this process is the chapter headings. Chapter 22 has the major sections Anatomy, Physiology, and Disease Overview, Pharmacology Overview, and Nursing Process. What is the importance of this heading structure? It tells you that the authors will focus on the pharmacologic aspects first and then explain how this relates to nursing. This does not tell the learner a great deal about what to anticipate in terms of chapter content, but it does make clear a structure that is consistent in most of the chapters in this text.

Heart failure drugs are broken down into subsections in this chapter. Spend several minutes considering the organization of these subsections. The first subtopic to consider is Mechanism of Action and Drug Effects. What is meant by mechanism of action? How do heart failure drugs act? On what do they act? It does not matter that you cannot answer these questions at this point. What is important is that you ask them as a means of fostering an active and participatory learning attitude when you begin to read the chapter. Think, question, anticipate, and then read. This sequence will enhance your learning.

Continue this process of looking at the subtopics and thinking ahead to what will be explained in the chapter. These subsections are the same in every chapter, and this thinking process should become automatic very quickly.

Glossary

The next chapter structure is one that has already been stressed in previous Study Skills Tips, and it is one that is essential to learning. The glossary is a minidictionary for each chapter. Words that have not been introduced earlier in the text and that are central to the content of this chapter are presented here. The listing is in alphabetical order, which means that the glossary terms will not necessarily occur in the same order in the body of the chapter.

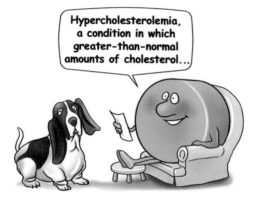

As you read the terms as presented in the glossary, be aware of the nature of the definition. A glossary definition is specific and brief. It is a very useful place to begin to learn the new terms in the chapter, but the definition presented may not be enough for full understanding. You will find that full understanding will come after reading the chapter and encountering the term within the fuller context of sentences and paragraphs of text that explain not only the term but how it applies in the particular situation.

Glossary and Text Relationship

The term *inotropic drugs* is defined in the Chapter 22 glossary. As I read it, I understand that inotropic has to do with force or energy of muscle contractions. Some of this information is clear, and some of it is still somewhat hazy. It should become clearer when connected with the chapter text. The first paragraph of the *Pharmacology Overview* section introduces inotropic drugs: "Drugs that increase the force of myocardial contraction are called positive **inotropic drugs,** and such drugs have a therapeutic role in the treatment of failing heart muscle."

With this sentence I find I have a much clearer understanding of what is meant by *inotropic drugs,* and I have the added benefit of knowing that there are positive inotropic drugs. This is what must happen to fully master the content-specific vocabulary. You must see the core definition as presented in the glossary, but you must also read to determine how that core definition is expanded and exemplified in the body of the text.

When preparing vocabulary cards, it is not a good idea simply to copy the definition from the glossary and assume that this definition will serve your purpose. Wait to fill out the card until after you encounter the same term in the body of the chapter, and then pick and choose the information from the glossary and the chapter body that will provide you with the clearest understanding of the term. Also, when placing information on vocabulary cards, it is always useful to include a chapter number and page numbers so that you can locate the source of your definition quickly should you find it necessary later.

These chapter structures can provide you with a clear picture of what you are expected to learn and the organizational pattern in which the material will be presented. Being aware of the structures and making use of them in this way will improve your concentration when you begin to read the chapter for understanding and memory. The time spent working with chapter structure is not wasted and does not significantly increase the study time for the chapter. In fact, the time you spend working with the objectives, headings, and glossary will generally save time when you are doing intensive reading and study.

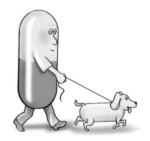

TEXT NOTATION

Highlighting or underlining text material is a tool that can be very helpful when rehearsing and reviewing materials after the study reading. The problem, as discussed in the *Study Guide,* is that it is often difficult to limit the quantity of material that is marked. Although a good general guideline is to try to limit yourself to marking no more than 20% to 25% of the total material, this guideline applies to large blocks of material. Some paragraphs contain essential information and must be marked extensively, whereas in other paragraphs only one or two sentences may need to be marked. In this Study Skills Tips section, the object is to look at how the author's structure and language can help you to select what should be marked.

Text Notation Application

Reproduced here are two paragraphs from Chapter 27 with my model underlining completed, followed by a discussion of the reasons for which I made the choices. You should not view the model underlining as a "perfect" example. The decision as to what to mark is very much an individual choice based on a number of factors, including prior experience with the subject matter and awareness of personal learning objectives and needs. These model paragraphs with accompanying discussion are intended to provide you with a basic model to adapt to your own learning style and needs.

Chapter 27, Paragraphs 1 and 2

Fluid and electrolyte management is one of the cornerstones of patient care. Most disease processes, tissue injuries, and surgical procedures greatly influence the physiologic status of fluids and electrolytes in the body. A prerequisite to the understanding of fluid and electrolyte management is knowledge of the extent and composition of the various body fluid compartments.

Approximately 60% of the adult human body is water. This is referred to as the *total body water* (TBW), and it is distributed in the three main compartments in the following proportions: **intracellular fluid (ICF), 67%; interstitial fluid (ISF), 25%; and plasma volume, 8%.** This distribution is illustrated in Figure 27-1. The actual volume of fluid that would normally be in each compartment in an average 70-kg man with a TBW content of 60% is shown in Table 27-1.

Discussion

The first thing you should notice is that the underlining I have done exceeds the 20% to 25% guideline. These are the first paragraphs in the chapter. First paragraphs are usually introductions to the topic and may vary a great deal in the quantity of important information. This chapter, in my view, contains a number of key points that must be considered. Because the content seems important, I have chosen to underline more.

The first sentence was chosen because of the word *cornerstones*. This word suggests that fluid management is extremely important in patient care and I must be sure to keep that focus throughout the chapter. Paying careful attention to the author's word choices plays a major role in selecting materials for text notation.

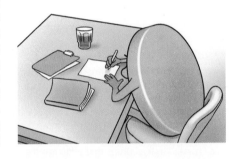

Paying attention to language led me to the third sentence, which begins, "A prerequisite to the understanding...." That phrase should immediately capture your attention. The phrase says that there is something that must be understood before anything else that follows will make complete sense. The phrase should also serve as an instant cue to generate a question for reading. "What is the prerequisite to understanding fluid and electrolyte management?" This question is answered directly by the sentence containing the phrase. The phrase serves as a language cue that there is something important. This in turn suggests that you probably will want to underline or highlight some information. The question helps you select what should be marked. Everything you do at this point serves as a guide to help you establish clear learning objectives and makes the process of selecting the best information for marking easier to accomplish.

The next segment was chosen because it stands out from the body of the paragraph. *Total body water* is italicized. This is a print convention used as a means of putting emphasis on something that the author believes to be of special importance. The decision to underline words and phrases that are already emphasized is a personal one. You may feel that, since the author has already marked

it, you have no need to add your own marks. I find that my own marking, even of italicized or bold print material, serves as a double reminder of the importance of the information. This is an excellent example of what I mean when I say that text notation is highly personal. Whether you choose to add your own marking or not, there is one aspect of this phrase that is essential. *Total body water* is part of the vocabulary of fluids and electrolytes. That means it is time to add to your vocabulary cards.

This term served as a lead-in to the next key point that I have marked. The next part of the sentence is, "it is distributed in the three main compartments." Whenever you see a phrase with a number and a word such as *main,* you should be aware that this is potentially important material. This phrase should generate a new question that will aid in your selection of material to mark. "What are the three main compartments?" You see immediately that the rest of this sentence answers that question, and therefore identifies what needs to be marked. This marking also identifies three additional vocabulary items to be added to your cards for this chapter. As you set up your cards, be careful. One fluid is *intra-* and the second is *inter-*. It would be easy to confuse the two, but they have very different meanings.

Chapter 27, Paragraph 3

The terms used to identify the various spaces within which the TBW is distributed can be quite confusing, and there are two basic approaches to distinguishing among the locations of the fluid. The TBW can be described as being in or out of the blood vessels, or vasculature. If this point of reference is used, then the term **intravascular fluid (IVF)** is used to describe the fluid inside the blood vessels and the term **extravascular fluid (EVF)** is used to refer to the fluid outside the blood vessels. Examples of EVF include lymph and cerebrospinal fluid. As these concepts are learned, the difference between the prefixes *intra-* (inside), *inter-* (between), and *extra-* (outside) should be recalled. The term **plasma** is used to describe the fluid that flows through the blood vessels (intravascular fluid). **Serum** is a closely related term (see glossary). The ISF is the fluid that is in the space between cells, tissues, and organs. Both plasma and ISF make up extracellular volume. Both ISF and ICF make up extravascular volume. These terms are often confused and misused. Table 27-1 lists these definitions for further clarity and understanding.

Discussion

The language conventions and the print conventions **(bold)** are the same that were used to help in the previous paragraph. This paragraph also makes a point about the possibility of confusing and/or misusing the terms introduced. Being told that there is confusing material suggests that it is crucial that you be able to identify, define, and explain each of the terms used, and that it will take some careful thought to do so. There is one additional point in this paragraph that is important. The last sentence points you to a table, Table 27-1. There are many tables in this text. Always remember that tables are often used in an effort to simplify complex material and to clarify the relationships between the items presented in the table. In these opening paragraphs, with the repeated reference to the confusing nature of the descriptions, Table 27-1 will almost certainly be important to your learning.

CHAPTER 22

Heart Failure Drugs

OBJECTIVES

When you reach the end of this chapter, you should be able to do the following:

1 Differentiate between the terms *inotropic, chronotropic,* and *dromotropic.*

2 Briefly discuss the pathophysiology of heart failure.

3 Identify the approach to treatment of heart failure as outlined by the 2005 American Heart Association and American College of Cardiology treatment guidelines.

4 Compare the mechanisms of action, pharmacokinetics, indications, dosages, dosage forms, routes of administration, cautions, contraindications, adverse effects, and toxicity of the following drugs used in treatment of heart failure: lisinopril, valsartan, carvedilol, metoprolol, dobutamine, nesiritide, hydralazine/isosorbide dinitrate, milrinone, and digoxin.

5 Briefly discuss the process of rapid versus slow digitalization as well as the use of the antidote digoxin immune Fab.

6 Identify significant drug-drug, drug–laboratory test, and drug-food interactions associated with digoxin and other heart failure drugs.

7 Develop a nursing care plan that includes all phases of the nursing process for patients undergoing treatment for heart failure and that complies with the 2005 American Heart Association and American College of Cardiology guidelines.

e-Learning Activities

NCLEX Review Questions • Animations • Nursing Care Plans • Audio Glossary • Category Catchers • Medication Errors Checklists • IV Therapy Checklists • Calculators • Frequently Asked Questions • Content Updates • Supplemental Resources • Answers to Case Studies and Critical Thinking Activities

Drug Profiles

- ◆ digoxin, p. 341
  digoxin immune Fab, p. 341
- ◆ dobutamine, p. 337
  hydralazine/isosorbide dinitrate, p. 337

- ◆ lisinopril, p. 336
- ◆ milrinone, p. 339
- ◆ nesiritide, p. 337
- ◆ valsartan, p. 336

———
◆ *Key drug.*

Glossary

Atrial fibrillation A common cardiac dysrhythmia involving atrial contractions that are so rapid that they prevent full repolarization of myocardial fibers between heartbeats. (p. 339)

Automaticity A property of specialized excitable tissue that allows self-activation through the spontaneous development of an action potential, as in the pacemaker cells of the heart. (p. 337)

Chronotropic drugs Drugs that influence the rate of the heartbeat. (p. 335)

Dromotropic drugs Drugs that influence the conduction of electrical impulses within tissues. (p. 335)

Ejection fraction The proportion of blood that is ejected during each ventricular contraction compared with the total ventricular filling volume. (p. 335)

Heart failure An abnormal condition in which cardiac pumping is impaired as a result of myocardial infarction, ischemic heart disease, or cardiomyopathy. (p. 335)

Inotropic drugs Drugs that influence the force or energy of muscular contractions, particularly contraction of the heart muscle. (p. 335)

Left ventricular end-diastolic volume The total amount of blood in the ventricle immediately before it contracts, or the preload. (p. 335)

Refractory period The period during which a *pulse generator* (e.g., the *sinoatrial node* of the heart) is unresponsive to an electrical input signal of specified amplitude and during which it is impossible for the myocardium to respond. This is the period during which the cardiac cell is readjusting its sodium and potassium levels and cannot be depolarized again. (p. 339)

● ● ●

Anatomy, Physiology, and Disease Overview

The anatomy of the heart, including its electrical conduction system, is illustrated in Figure 22-1. Estimates are that more than 5 million people in the United States have heart failure. Heart failure results in more than 3.5 million hospitalizations annually. Furthermore, it is the most common admitting diagnosis for elderly patients. The findings of one of the largest and most frequently cited studies involving patients with heart failure, the Framingham study, show that the 5-year survival rate in patients with heart failure is approximately 50%.

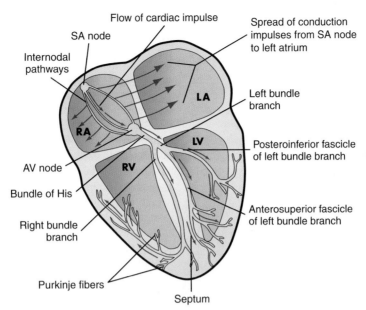

FIGURE 22-1 Conduction system of the heart. *AV,* Atrioventricular; *LA,* left atrium; *LV,* left ventricle; *RA,* right atrium; *RV,* right ventricle; *SA,* sinoatrial. (Modified from Kinney M et al: *Comprehensive cardiac care,* ed 8, St Louis, 1996, Mosby; Lewis SM et al: *Medical-surgical nursing: assessment and management of clinical problems,* ed 7, St Louis, 2007, Mosby.)

Heart failure is a pathologic state in which the heart is unable to pump blood in sufficient amounts from the ventricles (i.e., cardiac output is insufficient) to meet the body's metabolic needs. The signs and symptoms typically associated with this insufficiency constitute the syndrome of heart failure. Failure of the ventricle(s) to eject blood efficiently results in volume overload, chamber dilation, and elevated intracardiac pressure. This syndrome can affect primarily the left ventricle, primarily the right ventricle, or both ventricles simultaneously. Left ventricular or "left-sided" heart failure often leads to pulmonary edema, coughing, shortness of breath, and dyspnea. Right ventricular heart failure typically involves systemic venous congestion, pedal edema, jugular venous distension, ascites, and hepatic congestion. Both syndromes occur due to retrograde transmission of increased hydrostatic pressure from the ventricles into the pulmonary and/or systemic circulation.

More specifically, heart failure occurs due to a reduced ratio of **ejection fraction** to **left ventricular end-diastolic volume.** The ejection fraction is the amount of blood ejected with each contraction, whereas the left ventricular end-diastolic volume is the total amount of blood in the ventricle just before contraction. Ventricular diastole actually begins with the onset of the *second* heart sound and ends with the onset of the first heart sound. The ejection fraction is an index of left ventricular function. Its normal value is approximately 65% (0.65) of the total volume in the ventricle.

It should be noted that in this chapter on heart failure the emphasis is on *systolic dysfunction* or inadequate ventricular contractions *(systole)* during the pumping of the heart. Less common but still important is *diastolic dysfunction,* or inadequate ventricular filling during ventricular relaxation *(diastole).* This condition is most commonly associated with left ventricular hypertrophy secondary to chronic hypertension. However, it may also result from cardiomyopathy (e.g., virus induced), pericardial disease, and diabetes.

When a person has heart failure, the heart cannot then meet the increased demands placed on it and the blood supply to certain organs is reduced. The organs most dependent on blood supply, the brain and heart, are the last to be deprived of blood. The kidney, an organ that is relatively less dependent on blood supply, has its blood supply shunted away. Therefore, the filtration of fluids and removal of waste products is impaired. This can lead to acute or chronic renal failure. It also contributes to conditions such as pulmonary edema, shortness of breath, and peripheral edema.

The physical defects producing heart failure are of two types: (1) a myocardial defect such as myocardial infarction or valve insufficiency, which leads to inadequate cardiac contractility and ventricular filling; and (2) a defect outside the myocardium (e.g., coronary artery disease, pulmonary hypertension, or diabetes), which results in an overload on an otherwise normal heart. Either or both of these defects may be present in a given patient. These and other common causes of myocardial deficiency and systemic defects are listed in Box 22-1.

Pharmacology Overview

Drugs that increase the force of myocardial contraction are called positive **inotropic drugs,** and have a therapeutic role in the treatment of failing heart muscle. Negative inotropic drugs reduce the force of contraction. Drugs that increase the rate at which the heart beats are called positive **chronotropic drugs.** Negative chronotropic drugs do the opposite. Drugs may also affect how quickly electrical impulses travel through the conduction system of the heart (the sinoatrial [SA] node, atrioventricular [AV] node, bundle of His, and Purkinje fibers). Drugs that accelerate conduction are referred to as positive **dromotropic drugs.** Negative dromotropic drugs do the opposite. This chapter focuses on two of the main classes of positive inotropic drugs, *phosphodiesterase inhibitors* and *cardiac glycosides,* as well as the newest class of medications for heart failure, *B-type natriuretic peptides.* Although several other drugs are used in the treatment of heart failure, they are discussed in detail in other chapters; for example, angiotensin-converting enzyme (ACE) inhibitors and angiotensin receptor blockers (ARBs) are covered in Chapter 25; beta-blockers are discussed in Chapters 19 and 25; and diuretics are treated in Chapter 26. These drugs are mentioned in this chapter as well, but for specifics, refer to the indicated chapters.

The treatment of heart failure has changed dramatically over the past decade. Digoxin used to be the mainstay in heart failure treatment, but because of adverse effects and drug interactions, it has been widely replaced by other drugs. According to the latest American Heart Association and American College of Cardiology (2005) guidelines, the approach to the treatment of chronic heart failure revolves around reducing the effects of the renin-angiotensin-aldosterone system and the sympathetic nervous system. Therefore, the drugs of choice at the start of therapy are the ACE inhibitors (lisinopril, enalapril, captopril, and others) or the angiotensin II receptor blockers (valsartan, candesartan, losartan) and certain beta-blockers (metoprolol, a cardioselective beta-blocker; carvedilol, a nonspecific beta-blocker). Loop diuretics (furosemide) are used to reduce the symptoms of heart failure secondary to fluid overload, and the aldosterone inhibitors (spironolactone, eplerenone) are added as the heart failure progresses. Only after these drugs are used is digoxin added. Dobutamine, a positive inotropic drug, has also been used to treat heart failure. In 2005, a combination drug containing hydralazine and isosorbide dinitrate, became the first drug approved for a specific ethnic group. Hydralazine/isosorbide dinitrate (BiDil) was approved specifically for use in the African American population.

ANGIOTENSIN-CONVERTING ENZYME INHIBITORS

The ACE inhibitors are a class of drugs that, as their name implies, inhibit ACE, which is responsible for converting angiotensin I (formed through the action of renin) to angiotensin II. Angiotensin II is a potent vasoconstrictor and induces aldosterone secretion by the adrenal glands. Aldosterone stimulates sodium and water resorption, which can raise blood pressure. Together, these processes are referred to as the *renin-angiotensin-aldosterone system.* The ACE inhibitors are beneficial in the treatment of heart failure because they prevent sodium and water resorption by inhibiting aldosterone secretion. This causes diuresis, which decreases blood volume and blood return to the heart. This in turn decreases preload, or the left ventricular end-diastolic volume, and the work required of the heart.

Numerous ACE inhibitors are available, including lisinopril, enalapril, fosinopril, quinapril, captopril, ramipril, trandolapril, and perindopril. These drugs are all very similar, and lisinopril will be used as the class representative.

DRUG PROFILE

◆ lisinopril

Lisinopril (Prinivil, Zestril) is a commonly used ACE inhibitor and is available in a generic form. It is used for hypertension, heart failure, and acute myocardial infarction. Like all ACE inhibitors it is classified as a category C drug for women in the first trimester of pregnancy and a category D drug for women in the second and third trimesters; it can cause fetal death when used in the last two trimesters. Hyperkalemia may occur with any ACE inhibitor, and potassium supplementation or potassium-sparing diuretics should be used with caution. Like all ACE inhibitors, lisinopril can cause a dry cough, which will not harm the patient but is annoying. Lisinopril (and all ACE inhibitors) may be associated with a decrease in renal function and hyperkalemia. For drug interactions, please see Chapter 25.

PHARMACOKINETICS

Route	Onset of Action	Peak Plasma Concentration	Elimination Half-life	Duration of Action
PO	1 hr	6 hr	11-12 hr	24 hr

ANGIOTENSIN II RECEPTOR BLOCKERS

The therapeutic effects of ARBs in heart failure are related to their potent vasodilating properties. They may be used alone or in combination with other drugs such as diuretics in the treatment of hypertension or heart failure. The beneficial hemodynamic effect of ARBs is their ability to decrease systemic vascular resistance (a measure of afterload). Three ARBs are currently available: valsartan, candesartan, and losartan. Valsartan will be used as the class representative.

DRUG PROFILE

◆ valsartan

Valsartan (Diovan) is a commonly used ARB. Like all ARBs, it is a pregnancy category D drug. Valsartan shares many of the same adverse effects as lisinopril, profiled earlier. The ARBs are not as likely to cause the cough associated with the ACE inhibitors. For drug interactions, see Chapter 25.

PHARMACOKINETICS

Route	Onset of Action	Peak Plasma Concentration	Elimination Half-life	Duration of Action
PO	2 wk	Unknown	6 hr	12 hr

BETA-BLOCKERS

Beta-blockers (also discussed in Chapters 19, 23, and 25) work by reducing or blocking sympathetic nervous system stimulation to the heart and the heart's conduction system. By doing this, beta-blockers prevent catecholamine-mediated actions on the heart. This is known as a *cardioprotective* quality of beta-blockers. The resulting cardiovascular effects include reduced heart rate, delayed AV node conduction, reduced myocardial contractility, and decreased myocardial **automaticity.** Metoprolol is the beta-blocker most commonly used to treat heart failure. Metoprolol is available as an immediate-release and a sustained-release product, as well as an intravenous formulation.

Carvedilol (Coreg) has many effects, including acting as a nonselective beta-blocker, an alpha₁-blocker, a calcium channel blocker, and possibly an antioxidant. It is used primarily in the treatment of heart failure but is also beneficial for hypertension and angina. It has been shown to slow the progression of heart failure and to decrease the frequency of hospitalization in patients with mild to moderate (class II or III) heart failure. Carvedilol is most commonly added to digoxin, furosemide, and ACE inhibitors when used to treat heart failure. Carvedilol is available only for oral use. A controlled-release formulation, called Coreg CR, was recently approved. The dosages are different from those for immediate-release Coreg, and the two dosage forms cannot be interchanged.

MISCELLANEOUS HEART FAILURE DRUGS

DRUG PROFILES

hydralazine/isosorbide dinitrate
Hydralazine/isosorbide dinitrate (BiDil) was the first drug approved for a specific ethnic group, namely African Americans. This combination of two older drugs contains 37.5 mg of hydralazine and 20 mg of isosorbide dinitrate. The individual drugs are discussed in detail in Chapter 24 (isosorbide) and Chapter 25 (hydralazine). Peak plasma levels of hydralazine/isosorbide dinitrate are achieved in 1 hour. The dose is 1 tablet 3 times a day, titrated up to a maximum of 2 tablets 3 times daily.

◆ dobutamine
Dobutamine (Dobutrex) is a beta₁-selective vasoactive adrenergic drug that is structurally similar to the naturally occurring catecholamine dopamine. Through stimulation of the beta₁ receptors on heart muscle (myocardium), it increases cardiac output by increasing contractility (positive inotropy), which increases the stroke volume, especially in patients with heart failure. Dobutamine is available only as an intravenous drug and is given by continuous infusion. See Chapter 18 for further discussion on this drug.

B-TYPE NATRIURETIC PEPTIDE

The newest class of medications for heart failure, the B-type natriuretic peptides, currently includes only one drug, nesiritide.

◆ nesiritide
Nesiritide (Natrecor) is classified as a synthetic *recombinant* version of *human B-type natriuretic peptide.* (A "recombinant" drug is one that is manufactured using recombinant DNA technology. This method is described in Chapter 5.) Nesiritide is a synthetic hormone that has vasodilating effects on both arteries and veins. This vasodilation takes place in the heart itself and throughout the body. A related hormone that occurs naturally in the body is *atrial natriuretic peptide,* which affects vascular permeability. *Vascular permeability* refers to the ability of plasma to flow between blood vessels and their surrounding tissues, which serves as one way for the body to regulate blood pressure. In contrast, the effects of nesiritide have been shown to include diuresis (urinary fluid loss), *natriuresis* (urinary sodium loss), and vasodilation. These properties lead to an indirect increase in cardiac output and suppression of neurohormonal systems such as the renin-angiotensin system.

At this time, nesiritide is generally used in the intensive care setting as a final effort to treat severe, life-threatening heart failure, often in combination with several other cardiostimulatory medications. The manufacturer recommends that nesiritide not be used as a first-line drug for this purpose. In 2005, an expert panel reviewed nesiritide at the request of the U.S. Food and Drug Administration in response to reports of worsened renal function and mortality. The expert panel stated that the use of nesiritide should be strictly limited to treatment of patients with acutely decompensated heart failure who have dyspnea at rest. It should not be used to replace diuretics and should not be used repetitively or to improve renal function. Its only current contraindication is drug allergy, although it is not recommended for use in patients with low cardiac filling pressures, as typically measured in the intensive care unit. Adverse effects include hypotension, cardiac dysrhythmias, insomnia, headache, and abdominal pain. Currently identified drug interactions include additive hypotensive effects with coadministration of ACE inhibitors and diuretics. This drug is available only in injectable form. Recommended dosages are given in the Dosages table on p. 338.

PHARMACOKINETICS

Route	Onset of Action	Peak Plasma Concentration	Elimination Half-life	Duration of Action
IV	15 min	1 hr	18 min	1 to several hr

PHOSPHODIESTERASE INHIBITORS

As the name implies, phosphodiesterase inhibitors (PDIs) are a group of inotropic drugs that work by inhibiting the action of an enzyme called *phosphodiesterase.* These drugs were discovered in the search for positive inotropic drugs with a better therapeutic window than digoxin. Presently only two drugs in this category are available in the United States: inamrinone and milrinone. Inamrinone was originally called *amrinone,* but its name was modified to prevent confusion with the antidysrhythmic drug *amiodarone.*

Mechanism of Action and Drug Effects

The mechanism of action of PDIs differs from that of other inotropic drugs such as digoxin and the catecholamines. PDIs actually share a similar pharmacologic action with methylxanthines such as theophylline. Both types of drug inhibit the action of phosphodiesterase, which results in an increase in intracellular cyclic adenosine monophosphate (cAMP). However, milrinone and inamrinone are more specific for phosphodiesterase type III, which is common in the heart and vascular smooth muscles.

DOSAGES

Selected Drugs for Heart Failure

Drug (Pregnancy Category)	Pharmacologic Class	Usual Dosage Range	Indications
◆ digoxin (Lanoxin) (C)	Digitalis cardiac glycoside	**Pediatric** Digitalizing dose: IV: 0.008-0.035 mg/kg depending on age from premature infant to child older than 10 yr PO: 0.010-0.060 mg/kg depending on age from premature infant to child older than 10 yr Usual maintenance dose: 20%-35% of digitalizing dose **Adult** PO/IV: Usual digitalizing dose: 1-1.5 mg/day; usual maintenance dose: 0.125-0.5 mg/day	Heart failure, supraventricular dysrhythmias
◆ milrinone (Primacor) (C)	Phosphodiesterase inhibitor	**Adult** IV loading dose: 50 mcg/kg IV continuous infusion dose: 0.375-0.75 mcg/kg/min	Heart failure
◆ nesiritide (Natrecor) (C)	Recombinant human B-type natriuretic peptide	**Adult only (pediatric use not yet established)** IV: Initial bolus of 2 mcg/kg, followed by continuous infusion of 0.01 mcg/kg/min	Acutely decompensated heart failure in patients with dyspnea at rest or with minimal activity

IV, Intravenous; *PO,* oral.

The beneficial effects of milrinone and inamrinone come from the intracellular increase in cAMP. This results in two very beneficial effects in an individual with heart failure: a positive inotropic response and vasodilation. For this reason this class of drugs may also be referred to as *inodilators* (inotropics and dilators). These inodilators have a 10 to 100 times greater affinity for the smooth muscle fibers surrounding pulmonary and systemic blood vessels than they do for cardiac muscle. This suggests that the primary beneficial effects of inodilators come from their vasodilating effects. This causes a reduction in the force against which the heart must pump to eject its volume of blood.

Finally, inhibition of phosphodiesterase results in the availability of more calcium for myocardial muscle contraction. This leads to an increase in the force of contraction (i.e., positive inotropic action). The increased calcium present in heart muscle is also taken back up into its storage sites in the sarcoplasmic reticulum at a much faster rate than normal. As a result, the heart muscle relaxes more than normal and is also more compliant. In summary, PDIs have positive inotropic and vasodilatory effects. They may also increase heart rate in some instances and therefore may also have positive chronotropic effects as well.

Indications

PDIs are primarily used in the intensive care unit setting for the short-term management of acute heart failure. For long-term treatment of heart failure, some physicians have advocated weekly infusions of milrinone or the catecholamine dobutamine. However, the 2005 revised treatment guidelines of the American Heart Association and the American College of Cardiology re-

port no improvement in clinical status with such therapy and advise against the practice.

Contraindications

Contraindications to the use of PDIs include known drug allergy and may include the presence of severe aortic or pulmonary valvular disease and heart failure resulting from diastolic dysfunction.

Adverse Effects

Although inamrinone and milrinone are both PDIs, they have very different adverse effect profiles. The adverse effect that is most worrisome with inamrinone is thrombocytopenia. Inamrinone-induced thrombocytopenia occurs at a rate of about 2.4% and is more frequent when high doses are given over long periods. The other adverse effects associated with inamrinone therapy include dysrhythmia, nausea, and hypotension. With long-term use, elevations in liver enzyme levels may occur.

The primary adverse effect seen with milrinone therapy is dysrhythmia. Milrinone-induced dysrhythmias are mainly ventricular. Ventricular dysrhythmias occur in approximately 12% of patients treated with this drug. Some other adverse effects associated with milrinone therapy are hypotension, angina (chest pain), hypokalemia, tremor, and thrombocytopenia.

Toxicity and Management of Overdose

No specific antidote exists for an overdose of either inamrinone or milrinone. Hypotension secondary to vasodilation is the primary effect seen with excessive dosages of both drugs. The recommendation is to reduce the dosage or temporarily discontinue the drug if excessive hypotension occurs. This should be done until the patient's condition has stabilized. Initiation of general measures for circulatory support is also recommended.

Interactions

Concurrent administration of diuretics may cause significant hypovolemia and reduced cardiac filling pressure. The patient should be appropriately monitored in an intensive care setting to detect and respond to these problems. Also, additive inotropic effects may be seen with coadministration of digoxin. Furosemide must not be injected into intravenous lines for inamrinone or milrinone because it will precipitate immediately. Glucose-containing solutions should not be used when mixing inamrinone, because a loss of inamrinone activity is noted over 24 hours.

Dosages

For dosage information for a representative PDI, see the Dosages table on p. 338.

▪ DRUG PROFILE

◆ milrinone

Milrinone (Primacor) is the newer of the two presently available PDIs. Inamrinone was the first of the two PDIs to be used clinically for the short-term treatment of heart failure. As noted earlier, milrinone and inamrinone are also referred to as *inodilators* because they exert both a positive inotropic effect and a vasodilatory effect. Both of these drugs are contraindicated in cases of known drug allergy. Adverse effects include cardiac dysrhythmias, headache, hypokalemia, tremor, thrombocytopenia, and elevated liver enzyme levels. Drugs with which they interact include diuretics (additive hypotensive effects) and digoxin (additive inotropic effects). Milrinone is available only in injectable form. Recommended dosages are given in the table on p. 338.

PHARMACOKINETICS

Route	Onset of Action	Peak Plasma Concentration	Elimination Half-life	Duration of Action
IV	5-15 min	Immediate	2-3 hr	8-10 hr

CARDIAC GLYCOSIDES

Cardiac glycosides are one of the oldest groups of cardiac drugs. Not only do they have beneficial effects on the failing heart but they also help control the ventricular response to **atrial fibrillation.** They were originally obtained from either the *Digitalis purpurea* or *Digitalis lanata* plant, both commonly known as *foxglove.* For this reason, cardiac glycosides are sometimes referred to as *digitalis glycosides.* Cardiac glycosides were the mainstay of therapy for heart failure for more than 200 years, but, as mentioned previously, they are no longer used as first-line drugs in the treatment of this disorder. Digoxin is the only cardiac glycoside currently available in the United States. Although digoxin is a powerful positive inotropic drug, it has not been shown to reduce mortality. That being said, the nurse will invariably see patients who have been maintained on digoxin for years, and thus it is important to review digoxin therapy.

Mechanism of Action and Drug Effects

The primary beneficial effect of digoxin is thought to be an increase in myocardial contractility—known as a *positive inotropic effect.* This occurs secondarily to the inhibition of the sodium-potassium adenosine triphosphatase pump. When the action of this enzyme-complex is inhibited, the cellular sodium and calcium concentration increase. The overall result is enhanced myocardial contraction. Digoxin also augments cholinergic (or parasympathetic) stimulation via the *vagus* nerve of the parasympathetic nervous system. This is more commonly referred to as *vagal tone* and results in increased diastolic filling between heartbeats secondary to reduced heart rate. Vagal tone is also believed to sensitize cardiac baroreceptors, which reduces sympathetic stimulation from the central nervous system. All of these processes further enhance cardiac efficiency and output.

Digoxin also changes the electrical conduction properties of the heart, and this markedly affects the conduction system and cardiac automaticity. Digoxin decreases the velocity (rate) of electrical conduction and prolongs the **refractory period** in the conduction system. The particular site in the conduction system where this occurs is the area between the atria and the ventricles (SA node to AV node). The cardiac cells remain in a state of depolarization longer and are unable to start another electrical impulse, which also reduces heart rate and improves cardiac efficiency.

The following is a summary of the inotropic, chronotropic, dromotropic, and other effects produced by digoxin:

- A positive inotropic effect—an increase in the force and velocity of myocardial contraction without a corresponding increase in oxygen consumption
- A negative chronotropic effect—reduced heart rate
- A negative dromotropic effect—decreased automaticity at the SA node, decreased AV nodal conduction, reduced conductivity at the bundle of His, and prolongation of the atrial and ventricular refractory periods
- An increase in stroke volume
- A reduction in heart size during diastole
- A decrease in venous blood pressure and vein engorgement
- An increase in coronary circulation
- Promotion of tissue perfusion and diuresis as a result of improved blood circulation
- Decrease in exertional and paroxysmal nocturnal dyspnea, cough, and cyanosis
- Improved symptom control, quality of life, and exercise tolerance, but no apparent reduction in mortality

Indications

Digoxin is primarily used in the treatment of systolic heart failure and atrial fibrillation. However, the latest heart failure treatment guidelines recommend that it be used as an adjunct to drugs of other classes, including beta-blockers, diuretics, ACE inhibitors, and ARBs.

Contraindications

Contraindications to the use of digoxin include known drug allergy and may include second- or third-degree heart block, atrial fibrillation, ventricular tachycardia or fibrillation, heart failure resulting from diastolic dysfunction, and subaortic stenosis (obstruction in the left ventricle below the aortic valve). However, digoxin may be used to treat some of these conditions, if recommended by a competent cardiologist, depending on the given clinical situation.

Adverse Effects

The common undesirable effects associated with digoxin use are cardiovascular, central nervous system, ocular, and gastrointestinal effects. These are outlined in Table 22-1.

Toxicity and Management of Overdose

Digoxin has a low *therapeutic index* (see Chapter 2). Digoxin levels are monitored when the patient first starts taking the drug. However, monitoring of digoxin levels after the drug reaches steady state is normally necessary only if there is suspicion of toxicity, noncompliance, or deteriorating renal function. Normal therapeutic levels for digoxin are 0.5 to 2 ng/mL. Low potassium levels can increase the potential for digoxin toxicity. Therefore, frequent serum electrolyte level checks are also important. Estimates are that as many as 20% of patients taking digoxin exhibit symptoms of toxicity. A decrease in renal function is also a common cause of digoxin toxicity, because digoxin is excreted almost exclusively via the kidneys. Many conditions can predispose patients to digoxin toxicity; these are listed in Table 22-2.

The treatment strategies for digoxin toxicity depend on the severity of the symptoms. These strategies can range from simply withholding the next dose to instituting more aggressive therapies. The steps usually taken in the management of digoxin toxicity are listed in Table 22-3.

When significant toxicity develops as a result of digoxin therapy, the administration of digoxin immune Fab may be indicated. Digoxin immune Fab is an antibody that recognizes digoxin as an antigen and forms an antigen-antibody complex with the drug, thus inactivating the free digoxin. Digoxin immune Fab therapy is not indicated for every patient who is showing signs of digoxin toxicity. The following are the clinical settings in which its use may be indicated:

- Hyperkalemia (serum potassium level higher than 5 mEq/L) in a patient with digoxin toxicity
- Life-threatening cardiac dysrhythmias, sustained ventricular tachycardia or fibrillation, and severe sinus bradycardia or heart block unresponsive to atropine treatment or cardiac pacing
- Life-threatening digoxin overdose: more than 10 mg digoxin in adults; more than 4 mg digoxin in children

Interactions

A wide variety of significant drug interactions are possible with digoxin. Common examples are given in Table 22-4. The most important drug-drug interactions occurring with digoxin are in-

teractions with amiodarone, quinidine, and verapamil. These three drugs can increase digoxin levels by 50%. When large amounts of bran are ingested, the absorption of oral digoxin may be decreased. Certain herbal supplements may interact with digoxin; for example, ginseng may increase digoxin levels, hawthorn may potentiate the effects of digoxin, licorice may increase the risk of cardiac toxicity due to potassium loss, and St. John's wort may reduce digoxin levels.

Dosages

For dosage information for digoxin, see the Dosages table on p. 338. Also see the Preventing Medication Errors box on p. 341.

TABLE 22-2 Conditions Predisposing to Digitalis Toxicity

Condition/Disease	Significance
Use of cardiac pacemaker	A patient with this device may exhibit digitalis toxicity at lower dosages than usual.
Hypokalemia	The patient's risk of serious dysrhythmias is increased and the patient is more susceptible to digitalis toxicity.
Hypercalcemia	The patient is at higher risk of experiencing sinus bradycardia, dysrhythmias, and heart block.
Atrioventricular block	Heart block may worsen with increasing levels or digitalis.
Dysrhythmias	Dysrhythmias may occur that did not exist before digitalis use and thus could be related to digitalis toxicity.
Hypothyroidism, respiratory or renal disease	Patients with these disorders require lower dosages because they cause delayed renal drug excretion.
Advanced age	Because of decreased renal function and the resultant diminished drug excretion along with decreased body mass in this patient population, a lower dosage than usual is needed to prevent toxicity. The practice of polypharmacy may also lead to toxicity.
Ventricular fibrillation	Ventricular rate may actually increase with digitalis use.

TABLE 22-3 Digoxin Toxicity: Step-by-Step Management

Step	Actions
1	Discontinue administration of drug.
2	Begin continuous electrocardiographic monitoring for cardiac dysrhythmias; administer any appropriate antidysrhythmic drugs as ordered.
3	Determine serum digoxin and electrolyte levels.
4	Administer potassium supplements for hypokalemia if indicated, as ordered.
5	Institute supportive therapy for gastrointestinal symptoms (nausea, vomiting, or diarrhea).
6	Administer digoxin antidote (i.e., digoxin immune Fab) if indicated, as ordered.

TABLE 22-1 Digoxin: Common Adverse Effects

Body System	Adverse Effects
Cardiovascular	Any type of dysrhythmia, including bradycardia or tachycardia; hypotension
Central nervous	Headache, fatigue, malaise, confusion, convulsions
Eye	Colored vision (i.e., green, yellow, or purple), halo vision, or flickering lights
Gastrointestinal	Anorexia, nausea, vomiting, diarrhea

Normal therapeutic level = 0.5-2 ng/mL.

TABLE 22-4 Digoxin: Drug Interactions

Interacting Drug	Mechanism	Result
Antidysrhythmics calcium (parenteral)	Increase cardiac irritability	Increased digoxin toxicity
amphotericin B chlorthalidone Loop diuretics Laxatives Steroids (adrenal) Thiazide diuretics	Produce hypokalemia	Increased digoxin toxicity
Antacids Antidiarrheals cholestyramine colestipol sucralfate Anticholinergics	Decrease oral absorption	Reduced therapeutic effect
Barbiturates	Increase oral absorption	Increased therapeutic effect
Beta-blockers	Induce enzyme	Reduced therapeutic effect
Calcium channel blockers	Block beta$_1$ receptors in heart	Enhanced bradycardic effect of digoxin
quinidine	Block calcium channels in myocardium	Enhanced bradycardic and negative inotropic effects of digoxin
verapamil amiodarone	Decrease clearance	Digoxin levels increased by 50%; digoxin dose should be reduced 50%

DRUG PROFILES

◆ digoxin

Digoxin (Lanoxin) is indicated for the treatment of both heart failure and atrial fibrillation and flutter. Digoxin use is contraindicated in patients who have shown a hypersensitivity to it and in those with ventricular tachycardia and fibrillation. Normal therapeutic drug levels of digoxin are between 0.5 and 2 ng/mL. However, levels higher than 2 ng/mL are used for the treatment of atrial fibrillation. Digoxin is available in oral and injectable forms. Because of digoxin's fairly long duration of action and half-life, a loading, or "digitalizing," dose is often given to bring serum levels of the drug up to a desirable therapeutic level more quickly. See the table on p. 338 for the recommended digitalizing doses and the daily oral and intravenous adult and pediatric dosages.

PHARMACOKINETICS

Route	Onset of Action	Peak Plasma Concentration	Elimination Half-life	Duration of Action
PO	1-2 hr	2-8 hr	35-48 hr	3-4 days
IV	5-30 min	1-4 hr	35-48 hr	3-4 days

digoxin immune Fab

Digoxin immune Fab (Digibind) is the antidote for severe digoxin overdose and is indicated for the reversal of such life-threatening cardiotoxic effects as severe bradycardia, advanced heart block, ventricular tachycardia or fibrillation, and severe hyperkalemia. Use of digoxin immune Fab is contraindicated in patients who have shown a hypersensitivity to it. It is available only in parenteral form as a 40-mg vial. It is commonly dosed based on the patient's serum digoxin level in conjunction with his or her weight. The recommended dosages vary according to the amount of cardiac glycoside ingested. One vial binds 0.5 mg of digoxin. It is important to bear in mind that after digoxin immune Fab is given, all subsequent measurements of serum digoxin level will be elevated

PREVENTING MEDICATION ERRORS

The Importance of Decimal Points

Incorrect decimal placement can be lethal when calculating digoxin dosages! According to the Institute for Safe Medication Practices (ISMP), trailing zeros should *not* be used after decimal points. In the case of digoxin, if a "1 mg" dose is ordered and is written as "1.0 mg," the order could be misread as "10 mg," and the patient would receive 10 times the ordered dose.

The ISMP also recommends that leading zeroes be used if a dose is less than a whole number. For example, ".25 mg" can look like "25 mg," which is a dose that is 100 times the ordered dose. Instead, the order should be written as "0.25 mg" to avoid any errors.

Of course, such an error hopefully would be caught when the nurse realizes how many 250-mcg digoxin tablets it would take to give a "25 mg" dose, or how many milliliters would be needed for an intravenous dose. However, such errors have occurred. Consider what would happen if a digoxin overdose leads to digoxin toxicity and the serious effects this would have on the patient!

Data from Institute for Safe Medication Practices: ISMP's list of error-prone abbreviations, symbols, and dose designations; Huntington Valley, PA, 2007, available at *http://www.ismp.org/Tools/errorproneabbreviations.pdf.*

for days to weeks. Therefore, after its administration, the clinical signs and symptoms of digoxin toxicity, rather than the digoxin serum levels, should be the primary focus in monitoring for the effectiveness of reversal therapy.

PHARMACOKINETICS

Route	Onset of Action	Peak Plasma Concentration	Elimination Half-life	Duration of Action
IV	Immediate	Immediate	14-20 hr	Days to weeks

NURSING PROCESS

Assessment

Before a drug used to treat heart failure is given, a thorough assessment is required, including assessment of the patient's past and present medical history, drug allergies and family medical history with emphasis on any history of cardiac, hypertensive, or renal diseases. This review may yield findings that either dictate very cautious use of the drug or even represent contraindications to its use. Clinical parameters and other data that need to be assessed include the following:

- Blood pressure
- Pulse rate—both apical and radial, measured for 1 full minute
- Peripheral pulse location and grading of strength
- Capillary refill
- Presence or absence of edema
- Heart sounds
- Breath sounds
- Weight
- Intake and output amounts
- Serum laboratory values such as potassium, sodium, magnesium, and calcium levels
- Electrocardiogram
- Results of renal function tests, including BUN and creatinine levels
- Results of liver function tests such as levels of AST, ALT, CPK, LDH, and ALP
- Medication history and profile, including all prescription drugs, over-the-counter drugs, herbals, and nutritional supplements taken; for example, herbal products (e.g., Siberian ginseng) may increase digitalis drug levels; consumption of large amounts of bran with digoxin will decrease the drug's absorption
- Dietary habits and all meals and snacks consumed over the previous 24 hours
- Smoking history
- Alcohol intake

Thorough monitoring of electrolytes is needed, and baseline and subsequent levels of *digoxin* must be measured because of the narrow range between the therapeutic and toxic levels of digoxin (also called a *low therapeutic index;* see Chapter 2). Because low levels of certain electrolytes (e.g., hypokalemia) may precipitate digoxin toxicity, close assessment of electrolyte levels is critical to preventing complications and further problems. Other laboratory test results that need assessing prior to and during therapy include serum calcium, magnesium, and sodium levels. Baseline weight must be measured and documented as well. The following systems should also be assessed carefully: (1) neurologic system, with notation of any headaches, depression, weakness, changes in level of consciousness, level of alertness and orientation (vs. confusion), restlessness, fatigue, lethargy, or occurrence of nightmares; (2) gastrointestinal system, with attention to changes in appetite, diarrhea or constipation, nausea, and vomiting; (3) cardiac system, with documentation of any irregularities, pulse rate of lower than 60 beats/min or higher than 100 beats/min, abnormal heart sounds, and abnormal electrocardiogram findings (if this test is ordered); and (4) visual and sensory system, with documenta-

tion of baseline vision as well as any changes, such as green-yellow halos surrounding the peripheral field of vision. See Table 22-1 for more information on adverse effects of digoxin. Cautions, contraindications, and drug interactions should also be assessed (see Table 22-2).

As mentioned earlier, metoprolol is the *beta-blocker* most commonly used to treat heart failure. Carvedilol also has many therapeutic effects. These drugs are often added to digoxin, furosemide (loop diuretic), and ACE inhibitor therapy in heart failure patients. Related assessment information for alpha- and beta-blocking drugs can be found in Chapter 19. Dobutamine, a $beta_1$-selective adrenergic, is also used to treat heart failure and is discussed further in Chapter 18. The status of the patient's veins is important when this drug is taken, because it is only given intravenously. The newer drug nesiritide requires careful assessment of all body functions, especially cardiac function, with attention to heart sounds, blood pressure, pulse rate, and the presence of any cardiac dysrhythmias or hypotension, which may be exacerbated with the use of this drug. See previous discussion for other cautions, contraindications, and drug interactions. With any medication regimen, it is always important to assess support systems at home, because safe and effective therapy depends on close observation, monitoring of appropriate parameters (e.g.,

---

LIFE SPAN CONSIDERATIONS: The Pediatric Patient

Heart Failure

The cause, symptoms, treatment, and prognosis of heart failure in children vary depending on age. In infants, the cause of heart failure is generally holes in the heart or other structural problems. In older children, the structure of the heart may be normal but the heart muscle may be weakened. Symptoms of heart failure differ depending on age and become worse with age because the heart must keep up with increased oxygen demands and energy demands (with increased growth).

- Symptoms may include poor growth, difficulty in feeding, and tachypnea; in older children, inability to tolerate exercise and other activities, the need to rest more often, and dyspnea with minimal exertion occur more frequently.
- Treatment is generally age and cause specific. For septal defects, surgery or medication may be indicated. For more complex problems, surgery may be needed within the first few weeks of life.
- Drug therapy may include furosemide (a loop diuretic), angiotensin-converting enzyme inhibitors, beta-blockers, and sometimes digoxin to help improve heart pumping efficiency.
- Correct calculation of dosages for any of the medications used is very important to safe and cautious nursing care. A one-decimal-point placement error will result in a tenfold dosage error, which could be fatal.
- All medication calculations should be double-checked by a second registered nurse because of the narrow margin for error, especially if digoxin is indicated. Toxicity is manifested in children by nausea, vomiting, bradycardia, anorexia, and dysrhythmias.
- The prescriber should be notified immediately should the following symptoms indicative of heart failure develop or worsen: fatigue, sudden weight gain (2 pounds or more in 24 hours), palpitations, tachycardia or bradycardia, and/or respiratory distress.

Modified from Signs and symptoms: congestive heart failure, 2006, Cincinnati Children's Hospital Medical Center, available at *http://www.cincinnatichildrens.org/health/heart-encyclopedia/signs/chf.htm.*

daily weight), attention to patient complaints, and evaluation of how the patient is feeling and functioning.

Nursing Diagnoses

- Ineffective tissue perfusion, cardiopulmonary, related to the pathophysiologic influence of heart failure
- Deficient knowledge related to the first-time use of a cardiac glycoside or other medication and lack of information about the chronic nature of heart failure and the need for lifelong treatment
- Risk for injury related to limited information on the pathologic impact of heart failure and the potential adverse effects of drug therapy
- Imbalanced nutrition, less than body requirements, related to gastrointestinal adverse effects of digoxin toxicity
- Noncompliance with therapy regimen related to lack of information about the drug's effects and adverse effects

Planning

Goals

- Patient exhibits improved cardiac output once therapy is initiated.
- Patient states use, action, adverse effects, and toxic effects of therapy.
- Patient is free from injury related to medication therapy.
- Patient's appetite is improved or appetite is maintained while taking digoxin and other medications.

In planning for the administration of these drugs, the nurse must check the dosage and always double-check dose calculations as well as the patient's laboratory values, especially before giving any of the intravenous medications or digoxin preparations. Preplanning must also be carried out before administration of parenteral dosage forms so that all necessary equipment can be gathered before the drug is given.

Outcome Criteria

- Patient has improved to strong peripheral pulses, increased endurance for activity, decreased fatigue, and pink, warm extremities.
- Patient has increased urinary output resulting from therapeutic effects of the drug.
- Patient has improved heart and lung sounds with decreased dysrhythmias and crackles.
- Patient loses appropriate amount of weight and has less edema due to the therapeutic effects of the drug (increased urinary output caused by increased cardiac output).
- Patient's skin and mucous membranes (color and temperature) are improved to pink and warm.
- Patient maintains appetite while receiving therapy and reports anorexia, nausea, or vomiting immediately to the prescriber.
- Patient is free of toxicity as evidenced by absence of bradycardia and complaints of anorexia, nausea, or vomiting.
- Patient demonstrates proper technique for measuring radial pulse for 1 full minute before taking medication.
- Patient is able to state drug-related problems to report to the prescriber, such as palpitations, dysrhythmias, chest pain, and pulse rate lower than 60 beats/min or higher than 100 beats/min.

CASE STUDY

Phosphodiesterase Inhibitor for Heart Failure

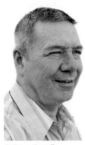
© Steve Carroll

Jim, a 58-year-old retired bus driver, has been in the hospital for a week for treatment of heart failure. He had a myocardial infarction a year earlier and tells the nurse that he "hasn't felt well for weeks." He is currently receiving carvedilol, lisinopril, furosemide, and potassium supplements (all orally), but he has had little improvement.

Today during morning rounds the nurse notes that Jim is having increased difficulty with breathing, and his heart rate is up to 120 beats/min. His weight has increased from 72 to 76 kg overnight, and his lower legs and ankles show edema rated as 3+. Crackles are heard over both lungs, and his pulse oximetry reading is 91% (down from 98% earlier). In addition, Jim is very restless. Oxygen is started, a Foley catheter is inserted, and Jim is transferred to the intensive care unit.

After examining Jim, Dr. Horne writes new medication orders as follows:

Change furosemide to 60 mg intravenously twice a day
Continue carvedilol and lisinopril
Start an infusion of milrinone as follows:
Loading dose: 50 mcg/kg over 10 minutes, followed by an infusion of 0.5 mcg/kg/min

1. Describe the drug effects of the medications Jim is receiving for the heart failure.
2. What laboratory values will you need to monitor while Jim is receiving the milrinone?

The charge nurse is in Jim's room when another nurse comes in to give Jim the intravenous dose of furosemide. As the nurse reaches for the tubing of the milrinone infusion to administer the diuretic, the charge nurse gently stops the nurse from giving the medication. Out in the hallway, the charge nurse speaks to the nurse.

3. What was the potential problem?

The next morning, Jim's breathing is better, his lungs are clearer, and his peripheral edema is now evaluated as trace edema. However, he complains of feeling his heart "skip" more than usual.

4. Is there a concern? What should the nurse do?

After a week, Jim's condition has improved greatly. The milrinone was stopped, he was transferred to a regular room, and today he is ready to go home.

5. In addition to receiving education regarding his medications, what should Jim be taught to monitor while recovering at home?

For answers, see *http://evolve.elsevier.com/Lilley.*

Implementation

First-Line Drugs

Nursing interventions associated with the use of angiotensin-converting enzyme inhibitors, angiotensin receptor blockers, nonspecific beta-blockers, and adrenergic drugs—all first-line drugs for treating heart failure—are discussed further in the chapters dealing with the corresponding drug classes, which have been listed previously. Nesiritide and hydralazine/isosorbide dinitrate, also first-line drugs, are discussed briefly here. Nesiritide must be given very cautiously and as ordered. This drug is usually given to very ill patients in an intensive care setting with cardiac monitoring. While the drug is being administered intravenously, the patient must be monitored for all of its severe adverse effects, such as hypotension, angina, dysrhythmias, bradycardia, and other cardiac irregularities. Hydralazine/isosorbide dinitrate, used to treat African American patients with heart failure, should also be given exactly as ordered. Syncope is a concern, and if it occurs, the drug will most likely be discontinued. If peripheral neuritis occurs, the prescriber may order pyridoxine. Blood pressure and other vital signs should be monitored, especially with the first few doses of hydralazine/isosorbide dinitrate. Drug interactions, cautions, and contraindications have been previously discussed.

Phosphodiesterase Inhibitors

Intravenous forms of inamrinone should not be mixed with dextrose. The true color of intravenous inamrinone solution is clear yellow (the majority of solutions are clear). Intake and output, heart rate, blood pressure, daily weight, respiration rate, heart sounds, and breath sounds should be recorded. Any evidence of hypokalemia should be noted and reported to the prescriber immediately. When heart failure drugs (e.g., digoxin, inamrinone, milrinone, digoxin immune Fab) are given parenterally, an infusion pump must be used unless the order is to administer them as an intravenous push.

Digoxin

Before administering any dose of digoxin (a cardiac glycoside), all electrolyte and drug levels should be checked to be sure they are within normal limits. The nurse should *always* measure the patient's apical pulse rate (auscultate the apical heart rate—found at the apical impulse located at the fifth left midclavicular intercostal space) for *1 full minute*. If the pulse rate is 60 beats/min or lower, or if it is higher than 100 beats/min, then the dose is generally withheld and the prescriber notified immediately of the problem. Although withholding of the dose is usually indicated, health care facilities and prescribers often have their own protocols that apply to individual patients. In addition, the prescriber should be contacted if the patient experiences any of the following signs and symptoms (which may indicate digitalis toxicity): anorexia, nausea, vomiting, diarrhea, or visual disturbances such as blurred vision or the perception of green or yellow halos around objects. Remember that most institutions and/or nursing units follow some protocol or policy with regard to digitalis and its administration.

Other nursing interventions include checking the dosage form and prescribed amounts and the prescriber's order carefully to make sure that the correct drug dosage has been dispensed (e.g., 0.125 or 0.25 mg). Oral digoxin may be administered with meals but not with foods high in fiber (bran), because the fiber will bind to the digitalis and lead to altered absorption and bioavailability of the drug. If the medication is to be given intravenously, the following interventions are critical to patient safety: infuse undiluted intravenous forms at around 0.25 mg/min or over longer than a 5-minute period, or as per hospital protocol. The administration of intramuscular forms of cardiac glycosides is extremely painful and is not indicated or recommended, because tissue necrosis and erratic absorption are often the outcome. Digoxin is incompatible with many other medications in solution or syringe, and compatibility must be double-checked before parenteral administration.

The nursing interventions for patients undergoing digitalization must be considered separately. Again, although digitalization is not commonly used in contemporary practice, it may still be performed in some areas of practice for the management of heart failure. Rapid digitalization (to achieve faster onset of action) is generally reserved for patients who have heart failure and are in acute distress. Such patients are hospitalized, because digitalis toxicities can appear quickly in this setting and are directly correlated with the high drug concentrations used. Should the patient undergoing rapid digitalization exhibit any of the manifestations of toxicity, the prescriber should be contacted immediately. These patients should be observed constantly with frequent measurement of vital signs and serum drug and potassium levels. Slow digitalization (rarely used) is generally performed on an outpatient basis in patients with heart failure who are not in acute distress. In this situation, it takes longer for toxic effects to appear (depending on the drug's half-life) than with rapid digitalization. The main advantages of slow digitalization are that it can be performed on an outpatient basis, oral dosage forms can be used, and it is safer than rapid digitalization. The disadvantages are that it takes longer for the therapeutic effects to occur and the symptoms of toxicity are more gradual in onset and therefore more insidious.

Should toxicity occur and digoxin rise to a life-threatening level, the antidote, digoxin immune Fab, should be administered as ordered. It is given parenterally over 30 minutes, and in some scenarios it is given as an intravenous bolus (e.g., if cardiac arrest is imminent). All vials of the drug should be refrigerated. The drug is stable for 4 hours after being mixed; it should be used immediately, and if not used within 4 hours, it should be discarded. Compatible solutions for dilution should be checked prior to infusion of the antidote. Blood pressure, apical pulse rate and rhythm, electrocardiogram, and serum potassium levels must be closely monitored and the findings recorded. The nurse must document baseline data and begin to observe closely for changes in assessment findings such as changes in muscle strength, occurrence of tremors and muscle cramping, changes in mental status, irregular cardiac rhythms (from hypokalemia), and confusion, thirst, and cold clammy skin (from hyponatremia). If the treatment does reduce the toxicity, these problems will improve considerably compared with the patient's baseline.

Evaluation

Monitoring patients after the administration of drugs to improve heart contractility, or positive inotropic drugs, is critical for identifying therapeutic effects and adverse effects. Because positive inotropic drugs increase the force of myocardial contractility; alter electrophysiologic properties, leading to a decrease in heart rate (negative chronotropic effect); and decrease AV node conduction properties (negative dromotropic effect), the therapeutic effects of these drugs include the following:

- Increased urinary output
- Decreased edema
- Decreased dyspnea and crackles
- Decreased fatigue
- Resolution of paroxysmal nocturnal dyspnea
- Improved peripheral pulses, skin color, and temperature

For patients taking lisinopril, valsartan, metoprolol, dobutamine, nesiritide, and hydralazine/isosorbide dinitrate, therapeutic effects include improvement in symptoms of heart failure and improved cardiac function. During therapy the evaluation must also monitor for the adverse effects of these medications, which have been discussed previously in the pharmacology section.

For patients receiving inamrinone, all vital signs and hemodynamic parameters (cardiac output, central venous pressure) must be constantly evaluated. Therapeutic effects of milrinone include an improvement in cardiac function with a corresponding improvement in the patient's heart failure. Adverse effects for which to monitor include hypotension, dysrhythmias, headache, ventricular fibrillation, chest pain, and hypokalemia. Patients taking milrinone should be evaluated for significant hypotension, and the drug should be discontinued or the infusion rate decreased per the prescriber's orders should this occur.

While the nurse is monitoring for the therapeutic effects of digoxin, it is essential to assess the patient for the development of toxicity because of the drug's low therapeutic index. Toxic effects associated with digoxin may include nausea, vomiting, and anorexia. Monitoring laboratory values such as serum creatinine, potassium, calcium, sodium, and chloride levels—as well as watching the serum levels of digoxin (which should normally be between 0.5 and 2 ng/mL)—is important to ensure safe and efficacious treatment.

PATIENT TEACHING TIPS

- Instruct the patient on how to take the radial pulse before each dose of digoxin or as indicated. Daily weights are important and should be done the same time every morning and with the exact amount of clothing. For elderly or physically or mentally challenged patients, it is important that home health care personnel or a heart failure/hospital-based clinic supervise the medication regimen. This is important because these individuals are at risk for adverse effects, toxicity and drug interactions. If the pulse rate is below 60 beats/min or is erratic, if the pulse rate is 100 beats/min or higher, or if there is anorexia, nausea, or vomiting, the healthcare provider should be contacted. The patient should also report any palpitations or a feeling that the heart is racing, change in heart rate, the occurrence of dizziness or fainting, any changes in vision and weight gain (2 pounds or more in 24 hours or 5 pounds or more in 1 week).
- A daily journal should be kept with notation of medications, daily weights, dietary intake and appetite, any adverse effects or changes in condition, and a rating of how the patient is feeling day to day.
- Every heart failure patient should wear a medical alert bracelet or necklace and keep a current medication and medical history card on his or her person at all times that lists allergies, medical diagnosis, and medications. Medical information and medication lists should be updated frequently or with each visit to prescriber.

- Digoxin is usually taken once a day, and the patient should be encouraged to take it at the same time every morning. If a dose is missed, the patient may take the omitted dose if no more than 12 hours have passed from the time the drug was to have been taken. The patient should be instructed that, if more than 12 hours have passed since the missed dose, the patient should *not* skip that dose, *not* double up on the next digoxin dose, and contact the prescriber immediately for further instructions.
- The patient should *never* abruptly stop any of the medications being taken for heart failure. If problems occur, the patient should always contact the prescriber.
- If potassium-depleting diuretics are being taken as part of the therapy, the patient should be encouraged to consume foods high in potassium and to report any weakness, fatigue, or lethargy. In addition, any worsening of dizziness or dyspnea or the occurrence of any unusual problems should be reported immediately.
- With medication regimens for heart failure, most patients should avoid using antacids or eating ice cream, milk products, yogurt, cheese (dairy products), or bran for 2 hours before or 2 hours after taking medication to avoid interference with the absorption of the oral dosage forms of these medications.

POINTS TO REMEMBER

- *Inotropic* drugs affect the force of myocardial contraction; positive inotropics (e.g., digoxin) increase the force of contractions and negative inotropics (e.g., beta-blockers, calcium channel blockers) decrease myocardial contractility. *Chronotropics* affect heart rate per minute, with positive chronotropics increasing heart rate and negative chronotropics decreasing the heart rate. *Dromotropic* drugs affect the conduction of electrical impulses through the heart; positive dromotropic drugs increase the speed of electrical impulses through the heart, whereas negative drugs have the opposite effect.
- Nurses need to be aware of the protocol for heart failure management, because digoxin, once the cornerstone of treatment for heart failure, is now used only after all other recommended drugs have been tried. The American Heart Association and American College of Cardiology (2005) guidelines provide the protocol guidelines of treatment for heart failure, including the following: Drugs of choice to initiate treatment are the ACE inhibitors (lisinopril, enalapril, captopril, and others) or the ARBs (valsartan, candesartan, losartan) and beta-blockers (metoprolol, a cardioselective beta-blocker; carvedilol, a nonspecific beta-

blocker). The loop diuretics (furosemide) are used to reduce the symptoms of heart failure secondary to fluid overload, and the aldosterone inhibitors (spironolactone, eplerenone) are added as the heart failure progresses. Only after these drugs are used is digoxin added. Hydralazine/isosorbide dinitrate became the first drug approved for use in the African-American population. Nesiritide is used in special situations in intensive care.
- Nurses need to be aware of some important physiologic concepts such as ejection fraction. A patient's ejection fraction reflects the contractility of the heart and is about 65% (0.65) in a normal heart. This value decreases as heart failure progresses; therefore, patients with heart failure have low ejection fractions because their hearts are failing to pump effectively.
- Nurses need to be informed regarding contraindications to the use of digoxin, which include a history of allergy to the digitalis medications, ventricular tachycardia and fibrillations, and AV block.
- Nurses must be aware that hypotension, dysrhythmias, and thrombocytopenia are major adverse effects of inamrinone and milrinone use.

NCLEX EXAMINATION REVIEW QUESTIONS

1 When teaching the patient about the signs and symptoms of cardiac glycoside toxicity, the nurse should alert the patient to watch for
  a visual changes such as photophobia.
  b flickering lights or halos around lights.
  c dizziness when standing up.
  d increased urine output.
2 During assessment of a patient who is receiving digoxin, the nurse monitors for findings that would indicate an increased possibility of toxicity, such as:
  a Apical pulse rate of 62 beats/min
  b Digoxin level of 1.5 ng/mL
  c Serum potassium level of 2.0 mEq/L
  d Serum potassium level of 4.8 mEq/L
3 When monitoring a patient who is receiving an intravenous infusion of inamrinone, the nurse will look for which adverse effect?
  a Thrombocytopenia
  b Proteinuria
  c Anemia
  d Decreased blood urea nitrogen and creatinine levels
4 A patient is taking a beta-blocker as part of the treatment plan for heart failure. The nurse knows that the purpose of the beta-blocker is to
  a increase urine output.
  b prevent stimulation of the heart by catecholamines.

  c increase the contractility of the heart muscle.
  d cause peripheral vasodilation.
5 The nurse is assessing a patient who is receiving a milrinone infusion and checks the patient's cardiac rhythm on the heart monitor. What adverse cardiac effect is most likely to occur in a patient who is receiving intravenous milrinone?
  a Tachycardia
  b Bradycardia
  c Atrial fibrillation
  d Ventricular dysrhythmia
6 The nurse is administering an intravenous infusion of a phosphodiesterase inhibitor to a patient who has heart failure. The nurse will evaluate the patient for which therapeutic effects? (Select all that apply.)
  a Positive inotropic effects
  b Vasodilation
  c Decreased heart rate
  d Increased blood pressure
  e Positive chronotropic effects

1. b, 2. c, 3. a, 4. b, 5. d, 6. a, b, e.

CRITICAL THINKING ACTIVITIES: BEST ACTION

1 A nurse administered 125 mg of digoxin instead of 0.125 mg of digoxin intravenously. The patient has developed a severe heart block dysrhythmia, and the slow heart rate has not responded to administration of atropine and other measures. What will the nurse expect to give next? How could this situation have been prevented?
2 The nurse is making morning medication rounds. One patient, a 78-year-old man, states that he has been nauseous and without an appetite and has experienced some diarrhea. He has been taking digoxin for the past few weeks for the treatment of recently diagnosed heart failure. What should the nurse do next? Explain.
3 A patient is receiving an ACE inhibitor, a diuretic, and a beta-blocker as treatment for mild heart failure. He has a history of hypothyroidism, which is controlled by thyroid replacement hor-

mones, and chronic bronchitis. He states that he stopped smoking a year ago after smoking two packs a day for 30 years. This morning he complains of a dry cough but says he does not feel short of breath, even when getting up to go to the bathroom. He is unable to produce any sputum. When the nurse listens to his lungs, his breath sounds are clear except for very few scattered rhonchi bilaterally. His weight is the same as yesterday's weight, and his ankles show only trace edema (2 days ago he had 21 edema on the edema scale). His temperature is 98.4° F (36.9° C), his pulse is 88 beats/min, and his blood pressure is 124/86. He says to the nurse, "This cough is awful! Is my heart failure getting worse, or am I getting pneumonia?" What is the nurse's best answer?

For answers, see *http://evolve.elsevier.com/Lilley*.

CHAPTER 23

Antidysrhythmic Drugs

OBJECTIVES

When you reach the end of this chapter, you should be able to do the following:

1 Describe the anatomy and physiology of the heart as well as cardiac electrophysiology, including normal conduction patterns, rate, and rhythm.

2 Briefly discuss the various disorders of cardiac electrophysiology and consequences to the patient.

3 Define the terms *dysrhythmia* and *arrhythmia*.

4 Identify the various causes of abnormal heart rhythms and their impact on the patient's health and activities of daily living.

5 Identify the most commonly encountered dysrhythmias.

6 Compare the various dysrhythmias with regard to their basic characteristics, impact on the structures of the heart, and related symptoms.

7 Contrast the various classes of antidysrhythmic drugs, citing prototypes in each class and describing their mechanisms of action, indications, routes of administration, dosing, any related drug protocols, adverse effects, cautions, contraindications, drug interactions, and any toxic reactions.

8 Develop a nursing care plan that includes all phases of the nursing process for patients receiving each class of antidysrhythmic drug.

e-Learning Activities

http://evolve.elsevier.com/Lilley

NCLEX Review Questions • Animations • Nursing Care Plans • Audio Glossary • Category Catchers • Medication Errors Checklists • IV Therapy Checklists • Calculators • Frequently Asked Questions • Content Updates • Supplemental Resources • Answers to Case Studies and Critical Thinking Activities

Drug Profiles

adenosine, p. 363
♦ amiodarone, p. 361
♦ atenolol, p. 361
♦ diltiazem, p. 363
♦ dofetilide, p. 362
esmolol, p. 361
flecainide, p. 360
ibutilide, p. 362

♦ lidocaine, p. 358
♦ metoprolol, p. 361
procainamide, p. 357
propafenone, p. 360
♦ propranolol, p. 361
quinidine, p. 358
♦ sotalol, p. 362
♦ verapamil, p. 363

♦ *Key drug.*

Glossary

Action potential Electrical activity consisting of a self-propagating series of polarizations and depolarizations that travel across the cell membrane of a nerve fiber during the transmission of a nerve impulse and across the cell membranes of a muscle cell during contraction or other activity of the cell. (p. 349)

Action potential duration For a cell membrane, the interval beginning with baseline (resting) membrane potential followed by depolarization and ending with repolarization to baseline membrane potential. (p. 350)

Arrhythmia Technically "no rhythm," meaning absence of heart rhythm (i.e., no heartbeat at all). More commonly used in clinical practice to refer to any variation from the normal rhythm of the heart. A synonymous term is *dysrhythmia,* which is the primary term used in this chapter and book. (p. 348)

Cardiac Arrhythmia Suppression Trial (CAST) The name of the major research study conducted by the National Heart, Lung, and Blood Institute to investigate the possibility of eliminating sudden cardiac death in patients with asymptomatic ectopy that has arisen after a myocardial infarction. (p. 360)

Depolarization The movement of positive and negative ions on either side of a cell membrane across the membrane in a direction that tends to bring the net charge to zero. (p. 349)

Dysrhythmia Any disturbance or abnormality in heart rhythm. (p. 348)

Effective refractory period The period after the firing of an impulse during which a cell may respond to a stimulus but the response will not be passed along or continued as another impulse. (p. 350)

Internodal pathways (Bachmann bundle) Special pathways in the atria that carry electrical impulses spontaneously generated by the sinoatrial node. These impulses cause the heart to beat. (p. 350)

Relative refractory period The time after generation of an action potential during which a nerve fiber will show a (reduced) response only to a strong stimulus. (p. 350)

Resting membrane potential (RMP) The transmembrane voltage that exists when the cell membranes of heart muscle (or other muscle or nerve cells) are at rest. (p. 348)

Sodium-potassium adenosine triphosphatase (ATPase) pump A mechanism for transporting sodium and potassium ions across the cell membrane against an opposing concentration gradient. Energy for this transport is obtained from the hydrolysis of adenosine triphosphate (ATP) by means of the enzyme ATPase. (p. 349)

Sudden cardiac death Unexpected, fatal cardiac arrest. (p. 360)

Threshold potential The critical state of electrical tension required for spontaneous depolarization of a cell membrane. (p. 350)

Torsades de pointes A rare ventricular arrhythmia that is associated with long QT interval and can degenerate into ventricular fibrillation and sudden death without medical intervention. (p. 354)

Vaughan Williams classification The system most commonly used to classify antidysrhythmic drugs. (p. 354; see also Table 23-3 on p. 354)

• • •

Anatomy, Physiology, and Disease Overview

DYSRHYTHMIAS AND NORMAL CARDIAC ELECTROPHYSIOLOGY

A **dysrhythmia** is any deviation from the normal rhythm of the heart. The term **arrhythmia** (literally "no rhythm") implies asystole, or no heartbeat at all. Thus, the more accurate term for an irregular heart rhythm is *dysrhythmia*. Dysrhythmias can develop in association with many conditions. Some of the more common ones arise after a myocardial infarction (MI), cardiac surgery, or as the result of coronary artery disease. These dysrhythmias are usually serious and may require treatment with an antidysrhythmic drug or nonpharmacologic therapies, although not all require

medical treatment. A cardiologist is usually consulted to make the judgment.

Disturbances in cardiac rhythm are the result of abnormally functioning cardiac cells. Thus, an understanding of the pathologic mechanism responsible for dysrhythmias first requires review of the electrical properties of these cells. Figure 22-1 on p. 335 shows the overall anatomy of the conduction system of the heart. Figure 23-1 illustrates some of the properties of this system from the standpoint of a single cardiac cell. Inside a resting cardiac cell there exists a net negative charge relative to the outside of the cell. This difference in the electronegative charge exists in all types of cardiac cells and is referred to as the **resting membrane potential (RMP).** The RMP results from an uneven distribution of ions (e.g., sodium, potassium, and calcium) across the cell membrane. This is known as *polarization.* Each ion moves primarily through its own specific *channel,* which is a specialized protein molecule that sits across the cell membrane. These proteins work continuously to restore the specific intracellular and extracellular concentrations of each ion. At RMP, the ionic concentration *gradient* (distribution) for the different ions is such that potassium ions are more highly concentrated intracellularly, whereas sodium and calcium ions are both more highly concentrated extracellularly. For this reason, potassium is generally thought of as an intracellular ion, whereas sodium and cal-

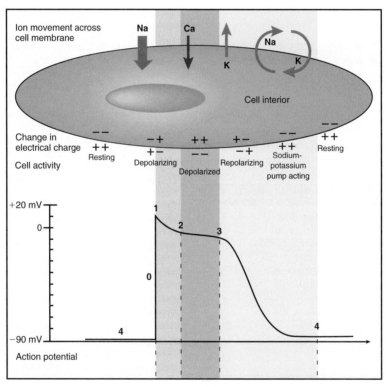

FIGURE 23-1 Phases of the action potential of a cardiac cell. In resting phase *(4)*, the cell membrane is polarized. The cell's interior has a net negative charge, and the membrane is more permeable to potassium ions (K) than to sodium ions (Na). When the cell is stimulated and begins to depolarize *(0)*, sodium ions enter the cell, potassium leaves the cell, calcium (Ca) channels open, and sodium channels close. In its depolarized phase *(1)*, the cell's interior has a net positive charge. In the plateau phase *(2)*, calcium and other positive ions enter the cell and potassium permeability declines, which lengthens the action potential. Then *(3)*, calcium channels close and sodium is pulled from the cell by sodium-potassium pump. The cell's interior then returns to its polarized, negatively charged state *(4)*. (From Monahan FD: *Phipps' medical-surgical nursing: health and illness perspectives,* ed 8, St Louis, 2006, Mosby.)

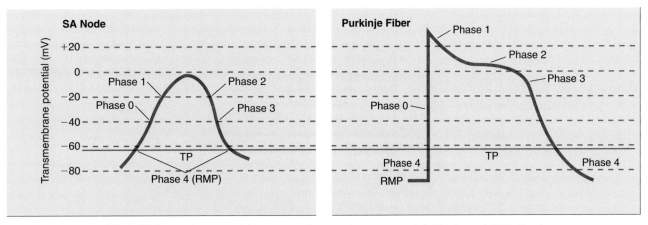

FIGURE 23-2   Action potentials. *RMP,* Resting membrane potential; *SA,* sinoatrial; *TP,* threshold potential.

cium are generally thought of as extracellular ions. Negatively charged intracellular and extracellular ions such as chloride (Cl^-) and bicarbonate (HCO_3^-) also contribute to this uneven distribution of ions, which is known as a *polarized* state. This polarized distribution of ions is maintained by the **sodium-potassium adenosine triphosphatase (ATPase) pump,** an energy-requiring ionic pump. The energy that drives this pump comes from molecules of *adenosine triphosphate (ATP),* which are a major source of energy in cellular metabolism.

Cardiac cells become excited when there is a change in this baseline distribution of ions across their membranes (RMP) that leads to the propagation of an electrical impulse. This change is known as an **action potential.** Action potentials normally occur in a continuous and regular manner in the cells of the cardiac conduction system, such as the *sinoatrial node (SA), atrioventricular node (AV),* and *His-Purkinje system.* This is because all of these tissues have the property of spontaneous electrical excitability known as *automaticity.* This excited state creates *action potentials,* which in turn generate electrical impulses that travel through the myocardium ultimately to create the heartbeat via contraction of cardiac muscle fibers.

An action potential has five phases. *Phase 0* is also called the *upstroke* because it appears as an upward line on the graph of an action potential, as shown in Figure 23-2, *A* and *B.* Both of these figures graphically illustrate the cycle of electrical changes that create an action potential. Note the variation in the shape of the curve of the graph depending on the relative conduction speed of the specific tissue involved (SA node vs. Purkinje fiber). A faster rate of conduction corresponds to a steeper slope on the graph. During phase 0, the resting cardiac cell membrane suddenly becomes highly permeable to sodium ions, which rush from the outside of the cell membrane to the inside *(influx)* through what are known as the *fast channels* or *sodium channels.* This disruption of the earlier *polarized* state of the membrane is known as **depolarization.** Depolarization can be thought of as a temporary equalization of positive and negative charges across the cell membrane. This releases spurts of electrochemical energy that drive the resulting electrical impulses through adjacent cells. *Phase 1* of the action potential begins a rapid process of *repolarization* that continues through *phases 2* and *3* to *phase 4,* which is the RMP. In phase 1, the sodium channels close and the con-

centrations of each ion begin to move back toward their ion-specific RMP levels. During *phase 2,* calcium ion influx occurs through the *slow channels* or *calcium channels.* They are called *slow channels* because the calcium influx occurs *relatively* more slowly than the earlier sodium influx. Potassium ions then flow from inside of the cell to outside *(efflux)* through specific *potassium channels* to offset the elevated positive charge caused by the influx of sodium and calcium ions. In the case of the Purkinje fibers, this causes a partial plateau (flattening on the graph) during which the overall membrane potential changes only slightly, as seen in Figure 23-2, *B.* In *phase 3,* the ionic flow patterns of phases 0 to 2 are changed by the sodium-potassium ATPase pump (or, more simply, the *sodium pump*), which reestablishes the baseline polarized state by restoring both intracellular and extracellular concentrations of sodium, potassium, and calcium (see Figure 23-1). As a result, the cell membrane is ultimately repolarized to its baseline level or RMP *(phase 4).* Note that this entire process occurs over roughly 400 *milliseconds*—that is, four hundred thousandths (less than one half) of *1* second.

There is some variation in this time period, however, between different parts of the conduction system. As an example, Figure 23-3 illustrates the pattern of movement of sodium, potassium, and calcium ions into and out of a Purkinje cell during the four phases of the action potential. Note that there are several differences in the action potentials of SA nodal cells and Purkinje cells. The level of the RMP for a given type of cell is an important determinant of the *rate* of its impulse conduction to other cells. The less negative (i.e., the closer to zero) the RMP at the onset of phase 0 of the action potential, the slower the upstroke *velocity* of phase 0. The *slope* of phase 0 is directly related to the impulse velocity. An upstroke with a steeper slope indicates faster conduction velocity. Thus, in the Purkinje cells, electrical conduction is relatively fast, and therefore electrical impulses are conducted quickly. These cells are referred to as *fast-response cells,* or *fast-channel cells,* and Purkinje fibers can therefore be thought of as fast-channel tissue. Many antidysrhythmic drugs affect the RMP and sodium channels, which in turn influences the rate of impulse conduction.

In contrast to Purkinje fibers, the cells of the SA node have a slower upstroke velocity, or a slower phase 0. This is illustrated in Figure 23-2, *A* as an upstroke curve that is less steep,

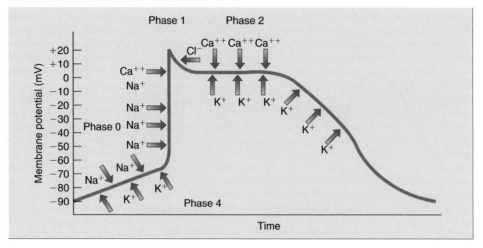

FIGURE 23-3 Purkinje fiber action potential.

which indicates a relatively slower rate of electrical conduction in these cells.

AV nodal cells are comparable to SA nodal cells in this regard. This slower upstroke in the SA and AV nodes is primarily dependent on the entry of calcium ions through the *slow channels* or *calcium channels*. This means that nodal action potentials are affected by calcium influx as early as phase 0. The nodes are therefore called *slow-channel tissue,* and conduction in these cells is slower than that in other parts of the conduction system. Drugs that affect calcium ion movement into or out of these cells (e.g., calcium channel blockers) tend to have significant effects on the SA and AV nodal conduction rates.

The interval between phase 0 and phase 4 is called the **action potential duration** (Figure 23-4). The period between phase 0 and midway through phase 3 is called the *absolute* or **effective refractory period.** During the effective refractory period the cardiac cell cannot be restimulated to depolarize and generate another action potential. During the remainder of phase 3 and until the return to the RMP (phase 4), the cardiac cell *can* be depolarized again if it receives a powerful enough impulse (such as one induced by drug therapy or supplied by an electrical *pacemaker*). This period is referred to as the **relative refractory period.** Figure 23-4 illustrates these various aspects of an action potential. Again, the actual shape of the action potential curve varies in different parts of the conduction system.

The RMP of certain cardiac cells gradually decreases (becomes less negative) over time in ongoing cycles, and this is probably secondary to small changes in the flux of sodium and potassium ions. Depolarization eventually occurs when a certain critical voltage is reached **(threshold potential).** This process of spontaneous depolarization is referred to as *automaticity,* or *pacemaker activity,* as mentioned earlier in this section. It is normal when it occurs in the SA node (see Figure 21-1). When spontaneous depolarizations occur elsewhere, however, dysrhythmias often result.

The SA node, the AV node, and His-Purkinje cells all possess the property of automaticity. The SA node is the natural pacemaker of the heart because it spontaneously depolarizes the most frequently. The SA node has an intrinsic rate of 60 to 100 depolarizations or beats per minute; that of the AV node is 40 to

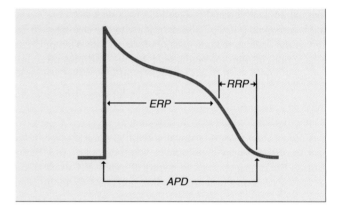

FIGURE 23-4 Aspects of an action potential. *APD,* Action potential duration; *ERP,* effective refractory period; *RRP,* relative refractory period.

60 beats/min; and that of the ventricular Purkinje fibers is 40 or fewer beats per minute. The action potentials and other properties in different areas of the heart are compared in Table 23-1.

As the pacemaker of the heart, the SA node, which is located near the top of the right atrium, generates the electrical impulse that ultimately produces the heartbeat. First, however, this impulse travels through the atria via specialized pathways called the **internodal pathways (Bachmann bundle).** This causes contraction of atrial myocardial fibers, which creates the first heart sound. Next, the impulse reaches the AV node, which is located near the bottom of the right atrium. The AV node slows this very fast moving electrical impulse just long enough to allow the ventricles to fill with blood. If the AV node did not slow the impulse in this way, ventricular contraction would overlap that of the atria, which would result in a smaller volume of ejected ventricular blood and reduced cardiac output.

Next, the AV nodal cells generate an electrical impulse that passes into the *bundle of His* (or *His bundle*), a band of cardiac muscle fibers located between the right and left ventricles in what is called the *ventricular septum* (wall between the ventricles). The bundle of His distributes the impulse into both ventricles via the *right* and *left bundle branches.* Each branch terminates in the *Purkinje fibers* that are located in the myocardium of the ventri-

TABLE 23-1 Comparison of Action Potentials in Different Cardiac Tissue

Tissue	Action Potential	Speed of Response	Threshold Potential (mV)	Conduction Velocity (m/sec)
SA node	⋀	Slow	260	Less than 0.05
Atrium	⋀	Fast	290	1
AV node	⋀	Slow	260	Less than 0.05
His-Purkinje system	⋀	Fast	295	3
Ventricle	⋀	Fast	290	1

AV, Atrioventricular; *SA,* sinoatrial.

cles. The stimulation of the Purkinje fibers causes ventricular contraction and ejection of blood from the ventricles. Blood from the right ventricle is pumped into the pulmonary circulation, whereas blood from the left ventricle is pumped into the systemic circulation to supply the rest of the body. The His bundle and Purkinje fibers are so named for the medical scientists who first identified them. Together, they are often referred to in the literature as the *His-Purkinje system.* Any abnormality in cardiac automaticity or impulse conduction often results in some type of dysrhythmia.

Electrocardiography

The electrophysiologic cardiac events described in detail earlier correspond more simply to the tracings of an electrocardiogram, abbreviated as *ECG* or *EKG* (Figure 23-5). The *P wave* corresponds to spontaneous impulse generation in the SA node followed immediately by depolarization of atrial myocardial fibers and their muscular contraction. This normally determines the heart rate and is affected by the balance between sympathetic and parasympathetic nervous system tone, the intrinsic automaticity of the SA nodal tissue, the mechanical stretch of atrial fibers due to incoming blood volume, and cardiac drugs. The *QRS complex* (or *QRS interval*) corresponds to depolarization and contraction of ventricular fibers. The *J point* marks the start of the *ST segment,* which corresponds to the beginning of ventricular repolarization. The *T wave* corresponds to completion of the repolarization of these ventricular fibers. As an analogy, depolarization can be thought of as discharge or contraction of cardiac muscle fibers, whereas repolarization can be thought of as a relaxation of just-contracted muscle fibers to prepare for the next contraction (heartbeat). Note that the repolarization of the atrial fibers is obscured on the ECG tracing by the QRS complex and thus has no corresponding deflection in the tracing. The *U wave* is not always present, and its physiologic basis is uncertain. When the U wave occurs it is generally correlated with electrophysiologic events such as repolarization of Purkinje fibers. These events may be a source of dysrhythmias caused by a triggered automaticity. Prominent U waves are often associated with sinus bradycardia, hypokalemia, use of quinidine and other class Ia antidysrhythmics, hyperthyroidism, and some cases of mitral valve prolapse. Abnormal U waves (inverted) are associated with serious conditions such as MI, acute angina, coronary artery spasms and ischemic heart disease. The PR and QT intervals and the ST segment are parts of the ECG tracing that are often altered in recognizable ways by disease or by the adverse effects of certain types of drug therapy or drug interactions, as discussed in later sections of this chapter.

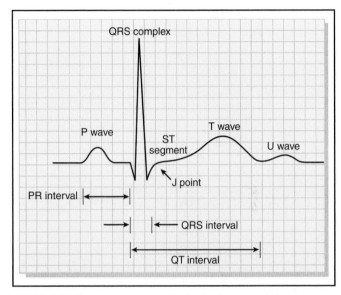

FIGURE 23-5 The waves and intervals of a normal electrocardiogram. (From Goldberger AL: *Clinical electrocardiography: a simplified approach,* ed 6, St Louis, 1999, Mosby.)

Common Dysrhythmias

A variety of cardiac dysrhythmias are recognized. Some are easier to treat than others using drug therapy and/or interventional cardiology procedures such as pacemaker implantation, catheter ablation, cardioversion, and implantation of cardioverters-defibrillators. Dysrhythmias are subdivided into several broad categories depending on their anatomic site of origin in the heart. *Supraventricular dysrhythmias* originate above the ventricles in the SA or AV node or atrial myocardium. *Ventricular dysrhythmias* originate below the AV node in the His-Purkinje system or ventricular myocardium. Dysrhythmias that originate outside the conduction system (i.e., in atrial or ventricular cells) are known as *ectopic,* and their specific points of origin are called *ectopic foci* (*foci* is the plural of the Latin-derived word *focus*). *Conduction blocks* are dysrhythmias that involve disruption of impulse conduction between the atria and ventricles through the AV node and may also originate in the His-Purkinje system, directly affecting ventricular function. Less commonly, impulse conduction between the SA and AV node is affected. Several of the most common dysrhythmias are described in Table 23-2, and corresponding ECG tracings are provided. They are also described further in the following text.

Among the supraventricular dysrhythmias, *atrial fibrillation* is a particularly common condition. It is characterized by rapid atrial contractions that only incompletely pump blood into the

Table 23-2 Common Dysrhythmias

Dysrhythmia	Description and ECG Tracing
Atrial flutter (AF)	Often progresses to atrial fibrillation 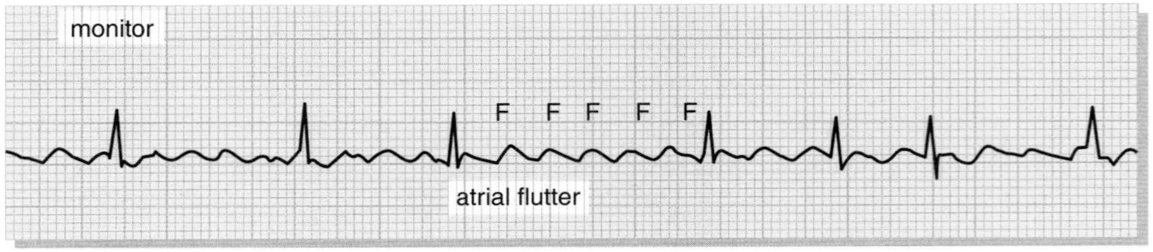
Atrial fibrillation (AF)	Rapid, ineffective atrial contractions 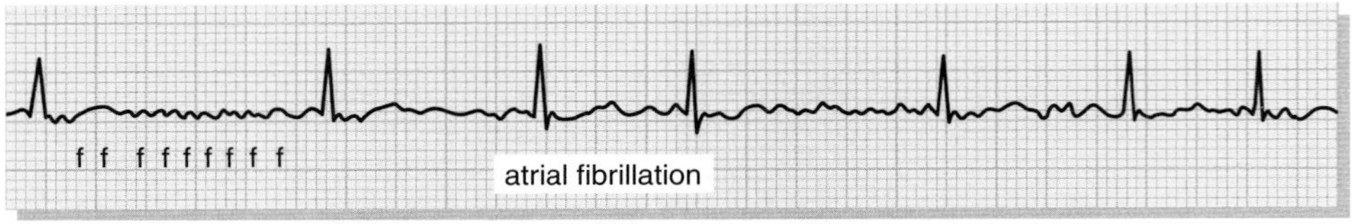
Paroxysmal supraventricular tachycardia (PSVT)	Heart rate of 180-200 beats/min or higher 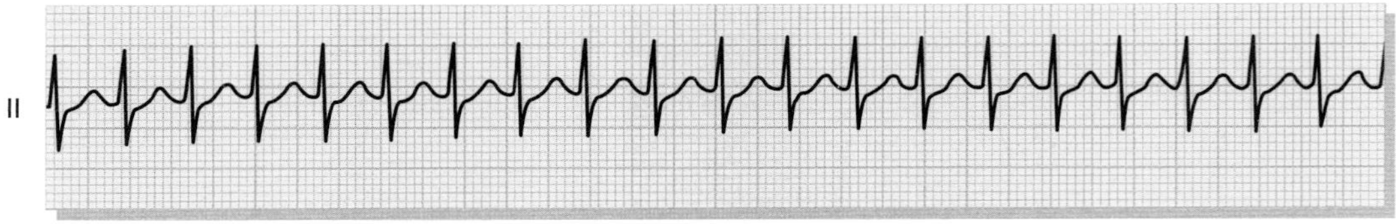
Premature ventricular contractions (PVCs)	Contractions generated by impulses arising from ectopic foci within ventricular myocardium 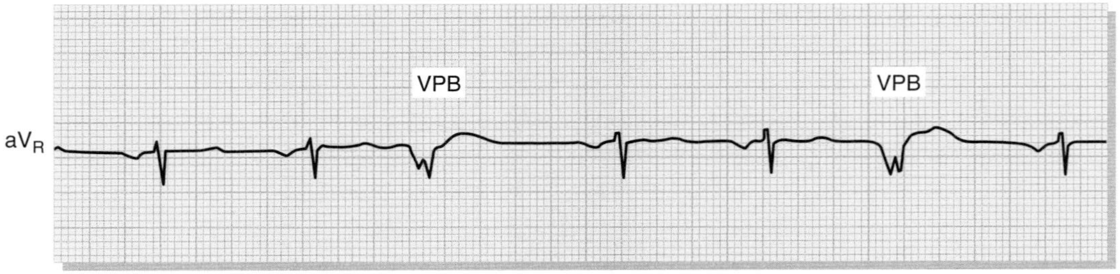
Nonsustained ventricular tachycardia (NSVT)	Relatively brief period (20 sec or less) in which ventricles contract rapidly on their own as well as in response to AV impulses 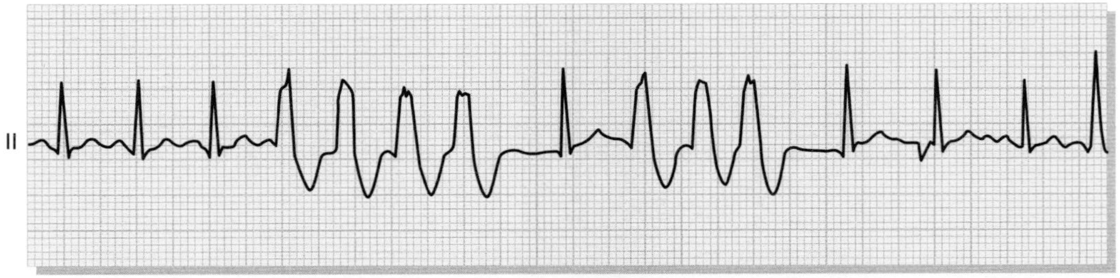

monitor

F F F F F

atrial flutter

f f f f f f f f

atrial fibrillation

II

VPB

VPB

aV$_R$

II

Sustained ventricular tachycardia (SVT)

Same as above but more prolonged

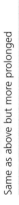

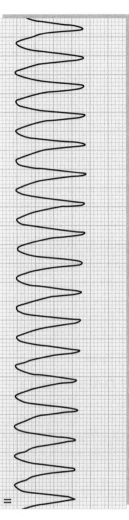

Torsades de pointes (TdP)

Rapid ventricular tachycardia preceded by QT interval prolongation (often progresses to ventricular fibrillation)

Monitor lead

Ventricular fibrillation (VF)

Rapid, ineffective ventricular contractions (fatal if not reversed)

Coarse VF

Fine VF

Coarse VF

ECG, Electrocardiogram.

ventricles. Atrial fibrillation is notable in that it predisposes the patient to stroke. This is due to the fact that the blood tends to stagnate in the incompletely emptied atria and is therefore more likely to clot. If such blood clots manage to make their way into the left ventricle, they may be embolized to the brain and cause a stroke. Although there would theoretically be a similar risk for pulmonary embolism, this seems to be of less clinical concern with atrial fibrillation than the risk for stroke. Patients with ongoing atrial fibrillation are often given anticoagulant therapy with warfarin (see Chapter 28) to reduce the likelihood of stroke. *AV nodal reentrant tachycardia (AVNRT)* is a conduction disorder that often gives rise to a dysrhythmia known as *paroxysmal supraventricular* tachycardia (PSVT). (The word *paroxysmal* means "sudden.") AVNRT occurs when electrical impulse transmission from the AV node into the His-Purkinje system of the ventricles is disrupted. As a result, some of the impulses circle backward *(retrograde impulses)* and reenter the atrial tissues to produce a tachycardic response. In Wolff-Parkinson-White syndrome, ectopic impulses that begin near the AV node actually bypass the AV node and reach the His-Purkinje system before the normal AV-generated impulses. This is one cause of ventricular tachycardia, although it is technically supraventricular in origin. Varying degrees of *AV block* (often called *heart block*) involve different levels of disrupted conduction of impulses from the AV node and His-Purkinje system to the ventricles. Although first-degree AV block is often asymptomatic, third-degree block, or *complete heart block,* often requires use of a cardiac pacemaker to ensure adequate ventricular function. There can also be blocks within the His-Purkinje system of the ventricles, known as *bundle branch blocks. Premature ventricular contractions (PVCs)* occur when impulses originate from ectopic foci within the ventricles (His-Purkinje system). PVCs probably occur periodically in many people; they become problematic when they occur frequently enough to compromise systolic blood volume. *Ventricular tachycardia* refers to a rapid heartbeat from impulses originating in the ventricles. It can be nonsustained (brief) or sustained, requiring definitive treatment. Worsening ventricular tachycardia can deteriorate into **torsades de pointes,** an intermediate dysrhythmia that often further deteriorates into *ventricular fibrillation.* Ventricular fibrillation is fatal if not reversed, which most often requires electrical defibrillation. Interestingly, torsades de pointes often responds preferentially to intravenous magnesium sulfate.

▌Pharmacology Overview
ANTIDYSRHYTHMIC DRUGS

Numerous drugs are available to treat dysrhythmias. These drugs are categorized according to where and how they affect cardiac cells. Although other classifications are described in the literature, the most commonly used system for this purpose is still the **Vaughan Williams classification.** This system is based on the electrophysiologic effect of particular drugs on the action potential. This approach identifies four major classes of drugs: I (including Ia, Ib, and Ic), II, III, and IV. The various drugs in these four classes are listed in Table 23-3. There is currently a gradual trend away from the use of class Ia drugs. The formerly available class Ic drug encainide was removed from the market after research indicated that the risk of fatal cardiac dysrhythmias associated with this drug overshadowed its dysrhythmia suppression effects. For similar reasons the other two class Ic drugs, flecainide and propafenone, are generally used in patients intolerant of other drugs. Nonetheless, several class I drugs remain available in the United States as therapeutic options. The class III drugs have emerged as among the most widely used antidysrhythmics at this time. The class IV drugs (calcium channel blockers) have limited usefulness in treating tachydysrhythmias (dysrhythmias involving tachycardia), unlike most of the other classes. The role of class II drugs (beta-blockers) continues to grow in the field of cardiology, including in dysrhythmia management. Digoxin, the cardiac glycoside discussed in Chapter 22, still has a place in dysrhythmia management, especially in the prevention of dangerous ventricular tachydysrhythmias secondary to atrial fibrillation.

Mechanism of Action and Drug Effects

Antidysrhythmic drugs work by correcting, to varying degrees and by various mechanisms, abnormal cardiac electrophysiologic function. As membrane-stabilizing drugs, class I drugs exert their actions on the sodium (fast) channels. However there are some slight differences in the actions of the drugs in this class, so they are divided into three subclasses. These subclasses are class Ia, Ib, and Ic drugs, and they are based on the magnitude of the effects of each drug on phase 0, the action potential duration, and the effective refractory period. Class Ia drugs (quinidine, procainamide, and disopyramide) block the sodium channels; more specifically, they delay repolarization and increase the action potential duration.

TABLE 23-3 Vaughan Williams Classification of Antidysrhythmic Drugs

Functional Class	Drugs
Class I: membrane-stabilizing drugs; fast sodium channel blockers	
Ia: ↑ blockade of sodium channel, delay repolarization, ↑ action potential duration	quinidine, disopyramide, procainamide
Ib: ↑ blockade of sodium channel, accelerate repolarization, ± action potential duration	lidocaine, phenytoin
Ic: ↑↑↑ blockade of sodium channel, ± repolarization; also suppress reentry	flecainide, propafenone
Class II: beta-blocking drugs	All beta-blockers
Class III: drugs whose principal effect on cardiac tissue is to ↑ action potential duration	amiodarone, sotalol,* ibutilide, dofetilide
Class IV: calcium channel blockers	verapamil, diltiazem
Other: antidysrhythmic drugs that have the properties of several classes and therefore cannot be placed in one particular class	digoxin, adenosine

↑, Increase; ±, increase or decrease.
*Sotalol also has class II properties.

Table **23-4** Antidysrhythmic Drugs: Mechanisms of Action

	Vaughan Williams Class			
	I	II	III	IV
Action	Blocks sodium channels, affects phase 0	Decreases spontaneous depolarization, affects phase 4	Prolongs action potential duration	Blocks slow calcium channels
Tissue	Fast	Slow	Fast	Slow
Effect on action potential				

Class Ib drugs (phenytoin, and lidocaine) also block the sodium channels, but unlike class Ia drugs, they accelerate repolarization and decrease the action potential duration. Phenytoin is more commonly used as an anticonvulsant (see Chapter 15) than as an antidysrhythmic drug. Class Ic drugs (flecainide, propafenone) have a more pronounced effect on the blockade of sodium channels but have little effect on repolarization or the action potential duration.

Class II drugs are the beta-adrenergic blockers (beta-blockers; see Chapter 19), and they are also commonly used as antianginal drugs (see Chapter 24) and as antihypertensives (see Chapter 25). They work by reducing or blocking sympathetic nervous system stimulation to the heart and, as a result, the transmission of impulses in the heart's conduction system. This results in depression of phase 4 depolarization. These drugs mostly affect slower-conducting cardiac tissues.

Class III drugs (amiodarone, sotalol, ibutilide, and dofetilide) increase the action potential duration by prolonging repolarization in phase 3. They affect fast tissue and are most commonly used to manage dysrhythmias that are difficult to treat. They are usually reserved for patients for whom other therapies have failed. Sotalol actually has properties of both class II and class III drugs, and it may be listed as a member of either one or the other class, depending on the specific reference used.

Class IV drugs are the calcium channel blockers, which, like beta-blockers, are also used as both antianginal drugs (see Chapter 24) and antihypertensives (see Chapter 25). As their name implies, they work specifically by inhibiting the calcium channels, which reduces the influx of calcium ions during action potentials. This results in depression of phase 4 depolarization. Diltiazem and verapamil are the calcium channel blockers most commonly used to treat cardiac dysrhythmias.

The mechanisms of action of the major classes of antidysrhythmics are summarized in Table 23-4. The effects of the various classes of drugs are presented in Box 23-1.

Indications

Antidysrhythmic drugs are effective in treating a variety of cardiac dysrhythmias. The antidysrhythmic drugs and the most common indications for their use are listed in Table 23-5.

Contraindications

As with all drugs, contraindications to the use of antidysrhythmic drugs include known drug allergy to a specific product. Other contraindications may include second- or third-degree AV block, bundle branch block, cardiogenic shock, sick sinus syndrome,

---

BOX **23-1** Effects of Antidysrhythmic Drugs

Class Ia (disopyramide, procainamide, quinidine)
- Depress myocardial excitability
- Prolong the effective refractory period
- Eliminate or reduce ectopic foci stimulation
- Decrease inotropic effect
- Have anticholinergic (vagolytic) activity

Class Ib (lidocaine, phenytoin)
- Decrease myocardial excitability in the ventricles
- Eliminate or reduce ectopic foci stimulation in the ventricles
- Have minimal effect on the SA node and automaticity
- Have minimal effect on the AV node and conduction
- Have minimal anticholinergic (vagolytic) activity

Class Ic (flecainide, propafenone)
- Produce dose-related depression of cardiac conduction, especially in the bundle of His–Purkinje system
- Have minimal effect on atrial conduction
- Eliminate or reduce ectopic foci stimulation in the ventricles
- Have minimal anticholinergic (vagolytic) activity
- Flecainide use now reserved for the most serious dysrhythmias

Class II (Beta-blockers [e.g., atenolol, esmolol, metoprolol])
- Block beta-adrenergic cardiac stimulation
- Reduce SA nodal activity
- Eliminate or reduce atrial ectopic foci stimulation
- Reduce ventricular contraction rate
- Reduce cardiac output and blood pressure

Class III (amiodarone, sotalol,* ibutilide, dofetilide)
- Prolong the effective refractory period
- Prolong the myocardial action potential
- Block both alpha- and beta-adrenergic cardiac stimulation

Class IV (diltiazem, verapamil)
- Prolong AV nodal effective refractory period
- Reduce AV nodal conduction
- Reduce rapid ventricular conduction caused by atrial flutter

AV, Atrioventricular; *SA,* sinoatrial.
*Sotalol also has class II properties.

---

and any other major ECG changes depending on the clinical judgment of a cardiologist, as well as concurrent use of certain drugs that interact with antidysrhythmics. The reason for these concerns is that antidysrhythmic drugs can potentially worsen existing dysrhythmias (also termed *dysrhythmogenic*). The risk of such an effect is greater in patients with structural heart damage (e.g., after MI). In particular, with AV block and bundle

TABLE 23-5 Antidysrhythmic Drugs: Indications

Drug Class	Indications
Class Ia	
disopyramide	Atrial fibrillation, premature atrial contractions,
procainamide	premature ventricular contractions, ventricular
quinidine	tachycardia, Wolff-Parkinson-White syndrome
Class Ib	
lidocaine	Ventricular dysrhythmias only (premature ventricular contractions, ventricular tachycardia, ventricular fibrillation)
phenytoin	Atrial and ventricular tachydysrhythmias caused by digitalis toxicity; long QT syndrome
Class Ic	
flecainide	Severe ventricular tachycardia and supraventricular
propafenone	tachycardia dysrhythmias, atrial fibrillation and flutter, Wolff-Parkinson-White syndrome
Class II	
Beta-blockers:	Both supraventricular and ventricular dysrhythmias
atenolol	(act as general myocardial depressants)
esmolol	
metoprolol	
propranolol	
Class III	
amiodarone	Life-threatening ventricular tachycardia or
dofetilide	fibrillation
ibutilide	Atrial fibrillation or flutter resistant to other drug
sotalol*	therapy
Class IV	
Calcium channel	Paroxysmal supraventricular tachycardia; rate
blockers:	control for atrial fibrillation and flutter
diltiazem	
verapamil	

*Sotalol also has class II properties.

branch block, there is a danger of drug-induced ventricular failure if a given drug should further compromise already existing AV conduction delays. The safe prescribing of antidysrhythmic drugs is an area that requires especially strong clinical expertise and careful judgment on a case-by-case basis.

Adverse Effects

Adverse effects common to most antidysrhythmics include hypersensitivity reactions, nausea, vomiting, and diarrhea. Other common effects include dizziness, headache, and blurred vision. In addition, at noted earlier, many antidysrhythmics are themselves capable of producing new dysrhythmias *(prodysrhythmic effect)*. Prolongation of the QTc interval is a potentially severe adverse effect shared by many antidysrhythmics. The concern with QTc prolongation is the potential for induction of torsades de pointes. As with any drug class, there are also cases of unpredictable or *idiosyncratic* (see Chapter 2) adverse effects that are not related to drug concentration in the body. Idiosyncratic reactions are unpredictable; however, it is thought that such effects will eventually be explained by genetic variations. Table 23-6 summarizes the most commonly reported adverse effects by specific drug.

Toxicity and Management of Overdose

The main toxic effects of the antidysrhythmics involve the heart, circulation, and central nervous system (CNS). Specific antidotes are not available, and the management of an overdose involves maintaining adequate circulation and respiration using general support measures and providing any required symptomatic treatment (Table 23-7).

Interactions

Antidysrhythmics can interact with many different categories of drugs. The most serious drug interactions are the ones that can result in dysrhythmias, hypotension or hypertension, respira-

TABLE 23-6 Antidysrhythmic Drugs: Common Adverse Effects

Class	Drug	Adverse Effects
Ia	procainamide	Hypotension, rash, diarrhea, nausea, agranulocytosis, SLE-like syndrome
	quinidine	Hypotension, syncope, QTc prolongation, lightheadedness, diarrhea, stomach cramping, bitter taste, anorexia, angina, palpitations, prodysrhythmic effect, blurred vision, tinnitus
Ib	lidocaine	Bradycardia, dysrhythmia, hypotension, agitation, anxiety, seizure, metallic taste
	phenytoin	Hypotension, bradycardia, thrombophlebitis, hypertrichosis, gingival hyperplasia
Ic	flecainide	Dizziness, visual disturbances, dyspnea, palpitations, nausea, vomiting, diarrhea, weakness
	propafenone	Prodysrhythmic effect, angina, tachycardia, syncope, AV block, dizziness, fatigue, dyspnea
II	Beta-blockers	Bradycardia, hypotension, dizziness, fatigue, AV block
III	amiodarone	Pulmonary toxicity, thyroid disorders, bradycardia, hypotension, SA node dysfunction, AV block, ataxia, QTc prolongation, torsades de pointes, dizziness, impaired memory, nausea, vomiting, constipation, photosensitivity, abnormal liver function test results, jaundice, visual disturbances, hyperglycemia or hypoglycemia, impotence, dermatologic reactions including rash, toxic epidermal necrolysis, vasculitis, blue-gray coloring of the skin (face, arms, neck)
	dofetilide	Headache, insomnia, ventricular tachycardia, chest pain, torsades de pointes, rash, back pain, nausea, diarrhea, abdominal pain
	ibutilide	Nonsustained ventricular tachycardia, ventricular extrasystoles, tachycardia, hypotension, AV block, headache, nausea
	sotalol*	Bradycardia, chest pain, palpitations, fatigue, dizziness, lightheadedness, weakness, dyspnea
IV	Calcium channel blockers	Constipation, bradycardia, heart block, hypotension, dizziness, dyspnea

*Sotalol also has class II properties.
AV, Atrioventricular; *SA,* sinoatrial; *SLE,* systemic lupus erythematosus.

TABLE 23-7 Selected Antidysrhythmic Drugs: Management of Overdose

Drug	Toxic Effect	Management
acebutolol	Bradycardia	1-3 mg IV atropine divided
	Bronchospasm	Beta$_2$-adrenergic or theophylline
	Cardiac failure	Digitalization
	Hypotension	Vasopressor
adenosine	Usually self-limiting due to a very short half-life	Competitive antagonists caffeine or theophylline
amiodarone	Bradycardia	Beta-adrenergic drug
	Hypotension	Positive inotropic drug or vasopressor
digoxin	Decreased clearance due to drug interactions with other antidysrhythmic drugs (e.g., quinidine, verapamil, amiodarone)	See Chapter 22 for more information
disopyramide	Loss of consciousness, cardiac and respiratory arrest	Neostigmine for anticholinergic effects, emesis induction, activated charcoal, and hemodialysis
esmolol	Same as for acebutolol	Same as for acebutolol
flecainide	Reduced heart rate	Dopamine or dobutamine; acidification of very alkaline urine
lidocaine	Convulsions	Diazepam or thiopental
moricizine	Hypotension, heart failure, myocardial infarction	Gastric evacuation and advanced life support measures
phenytoin	Circulatory and respiratory arrest, convulsions	Life support measures when required
procainamide	Cardiac depression	IV pressor drugs and supportive measures
	Convulsions	Diazepam and mechanically assisted respiration
propafenone	Same as for acebutolol	Same as for acebutolol
propranolol	Cardiac dysrhythmias	Sodium lactate (reduces toxicity except in alkalosis); lidocaine
quinidine	Same as for acebutolol	Same as for acebutolol
sotalol*	Convulsions	Diazepam or short-acting barbiturate
verapamil	Cardiac failure	Dopamine or dobutamine
	Conduction problems	Cardiac pacing
	Hypotension	Vasopressors, 10% calcium chloride solution

*Sotalol also has class II properties.
IV, Intravenous.

tory distress, or any excessive therapeutic or toxic drug effects. Drug interactions occur when the presence of one drug strengthens or weakens the pharmacologic effects of another. This is most commonly seen when the first drug affects the activity of the enzymes that metabolize the second drug, either speeding or slowing its elimination. One particular interaction common to many antidysrhythmics is the potentiation of anticoagulant activity with warfarin (Coumadin). Because many patients receiving antidysrhythmic therapy also need warfarin, prothrombin time and international normalized ratio (INR) should be monitored appropriately and necessary adjustments made to the warfarin dosage. This is especially true with amiodarone. The INR will increase by 50% in almost 100% of patients receiving amiodarone and warfarin. Grapefruit juice can also inhibit the metabolism of several antidysrhythmics such as amiodarone, disopyramide, and quinidine. Other common interactions are summarized in Table 23-8. To explain the mechanism for each interaction is beyond the scope of this text. Readers needing more detailed information are encouraged to consult other appropriate references.

Dosages

For the recommended dosages of selected antidysrhythmic drugs, see the Dosages table on p. 359.

Because the four classes of antidysrhythmics produce a variety of effects on the action potential of the cardiac cell, they exert a major influence on cardiac electrophysiologic function. The diversity of therapeutic effects and the adverse effects pose a special challenge to the nurse, who is responsible for ensuring the safe and efficacious use of these drugs. Because the aspects of the nursing process that relate to the administration of these drugs differ for each of the four classes of drug, each group is discussed separately.

CLASS IA DRUGS

Class Ia drugs are considered membrane-stabilizing drugs because they possess local anesthetic properties. They stabilize the membrane and have depressant effects on phase 0 of the action potential. These drugs include procainamide, quinidine, and disopyramide.

procainamide

The electrophysiologic effect of procainamide (Pronestyl) is similar to that of quinidine. Procainamide is useful in the management of atrial and ventricular tachydysrhythmias. Procainamide is chemically related to the local anesthetic procaine. Significant adverse effects of the drug include ventricular dysrhythmias and blood disorders. It can cause a systemic lupus erythematosus–like syndrome, which occurs in about 30% of patients on long-term therapy. It can also cause gastrointestinal effects such as nausea,

TABLE 23-8 Selected Antidysrhythmic Drugs: Common Drug Interactions

Drug (Class)	Interacting Drugs	Effects*
quinidine (Ia)	amiodarone, amitriptyline, bepridil, erythromycin, haloperidol, sotalol, moxifloxacin	Additive QTc prolongation
	digoxin	Increase in digoxin levels by 50%
lidocaine (Ib)	amiodarone, azole antifungals, beta-blockers, erythromycin, verapamil, cimetidine	Increased serum levels of lidocaine
	aminophylline, calcium channel blockers, cyclosporine, selected HMG-CoA reductase inhibitors, SSRI antidepressants	Increase in effects of interacting drugs
propafenone (Ic)	cimetidine, quinidine	Increase in propafenone levels; use is contraindicated
	digoxin, warfarin, beta-blockers	Increase in level of interacting drugs; digoxin dose should be reduced by 50%
	Class Ia and III antidysrhythmics, erythromycin	QTc prolongations
amiodarone (III)	amitriptyline, azole antifungals, bepridil, clarithromycin, disopyramide, erythromycin, haloperidol, moxifloxacin, quinidine, procainamide	Prolonged QTc interval
	digoxin, diltiazem, verapamil, beta-blockers	AV block
	warfarin, digoxin	Increase in INR by 50% in almost 100% of patients, increase in levels of digoxin by 50%
	cyclosporine	Increased cyclosporine levels and toxicity
dofetilide (III)	cimetidine, verapamil, hydrochlorothiazide (HCTZ), ketoconazole, trimethoprim	Increased dofetilide concentrations—use is contraindicated
	bepridil, clarithromycin, erythromycin, tricyclic antidepressants, phenothiazines, moxifloxacin	Prolonged QTc interval
sotalol (III)†	Calcium channel blockers	Additive effects on AV conduction, bradycardia
	Class I antidysrhythmics, erythromycin, bepridil, moxifloxacin, amiodarone	Prolonged QT interval, bradycardia
	Antacids, NSAIDs, rifampin	Decreased sotalol effectiveness
verapamil, diltiazem (IV)	amiodarone, beta-blockers, flecainide, digoxin	Bradycardia, decreased cardiac output, hypotension
	Azole antifungals, clarithromycin, erythromycin, isoniazid, HIV drugs	Increased verapamil effects

AV, Atrioventricular; *HIV*, human immunodeficiency virus; *HMG-CoA*, hydroxymethylglutaryl–coenzyme A; *INR*, international normalized ratio; *NSAIDs*, nonsteroidal antiinflammatory drugs; *SSRIs*, selective serotonin reuptake inhibitors.
*Note that enhanced activity of any antidysrhythmic drug may reach the level of drug toxicity, including potentially fatal cardiac dysrhythmias.
†Sotalol also has class II properties.

vomiting, and diarrhea. Other adverse effects include fever, leukopenia, maculopapular rash, urticaria, pruritus, flushing, and torsades de pointes resulting from prolongation of the QT interval. Use of procainamide is contraindicated in patients who have shown hypersensitivity reactions to its use and in those with heart block and lupus erythematosus. It is available in both oral and injectable form.

PHARMACOKINETICS

Route	Onset of Action	Peak Plasma Concentration	Elimination Half-life	Duration of Action
IV/IM	10-30 min	10-60 min	3 hr	3 hr
PO	0.5-1 hr	1-2 hr	3 hr	3-8 hr

quinidine

Quinidine (Quinidex) has both a direct action on the electrical activity of the heart and an indirect (anticholinergic) effect. Significant adverse effects of the drug include cardiac asystole and ventricular ectopic beats. Quinidine can cause cinchonism. Symptoms of mild cinchonism include tinnitus, loss of hearing, slight blurring of vision, and gastrointestinal upset. Contraindications to the use of the drug include hypersensitivity, thrombocytopenic purpura resulting from previous therapy, AV block, intraventricular conduction defects, and torsades de pointes. Quinidine is available in both oral and paren-

teral (injectable) forms and in three different salt forms. The oral preparations include sulfate and gluconate salts.

PHARMACOKINETICS

Route	Onset of Action	Peak Plasma Concentration	Elimination Half-life	Duration of Action
PO	1-3 hr	0.5-6 hr	6-7 hr	6-12 hr

CLASS IB DRUGS

Class Ib drugs share many characteristics with class Ia drugs but are grouped together because they act preferentially on ischemic myocardial tissue. They have little effect on conduction velocity in normal tissue. Class Ib drugs have a weak depressive effect on phase 0 depolarization, the action potential duration, and the effective refractory period. They include lidocaine and phenytoin.

◆ lidocaine

Lidocaine (Xylocaine) is the prototypical Ib drug. It is one of the most effective drugs for the treatment of ventricular dysrhythmias, but it can only be administered intravenously because it has an extensive first-pass effect (i.e., when it is taken orally, the liver metabolizes most of it to inactive metabolites). Because of its extensive hepatic metabolism, dosage reduction by 50% is recommended for patients with frank liver failure or cirrhosis. Dosage

DOSAGES

Selected Antidysrhythmic Drugs

Drug Name (Pregnancy Category)	Pharmacologic Class	Usual Dosage Range
adenosine (Adenocard) (C)	Unclassified antidysrhythmic	**Adult** IV: 6-mg bolus over 1-2 sec; second rapid bolus of 12 mg as needed, which may be repeated a second time as needed
◆ amiodarone (Cordarone) (D)	Class III antidysrhythmic	**Adult** IV: 150 mg over 10 min, then 60 mg/hr for 6 hr, then 30 mg/hr as maintenance dose PO: 800-1600 mg/day for 1-3 wk, reduced to 400-800 mg/day for 5 wk; usual maintenance dose 200-400 mg/day PO: 200-400 mg/day
◆ atenolol (Tenormin) (D)	Beta$_1$-blocker (class II antidysrhythmic)	**Adult** IV: 5 mg over 5 min followed by 5 mg over 10 min followed by 50 mg PO 10 min after last IV injection and another 50 mg PO 12 hr later, then 100 mg/day PO for a further 6-9 days PO (maintenance): 12.5 to 100 mg once daily
◆ diltiazem (Cardizem)	Calcium channel blocker (class IV antidysrhythmic)	**Adult** IV: Bolus dose 0.25 mg/kg over 2 min, second dose 0.35 mg/kg over 2 min after 15 min as needed, then 5-10 mg/hr or more by continuous infusion
◆ dofetilide (Tikosyn) (C)	Class III antidysrhythmic	**Adult** PO: 125-500 mg bid (note dose is individualized)
ibutilide (Corvert) (C)	Class III antidysrhythmic	**Adult** IV: 1-mg infusion over 10 min (if less than 60 kg, then 0.1 mL/kg)
◆ lidocaine (Xylocaine) (B)	Class Ib antidysrhythmic	**Pediatric** IV: Suggested bolus dose, 1 mg/kg; usual maintenance infusion rate, 20-50 mcg/kg/min **Adult** IV: Bolus dose 50-100 mg; may be repeated in 5 min; do not exceed 200-300 mg over 1 hr; usual maintenance infusion rate 1-4 mg/min
◆ metoprolol (Lopressor) (D)	Beta$_1$-blocker (class II antidysrhythmic)	**Adult** IV/PO: 3 bolus injections of 5 mg at 2-min intervals followed by 50 mg PO q6h for 48 hr, thereafter 10 mg bid PO: 12.5-100 mg bid
propafenone (Rythmol) (C)	Class Ic antidysrhythmic	**Adult** PO: Start with 150 mg q8h and increase q3-4d; usual range, 450-900 mg/day divided
◆ propranolol (Inderal) (D)	Beta-blocker (class II antidysrhythmic)	**Adult** IV: 1-3 mg; if needed, repeat in 2 min with additional doses as needed q4h or longer; switch to PO as soon as possible PO: 10-30 mg q6-8h PO: 80-320 mg/day divided bid-qid
quinidine (Quinidex [sulfate], Cardioquin [polygalacturonate], Quinaglute, Dura-Tab [gluconate]) (C)	Class Ia antidysrhythmic	**Adult** *Gluconate* PO: 324-648 mg q8-12h IM: 600 mg followed by 400 mg q2-6h or more if needed IV: 200-750 mg infused at up to 10 mg/min *Sulfate* PO: 200-mg load; 100-600 mg q4-6h 300-600 mg tid-qid
◆ sotalol* (Betapace) (B)	Class III antidysrhythmic	**Adult** PO: 160-320 mg/day divided into 2-3 doses
◆ verapamil (Calan, Isoptin, Verelan) (C)	Calcium channel blocker (class IV antidysrhythmic)	**Pediatric** IV: 1 yr or younger: 0.1-0.2 mg/kg bolus over 2 min; repeat dose after 30 min IV: 1-15 yr: 0.1-0.3 mg/kg bolus over 2 min; do not exceed 5-mg dose; repeat dose not exceeding 10 mg may be given after 30 min **Adult** PO: Start with 80 mg tid-qid; daily range 240-480 mg IV: 2.5-5 mg bolus over 2 min; repeat dose of 5-10 mg may be given after 30 min

IM, Intramuscular; *IV,* intravenous; *PO,* oral.
*Sotalol also has Class II properties.

reductions may also be necessary in patients with renal impairment because of extensive excretion of the drug and its metabolites by the kidney.

Lidocaine exerts its effects on the conduction system of the heart by making it difficult for the ventricles to develop a dysrhythmia, an action known as *raising the ventricular fibrillation threshold*. It does this by decreasing the sensitivity of the cardiac cell membrane to impulses and decreasing the cell's ability to depolarize on its own (decreasing automaticity). Many of these effects are accomplished by blockade of fast sodium channels.

Significant adverse effects include CNS toxic effects such as twitching, convulsions, and confusion; respiratory depression or arrest; and the cardiovascular effects of hypotension, bradycardia, and dysrhythmias. Use of the drug is contraindicated in patients who are hypersensitive to it, who have severe SA or AV intraventricular block, or who have Stokes-Adams or Wolff-Parkinson-White syndrome. Lidocaine is available only in parenteral form for intramuscular or intravenous administration. Intramuscular administration is recommended only in extenuating circumstances, such as when the patient is symptomatic and no intravenous or ECG equipment is available.

PHARMACOKINETICS

Route	Onset of Action	Peak Plasma Concentration	Elimination Half-life	Duration of Action
IV	2-15 min	5-10 min	8 min	20 min–1.5 hr

CLASS IC DRUGS

Class Ic drugs (flecainide, propafenone) produce a more pronounced sodium channel blockade than class Ia and Ib drugs but have little effect on repolarization or the action potential duration. These drugs significantly slow conduction in the atria, AV node, and ventricles. Because of their marked effect on conduction, these drugs strongly suppress PVCs, reducing or eliminating them in a large number of patients.

flecainide

Flecainide (Tambocor) is a chemical analogue of procainamide. A large multicenter double-blind placebo-controlled study called the **Cardiac Arrhythmia Suppression Trial (CAST)** was conducted by the National Heart, Lung, and Blood Institute to determine whether the incidence of **sudden cardiac death** could be reduced in post-MI patients with asymptomatic ectopy through the use of flecainide. The findings showed that mortality and nonfatal cardiac arrest rates in patients treated with this drug were actually comparable to or higher than those seen in patients who received the placebo. Because of these findings, the U.S. Food and Drug Administration (FDA) required that the labeling of flecainide be revised to indicate that its use should be limited to the treatment of documented life-threatening ventricular dysrhythmias such as sustained ventricular tachycardia. Treatment with this drug should be initiated in the hospital. This drug is not indicated for the management of less severe dysrhythmias such as nonsustained ventricular tachycardia or frequent PVCs.

Although flecainide is better tolerated than quinidine or procainamide, it is also more prodysrhythmic. It is this prodysrhythmic potential that limits its use to the management of life-threatening dysrhythmias. Flecainide has a negative inotropic effect and depresses left ventricular function. Less serious but more common noncardiac adverse effects include dizziness, visual disturbances, and dyspnea. Contraindications to its use include hypersensitivity, cardiogenic shock, second- or third-degree AV block, and non–life-threatening dysrhythmias. It is available only for oral use.

PHARMACOKINETICS

Route	Onset of Action	Peak Plasma Concentration	Elimination Half-life	Duration of Action
PO	3 hr	1.5-3 hr	11-12 hr	12-27 hr

propafenone

Propafenone (Rythmol) is similar in action to flecainide. It reduces the fast inward sodium current in Purkinje fibers and to a lesser extent in myocardial fibers. Unlike other class I drugs, propafenone has mild beta-blocking effects. This may contribute to its overall effects on the conduction system. It is also believed to have calcium channel blocking effects, which may contribute to its mild negative inotropic effects.

Until recently, propafenone's use was limited to the treatment of documented life-threatening ventricular dysrhythmias such as sustained ventricular tachycardia. Recent findings suggest that at low dosages it has benefit in the treatment of atrial fibrillation as well. Treatment should be started while the patient is in the hospital. Unlike flecainide, however, propafenone can be given to patients with depressed left ventricular function and may be a better drug than disopyramide, procainamide, and quinidine in these patients. It should be used with caution in patients with heart failure, because it has some beta-blocking properties and dose-dependent negative inotropic effects.

Propafenone is generally well tolerated. The most commonly reported adverse reaction is dizziness. Patients may also complain of a metallic taste, constipation, and headache, along with nausea and vomiting. These gastrointestinal adverse effects may be reduced by taking propafenone with food. Propafenone use is contraindicated in patients with a known hypersensitivity to it and in those with bradycardia, bronchial asthma, significant hypotension, uncontrolled heart failure, cardiogenic shock, and various conduction disorders. It is available only for oral use.

PHARMACOKINETICS

Route	Onset of Action	Peak Plasma Concentration	Elimination Half-life	Duration of Action
PO	2 hr	3-5 hr	2-10 hr	Unknown

CLASS II DRUGS

Class II antidysrhythmics are also known as *beta-blockers* (see Chapter 19). These drugs work by reducing or blocking sympathetic nervous system stimulation to the heart and the heart's conduction system. By doing this, beta-blockers prevent catecholamine-mediated actions on the heart. This is known as a *cardioprotective* quality of beta-blockers. The resulting cardiovascular effects include a reduced heart rate, delayed AV node conduction, reduced myocardial contractility, and decreased myocardial automaticity. The pharmacologic effects of the beta-blockers are especially beneficial after an MI because of the many catecholamines released at this time, which make the heart hyperirritable and predisposed to many types of dysrhythmias. The beta-blockers offer protection from these potentially very dangerous complications. Several studies have demonstrated a significant reduction (on the average of 25%) in the incidence of sudden cardiac death after MI in patients treated with beta-blockers on an ongoing basis.

Although there are several beta-blockers, only a few are commonly used as antidysrhythmics. Those currently approved by the FDA for this purpose are acebutolol, esmolol, propranolol, and sotalol (which has both class II and class III properties). Selected drugs are described here. The class II drugs are classified as pregnancy category C drugs except acebutolol, pindolol, and sotalol, which are all category B drugs.

◆ atenolol

Atenolol (Tenormin) is a cardioselective beta-blocker, which means that it preferentially blocks the beta$_1$-adrenergic receptors that are located primarily in the heart. Noncardioselective beta-blockers block not only the beta$_1$-adrenergic receptors in the heart but also the beta$_2$-adrenergic receptors in the lungs and therefore can exacerbate preexisting asthma or chronic obstructive pulmonary disease. In addition to having class II antidysrhythmic properties, atenolol is useful in the treatment of hypertension and angina. Its use is contraindicated in patients with severe bradycardia, second- or third-degree heart block, heart failure, cardiogenic shock, or a known hypersensitivity to it. This drug is available in both oral and injectable forms.

PHARMACOKINETICS

Route	Onset of Action	Peak Plasma Concentration	Elimination Half-life	Duration of Action
IV	Immediate	Less than 5 min	6-7 hr	Less than 12 hr
PO	1 hr	2-4 hr	6-7 hr	24 hr

esmolol

Esmolol (Brevibloc) is an ultra-short-acting beta-blocker with pharmacologic and electrophysiologic effects on the heart's conduction system similar to those of atenolol. Esmolol is also a cardioselective beta-blocker that primarily and preferentially blocks the beta$_1$-adrenergic receptors in the heart. It is used in the acute treatment of supraventricular tachydysrhythmias or dysrhythmias that originate above the ventricles. It is also used to control hypertension and tachydysrhythmias that develop after an acute MI. Use of esmolol is contraindicated in patients with a known hypersensitivity to it or those with severe bradycardia, second- or third-degree heart block, heart failure, cardiogenic shock, or severe asthma. It is available only in injectable form and is most commonly used in anesthesia.

PHARMACOKINETICS

Route	Onset of Action	Peak Plasma Concentration	Elimination Half-life	Duration of Action
IV	Immediate	6 min	9 min	15-20 min

◆ metoprolol

Metoprolol (Lopressor) is another cardioselective beta-blocker commonly given after an MI to reduce the risk of sudden cardiac death. It is also used in the treatment of hypertension and angina. The contraindications to metoprolol use are the same as those for the use of both atenolol and esmolol. It is available in both oral and injectable forms.

PHARMACOKINETICS

Route	Onset of Action	Peak Plasma Concentration	Elimination Half-life	Duration of Action
IV	1 min	20 min	3-8 hr	5-8 hr
PO	1 hr	2-4 hr	3-8 hr	10-20 hr

◆ propranolol

Propranolol (Inderal), approved in 1967, was one of the first beta-blockers introduced into clinical practice. Propranolol is a nonspecific beta-blocker that blocks both beta$_1$- and beta$_2$-adrenergic receptors in the heart and lungs. Its primary effect on the heart is the blockade of cardiac beta$_1$-adrenergic receptors, which prevents catecholamine-mediated stimulation of the heart. The resulting cardiovascular effects are a reduced heart rate, delayed AV node conduction, reduced myocardial contractility, and decreased myocardial automaticity. Propranolol is also believed to have membrane-stabilizing properties that may play a small role in its overall antidysrhythmic effect.

Because propranolol is the oldest of this class of drugs, there are now many indications for its use. Hypertension, angina, supraventricular dysrhythmias, ventricular tachycardia, the tachydysrhythmias associated with cardiac glycoside toxicity, hypertrophic subaortic stenosis, pheochromocytoma, thyrotoxicosis, migraines, post-MI status, and essential tremor are just some of the conditions it is used to treat. The contraindications for propranolol are the same as those for atenolol. It is available in both oral and parenteral dosage forms.

PHARMACOKINETICS

Route	Onset of Action	Peak Plasma Concentration	Elimination Half-life	Duration of Action
IV	2 min	1-4 hr	3-5 hr	3-6 hr
PO	1-2 hr	1-4 hr	3-5 hr	6-12 hr

CLASS III DRUGS

Class III drugs consist of amiodarone, sotalol (which also has class II properties), ibutilide, and dofetilide. Amiodarone controls dysrhythmias by inhibiting repolarization and markedly prolonging refractoriness and the action potential duration. Ibutilide and dofetilide are both indicated for conversion of atrial fibrillation or flutter to a normal sinus rhythm. Amiodarone is indicated for the management of life-threatening ventricular tachycardia or ventricular fibrillation that is resistant to other drug therapy. This drug has also been very effective in the treatment of sustained ventricular tachycardias. Amiodarone has recently been used more frequently to treat atrial dysrhythmias as well.

◆ amiodarone

Amiodarone (Cordarone) markedly prolongs the action potential duration and the effective refractory period in all cardiac tissues. Besides exerting these dramatic effects, it is also known to block both the alpha- and beta-adrenergic receptors of the sympathetic nervous system. Clinically it is one of the most effective antidysrhythmic drugs for controlling supraventricular and ventricular dysrhythmias. It is indicated for the management of sustained ventricular tachycardia, ventricular fibrillation, and nonsustained ventricular tachycardia. It is reported to be effective in 40% to 60% of all patients with ventricular tachycardia. It is now the drug of choice for ventricular dysrhythmias according to the Advanced Cardiac Life Support guidelines. Recently it has shown promise in the management of atrial dysrhythmias that are difficult to treat with other less toxic drugs.

Amiodarone has many unwanted adverse effects, and these can be attributed to its chemical properties. Amiodarone is very lipophilic, or fat loving. Therefore, it can penetrate and concentrate in the adipose tissue of any organ in the body, where it may cause unwanted effects. It also has iodine in its chemical structure. One organ that sequesters iodine from the diet is the thyroid gland. As a result, amiodarone can cause either hypothyroidism or hyperthyroidism. Adverse reactions occur in approximately 75% of patients treated with this drug, but the incidence is higher and the severity greater with higher dosages (those exceeding 400 mg/day) and prolonged therapy. One of the most common adverse effect is corneal microdeposits, which may cause visual halos, photophobia, and dry eyes. This occurs in virtually all adults who take the drug for longer than 6 months. Photosensitivity is also very common, reported in 10% to 75% of patients taking amiodarone.

The most serious adverse effect is pulmonary toxicity, which is fatal in about 10% of patients and involves a clinical syndrome of progressive dyspnea and cough accompanied by damage to the alveoli. The result can be pulmonary fibrosis. Another serious complication of amiodarone therapy is that it not only may treat the dysrhythmias but also may provoke them.

Amiodarone has an exceptionally long half-life, approaching many days. As a result, the therapeutic as well as any adverse effects of amiodarone may linger long after the drug has been discontinued. In fact, it may take as long as 2 to 3 months after the drug has been stopped for some adverse effects to subside. Therapy is usually started in the hospital and is closely monitored until the patient's serum levels are within a therapeutic range.

Amiodarone has two very significant drug interactions, namely with digoxin and warfarin. It is reported that digoxin levels will increase by 50% and that the INR will increase by 50% in 100% of patients taking the these drugs in combination with amiodarone. When amiodarone is started in patients who are already taking one of these drugs, the dose of digoxin or warfarin should be reduced by 50% at the start of amiodarone therapy.

Use of amiodarone is contraindicated in patients who have a known hypersensitivity to it and in those with severe sinus bradycardia or second- or third-degree heart block. For cases in which the patient is maintained on long-term oral amiodarone therapy after intravenous amiodarone administration is discontinued, recommended conversions are available (Table 23-9). This drug is marketed in both oral and injectable forms.

PHARMACOKINETICS

Route	Onset of Action	Peak Plasma Concentration	Elimination Half-life	Duration of Action
PO	1-3 wk	2-10 hr	15-100 days	10-150 days

ibutilide

Ibutilide (Corvert) is a class III antidysrhythmic drug. Unlike the other two class III antidysrhythmics, ibutilide is indicated for atrial dysrhythmias. Atrial fibrillation and atrial flutter cause irregular contractions of the heart and can lead to serious conditions such as decreased cardiac output, heart failure, low blood pressure, and stroke. Although other pharmacologic therapies are used to treat atrial fibrillation and flutter, ibutilide and dofetilide are the only drugs available for rapid conversion of these two conditions to normal sinus rhythm. The only other treatment that can produce rapid conversion is electrical cardioversion. Although it is effective, electrical cardioversion carries the risk, expense, and inconvenience of both the procedure itself and the anesthesia it requires.

Ibutilide is dosed based on patient weight. Use of ibutilide is contraindicated in patients who have previously demonstrated hypersensitivity to it. As with other antidysrhythmic drugs, ibutilide should be used with caution, because it can itself produce dysrhythmias, most significantly ventricular tachycardia and torsades de pointes. Class Ia antidysrhythmic drugs (e.g., disopyramide, quinidine, and procainamide) and other class III drugs (e.g., amiodarone and sotalol) should not be administered with ibutilide, nor should they be given within 4 hours after infusion of ibutilide because of their potential to prolong refractoriness. Ibutilide is available only in injectable form.

PHARMACOKINETICS

Route	Onset of Action	Peak Plasma Concentration	Elimination Half-life	Duration of Action
IV	10 min	30 min	6 hr	4 hr

◆ dofetilide

Dofetilide (Tikosyn) is the newest antidysrhythmic drug. Because dofetilide can cause serious toxicity, specifically torsades de pointes, only physicians who have received special training are allowed to prescribe it. Dofetilide therapy must be initiated in the hospital, and the patient must have continuous ECG monitoring

TABLE 23-9 Recommendations for Oral Dosage After Intravenous Infusion of Amiodarone

Duration of Amiodarone IV Infusion	Initial Daily Dose of Oral Amiodarone
Less than 1 wk	800-1600 mg
1-3 wk	600-800 mg
More than 3 wk	400 mg

IV, Intravenous.

for the first 3 days. Any dosage adjustment or reinitiation of therapy also requires hospitalization.

Dofetilide is contraindicated in patients with hypersensitivity to it, as well as patients with congenital or acquired long QTc intervals or in whom the QTc interval is longer than 440 msec. It is also contraindicated in patients with severe renal impairment and in those taking the following drugs: verapamil, cimetidine, hydrochlorothiazide, trimethoprim, itraconazole, ketoconazole, prochlorperazine, and megestrol. Other drugs that can prolong the QTc interval must be used with great caution during dofetilide therapy. Dofetilide is also contraindicated in patients with hypokalemia and/or hypomagnesemia, because these two states predispose patients to toxicity.

The most common adverse effects are torsades de pointes, supraventricular dysrhythmias, headache, dizziness, and chest pain.

PHARMACOKINETICS

Route	Onset of Action	Peak Plasma Concentration	Elimination Half-life	Duration of Action
PO	1 hr	2-3 hr	10 hr	12 hr

◆ sotalol

Sotalol (Betapace) is a selective beta-blocker that is used to treat dysrhythmias. It is unique in that it possesses antidysrhythmic properties similar to those of the class III drugs (such as amiodarone) while simultaneously exerting beta-blocker or class II effects on the conduction system of the heart. In addition, sotalol has prodysrhythmic properties similar to those of the class Ic drugs. This means that while patients are taking sotalol, it can cause serious dysrhythmias such as torsades de pointes or a new ventricular tachycardia or fibrillation. For this reason, sotalol is usually reserved for the treatment of documented life-threatening ventricular dysrhythmias such as sustained ventricular tachycardia.

Contraindications to sotalol use include hypersensitivity to it, bronchial asthma, cardiogenic shock, and sinus bradycardia. Sotalol is available only in oral form.

PHARMACOKINETICS

Route	Onset of Action	Peak Plasma Concentration	Elimination Half-life	Duration of Action
PO	1-2 hr	2.5-4 hr	12 hr	8-16 hr

CLASS IV DRUGS

Class IV antidysrhythmic drugs are calcium channel blockers. Although more than nine such drugs are currently available, only a few are commonly used as antidysrhythmics. Besides being effective antidysrhythmics, calcium channel blockers are useful in the treatment of hypertension (see Chapter 25) and angina. Verapamil and diltiazem are the two calcium channel blockers most commonly used for the following:

- Treating dysrhythmias, specifically those that arise above the ventricles (PSVT)

- Controlling the ventricular response to atrial fibrillation and flutter by slowing conduction and prolonging refractoriness of the AV node (i.e., preventing the ventricles from beating as fast as the atria)

These drugs block the slow inward flow of calcium ions into the slow (calcium) channels in cardiac conduction tissue. The conduction effects of these drugs are limited to the atria and the AV node, where conduction is prolonged and the tissues are made more refractory to stimulation. These drugs have little effect on the ventricular tissues.

◆ diltiazem

Diltiazem (Cardizem) is primarily indicated for the temporary control of a rapid ventricular response in a patient with atrial fibrillation or flutter and PSVT. Its use is contraindicated in patients with hypersensitivity, acute MI, pulmonary congestion, Wolff-Parkinson-White syndrome, severe hypotension, cardiogenic shock, sick sinus syndrome, or second- or third-degree AV block. Diltiazem is available in both oral and parenteral forms.

PHARMACOKINETICS

Route	Onset of Action	Peak Plasma Concentration	Elimination Half-life	Duration of Action
PO	0.5-1 hr	2-3 hr	3.5-9 hr	4-12 hr

◆ verapamil

Verapamil (Calan) has actions similar to those of diltiazem in that it also inhibits calcium ion influx across the slow calcium channels in cardiac conduction tissue. This results in dramatic effects on the AV node. Verapamil is used to prevent and convert recurrent PSVT and to control ventricular response in atrial flutter or fibrillation. It can also temporarily control a rapid ventricular response to these frequent atrial stimulations, usually decreasing the heart rate by at least 20%. Verapamil is not only used for the management of various dysrhythmias but is also used to treat angina, hypertension, and hypertrophic cardiomyopathy. The contraindications that apply to diltiazem apply to verapamil as well. It is also available in both oral and parenteral forms.

PHARMACOKINETICS

Route	Onset of Action	Peak Plasma Concentration	Elimination Half-life	Duration of Action
PO	1-2 hr	3 hr	4.5-12 hr	6-8 hr

UNCLASSIFIED ANTIDYSRHYTHMIC
adenosine

Adenosine (Adenocard) is an unclassified antidysrhythmic drug. It slows the electrical conduction time through the AV node and is indicated for the conversion of PSVT to sinus rhythm. It is particularly useful when the PSVT has failed to respond to verapamil or when the patient has coexisting conditions such as heart failure, hypotension, or left ventricular dysfunction that limit the use of verapamil. Its use is contraindicated in patients with second- or third-degree heart block, sick sinus syndrome, atrial flutter or fibrillation, or ventricular tachycardia, as well as in those with a known hypersensitivity to it. It has an extremely short half-life of less than 10 seconds. For this reason, it is administered only intravenously and only as a fast intravenous push. It commonly causes asystole for a period of seconds. All other adverse effects are minimal because of its very short duration of action. Adenosine is available only in parenteral form.

PHARMACOKINETICS

Route	Onset of Action	Peak Plasma Concentration	Elimination Half-life	Duration of Action
IV	Immediate	Immediate	Less than 10 sec	Very brief

Antidysrhythmic Medications

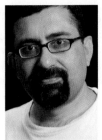

© YellowCrest Media

A 46-year-old patient, Mr. V.T., is admitted to the intensive care unit after going to the hospital with complaints of chest pain. He is diagnosed with coronary artery disease with a partial block of one of his coronary arteries and is awaiting an angioplasty procedure. He has a history of alcoholism but states that he has not had a drink for 2 years, thanks to Alcoholics Anonymous. In the intensive care unit, his heart monitor indicates increased episodes of premature ventricular contractions. When a 20-second run of ventricular tachycardia is noted, the nurse decides to implement the standing orders for a lidocaine infusion. The standing order reads: "For episodes of ventricular tachycardia, give a loading dose of 75 mg of lidocaine intravenous (IV) push; repeat this dose in 5 minutes, then begin a continuous infusion of 2 mg/min IV."

1. What factors should the nurse consider before beginning the lidocaine infusion?
2. What should the nurse monitor while V.T. is receiving this infusion?

Three days later, V.T. is ready for discharge. He has had the angioplasty procedure, which was deemed a success, and the lidocaine infusion was discontinued yesterday. He has been started on oral quinidine, 324 mg, every 6 hours. One month later, he calls the office and tells the nurse that he is hearing a "ringing sound" in his ears, even when the television and radio are turned off.

3. Is this ringing sound significant?

The physician decides to change V.T.'s medication to procainamide. V.T. asks the nurse, "What should I worry about with this drug? It seems that they all have bad side effects."

4. What is the nurse's best answer to this question?

For answers, see *http://evolve.elsevier.com/Lilley.*

PHARMACOKINETIC BRIDGE
to Nursing Practice

A study of long-term oral amiodarone therapy for the treatment of dysrhythmias provides a different perspective on pharmacokinetics. To aid in evaluating the complex pharmacokinetic properties of amiodarone and developing an optimal dosing schedule for the drug in long-term oral drug therapy, serum concentrations of the drug and its metabolite, desethylamiodarone, were monitored in 345 Japanese patients receiving amiodarone. Serum concentrations of the drug and its metabolite were determined by an analysis called *chromatography*. In 245 participants who took fixed maintenance dosages of the drug for 6 months, there were small variations in the ratio of the serum level of the actual drug to the serum level of its metabolite. (The concept of metabolism as it relates to pharmacokinetics is discussed in Chapter 2.) Other pharmacokinetic properties of amiodarone included a slightly higher average clearance in women than in men, even though there was no differences between men and women with regard to age, dosage, or duration of action of the dose. Japanese patients showed little variation in the pharmacokinetics of the drug. From this study, one can see how important it is to fully understand basic pharmacokinetic parameters (e.g., dosing, clearance, drug metabolism, serum concentrations) and to recognize that they are very critical components of drug therapy and the nursing process. It is also important to note that culture, gender, age, and racial or ethnic group have an impact on how each person responds to a drug and how each drug may vary in its action.

NURSING PROCESS

Assessment

Before administering any *antidysrhythmic* to a patient, a thorough nursing assessment should be conducted as well as a head-to-toe physical assessment, and a complete medical history and medication profile. Contraindications, cautions, and drug interactions for all of the antidysrhythmic drugs have been previously discussed in the pharmacology section. Other focused areas of assessment include the review of any baseline ECGs and interpretation of the results and measurement of the patient's vital signs with attention to heart sounds, heart rate, rhythm, and quality. Postural blood pressures should also be measured before and during the administration of these drugs. Other signs and symptoms for which to assess in relation to cardiac functioning include apical-radial pulse deficits, jugular vein distension, edema, prolonged capillary refill (longer than 5 seconds), decreased urinary output, activity intolerance, chest pain or pressure, dyspnea, and fatigue. Baseline neurologic functioning should be documented, and any neuromuscular deficits, such as muscle weakness, should be identified. These problems may be exacerbated or worsened by some of the antidysrhythmics (e.g., amiodarone, procainamide). Any changes in alertness, increase in anxiety levels, syncope, or dizziness should be noted and documented. Laboratory studies generally include renal and hepatic function tests because abnormal functioning may call for a decrease in the drug dosage by the prescriber to prevent toxicity. Other laboratory studies should include complete blood cell counts and measurement of baseline thrombocyte counts and clotting factor levels because of the adverse effect of thrombocytopenia. Because of the potential for clotting problems, there should also be assessment for any bleeding, such as bleeding gums, easy bruising or bleeding of skin, black tarry stools, hematuria (blood in the urine), or hematemesis (blood in the vomit). One very important drug interaction to emphasize is the interaction with grapefruit juice, which inhibits metabolism by cytochrome P-450 3A4 hepatic enzymes (see Chapter 2 for a more in-depth discussion of this topic). The interaction of grapefruit juice with quinidine, an antidysrhythmic, leads to increased blood levels of the drug and risk of cinchonism (see Table 23-8). Other drug interactions have been previously discussed and are presented in Table 23-8.

Use of *lidocaine* requires assessment of the central nervous and cardiovascular systems, with attention to heart rate and blood pressure. Further assessment of respiratory, thyroid, hepatic, and/or hypertensive conditions is needed with use of amiodarone. This drug is associated with many drug interactions (see previous discussion and Table 23-8) and requires very cautious assessment for these interactions as well as contraindications and cautions. In addition, serum potassium and magnesium levels should be noted, because hypokalemia and/or hypomagnesemia may precipitate dofetilide toxicity.

Nursing Diagnoses

- Decreased cardiac output related to the pathology of the dysrhythmia
- Ineffective cerebral and peripheral tissue perfusion related to the physiologic impact of the dysrhythmia
- Risk for injury to self related to adverse effects of the medications, such as hypotension and dizziness
- Deficient knowledge related to lack of experience with medication therapy
- Impaired gas exchange (decreased) related to adverse effects associated with some of the antidysrhythmics
- Disturbed body image related to changes in lifestyle and sexual functioning caused by the disease process and the adverse effects of medications
- Noncompliance with the medication regimen due to unpleasant adverse effects and lack of knowledge

Planning
Goals

- Patient is free of injury to self during the duration of drug therapy.
- Patient demonstrates adequate knowledge about drug therapy and related instruction.
- Patient regains normal respiratory patterns and experiences minimal respiratory adverse effects during drug therapy.
- Patient regains normal or near-normal cardiac output and tissue perfusion.
- Patient has improved tolerance of activity and improved general sense of well-being.
- Patient is free of complications associated with drug therapy.
- Patient maintains intact self-esteem and body image during drug therapy.
- Patient demonstrates adequate knowledge of drug therapy and its adverse effects.

Outcome Criteria

- Patient's symptoms of dysrhythmia, such as shortness of breath and chest pain, are decreased or alleviated by drug and/or nondrug therapy.
- Patient has normal breathing patterns (rate and rhythm) and no shortness of breath, cough, or chest pain.
- Patient exhibits signs and symptoms of improved cardiac output and tissue perfusion as evidenced by regular apical and radial pulses, vital signs within normal limits, and a decrease in weight, edema, crackles, and shortness of breath, attributable to compliance with therapy.
- Patient states the common adverse effects of the medication being taken, such as constipation, dry mouth, and dizziness.
- Patient experiences increase in energy and stamina and is able to carry out activities of daily living without symptoms.
- Patient states the importance of complying with the medication regimen and of scheduling and attending follow-up visits with the prescriber or other health care provider.
- Patient openly discusses feelings of inadequacy and low self-esteem, fears, and negative feelings about self.

Implementation

When *antidysrhythmics* are administered, pulse rates (and other vital signs) should continue to be monitored; if pulse rate is lower than 60 beats/min, the prescriber should be notified. Initially, the electrocardiogram and vital signs must be monitored closely because of possible prolongation of the QT interval by more than 50%. The end result may be the occurrence of a variety of conduction disturbances; thus very close monitoring is needed during the

EVIDENCE-BASED PRACTICE

Antidysrhythmics and the Elderly Patient

■ *Review*

A review article presented a thorough examination of various research studies and clinical trials investigating the management of dysrhythmias in elderly patients. As noted in the article, the most interesting and recent application of pacemaker implantation has been for cardiac resynchronization in patients with advanced heart failure. Chronic heart failure is increasing in prevalence, with about 5 million individuals affected. Because elderly patients are more susceptible to atrial fibrillation, life-threatening ventricular dysrhythmias, and symptomatic bradycardia, it is very important for the clinician to be able to identify abnormal rhythms and initiate appropriate therapies to help prevent stroke and improve quality of life and survival. Data are reviewed in this article, but it is the summary of the various treatment modalities that is noteworthy.

■ *Type of Evidence*

This article provided a review of clinical trials and management of irregularities in heart rate in the elderly. It also presented a review of various treatment regimens.

■ *Results of Study*

Elderly patients are at increased risk for both atrial and ventricular irregularities even though they may be clinically healthy, and the occurrence of such irregularities increases the risk of other problems in these patients. This study discussed the options of a new generation of oral anticoagulants and percutaneously implanted devices that may soon play a more expanded role in the management of atrial fibrillation.

Large clinical trial data have shown that the use of automatic implantable cardioverters-defibrillators to treat ventricular tachydysrhythmias improves the survival of these patients in the appropriate setting. Biventricular pacing is also a treatment modality with an identifiable role in reducing morbidity in patients with heart failure. Other studies and trials evaluating the role of various treatment modalities in the management of cardiac irregularities in the elderly were also reviewed in this article. The treatment methods examined have provided elderly patients with the possibility of improved quality of life, decreased morbidity, and longer survival.

■ *Link of Evidence to Nursing Practice*

Elderly patients are subject to a variety of insults to their physiologic and psychologic status, and even if they are in normal health for their age, the risk for abnormal cardiac conditions and rhythms is high. The studies reviewed in this article provide evidence of improved quality of life and reduced morbidity and mortality with the use of these treatment modalities. It is important for the nurse to be aware of reliable, valid clinical trial data such as those examined in the article so that the nurse can support the patient and family throughout implementation of new treatment plans, including the use of antidysrhythmics, anticoagulants, implanted pacemakers and cardioverters/defibrillators, and biventricular pacing. Research findings, such as the trial data reviewed in this article, may continue to improve patient care and lead to sound, evidence-based medical and nursing practice.

Data from Hanna IR et al: Approaching cardiac arrhythmias in the elderly patient, *MedGenMed* 7(4):24, 2005.

initiation of therapy. Oral dosage forms should be taken as ordered and with food and fluids to help minimize gastrointestinal upset. *Quinidine* comes in different salt forms, and these are not interchangeable. During treatment with quinidine (or with any of the antidysrhythmics), any chest pain, hypotension, severe gastrointestinal distress, dizziness, syncope, blurred vision, change in respiratory status, or edema (weight gain of 2 pounds or more in 24 hours or 5 pounds or more in 1 week), should be reported to the prescriber immediately. Hypersensitivity to these drugs may not occur for up to 3 to 20 days and is commonly manifested by fever. An infusion pump should be used for intravenous dosing of any of the classes of antidysrhythmics, with proper solution and dilution.

With *lidocaine*, vials of clear solution are labeled as either for cardiac or *not* for cardiac use. This is important to remember when reading the vial's label so that the wrong drug is not given. It is also important to remember that lidocaine solutions need to be used with extreme caution and that it is the plain solution that is used to treat various cardiac conditions. Parenteral solutions of these drugs are usually stable only for 24 hours. Lidocaine is also used as an anesthetic, and so the different concentrations of the drug should be double-checked—if not triple-checked. In addition, lidocaine comes in a solution with epinephrine, a potent vasoconstrictor. This combined solution is indicated when the surgeon or physician is suturing or repairing wounds, with the lidocaine acting as an anesthetic and the epinephrine causing vasoconstriction of the local blood vessels and helping to control bleeding of the area, or in dental or oral situations. It must be emphasized that the solution with epinephrine must *never* be used intravenously, but only as a topical anesthetic!

Amiodarone may lead to gastrointestinal upset, which may be prevented or decreased by taking the drug with food or a snack. Photosensitivity (sunburn and other exaggerated skin reactions to the sunlight) and photophobia (light sensitivity) are other concerns with this drug. With photosensitivity, protective clothing/hat and sunscreen are needed. Protection of the eyes, with wearing of sunglasses and/or tinted contact lenses, is important to emphasize to patients on this medication. Consumption of a high-fiber diet and forcing of fluids are also recommended to minimize the constipation that is a common adverse effect of antidysrhythmic drugs. The drug amiodarone should *not be confused* with amrinone, now called inamrinone. When a beta-blocker is used with the antidysrhythmic, any shortness of breath, weight gain (see earlier) or rash should be reported to the prescriber immediately. Beta-blockers are discussed further in Chapters 19 (antiadrenergics) and 25 (antihypertensives). *Beta-blockers, diltiazem,* and *verapamil* may all be used to manage abnormal rhythms and should be given only after checking and documenting pulse rates and blood pressures. The prescriber should be contacted and the drug withheld—if supported by facility policy and the prescriber's guidelines—if the pulse rate is 60 beats/min or lower or 100 beats/min or higher and/or systolic blood pressure is 90 mm Hg or lower.

With the use of *dofetilide*, a newer antidysrhythmic drug, the patient should be continually monitored for any changes in the ECG, especially over the first 3 days of treatment. This drug requires specialized monitoring once ordered by the prescriber, who must have received special prescription training. The patient should be encouraged to report any difficulty such as headache, dizziness, chest pain, or palpitations to the prescriber immediately. Should a dosage amount require adjustment, hospitalization is necessary.

Evaluation

The monitoring of patients receiving all classes of antidysrhythmics is important to confirm the therapeutic effects as well as identify the adverse and toxic effects. Class I through class IV drugs have many overlapping therapeutic effects, adverse effects, and toxicities. Therapeutic effects include improved cardiac output; decreased chest discomfort; decreased fatigue; improved vital signs, skin color, and urinary output; and conversion of irregularities to normal rhythm. Adverse effects include bradycardia, dizziness, headache, cinchonism (class I drugs; see pharmacology discussion), chest pain, heart failure, peripheral edema, and conduction disorders; bronchospasms with class I and II drugs; heart failure with class I, II, and IV drugs; corneal microdeposits and visual disturbances, extrapyramidal symptoms, hepatic dysfunction, pneumonitis, and pulmonary fibrosis with class III drugs; and ventricular asystole with class IV drugs. Toxic effects range from cardiac failure and bradycardia to hypotension, hypertension, and CNS-related effects such as confusion and convulsions.

PATIENT TEACHING TIPS

- Any oral dosage form that is identified as sustained released should not be crushed or chewed. In these cases, the original form of the drug should not be altered in any way.
- Some dosage forms are delivered in a sustained-released tablet or capsule that may be composed of a wax matrix and that this matrix may be visible in the patient's stool. This extended-release dosage form provides for a slow release of the medicine, and the wax substance may then be passed out of the body through the stool. The passing of the matrix through the stool occurs after the drug has been absorbed, and although the matrix is often visible to the naked eye, it is of no major concern.
- If the use of an oral preparation is associated with continual and moderate or severe gastrointestinal upset, the patient should be told to take the drug with food and to contact the prescriber if nausea and vomiting worsen.
- If an antacid is needed, it should be taken either 2 hours before or 2 hours after the drug to avoid interference with drug absorption.
- A well-balanced diet is recommended without an excess of alkaline ash foods (e.g., citrus fruits, vegetables, and milk). Fluid intake should be increased to up to 3 L/day (unless contraindicated).
- Caffeine intake should be limited or avoided (see Chapter 14 for a listing of foods and beverages containing caffeine).
- Medications should be taken exactly as prescribed without doubling up or omitting doses. If the patient forgets a dose or is ill and cannot take a dose, the prescriber should be contacted for further instructions.
- The patient should receive instructions and provide return demonstrations on how to measure the pulse and blood pressure and should be encouraged to keep a daily journal of these readings. Should this be problematic for the patient, the patient may be able to go to the local fire and rescue station or the prescriber's office for pulse and blood pressure checks.
- Journaling is important to document how the patient feels each day. The journal should record any worsening or improvement of symptoms, adverse effects, daily weights, activity tolerance, blood pressure, and pulse rate.
- The patient's weight should be measured daily at the same time every day and while the patient is wearing the same amount of clothing.

- The prescriber should be contacted immediately if there is a weight gain of 2 pounds or more in 24 hours or 5 pounds or more in 1 week.
- The patient should be told to change positions purposefully and with caution because of the common adverse effect of postural hypotension. Moving too quickly may lead to dizziness, syncope, and subsequent injury or falls.
- At the beginning of therapy and after any dosage increase, the patient should be encouraged to avoid driving and other hazardous activities until sedating adverse effects have resolved.
- Dry mouth may be helped by frequent mouth care, drinking fluids, sucking on sugarless gum or candy, and/or eating ice chips. Artificial saliva and special toothpaste made specifically for dry mouth and its management are available over the counter. Frequent dental visits are also encouraged.
- Exertion, hot temperatures, saunas, and hot tubs should be avoided because of the heat-induced vasodilation, which can lead to postural hypotension with dizziness and/or syncope and a subsequent risk for falls or injury.
- The patient needs to thoroughly understand the need to carry a medical alert identification card at all times. Medical alert jewelry is also available to provide information on medical diagnoses, allergies, and medications.
- Any dizziness, shortness of breath, chest pain, and/or worsening of symptoms or occurrence of new symptoms should be reported immediately to the prescriber.
- The patient should *never* stop taking these medications without specific instructions to do so; an abrupt discontinuation of these drugs may lead to severe or life-threatening complications.
- With amiodarone, photosensitivity is an adverse effect, so the patient should avoid sun exposure and wear sun-protective clothing and dark glasses when going outside. Sunscreens are ineffective because they do not block ultraviolet B light, to which the patient may react while taking this medications. Instead, barrier sunblocks, such as zinc or titanium chloride, are recommended.
- With amiodarone, the patient should immediately report any blue-gray discoloration of the skin (often after 1 year, and especially on the face, neck, and arms) as well as any jaundice, unusual rash or skin reactions, nausea, vomiting, or dizziness.

POINTS TO REMEMBER

- The SA node, AV node, and His-Purkinje system are all areas in which there is automaticity (cells can depolarize spontaneously). The SA node is the pacemaker because it can spontaneously depolarize easier and faster than the other areas.
- Any disturbance or abnormality in the normal pattern of the heartbeat and pulse rate is termed a *dysrhythmia*.
- Antidysrhythmic drugs are used to correct dysrhythmias; however, they may also cause dysrhythmias, and for this reason are said to be *prodysrhythmic*. The Vaughan Williams classification is the system most commonly used to categorize antidysrhythmic drugs. It classifies drugs into the following groups according to where and how they affect cardiac cells and what their mechanisms of action is:
  - *Class I:* membrane-stabilizing drugs (examples are class Ia, quinidine; class Ib, lidocaine; class Ic, flecainide)
  - *Class II:* beta-adrenergic blockers that depress phase 4 depolarization (e.g., propranolol)
  - *Class III:* drugs that prolong repolarization in phase 3 (e.g., amiodarone and dofetilide
  - *Class IV:* calcium channel blockers that depress phase 4 depolarization (e.g., verapamil)
- Nursing actions for the various antidysrhythmics include skillful nursing assessment and close monitoring of heart rate, blood pressure, heart rhythms, general well-being, skin color, temperature, and heart and breath sounds.
- The therapeutic responses to antidysrhythmics include a decrease in blood pressure in hypertensive patients, a decrease in edema, and restoration of a regular pulse rate or a pulse rate without major irregularities or with improved regularity compared with the irregularity that existed before therapy.

NCLEX EXAMINATION REVIEW QUESTIONS

1 A patient with a rapid, irregular heart rhythm is being treated in the emergency department with adenosine. During administration of this drug, the nurse should be prepared to monitor the patient for which effect?
   a Nausea and vomiting
   b Transitory asystole
   c Muscle tetany
   d Hypertension

2 When assessing a patient who has been taking amiodarone for 6 months, the nurse monitors for which potential adverse effect?
   a Glycosuria
   b Dysphagia
   c Photophobia
   d Urticaria

3 The nurse is assessing a patient who has been taking quinidine and asks about adverse effects. Adverse effects associated with the use of this drug include:
   a Muscle pain
   b Tinnitus
   c Chest pain
   d Excessive thirst

4 A patient calls the family practice office to report that he has seen his pills in his stools when he has a bowel movement. What should be the nurse's response?
   a "The pills are not being digested properly. You should be taking them on an empty stomach."

   b "The pills are not being digested properly. You should be taking them with food."
   c "What you are seeing is the waxy matrix that contained the medication, but the drug has been absorbed."
   d "This indicates that you are not tolerating this medication and will need to switch to a different form."

5 The nurse is administering a class I antidysrhythmic and considers which condition, if present in the patient, a caution for the use of this drug?
   a Tachycardia
   b Hypertension
   c Ventricular dysrhythmias
   d Renal dysfunction

6 When the nurse is teaching a patient about taking an antidysrhythmic drug, which statements by the nurse are correct? (Select all that apply.)
   a "Take the medication with an antacid if stomach upset occurs."
   b "Do not chew sustained-release capsules."
   c "If weight gain of 5 pounds within 1 week occurs, notify your physician at the next office visit."
   d "If you experience severe adverse effects, stop the drug and notify your physician."
   e "You may take the medication with food if stomach upset occurs."

1. b, 2. c, 3. b, 4. c, 5. d, 6. b, e.

CRITICAL THINKING ACTIVITIES: BEST ACTION

1 A patient who was admitted to the hospital for treatment of atrial fibrillation is about to go home with a new prescription for diltiazem (Cardizem). As the nurse goes over the patient's medication list, the patient complains, "I'm feeling very tired. And when I stand up, I can hardly walk because I'm so dizzy." What should be the nurse's first action?

2 A patient will be discharged from the hospital with a prescription for amiodarone (Cordarone). He has been ill for some time and tells the nurse, "I cannot wait to get to my beach house and

relax outside by the ocean. I'm sure the fresh air will be good for me." What is the best action by the nurse at this time?

3 A patient has been admitted to the emergency department and is experiencing PSVT that has not responded to treatment with calcium channel blockers. Immediately after the patient receives a dose of adenosine (Adenocard) by intravenous push, the monitor shows asystole. What is the best action by the nurse?

For answers, see *http://evolve.elsevier.com/Lilley.*

CHAPTER 24

Antianginal Drugs

OBJECTIVES

When you reach the end of this chapter, you should be able to do the following:

1 Briefly describe the pathophysiology of myocardial ischemia and the subsequent occurrence of angina.

2 Describe the various factors that may precipitate angina as well as measures that decrease its occurrence.

3 Contrast the major classes of antianginal drugs (nitrates, calcium channel blockers, and beta-blockers) with regard to their mechanisms of action, dosage forms, routes of administration, cautions, contraindications, drug interactions, adverse effects, patient tolerance, toxicity, and patient education requirements.

4 Develop a nursing care plan incorporating all phases of the nursing process related to the administration of antianginal drugs.

e-Learning Activities

http://evolve.elsevier.com/Lilley

NCLEX Review Questions • Animations • Nursing Care Plans • Audio Glossary • Category Catchers • Medication Errors Checklists • IV Therapy Checklists • Calculators • Frequently Asked Questions • Content Updates • Supplemental Resources • Answers to Case Studies and Critical Thinking Activities

Drug Profiles

amlodipine, p. 375
◆ atenolol, p. 373
◆ diltiazem, p. 375
◆ isosorbide dinitrate, p. 371

◆ isosorbide mononitrate, p. 371
◆ metoprolol, p. 373
◆ nitroglycerin, p. 371
  ranolazine, p. 375

◆ *Key drug.*

Glossary

Angina pectoris Chest pain that occurs when the heart's supply of blood carrying oxygen and energy-rich nutrients is insufficient to meet the demands of the heart. (p. 368)

Atherosclerosis A common form of arteriosclerosis involving deposits of fatty, cholesterol-containing material *(plaques)* within arterial walls. (p. 368)

Chronic stable angina Chest pain that has as its primary cause atherosclerosis, which results in a long-term but relatively stable level of obstruction in one or more coronary arteries. (p. 369)

Coronary arteries Arteries that deliver oxygen to the heart muscle. (p. 368)

Coronary artery disease (CAD) Any one of the abnormal conditions that can affect the arteries of the heart and produce various pathologic effects, especially a reduced supply of oxygen and nutrients to the myocardium. (p. 368)

Ischemia Poor blood supply to an organ. (p. 368)

Ischemic heart disease Poor blood supply to the heart via the coronary arteries. (p. 368)

Myocardial infarction (MI) Gross necrosis of the myocardium following interruption of blood supply; it is almost always caused by atherosclerosis of the coronary arteries and is commonly called *heart attack.* (p. 368)

Reflex tachycardia A rapid heartbeat caused by a variety of autonomic nervous system effects, such as blood pressure changes, fever, or emotional stress. (p. 370)

Unstable angina Early stage of progressive coronary artery disease. (p. 369)

Vasospastic angina Ischemia-induced myocardial chest pain caused by spasms of the coronary arteries. (p. 369)

• • •

Anatomy, Physiology, and Disease Overview

The heart is a very efficient organ, but it is very demanding in an aerobic sense because it requires a large supply of oxygen to meet the incredible demands placed on it. Pumping blood to all the tissues and organs of the body is a difficult job. The heart's much-needed oxygen supply is delivered to the heart muscle by means of the **coronary arteries.** When the heart's supply of blood carrying oxygen and energy-rich nutrients is insufficient to meet the demands of the heart, the heart muscle (or myocardium) aches. This is called **angina pectoris,** or chest pain. Poor blood supply to an organ is referred to as **ischemia.** When the organ involved is the heart, the condition is called **ischemic heart disease.**

Ischemic heart disease is the number one killer in the United States today, and the primary cause is a disease of the coronary arteries known as **atherosclerosis** (fatty plaque deposits in the arterial walls). When atherosclerotic plaques project from the walls into the lumens of these vessels, the vessels become narrow. The supply of oxygen and energy-rich nutrients needed for the heart to meet the demands placed on it is then decreased. This disorder is called **coronary artery disease (CAD).** An acute result of CAD and of ischemic heart disease is **myocardial infarction (MI),** or heart attack. It occurs when blood flow through the coronary arteries to the myocardium is completely blocked so that part of the heart muscle cannot receive any of the blood-borne nutrients (especially oxygen) necessary for normal function. If this process is not reversed immediately, that area of the heart will die and become *necrotic* (dead or nonfunctioning).

Damage to a large enough area of the myocardium can be disabling or fatal.

The rate at which the heart pumps and the strength of each heartbeat (contractility) also influence oxygen demands on this organ. There are many substances and situations that can increase heart rate and contractility and thus increase oxygen demand. These include caffeine, exercise, and stress. These substances or situations result in stimulation of the sympathetic nervous system, which leads to increased heart rate and contractility. In an already overburdened heart, such as one in a patient with CAD, this can worsen the balance between myocardial oxygen supply and demand and result in angina. Some drugs that are used to treat angina are aimed at correcting the imbalance between myocardial oxygen supply and demand by decreasing heart rate and contractility. The beta-blockers and the calcium channel blockers (CCBs) are two examples of classes of drugs used to treat angina.

The pain of angina is a result of the following process: Under ischemic conditions when the myocardium is deprived of oxygen, the heart shifts to anaerobic metabolism to meet its energy needs. One of the by-products of anaerobic metabolism is lactic acid. The accumulation of lactic acid and other metabolic by-products causes the pain receptors surrounding the heart to be stimulated, which produces the heart pain known as *angina*. It is the same pathophysiologic mechanism responsible for causing the soreness in skeletal muscles after vigorous exercise.

There are three classic types of chest pain, or angina pectoris. **Chronic stable angina** has atherosclerosis as its primary cause. *Classic angina* and *effort angina* are other names for it. Chronic stable angina can be triggered by exertion or other stress (e.g., cold, emotions). The nicotine in tobacco as well as alcohol, coffee, and other drugs that stimulate the sympathetic nervous system can also exacerbate it. The pain of chronic stable angina is commonly intense but subsides within 15 minutes of either rest or appropriate antianginal drug therapy. **Unstable angina** is usually the early stage of progressive CAD. It often culminates in MI in subsequent years. For this reason, unstable angina is also called *preinfarction angina*. Another term for this type of angina is *crescendo angina*, because the pain increases in severity, as does the frequency of attacks. In the later stages, pain may even occur while the patient is at rest. **Vasospastic angina** results from spasms in the layer of smooth muscle that surrounds atherosclerotic coronary arteries. In contrast to chronic stable angina, this type of pain often occurs at rest and without any precipitating cause. It does seem to follow a regular pattern, however, usually occurring at the same time of day. This type of angina is also called *Prinzmetal angina* or *variant angina*. Dysrhythmias and electrocardiogram (ECG) changes often accompany these different types of anginal attacks.

Pharmacology Overview

The three main classes of drugs used to treat angina pectoris are the nitrates and nitrites, the beta-blockers, and the CCBs. Their various therapeutic effects are summarized and compared in Table 24-1. There are three main therapeutic objectives of antianginal drug therapy. It must (1) minimize the frequency of attacks and decrease the duration and intensity of the anginal pain; (2) improve the patient's functional capacity with as few adverse effects as possible; and (3) prevent or delay the worst possible outcome, MI. The overall goal of antianginal drug therapy is to increase blood flow to ischemic myocardium, decrease myocardial oxygen demand, or both. Figure 24-1 illustrates how drug therapy works to alleviate angina. Evidence exists to suggest that drug therapy may be at least as effective as angioplasty in treating this condition.

NITRATES AND NITRITES

Nitrates have long been the mainstay of both the prophylaxis and treatment for angina and other cardiac problems. Today there are several chemical derivatives of the early precursors, all of which are organic nitrate esters. They are available in a wide variety of preparations, including sublingual, chewable, and oral tablets; capsules; ointments; patches; a translingual spray; and intravenous solutions. The following are the rapid- and long-acting nitrates available for clinical use:

- amyl nitrite (rapid acting)
- nitroglycerin (both rapid and long acting)
- isosorbide dinitrate (both rapid and long acting)
- isosorbide mononitrate (primarily long acting)

Mechanism of Action and Drug Effects

Medicinal nitrates and nitrites, more commonly referred to simply as *nitrates,* dilate all blood vessels. They predominantly affect venous vascular beds; however, they also have a dose-dependent

TABLE 24-1 Antianginal Drugs: Therapeutic Effects

Therapeutic Effect	Nitrates	Beta-Blockers*	Amlodipine	Verapamil	Diltiazem
Supply					
Blood flow	↑↑	↑	↑↑↑	↑↑↑	↑↑↑
Duration of diastole	0	↑↑↑	0/↑	↑↑↑	↑↑
Demand					
Preload†	↓↓	↑	↓/0	0	0/↓
Afterload	↓	0/↓	↓↓↓	↓↓	↓↓
Contractility	0	↓↓↓	↓	↓↓↓	↓↓
Heart rate	0/↑	↓↓↓	0/↓	↓↓	↓↓

↑, Increase; ↓, decrease; *0*, little or no effect.
*In particular, those that are cardioselective and do not have intrinsic sympathomimetic activity.
†*Preload* is pressure in the heart caused by blood volume. The nitrates effectively move part of this blood out of the heart and into blood vessels, thereby decreasing preload or filling pressure.

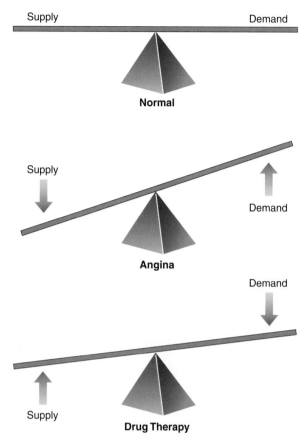

FIGURE 24-1   Benefit of drug therapy for angina through increasing oxygen supply and decreasing oxygen demands.

arterial vasodilator effect. These vasodilatory effects are the result of relaxation of the smooth muscle cells that are part of the wall structure of veins and arteries. Particularly notable, however, is the potent dilating effect of nitrates on the coronary arteries, both large and small. This causes redistribution of blood and therefore of oxygen to previously ischemic myocardial tissue and reduction of anginal symptoms. By causing venous dilation, the nitrates reduce venous return and, in turn, reduce the *left ventricular end-diastolic volume* (or *preload*), which results in a lower left ventricular pressure. Left ventricular systolic wall tension is thus reduced, as is myocardial oxygen demand. These and other nitrate drug effects are summarized in Table 24-1.

Coronary arteries that have been narrowed by atherosclerosis can still be dilated as long as there remains smooth muscle surrounding the coronary artery and the atherosclerotic plaque does not completely obstruct the arterial lumen. Exercise-induced spasms in atherosclerotic coronary arteries can also be reversed or prevented by administration of nitrates, which encourages healthy physical activity in patients.

Indications

The nitrates are used to treat stable, unstable, and vasospastic (Prinzmetal) angina. Long-acting dosage forms are used more for *prevention* of anginal episodes. Rapid-acting dosage forms, most often sublingual nitroglycerin tablets, or an intravenous drip in the hospital setting, are used to treat acute anginal attacks.

Contraindications

Contraindications to the use of nitrates include known drug allergy, as well as severe anemia, closed-angle glaucoma, hypotension, and severe head injury. This is because the vasodilatory effects of nitrates can worsen these latter conditions. In anemia, a drug-induced hypotensive episode can further compromise already reduced tissue oxygenation. Nitrates are also contraindicated with the use of the erectile dysfunction drugs sildenafil (Viagra), tadalafil (Cialis), and vardenafil (Levitra).

Adverse Effects

Nitrates are well tolerated, and most adverse effects are usually transient and involve the cardiovascular system. The most common undesirable effect is headache, which generally diminishes soon after the start of therapy. Other cardiovascular effects include tachycardia and postural hypotension. If nitrate-induced vasodilation occurs too rapidly, the cardiovascular system overcompensates and increases the heart rate, a condition referred to as **reflex tachycardia.** This may occur with significant vasodilation that involves the systemic veins. When this happens, there is a large shift in blood volume toward the systemic venous circulation and away from the heart. Baroreceptors (blood pressure receptors) in the heart then falsely sense that there has been a dramatic loss of blood volume. At this point, the heart begins beating more rapidly to move the apparently smaller volume of blood more quickly throughout the body, especially toward the vital organs (including the heart itself). However, the same baroreceptors soon sense that there has not been a loss of blood volume but that the volume of blood missing in the heart is now in the periphery (e.g., venous system), and the heart rate slows back to normal.

Topical nitrate dosage forms can produce various types of contact dermatitis (skin inflammation), but these are actually reactions to the dosage delivery system and not to the nitroglycerin itself; thus, it is not a true drug allergy. It is important for the nurse to document the type of allergic reaction, so that clinicians do not avoid this important drug class if the reaction is only a contact dermatitis.

Tolerance to the antianginal effects of nitrates can occur surprisingly quickly in some patients, especially those taking long-acting formulations or taking nitrates around the clock. In addition, cross-tolerance can arise when a patient receives more than one nitrate dosage form. To prevent this, a regular nitrate-free period is arranged to allow certain enzymatic pathways to replenish themselves. A common regimen with transdermal patches is to remove them at night for 8 hours and apply a new patch in the morning. This has been shown to prevent tolerance to the beneficial effects of nitrates.

Interactions

Nitrate antianginal drugs can produce additive hypotensive effects when taken in combination with alcohol, beta-blockers, CCBs, phenothiazines, and erectile-dysfunction drugs such as sildenafil, tadalafil, and vardenafil. In fact, numerous deaths have been reported due to interactions with erectile-dysfunction drugs.

Dosages

The organic nitrates are available in an array of forms and doses. See the Dosages table on p. 371 for more information.

DOSAGES

Selected Antianginal Nitrate Coronary Vasodilators

Drug (Pregnancy Category)	Usual Dosage Range	Indications
◆ isosorbide dinitrate (Isordil, Sorbitrate, Dilatrate-SR) (C)	**Adult** Chewable/SL: 2.5-10 mg q4-6h prn PO: 5-30 mg bid-tid and 40-80 mg at 8 AM and 2 PM for SR formulations	
◆ isosorbide mononitrate (Imdur, Monoket, Ismo) (C)	**Adult** PO: 20 mg bid given 7 hr apart and 30-120 mg daily for SR formulations	Angina
◆ nitroglycerin (Nitro-Bid, Nitrostat, Nitrol, others) (C)	**Adult** IV (continuous infusion): 5-20 mcg/min Ointment, 2%: 1-2 inch ribbon q8h, up to 4-5 inch ribbon q4h PO: 2.5-6.5 mg bid-tid during the day Spray: 1-2 sprays onto or under tongue at onset of attack; repeat as needed to max of 3 sprays in 15 min Sublingual: 1 tab under tongue at first sign of chest pain; if pain not relieved after 1 dose, call 911; may repeat up to 3 tablets Patch: 0.1 to 0.8 mg/hr applied once daily	

IV, Intravenous; *PO,* oral; *SL,* sublingual; *SR,* sustained release.

DRUG PROFILES

◆ isosorbide dinitrate
Isosorbide dinitrate (Isordil) is an organic nitrate. It exerts the same effects as the other nitrates. When isosorbide dinitrate is metabolized in the liver, it is broken down into two active metabolites, both of which have the same therapeutic actions as isosorbide dinitrate itself. This drug is available in rapid-acting sublingual tablets, immediate-release tablets, and long-acting oral dosage forms.

PHARMACOKINETICS

Route	Onset of Action	Peak Plasma Concentration	Elimination Half-life	Duration of Action
PO	1 hr	Unknown	3-5 hr	4-6 hr

◆ isosorbide mononitrate
Isosorbide mononitrate (Imdur) is one of the two active metabolites of isosorbide dinitrate, but it has no active metabolites. Because of these qualities, it produces a more consistent, steady therapeutic response, with less variation in response within the same patient and between patients. It is available in both immediate- and sustained-release oral dosage forms but is most commonly used in the sustained-release form.

PHARMACOKINETICS

Route	Onset of Action	Peak Plasma Concentration	Elimination Half-life	Duration of Action
PO	15-30 min	0.5-1 hr	5 hr	5-12 hr

◆ nitroglycerin
Nitroglycerin is the prototypical nitrate and is manufactured by many pharmaceutical companies; therefore, it goes by many different trade names (e.g., Nitro-Bid, Nitrostat). It is often abbreviated as NTG or TNG. It has traditionally been the most important drug used in the symptomatic treatment of ischemic heart conditions such as angina. When given orally, nitroglycerin goes to the liver to be metabolized before it can become active in the body. During this process, a very large amount of the nitroglycerin is removed from the circulation. This is called a *large first-pass effect* (see Chapter 2). For this reason, nitroglycerin is administered by many other routes to bypass the first-pass effect. It also is available

in many formulations and has proved useful for the treatment of a variety of cardiovascular conditions. Tablets administered by the sublingual route are used for the treatment of chest pain or angina of acute onset and for the prevention of angina when patients find themselves in situations likely to provoke an attack. Use of these routes is advantageous for relieving these acute conditions because the area under the tongue and inside the cheek is highly vascular. This means that the nitroglycerin is absorbed quickly and directly into the bloodstream, and hence its therapeutic effects occur rapidly. Sublingual nitroglycerin tablets must be stored in their original container, because exposure to air and moisture inactivates them. Nitroglycerin also comes as a metered-dose aerosol that is sprayed under the tongue. Nitroglycerin is available in an intravenous form that is used for blood pressure control in hypertensive patients perioperatively; for the treatment of ischemic pain, heart failure, and pulmonary edema associated with acute MI; and in hypertensive emergency situations. Oral and topical dosage formulations are used for the long-term prophylactic management of angina pectoris. The topical formulation offers the same advantages as the sublingual formulation in that it also bypasses the liver and the first-pass effect. They also allow for the continuous slow delivery of nitroglycerin, so that a steady dose of nitroglycerin is supplied to the patient. See the Preventing Medication Errors box on p. 372.

PHARMACOKINETICS

Route	Onset of Action	Peak Plasma Concentration	Elimination Half-life	Duration of Action
Sublingual	2-3 min	Unknown	1-4 min	0.5-1 hr

BETA-BLOCKERS

The beta-adrenergic blockers, more commonly referred to as *beta-blockers,* have become the mainstay in the treatment of several cardiovascular diseases. These include angina, MI, dysrhythmias (see Chapter 23), and hypertension (see Chapter 25). Most available beta-blockers demonstrate antianginal efficacy, although not all have been approved for this use. Those beta-blockers approved as antianginal drugs are atenolol, metoprolol, nadolol, and propranolol.

Mechanism of Action and Drug Effects

The primary drug effects of the beta-blockers are related to the cardiovascular system. As discussed in previous chapters, the predominant beta-adrenergic receptors in the heart are the beta$_1$ receptors, located in the heart's conduction system and throughout the myocardium. The beta-adrenergic receptors are normally stimulated by the binding of the neurotransmitters epinephrine and norepinephrine. These catecholamines are released in greater quantities during times of exercise or other stress to stimulate the heart muscle to contract more strongly. At the normal heart rate of 60 to 80 beats/min, the heart spends 60% to 70% of its time in diastole. As the heart rate increases during stress or exercise, the heart spends more time in systole and less time in diastole. The physiologic consequence is that the coronary arteries receive increasingly less blood, and eventually the myocardium becomes ischemic. In an ischemic heart, the increased oxygen demand from increasing contractility (systole) also leads to increasing degrees of ischemia and chest pain. The physiologic act of systole requires energy in the form of adenosine triphosphate (ATP) and oxygen. Therefore, any decrease in the energy demands on the heart is beneficial for alleviating conditions such as angina. When beta receptors are blocked by beta-blockers, the rate at which the pacemaker (sinoatrial, or SA, node) fires decreases, and the time it takes for the node to recover increases. The beta-blockers also slow conduction through the atrioventricular (AV) node and reduce myocardial contractility (negative inotropic effect). Both of these effects serve to slow the heart rate (negative chronotropic effect). These effects reduce myocardial oxygen demand, which aids in the treatment of angina by reducing the workload of the heart. Slowing the heart rate is also beneficial in patients with ischemic heart disease, because the coronary arteries have more diastolic time to fill with oxygen- and nutrient-rich blood and deliver these substances to the myocardial tissues.

The beta-blockers also have many therapeutic effects after an MI. After a patient has experienced an MI, there is a high level of circulating catecholamines (norepinephrine and epinephrine). These catecholamines will produce harmful consequences if their actions go unopposed. They cause the heart rate to increase, which leads to a further imbalance in the supply and demand ratio, and they irritate the conduction system of the heart, which can result in dysrhythmias that can be fatal. The beta-blockers block all of these harmful effects, and their use has been shown to improve the chances for survival in patients after MI. Unless strongly contraindicated, they should be given to all patients in the acute stages after an MI.

The beta-blockers also suppress the activity of the hormone *renin*, which is the first step in the renin-aldosterone-angiotensin system. Renin is a potent vasoconstrictor released by the kidneys when they sense that they are not being adequately perfused. When beta-blockers inhibit the release of renin, the blood vessels to and in the kidney dilate, which reduces blood pressure (see Chapter 25).

Indications

The beta-blockers are most effective in the treatment of typical *exertional* angina (i.e., that caused by exercise). This is because the usual physiologic increase in the heart rate and systolic blood pressure that occurs during exercise or stress is blunted by the beta-blockers, which thereby decreases the myocardial oxygen demand. It should be kept in mind that for an individual (often elderly) with significant angina, "exercise" may simply be carrying out the activities of daily living, such as bathing, dressing, cooking, housekeeping, and so on. Performing such activities with significant angina can become a major stressor for these patients. The beta-blockers are also approved for the treatment of MI, hypertension (see Chapter 25), cardiac dysrhythmias (see Chapter 23), and essential tremor. Some uses that are common but are not U.S. Food and Drug Administration (FDA) approved are treatment of migraine headache and, in low dosages, even treatment of the tachycardia associated with stage fright.

Contraindications

There are a number of contraindications to the use of beta-blockers, including systolic heart failure and serious conduction disturbances, because of the effects of beta receptor blockade on heart rate and myocardial contractility. These drugs should also be used with caution in patients with bronchial asthma, because any level of blockade of beta$_2$ receptors can promote bronchoconstriction. These contraindications are relative rather than absolute and depend on patient-specific risks and expected benefits of this drug therapy. Other relative contraindications include diabetes mellitus (due to masking of hypoglycemia-induced tachycardia), reduced mental alertness, and peripheral vascular disease (the drug may further compromise cerebral or peripheral blood flow).

Adverse Effects

The adverse effects of the beta-blockers result from the ability of these drugs to block beta-adrenergic receptors (beta$_1$ and beta$_2$ receptors) in various areas of the body. Blocking of beta$_1$ receptors may lead to a decrease in heart rate, cardiac output, and cardiac contractility, whereas blocking of beta$_2$ receptors may result in bronchoconstriction and increased airway resistance in patients with asthma or chronic obstructive pulmonary disease. Beta-blockers may lead to cardiac rhythm problems, decreased SA and AV nodal conduction, a decrease in systolic and diastolic blood pressures, and possible peripheral receptor blockade and/or decreased renin release from the kidneys. Beta-blockers can mask the tachycardia associated with hypoglycemia. Fatigue, insomnia, and weakness may occur because of the negative effects on the cardiac and central nervous systems. The beta-blockers can also cause both hypoglycemia and hyperglycemia, which is of particular concern in diabetic patients. Other common beta-blocker–related adverse effects are listed in Table 24-2.

Interactions

There are many important drug interactions that involve the beta-blockers. The more common and important of these are listed in Table 24-3.

Dosages

For information on the dosages of selected beta-blockers, see the Dosages table on p. 374.

DRUG PROFILES

Beta-blockers are the mainstay in the treatment of a wide range of cardiovascular diseases, mainly hypertension, angina, and the acute stages of MI. The three most commonly used beta-blockers are carvedilol, metoprolol, and atenolol. Carvedilol (Coreg) is not indicated for angina per se, but it is instead indicated for heart failure, essential hypertension, and left ventricular dysfunction. The newest beta-blocker, nebivolol (Bystolic), is used to treat hypertension. Atenolol, metoprolol, nadolol, and propranolol all are indicated for angina. The drug profile for carvedilol appears in Chapter 19 on p. 306.

◆ atenolol

Atenolol (Tenormin) is a cardioselective beta$_1$-adrenergic receptor blocker and is indicated for the prophylactic treatment of angina pectoris. Use of atenolol after MI has been shown to decrease mortality. It is available in a parenteral form, which is an advantage

because often during and immediately after an MI, blood flow to the gastrointestinal tract is poor and patients may be intubated, which rules out enteral administration of a drug. It is available in oral and injectable forms.

PHARMACOKINETICS

Route	Onset of Action	Peak Plasma Concentration	Elimination Half-life	Duration of Action
PO	1 hr	2-4 hr	6-7 hr	24 hr

◆ metoprolol

Metoprolol (Lopressor) is also a cardioselective beta$_1$-adrenergic receptor blocker that is used for the prophylactic treatment of angina and has many of the same characteristics as atenolol. It has shown similar efficacy in reducing mortality in patients after MI and in treating angina. It is available in both oral (immediate-release and long-acting) and parenteral (injectable) forms. Intravenous metoprolol is commonly administered to hospitalized patients after an MI and is used for treatment of hypertension in patients unable to take oral medicine.

PHARMACOKINETICS

Route	Onset of Action	Peak Plasma Concentration	Elimination Half-life	Duration of Action
IV	1 min	20 min	3-8 hr	5-8 hr
PO	1 hr	2-4 hr	3-8 hr	10-20 hr

CALCIUM CHANNEL BLOCKERS

The three chemical classes of CCBs are phenylalkylamines, benzothiazepines, and dihydropyridines, commonly represented by verapamil, diltiazem, and amlodipine, respectively (Table 24-4). Although they all block calcium channels, their chemical structures and therefore their mechanisms of action differ slightly. More than nine CCBs are available today, with more on the way. Those that are used for the treatment of chronic stable angina are amlodipine, diltiazem, nicardipine, nifedipine, and verapamil.

Mechanism of Action and Drug Effects

Calcium plays an important role in the excitation-contraction coupling process that occurs in the heart and vascular smooth muscle cells, as well as in skeletal muscle. Preventing calcium from entering into this process therefore prevents muscle contraction and promotes muscle relaxation. Relaxation of the smooth muscles that surround the coronary arteries causes them to dilate. This increases blood flow to the ischemic heart, which in turn increases the oxygen supply and helps shift the supply/

TABLE 24-2 Beta-Blockers: Adverse Effects

Body System	Adverse Effects
Cardiovascular	Bradycardia, hypotension, atrioventricular block, heart failure, peripheral vascular insufficiency
Central nervous	Dizziness, fatigue, mental depression, lethargy, drowsiness, unusual dreams
Metabolic	Hyperglycemia and/or hypoglycemia, hyperlipidemia
Other	Wheezing, dyspnea, impotence

TABLE 24-3 Beta-Blockers: Common Drug Interactions

Interacting Drug	Mechanism	Result
Anticholinergics, cimetidine	Antagonistic effects	Decreased level of beta-blocker
	Decreased metabolism	Increased levels and pharmacodynamic effects of propranolol and metoprolol
Diuretics and antihypertensives	Additive effects	Hypotension
phenothiazine	Additive hypotensive effects	Hypotension and cardiac arrest
Calcium channel blockers (diltiazem, verapamil)	Additive atrioventricular node suppression	Hypotension, bradycardia, heart block
insulin and oral antidiabetic drugs	Additive hypoglycemic effects	Hypoglycemia, possibly requiring dosage adjustment of beta-blocker or antidiabetic drugs

DOSAGES

Selected Beta₁-Adrenergic–Blocking Drugs

Drug (Pregnancy Category)	Pharmacologic Class	Usual Dosage Range	Indications
◆ atenolol (Tenormin) (C)	Beta₁-blocker	**Adult** PO: 50-200 mg/day as a single dose IV: 1.25-5 mg every 6 to 12 hr	Angina
◆ metoprolol (Lopressor, Toprol-XL) (C)		**Adult** PO: 100-400 mg/day in 2 divided doses IV: 5 mg every 2 min × 3 doses, then PO therapy as indicated	

IV, Intravenous; *PO,* oral.

TABLE 24-4 Classification of Calcium Channel Blockers

Generic Name	Trade Name	Available Routes
Benzothiazepines		
diltiazem	Cardizem, Dilacor, Tiazac, others	PO/IV
Dihydropyridines		
amlodipine	Norvasc	PO
felodipine	Plendil	PO
isradipine	DynaCirc	PO
nicardipine	Cardene	PO/IV
nifedipine	Adalat, Procardia	PO
nimodipine	Nimotop	PO
Phenylalkylamines		
verapamil	Calan, Isoptin, Verelan	PO/IV

IV, Intravenous; *PO,* oral.

TABLE 24-5 Calcium Channel Blockers: Adverse Effects

Body System	Adverse Effects
Cardiovascular	Hypotension, palpitations, tachycardia or bradycardia, heart failure
Gastrointestinal	Constipation, nausea
Other	Dermatitis, dyspnea, rash, flushing, peripheral edema, wheezing

demand ratio back to normal. This dilation also occurs in the arteries throughout the body, which results in a decrease in the force (systemic vascular resistance) against which the heart must exert itself when delivering blood to the body (afterload). Decreasing the afterload reduces the workload of the heart and therefore reduces myocardial oxygen demand. This is the primary beneficial antianginal effect of the dihydropyridine CCBs such as amlodipine and nifedipine. These drugs have a less negative inotropic effect than do verapamil and diltiazem.

Another cardiovascular effect of the CCBs is depression of the automaticity of and conduction through the SA and AV nodes. For this reason, they are useful in treating cardiac dysrhythmias (see Chapter 23). Finally, the CCBs reduce myocardial contractility and peripheral and coronary artery tone. Verapamil and diltiazem also decrease heart rate. Their strongest antianginal properties are secondary to their effects on myocardial contractility and the smooth muscle tone of peripheral and coronary arteries.

Indications

The therapeutic benefits of the CCBs are numerous. Because of their very acceptable adverse effect and safety profiles, they are considered first-line drugs for the treatment of such conditions as angina, hypertension, and supraventricular tachycardia. They are often effective for the treatment of coronary artery spasms (vaso-spastic or Prinzmetal angina). However, they may not be as effective as the beta-blockers in blunting exercise-induced elevations in heart rate and blood pressure. They are also used for the short-term management of atrial fibrillation and flutter (see Chapter 23), migraine headaches (see Chapter 14), and Raynaud's disease (a type of peripheral vascular disease). The dihydropyridine CCB nimodipine is indicated solely for cerebral artery spasms associated with aneurysm rupture.

Contraindications

Contraindications include known drug allergy, acute MI, second- or third-degree AV block (unless the patient has a pacemaker), and hypotension.

Adverse Effects

The adverse effects of the CCBs are limited and primarily relate to overexpression of their therapeutic effects. The most common adverse effects are listed in Table 24-5. Historically, immediate-release nifedipine was used to lower blood pressure in acute hypertensive emergencies (the capsule was punctured and given sublingually). However, negative outcomes were reported with the rapid, dramatic reduction in blood pressure. For this reason, only the extended-release form of nifedipine is used today. (The exception is the use of immediate-release nifedipine for the treatment of premature labor.)

Interactions

Important drug interactions are listed in Table 24-6. A particular food interaction of note is the interaction with grapefruit juice, which can reduce the metabolism of the CCBs, especially nifedipine.

Dosages

For information on the dosages of selected CCBs, see the Dosages table below.

◆ diltiazem

Diltiazem (Cardizem) is the only benzothiazepine CCB. It has a particular affinity for the cardiac conduction system and is very effective for the oral treatment of angina pectoris resulting from coronary insufficiency and hypertension. It is one of the few CCBs that are also available in parenteral form, for which it is used for the treatment of atrial fibrillation and flutter along with paroxysmal supraventricular tachycardia. Verapamil is another CCB with similar indications. Several sustained-delivery formulations of diltiazem are available, which can be confused with each other. For example, there is Cardizem SR, which is taken twice a day, and Cardizem CD, which is taken once a day. In addition to other brands of these two dosage forms, the drug is also available in several strengths of immediate-release capsule as well as in intravenous form.

PHARMACOKINETICS

Route	Onset of Action	Peak Plasma Concentration	Elimination Half-life	Duration of Action
PO	0.5-1 hr	2-3 hr	3.5-9 hr	4-12 hr

TABLE 24-6 Calcium Channel Blockers: Common Drug Interactions

Interacting Drug	Mechanism	Result
Beta-blockers	Additive effects	Bradycardia and atrioventricular block
digoxin	Interference with drug elimination	Possible increased digoxin levels
H₂ blockers	Decreased clearance	Elevated levels of calcium channel blockers
Amiodarone	Decreased metabolism	Bradycardia and decreased cardiac output
Azole antifungals, clarithromycin, erythromycin, HIV drugs	Decreased metabolism	Elevated levels and effects of calcium channel blockers

amlodipine

Amlodipine (Norvasc) is currently the most popular CCB of the dihydropyridine subclass. It is indicated for both angina and hypertension and is available only for oral use.

PHARMACOKINETICS

Route	Onset of Action	Peak Plasma Concentration	Elimination Half-life	Duration of Action
PO	30-50 min	6-12 hr	30-50 hr	24 hr

MISCELLANEOUS ANTIANGINAL DRUG

ranolazine

Ranolazine (Ranexa) is the newest antianginal drug, approved by the FDA in 2006 for chronic angina. Its mechanism of action is unknown, but unlike other antianginal drugs, it has antianginal and antiischemic effects that do not involve reductions in heart rate or blood pressure. Ranolazine is known to prolong the QT interval on the ECG. For this reason, this drug is reserved for patients who have failed to benefit from other antianginal drug therapy. In fact, ranolazine is contraindicated in patients with preexisting QT prolongation or hepatic impairment, in those taking other QT-prolonging drugs (see Chapter 23 for examples), and in patients taking moderately potent cytochrome P-450 enzyme 3A4 inhibitors such as diltiazem. Other significant drug interactions include interactions with ketoconazole and verapamil, both of which can raise ranolazine levels. Ranolazine can also raise digoxin levels. The usual dose of ranolazine is 500 mg orally twice daily, which may be advanced to 1000 mg orally twice daily based on clinical symptoms. The drug is available only for oral use.

SUMMARY OF ANTIANGINAL PHARMACOLOGY

In patients with CAD, the clinical symptoms result from a lack or inadequate delivery of blood carrying oxygen and nutrients to the heart, which results in ischemic heart disease. Antianginal drugs such as nitrates, nitrites, beta-blockers, and CCBs are used to reduce ischemia by increasing the delivery of oxygen- and nutrient-rich blood to cardiac tissues or by reducing oxygen consumption by the coronary vessels. Either of these mechanisms can reduce ischemia and lead to a decrease in anginal

DOSAGES

Selected Calcium Channel–Blocking Drugs

Drug (Pregnancy Category)	Usual Dosage Range	Indications
amlodipine (Norvasc) (C)	**Adult** PO: 5-10 mg daily	Angina
◆ diltiazem (Cardizem, Dilacor, Tiazac) (C)	**Adult** PO: Initial dose 30 mg qid before meals and at bedtime; range of 180-360 mg divided in 3-4 doses, or 1 daily for extended-release capsule; dosages of 480 mg/day may be needed	

PO, Oral.

pain. Nitrates and nitrites work mainly by decreasing venous return to the heart (preload) and decreasing systemic vascular resistance (afterload). The CCBs decrease calcium influx into the smooth muscle, causing vascular relaxation. This either reverses or prevents the spasms of coronary vessels that cause the anginal pain associated with Prinzmetal or chronic angina. The beta-blockers help by slowing the heart rate and decreasing contractility, thereby decreasing oxygen demands. Although these groups of drugs have similar clinical effects, the nursing process required for each is somewhat specific because of the characteristics and effects of the drugs and the indications for and contraindications to their use.

PHARMACOKINETIC BRIDGE
to Nursing Practice

Not only are the pharmacokinetic properties of the nitrates very interesting, but knowledge of these specific properties is critical to safe and accurate nursing care. Moreover, the patient's understanding of nitrate pharmacokinetics is also important, because the level of the patient's knowledge may strongly influence adherence to the drug regimen and the effectiveness of treatment for angina. The pharmacokinetics differ for the various dosage forms of nitroglycerin and are as follows:

Intravenous infusion: onset within 1 to 2 minutes (fastest of all dosage forms), peak time not applicable, duration of action 3 to 5 minutes

Sublingual tablet: onset of action 2 to 3 minutes, peak action unknown, duration of action 0.5 to 1 hour

Extended-release tablet: onset in 20 to 45 minutes, peak action varies, duration of action between 3 and 8 hours

Topical ointment: onset 15 to 60 minutes, peak within ½ to 2 hours, duration of action 3 to 8 hours

Transdermal patch: onset 30 to 60 minutes, peak 1 to 3 hours, duration of action 8 to 12 hours

If the goal of treatment is to abort or treat a sudden attack of angina, then *rapid* onset of action is needed, so the clinical decision (by the prescriber) would be to order either intravenous infusion, sublingual tablet (and/or translingual spray, which has a similar onset time). These dosage forms have pharmacokinetics that allow quick entry of the drug into the bloodstream and lead to more rapid vasodilation. This provides more oxygenated blood to the myocardium and aborts acute attacks. If symptoms persist, more drastic medical management would be indicated. The quick-onset nitroglycerin dosage forms may also be used by the patient before engaging in activities known to provoke angina, such as increased physical activity, sexual intercourse, or other forms of physical exertion. If the purpose of treatment is maintenance therapy, the nitrate form must have other pharmacokinetic properties, such as a longer duration of action to provide protection against angina; a longer onset of action is acceptable because stopping an attack is not needed in this situation. Use of ointments, transdermal patches, or extended-release preparations would be appropriate in such cases. If an acute episode of angina occurs while the patient is taking maintenance therapy, a dosage form with a rapid onset of action is indicated (as ordered). It is easy to see that thorough knowledge of a drug and its pharmacokinetics will allow the nurse to make safe and sound decisions about drug therapy for patients with angina.

NURSING PROCESS

Assessment

Before antianginal drugs are administered, a thorough past and present medical-health history and medication history (e.g., listing of all prescription drugs, over-the-counter products, herbals, vitamins, and supplements being taken) should be obtained and documented. Weight, height, and vital signs, with attention to supine, sitting, and standing blood pressures, should also be measured. A systolic blood pressure reading of less than 90 mm Hg should be reported to the prescriber before a dose of any of these drugs is given. With use of any drugs affecting blood pressure or pulse rate, such as antianginals, taking the apical pulse is preferred over taking the radial pulse, and pulse rates should be measured for one full minute. If the pulse rate is 60 beats/min or less, the prescriber should be contacted for further instructions. In addition to rate, the quality and rhythm of the heartbeat should also be assessed and documented prior to the administration of antianginal drugs. The patient's chest pain should also be thoroughly assessed, with documentation about onset, character (e.g., sharp, dull, piercing, squeezing, radiating), intensity, location, duration, precipitating factors (e.g., physical exertion, exercise, eating, stress, sexual intercourse), alleviating factors, and presence of nausea or vomiting. The prescriber may order an ECG, and these results should be documented. Contraindications, cautions, and any drug interactions should be assessed for and noted. Drugs leading to significant interactions include sildenafil, tadalafil, and vardenafil (used for erectile dysfunction); taking these drugs with nitrates will result in worsening of hypotensive responses, paradoxical bradycardia, and a resultant increase in angina and subsequent significant risk of cardiac or cerebrovascular complications due to decreased perfusion. Elderly patients often have difficulty with blood pressure control because of the occurrence of normal age-related periods of hypotension, and the use of antianginals may lead to worsening of hypotensive responses, paradoxical bradycardia, and increased angina. If patients are taking nitrates on a long-term basis, it is important to assess continued therapeutic responses because of the development of tolerance to the drug's effects. During assessment and initiation of drug therapy, it is critical to patient safety to notify the prescriber of any increased angina, because another antianginal or vasodilating drug may be needed.

Concerns arise with the use of *nonselective beta-blockers* and *beta₂-blockers* (as vasodilators) in patients with bronchospastic disease because of the drug-related effects of bronchoconstriction and increased airway resistance. Therefore, if asthma or other respiratory problems are present, beta-blockers would not be indicated because bronchoconstriction could be exacerbated. In addition, there are also concerns about the use of beta-blockers in patients with hyperthyroidism, impaired renal or liver function, peripheral vascular disease, or diabetes. Hypoglycemia may occur in patients with previously controlled diabetes, and nonselective beta-blockers may also exacerbate preexisting heart failure. Assessment for edema is important because of drug-related edema. Weight gain of 2 pounds or more over 24 hours or 5 pounds or more in 1 week should be reported immediately to the prescriber.

Nursing Diagnoses

- Decreased cardiac output related to the pathology of coronary artery disease
- Ineffective tissue perfusion related to the physiologic impact of CAD
- Risk for injury to self related to the drug-related adverse effects of hypotension with subsequent dizziness and/or syncope possible causing falls
- Acute pain related to the pathologic impact of CAD and cardiac tissue ischemia
- Impaired physical mobility related to the impact of cellular ischemia
- Deficient knowledge related to first-time use of antianginal drugs and a new diagnosis of CAD

Planning

Goals

- Patient experiences fewer episodes of chest pain because of appropriate use of antianginal medication.
- Patient is able to perform activities of daily living and increase mobility with greater comfort, less chest pain, and increased stamina and energy.
- Patient tolerates moderate, supervised exercise while taking antianginals.
- Patient remains free of injury while receiving drug therapy.
- Patient states the rationale for medication therapy as well as adverse effects to report.

Outcome Criteria

- Patient states that there are more frequent periods of comfort while carrying out activities of daily living, engaging in supervised exercise, and performing moderate activity without reoccurring angina and without major adverse effects on follow-up with the prescriber.
- Patient states measures to decrease risk of injury, such as changing positions slowly, keeping legs moving when in a still position, increasing fluid intake with medication regimen, and removing rugs or carpets that can cause tripping or slipping.
- Patient states symptoms that should be reported to the prescriber, such as syncope, excessive dizziness, severe headache, or increase in the number of episodes of chest pain and/or in its severity.

Implementation

It is crucial for the nurse to always review and/or record the patient's vital signs and description of chest pain for the duration of therapy. The following are nursing considerations associated with the use of the various dosage forms and routes of administration: (1) *For any dosage form:* The drug should always be administered while the patient is seated to avoid falls or injury from drug-induced hypotension. This hypotension may last for up to 30 minutes after dosing of the drug. When nitrates are given, the patient's chest pain should be monitored, and the pain should be rated on a scale of 1 to 10 before, during, and after therapy. The patient's response to drug therapy should also be monitored by measurement of the patient's blood pressure and pulse rate and assessment for the presence of headache, dizziness, and/or lightheadedness. When the patient is in a supine position, an appropriate dose of a nitrate should produce a clinical response of a fall in blood pressure of

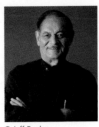

CASE STUDY

Nitroglycerin for Angina

© Jeff Banke

Mr. M.S., a 68-year-old accountant, has been diagnosed with coronary artery disease (CAD) after experiencing chest pain at times when he jogs. After undergoing a thorough physical examination, including cardiac catheterization, he is given a prescription for extended-release nitroglycerin capsules, 6 mg, three times a day. He also has a prescription for 0.4-mg sublingual nitroglycerin tablets to take as needed for chest pain.

1. What type of angina is he experiencing, and what are the therapeutic goals of the drug therapy he has received?

   M.S. asks you, "Why do I have two prescriptions for the same drug? It doesn't make sense to me!"

2. What is the best answer to his question?

3. Two days after he begins the nitroglycerin, M.S. calls the office and says, "I'm having awful headaches. What is wrong?"

   What is the best explanation, and what can he do about the headaches?

   After a month, M.S. is switched from the extended-release capsules to a transdermal nitroglycerin patch. He says that he is glad he does not have to remember to "take those pills" three times a day. However, 2 months later, he calls and says, "I don't think this patch is working. I'm having more episodes of chest pain now when I jog."

4. What could be the explanation for this, and what can be done?

For answers, see *http://evolve.elsevier.com/Lilley*.

about 10 mm Hg and/or a rise in heart rate of 10 beats/min. However, the following parameters should alert the nurse that there may be a problem and that the prescriber should be contacted: a systolic blood pressure of 90 mm Hg systolic or less and/or pulse rate of 60 beats/min or less or pulse rate greater than 100 beats/min. (2) *For oral dosage forms:* These forms should be taken as ordered before meals and with 6 oz of water. Extended-release preparations should not be crushed, chewed, or altered in any way. Acetaminophen may be given if there is a drug-related headache. (3) *For sublingual forms:* Tablets are to be placed under the tongue as directed and *not* swallowed until the drug is completely dissolved. Metered-dose aerosol sprays are applied onto or under the tongue (see Dosages table). Nitrates should be kept in their original packaging or container (e.g., sublingual tablets come in a small amber-colored glass container with a metal lid). Exposure to light, plastic, cotton filler, and moisture should be avoided. (4) *For ointment:* The proper dosing paper supplied by the drug company should be used to apply a thin layer on clean, dry, hairless skin of the upper arms or body. Areas below the knees and elbows should be avoided. The ointment should not be applied with the fingers unless a glove is worn to avoid contact with the skin and subsequent absorption. A tongue depressor may also be used, but in most situations the ointment may be squeezed directly from the tube onto the proper dosing paper. Once the ointment is in place, it should *not* be rubbed into the skin, and the area should be covered with an occlusive dressing if not provided (e.g., plastic wrap). Application sites should be rotated, and all residue from the previous dose of ointment should be gently removed with soap and water and the area patted dry. (5) *For transdermal forms:* The patch should be applied to a clean, residue-free, hairless area, and sites should be rotated. If cardioversion or use of an automated electrical defibrillator is required, the patch should be removed to avoid burning of the skin and damage to the defibrillator paddles. Before a new patch is applied, the old patch should be located and removed and the skin cleansed of any residual drug. Used, unneeded, or defective transdermal patches of any medication should be disposed of by folding the sticky side of the patch together (until it sticks to itself) and flushing the patch down the toilet or cutting it into several, small pieces before disposing of it in the commode (see *http://www.fda. gov/cder/drug/MedErrors/transdermal.pdf.*) (6) *For intravenous forms:* Intravenous dosing is for use in emergency situations only and in settings providing close automatic monitoring of the blood pressure and pulse and constant ECG monitoring. Intravenous administration of nitrates may lead to sudden and severe hypotension, cardiovascular collapse, and shock. The nurse must always check for incompatibilities and the proper diluent. Intravenous solutions should be given only through an infusion pump and as ordered. Intravenous dosage forms are available as ready-to-use injectable doses and are administered using *specific nonpolyvinylchloride* (non-PVC) plastic intravenous bags and tubing. The non-PVC infusion kits are used to avoid absorption or uptake of the nitrate by the intravenous tubing and bag. This prevents decomposition of the nitrate with breakdown into cyanide when the drug is exposed to light. Intravenous forms of nitroglycerin are stable for about 96 hours after preparation. If parenteral solutions are not clear and are discolored, the solution should be discarded.

With *isosorbide,* tablets are best taken on an empty stomach; however, if the patient complains of headache or gastrointestinal upset, the medicine should be taken with meals. Oral tablets of isosorbide can be crushed; however, the sublingual and extended-release forms should *not* be crushed or chewed. In addition, if a "chewable" form is to be given, it should *not* be crushed, even though it is chewable. As with sublingual nitroglycerin, the patient should not swallow the medication until it is completely dissolved. If dizziness or lightheadedness occurs, the patient should be assisted and encouraged to change positions slowly. The patient's blood pressure, including orthostatic blood pressures, should be closely monitored. The occurrence of anginal episodes should be documented, and their character, precipitating factors, severity, and frequency should be noted.

CCBs should be taken as ordered and without sudden withdrawal. Abrupt withdrawal can precipitate rebound hypertension and worsening of tissue ischemia. Weight should be measured daily (see later discussion), and the patient should be constantly monitored for edema and shortness of breath. The patient should be instructed to move and change positions slowly and cautiously to prevent syncope. Constipation may be prevented by forcing fluids and increasing fiber and roughage in the daily diet. Should the patient experience cardiac irregularities, pronounced dizziness, nausea, or dyspnea, the prescriber should be contacted immediately. Intravenous administration of any CCB requires the

use of an infusion pump and careful monitoring. (See Chapter 25 for further information.)

Beta-blockers should be given as ordered and taken with or without food, and abrupt withdrawal should be avoided. Weight should be measured every day at the same time and with the patient wearing the same amount of clothing. Should there be a gain of 2 pounds or more in 24 hours or 5 pounds or more in 1 week, the prescriber should be contacted immediately. When these drugs are used, measures should be taken to reduce the incidence of orthostatic hypotension, such as advising the patient dangle the legs on the side of the bed before standing and to move slowly and purposefully. Any dizziness, lightheadedness, mental depression, confusion, rash, or unusual bleeding or bruising should be reported immediately to the prescriber. (See Chapter 25 for further information.)

Patients taking vasodilators should avoid alcohol, saunas, hot tubs, hot showers, and hot weather or a hot environment. These conditions will exacerbate vasodilation and increase the occurrence of orthostatic hypotension, which will raise the risk for dizziness, syncope, and falls. The patient should be warned that with certain sustained-release forms of medication, the wax matrix may appear in the stool, and if this occurs it is possible that the medication is moving too rapidly through the gastrointestinal tract. The prescriber should be contacted, because use of a different dosage form may be indicated. The patient should be taught how to self-monitor blood pressure and pulse rate, and should document the findings in a journal so that the information can be shared with health care providers. The journal can also list daily weights, response to the medication regimen, and any adverse effects. If the patient is taking beta-blockers, the patient should be advised that it may take up to 1 to 2 weeks for therapeutic effects to occur. See Patient Teaching Tips for more information.

Evaluation

Patients taking antianginals must be monitored carefully for the occurrence of an allergic reaction, which may be manifested by dyspnea, swelling of the face, or hives. Evaluation of therapeutic effects includes a review for accomplishment of goals and outcomes, such as appropriate decrease in blood pressure, increase in cardiac output and tissue perfusion with decrease in angina, and a gradual increase in activity and performance of activities of daily living without exacerbation of anginal episodes. In addition, the patient must be monitored for adverse reactions such as headache, lightheadedness, dizziness, and decreased blood pressure, which may indicate the need to decrease the dosage. If the patient is receiving intravenous nitroglycerin, the nurse should evaluate for the development of pedal edema, abnormal skin turgor, nausea, vomiting, crackles, dyspnea, and orthopnea. If the patient experiences blurred vision, dry mouth, excessive drop in blood pressure and pulse rate, excessive facial or neck flushing, and/or worsening of angina, the prescriber should be notified immediately.

PATIENT TEACHING TIPS

Nitroglycerin

- The importance of keeping a daily journal should be emphasized with documentation of how the patient feels; number of anginal episodes with attention to their intensity, frequency, duration, character, and precipitating and relieving factors. Tolerance of medication is also important.
- *Capsules* or *extended-release* dosage forms should never be chewed, crushed, or altered in any way.
- The patient taking *aerosol* (spray) dosage forms should be instructed not to shake the canister before lingual spraying and to avoid inhaling or swallowing the lingual aerosol until the drug is dispersed. With *sublingual* forms, the medication should be taken at the first sign of chest pain and not delayed until the pain is severe. The patient should sit or lie down and take one sublingual tablet. According to current guidelines, if the chest pain or discomfort is not relieved in 5 minutes, after *one* dose, the patient (or family member) should call 911 immediately. The patient can take one more tablet while awaiting emergency care and a third tablet 5 minutes later, but no more than three tablets total. These guidelines reflect the fact that angina pain that does not respond to nitroglycerin may indicate a myocardial infarction. The sublingual dose should be placed under the tongue and the patient should avoid swallowing until the tablet is dissolved. The patient should not eat or drink until the drug has completely dissolved.
- Educate about the best place to store the medication, such as keeping medicine away from moisture, light, heat, and cotton filler material. The *sublingual* dosage form of nitroglycerin should be kept in its original amber-colored glass container with metal lid to avoid loss of potency from exposure to the aforementioned environmental factors.
- Potency of the sublingual nitroglycerin is noted if there is burning or stinging once the medication is placed under the tongue; if the medication does not burn, then the drug has lost its potency, and a new prescription must be obtained.
- It is important to emphasize that the medication is potent only for 3 to 6 months. The patient should be reminded always to have a fresh supply of the drug on hand, to plan ahead if traveling, and (no matter the dosage form) to sit or lie down when taking the medication to avoid falls secondary to a drop in blood pressure.
- With *all forms of nitrates,* the patient should be educated about adverse effects such as flushing of the face, dizziness, fainting, brief throbbing headache, increase in heart rate, and lightheadedness. Headaches associated with nitrates last approximately 20 minutes (with sublingual forms) and may be easily managed with acetaminophen. If headaches are bothersome when an oral dosage form is used, the drug should be taken with meals, and the patient should contact the prescriber if adverse effects continue. Blurred vision, dry mouth, or severe headaches may indicate drug overdose and require immediate medical attention.
- While taking an antianginal, the patient should avoid alcohol, hot environmental temperatures, saunas, hot tubs, and excessive exertion. These increase vasodilation with subsequent worsening of hypotension, which possibly can lead to syncope (fainting) and/or other cardiac events.

- In many situations, the prescriber specifies that nitroglycerin be taken *before* stressful activities or events such as emotional situations, consumption of large meals, smoking, or sudden increase in activity (e.g., sexual intercourse). The patient should follow the prescriber's directions regarding prophylactic dosing very closely.
- With *ointment* forms, the patient should be reminded to use the appropriate dosage paper for application of the ointment and not to use the fingers to apply the medicine. The medication can be pressed evenly and directly from the tube onto the printed dosing line on the paper. The patient should squeeze a thin line of ointment onto the paper and follow instructions regarding its application, such as measuring and applying ½ inch of ointment. An occlusive covering should be used, such as applying a piece of plastic wrap taped around the edges to adhere the dose to the skin. Only clean, nonirritated, and nonhairy areas free of residual medication should be used for these ointments.
- With *transdermal nitrate* use, the patient should be instructed to apply the patch at the same time each day and to be sure to have only one patch in place at a time, cleansing all residue off the skin before applying a new patch. Skinfolds, hairy areas, and any area distal to the knees or elbows should be avoided as application sites. A transdermal patch should not be applied to irritated or open skin and if the patch becomes loose the patient should remove it and gently wash off the residue with lukewarm soap and water, *pat* the area dry, and place another patch in another area. Rotation of sites is encouraged to prevent irritation (with ointments, too). The prescriber may order the removal of the patch for an 8-hour period on specific days to help decrease or prevent drug tolerance, which may develop over time. Emphasize all instructions with both written and verbal instructions.

Isosorbide Dinitrate or Isosorbide Mononitrate

- Educate about the basic differences in oral nitrates (e.g., the mononitrate form is well absorbed after oral dosing; the dinitrate form is poorly absorbed, but its metabolite, isosorbide mononitrate, is active and well absorbed). It is important that the patient know that these drugs are *not interchangeable.*
- The patient should be told to take the medication exactly as ordered with understanding that emphasis on the need to lie down when doses are taken to avoid injury from the sudden drop in blood pressure, which can cause dizziness, lightheadedness, and fainting.
- Isosorbide dinitrate is generally given three times a day with a 12-hour drug-free interval, such as dosing at 0700, 1300, and 1900. The 12-hour drug-free interval helps prevent the development of tolerance.
- Oral dosage forms should not be altered in any way and taken with at least 6 to 8 oz of water.
- The patient should be cautious while taking these drugs and move slowly and purposefully. The patient should be encouraged to rise slowly and move the legs about before standing up from a lying or sitting position to help prevent dizziness, possible fainting, and falls. See earlier patient teaching tips regarding the avoidance of alcohol, heat, and saunas.
- These and other antianginals should not be stopped abruptly.

POINTS TO REMEMBER

- Angina pectoris (chest pain) occurs because of a mismatch between the oxygen supply and oxygen demand, with either too high a demand for oxygen or too little oxygen delivery.
- The heart is a very aerobic (oxygen-requiring) muscle, and when it does not receive enough oxygen, pain (angina) occurs. When the coronary arteries that deliver oxygen to the heart muscle become blocked, a heart attack or MI occurs.
- Coronary artery disease is an abnormal condition of the arteries (blood vessels) that deliver oxygen to the heart muscle. These arteries may become narrowed, which results in reduced flow of oxygen and nutrients to the myocardium.
- Nitrates, CCBs, and beta-blockers may be used to treat the symptoms of angina.
- Nitroglycerin is the prototypical nitrate. Nitrates dilate constricted coronary arteries, helping to increase the supply of oxygen and nutrients to the heart muscle. Nitrates also dilate all other blood vessels. The venous dilation results in a decrease in blood return to the heart (decreased preload), whereas the arterial dilation results in a decrease of peripheral resistance (decreased afterload—that is, the pressure or force against which the left ventricle must pump). Isosorbide dinitrates were the first group of oral drugs used to treat angina; isosorbide mononitrates are new and improved nitrates used for angina therapy. Beta-blockers are also used to relieve angina and do so by decreasing the heart rate, reducing workload on the heart and decreasing oxygen demands.

- Dosage forms for nitrates include conventional tablets, translingual spray, controlled-release and sustained-release capsules, transdermal patch, topical ointment, and intravenous injection.
- Quick-onset nitrates should be used to treat acute anginal attacks while longer-onset nitrates are used for prophylaxis.
- CCBs and beta-blockers may be associated with the adverse effects of postural hypotension, dizziness, headache, and edema. The nonselective beta-blockers may exacerbate congestive heart failure, problems related to respiratory bronchospasm, and hypoglycemia. The patient's pulse rate should be checked before drug administration, and if pulse rate is 60 beats/min or lower, the prescriber should be contacted for further instructions.
- Patients should be instructed always to keep a fresh supply of sublingual nitroglycerin on their person and in their home, because the drug is only stable for 3 to 6 months.

NCLEX EXAMINATION REVIEW QUESTIONS

1 A patient has a new prescription for transdermal nitroglycerin patches. The nurse teaches the patient that these patches are most appropriately used
  a to relieve exertional angina.
  b to prevent palpitations.
  c to prevent the occurrence of angina.
  d to reduce the severity of anginal episodes.

2 A nurse with adequate knowledge about the administration of intravenous nitroglycerin will recognize that which statement is correct?
  a The intravenous form is given by bolus injection.
  b Because the intravenous forms are short-lived, the dosing must be every 2 hours.
  c Intravenous nitroglycerin must be protected from exposure to light through use of special tubing.
  d Intravenous nitroglycerin can be given via gravity drip infusions.

3 Which statement by the patient reflects the need for additional patient education about the calcium channel blocker diltiazem (Cardizem)?
  a "I can take this drug to stop acute anginal attacks."
  b "I understand that food and antacids alter the absorption of this oral drug."
  c "When the long-acting forms are taken, the drug cannot be crushed."
  d "This drug may cause my blood pressure to drop, so I should be careful when getting up."

4 While assessing a patient with angina who is to start beta-blocker therapy, the nurse is aware that the presence of which condition may be a problem if these drugs are used?

  a Hypertension
  b Essential tremors
  c Exertional angina
  d Asthma

5 A 68-year-old man has been taking the nitrate isosorbide dinitrate for 2 years for angina. He recently has been experiencing erectile dysfunction and wants a prescription for sildenafil (Viagra). Which response would the nurse most likely hear from the prescriber?
  a "He will have to be switched to isosorbide mononitrate if he wants to take sildenafil."
  b "Taking sildenafil with the nitrate may result in severe hypotension, so a contraindication exists."
  c "I'll write a prescription, but if he uses it, he needs to stop taking the isosorbide for one dose."
  d "These drugs are compatible with each other, and so I'll write a prescription."

6 The nurse is reviewing drug interactions with a male patient who has a prescription for isosorbide dinitrate (Isordil) as treatment for angina symptoms. Which substances listed below could potentially result in a drug interaction? (Select all that apply.)
  a A glass of wine
  b Thyroid replacement hormone
  c Sildenafil (Viagra), an erectile dysfunction drug
  d Metformin (Glucophage), an antidiabetic drug
  e Carvedilol (Coreg), a beta-blocker

CRITICAL THINKING ACTIVITIES: BEST ACTION

1 Mrs. A. has been shoveling snow all morning. As you work on the snow in your yard, you see her suddenly sit down in her driveway. When you go over to check on her, she says that she has nitroglycerin tablets in her jacket pocket but she forgot how to take them. What is the best action at this time?

2 Your patient has been switched from oral nitroglycerin capsules to a transdermal form. What are the priorities for patient teaching regarding transdermal nitroglycerin therapy?

3 Mr. J. is a 45-year-old man with stable angina who has recently been prescribed sublingual nitroglycerin tablets for the relief of his anginal attacks. He asks you how many milligrams of nitroglycerin are in his tablets. All the bottle says is "$\frac{1}{150}$ grain tablets." How many milligrams of nitroglycerin are in Mr. J.'s $\frac{1}{150}$ grain tablets?

For answers, see *http://evolve.elsevier.com/Lilley*.

CHAPTER 25

Antihypertensive Drugs

OBJECTIVES

When you reach the end of this chapter, you should be able to do the following:

1 Briefly discuss the normal anatomy and physiology of the autonomic nervous system, including the events that take place within the sympathetic and parasympathetic divisions and the way they relate to long-term and short-term control of blood pressure.

2 Define *hypertension* and compare primary and secondary hypertension and their related manifestations.

3 Describe the protocol for treating hypertension as detailed in the *Seventh Report of the Joint National Committee on Prevention, Detection, Evaluation, and Treatment of High Blood Pressure* (JNC 7), including the rationale for its use.

4 List the criterion pressure values (in millimeters of mercury) for the new hypertension categories of normal blood pressure, prehypertension, hypertension stage 1, and hypertension stage 2 as defined in *JNC 7*.

5 Using the most recent guidelines, compare the various drugs used in the pharmacologic management of hypertension with regard to mechanism of action, specific indications, adverse effects, toxic effects, cautions, drug interactions, contraindications, dosages, and routes of administration.

6 Discuss the rationale for the nonpharmacologic management of hypertension.

7 Develop a nursing care plan that includes all phases of the nursing process for patients receiving antihypertensive drugs.

e-Learning Activities

http://evolve.elsevier.com/Lilley

NCLEX Review Questions • Animations • Nursing Care Plans • Audio Glossary • Category Catchers • Medication Errors Checklists • IV Therapy Checklists • Calculators • Frequently Asked Questions • Content Updates • Supplemental Resources • Answers to Case Studies and Critical Thinking Activities

Drug Profiles

aliskiren, p. 395
bosentan, p. 394
◆ captopril, p. 390
carvedilol, p. 388
◆ clonidine, p. 388
doxazosin, p. 388
enalapril, p. 391

eplerenone, p. 394
◆ hydralazine, p. 393
◆ losartan, p. 392
nebivolol, p. 389
sodium nitroprusside, p. 394
treprostinil, p. 395

◆ *Key drug.*

Glossary

Alpha₁-blockers Drugs that primarily cause arterial and venous dilation through their action on peripheral sympathetic neurons. (p. 385)
Antihypertensive drugs Medications used to treat hypertension. (p. 382)
Cardiac output The amount of blood ejected from the left ventricle, measured in liters per minute. (p. 383)
Centrally acting adrenergic drugs Drugs that modify the function of the sympathetic nervous system in the brain by stimulating alpha₂ receptors, which has a reverse sympathetic effect that causes decreased blood pressure. (p. 384)

Essential hypertension Elevated systemic arterial pressure for which no cause can be found and which is often the only significant clinical finding; also called *primary* or *idiopathic hypertension.* (p. 393)
Hypertension A common, often asymptomatic disorder in which blood pressure persistently exceeds 140/90 mm Hg. (p. 382)
Orthostatic hypotension A common adverse effect of adrenergic drugs involving a sudden drop in blood pressure when a person changes position, especially when rising from a seated or horizontal position. (p. 386)
Prodrug A drug that is inactive in its administered form and must be metabolized to its active form in the body, generally by the liver, to be effective. (p. 389)
Secondary hypertension High blood pressure associated with a primary disease such as renal, pulmonary, endocrine, or vascular disease. (p. 383)

• • •

Anatomy, Physiology, and Disease Overview

Significant advances have been made in the detection, evaluation, and treatment of high blood pressure, or **hypertension.** Over the past 40 years the development of new antihypertensive medications has had an enormous impact on the quality of life of affected persons by reducing the incidence of the various complications associated with hypertension and decreasing the adverse effects associated with these medications. Drug therapy for hypertension first became available in the early 1950s with the introduction of *ganglionic blocking drugs.* However, unpleasant adverse effects and inconsistent therapeutic effects were common problems with these **antihypertensive drugs.** In 1953 the vasodilator hydralazine was introduced, and in 1958 the thiazide diuretics became available. These drugs offered important advantages over the previous antihypertensive drug therapies. In addition, with the discovery of these newer drugs came a better understanding of the disease process itself.

Since that time, several additional drug categories have emerged, including loop diuretics (also called *potassium-wasting diuretics*), potassium-sparing diuretics, beta-blockers (beta receptor antagonists), angiotensin-converting enzyme (ACE) inhibitors, alpha$_1$ antagonists, alpha$_2$ agonists, angiotensin II receptor blockers (ARBs), calcium channel blockers (CCBs), vasodilators, and the newest class, the direct renin inhibitors. Although some of the medications mentioned in this chapter represent older classes of drugs, all are current therapeutic options listed in the treatment guidelines for hypertension published by the National Heart, Lung, and Blood Institute.

HYPERTENSION

As many as 50 million people in the United States have some form of hypertension, which makes it the most common disease in the population of the Western hemisphere. Not only does hypertension affect a large portion of our society, but it has many severe consequences if left untreated. Hypertension is a major risk factor for coronary artery disease, cardiovascular disease, and death resulting from cardiovascular causes. It is the most important risk factor for stroke and heart failure, and it is also a major risk factor for renal failure and peripheral vascular disease.

The diagnosis and treatment of hypertension have varied considerably over the years. The *Seventh Report of the Joint National Committee on Prevention, Detection, Evaluation, and Treatment of High Blood Pressure (JNC 7)* was released in May 2003. This report provides treatment guidelines for hypertension assembled by two large expert panels based on a review of the latest clinical research publications on the disease. As with previous such reports, the development of *JNC 7* was sponsored by the National Heart, Lung, and Blood Institute of the National Institutes of Health, the major governmental health research entity of the United States. The efforts of the Joint National Committee are intended to educate both health care professionals and the general public about the dangers of the disease and the importance of its treatment. The *Eighth Report of the Joint National Committee on Prevention, Detection, Evaluation, and Treatment of High Blood Pressure (JNC 8)* is scheduled to be published in spring 2010 and can be found at *http://www.nhlbi.nih.gov/guidelines/hypertension.* See *http://evolve.elsevier.com/Lilley* for further information on new JNC 8 guidelines.

One of the major changes that appeared in the earlier guideline *Sixth Report of the Joint National Committee on Prevention, Detection, Evaluation, and Treatment of High Blood Pressure (JNC 6)* in 1997 was a new classification system for blood pressure. The previously applied term *mild hypertension* did not adequately reflect the serious nature of this condition. This became evident when it was found that, although the overwhelming majority of patients with hypertension have so-called mild hypertension, most of the morbidity and mortality actually occur in this group. In addition, whereas pre–*JNC 6* reports had recommended a stepped-care pharmacologic approach to treating the illness, many practitioners believed that this approach

no longer adequately reflected the current range of pharmacologic alternatives or furnished the type of care dictated by the current level of scientific understanding of the disorder. In *JNC 6*, individualized therapy was proposed as a more appropriate treatment strategy, because it allowed specific patient circumstances to be addressed and pharmacologic alternatives to be considered. This individualized approach continues to be emphasized in *JNC 8*, with the recognition that some patients may require two or more medications, even as initial therapy, depending on their individual cardiovascular risk factors such as obesity, diabetes, and family history. Prescribers are therefore encouraged to adopt an individualized approach to the planning of drug therapy that takes into consideration the demographic concerns for the given patient, the presence of more than one disease, the use of concurrent therapies, and the patient's quality of life.

The classification scheme used to categorize individual cases of hypertension has been simplified to the following four stages based on blood pressure measurements: normal, prehypertension, stage 1 hypertension, and stage 2 hypertension. (The reader is referred to *JNC 8* at *http://www.nhlbi.nih.gov/guidelines/hypertension.*)

Hypertension can also be defined by its cause. When the specific cause of hypertension is unknown, it may be called *essential, idiopathic,* or *primary hypertension*. About 90% of cases of hypertension are of this type. **Secondary hypertension** accounts for the other 10%. Secondary hypertension is most commonly the result of another disease such as pheochromocytoma (adrenal tumor), preeclampsia of pregnancy (a pregnancy complication involving acute hypertension, among other symptoms), or renal artery disease. It may also result from the use of certain medications. If the cause of secondary hypertension can be eliminated, blood pressure usually returns to normal.

Blood pressure is determined by the product of **cardiac output** (4 to 8 L/min) and systemic vascular resistance (SVR). Cardiac output is the amount of blood that is ejected from the left ventricle and is measured in liters per minute. SVR is the force (resistance) the left ventricle has to overcome to eject its volume of blood. Numerous factors interact to regulate these two major variables and keep the blood pressure within normal limits. These are illustrated in Figure 25-1. These are the same factors that can cause high blood pressure and are the targets of action of many of the antihypertensive drugs.

▌Pharmacology Overview

The drug therapy for hypertension should be individualized. Important considerations in planning drug therapy are whether the patient has multiple medical problems and what impact drug therapy will have on the patient's quality of life. For example, one very common adverse effect of almost any antihypertensive drug is sexual dysfunction in male patients, which is the most common reason for nonadherence to drug therapy. Demographic factors, cultural implications, the ease of medication administration (e.g., a once-a-day dosing schedule or transdermal administration), and cost are other important considerations.

There are essentially seven main categories of pharmacologic drugs: diuretics, adrenergic drugs, vasodilators, ACE inhibitors, ARBs, CCBs, and direct renin inhibitors. Because all antihypertensive drugs (with the exception of diuretics) have

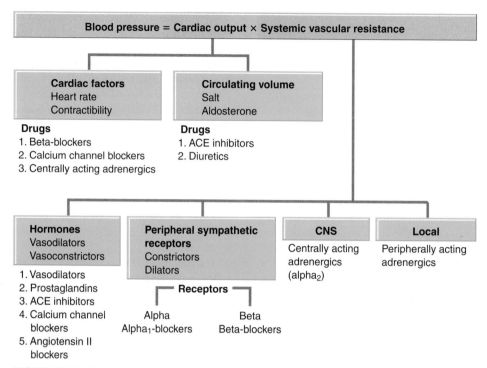

FIGURE 25-1 Normal regulation of blood pressure and corresponding medications. *ACE,* Angiotensin-converting enzyme; *CNS,* central nervous system.

some vasodilatory action, those in the vasodilator category are also called *direct vasodilators* to differentiate them. Drugs in these classes may be used either alone or in combination. The various categories and subcategories of antihypertensive drugs are listed in Box 25-1. The diuretics are discussed in detail in Chapter 26 and therefore are not covered here.

REVIEW OF AUTONOMIC NEUROTRANSMISSION

The stimulation of the two divisions of the autonomic nervous system (ANS), the parasympathetic nervous system (PSNS) and sympathetic nervous system (SNS), is controlled by the neurotransmitters acetylcholine and norepinephrine. The receptors for both divisions of the ANS are located throughout the body in a variety of tissues. ANS physiology is reviewed in greater detail in the introductory sections of Chapters 18 through 21. The receptor located between the postganglionic fiber and the effector cells (i.e., the postganglionic receptor) is called the *muscarinic* or *cholinergic receptor* in the PSNS and the *adrenergic* or *noradrenergic receptor* (i.e., alpha or beta receptor) in the SNS. Physiologic activity at muscarinic receptors is stimulated by acetylcholine and cholinergic agonist drugs (see Chapter 20) and is inhibited by cholinergic antagonists (anticholinergic drugs; see Chapter 21). Similarly, physiologic activity at adrenergic receptors is stimulated by norepinephrine and epinephrine and adrenergic agonist drugs (see Chapter 18) and inhibited by antiadrenergic drugs (adrenergic blockers, i.e., alpha or beta receptor blockers; see Chapter 19). Figure 25-2 shows how these various receptors are arranged in both the PSNS and SNS and indicates their corresponding neurotransmitters.

ADRENERGIC DRUGS

Adrenergic drugs are a large group of antihypertensive drugs, as shown in Box 25-1. The alpha-blockers and combined alpha/beta-blockers were described in detail in Chapter 19. The adrenergic drugs discussed here exert their antihypertensive action at different sites.

Mechanism of Action and Drug Effects

Five specific drug subcategories are included in the adrenergic antihypertensive drugs as indicated in Box 25-1. Each of these subcategories of drugs can be described as having central action (in the brain) or peripheral action (at the heart and blood vessels). These drugs include the adrenergic neuron blockers (central and peripheral), the alpha$_2$ receptor agonists (central), the alpha$_1$ receptor blockers (peripheral), the beta receptor blockers (peripheral), and the combination alpha$_1$ and beta receptor blockers (peripheral).

The centrally acting alpha$_2$-adrenergic drugs clonidine and methyldopa both act by modifying the function of the SNS. Because SNS stimulation leads to an increase in heart rate and force of contraction, the constriction of blood vessels, and the release of renin from the kidney, the result is hypertension. The **centrally acting adrenergic drugs** work by stimulating the alpha$_2$-adrenergic receptors in the brain. The alpha$_2$-adrenergic receptors are unique in that receptor stimulation actually reduces sympathetic outflow, in this case from the central nervous system (CNS). The resulting lack of norepinephrine production reduces blood pressure. This stimulation of the alpha$_2$-adrenergic receptors also affects the kidneys, reducing the activity of renin. Renin is the hormone and enzyme that converts the protein precursor angiotensinogen to the protein angiotensin I, the precursor of angiotensin II (AII), a potent vasoconstrictor that raises blood pressure.

BOX 25-1 Categories and Subcategories of Antihypertensive Drugs

Adrenergic Drugs
- Centrally and peripherally acting adrenergic neuron blockers
- Centrally acting alpha$_2$ receptor agonists
- Peripherally acting alpha$_1$ receptor blockers
- Peripherally acting beta receptor blockers (beta-blockers)
  - Cardioselective (beta$_1$ receptor blockers)
  - Nonselective (beta$_1$ and beta$_2$ receptor blockers)
- Peripherally acting dual alpha$_1$ and beta receptor blockers

Angiotensin-Converting Enzyme Inhibitors
Angiotensin II Receptor Blockers
Calcium Channel Blockers
- Benzothiazepines
- Dihydropyridines
- Phenylalkylamines

Diuretics
- Loop diuretics
- Potassium-sparing diuretics
- Thiazides and thiazide-like diuretics

Vasodilators
Act directly on vascular smooth muscle cells, *not* through alpha or beta receptors.

Direct Renin Inhibitors

In the periphery the **alpha$_1$-blockers** doxazosin, prazosin, and terazosin also modify the function of the SNS. However, they do so by blocking the alpha$_1$-adrenergic receptors. When alpha$_1$-adrenergic receptors are stimulated by circulating norepinephrine, they produce increased blood pressure. Thus, when these receptors are blocked, blood pressure is decreased. The drug effects of the alpha$_1$-blockers are primarily related to their ability to dilate arteries and veins, which reduces peripheral vascular resistance and subsequently decreases blood pressure. This produces a marked decrease in the systemic and pulmonary venous pressures and an increase in cardiac output. The alpha$_1$-blockers also increase urinary flow rates and decrease outflow obstruction by preventing smooth muscle contractions in the bladder neck and urethra. This can be beneficial in cases of benign prostatic hyperplasia (BPH; see later).

The beta-blockers also act in the periphery and include propranolol and atenolol as well as several other drugs. These drugs are discussed in more detail in Chapter 23 because they also have antidysrhythmic properties. Their antihypertensive effects are related to their reduction of the heart rate through beta$_1$ receptor blockade. Furthermore, beta-blockers also cause a reduction in the secretion of the hormone *renin* (see section on ACE inhibitors), which in turn reduces both AII-mediated vasoconstriction and aldosterone-mediated volume expansion. Long-term use of beta-blockers also reduces peripheral vascular resistance.

CULTURAL IMPLICATIONS

Antihypertensive Drug Therapy

The following are some important generalizations about demographics and the drugs used to treat hypertension:
- Beta-blockers and angiotensin-converting enzyme (ACE) inhibitors have been found to be more effective in lowering blood pressure in whites than in African Americans.
- Calcium channel blockers and diuretics have been shown to be more effective in African American patients than in white patients.
- Captopril used as monotherapy to treat hypertension has been found to elicit a lesser response in African American patients, who are considered to be low-renin hypertensives, than in the general treatment population.
- Losartan used as monotherapy for hypertension has been found to be less effective in African American patients than in other racial groups because African American patients are low-renin hypertensives.

These findings are important to remember in the care of patients, whether they are in an inpatient setting; are being seen by a physician, physician's assistant, or a nurse practitioner; or are being screened by a nurse in the community. The significance of these cultural-ethnic factors is that they allow a better understanding of the dynamics of pharmacologic treatment in hypertensive patients of different ethnic groups and also underscore the importance of a thorough nursing assessment that includes attention to cultural influences. These factors also allow an appreciation of individual responses to drug therapy and aid in achieving more successful treatment of the disease. These responses are often considered by health care providers in selecting first-line therapy.

Results of many studies have supported a difference between African Americans and whites in response to antihypertensive drugs; however, conflicting findings in this area should be mentioned for balance. Although researchers have reported that, on average, African Americans and whites differ slightly in their responses to antihypertensive drugs, a meta-analysis published in the March 2004 issue of *Hypertension* found that the majority of African Americans and whites in the studies analyzed had similar responses to some of the more commonly used antihypertensives such as diuretics, beta-blockers, calcium channel blockers, and ACE inhibitors. In this analysis, which pooled data on the use of common antihypertensives in some 9300 whites and 2900 African Americans, 81% to 95% of African Americans and whites were found to experience similar changes in blood pressure in response to each of the four groups of commonly used drugs. This analysis concluded that race, as examined in this context, had little value in predicting response to these drugs and that the responses of the two groups were overlapping. The reason to mention this research is that clinical decisions may be more efficient and of greater therapeutic value if drug treatment is based on considerations relevant to the given individual, such as indications and medical history, rather than being based solely on race. In summary, it is important for nurses to fully understand all the cultural and multifactor influences on pharmacologic therapies so that the nursing process can be implemented thoroughly and effectively.

Modified from Rakel RE, Bope ET: *Conn's current therapy 2004*, Philadelphia, 2004, Saunders; Sehgal A: Overlap between whites and blacks in response to antihypertensive drugs, *Hypertension* 43:566-572, 2004.

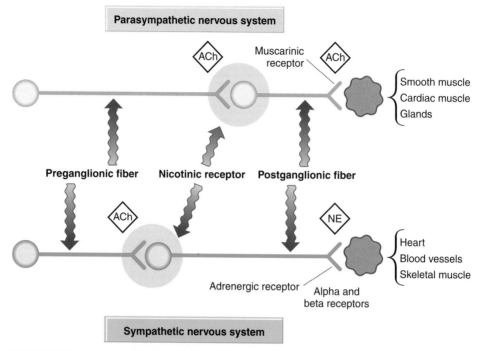

FIGURE 25-2 Location of the nicotinic receptors in the parasympathetic and sympathetic nervous systems. *ACh,* Acetylcholine; *NE,* norepinephrine.

Two dual-action alpha$_1$ and beta receptor blockers, which also act in the periphery at the heart and blood vessels, are currently available. These two drugs are labetalol and carvedilol. They have the dual antihypertensive effects of reduction in heart rate (beta$_1$ receptor blockade) and vasodilation (alpha$_1$ receptor blockade). Figure 25-3 illustrates the site and mechanisms of action of the various antihypertensive drugs.

Indications

All of the drugs mentioned are used primarily for the treatment of hypertension, either alone or in combination with other antihypertensive drugs. Various forms of glaucoma may also respond to treatment with some of these drugs. Clonidine also has several off-label uses (not approved by the U.S. Food and Drug Administration but still common in practice), including prophylaxis against migraine headaches and treatment of severe dysmenorrhea or menopausal flushing. It is also useful in the management of withdrawal symptoms in persons with opioid, nicotine, or alcohol dependency. The alpha$_1$-blockers doxazosin, prazosin, and terazosin have been used to relieve the symptoms associated with BPH. They have also proved effective in the management of severe heart failure when used with cardiac glycosides (see Chapter 22) and diuretics (see Chapter 26).

Contraindications

Contraindications to the use of the adrenergic antihypertensive drugs include known drug allergy and may also include acute heart failure, concurrent use of monoamine oxidase inhibitors (see Chapter 17), severe mental depression, peptic ulcer, colitis, and severe liver or kidney disease. Asthma may also be a contraindication to the use of any noncardioselective beta-blocker (e.g., carvedilol). As mentioned in Chapter 22, the use of vasodilating

drugs may also be contraindicated in cases of heart failure that is secondary to diastolic dysfunction.

Adverse Effects

The most common adverse effects of adrenergic drugs are bradycardia with reflex tachycardia, postural and postexercise hypotension, dry mouth, drowsiness, sedation, dizziness, edema, constipation, and sexual dysfunction (e.g., impotence). Other effects include headaches, sleep disturbances, nausea, rash, peripheral pooling of blood, and cardiac disturbances such as palpitations. There is also a high incidence of **orthostatic hypotension** (a sudden drop in blood pressure during changes in position) in patients taking these drugs. Orthostatic hypotension is commonly referred to as postural hypotension. This can lead to a situation known as *first-dose syncope,* in which the hypotensive effect is severe enough to cause the patient to lose consciousness with even the first dose of medication. This is especially true with alpha-blockers. Patients should be educated to change positions slowly. In addition, the abrupt discontinuation of the centrally acting alpha$_2$ receptor agonists can result in rebound hypertension. This may also be true for other antihypertensive drug classes, especially beta-blockers. Nonselective blocking drugs are also more commonly associated with bronchoconstriction (due to unrestrained parasympathetic tone) as well as metabolic inhibition of glycogenolysis in the liver, which can lead to hypoglycemia. However, hyperglycemic episodes are also among the adverse effects reported for this drug class. Any change in the dosing regimen for cardiovascular medications should be undertaken gradually and with appropriate patient monitoring and follow-up. Although the same is also true for most other classes of medications, abrupt dosage changes of cardiovascular medications, either up or down, can be especially hazardous for the

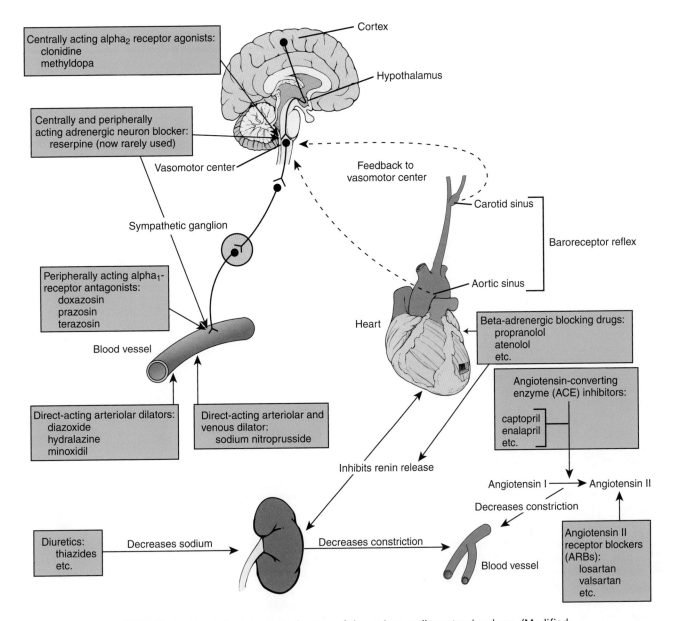

FIGURE 25-3 Site and mechanism of action of the various antihypertensive drugs. (Modified from Lewis SM et al: *Medical-surgical nursing: assessment and management of clinical problems,* ed 7, St Louis, 2007, Mosby.)

patient. Some of these drugs can also cause disruptions in blood count as well as in serum electrolyte levels and renal function. Periodic monitoring of white blood cell count, serum potassium and sodium levels, and urinary protein levels is recommended.

Interactions

Adrenergic drugs interact primarily with CNS depressants such as alcohol, benzodiazepines, and opioids. The additive effects of these combinations of drugs increase CNS depression. Other drug interactions that can occur with selected adrenergic drugs are summarized in Table 25-1. This list is merely representative and is not exhaustive. The nurse should always keep a drug information handbook available to check in cases in which a specific drug interaction is suspected. Hospital pharmacists are also excellent resources for the nurse.

Dosages

For information on the dosages of selected adrenergic antihypertensive drugs, see the Dosages table on p. 388.

DRUG PROFILES

ALPHA₂-ADRENERGIC RECEPTOR STIMULATORS (AGONISTS)

Of the available alpha₂ receptor agonists—clonidine and methyldopa—clonidine is by far the most commonly used and the prototypical drug for this class. Methyldopa is also administered for the treatment of hypertension and is commonly used to treat hypertension in pregnancy. However, these drugs are not typically prescribed as first-line antihypertensive drugs, because their use is associated with a high incidence of unwanted adverse effects such as orthostatic hypotension, fatigue, and dizziness. They may be

TABLE 25-1 Adrenergic Drugs: Drug Interactions

Drug	Interacts with	Mechanism	Result
Clonidine	Opioids, sedatives, hypnotics, anesthetics, alcohol	Additive	Increased CNS depression
	TCAs, MAOIs, appetite suppressants, amphetamines	Opposing actions	Decreased hypotensive effects
	Diuretics, nitrates, other antihypertensive drugs	Additive	Increased hypotensive effects
	Beta-blockers	Additive	May potentiate bradycardia and increase the rebound hypertension in clonidine withdrawal
Doxazosin	Diuretics, other hypotensive drugs	Additive	Increased hypotension
	indomethacin	Opposing effects	Decreased hypotensive effect
	verapamil	Increased serum prazosin levels	Increased hypotension

CNS, Central nervous system; *MAOIs,* monoamine oxidase inhibitors; *TCAs,* tricyclic antidepressants.

DOSAGES

Selected Antihypertensive Drugs: Adrenergic Agonist and Antagonists

Drug (Pregnancy Category)	Pharmacologic Class	Usual Dosage Range	Indications/Uses
carvedilol (Coreg) (C)	Peripherally acting alpha$_1$, beta$_1$, and beta$_2$ receptor antagonist (blocker)	PO: 3.125-25 mg bid	Hypertension (also used in heart failure)
◆ clonidine (Catapres, Catapres-TTS) (C)	Centrally acting alpha$_2$ receptor agonist	PO: Initial dose 0.1 mg daily-bid; may titrate up to a maximum of 2.4 mg/day, divided bid-qid. Transdermal patch: 0.1, 0.2, or 0.3 mg/24 hr, applied weekly	Hypertension (may have other unlabeled uses including treatment of psychiatric, cardiovascular, and gastrointestinal problems)
doxazosin (Cardura) (C)	Peripherally acting alpha$_1$ receptor antagonist	PO: Initial dose 1 mg daily; may titrate up to maximum of 16 mg/day	Hypertension

PO, Oral.

used as adjunct drugs in the treatment of hypertension after other drugs have failed or may be used in conjunction with other antihypertensives such as diuretics.

◆ clonidine

Clonidine (Catapres) is used primarily for its ability to decrease blood pressure. It is also useful in the management of opioid withdrawal. It has a better safety profile than the other centrally acting adrenergics and has the advantage of being available in several dosage formulations, including both topical and oral preparations. When the patch dosage form is used, it is important to remove the old patch before applying a new one. Clonidine should not be discontinued abruptly, because this will lead to severe rebound hypertension. Its use is contraindicated in patients who have shown hypersensitivity reactions to it. See the table above for recommended dosages.

PHARMACOKINETICS

Route	Onset of Action	Peak Plasma Concentration	Elimination Half-life	Duration of Action
PO	30-60 min	3-5 hr	6-20 hr	8 hr

ALPHA$_1$-BLOCKERS

The alpha$_1$-blockers are doxazosin (Cardura), prazosin (Minipress), tamsulosin (Flomax), and terazosin (Hytrin). They are the newest of the adrenergics and have the best safety and efficacy profiles, but they are not free of adverse effects. Their use is contraindicated in patients who have shown a hypersensitivity to them. They

are classified as pregnancy category C drugs. They are available only as oral preparations. Tamsulosin is not used to control blood pressure but is indicated solely for symptomatic control of BPH. This use is described further in Chapter 35.

doxazosin

Doxazosin (Cardura) is the most commonly used alpha$_1$-blocker. It reduces peripheral vascular resistance and blood pressure by dilating both arterial and venous blood vessels. It has been shown to be beneficial in the treatment of hypertension and the relief of the symptoms of obstructive BPH. It is available in immediate- and extended-release formulations. When the drug is released from the extended-release form, the matrix of the capsule is expelled in the stool. Patients should be educated about this and reassured that the active drug has been absorbed. Confusion over this fact could cause patients to take more than the prescribed dosage. Recommended dosages are given in the table above.

PHARMACOKINETICS

Route	Onset of Action	Peak Plasma Concentration	Elimination Half-life	Duration of Action
PO	1-2 hr	2-3 hr	15-22 hr	Less than 24 hr

DUAL-ACTION ALPHA$_1$ AND BETA RECEPTOR BLOCKERS
carvedilol

Carvedilol (Coreg) is a widely used drug and seems to be well tolerated by most patients. In addition to treatment of hypertension, it is also indicated for treatment of mild to moderate heart failure in conjunction with digoxin, diuretics, and ACE inhibitors. Its contraindications include known drug allergy, cardiogenic shock, severe bradycardia or heart failure, bronchospastic conditions such as asthma, and various cardiac problems involving the conduction system. Dosage information appears in the table on p. 388.

PHARMACOKINETICS

Route	Onset of Action	Peak Plasma Concentration	Elimination Half-life	Duration of Action
PO	20-120 min	1-4 hr	6-8 hr	8-24 hr

NEW BETA RECEPTOR BLOCKER
nebivolol

Nebivolol (Bystolic) is the newest beta-blocker, released in 2008. It is a beta$_1$-selective beta blocker approved for use in hypertension. It is also being used for treatment of heart failure. Nebivolol is similar to other beta$_1$-selective blockers; however, in addition to blocking beta$_1$ receptors, it also produces an endothelium-derived nitric oxide–dependent vasodilatation, which results in a decrease in SVR. It is promoted as causing less sexual dysfunction. Like other beta-blockers, it should not be stopped abruptly but must be tapered over 1 to 2 weeks. Dosing starts at 5 mg/day and may be increased at 2-week intervals to a maximum of 40 mg/day.

ANGIOTENSIN-CONVERTING ENZYME INHIBITORS

The ACE inhibitors are a large group of antihypertensive drugs. Currently 10 ACE inhibitors are available for clinical use, in addition to various combination drug products in which a thiazide diuretic or a CCB is combined with an ACE inhibitor. Combination products tend to increase adherence as the patient is taking less number of drugs. The available ACE inhibitors are captopril (Capoten), benazepril (Lotensin), enalapril (Vasotec), fosinopril (Monopril), lisinopril (Prinivil), moexipril (Univasc), perindopril (Aceon), quinapril (Accupril), ramipril (Altace), and trandolapril (Mavik). These drugs are very safe and efficacious and are often used as the first-line drugs in the treatment of both heart failure and hypertension. Some of the available drug combinations and dosing schedules for the various drugs that make up this large class of antihypertensives are summarized in Table 25-2. The ACE inhibitors as a class are very similar and differ in only a few of their chemical properties, but there are some significant differences among them in their clinical properties. Knowing these differences can help the practitioner select the proper drug for a particular patient.

Captopril has the shortest half-life and therefore must be dosed more frequently than any of the other ACE inhibitors. This may be an important drawback to its use in a patient who has a history of being noncompliant with his or her medication regimen. On the other hand, it may be best to start with a drug that has a short half-life in a patient who is still very critically ill and may not tolerate medications well, so that if problems arise they will be short lived. Both captopril and enalapril can be dosed multiple times a day.

Captopril and lisinopril are the only two ACE inhibitors that are not prodrugs. A **prodrug** is a drug that is inactive in its administered form and must be metabolized to its active form in the body, generally by the liver, to be effective. This characteristic of

TABLE 25-2 ACE Inhibitors

Drug (Trade Name)	Combination with Hydrochlorothiazide	Dosing Schedule
benazepril (Lotensin)	Lotensin HCT	Once a day
captopril (Capoten)	Capozide	Multiple
enalapril (Vasotec)	Vaseretic	Multiple
fosinopril (Monopril)	None	Once a day
lisinopril (Prinivil)	Prinzide	Once a day
lisinopril (Zestril)	Zestoretic	Once a day
moexipril (Univasc)	None	Once a day
perindopril (Aceon)	None	Once to twice daily
quinapril (Accupril)	None	Once a day
ramipril (Altace)	None	Once a day
trandolapril (Mavik)	None	Once a day

ACE, Angiotensin-converting enzyme.

captopril and lisinopril is an important advantage in treating a patient with liver dysfunction; because all of the other ACE inhibitors are prodrugs, their transformation to active form in such patients is hindered.

Enalapril is the only ACE inhibitor that is available in a parenteral preparation. All of the newer ACE inhibitors, such as benazepril, fosinopril, lisinopril, quinapril, and ramipril, have long half-lives and long durations of action, which allows them to be given only once a day. A once-a-day medication regimen promotes better patient adherence.

All ACE inhibitors have detrimental effects on the unborn fetus and neonate. They are classified as pregnancy category C drugs for women in their first trimester and as pregnancy category D drugs for women in their second or third trimester. ACE inhibitors should be used by pregnant women only if there are no safer alternatives. Fetal and neonatal morbidity and mortality have been reported to have occurred in at least 50 cases in which women received ACE inhibitors during their pregnancies.

Mechanism of Action and Drug Effects

As is often the case with pharmaceutical innovations, the development of the ACE inhibitors was spurred by the discovery of an animal substance found to have beneficial effects in humans. This particular substance was the venom of a South American viper, which was found to inhibit kininase activity. Kininase is an enzyme that normally breaks down bradykinin, a potent vasodilator in the human body.

The ACE inhibitors have several beneficial cardiovascular effects. As their name implies, they inhibit angiotensin-converting enzyme, which is responsible for converting AI (formed through the action of renin) to AII. AII is a potent vasoconstrictor and induces aldosterone secretion by the adrenal glands. Aldosterone stimulates sodium and water resorption, which can raise blood pressure. Together, these processes are referred to as the renin-angiotensin-aldosterone system.

The primary effects of the ACE inhibitors are cardiovascular and renal. Their cardiovascular effects are due to their ability to reduce blood pressure by decreasing SVR. They do this by preventing the breakdown of the vasodilating substance bradykinin and also of substance P (another potent vasodilator), and preventing the

TABLE 25-3 ACE Inhibitors: Therapeutic Effects

Body Substance	Effect in Body	ACE Inhibitor Action	Resulting Hemodynamic Effect
Aldosterone	Causes sodium and water retention	Prevents its secretion	Diuresis = ↓ plasma volume = ↓ filling pressures or ↓ preload
Angiotensin II	Potent vasoconstrictor	Prevents its formation	↓ SVR = ↓ afterload
Bradykinin	Potent vasodilator	Prevents its breakdown	↓ SVR = ↓ afterload

↓, Decreased; *ACE,* angiotensin-converting enzyme; *SVR,* systemic vascular resistance.

formation of AII. These combined effects decrease afterload, or the resistance against which the left ventricle must pump to eject its volume of blood during contraction. The ACE inhibitors are beneficial in the treatment of heart failure because they prevent sodium and water resorption by inhibiting aldosterone secretion. This causes diuresis, which decreases blood volume and return to the heart. This in turn decreases preload, or the left ventricular end-diastolic volume, and the work required of the heart.

Indications

The therapeutic effects of the ACE inhibitors are related to their potent cardiovascular effects. They are excellent antihypertensives and adjunctive drugs for the treatment of heart failure. They may be used alone or in combination with other drugs such as diuretics in the treatment of hypertension or heart failure.

The beneficial hemodynamic effects of the ACE inhibitors have been studied extensively. Because of their ability to decrease SVR (a measure of afterload) and preload, ACE inhibitors can stop the progression of left ventricular hypertrophy, which is sometimes seen after a myocardial infarction (MI). This pathologic process is known as *ventricular remodeling.* The ability of ACE inhibitors to prevent it is termed a *cardioprotective effect.* ACE inhibitors have been shown to decrease morbidity and mortality in patients with heart failure. They should be considered the drugs of choice for hypertensive patients with heart failure. ACE inhibitors have also have been shown to have a protective effect on the kidneys, because they reduce glomerular filtration pressure. This is one reason that they are among the cardiovascular drugs of choice for diabetic patients. Numerous studies have shown that the ACE inhibitors reduce proteinuria, and they are considered by many to be standard therapy for diabetic patients to prevent the progression of diabetic nephropathy. The various therapeutic effects of the ACE inhibitors are listed in Table 25-3, which lists the biochemicals on which ACE inhibitors act and the resulting beneficial hemodynamic effects.

Contraindications

Contraindications to the use of ACE inhibitors include known drug allergy, especially a previous reaction of angioedema (e.g., laryngeal swelling) to an ACE inhibitor. Patients with a baseline potassium level of 5 mEq/L or higher may not be suitable candidates for ACE inhibitor therapy, because these drugs can promote hyperkalemia (see later). All ACE inhibitors are contraindicated in lactating women, children, and patients with bilateral renal artery stenosis.

Adverse Effects

Major CNS effects of the ACE inhibitors include fatigue, dizziness, mood changes, and headaches. A characteristic dry, nonproductive cough may occur that is reversible with discontinua-

tion of the therapy. A first-dose hypotensive effect can cause a significant decline in blood pressure. Other adverse effects include loss of taste, hyperkalemia, rash, pruritus, anemia, neutropenia, thrombocytosis, and agranulocytosis. In patients with severe heart failure whose renal function may depend on the activity of the renin-angiotensin-aldosterone system, treatment with ACE inhibitors may cause acute renal failure. ACE inhibitors tend to promote potassium resorption in the kidney, although they also promote sodium excretion due to their reduction of aldosterone secretion. For this reason, serum potassium levels should be monitored regularly. This is especially true when there is concurrent therapy with potassium-sparing diuretics, although many patients tolerate both types of drug therapy with no major problems. One rare, but potentially fatal, adverse effect is *angioedema.* This is a strong vascular reaction involving inflammation of submucosal tissues, which can progress to anaphylaxis.

Toxicity and Management of Overdose

The most pronounced symptom of an overdose of an ACE inhibitor is hypotension. Treatment is symptomatic and supportive and includes the administration of intravenous fluids to expand the blood volume. Hemodialysis is effective for the removal of captopril and lisinopril.

Interactions

Nonsteroidal antiinflammatory drugs (NSAIDs), such as ibuprofen, can reduce the antihypertensive effect of ACE inhibitors. The use of NSAIDs and ACE inhibitors may also predispose patients to the development of acute renal failure. Concurrent use of ACE inhibitors and other antihypertensives or diuretics can have hypotensive effects. Giving lithium and ACE inhibitors together can result in lithium toxicity. Potassium supplements and potassium-sparing diuretics, when administered with ACE inhibitors, may result in hyperkalemia. The monitoring of serum potassium levels becomes important in these cases. False-positive results on tests for acetone in the urine may occur in patients taking captopril.

Dosages

For information on the dosages for selected ACE inhibitors, see the Dosages table on p. 391.

DRUG PROFILES

◆ captopril

Captopril (Capoten) was the first ACE inhibitor to become available and is considered the prototypical drug for the class. Several large multicenter studies have shown its clinical efficacy in minimizing or preventing the left ventricular dilatation and dysfunction (also called *ventricular remodeling*) that can arise in the acute period after an

DOSAGES

Selected Antihypertensive Drugs: ACE Inhibitors and Angiotensin II Receptor Blockers

Drug (Pregnancy Category)	Pharmacologic Class	Usual Dosage Range	Indications
◆ captopril (Capoten, Capozide*) (C, first trimester; D, second and third trimesters)	ACE inhibitor	**Adult** PO: 25-150 mg bid-tid PO (Capozide*): Usual dosage 1-2 tabs/bid-tid or more based on ratio of the two drugs	Hypertension, heart failure Hypertension
enalapril (Vasotec, Vaseretic*) (C, first trimester; D, second and third trimesters)	ACE inhibitor	**Adult** PO: 10-40 mg/day as a single dose or in 2 equal doses PO: 10-20 mg bid as a single dose with digoxin and diuretic IV: 1.25 mg q6h over a 5-min period	Hypertension Heart failure Hypertension
◆ losartan (Cozaar) (C, first trimester; D, second and third trimesters)	Angiotensin II receptor blocker	**Adult** PO: 25-100 mg as a single dose or divided bid	Hypertension, heart failure

ACE, Angiotensin-converting enzyme; *IV*, intravenous; *PO*, oral.
*Fixed-combination tablet with hydrochlorothiazide.

MI and thereby improving the patient's chances of survival. It can also reduce the risk of heart failure in these patients and thus the need for subsequent hospitalizations for the treatment of heart failure. Because it has the shortest half-life of all of the currently available ACE inhibitors, it must be given three or four times a day. Recommended dosages are given in the table above.

PHARMACOKINETICS

Route	Onset of Action	Peak Plasma Concentration	Elimination Half-life	Duration of Action
PO	15 min	1-2 hr	2 hr	2-6 hr

enalapril

Enalapril (Vasotec) is the only ACE inhibitor currently marketed that is available in both oral and parenteral preparations. The parenteral formulation (enalaprilat) is an active drug. It offers the hemodynamic benefit of inhibiting ACE activity in an acutely ill patient who cannot tolerate oral medications. The other benefit to intravenous enalapril is that it does not require cardiac monitoring as do the intravenous beta-blockers and CCBs. Although its half-life is slightly longer than that of captopril, it may in some instances still have to be given twice a day. The oral form of enalapril differs from captopril in that it is a prodrug, and the patient must have a functioning liver for the drug to be converted into its active form. As with captopril, it has been shown in many large studies to improve a patient's chances of survival after an MI and to reduce the incidence of heart failure. Recommended dosages are given in the table above.

PHARMACOKINETICS

Route	Onset of Action	Peak Plasma Concentration	Elimination Half-life	Duration of Action
PO	1 hr	4-6 hr	2 hr	12-24 hr

ANGIOTENSIN II RECEPTOR BLOCKERS

ARBs are one of the newer classes of antihypertensives. The class includes Losartan (Cozaar), eprosartan (Teveten), valsartan (Diovan), irbesartan (Avapro), candesartan (Atacand), olmesartan (Benicar), and telmisartan (Micardis).

Mechanism of Action and Drug Effects

ARBs block the binding of AII to type 1 AII receptors. ACE inhibitors such as enalapril block conversion of AI to AII, but AII also may be formed by other enzymes that are not blocked by ACE inhibitors. For comparison, recall that ACE inhibitors block the breakdown of bradykinins and substance P, which accumulate and may cause adverse effects such as cough but might also contribute to the drugs' antihypertensive and cardiac and nephroprotective effects. Bradykinins are potent vasodilators and help to reduce blood pressure by dilating arteries and decreasing SVR.

In contrast to ACE inhibitors, ARBs affect primarily vascular smooth muscle and the adrenal gland. By selectively blocking the binding of AII to the type 1 AII receptors in these tissues, ARBs block vasoconstriction and the secretion of aldosterone. AII receptors have been found in other tissues throughout the body, but the effects of ARB blocking of these receptors is unknown.

Clinically, ACE inhibitors and ARBs appear to be equally effective for the treatment of hypertension. Both are well tolerated, but ARBs do not cause cough. There is evidence that ARBs are better tolerated and are associated with lower mortality after MI than ACE inhibitors. It is not yet clear whether ARBs are as effective as ACE inhibitors in treating heart failure (cardioprotective effects) or in protecting the kidneys, as in diabetes. Both types of drugs are contraindicated for use in the second or third trimester of pregnancy. Whether one or more of these drugs, particularly the newer drugs, could prove to have unique adverse effects with long-term use is unknown.

Indications

The therapeutic effects of ARBs are related to their potent vasodilating properties. They are excellent antihypertensives and adjunctive drugs for the treatment of heart failure. They may be used alone or in combination with other drugs such as diuretics in the treatment of hypertension or heart failure. The beneficial hemodynamic effect of ARBs is their ability to decrease SVR (a measure of afterload). Their use is rapidly growing, and more and more studies are verifying their beneficial effects. Currently these drugs are used primarily in patients who have been intolerant of ACE inhibitors.

Contraindications

The only usual contraindications to the use of ARBs are known drug allergy, pregnancy, and lactation. They should be used very cautiously in elderly patients and in patients with renal dysfunction because of increased sensitivity to its effects and risk for more adverse effects in these patients. As with other antihypertensives, blood pressure and apical pulse rate should be assessed before and during drug therapy.

Adverse Effects

The most common adverse effects of ARBs are upper respiratory infections and headache. Occasionally dizziness, inability to sleep, diarrhea, dyspnea, heartburn, nasal congestion, back pain, and fatigue can occur. Rarely, anxiety, muscle pain, sinusitis, weight gain, dyspnea, chest pain, cough, and insomnia can also occur. Hyperkalemia is much less likely to occur than with the ACE inhibitors.

Toxicity and Management of Overdose

Overdose may manifest as hypotension and tachycardia; bradycardia occurs less often. Treatment is symptomatic and supportive, and includes the administration of intravenous fluids to expand the blood volume.

Interactions

The drugs that interact with ARBs, the mechanism responsible, and the result of the interaction are summarized in Table 25-4. In addition, as is the case with ACE inhibitors, ARBs can promote hyperkalemia, especially when taken concurrently with potassium supplements (although this occurs much less frequently than with ACE inhibitors). Patients' individual chemistries vary widely, however, so monitoring of the serum potassium level is necessary for all patients. Potassium supplements may still be indicated for those patients with a tendency toward hypokalemia (whether acute or chronic).

Dosages

For information on the dosages for selected ARBs, see the table on p. 391.

TABLE 25-4 Angiotensin II Receptor Blockers: Drug Interactions

Drug	Mechanism	Result
Cimetidine	Competes for metabolism	Increased ARB effect
Lithium	Inhibits lithium elimination	Increased lithium concentrations
phenobarbital, rifampin	Increased metabolism	Decreased ARB effect

ARB, Angiotensin II receptor blocker.

DRUG PROFILE

◆ **losartan**

Losartan (Cozaar) has been shown to be beneficial in patients with hypertension and heart failure. Studies indicate that ARBs are better tolerated and produce a marginally lower mortality rate after MI than treatment with ACE inhibitors.

The use of losartan is contraindicated in patients who are hypersensitive to any component of this product. It should be used with caution in patients with renal or hepatic dysfunction and in patients with renal artery stenosis. Breast-feeding women should not take losartan, because it can cause serious adverse effects on the nursing infant. Recommended dosages are given in the table on p. 391.

PHARMACOKINETICS

Route	Onset of Action	Peak Plasma Concentration	Elimination Half-life	Duration of Action
PO	1 hr	6 hr	6-9 hr	24 hr

CALCIUM CHANNEL BLOCKERS

CCBs have been discussed in some detail in the two previous chapters on antidysrhythmic drugs (see Chapter 23) and antianginal drugs (see Chapter 24). As a class, they are used for several indications and have many beneficial effects and relatively few adverse effects. Their primary use is for the treatment of hypertension and angina. Their effectiveness in treating hypertension is related to their ability to cause smooth muscle relaxation by blocking the binding of calcium to its receptors, which thereby prevents contraction. Because of their effectiveness and safety, they have been added to the list of first-line drugs for the treatment of hypertension. Amlodipine (Norvasc) is the CCB most commonly used for hypertension. They are effective antidysrhythmics and they can prevent the cerebral artery spasms that can occur after a subarachnoid hemorrhage (nimodipine). They are also sometimes used in the treatment of Raynaud's disease and migraine headache. They are also used in combination with other drugs. Some examples are amlodipine/atorvastatin (Caduet), which is both an antihypertensive and a cholesterol-lowering drug (see Chapter 29); amlodipine/benazepril (Lotrel); amlodipine/olmesartan (Azar); and amlodipine/valsartan (Exforge).

DIURETICS

The diuretics are a highly effective class of antihypertensive drugs. They are listed as the current first-line antihypertensives in the *JNC 7* guidelines for the treatment of hypertension. They may be used as monotherapy (single-drug therapy) or in combination with drugs of other antihypertensive classes. Their primary therapeutic effect is decreasing the plasma and extracellular fluid volumes, which results in decreased preload. This leads to a decrease in cardiac output and total peripheral resistance, all of which decrease the workload of the heart. This large group of antihypertensives is discussed in detail in Chapter 26. The thiazide diuretics (e.g., hydrochlorothiazide) are the most commonly used diuretics for treatment of hypertension.

VASODILATORS

Vasodilators act directly on arteriolar and/or venous smooth muscle to cause relaxation. They do not work through adrenergic receptors.

Mechanism of Action and Drug Effects

Direct-acting vasodilators are useful as antihypertensive drugs because of their ability to directly elicit peripheral vasodilation. This results in a reduction in SVR. In general, the most notable effect of the vasodilators is their hypotensive effect. However, in recent years minoxidil (in its topical form) has also received increasing attention because of its effectiveness in restoring hair growth. This application is described further in Chapter 56. Diazoxide, hydralazine, and minoxidil work primarily through arteriolar vasodilation, whereas nitroprusside has both arteriolar and venous effects.

Indications

All of the vasodilators can be used to treat hypertension, either alone or in combination with other antihypertensives. Sodium nitroprusside and intravenous diazoxide are reserved for the management of hypertensive emergencies, in which blood pressure is severely elevated. Minoxidil in its topical form is used to restore hair growth.

Contraindications

Contraindications include known drug allergy and may also include hypotension, cerebral edema, head injury, acute MI, and coronary artery disease.

As mentioned in Chapter 22, vasodilating drugs may also be contraindicated in cases of heart failure that is secondary to diastolic dysfunction.

Adverse Effects

Undesirable effects of diazoxide include dizziness, headache, orthostatic hypotension, dysrhythmias, sodium and water retention, nausea, vomiting, acute pancreatitis (rare), and hyperglycemia in diabetic patients. These adverse effects have dramatically reduced the use of diazoxide. The adverse effects of hydralazine include dizziness, headache, anxiety, tachycardia, edema, nasal congestion, dyspnea, anorexia, nausea, vomiting, diarrhea, anemia, agranulocytosis, hepatitis, peripheral neuritis, systemic lupus erythematosus (SLE), and rash. Minoxidil adverse effects include T-wave electrocardiographic changes, pericardial effusion or tamponade, angina, breast tenderness, rash, and thrombocytopenia. Sodium nitroprusside effects include bradycardia, decreased platelet aggregation, rash, hypothyroidism, hypotension, methemoglobinemia, and, rarely, cyanide toxicity. Cyanide ions are a by-product of nitroprusside metabolism. Cyanide and thiocyanate toxicity are seen clinically when nitroprusside is used at high dosages for long periods of time and/or in patients with renal insufficiency.

Toxicity and Management of Overdose

The main symptom of diazoxide overdose or toxicity is hypotension, which can usually be controlled by placing the patient's bed in the Trendelenburg position. Sympathomimetics such as dopamine or norepinephrine may also be required. Hydralazine toxicity or overdose produces hypotension, tachycardia, headache, and generalized skin flushing. Treatment is supportive and symptomatic and includes the administration of intravenous fluids, digitalization if needed, and the administration of beta-blockers for the control of tachycardia.

Minoxidil overdose or toxicity can precipitate excessive hypotension. Treatment is supportive and symptomatic and includes the administration of intravenous fluids. Norepinephrine and epinephrine should not be used to reverse the hypotension because of the possibility of causing excessive cardiac stimulation.

The main symptom of sodium nitroprusside overdose or toxicity is excessive hypotension. This drug is normally administered only to patients receiving intensive care. Under these conditions the infusion rate is usually carefully titrated to immediately visible results on a cardiovascular monitor that provides constant measurements of blood pressure from centrally placed venous or arterial catheters. For this reason excessive hypotension is usually avoidable. When it does occur, discontinuation of the infusion has an immediate effect, because the drug is metabolized very rapidly (half-life of 10 minutes). Treatment for the hypotension is supportive and symptomatic; if necessary, pressor drugs can be infused to quickly raise blood pressure. The chemical structure of nitroprusside does contain cyanide groups, which are released upon its metabolism in the body and can result in cyanide or thiocyanate toxicity. As noted earlier, this usually occurs clinically when the drug is used at high dosages for prolonged periods and/or in patients with renal failure. Should this occur, treatment can be administered using a standard cyanide antidote kit that includes sodium nitrite and sodium thiosulfate for injection and amyl nitrite for inhalation.

Interactions

The incidence of drug interactions is low for the direct-acting vasodilators as a class. Hydralazine can produce additive hypotensive effects when given with adrenergic or other antihypertensive drugs.

Dosages

For dosage information for selected vasodilator drugs, see the Dosages table on p. 394.

DRUG PROFILES

◆ hydralazine

Hydralazine (Apresoline) is less commonly used now than when it first became available, but it is still effective for selected patients. It can be taken orally to treat routine cases of **essential hypertension.** It is also available in injectable form for hypertensive emergencies and is useful for patients who cannot tolerate oral therapy in the hospital. Hydralazine may be given intravenously without the need for cardiac monitoring. Contraindications, in addition to drug allergy, include coronary artery disease and mitral valve dysfunction, such as that related to childhood rheumatic fever. A new combination drug product is a tablet that contains both 37.5 mg of hydralazine and 20 mg of the antianginal drug isosorbide dinitrate (see Chapter 24). This drug combination is known as BiDil, and it is specifically indicated as an adjunct for treatment of heart failure in self-identified African American patients. This drug combination has been shown to improve patient survival and prolong time to hospitalization for heart failure in African American patient populations.

PHARMACOKINETICS

Route	Onset of Action	Peak Plasma Concentration	Elimination Half-life	Duration of Action
IV	5-20 min	30-45 min	2-8 hr	1-4 hr
PO	20-30 min	1-2 hr	2-8 hr	8 hr

DOSAGES

Selected Antihypertensive Drugs: Vasodilators

Drug (Pregnancy Category)	Pharmacologic Class	Usual Dosage Range	Indications
◆ hydralazine (Apresoline) (C)	Direct-acting peripheral vasodilators	**Pediatric** PO: 0.75-7.5 mg/kg/day to a max of 200 mg/day **Adult** PO: 10 mg qid for 2-4 days, followed by 25 mg qid for balance of week; second and subsequent weeks 50 mg qid, then adjust to lowest effective dose for maintenance IV: 20-40 mg prn	Hypertension
sodium nitroprusside (Nipride, Nitropress) (C)		**Pediatric and adult** IV: 0.25 mcg/kg/min	

IV, Intravenous; *PO,* oral.

DOSAGES

Miscellaneous Antihypertensive Drugs

Drug (Pregnancy Category)	Pharmacologic Class	Usual Dosage Range	Indications
aliskiren (Tekturna)	Direct renin inhibitor	150-300 mg daily	Hypertension
bosentan (Tracleer) (X)	Endothelin receptor antagonist	**Adult only** PO: Initial dose of 62.5 mg bid ×4 wk, then increase as tolerated to maintenance dose of 125 mg bid	Pulmonary artery hypertension in patients with moderate to severe heart failure
eplerenone (Inspra) (B)	Aldosterone receptor antagonist	**Adult only** PO: Initial dose of 50 mg once daily ×4 wk, then increase as tolerated to max dose of 50 mg bid	Hypertension and post-MI status (to improve post-MI survival in patients with stable heart failure)
treprostinol (Remodulin) (B)	Vasodilator and platelet aggregation inhibitor	**Adult only** Continuous subcutaneous infusion: 0.625-2.5 ng/kg/min	Pulmonary artery hypertension in patients with severe heart failure

MI, Myocardial infarction; *PO,* oral.

sodium nitroprusside

Sodium nitroprusside (Nitropress), like diazoxide, is normally used in the intensive care setting for severe hypertensive emergencies and is titrated to effect by intravenous infusion. Its use is contraindicated in patients with a known hypersensitivity to the drug, severe heart failure, and known inadequate cerebral perfusion (especially during neurosurgical procedures). See the table above for dosage information.

PHARMACOKINETICS

Route	Onset of Action	Peak Plasma Concentration	Elimination Half-life	Duration of Action
IV	Less than 2 min	2-5 min	2 min	1-10 min

MISCELLANEOUS ANTIHYPERTENSIVE DRUGS

DRUG PROFILES

Four newer medications exemplify some of the antihypertensive drugs most recently made available in the United States. These include eplerenone, bosentan, treprostinil, and aliskiren. All of these drugs are currently indicated for adult use only.

eplerenone

Eplerenone (Inspra) is currently the only drug in a new class of antihypertensive drugs called *selective aldosterone blockers.* It reduces blood pressure by blocking the actions of the hormone aldosterone at its corresponding receptors in the kidney, heart, blood vessels, and brain. Eplerenone is indicated for both routine treatment of hypertension and for post-MI heart failure. Its use is contraindicated in patients with known drug allergy, elevated serum potassium levels (higher than 5.5 mEq/L), or severe renal impairment and in those using a medication that inhibits the action of cytochrome P-450 enzyme 3A4. Many commonly used medications inhibit the action of this enzyme, including several antibiotic, antifungal, and antiviral drugs. The prescriber is advised to review the known drug interactions of all of the patient's concurrently used drugs before administering this medication. Recommended dosages are given in the Dosages table above.

bosentan

Bosentan (Tracleer) is also currently the single drug in a new drug class and works by blocking the receptors of the hormone endothelin. Normally this hormone acts to stimulate the narrowing of blood vessels by binding to endothelin receptors (ET_A and ET_B) in the endothelial (innermost) lining of blood vessels and in vascular smooth muscle. Bosentan reduces blood pressure by blocking this action. However, currently it is specifically indicated only for the treatment of pulmonary artery hypertension in patients with moderate to severe heart failure. It is available only through a limited distribution program directly from the manufacturer. Its use is contraindicated in patients with known drug allergy, pregnancy, or significant liver impairment, and in patients receiving concurrent drug therapy with cyclosporine or glyburide. Recommended dosages are given in the table on p. 394.

treprostinil

Treprostinil (Remodulin) lowers blood pressure through a combined mechanism of action by dilating both pulmonary and systemic blood vessels and by inhibiting platelet aggregation. Like bosentan, it is indicated specifically for treatment of pulmonary artery hypertension in patients with moderate to severe heart failure. Its only current contraindication is known drug allergy. It is also unique to date in being the only drug diluted to the nanogram level for administration. Recommended dosages are given in the table on p. 394.

aliskiren

Aliskiren (Tekturna) is a member of the newest class of antihypertensives, called *direct renin inhibitors*. It is used for the treatment of hypertension, either alone or in combination with other antihypertensive drugs. As a direct renin inhibitor, it blocks the conversion of angiotensinogen to AI, which then decreases the level of AII and activation of the renin-angiotensin-aldosterone system to further decrease the release of renin (see previous discussion on ACE inhibitors for more information on the renin-angiotensin-aldosterone sys-

tem). Before aliskiren is started, hypovolemia must be corrected and volume status must be carefully monitored in patients taking concurrent diuretics. Aliskiren is a pregnancy category D drug and must be stopped immediately if pregnancy is suspected or confirmed. Recommended dosages are given in the table on p. 394.

NURSING PROCESS

Over the last several decades, the diagnosis and treatment of hypertension has changed greatly from a stepped approach to a medical regimen that is now based on guidelines from the National Institutes of Health (issued in May 2003). These guidelines apply to adults aged 18 years and older and describe evaluation, classification, diagnosis, risk factors, identifiable causes, and blood pressure measurement techniques. One of the major differences in these guidelines, contained in *JNC 7*, is the creation of a "prehypertension" category, defined as a systolic blood pressure of 120 to 139 mm Hg and/or a diastolic blood pressure of 80 to 89 mm Hg. This is a change from previous guidelines and provides a more aggressive approach to the identification and subsequent management of the disease process, instead of a later diagnosis and treatment when multiple organ damage may be present. The nursing process discussion that follows provides both general and specific information related to the pharmacologic and nonpharmacologic treatment of all stages of hypertension.

EVIDENCE-BASED PRACTICE

Effects of Exercise on Blood Pressure in Those 55 Years of Age and Older

■ Review

The Senior Hypertension and Physical Exercise (SHAPE) study examined the effects of exercise on blood pressure in men and women 55 years of age or older with a diagnosis of mild hypertension. Those who participated in a 6-month exercise program showed greater reductions in diastolic (but not systolic) blood pressure than did subjects who did not exercise.

■ Type of Evidence

The participants were between 55 and 75 years of age, had systolic blood pressures (SBP) of 130 to 159 mm Hg or diastolic blood pressures (DBP) of 85 to 89 mm Hg, and were not taking any antihypertensive drugs. Fifty-three control subjects were asked to follow the standard recommendations for physical activity contained in the National Institute of Aging guidelines for exercise. They were also given dietary advice based on the American Heart Association Step 1 diet. In addition to receiving the same standard advice regarding diet and activity, the experimental group followed an exercise regimen based on the American College of Sports Medicine guidelines and participated in three supervised exercise sessions per week that included both resistance and aerobic training. Fifty-one individuals completed the exercise program between 1999 and 2003. The nonexercise group was not a true control group because these subjects may have made unreported lifestyle changes in response to the diet and exercise advice they received. SHAPE investigators were based at the Johns Hopkins School of Medicine and the National Institute on Aging.

■ Results of Study

The study reported significant mean decreases in SBP and DBP of 5.3 and 3.7 mm Hg, respectively, in the exercise group and 4.5 and 1.5 mm Hg, respectively, in the control group. The mean decrease in DBP was significantly greater in the exercisers than in the control group, but the difference in SBP in the two groups was not statistically significant. There was no difference between men and women in blood pressure reductions. The investigators pointed out that the main reason the decrease in SBP in the exercise group was smaller than anticipated was that increased arterial stiffness contributes to systolic hypertension in older patients. This age-related change may not be amenable to modification by exercise.

■ Link of Evidence to Nursing Practice

For older patients with hypertension, exercise has always been considered to be a lifestyle change that may help to decrease both SBP and DBP. Although this study did not find a larger decrease in blood pressure in the group that participated in the exercise program, as had been anticipated, other benefits were noted in this group: improvement in aerobic ability and fitness, increased strength, increase in lean body mass, and decrease in overall and abdominal obesity. Improved body composition accounted for 8% of the reduction in SBP and 17% of the reduction in DBP among the exercisers. This study may be helpful in establishing the importance of exercise training as a means of improving cardiovascular health in older men and women, as suggested by the SHAPE investigators. More research is needed to demonstrate the benefits of lifestyle changes for individuals in all age groups so that patients with hypertension can be educated regarding the importance of nonpharmacologic and pharmacologic treatment regimens for management of hypertension.

Modified from Stewart KJ et al: Effect of exercise on blood pressure in older persons: a randomized controlled trial, *Arch Intern Med* 165:756-762, 2005.

Assessment

Before any antihypertensive drug is given to a patient, a thorough health history should be obtained and a head-to-toe physical assessment should be performed. Parameters to measure and document include blood pressure, pulse rate, respirations, and pulse oximetry readings. Results of laboratory tests—especially those indicative of fluid and electrolyte imbalances, heart function, heart tissue damage, renal function, and liver function—should be monitored. These laboratory tests may include the following: (1) serum sodium, potassium, chloride, magnesium, and calcium levels; (2) serum level of troponin, which is usually elevated within 4 to 6 hours after a heart attack begins and may be a reliable indicator up to 14 days after a heart attack; (3) renal function studies, including BUN level and serum and urinary creatinine levels; and (4) hepatic function studies, including serum levels of ALT and AST.

Laboratory tests will most likely be complemented by more sophisticated scans and imaging studies. Noninvasive ophthalmoscopic examination of the eye structures (e.g., optic nerve, optic disk, vessels) by a professionally trained health care practitioner (e.g., nurse practitioner, physician assistant, physician, ophthalmologist, optometrist) allows easy visualization of the structures impacted by hypertension. If hypertensive retinopathy is present, the examination will reveal narrowing of blood vessels in the eye, oozing of fluid from these blood vessels, spots on the retina, swelling of the macula and optic nerve, and/or bleeding in the back of the eye. These problems may be prevented by controlling the blood pressure or treating hypertension with appropriate follow-up once it is diagnosed.

The nurse must also assess for conditions, factors, or variables that may be underlying causes of a patient's hypertension, such as the following:

- Addison's disease
- Coarctation of the aorta
- Coronary heart disease
- Culture and race or ethnicity
- Cushing's disease
- Family history of hypertension
- Nicotine use
- Obesity
- Peripheral vascular disease
- Pheochromocytoma
- Renal artery stenosis
- Renal or liver insufficiency
- Stressful lifestyle

Many of these factors demand very cautious use of antihypertensive drugs. Cautions and contraindications have been discussed previously, but it should be emphasized that the use of these drugs in the elderly and those with chronic illnesses raises special concerns because of further compromise of the physical condition of these patients due to uncontrolled or untreated hypertension or the adverse effects of antihypertensives (e.g., fluid loss, dehydration, electrolyte imbalances, hypotension). For a complete listing of adverse effects as well as drug interactions associated with antihypertensives, see the pharmacology section of this chapter.

Use of *alpha-adrenergic agonists* demands close assessment of the patient's blood pressure, pulse rate, and weight before and during treatment because of their strong vasodilating properties and subsequent hypotensive adverse effects. These drugs may also be associated with fluid retention and edema, and thus there is a need for assessment of heart and breath sounds as well as intake and output, and examination for dependent edema and fluid retention. The *alpha-adrenergic antagonists* should also be used cautiously, because of the potential for hypotension-induced dizziness and syncope. The use of either of these groups of drugs requires close assessment of all parameters, especially in the elderly or other patients with preexisting dizziness or syncope, or a debilitated state. With doxazosin, first-dose orthostatic hypotension may occur within 2 to 6 hours; therefore, careful assessment of blood pressures (supine and standing) and measurement of corresponding pulse rates are needed before the first dose and 2 to 6 hours afterward, as well as with any subsequent increase in the dosage. When any antihypertensive drug is used, blood pressures and pulse rates (supine and standing) should be measured, and assessment for cautions, contraindications, and drug interactions should be performed. *Centrally acting alpha-blockers* require additional assessment of white blood cell counts, serum potassium and sodium levels, and level of protein in the urine (to identify proteinuria). The route of administration specified in the drug order should also be noted, because concerns differ depending on the specific route (e.g., skin sites must be assessed for readiness for transdermal application of a drug, such as clonidine).

Beta-blockers and their mechanisms of action are important to remember before these drugs are administered to a patient because of the risk for complications in certain patient populations. If the drug is a nonselective beta-blocker, it blocks both beta$_1$ and beta$_2$ receptors and will have both cardiac and respiratory effects, whereas if a drug is only a beta$_1$-blocking drug, the cardiac system will be affected (pulse rate and blood pressure will decrease) but there will be no beta$_2$ effects, which limits any concern regarding respiratory problems (e.g., bronchoconstriction). Therefore, if a patient needs a beta-blocker but has restrictive airway problems nonselective beta-blockers should be chosen (to avoid bronchoconstriction). A beta$_1$-specific blocker should be used to avoid a negative impact on the lungs. If there is no history of respiratory illness or concerns, however, the nonselective beta-blockers may be very effective as antihypertensives. In addition, for patients with heart failure, it is important to understand that beta-blockers also have a negative inotropic effect on the heart (decreased contractility); their use would lead to worsening of heart failure, which calls for a completely different class of antihypertensive.

With the use of beta blockers, assessment should include measurement of blood pressure and apical pulse rate immediately before each dose; if the systolic blood pressure is less than 90 mm Hg or the pulse rate is less than 60 beats/min, the prescriber should be notified because of the risk of adverse effects (e.g., hypotension, bradycardia). In such cases the drug would usually be withheld, as ordered or per protocol. These blood pressure and pulse rate parameters are also applicable with use of other antihypertensives. Breath sounds and heart sounds should also be assessed before and during drug therapy.

PREVENTING MEDICATION ERRORS

Oral Nimodipine Given Intravenously

The Institute for Safe Medication Practices (ISMP) reports that oral nimodipine has been given intravenously, which resulted in patient death on several occasions.

Oral nimodipine comes in capsule form, and the drug's manufacturer indicates in the product labeling that the drug may be extracted from the capsule into a syringe, using an 18-gauge needle, and then administered via an enteric tube to patients who cannot swallow the drug. Using a parenteral syringe for an oral dose is potentially dangerous, however, as noted by the ISMP in a newsletter article dated August 25, 1999.

One fatal incident occurred when the pharmacy dispensed the nimodipine capsules without knowing that the patient could not swallow and thus did not provide instructions on how to prepare the capsule contents for feeding tube administration. The nurse used a parenteral syringe to draw up the medication from the capsule, and the dose was later administered into an intravenous (IV) line instead of the feeding tube. As a result, the patient died.

Many procedures can be used to prevent inadvertent IV administration of oral solutions. The pharmacy can prepare oral doses of nimodipine in amber oral syringes, labeling the syringes with a "use by" date, the notation "For Oral Use Only," and the drug information. The pharmacy should also communicate to the nurse the potential danger of inadvertent IV injection of this drug. It is also important for the nurse to communicate to the pharmacy that a given patient is unable to swallow oral doses so that the correct dosage form is sent for administration. Most importantly, parenteral syringes should *never* be used to prepare and administer oral medications.

For more information, see Institute for Safe Medication Practices: ISMP medication safety alert: take steps to avoid inadvertent IV administration of nimodipine, 2005, available at *http://www.ismp.org/Newsletters/acutecare/articles/20050728_1.asp.*

The use of *ACE inhibitors* requires assessment of blood pressure, apical pulse rate, and respiratory status (because of the adverse effect of a dry, hacking, chronic cough). Blood pressure should be taken immediately before initial and subsequent doses of the drug so that extreme fluctuations may be identified early. Serum potassium, sodium, and chloride levels should also be assessed. Tests of baseline cardiac functioning will most likely be ordered prior to initiation of therapy. Because of the potential adverse effects of neutropenia and other blood disorders, a complete blood count should be performed before and during therapy, as ordered. *Angiotensin receptor blockers (ARBs)* should be used very cautiously in elderly patients and in patients with renal dysfunction. These patients have shown increased sensitivity to the drug's effects and increased risk for adverse effects.

Vasodilators require baseline neurologic assessment, with attention to level of consciousness and cognitive ability. These drugs should be used with extreme caution with the elderly, because they are more sensitive to the drugs' blood pressure–lowering effects and consequently experience more problems with hypotension, dizziness, and syncope. See Chapters 23, 24, and 26 for discussion of other antihypertensives.

In summary, many assessment parameters are similar for the various groups of antihypertensives. The difference in the level of assessment depends on the drug's impact on blood pressure as well as the individual's response to the medication and any preexisting illness or condition. Other factors to be assessed in any patient receiving these drugs, as well as most other drugs, include the patient's cultural background, racial or ethnic group, reading level, learning needs, developmental and cognitive status, financial status, mental health status, available support systems, and overall physical health. Patients should always be encouraged to learn how to assess and monitor themselves and their individual responses to drug therapy.

Nursing Diagnoses

- Deficient knowledge related to new prescribed drug regimen and lack of familiarity with medications and lifestyle changes associated with the use of antihypertensives
- Noncompliance with drug therapy related to lack of familiarity with or acceptance of the disease process
- Sexual dysfunction related to adverse effects of some antihypertensive drugs
- Acute pain related to headache as an adverse effect of drug therapy
- Ineffective tissue cerebral and peripheral perfusion related to the impact of the hypertensive disease process and/or possible severe hypotensive adverse effects associated with antihypertensive drug therapy
- Excess fluid volume related to adverse effects of fluid retention associated with some antihypertensive drugs
- Imbalanced nutrition, less than body requirements, related to the drug's adverse effects of impaired taste or loss of appetite
- Constipation related to the adverse effects of antihypertensive drugs
- Risk for injury (e.g., possible falls) related to possible antihypertensive drug–induced orthostatic hypotension with dizziness and syncope
- Risk for injury (e.g., possible falls) related to possibly antihypertensive drug–induced CNS adverse effects such as paresthesia, sedation, tremors, weakness, and seizures
- Risk for injury to mucous membranes related to the adverse effects of decreased saliva production and dry mouth associated with antihypertensive drug therapy
- Disturbed body image related to the undesired adverse effects associated with the use of antihypertensives, such as impotence, sexual dysfunction, weight gain, and fatigue

Planning

Nursing goals for antihypertensive therapy should focus on educating the patient and his or her family on the need for adequate management to prevent end-organ damage. These goals include making sure the patient understands the nature of the disease, its symptoms and treatment, and the importance of adhering to the treatment regimen. The patient must also come to terms with the diagnosis as well as with the fact that there is no cure for the disease and treatment will be lifelong. The influence of chronic illness and the importance of nonpharmacologic therapy, stress reduction, and follow-up care must also be emphasized. The nurse needs to plan for ongoing assessment of blood pressure, weight, diet, exercise, smoking habits, alcohol intake, compliance with therapy, and sexual function in the patient receiving therapy for hypertension.

Goals

- Patient takes the drug exactly as prescribed.
- Patient experiences relief of symptoms for which the medication was prescribed (e.g., a decrease in blood pressure).
- Patient demonstrates adequate knowledge about the use of the specific medication, its adverse effects, and the appropriate dosing at home.
- Patient is free of self-injury resulting from adverse effects of drug therapy.
- Patient states the rationale for and importance of antihypertensive therapy.
- Patient describes measures to implement to decrease the impact of the adverse effects of antihypertensive therapy.
- Patient reports any change in sexual patterns and function, bowel pattern changes, and activity intolerance.
- Patient remains compliant with the therapy regimen.

Outcome Criteria

- Patient states the risks and complications of potent antihypertensive drugs, such as tremors, decreased sweating, tachycardia, and hypotension.
- Patient states conditions to report to the prescriber, such as syncope and chest pain.
- Patient states the importance of lifelong adherence to the drug regimen for hypertension to decrease end-organ damage and complications.
- Patient follows instructions to change position slowly, monitor blood pressure, keep follow-up appointments with the prescriber, and maintain a journal to help monitor the effects of therapy.
- Patient communicates openly with nurses and other members of the health care team regarding the disease, its treatment, and any concerns related to changes in body image.
- Patient reports to the prescriber immediately any pitting edema of the feet, hands, or sacral area or a weight gain of 2 pounds or more within 24 hours or 5 pounds or more in 1 week.
- Patient maintains normal nutritional status through adherence to a prescribed diet high in fiber and fluids and avoidance of alcohol.

Implementation

Nursing interventions may help patients achieve stable blood pressure while minimizing adverse effects during treatment with antihypertensives. Many patients have problems complying with treatment because the disease itself is silent or without symptoms. Because of this, some patients are unaware of their increased blood pressure or think that if they do not feel bad there is nothing wrong with them, which poses many problems for treatment. Also, the antihypertensives are often associated with multiple adverse effects that may impact patients' self-concept and/or sexual integrity. These adverse effects may lead patients to abruptly stop taking the medication. It is important to inform patients that any abrupt withdrawal is a serious concern because of the risk of developing rebound hypertension. Rebound hypertension is characterized by a sudden and very high elevation of blood pressure. This places the patient at risk for a cerebrovascular accident or other cerebral or cardiac adverse events. It is important to understand that with *all* antihypertensives there is a risk of rebound hypertension (with abrupt withdrawal), and prevention of this through patient educa-

CASE STUDY

Aliskiren for Hypertension

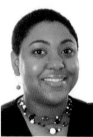

Hypertension was diagnosed in Gina S., who is 30 years old. Both her mother and her sister have hypertension, and both were also in their thirties when it was diagnosed. Gina's most current blood pressure reading is 150/96 mm Hg, and for this reason the nurse practitioner has recommended therapy with aliskiren (Tekturna), light exercise in the form of walking, and relaxation therapy. After 1 month of therapy, Gina's blood pressure is 145/86 mm Hg. Stress reduction has been the biggest obstacle in her treatment, because she is a lawyer with a prominent law firm and has found that her blood pressure is consistently elevated (160/100 mm Hg) whenever she measures it at work. At this follow-up visit, she is also given a prescription for a diuretic to help with her blood pressure control.

© Flashon Studio

1. How does aliskiren reduce blood pressure?
2. What precautions should Gina be aware of while taking this drug?
3. Gina states that she and her husband are planning to start a family in a year. What should you, as her nurse, tell her about pregnancy and therapy with aliskiren?
4. What lifestyle changes would you, as her nurse, recommend that she make and, even more important, what information would you give her to help her change her lifestyle and more effectively reduce the stress in her life?

For answers, see *http://evolve.elsevier.com/Lilley.*

tion is critical to patient safety. Other interventions related to each major group of drugs are discussed in the following paragraphs. See the Patient Teaching Tips for more information.

Because of the potential for drug-related orthostatic hypotensive effects, patients taking *alpha-adrenergic agonists* will need to monitor their blood pressure and pulse rate at home or else have these parameters measured for them by a family member who has received instructions or by local fire department, rescue, or emergency medical personnel or another health care provider. The blood pressure machines found in grocery stores do not provide as accurate readings as measurement in the aforementioned ways. *Alpha-adrenergic antagonist drugs* are associated with first-dose syncope, so to avoid injury, patients must be told to remain supine for the first dose of the drug. More than likely, these drugs will be prescribed to be given at bedtime to allow the patient to sleep through the drug's first-dose syncope. It may take 4 to 6 weeks for the drug to achieve its full therapeutic effects, so education about delayed onset of action and bedtime dosing is important to avoid injury. The patient should also receive continued monitoring for dizziness, syncope, edema, and other adverse effects (e.g., shortness of breath, exacerbation of preexisting cardiac disorders). Diuretics may be ordered as adjunctive therapy to minimize the adverse effects of edema, but they may lead to more dizziness and electrolyte problems. *Centrally acting alpha-blockers* require the same type of nursing interventions as other alpha-blockers; however, as their name indicates, the mechanism of action of these drugs is central, so adverse effects are often more pronounced (e.g., hypotension, sedation, bradycardia, edema). See the Patient Teaching Tips for more information.

The *beta-blockers* are either nonselective (block both $beta_1$ and $beta_2$ receptors; e.g., propranolol) or cardioselective (block mainly $beta_1$ receptors; e.g., atenolol). With any beta-blocker, careful adherence to the drug regimen is critical to patient safety. Patients taking beta-blockers may experience an exacerbation of respiratory diseases such as asthma, bronchospasm, and chronic obstructive pulmonary disease (because of increased broncho-constriction due to $beta_2$ blocking) or an exacerbation of heart failure because of the drug's negative inotropic effects (decreased contractility due to $beta_1$ blocking). Instructions about reporting adverse effects and instructions for taking blood pressure and pulse rates must be clear and concise. If a $beta_1$-blocker causes shortness of breath, it is most likely due to edema and/or exacer-bation of heart failure. Any dizziness, depression, confusion, or unusual bleeding or bruising should also be reported to the pre-scriber immediately. See the Patient Teaching Tips for more in-formation.

ACE inhibitors must also be taken exactly as prescribed. If angioedema occurs, the prescriber should be contacted immedi-ately. If the drug must be discontinued, weaning is recommended (as with all antihypertensives) to avoid rebound hypertension. Serum sodium and potassium levels should be monitored during therapy. Serum potassium levels increase as an adverse effect of these drugs, resulting in hyperkalemia and possible complica-tions. Impaired taste may occur as an adverse effect and last up to 2 to 3 months after the drug has been discontinued. It is also important to educate the patient that it takes several weeks to see the full therapeutic effects and that potassium supplements should not be used with these drugs (due to the adverse effect of hyperkalemia).

Angiotensin receptor blockers (ARBs) must also be taken ex-actly as prescribed. They are often tolerated best with meals, as with many antihypertensives. The dosage should not be changed nor the medication discontinued except on the order of the pre-scriber. With ARBs, if the patient has hypovolemia or hepatic dysfunction, the dosage may need to be reduced. A diuretic such as hydrochlorothiazide may be ordered in combination with an ARB for patients who have hypertension with left ventricular hypertrophy. Losartan is also an option for patients at risk for stroke and for those who are hypertensive and have left ventricu-lar hypertrophy. Most importantly, with ARBs, any unusual shortness of breath, dyspnea, weight gain, chest pain, or palpita-tions should be reported to the prescriber immediately.

Nursing considerations for *vasodilators* are similar to those for other antihypertensives; however, the impact of the vasodila-tors on blood pressure may be more drastic, depending on the specific drug and dosage. Hydralazine given by injection may result in reduced blood pressure within 10 to 80 minutes after administration and requires very close monitoring of the patient. With hydralazine, SLE may be an adverse effect if the patient is taking more than 200 mg/day orally. If signs and symptoms of SLE occur, such as glomerulonephritis, photosensitivity, charac-teristic skin rashes, CNS changes, or various blood dyscrasias (hemolytic anemia, leukopenia, thrombocytopenia), the drug should be discontinued, the prescriber should be contacted im-mediately, and the patient should be closely monitored. Electro-cardiographic changes, cardiovascular inadequacies, and hypo-tension may have pronounced effects on the patient's cardiac status, and therefore the drug should *never* be given without ad-equate monitoring and frequent assessment. Pyridoxine may help to diminish the adverse effect of peripheral neuritis.

Sodium nitroprusside must always be diluted per manufactur-er's guidelines. Because this drug is a potent vasodilator, it may lead to extreme decreases in the patient's blood pressure. Close monitoring is therefore important to prevent further complications. Severe drops in blood pressure may lead to irreversible ischemic injury and even death. The nurse must remember that sodium ni-troprusside should never be infused at the maximum dose rate for more than 10 minutes. If this drug does not control a patient's blood pressure after 10 minutes, it will most likely be ordered to be discontinued. To help prevent complications of cyanide and thio-cyanate toxicity, the nurse should (1) dilute the medication prop-erly and avoid use of any solution that has turned blue, green, or red; (2) infuse only using a volumetric infusion pump, not through ordinary intravenous sets; (3) continuously monitor blood pressure during the infusion (often by invasive measures); and (4) when more than 500 mcg/kg of sodium nitroprusside is administered at a rate faster than 2 mcg/kg/min, be aware that this may result in production of cyanide at a faster rate than it can be eliminated by the patient unaided. (See the Laboratory Values Related to Drug Therapy box on p. 400 for more information.)

Calcium channel blockers and related nursing interventions are discussed only briefly here, because these drugs are covered in other chapters. Drugs like enalapril are to be taken exactly as prescribed with a warning to the patient not to puncture, open, or crush the extended-release or sustained-release tablets and cap-sules. The nurse must be aware that CCBs are negative inotropic drugs (decrease cardiac contractility), because this action may induce more signs of heart failure if these drugs are given with drugs that are used to increase cardiac contractility, such as digi-talis glycosides. Monitoring of blood pressure and pulse rate before and during therapy will aid in prevention or early detec-tion of any problems related to the negative inotropic effects, negative chronotropic effects (decreased heart rate), and negative dromotropic effects (decreased conduction).

The nurse must remember always to base nursing interven-tions on a thorough assessment and plan of care that also includes consideration of the patient's cultural and ethnic group. This is particularly important with antihypertensives, because research studies have documented differences in responses to antihyper-tensives among different racial and ethnic groups. Some ethnic groups respond less favorably to certain drugs than to others. As for patients with any disease, patients with hypertension must be treated with respect and with an appreciation for a holistic ap-proach to health care in which all physical, psychosocial, and spiritual needs are taken into consideration (see Cultural Implica-tions box on p. 000). In summary, some educational information to be conveyed to the patient has been mentioned for particular groups of drugs or specific drugs. The nurse must remember that patient education is of critical importance and plays an important role in ensuring adherence to the drug regimen and in decreasing the incidence of problems related to these medications.

Evaluation

Because patients with hypertension are at high risk for cardiovas-cular injury, it is critical for them to adhere to both their pharma-cologic and nonpharmacologic treatment regimens. Monitoring patients for the adverse effects (e.g., orthostatic hypotension, diz-

LABORATORY VALUES RELATED TO DRUG THERAPY

Sodium Nitroprusside

Laboratory Test	Normal Ranges	Rationale for Assessment
Serum methemoglobin and serum cyanide levels	Normally there are no detectable amounts with appropriate drug levels of sodium nitroprusside	Use of sodium nitroprusside may be associated with sequestration of hemoglobin as methemoglobin. The appearance of this clinically significant adverse effect of methemoglobinemia is rare (less than 10% of cases). For a patient receiving this drug at the maximum rate of 10 mcg/kg/min, 16 or more hours would be required for the patient to reach a total accumulated dose of 10 mg/kg, so serum laboratory testing is used to measure the amount of methemoglobin. One significant clinical sign of this adverse effect is impaired oxygen delivery despite adequate cardiac output. When the sequestration is diagnosed, the treatment of choice is 1 to 2 mg/kg of methylene blue given intravenously over several minutes to allow binding of the metabolic by-product of cyanide to methemoglobin as cyanmethemoglobin, but this should be given only as ordered and with extreme caution. In addition, sodium nitroprusside may lead to toxic reactions, even at dosages that are within the recommended ranges. Toxic reactions are manifested by extreme hypotension, cyanide toxicity, or thiocyanate toxicity. Cyanide assays are performed to detect cyanide in body fluids, but the results of this test are difficult to interpret and so it is not the most reliable method of monitoring. Other laboratory tests that may be helpful in diagnosing cyanide toxicity are alterations of acid-base balance and venous oxygen concentrations. Actual cyanide levels in the blood may lag behind peak cyanide levels by an hour or longer. Signs of thiocyanate toxicity include ringing of the ears (tinnitus), miosis, and hyperreflexia as well as methemoglobinemia.

ziness, fatigue) and toxic effects of the various types of antihypertensive drugs helps the nurse to identify potentially life-threatening complications. The most important aspect of the evaluation process is collecting data and monitoring patients for evidence of controlled blood pressure. Blood pressure should be maintained at values lower than the parameters established by the Joint National Committee or below the levels set by the Joint National Committee for "prehypertension," namely, a systolic blood pressure of 120 to 139 mm Hg and/or a diastolic blood pressure of 80 to 89 mm Hg. If compelling indications are present, such as diabetes mellitus or kidney disease, then the blood pressure goal is often lower. Blood pressure should be monitored at periodic intervals, and patient education about self-monitoring is very important to the safe use of these drugs. Updated information on hypertension and its diagnosis, treatment, and evaluation is available at the National Heart, Lung, and Blood Institute website at *http://www.nhlbi.nih.gov/guidelines/hypertension.* In addition to measuring blood pressure, the prescriber will examine the fundus of the patient's eye. Changes in the fundus have been found to be a more reliable indicator of the long-term effectiveness of treatment than blood pressure readings because of the changes in the vasculature of the eye caused by high blood pressure. The patient must also be monitored continually for the development of end-organ damage and for the presence of the specific problems that the medication can cause. Male patients receiving antihypertensives should be counseled and constantly monitored for any sexual dysfunction. This is important, because the patient may experience sexual dysfunction, and if the patient is not expecting it, he or she may not report the problem and decide to stop taking the medication abruptly, which places the patient at high risk for rebound hypertension and possible stroke or other complications. Communication is critical in these situations. Follow-up visits to the prescriber are important for monitoring these and other adverse effects and checking patient adherence to the drug regimen. Therapeutic effects of antihypertensives in general include an improvement in blood pressure and in the disease process. Patients should report a return to a normal baseline level of blood pressure with improved energy levels and decreased signs and symptoms of hypertension, such as less edema, improved breath sounds, no abnormal heart sounds, capillary refill in less than 5 seconds, and less shortness of breath (dyspnea). Adverse effects for which to monitor include all of the specific adverse effects discussed in the pharmacology section of the chapter as well as those described for each group of drugs earlier in the nursing process section.

PATIENT TEACHING TIPS

Antihypertensives in General

- Medications should be taken exactly as ordered with avoidance of doubling up or omitting doses.
- Successful therapy requires adherence to the medication regimen as well as to any dietary restrictions (e.g., decreasing consumption of fatty or high-cholesterol foods).
- The patient should always monitor stress levels and use biofeedback, imagery, and/or relaxation techniques or massage, as needed. Exercise, if approved by the prescriber, may also help in the management of hypertension and serves to relieve stress; supervised, prescribed exercise is usually ordered.
- The importance of safety and the need to avoid smoking and excessive alcohol intake as well as excessive exercise, hot climates, saunas, hot tubs, and hot environments should be emphasized. Heat may precipitate vasodilation and lead to worsening of hypotension with the risk of fainting and injury to self.
- Frequent laboratory tests may be needed for the duration of therapy, so the importance of keeping follow-up appointments must be emphasized to the patient.
- All medications should be kept out of the reach of children because of the potential for extreme toxicity. If a transdermal patch is used, the patient should be taught to check periodically to make sure the patch is in place and intact. There have been cases in which a patch that was placed on an adult later dropped off and was accidentally picked up on the skin of a crawling infant, with severe consequences.
- Encourage the wearing of a medical alert bracelet or necklace and to carry a medical identification card specifying the patient's diagnosis, noting allergies, and listing all medications (e.g., prescribed drugs, over-the-counter medications, herbals, vitamins, and supplements). The same information should be kept in a visible location in the patient's car as well as in the patient's home on the refrigerator for emergency medical personnel.
- It is recommended that the patient's weight be measured daily each morning before breakfast, at the same time and with the same amount of clothing worn. This information should be recorded in a daily journal along with blood pressure readings. The patient should be instructed to report to the prescriber an increase in weight by 2 pounds or more over a 24-hour period or 5 pounds or more in 1 week.
- Blood pressure should be recorded, including postural blood pressures. The patient should be sure he or she feels comfortable in taking his or her own blood pressure and pulse rate. The patient should practice as needed and should never hesitate to ask for assistance.
- The patient should inform all health care providers (e.g., dentist, surgeon) that he or she is taking an antihypertensive drug.
- Encourage careful, purposeful and cautious changing of positions because of the possible adverse effect of postural hypotension and associated risk for dizziness, lightheadedness, and possible fainting and falls.
- Adequate supply of antihypertensive medications should be kept on hand, especially while traveling.
- Scheduling of periodic eye examinations (e.g., every 6 months) should be emphasized because of the need to evaluate treatment effectiveness and the impact of hypertension on the vasculature of the eyes.

- With successful therapy, the patient's condition will improve; however, the patient should be cautioned not to stop taking the medication just because he or she is feeling better. Lifelong therapy is usually required.
- Saliva substitutes, use of sugar-free hard candy/gum, and forcing fluids (unless contraindicated) may help with dry mouth. Forcing fluids and increasing dietary fiber and roughage may help with preventing constipation. If it remains a problem, the prescriber should be contacted.
- Sexual dysfunction may occur with antihypertensives, so the patient should be encouraged to be open in reporting and discussing any problems or concerns. The patient should be told that, should this adverse effect occur, options are available to help alleviate the problem, such as combination therapy that allows lower dosages of drugs to be used, as well as a change to other types of antihypertensives. The patient should always report any problems to the prescriber, because solutions are usually available.
- Medications should never be stopped abruptly for any reason, including sexual problems, because of the risk of severe hypertensive rebound. Avoiding abrupt withdrawal of *any* of the antihypertensives is critical to patient safety.
- The patient should be aware that antihypertensives may lead to depression, so any change in emotional status should be reported to the prescriber.

Alpha-Adrenergic Agonists

- First-dose syncope is related to the alpha adrenergic agonists and so patients should avoid conditions/situations/drugs that would exacerbate this.
- The patient should be cautioned to be careful at first with driving and other activities requiring alertness. The patient may have to postpone driving and other activities until the drug-related drowsiness subsides.
- The patient should report any jaundice, unexplained fever, or flulike symptoms to the prescriber immediately.
- Because centrally acting blockers may also affect the patient's sexual functioning (e.g., causing impotence or decreased libido), the patient should be informed of these possible adverse effects and should be told to contact the prescriber if these effects are problematic for them. Other treatment options may be indicated.
- Transdermal patches of clonidine should be applied to nonhairy areas of the skin as ordered, and application sites should be rotated. All residual drug on the skin should be cleansed with a cloth soaked in lukewarm water before applying a new patch.

Beta-Blockers

- The patient should be cautioned to move and change positions slowly to avoid possible dizziness, fainting, and falls and should be instructed to report a pulse rate lower than 60 beats/min, any peripheral numbness, dizziness, weight gain (see earlier), or a systolic blood pressure of 90 mm Hg or lower to the prescriber.
- Prolonged sitting or standing and excessive physical exercise may also lead to exacerbation of hypotensive effects, so the patient should be encouraged to avoid these activities or counteract them with healthy practices such as pumping the feet up and down while sitting.

POINTS TO REMEMBER

- All antihypertensives in some way affect cardiac output. Cardiac output is the amount of blood ejected from the left ventricle and is measured in liters per minute.
- The major groups of antihypertensives are diuretics (see Chapter 26), alpha-blockers, centrally active alpha-blockers, beta-blockers, ACE inhibitors, vasodilators, CCBs, and ARBs.
- ACE inhibitors work by blocking a critical enzyme system responsible for the production of AII (a potent vasoconstrictor). They (1) prevent vasoconstriction caused by AII, (2) prevent aldosterone secretion and therefore sodium and water resorption, and (3) prevent the breakdown of bradykinin (a potent vasodilator) by AII.
- ARBs work by blocking the binding of angiotensin at the receptors; the end result is a decrease in blood pressure.
- Calcium channel blockers may be used to treat angina, dysrhythmias, and hypertension and help to reduce blood pressure by causing smooth muscle relaxation and dilatation of blood vessels. If calcium is not present, then the smooth muscle of the blood vessels cannot contract.

- A thorough nursing assessment should include finding out whether the patient has any underlying causes of hypertension, such as renal or liver dysfunction, a stressful lifestyle, Cushing's disease, Addison's disease, renal artery stenosis, peripheral vascular disease, or pheochromocytoma.
- The nurse should always assess for the presence of contraindications, cautions, and potential drug interactions before administering any of the antihypertensive drugs. Contraindications include a history of MI or chronic renal disease. Cautious use is recommended in patients with renal insufficiency or glaucoma. Drugs that interact with antihypertensive drugs include other antihypertensive drugs, anesthetics, and diuretics.
- Patients' hypertension should be managed by both pharmacologic and nonpharmacologic means. Patients should be encouraged to consume a diet low in fat, make any other necessary modifications in their diet (such as possibly decrease the intake of sodium and increase fiber intake), engage in regular supervised exercise, and reduce the amount of stress in their lives.

NCLEX EXAMINATION REVIEW QUESTIONS

1 The nurse is administering antihypertensive drugs to older adult patients. The nurse knows that which adverse effect is of most concern for these patients?
   a Dry mouth
   b Hypotension
   c Restlessness
   d Constipation
2 When giving antihypertensive drugs, the nurse must consider giving the first dose at bedtime for which class of drugs?
   a Alpha-blockers such as doxazosin (Cardura)
   b Diuretics such as furosemide (Lasix)
   c ACE inhibitors such as captopril (Capoten)
   d Vasodilators such as hydralazine (Apresoline)
3 A 56-year-old man started antihypertensive drug therapy 3 months earlier and is in the office for a follow-up visit. While the nurse is taking his blood pressure, he informs the nurse that he has had some problems with sexual intercourse. Which would be the most appropriate response by the nurse?
   a "Not to worry. Eventually, tolerance will develop."
   b "The physician can work with you on changing the dose and/ or drugs."

   c "Sexual dysfunction happens with this therapy, and you must learn to accept it."
   d "This is an unusual occurrence, but it is important to stay on your medications."
4 When a patient is being taught about the potential adverse effects of an ACE inhibitor, which of the following should the nurse mention as possibly occurring when this drug is taken to treat hypertension?
   a Hypokalemia
   b Nausea
   c Dry, nonproductive cough
   d Sedation
5 A patient has a new prescription for a beta-blocker. During a review of the patient's list of current medications, which would cause concern for a possible interaction with this new prescription? (Select all that apply.)
   a A benzodiazepine taken as needed for allergies
   b A multivitamin with iron taken daily
   c An oral anticoagulant taken daily
   d An opioid used for occasional severe pain
   e An NSAID taken as needed for headaches

1. b, 2. a, 3. b, 4. c, 5. a, d.

CRITICAL THINKING ACTIVITIES: BEST ACTION

1 Primary hypertension has been diagnosed in a 53-year-old woman who has a history of hypothyroidism and asthma. The nurse is reviewing the new orders and notes an order for carvedilol (Coreg) as part of the treatment for hypertension. Considering the patient's history, what is the nurse's best action at this time?
2 A 79-year-old woman has been admitted to the emergency department after experiencing severe headaches and "feeling faint." Upon admission, her blood pressure is measured as 286/190 mm Hg. A sodium nitroprusside infusion is started, and

the nurse is monitoring the patient closely. After 8 minutes of infusion, the nurse notes that the patient's blood pressure suddenly drops to 100/60. What is the best action of the nurse at this time?
3 During a follow-up appointment, a 58-year-old man is pleased to hear that his blood pressure is 118/64 mm Hg. He says, "I've been hoping to hear this good news! Now I can stop the medication, right?" What would be the nurse's best answer?

For answers, see *http://evolve.elsevier.com/Lilley.*

CHAPTER 26

Diuretic Drugs

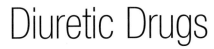

OBJECTIVES

When you reach the end of this chapter, you should be able to do the following:

1 Describe the normal anatomy and physiology of the renal system.

2 Briefly discuss the impact of the renal system on blood pressure regulation.

3 Describe how diuretics work in the kidneys and how they lower blood pressure.

4 Distinguish among the different classes of diuretics with regard to mechanisms of action, indications, dosages, routes of administration, adverse effects, toxicity, cautions, contraindications, and drug interactions.

5 Develop a nursing care plan that includes all phases of the nursing process for patients receiving diuretics.

e-Learning Activities

http://evolve.elsevier.com/Lilley

NCLEX Review Questions • Animations • Nursing Care Plans • Audio Glossary • Category Catchers • Medication Errors Checklists • IV Therapy Checklists • Calculators • Frequently Asked Questions • Content Updates • Supplemental Resources • Answers to Case Studies and Critical Thinking Activities

Drug Profiles

acetazolamide, p. 406
amiloride, p. 409
◆ furosemide, p. 407
◆ hydrochlorothiazide, p. 411

◆ mannitol, p. 417
metolazone, p. 411
◆ spironolactone, p. 410
triamterene, p. 410

◆ *Key drug.*

Glossary

Afferent arterioles The small blood vessels approaching the glomerulus (proximal part of the nephron). (p. 404)

Aldosterone A mineralocorticoid steroid hormone produced by the adrenal cortex that mediates the actions of the renal tubule in the regulation of sodium and potassium balance in the blood. (p. 404)

Ascites An abnormal intraperitoneal accumulation of fluid (defined as a volume of 500 mL or more) containing large amounts of protein and electrolytes. (p. 407)

Collecting duct The most distal part of the nephron between the distal convoluted tubule and the ureters, which lead to the urinary bladder. (p. 404)

Distal convoluted tubule The part of the nephron immediately distal to the ascending loop of Henle and proximal to the collecting duct. (p. 404)

Diuretics Drugs or other substances that tend to promote the formation and excretion of urine. (p. 403)

Efferent arterioles The small blood vessels exiting the glomerulus. At this point blood has completed its filtration in the glomerulus. (p. 404)

Filtrate The material that passes through a filter. In the case of the kidney, the filter is the glomerulus and the filtrate is the material extracted from the blood (normally liquid) that ultimately becomes urine. (p. 404)

Glomerular capsule The open, rounded, and most proximal part of the proximal convoluted tubule that surrounds the glomerulus and receives the filtrate from the blood. (p. 404)

Glomerular filtration rate (GFR) The volume of ultrafiltrate extracted per unit of time from the plasma flowing through the glomeruli of the kidney. (p. 404)

Glomerulus The cluster of kidney capillaries that marks the beginning of the nephron and is immediately proximal to the proximal convoluted tubule. (p. 404)

Loop of Henle The part of the nephron between the proximal and distal convoluted tubules. (p. 404)

Nephron The microscopic functional filtration unit of the kidney, consisting of (in anatomical order from proximal to distal) the glomerulus, proximal convoluted tubule, loop of Henle, distal convoluted tubule, and collecting duct, which empties urine into the ureters. There are approximately 1 million nephrons in each kidney. (p. 404)

Open-angle glaucoma A condition in which pressure is elevated in the eye because of obstruction of the outflow of aqueous humor, but access to the trabecular meshwork remains open. (p. 405)

Proximal convoluted (twisted) tubule The part of the nephron that is immediately distal to the glomerulus and proximal to the loop of Henle. (p. 404)

• • •

Anatomy and Physiology Overview

Diuretics are drugs that accelerate the rate of urine formation via a variety of mechanisms. The result is the removal of sodium and water from the body. Diuretics were discovered by accident when it was noticed that a mercury-based antibiotic had a very potent diuretic effect. All the major classes of diuretic drugs in use today were developed between 1950 and 1970, and they remain among the most commonly prescribed drugs in the world. The Seventh Joint National Committee on the Detection, Evaluation, and Treatment of Hypertension recently reaffirmed the role of diuretics, especially the thiazides, as the first-line drugs in the treatment of hypertension. The hypotensive activity of diuretics is due to many different mechanisms. They cause direct arteriolar dilation, which decreases peripheral vascular resistance. They also reduce extracellular fluid volume, plasma volume, and cardiac output, which may account for the decrease in blood pressure. They have long been the mainstay of therapy not only for hypertension but also for heart failure. Two of their advantages are their relatively low cost and their favorable safety profile. The main problem with their use is the metabolic adverse effects that can result from excessive fluid and electrolyte loss. These effects are usually dose related and are therefore controllable with dosage *titration* (careful adjustment).

This chapter reviews the essential properties and actions of the following important classes of diuretic drugs: carbonic anhydrase inhibitors, loop diuretics, osmotic diuretics, potassium-sparing diuretics, and thiazide and thiazide-like diuretics. Before these drug classes are discussed in detail, however, it is important to quickly review kidney function, because all diuretics work primarily in the kidneys.

The kidney plays a very important role in the day-to-day functioning of the body. It filters out toxic waste products from the blood while simultaneously conserving essential substances. This delicate balance between elimination of toxins and retention of essential chemicals is maintained by the **nephron.** The nephron is the main structural unit of the kidney, and each kidney contains approximately 1 million nephrons. Diuretics exert their effect in the nephron. The initial filtering of the blood takes place in the **glomerulus,** a cluster of capillaries surrounded by the **glomerular capsule.** The rate at which this filtering occurs is referred to as the **glomerular filtration rate (GFR),** and it is used as a gauge of how well the kidneys are functioning as filters. The GFR can be estimated mathematically by calculating creatinine clearance. This is typically calculated by hospital pharmacists and is used to adjust drugs based on the patient's renal function. Normally about 180 L of blood are filtered through the nephrons every day. The GFR, which can also be thought of as the rate at which blood flows into and out of the glomerulus, is regulated by the small blood vessels approaching the glomerulus (**afferent arterioles**) and the small blood vessels exiting the glomerulus (**efferent arterioles**). A mnemonic (memory aid) for remembering which arteriole is which is "*A* for *approach* and *afferent*" and "*E* for *exit* and *efferent*." Alterations in blood flow such as those that occur in a patient in shock can therefore have a dramatic effect on kidney (renal) function. Diuretics may have diminished effects in situations of low blood flow, because the kidney receives less blood, and therefore less diuretic gets to its site of action

The **proximal convoluted (twisted) tubule** or, more simply, *proximal tubule,* anatomically follows the glomerulus and returns 60% to 70% of the sodium and water from the filtered fluid back into the bloodstream. Blood vessels surround the nephrons and allow substances to be directly resorbed from or secreted into the bloodstream. This process is one of active transport that requires energy in the form of adenosine triphosphate molecules. The active transport of sodium and potassium ions back into the blood causes the passive resorption of chloride and water. The chloride ions (Cl^-) and water passively follow the sodium ions (Na^+) and, to a lesser extent, potassium ions (K^+) by osmosis. Another 20% to 25% of sodium is resorbed back into the bloodstream in the

ascending **loop of Henle.** Here it is the chloride that is actively resorbed, and the sodium passively follows it.

The remaining 5% to 10% of sodium resorption takes place in the **distal convoluted tubule,** often called simply the *distal tubule,* which anatomically follows the ascending loop of Henle. In the distal tubule, sodium is actively filtered in exchange for potassium or hydrogen ions, a process regulated by the hormone **aldosterone.** The **collecting duct** is the final common pathway for the **filtrate** that started in the glomerulus. It is here that antidiuretic hormone acts to increase the absorption of water back into the bloodstream, thereby preventing it from being lost in the urine. The entire nephron, along with the sites of action of the different classes of diuretics, is shown in Figure 26-1.

Pharmacology Overview

The various diuretics are classified according to their sites of action within the nephron, their chemical structure, and their diuretic potency. The sites of action of the various diuretics are determined by the way in which they affect the various solute (electrolyte) and water transport systems located along the nephron (see Figure 26-1). The commonly used classes of drugs and the individual drugs in these classes are listed in Table 26-1. The most potent diuretics are the loop diuretics, followed by mannitol, metolazone (a thiazide-like diuretic), the thiazides, and the potassium-sparing diuretics. The potency of these diuretics is a function of where they work in the nephron to inhibit sodium and water resorption. The more sodium and water they inhibit from resorption, the greater the amount of diuresis and therefore greater the potency.

CARBONIC ANHYDRASE INHIBITORS

Carbonic anhydrase inhibitors (CAIs) are chemical derivatives of sulfonamide antibiotics. As their name implies, CAIs inhibit the activity of the enzyme carbonic anhydrase, which is found in the kidneys, eyes, and other parts of the body. The site of action of the CAIs is the location of the carbonic anhydrase enzyme system along the nephron, primarily in the proximal tubule. Acetazolamide is the CAI most commonly used today,

Mechanism of Action and Drug Effects

The carbonic anhydrase system in the kidney is located just distal to the glomerulus in the proximal tubules, where roughly two thirds of all sodium and water is resorbed into the blood. In the proximal tubules, an active transport system operates that exchanges sodium for hydrogen ions. For sodium and thus water to be resorbed back into the blood, hydrogen must be exchanged for it. Without hydrogen, this cannot occur, and the sodium and water will be eliminated with the urine. Carbonic anhydrase helps to make the hydrogen ions available for this exchange. When its actions are inhibited by a CAI such as acetazolamide, little sodium and water can be resorbed into the blood and they are eliminated with the urine. The CAIs reduce the formation of hydrogen (H^+) and bicarbonate (HCO_3^-) ions from carbon dioxide and water by the noncompetitive, reversible inhibition of carbonic anhydrase activity. This results in a reduction in the availability of these ions, mainly hydrogen, for use by active electrolyte transport systems.

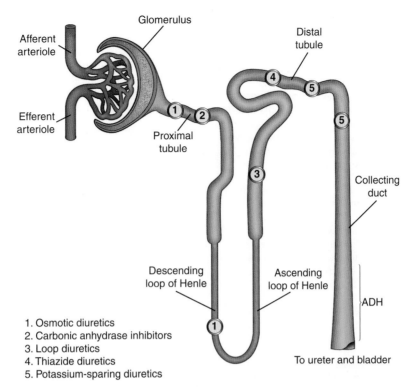

1. Osmotic diuretics
2. Carbonic anhydrase inhibitors
3. Loop diuretics
4. Thiazide diuretics
5. Potassium-sparing diuretics

FIGURE 26-1 The nephron and diuretic sites of action. *ADH,* Antidiuretic hormone.

TABLE 26-1 Classification of Diuretics

Class	Drugs
Carbonic anhydrase inhibitors	acetazolamide, dichlorphenamide, methazolamide
Loop diuretics	bumetanide, ethacrynic acid, furosemide, torsemide
Osmotic diuretics	Mannitol
Potassium-sparing diuretics	amiloride, spironolactone, triamterene
Thiazide and thiazide-like diuretics	bendroflumethiazide, chlorthalidone, chlorothiazide, hydrochlorothiazide, indapamide, metolazone

The reduction in the formation of bicarbonate and hydrogen ions can have many effects on other parts of the body. CAIs can induce metabolic acidosis, which is beneficial in the prevention of certain seizure conditions. In addition, CAIs can induce respiratory acidosis, and both the respiratory and metabolic acidosis can increase oxygenation during hypoxia by increasing ventilation, cerebral blood flow, and the dissociation of oxygen from oxyhemoglobin, all of which is usually beneficial to the patient. An undesirable effect of CAIs is elevation of the blood glucose level and glycosuria in diabetic patients. This may be due in part to CAI-enhanced potassium loss through the urine.

Indications

The therapeutic applications of CAIs include the treatment of glaucoma, edema, and high-altitude sickness and rare use as an antiepleptic. Although there are three CAIs, acetazolamide is the drug used most commonly.

CAIs are used as adjunct drugs in the long-term management of **open-angle glaucoma** that cannot be controlled by topical miotic drugs or epinephrine derivatives alone. Simply put, glaucoma is caused by the obstruction of the outflow of aqueous humor. When CAIs are given with the above-mentioned drugs, an increase in the outflow of aqueous humor results. They are also used short term in conjunction with miotics to lower intraocular pressure in preparation for ocular surgery in patients with acute ocular disorders or angle-closure glaucoma and as an adjunct in the treatment of secondary glaucoma.

Acetazolamide is also used to manage edema secondary to heart failure that has become resistant to other diuretics. However, as a class, CAIs are much less potent diuretics than loop diuretics or thiazides, and the metabolic acidosis they induce diminishes their diuretic effect in 2 to 4 days.

Acetazolamide is also effective in both the prevention and treatment of the symptoms of high-altitude sickness. These symptoms include headache, nausea, shortness of breath, dizziness, drowsiness, and fatigue.

Contraindications

Contraindications to the use of CAIs include known drug allergy, hyponatremia, hypokalemia, severe renal or hepatic dysfunction, adrenal gland insufficiency, and cirrhosis.

Adverse Effects

The more common undesirable effects of CAIs are metabolic abnormalities such as acidosis—which, as stated earlier, may be beneficial in some patients—and hypokalemia. Drowsiness, anorexia, paresthesias, hematuria, urticaria, photosensitivity, and melena (blood in the stool) can also occur.

Interactions

Because CAIs can cause hypokalemia, an increase in digitalis toxicity may occur when they are combined with this drug. Use with corticosteroids may also cause hypokalemia. The effects of amphetamines, carbamazepine, cyclosporine, phenytoin, and quinidine may be increased when these drugs are taken concurrently with CAIs.

Dosages

For information on the dosages of acetazolamide, see the following drug profile.

DRUG PROFILE

acetazolamide
Use of acetazolamide (Diamox) is contraindicated in patients who have shown a hypersensitivity to it as well as in those with significant liver or kidney dysfunction, low serum potassium or sodium levels, acidosis, or adrenal gland failure. Acetazolamide is available in both oral and parenteral forms. Pregnancy category C.

PHARMACOKINETICS

Route	Onset of Action	Peak Plasma Concentration	Elimination Half-life	Duration of Action
PO	1 hr	2-4 hr	10-15 hr	8-12 hr

LOOP DIURETICS

Loop diuretics (bumetanide, ethacrynic acid, furosemide, and torsemide) are very potent diuretics. Bumetanide, furosemide, and torsemide are chemically related to the sulfonamide antibiotics. Because they are structurally related to the sulfonamides,

they are often listed as contraindicated in sulfa-allergic patients. However, analysis of the literature indicates that cross-reaction is unlikely to occur. Loop diuretics are commonly given to patients with sulfa allergy with no problems; however, the nurse should always be aware of the potential of allergy.

Mechanism of Action and Drug Effects

Loop diuretics have renal, cardiovascular, and metabolic effects. These drugs act primarily along the thick ascending limb of the loop of Henle, blocking chloride and, secondarily, sodium resorption. They are also believed to activate renal prostaglandins, which results in dilatation of the blood vessels of the kidneys, the lungs, and the rest of the body (i.e., reduction in renal, pulmonary, and systemic vascular resistance). The beneficial hemodynamic effects of loop diuretics are a reduction in both the preload and central venous pressures, which are the filling pressures of the ventricles. These actions make them very useful in the treatment of the edema associated with heart failure, hepatic cirrhosis, and renal disease.

Loop diuretics are particularly useful when rapid diuresis is needed, because of their rapid onset of action. In addition, the diuretic effect lasts at least 2 hours. A distinct advantage they have over thiazide diuretics is that their diuretic action continues even when creatinine clearance decreases below 25 mL/min. This means that even when the function of the kidney diminishes, loop diuretics can still work. Because of their potent diuretic effect and the duration of this effect, loop diuretics are often effective when given in a single daily dose. This allows the renal tubule time to partially compensate for the potassium depletion and other electrolyte derangements that often accompany around-the-clock diuretic therapy. Despite this, the major adverse effect of loop diuretics is electrolyte disturbances. Prolonged administration of high dosages can also result in hearing loss stemming from ototoxicity, although this is rare.

Summary of Major Drug Effects of Loop Diuretics

Loop diuretics produce a potent diuresis and subsequent loss of fluid. The resulting decreased fluid volume leads to a decreased return of blood to the heart, or decreased filling pressures. This has the following cardiovascular effects:
- Reduces blood pressure
- Reduces pulmonary vascular resistance
- Reduces systemic vascular resistance
- Reduces central venous pressure
- Reduces left ventricular end-diastolic pressure

The metabolic effects of the loop diuretics are secondary to the electrolyte losses resulting from the potent diuresis. Major electrolyte losses include loss of sodium and potassium and, to a lesser extent, calcium. Changes in the plasma levels of insulin, glucagon, and growth hormone have also been observed in association with loop diuretic therapy.

Indications

Loop diuretics are used to manage the edema associated with heart failure and hepatic or renal disease, to control hypertension, and to increase the renal excretion of calcium in patients with hypercalcemia. As with certain other classes of diuretics, they may also be indicated in cases of heart failure resulting from diastolic dysfunction.

Contraindications

Contraindications to the use of loop diuretics include known drug allergy, hepatic coma, and severe electrolyte loss. Although allergy to sulfonamide antibiotics is listed as a contraindication, as noted earlier, analysis of the literature indicates that cross-reaction with the loop diuretics is unlikely to occur. Loop diuretics are commonly given to such patients in clinical practice.

Adverse Effects

Common undesirable effects of the loop diuretics are listed in Table 26-2. Hypokalemia is of serious clinical importance. Many times patients will receive potassium supplements along with furosemide. Furosemide can produce erythema multiforme, exfoliative dermatitis, photosensitivity, and in rare cases aplastic anemia. Torsemide may rarely cause blood disorders, including, thrombocytopenia, agranulocytosis, leukopenia, and neutropenia. It may also cause a severe skin disorder called *Stevens-Johnson syndrome.*

Toxicity and Management of Overdose

Electrolyte loss and dehydration, which can result in circulatory failure, are the main toxic effects of loop diuretics that require attention. Treatment involves electrolyte and fluid replacement.

Interactions

Loop diuretics exhibit both neurotoxic and nephrotoxic properties, and they produce additive effects when given in combination with drugs that have similar toxicities. The drug interactions are summarized in Table 26-3.

Loop diuretics also affect certain laboratory results. They cause increases in the serum levels of uric acid, glucose, alanine aminotransferase, and aspartate aminotransferase. Their combined use with a thiazide (especially metolazone) results in the blockade of sodium and water resorption at multiple sites in the nephron, a property referred to as *sequential nephron blockade,* which increases their effects. Nonsteroidal antiinflammatory drugs (NSAIDs) may impede the reduction in vascular resistance induced by loop diuretics because these two drug classes have opposite effects on prostaglandin activity.

Dosages

For the recommended dosages of loop diuretics, see the Dosages table on p. 408.

DRUG PROFILE

The currently available loop diuretics are bumetanide, ethacrynic acid, furosemide, and torsemide. Ethacrynic acid is rarely used clinically. As a class they are very potent diuretics, but potency varies for the different drugs. The equipotent doses of the drugs are as follows:

bumetanide	ethacrynic acid	furosemide	torsemide
1 mg	50 mg	40 mg	10 mg

◆ furosemide

Furosemide (Lasix) is by far the most commonly used loop diuretic in clinical practice and the prototypical drug in this class. It has all the therapeutic and adverse effects of the loop diuretics mentioned earlier. It is used in the management of pulmonary edema and the edema associated with heart failure, liver disease, ne-

TABLE 26-2 Loop Diuretics: Common Adverse Effects

Body System	Adverse Effects
Central nervous	Dizziness, headache, tinnitus, blurred vision
Gastrointestinal	Nausea, vomiting, diarrhea
Hematologic	Agranulocytosis, thrombocytopenia, neutropenia
Metabolic	Hypokalemia, hyperglycemia, hyperuricemia

TABLE 26-3 Loop Diuretics: Common Drug Interactions

Interacting Drug	Mechanism	Results
Aminoglycosides chloroquine Vancomycin	Additive effect	Increased neurotoxicity, especially ototoxicity
Corticosteroids Digoxin	Hypokalemia	Additive hypokalemia Increased digoxin toxicity
Lithium	Decrease in renal excretion	Increased lithium toxicity
NSAIDs	Inhibition of renal prostaglandins	Decreased diuretic activity
Sulfonylureas	Decrease in glucose tolerance	Hyperglycemia

NSAIDs, Nonsteroidal antiinflammatory drugs.

phrotic syndrome, and **ascites.** It has also been used in the treatment of hypertension, usually that caused by heart failure.

Furosemide use is contraindicated in patients who have shown a hypersensitivity to it or the sulfonamides; in infants and lactating women; and in patients with anuria, hypovolemia, or electrolyte depletion. As stated previously, although allergy to sulfonamides is listed as a contraindication, clinical evidence and practice has shown the use of furosemide in such patients to be safe and effective. It is available in oral form as a solution, tablets and an injectable form. Pregnancy category C. Recommended dosages are given in the Dosages table on p. 408.

PHARMACOKINETICS

Route	Onset of Action	Peak Plasma Concentration	Elimination Half-life	Duration of Action
IV	5 min	15 min	1-2 hr	2 hr
PO	30-60 min	1-2 hr	1-2 hr	6-8 hr

OSMOTIC DIURETICS

The osmotic diuretics include mannitol, urea, organic acids, and glucose. Mannitol, a nonabsorbable solute, is the most commonly used of these drugs.

Mechanism of Action and Drug Effects

Mannitol works along the entire nephron. Its major site of action, however, is the proximal tubule and descending limb of the loop of Henle. Because it is nonabsorbable, it produces osmotic pres-

DOSAGES

Selected Loop Diuretics and Osmotic Diuretics

Drug	Pharmacologic Class	Usual Dosage Range	Indications
◆ furosemide (Lasix)	Loop diuretic	**Pediatric** IM/IV: 1 mg/kg/dose; do not exceed 6 mg/kg/day PO: 1-2 mg/kg as a single dose; do not exceed 6 mg/kg/day **Adult** IM/IV: 20-40 mg/dose; max 600 mg/day; administer high-dose IV therapy as a controlled infusion at a rate of 4 mg/mL or less PO: 20-80 mg/day as a single dose	Heart failure, hypertension, renal failure, pulmonary edema, cirrhosis
◆ mannitol (Osmitrol)	Osmotic diuretic	**Adult** IV infusion: 50-200 g/day, 1.5-2 g/kg over 30-60 min Test dose of 25 g, followed by an infusion rate to produce a urine flow of 100-500 mL/hr	Renal failure, abnormally high intraocular or intracranial pressure Drug intoxication (to induce diuresis)

IM, Intramuscular; *IV*, intravenous; *PO*, oral.

sure in the glomerular filtrate, which in turn pulls fluid, primarily water, into the renal tubules from the surrounding tissues. This process also inhibits the tubular resorption of water and solutes, which produces a rapid diuresis. Ultimately this reduces cellular edema and increases urine production, causing diuresis. However, it produces only a slight loss of electrolytes, especially sodium. Therefore, mannitol is not indicated for patients with peripheral edema because it does not promote sufficient sodium excretion.

Mannitol may induce vasodilation and in doing so increase both glomerular filtration and renal plasma flow. This makes it an excellent drug for preventing kidney damage during acute renal failure. It is also often used to reduce intracranial pressure and cerebral edema resulting from head trauma. In addition, mannitol treatment may be tried when elevated intraocular pressure is unresponsive to other drug therapies.

Indications

Mannitol is the osmotic diuretic of choice. It is commonly used in the treatment of patients in the early, oliguric phase of acute renal failure. For it to be effective in this setting, however, enough renal blood flow and glomerular filtration must still remain to enable the drug to reach the renal tubules. Increased renal blood flow resulting from the dilatation of blood vessels supplying blood to the kidneys is another therapeutic benefit of mannitol therapy in such patients. It can also be used to promote the excretion of toxic substances, reduce intracranial pressure, and treat cerebral edema. In addition, it can be used as a genitourinary irrigant in the preparation of patients for transurethral surgical procedures and as supportive treatment in patients with edema induced by other conditions.

Contraindications

Contraindications to the use of mannitol normally include known drug allergy, severe renal disease, pulmonary edema (loop diuretics are used instead), and active intracranial bleeding.

Adverse Effects

The significant undesirable effects of mannitol include convulsions, thrombophlebitis, and pulmonary congestion. Other less significant effects are headaches, chest pains, tachycardia, blurred vision, chills, and fever.

Interactions

There are no drugs that interact significantly with mannitol.

Dosages

For the recommended dosages of mannitol, see the Dosages table above.

DRUG PROFILE

◆ mannitol

Mannitol (Osmitrol) is the prototypical osmotic diuretic. Its use is contraindicated in patients with a hypersensitivity to it as well as in those with anuria, severe dehydration, pulmonary congestion, or cerebral hemorrhage. Treatment should be terminated if severe cardiac or renal impairment develops after the initiation of therapy. It is available only in parenteral form as 5%, 10%, 15%, 20%, and 25% solutions for intravenous injection. Mannitol may crystallize when exposed to low temperatures. This is more likely to occur when concentrations exceed 15%. Because of this, mannitol should always be administered intravenously through a filter, and vials of the drug are often stored in a warmer in the pharmacy. Before administering mannitol, the nurse should visually inspect the mannitol container for precipitants. Pregnancy category C. Recommended dosages are given in the Dosages table above.

PHARMACOKINETICS

Route	Onset of Action	Peak Plasma Concentration	Elimination Half-life	Duration of Action
IV	0.5-1 hr	0.25-2 hr	1.5 hr	6-8 hr

POTASSIUM-SPARING DIURETICS

The currently available potassium-sparing diuretics are amiloride, spironolactone, and triamterene. These diuretics are also referred to as *aldosterone-inhibiting diuretics* because they block the aldosterone receptors. In fact, spironolactone is a competitive antagonist of aldosterone and for this reason causes sodium and water to be excreted and potassium to be retained. It is the most commonly used of the three drugs.

Mechanism of Action and Drug Effects

These drugs work in the collecting ducts and distal convoluted tubules, where they interfere with sodium-potassium exchange. Spironolactone competitively binds to aldosterone receptors and therefore blocks the resorption of sodium and water that is induced by aldosterone secretion. These receptors are found primarily in the distal tubule. Amiloride and triamterene do not bind to aldosterone receptors. However, they inhibit both aldosterone-induced and basal sodium reabsorption, working in both the distal tubule and collecting ducts. They are often prescribed for children with heart failure, because pediatric cardiac problems are frequently accompanied by an excess secretion of aldosterone, and the loop and thiazide diuretics are often ineffective in their management.

The potassium-sparing diuretics are relatively weak compared with the thiazide and loop diuretics. When diuresis is needed, they are generally used as adjuncts to thiazide treatment. This combination is beneficial in two respects. First, the drugs have synergistic diuretic effects; second, the two drugs counteract the adverse metabolic effects of one another. The thiazide diuretics cause potassium, magnesium, and chloride to be lost in the urine, and the potassium-sparing diuretics counteract this by elevating the potassium and chloride levels.

Indications

The therapeutic applications of the potassium-sparing diuretics vary depending on the particular drug. Spironolactone and triamterene are used to treat hyperaldosteronism and hypertension and to reverse the potassium loss caused by the potassium-wasting (e.g., loop, thiazide) diuretics. One common feature of various types of heart failure is a hyperactive renin-angiotensin-aldosterone system. Research has identified this hyperactivity as a causative factor in permanent ventricular myocardial wall damage, known as *remodeling*, following myocardial infarction. Various clinical drug trials are increasingly demonstrating a cardioprotective benefit of spironolactone in preventing this remodeling process, owing to its aldosterone-inhibiting activity. The uses for amiloride are similar to those for spironolactone and triamterene, but amiloride is less effective in the long term. It may be more effective than spironolactone or triamterene in the treatment of metabolic alkalosis, however. It is primarily used in the management of heart failure. As with certain other classes of diuretics, potassium-sparing diuretics may also be indicated in cases of heart failure due to diastolic dysfunction.

Contraindications

Contraindications to the use of potassium-sparing diuretics include known drug allergy, hyperkalemia (i.e., serum potassium level exceeding 5.5 mEq/L), and severe renal failure or anuria. Triamterene use may also be contraindicated in cases of severe hepatic failure.

TABLE 26-4 Potassium-Sparing Diuretics: Common Adverse Effects

Body System	Adverse Effects
Central nervous	Dizziness, headache
Gastrointestinal	Cramps, nausea, vomiting, diarrhea
Other	Urinary frequency, weakness, hyperkalemia

Adverse Effects

Potassium-sparing diuretics have several common undesirable effects, which are listed in Table 26-4. There are also some significant adverse effects that are specific to individual drugs. Spironolactone can cause gynecomastia, amenorrhea, irregular menses, and postmenopausal bleeding. Triamterene may reduce folic acid levels and cause the formation of kidney stones and urinary casts. It may also precipitate megaloblastic anemia. However, adverse effects from triamterene use are rare. Hyperkalemia may occur when potassium-sparing diuretics are used in combination with each other and/or with other potassium-sparing drugs such as angiotensin-converting enzyme (ACE) inhibitors (see Chapter 25, as well as the Interactions section, which follows).

Interactions

Concurrent use of potassium-sparing diuretics and lithium, ACE inhibitors, or potassium supplements can result in significant drug interactions. The administration of ACE inhibitors or potassium supplements in combination with potassium-sparing diuretics can result in hyperkalemia. When lithium and potassium-sparing diuretics are given together, lithium toxicity can result. NSAIDs can inhibit renal prostaglandins, which decreases blood flow to the kidneys and therefore decreases the delivery of diuretic drugs to this site of action. This in turn can lead to a diminished diuretic response.

Dosages

For the recommended dosages of potassium-sparing diuretics, see the Dosages table on p. 410.

DRUG PROFILES

amiloride

Amiloride (Midamor) is generally used in combination with a thiazide or loop diuretic in the treatment of heart failure. Hyperkalemia may occur in as many as 10% of the patients who take amiloride alone. It should be used with caution in patients who have renal impairment or diabetes mellitus and in elderly patients. It has only weak antihypertensive properties. Amiloride is available only in oral form. It is also available in combination with hydrochlorothiazide. Pregnancy category B. Recommended dosages are given in the dosages table on p. 410.

PHARMACOKINETICS

Route	Onset of Action	Peak Plasma Concentration	Elimination Half-life	Duration of Action
PO	2 hr	6-10 hr	6-9 hr	24 hr

DOSAGES

Selected Potassium-Sparing Diuretic Drugs

Drug	Usual Dosage Range	Indications
amiloride (Midamor)	**Adult** PO: 5-20 mg/day	Edema, heart failure (as an adjunct to loop diuretics)
◆ spironolactone (Aldactone)	**Pediatric** PO: 3.3 mg/kg/day in single or divided doses **Adult** PO: 25-200 mg/day; given once or divided twice daily	Edema, hypertension, heart failure, ascites
triamterene (Dyrenium)	**Adult** PO: 100 mg bid; do not exceed 300 mg/day	

PO, Oral.

◆ spironolactone

Structurally, spironolactone (Aldactone) is a synthetic steroid that blocks aldosterone receptors. It is used in high dosages for the treatment of ascites, a condition commonly associated with cirrhosis of the liver. The serum potassium level should be monitored frequently in patients who have impaired renal function or who are currently taking potassium supplements, because hyperkalemia is a common complication of spironolactone therapy. It is the potassium-sparing diuretic most commonly prescribed for children who have heart failure. Recently spironolactone has been shown to reduce morbidity and mortality in patients with severe heart failure when added to standard therapy. Of the three commonly used potassium-sparing diuretics, spironolactone has the greatest antihypertensive activity. It is available only in oral form. It also is available in combination with hydrochlorothiazide. Pregnancy category D. Recommended dosages are given in the Dosages table above.

PHARMACOKINETICS

Route	Onset of Action	Peak Plasma Concentration	Elimination Half-life	Duration of Action
PO	1-3 days	2-3 days	13-24 hr	2-3 days

triamterene

The pharmacologic properties of triamterene (Dyrenium) are similar to those of amiloride. Like amiloride, triamterene acts directly on the distal renal tubule of the nephron to depress the resorption of sodium and the excretion of potassium and hydrogen, processes otherwise stimulated at that site by aldosterone. It has little or no antihypertensive effect. Triamterene is available only in oral form and is also available in combination with hydrochlorothiazide. Pregnancy category D. Recommended dosages are given in the Dosages table above.

PHARMACOKINETICS

Route	Onset of Action	Peak Plasma Concentration	Elimination Half-life	Duration of Action
PO	2-3 hr	6-8 hr	2-3 hr	12-16 hr

THIAZIDES AND THIAZIDE-LIKE DIURETICS

Thiazide and thiazide-like diuretics are generally considered equivalent in their effects. Thiazide diuretics, like several of the loop diuretics, are benzothiadiazines, chemical derivatives of sulfonamide antibiotics. The thiazide diuretics include chlorothiazide, hydrochlorothiazide, and bendroflumethiazide. Hydrochlorothiazide is undoubtedly the most commonly prescribed and the least expensive of the thiazide diuretics. Hydrochlorothiazide is included in numerous combination products with antihypertensive drugs. The thiazide-like diuretics are very similar to the thiazides and include chlorthalidone, indapamide, and metolazone. Metolazone may be more effective than other drugs in this class in the treatment of patients with renal dysfunction.

Mechanism of Action and Drug Effects

The primary site of action of thiazides and thiazide-like diuretics is the distal convoluted tubule, where they inhibit the resorption of sodium, potassium, and chloride. This results in osmotic water loss. Thiazides also cause direct relaxation of the arterioles (small blood vessels), which reduces peripheral vascular resistance (afterload). Decreased preload (filling pressures) and decreased afterload (the force the ventricles must overcome to eject the volume of blood they contain) are the beneficial hemodynamic effects. This makes them very effective for the treatment of both heart failure and hypertension.

As renal function decreases, the efficacy of thiazides diminishes, probably because delivery of the drug to the site of activity is impaired. Thiazides generally should not be used if creatinine clearance is less than 30 to 50 mL/min. Normal creatinine clearance is 125 mL/min. The only exception is metolazone, which remains effective to a creatinine clearance of 10 mL/min, and thus is used in cases of renal failure. The major adverse effects of the drugs stem from the electrolyte disturbances they produce. They are noted for precipitating hypokalemia and hypercalcemia, as well as metabolic disturbances such as hyperlipidemia, hyperglycemia, and hyperuricemia.

Indications

The thiazide and thiazide-like diuretics are used in the treatment of edema of various origins, idiopathic hypercalciuria, and diabetes insipidus, in addition to hypertension. They are also used as adjunct drugs in the management of heart failure and hepatic cirrhosis. Any of these drugs can be used either as monotherapy or in combination with other drugs. As with certain other classes of diuretics, they may also be indicated in cases of heart failure due to diastolic dysfunction.

Contraindications

Contraindications to the use of thiazides and thiazide-like diuretics include known drug allergy, hepatic coma (metolazone), anuria, and severe renal failure.

Adverse Effects

The major adverse effects of the thiazide and thiazide-like diuretics relate to the electrolyte and metabolic disturbances they cause. These are mainly reduced potassium levels and elevated levels of calcium, lipids, glucose, and uric acid. Other effects, such as gastrointestinal disturbances, skin rashes, photosensitivity, thrombocytopenia, pancreatitis, and cholecystitis, are less common. Dizziness and vertigo are common adverse effects of metolazone therapy and are attributed to sudden shifts in the plasma volume brought about by the drug. Headache, impotence, and decreased libido are other important adverse effects of these drugs. Many of these adverse effects are dose related and are seen at higher doses, especially those above 25 mg. The more common adverse effects of the thiazide and thiazide-like diuretics are listed in Table 26-5.

Toxicity and Management of Overdose

An overdose of these drugs can lead to an electrolyte imbalance resulting from hypokalemia. Symptoms include anorexia, nausea, lethargy, muscle weakness, mental confusion, and hypotension. Treatment involves electrolyte replacement.

TABLE 26-5 Thiazide and Thiazide-Like Diuretics: Potential Adverse Effects

Body System	Adverse Effects
Central nervous	Dizziness, headache, blurred vision, paresthesia, decreased libido
Gastrointestinal	Anorexia, nausea, vomiting, diarrhea, pancreatitis, cholecystitis
Genitourinary	Impotence
Hematologic	Jaundice, leukopenia, purpura, agranulocytosis, aplastic anemia, thrombocytopenia
Integumentary	Urticaria, photosensitivity
Metabolic	Hypokalemia, glycosuria, hyperglycemia, hyperuricemia, hypochloremic alkalosis

Interactions

Thiazides and related drugs interact with corticosteroids, diazoxide, digitalis, and oral hypoglycemics. The mechanisms and results of these interactions are summarized in Table 26-6. Excessive consumption of licorice can lead to an additive hypokalemia in patients taking these drugs.

Dosages

For information on the dosages for thiazides and thiazide-like diuretics, see the Dosages table on p. 412.

DRUG PROFILES

◆ hydrochlorothiazide

Hydrochlorothiazide (HydroDIURIL), which is considered the prototypical thiazide diuretic, is a very commonly prescribed and inexpensive thiazide diuretic. It is also a very safe and effective diuretic. Hydrochlorothiazide is used in combination with many other drugs, including methyldopa, propranolol, spironolactone, triamterene, hydralazine, ACE inhibitors, beta-blockers, and labetalol. Dosages exceeding 50 mg/day rarely produce additional clinical results and may only increase drug toxicity. This property is known as a *ceiling effect.*

Hydrochlorothiazide is available only in oral form. Pregnancy category B. Recommended dosages are given in the Dosages table on p. 412.

PHARMACOKINETICS

Route	Onset of Action	Peak Plasma Concentration	Elimination Half-life	Duration of Action
PO	2 hr	4-6 hr	5-15 hr	6-12 hr

metolazone

Metolazone (Zaroxolyn) is a thiazide-like diuretic that appears to be more potent than the thiazide diuretics. This greater potency is most visible in patients with renal dysfunction. One striking advantage of metolazone is that, as noted earlier, it remains effective to a creatinine clearance as low as 10 mL/min. It may also be given in combination with loop diuretics to produce potent diuresis in patients with severe symptoms of heart failure. It is available only in oral form. Pregnancy category B. Recommended dosages are given in the Dosages table on p. 412.

PHARMACOKINETICS

Route	Onset of Action	Peak Plasma Concentration	Elimination Half-life	Duration of Action
PO	1 hr	1-2 hr	6-20 hr	24 hr

TABLE 26-6 Thiazide and Thiazide-Like Diuretics: Common Drug Interactions

Interacting Drug	Mechanism	Results
Corticosteroids	Additive effect	Hypokalemia
diazoxide	Additive effect	Hyperkalemia
digoxin	Hypokalemia	Increased digoxin toxicity
lithium	Decreased clearance	Increased lithium toxicity
NSAIDs	Inhibition of renal prostaglandins	Decreased diuretic activity
Oral hypoglycemics	Antagonism	Reduced therapeutic hypoglycemic effect (i.e., increased blood glucose levels)

NSAIDs, Nonsteroidal antiinflammatory drugs.

DOSAGES

Selected Thiazide and Thiazide-Like Diuretic Drugs

Drug	Pharmacologic Class	Usual Dosage Range	Indications
◆ hydrochlorothiazide (Esidrix, HydroDIURIL)	Thiazide diuretic	**Pediatric** Less than 6 mo, 3 mg/kg/day; 6 mo-2 yr, 12.5-37.5 mg/day in 2 doses; 2-12 yr, 37.5-100 mg/day in 2 doses **Adult** 25-200 mg/day, usually divided **Elderly** 12.5-25 mg/day	Edema, heart failure (as an adjunct to loop diuretics)
metolazone (Mykrox, Diulo, Zaroxolyn)	Thiazide-like diuretic	**Adult** PO: 2.5-20 mg/day	

PO, Oral.

NURSING PROCESS

Assessment

Before giving a patient any type of diuretic, the nurse should obtain a complete patient history and thorough medication history. A physical assessment should also be completed and all findings documented, with an emphasis on those body systems affected by the disease process or indication for the diuretic as well as by potential drug-related adverse effects. This would most likely include assessing baseline breath sounds, heart sounds, and neurologic status, as well as checking skin turgor (for edema), moisture levels of mucus membranes, and capillary refill. Because fluid volume levels and electrolyte concentrations (see later) are affected by diuretics, the patient's baseline fluid volume status (as indicated by vital signs, weight, and intake-output measurements) should be assessed and documented. Postural blood pressures (e.g., lying, sitting, standing) should be assessed before and during drug therapy because of diuretic-induced fluid volume loss, which may lead to postural or orthostatic hypotension. Postural or orthostatic hypotension is a drop in blood pressure of 20 mm Hg or more upon standing.

In addition to performing a thorough physical assessment and taking a history, it is important to assess specific laboratory values associated with renal and hepatic functioning; for example, BUN level (normal range, 8 to 25 mg/100 mL) and creatinine level (normal range, 0.6 to 1.5 mg/100 mL) for renal function, and ALP (normal range, 13 to 39 units/L), AST (normal range, 8 to 46 units/L in males, 7 to 34 units/L in females), and LDH (normal range, 45 to 90 units/L) for hepatic function. It is important to note, however, that normal ranges of these laboratory values may vary somewhat from facility to facility. Serum electrolyte levels are also critical to assess before and during diuretic therapy because of the subsequent loss of electrolytes through the urine and their relationship to fluid volume status. Specifically, serum potassium, sodium, chloride, magnesium, calcium, uric acid, and creatinine levels should be obtained and documented, as ordered. Other laboratory studies may include arterial blood gas levels. Additional concerns call for monitoring fluid volume status and electrolyte levels as well as measuring vital signs frequently in patients with hypokalemia, hypovolemia, renal disease, liver disease, lupus erythematosus, diabetes, chronic obstructive pulmonary disease, and gout. *Loop diuretics* are more potent than thiazide diuretics, combination products, and/or potassium-sparing diuretics, so these drugs may pose more problems for the elderly or those with the above-listed disorders. An additional and significant concern for patients taking loop diuretics is the interaction with other medications that are ototoxic or nephrotoxic (see Table 26-3). With *potassium-*

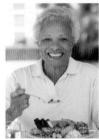

LIFE SPAN CONSIDERATIONS: The Elderly Patient

Diuretic Therapy

- Before and during diuretic drug therapy, the patient's height, weight, intake and output, blood pressure, pulse rate, respiratory rate, and temperature should be measured; breath and heart sounds and edematous areas should be assessed; and serum sodium, potassium, and chloride levels should be monitored, so that adverse effects and/or complications can be minimized or identified early.

- It should be emphasized to the elderly patient that diuretics should be taken at the same time every day. These drugs are generally ordered to be taken in the morning to help prevent nocturia (voiding at night), which can result in lack of sleep. More importantly, nocturia can lead to injury if the individual needs to get out of bed to void, becomes dizzy and/or confused, and falls. A bedside commode may be used to decrease the risk of injury.

- If the elderly patient is living alone and has minimal or no assistance with the medication regimen, visits from a home health aide or other health care professional may help ensure safety, efficacy, and compliance not only in taking the medication but also in following all aspects of the therapeutic regimen.

- Caution should be exercised in administering diuretics to the elderly, because they are more sensitive to the therapeutic effects of these drugs (often reacting to smaller dosages of medication than are required by other patients) and are also more likely to experience the adverse effects of diuretics such as dehydration, electrolyte loss, dizziness, and syncope.

- The patient should be encouraged to change positions slowly because of the risk of orthostatic hypotension and subsequent falls and injury. Weight, blood pressure, and overall well-being should be recorded daily.

- Carrying a card containing a brief medical history, blood pressure readings, names and telephone numbers of contact persons, and a list of medications is important to ensure safety and minimize complications. The card should be formatted so that it can fit in a wallet, and a copy should be placed in the kitchen on the refrigerator door or in another visible location so that it will be easily available to emergency personnel. Copies of the card should be given to the caregiver(s), family members, significant others, prescribers, dentist, and relevant health care personnel. The card should be updated at regular intervals by the patient or another adult or by a prescriber involved in the patient's care. Such a card can be made easily using standard card stock or an index card. It can be placed in a wallet sleeve or can even be laminated and information entered using an erasable pen or pencil. The following sample shows suggested headings and content for such a card:

1. Name: _____
2. Age: _____   3. Blood type: _____   4. Drug/food allergies: _____
5. Medical history (circle all that apply and write in any not listed):

Anemia	Depression	Nerve problems
Asthma	Diabetes	Pacemaker or defibrillator device
Bleeding problems	Difficulty swallowing	Recent weight gain
Blood clots	Heart problems	Recent weight loss
Breathing problems	High blood pressure	Stroke
Cancer	Low blood pressure	Thyroid problems

   Others: _____
6. Current medications:
   Prescription drugs
   Name of drug: _____
   Dose amount: _____
   Frequency of doses: _____
   Condition for which drug is taken: _____
   Over-the-counter drugs
   Name of drug: _____
   Dose amount: _____
   Frequency of doses: _____
   Condition for which drug is taken: _____
   Herbals, vitamins, and other preparations
   Name of drug: _____
   Dose amount: _____
   Frequency of doses: _____
   Condition for which substance is taken: _____
7. Surgery (list all):
   Date: _____ Type and purpose: _____
   Any complications: _____
8. Prosthetics used: _____
9. Dental problems or concerns: _____
10. Wear glasses _____ Use hearing aid(s) _____ Need help with mobility _____
11. Other important information that should be known in case of emergency: _____
12. Contact names and telephone numbers: _____

sparing diuretics, hyperkalemia may be an adverse effect and thus the patient's serum levels of potassium must be assessed. See the pharmacology section of this chapter for further discussion of additional cautions, contraindications, and drug interactions associated with diuretic use.

Nursing Diagnoses

- Decreased cardiac output related to drug effects and adverse effects of diuretics (e.g., fluid and electrolyte loss)
- Deficient fluid volume related to drug effects and adverse effects of diuretics
- Risk for injury related to postural hypotension and dizziness
- Deficient knowledge related to lack of experience with newly prescribed medication regimen
- Acute pain related to occurrence of headache and other adverse effects of diuretics
- Noncompliance with the treatment regimen related to lack of information and experience with the drug regimen and adverse effects

Planning

Goals

- Patient regains fluid and electrolyte balance.
- Patient remains free of the complications associated with diuretic use.
- Patient remains free of injury to self while taking diuretics.
- Patient remains compliant with the therapy regimen.

Outcome Criteria

- Patient maintains normal levels of electrolytes (sodium, potassium, and chloride) while taking diuretics.
- Patient continues to show or regains normal cardiac output while receiving diuretic therapy as evidenced by vital signs, adequate intake, and output within normal limits (pulse between 60 and 100 beats/min; blood pressure 120/80 mm Hg or within normal parameters; urine output 30 mL/hr or higher).
- Patient's skin is pliable and without edema or dryness.
- Patient rises slowly and changes positions slowly and cautiously while receiving diuretics to avoid postural orthostatic hypotension and subsequent dizziness and possible syncope.
- Patient states the importance of and rationale for follow-up visits with the prescriber, such as monitoring for adverse effects, dehydration, and fluid and electrolyte imbalances.
- Patient reports dizziness, fainting, palpitations, tingling, confusion, or disorientation to the prescriber immediately.

Implementation

Blood pressure, pulse rate, intake and output, and daily weights should continue to be measured and recorded during diuretic therapy. Changes from the initial assessment data (see earlier) that would alert the nurse to possible problems with the drug therapy include the presence of dizziness, fainting, lightheadedness on standing or changing positions, weakness, fatigue, tremor, muscle cramping, changes in mental status, or cold clammy skin. Diuretic therapy may also precipitate cardiac ir-

regularities or palpitations, and thus heart rate and rhythm must continue to be monitored. Fluid loss from the action of the diuretic may lead to the adverse effect of constipation so that preventative measures are required, such as increased intake of fluids, bulk, and fiber (unless contraindicated) and/or the use of natural bulk-forming products. If constipation continues, the prescriber may need to provide alternatives to psyllium-based bulk-forming laxatives. Diuretics should always be given exactly as directed but with consideration of the patient's age and related needs. Dosing and timing of the drugs are often very important to enhance therapeutic effects and minimize adverse effects. Because diuretics taken late in the afternoon or evening may lead to nocturia (urination at night) and subsequent loss in sleep, these medications should be scheduled for morning dosing. Safety concerns exist with nocturia, especially in the elderly, because possible confusion and dizziness associated with getting up in the middle of the night may create the potential for falls and injury.

Loop diuretics (if taken at high dosages as ordered) may put patients at greater risk for fluid volume and electrolyte depletion (e.g., hypokalemia, hyponatremia, dehydration). Monitoring of therapy should include frequent assessment of blood pressure and pulse rate, including orthostatic blood pressures and pulse rates (supine and standing); hydration status; and capillary refill, as well as daily measurement of weight. Acute hypotensive episodes may occur with higher dosages of loop diuretics and precipitate syncope and falls; therefore, the patient should be educated about safety measures to prevent falls. Generally speaking, most oral diuretics should be taken with food to help minimize gastric upset. If intravenous dosage forms are given, it is crucial to check for proper diluents, drug incompatibilities, and intactness of the intravenous site. Rates of infusion should be confirmed, and an infusion pump used, as deemed necessary. With *potassium-sparing diuretics,* potassium is reabsorbed and not excreted (as previously discussed), so hyperkalemia, rather than hypokalemia, may become problematic. Signs and symptoms of hyperkalemia include nausea, vomiting, diarrhea, and abdominal cramping (see Chapter 27) and should be reported immediately. See the Patient Teaching Tips for more information.

Evaluation

The therapeutic effects of diuretics include the resolution of or reduction in edema, fluid volume overload, heart failure, or hypertension, or a return to normal intraocular pressures (if used for that purpose). The patient must also be monitored for the occurrence of adverse reactions to the diuretics, such as metabolic acidosis (arterial blood gas values should be monitored), drowsiness (with CAIs), hypokalemia, tachycardia (less significant with mannitol) and hypotension (from loss of volume). Hypokalemia may be manifested by leg cramps with restlessness and decreased mental alertness associated with toxicity. With potassium-sparing diuretics, hyperkalemia may be the adverse effect for which to monitor in assessing the effects of the therapeutic regimen. All goals and outcome criteria should be reviewed in the evaluation process.

PATIENT TEACHING TIPS

- Patients taking diuretics should maintain proper nutritional intake and fluid volume and should eat potassium-rich foods, except when contraindicated or when potassium-sparing diuretics are used. Foods high in potassium include bananas, oranges, apricots, dates, raisins, broccoli, green beans, potatoes, tomatoes, meats, fish, wheat bread, and legumes.
- Potassium supplementation may be recommended by a prescriber when the potassium level is below 3 mEq/L (see Chapter 27; always refer to laboratory guidelines for normal ranges).
- Frequent laboratory tests may be indicated at the beginning of and during therapy with diuretics. These tests may include measurement of electrolytes, uric acid, and blood gases.
- Encourage patients to change positions slowly and to rise slowly after sitting or lying to prevent dizziness and possible fainting (syncope).
- Forcing of fluids may be needed (if not contraindicated) to prevent dehydration and minimize constipation. Increased consumption of fiber, bulk, and roughage may also help with constipation.
- Any unusual adverse effects or problems, such as excessive dizziness, syncope, weakness, or muscle aches, should be reported immediately to the prescriber.

- Keeping a daily journal should include weight, how the patient feels each day, and any other important information related to the diagnosis and medical treatment.
- The patient should be educated about the signs and symptoms of hypokalemia, such as weakness, leg cramps, and other muscle cramps. In addition, the patient should be cautioned to avoid hot climates, excessive sweating, fever, and the use of saunas or hot tubs. Heat raises core body temperature and causes further loss of potassium, sodium, and water through sweat, which can lead to potential problems with hypotension and fluid-electrolyte imbalances. Fluid volume and electrolyte loss may also occur with vomiting and diarrhea.
- If the patient is taking a diuretic along with a digitalis preparation, the patient, family members, and anyone involved in the patient's care should be educated about how to monitor pulse rate. The warning signs and symptoms of digitalis toxicity should be emphasized, such as anorexia, nausea, vomiting, and bradycardia (a pulse rate of 60 beats/min or lower; always check facility policy or guidelines).
- Diabetic patients who are taking thiazide and/or loop diuretics require education about the need for close monitoring of blood glucose levels.

POINTS TO REMEMBER

- The five main types of diuretics are CAIs and loop, osmotic, potassium-sparing, and thiazide and thiazide-like diuretics.
- The loop, potassium-sparing, and thiazide and thiazide-like diuretics are the most commonly used. The nurse must remember that the loop diuretics are more potent than the thiazides, combination diuretics, and potassium-sparing diuretics.
- Thiazide diuretics are the most frequently prescribed diuretics and are the least expensive, because several generic preparations are available. Hydrochlorothiazide is considered the prototypical thiazide diuretic and is used as adjunctive therapy to manage hepatic cirrhosis, edema, and heart failure. Related adverse metabolic effects for which the nurse needs to monitor are hypokalemia, hypercalcemia, hyperlipidemia, hyperglycemia, and hyperuricemia.

- Nurses must have a thorough knowledge of renal anatomy and physiology and how it relates to the action of the various diuretics; for example, if a loop diuretic is given, its site of action is the loop of Henle and it causes the excretion of sodium, potassium, and chloride into the urine.
- Methods for monitoring excess and deficit fluid volume states include assessment of skin and mucous membranes, blood pressure, pulse rate, intake and output, and daily weights.
- The nurse should always be concerned about the more vulnerable patient populations, such as the elderly, those with chronic illnesses, and patients with altered renal or liver function.

NCLEX EXAMINATION REVIEW QUESTIONS

1 The nurse is reviewing the medications that have been ordered for a patient for whom a loop diuretic has just been prescribed. The loop diuretic may have a possible interaction with which of the following?
   a Vitamin C
   b Warfarin
   c Penicillins
   d NSAIDs
2 When monitoring laboratory test results for patients receiving loop and thiazide diuretics, the nurse knows to look for
   a decreased serum levels of potassium.
   b increased serum levels of calcium.
   c decreased serum levels of glucose.
   d increased serum levels of sodium.
3 When the nurse is checking the laboratory data for a patient taking spironolactone (Aldactone), which result would be a potential concern?
   a Serum sodium level of 140 mEq/L
   b Serum calcium level of 10.2 mg/dL
   c Serum potassium level of 5.8 mEq/L
   d Serum magnesium level of 2.0 mg/dL
4 Which statement should be included in patient education for a patient with heart failure who is taking daily doses of spironolactone (Aldactone)?
   a "Be sure to eat foods that are high in potassium."
   b "Avoid foods that are high in potassium."

c "While you are taking this medication you need to avoid grapefruit juice."
d "A low-fiber diet will help prevent adverse effects of this medication."
5 A patient with diabetes has a new prescription for a thiazide diuretic. Which statement should the nurse include when teaching the patient about the thiazide drug?
   a "There is nothing for you to be concerned about when you are taking the thiazide diuretic."
   b "Be sure to avoid foods that are high in potassium."
   c "You should take the thiazide at night to avoid interactions with the diabetes medicine."
   d "Monitor your blood glucose level closely, because the thiazide diuretic may cause the levels to increase."
6 An elderly patient has been discharged following treatment for a mild case of heart failure. He will be taking a loop diuretic. Which instruction(s) from the nurse are appropriate? (Select all that apply.)
   a "Take the diuretic at the same time each morning."
   b "Take the diuretic only if you notice swelling in your feet."
   c "Be sure to stand up slowly because the medicine may make you feel dizzy if you stand up quickly."
   d "Drink at least 8 glasses of water each day."
   e "Here is a list of foods that are high in potassium—you should avoid these."
   f "Please call your doctor immediately if you notice muscle weakness or increased dizziness."

1. d, 2. a, 3. c, 4. b, 5. d, 6. a, c, f

CRITICAL THINKING ACTIVITIES: BEST ACTION

1 While assessing a patient who is taking a diuretic, the nurse notes the following blood pressure (BP) readings:
   BP while lying in bed: 134/86
   BP while sitting on the side of the bed: 130/82
   BP while standing: 108/62
   In addition, the patient commented that he felt "woozy" while standing. What has happened, and what is the nurse's priority at this time?
2 A patient has been given a new order for spironolactone (Aldactone), 50 mg daily. While reviewing the patient's orders, the

nurse notes that the patient has an existing order for potassium chloride (K-Dur), 20 mEq daily. The patient's potassium level is 3.9 mEq/L. What is the nurse's best action at this time?
3 The nurse is administering a thiazide diuretic to a patient who has been receiving digoxin for several months as part of treatment for a cardiac dysrhythmia. What concerns should the nurse be aware of regarding these medications?

For answers, see *http://evolve.elsevier.com/Lilley.*

CHAPTER 27

Fluids and Electrolytes

OBJECTIVES

When you reach the end of this chapter, you should be able to do the following:

1 Review the function of fluid volume and compartments within the body as well as the role each of the major electrolytes plays in maintaining homeostasis.

2 Identify the various electrolytes and give normal serum values for each.

3 Briefly discuss the various fluid and electrolyte disorders that commonly occur in the body with attention to fluid volume and/or electrolyte deficits and excesses.

4 Identify the fluid and electrolyte solutions commonly used to correct states of deficiency or excess.

5 Discuss the mechanisms of action, indications, dosages, routes of administration, contraindications, cautions, adverse effects, toxicity, and drug interactions of the various fluid and electrolyte solutions.

6 Compare the various solutions used to expand and/or decrease a patient's fluid volume and electrolytes with regard to how they work, why they are used, and specific antidotes available to counter any toxic effects.

7 Develop a nursing care plan that includes all phases of the nursing process for patients receiving fluid and electrolyte solutions.

e-Learning Activities

http://evolve.elsevier.com/Lilley

NCLEX Review Questions • Animations • Nursing Care Plans • Audio Glossary • Category Catchers • Medication Errors Checklists • IV Therapy Checklists • Calculators • Frequently Asked Questions • Content Updates • Supplemental Resources • Answers to Case Studies and Critical Thinking Activities

Drug Profiles

albumin, p. 421
dextran, p. 422
fresh frozen plasma, p. 423
packed red blood cells, p. 423

potassium, p. 425
sodium chloride, pp. 420, 426
sodium polystyrene sulfonate, p. 425

Glossary

Blood The fluid that circulates through the heart, arteries, capillaries, and veins, carrying nutriment and oxygen to the body cells. It consists of *plasma,* its liquid component, plus three major solid components: *erythrocytes* (red blood cells or RBCs), *leukocytes* (white blood cells or WBCs), and *platelets.* (p. 418)

Colloids Protein substances that increase the colloid oncotic pressure (p. 421)

Colloid oncotic pressure Another name for oncotic pressure. It is a form of osmotic pressure exerted by protein in blood plasma that normally tends to pull water into the circulatory system. (p. 418)

Crystalloids Substances in a solution that diffuse through a semipermeable membrane. (p. 419)

Dehydration Excessive loss of water from the body tissues. It is accompanied by an imbalance in the concentrations of essential electrolytes, particularly sodium, potassium, and chloride. (p. 419)

Edema The abnormal accumulation of fluid in interstitial spaces. (p. 419)

Extracellular fluid (ECF) That portion of the body fluid comprising the interstitial fluid and blood plasma. (p. 418)

Extravascular fluid (EVF) Fluid in the body that is outside the blood vessels. (p. 418)

Gradient A difference in the concentration of a substance on two sides of a permeable barrier. (p. 419)

Hydrostatic pressure (HP) The pressure exerted by a liquid. (p. 419)

Hyperkalemia An abnormally high potassium concentration in the blood; most often due to defective renal excretion but can also be due to excessive dietary potassium. (p. 423)

Hypernatremia An abnormally high sodium concentration in the blood; may be due to defective renal excretion but is more commonly caused by excessive dietary sodium or replacement therapy. (p. 425)

Hypokalemia A condition in which there is an inadequate amount of potassium, the major intracellular cation, in the bloodstream. (p. 423)

Hyponatremia A condition in which there is an inadequate amount of sodium, the major extracellular cation, in the bloodstream, caused either by inadequate excretion of water or by excessive water intake. (p. 425)

Interstitial fluid (ISF) The extracellular fluid that fills in the spaces between most of the cells of the body. Note also: an *interstice* is defined as a small space within a tissue. (p. 418)

Intracellular fluid (ICF) The fluid located within cell membranes throughout most of the body. It contains dissolved solutes that are essential to maintaining electrolyte balance and healthy metabolism. (p. 418)

Intravascular fluid (IVF) The fluid inside blood vessels. (p. 418)

Isotonic Having the same concentration of a solute as another solution and hence exerting the same osmotic pressure as that solution, such as an isotonic saline solution that contains an amount of salt equal to that found in the intracellular and extracellular fluid. (p. 418)

Osmotic pressure The pressure produced by a solution necessary to prevent the osmotic passage of solvent into it when the solution and solvent are separated by a semipermeable membrane. (p. 418)

Plasma The watery, straw-colored fluid component of lymph and blood in which the leukocytes, erythrocytes, and platelets are suspended. (p. 418)

Serum The clear, cell-free portion of the blood from which fibrinogen has also been separated during the clotting process, as typically carried out with a laboratory sample. (p. 418)

• • •

Anatomy, Physiology, and Disease Overview

Fluid and electrolyte management is one of the cornerstones of patient care. Most disease processes, tissue injuries, and surgical procedures greatly influence the physiologic status of fluids and electrolytes in the body. A prerequisite to the understanding of fluid and electrolyte management is knowledge of the extent and composition of the various body fluid compartments.

Approximately 60% of the adult human body is water. This is referred to as the *total body water (TBW),* and it is distributed in the three main compartments in the following proportions: **intracellular fluid (ICF),** 67%; **interstitial fluid (ISF),** 25%; and plasma volume, 8%. This distribution is illustrated in Figure 27-1. The actual volume of fluid that would normally be in each compartment in an average 70-kg man with a TBW content of 60% is shown in Table 27-1.

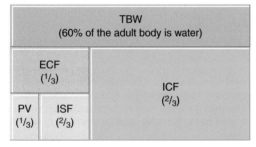

FIGURE 27-1 Distribution of total body water (TBW). *ECF,* Extracellular fluid; *ICF,* intracellular fluid; *ISF,* interstitial fluid; *PV,* plasma volume.

The terms used to identify the various spaces within which the TBW is distributed can be quite confusing, and there are two basic approaches to distinguishing among the locations of the fluid. The TBW can be described as being in or out of the **blood** vessels, or vasculature. If this point of reference is used, then the term **intravascular fluid (IVF)** is used to describe the fluid inside the blood vessels and the term **extravascular fluid (EVF)** is used to refer to the fluid outside the blood vessels. Examples of EVF include lymph and cerebrospinal fluid. As these concepts are learned, the difference between the prefixes *intra-* (inside), *inter-* (between), and *extra-* (outside) should be recalled. The term **plasma** is used to describe the fluid that flows through the blood vessels (intravascular fluid). **Serum** is a closely related term (see glossary). The ISF is the fluid that is in the space between cells, tissues, and organs. Both plasma and ISF make up extracellular volume. Both ISF and ICF make up extravascular volume. These terms are often confused and misused. Table 27-1 lists these definitions for further clarity and understanding.

What, then, keeps fluid inside the blood vessels? All the fluid outside the cells, the **extracellular fluid (ECF),** which consists of both the plasma and the ISF, has about the same concentration of electrolytes. However, there is one big difference between the plasma and the ISF. The plasma has a protein concentration four times greater than that of the ISF. These proteins consist primarily of albumin but also include globulin and fibrinogen. The reason for this higher intravascular concentration of protein is that these solutes (proteins) have a molecular weight that exceeds 69,000 daltons, and this makes them too large to pass through the walls of the blood vessels. Because of the difference in the concentration of plasma proteins, fluid flows from the area of low protein concentration in the interstitial compartment to the area of high concentration inside the blood vessel to try to create an **isotonic** environment on either side of the blood vessel wall. (*Isotonic* means an equal concentration of solutes across a membrane.) The protein in the blood vessels therefore exerts a constant **osmotic pressure** that prevents the leakage of too much plasma through the capillaries into the tissues. Because proteins suspended in plasma are in a *colloidal* state, this particular pressure is called **colloid oncotic pressure,** and normally it is 24 mm Hg. The opposing pressure, that exerted by the ISF, is called **hydrostatic pressure (HP),** and

TABLE **27-1** Fluid Location: Descriptive Terms and Actual Volumes

Term	Location	Actual Volumes (in a 70-kg Man with a TBW Content of 60% of Total Body Weight)
If the Point of Reference Is the Cells, These Terms Are Used		
Intracellular fluid (ICF)	Inside of cells	28,000 mL
Extracellular fluid (ECF)	Outside of cells	14,000 mL (composed of both intravascular plasma and interstitial fluid)
If the Point of Reference Is the Blood Vessels, These Terms Are Used		
Intravascular fluid or plasma volume (PV)	In blood vessels	3500 mL
Extravascular fluid (EVF)	Out of blood vessels	38,500 mL
If the Point of Reference Is the Tissues, These Terms Are Used		
Interstitial fluid (ISF)	In the spaces between cells, tissues, and organs but not in the plasma or the cells	10,500 mL

TBW, Total body water.

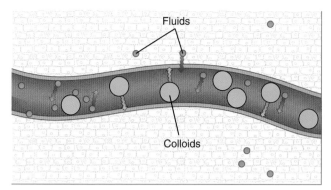

FIGURE 27-2 Colloid osmotic pressure (oncotic pressure). As shown, the colloids inside the blood vessel are too large to pass through the vessel wall. The resulting oncotic pressure exerted by the colloids draws fluid from the surrounding tissues and other extravascular spaces into the blood vessels and also keeps fluid inside the blood vessel.

TABLE 27-2 Types of Dehydration

Type of Dehydration	Characteristics
Hypertonic	Occurs when water loss is greater than sodium loss, which results in a concentration of solutes outside the cells and causes the fluid inside the cells to move to the extracellular space, thus dehydrating the cells. Example: Elevated temperature resulting in perspiration.
Hypotonic	Occurs when sodium loss is greater than water loss, which results in higher concentrations of solute inside the cells and causes fluid to be pulled from outside the cells (plasma and interstitial spaces) into the cells. Examples: Renal insufficiency and inadequate aldosterone secretion.
Isotonic	Caused by a loss of both sodium and water from the body, which results in a decrease in the volume of extracellular fluid. Examples: Diarrhea and vomiting.

normally it is 17 mm Hg—which, of course, is less than the colloid oncotic pressure. The phenomenon of colloid oncotic pressure is illustrated in Figure 27-2.

This regulation of the volume and composition of body water is essential for life, because body water is the medium in which all metabolic reactions occur. The body maintains the volume and composition remarkably constant by preserving the balance between intake and excretion. The amount of water gained each day is kept roughly equal to the amount of water lost. When, for some reason, the body cannot maintain this equilibrium, therapy with various agents becomes necessary. If the amount of water gained exceeds the amount of water lost, a water excess or overhydration occurs. Such fluid excesses often accumulate in interstitial spaces, such as in the pericardial sac, intrapleural space, peritoneal cavity, joint capsules, and lower extremities. This is referred to as **edema.** If the quantity of water lost exceeds that gained, a water deficit, or **dehydration,** occurs. Death often occurs when 20% to 25% of TBW is lost.

TABLE 27-3 Conditions Leading to Fluid Loss or Dehydration and Associated Corresponding Symptoms*

Condition	Associated Symptoms
Bleeding	Tachycardia and hypotension
Bowel obstruction	Reduced perspiration and mucous secretions
Diarrhea	Reduced urine output (oliguria)
Fever	Dry skin and mucous membranes
Vomiting	Reduced lacrimal (tears) and salivary secretions

*There may be overlap involving more than one of the symptoms depending on the patient's specific condition.

Dehydration leads to a disturbance in the balance between the amount of fluid in the extracellular compartment and that in the intracellular compartment. Sodium is the principle extracellular electrolyte and plays a primary role in maintaining water concentration in the body due to its highly osmotic chemistry. In the initial stages of dehydration, water is lost first from the extracellular compartments. The nature of further fluid losses, colloid oncotic pressure changes, or both depends on the type of clinical dehydration (Table 27-2). Clinical conditions that can result in dehydration and fluid loss, as well as the symptoms of dehydration and fluid loss, are presented in Table 27-3.

When fluid that has been lost must be replaced, there are three categories of agents that can be used to accomplish this: crystalloids, colloids, and blood products. The clinical situation dictates which category of agents is most appropriate.

Pharmacology Overview

CRYSTALLOIDS

Crystalloids are fluids given by intravenous (IV) injection that supply water and sodium to maintain the osmotic **gradient** between the extravascular and intravascular compartments. Their plasma volume–expanding capacity is related to their sodium concentration. The different crystalloids are listed in Table 27-4.

Mechanism of Action and Drug Effects

Crystalloid solutions contain fluids and electrolytes that are normally found in the body. They do not contain proteins (colloids), which are necessary to maintain the colloid oncotic pressure and prevent water from leaving the plasma compartment. In fact, the administration of large quantities of crystalloid solutions for fluid resuscitation decreases the colloid oncotic pressure, due to a dilutional effect. Crystalloids are distributed faster into the interstitial and intracellular compartments than colloids. This makes crystalloids better for treating dehydration than for expanding the plasma volume alone, such as in hypovolemic shock.

Indications

Crystalloid solutions are most commonly used as maintenance fluids. They are used to compensate for insensible fluid losses, to replace fluids when there are body-fluid deficits, and to manage specific fluid and electrolyte disturbances. Crystalloids also promote urinary flow. They are much less expensive than

TABLE 27-4 Crystalloids

Product	Composition (mEq/L)							
	Na	Cl	K	Ca	Mg	Lactate	Volume (mL)	Cost*
NS	154	154	0	0	0	0	1000	1
Hypertonic saline	513	513	0	0	0	0	500	1
Lactated Ringer's	130	109	4	3	0	28	1000	2.5
D₅W	0	0	1	0	0	0	1000	2

Ca, Calcium; *Cl*, chloride; *D₅W*, 5% dextrose in water; *K*, potassium; *Mg*, magnesium; *Na*, sodium; *NS*, normal saline.
*Relative cost compared with the cost of normal saline; for example: D₅W is two times the cost of normal saline.

colloids and blood products. In addition, there is no risk for viral transmission or anaphylaxis and no alteration in the coagulation profile associated with their use, unlike with blood products. The choice of whether to use a crystalloid or a colloid depends on the severity of the condition. The following are the common indications for either crystalloid or colloid replacement therapy:

- Acute liver failure
- Acute nephrosis
- Adult respiratory distress syndrome
- Burns
- Cardiopulmonary bypass
- Hypoproteinemia
- Reduction of the risk for deep vein thrombosis
- Renal dialysis
- Shock

Contraindications

Contraindications to the use of crystalloids include known drug allergy to a specific product and hypervolemia, and may include severe electrolyte disturbance, depending on the type of crystalloid used.

Adverse Effects

Crystalloids are a very safe and effective means of replacing needed fluid. They do, however, have some unwanted effects. Because they contain no large particles, such as proteins, they do not stay within the blood vessels and can leak out of the plasma into the tissues and cells. This may result in edema anywhere in the body. Peripheral edema and pulmonary edema are two common examples. Crystalloids also dilute the proteins that are in the plasma, which further reduces the colloid oncotic pressure. Because crystalloids cannot carry oxygen, their use may result in decreased oxygen tension due to a dilutional effect on erythrocyte concentration. Typically, large volumes (liters of fluid) are required for crystalloids to be effective. As a result, large or prolonged infusions may worsen acidosis or alkalosis, or adversely affect central nervous system function, due to fluid overload. Another disadvantage of crystalloids is that their effects are relatively short lived.

Interactions

Interactions with crystalloid solutions are rare because they are very similar if not identical to normal physiologic substances. Certain electrolytes contained in lactated Ringer's solution may

TABLE 27-5 Crystalloids and Colloids: Dosing Guidelines

	Crystalloids and Colloids			
	0.9% Saline	3% Saline	5% Colloid*	25% Colloid†
To Raise Plasma Volume by 1 L, Administer:				
	5-6 L	1.5-2 L	1 L	0.5 L
Compartment to Which Fluid Is Distributed:				
Plasma	25%	25%	100%	200%-300%
Interstitial space	75%	75%	0	Decreased fluid levels
Intracellular space	0	0	0	Decreased fluid levels

*Iso-oncotic solutions such as 5% albumin, dextran 70, and hetastarch.
†Hyperoncotic solutions such as 25% albumin.

be incompatible with other electrolytes, forming a chemical precipitate.

Dosages

For the recommended dosages of crystalloids, see Table 27-5.

DRUG PROFILE

The most commonly used crystalloid solutions are normal saline (NS or 0.9% sodium chloride) and lactated Ringer's solution. The available crystalloid solutions and their compositions are summarized in Table 27-4. Sodium chloride is also discussed briefly in the section on electrolytes and in the nursing process section under electrolytes.

sodium chloride
Sodium chloride (NaCl) is available in several concentrations, the most common being 0.9%. This is the physiologically normal concentration of sodium chloride, and for this reason it is referred to as *normal saline* (NS). Other concentrations are 0.45% ("half-normal"), 0.2% ("quarter-normal"), 3% (hypertonic saline), and 5%. These solutions have different indications, and they are used in different situations, depending on how urgently fluid volume restoration is needed and/or the extent of the sodium loss.

Sodium chloride is a physiologic electrolyte that is present throughout the body's water. For this reason, there are no hypersensitivity reactions to it. It is safe to administer it during any stage of pregnancy, but it is contraindicated in patients with hypernatremia and/or hyperchloremia. Hypertonic saline injections (3% and 5%) are contraindicated in the presence of increased, normal, or only slightly decreased serum electrolyte concentrations. Hypertonic saline is considered a high-risk drug because deaths have occurred when it is infused inappropriately. Sodium chloride is also available as a 650-mg tablet and as 0.45%, 0.9%, 3%, and 5% solutions.

The dose of sodium chloride administered depends on the clinical situation. The volume of crystalloid or colloid needed to expand the plasma volume by 1 L (1000 mL) is given in Table 27-5, and this can be used as a general guide to dosing.

PHARMACOKINETICS

Plasma Volume Expansion*	Colloid Oncotic Pressure	Duration of Expansion
60-70 mL	30 mm Hg	Few hours

*500 mL of normal saline will expand the plasma volume by 60 to 70 mL.

COLLOIDS

Colloids are protein substances that increase the colloid oncotic pressure and effectively move fluid from the interstitial compartment to the plasma compartment by pulling the fluid into the blood vessels. Normally, this task is performed by the three blood proteins: albumin, globulin, and fibrinogen. However, for colloids to be effective, the total protein level must be in the range of 7.4 g/dL. If this level drops below 5.3 g/dL, fluid shifts out of blood vessels into the tissues. When this happens, colloid replacement therapy is required to reverse this process by increasing the colloid oncotic pressure. The colloid oncotic pressure decreases with age and also with hypotension and malnutrition. The commonly used colloids are listed in Table 27-6.

Mechanism of Action and Drug Effects

The mechanism of action of colloids is related to their ability to increase the colloid oncotic pressure. As previously explained, because the colloids cannot pass into the extravascular space, there is ordinarily a higher concentration of colloid solutes (solid particles) inside the blood vessels (intravascular space) than outside the blood vessels. Fluid thus moves toward this hypertonic area, from the extravascular space, in an attempt to make it isotonic. Because colloids increase the blood volume, they are sometimes called *plasma expanders*. They also make up part of the total plasma volume.

TABLE 27-6 Commonly Used Colloids

Product	Composition (mEq/L)		Volume (mL)	Cost*
	Na	**Cl**		
Dextran 70†	154	154	500	1
Dextran 40†	154	154	500	2
Hetastarch	154	154	500	5
5% Albumin	145	145	500	10
25% Albumin	145	145	100	10

Cl, Chloride; *Na*, sodium.
*Relative cost compared with the cost of dextran 70.
†Dextran is available in NaCl, which has 154 mEq/L of both Na and Cl. It is also available in 5% dextrose in water, which contains no Na or Cl.

Administered colloids increase the colloid oncotic pressure and move fluid from outside the blood vessels to inside the blood vessels. They can maintain the colloid oncotic pressure for several hours. They are naturally occurring products and consist of proteins (albumin), carbohydrates (dextrans or starches), fats (lipid emulsion), and animal collagen (gelatin). Usually they contain a combination of both small and large particles. The small particles are eliminated quickly and promote diuresis and perfusion of the kidneys; the larger particles maintain the plasma volume. Albumin is the one exception in that it contains particles that are all the same size.

Indications

Colloids are used to treat a wide variety of conditions (see the list on p. 420). Clinically, colloids are superior to crystalloids because of their ability to maintain the plasma volume for a longer time. However, crystalloids are less expensive and are less likely to promote bleeding. Crystalloids are more likely to cause edema because of the larger volumes needed to achieve the desired clinical effect. Crystalloids are better than colloids for emergency short-term plasma volume expansion.

Contraindications

Contraindications to the use of colloids include known drug allergy to a specific product and hypervolemia, and may include severe electrolyte disturbance.

Adverse Effects

Colloids are relatively safe agents, although there are some disadvantages to their use. They have no oxygen-carrying ability and contain no clotting factors, unlike blood products. Because of this, they can alter the coagulation system through a dilutional effect, which results in impaired coagulation and possibly bleeding. They may also dilute the plasma protein concentration, which, in turn, may impair the function of platelets. Rarely, dextran therapy causes anaphylaxis or renal failure.

Interactions

No drug interactions occur with colloids.

Dosages

For the recommended dosages of colloids, see Table 27-5.

DRUG PROFILES

The specific colloid used for replacement therapy varies from institution to institution. The three most commonly used are 5% albumin, dextran 40, and hetastarch. They all have a very rapid onset of action as well as a long duration of action. They are metabolized in the liver and excreted by the kidneys. Albumin is the one exception: it is metabolized by the reticuloendothelial system and excreted by the kidneys and the intestines. Hetastarch is a synthetic colloid with properties similar to those of albumin and dextran.

albumin

Albumin (Albuminar) is a natural protein that is normally produced by the liver. It is responsible for generating approximately 70% of the colloid oncotic pressure. Human albumin is a sterile solution of serum albumin that is prepared from pooled blood, plasma, serum, or placentas obtained from healthy human donors. It is pasteurized (heated at 140° F [60° C] for 10 hours) to destroy any contaminants. Unfortunately, because it is derived from human donors, the supply is limited. Many institutions have specific indications for the use of albumin.

Albumin is contraindicated in patients with a known hypersensitivity to it and in those with heart failure, severe anemia, or renal insufficiency. Albumin is available only in parenteral form in concentrations of 5% and 25%. Pregnancy category C. See Table 27-5 for dosing guidelines.

PHARMACOKINETICS

Route	Onset of Action	Peak Plasma Concentration	Elimination Half-life	Duration of Action
IV	Less than 1 min	Unknown	16 hr	Less than 24 hr

dextran

Dextran (Gentran) is a solution of glucose. It is available in three concentrations, dextran 40 and the more concentrated dextran 70 and dextran 75, and it has a molecular weight similar to that of albumin. Dextran 40 is the more commonly used of the two and is a low-molecular-weight polymer of glucose. It is a derivative of sugar that has actions similar to those of human albumin in that it expands the plasma volume by drawing fluid from the interstitial space to the intravascular space.

Dextran is contraindicated in patients with hypersensitivity to it and in those with heart failure, renal insufficiency, and extreme dehydration. It is available only in parenteral form in either a 5% dextrose solution or a 0.9% sodium chloride solution. Pregnancy category C. See Table 27-5 for dosing guidelines.

PHARMACOKINETICS

Route	Onset of Action	Peak Plasma Concentration	Elimination Half-life	Duration of Action
IV	5 min	Unknown	2-6 hr	4-6 hr

BLOOD PRODUCTS

Blood products can be thought of as biologic drugs. All of them can augment the plasma volume. Red blood cell (RBC)–containing products can also improve tissue oxygenation, as well as augment plasma volume. Blood products are also more expensive than crystalloids and colloids and are less available because they are natural products and require human donors. The available blood products are listed in Table 27-7. They are most often indicated when a patient has lost 25% or more blood volume.

Mechanism of Action and Drug Effects

The mechanism of action of blood products is related to their ability to increase the colloid oncotic pressure, and hence the plasma volume. They do so in the same manner as colloids and crystalloids, by pulling fluid from the extravascular space to the intravascular space. Because of this they are also considered plasma expanders. RBC products also have the ability to carry oxygen. They can maintain the colloid oncotic pressure for several hours to days, and because they come from human donors, they have all the benefits (and hazards) that human blood products have. They are administered when a person's body is deficient in these products.

TABLE 27-7 Blood Products

Product	Dosage	Cost*
Cryoprecipitate	1 unit	1
FFP	1 unit	1.7
PRBCs	1 unit	2.2
PPF	1 unit	1
Whole blood	1 unit	3.33

FFP, Fresh frozen plasma; *PPF*, plasma protein fraction; *PRBCs*, packed red blood cells.
*Relative cost compared with the cost of cryoprecipitate.

TABLE 27-8 Blood Products: Indications

Blood Product	Indication
Cryoprecipitate and PPF	To manage acute bleeding (over 50% blood loss slowly or 20% rapidly)
FFP	To increase clotting factor levels in patients with a demonstrated deficiency
PRBCs	To increase oxygen-carrying capacity in patients with anemia, in patients with substantial hemoglobin deficits, and in patients who have lost up to 25% of their total blood volume
Whole blood	Same as for PRBCs, except that whole blood is more beneficial in cases of extreme (over 25%) loss of blood volume because whole blood also contains plasma, the chief fluid volume of the blood; it also contains plasma proteins, the chief osmotic component, which help draw fluid back into blood vessels from surrounding tissues

FFP, Fresh frozen plasma; *PPF*, plasma protein fraction; *PRBCs*, packed red blood cells.

Indications

Blood products are used to treat a wide variety of clinical conditions, and the blood product used depends on the specific indication. The available blood products and the specific conditions they are used to treat are listed in Table 27-8.

Contraindications

There are no absolute contraindications to the use of blood products. However, because there is risk for transfer of infectious disease, although remote, their use should be based on careful clinical evaluation of the patient's condition.

Adverse Effects

Blood products can produce undesirable effects, some potentially serious. Because these products come from other humans, they can be incompatible with the recipient's immune system. These incompatibilities are tested for before the administration of the particular blood product by determining the respective blood types of the donor and recipient and by performing cross-matching tests to screen for incompatibility between selected blood proteins. This helps reduce the likelihood that the recipient will reject the blood product, which would precipitate transfusion reactions and anaphylaxis. These products can also transmit pathogens from the donor to the recipient. Examples of such pathogens are hepatitis virus and human immunodeficiency virus. Various preparation techniques are now used to reduce the risk for pathogen transmission, and these have resulted in a drastic reduction in the incidence of such problems.

Interactions

As with crystalloids and colloids, blood products are very similar if not identical to normal physiologic substances; therefore, they are involved in very few interactions. Calcium and drugs such as aspirin that normally affect coagulation may interact with these substances when infused in the body in much the same way that they interact with the body's own blood components. Blood must not be administered with any solution other than NS.

Dosages

For the dosage guidelines pertaining to blood products, see Table 27-9.

DRUG PROFILES

Packed red blood cells (PRBCs) and fresh frozen plasma (FFP) are among the most commonly used blood products. All of the blood products are derived from pooled blood from human donors. Other less commonly used, but still important, blood products are whole blood, plasma protein fraction, cryoprecipitate, and platelets.

packed red blood cells

PRBCs are obtained by the centrifugation of whole blood and the separation of RBCs from plasma and the other cellular elements. The advantage of PRBCs is that their oxygen-carrying capacity is better than that of the other blood products, and they are less likely to cause cardiac fluid overload. Their disadvantages include high cost, limited shelf life, and fluctuating availability, as well as their ability to transmit viruses, trigger allergic reactions, and cause bleeding abnormalities. The suggested guidelines for their use are given in Table 27-9.

fresh frozen plasma

FFP is obtained by centrifuging whole blood and thereby removing the cellular elements. The resulting plasma is then frozen at −0.4° F (−18° C). FFP is not recommended for routine fluid resuscitation, but it may be used as an adjunct to massive blood transfusion in the treatment of patients with underlying coagulation disorders. The plasma-expanding capability of FFP is similar to that of dextran but slightly less than that of hetastarch. The disadvantage of FFP use is that it can transmit pathogens. The suggested guidelines for use are given in Table 27-9.

Physiology of Electrolyte Balance

The chemical composition of the fluid compartments varies from compartment to compartment. The principal electrolytes in the extracellular fluid are sodium cations (Na^+) and chloride anions (Cl^-); the major electrolyte in the ICF is the potassium cation (K^+). Other important electrolytes are calcium, magnesium, and phosphorus. These different chemical components are vital to the normal function of all body systems. They are controlled by the renin-angiotensin-aldosterone system, antidiuretic hormone system, and sympathetic nervous system. When these neuroendocrine systems are out of balance, adverse electrolyte imbalances commonly result.

TABLE 27-9   Suggested Guidelines for Blood Products: Management of Bleeding

Amount of Blood Loss	Fluid of Choice
20% or less (slow loss)	Crystalloids
20%-50% (slow loss)	Nonprotein plasma expanders (dextran and hetastarch)
Over 50% (slow loss) or 20% (acutely)	Whole blood or PRBCs, and/or PPF and FFP
80% or more	As above, but for every 5 units of blood given, administer 1-2 units of FFP and 1-2 units of platelets to prevent the hemodilution of clotting factors and bleeding

FPP, Fresh frozen plasma; *PPF,* plasma protein fraction; *PRBCs,* packed red blood cells.

POTASSIUM

Potassium is the most abundant cationic (positively charged) electrolyte inside cells (the intracellular space), where the normal concentration is approximately 150 mEq/L. Approximately 95% of the potassium in the body is intracellular. In contrast, the potassium content outside the cells in the plasma ranges from 3.5 to 5 mEq/L. These plasma levels are critical to normal body function.

Potassium is obtained from a variety of foods, the most common being fruit and juices, vegetables, fish, and meats. It has been estimated that for normal body functions to be maintained, a person must consume 5 to 10 mEq of potassium per day. Fortunately, the average daily diet usually provides 35 to 100 mEq of potassium, which is well above the required daily amount. Excess dietary potassium is usually excreted by the kidneys in the urine. However, if the kidneys lose their ability to filter and secrete waste products, potassium can accumulate so that toxic levels are reached, and these, in turn, can precipitate ventricular fibrillation and cardiac arrest. Hyperaldosteronism and use of potassium-sparing diuretics can alter normal potassium balance as well. **Hyperkalemia** is the term for an excessive serum potassium level and is defined as a serum potassium level exceeding 5.5 mEq/L. There are several causes of hyperkalemia. One, renal failure, was just mentioned. Others are as follows:

- Angiotensin-converting enzyme (ACE) inhibitor use
- Burns
- Excessive loss from cells
- Infections
- Metabolic acidosis
- Potassium supplementation
- Potassium-sparing diuretic use
- Trauma

The opposite of hyperkalemia is **hypokalemia,** or a deficiency of potassium. This condition is more often the result of excessive potassium loss than of poor dietary intake, however. As with hyperkalemia, there are many clinical conditions and other situations that can cause it. These include the following:

- Alkalosis
- Increased secretion of mineralocorticoids (hormones of the adrenal cortex)

- Burns*
- Corticosteroid use
- Crash diets
- Diarrhea
- Hyperaldosteronism
- Ketoacidosis
- Consumption of large amounts of licorice
- Loop diuretic use
- Malabsorption
- Prolonged laxative misuse
- Thiazide diuretic use
- Thiazide-like diuretic use
- Vomiting

A low serum potassium level can also greatly increase the toxicity associated with digitalis preparations, and this can precipitate serious ventricular dysrhythmias.

The early detection of hypokalemia is important to prevent the serious, life-threatening consequences of this metabolic disturbance if it goes untreated. The key to early detection is knowing its early symptoms, which are generally mild and can easily go unnoticed. Both the early (mild) symptoms and late (severe) symptoms of hypokalemia are listed in Box 27-1. The treatment of hypokalemia involves both identifying and treating the cause and restoring the serum potassium levels to normal (higher than 3.5 mEq/L). The consumption of potassium-rich foods can usually correct mild hypokalemia, but clinically significant hypokalemia requires the oral or parenteral administration of a potassium supplement, which usually contains potassium chloride.

Mechanism of Action and Drug Effects

The importance of potassium as the primary intracellular electrolyte is highlighted by the enormous number of life-sustaining physiologic functions that require it. Muscle contraction, the transmission of nerve impulses, and the regulation of heartbeats (the pacemaker function of the heart) are just a few of these functions.

Potassium is also essential for the maintenance of acid-base balance, isotonicity, and the electrodynamic characteristics of the cell. It plays a role in many enzymatic reactions, and it is an essential component in gastric secretion, renal function, tissue synthesis, and carbohydrate metabolism.

Indications

Potassium replacement therapy is called for in the treatment or prevention of potassium depletion in patients whenever dietary measures prove inadequate. Potassium salts commonly used for this purpose include potassium chloride, potassium phosphate, and potassium acetate. The chloride is required to correct the hypochloremia (low level of chloride in the blood) that commonly accompanies potassium deficiency, and phosphate is used to correct hypophosphatemia. The acetate salt may be used to raise the blood pH in acidotic conditions.

Other therapeutic effects of potassium are related to its role in the contraction of muscles and the maintenance of the electrical characteristics of cells. Potassium salts may be used to stop irregular heartbeats (dysrhythmias) and to manage the tachydysrhythmias that can occur after cardiac surgery.

---

*Burn patients can exhibit either hyperkalemia or hypokalemia.

BOX 27-1 Symptoms of Hypokalemia
Early
Anorexia
Hypotension
Lethargy
Mental confusion
Muscle weakness
Nausea
Late
Cardiac dysrhythmias
Neuropathy
Paralytic ileus
Secondary alkalosis

Contraindications

Contraindications to potassium replacement products include known allergy to a specific drug product, hyperkalemia from any cause, severe renal disease, acute dehydration, untreated Addison's disease, severe hemolytic disease, and conditions involving extensive tissue breakdown (e.g., multiple trauma, severe burns).

Adverse Effects

The adverse effects of potassium therapy are primarily limited to the gastrointestinal (GI) tract and occur with the oral administration of potassium preparations. These GI effects include diarrhea, nausea, and vomiting. More significant effects include GI bleeding and ulceration. The parenteral administration of potassium usually produces pain at the injection site. Cases of phlebitis have been associated with IV administration, and the excessive administration of potassium salts can lead to hyperkalemia and toxic effects. If IV potassium is administered too rapidly, cardiac arrest may occur. IV potassium should be given no faster than 10 mEq/hr to patients who are not on cardiac monitors. For critically ill patients on cardiac monitors, rates of 20 mEq/hr or more may be used.

Toxicity and Management of Overdose

The toxic effects of potassium are the result of hyperkalemia. Symptoms include muscle weakness, paresthesia, paralysis, cardiac rhythm irregularities that can result in ventricular fibrillation, and cardiac arrest. The treatment instituted depends on the degree of the hyperkalemia and ranges from regimens for reversal of life-threatening problems to simple dietary restrictions. In the event of severe hyperkalemia, the IV administration of sodium bicarbonate, calcium gluconate or chloride, or dextrose solution with insulin is often required. These drugs correct severe hyperkalemia by causing a rapid intracellular shift of potassium ions, which reduces the serum potassium concentration. Such interventions are often followed with orally or rectally administered sodium polystyrene sulfonate (Kayexalate) or hemodialysis to eliminate the extra potassium from the body. Less critical levels can be reduced with dietary restrictions.

Interactions

Concurrent use of potassium-sparing diuretics and ACE inhibitors can produce a hyperkalemic state. Concurrent use of non–potassium-sparing diuretics, amphotericin B, and mineralocorticoids can produce a hypokalemic state.

Dosages

Fluid and electrolyte therapy involves replacing any deficits or losses and/or providing maintenance levels for specific patient requirements. Accordingly, specific dosage amounts of fluids or electrolytes depend on several clinical factors, including the following:

- Specific patient losses
- Efficacy of patient physiologic systems involved in fluid and electrolyte metabolism, especially adrenal, cardiovascular, and kidney functions
- Current drug therapy for pathologic conditions that complicate the amount and duration of replacement
- Selection of oral or parenteral replacement formulations

Suggested dosage guidelines for potassium with subsequent adjustments are 10 to 20 mEq administered orally several times a day or parenteral administration of 30 to 60 mEq every 24 hours.

DRUG PROFILES

potassium

Potassium supplements are administered either to prevent or to treat potassium depletion. The acetate, bicarbonate, chloride, citrate, and gluconate salts of potassium are available for oral administration, including tablets, solutions, elixirs, and powders for solution. The parenteral salt forms of potassium for IV administration are acetate, chloride, and phosphate. The dosage of potassium supplements is usually expressed in milliequivalents of potassium and depends on the requirements of the individual patient. Different salt forms of potassium deliver varying milliequivalent amounts of potassium.

Potassium is contraindicated in patients with severe renal disease, severe hemolytic disease, or Addison's disease and in those with hyperkalemia, acute dehydration, or extensive tissue breakdown stemming from multiple traumas. Pregnancy category A.

PHARMACOKINETICS

Route	Onset of Action	Peak Plasma Concentration	Elimination Half-life	Duration of Action
IV	Immediate	Rapid	Variable	Variable

sodium polystyrene sulfonate (potassium exchange resin)

Sodium polystyrene sulfonate (Kayexalate) is known as a *cation exchange resin* and is used to treat hyperkalemia. For this purpose it is usually administered orally via nasogastric tube or as an enema. It works in the intestine, where potassium ions from the body are exchanged for sodium ions in the resin. Although the drug effects in each case are unpredictable, approximately 1 mEq of potassium is lost from the body per gram of resin administered. It has no listed contraindications per se, but it can cause disturbances in electrolytes other than potassium, such as calcium and magnesium. For this reason, patients' electrolytes should be closely monitored during treatment with sodium polystyrene sulfonate. It is typically dosed in multiples of 15 to 30 grams until the desired effect on serum potassium occurs. Onset of action varies from 2 to 12 hours and is generally faster with the oral route than with rectal administration. It is available in 15 g/60 mL suspensions and in a powder for reconstitution. Pregnancy category C.

SODIUM

Although sodium was discussed under colloids earlier in this chapter, it is also presented here in the electrolyte section because it is most commonly given for replenishing purposes. Sodium is the counterpart of potassium in that potassium is the principal cation inside cells, whereas sodium is the principal cation outside cells. The normal concentration of sodium outside cells is 135 to 145 mEq/L, and it is maintained through the dietary intake of sodium in the form of sodium chloride, which is obtained from salt, fish, meats, and other foods flavored, seasoned, or preserved with salt.

Hyponatremia is a condition of sodium loss or deficiency and occurs when the serum levels decrease below 135 mEq/L. It is manifested by lethargy, hypotension, stomach cramps, vomiting, diarrhea, and seizures. Some of the same conditions that cause hypokalemia can also cause hyponatremia, and these are listed on pp. 423-424. Other causes of hyponatremia are excessive perspiration, occurring during hot weather or physical work; prolonged diarrhea or vomiting, especially in young children; renal disorders; and adrenocortical impairment.

Hypernatremia is the condition of sodium excess and occurs when the serum levels of sodium exceed 145 mEq/L. Some of the symptoms are water retention (edema) and hypertension. The most common cause is poor renal excretion stemming from kidney malfunction. Inadequate water consumption and dehydration are other causes. Symptoms of hypernatremia include red, flushed skin; dry, sticky mucous membranes; increased thirst; temperature elevation; and decreased or absent urination.

Mechanism of Action and Drug Effects

As one of the body's electrolytes, sodium performs many physiologic roles necessary for the normal function of the body. It is the major cation in ECF and is principally involved in the control of water distribution, fluid and electrolyte balance, and osmotic pressure of body fluids. Sodium also participates along with both chloride and bicarbonate in the regulation of acid-base balance. Chloride, the major extracellular anion (negatively charged substance), closely complements the physiologic action of sodium. Sodium is also capable of causing diuresis.

Indications

Sodium is primarily administered for the treatment or prevention of sodium depletion when dietary measures have proved inadequate. Sodium chloride is the primary salt used for this purpose. Mild hyponatremia is usually treated with the oral administration of sodium chloride tablets and/or fluid restriction. Pronounced sodium depletion is treated with NS or lactated Ringer's solution administered IV. These drugs were discussed earlier in this chapter.

Contraindications

The only usual contraindications to the use of sodium replacement products are known drug allergy to a specific product and hypernatremia.

Adverse Effects

The oral administration of sodium chloride can cause gastric upset consisting of nausea, vomiting, and cramps. Venous phlebitis can be a consequence of its parenteral administration. Hypertonic saline (3% or 5%) can cause death by cerebral edema if administered too rapidly.

Toxicity and Management of Overdose

Hypernatremia leads to hypertension, edema, thirst, tachycardia, weakness, convulsions, and possibly coma. Treatment consists of increased fluid intake and dietary restrictions. In more serious cases, diuretics may be required to enhance urinary sodium excretion. IV administration of dextrose in water solution (e.g., %5 or 10% dextrose in water) may also be helpful by producing both intravascular sodium dilution and enhanced urine volume output.

Interactions

Sodium is not known to interact significantly with any drugs with the exception of the antibiotic Synercid, with which it is incompatible.

Dosages

Fluid and electrolyte therapy involves replacing any deficit losses and/or providing maintenance levels for specific patient requirements. Accordingly, specific dosage amounts of fluids or electrolytes depend on several clinical factors, as follows:

- Specific patient losses
- Efficacy of patient physiologic systems involved in fluid and electrolyte metabolism, especially adrenal, cardiovascular, and kidney functions
- Current drug therapy for pathologic conditions that complicate the amount and duration of replacement
- Selection of oral or parenteral replacement formulations

Suggested dosage guidelines for sodium chloride with subsequent adjustments are 1 to 2 g administered orally several times a day or parenteral administration of 1 L of sodium chloride injection (NS).

DRUG PROFILE

sodium chloride

Sodium chloride is primarily used as a replacement electrolyte for either the prevention or treatment of sodium loss. It is also used as a diluent for the infusion of compatible drugs and in the assessment of kidney function after a fluid challenge. Sodium chloride is contraindicated in patients who are hypersensitive to it. It is available in many IV preparations and in oral form as 650-mg tablets. Pregnancy category C.

PHARMACOKINETICS

Route	Onset of Action	Peak Plasma Concentration	Elimination Half-life	Duration of Action
IV	Immediate	Rapid	Unknown	Variable

NURSING PROCESS

Assessment

For fluid replacement, patient needs vary, and any medications or solutions ordered should be given exactly as prescribed and without substitution. However, the prescriber's order should never be taken at face value without confirming the order against authoritative resources (e.g., recent drug reference guide, *Physicians Desk Reference,* nursing pharmacology textbook, manufacturer's drug insert) or speaking with a pharmacist. Important to remember is that the nurse is responsible for making sure that the drug therapy administration process—beginning with the assessment phase of the nursing process and through to evaluation—is accurate and safe, and meets professional standards of care. For fluid replacement or solutions ordered, they should be given exactly as ordered and without substitution. To assist in the development of a thorough assessment plan, a brief review of the various solutions is needed. Parenterally administered hydrating and hypotonic solutions include 0.2% NaCl and 0.45% NS/D_5W. These are used mainly for the prevention and/or treatment of dehydration. D_5W alone in an IV bag is considered isotonic but acts as a hypotonic solution once in the blood stream. Isotonic solutions (e.g., 0.9% NaCl [normal saline] and lactated Ringer's) are customarily used to augment extracellular volume in patients experiencing blood loss, severe vomiting, or any condition that leads to a chloride loss equal to or greater than the sodium loss. Isotonic solutions include 0.9% NaCl (normal saline) and are used to augment extracellular volume in patients suffering from blood loss, severe vomiting, or any condition that leads to a chloride loss equal to or greater than the sodium loss. Isotonic NaCl is also used as diluting fluid for blood transfusions because D_5W results in hemolysis of red blood cells (in transfusions). Hypertonic solutions, such as 3% NaCl, 5% NaCl, albumin, and blood products, are used for replacement of special fluids and electrolytes (see previous discussion).

Because of the potential risks related to the use of these solutions, they are rarely administered outside of the hospital setting. After all prescriber orders are verified and checked for accuracy and completeness (as with all drugs), assessment of the solution or product, the patient, and the IV site (if applicable) should be performed. The nurse must also assess the following for IV infusions of fluids and/or electrolytes: the solution to be infused, infusion equipment, infusion rate of the solution, concentration of the parenteral solution, related mathematical calculations, laboratory values (e.g., sodium, chloride, potassium), and parenteral compatibilities. More specific assessment of the patient who is to receive a parenteral replacement solution should focus on gathering information about the patient's medical history, including diseases of the GI, renal, cardiac, and/or hepatic systems. A medication history should be obtained that includes a listing of prescription drugs, over-the-counter medications, supplements, and herbals. A dietary history is also important and should include specific dietary habits and recall of all foods consumed during the previous 24 hours. Fluid volume and electrolyte status should be assessed (through laboratory testing and measurement of urinary specific gravity, vital signs, and intake and output) and should be documented. The skin and mucous membranes also reflect a patient's hydration status and are important to assess, including skin turgor and/or rebound elasticity of skin over the top of the hand and other areas over the body. The findings should be documented as "immediate" rebound or "delayed" rebound. It would be appropriate to count the number of seconds that the patient's skin stays in the pinched-up position, with normal return being immediately or within 3 to 5 seconds.

Potassium is presented first in the discussion of electrolytes, and one important place to begin assessment is knowing the normal range, which is 3.5 to 5 mEq/L. Levels below 3.5 mEq/L (hypokalemia) may result in a variety of problems, such as cardiac irregularities and muscle weakness. Tartrazine sensitivity, mostly noted in patients with aspirin allergies, should be

LABORATORY VALUES RELATED TO DRUG THERAPY

Calcium

Laboratory Test	Normal Ranges	Rationale for Assessment
Serum calcium level	9-10.5 mg/dL or 4.65-5.28 mg/dL (ionized level)	Calcium supplementation may be deemed necessary whenever the level of calcium drops below the normal range. In addition to normal serum calcium level, ionized calcium level is reported. Serum ionized calcium is the amount of calcium not bound to protein. Clinical signs and symptoms of hypocalcemia include abnormal neuromuscular contractions and tremors. There are assessment tests for the presence of abnormal neuromuscular contractions. The two classic tests are the Chvostek's and Trousseau's signs. The Chvostek's sign is elicited by gently tapping the face at a point just anterior to the ear and below the zygomatic bone with the blunt end of a reflex hammer. A positive response for hypocalcemia is twitching of the ipsilateral facial muscles and is suggestive of neuromuscular excitability secondary to hypocalcemia. The Trousseau's sign is elicited by inflating a sphygmomanometer cuff (blood pressure cuff) for several minutes. A positive response is muscle contraction with flexion of the wrist and metacarpophalangeal joints, hyperextension of the fingers, and flexion of the thumb on the palm. This muscle contraction is indicative of neuromuscular excitability secondary to hypocalcemia. These tests, in addition to serum calcium measurement, may be helpful in confirming the presence of hypocalcemia.

Modified from Urbano FL: Signs of hypocalcemia: Chvostek's and Trousseau's signs, *Hosp Physician*, p 43, March 2000.

---

assessed carefully if the patient is taking potassium chloride because of the risk of cross-sensitivity. Potassium supplementation should be avoided or used with extreme caution in patients taking ACE inhibitors or potassium-sparing diuretics (such as spironolactone). These drugs are associated with adverse effects of hyperkalemia and, if given with potassium supplementation, could worsen hyperkalemia and possibly result in severe cardiac compromise and possible cardiac arrest. Oral potassium supplements are irritants and can be ulcerogenic, and thus a thorough GI tract assessment is needed. If the patient has a history of ulcers or GI bleeding, the supplementation should not be given orally, and the prescriber should be contacted for further instructions.

The range of serum potassium levels defined as normal often vary depending on the institution and/or the prescriber. For identification and treatment of hyperkalemia, the normal range of potassium must be established. The nurse must realize that potassium levels of 5.3 mEq/L may be identified as abnormally high by some laboratories, whereas other laboratories may categorize 5.0 mEq/L as being abnormally high. Be sure to check hospital policy and laboratory guidelines for normal ranges and report any elevations or decreases in serum potassium. However, a serum level exceeding 5.5 mEq/L is considered by most sources to be toxic and dangerous to the patient, and should be reported immediately to the prescriber. With close monitoring of patients, the dangerous effects of hyperkalemia will hopefully be prevented or at least identified early and treated appropriately to prevent potentially life-threatening complications (see previous discussion of hyperkalemia).

Venous access is an issue with parenteral potassium supplementation, because the vein can be irritated if infiltration occurs or if the solution has not been mixed thoroughly. The following are some important considerations regarding peripheral venous access (for potassium, sodium, fluid, and any other type of medication given by the IV route): (1) Try to use distal veins first. (2) Know the purpose of administering potassium and other electrolytes. (3) Set the rate as ordered and recalculated for infusion. (4) Know the anticipated duration of therapy. (5) Assess the overall condition of the veins. (6) Know the restrictions imposed by the patient's history (e.g., affected arm of a patient who has undergone a mastectomy and lymph node dissection). In postmastectomy patients and patients who have experienced stroke, limb circulation may be inadequate, which can lead to edema and other complications.

Sodium is another electrolyte that is an ingredient in various IV replacement solutions. Hyponatremia, or serum sodium level below 135 mEq/L, if not resolved with dietary and/or oral intake, may need to be treated with parenteral infusions. Venous access sites should be carefully chosen because of possible irritation of the vein and subsequent phlebitis. If replacement to correct hyponatremic states is overzealous, the result may be hypernatremia and fluid overload, edema, worsening of heart failure, dyspnea, and crackles. Continual monitoring of vital signs, hydration status of the skin and mucous membranes, and level of consciousness is important to safe replacement and prevention of further complications.

Hypernatremia also requires careful assessment. Identification of any precipitating events, medical concerns, and risk-prone patient situations is important to finding early solutions for treatment. The populations at risk for hypernatremia include the elderly, those with renal and cardiovascular diseases, patients who are receiving sodium supplements or who have increased sodium intake, and those with decreased fluid intake. Administration of any electrolyte requires assessment for cautions, contraindications, and drug interactions.

Albumin and other colloids have associated cautions, contraindications, and drug interactions that need to be assessed. It is also important to assess the patient's hematocrit, hemoglobin levels, and serum protein levels. The patient's blood pressure, pulse rate, respiratory status, and intake and output should be monitored and documented. Assessment for dyspnea or hypoxia should also be performed and the findings reported prior to the use of these drugs. Laboratory interference is seen with measurement of alkaline phosphatase (ALP) levels, which are increased when albumin is given.

Fluid infusions may include the giving of blood or blood components. The nurse should obtain a thorough history regarding any transfusions received previously and the patient's response. Any history of adverse reactions to transfusions should be reported to the prescriber and the nature of these reactions documented. It is also important to assess the status of venous access areas as well as to check the patient's laboratory values (e.g., hematocrit, hemoglobin, white blood cells [WBCs], RBCs, platelets, and clotting factors). Baseline vital signs should be noted before infusing the blood or blood product. Even the general appearance of the patient, energy levels, ability to carry out activities of daily living, and color of extremities are important to note. During the infusion of blood components, the nurse should be alert to the occurrence of fever and blood in the urine, which are both indicative of an adverse reaction.

In summary, safety and caution are top priorities when patients receive any drug, including fluid and electrolyte replacements. Excess levels of fluid and electrolytes as well as deficits may pose tremendous risks to patients, and therefore the nurse must assess thoroughly so that safety and caution are maintained. In addition, because so many patients receive therapies in the home setting, the nurse has even more accountability and responsibility for performing skillful and thorough assessment before, during, and after therapy.

Nursing Diagnoses

- Risk for falls related to fluid and electrolyte imbalances
- Risk for imbalanced fluid volume related to drug-induced fluid excess or deficits and electrolyte excesses or deficits
- Risk for injury related to complications of the transfusion or infusion of blood products, blood components, or related agents
- Deficient knowledge about the treatment regimen related to the lack of patient education about electrolyte disturbances and the influence of treatment

Planning
Goals

- Patient has minimal problems with volume overload related to the transfusion or infusion.
- Patient begins minimal exercise and shows increased tolerance daily.
- Patient participates in activities as he or she can tolerate them.
- Patient states measures to implement to minimize self-injury related to altered blood component levels or altered fluid and electrolyte levels.
- Patient states the rationale for treatment and the adverse effects of replacement agents.
- Patient states symptoms and problems to report to the prescriber.

Outcome Criteria

- Patient remains free of self-injury as a result of adverse reactions (dizziness, volume overload, hypersensitivity) to the transfusion or infusion or an allergic reaction.

CASE STUDY

Fluid and Electrolyte Replacement

© Dundanim

M.S., an 85-year-old retired engineer, seemed somewhat confused when his daughter came home from work. When she brings him to the emergency department, his blood pressure is 90/62 mm Hg, his heart rate is 114 beats/min, and his skin is dry but cool. His daughter says that he seems "much weaker" than usual, and he is unable to answer questions clearly. His daughter reports that he has "lost his appetite" lately and has not taken in much food or drink. The nurse starts an IV infusion of 0.9% sodium chloride (NS) at 100 mL/hr.

1. What do you think is M.S.'s main medical problem at this time?
   The emergency department is very busy, and when the nurse returns, she is shocked to see that almost the entire 500-mL bag of NS has infused within an hour's time.
2. What should the nurse do first? What should the nurse watch for at this time?
3. When monitoring his fluid status, which indicators should the nurse consider the most reliable?
   Twenty-four hours after his admission, M.S. is much less confused and is able to move to a chair for lunch without much difficulty. He is receiving 5% dextrose/½ NS with 20 mEq of potassium chloride at a rate of 75 mL/hr via an infusion pump. His daughter notices that the area above the IV insertion site is red, and M.S. complains that the area is "very sore."
4. What is the possible problem with the IV line? What should be done at this time?

For answers, see *http://evolve.elsevier.com/Lilley*.

- Patient regains the ability to engage in normal or near-normal exercise, showing increased tolerance daily as evidenced by walking small distances and increasing to regular supervised exercise.
- Patient participates in activities according to his or her ability to tolerate them without dyspnea or chest pain.
- Patient demonstrates a return to normal or near-normal values of blood components or fluid and electrolyte levels.
- Patient sees the prescriber for follow-up as ordered to monitor laboratory values pertinent to treatment.

Implementation

Continued monitoring of the patient during fluid or electrolyte therapy is crucial to ensure safe and effective treatment. It is also important to continue monitoring so that adverse effects can be identified early and complications of overzealous treatment and/or undertreatment can be prevented. No serum electrolyte levels should exceed normal ranges (see the pharmacology section).

With parenteral dosing, the nurse must monitor infusion rates as well as the appearance of the fluid or solution (i.e., potassium and saline solutions are clear, whereas albumin is brown, clear, and viscous). The IV site must also be monitored frequently as per facility policy and nursing standards of care for evidence of infiltration (e.g., swelling, coolness of skin to the touch around IV site, no or decreased flow rate, and no blood return from IV catheter) or thrombophlebitis (e.g., swelling, redness, heat, and pain at site). Volume overload, drug toxicity, fever, infection, and emboli are other complications of IV therapy.

With the administration of any fluid or electrolyte solution, a steady and even flow rate must be maintained to prevent complications. Infusion rates must follow the prescriber's orders, and calculations must be rechecked for accuracy. The IV site, tubing, IV bag, fluids, and/or solutions as well as expiration dates should all be checked with infusion of both replacement fluids and electrolytes. The nurse should always behave in a prudent, safe, and thorough manner when administering fluids and electrolyte solutions and remember that elderly and/or pediatric patients have increased sensitivity to these solutions and fluids (as well as to most medications). Patients at risk for volume deficits, especially the elderly, should be informed of the effect of a hot, humid environment on physiologic functioning and the danger of exacerbation by excessive perspiration. Water is at the crux of every metabolic reaction that occurs within the body, and when there are deficits, physiologic reactions are negatively impacted and the composition of fluids and electrolytes altered. For any age group, staying hydrated at all times is a preventative measure.

With the various IV solutions, knowing their osmolality and concentrations is important to their safe use. Administration of isotonic solutions (e.g., 0.9% sodium chloride, lactated Ringer's solution) requires constant monitoring during and after therapy for possible fluid overload (potentially pulmonary edema), and patients with heart failure are at even higher risk. It is important to remember that 5% dextrose/0.2% saline solutions, even though initially isotonic, should not be used to maintain vascular volume in a patient who is hypovolemic and hypotensive, because the solutions rapidly become hypotonic when dextrose is metabolized. Hypotonic solutions (e.g., 0.2% or 0.45% sodium chloride), although useful in conditions of cellular dehydration, may lead to a sudden shift of fluids if given too rapidly. Hypertonic solutions are used rarely because of the risk of cellular dehydration and vascular volume overload. These solutions are also associated with phlebitis and spasm if IV infiltration and/or extravasation in the peripheral veins occurs. Therefore, if indicated, these solutions may be administered through a larger bore vein (e.g., central line) but only with close monitoring of the patient's vital signs and cardiac status.

Oral preparations of potassium, rather than parenteral dosage forms, should be prescribed whenever possible. The oral dosage forms should be prepared per the manufacturer's inserts or per policy and standard of care. Generally, oral forms of potassium must be taken with food to minimize gastric distress or irritation. Powder or effervescent forms should be prepared according to the package guidelines and mixed thoroughly with at least 4 to 6 oz of fluid before the medication is taken. Enteric-coated and sustained-released forms may still result in gastric upset and lead to ulcer development (ulcerogenic). The safest and most effective intervention is frequent and close monitoring for complaints of nausea, vomiting, abdominal pain, or bleeding (such as blood in the stool and/or the occurrence of hematemesis or blood in the vomitus). Should abnormalities be noted, vital signs and other parameters should continue to be monitored and the findings reported to the prescriber immediately. Serum levels of potassium should be monitored during therapy as well.

For the patient who is at risk for hypokalemia, educational materials and patient teaching should encourage consumption of certain foods high in potassium. The minimal daily requirement for potassium is between 40 and 50 mEq for adults and 2 to 3 mEq/kg of body weight for infants. A list of foods containing potassium should be shared with the patient. Two medium-sized bananas or an 8-oz glass of orange juice contains 45 mEq; 20 large dried apricots contain 40 mEq; and a level teaspoon of salt substitute (KCl) contains 60 mEq of potassium. Conversely, if the patient is already hyperkalemic, these are food items that should be avoided. Refer to the previous discussion concerning the use of sodium polystyrene sulfonate to treat hyperkalemia. See the Patient Teaching Tips for more information.

Potassium chloride is the salt customarily used for IV infusions. The concern and caution with potassium chloride use is to avoid overdosage, because it can lead to cardiac arrest. IV dosage forms of potassium must ALWAYS be given in a DILUTED form. There is NO use or place for UNDILUTED potassium, because undiluted potassium is associated with cardiac arrest. Therefore, parenteral forms of potassium should be diluted properly. Nowadays, most pharmacies premix the infusion; however, it is still imperative to double-check the concentration and amount of diluent. The nurse should never assume that what was premixed is 100% correct, because the nurse is ultimately responsible for whatever he or she administers. Diluted potassium should also be given only when there is adequate urine output of at least 30 mL/hr. Manufacturer instructions and policy protocols generally recommend that IV solutions be given at concentrations of less than 40 mEq/L of potassium and a rate not exceeding 20 mEq/hr. Another precautionary measure that must be followed is to avoid adding potassium chloride to an already existing IV solution, because the exact concentration cannot be accurately calculated and thus there is a risk of complications, overdosage, or toxicity. The nurse must make sure that all IV fluids are labeled appropriately and documented, as with any medication. If the IV fluid rate must be monitored very closely, an infusion pump may be used. There is *no* place for IV push or IV bolus potassium replacement!

Replacement of sodium carries the same concern regarding dosing and route of administration. When the patient is only mildly depleted, an increase in oral intake of sodium should be tried. Food items high in sodium include catsup, mustard, cured meats, cheeses, potato chips, peanut butter, popcorn, and table salt. In some situations, salt tablets may be necessary. If the patient is given salt tablets, it is very important that the patient also take plenty of fluids, up to 3000 mL/24 hr, unless contraindicated. If the sodium deficit requires IV replacement, venous access issues and drip rate are as important as with volume and potassium infusions (see previous discussion regarding IV infusion and IV sites).

IV infusion of albumin and other colloids should always be carried out slowly and cautiously and with careful monitoring to prevent fluid overload and heart failure, especially in those patients who are at particular risk for heart failure. Fluid overload would be evidenced by shortness of breath, crackles at the bases of the lungs, decreased pulse oximeter readings, edema of dependent areas, and increase in weight (see the previous parameters). Serum hematocrit and hemoglobin values should also be determined in advance of therapy—as well as during and after therapy—so that any dilutional effects can be determined. For example, if a patient has received albumin and other colloids too quickly, and hypervolemia results, the patient's hemoglobin and hematocrit may actually be decreased. This decrease would be due to a dilutional factor from too much volume in relation to the concentration of solutes. Clinically, the patient would appear to be anemic, but in fact the deficit would be attributable to the increase in volume. It is also important to remember that albumin is to be given at room temperature.

For infusion of blood, it is essential always to check the expiration date of blood and/or blood components to make sure that the blood is not outdated. Under NO circumstances should outdated blood be used! Policies at most hospitals and other health care agencies require that blood and blood products be double-checked by another registered nurse BEFORE the blood is hung and infused. This is important to prevent a mixup in blood types. Blood types should always be a major concern because of the possible complications that can occur, some life threatening, if the wrong blood type is given or if the blood is given to the wrong person. The "Six Rights" of drug administration remain critical in all that nurses do with medications, and administering blood is no exception.

When blood and blood products are infused, all vital signs and related parameters should be documented before, during, and after administration of the blood product, component (e.g., plasma protein fractions, platelets, FFP), or solution. The patient should then be assessed and the findings documented. Vital signs should also be monitored and recorded frequently during and after administration. A transfusion reaction would most likely be manifested by the occurrence of the following: apprehension, restlessness, flushed skin, increased pulse and respirations, dyspnea, rash, joint or lower back pain, swelling, fever and chills (a febrile reaction beginning 1 hour after the start of administration and possibly lasting up to 10 hours), nausea, weakness, and jaundice. These signs and symptoms should be reported to the prescriber immediately, and regardless of when the reaction occurs, the blood or product should be stopped and the IV line kept patent with isotonic NS solution in-

fusing at a slow rate. The facility's protocol for transfusion reactions should always be followed.

In summary, patients receiving any type of fluid or electrolyte substance, colloid, or blood component should be encouraged to immediately report unusual adverse effects to their prescriber. Such complaints include chest pain, dizziness, weakness, and shortness of breath.

Evaluation

The therapeutic response to fluid, electrolyte, and blood or blood component therapy includes normalization of fluid volume and laboratory values, including RBC and WBC counts, hemoglobin level, hematocrit, and sodium and potassium levels. In addition to review of these laboratory values, evaluation of the patient's cardiac, respiratory, musculoskeletal, and GI functioning is also important. Energy levels and tolerance of activities of daily living should return to normal. There should be improved skin color and minimal to no dyspnea, chest pain, weakness, or fatigue. Correct treatment of blood volume problems will be evidenced by a return of laboratory values to the normal range, improved vital signs, an increase in energy, and near normal oxygen saturation levels. The therapeutic response to albumin therapy includes an elevation of blood pressure, decreased edema, and increased serum albumin levels. Monitoring for the adverse effects of any of these drugs and/or solutions should occur frequently and should include checking for distended neck veins; shortness of breath; anxiety; insomnia; expiratory crackles; frothy, blood-tinged sputum; and cyanosis.

PATIENT TEACHING TIPS

- As needed, the patient should be educated about the difference in the signs and symptoms of hyponatremia and hypernatremia. Hyponatremia is manifested by lethargy, hypotension, stomach cramps, vomiting, diarrhea, and possibly seizures. Hypernatremia is manifested by red, flushed skin; dry, sticky mucous membranes; increased thirst; temperature elevation; and a decrease in or absence of urination.
- The patient should be given information about how to take oral potassium chloride. Directions should include mixing any powdered or liquid solutions in at least 4 to 8 oz of cold water/juice and to drink the entire mixture slowly. Oral doses should be taken with food/snack. Patients taking potassium supplements should report any complaints of GI upset, abdominal pain, muscle cramps or weakness, fatigue, or irregular heartbeat to the prescriber immediately. The patient should be told about the many drugs with which potassium interacts, including antacids, diuretics, and digitalis drugs.
- Educate patients about drug interactions with potassium such as antacids, diuretics and digitalis drugs. Foods high in potassium include bananas, oranges, apricots, dates, raisins, broccoli, green beans, potatoes, tomatoes, meats, fish, wheat bread, and legumes.
- Sustained-release capsules and tablets must be swallowed whole and should not be crushed, chewed, or allowed to dissolve in the mouth.
- The patient should be encouraged to report any difficulty in swallowing, painful swallowing, or feeling that the capsule or tablet is getting stuck in the throat. Other serious adverse effects

that need to be reported include vomiting of coffee ground–like material, stomach or abdominal pain or swelling, and black tarry stools.
- Extended-release dosage forms should be taken in full. If the patient has difficulty swallowing the whole tablet, and if approved by the prescriber, the patient can break the tablet in half and take each half separately, drinking half a glass of water (4 oz) with each half and taking the entire dose within a few minutes. The patient should be encouraged not to save a half to take later. If the tablet must be dissolved as prescribed, the patient should be told to allow 2 minutes for the tablet to dissolve in 4 oz of water, to stir for 30 seconds, and then to drink immediately. Adding 1 oz of water to the glass, swirling it, and then drinking the residual will allow adequate dosing. Water is recommended as the fluid for mixing the extended-release dosage form.
- Effervescent tablets should be dissolved as directed, and the patient should be told to use at least 3 oz of cold water per tablet. The patient should be instructed to take the dose as soon as it is fully dissolved, sipping the mixture over 5 to 10 minutes and taking the dose after food to minimize GI upset.
- The patient should be informed that salt substitutes contain potassium, so another alternative should be recommended if the patient is hyperkalemic.
- The patient should be told to report any feelings of irritation (e.g., burning) at the IV site at any time.
- Salt tablets should be taken as prescribed, with caution, and with adequate fluid intake.

POINTS TO REMEMBER

- TBW is divided into intracellular (inside the cell) and extracellular (outside the cell) compartments. Fluid volume outside cells is either in the plasma (intravascular volume) or between the tissues, cells, or organs.
- Colloids are large protein particles that cannot leak out of the blood vessels. Because of their greater concentration inside blood vessels, fluid is pulled into the blood vessels. Examples of colloids include albumin, hetastarch, and dextran. Albumin must be administered with caution because of the high risk for hypervolemia and possibly heart failure. The nurse needs to monitor intake and output, weights, heart and breath sounds, and appropriate laboratory values.
- Blood products are the only fluids that are able to carry oxygen because they are the only fluids that contain hemoglobin. Patients should show improved energy and increasing tolerance for activities of daily living. The nurse should also monitor pulse oximeter readings.
- Dehydration may be hypotonic, resulting from the loss of salt; hypertonic, resulting from fever with perspiration; or isotonic, resulting from diarrhea or vomiting. Each form of dehydration is treated differently. The nurse should carefully assess intake and output as well as skin turgor, urine specific gravity, and blood levels of potassium, sodium, and chloride.
- Hypertonic solutions should be given slowly because of the risk for hypervolemia from overzealous replacement.
- Symptoms of hypokalemia include lethargy, weakness, fatigue, respiratory difficulty, paralysis, and even possible paralytic ileus. Caution: When replacing potassium via IV infusion, the nurse should never give undiluted potassium chloride because it can result in ventricular fibrillation and cardiac arrest due to hyperkalemia. Nursing units should use only diluted potassium/premixed IV fluids containing potassium.
- Hyperkalemia is treated with the use of sodium polystyrene sulfonate.
- With administration of blood products, measurement of vital signs and frequent monitoring of the patient before, during, and after infusions are critical to patient safety. Blood products should be given only with normal saline (0.9% sodium chloride), because D_5W will also cause hemolysis of the blood product.

NCLEX EXAMINATION REVIEW QUESTIONS

1 Which action by the nurse is more appropriate for the patient receiving an infusion of packed red blood cells?
   a Flush the IV line with NS before the blood is added to the infusion.
   b Flush the IV line with dextrose before the blood is added to the infusion.
   c Check the patient's vital signs once the infusion is completed.
   d Anticipate that flushed skin and fever are expected reactions to a blood transfusion.
2 When preparing an IV solution that contains potassium, the nurse knows that a contraindication to the potassium infusion would be
   a diarrhea.
   b serum sodium level of 145 mEq/L.
   c serum potassium level of 5.6 mEq/L.
   d dehydration.
3 When assessing a patient for whom an order for albumin has been written, the nurse knows that a contraindication for albumin would be
   a acute liver failure.
   b heart failure.
   c severe burns.
   d fluid-volume deficit.

4 The nurse is preparing an infusion for a patient who has a deficiency in clotting factors. Which type of infusion is most appropriate?
   a Albumin 5%
   b Packed RBCs
   c Whole blood
   d Fresh frozen plasma
5 While monitoring a patient who is receiving an infusion of a crystalloid solution, the nurse should look for which potential problem?
   a Bradycardia
   b Hypotension
   c Decreased skin turgor
   d Fluid overload
6 The nurse is administering an IV solution that contains potassium chloride to a patient who has a severely decreased serum potassium level. Which action(s) by the nurse are appropriate? (Select all that apply.)
   a Administer the potassium by slow IV bolus
   b Administer the potassium at a rate no faster than 20 mEq/hr
   c Monitor the patient's cardiac rhythm with a heart monitor
   d Use an infusion pump for the administration of IV potassium chloride
   e Administer the potassium IV push for quick results

1. a, 2. c, 3. b, 4. d, 5. d, 6. b, c, d.

CRITICAL THINKING ACTIVITIES: BEST ACTION

1 After having vomiting and diarrhea from the flu for the previous 24 hours, a patient is admitted for treatment of dehydration. The nurse's best action is to prepare to administer what type of fluid? Explain.
2 During a transfusion of PRBCs, the patient complains that his back is starting to "hurt" and he feels anxious. His temperature is 98.8° F (37.1° C). What is the nurse's best action?
3 The latest potassium level of a patient with hyperkalemia is 6.1 mEq/L, and the physician has ordered two doses of sodium polystyrene sulfonate via enema, 30 g per dose. The patient questions the nurse when he hears he is to receive two enemas, saying, "How in the world is an enema going to help me?" What is the nurse's best answer?

For answers, see *http://evolve.elsevier.com/Lilley.*

CHAPTER 28

Coagulation Modifier Drugs

OBJECTIVES

When you reach the end of this chapter, you should be able to do the following:

1 Briefly review the coagulation process and the impact of coagulation modifiers, including anticoagulants, antiplatelets, antifibrinolytics, and thrombolytics.

2 Compare the mechanisms of action, indications, cautions, contraindications, drug interactions, adverse effects, routes of administration, and dosages of the various anticoagulants, antiplatelets, antifibrinolytics, and thrombolytics.

3 Discuss the administration procedures and techniques as well as related standards of care for the various coagulation modifiers.

4 Identify any available antidotes for the coagulation modifiers.

5 Compare the laboratory tests used in conjunction with treatment with the various coagulation modifiers and their implications for therapeutic use of these drugs and monitoring for adverse reactions.

6 Develop a nursing care plan that includes all phases of the nursing process for patients receiving anticoagulants, antiplatelets, antifibrinolytics, and thrombolytics.

e-Learning Activities

http://evolve.elsevier.com/Lilley

NCLEX Review Questions • Animations • Nursing Care Plans • Audio Glossary • Category Catchers • Medication Errors Checklists • IV Therapy Checklists • Calculators • Frequently Asked Questions • Content Updates • Supplemental Resources • Answers to Case Studies and Critical Thinking Activities

Drug Profiles

- alteplase, p. 446
  aminocaproic acid, p. 444
  argatroban, p. 440
- aspirin, p. 442
- clopidogrel, p. 443
  desmopressin, p. 444

- enoxaparin, p. 438
- eptifibatide, p. 443
- heparin, p. 439
  lepirudin, p. 440
- warfarin, p. 438

  ◆ *Key drug.*

Glossary

Anticoagulants Substances that prevent or delay coagulation of the blood. (p. 434)

Antifibrinolytic drugs Drugs that prevent the lysis of fibrin and in doing so promote clot formation. (p. 435)

Antiplatelet drugs Substances that prevent platelet plugs from forming, which can be beneficial in defending the body against heart attacks and strokes. (p. 434)

Antithrombin III A substance that inactivates ("turns off") three major activating factors of the clotting cascade: activated factor II (thrombin), activated factor X, and activated factor IX. (p. 436)

Clot Insoluble solid elements of blood (cells, fibrin threads, etc.) that have chemically separated from the liquid (plasma) component of the blood. (p. 433)

Coagulation The process of blood clotting. More specifically, the sequential process by which the multiple coagulation factors of the blood interact in the *coagulation cascade,* ultimately forming an insoluble fibrin clot. (p. 433)

Coagulation cascade The series of steps beginning with the *intrinsic* or *extrinsic* pathways of coagulation and proceeding through the formation of a *fibrin clot.* (p. 433)

Deep vein thrombosis (DVT) The formation of a thrombus in one of the deep veins of the body. The deep veins most commonly affected are the iliac and femoral veins. (p. 436)

Embolus A blood clot *(thrombus)* that has been dislodged from the wall of a blood vessel and is traveling throughout the bloodstream. Emboli that lodge in critical blood vessels can result in ischemic injury to a vital organ (e.g., heart, lung, brain) and result in disability or death. (p. 433)

Enzyme A protein molecule that catalyzes chemical reactions of other substances without being altered or destroyed in the process. (p. 437)

Fibrin A stringy, insoluble protein produced by the action of thrombin on fibrinogen during the clotting process; a major component of blood *clots* or *thrombi* (see *thrombus*). (p. 433)

Fibrin specificity The property of newer thrombolytic drugs of activating the conversion of plasminogen to plasmin only in the presence of established clots having fibrin threads rather than inducing systemic plasminogen activation throughout the body, which increases bleeding risk. (p. 445)

Fibrinogen A plasma protein that is converted into fibrin by thrombin in the presence of calcium ions. (p. 440)

Fibrinolysis The continual process of fibrin decomposition produced by the actions of the enzymatic protein *fibrinolysin.* It is the normal mechanism for removing small fibrin clots and is stimulated by anoxia, inflammatory reactions, and other kinds of stress. (p. 434)

Fibrinolytic system An area of the circulatory system undergoing fibrinolysis. (p. 434)

Hemophilia A rare, inherited blood disorder in which the blood does not clot normally. (p. 434)

Hemorheologic drugs Drugs that alter the function of platelets without compromising their blood-clotting properties. (p. 434)

Hemostasis The arrest of bleeding, either by the physiologic properties of vasoconstriction and coagulation or by mechanical, surgical, or pharmacologic means. (p. 433)

Hemostatic Refering to any procedure, device, or substance that arrests the flow of blood. (p. 435)

Plasmin The enzymatic protein that breaks down fibrin into fibrin degradation products; it is derived from plasminogen. (p. 434)

Plasminogen A plasma protein that is converted to plasmin. (p. 434)

Pulmonary embolism The blockage of a pulmonary artery by foreign matter such as fat, air, tumor, or a thrombus (which usually arises from a peripheral vein). (p. 436)

Stroke Occlusion of the blood vessels of the brain by an embolus, thrombus, or cerebrovascular hemorrhage, resulting in ischemia of the brain tissue. (p. 436)

Thromboembolic events Events in which a blood vessel is blocked by an embolus carried in the bloodstream from the site of its formation. The tissue supplied by an obstructed artery may tingle and become cold, numb, cyanotic, and eventually necrotic (dead). (p. 436)

Thrombolytic drugs Drugs that dissolve thrombi by functioning similarly to *tissue plasminogen activator*. (p. 435)

Thrombus The technical term for a blood clot (plural: *thrombi*); an aggregation of platelets, fibrin, clotting factors, and the cellular elements of the blood that is attached to the interior wall of a vein or artery, sometimes occluding the vessel lumen. (p. 433)

Tissue plasminogen activator A naturally occurring plasminogen activator secreted by vascular endothelial cells in the walls of blood vessels. Thrombolytic drugs are based on this blood component. (p. 433)

• • •

Anatomy, Physiology, and Disease Overview

Hemostasis is a general term for any process that stops bleeding. This can be accomplished by mechanical means (e.g., compression to the bleeding site) or even surgical means (e.g., surgical clamping or cauterization of a blood vessel). When hemostasis occurs due to physiologic clotting of blood, it is called **coagulation**, which is the process of blood clot formation. The technical term for a blood clot is a **thrombus**, and a thrombus that is not stationary but moves through blood vessels from its point of origin is called an **embolus**. Normal hemostasis involves the complex interaction of substances that promote **clot** formation and substances that either inhibit coagulation or dissolve the formed clot. Substances that promote coagulation include *platelets, von Willebrand factor, activated clotting factors,* and *tissue thromboplastin.* Substances that inhibit coagulation include *prostacyclin, antithrombin III,* and *proteins C* and *S.* In addition, **tissue plasminogen activator** is a natural substance that dissolves clots that are already formed.

The coagulation system is illustrated in Figures 28-1 and 28-2. It is called a *cascade* (or **coagulation cascade**) because each activated clotting factor serves as a catalyst that amplifies the next reaction. The result is a large concentration of a clot-forming substance called **fibrin.** The coagulation cascade is typically divided into the intrinsic and extrinsic pathways, and these pathways are activated by different types of injury. When blood vessels are damaged by penetration from the outside (e.g., knife or bullet wound), thromboplastin, a substance contained in

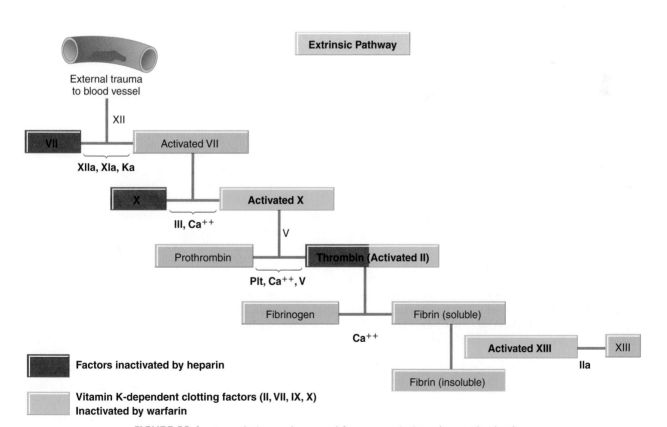

FIGURE 28-1 Coagulation pathway and factors: extrinsic pathway. *Plt,* Platelets.

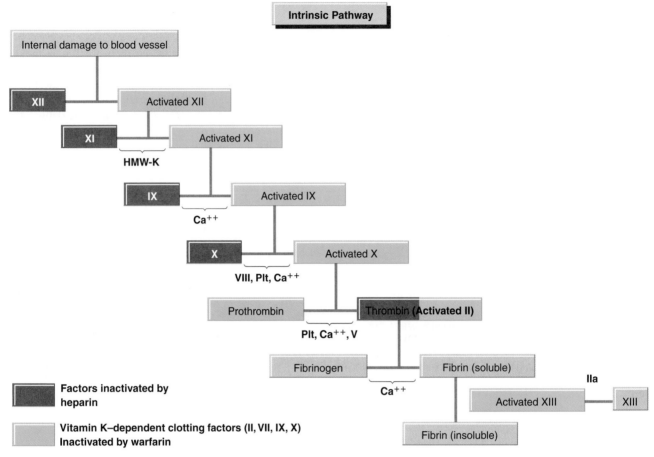

FIGURE 28-2 Coagulation pathway and factors: intrinsic pathway. *HMW-K,* High molecular weight kininogen; *Plt,* platelets.

the walls of blood vessels, is released. This initiates the *extrinsic pathway* by activating factors VII and X (see Figure 28-1). All of the components of the *intrinsic pathway* are present in the blood in their inactive forms (see Figure 28-2). This pathway is activated when factor XII comes in contact with exposed collagen on the *inside* of damaged blood vessels. Figures 28-1 and 28-2 illustrate the steps that occur in the extrinsic and intrinsic pathways, respectively, and the coagulation factors involved. They also illustrate the site of action of two commonly used anticoagulant drugs: warfarin and heparin.

Once a clot is formed and fibrin is present, the **fibrinolytic system** is activated. This is the system that initiates the breakdown of clots and serves to balance the clotting process. **Fibrinolysis** is the reverse of the clotting process. It is the mechanism by which formed thrombi are *lysed* (broken down) to prevent excessive clot formation and blood vessel blockage. It is the fibrin in the clot that binds to a circulating protein known as **plasminogen.** This converts plasminogen to **plasmin.** Plasmin is the enzymatic protein that eventually breaks down the fibrin thrombus into *fibrin degradation products.* This keeps the thrombus localized to prevent it from becoming an embolus that can travel to obstruct a major blood vessel in the lung, heart, or brain. Figure 28-3 illustrates the fibrinolytic system.

Hemophilia is a rare genetic disorder in which the above-mentioned natural coagulation and hemostasis factors are limited or absent. Hemophilia is categorized into two main types depend-

ing on which of the coagulation factors is absent (factor VII, factor VIII, and/or factor IX). Patients with hemophilia can bleed to death if coagulation factors are not given.

Pharmacology Overview

Drugs that affect coagulation are some of the most dangerous drugs used today. As is discussed throughout this chapter, numerous factors can affect their action. These drugs are among the most commonly associated with adverse drug reactions. In fact, the Joint Commission, a hospital accreditation agency, has made safe use of coagulation-modifying drugs a national patient safety goal. This goal requires hospitals to make preventing adverse events associated with these drugs a top priority. Further information on this national patient safety goal may be found at *http://www.jointcommission.org/PatientSafety/NationalPatientSafetyGoals.*

The drugs discussed in this chapter aid the body in reversing or achieving hemostasis, and they can be broken down into several main categories based on their actions. **Anticoagulants** inhibit the action or formation of clotting factors and therefore prevent clots from forming. **Antiplatelet drugs** prevent platelet plugs from forming by inhibiting platelet aggregation, which can be beneficial in preventing heart attacks and strokes. Other drugs alter platelet function without preventing them from working. These are sometimes referred to as **hemorheologic drugs.** Sometimes clots form and totally block a blood vessel. When this

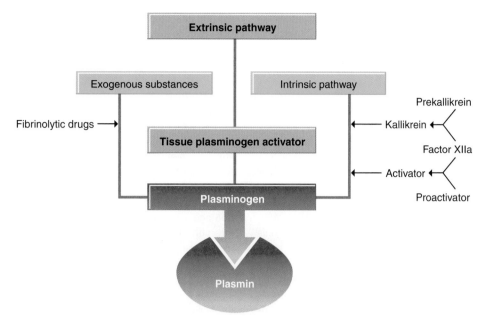

FIGURE 28-3   The fibrinolytic system.

TABLE 28-1 Coagulation Modifiers: Comparison of Drug Subclasses

Type of Coagulation Modifier and Mechanism of Action	Drug Class	Individual Drugs
Prevent Clot Formation **Anticoagulants**		
Inhibit clotting factors IIa (thrombin) and Xa	Heparins	unfractionated heparin ("heparin") and low molecular weight heparins (enoxaparin [Lovenox], dalteparin [Fragmin], tinzaparin [Innohep])
Inhibit vitamin K–dependent clotting factors II, VII, IX, and X	Coumarins	warfarin (Coumadin)
Inhibit thrombin (factor IIa)	Direct thrombin inhibitors	human antithrombin III (Thrombate), lepirudin (Refludan), argatroban (Argatroban), bivalirudin (Angiomax)
Inhibits factor Xa	Selective factor Xa inhibitor	fondaparinux (Arixtra)
Antiplatelet Drugs		
Interfere with platelet function	Aggregation inhibitors Aggregation inhibitors/vasodilators Glycoprotein IIb/IIIa inhibitors Miscellaneous	cilostazol (Pletal), clopidogrel (Plavix) treprostinil (Remodulin) abciximab (ReoPro), eptifibatide (Integrilin), tirofiban (Aggrastat) anagrelide (Agrylin), dipyridamole (Persantine)
Promote Clot Formation **Antifibrinolytics**		
Prevent lysis of fibrin	Systemic hemostatics	aminocaproic acid (Amicar), tranexamic acid (Cyklokapron)
Reduce Blood Viscosity	Hemorheologic	pentoxifylline (Trental)
Lyse a Preformed Clot **Thrombolytics**		
Dissolve thrombi	Tissue plasminogen activators	alteplase (Activase, Cathflo Activase), reteplase (Retavase), tenecteplase (TNKase)
Reversal Drugs	Heparin antagonist Warfarin antagonist	protamine sulfate vitamin K

happens in one of the coronary arteries, a heart attack occurs, and the clot blocking the blood vessel must be lysed to prevent or minimize damage to the myocardial muscle. The **thrombolytic drugs** lyse (break down) clots, or *thrombi,* that have already formed. This is a unique difference between thrombolytics and the anticoagulants, which can only prevent the formation of a clot. **Antifibrinolytic drugs,** also known as **hemostatic** drugs, have the opposite effect of these other classes of drugs; they actually *promote* blood coagulation and are helpful in the management of conditions in which excessive bleeding would be harmful. The various drugs in each category of coagulation modifiers are listed in Table 28-1. Understanding the individual coagulation modifiers and their mechanisms of action requires a basic working knowledge of the coagulation pathway and coagulation factors, which is provided in the next section.

ANTICOAGULANTS

Drugs that prevent the formation of a clot by inhibiting certain clotting factors are called *anticoagulants.* These drugs are only given prophylactically because they have no direct effect on a blood clot that has already formed. By decreasing blood coagulability, anticoagulants prevent intravascular thrombosis. Their uses vary from preventing clot formation to preventing the extension of an established clot, or a thrombus.

Once a clot forms on the wall of a blood vessel, it may dislodge and travel through the bloodstream. This is referred to as an *embolus.* If it lodges in a coronary artery, it causes a myocardial infarction (MI); if it obstructs a brain vessel, it causes a **stroke;** if it goes to the lungs, it is a **pulmonary embolism;** and if it goes to a vein in the leg, it is a **deep vein thrombosis (DVT).** Collectively, these complications are called **thromboembolic events,** because they involve a thrombus that becomes an embolus and causes an adverse cardiovascular "event." Anticoagulants can prevent all of these from occurring if used in the correct manner. Both orally and parenterally administered anticoagulants are available, and each drug has a slightly different mechanism of action and indications. All of them have their own risks, mainly the risk for causing bleeding. The mechanisms of action of the anticoagulants vary depending on the drug. Drug classes of anticoagulants include older drugs such as unfractionated heparin and warfarin. There are also several newer drug classes, including low molecular weight heparins (LMWHs), direct thrombin inhibitors, and a selective factor Xa inhibitor. Dosages, indications, and other information appear in the Dosages table on p. 439.

Mechanism of Action and Drug Effects

Anticoagulants are also called *antithrombotic* drugs because they all work to prevent the formation of a clot or thrombus, a condition known as *thrombosis.* All anticoagulants work in the clotting cascade but do so at different points. As shown in Figures 28-1 and 28-2, heparin works by binding to a substance called **antithrombin III,** which turns off three main activating factors: activated factor II (also called *thrombin*), activated factor X, and activated factor IX. (Factors XI and XII are also inactivated but do not play as important a role as the other three factors.) Of these, the thrombin is the most sensitive to the actions of heparin. Antithrombin III is the major natural inhibitor of thrombin in the blood. The overall effect of heparin is that it turns off the coagulation pathway and prevents clots from forming. As previously noted, however, it cannot lyse a clot. The drug name heparin usually refers to *unfractionated* heparin, which is a relatively large molecule and is derived from various animal sources. In contrast, LMWHs are synthetic and have a smaller molecular structure. These include enoxaparin (Lovenox), dalteparin (Fragmin), and tinzaparin (Innohep). All three work similarly to heparin. Heparin primarily binds to activated factors II, X, and IX. LMWHs differ from heparin in that they are much more specific for activated factor X (Xa) than for activated factor II (IIa, or thrombin). This property confers on LMWHs a much more predictable anticoagulant response. As a result, frequent laboratory monitoring of bleeding times using tests such as activated partial thromboplastin time (aPTT), which is imperative with unfractionated heparin, is not required with LMWHs.

Warfarin (Coumadin) works by inhibiting vitamin K synthesis by bacteria in the gastrointestinal tract. This, in turn, inhibits production of clotting factors II, VII, IX, and X. These four factors are normally synthesized in the liver and are known as *vitamin K–dependent clotting factors.* As with heparin, the final effect is the prevention of clot formation. Figures 28-1 and 28-2 show where in the clotting cascade this occurs.

Fondaparinux (Arixtra) inhibits thrombosis by its specific action against factor Xa alone. There are also currently four antithrombin drugs that inhibit the thrombin molecules directly, one natural and three synthetic. The natural drug is human antithrombin III (Thrombate), which is isolated from the plasma of human donors. The three synthetic drugs are lepirudin (Refludan), argatroban (Argatroban), and bivalirudin (Angiomax). All of these drugs work similarly to inhibit thrombus formation by inhibiting thrombin.

Indications

The ability of anticoagulants to prevent clot formation is of benefit in certain settings in which there is a high likelihood of clot formation. These include MI, unstable angina, atrial fibrillation, use of indwelling devices such as mechanical heart valves, and conditions in which blood flow may be slowed and blood may pool, such as major orthopedic surgery or prolonged periods of immobilization like hospitalization or even long plane rides. As previously mentioned, the ultimate consequence of a clot can be a stroke or a heart attack, DVT, or PE; therefore, the prevention of these serious events is the ultimate benefit of these drugs. Warfarin is indicated for *prevention* of any of these events, whereas both unfractionated heparins and LMWHs are used for both prevention and treatment. Patients at risk for clots are given DVT prophylaxis while in the hospital and after major surgery. LMWHs, especially enoxaparin, are also routinely used as anticoagulant bridge therapy in situations in which a patient must stop warfarin for surgery or other invasive medical procedures. The term *bridge therapy* refers to the fact that enoxaparin acts as a bridge to provide anticoagulation while the patient must be off of his or her warfarin therapy. The remainder of the antithrombotic drugs have similar but more restricted indications, which are listed in the Dosages table for anticoagulants.

Contraindications

Contraindications to the use of anticoagulants are generally similar for all of the different drugs. They include known drug allergy to a specific product and usually include any acute bleeding process or high risk for such an occurrence, as well as thrombocytopenia. Warfarin is strongly contraindicated in pregnancy, whereas the other anticoagulants are rated in lower pregnancy categories (B or C). LMWHs are contraindicated in patients with an indwelling epidural catheter, they can be given 2 hours after the epidural is removed. This is very important for nurses to remember, because giving an LMWH with an epidural has been associated with epidural hematoma.

Adverse Effects

Bleeding is the main complication of anticoagulation therapy, and the risk increases with increasing dosages. Such bleeding may be localized (e.g., hematoma at the site of injection) or systemic. It also depends on the nature of the patient's underlying clinical disorder and is increased in patients also taking high doses of aspirin or other drugs that impair platelet function. One particularly notable adverse effect of heparin is *heparin-induced thrombocytopenia (HIT)*, which is also called *heparin-associated thrombocytopenia*. There are two types of HIT. Type I is characterized by a more gradual reduction in platelets. In this type, heparin therapy can generally be continued. In contrast, in type II HIT there is an acute fall in the number of platelets (more than 50% reduction from baseline). Heparin therapy must be discontinued in patients with type II HIT. The greatest risk to the patient with HIT is the paradoxical occurrence of thrombosis, something that heparin normally prevents or alleviates. Thrombosis that occurs in the presence of HIT can be fatal. The incidence of this disorder ranges from 5% to 15% of patients and is higher with *bovine* (cow-derived) than with *porcine* (pig-derived) heparins. The direct thrombin inhibitors lepirudin and argatroban are both specifically indicated for treatment of HIT. Warfarin can cause skin necrosis and "purple toes" syndrome. Other adverse effects are listed in Table 28-2.

Toxicity and Management of Overdose

Treatment of the toxic effects of anticoagulants is aimed at reversing the underlying cause. Although the toxic effects of heparin, LMWH, and warfarin are hemorrhagic in nature, the management is different for each drug. Symptoms that may be attributed to toxicity or an overdose of anticoagulants are hematuria, melena (blood in the stool), petechiae, ecchymoses, and gum or mucous membrane bleeding. In the event of heparin or warfarin toxicity, the drug should be discontinued immediately. In the case of heparin, stopping the drug alone may be enough to reverse the toxic effects because of the drug's short half-life (1 to 2 hours). In severe cases or when large doses have been given intentionally (i.e., during cardiopulmonary bypass for heart surgery), IV injection of protamine sulfate is indicated. This drug is a specific heparin antidote and forms a complex with heparin, completely reversing its anticoagulant properties. This occurs in as few as 5 minutes. In general, 1 mg of protamine can reverse the effects of 100 units of heparin. Protamine may also be used to reverse the effects of LMWHs. A 1-mg dose of protamine should be administered for each milligram of LMWH given, (e.g., 1 mg protamine for 1 mg enoxaparin). If the heparin overdose has resulted in a large blood loss, replacement with packed red blood cells may be necessary.

In the event of warfarin toxicity or overdose, the first step is to discontinue the warfarin. As with heparin, the toxicity associated with warfarin is an extension of its therapeutic effects on the clotting cascade. However, because warfarin inactivates the vitamin K–dependent clotting factors and because these clotting factors are synthesized in the liver, it may take 36 to 42 hours before the liver can resynthesize enough clotting factors to reverse the warfarin effects. An IV injection of vitamin K (phytonadione) can hasten the return to normal coagulation. The dose and route of administration of the vitamin K depend on the clinical situation and its acuity (i.e., how quickly the warfarin-

TABLE 28-2 Anticoagulants: Common Adverse Effects

Drug Subclass	Adverse Effects
Heparins (unfractionated heparin, low molecular weight heparin)	Bleeding, hematoma, nausea, anemia, thrombocytopenia, fever, edema
Direct thrombin inhibitors (lepirudin, argatroban, bivalirudin)	Bleeding, dizziness, chest discomfort, nausea, constipation, chills, shortness of breath, fever, urticaria, heart and kidney failure (lepirudin, argatroban), cardiac dysrhythmias (argatroban), hypotension (argatroban and bivalirudin)
Selective factor Xa inhibitor (fondaparinux)	Bleeding, hematoma, dizziness, confusion, rash, gastrointestinal distress, urinary tract infection, urinary retention, anemia

induced effects must be reversed and whether the patient is having significant bleeding). High doses of vitamin K (10 mg) given IV should reverse the anticoagulation within 6 hours. Current recommendations are to use the lowest amount of vitamin K possible, based on the clinical situation. This is because once vitamin K is given, warfarin resistance will occur for up to 7 days; thus the patient cannot be anticoagulated by warfarin during this period. In such cases, either heparin or an LMWH may need to be added to provide adequate anticoagulation. In acute situations in which bleeding is severe and the time it would take for the vitamin K to take effect is too long, it may be necessary to administer transfusions of human plasma or clotting factor concentrates. Vitamin K can cause anaphylaxis when given by the IV route. Because of this, the oral route is preferred. If the IV route is necessary, the risk of reaction can be lowered by diluting the drug and administering it over 30 minutes. There is some controversy as to whether vitamin K may be given by IV push, and many institutions have specific guidelines for its administration. Vitamin K is available in 5-mg tablets and in 10-mg and 1-mg injections. It is quite common to give the injectable form orally.

Transfusions may be indicated for overdoses of direct thrombin inhibitors and the selective factor Xa inhibitor fondaparinux, which both lack specific antidotes. These drugs may also be removed with hemodialysis.

Interactions

The drug interactions involving the oral anticoagulants are profound and complicated. The main interaction mechanisms responsible for increasing anticoagulant activity include the following:

- **Enzyme** inhibition of metabolism
- Displacement of the drug from inactive protein-binding sites
- Decrease in vitamin K absorption or synthesis by the bacterial flora of the large intestines
- Alteration in the platelet count or activity

The drugs that interact with warfarin and heparin are listed in Table 28-3 and more specifics on significant drug interactions are discussed under the drug profiles. Although both aspirin and warfarin increase the risk of bleeding when given with heparin,

TABLE 28-3 Anticoagulants: Drug Interactions

Drug	Mechanism	Result
Warfarin		
acetaminophen (high doses) amiodarone bumetanide furosemide	Displacement from inactive protein-binding sites	
aspirin, other NSAIDs Broad-spectrum antibiotics cephalosporin	Decrease in platelet activity	Increased anticoagulant effect
Mineral oil vitamin E	Interference with vitamin K	
Barbiturates carbamazepine rifampin phenytoin	Enzyme induction	Decreased anticoagulant effect
amiodarone cimetidine ciprofloxacin erythromycin ketoconazole metronidazole omeprazole Sulfonamides Macrolides	Enzyme inhibition	Increased anticoagulant effect
cholestyramine sucralfate	Impairment of warfarin absorption	Decreased anticoagulant effect
Heparin		
aspirin, other NSAIDs	Decrease in platelet activity	Increased risk of bleeding
Oral anticoagulants Thrombolytics Cephalosporins Penicillins	Additive	Increased anticoagulant effect
Any other anticoagulant, antiplatelet, or thrombolytic drug	Additive	Increased bleeding risk

NSAIDs, Nonsteroidal antiinflammatory drugs.

they are commonly given together in clinical practice. In fact, when a patient is placed on IV heparin, it is recommended that warfarin be started at the same time. Heparin is continued until the warfarin effect is therapeutic for at least 2 days.

Dosages

For the recommended dosages of selected anticoagulants, see the Dosages table on p. 439.

DRUG PROFILES

Of the anticoagulants, warfarin is available only for oral use. The rest are given by IV and/or subcutaneous injection only. Intramuscular (IM) injection of these drugs is contraindicated due to their propensity to cause large hematomas at the site of injection.

◆ warfarin

Warfarin sodium (Coumadin) is a pharmaceutical derivative of the natural plant anticoagulant known as *coumarin*. Warfarin is the most commonly prescribed oral anticoagulant and is available only for oral use. Use of this drug requires careful monitoring of the prothrombin time/international normalized ratio (PT/INR), which is a standardized measure of the degree to which a patient's blood coagulability has been reduced by the drug. A normal INR (without warfarin) is 1.0, whereas a therapeutic INR (with warfarin) ranges from 2 to 3.5, depending on the indication for use of the drug (e.g., atrial fibrillation, thromboprevention, prosthetic heart valve). Patients older than 65 years may have a lower INR threshold for bleeding complications and should be monitored accordingly. Elderly patients should be started on lower dosages initially. Recently, it has been shown that about one third of patients receiving warfarin metabolize it differently than what would be expected, based on variations in certain genes, CYP2CP and VKORC1. Genetic testing for these genes is helpful in determining the appropriate initial dosage of warfarin. The maintenance dosage is still determined by the INR.

Warfarin has significant interactions with many drugs, including amiodarone, fluconazole, erythromycin, metronidazole, sulfonamide antibiotics, and cimetidine. Although many more drugs can interact with warfarin, the aforementioned are by far the most common. Combining warfarin and amiodarone will lead to a 50% increase in the INR. When amiodarone is added to warfarin therapy, the warfarin dose should be cut in half.

Because warfarin inhibits vitamin K–dependent clotting factors, foods that are high in vitamin K may reduce warfarin's ability to prevent clots. Common foods rich in vitamin K include leafy green vegetables (kale, spinach, collard greens). The most important aspect of these food-drug interactions is consistency in diet. Patients should be educated to maintain consistency in their intake of leafy green vegetables. Many patients are under the misconception that they must avoid all leafy green vegetables. This is not true. What patients must understand is that once their maintenance warfarin dose is established, they should continue their regular diet of greens and neither increase nor decrease their intake, because this can affect the INR. Herbals that interact with warfarin and result in increased risk of bleeding include capsicum, chamomile, feverfew, garlic, ginger, ginkgo, licorice, passion flower, red clover, and willow.

PHARMACOKINETICS

Route	Onset of Action	Peak Plasma Concentration	Elimination Half-life	Duration of Action
PO	24-72 hr	4 hr	0.5-3 days	2-5 days

◆ enoxaparin

Enoxaparin (Lovenox) is the prototypical LMWH and is obtained by enzymatically cleaving large unfractionated heparin molecules into small fragments. These smaller fragments of heparin have a greater affinity for factor Xa than for factor IIa and have a higher degree of bioavailability and a longer elimination half-life than unfractionated heparin. Laboratory monitoring, as done with heparin therapy, is not necessary when enoxaparin is given because of its greater affinity for factor Xa. It is available only in injectable form. Other anticoagulants with comparable pharmacology and indications include danaparoid and dalteparin. Enoxaparin is the most frequently used LMWH and is commonly given for both prophylaxis and treatment. All LMWHs have a distinct advantage over heparin in that it does not require any laboratory monitoring and can be given at home for the treatment of DVT or

DOSAGES

Selected Anticoagulant Drugs

Drug (Pregnancy Category)	Pharmacologic Class	Usual Dosage Range	Indications/Uses
argatroban (Argatroban) (B)	Synthetic thrombin inhibitor	**Adult** IV: 350 mcg/kg bolus then 5-30 mcg/kg/min until ACT in desired range	Thromboprevention and treatment in HIT and with PCI in patients at risk for HIT
◆ enoxaparin (Lovenox) (B)	LMWH	**Adult** Subcut: 30-40 mg every 12 hr for prophylaxis or 1 mg/kg every 12 hr for treatment	Prevention and treatment of thromboembolic and ischemic processes in unstable angina and postoperative and post-MI situations
◆ heparin (generic only) (C)	Natural anticoagulant	**Pediatric** IV: Initial 50 units/kg, then 12-25 units/kg/hr, increased by 2-4 units/kg/hr q6-8h prn **Adult** Subcut: 5000 units q8-12hr for prophylaxis IV infusion: 20,000-40,000 units/day usually given as 80 unit/kg bolus then 18 units/kg/hr aPTT determines maintenance dosage	Thrombosis/embolism, coagulopathies (e.g., DIC), DVT and PE prophylaxis, clotting prevention (e.g., open heart surgery, dialysis)
lepirudin (Refludan) (B)	Synthetic thrombin inhibitor	**Adult** IV: 0.4 mg/kg bolus, then 0.15 mg/kg continuous infusion × 2-10 days	Thromboprevention in patients with HIT
◆ warfarin (X)	Coumarin anticoagulant	PT or INR determines maintenance dose, usually 2-10 mg/day orally	Thromboprevention and treatment in DVT, PE, atrial fibrillation, post-MI status

ACT, Activated clotting time; *aPTT,* activated partial thromboplastin time; *DIC,* disseminated intravascular coagulation; *DVT,* deep vein thrombosis; *HIT,* heparin-induced thrombocytopenia; *INR,* international normalized ratio; *IV,* intravenous; *LMWH,* low molecular weight heparin; *MI,* myocardial infarction; *PCI,* percutaneous coronary intervention; *PE,* pulmonary embolism; *PT,* prothrombin time; *subcut,* subcutaneous.

---

pulmonary embolism. This allows patients to be discharged from the hospital sooner. It is also used at home after major orthopedic surgery.

A potentially deadly medication error is to give heparin in combination with enoxaparin (or any LMWH). The nurse should always double-check that enoxaparin and heparin are never given to the same patient.

PHARMACOKINETICS

Route	Onset of Action	Peak Plasma Concentration	Elimination Half-life	Duration of Action
Subcut	3-5 hr	4-5 hr	4-5 hr	12 hr

◆ heparin

Heparin (generic only) is a natural mucopolysaccharide anticoagulant obtained from the lungs, intestinal mucosa, or other suitable tissues primarily of pigs. One brand name for some of the commonly used heparin products is Hep-Lock. This brand name refers only to small vials of aqueous heparin IV flush solutions used to maintain the patency of heparin-lock IV insertion sites. Because of the risk for the development of HIT, however, most institutions routinely use normal saline (0.9% sodium chloride) as a flush for heparin-lock IV ports and have moved away from using heparin flush solutions per se for this purpose. Heparin flushes are still used for central catheters.

Heparin is commonly used for DVT prophylaxis in a dose of 5000 units two or three times a day given subcutaneously, and it does not need to be monitored when used for prophylaxis. When heparin is used therapeutically (for treatment) it is given by continuous IV infusion. Most hospitals have weight-based protocols for heparin administration. Because the dosage is based on the patient's weight in kilograms, it is incumbent upon the nurse to ensure that the appropriate weight is recorded and that only kilograms are used, not pounds. A potential double-dose medication error can occur if pounds and kilograms are mixed. This is also true for enoxaparin, because it is dosed on body weight when used therapeutically. When heparin is given by IV infusion, monitoring by frequent measurement of aPTT (usually every 6 hours until therapeutic effects are seen) is necessary. Because the required monitoring is very time consuming, many institutions now use enoxaparin in place of heparin.

Other drugs that affect the coagulation cascade can have additive effects with heparin, which may lead to bleeding. Even though warfarin can cause additive effects, it is combined with IV heparin therapy. In fact, it is usually started within the first day or two of heparin infusion.

Heparin is available only in injectable form in multiple strengths ranging from 10 to 40,000 units/mL. The vials of different strengths of heparin are very similar and look very much alike. In fact, several newborns have died when a vial of more concentrated heparin was mistaken for a more dilute solution. Nurses should take great care in checking and double-checking the concentration of heparin before administering it.

PHARMACOKINETICS

Route	Onset of Action	Peak Plasma Concentration	Elimination Half-life	Duration of Action
IV	Immediate	Immediate	1-2 hr	Dependent on infusion duration
Subcut	20-30 min	2-4 hr	1-2 hr	8-12 hr

lepirudin

Lepirudin (Refludan) is a recombinant, yeast-derived inhibitor of thrombin. It is used specifically for the treatment of HIT and is available only for IV use. As with heparin, its effects are monitored by measuring the aPTT. Argatroban is another drug in this class with the same indication. Other drugs in this class with more variable indications are human antithrombin III (for hereditary deficiency), and bivalirudin (for unstable angina).

PHARMACOKINETICS

Route	Onset of Action	Peak Plasma Concentration	Elimination Half-life	Duration of Action
IV	Immediate	Immediate	1.3 hr	Dependent on infusion duration

argatroban

Argatroban, which has the same trade name, is a synthetic direct thrombin inhibitor that is derived from the amino acid L-arginine. It is indicated both for treatment of active HIT and for *percutaneous coronary intervention* procedures in patients at risk for HIT (i.e., those with a history of the disorder). It is given only by the IV route. A lower dosage must be used in patients with severe hepatic dysfunction.

PHARMACOKINETICS

Route	Onset of Action	Peak Plasma Concentration	Elimination Half-life	Duration of Action
IV	Immediate	1-3 hr	30-50 min	Dependent on infusion duration

ANTIPLATELET DRUGS

Another class of coagulation modifiers that prevent clot formation is the antiplatelet drugs. The anticoagulants work in the clotting cascade. In contrast, antiplatelet drugs work to prevent platelet *adhesion* to the site of blood vessel injury, which actually occurs before the clotting cascade. A knowledge of the role of platelets in the clotting process is essential to understanding how antiplatelet drugs work.

Platelets normally flow through blood vessels without adhering to their surfaces. Blood vessels can be injured by a disruption of blood flow, trauma, or the rupture of plaque from a vessel wall. When such events occur, substances such as collagen and fibronectin, which are present in the walls of blood vessels, become exposed. Collagen is a potent stimulator of platelet adhesion, as is a prevalent component of the platelet membranes themselves, *glycoprotein IIb/IIIa* (GP IIb/IIIa). Once platelet adhesion occurs, stimulators (compounds such as adenosine diphosphate [ADP], thrombin, thromboxane A_2 [TXA_2], and prostaglandin H_2) are released from the activated platelets. These cause the platelets to *aggregate* (accumulate) at the site of injury. Once at the site of vessel injury, the platelets change shape and release their contents, which include

ADP, serotonin, and platelet factor 4. The hemostatic function of these substances is twofold. First, they act as platelet recruiters, attracting additional platelets to the site of injury; second, they are potent vasoconstrictors. Vasoconstriction limits blood flow to the damaged blood vessel to reduce blood loss.

A platelet plug that has formed at a site of vessel injury is not stable and can be dislodged. The clotting cascade is therefore stimulated to form a more permanent *fibrin* plug (blood clot). The role of platelets and their relationship to the clotting cascade are illustrated in Figure 28-4.

Mechanism of Action and Drug Effects

Many of the antiplatelet drugs affect the *cyclooxygenase* pathway, which is one of the common final enzymatic pathways in the complex *arachidonic acid* pathway that operates within platelets and on blood vessel walls. This pathway as it functions in both platelets and blood vessel walls is illustrated in Figure 28-5.

Aspirin is also widely used for its analgesic, antiinflammatory, and antipyretic (antifever) properties (see Chapter 44). In terms of its anticoagulant effects, aspirin (acetylsalicylic acid) acetylates and inhibits cyclooxygenase in the platelet irreversibly so that the platelet cannot regenerate this enzyme. Therefore, the effects of aspirin last the life span of a platelet, or 7 days. This irreversible inhibition of cyclooxygenase in the platelet prevents the formation of TXA_2, a substance that causes blood vessels to constrict and platelets to aggregate. Thus, by preventing TXA_2 formation, aspirin prevents these actions, which results in dilation of the blood vessels and prevention of platelets from aggregating or forming a clot.

Dipyridamole, another antiplatelet drug, also works to inhibit platelet aggregation by preventing the release of ADP, platelet factor 4, and TXA_2, all substances that stimulate platelets to aggregate or form a clot. Figure 28-4 shows how these substances accomplish this. Dipyridamole may also directly stimulate the release of prostacyclin and inhibit the formation of TXA_2 (see Figure 28-5).

Clopidogrel is a drug that belongs to the class of antiplatelet drugs called the *ADP inhibitors*. Its use has largely superseded that of the original ADP inhibitor ticlopidine. Its mechanism of action is entirely different from that of aspirin in that it inhibits platelet aggregation by altering the platelet membrane so that it can no longer receive the signal to aggregate and form a clot. This signal is in the form of **fibrinogen** molecules, which attach to glycoprotein receptors (GP IIb/IIIa) on the surface of the platelet. Clopidogrel inhibits the activation of this receptor. Clopidogrel has been shown to be somewhat better than aspirin at reducing the number of heart attacks, strokes, and vascular deaths in patients at risk. The combination of aspirin and clopidogrel has been shown to be effective in patients with known cardiovascular disease, but not in patients who only have risk factors.

Pentoxifylline, another antiplatelet drug, is a methylxanthine derivative with properties similar to those of other methylxanthines, such as caffeine and theophylline (see Chapter 37). It was one of the earliest antiplatelet drugs but is now much less commonly used. It reduces the viscosity of blood by increasing the flexibility of red blood cells and reducing the aggregation of platelets. It is sometimes referred to as a *hemorheologic drug,* or a drug that alters the fluid dynamics of the blood. The antiplatelet effects of pentoxifylline are attributed to its inhibition of ADP, serotonin, and platelet factor 4 (see Figure 28-4). Pentoxifylline also stimulates the synthesis and release of prostacyclin from

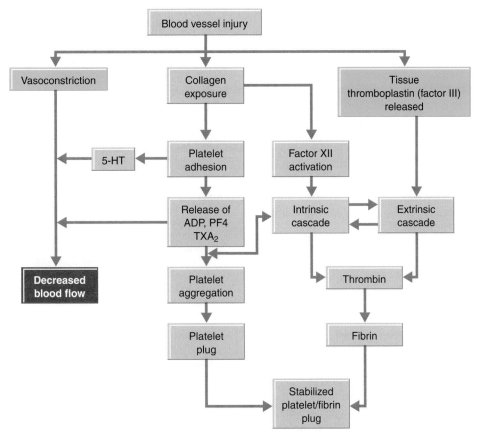

FIGURE 28-4 Relationship between platelets and the clotting cascade. *ADP,* Adenosine diphosphate; *5-HT,* serotonin; *PF4,* platelet factor 4; *TXA₂,* thromboxane A₂.

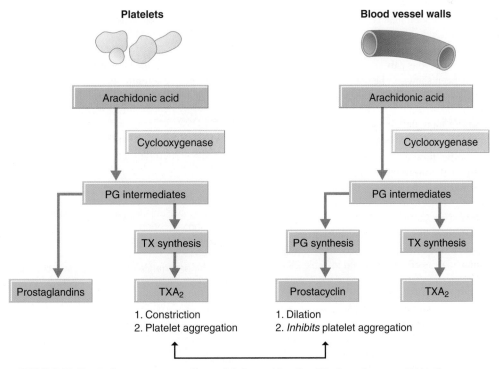

FIGURE 28-5 Cyclooxygenase pathway. *PG,* Prostaglandin; *TX,* thromboxane; *TXA₂,* thromboxane A₂.

blood vessels (see Figure 28-5). In addition, it may have effects on the fibrinolytic system by raising the plasma concentrations of tissue plasminogen activator (see Figure 28-3).

Cilostazol is another antiplatelet drug, which works through inhibition of *type 3 phosphodiesterase* in the platelets and primarily lower-extremity blood vessels. Its effects are to reduce platelet aggregation and promote vasodilation.

The newest available antiplatelet class of drugs is the GP IIb/IIIa inhibitors. They work by blocking the receptor protein by the same name that occurs in the platelet wall membranes. This protein plays a role in promoting the aggregation of platelets in preparation for fibrin clot formation. There are currently three available drugs in this class: tirofiban (Aggrastat), eptifibatide (Integrilin), and abciximab (ReoPro). The GP IIb/IIIa inhibitors are available only for IV infusion.

Indications

The therapeutic effects of the antiplatelet drugs depend on the particular drug. Aspirin has multiple therapeutic effects, but many of them vary depending on the dosage. Aspirin is officially recommended for stroke prevention by the American Stroke Society in daily doses of 50 to 325 mg. (However, in clinical practice, dosages may vary.) Clopidogrel is also given to reduce the risk for fatal and nonfatal thrombotic stroke, and is used for prophylaxis against *transient ischemic attacks* as well for post-MI prevention of thrombosis. Dipyridamole is used as an adjunct to warfarin in the prevention of postoperative thromboembolic complications. It is also used to decrease platelet aggregation in various other thromboembolic disorders. The GP IIb/IIIa inhibitors are used to treat acute unstable angina and MI, and are given during percutaneous coronary intervention procedures, such as angioplasty. Their purpose is to prevent the formation of thrombi. This is known as *thromboprevention*. This treatment approach is based on the fact that *prevention* of thrombus formation is easier and less risky overall from a pharmacologic standpoint than is lysing a formed thrombus. Pentoxifylline is indicated for peripheral vascular disease, whereas cilostazol is indicated specifically for *intermittent claudication* (pain and cramping in the calf muscles associated with walking). Cilostazol has been shown to be superior to pentoxifylline in improving exercise tolerance in elderly patients.

Contraindications

Contraindications to the use of antiplatelet drugs include known drug allergy to a specific product, thrombocytopenia, active bleeding, leukemia, traumatic injury, gastrointestinal ulcer, vitamin K deficiency, and recent stroke.

Adverse Effects

The potential adverse effects of the various antiplatelet drugs can be serious, and they all pose a risk for inducing a serious bleeding episode. The most common adverse effects are listed in Table 28-4.

Interactions

Some potentially dangerous drug interactions can occur with antiplatelet drugs. The use of dipyridamole with clopidogrel, aspirin, and/or other nonsteroidal antiinflammatory drugs (NSAIDs) produces additive antiplatelet activity and increased bleeding potential. There is allergic cross-reactivity between aspirin and other NSAIDs. Patients with documented aspirin allergy should not re-

TABLE 28-4 Selected Antiplatelet Drugs: Adverse Effects

Body System	Adverse Effects
Aspirin	
Central nervous	Stimulation, drowsiness, dizziness, confusion, flushing
Gastrointestinal	Nausea, vomiting, gastrointestinal bleeding, diarrhea, heartburn
Hematologic	Thrombocytopenia, agranulocytosis, leukopenia, neutropenia, hemolytic anemia, bleeding
Clopidogrel	
Cardiovascular	Chest pain, hypertension, edema
Central nervous	Flulike symptoms, headache, dizziness, fatigue
Gastrointestinal	Abdominal pain, dyspepsia, diarrhea, nausea
Miscellaneous	Epistaxis and integumentary disorders, including rash and pruritus (itching)
Glycoprotein IIb/IIIa Inhibitors	Bleeding, bradycardia, dizziness, edema, leg pain, pelvic pain, chills

ceive other NSAIDs. The combined use of steroids or nonaspirin NSAIDs with aspirin can increase the ulcerogenic effects of aspirin. The combined use of aspirin and heparin with GP IIb/IIIa inhibitors also further enhances antiplatelet activity and increases the likelihood of a serious bleeding episode. In spite of all of these interactions, it is not uncommon to see patients taking daily maintenance doses of aspirin for thrombopreventive purposes, sometimes in combination with other antiplatelet drugs. The most commonly used dose is the "baby aspirin" dose of 81 mg (the standard adult dose is 325 mg). Even though GP IIb/IIIa and heparin have additive therapeutic effects when given concurrently and are listed as interacting drugs, it is very common to see both used together. However, the therapeutic goal of heparin treatment, and thus the dose, is lower when used with a GP IIb/IIIa inhibitor.

Dosages

For the recommended dosages of selected antiplatelet drugs, see the Dosages table on p. 443.

DRUG PROFILES

Antiplatelet drugs are extremely useful in the management of thromboembolic disorders. Each has unique pharmacologic properties, and therefore they all are somewhat different from one another.

♦ aspirin

Aspirin is available in many combinations with other prescription and nonprescription drugs and goes by many product names. One unique contraindication for aspirin is flulike symptoms in children and teenagers. The use of aspirin in this situation is associated with the occurrence of Reye's syndrome, a rare, acute, and sometimes fatal condition involving hepatic and central nervous system damage (see Chapter 44). Aspirin is available in both oral and rectal forms.

PHARMACOKINETICS

Route	Onset of Action	Peak Plasma Concentration	Elimination Half-life	Duration of Action
PO	15-30 min	0.25-2 hr	2-3 hr	4-6 hr

DOSAGES

Selected Antiplatelet Drugs

Drug (Pregnancy Category)	Pharmacologic Class	Usual Dosage Range	Indications/Uses
◆ aspirin (C/D)	Salicylate antiplatelet	**Adult** PO: 81-325 mg once daily PO: 40-325 mg once daily	MI prophylaxis TIA prophylaxis
◆ clopidogrel (Plavix) (B)	ADP inhibitor	**Adult** PO: 75 mg once daily; 300 mg may be given as a one-time loading dose after coronary stent implantation	Reduction of atherosclerotic events; acute coronary syndrome without ST segment elevation
◆ eptifibatide (Integrilin) (B)	GP IIb/IIIa inhibitor	IV: Single bolus followed by continuous infusion; specific doses are based on patient weight from 37 to more than 121 kg*	Unstable angina, MI, percutaneous coronary procedures

ADP, Adenosine diphosphate; *GP*, glycoprotein; *IV*, intravenous; *MI*, myocardial infarction; *PO*, oral; *TIA*, transient ischemic attack.
*See table in package insert for specific dose.

◆ clopidogrel

Clopidogrel (Plavix) is currently the most widely used ADP inhibitor on the market. It has superseded ticlopidine (Ticlid) due to the associated serious adverse reactions to the latter drug, including life-threatening neutropenia and agranulocytosis. It was initially believed that clopidogrel might be free from such adverse effects. However, some case reports are emerging of clopidogrel-associated hematologic adverse effects. It is available only for oral use.

PHARMACOKINETICS

Route	Onset of Action	Peak Plasma Concentration	Elimination Half-life	Duration of Action
PO	1-2 hr	1 hr	8 hr	7-10 days

◆ eptifibatide

Eptifibatide (Integrilin) is a GP IIb/IIIa inhibitor, along with tirofiban (Aggrastat) and abciximab (ReoPro). These drugs are usually administered in intensive care or cardiac catheterization laboratory settings where continuous cardiovascular monitoring is the norm. All are available only for IV use.

PHARMACOKINETICS

Route	Onset of Action	Peak Plasma Concentration	Elimination Half-life	Duration of Action
IV	1 hr	Unknown	2-2.5 hr	4 hr

ANTIFIBRINOLYTIC DRUGS

The individual antifibrinolytic drugs have varying mechanisms of action, but all prevent the lysis of fibrin. Fibrin is the substance that helps make a platelet plug insoluble and anchors the clot to the damaged blood vessel (see Figures 28-1 and 28-2). The term *antifibrinolytic* refers to what these drugs do, which is to prevent the lysis of fibrin; in doing so, they actually *promote* clot formation. For this reason, they are also called *hemostatic* drugs. Their effects are opposite to those of anticoagulant and antiplatelet drugs, which *prevent* clot formation. Three synthetic antifibrinolytics are available—aminocaproic acid, tranexamic acid, and desmopressin. Dosages, indications, and other information ap-

pear in the associated Dosages table. There are also hemostatic drugs that are used *topically* (on the skin or tissue surface) in surgical settings to stop excessive bleeding. These include topical thrombin, microfibrillar collagen, absorbable gelatin, and oxidized cellulose.

Although not technically antifibrinolytic drugs, there are three drugs used for the treatment of hemophilia. These are produced by recombinant DNA technology, which eliminates the risk associated with obtaining them from human blood. Products currently available include rVII, rVIII, and rIX. As mentioned earlier, factors VII, VIII, and IX are important in the coagulation pathway. Warfarin also inhibits these factors. These products are used in patients with hemophilia and are also used in patients with severe bleeding due to warfarin therapy.

Mechanism of Action and Drug Effects

The antifibrinolytic drugs vary in several ways. The various antifibrinolytic drugs and their proposed mechanisms of action are described in Table 28-5.

The drug effects of the antifibrinolytics are very specific and limited. They do not have many effects outside of their hematologic ones. Aminocaproic acid and tranexamic acid inhibit the breakdown of fibrin, which prevents the destruction of the formed platelet clot. Desmopressin causes a dose-dependent increase in the concentration of plasma factor VIII (von Willebrand factor), along with an increase in the plasma concentration of tissue plasminogen activator. The overall effect of this is increased platelet aggregation and clot formation. This drug is also an analogue of antidiuretic hormone and is discussed further in Chapter 30.

Indications

Antifibrinolytics are useful in both the prevention and treatment of excessive bleeding resulting from systemic hyperfibrinolysis or surgical complications. They have also proved successful in arresting excessive oozing from surgical sites such as chest tubes as well as in reducing the total blood loss and the duration of bleeding in the postoperative period.

TABLE 28-5 Antifibrinolytics: Mechanisms of Action

Antifibrinolytic Drug	Mechanism of Action
aminocaproic acid (Amicar) and tranexamic acid (Cyklokapron)	Form a reversible complex with plasminogen and plasmin. By binding to the lysine-binding site of plasminogen, these drugs displace plasminogen from the surface of fibrin. This prevents plasmin from lysing the fibrin clot. Therefore, these drugs can work only if a clot has formed.
desmopressin (DDAVP)	Works by increasing the level of factor VII (von Willebrand factor), which anchors platelets to damaged vessels via the glycoprotein Ib platelet receptor. It appears that desmopressin acts as a general endothelial stimulant, promoting the release of factor VIII, prostaglandin I_2, and plasminogen activator.

TABLE 28-6 Antifibrinolytics: Adverse Effects

Body System	Adverse Effects
Cardiovascular	Dysrhythmias, orthostatic hypotension, bradycardia
Central nervous	Headache, dizziness, fatigue, hallucinations, psychosis, convulsions
Gastrointestinal	Nausea, vomiting, abdominal cramps, diarrhea

Desmopressin may also be used in patients who have hemophilia A or type I von Willebrand disease. As stated earlier, recombinant factors VII, VIII, and IX are used to treat hemophilia or to stop the bleeding from excessive warfarin therapy.

Contraindications

Contraindications to the use of antifibrinolytic drugs include known drug allergy to a specific product and disseminated intravascular coagulation, which could be worsened by these drugs.

Adverse Effects

The adverse effects of antifibrinolytic drugs occur uncommonly and are mild. However, there have been rare reports of these drugs' causing thrombotic events, such as acute cerebrovascular thrombosis and acute MI. The common adverse effects of antifibrinolytics are listed in Table 28-6.

Interactions

When drugs such as estrogens or oral contraceptives are used concurrently with aminocaproic acid or tranexamic acid, additive effects may occur, resulting in increased coagulation. Few specific interactions have been reported for desmopressin, although it should be given cautiously in patients receiving lithium, large doses of epinephrine, demeclocycline, heparin, or alcohol. Drugs such as chlorpropamide and fludrocortisone may potentiate the antidiuretic response, which may lead to edema.

Dosages

For the recommended dosages of aminocaproic acid and desmopressin, see the Dosages table on p. 445.

DRUG PROFILES

aminocaproic acid

Aminocaproic acid (Amicar) is a synthetic antifibrinolytic drug used to prevent and control the excessive bleeding that can result from surgery or overactivity of the fibrinolytic system. It is available in both oral and parenteral preparations.

PHARMACOKINETICS

Route	Onset of Action	Peak Plasma Concentration	Elimination Half-life	Duration of Action
IV	Unknown	1.2 hr	2 hr	3 hr

desmopressin

Desmopressin (DDAVP) is a synthetic polypeptide. It is structurally very similar to vasopressin, which is antidiuretic hormone, the natural human posterior pituitary hormone (see Chapter 30). Because of these physical characteristics, it is most often used to increase the resorption of water by the collecting ducts in the kidneys to prevent or control polydipsia, polyuria, and dehydration in patients with diabetes insipidus due to a deficiency of endogenous posterior pituitary vasopressin or in patients with polyuria and polydipsia resulting from trauma or surgery in the pituitary region.

Desmopressin also causes a dose-dependent increase in plasma factor VIII (von Willebrand factor), along with an increase in tissue plasminogen activator, which results in increased platelet aggregation and clot formation. Desmopressin is contraindicated in patients with a known hypersensitivity to it and in those with nephrogenic diabetes insipidus. It is available in both injectable and intranasal dosage forms. Desmopressin nasal spray is used for primary nocturnal enuresis.

PHARMACOKINETICS

Route	Onset of Action	Peak Plasma Concentration	Elimination Half-life	Duration of Action
IV	15-30 min	1-2 hr	2 hr	Unknown

THROMBOLYTIC DRUGS

Thrombolytics are coagulation modifiers that lyse thrombi in the blood vessels that supply the heart with blood, the coronary arteries. This reestablishes blood flow to the blood-starved heart muscle. If the blood flow is reestablished early, the heart muscle and left ventricular function can be saved. If blood flow is not reestablished early, the affected area of the heart muscle becomes ischemic, and eventually necrotic and nonfunctional.

Thrombolytic therapy made its debut in 1933 when a substance that would break down fibrin clots was isolated from a patient's blood. This substance was determined to be produced by certain bacteria growing in the patient's blood. The bacteria were found to be *beta-hemolytic streptococci (group A)*, and the substance was eventually called *streptokinase*.

Streptokinase was first used in a patient in 1947 to dissolve a clotted hemothorax, but it was not until 1958 that it was given to a patient with an acute MI. In 1960, a naturally occurring human plasminogen activator called *urokinase*, which was found to exert fibrinolytic effects on pulmonary emboli (clots in

DOSAGES

Selected Antifibrinolytic Drugs

Drug (Pregnancy Category)	Pharmacologic Class	Usual Dosage Range	Indications/Uses
aminocaproic acid (Amicar) (C)	Hemostatic	**Adult** IV infusion: 4-5 g during first hour, then 1-1.25 g at 1-hr intervals up to a daily max of 30 g	Excessive bleeding caused by systemic hyperfibrinolysis or urinary fibrinolysis
desmopressin (DDAVP) (B)	Synthetic posterior pituitary hormone	**Adult** IV: 0.3 mcg/kg infused over 15-30 min; preoperative use: drug is administered 30 min before surgery	Surgical and postoperative hemostasis and management of bleeding in patients with hemophilia A or type I von Willebrand disease

IV, Intravenous.

the lungs), became available. However, the results of the early thrombolytic trials conducted during the 1960s and 1970s that enrolled patients who had had an acute MI were not taken seriously by the medical community. In the 1980s the underlying cause of acute MI was determined to be due to coronary artery occlusion. This marked the start of rapid growth in the use of thrombolytic drugs for the early treatment of acute MI. Since that time, several new thrombolytics have become available for this and other clinical uses. *Tissue plasminogen activator (t-PA)* and *anisoylated plasminogen streptokinase activator complex (APSAC)* are two of these drugs. Following the advent of these new thrombolytics came the results of several large landmark thrombolytic research studies. These studies showed that early thrombolytic therapy could bring about a 50% reduction in mortality, a reduction in the infarct size, an improvement in left ventricular function, and a reduction in the incidence and severity of congestive heart failure. These findings and developments, along with a better understanding of the pathogenesis of acute MI, have led the way to the advancements made in the treatment of acute MI. However, the use of thrombolytics has almost completely been replaced by interventional cardiologic procedures, such as percutaneous coronary intervention. Thrombolytics are still a viable option in hospitals that do not offer percutaneous coronary intervention. Currently available thrombolytic drugs include t-PAs (anistreplase [Eminase], alteplase [Activase], reteplase [Retavase], and tenecteplase [TNKase]). Dosages, indications, and other information appear in the Dosages table for thrombolytics.

Mechanism of Action and Drug Effects

There is a fine balance between the formation and dissolution of a clot. The coagulation system is responsible for forming clots, whereas the fibrinolytic system is responsible for dissolving clots. The natural fibrinolytic system within the blood takes several days to break down a clot (thrombus). This is of little value in the case of a clotted blood vessel that supplies blood to the heart muscle. Necrosis of the myocardium would not be prevented by these natural means, but thrombolytic drug therapy activates the fibrinolytic system to break down the thrombus in the blood vessel quickly so that the delivery of blood to the heart muscle via the coronary arteries is quickly reestab-

lished. This prevents myocardial tissue (heart muscle) and heart function from being destroyed. Thrombolytics accomplish this by activating the conversion of plasminogen to plasmin, which breaks down, or lyses, the thrombus (see Figure 28-3). Plasmin is a proteolytic enzyme, which means that it breaks down proteins. It is a relatively nonspecific serine protease that is capable of degrading proteins such as fibrin, fibrinogen, and other procoagulant proteins like factors V, VIII, and XII. In other words, the substances that form clots are destroyed by plasmin. Essentially, thrombolytic drugs work by mimicking the body's own process of clot destruction. Although the individual thrombolytic drugs are somewhat diverse in their actions, they all have this common result.

Streptokinase, the original thrombolytic enzyme, and the naturally occurring urokinase have been removed from the U.S. market, primarily due to their adverse effects—namely, they were not fibrin specific. The newer thrombolytics have chemical specificity for fibrin threads (**fibrin specificity**) and work primarily at the site of a clot. They still carry some bleeding risk, but much less than that of the thrombolytic enzymes.

Tissue plasminogen activator is a naturally occurring plasminogen activator secreted by vascular endothelial cells (the walls of blood vessels). However, the amount secreted naturally is not sufficient to dissolve a coronary thrombus quickly enough to restore circulation to the heart and save the heart muscle. Recombinant DNA techniques are now used to produce t-PA, and thus it can be administered in quantities sufficient to dissolve a coronary thrombus quickly. Again, it is fibrin specific (clot specific); that is, only the fibrin clot stimulates t-PA to convert plasminogen to plasmin. Therefore, it has a lower propensity to induce a systemic thrombolytic state, compared to the thrombolytic enzymes.

Indications

The purpose of all the thrombolytic drugs is to activate the conversion of plasminogen to plasmin, the enzyme that breaks down a thrombus. The presence of a thrombus that interferes significantly with normal blood flow on either the venous or the arterial side of the circulation is an indication for the use of thrombolytic therapy. An exception may be a thrombus that has formed in blood vessels that connect directly with the central nervous system. The indications for thrombolytic therapy include acute MI,

DOSAGES

Selected Thrombolytic Drug

Drug (Pregnancy Category)	Pharmacologic Class	Usual Dosage Range	Indications
◆ alteplase (Activase) (C)	Tissue plasminogen activator	**Adult** IV: 100 mg over 90 min given as a 15-mg IV bolus, then 50 mg over 30 min, then 35 mg over 60 min	Acute myocardial infarction
		IV: 100 mg over 2 hr or 30-50 mg over 1.5-2 hr via pulmonary artery	Pulmonary embolism
		IV: 0.9 mg/kg (total dose not to exceed 90 mg) 10% given as an IV bolus over 1 min, remainder over 60 min; must be given within 3 hr of onset of symptoms	Acute ischemic stroke

IV, Intravenous.

arterial thrombosis, DVT, occlusion of shunts or catheters, pulmonary embolism, and acute ischemic stroke.

Contraindications

Contraindications to the use of thrombolytic drugs include known drug allergy to the specific product and any preservatives, and concurrent use of other drugs that alter clotting.

Adverse Effects

The most common undesirable effect of thrombolytic therapy is internal, intracranial, and superficial bleeding. Other problems include hypersensitivity, anaphylactoid reactions, nausea, vomiting, and hypotension. These drugs can also induce cardiac dysrhythmias.

Toxicity and Management of Overdose

Acute toxicity primarily causes an extension of the adverse effects of the thrombolytic drug. Treatment is symptomatic and supportive, because thrombolytic drugs have a relatively short half-life and no specific antidotes.

Interactions

The most common effect of drug interactions is an increased bleeding tendency resulting from the concurrent use of anticoagulants, antiplatelets, or other drugs that affect platelet function.

A laboratory test interaction that can occur with thrombolytic drugs is a reduction in the plasminogen and fibrinogen levels.

Dosages

For the recommended dosages of alteplase, see the Dosages table above.

▌ DRUG PROFILE

All thrombolytic drugs exert their effects by activating plasminogen and converting it to plasmin, which is capable of digesting fibrin, a major component of clots.

◆ alteplase

Alteplase (Activase) is a naturally occurring t-PA secreted by vascular endothelial cells. The pharmaceutically available t-PA is made through recombinant DNA techniques, and modified mammalian

hamster ovary cells produce the substance. It is clot (fibrin) specific and therefore does not produce a systemic lytic state. In addition, because it is present in the human body in a natural state, its administration for therapeutic use does not induce an antigen-antibody reaction. Therefore, it can be readministered immediately in the event of reinfarction. The drug t-PA has a very short half-life of 5 minutes. It is believed to open the clogged artery rapidly, but its action is short-lived. Therefore, it is given with heparin to prevent reocclusion of the infarcted blood vessel. Alteplase is available only in parenteral form. There is also a smaller dosage form known as Cathflo Activase that is used to flush clogged IV or arterial lines. Tenecteplase (TNKase) is a newer form of alteplase that is given by IV push after MI.

PHARMACOKINETICS

Route	Onset of Action	Peak Plasma Concentration	Elimination Half-life	Duration of Action
IV	30 min	60 min	26-50 min	Dependent on infusion duration

NURSING PROCESS

Coagulation modifiers have a variety of uses, including the following: (1) prevention or elimination of clotting in a peripherally inserted catheter (PIC, or PICC—a *peripherally inserted central catheter*), (2) maintenance of patency (without clotting) of central venous catheters, (3) clot prevention in coronary artery bypass grafting, (4) prevention of clotting after major vessel injury, (5) treatment of thrombophlebitis to prevent venous and/or arterial thromboembolism, and (6) prevention of clotting with use of prosthetics (e.g., heart valve replacements) and in atrial fibrillation. The drugs that are used for these different indications are varied in their mechanisms of action and the related general and specific nursing process issues will be discussed.

Assessment

Nursing assessment associated with the use of all *coagulation-modifying* drugs should begin with taking a thorough nursing history and medication history, and performing a brief physical examination. A thorough patient health history should include the assessment of the following: any drug or food allergies, current medical problems, underlying systemic disease processes, past and present medical history, family health history, dietary habits, changes in body weight over time, ability to perform activities of daily living, level of exercise and/or degree of sedentary lifestyle, employment activities, success of previous treatment regimens, blood pressure, pulse rate, respirations, body weight, height, dietary intake, and fluid intake. A thorough patient assessment to identify the presence of the following risk factors is also needed: immobility; history of limited activity or prolonged bed rest (e.g., generally for longer than 3 to 5 days); dehydration; obesity; smoking; congestive heart failure; mitral or aortic stenosis; coronary heart disease with documented atherosclerosis or arteriosclerosis; peripheral vascular disease; pelvic, gynecologic-genitourinary, abdominal, orthopedic, or vascular major surgery; history of thrombophlebitis, DVT, thromboembolism including pulmonary embolism, myocardial infarct, atrial fibrillation; edema of the periphery; trauma to the lower extremities; use of oral contraceptives; and/or recent extended airline travel time. If the patient has a history of clotting disorders and/or thromboembolism, the following must also be assessed and documented: presenting signs and symptoms of thrombophlebitis of the leg such calf edema; pain, warmth, or redness directly over the vessel (more indicative of a superficial clot); increased diameter of the calf of the affected leg; pain in the calf with dorsiflexion (often called the Homans sign; however, this is a very controversial method of assessment) or pain upon gentle compression of the calf muscle against the tibial bone; and presenting signs and symptoms of pulmonary embolism such as chest pain, cough, dyspnea, tachypnea, drop in oxygen saturation (by oximetry or blood gas measurement), hemoptysis, tachycardia, drop in blood pressure, and possible shock. All contraindications, cautions, and drug interactions should also be assessed (see pharmacology discussion) and documented.

Because of the effects of coagulation modifiers it is also important to assess the skin, oral mucous membranes, gums, urine, and stool for any evidence of bleeding. Patients should be assessed for any blood in the urine or stool, easy bruising, excessive bleeding from tooth brushing or shaving, or unexplained nosebleeds while receiving these medications, and any such findings reported. Cautions and contraindications should be noted (see previous discussion). Drugs and herbals that may exacerbate bleeding because of their effects on clotting have been previously discussed and should be assessed and documented. Laboratory tests performed before and during therapy with these drugs usually include, but are not limited to, baseline complete blood counts, hemoglobin level, hematocrit, lipoprotein fractionation, triglyceride and cholesterol levels, various clotting studies, and liver function tests. The serum laboratory tests that should be performed with anticoagulant therapy are presented in the Laboratory Values Related to Drug Therapy box.

With *heparin* and *LMWHs*, it is critical to patient safety to continually assess the skin to identify potential subcutaneous injection sites. For these injection sites, the standard is to *avoid* any area within 2 inches of the umbilicus, open wounds, scars, open or abraded areas, incisions, drainage tubes, stomas, or areas of bruising or oozing, because these sites would be at higher risk for further tissue damage with injection of the anticoagulant. Appropriate sites for injection of subcutaneous

heparin and LMWHs include the upper, outer area of the arms, the thigh, and the subcutaneous fatty area across the lower abdomen and between the iliac crests (see Chapter 10 for more information).

With use of the *parenteral anticoagulant* heparin, to ensure patient safety and prevent injury the nurse should assess for allergies, contraindications, cautions, drug interactions (see pharmacology discussion), severe hypertension, ulcer disease, ulcerative colitis, aneurysms, malignant hypertension, alcoholism, and head injuries. An important caution for heparin use is pregnancy or lactation; however, should there be a need for an anticoagulant during pregnancy, heparin is the drug of choice, not warfarin. Other information is presented in Table 28-1. It is crucial to patient safety that the nurse remember that heparin is *not* interchangeable unit for unit with drugs in another class of anticoagulants, the LMWHs. It is important to know that heparin sodium contains benzyl alcohol; therefore, assessment for allergy to this additional component is required. Although the use of *LMWHs* leads to fewer adverse reactions in some patients, these drugs are still associated with specific contraindications, cautions, and drug interactions (see previous discussion). The same assessment parameters discussed earlier for heparin are also appropriate for LMWHs. In addition, LMWHs contain sulfites and benzyl alcohol, and so the patient should be assessed for allergies to these substances. It is important to note again that the LMWHs differ from standard heparin and also from each other, and for this reason they are not interchangeable. LMWHs may be used for outpatient anticoagulant therapy, because these drugs usually require less close monitoring than standard heparin. Results of clotting studies should also be assessed prior to therapy.

The *oral anticoagulant* warfarin and its related contraindications, cautions, and drug interactions have been discussed earlier in this chapter. All of the previously mentioned assessment parameters and laboratory studies are applicable to warfarin. Because of the drug's action, warfarin (as with all drugs altering bleeding/clotting) should be withdrawn—as ordered—before the patient undergoes any dental procedures or if there is any evidence of tissue necrosis, gangrene, diarrhea, intestinal flora imbalances, or steatorrhea; thus, close assessment is needed. Important to emphasize with this drug is the fact that warfarin is indicated for prophylaxis and long-term treatment of a variety of thromboembolic disorders (see previous pharmacology discussion), and constant and skillful assessment of the patient and clotting results is required. Most prescribers use standard protocols for warfarin to assist in dosing the drug based on PT/INR (the standardized measures of blood coagulability). The most common starting dosage for warfarin is 5 mg daily. However, the dose can range from 1 to 10 mg, and occasionally even higher (e.g., 12 mg) depending on individual patient response. In most situations, dosage for adults is between 1 and 5 mg orally every day. In addition, the pharmacokinetics of warfarin are important to assess and understand, because it takes about 3 days for the drug to reach a steady state. Patients taking heparin may receive warfarin before discontinuation of heparin for anticoagulation.

With *antiplatelet* drugs, a thorough nursing history and medication history should be obtained, and a physical assessment should be performed. Possible drug interactions, cautions,

LABORATORY VALUES RELATED TO DRUG THERAPY

Anticoagulants

Laboratory Test	Normal Ranges	Rationale for Assessment
Activated partial thromboplastin time (aPTT), partial thromboplastin time (PTT)*	With heparin therapy, aPTT values should fall between 1.5 and 2.5 times the control or baseline value. Normal control values are 25 to 35 sec, so therapeutic values should then be between approximately 45 and 70 sec.	Therapeutic levels of aPTT indicate decreased levels of clotting factors and subsequent clotting activity. aPTT is a more sensitive part of PTT and often replaces it. It is used to determine whether there are deficiencies in the patient's intrinsic coagulation pathway and to monitor heparin therapy. aPTT is sensitive to changes in blood clotting factors, except for factor VII. Therefore, it is used to assess for normal blood coagulation. With continuous IV infusions of heparin, blood samples for aPTT testing can be drawn at any time, but with intermittent infusions the blood sample should be drawn approximately 1 hr before a dose of heparin is scheduled to be given.
Prothrombin time (PT)	The normal control PT value ranges from 11 to 13 sec; target therapeutic level of anticoagulation is 1.5 times the control value, or about 18 sec.	Prothrombin is a vitamin K–dependent protein, a major component of the clotting process. It reflects clotting activity and is used to monitor the effectiveness of warfarin therapy. PT values vary for each laboratory center and are based on the specifics of the testing procedure.
International normalized ratio (INR)	Target levels of INR range from 2 to 3 or an average of 2.5. For individuals taking warfarin for treatment of recurring systemic clots or emboli and those with mechanical heart valves, the target INR may be 2.5 to 3.5, with a middle value of 3.	INR determination is a routine test to evaluate coagulation while patients are taking warfarin. When the therapy is initiated, the INR and PT should be measured daily until a stable daily dose is reached (the dose maintains the PT and INR within therapeutic ranges and does not cause bleeding). INR values actually reflect the dose of warfarin given 36 to 72 hr prior to the testing. Advantages of INR testing include the fact that there is more consistency among laboratories and a more consistent warfarin dosage is achieved. Some laboratories report INR and PT together.

IV, Intravenous.
These terms are used interchangeably.

and contraindications have been discussed, but close assessment of any bleeding is most important to patient safety. Because aspirin, other NSAIDs, and other antiplatelet drugs alter bleeding times, these drugs should be withheld for 5 to 7 days before the patient undergoes surgical procedures. Specific guidelines are generally given by the prescriber to avoid the concurrent use of other anticoagulants, antiplatelets, and fibrinolytics. Because of the ototoxicity of aspirin, other drugs that have the same adverse effect, such as the aminoglycosides (e.g., vancomycin), should not be given at the same time. Baseline cardiovascular assessment is needed, with documentation of general history, history of chest pain, complete blood count, hemoglobin level and hematocrit, platelet counts, and PT and INR values. This provides baseline values with which therapy values can be compared. If platelet counts are at or fall below 80,000 cells/mm³, the prescriber should be notified, and antiplatelet therapy most likely will not be initiated (or will be discontinued). In addition, it is important to patient safety to reemphasize the fact that aspirin is not to be used in children and teenagers, in patients with any bleeding disorder, in pregnant or lactating women, or in patients with vitamin K deficiency or peptic ulcer disease. These are situations in which major consequences could occur if aspirin were used; for example, Reye's syndrome in children and teenagers, teratogenic effects in pregnant women, and ulcers or bleeding tendencies in patients with vitamin K deficiency or peptic ulcer disease. In addition, it is always important to know how each of the drugs works in the body so that a sound knowledge base exists for critical thinking and decision making: for example, the decision to call the prescriber and not to administer two antiplatelets at

the same time or not to give a thrombolytic with heparin, warfarin, or aspirin or other NSAIDs. This type of critical drug information is very important to make sure the patient receives the safest and most appropriate care during all phases of the nursing process.

The *GP IIb/IIIa inhibitors*—for example, eptifibatide, tirofiban, and abciximab—require the same baseline assessment information (e.g., vital signs, medical history, history of chest pain or cardiac disease, complete blood cell counts, hemoglobin level, hematocrit, renal function tests, platelet counts). Before or during therapy, if the platelet count is below 90,000/mm³ the prescriber should be contacted for further orders. *Antifibrinolytics* require the same skillful assessment of baseline parameters and laboratory testing; however, there are additional concerns for patients with altered cardiac, renal, or hepatic functioning. These are situations in which the prescriber may need to decrease the dosage of medication. Serum potassium levels should be noted prior to therapy, because of the potential for drug-induced hyperkalemia.

Thrombolytics require similar assessments, including attention to baseline complete blood cell counts and results of clotting studies. The use of alteplase and other thrombolytics always carries major concerns/cautions, contraindications and drug interactions (see previous pharmacology discussion). Any arterial punctures, venous cut-down sites, peripherally inserted central catheter sites, and central infusion ports or sites should be constantly assessed for bleeding. IM injections are not to be used in any situation and pose problems with bleeding. As with any drugs that alter clotting and platelet activity, the thrombolytics are associated with the risk of bleeding from wounds or from the gastrointestinal, genitourinary, or respiratory tract, so any drainage, urine, stool, emesis, sputum, and secretions should be assessed for the presence of blood.

Nursing Diagnoses

- Ineffective cardiac, cerebral, and peripheral tissue perfusion related to the clotting disorder, such as thrombus formation
- Impaired physical mobility related to tissue injury or decreased tissue perfusion caused by various coagulation disorders
- Risk for injury related to possible adverse reactions to any of the drugs that alter blood clotting
- Deficient knowledge of the medication treatment regimen related to lack of information and/or lack of experience with drug therapy
- Acute pain related to symptoms of the underlying clotting disorder or tissue ischemia
- Deficient knowledge related to the new medication regimen and the need for altered lifestyle
- Activity intolerance related to the underlying clotting disorder or ischemia

Planning

Goals

- Patient experiences increased comfort and relief of pain.
- Patient exhibits improved blood flow as a result of the therapeutic effects of the anticoagulant.
- Patient remains free from injury resulting from either the disease or the medication being taken.
- Patient is compliant with the lifestyle changes required and with the medication regimen.
- Patient demonstrates adequate knowledge regarding medication therapy and its potential adverse effects.

Outcome Criteria

- Patient experiences relief of symptoms such as decreased pain, swelling, and edema once tissue perfusion is regained as a result of medication therapy.
- Patient shows improved circulation with warm extremities or strong pedal pulses or experiences a return to his or her predisease state of tissue perfusion.
- Patient is free of bruising, bleeding problems, and any other adverse reaction to the medication.
- Patient states the rationale for the use of the medication regimen, such as decreased clotting or clot formation.
- Patient states the nature of and rationale for the lifestyle changes needed, such as improved diet, exercise, and avoidance of smoking.
- Patient states the adverse effects of the drug therapy, the way to monitor for complications of the anticoagulants, the importance of scheduling follow-up appointments with the prescriber and of frequent laboratory studies, and the circumstances under which to contact the prescriber to prevent complications such as hemorrhage.

Implementation

Vital signs, heart sounds, peripheral pulses, and neurologic status are routinely monitored in all patients during and immediately after anticoagulant therapy. The various laboratory values to be monitored are presented in the Laboratory Values Related to Drug Therapy box on p. 448. If there is any change in pulse rate or rhythm, blood pressure, or level of consciousness, and/or unexplained restlessness occurs, the prescriber should be contacted immediately. These changes may indicate bleeding or hemorrhage.

Knowledge of the proper techniques of administration is crucial for safe and effective use of *heparin* and the *LMWHs* (see Box 28-1 for other dosing and route information). Heparin may be given by the subcutaneous or IV routes but *not* IM. Inadvertent IM injection can be easily avoided if the nurse uses only subcutaneous syringes, which are usually made available in prefilled syringes that include a $\frac{1}{2}$-inch (1.5-cm) 25- to 28-gauge needle. No major harm would result if a subcutaneous dose were inadvertently administered IV. If rapid anticoagulation is needed, IV heparin by continuous or intermittent infusion may be prescribed. Whether the drug is given by IV infusion or subcutaneous injection, monitoring of daily clotting study results will be needed, and these studies should be performed as ordered. The drug effects can be reversed with the IV administration of protamine sulfate. With subcutaneous heparin, several doses of protamine sulfate may be needed to reverse the anticoagulant effect because of the variable rates of absorption of this dosage form. See Box 28-1 for the procedure for the intermittent or continuous IV administration of heparin.

LMWHs are given by subcutaneous injection deep into the injection site (see previous discussion) using the same techniques as for heparin. Sites should be rotated frequently. There should be no aspiration with the subcutaneous injection, nor should the area be massaged after the injection. Prefilled syringes of LMWHs are available for inpatient use and for at-home treatment. Solutions may be clear to pale yellow. The usual length of therapy is approximately 5 to 10 days, and it is important to constantly be aware of any bleeding problems while the patient is taking this or other clotting-altering drugs. Complete blood counts, platelet counts, and stool tests for occult blood are tests that will probably be performed during therapy for monitoring purposes. Tests for occult blood in the stool can be done simply if occult blood test paper and developer are available. Blood in the stool may occur as an adverse effect of LMWHs or any clotting-altering drug.

When the *oral anticoagulant* warfarin is prescribed, therapy is often initiated while the patient is still receiving heparin. This overlapping is done purposefully to allow time for the blood levels of warfarin to rise, so that when the heparin is eventually discontinued, therapeutic anticoagulation levels of warfarin will have been achieved. The full therapeutic effect of warfarin does not occur until 4 to 5 days after the first dose. This overlap of activity is required in patients who have been receiving heparin for anticoagulation and are to be switched to warfarin so that prevention of clotting is continuous. Monitoring results of the various clotting studies is still of utmost priority, as is watching for any clotting or bleeding problems. The administration procedures for warfarin are outlined in Box 28-1. For conversion from heparin to an oral anticoagulant such as warfarin, the dose of the oral drug should be the usual initial amount, with PT/INR levels then used to help the prescriber determine the next appropriate dosage of warfarin. Once there is continuous therapeutic anticoagulation coverage and warfarin has reached therapeutic levels, the heparin or

BOX 28-1 Anticoagulation Therapy and Related Nursing Considerations

Subcutaneous Heparin Injections

- After thoroughly checking the prescriber's order, assess the patient for the existence of any allergies, contraindications, cautions, or drug interactions.
- Wash hands thoroughly. Prefilled syringes are available for convenience as well as accurate technique and dosing, and should be used whenever possible. As a point of reference, the prefilled syringe comes with a tuberculin syringe to draw up the exact dose of heparin. For a 25- to 28-gauge needle, the length of the needle is ½ to ⅝ inch. When the medication is not available in a prefilled or premeasured syringe, a tuberculin syringe is used because it is the correct gauge and needle length. See Chapter 10 for more information on the technique associated with heparin and LMWH administration. Check site for bleeding or bruising and do *not* massage/rub the site before or after the injection. *Do not aspirate* before injecting to prevent hematoma formation.
- Make sure the patient is comfortable, then remove gloves and wash hands. Monitor patient and document.

Intravenous Heparin Administration

- Always double-check the specific prescriber's order for dosage, rate of infusion, and time and route before beginning therapy and always follow the "Six Rights" of medication administration to prevent overdosing or erroneous dosing. Make sure the proper diluent is used and check the compatibility of solutions or other drugs before beginning the infusion.
- For continuous intravenous (IV) administration of heparin, an IV pump must be used to ensure a precise rate of infusion.
- Continuous dosing is preferred over intermittent dosing because continuous dosing helps maintain blood levels of the drug and because intermittent IV dosing is associated with a higher risk for bleeding abnormalities.
- Treatment by continuous IV infusion generally begins with a loading dose and is followed by a maintenance dose. Be aware that dosage adjustments are made exactly as ordered. The patient's activated partial thromboplastin time (aPTT) and/or results of other related clotting studies are used as parameters for dosing of standard heparin.
- For intermittent infusions, a heparin lock was used in the past. Heparin locks are now referred to as *intermittent infusion locks* or *saline*

locks (because the locks are flushed with isotonic saline and not with heparin).
- Intermittent infusions of heparin are usually ordered to be given every 4 to 6 hours because of heparin's short half-life. Needleless systems are used for intermittent infusions and all other types of IV infusions.
- Regardless of the type of IV infusion (e.g., intermittent or continuous IV infusion), it is crucial to check the site to determine whether infiltration has occurred so that hematoma formation may be prevented. If infiltration is suspected, the lock should be removed and replaced at a new site before the next scheduled infusion. Document your actions in the nurse's notes.
- The therapeutic dosage of heparin is guided by aPTT with a targeted level of 1.5 to 2.5 times the control (normal) value. The aPTT is measured within 24 hours of beginning therapy, 24 to 48 hours after therapy starts, and 1 to 2 times weekly for about 3 to 4 weeks on average. With long-term therapy, aPTT is monitored 1 to 2 times per month.

Oral Anticoagulant Administration

- It is important to recheck the prescriber's orders and the patient's medication and medical history before administering the drug. Always check to make sure the patient has no known hypersensitivity to the drug.
- Scored tablets may be crushed and may be given with or without food.
- Many more drugs can interact with oral anticoagulants than with heparin, especially those that are highly protein bound (such as the ones listed in Table 28-3). Always check the patient's medication list before initiating therapy with warfarin.
- Dosages of warfarin are calculated based on international normalized ratio (INR) blood values. INRs are also used to monitor the effectiveness of therapy. Remember, however, that dosing is highly individualized!
- Oral anticoagulants should be administered at the same time every day to maintain steady blood levels.
- Document the dose, time of administration, and any other pertinent facts.

LMWH may be discontinued without tapering. Should uncontrolled bleeding occur with any of these medications, the nurse must take action to control bleeding as well as institute emergency measures to stabilize the patient's condition, and the prescriber should be contacted immediately.

Of benefit to counter toxic effects of *anticoagulants* is the use of antidotes. The antidote to hemorrhage or uncontrolled bleeding resulting from heparin or LMWH therapy is protamine sulfate. This antidote is given IV and may be administered in an undiluted form over a 10-minute period at a rate *not to exceed* 5 mg/min or 50 mg in any 10-minute period. The benchmark dose is based on the fact that 1 mg of protamine sulfate neutralizes 90 to 115 units of heparin. It is important to note that too-rapid an infusion may lead to acute hypotensive episodes, bradycardia, dyspnea, and transient feelings of warmth and flushing. The aPTT ranges and hematocrit levels are generally used at this point to monitor bleeding, clotting, and risk for bleeding. The patient should always be watched,

especially for any changes in blood pressure and pulse rate. The antidote to oral anticoagulant (warfarin sodium) therapy is vitamin K, which is preferably given via the subcutaneous route, although oral, IV, and IM dosage forms are available. This drug may lead in rare cases to severe reactions such as dyspnea, dizziness, rapid or weak pulse, chest pain, and hypotension, which may progress to shock and cardiac arrest. Continual monitoring of the patient's vital signs, cardiac parameters, and bleeding times and other clotting study results are very important.

The patient being treated with *antiplatelet* drugs (or any clotting-altering drug) should be constantly monitored for signs and symptoms of bleeding during and after their use, including epistaxis, hematuria, hematemesis, easy or excessive bruising, blood in the stools, and bleeding of the gums. If invasive procedures must be performed or injections given, appropriate pressure should be applied to bleeding sites, and all areas of venous or arterial catheter insertion should be closely watched for

Heparin Therapy

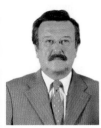

© Martin Allinger

In the past 2 years, Mr. L., a 56-year-old archi-tect, has experienced three episodes of deep vein thrombosis. All occurred without compli-cations and all were treated successfully with anticoagulant therapy and bed rest. He now arrives at the urgent care center because of increased pain and swelling in his left calf that has lasted for the past 3 days. Initially he is given 5000 units of heparin IV. On admis-sion to the hospital for anticoagulant therapy he is started on a continuous infusion of 25,000 units of heparin in 1000 mL of 0.9% sodium chloride.

1. What nursing actions should be implemented to ensure the accu-racy and safety of the continuous heparin infusion?
2. What patient findings would indicate a therapeutic response to the heparin therapy?

  During Mr. L.'s hospital stay, the physician orders an extra bolus of 10,000 units of heparin, IV push, because the results of Mr. L.'s labora-tory tests indicated that his activated partial thromboplastin time (aPTT) was not at a therapeutic level. After giving the dose, the nurse notices that a dose of 50,000 units was given instead of 10,000 units.

3. What should the nurse do first, and what subsequent orders should the nurse prepare to carry out?

For answers, see *http://evolve.elsevier.com/Lilley*.

---

bleeding. Extended-release dosage forms should be taken in their entirety and without chewing or crushing. Enteric-coated aspirin should be taken with 6 to 8 oz of water and with food to help decrease gastrointestinal upset. To avoid irritation to the esophagus, the patient should remain upright and not lie down for up to 30 minutes after the dose of aspirin. If the aspirin has a strong, vinegar-like odor, the drug should be discarded. Inter-ventions with clopidogrel therapy are similar to those for aspi-rin. The patient should report any of the following: aches in the joints, back pain, dizziness, severe headache, dyspepsia, flulike signs and symptoms, and epigastric pain. These drugs are often discontinued for 7 days prior to surgery, as ordered. However, some surgical procedures (e.g., cardiovascular surgery) may warrant that the patient remain in an anticoagulated state intra-operatively. Oral forms of dipyridamole are recommended to be taken on an empty stomach; however, if this is not tolerated, the drug may be taken with food. If nausea occurs, cola, unsalted crackers, or dry toast may help to alleviate this adverse effect. In addition, it may take up to 2 to 3 months of continuous therapy for the drug to reach therapeutic levels. Patients should be encouraged to change positions slowly and to take their time in going from lying to sitting to standing because of the adverse effects of dizziness and postural hypotension with antiplatelets and all other drugs covered in this chapter.

Nursing considerations associated with the *GP IIb/IIIa in-hibitors*, such as abciximab, eptifibatide, and tirofiban, include some similar, yet different, nursing actions. Close monitoring of all vital signs, electrocardiogram readings, peripheral pulses, heart sounds, skin color, and temperature is an important part of nursing care during and after the use of these drugs. Because these drugs are used in combination with heparin to treat indi-viduals suspected of having acute coronary syndrome or those undergoing percutaneous transluminal coronary angioplasty (PTCA), there is always concern for the stability of the patient as well as a high risk for serious bleeding and/or extension of an acute MI. The patient in this situation is at risk for other medical complications, and this risk may be intensified by the drug. Avoidance of further invasive procedures while the pa-tient is taking these drugs is important to help prevent bleeding. If invasive procedures are required, it is crucial to monitor con-stantly for bleeding and to measure all vital parameters before, during, and after the procedure. IV tirofiban should be pro-tected from light, and any unused solutions should be discarded 24 hours after an infusion has been started. No other drugs should be given with this drug except for heparin, which may be administered through the same IV line. For PCTA, abcix-imab can be given by bolus or by continuous infusion, with infusion rates monitored closely. Manufacturer guidelines call for the use of a sterile, nonpyrogenic, low protein-binding 0.2- or 0.22-micron filter, and while the vascular shield is in posi-tion, the patient should remain on complete bed rest with the head of the bed elevated 30 degrees. The affected extremity should be maintained in a straight position with constant moni-toring of peripheral pulses and the color and temperature of the distal extremities. Once the sheath is removed, application of pressure to the femoral artery is required for at least 30 min-utes, either by manual or mechanical pressure. A pressure dressing should be applied once bleeding has stopped. The site should be closely monitored for any oozing or bleeding.

If serious bleeding occurs, the GP IIb/IIIa inhibitor and hepa-rin (the usual protocol for PTCA) should be discontinued imme-diately, the patient should be monitored closely, and the pre-scriber should be notified immediately for initiation of emergency treatment. These patients should always be moved and handled with caution and unnecessary trauma avoided because of the risk for hematoma formation or bleeding. Blood pressure SHOULD NOT be taken in the lower extremities, but a close and constant watch should be kept on the patient's blood pressure (for hypo-tension) and pulse rate (for tachycardia), and the patient should be monitored for any complaints of abdominal or back pain, se-vere headache, and any other signs or symptoms of hemorrhage. When adhesive or sticky tape is removed, care should always be taken to avoid tearing or ripping the skin, which would lead to tissue trauma and further risk for bleeding. The aPTT levels should be monitored after the procedure, and the patient should be very closely observed for bleeding, with attention to IM injec-tion sites, arterial or venous puncture sites, and bleeding from nasogastric tubes and/or urinary catheters. Such invasive proce-dures should be avoided, if at all possible, during and immedi-ately after the angioplasty.

With *antifibrinolytics,* it is important to understand the rea-sons for the use of these drugs, such as to stop bleeding from overdosages of thrombolytic drugs or to control bleeding dur-ing cardiac surgery. Aminocaproic acid and tranexamic acid are usually given IV until bleeding is controlled. Use of these drugs requires very close patient monitoring, and if there is any change in motor strength or level of consciousness, the prescriber should be notified. Nurses have to apply their knowledge of certain adverse effects of drugs like these, so that nursing care can be focused on prevention of complications, maintenance of safety, and return of the patient to a healthier state. Because of the possibility of drug-induced skeletal myopathies, creatine kinase level and results of liver function studies should be monitored. It is also important to monitor heart rate and blood pressure with attention to the quality and strength of peripheral pulses. For the patient with hemophilia, tranexamic acid may be used to help decrease bleeding from dental extractions. Close monitoring of these patients for any oral bleeding is important during postdental care at home.

Nursing considerations related to *thrombolytics* are very similar to those for the other drugs discussed previously. Specifically, preparation for their IV administration should be carried out per manufacturer guidelines and per protocol. Invasive procedures should be avoided during the use of these drugs, as should the simultaneous use of anticoagulants or antiplatelets. IV infusion sites should be monitored frequently for bleeding, redness, and pain. IM injections of other drugs are contraindicated to prevent tissue damage and bleeding. Any bleeding from gums or mucous membranes or the occurrence of epistaxis or increased pulse (higher than 100 beats/min) should be reported to the prescriber immediately, and all vital signs should be monitored frequently. Other nursing considerations include monitoring for hypotension, restlessness, and a decrease in hemoglobin level or hematocrit, which should be reported to the prescriber immediately. Patients should be instructed to report pink, red, or cloudy urine; black, tarry stools or frank red blood in the stools; abdominal or chest pain; dizziness; and severe headache. The drug should be reconstituted for IV dosing with sodium chloride or 5% dextrose in water. Solutions should be rolled gently to mix and not shaken to maintain a stable solution. INR, aPTT, platelet counts, and fibrinogen levels should be monitored continually, beginning no later than 2 to 3 hours after the administration of thrombolytics. The patient's fibrinogen level may be measured to check for the occurrence of fibrinolysis. With the breakdown of fibrin (or fibrinolysis), INR will increase and aPTT will be prolonged. Should bleeding occur, the prescriber will most likely discontinue the drug and replace fibrinogen through infusions of whole blood plasma or cryoprecipitate. The above-mentioned antifibrinolytics (e.g., aminocaproic acid and tranexamic acid) may also be given. Patient teaching tips for several clotting-altering drugs are listed in the box on p. 453.

Evaluation

Monitoring for the therapeutic and adverse effects of clotting-altering drugs is crucial for their safe administration. Because these drugs are used for a variety of purposes, therapeutic responses vary. Some of the therapeutic effects include decreased chest pain and a decrease in dizziness, as well as in other neurologic symptoms. Adverse effects may include drops in blood pressure, headache, hematoma formation, irritation and pain at the injection site, hemorrhage, thrombocytopenia, shortness of breath, chills, and fever. Early signs of drug overdose for any of the clotting-altering drugs include bleeding of the gums while brushing the teeth, unexplained nosebleeds or bruising, and heavier-than-usual menstrual bleeding. Abdominal pain, back pain, bloody or tarry stools, bloody urine, constipation, blood in the sputum, severe or continuous headaches, and the vomiting of frank red blood or a coffee ground–like substance (old blood) are all possible indications of internal bleeding. The adverse effects of aspirin use include gastrointestinal upset or bleeding, heartburn, headache, hepatitis, thrombocytopenia, agranulocytosis, leukopenia, neutropenia, hemolytic anemia, prolonged PT, tinnitus, hearing loss, rapid pulse, wheezing, hypoglycemia, hyponatremia, and hypokalemia. Adverse effects of antiplatelets include postural hypotension, headache, weakness, syncope, gastrointestinal upset, rash, flushing of the face, and dizziness. It is necessary to continually monitor liver, renal, and clotting function in patients receiving long-term therapy with aspirin and other anticlotting drugs. Therapeutic effects of clopidogrel and similar drugs include a decrease in the occurrence of clotting events such as transient ischemic attacks and strokes. Adverse effects for which to monitor with these drugs include increased bleeding tendencies, flulike symptoms, headache, fatigue, chest pain, and epistaxis. Therapeutic levels of anticoagulants and other clotting-altering drugs are also monitored by laboratory studies such as aPTT, PT, and INR, which are described in the Laboratory Values Related to Drug Therapy box on p. 448. It should be remembered, however, that aPTT levels are measured with heparin, whereas PT and INR are measured with warfarin. Once the level of the particular drug stabilizes and maintenance therapy is ongoing, the clotting studies may be performed at 1- to 4-week intervals, depending on the specific drug, the patient's response, and the patient's overall physical condition. Should a heparin or LMWH overdose occur, the antidote is protamine sulfate, whereas vitamin K, or phytonadione, is the antidote to oral anticoagulant overdose (see nursing considerations earlier).

The continuous monitoring of the patient for the signs and symptoms of internal or external bleeding is critical during both the initiation and maintenance of therapy. Therapeutic effects of antifibrinolytics include the arrest of oozing of blood from a surgical site or a decrease in blood loss. Because of the complexity and life-threatening nature of the conditions for which these drugs are used, the nurse must continually monitor and reevaluate the patient's response to the treatment, document this response accordingly, and always keep goals and outcome criteria within the plan of care to serve as a benchmark. From the evaluation phase, the patient will hopefully emerge experiencing full therapeutic effects and minimal adverse and/or toxic effects related to drug therapy.

PATIENT TEACHING TIPS

- The use of coagulation-modifying drugs to prevent serious complications related to clotting, such as strokes, heart attacks, clot formation (deep vein thrombosis of the legs) with heart valve replacements, and mini-strokes/TIAs (transient ischemic attacks), requires frequent and close monitoring. The patient must understand that a healthy lifestyle is an important part of therapy and will most likely include eating the right foods, weight reduction if needed, smoking cessation, control of blood pressure, and stress reduction. A listing of all medications should be given to all possible prescribers, e.g., dentists.
- All of the clotting altering drugs must be taken exactly as prescribed because too little of the drug may lead to clot formation and too much of the drug may lead to bleeding. Regular follow-up appointments are an important part of patient care, with frequent blood tests to monitor for therapeutic effects and adverse effects of the medication. The results of the blood tests will help the prescriber determine the proper dosage.
- An identification card should be carried or a medical alert bracelet or necklace worn at all times stating allergies, medical diagnosis, list of drugs, prescriber's name and phone number as well as an emergency contact name and number.
- Home heparin therapy may require injections for a period of time, and LMWHs are generally used. If there is a switch from heparin to warfarin (Coumadin), there may be an overlap period of approximately 3 to 5 days during which both drugs are taken to allow therapeutic levels of the oral warfarin to be reached before the heparin is discontinued. This process may occur in the hospital or at home. Complete and thorough instructions and return demonstrations are an important part of patient education (see Chapter 10).
- The patient should report any unusual bleeding from anywhere on the body or the occurrence of a severe headache, blurred vision, vomiting of blood, dizziness, fainting, fever, muscular or limb weakness, rash, nosebleeds, or excessive vaginal or menstrual bleeding to the prescriber.
- If bleeding occurs, the patient should know to apply direct pressure to the site for 3 to 5 minutes or longer, as needed.
- Journal keeping by the patient with daily notation of how the patient is feeling as well as how the patient is tolerating the medication and any adverse effects is beneficial to ensure safe, effective treatment.

- To reduce risk factors for cardiovascular disease, the prescriber may recommend consumption of a low-fat, low-cholesterol diet; cholesterol-lowering drug therapy; weight reduction; control of blood pressure if hypertension is present; avoidance of smoking; management of stress; and regular exercise.
- Teaching about clot-preventative measures is encouraged, including situations to minimize sluggish circulation (e.g., avoid tight-fitting clothing, minimize sitting for prolonged periods of time, avoid crossing the legs at the knees and wearing of tight-fitting socks/stockings, avoid prolonged bed rest, make stops during long trips to walk around every 1 to 2 hours, keep well hydrated).
- When taking any of the anticoagulants (oral drugs and/or heparin or LMWHs) or clotting-altering drugs, the patient should be encouraged to avoid brushing the teeth with a hard-bristled toothbrush, shaving with a straight razor, and/or engaging in any activity that would increase the risk of tissue injury. Caution with shaving, nail trimming, gardening, and/or participating in rough or contact sports should be emphasized.
- While taking an anticoagulant, ingesting large amounts of foods high in vitamin K (e.g., broccoli, Brussels sprouts, collard greens, kale, lettuce, mustard greens, tomatoes) should be avoided to minimize food/drug interactions.
- Capsicum (red pepper), feverfew, garlic, ginger, and ginkgo are some herbals that have potential interactions, especially with warfarin. Educate about these and other interactions.
- Any decrease in urine output; constant ringing in the ears; swelling of the feet, ankles, or legs; dark urine; clay-colored stools; abdominal pain; rash (use should be discontinued if rash occurs); and/or blurred vision should be reported to the prescriber immediately.
- If doses of medications are omitted, the patient should contact the prescriber for further instructions.
- Oral dosage forms of any of these medications should be taken with at least 8 oz of water and/or with food to help minimize stomach upset.
- Keep all medication containers out of the reach of children, and use childproof tops. All syringes, needles, and other equipment should be kept out of the reach of children and other individuals as well.

POINTS TO REMEMBER

- Coagulation modifiers work by preventing/promoting clot formation, lysing a preformed clot, and/or reversing the action of anticoagulants. Coagulation modifiers include anticoagulants, antiplatelets, antifibrinolytics, thrombolytics, and reversal drugs.
- Warfarin prevents clot formation by inhibiting vitamin K–dependent clotting factors (factors II, VII, IX, and X) and is used prophylactically to prevent clots from forming; it cannot lyse preformed clots.
- The degree of anticoagulation (for any of these medications) is monitored by the PT.
- Heparin, given IV or subcutaneously, prevents clot formation by binding to antithrombin III, which turns off certain activating factors. The overall effect is to inactivate the coagulation pathway and prevent clots from forming. Heparin does not lyse (break down) a clot.
- Antiplatelet drugs prevent clot formation by preventing platelet involvement in clot formation.

- Antifibrinolytics prevent the lysis of fibrin, thus promoting clot formation, and have an effect opposite to that of the anticoagulants.
- Thrombolytics are able to break down or lyse preformed clots in blood vessels such as those that supply the heart with blood. Therapeutic effects for which the nurse should monitor include improved tissue perfusion, decreased chest pain, and prevention of further myocardial damage. The therapeutic effects of most coagulation modifier drugs include improved circulation, improved tissue perfusion, decreased pain, and prevention of further tissue damage. Before giving these drugs, a thorough physical assessment should be performed as well as checking of pertinent laboratory values (e.g., INR, aPTT, PT).
- Nursing care is very individualized and is based on the characteristics of the patient, thorough assessment data, existing medical conditions, and the specific drug.

1 The nurse is monitoring a patient who is receiving antithrombolytic therapy in the emergency department because of a possible MI. Which adverse effect would be of the greatest concern at this time?
a Dizziness
b Blood pressure of 130/98 mm Hg
c Slight bloody oozing from the IV insertion site
d Irregular heart rhythm

2 A patient is receiving instructions regarding warfarin therapy and asks the nurse about what medications she can take for headaches. The nurse should tell her to avoid which type of medication?
a Opioids
b Acetaminophen (Tylenol)
c NSAIDs
d There are no restrictions while taking warfarin.

3 The nurse is teaching a patient about self-administration of enoxaparin (Lovenox). Which statement should be included in this teaching session?
a "We will need to teach a family member how to give this drug in your arm."
b "This drug is given in the folds of your abdomen, but at least 2 inches away from your navel."
c "This drug needs to be taken at the same time every day with a full glass of water."
d "Be sure to massage the injection site thoroughly after giving the drug."

4 A patient is receiving heparin therapy as part of the treatment for a pulmonary embolism. The nurse monitors the results of which laboratory test to check the drug's effectiveness?
a PT-INR
b aPTT
c Vitamin K levels
d Platelet counts

5 A patient has received a double dose of heparin during surgery and is bleeding through the incision site. While the surgeons are working to stop the bleeding at the incision site, the nurse will prepare to take what action at this time?
a Give IV vitamin K as an antidote
b Give IV protamine sulfate as an antidote
c Call the blood bank for an immediate platelet transfusion
d Obtain an order for packed red blood cells

6 A patient is starting warfarin (Coumadin) therapy as part of treatment for atrial fibrillation. The nurse will follow which principles of warfarin therapy? (Select all that apply.)
a Teach proper subcutaneous administration
b Administer the oral dose at the same time every day
c Assess carefully for excessive bruising or unusual bleeding
d Monitor laboratory results for a target INR of 2 to 3
e Monitor laboratory results for a therapeutic aPTT value of 1.5 to 2.5 times the control value

1 After a patient undergoes total hip replacement, the nurse reviews the new postoperative orders and notes an order for enoxaparin (Lovenox) 30 mg subcutaneously twice a day. When assessing the patient before administering the drug, the nurse sees that the patient has an epidural catheter for administration of pain medication. What is the nurse's best action regarding the administration of the enoxaparin?

2 A patient is going home and will be taking warfarin (Coumadin). While discussing his medications just before his discharge to home, the patient says, "I want to get back to taking my vita-mins with gingko. They really help my memory." What is the nurse's best reply to this patient?

3 A patient who has been receiving a heparin infusion for DVT has a new order for warfarin (Coumadin). When the nurse explains that the warfarin is another drug to prevent blood clot formation, the patient asks if it is safe to be taking "two blood thinners at the same time." What is the nurse's best response to this patient's question?

For answers, see *http://evolve.elsevier.com/Lilley*.

CHAPTER 29

Antilipemic Drugs

OBJECTIVES

When you reach the end of this chapter, you should be able to do the following:

1 Explain the pathology of primary and secondary hyperlipidemia, including causes and risk factors.
2 Discuss the different types of lipoproteins and their role in cardiovascular diseases and in hyperlipidemia.
3 List the overall drug classes and specific drugs that are used to treat hyperlipidemia.
4 Compare the various drugs used to treat hyperlipidemia with regard to the rationale for treatment, indications, mechanisms of action, dosages, routes of administration, adverse effects, toxicity, cautions, contraindications, and associated drug interactions.
5 Develop a nursing care plan that includes all phases of the nursing process for patients receiving antilipemic drugs.

e-Learning Activities

NCLEX Review Questions • Animations • Nursing Care Plans • Audio Glossary • Category Catchers • Medication Errors Checklists • IV Therapy Checklists • Calculators • Frequently Asked Questions • Content Updates • Supplemental Resources • Answers to Case Studies and Critical Thinking Activities

Drug Profiles

♦ atorvastatin, p. 461
♦ cholestyramine, p. 462
   ezetimibe, p. 464
   gemfibrozil, p. 464
♦ niacin, p. 463

    ♦ *Key drug.*

Glossary

Antilipemic A drug that reduces lipid levels. (p. 455)
Apolipoproteins The protein components of lipoproteins. (p. 456)
Cholesterol A fat-soluble crystalline steroid alcohol found in animal fats and oils and egg yolk and widely distributed in the body, especially in the bile, blood, brain tissue, liver, kidneys, adrenal glands, and myelin sheaths of nerve fibers. (p. 455)
Chylomicrons Minute droplets of lipoproteins; the forms in which dietary fats are absorbed from the small intestine. Chylomicrons consist of about 90% triglycerides and small amounts of cholesterol, phospholipids, and proteins. (p. 456)
Exogenous lipids Lipids originating outside the body or an organ (e.g., dietary fats) or produced as the result of external factors, such as a disease caused by a bacterial or viral agent foreign to the body. (p. 456)
Foam cells The characteristic initial lesion of atherosclerosis, also known as a *fatty streak*. (p. 457)
Hydroxymethylglutaryl–coenzyme A (HMG–CoA) reductase inhibitors A class of cholesterol-lowering drugs that work by inhibiting the rate-limiting step in cholesterol synthesis; also commonly referred to as *statins*. (p. 459)

Hypercholesterolemia A condition in which higher than normal amounts of cholesterol are present in the blood. High levels of cholesterol and other lipids may lead to the development of atherosclerosis and serious illnesses such as coronary heart disease. (p. 456)
Lipoprotein A conjugated protein in which lipids form an integral part of the molecule. Lipoproteins are synthesized primarily in the liver; contain varying amounts of triglycerides, cholesterol, phospholipids, and protein; and are classified according to their composition and density. (p. 456)
Statins A class of cholesterol-lowering drugs that are more formally known as *HMG–CoA reductase inhibitors*. (p. 459)
Triglycerides Compounds consisting of fatty acids and a type of alcohol known as *glycerol*. Triglycerides make up most animal and vegetable fats and are the principal lipids in the blood, where they circulate bound to a protein, forming high-density and low-density lipoproteins (HDLs and LDLs). (p. 455)

• • •

Anatomy, Physiology, and Disease Overview

An understanding of **antilipemic** drugs begins with an understanding of how **cholesterol** and **triglycerides** are transported and used in the human body and how lipoproteins, apolipoproteins, receptors, and enzyme systems are involved in these processes. Also essential is a comprehension of the basic mechanisms underlying lipid abnormalities and the link between hyperlipidemia and coronary heart disease (CHD). Armed with this knowledge, the clinician can develop and implement a rational approach to treatment using both nonpharmacologic and pharmacologic interventions. Some patients also use dietary supplements for control of hyperlipidemia (see the Herbal Therapies and Dietary Supplements boxes on p. 456).

LIPIDS AND LIPID ABNORMALITIES

Primary Forms of Lipids

Triglycerides and cholesterol are the two primary forms of lipids in the blood. Triglycerides function as an energy source and are stored in adipose (fat) tissue. Cholesterol is primarily used to make steroid hormones, cell membranes, and bile acids. Triglycerides and cholesterol are both water-insoluble fats that must be bound to specialized lipid-carrying proteins called **apolipoproteins.** This combination of triglycerides and cholesterol with an apolipoprotein is referred to as a **lipoprotein.** Lipoproteins transport lipids via the blood. There are various types of lipoproteins, and they are classified according to their density and the type of apolipoproteins they contain. These various types of lipoproteins and their classifications are presented in Table 29-1.

Cholesterol Homeostasis

There is a complex array of biochemical factors and reactions that are all part of physiologic (normal) cholesterol homeostasis. Figure 29-1 summarizes the major concepts that are described. Fats are taken into the body through the diet and are broken down in the small intestine to form triglycerides. These triglycerides are in turn incorporated into **chylomicrons** in the cells of the intestinal wall, which are then absorbed into the lymphatic system. The primary purpose of chylomicrons is to transport lipids obtained from dietary sources (**exogenous lipids**) from the intestines to the liver to be used to make steroid hormones, lipid structural components for peripheral body cells, and bile acids.

The liver is the major organ where lipid metabolism occurs. The liver produces very-low-density lipoprotein (VLDL) from both endogenous and exogenous sources. The major role of VLDL is the transport of endogenous lipids to peripheral cells. Once VLDL is circulating, it is enzymatically cleaved by lipoprotein lipase and loses triglycerides. This creates intermediate-

TABLE 29-1   Lipoprotein Classification

Lipid Content	Lipoprotein Classification	Protein Content
Most	Chylomicron	Least
	VLDL	
↓	LDL	↑
	IDL	
Least	HDL	Most

HDL, High-density lipoprotein; *IDL,* intermediate-density lipoprotein; *LDL,* low-density lipoprotein; *VLDL,* very-low-density lipoprotein.

density lipoprotein (IDL), which is soon also cleaved by lipoprotein lipase to create low-density lipoprotein (LDL). Cholesterol is almost all that is left in LDL after this process. Any tissues that require LDL, such as endocrine cells, possess LDL receptors. LDL and about half of IDL are reabsorbed from the circulation into the liver by means of LDL receptors on the liver.

High-density lipoprotein (HDL) is produced in the liver and intestines and is also formed when chylomicrons are broken down. Lipids that are not used by peripheral cells are transferred as cholesterol esters to HDL. HDL then transfers the cholesterol esters to IDL to be returned to the liver. HDL is responsible for the "recycling" of cholesterol. HDL is sometimes referred to as the *good lipid* (or *good cholesterol*) because it is believed to be cardioprotective.

If the liver has an excess amount of cholesterol, the number of LDL receptors on the liver decreases, which results in an accumulation of LDL in the blood. One explanation for **hypercholesterolemia** (cholesterol in the blood), therefore, is this downregulation (reduced production) of hepatic LDL receptors. A major function of the liver is to manufacture cholesterol, a process that requires acetyl coenzyme A (CoA) reductase. Inhibition of this enzyme thus results in decreased cholesterol production by the liver.

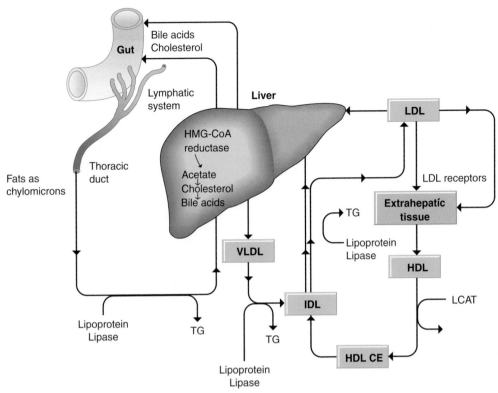

FIGURE 29-1 Cholesterol homeostasis. *CE,* Cholesterol ester; *HDL,* high-density lipoprotein; *HMG-CoA,* hydroxymethylglutaryl-coenzyme A; *IDL,* intermediate-density lipoprotein; *LCAT,* lecithin cholesterol acetyltransferase; *LDL,* low-density lipoprotein; *TG,* triglyceride; *VLDL,* very-low-density lipoprotein.

ATHEROSCLEROTIC PLAQUE FORMATION

Fundamental to the study of hyperlipidemia is an understanding of the processes by which lipids and lipoproteins participate in the formation of atherosclerotic plaque and subsequently the development of CHD. When the serum cholesterol levels are elevated, circulating monocytes adhere to the smooth endothelial surfaces of the coronary vasculature. These monocytes burrow into the next layer of the blood vessel (subendothelial tissue) and change into macrophage cells, which then take up cholesterol from circulating lipoproteins until they become filled with fat. Soon they become what are known as **foam cells,** the characteristic precursor lesion of atherosclerosis, also known as a *fatty streak.* Once this process is established, it is usually present throughout the coronary and systemic circulation.

LINK BETWEEN CHOLESTEROL AND CORONARY HEART DISEASE

Numerous epidemiologic trials have shown that as blood cholesterol levels increase in the members of a population, the incidence of death and disability related to CHD also increases. The risk for CHD in patients with cholesterol levels of 300 mg/dL is three to four times greater than that in patients with levels of less than 200 mg/dL. The incidence of CHD in premenopausal women. This is thought to be secondary to the effects of estrogen, because the risk for CHD climbs considerably in postmenopausal women. There has been emerging controversy, however, regarding this longstanding belief, because two recent trials of estrogen replacement therapy (ERT) did not demonstrate prevention of cardiovascular events in women receiving ERT. Other experimental studies that looked for any benefits of low-dose estrogen therapy in *male* patients also failed to demonstrate significant cardioprotective efficacy.

Statistics show that half of all Americans, both male and female, will die of a heart attack. Thus the thrust of treatment is two-pronged: primary prevention of cardiac events in patients with risk factors and secondary prevention of subsequent cardiac events in individuals who have previously experienced a cardiac event (e.g., myocardial infarction). The benefits of cholesterol reduction for primary prevention have been illustrated in a number of recent trials. Results of some of the larger and more recent investigations support the view that, in patients with known risk factors for CHD, therapy with an antilipemic drug can reduce the occurrence of CHD. First-time heart attack and death caused by heart disease can be reduced with drug therapy.

The benefits of cholesterol reduction for secondary prevention have been illustrated in a variety of recent trials as well. In patients with documented CHD, treatment with a cholesterol-lowering drug has many positive outcomes. Three of these are decreased coronary events, regression of coronary atherosclerotic lesions, and prolonged survival.

Measures taken early in a person's life to reduce and maintain cholesterol levels in a desirable range should have a dramatic effect in terms of preventing CHD and the death and disability it causes. These include lifestyle modifications related to diet,

BOX 29-1 Coronary Heart Disease: Risk Factors

Positive Risk Factors
- Age: Males: 45 years or older
- Family history: History of premature CHD (e.g., MI or sudden death before age 55 years in father or other male first-degree relative, or before age 65 years in mother or other female first-degree relative)
- Current cigarette smoking
- Hypertension: blood pressure higher than 140/90 mm Hg or current antihypertensive drug therapy
- Low HDL cholesterol level: lower than 40 mg/dL
- Diabetes mellitus

Negative Risk Factor
- High HDL cholesterol: 60 mg/dL or higher—if the HDL cholesterol is 60 mg/dL or higher, subtract one risk factor

CHD, Coronary heart disease; *HDL,* high-density lipoprotein; *MI,* myocardial infarction.

weight, and activity level. Diets lower in saturated fat and higher in fiber and plant chemicals known as sterols and stanols, and possibly the substitution of soy-based proteins for animal proteins, appear to promote healthier lipid profiles. These are among the dietary recommendations made in 2001 by the National Cholesterol Education Program (NECP) Adult Treatment Panel III (ATP III) of the National Institutes of Health. The consumption of fatty fish or dietary supplements containing omega-3 fatty acids appears to have beneficial effects on triglyceride and HDL levels and is currently recommended by the American Heart Association (AHA). The AHA also strongly emphasizes the substantial therapeutic benefits of even modest weight reduction and exercise in both improvement of lipid profiles and reduction of the likelihood of heart disease.

HYPERLIPIDEMIAS AND TREATMENT GUIDELINES

The decision to prescribe hyperlipemic drugs as an adjunct to dietary therapy in patients with an elevated cholesterol level should be based on the patient's clinical profile. This includes the patient's age, sex, menopausal status for women, family history, and response to dietary treatment, as well as the presence of risk factors (other than hyperlipidemia) for premature CHD and the cause, duration, and phenotypic pattern of the patient's hyperlipidemia.

A major source of guidance for antilipemic treatment at the disposal of health care professionals in the United States has been the NCEP, which has been developed in close cooperation with major professional organizations such as the AHA. This program has two main thrusts, both aimed at reducing the total risk for CHD in the population of the United States. One is focused on the entire population and consists of general guidelines for the prevention of CHD. It emphasizes the appropriate dietary intake of total cholesterol and saturated fat, weight control, physical activity, and the control of other lifestyle risk factors. The other focus is on the management of individual patients who

are at increased risk for CHD. The original guidelines for the detection, evaluation, and treatment of high serum cholesterol levels in adults were published in 1988 and 2001. They were updated again in July 2004. In these guidelines, the selection of dietary and drug therapy options is determined by the presence of certain risk factors. The latest guidelines are the first to include CHD risk equivalents. CHD risk equivalents have been statistically calculated to equate a person's 10-year risk for a major coronary event (e.g., myocardial infarction) for those patients who do not currently have CHD, but may have other diseases such as diabetes. These risk factors and risk equivalents are listed in Box 29-1.

When the decision to institute drug therapy has been made, the choice of drug should then be determined by the specific lipid profile of the patient. Five patterns or phenotypes of hyperlipidemia have been identified, and these are defined by the plasma (serum) concentrations of total cholesterol, triglycerides, and lipoprotein fractions (HDL, LDL, IDL, VLDL). These various types of hyperlipidemia are listed in Table 29-2. The process of characterizing a patient's specific lipid profile in this way is referred to as *phenotyping*.

One of the basic tenets of the NCEP guidelines is that all reasonable nonpharmaceutical means of controlling the blood cholesterol level (e.g., diet, exercise) should be tried for at least 6 months and found to fail before drug therapy is considered. Because the drug treatment for hyperlipidemias entails a long-term commitment to the therapy, factors that should be considered before the initiation of therapy are the type and magnitude of dyslipidemia, the age and lifestyle of the patient, the relative indications and contraindications of different drugs and drug categories for a given patient, potential drug interactions, adverse effects, and the overall cost of therapy. The 2004 updated NCEP guidelines recommend that all patients with LDL cholesterol levels exceeding 190 mg/dL and those with LDL cholesterol levels between 160 and 190 mg/dL who have CHD or two or more risk factors for heart disease be considered for drug therapy after an adequate trial of dietary and other nondrug therapies has proved ineffective. The treatment decisions that should be made based on the LDL cholesterol levels are listed in Table 29-3. The

TABLE 29-2 Types of Hyperlipidemias

Phenotype	Lipoprotein Elevated	Lipid Composition	
		Cholesterol (mg/dL)	Triglyceride
I	Chylomicrons	Greater than or equal to 300	Greater than 3000
IIa	LDL	Greater than 300	Normal $\cong$ 148
IIb	LDL, VLDL	Greater than 300	Normal $\cong$ 148
III	IDL	Greater than 400	Greater than 600 (1-3$\times$ higher than cholesterol)
IV	VLDL	Normal or mildly elevated approximately equal to 250	Greater than 400
V	VLDL, chylomicrons	Greater than 300	Greater than 2000

$\cong$, Approximately equal to; *IDL,* intermediate-density lipoprotein; *LDL,* low-density lipoprotein; *VLDL,* very-low-density lipoprotein.

TABLE 29-3 Treatment Decisions Based on LDL Cholesterol Level

Patient Category	Initiation Level	LDL Goal
Dietary Therapy		
Without CHD and with less than 2 risk factors (low risk)	Greater than or equal to 160 mg/dL (4.1 mmol/L)	Less than 160 mg/dL (4.1 mmol/L)
Without CHD and with greater than or equal to 2 risk factors (moderately high risk)	Greater than or equal to 130 mg/dL (3.4 mmol/L)	Less than 130 mg/dL (3.4 mmol/L)
With CHD (high or very high risk)	Greater than or equal to 100 mg/dL (2.6 mmol/L)	Less than 100 mg/dL (2.6 mmol/L)
Drug Therapy		
Without CHD and with less than 2 risk factors (low risk)	Greater than or equal to 190 mg/dL (4.9 mmol/L)	Less than 160 mg/dL (4.1 mmol/L)
Without CHD and with greater than or equal to 2 risk factors (moderately high risk)	Greater than or equal to 160 mg/dL (4.1 mmol/L)	Less than 130 mg/dL (3.4 mmol/L)
With CHD (high or very high risk)	Greater than or equal to 130 mg/dL (3.4 mmol/L)	Less than 100 mg/dL (2.6 mmol/L)

CHD, Coronary heart disease; *LDL,* low-density lipoprotein.

BOX 29-2 Identifying Features of the Metabolic Syndrome

- Waist circumference greater than 40 inches in men or 30 inches in women
- Serum triglyceride level of 150 mg/dL or more
- High-density lipoprotein cholesterol level of less than 40 mg/dL in men or less than 50 mg/dL in women
- Blood pressure of 130/85 mm Hg or higher
- Fasting serum glucose level higher than 110 mg/dL

fibric acid derivatives (fibrates). In addition to all of these drugs, the new drug *ezetimibe (Zetia)* is now available that is a cholesterol absorption inhibitor. In many cases, patient outcomes are improved when various combinations of these drugs are used. One of the newest examples of this is the combination tablet Vytorin, which contains both the statin drug atorvastatin and ezetimibe.

▌Pharmacology Overview

HYDROXYMETHYLGLUTARYL–COENZYME A REDUCTASE INHIBITORS

The rate-limiting enzyme in cholesterol synthesis is known as HMG–CoA reductase. The class of medications that competitively inhibit this enzyme, called the **hydroxymethylglutaryl–coenzyme A (HMG–CoA) reductase inhibitors,** are the most potent of the drugs available for reducing plasma concentrations of LDL cholesterol. Lovastatin was the first drug in this class to be approved for use, which occurred in 1987. Since that time, five other HMG–CoA reductase inhibitors have become available on the U.S. market: pravastatin, simvastatin, atorvastatin, fluvastatin, and rosuvastatin. Because of the shared suffix of their generic names, these drugs are often collectively referred to as *statins.* When these drugs are taken, lipid levels may not be lowered to their maximum extent until 6 to 8 weeks after the start of therapy. Few direct comparisons of the statins have been reported in the literature. The following doses of drugs are considered to be "therapeutically equivalent," meaning they produce the same therapeutic effect: simvastatin 10 mg; pravastatin 20 mg; lovastatin 20 mg, atorvastatin 10 mg, fluvastatin 40 mg, and rosuvastatin 5 mg.

updated guidelines even recommend optional use of drug therapy to reduce LDL to less than 70 mg/dL in patients at very high risk and to less than 100 mg/dL in patients at moderately high risk. "Very high risk" patients include those with active cardiovascular disease with other major risk factors such as diabetes, continued smoking, or *metabolic syndrome.* Metabolic syndrome is a set of risk factors associated with obesity, including hypertriglyceridemia and low HDL level. "Moderately high risk" patients include those without cardiovascular disease but with two or more risk factors. Box 29-2 lists the identifying features of patients with metabolic syndrome.

There are currently four established classes of drugs used to treat dyslipidemia: hydroxymethylglutaryl–coenzyme A (HMG–CoA) reductase inhibitors **(statins),** bile acid sequestrants, the B vitamin niacin (vitamin B$_3$, also known as *nicotinic acid*), and the

Mechanism of Action and Drug Effects

Statins lower the blood cholesterol level by decreasing the rate of cholesterol production. The liver requires HMG–CoA reductase to produce cholesterol. It is the rate-limiting enzyme in the reactions needed to make cholesterol. The statins inhibit this enzyme, thereby decreasing cholesterol production. When less cholesterol is produced, the liver increases the number of LDL receptors to augment the recycling of LDL from the circulation back into the liver, where it is needed for the synthesis of other required substances such as steroids, bile acids, and cell membranes. Lovastatin and simvastatin are administered as inactive drugs or prodrugs that must be biotransformed into their active metabolites in the liver. In contrast, pravastatin is administered in its active form.

Indications

The statins are still recommended by the latest NCEP ATP III guidelines as first-line drug therapy for hypercholesterolemia (especially elevated levels of LDL cholesterol), the most common and dangerous form of dyslipidemia. More specifically, they are indicated for the treatment of type IIa and IIb hyperlipidemia and have been shown to reduce the plasma concentrations of LDL cholesterol by 30% to 40%. Their cholesterol-lowering properties are dose dependent; that is, the larger the dose, the greater the cholesterol-lowering effects. A 10% to 30% decrease in the concentrations of plasma triglycerides has also been observed in patients receiving any of these drugs. Another very important therapeutic effect of the statins is an overall tendency for the HDL cholesterol level to increase by 2% to 15%, a known beneficial factor that reduces risk (i.e., a negative risk factor) for cardiovascular disease.

These drugs appear to be equally effective in their ability to reduce LDL cholesterol concentrations. However, simvastatin and atorvastatin are more potent on a milligram basis. Atorvastatin appears to be more effective in lowering triglyceride levels than other HMG–CoA reductase inhibitors. Combined drug therapy with more than one class of antilipemic drug may be necessary for desired results, and the statins are often combined with niacin or fibrates for this purpose, though this combination can increase the risk of adverse drug effects (see Adverse Effects).

Contraindications

Contraindications to the use of HMG–CoA reductase inhibitors (statins) include known drug allergy and pregnancy. Other contraindications may include liver disease or elevation of liver enzyme levels.

Adverse Effects

Generally speaking, the HMG–CoA reductase inhibitors available for clinical use have proved to be well tolerated, and significant adverse effects are fairly uncommon. Mild, transient gastrointestinal disturbances, rash, and headache have been the most common problems. These and other less common adverse effects are listed in Table 29-4. Elevations in liver enzyme levels may also occur, and the patient should be monitored for excessive elevations, which may indicate the need for alternative drug therapy. Dose-dependent elevations in liver enzyme levels to

TABLE 29-4 HMG-CoA Reductase Inhibitors: Adverse Effects

Body System	Adverse Effects
Central nervous	Headache, dizziness, blurred vision, fatigue, nightmares, insomnia
Gastrointestinal	Constipation, diarrhea, nausea, changes in bowel function
Other	Myalgias, skin rashes

HMG-CoA, Hydroxymethylglutaryl–coenzyme A.

values of more than three times the upper limit of normal have been noted in 0.4% to 1.9% of patients taking HMG–CoA reductase inhibitors. Serum creatine phosphokinase concentrations may be increased to more than 10 times the normal level in patients receiving these drugs. Most of these patients have remained asymptomatic, however.

A less common but still clinically important adverse effect is myopathy (muscle pain), which may progress to a serious condition known as *rhabdomyolysis*. Rhabdomyolysis is the breakdown of muscle protein accompanied by myoglobinuria, which is the urinary elimination of the muscle protein myoglobin, the oxygen-carrying pigment of muscle tissue that is similar to a single subunit of hemoglobin. This abnormal urinary excretion of protein can place a severe strain on the kidneys, possibly leading to acute renal failure and even death. This myopathy is uncommon during monotherapy with statins. It appears to be dose dependent and is more common in patients receiving a statin in combination with cyclosporine, niacin, gemfibrozil (a fibrate), or erythromycin. Patients receiving statin therapy should be advised to immediately report to the prescriber any unexplained muscular pain or discomfort. When recognized reasonably early, rhabdomyolysis is usually reversible with discontinuation of the statin drug. In June 2004, the U.S. Food and Drug Administration (FDA) published a public health advisory summarizing recent reports of myopathy and rhabdomyolysis cases associated with the use of rosuvastatin (Crestor), one of the newer statin drugs. The manufacturer of this drug altered its labeling for the drug, listing risk factors for myopathy symptoms. These include age older than 65 years, hypothyroidism, renal insufficiency, and concurrent use of the immunosuppressant drug cyclosporine or the antihyperlipidemic drug gemfibrozil. The FDA also required the manufacturer to make a 5-mg tablet available for those patients with significant risk factors for drug toxicity, with a maximum recommended daily dose of 10 mg for these patients. In March 2005, the FDA published a second public health advisory regarding reports of both myopathy and renal failure associated with the use of rosuvastatin as well as other statin drugs. Although these adverse effects are relatively uncommon, and although much benefit is often derived from the use of statin drugs, prescribers are advised to use minimal effective doses, with regular laboratory blood monitoring of liver and kidney function (every 3 to 6 months). Patients should also be educated regarding these serious, although uncommon, adverse drug ef-

DOSAGES

Selected Antilipemic Drugs

Drug (Pregnancy Category)	Pharmacologic Class	Usual Dosage Range	Indications
◆ atorvastatin (Lipitor) (X)	HMG–CoA reductase inhibitor	**Adult** PO: 10-80 mg/day	
◆ cholestyramine (Questran) (C)	Bile acid sequestrant	**Adult** PO: Powder, 9 g 1-6×/day	
ezetimibe (Zetia) (C)	Cholesterol absorption inhibitor	**Adult** PO: 10 mg 1×/day	Hyperlipidemia
gemfibrozil (Lopid) (C)	Fibric acid derivative	**Adult** PO: 600 mg bid 30 min ac in AM and PM	
◆ niacin (nicotinic acid, vitamin B$_3$) (A; C if dose exceeds RDA)	B vitamin	**Adult** PO: 1.5 to 6 gm/day in 2-4 divided doses.	

HMG–CoA, Hydroxymethylglutaryl–coenzyme A; *PO,* oral; *RDA,* recommended daily allowance.

fects and instructed to immediately report any signs of toxicity, including muscle soreness, changes in urine color, fever, malaise, nausea, or vomiting.

Toxicity and Management of Overdose

Very limited data are available on the nature of toxicity and overdose in patients taking HMG–CoA reductase inhibitors. Treatment, if needed, is supportive and based on presenting symptoms.

Interactions

HMG–CoA reductase inhibitors should be used cautiously in patients taking oral anticoagulants. In addition, the coadministration of the statins with drugs in other antilipemic classes (such as gemfibrozil), oral antidiabetic drugs, erythromycin, insulin, niacin, amiodarone, and even grapefruit juice has been observed in rare cases to lead to the development of rhabdomyolysis. Patients are advised to limit grapefruit juice to less than 1 quart daily, which is probably more than most people drink. The mechanism for most significant drug interactions involves inhibition of the metabolic protein *cytochrome P-450* enzyme 3A4 (CYP3A4). The following example involving grapefruit juice illustrates the interaction. Components in grapefruit juice inactivate CYP3A4 in both the liver and intestines. This enzyme plays a key role in statin metabolism. The presence of grapefruit juice in the body may therefore result in sustained levels of unmetabolized statin drug, which increases the risk for major drug toxicity (e.g., rhabdomyolysis). Pravastatin and fluvastatin inhibit CYP3A4 to a much smaller degree than the other statins, whereas lovastatin and simvastatin are the most potent inhibitors of this enzyme.

Laboratory Test Interactions

Laboratory interactions that can occur include increases in ALT levels and activated clotting time, thrombocytopenia, and transient eosinophilia.

Dosages

For dosage information on atorvastatin, see the following drug profile and the Dosages table above.

DRUG PROFILE

The HMG–CoA reductase inhibitors, or statins, are all potent inhibitors of the enzyme that catalyzes the rate-limiting step in the synthesis of cholesterol. Six statins are currently on the market in the United States: atorvastatin (Lipitor), fluvastatin (Lescol), lovastatin (Mevacor), pravastatin (Pravachol), simvastatin (Zocor), and rosuvastatin (Crestor). There are some minor differences between drugs in this class of antilipemics; the most dramatic difference is that of potency. All six medications are prescription-only drugs and are contraindicated in those with active liver dysfunction or elevated serum transaminase levels of unknown cause. They are pregnancy category X drugs and should be avoided during pregnancy and lactation. There is little evidence to recommend one drug over another, except that fluvastatin may be somewhat less effective than the others.

◆ atorvastatin

Atorvastatin (Lipitor) has become the most commonly used drug in this class of cholesterol-lowering drugs. It is used primarily to lower total and LDL cholesterol levels as well as levels of triglycerides. Atorvastatin has also been shown to raise levels of "good" cholesterol, the HDL component. All statins are generally dosed once daily, usually with the evening meal or at bedtime. One particular advantage of atorvastatin is that it can be dosed at any time of day. However, bedtime dosing provides peak drug levels in a time frame that correlates better with the natural *diurnal* (daytime) rhythm of cholesterol production in the body. The recommended dosage for atorvastatin is 10 to 80 mg daily. It is available only in tablet form in strengths of 10, 20, 40, and 80 mg. Pregnancy category X.

PHARMACOKINETICS

Route	Onset of Action	Peak Plasma Concentration	Elimination Half-life	Duration of Action
PO	0.5 hr	1-2 hr	7-14 hr	Unknown

BILE ACID SEQUESTRANTS

Bile acid sequestrants, also called *bile acid–binding resins* and *ion-exchange resins,* include cholestyramine, colestipol, and colesevelam. The first two of these drugs have been used widely for more than 20 years and have been evaluated extensively in well-controlled clinical trials. They have proven efficacy, but their powdered forms are somewhat messy to use. Colestipol is also available in tablet form. Colesevelam is a newer drug with a similar mechanism of action but is available only in tablet form. These drugs are now considered second-line drugs in most cases, less preferred than the more potent *statins*. However, they are still a suitable alternative in patients intolerant of the statins. Generally these drugs lower the plasma concentrations of LDL cholesterol by 15% to 30%. They also increase the HDL cholesterol level by 3% to 8% and increase hepatic triglyceride and VLDL production, which may result in a 10% to 50% increase in the triglyceride level.

Mechanism of Action and Drug Effects

Bile acid sequestrants bind bile, preventing the resorption of the bile acids from the small intestine. Instead, an insoluble bile acid and resin (drug) complex is excreted in the bowel movement. Bile acids are necessary for the absorption of cholesterol from the small intestine and are also synthesized from cholesterol by the liver. This is one natural way that the liver excretes cholesterol from the body. The more that bile acids are excreted in the feces, the more the liver converts cholesterol to bile acids. This reduces the level of cholesterol in the liver and thus in the circulation as well. The liver then attempts to compensate for the loss of cholesterol by increasing the number of LDL receptors on its surface. Circulating LDL molecules bind to these receptors to be taken up into the liver, which also has the benefit of reducing circulating LDL in the bloodstream.

Indications

Bile acid sequestrants may be used as primary or adjunct drug therapy in the management of type II hyperlipoproteinemia. One common strategy is to use them along with statins for an additive drug effect in reducing LDL cholesterol levels. In addition, cholestyramine is used to relieve the pruritus associated with partial biliary obstruction. The newest drug in this class, colesevelam, may be better tolerated by higher risk patients who are intolerant of other antihyperlipemic therapy, including organ transplant recipients and those with serious liver or kidney disease.

Contraindications

Contraindications to the use of bile acid sequestrants include known drug allergy, biliary or bowel obstruction, and phenylketonuria (PKU).

Adverse Effects

The adverse effects of colestipol, cholestyramine, and colesevelam are similar; however, colesevelam is reported to have fewer gastrointestinal adverse effects and drug interactions. Constipation is a common problem and may be accompanied by heartburn, nausea, belching, and bloating. These adverse effects tend to disappear over time, however. Many patients require extra education and support to help them deal with the gastrointestinal effects and comply with the medication regimen. It is important that therapy be initiated with low dosages and that patients be instructed to take the drugs with meals to reduce the adverse effects. Increasing dietary fiber intake or taking a fiber supplement such as psyllium (Metamucil and others), as well as increasing fluid intake, may relieve constipation and bloating. These drugs

TABLE 29-5 Bile Acid Sequestrants: Adverse Effects

Body System	Adverse Effects
Gastrointestinal	Constipation, heartburn, nausea, belching, bloating
Other	Bleeding, headache, tinnitus, burnt odor of urine

may also cause mild increases in the triglyceride levels. The most common adverse effects of the bile acid sequestrants are listed in Table 29-5.

Toxicity and Management of Overdose

Because the bile acid sequestrants are not absorbed, an overdose can cause obstruction of the gastrointestinal tract. Therefore, treatment of an overdose involves restoring gut motility.

Interactions

The significant drug interactions associated with the use of bile acid sequestrants are limited to effects on the absorption of concurrently administered drugs. All drugs should be taken at least 1 hour before or 4 to 6 hours after the administration of bile acid sequestrants. In addition, high doses of a bile acid sequestrant decrease the absorption of fat-soluble vitamins (A, D, E, and K).

Dosages

For the recommended dosages of a selected bile acid sequestrant, see the Dosages table on p. 461.

DRUG PROFILE

The bile acid sequestrants cholestyramine, colestipol, and colesevelam are indicated for the treatment of type IIa and IIb hyperlipidemia. They lower the cholesterol level, in particular the LDL cholesterol level, by increasing the destruction of LDL. However, their use may result in increases in the VLDL cholesterol level. Because of the high incidence of gastrointestinal adverse effects in patients taking these drugs, adherence to the prescribed dosage schedules is often poor. However, educating patients about the purpose and expected adverse effects of therapy can foster improved adherence. Patients must be warned not to take bile acid sequestrants concurrently with other drugs, because the drug interactions can be very pronounced. Other drugs must be taken at other times of the day. This requirement cannot be overemphasized.

♦ **cholestyramine**

Cholestyramine (Questran) is a prescription-only drug that is contraindicated in patients with a known hypersensitivity to it and in those who have complete biliary obstruction or PKU. It may interfere with distribution of the proper amounts of fat-soluble vitamins to the fetus or nursing infant of a pregnant or nursing woman taking the drug. Cholestyramine is now being used for its constipating effect, often given as needed for loose bowel movements.

NIACIN

Niacin, or nicotinic acid, is not only a very unique lipid-lowering drug, it is also a vitamin. For its unique lipid-lowering properties to be realized, much larger doses of the drug are required than are commonly given when it is used as a vitamin. Niacin is a

B vitamin, specifically vitamin B_3. It is an effective and inexpensive medication that exerts favorable effects on the plasma concentrations of all lipoproteins. Niacin is often given in combination with other antilipemic drugs to enhance the lipid-lowering effects.

Mechanism of Action and Drug Effects

Although the exact mechanism of action of niacin is unknown, the beneficial effects are believed to be related to its ability to inhibit lipolysis in adipose tissue, decrease esterification of triglycerides in the liver, and increase the activity of lipoprotein lipase. The drug effects of niacin are primarily limited to reduction of the metabolism or catabolism of cholesterol and triglycerides. Niacin decreases the LDL levels moderately (10% to 20%), decreases the triglyceride levels (30% to 70%), and increases the HDL levels moderately (20% to 35%). Niacin is also a vitamin needed for many bodily processes. In large doses, it may produce vasodilatation that is limited to the cutaneous vessels. This effect seems to be induced by prostaglandins. Niacin also causes the release of histamine, which results in an increase in gastric motility and acid secretion. Niacin may also stimulate the fibrinolytic system to break down fibrin clots.

Indications

Niacin has been shown to be effective in lowering lipid levels, including triglyceride, total serum cholesterol, and LDL cholesterol levels. It also brings about an increase in the HDL cholesterol levels. Niacin may also lower the levels of lipoprotein (a), except in patients with severe hypertriglyceridemia. It has been shown to be effective in the treatment of type IIa, IIb, III, IV, and V hyperlipidemia. Niacin's effects on triglyceride levels begin to be noticed after 1 to 4 days of therapy, with the maximum effects seen after 3 to 5 weeks of continuous therapy.

Contraindications

Contraindications to the use of niacin include known drug allergy and may include liver disease, hypertension, peptic ulcer, and the presence of any active hemorrhagic process.

Adverse Effects

Niacin can cause flushing, pruritus, and gastrointestinal distress. Small doses of aspirin or nonsteroidal antiinflammatory drugs (NSAIDs) may be taken 30 minutes before the niacin dose to minimize the cutaneous flushing. These undesirable effects can also be minimized by starting patients on a low initial dosage and increasing it gradually, and by having patients take the drug with meals. The most common adverse effects associated with niacin therapy are listed in Table 29-6.

Interactions

The major drug interactions associated with niacin are minimal. One interaction of note: when niacin is taken with an HMG–CoA reductase inhibitor, the likelihood of myopathy development is greatly increased, although it is not uncommon to see these drugs used together.

Dosages

For dosage information on niacin, see the following drug profile for this drug and the Dosages table on p. 461.

TABLE 29-6 Niacin (Nicotinic Acid): Adverse Effects

Body System	Adverse Effects
Gastrointestinal	Abdominal discomfort, gastrointestinal distress
Integumentary	Cutaneous flushing, pruritus, hyperpigmentation
Other	Blurred vision, glucose intolerance, hyperuricemia, hepatotoxicity

---

DRUG PROFILE

◆ niacin

Used alone or in combination with other lipid-lowering drugs, niacin (nicotinic acid, vitamin B_3) (Nicobid) is a very effective, inexpensive medication that, as previously mentioned, has beneficial effects on LDL cholesterol, triglyceride, and HDL cholesterol levels. Drug therapy with niacin is usually initiated at a small daily dose taken with or after meals to minimize the adverse effects previously discussed. Liver dysfunction has been observed in individuals taking sustained-release forms of niacin, but not immediate-release forms. However, newer extended-release dosage forms, which dissolve more slowly than the immediate-release forms but faster than the sustained-release forms, appear to have even better adverse effect profiles, including less hepatotoxicity and flushing of the skin. Niacin is contraindicated in patients who have shown a hypersensitivity to it; in those with peptic ulcer, hepatic disease, hemorrhage, or severe hypotension; and in lactating women. It is also not recommended for patients with gout. Niacin is available over the counter and by prescription.

PHARMACOKINETICS

Route	Onset of Action	Peak Plasma Concentration	Elimination Half-life	Duration of Action
PO	Rapid	30-60 min	45 min	Unknown

FIBRIC ACID DERIVATIVES AND CHOLESTEROL ABSORPTION INHIBITOR

Current fibric acid derivatives include gemfibrozil and fenofibrate. These drugs primarily affect the triglyceride levels but may also lower the total cholesterol and LDL cholesterol levels and raise the HDL cholesterol level. They are often collectively referred to as *fibrates*.

Mechanism of Action and Drug Effects

Fibric acid drugs are believed to work by activating lipoprotein lipase, an enzyme responsible for the breakdown of cholesterol. This enzyme usually cleaves off a triglyceride molecule from VLDL or LDL, leaving behind lipoproteins. Fibric acid derivatives can also suppress the release of free fatty acid from adipose tissue, inhibit the synthesis of triglycerides in the liver, and increase the secretion of cholesterol into bile. They have been shown to reduce triglyceride levels and serum VLDL and LDL concentrations. Independent of their lipid-lowering actions, fibric acid derivatives can also induce changes in blood coagulation. This involves a tendency toward a decrease in platelet adhesiveness. They can also increase plasma fibrinolysis, the process that causes fibrin, and therefore clots, to be broken down.

TABLE 29-7 Fibric Acid Derivatives: Adverse Effects

Body System	Adverse Effects
Gastrointestinal	Nausea, vomiting, diarrhea, gallstones
Genitourinary	Impotence, decreased urine output, hematuria, increased risk for urinary tract infections and viral infections
Other	Drowsiness, dizziness, rash, pruritus, alopecia, eczema, vertigo, headache

Indications

The fibric acid derivatives gemfibrozil and fenofibrate all decrease the triglyceride level and increase the HDL cholesterol level by as much as 25%. Both decrease the LDL concentrations in patients with type IIa and IIb hyperlipidemia but increase the LDL levels in patients with type IV and V hyperlipemia. They are indicated for the treatment of type III, IV, and V hyperlipidemia, and in some cases the type IIb form, although other classes of antilipemics are usually tried first.

Contraindications

Contraindications to the use of fibrates include known drug allergy and may include severe liver or kidney disease, cirrhosis, and gallbladder disease.

Adverse Effects

The most common adverse effects of the fibric acid derivatives as a class are abdominal discomfort, diarrhea, nausea, headache, blurred vision, increased risk for gallstones, and prolonged prothrombin time. Liver function tests may also show increased enzyme levels. The more common adverse effects are listed in Table 29-7.

Toxicity and Management of Overdose

The management of fibrate overdose, which is uncommon, is supportive care based on presenting symptoms. Gastrointestinal decontamination or use of gastric lavage may be indicated for large overdoses.

Interactions

Gemfibrozil can enhance the action of oral anticoagulants, so that careful adjustment of the dosage of these latter drugs is required. The risk for myositis, myalgias, and rhabdomyolysis is increased when either gemfibrozil or fenofibrate is given with a statin. Combining gemfibrozil with a statin is generally not recommended. Fenofibrate may also raise the blood level of ezetimibe if the two are taken concurrently.

Laboratory test interactions that can occur in patients taking gemfibrozil include a decrease in the hemoglobin level, hematocrit value, and white blood cell count. In addition, the aspartate aminotransferase level, activated clotting time, lactate dehydrogenase level, and bilirubin level can be increased.

Dosages

For the recommended dosage of gemfibrozil, see the table on p. 461.

FIBRIC ACID DERIVATIVES (FIBRATES)

The fibric acid derivatives gemfibrozil and fenofibrate are prescription-only drugs and are now the only two drugs available in this class. They are both pregnancy category C drugs and are contraindicated in patients with hypersensitivity, preexisting gallbladder disease, significant hepatic or renal dysfunction, and primary biliary cirrhosis. Both drugs decrease the triglyceride levels and increase the HDL levels by as much as 25%. They are good drugs for the treatment of mixed hyperlipidemias.

gemfibrozil

Gemfibrozil (Lopid) is a fibric acid derivative that decreases the synthesis of apolipoprotein B and lowers the VLDL level. It can also increase the HDL level. In addition, it is highly effective for lowering plasma triglyceride levels. In a landmark study reported in 1987 in the *New England Journal of Medicine,* known as the Helsinki study, the triglyceride levels of the group receiving gemfibrozil were reduced by as much as 43% compared with those in the control group. The total cholesterol and LDL cholesterol levels were reduced by 11% and 10%, respectively, and the HDL level was increased by 10%. Gemfibrozil is indicated for treatment of type IV and V hyperlipidemia, and, in some cases, the type IIb form. Specific dosing recommendations are given in the table on p. 461.

PHARMACOKINETICS

Route	Onset of Action	Peak Plasma Concentration	Elimination Half-life	Duration of Action
PO	Several days	1-2 hr	1.3-1.5 hr	Unknown

CHOLESTEROL ABSORPTION INHIBITOR
ezetimibe

Ezetimibe (Zetia) is currently the only cholesterol absorption inhibitor and was approved by the FDA in 2002. Ezetimibe has a novel mechanism of action in that it selectively inhibits absorption in the small intestine of cholesterol and related sterols. The result is a reduction in several blood lipid parameters: total cholesterol level, LDL cholesterol level, apolipoprotein B level, and level of triglycerides. However, serum levels of HDL cholesterol, the so-called good cholesterol, have been shown actually to increase with the use of ezetimibe. These beneficial effects appear to be further enhanced when ezetimibe is taken with a statin drug. Ezetimibe may be used as monotherapy. Recent studies have shown that, although the combination of ezetimibe and a statin is effective in reducing LDL, the rate of atherosclerotic progression is no different than when a statin is given alone. A large multicenter trail is currently underway that will provide further information in defining the role of ezetimibe. Until the results are available, current recommendations are to reserve ezetimibe for patients who have not responded to or are intolerant of other therapy. Ezetimibe has not been shown to interact significantly with cimetidine, warfarin, digoxin, oral contraceptives, or antacids. However, fibric acid derivatives (fibrates) have been shown to significantly increase the serum levels of ezetimibe. It is not yet known whether this is harmful, but currently, concurrent use of ezetimibe and fibrates is not recommended. The use of ezetimibe with bile acid sequestrants has been shown to reduce the serum level of ezetimibe by 55% to 80%. Concurrent use of these two types of drugs is not yet contraindicated, but it should be recognized that the extent of LDL reduction normally promoted by ezetimibe is likely to be reduced when this drug combination is used. Ezetimibe is contraindicated in cases of demonstrated allergy to the drug, or active liver disease or unexplained elevations in serum liver enzyme levels. It may be taken with or without food and, for patient convenience, may be dosed at the same time as a statin drug, if prescribed.

PHARMACOKINETICS

Route	Onset of Action	Peak Plasma Concentration	Elimination Half-life	Duration of Action
PO	Unknown	4-12 hr	22 hr	Unknown

NURSING PROCESS

Assessment

Before initiating therapy with any *antilipemic* drug, the nurse should obtain a thorough health and medication history with a listing of allergies and any prescription drugs, over-the-counter drugs, herbals, or supplements the patient is taking. It is important to assess the patient's dietary patterns, exercise program and frequency, weight, height, and vital signs, and to document these parameters—especially food intake—over time, such as for several weeks. Also, the patient's use of tobacco, alcohol, and/or social drugs, along with information about frequency, amount, and duration of use, should be documented. Some of the lipid disorders are hereditary, and therefore a thorough assessment of the family history is required. Some positive risk factors for CHD for which the patient should be assessed are the following:

- Age (male 45 years of age or older; female 55 years of age or older)
- Smoking
- HDL levels of 29 mg/dL or less
- Diabetes mellitus
- Family history of premature CHD

Assessment to identify any cautions, contraindications, and potential drug interactions should be performed before initiating use of any of the antilipemics. Serum lipid values and lipoprotein levels also need to be assessed. The following are the normal ranges: (1) lipids—cholesterol level less than or equal to 200 mg/dL, (2) triglyceride level less than 150 mg/dL, and (3) lipoproteins— low density lipoprotein cholesterol levels (LDL) less than 100 mg/dL and high density lipoprotein cholesterol levels (HDL) of 60 mg/dL or higher. With the use of cholestyramine, which contains aspartame, it is of particular interest to know if there is a history of PKU. Patients with PKU cannot properly process the amino acid phenylalanine, a component of protein. It is known that high levels of phenylalanine lead to behavioral, cognitive, and learning dysfunction as early as 3 weeks of age in such patients. Dietary restrictions must continue throughout life, and adult patients require monthly testing of phenylalanine levels. Because of the aspartame in cholestyramine, another class of an antilipemics would be indicated for such patients, as ordered, to prevent further complications from this disorder.

HMG–CoA reductase inhibitors (the statins) must not be used in patients younger than 10 years of age. Other contraindications, cautions, and drug interactions have been previously discussed in the pharmacology section of this chapter. The patient's intake of alcohol is also important to assess, including the amount consumed and the period of time that alcohol has been used, because of the potential for liver dysfunction associated with the majority

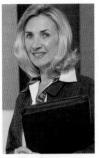
of lipid-lowering drugs. These drugs may have more adverse effects on an already damaged liver. Levels of liver enzymes that are indicative of liver function should also be assessed, including AST, CPK, and/or ALT. Lipid and lipoprotein levels also need to be reviewed before, during, and after drug therapy with the statins as well as with other antilipemic drugs. The patient should also be assessed for myopathies and rhabdomyolysis during and after drug therapy. Should AST or ALT blood levels increase and myopathy and/or rhabdomyolysis occur, the drug will most likely be discontinued by the prescriber. Also, with statin drugs, cultural influences need to be assessed with a focus on the individual's beliefs about how to control diet and cholesterol levels. Cultural practices also need to be considered because the patient may be using herbal and/or homeopathic therapies. *Bile acid sequestrants, niacin,* and *fibric acid derivatives* and their related contraindications, cautions, and drug interactions have been discussed previously, but the nurse should always check for the numerous drug interactions.

Nursing Diagnoses

- Imbalanced nutrition, more than body requirements, related to poor dietary habits of high fat intake
- Deficient knowledge related to a lack of information about the disease and related complications
- Deficient knowledge related to a lack of understanding of drug therapy and need for lifestyle changes

LABORATORY VALUES RELATED TO DRUG THERAPY

Coronary Heart Disease

Laboratory Test	Normal Ranges*	Rationale for Assessment
Serum lipid panel with cholesterol, triglycerides, and various lipids	• Serum cholesterol level: less than or equal to 200 mg/dL (less than 5.17 mmol/L) • Triglyceride level: less than 150 mg/dL • Low-density lipoprotein (LDL) cholesterol level: less than 100 mg/dL (less than 2.6 mmol/L) • High-density lipoprotein (HDL) cholesterol level: greater than or equal to 60 mg/dL (1.56 mmol/L[CB8]) • Very-low-density lipoprotein (VLDL) level: less than 130 mg/dL (less than 3.4 mmol/L)	A lipid panel is a serum test that measures the levels of lipids, fats, and fatty substances used as a source of energy in the body. Lipids include cholesterol, triglycerides, HDL, and LDL. When a lipid panel is ordered, the levels of all of the following are reported: total cholesterol, triglycerides, HDL, LDL, VLDL, ratio of total cholesterol to HDL, and ratio of LDL to HDL. Lipid levels are important to health status and are indicators of health; if there are abnormalities (e.g., high cholesterol, triglyceride, VLDL, and LDL levels and low HDL level), the individual is at increased risk for heart disease and stroke. Dietary and other lifestyle changes may be implemented to help decrease the levels of "bad" cholesterols (LDL and VLDL) and elevate the levels of "good" cholesterol (HDL). Medical treatment protocols may also be implemented to help prevent heart attack and strokes.

*The values in this table are from the National Cholesterol Education Program of the National Institutes of Health.

- Impaired home maintenance related to lack of experience with lifestyle changes and unfamiliar medication therapy
- Imbalanced nutrition, less than body requirements, related to vitamin A, D, E, and K deficits from adverse effects of antilipemics

Planning

Goals

- Patient remains compliant with both nonpharmacologic and pharmacologic therapy.
- Patient remains free of the complications associated with antilipemics because of appropriate use of the drug.
- Patient sees the prescriber regularly and as indicated for the treatment of hyperlipidemia and for repetition of laboratory studies until normal values return.
- Patient maintains homeostasis and nutritional well-being while taking the antilipemic drug.

Outcome Criteria

- Patient states the importance of pharmacologic and nonpharmacologic therapy for his or her overall health and safety, such as for decreasing the risk for CHD.
- Patient states the rationale for therapy as well as its adverse effects and expected therapeutic effects (i.e., decreasing lipid levels, gastrointestinal adverse effects, and therapeutic response of improved lipid profile).
- Patient states the conditions that may arise of which the prescriber should be notified, such as jaundice and abdominal pain.
- Patient states that cholesterol levels should return to a value of less than 200 mg/dL within approximately 6 to 8 weeks.
- Patient states the importance of follow-up care with the prescriber to monitor for changes in liver function as well as to monitor lipid levels.
- Patient states measures to maintain adequate levels of fat-soluble vitamins.

Implementation

Patients who are taking *antilipemics* for a long period may have altered levels of the fat-soluble vitamins and may then require supplementation of vitamins A, D, and K. Antilipemics may also cause problems with the liver and biliary systems, and they may cause gastrointestinal tract problems such as constipation. Appropriate actions need to be taken to avoid or minimize constipation, such as increasing intake of fiber and fluids. Monitoring the results of blood studies per the prescriber's instructions often includes reviewing levels of serum transaminases and results of other tests of liver function.

With the *HMG-CoA reductase inhibitors,* serum levels of the aforementioned components are often measured every 6 to 8 weeks for the first 6 months of statin therapy and then every 3 to 6 months. If a lipid profile is ordered, the patient should be instructed to fast for 12 to 14 hours before the blood sample is drawn and should be told that the following are the desired levels to achieve: cholesterol level of less than 200 mg/dL; triglyceride level of less than 150 mg/dL; LDL level of less than 130 mg/dL; and HDL level of more than 60 mg/dL (HDLs are the "good" lipids). Because severe cardiovascular diseases and cerebral vascular accidents (also known as *strokes*) are associated with cholesterol levels higher than 240 mg/dL, LDL levels higher than 160 mg/dL, and HDL levels lower than 35 mg/dL, it is critical to the maintenance of health and the prevention of complications that the patient continue with any prescribed nonpharmacologic and/or pharmacologic therapies, regardless of the specific antilipemic used. These drugs should never be discontinued abruptly.

Bile acid sequestrants often come in powder form and should be mixed thoroughly with fruit (e.g., crushed pineapple) or other food or fluids (at least 4 to 6 oz of fluid). The powder may not mix completely at first, but patients should be sure to mix the dose as much as possible and then dilute any undissolved portion with additional fluid. The powder should be dissolved for at least 1 full minute. Powder and/or granule dosage forms are *never* to be taken in dry form. It is important that colestipol and any of these drugs should be taken 1 hour before or 4 to 6 hours after any other oral medication and/or meals because of the high risk for drug-drug and drug-food interactions. Cholestyramine should be taken just before meals or with meals and should never be given to a patient with PKU because it contains aspartame (see previous discussion). To prevent injuries from falls, patients should be encouraged to change positions slowly and to lie down should they get dizzy (due to orthostatic changes).

Statins and Stroke Reduction in Patients With and Without Coronary Heart Disease

■ Review

A meta-analysis was conducted to examine the management of lipid levels as an important component of stroke prevention. Randomized clinical trials were reviewed to determine the effects of lipid-lowering interventions (statins, fibrates, resins, omega-3 fatty acids, and dietary measures) for the prevention of nonfatal and fatal strokes.

■ Type of Evidence

To select studies for the meta-analysis, a review of the literature was conducted using MEDLINE, EMBASE/Excerpta Medica, Pascal, and Index Medicus. Sixty-five randomized, controlled trials that had a follow-up of at least 6 months (range: 6 months to 6.1 years) and provided data on nonfatal and fatal strokes and total mortality were included in the meta-analysis, which pooled the intervention and control groups. The goal of the analysis was to compare dietary or pharmaceutical lipid-lowering interventions with "usual" diet or placebo to study their effectiveness of these interventions in reducing strokes.

■ Results of Study

The analysis found that statins reduced the risk of nonfatal and fatal stroke more than the control interventions in patients with and without coronary heart disease combined. Fibrates, resins, omega-3 fatty acids, and dietary interventions were found to be no more effective than the control interventions in reducing the risk for nonfatal and fatal stroke. Several research studies quoted in the commentary of

this study pointed out that the findings of Briel and collegues show the importance of statin treatment in helping to reduce the incidence of stroke in patients with and without heart disease. It is thought that statins are pleiotropic (have multiple effects) and produce their benefits through antiinflammatory action and endothelial protection. Although this meta-analysis did not confirm the benefits of nonstatin lipid-lowering therapy, the authors did not dismiss the merits of such treatments. The fact that no significant treatment effects were found for the nonstatins could be attributable to small cohorts and other variables.

■ Link of Evidence to Nursing Practice

The results of this meta-analysis emphasize the importance of looking at different treatment options such as the use of statins to reduce nonfatal and fatal strokes in patients with and without coronary heart disease. Although the benefits of statins are known, many patients remain inadequately treated. Nurses play a major role in performing assessments and interventions for patients with cardiovascular disorders as well as in monitoring the pharmacologic management of these patients. Nurses also continue to play an important part in the education of patients and the community about the risk factors for stroke, including coronary artery disease and hyperlipidemia, as well as in education about the need to comply with all types of interventions and therapies to reduce cardiovascular risk.

Modified from Briel M et al: Effects of statins on stroke prevention in patients with and without coronary heart disease: a meta-analysis of randomized clinical trials, *Am J Med* 117:596-606, 2004; Briel M et al: Review: statins reduce non-fatal and fatal strokes in patients with and without coronary heart disease, *Evid Based Nurs* 8:86, 2005.

With *niacin,* flushing of the face may occur, and the patient should be aware of this adverse effect. Postural hypotensive adverse effects require that the patient change positions slowly and with caution, as well as lie down should dizziness occur. To minimize gastrointestinal upset, patients should take these medications with fluids or food. Of the different dosage forms available, the extended-release dosage forms, which dissolve more slowly than the immediate-release forms but faster than the sustained-release forms, appear to be associated with less liver toxicity and flushing of the skin. Other actions that may help to minimize flushing of the skin and hyperuricemia include titrating the drug dosage and taking aspirin or NSAIDs as ordered.

Evaluation

Evaluation of goals and outcome criteria is the best place to begin when trying to evaluate for the therapeutic versus adverse effects of these medications. In addition, cholesterol and triglyceride levels are used to monitor the patient's response to the medication regimen, and specific target levels were mentioned in the nursing assessment section. While taking antilipemics, patients remain on a low-fat, low-cholesterol diet as an integrated

part of a change in lifestyle. Patients receiving antilipemic drugs need to be monitored for therapeutic and adverse effects during their therapy. The therapeutic effects of both nonpharmacologic and pharmacologic measures are evidenced by a decrease in cholesterol and triglyceride levels to within the normal ranges (see previous serum laboratory values). Another marker commonly monitored as a risk factor for atherosclerotic heart disease is C-reactive protein level. Any elevation in the level of this protein is associated with greater risk for major ischemic heart disease (e.g., myocardial infarction). Nonpharmacologic measures include a low-fat, low-cholesterol diet; supervised, moderate exercise; weight loss; cessation of smoking and drinking; and relaxation therapy. If there is no response to pharmacologic therapy after about 3 months, the medication is generally withdrawn. Fenofibrate dosage may be increased at 4- to 8-week intervals depending on the triglyceride levels. Adverse effects for which to monitor include gastrointestinal upset, increased liver enzyme levels, hepatomegaly, myalgias, and other effects mentioned earlier in the chapter. Patients' renal and liver function should be closely monitored before and throughout treatment to detect the development of liver or renal dysfunction.

PATIENT TEACHING TIPS

- The prescriber should be notified if there are any new or troublesome symptoms or if there is persistent gastrointestinal upset, constipation, gas, bloating, heartburn, nausea, vomiting, abnormal or unusual bleeding, or yellow discoloration of the skin. Other symptoms to report include muscle pain, decreased sex drive, impotence, and difficulty urinating.
- These and all medications should be kept out of the reach of children and protected with childproof lids.
- Encourage a diet that is plentiful in raw vegetables, fruit, and bran. Forcing fluids (up to 3000 mL/day unless contraindicated) may also help prevent the constipation.
- The patient should be told to inform all health care providers about all medications the patient is taking, including antilipemics. These drugs are highly protein bound and are therefore associated with many drug interactions, including drugs that a dentist may prescribe. In addition, these drugs may alter clotting if taken on a long-term basis, so bleeding with dental work may occur.
- Exercise should be done with moderation and often with supervision as indicated.
- These medications should be kept away from heat and moisture to avoid alteration in the drug composition.
- When taking an HMG–CoA reductase inhibitor, it should be taken with at least 6 oz of water or with meals to help minimize gastric upset and with the knowledge that it may take several weeks before therapeutic results are seen.
- An ophthalmologic examination is needed prior to and during therapy with statin drugs because of the reported drug-related problems with visual acuity.
- If taking a bile acid sequestrant, the patient should contact the prescriber immediately if stools appear black and tarry.
- These medications should never be abruptly discontinued.

POINTS TO REMEMBER

- There are two primary forms of lipids: triglycerides and cholesterol. Triglycerides function as an energy source and are stored in adipose (fat) tissue. Cholesterol is primarily used to make steroid hormones, cell membranes, and bile acids.
- Lipids and lipoproteins participate in the formation of atherosclerotic plaque, which leads to CHD, and nurses need to understand the pathology of this disease process so that appropriate patient education may be delivered.
- When plaque forms in the blood vessels that supply the heart with needed oxygen and nutrients, the lumens of these blood vessels will eventually decrease in size and the amount of oxygen and nutrients that can reach the heart will be reduced.
- Antilipemic drugs are used to lower the high levels of lipids in the blood (triglycerides and cholesterol).
- The major classes of antilipemics include HMG–CoA reductase inhibitors, bile acid sequestrants, niacin, fibric acid derivatives, and cholesterol absorption inhibitors, with each having their own mechanism of action.
- While taking a nursing history, it is important for the nurse to assess the patient for any possible cautions, contraindications, and drug interactions.
- Fat-soluble vitamins may need to be prescribed for patients taking these medications for long periods, because the antilipemics have long-term effects on the liver's production of these vitamins.
- When the powder or granule oral forms of these drugs are used, they must be mixed with noncarbonated liquids and *never* taken dry.
- Monitoring for adverse effects of the antilipemics includes periodic liver and renal function studies.
- The statins have gained much attention for their adverse effects of muscle aches and pain due to breakdown of muscle tissue. Some patients experience irreversible renal damage and severe pain and may have to alter dosages or change drugs as ordered by the prescriber.

NCLEX EXAMINATION REVIEW QUESTIONS

1 A nurse administering niacin would implement which action to help to reduce adverse effects?
 a Give the medication with grapefruit juice
 b Administer a small dose of aspirin or an NSAID 30 minutes before the niacin dose
 c Administer the medication on an empty stomach
 d Have the patient increase dietary fiber intake

2 When administering niacin, the nurse needs to monitor for which adverse effect?
 a Cutaneous flushing
 b Low back pain
 c Headache
 d Constipation

3 Which point is appropriate to emphasize to a patient taking an antilipemic medication?
 a The drug should be taken on an empty stomach before meals.
 b A low-fat diet is not necessary while taking these medications.
 c It is important to report muscle pain immediately.
 d Improved cholesterol levels should be evident within 2 weeks.

4 A patient is being assessed before a newly ordered antilipemic medication is given. Which condition would be a potential contraindication?

 a Diabetes insipidus
 b Pulmonary fibrosis
 c Liver cirrhosis
 d Myocardial infarction

5 A patient is currently taking a statin. The nurse considers that the patient may have a higher risk of developing rhabdomyolysis when also taking which product?
 a NSAIDs
 b Gemfibrozil
 c Orange juice
 d Fat soluble vitamins

6 The nurse is administering cholestyramine (Questran), a bile acid sequestrant. Which nursing intervention(s) is appropriate? (Select all that apply.)
 a Administering the drug on an empty stomach
 b Administering the drug with meals
 c Instructing the patient to follow a low-fiber diet while taking this drug
 d Instructing the patient to take a fiber supplement while taking this medication
 e Increasing fluid intake if possible
 f Not administering this drug at the same time as other drugs

1. b, 2. a, 3. c, 4. c, 5. b, 6. b, d, e, f

CRITICAL THINKING ACTIVITIES: BEST ACTION

1 A patient has started taking niacin (nicotinic acid) as part of treatment for high cholesterol levels. After the first dose, he tells the nurse that he feels "hot" and that his face and neck are flushed. He says that he thinks he is having an allergic reaction. What is the nurse's best response at this time?

2 While reviewing instructions for newly prescribed anticholesterol medications, a patient informs the nurse that he "hates to mix powdered medicines" and plans to take his Cholestyramine (Questran) powder dry. What is the nurse's best response to this patient?

3 A patient has been taking simvastatin (Zocor) for 6 months. Today he received a call that he needs to come to the office for a "laboratory check." What laboratory studies would need to be done at this time?

For answers, see *http://evolve.elsevier.com/Lilley.*

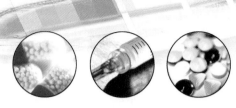
Drugs Affecting the Endocrine System

QUESTIONING STRATEGY

One of the most important activities for learning is to become actively involved with the text. The best way to achieve this involvement is to develop the habit of asking questions. These questions can be generated using a number of different cues and elements that are part of the part and chapter structure. Some of what you anticipate as related material will not be correct, so you will adjust your expectations as you read the material. For now, focus on asking a lot of questions and making use of everything you know, which can help start the process of answering your questions.

Part Title

As you begin each new part, ask a question to focus your attention, seeking to learn what all the chapters in this part have in common. In Part 5, this question is, "What is the endocrine system?" This same question could be asked of Parts 2 through 9 by simply replacing *endocrine* with the appropriate system for the specific part. Looking at the chapter titles in the part tells you that the endocrine system has to do with the pituitary drugs, thyroid and antithyroid drugs, antidiabetic drugs, adrenal drugs, women's health drugs, and men's health drugs. Although this answer is far too general to demonstrate any real understanding of the endocrine system, it is a beginning and helps keep you aware of what you need to learn from each chapter.

Chapter Titles

Chapter titles provide the first mechanism that can be used to generate questions. The first question to ask about each chapter is a very basic one, involving what the chapter is about. That question is also answered immediately. "What is Chapter 30 about?" It is about pituitary drugs.

The next question is equally obvious but also extremely important. The question to ask next is, "To what do pituitary (see Chapter 30), thyroid and antithyroid (see Chapter 31), antidiabetic (see Chapter 32), adrenal (see Chapter 33), women's health (see Chapter 34), and men's health (see Chapter 35)

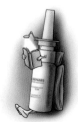

refer?" Take the chapter title and state it as a question. What do you know about these subjects?

Chapter Objectives

To enhance your study, turn each chapter objective into one or more questions. Here are some possible questions using the objectives from Chapter 32.

Objective 1: Discuss the normal actions and functions of the pancreas.

* What are the normal actions and functions of the pancreas?

Objective 2: Contrast type 1 and type 2 diabetes mellitus with regard to age of onset, signs and symptoms, pharmacologic and nonpharmacologic treatment, incidence, and etiology.

* What is type 1 diabetes mellitus?
* What is type 2 diabetes mellitus?
* How do types 1 and 2 diabetes mellitus differ in age of onset, signs and symptoms, treatment, incidence, and etiology?

Because the objectives tell you what the authors expect you to know at the end of the chapter, starting out with questions based on the objectives will improve your learning and probably save you time.

Chapter Headings

The same principle can be applied to each of the topic headings set out in the chapter. Continuing to use Chapter 32 as a model, here are some samples of questions that might be useful as preparation for reading.

Type 1 Diabetes Mellitus

* What is type 1 diabetes?
* What is mellitus?

As you start to process the chapter headings, you should also notice that they begin to answer some of the questions from the chapter objectives. This is a good time to begin setting up vocabulary cards.

Mechanism of Action and Drug Effects

* What is the mechanism of action of insulin?
* Is there more than one mechanism?
* What are the most important drug effects of insulin?

- Where do these effects take place?
- What is the evidence of these effects?

The idea is to focus on the major content of the chapter and establish a guide for learning as you read.

Print Conventions Within the Body of the Chapter

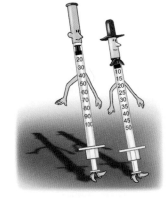

Print conventions are useful in this study skills strategy. The use of *italics,* **bold,** <u>underlining,</u> and multiple colors of ink are examples of print conventions. They are designed to catch your attention. Use them as a basis for questions.

In the first paragraph of Chapter 32, the first obvious print convention is the word **insulin.** It is printed in bold. If you let your eyes float down the page and do not read anything, this word stands out. It must be important.

- What is insulin?
- What is the relationship between insulin and type 1 diabetes mellitus?

There are more words on the first page of the chapter text that are in the same print style. Apply the same procedure to these terms. Also, notice that two of the terms, **glycogen** and **glycogenolysis,** must have some direct relationship, because the second term contains the first term. The basic question in each case is, "What does the term mean?" However, there should be more to your questions than just the basics. *Glycogenolysis* seems to mean that there is some operation or activity taking place. Ask yourself the following:

- What happens in glycogenolysis?
- Where does glycogenolysis occur?

- When does glycogenolysis occur?
- How does it relate to type 1 diabetes mellitus?

Chapter Tables

Tables serve as a summary of information discussed in the chapter. You can learn a great deal from tables if you take the time.

Look at Table 32-2. The table summarizes characteristics of type 1 and type 2 diabetes. There are two obvious questions for each type.

- What is type 1 (and type 2) diabetes?
- What are its characteristics?

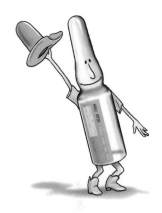

Use these questions to study Table 32-2 and you will find that all the information you need to respond to these questions is found here. It may be useful to make a first pass through the chapter focusing only on the tables before you begin to read. You will learn a great deal about some of the topics, and you will have established background information that will help you ask better questions and read with better understanding.

The time you spend asking questions makes the reading and learning go more quickly. Another benefit is that some of the questions you ask appear on tests. These questions will be easy for you to answer. This promotes test-taking confidence, and better test scores result in better grades. If you have not been using questioning strategy up to this point in your text, begin now. After you use the strategy for two or three chapters, you will find that the benefits far outweigh the time it takes.

CHAPTER **30**

Pituitary Drugs

OBJECTIVES

When you reach the end of this chapter, you should be able to do the following:

1 Describe the normal function of the anterior and posterior lobes of the pituitary gland and the impact of the pituitary gland on the human body.

2 Compare the various pituitary drugs with regard to their indications, mechanisms of action, dosages, routes of administration, adverse effects, cautions, contraindications, and drug interactions.

3 Develop a nursing care plan that includes all phases of the nursing process for patients receiving pituitary drugs, such as desmopressin, octreotide, somatropin, and vasopressin.

---

e-Learning Activities

http://evolve.elsevier.com/Lilley

NCLEX Review Questions • Animations • Nursing Care Plans • Audio Glossary • Category Catchers • Medication Errors Checklists • IV Therapy Checklists • Calculators • Frequently Asked Questions • Content Updates • Supplemental Resources • Answers to Case Studies and Critical Thinking Activities

Drug Profiles

♦ octreotide, p. 475　　　　　♦ vasopressin, p. 475

　　♦ *Key drug.*

Glossary

Hypothalamus The gland above and behind the pituitary gland and the optic chiasm. Both glands are suspended beneath the middle area of the bottom of the brain. The hypothalamus secretes the hormones vasopressin and oxytocin, which are stored in the posterior pituitary. The hypothalamus also secretes several hormone-releasing factors that stimulate the anterior pituitary to secrete a variety of hormones that control many body functions. (p. 472)

Negative feedback loop A system in which the production of one hormone is controlled by the levels of a second hormone in a way that reduces the output of the first hormone. A gland produces a hormone that stimulates a second gland to produce a second hormone. In response to the increased levels of the second hormone, the source gland of the first hormone reduces production of that hormone, until blood levels of the second hormone fall below a certain minimum level needed; then the cycle begins again. (See simplified example on p. 473.) (p. 473)

Neuroendocrine system The system that regulates the reactions to both internal and external stimuli and involves the integrated activities of the endocrine glands and nervous system. (p. 472)

Pituitary gland An endocrine gland suspended beneath the brain which supplies numerous hormones that control many vital processes. (p. 472)

• • •

Anatomy and Physiology Overview

ENDOCRINE SYSTEM

The maintenance of physiologic stability is the main goal of the endocrine system. The endocrine system must accomplish this task despite constant changes in the internal and external environments. Every cell, and hence organ, in the body comes under the influence of the endocrine system. It communicates with the nearly 50 million target cells in the body using a chemical "language" called *hormones*. Hormones are a large group of natural substances that cause highly specific physiologic effects in the cells of their target tissues. They are secreted into the bloodstream in response to the body's needs and travel through the blood to their site of action—the target cell.

For decades the pituitary gland was believed to be the master gland that regulated and controlled the other endocrine glands. However, evidence now suggests that the central nervous system (CNS), specifically the **hypothalamus,** controls the pituitary. The hypothalamus and pituitary are now viewed as functioning together as an integrated unit, with the primary direction coming from the hypothalamus. For this reason, these structures are now commonly referred to as the **neuroendocrine system.** In fact, the endocrine system can be considered in much the same way as the CNS. Each is basically a system for signaling, and each operates in a stimulus-and-response manner. Together these two systems essentially govern all bodily functions.

The **pituitary gland** is made up of two distinct lobes—the anterior pituitary (adenohypophysis) and posterior pituitary (neurohypophysis). They are individually linked to and communicate with the hypothalamus, and each lobe secretes its own different set of hormones. These various hormones are listed in Box 30-1 and shown in Figure 30-1.

Hormones are either water or lipid soluble. The water-soluble hormones are protein-based substances such as the catecholamines norepinephrine and epinephrine. The lipid-soluble hormones consist of the steroid and thyroid hormones.

The activity of the endocrine system is regulated by a system of surveillance and signaling usually dictated by the body's ongoing needs. Hormone secretion is commonly regulated by a

472

negative feedback loop. This is best explained using a fictional example: When gland X releases hormone X, this stimulates target cells to release hormone Y. When there is an excess of hormone Y, gland X senses this excess and decreases its release of hormone X.

Pharmacology Overview

PITUITARY DRUGS

A variety of drugs affect the pituitary gland. They are generally used either as replacement drug therapy to make up for a hormone deficiency or as diagnostic aids to determine the status of the patient's hormonal functions. The currently identified anterior and posterior pituitary hormones and the drugs that mimic or antagonize their actions are listed in Table 30-1. Many of these hormones have been synthesized, and some of them have already been discussed in other chapters.

The anterior pituitary drugs discussed in this chapter are cosyntropin, somatotropin, somatrem, and octreotide; the pos-

---

BOX 30-1   Hormones of the Anterior and Posterior Pituitary

Anterior Pituitary (Adenohypophysis)
Adrenocorticotropic hormone (ACTH)
Follicle-stimulating hormone (FSH)
Growth hormone (GH)
Luteinizing hormone (LH)
Prolactin (PH)
Thyroid-stimulating hormone (TSH)

Posterior Pituitary (Neurohypophysis)
Antidiuretic hormone (ADH)
Oxytocin

---

terior pituitary drugs discussed in this chapter are vasopressin and desmopressin.

Mechanism of Action and Drug Effects

The mechanisms of action of the various pituitary drugs differ depending on the drug, but overall they either augment or antagonize the natural effects of the pituitary hormones. Exogenously administered corticotropin elicits all of the same pharmacologic responses as those elicited by endogenous corticotropin (also known as *adrenocorticotropic hormone,* or *ACTH*). Exogenous corticotropin is no longer manufactured. It has been replaced by cosyntropin (Cortrosyn). Cosyntropin travels to the adrenal cortex, located just above the kidney, and stimulates the secretion of cortisol (the drug form of which is hydrocortisone [Solu-Cortef]). Cortisol has many antiinflammatory effects, including reduction of inflammatory leukocyte functions and scar tissue formation. Cortisol also promotes renal retention of sodium, which can result in edema and hypertension.

The drugs that mimic growth hormone (GH) are somatropin and somatrem. These drugs promote growth by stimulating various anabolic (tissue-building) processes, liver glycogenolysis (to raise blood sugar levels), lipid mobilization from body fat stores, and retention of sodium, potassium, and phosphorus. Both drugs promote linear growth in children who lack normal amounts of the endogenous hormone.

Octreotide is a drug that antagonizes the effects of natural GH. It does so by inhibiting GH release. Octreotide is a synthetic polypeptide that is structurally and pharmacologically similar to GH release–inhibiting factor, which is also called *somatostatin.* It also reduces plasma concentrations of vasoactive intestinal polypeptide (VIP), a protein secreted by a type of tumor known as a *VIPoma* that causes profuse watery diarrhea.

The drugs that affect the posterior pituitary, such as vasopressin and desmopressin, mimic the actions of the naturally occurring antidiuretic hormone (ADH). They increase water resorption

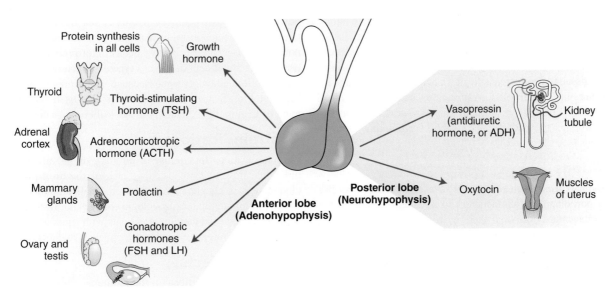

FIGURE 30-1 Pituitary hormones. *FSH,* Follicle-stimulating hormone; *LH,* luteinizing hormone. (From McKenry LM, Tessier E, Hogan MA: Mosby's pharmacology in nursing, ed 22, St Louis, 2006, Mosby.)

TABLE 30-1 Anterior and Posterior Pituitary Hormones and Drugs

Hormone	Function and Mimicking Drug
Anterior Pituitary	
Adrenocorticotropic hormone	Targets adrenal gland; mediates adaptation to physical and emotional stress and starvation; redistributes body nutrients; promotes synthesis of adrenocortical hormones (glucocorticoids, mineralocorticoids, androgens); involved in skin pigmentation *cosyntropin:* Used for diagnosis of adrenocortical insufficiency
Follicle-stimulating hormone (FSH)	Stimulates oogenesis and follicular growth in females and spermatogenesis in males *Menotropins:* Same pharmacologic effects as FSH; many of the other gonadotropins also stimulate FSH (see Chapter 34)
Growth hormone (GH)	Regulates anabolic processes related to growth and adaptation to stressors; promotes skeletal and muscle growth; increases protein synthesis; increases liver glycogenolysis; increases fat mobilization *somatropin, somatrem:* Human GH for treatment of hypopituitary dwarfism *octreotide:* A synthetic polypeptide structurally and pharmacologically similar to GH release–inhibiting factor; inhibits GH
Luteinizing hormone (LH)	Stimulates ovulation and estrogen release by ovaries in females; stimulates interstitial cells in males to promote spermatogenesis and testosterone secretion *Gonadotropins:* Many of the drugs discussed in Chapter 34 stimulate LH
Prolactin	Targets mammary glands; stimulates lactogenesis and breast growth *bromocriptine:* Inhibits action of prolactin and therefore inhibits lactogenesis (see Chapter 16)
Thyroid-stimulating hormone	Stimulates secretion of thyroid hormones T_3 and T_4 by the thyroid *thyrotropin:* Increases the production and secretion of thyroid hormones (see Chapter 31)
Posterior Pituitary	
Antidiuretic hormone (ADH)	Increases water resorption in distal tubules and collecting duct of nephron; concentrates urine; causes potent vasoconstriction *vasopressin:* ADH; performs all the physiologic functions of ADH *desmopressin:* A synthetic vasopressin
Oxytocin	Targets mammary glands; stimulates ejection of milk and contraction of uterine smooth muscle *Pitocin:* Has all the physiologic actions of oxytocin (see Chapter 34)

T_3, Triiodothyronine; T_4, thyroxine.

in the distal tubules and collecting ducts of the nephrons, and concentrate urine, reducing water excretion by up to 90%. Vasopressin is also a potent vasoconstrictor in larger doses and is therefore used in certain hypotensive emergencies, such as vasodilatory shock (septic shock). Its use is also called for in the Advanced Cardiac Life Support (ACLS) guidelines for treatment of pulseless cardiac arrest. Vasopressin is also used to stop bleeding of esophageal varices. Desmopressin causes a dose-dependent increase in the plasma levels of factor VIII (antihemophilic factor), von Willebrand factor (acts closely with factor VIII), and tissue plasminogen activator. These properties make it useful in treating certain blood disorders. Desmopressin is also used for management of nocturnal enuresis. The drug form of oxytocin mimics the endogenous hormone, promoting uterine contractions (see Chapter 34).

Indications

Cosyntropin is used in the diagnosis of adrenocortical insufficiency. Upon diagnosis, the actual drug treatment generally involves replacement hormonal therapy using drug forms of the deficient corticosteroid hormones. These drugs are discussed in more detail in Chapter 33. Somatropin and somatrem are human GH produced by recombinant technology. They are effective in stimulating skeletal growth in patients with an inadequate secretion of normal endogenous GH, such as those with hypopituitary dwarfism, and are also used for wasting associated with human

immunodeficiency virus infection. Octreotide is of benefit in alleviating certain symptoms of carcinoid tumors stemming from the secretion of VIP, including severe diarrhea and flushing and potentially life-threatening hypotension associated with a carcinoid crisis. It is also used for the treatment of esophageal varices. Vasopressin and desmopressin are used to prevent or control polydipsia (excessive thirst), polyuria, and dehydration in patients with diabetes insipidus caused by a deficiency of endogenous ADH. Because of their vasoconstrictor properties, they are useful in the treatment of various types of bleeding, in particular gastrointestinal hemorrhage. Because of its effects on various blood-clotting factors, desmopressin is also useful in the treatment of hemophilia A and type I von Willebrand's disease.

Contraindications

Contraindications for the use of pituitary drugs vary with each individual drug and are listed in each of the drug profiles included in this chapter. Because even small amounts of these drugs can initiate major physiologic changes, all of them should be used with special caution in patients with acute or chronic illnesses such as migraine headaches, epilepsy, and asthma.

Adverse Effects

Most of the adverse effects of the pituitary drugs are specific to the individual drug. Those drugs possessing similar hormonal effects generally have similar adverse effects. The most common

TABLE 30-2 Octreotide: Common Adverse Effects

Body System	Adverse Effects
Central nervous	Fatigue, malaise, headache
Endocrine	Increase or decrease in blood glucose levels
Gastrointestinal	Diarrhea, nausea, vomiting
Respiratory	Dyspnea
Musculoskeletal	Arthralgia
Cardiovascular	Conduction abnormalities

TABLE 30-3 Desmopressin and Vasopressin: Common Adverse Effects

Body System	Adverse Effects
Cardiovascular	Increased blood pressure
Central nervous	Fever, vertigo, headache
Gastrointestinal	Nausea, heartburn, cramps
Genitourinary	Uterine cramping
Other	Nasal irritation and congestion, tremor, sweating, vertigo

TABLE 30-4 Growth Hormone Analogues: Common Adverse Effects

Body System	Adverse Effects
Central nervous	Headache
Endocrine	Hyperglycemia, hypothyroidism
Genitourinary	Hypercalciuria
Other	Rash, urticaria, development of antibodies to growth hormone, inflammation at injection site, flulike syndrome

TABLE 30-5 Pituitary Drugs: Selected Drug Interactions

Pituitary Drug	Interacting Drug	Potential Result
desmopressin	carbamazepine	Enhanced desmopressin effects
	lithium, alcohol, demeclocycline	Reduced desmopressin effects
octreotide	cyclosporine	Case report of transplant rejection
	thioridazine, ciprofloxacin	Prolongation of QTc interval
somatropin and somatrem	Glucocorticoids	Reduction of growth effects
vasopressin	carbamazepine, fludrocortisone	Enhanced antidiuretic effect
	demeclocycline, norepinephrine, lithium	Reduced antidiuretic effect

adverse effects of the pituitary drugs described here are listed in Tables 30-2 to 30-4.

Interactions

Selected interactions involving pituitary drugs are summarized in Table 30-5.

Dosages

For the recommended dosages of pituitary drugs, see the Dosages table on p. 476.

DRUG PROFILES

◆ octreotide

Octreotide (Sandostatin) is contraindicated in patients who have shown a hypersensitivity to it or any of its components. It may impair gallbladder function and should be used with caution in patients with renal impairment. It may affect glucose regulation, and severe hypoglycemia may occur in patients with type 1 diabetes. It may cause hyperglycemia in patients with type 2 diabetes or in patients without diabetes. It may enhance the toxic effects of drugs that prolong the QTc interval. Ciprofloxacin may enhance the QTc-prolonging effects of octreotide. Octreotide can be given intravenously (IV), intramuscularly (IM), or subcutaneously. Pregnancy category B. Common dosages are listed in the Dosages table on p. 476.

PHARMACOKINETICS

Route	Onset of Action	Peak Plasma Concentration	Elimination Half-life	Duration of Action
PO	Rapid	0.4-1 hr	1.7-1.9 hr	6-12 hr

◆ vasopressin

Vasopressin (Pitressin) is contraindicated in patients with known hypersensitivity. It is pregnancy category C. It should be used with caution in patients with seizure disorders, asthma, cardiovascular disease, and renal disease. IV infiltration may lead to severe vasoconstriction and localized tissue necrosis. Nurses should watch the IV site closely for any signs of infiltration. Vasopressin is available as a nasal spray or injection for IM or IV use. When used to treat septic shock, it is given by continuous IV infusion.

PHARMACOKINETICS

Route	Onset of Action	Peak Plasma Concentration	Elimination Half-life	Duration of Action
IV	Rapid	1 hr	0.5 hr	2-8 hr

NURSING PROCESS

Assessment

Before administering any of the pituitary drugs, the nurse should perform a thorough nursing assessment with documentation of the patient's height, weight, and vital signs, as well as obtain a complete medication history with notation of allergies, prescription drug use, and use of over-the-counter drugs and herbals. Serum glucose, cholesterol, and electrolyte levels should be checked as they are ordered and documented with the use of the majority of these medications. Specifically, adminis-

DOSAGES

Selected Pituitary Drugs

Drug	Pharmacologic Class	Usual Dosage Range	Indications/Uses
◆ octreotide (Sandostatin, Sandostatin LAR Depot)	Somatostatin (GH inhibitor) analogue	**Adult*** IV/subcut: Initial dose of 50 mcg bid-tid; may titrate up to 500 mcg tid IV/subcut: 100-750 mcg/day divided bid-qid Depot IM: 10-30 mg q4wk	Acromegaly Metastatic carcinoid tumor (to control flushing and diarrhea symptoms) VIPoma Small bowel fistula Esophageal varices
◆ vasopressin (Pitressin)	Natural or synthetic ADH	**Adult** IM/subcut: 5-10 units bid-qid IV: 0.5 milliunits/kg/hr titrated to a maximum of 0.01 units/kg/hr **Pediatric** IV: 2.5-10 units bid-qid IV: 0.01-0.04 units/min **Adult** IV: 0.02-0.04 unit/min **Pediatric** IV: 0.002-0.005 units/kg/min	Diabetes insipidus; prevention or treatment of postoperative abdominal distension; dispersal of abdominal gas to improve imaging in abdominal radiographic studies Vasodilatory shock (septic shock) GI hemorrhage Esophageal varices Vasodilatory shock (septic shock) GI hemorrhage Esophageal varices

ADH, Antidiuretic hormone; *GH,* growth hormone; *GI,* gastrointestinal; *IM,* intramuscular; *IV,* intravenous; *subcut,* subcutaneous; *VIPoma,* vasoactive intestinal peptide–producing tumor.
*Normally used only in adults.

tration of desmopressin requires the checking of vital signs, including supine and standing blood pressures; weekly measurement of weight; and review of baseline complete blood counts, cardiac enzyme levels, and leukocyte counts. The prescriber may also order an electrocardiogram. Cautions, contraindications, and drug interactions are discussed in the pharmacology section. Octreotide acetate use requires assessment of baseline thyroid function test results and plasma serotonin levels. Baseline gallbladder functioning should be noted because of the risk of gallstone formation (cholelithiasis). Patients taking octreotide may require special dosing if they have decreased liver and kidney function, so baseline levels should always be assessed before administering these drugs. The prescriber may also order thyroid function tests and serum glucose and electrolyte levels. Urine specific gravity should also be tested. It is also important to be sure that assessment includes steps to prevent medication errors and awareness of concerns regarding look-alike sound-alike drugs. Octreotide acetate, or Sandostatin and Sandostatin LAR, should not be confused with Sandimmune (cyclosporine) or Sandoglobulin (IV immune globulin).

Use of somatropin requires attention to the growth, motor skills, height, and weight of the pediatric patient. Measurement of serum glucose levels and thyroid hormone levels is often ordered, with the results of these tests assessed and noted prior to use of the drug. Vasopressin therapy requires assessment for the usual cautions, contraindications, and drug interactions (see previous discussion), as well as measurement of vital signs with attention to blood pressure and documentation of baseline weight. Patient groups for which there are specific concerns and cautions include the elderly and those with liver or kidney dysfunction. See previous discussion for more information on cautions, contraindications, and drug interactions. Further assessment may

possibly include electrocardiography (ECG), neurologic testing, and ruling out of seizure activity.

Nursing Diagnoses

- Disturbed body image related to the specific disease process and/or drug adverse effects and their impact on the patient's physical characteristics
- Excess fluid volume related to adverse effects of the various pituitary drugs
- Fatigue related to adverse effects of pituitary drug therapy
- Acute pain related to gastrointestinal adverse effects associated with the use of various pituitary drugs
- Deficient knowledge related to lack of information and experience with pituitary drug treatment

Planning

Goals

- Patient maintains positive body image and remains positive about drug therapy.
- Patient maintains normal fluid volume and electrolyte status while taking the particular pituitary drug.
- Patient returns to normal or near normal levels of activity.
- Patient experiences little to no pain related to medication-induced gastrointestinal upset or epigastric distress.
- Patient remains compliant with medication therapy.
- Patient is without self-injury related to adverse effects of medications.

Outcome Criteria

- Patient openly verbalizes fears, anxieties, and concerns to health care professionals regarding changes in body image related to disease process and the adverse effects of drug therapy.

- Patient's sodium level remains within normal limits while medication is taken.
- Patient states ways to decrease fluid retention (edema) caused by medication, such as dietary precautions.
- Patient experiences minimal gastrointestinal upset and gastric distress by taking medication with food or at mealtimes.
- Patient states ways to help minimize risk for falls, such as changing positions slowly and reporting drug-related musculoskeletal and neurologic adverse effects to the prescriber.
- Patient performs activities of daily living and other normal activity without difficulty and with proper caution.
- Patient keeps follow-up appointments with the prescriber and understands their importance (e.g., to monitor adherence to the drug regimen, drug therapeutic effects, and adverse reactions).

Implementation

Desmopressin should be administered per the prescriber's orders because dosage and route may vary with the indication (i.e., diabetes insipidus vs. other forms of pituitary dysfunction). Dosage forms include oral, IV, intranasal, and subcutaneous. Subcutaneous injection sites for desmopressin and somatropin (also given IM, in ventral gluteal site) should be rotated to avoid tissue damage. Injectable solutions should be mixed by gently swirling the liquid, with use of only clear solutions. Morning and evening doses are often adjusted separately for adequate diurnal rhythm of water turnover. Intranasal use may lead to changes in the nasal mucosa with unpredictable absorption and so if the condition is worsening the prescriber needs to be contacted immediately. Fluid intake may be adjusted according to the predicted risk of water intoxication and sodium deficit. The elderly and children may have more problems with these risks. When giving this drug be cautious to the look alike-sound alike drug, vasopressin, to avoid medication error. Somatropin may also be confused with somatrem or sumatriptan. See patient teaching for more information on dosage administration.

Octreotide should be given as ordered with attention to the injectable solution. To be sure to avoid giving the wrong medication, be careful not to confuse octreotide acetate injection with injectable depot suspension product. Use only clear solutions and always check for incompatibilities, e.g., total parenteral nutrition. Make sure patients understand the importance of reporting abdominal discomfort to the prescriber immediately. Stress the importance of follow-up appointments for laboratory testing during treatment with this drug.

Vasopressin is available as a nasal spray or as an injection for IM or IV use. The clarity of parenteral solutions should always be checked before the medication is used and the solution discarded if there are visible particles or any fluid discoloration. The nurse should be alert to the adverse effects of nausea, diarrhea, pallor, abdominal pain, and flatus (gas). If these worsen or persist, the prescriber should be notified immediately. Severe headache, sweating, chest pain, tremors, heart irregularities, unexplained weight gain, blood in the stool, black tarry stools, and/or seizure activity should be reported to the prescriber.

CASE STUDY

Octreotide for VIPoma-Related Diarrhea

J.R., a 56-year-old beautician, has been diagnosed with a VIPoma (vasoactive intestinal peptide–producing tumor). She was scheduled for surgery but developed severe diarrhea. She has been hospitalized because, after 2 days of profuse, watery diarrhea, she became dehydrated. She has not eaten for several days. In addition to having diarrhea, she is nauseated, has facial flushing, and has lost 5 pounds in 2 days. Intravenous fluid replacement with normal saline has been started, and she will be receiving octreotide (Sandostatin). She had her gallbladder removed 8 years ago but has no history of other illnesses.

© Junial Enterprises

1. How does the octreotide work to control the VIPoma-related diarrhea?
2. As J.R. begins therapy with octreotide, the nurse should continue to assess what parameters?

After 2 days of treatment, the episodes of diarrhea have become less frequent. However, the nurse notes that J.R.'s blood glucose levels are elevated.

3. What is the best explanation for this elevation?

For answers, see *http://evolve.elsevier.com/Lilley.*

Evaluation

Once goals and outcome criteria have been reviewed, therapeutic responses to these drugs should be evaluated. For desmopressin and vasopressin, severe thirst should be decreased or eliminated and urinary output improved. For somatropin, increased growth is expected in patients for whom it is indicated. With octreotide, therapeutic effects should include improved symptoms related to carcinoid tumors, acromegaly, or carcinoid crisis. Improvement of diarrhea in those receiving chemotherapy, radiation, or acquired immunodeficiency-related drugs should be expected. Somatropin may increase serum calcium levels. The patient should be monitored for the adverse effects of desmopressin and vasopressin, such as hypertension, nausea, gastrointestinal upset, tremors, respiratory distress, and drowsiness (see previous discussion). Octreotide may result in abdominal discomfort, and this should be reported immediately to the prescriber. Allergic reactions to these drugs may include rash, urticaria, fever, and dyspnea. If these problems occur, the drug should be discontinued and the prescriber notified.

PATIENT TEACHING TIPS

- The patient should avoid alcohol while taking any of the pituitary drugs. There should also be instructions about not abruptly discontinuing this drug due to possible negative consequences to the patient and levels of pituitary hormones.
- Counsel the patient that the medication does not lead to a cure but does help alleviate the symptoms of the disease for which it is being given.
- Routes and techniques of administration should be carefully discussed with the patient and anyone else involved in the patient's care. With pediatric patients, the technique of administration should be demonstrated to the family or caregiver before discharge and comprehension evaluated with return demonstrations. Written instructions should always be provided, as age appropriate. The patient should be encouraged to keep a journal about the drug therapy and to record how the drugs are being tolerated.
- As for any medication or illness, the patient should keep a medical alert bracelet, necklace, or wallet card on the person at all times.

- Any fever, sore throat, joint pain, or muscular pain should be reported to the prescriber immediately.
- Intranasal dosage forms should be given only after the nasal passages have been cleared. With desmopressin, the pump should be pressed down four times to help prime the pump. The level of drug left in the pump should be carefully monitored so that there is always enough medication on hand. The pump may not have enough medication left after 25 doses (at 150 mcg per spray) or 50 doses (at 10 mcg per spray).
- Parents should be educated about the fact that children with endocrine disorders may have an increased risk of bone problems and instructed that if they notice their child limping, this should be reported immediately to the prescriber.
- Diabetic patients need to be monitored closely for changes in serum glucose levels.
- Ophthalmologic examinations are recommended.
- Water restriction will be needed. Exact amounts must be determined for each patient.

POINTS TO REMEMBER

- The pituitary gland is composed of two distinct lobes: anterior and posterior. Each lobe secretes its own set of hormones: *anterior:* thyroid-stimulating hormone, GH, ACTH, prolactin, follicle-stimulating hormone, luteinizing hormone; *posterior:* ADH, oxytocin.
- Pituitary drugs are used to either mimic or antagonize the action of endogenous pituitary hormones.
- Drugs that mimic the action of endogenous pituitary hormones include cosyntropin somatropin, somatrem, vasopressin, and desmopressin. A drug that antagonizes the actions of endogenous pituitary hormones is octreotide, which suppresses or inhibits certain symptoms related to carcinoid tumors.
- Nursing assessment of patients receiving pituitary hormones should include measurement of baseline vital signs; review of

electrolyte values (sodium, potassium, chloride), blood glucose levels, and chest radiographs; and measurement of weight. For patients taking desmopressin, vital signs should be measured with documentation of both supine and standing blood pressures and pulse rates. Other assessment data should include complete blood count, cardiac and liver enzyme activity, electrocardiogram, and weight.

- For patients receiving somatropin, levels of thyroid hormones and GH should be assessed and documented. Assessment should include measurement of vital signs, intake and output, and weight, and examination for the presence of edema.

NCLEX EXAMINATION REVIEW QUESTIONS

1 A patient is experiencing severe diarrhea, flushing, and life-threatening hypotension associated with carcinoid crisis. The nurse will prepare to administer which drug?
 a Octreotide
 b Vasopressin
 c Somatotropin
 d Cosyntropin

2 A patient is suspected of having adrenocortical insufficiency. The nurse expects to administer which drug to aid in the diagnosis of this condition?
 a Octreotide
 b Vasopressin
 c Somatropin
 d Cosyntropin

3 The nurse is reviewing the medication list for a patient who will be starting therapy with somatropin. Which drug would raise a concern that would need to be addressed before the patient starts this new drug?
 a Nonsteroidal antiinflammatory drug for arthritis
 b Antidepressant drug
 c Penicillin
 d Thyroid hormone

4 A patient who is about to be given octreotide is also taking a diuretic, IV heparin, ciprofloxacin, and an opioid as needed for pain. The nurse should be watchful for what possible interaction?
 a Hypokalemia due to an interaction with the diuretic
 b Decreased anticoagulation due to an interaction with the heparin
 c Prolongation of the QTc interval due to an interaction with ciprofloxacin
 d Increased sedation if the opioid is given

5 When monitoring for the therapeutic effects of intranasal desmopressin in a patient who has diabetes insipidus, which assessment finding would the nurse look for as an indication that the medication therapy is successful?
 a Increased insulin levels
 b Decreased diarrhea
 c Improved nasal patency
 d Decreased thirst

6 Which drugs have an action similar to that of the naturally occurring hormone ADH? (Select all that apply.)
 a cosyntropin
 b desmopressin
 c somatropin
 d vasopressin
 e octreotide

1. a, 2. d, 3. d, 4. c, 5. d, 6. b, d.

CRITICAL THINKING ACTIVITIES: BEST ACTION

1 When the nurse checks the insertion site of a patient who is receiving an IV infusion of vasopressin, the site is swollen and cool to the touch. What is the first action the nurse should take? Explain.

2 A child is experiencing delayed growth due to an endocrine disorder. Which pituitary drugs are used to treat this condition, and how do they work? What is the best way for the nurse to measure the patient's response to the drug therapy?

3 A patient will be receiving intranasal desmopressin, and the nurse is teaching the patient how to self-administer the drug. After the nurse explains how the pump works and how to prime the pump, what is important for the nurse to tell the patient to do just before taking the medication?

For answers, see *http://evolve.elsevier.com/Lilley*.

CHAPTER 31

Thyroid and Antithyroid Drugs

OBJECTIVES

When you reach the end of this chapter, you should be able to do the following:

1   Briefly describe the normal anatomy and physiology of the thyroid gland.
2   Discuss the various functions of the thyroid gland and related hormones.
3   Describe the differences in the diseases resulting from the hyposecretion and hypersecretion of thyroid gland hormones.
4   Identify the various drugs used to treat the hyposecretion and hypersecretion states of the thyroid gland.
5   Discuss the mechanisms of action, indications, dosages, routes of administration, contraindications, cautions, drug interactions, and adverse effects of the various drugs used to treat hypothyroidism and hyperthyroidism.
6   Develop a nursing care plan that includes all phases of the nursing process for patients receiving thyroid replacement therapy as well as for patients receiving antithyroid drugs.

e-Learning Activities

NCLEX Review Questions • Animations • Nursing Care Plans • Audio Glossary • Category Catchers • Medication Errors Checklists • IV Therapy Checklists • Calculators • Frequently Asked Questions • Content Updates • Supplemental Resources • Answers to Case Studies and Critical Thinking Activities

Drug Profiles

◆ levothyroxine, p. 482

◆ propylthiouracil, p. 484

◆ *Key drug.*

Glossary

Euthyroid Referring to normal thyroid function. (p. 481)
Hyperthyroidism A condition characterized by excessive production of the thyroid hormones. A severe form of this disorder is called *thyrotoxicosis.* (p. 482)
Hypothyroidism A condition characterized by diminished production of the thyroid hormones. (p. 481)
Thyroid-stimulating hormone (TSH) An endogenous substance secreted by the pituitary gland that controls the release of thyroid gland hormones and is necessary for the growth and function of the thyroid gland (also called *thyrotropin*). As a drug preparation, TSH increases the uptake of radioactive iodine in the thyroid and the secretion of thyroxine by the thyroid gland. (p. 481)
Thyroxine (T$_4$) The principle thyroid hormone that influences the metabolic rate. (p. 480)
Triiodothyronine (T$_3$) A secondary thyroid hormone that also affects body metabolism. (p. 480)

• • •

Anatomy, Physiology, and Disease Overview

THYROID FUNCTION

The thyroid gland lies across the larynx in front of the thyroid cartilage ("Adam's apple"). Its lobes extend laterally on both sides of the front of the neck. It is responsible for the secretion of three hormones essential for the proper regulation of metabolism: **thyroxine (T$_4$), triiodothyronine (T$_3$),** and calcitonin (see Chapter 34). It is also close to and communicates with the parathyroid glands, which lie just above and behind it. The parathyroid glands are two pairs of bean-shaped glands. These glands are made up of encapsulated cells, which are responsible for maintaining adequate levels of calcium in the extracellular fluid, primarily by mobilizing calcium from bone.

T$_4$ and T$_3$ are produced in the thyroid gland through the iodination and coupling of the amino acid tyrosine. The iodide (I$^-$, the ionized form of iodine) needed for this process is acquired from the diet, and about 1 mg of iodide is needed per week. This iodide is sequestered by the thyroid gland, where it is absorbed from the blood and concentrated to 20 times its blood level. Here it is also converted to iodine (I$_2$), which is combined with tyrosine to make diiodotyrosine. The combination of two molecules of diiodotyrosine causes the formation of thyroxine, which therefore has four iodine molecules in its structure (T$_4$). Triiodothyronine is formed by the coupling of one molecule of diiodotyrosine with one molecule of monoiodotyrosine; thus it has three iodine molecules in its structure (T$_3$). The biologic potency of T$_3$ is about four times greater than that of T$_4$, but T$_4$ is present in much greater quantities. After the synthesis of these two thyroid hormones, they are stored in the follicles in the thyroid gland in a complex with thyroglobulin (a protein that contains tyrosine and an amino acid), called the *colloid.* When the thyroid gland is signaled to do so, the thyroglobulin–thyroid hormone complex is enzymatically broken down to release T_3 and T_4 into the circulation. This entire process is triggered by **thyroid-stimulating hormone (TSH),** also called *thyrotropin.* Its release from the anterior pituitary is stimulated when the blood levels of T_3 and T_4 are low.

The thyroid hormones are involved in a wide variety of bodily processes. They regulate lipid and carbohydrate metabolism, are essential for normal growth and development, control the heat-regulating system (thermoregulatory center in the brain), and have various effects on the cardiovascular, endocrine, and neuro-muscular systems. Therefore, hyperfunction or hypofunction of the thyroid gland can lead to a wide range of serious conse-quences.

HYPOTHYROIDISM

There are three types of **hypothyroidism.** Primary hypothyroid-ism stems from an abnormality in the thyroid gland itself and occurs when the thyroid gland is not able to perform one of its many functions, such as releasing the thyroid hormones from their storage sites, coupling iodine with tyrosine, trapping iodide, converting iodide to iodine, or any combination of these defects. Primary hypothyroidism is the most common of the three types of hypothyroidism. Secondary hypothyroidism begins at the level of the pituitary gland and results from reduced secretion of TSH. TSH is needed to trigger the release of the T_3 and T_4 stored in the thyroid gland. Tertiary hypothyroidism is caused by a reduced level of the thyrotropin-releasing hormone from the hypothala-mus. This reduced level, in turn, reduces TSH and thyroid hor-mone levels.

Hypothyroidism can also be classified by when it occurs in the life span. Hyposecretion of thyroid hormone during youth may lead to cretinism. Cretinism is characterized by low metabolic rate, retarded growth and sexual development, and possibly men-tal retardation. Hyposecretion of thyroid hormone as an adult may lead to myxedema. Myxedema is a condition manifested by decreased metabolic rate, but it also involves loss of mental and physical stamina, weight gain, hair loss, firm edema, and yellow dullness of the skin.

Some forms of hypothyroidism may result in the formation of a goiter, which is an enlargement of the thyroid gland resulting from its overstimulation by elevated levels of TSH. The TSH level is elevated because there is little or no thyroid hormone in the circulation.

▮ Pharmacology Overview
THYROID REPLACEMENT DRUGS

All three types of hypothyroidism are amenable to treatment by thyroid hormone replacement using various thyroid preparations. These drugs can be either natural or synthetic in origin. The natural thyroid preparations are derived from the thyroids of ani-mals such as cattle and hogs. Currently only one natural prepara-tion is available in the United States, and it is called simply *thy-roid* or *thyroid, desiccated.* Desiccation is the term for the drying process used to prepare this drug form. All natural preparations are standardized for their iodine content. The synthetic thyroid

TABLE 31-1 Thyroid Drugs: Clinically Equivalent Doses

Thyroid Drug	Approximate Equivalent Dose
Natural Thyroid Preparation	
Thyroid	60-65 mg (1 grain)
Synthetic Thyroid Preparations	
levothyroxine	100 mcg or more
liothyronine	25 mcg
liotrix	50 mcg/12.5 mcg (T_4/T_3)

T3, Triiodothyronine; *T4,* thyroxine.

preparations are levothyroxine (T_4), liothyronine (T_3), and liotrix (which contains a combination of T_4 and T_3 in a 4:1 ratio). The approximate clinically equivalent doses of the drugs are given in Table 31-1. This information is useful for guiding dosage adjust-ments when a patient is switched from one thyroid hormone to another.

Mechanism of Action and Drug Effects

The thyroid drugs work in the same manner as the endogenous thyroid hormones, affecting many body systems. At the cellular level they work to induce changes in the metabolic rate, including the rate of protein, carbohydrate, and lipid metabolism, and to increase oxygen consumption, body temperature, blood volume, and overall cellular growth and differentiation. These drugs also stimulate the cardiovascular system by increasing the number of myocardial beta-adrenergic receptors. This, in turn, increases the sensitivity of the heart to catecholamines and ultimately increases cardiac output. In addition, thyroid hormones increase renal blood flow and the glomerular filtration rate, which results in a diuretic effect.

Indications

The thyroid preparations are given to replace what the thyroid gland itself cannot produce to achieve normal thyroid hormone levels (**euthyroid** condition). The various thyroid preparations are used in the treatment of all three forms of hypothyroidism, although levothyroxine is generally the preferred drug because its hormonal content is standardized and its effect is therefore predictable. The thyroid drugs can also be used for the diagnosis of suspected hyperthyroidism (as in a TSH-suppression test) and in the prevention or treatment of various types of goiters. They are also used for replacement hormonal therapy in patients whose thyroid glands have been surgically removed or destroyed by ra-dioactive iodine in the treatment of thyroid cancer or hyperthy-roidism. Hypothyroidism during pregnancy should also be treated, with the dose of prescribed thyroid hormones adjusted every 4 weeks to maintain the TSH level at the lower end of the normal range. Fetal growth may be retarded if maternal hypothy-roidism remains untreated during pregnancy.

Contraindications

Contraindications to thyroid preparations include known drug allergy to a given drug product, recent myocardial infarction, adrenal insufficiency, and hyperthyroidism.

TABLE 31-2 Thyroid Drugs: Common Adverse Effects

Body System	Adverse Effects
Cardiovascular	Tachycardia, palpitations, angina, dysrhythmias, hypertension, cardiac arrest
Central nervous	Insomnia, tremors, headache, anxiety
Gastrointestinal	Nausea, diarrhea, increased or decreased appetite, cramps
Other	Menstrual irregularities, weight loss, sweating, heat intolerance, fever

TABLE 31-3 Thyroid Drugs: Interactions

Drug	Action
insulin	Decreased efficacy of insulin (resulting in increased blood glucose levels)
Antidiabetic oral drugs	Decreased efficacy of antidiabetic drugs (resulting in increased blood glucose levels)
estrogen	Reduced thyroid drug activity
digoxin	Decreased digoxin effectiveness
phenytoin and fosphenytoin	Reduced levothyroxine effectiveness
phenobarbital	Reduced levothyroxine effectiveness

Adverse Effects

The adverse effects of thyroid medications are usually the result of overdose. The most significant adverse effect is cardiac dysrhythmia with the risk for life-threatening or fatal irregularities. Other more common undesirable effects are listed in Table 31-2.

Interactions

Thyroid drugs may enhance the activity of oral anticoagulants, the dosages of which may need to be reduced. Taking thyroid preparations concurrently with digitalis glycosides may decrease serum digitalis levels. Cholestyramine binds to thyroid hormone in the gastrointestinal tract, which possibly reduces the absorption of both drugs. Diabetic patients taking a thyroid drug may require increased dosages of their hypoglycemic drugs. In addition, the use of thyroid preparations with epinephrine in patients with coronary disease may induce coronary insufficiency. See Table 31-3 for more drug interactions.

Dosages

For the recommended dosages of the thyroid drugs, see the Dosages table on p. 483.

DRUG PROFILE

There are several drugs that may be administered to treat hypothyroidism. The most commonly used are the synthetic drugs, although some patients experience better results with the animal-derived products. Many factors must be considered before the initiation of drug therapy with a thyroid drug. These include the desired ratio of T_3 to T_4, the cost, and the desired duration of effect. The thyroid hormone replacement drugs are classified as pregnancy category A drugs. They are all contraindicated in patients who have had a hypersensitivity reaction to them in the past and in those with adrenal insufficiency, previous myocardial infarction, or hyperthyroidism.

◆ levothyroxine

Levothyroxine (Levoxyl, Levothroid, Synthroid, others), or T_4, is the most commonly prescribed synthetic thyroid hormone and is generally considered the drug of choice. One advantage it has over the natural thyroid preparations is that it is chemically pure, being 100% T_4 (thyroxine); this makes its effects more predictable than those of both natural thyroid products, which contain T_3 and T_4 in varying ratios (depending on the animal source), and synthetic T_3/T_4 combination drugs (e.g., liotrix). Its half-life is long enough that it only needs to be administered once a day. It is available in oral form and in parenteral form. Pregnancy category A. Liothyronine, liotrix, and desiccated thyroid ("thyroid") are other drug examples. Switching between different brands of levothyroxine during treatment can destabilize the course of treatment and should be minimized. Thyroid function test results should be monitored more carefully when switching is necessary due to cost concerns or drug availability, such as because of drug formulary requirements of the patient's insurance provider. Common dosages are given in the table on p. 483. Levothyroxine is dosed in micrograms. A common medication error is to write the intended dose in milligrams instead of micrograms. If not caught, this error would result in a thousandfold overdose. Doses higher than 200 mcg should be questioned in case this error occurred. Levothyroxine is available in an intravenous form. The intravenous dose is generally 50% of the oral dose.

PHARMACOKINETICS

Route	Onset of Action	Peak Plasma Concentration	Elimination Half-life	Duration of Action
PO	3-5 days	24 hr	6-10 days	24 hr

▌Disease Overview
HYPERTHYROIDISM

The excessive secretion of thyroid hormones, or **hyperthyroidism,** may be caused by several different diseases and drugs. Some of the causative diseases are Graves disease, which is the most common cause; Plummer disease, also known as *toxic nodular disease,* which is the least common cause; multinodular disease; and thyroid storm, which is a severe and potentially life threatening exacerbation of the symptoms of hyperthyroidism that is usually induced by stress or infection.

Hyperthyroidism can affect multiple body systems, resulting in an overall increase in metabolism. Commonly reported symptoms are diarrhea, flushing, increased appetite, muscle weakness, fatigue, palpitations, irritability, nervousness, sleep disorders, heat intolerance, and altered menstrual flow.

▌Pharmacology Overview
ANTITHYROID DRUGS

The treatment of hyperthyroidism may be aimed at treating either the primary cause or the symptoms of the disease. Antithyroid drugs, iodides, ionic inhibitors, surgery, and radioactive

DOSAGES

Selected Thyroid Drug

Drug (Pregnancy Category)	Pharmacologic Class	Usual Dosage Range	Indications
◆ levothyroxine (Synthroid, Levoxyl, others) (A)	Synthetic levothyroxine (thyroid hormone T_4)	**Adult** PO: 25-300 mcg/day (25-200 mcg/day most common) IM/IV: 50% of oral dose IV: 200-500 mcg in a single dose; repeat next day 100-300 mcg if necessary	Hypothyroidism Myxedema coma
		Pediatric 0-12 yr PO: 25-150 mcg/day	Congenital hypothyroidism

IM, Intramuscular; *IV*, intravenous; *PO*, oral.

isotopes of iodine are used to treat the underlying cause, and drugs such as beta-blockers are used to treat the symptoms. The focus of the discussion here is on the antithyroid drugs called the *thioamide* derivatives, namely methimazole and propylthiouracil. In addition to the thioamides, radioactive iodine (iodine 131) may be used to treat hyperthyroidism. Radioactive iodine works by destroying the thyroid gland, in a process known as *ablation*. It does this by emitting destructive beta rays once it is taken up into the follicles of the thyroid gland. It is a commonly used treatment for both hyperthyroidism and thyroid cancer. Thyroid surgery involves removal of part or all of the thyroid gland. It is usually a very effective way to treat hyperthyroidism, but lifelong hormone replacement therapy is normally required after thyroid surgery.

Mechanism of Action and Drug Effects

Methimazole and propylthiouracil act by inhibiting the incorporation of iodine molecules into the amino acid tyrosine, a process required to make both monoiodotyrosine and diiodotyrosine, the precursors of T_3 and T_4. By doing so, these drugs impede the formation of thyroid hormone. Propylthiouracil has the added ability to inhibit the conversion of T_4 to T_3 in the peripheral circulation. Neither drug can inactivate already existing thyroid hormone, however.

The drug effects of methimazole and propylthiouracil are primarily limited to the thyroid gland, and their overall effect is a decrease in the thyroid hormone level. The administration of these medications to patients with hyperthyroidism lowers the high levels of thyroid hormone, thereby normalizing the overall metabolic rate.

Indications

Antithyroid drugs are used to treat hyperthyroidism and to prevent the surge in thyroid hormones that occurs after the surgical treatment of or during radioactive iodine therapy for hyperthyroidism or thyroid cancer. In some types of hyperthyroidism, such as that seen in the Graves disease, the long-term administration of these drugs (for several years) may induce a spontaneous remission. Surgical resection of the thyroid (*thyroidectomy*) is often used both in patients who are intolerant of antithyroid drug therapy and in pregnant women, in whom both antithyroid drugs and radioactive iodine therapy are usually contraindicated.

TABLE 31-4 Antithyroid Drugs: Common Adverse Effects

Body System	Adverse Effects
Central nervous	Drowsiness, headache, vertigo, fever, paresthesia
Gastrointestinal	Nausea, vomiting, diarrhea, jaundice, hepatitis, loss of taste
Genitourinary	Smoky urine, decreased urine output
Hematologic	Agranulocytosis, leukopenia, thrombocytopenia, hypothrombinemia, lymphadenopathy, bleeding
Integumentary	Rash, pruritus, hyperpigmentation
Musculoskeletal	Myalgia, arthralgia, nocturnal muscle cramps
Renal	Increased blood urea nitrogen and serum creatinine levels
Other	Enlarged thyroid, nephritis

Contraindications

The only usual contraindications to the use of the two antithyroid drugs is known drug allergy. These drugs should be avoided in pregnancy whenever possible, and in fact both are rated pregnancy category D. However, they are sometimes used in the lowest effective dosage to treat hyperthyroidism that is exacerbated by the metabolic demands of pregnancy.

Adverse Effects

The most damaging or serious adverse effects of the antithyroid medications are liver and bone marrow toxicity. These and the more common adverse effects of methimazole and propylthiouracil are listed in Table 31-4.

Interactions

Drug interactions that occur with antithyroid drugs include additive leukopenic effects when they are taken in conjunction with other bone marrow depressants and an increase in the activity of oral anticoagulants.

Dosages

For the recommended dosages of propylthiouracil, see the Dosages table on p. 484.

DOSAGES

Selected Antithyroid Drug

Drug (Pregnancy Category)	Pharmacologic Class	Usual Dosage Range	Indications
◆ propylthiouracil* (generic only) (D)	Antithyroid	**Adult** 300-900 mg/day **Pediatric 6-10 yr** PO: 50-150 mg/day **Pediatric older than 10 yr** PO: 150-300 mg/day	Hyperthyroidism

PO, Oral.
*Often abbreviated PTU.

DRUG PROFILE

◆ propylthiouracil

Propylthiouracil (PTU) is a thioamide antithyroid drug and is rated as a pregnancy category D drug. Approximately 2 weeks of therapy with propylthiouracil may be necessary before symptoms improve. It is available only in oral form as a 50-mg tablet. Methimazole is the only alternative drug in this class and is rarely used clinically. Common dosages are given in the table above.

PHARMACOKINETICS

Route	Onset of Action	Peak Plasma Concentration	Elimination Half-life	Duration of Action
PO	24-36 hr	1 hr	1.5-5 hr	2-3 hr

PHARMACOKINETIC BRIDGE
to Nursing Practice

Thyroid replacement drugs possess very specific pharmacokinetic characteristics, as do many drugs. Nurses must understand the pharmacokinetics to think their way critically through clinical situations involving patients who are taking thyroid replacement drugs. For the drug levothyroxine (Synthroid, Levothroid, Levoxyl, Novothyrox), the pharmacokinetic characteristics include an onset of action of 3 to 5 days, peak plasma concentrations within 24 hours, elimination half-life of 6 to 10 days, and a duration of action of 24 hours. Due to the prolonged half-life (see Chapter 2) of this drug, there is an increased risk of toxicity. Toxicity is manifested by the following: weight loss, tachycardia, nervousness, tremors, hypertension, headache, insomnia, menstrual irregularities, and cardiac irregularities or palpitations. Another important pharmacokinetic property is that the drug is more than 99% protein bound. A highly protein-bound drug acts like a biologic sustained-release drug and remains in the body longer, with increased risk of more interactions with other highly protein-bound drugs as well as greater potential for toxicity. This is yet another example of the importance a current and thorough knowledge base about drugs—and specifically about their pharmacokinetics—is to their safe and efficient administration.

NURSING PROCESS

Assessment

Assessment of the patient taking *thyroid replacement drugs* for hypothyroidism includes baseline monitoring of vital signs for comparative purposes. Levels of T_3, T_4, and TSH should also be assessed before and during drug therapy, as ordered. It is also important to thoroughly assess and document any past and present medical problems or concerns with a thorough physical assessment. A medication history should be taken that includes drug allergies and a list of all prescription, over-the-counter drugs, herbals, and supplements the patient is taking. Cautions, contraindications, and drug interactions associated with the use of thyroid hormone have been previously discussed, and the patient should be assessed for these before these medications are given. For the female patient, a thorough assessment of the reproductive system is needed due to the impact of thyroid hormones on this system. It is also important to remember that certain thyroid hormones may work faster than others because of their dosage form and properties (see Pharmacokinetic Bridge to Nursing Practice). Drug interactions that deserve emphasis because of their importance for patient safety and because they involve commonly used medications include the interactions with estrogens, fosphenytoin and phenytoin, insulin, oral antidiabetic drugs, digoxin, phenobarbital, and warfarin (see Table 31-3). If the patient is taking an oral anticoagulant, it is suggested that blood levels of the anticoagulant be monitored. Life span considerations include increased sensitivity to the effects of thyroid medications in the elderly. Individualization of drug therapy is important with thyroid replacement, because different patients may respond very differently to the same drug and/or dosage.

For *antithyroid drugs,* such as propylthiouracil and methimazole (rarely used), it is important first to measure vital signs and to assess for signs and symptoms of thyroid crisis, or what is often called *thyroid storm.* These include tachycardia, cardiac irregularities, fever, heart failure, flushed skin, confusion, apathetic attitude, behavioral changes, possible hypotension, and vascular collapse. Baseline weight and intake and output should also be assessed in patients receiving antithyroid and thyroid preparations. Assessing for thyroid storm also means assessing for potential causes, including thyroidectomy or abrupt withdrawal of antithyroid drugs. Other causes include excess thyroid replacement or failure to give antithyroid medications before thyroid surgery. Related cautions and contraindications have been discussed previously but some important drug interactions to reemphasize include the interactions with oral anticoagulants (which can cause an increase in anticoagulation and thus risk for bleeding) and any

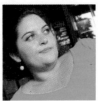
medications that may lead to bone marrow suppression or cause leukopenia.

Nursing Diagnoses

- Risk for injury related to the adverse effects of the medication
- Risk for infection related to the bone marrow depression caused by antithyroid medication
- Acute pain related to the adverse effects of the medication
- Decreased cardiac output related to the adverse effects of the thyroid drugs
- Deficient knowledge related to lack of experience with self-administration of the medication

Planning

Goals

- Patient remains free of injury caused by the adverse effects of the medication.
- Patient is monitored closely (e.g., by measuring thyroid hormone levels) while taking the medication.
- Patient remains free of infection while receiving antithyroid medication.
- Patient maintains normal energy levels while taking thyroid drugs.
- Patient experiences minimal adverse effects resulting from the medication.
- Patient demonstrates an understanding of the use of the thyroid drug and its adverse effects and the need for compliance with the drug regimen by stating this information.

Outcome Criteria

- Patient states the importance of follow-up appointments with the prescriber for frequent blood studies and monitoring of therapeutic effects.
- Patient states ways to decrease the risk for infection while receiving an antithyroid medication, such as avoiding persons with infections, eating a proper diet, and getting adequate rest.
- Patient uses relaxation techniques to deal with the nervousness and irritability caused by the drug or the disease.

Implementation

When *thyroid drugs* are administered, it is important that the drug be given at the same time every day to help maintain consistent blood levels of the drug. If possible, it is best to administer thyroid drugs once daily in the morning to decrease the likelihood of insomnia, which may result from evening dosing and the subsequent increase in energy level. It is also very important to avoid interchanging brands because of problems with the bioequivalence of drugs from different manufacturers. If needed, tablets may be crushed. If the patient is scheduled to undergo radioactive iodine isotope studies, the thyroid medication is usually discontinued about 4 weeks before the test, but only on the prescriber's order. The elderly may require alteration of the dosage amount, with a decrease of 25% for patients 60 years of age or older. See Patient Education Tips for more information.

Use of the *antithyroid drug* propylthiouracil requires education about taking the medication with meals to help decrease stomach upset. Any fever, sore throat, mouth ulcers or sores, or skin eruptions, as well as any unusual bleeding or bruising, should be reported to the prescriber immediately. Patients should be educated not to use iodized salt or eat shellfish because of their potential for altering the drug's effectiveness. Patients should be aware of the signs and symptoms of hypothyroidism, including unexplained weight gain, fatigue, mental depression, and cold intolerance, and should be told to report these should they occur. Frequent monitoring of complete blood counts is needed to watch for potential problems with leukopenia and thrombocytopenia. Monitoring of the results of liver function studies is also important during follow-up visits with the prescriber.

Evaluation

A therapeutic response to *thyroid drugs* is manifested by the disappearance of the symptoms of hypothyroidism, including depression, constipation, loss of appetite, weight gain, cold intolerance, syncope, and dry and brittle hair. Increased nervousness, irritability, mood changes, angina, and palpitations are adverse effects that need to be reported to the prescriber immediately. Clues that a patient is receiving inadequate doses of the thyroid medication include a return of the symptoms of hypothyroidism (see previous discussion). Long-term use of thyroid replacement therapy may cause some bone loss in premenopausal or post-menopausal women, and so a baseline bone density measurement should be documented and bone density evaluated closely during therapy.

A therapeutic response to *antithyroid medications* is manifested by weight gain, decreased pulse, a return to a normal blood pressure, and decreased serum levels of T_4. Symptoms of overdose include cold intolerance, depression, and edema. The patient should be encouraged to report the development of any swelling, sore throat, lesions, or other signs of inflammation. Clues that a patient is not receiving adequate doses include tachycardia, insomnia, irritability, fever, and diarrhea.

PATIENT TEACHING TIPS

- Thyroid replacement drugs should be taken ½ to 1 hour before breakfast to maintain constant hormone levels and to help prevent insomnia.
- These medications should never be abruptly discontinued, and lifelong therapy is usually the norm.
- The importance of keeping follow-up visits so the prescriber can monitor thyroid hormone levels, complete blood counts, and results of liver function studies should be emphasized to the patient.
- Brands of thyroid replacement drugs cannot be interchanged. Patients should always check to be sure that the pharmacy has provided the correct brand of thyroid replacement drug.
- Patients should report any chest pain, weight loss, palpitations, tremors, sweating, nervousness, shortness of breath, or insomnia to the prescriber immediately.
- Keeping a daily journal is encouraged, with notations about how the patient is feeling, energy levels, appetite, and any adverse effects.

- It may take up to 3 to 4 weeks to see the full therapeutic effects of thyroid drugs.
- All thyroid tablets should be protected from light.
- Antithyroid medications are better tolerated when taken with meals or a snack. These drugs should also be given at the same time every day to maintain consistent blood levels of the drug, and they should never be withdrawn abruptly.
- Patients taking thyroid or antithyroid drugs should be instructed not to take any over-the-counter medications without first consulting with the prescriber or pharmacist.
- Patients taking antithyroid medications should avoid eating foods high in iodine, such as tofu and other soy products, turnips, seafood, iodized salt, and some breads. These foods may interfere with the effectiveness of the antithyroid drug.
- Illnesses, weight gain, cold intolerance, and depression should be reported to the prescriber immediately.

POINTS TO REMEMBER

- T_4 and T_3 are the two hormones produced by the thyroid gland; thyroid hormones are made by iodination and coupling with the amino acid tyrosine.
- Thyroid hormone replacement is generally carried out carefully by the prescriber with frequent monitoring of serum levels until stabilization appears to have occurred. Nurses must monitor and review laboratory values to be sure that serum levels are within normal limits to avoid possible toxicity.

- Hyperthyroidism is caused by excessive secretion of thyroid hormone by the thyroid gland and may be caused by different diseases (Graves disease, Plummer disease, and multinodular disease) or drugs. Important information about the patient's medical history should always be assessed and documented appropriately.
- Patients receiving levothyroxine should report the occurrence of excitability, irritability, or anxiety to the prescriber, because these symptoms may indicate toxicity.

NCLEX EXAMINATION REVIEW QUESTIONS

1 When monitoring the laboratory values of a patient who is taking antithyroid drugs, the nurse knows to watch for
  a increased platelet counts.
  b decreased white blood cell counts.
  c decreased blood urea nitrogen level.
  d increased blood glucose levels.

2 The pharmacy has called a patient to notify her that the current brand of thyroid replacement hormone is on back order. The patient calls the clinic to ask what to do. Which is the best response by the nurse?
  a "Go ahead and take the other brand that the pharmacy has available for now."
  b "You should stop the medication until your current brand is available."
  c "You can split the thyroid pills that you have left so that they will last longer."
  d "Let me ask your physician what should be done; we will need to watch how you do if you switch brands."

3 When assessing the older adult patient, the nurse keeps in mind that certain nonspecific symptoms may represent hypothyroidism in older patients, such as:
  a Leukopenia, anemia
  b Loss of appetite, polyuria

  c Weight loss, dry cough
  d Cold intolerance, depression

4 To help with the insomnia associated with thyroid hormone replacement therapy, the nurse should teach the patient to
  a take half the dose at lunchtime and the other half 2 hours later.
  b use a sedative to assist with falling asleep.
  c take the dose first thing in the morning.
  d reduce the dosage as needed if sleep is impaired.

5 When teaching a patient who has a new prescription for thyroid hormone, the nurse should instruct the patient to notify the physician if which adverse effect is noted?
  a Palpitations
  b Headache
  c Anxiety
  d Appetite changes

6 The nurse is giving an intravenous dose of levothyroxine. The order reads: "Give 0.1 mg IV push now." The vial of reconstituted levothyroxine contains 200 mcg. What is the ordered dose in micrograms?

1. b, 2. d, 3. d, 4. c, 5. a, 6. 100 mcg.

CRITICAL THINKING ACTIVITIES: BEST ACTION

1 A patient has been taking thyroid drugs for about 16 months and has recently noted palpitations and some heat intolerance. What is the nurse's best action at this time?

2 A patient with a history of hypothyroidism is in her first trimester of pregnancy. She asks the nurse, "How often will they check my thyroid hormone levels? I'm very worried about how this will affect my baby." What would be the nurse's best response?

3 A 33-year-old man, newly admitted to the medical-surgical unit from the step-down intensive care unit, underwent a thyroidec-

tomy 2 days earlier. While reviewing the orders the nurse notices that the patient is to start receiving his thyroid medication upon transfer to the medical-surgical unit. The written orders specify that 25 mcg of levothyroxine should be given once daily. However, the automated drug-dispensing machine on the unit has 25 mcg of liothyronine stocked. What is the nurse's best action at this time?

For answers, see *http://evolve.elsevier.com/Lilley.*

CHAPTER 32

Antidiabetic Drugs

Tom Lynch, PharmD, BCPS

OBJECTIVES

When you reach the end of this chapter, you should be able to do the following:

1 Discuss the normal actions and functions of the pancreas.

2 Contrast type 1 and type 2 diabetes mellitus with regard to age of onset, signs and symptoms, pharmacologic and nonpharmacologic treatment, incidence, and etiology.

3 Discuss the various factors influencing blood glucose level in nondiabetic individuals and in patients with either type of diabetes mellitus.

4 Identify the various drugs used to manage type 1 and type 2 diabetes mellitus.

5 Discuss the mechanisms of action, indications, contraindications, cautions, drug interactions, and adverse effects of insulin, traditional oral hypoglycemic drugs, and newer antidiabetic drugs.

6 Compare rapid-, short-, intermediate-, and long-acting insulins with regard to their onset of action, peak effects, and duration of action.

7 Compare the signs and symptoms of hypoglycemia and hyperglycemia and their related treatments.

8 Develop a nursing care plan that include all phases of the nursing process for patients with type 1 or type 2 diabetes with a focus on drug therapies.

e-Learning Activities

NCLEX Review Questions • Animations • Nursing Care Plans • Audio Glossary • Category Catchers • Medication Errors Checklists • IV Therapy Checklists • Calculators • Frequently Asked Questions • Content Updates • Supplemental Resources • Answers to Case Studies and Critical Thinking Activities

Drug Profiles

acarbose, p. 500
♦ glipizide, p. 500
♦ insulin glargine and insulin detemir, p. 496
insulin isophane suspension (NPH), p. 496

insulin lispro, p. 495
♦ metformin, p. 500
♦ pioglitazone, p. 500
♦ regular insulin, p. 496
♦ repaglinide, p. 500
♦ sitagliptin, p. 501

♦ *Key drug.*

Glossary

Diabetes mellitus A complex disorder of carbohydrate, fat, and protein metabolism resulting primarily from the lack of insulin secretion by the beta cells of the pancreas or from defects of the insulin receptors; it is commonly referred to simply as *diabetes*. There are two major types of diabetes: type 1 and type 2. (p. 489)

Diabetic ketoacidosis (DKA) A severe metabolic complication of uncontrolled diabetes that, if untreated, leads to diabetic coma and death. (p. 491)

Gestational diabetes Diabetes that develops during pregnancy. It may resolve after pregnancy but may also be a precursor of type 2 diabetes in later life. (p. 492)

Glucagon A hormone produced by the alpha cells in the islets of Langerhans that stimulates the conversion of glycogen to glucose in the liver. (p. 489)

Glucose One of the simple sugars that serves as a major source of energy. It is found in foods (e.g., fruits, refined sweets) and also is the final breakdown product of complex carbohydrate metabolism in the body; it is also commonly referred to as *dextrose*. (p. 489)

Glycogen A polysaccharide that is the major carbohydrate stored in animal cells. (p. 489)

Glycogenolysis The breakdown of glycogen to glucose. (p. 489)

Hemoglobin A1C (A1C) Hemoglobin molecules to which glucose molecules are bound; blood levels of hemoglobin A1C are used as a diagnostic measure of average daily blood glucose levels in the monitoring of diabetes; it is also called *glycosylated hemoglobin* or *glycated hemoglobin*. (p. 493)

Hyperglycemia A fasting blood glucose level of 126 mg/dL or higher or a nonfasting blood glucose level of 200 mg/dL or higher. (p. 489)

Hyperosmolar nonketotic syndrome (HNKS) A metabolic complication of uncontrolled diabetes, similar in severity to diabetic ketoacidosis but without ketosis and acidosis. (p. 492)

Hypoglycemia A blood glucose level of less that 50 mg/dL. (p. 501)

Impaired fasting glucose level A fasting glucose level of at least 110 mg/dL but lower than 126 mg/dL; it defines a prediabetic state that is sometimes called *prediabetes*. (p. 493)

Insulin A naturally occurring hormone secreted by the beta cells of the islets of Langerhans in the pancreas in response to increased levels of glucose in the blood. (p. 489)

Ketones Organic chemical compounds produced through the oxidation of secondary alcohols (e.g., fat molecules), including dietary carbohydrates. (p. 489)

Polydipsia Chronic excessive intake of water; it is a common symptom of diabetes. (p. 489)

Polyphagia Excessive eating; it is a common symptom of diabetes. (p. 489)

Polyuria Increased frequency or volume of urinary output; it is a common symptom of diabetes. (p. 489)

Type 1 diabetes mellitus Diabetes mellitus that is a genetically determined autoimmune disorder characterized by a complete or nearly complete lack of insulin production; it most commonly arises in children or adolescents. (p. 490)

Type 2 diabetes mellitus A type of diabetes mellitus that most commonly presents in adults. The disease may be controlled by lifestyle modifications, oral drug therapy, and/or insulin, but patients are not necessarily dependent on insulin. (p. 492)

• • •

Anatomy, Physiology, and Disease Overview

PANCREAS

The pancreas is a large, elongated organ that is located behind the stomach. It is both an exocrine gland (secreting digestive enzymes through the pancreatic duct) and an endocrine gland (secreting hormones directly into the bloodstream and not through a duct). The endocrine functions of the pancreas are the focus of this chapter. Two main hormones are produced by the pancreas: **insulin** and **glucagon.** Both hormones play an important role in the regulation of glucose homeostasis, specifically the use, mobilization, and storage of glucose by the body. **Glucose** is one of the primary sources of energy for the cells of the body. It is also the simplest form of carbohydrate (sugar) found in the body and is often referred to by the name of its D-isomer form, *dextrose.* There is a normal amount of glucose that circulates in the blood to meet requirements for quick energy. However, not all of the glucose consumed is needed. When the quantity of glucose in the blood is sufficient, the excess is stored as **glycogen** in the liver and, to a lesser extent, in skeletal muscle tissue, where it remains until the body needs it. Glucose is also stored in adipose tissue as triglyceride body fat.

When more circulating glucose is needed, glycogen—primarily that stored in the liver—is converted back to glucose through a process called **glycogenolysis.** The hormone responsible for initiating this process is glucagon. Glucagon has only minimal effects on muscle glycogen and adipose tissue triglyceride stores.

Glucagon is a protein hormone consisting of a single chain of amino acids (polypeptide chain). Its molecules are about half the size of those of insulin. Glucagon is released from the alpha cells of the islets of Langerhans in the pancreas. The beta cells of these same islets secrete insulin, a protein hormone composed of two amino acid chains (acidic A chain and basic B chain) joined by a disulfide linkage. There is a continuous homeostatic balance in the body between the actions of insulin and those of glucagon. This natural balance serves to maintain physiologically optimal blood glucose levels, which normally range between 70 and 100 mg/dL. Because of the critical role of the pancreas in producing and maintaining these two hormones, the drastic measure of *pancreatic transplant* is now sometimes undertaken to treat type 1 diabetes that has not been successfully controlled by other means. Another treatment, which is becoming more common, is continuous insulin administration via a mechanized *insulin pump.*

Insulin serves several important metabolic functions in the body. It stimulates carbohydrate metabolism in skeletal and cardiac muscle and in adipose tissue by facilitating the transport of glucose into these cells. In the liver, insulin facilitates the phosphorylation of glucose to glucose-6-phosphate, which is then converted to glycogen for storage. By causing glucose to be stored in the liver as glycogen, insulin keeps the kidney free of glucose. Without insulin, the kidneys are unable to reabsorb the excess glucose and then excrete large amounts of glucose (a critical body nutrient and energy source), **ketones,** and other solutes into the urine. This loss of nutrient energy sources eventually leads to **polyphagia,** weight loss, and malnutrition. The presence of these solutes in the distal renal tubules and collecting ducts also draws large volumes of water into the urine through *osmotic diuresis,* which leads to **polyuria,** dehydration, and **polydipsia.** Insulin also has a direct effect on fat metabolism. It stimulates lipogenesis and inhibits lipolysis and the release of fatty acids from adipose cells. In addition, insulin stimulates protein synthesis and promotes the intracellular shift of potassium and magnesium, thereby decreasing elevated blood concentrations of these electrolytes. Other substances such as cortisol, epinephrine, and growth hormone work synergistically with glucagon to counter the effects of insulin and cause increases in the blood glucose level.

DIABETES MELLITUS

Hyperglycemia is a state involving excessive concentrations of glucose in the blood and results when the normal counterbalancing actions of glucagon and insulin fail to maintain normal glucose homeostasis (i.e., serum levels of 70 to 100 mg/dL). Complications in protein and fat metabolism (*dyslipidemia;* see Chapter 29) are also involved. The current key diagnostic criterion for **diabetes mellitus** is hyperglycemia with a fasting plasma glucose level of higher than 126 mg/dL. Diagnostic indicators are described in more detail in Box 32-1. It is important to note that the definition of diabetes established by the American Diabetes Association (ADA) differs from that issued by the American College of Endocrinology. This text uses the ADA as a reference.

Diabetes mellitus, more commonly referred to simply as *diabetes,* is primarily a disorder of carbohydrate metabolism that involves either a deficiency of insulin, a resistance of tissue (e.g., muscle, liver) to insulin, or both. Whatever the cause of the diabetes, the result is hyperglycemia. Uncontrolled hyperglycemia correlates strongly with serious long-term *macrovas-*

BOX 32-1 Criteria for Diagnosis of Diabetes

Fasting plasma glucose level of 126 mg/dL or higher. "Fasting" is defined as no caloric intake for at least 8 hours.
OR
Symptoms of diabetes plus casual plasma glucose level of 200 mg/dL or higher. "Casual" means measured at any time of day without regard to time since last meal. The classic symptoms of hyperglycemia include polyuria, polydipsia, and unexplained weight loss.
OR
Two-hour plasma glucose level of 200 mg/dL or higher during an *oral glucose tolerance test (OGTT).* The glucose load should contain the equivalent of 75 gm of glucose dissolved in water. Note that the OGTT is not recommended for routine clinical use.

Any positive finding for the above assessments should be confirmed by repeat testing on a different day.

TABLE 32-1 Major Long-Term Consequences of Type 1 and Type 2 Diabetes

Pathology	Possible Consequences
Macrovascular (Atherosclerotic Plaque)	
Coronary arteries	Myocardial infarction
Cerebral arteries	Stroke
Peripheral vessels	Peripheral vascular disease (e.g., neuropathies [see below], foot ulcers, possible amputations)
Microvascular (Capillary Damage)	
Retinopathy (retinal damage)	Partial or complete blindness
Neuropathy (autonomic and somatic nerve damage, due to both metabolic alterations and compromised circulation)	Autonomic nerve damage: For example, diabetic gastroparesis, bladder dysfunction, unawareness of hypoglycemia
	Somatic nerve damage: For example, diabetic foot ulcer and/or leg or foot amputation (resulting from undetected injuries due to loss of sensation and also from compromised circulation)
Nephropathy (kidney damage)	Proteinuria (microalbuminuria), chronic renal failure (may require dialysis or kidney transplantation)

Data from American Diabetes Association. Available at *www.diabetes.org*.

cular and *microvascular* complications. Macrovascular complications are usually secondary to large vessel damage caused by deposition of atherosclerotic plaque. This compromises both central and peripheral circulation. In contrast, microvascular complications are secondary to damage to the capillary vessels, which impairs peripheral circulation. In addition, both autonomic and somatic nerve damage occur, caused primarily by the metabolic changes themselves and to a lesser degree by the compromised circulation. Table 32-1 lists common long-term complications of diabetes.

Diabetes mellitus has been recognized since 1550 BC, when Egyptians wrote of a malady they called *honeyed urine*. The first step toward discerning the cause of diabetes mellitus occurred in 1788 when Thomas Cawley, an English physician, voiced his suspicion that the source of the illness lay in the pancreas. However, it took over a century to prove this conjecture correct, and it took even longer to discover the active substance, insulin, that is secreted from the pancreas. Not until the early 1920s was insulin finally isolated. Its discovery is now considered one of the greatest triumphs of twentieth-century medicine, and its use in the treatment of diabetes mellitus has proved to be life saving for millions of people affected by the disease.

Diabetes mellitus actually is not a single disease, but a group of diseases. For this reason, it is often regarded as a syndrome rather than a disease. In some cases, diabetes is caused by a relative or absolute lack of insulin that is believed to result from the destruction of beta cells in the pancreas. As a result, insulin cannot be produced. However, hyperglycemia can also be caused by defects in insulin receptors that results in *insulin resistance*. The proteins that serve as insulin receptors are attached to the surface of cells in the liver, muscle, and adipose tissue. These proteins are stimulated by insulin molecules to remove glucose molecules

from the blood. When these proteins become defective, they no longer respond normally to insulin molecules. The result is that glucose molecules remain in the blood, rather than being stored in the tissues.

Two major types of diabetes mellitus are currently recognized and designated by the ADA: type 1 and type 2. Type 1 diabetes was previously called *insulin-dependent diabetes mellitus (IDDM)* or *juvenile-onset diabetes*. Type 2 diabetes was previously called *non–insulin-dependent diabetes mellitus (NIDDM)* or *adult-onset diabetes*. The numerical designations for both conditions were adopted by the ADA as the preferred terms in 1995. The previous designations were abandoned for several reasons. One reason is that many patients with type 2 diabetes *do* eventually become dependent on insulin therapy for control of their illness. A second reason is that the current epidemic of both child and adult obesity in the United States is increasing the incidence of type 2 diabetes in children and adolescents. This condition is now called *maturity-onset diabetes of youth (MODY)* and refers in general to hyperglycemia in persons younger than 25 years of age. Obesity is one of the major risk factors for the development of type 2 diabetes. Nonwhite ethnic groups, including African, Asian, and Hispanic Americans and Native Americans, are all at higher risk for the disease than are whites. The usual differences between type 1 and type 2 diabetes mellitus are listed in Table 32-2. Interestingly, approximately 10% of patients with type 2 diabetes have circulating antibodies that suggest an autoimmune origin for the disease. This condition is known as *latent autoimmune diabetes in adults (LADA)* and is basically a more slowly progressing form of type 1 diabetes.

The most common signs and symptoms of diabetes are elevated blood glucose level (fasting glucose level higher than 126 mg/dL) and polyuria, polydipsia, polyphagia, glucosuria, weight loss, and fatigue.

Type 1 Diabetes Mellitus

Type 1 diabetes mellitus is characterized by a lack of insulin production or by the production of defective insulin, which results in acute hyperglycemia. Affected patients require exogenous insulin to lower the blood glucose level and prevent diabetic complications. It is believed that a genetically determined autoimmune reaction gradually destroys the insulin-producing beta cells of the pancreatic islets of Langerhans (Figure 32-1). The *preclinical* phase of beta cell destruction may be prolonged, possibly lasting several years. At some critical point, a rapid transition from preclinical to clinical type 1 diabetes occurs. This transition is believed to be triggered by a specific event such as an acute illness or major emotional stress. An unidentified viral infection is also strongly suspected as an environmental trigger. The stressor triggers the release of the counter-regulatory hormones cortisol and epinephrine. These hormones then mobilize glucagon to release glucose from the storage sites in the liver. This further increases the already rising levels of glucose in the blood secondary to islet cell damage. At some point during this critical cascade of events an autoimmune reaction may be initiated that destroys the insulin-producing beta cells of the pancreatic islets of Langerhans. The result is essentially a complete lack of endogenous insulin production by the pancreas, which necessitates long-term insulin replacement therapy. Fortunately, type 1 diabetes accounts for fewer than 10% of all diabetes cases.

TABLE 32-2 Characteristics of Type 1 and Type 2 Diabetes

Characteristic	Type 1	Type 2
Etiology	Autoimmune destruction of beta cells in the pancreas	Multifactorial genetic defects; strong association with obesity and insulin resistance resulting from a reduction in the number or activity of insulin receptors
Incidence	10% of cases	90% of cases
Onset	Juvenile onset, age younger than 20 yr	Previously maturity onset, age older than 40 yr; now increasingly seen in younger adults and even adolescents—attributed to obesity epidemic
Endogenous insulin	Little or none	Normal levels
Insulin receptors	Normal	Decreased or defective
Body weight	Usually nonobese	Obese (80% of cases)
Treatment	Insulin	Weight loss, diet and exercise, and oral hypoglycemics; only about one third of all patients need insulin

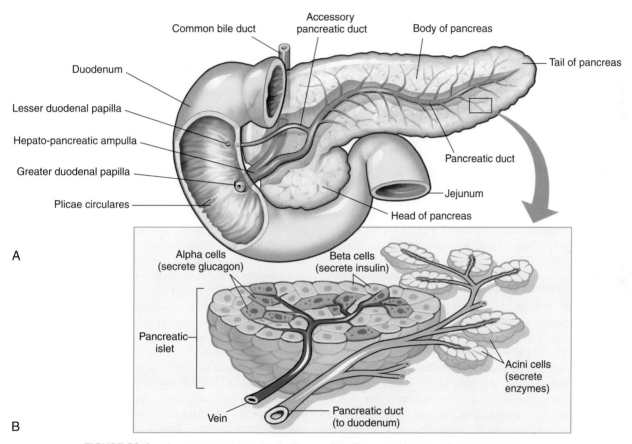

FIGURE 32-1 The pancreas. **A,** Pancreas dissected to show main and accessory ducts. **B,** Exocrine glandular cells (around small pancreatic ducts) and endocrine glandular cells of the pancreatic islets (adjacent to blood capillaries). Exocrine pancreatic cells secrete pancreatic enzymes, alpha endocrine cells secrete glucagon, and beta endocrine cells secrete insulin. (From Thibodeau GA, Patton K: *Anatomy and physiology,* ed 6, St Louis, 2007, Mosby.)

Acute Diabetic Complications: Diabetic Ketoacidosis and Hyperosmolar Nonketotic Syndrome

When blood glucose levels are high but no insulin is present to allow glucose to be used for energy production, the body may break down fatty acids for fuel, producing ketones as a metabolic by-product. If this occurs to a sufficient degree, **diabetic ketoacidosis (DKA)** may result. DKA is a complex multisystem complication of uncontrolled diabetes. Without treatment, DKA will lead to coma and death. DKA is characterized by extreme hyperglycemia, the presence of ketones in the serum, acidosis, dehydration, and electrolyte imbalances. Approximately 25% to

TABLE 32-3 Comparison of Features of Diabetic Ketoacidosis and Hyperosmolar Nonketotic Syndrome

	Condition	
Feature	Diabetic Ketoacidosis	Hyperosmolar Nonketotic Syndrome
Age of patient	Usually younger than 40 yr	Usually older than 40 yr
Duration of symptoms	Usually less than 2 days	Usually longer than 5 days
Serum glucose level	Usually less than 800 mg/dL	Usually higher than 800 mg/dL
Serum Na level	More likely to be normal or low	More likely to be normal or high
Serum K level	High, normal, or low	High, normal, or low
Serum HCO₃ level	Low	Normal
Ketone bodies	At least 4+ in 1:1 dilution	Less than 2+ in 1:1 dilution
pH	Low	Normal
Serum osmolality	Usually less than 350 mOsm/kg	Usually more than 350 mOsm/kg
Cerebral edema	Often subclinical; occasionally clinical	Not evaluated if subclinical; rarely clinical
Prognosis	3% to 10% mortality	10% to 20% mortality
Subsequent course	Insulin therapy required in virtually all cases	Insulin therapy not required in many cases

From Harmel AP, Mathur R: *Davidson's diabetes mellitus: diagnosis and treatment,* ed 5, Philadelphia, 2004, Saunders.

30% of patients with newly diagnosed type 1 diabetes mellitus present with DKA. Another complication of comparable severity that is also triggered by extreme hyperglycemia is **hyperosmolar nonketotic syndrome (HNKS).** The most common precipitator of DKA and HNKS is some type of physical or emotional stress. It was formerly believed that DKA occurred only in type 1 diabetes and HNKS occurred only in type 2 diabetes. However, it is now recognized that both disorders can occur with diabetes of either type, and this overlap is increasingly common with the rapidly decreasing age of patients with type 2 diabetes.

Table 32-3 describes the subtle differences between these two acute diabetic complications. Treatment for either involves fluid and electrolyte replacement as well as intravenous insulin therapy (more common for DKA).

Type 2 Diabetes Mellitus

Type 2 diabetes mellitus is by far the most common form of diabetes, accounting for at least 90% of all cases of diabetes mellitus and affecting as much as 20% of the population over 70 years of age. Over 17 million people in the United States have this disease. In part because this form of diabetes does not always require insulin therapy, there are many common and dangerous misconceptions regarding type 2 diabetes mellitus: that it is a mild diabetes; that it is easy to treat; and that tight metabolic control is unnecessary because these patients, who are mostly older adults, will die before diabetic complications develop. The clinical realities of this disease demonstrate otherwise, however.

Type 2 diabetes mellitus is caused by both insulin resistance and insulin deficiency, but there is not an absolute lack of insulin as in type 1 diabetes. One of the normal roles of insulin is to facilitate the uptake of circulating glucose molecules into tissues to be used as energy. In type 2 diabetes all of the main target tissues of insulin (muscle, liver, and adipose tissue) are hyporesponsive (resistant) to the effects of the hormone. Not only is the absolute number of insulin receptors in these tissues reduced, but their individual sensitivity and responsiveness to insulin is decreased as well. Therefore, it is possible for a patient with type 2 diabetes mellitus to have normal or even elevated levels of insulin yet still have high blood glucose levels. Another reason for this para-doxical situation is that the altered insulin receptor dynamics also cause the liver to overproduce glucose, which exacerbates the already present hyperglycemic condition. All of these processes also result in impaired postprandial (after a meal) glucose metabolism. This is another problematic feature of type 2 diabetes that contributes to the hazardous hyperglycemic state.

In addition to the reduction in the number and sensitivity of insulin receptors in type 2 diabetes, there is often reduced insulin secretion by the pancreas. This insulin deficiency results from a loss of the normal responsiveness of the beta cells in the pancreas to elevated blood glucose levels. When the beta cells do not recognize glucose, they do not secrete insulin, and the normal insulin-facilitated transport of glucose into cells of muscle, liver, and adipose tissue does not occur. This situation is analogous to the loss of responsiveness of insulin receptors to insulin described earlier.

Type 2 diabetes is a multifaceted disorder. Although loss of blood glucose control is its primary hallmark, several other significant conditions are strongly associated with the disease. These include obesity, coronary heart disease, dyslipidemia, hypertension, microalbuminuria (spilling of protein into the urine), and an increased risk for thrombotic (blood clotting) events. For patients with type 2 diabetes, the ADA recommends the regular use of aspirin for prevention of coronary artery heart disease and antihyperlipidemic drug therapy (see Chapter 29), when applicable, in addition to any necessary antidiabetic drug therapy. These comorbidities are strongly associated with the development of type 2 diabetes and are collectively referred to as *metabolic syndrome* (also known as *insulin-resistance syndrome* and *syndrome X*). Roughly 90% of patients with diabetes are obese at the time of initial diagnosis. Obesity serves only to worsen the insulin resistance, because adipose tissue is often the site of a large proportion of the body's defective insulin receptors.

Gestational Diabetes

Gestational diabetes is a type of hyperglycemia that develops during pregnancy. Relatively uncommon, it occurs in about 4% of pregnancies. The use of insulin is necessary to decrease the risk of birth defects. In most cases gestational diabetes subsides after delivery. However, as many as 30% of patients who experience gestational diabetes are estimated to develop type 2 diabetes within 10 to 15 years.

All pregnant women should have blood glucose screenings at regular prenatal visits. Women who develop gestational diabetes should be screened for lingering diabetes 6 to 8 weeks postpartum. They should also be advised of their increased risk for recurrent diabetes and of the importance of regular medical checkups. Finally, women who are known to be diabetic before pregnancy should ideally have detailed prepregnancy counseling (and therefore preferably a planned pregnancy) and prenatal care from a prescriber experienced in managing pregnancies in diabetic women. Specific drug therapy issues pertaining to gestational diabetes are discussed further in the section on insulins.

Prevention and Screening

Both macrovascular and microvascular problems are now recognized to occur at fasting plasma glucose (FPG) levels as low as 126 mg/dL, where "fasting" is defined loosely as an overnight fast (no food from midnight until after the blood sample is taken in the morning). **Impaired fasting glucose level** is defined as an FPG level higher than or equal to 100 mg/dL but less than 126 mg/dL. This condition often proves to be a precursor to diabetes and is therefore sometimes referred to as *prediabetes.* Another recognized prediabetic condition is *impaired glucose tolerance,* which is identified using an oral glucose challenge test (see Box 32-1). The ADA, the National Institute of Diabetes and Digestive and Kidney Diseases, and the Centers for Disease Control and Prevention recommend that all adults 45 years of age and older be screened for elevated FPG levels every 3 years. Several preventive measures are also recommended. Reducing alcohol consumption is helpful, because alcohol is broken down in the body to simple carbohydrates, which leads to increases in blood glucose levels. Regular exercise, in addition to having beneficial effects on weight and high blood pressure, also lowers blood glucose levels by increasing insulin receptor sensitivity.

Nonpharmacologic Treatment Interventions

Patients diagnosed with type 1 diabetes almost always require insulin therapy. For patients with new-onset type 2 diabetes, lifestyle changes should always be initiated as a first step in treatment. The benefits of weight loss, as noted earlier, are that it not only lowers the blood glucose and lipid levels of these patients, but it also reduces another common comorbidity, hypertension. Other recommended lifestyle changes include improved dietary habits (e.g., consumption of a diet higher in protein and lower in fat and carbohydrates), smoking cessation, reduced alcohol consumption, and regular physical exercise. Cigarette smoking doubles the risk of cardiovascular disease in diabetic patients, largely because of its effects on peripheral vascular circulation and respiratory function. In fact, smoking cessation would probably save far more lives than antihypertensive, antilipemic, and antidiabetic drug treatment combined!

Glycemic Goal of Treatment

The glycemic goal recommended by the ADA for diabetic patients is a **hemoglobin A1C (A1C)** level of less than 7%. The HbA1C test measures the percentage of hemoglobin A that is irreversibly glycosylated. A1C is an indicator of glycemic control in a patient over the preceding 2 to 3 months (the average life span of a red blood cell) and is not affected by recent fluctuations in blood glucose levels.

Pharmacology Overview

ANTIDIABETIC DRUGS

Two major classes of drugs traditionally used to treat diabetes mellitus are the insulins and the oral hypoglycemic drugs. In addition, several new classes of drugs with unique mechanisms of action have been developed that may be used in addition to insulins or oral hypoglycemic drugs to treat resistant diabetes. All of these drugs are more broadly referred to as *antidiabetic drugs,* and they are aimed at producing a normoglycemic or euglycemic (normal blood glucose) state.

INSULINS

Patients with type 2 diabetes are not generally prescribed insulin until other measures—namely, lifestyle changes and oral drug therapy—no longer provide adequate glycemic control. Currently insulin is synthesized in laboratories using recombinant deoxyribonucleic acid (DNA) technology and is referred to as *human insulin.* Insulin was originally isolated from cattle or pigs, but bovine (cow) and porcine (pig) insulins are associated with a higher incidence of allergic reactions and insulin resistance than human insulin and are no longer available on the U.S. market. Recombinant insulin is produced by bacteria or yeast that have been altered to contain the genetic information necessary for them to reproduce an insulin that is exactly like human insulin. The pharmacokinetic properties of insulin (onset of action, peak effect, and duration of action) can also be altered by making various minor modifications to either the insulin molecule itself or the drug formulation (final product). This practice has led to the development of many different insulin preparations, including several combination insulin products that contain more than one type of insulin in the same solution. Chemical manipulation of insulin activity in this way helps to meet the often very individual time-oriented metabolic demands for insulin of diabetic patients. Further modifications can be accomplished by mixing compatible insulin preparations in the syringe before administration. The latest syringe compatibility data for currently available insulin products are given in Table 32-4. Patients should be thoroughly educated regarding how, when, and whether they should (or should not) mix different types of insulin. Some combinations are chemically incompatible and can result in undesirable alteration of glycemic effects.

Mechanism of Action and Drug Effects

Exogenously administered insulin functions as a substitute for the endogenous hormone. It serves to replace the insulin that is either not made at all or is made defectively in the body of a diabetic patient. The drug effects of exogenously administered insulin are many and involve many body systems. They are the same as those of normal endogenous insulin. That is, exogenously administered insulin restores the diabetic patient's ability to metabolize carbohydrates, fats, and proteins; to store glucose in the liver; and to convert glycogen to fat stores. Insulin pumps are a

TABLE 32-4 Insulin Mixing Compatibilities

Type of Insulin	Compatible with
regular insulin (Humulin R, Novolin R)	All insulins except glargine, and glulisine
insulin glulisine (Apidra)	NPH only
insulin lispro (Humalog), insulin aspart (NovoLog)	Regular, NPH insulins
insulin detemir (Levemir)	Must be given alone
insulin glargine (Lantus)	Must be given alone due to low pH of diluent
NPH 70% and regular insulin 30% (Humulin 70/30, Novolin 70/30) NPH 50% and regular insulin 50% (Humulin 50/50) insulin aspart protamine suspension 75% and insulin aspart 25% (NovoLog Mix 75/25) insulin lispro protamine suspension 75% and insulin lispro 25% (Humalog Mix 75/25)	Premixed; do not mix with other insulins

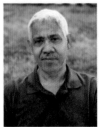
very attractive way to administer insulin to patients. The insulin pump provides an alternative to multiple daily subcutaneous injections and allows patients to match their insulin intake to their lifestyle. When an insulin pump is used, insulin is administered constantly over a 24-hour period, and the patient is then allowed to give bolus injections based on the amount of food ingested. Insulin pumps are described further in the nursing section.

Indications

All insulin preparations can be used to treat both type 1 and type 2 diabetes, but each patient requires careful customization of the dosing regimen for optimal glycemic control. Additional therapeutic approaches such as lifestyle modifications (e.g., improved dietary and exercise habits) are also indicated and, for type 2 diabetes, oral drug therapy as well.

Contraindications

Contraindications to the use of all insulin products include known drug allergy to the specific product. Insulin also should never be administered to an already hypoglycemic patient.

Adverse Effects

Hypoglycemia resulting from excessive insulin dosing can result in shock and possibly death. This is the most immediate and serious adverse effect of insulin. Other adverse effects of insulin therapy include weight gain, lipodystrophy at the site of repeated injections, and in rare cases allergic reactions.

Interactions

Drug interactions that can occur with the insulins are significant. Corticosteroids, niacin, thiazide and loop diuretics, sympathomimetic drugs, and thyroid hormones (both endogenous and exogenous) all can antagonize the hypoglycemic effects of insulin (which results in elevated blood glucose levels). Alcohol, anabolic steroids, sulfa drugs, clofibrate, monoamine oxidase inhibitors, and salicylates all can increase insulin's hypoglycemic effects, which leads to lower blood glucose levels. Nonselective beta-blockers (see Chapter 19) may mask the tachycardia from hypoglycemia caused by insulin and the sulfonylureas, and the hypoglycemic effect of insulin and the sulfonylureas may be enhanced. Insulin increases the risk of hypoglycemia when administered with other hypoglycemic drugs.

Dosages

For the recommended dosages of the various insulin products, see the Dosages table on p. 495. The concentration of insulin is expressed as the number of units of insulin per milliliter. Insulin is usually given by subcutaneous injection or via a subcutaneous infusion pump. In emergency situations requiring prompt insulin action, regular insulin can be given intravenously.

Insulin Use in Special Populations

Two special patient populations for whom careful attention is required during insulin therapy are pediatric patients and pregnant women. Insulin dosages for both are calculated by weight as they are for the general adult population. The usual dosage range is 0.5 to 1 units/kg/day as a total daily dose. The nurse must be aware of a few important differences regarding the use of some insulin products in pediatric populations. The rapid-acting insulin lispro is approved for use in children older than 3 years of age and is often used in combination with oral sulfonylurea therapy (discussed later in the chapter). However, the combination lispro product Humalog 75/25, which contains 75% insulin lispro protamine (an intermediate-acting insulin) and 25% insulin lispro (a rapid-acting insulin), is *not* currently approved for use in children younger than 18 years of age. Children need age-appropriate education and supervision by health

DOSAGES

Selected Human-Based Insulin Products

Drug (Pregnancy Category)	Pharmacologic Class	Usual Dosage Range	Indications
Rapid Acting insulin lispro (Humalog) (B)	Human recombinant rapid-acting insulin analogue	Subcut: 0.5-1 unit/kg/day; doses are highly individualized to desired glycemic control; rapid-acting insulins are best given 15 min before a meal May be given per sliding scale; may also be given via continuous subcutaneous infusion pump	
Short Acting ◆ regular insulin (Humulin R, Novolin R) (B)	Human recombinant short-acting insulin	Subcut: Same dosage as insulin lispro; subcut doses of regular insulin are best given 30 to 60 min before a meal Regular insulin may also be given per sliding scale and is the insulin usually given IV as a continuous infusion	Diabetes mellitus type 1 and type 2
Long Acting insulin glargine (Lantus) (C)	Human recombinant long-acting insulin analogue	Subcut only: Same dosage as others but is approved only for once- or twice-daily dosage (basal dosing)	

IV, Intravenous; *Subcut,* subcutaneous.

care professionals and parents, which includes a safe and gradual transfer of responsibility for self-management of their illness.

Pregnant women also require special care with regard to diabetes management. Gestational diabetes reportedly occurs in approximately 4% of pregnancies in the United States. Although most of these mothers will return to a normal glycemic state after pregnancy, they are at risk of developing diabetes again in later life. All currently available oral and injectable antidiabetic drugs are classified as pregnancy category B or C. Oral medications are generally not recommended for pregnant patients because of a lack of firm safety data. For this reason, insulin therapy is the only currently recommended drug therapy for pregnant women with diabetes. Roughly 15% of women who develop gestational diabetes require insulin therapy during pregnancy. Insulins, both endogenous and exogenous, do not normally cross the placenta. However, insulin is normally excreted into human milk. It is currently unknown whether insulin glargine is excreted in breast milk, and thus it should not be used in women while they are breast-feeding. It is very important that insulin therapy and diet be well controlled for a nursing mother, because inadequate or excessive glycemic control may reduce milk production. Effective glycemic control during pregnancy is also essential, because infants born to women with gestational diabetes have a twofold to threefold greater risk of congenital anomalies. In addition, the incidence of stillbirth is directly related to the degree of maternal hyperglycemia. Weight reduction is generally *not* advised for these women, because it can jeopardize fetal nutritional status.

DRUG PROFILES

There are currently four major classes of insulin, as determined by their pharmacokinetic properties: rapid acting, short acting, intermediate acting, and long acting. The duration of action ranges from several hours to over 24 hours depending on the insulin class (Figure 32-2). The insulin dosage regimen for all diabetic patients is highly individualized and may consist of one or more classes of insulin administered at either fixed dosages or variable dosages in response to self-measurements of blood glucose level. With insulins, color and appearance is important to understand for patient safety and for the prevention of adverse effects and complications. Several insulins are clear, colorless solutions. These include regular insulin, insulin lispro (Humalog), and insulin glargine (Lantus). Other insulins, such as NPH insulin (insulin isophane) are white opaque (cloudy) solutions. This issue is discussed further in the Implementation subsection under Nursing Process.

RAPID-ACTING INSULINS
insulin lispro
There are currently three insulin products that are classified as rapid acting: insulin lispro (Humalog), insulin aspart (NovoLog), and the most recently developed, insulin glulisine (Apidra). These have the most rapid onset of action (roughly 15 minutes) as well as a shorter duration of action than other insulin categories. The effect of insulin lispro is most like that of the endogenous insulin produced by the pancreas in response to a meal. After a meal, the glucose that is ingested stimulates the pancreas to secrete insulin. This insulin then chemically facilitates uptake of the excess glucose at hepatic insulin receptor sites for storage in the liver as glycogen. In people with diabetes mellitus, the insulin response to meals is deficient; therefore, a rapid-acting insulin product is often used

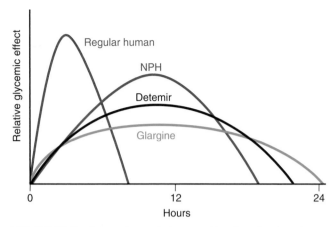

FIGURE 32-2   Comparison of pharmacokinetics of various insulins. (Modified from McMahon GT, Dluhy RG: Intention to treat—initiating insulin and the 4-T Study, *N Engl J Med* 357:1759-1761, 2007.)

within 15 minutes of mealtime. This corresponds to the time required for the onset of action of these products. It is essential that a diabetic patient eat a meal after injection. Otherwise profound hypoglycemia may result. Insulin lispro was approved by the U.S. Food and Drug Administration (FDA) in 1996, becoming the first new insulin product to appear on the U.S. market in 14 years.

PHARMACOKINETICS

Route	Onset of Action	Peak Plasma Concentration	Elimination Half-life	Duration of Action
Subcut	15 min	1-2 hr	80 min	3-5 hr

SHORT-ACTING INSULIN
◆ regular insulin
Regular insulin (Humulin R) is currently the only insulin that is classified as a short-acting insulin. Regular insulin is the usual insulin product to be dosed via intravenous bolus, intravenous infusion, or even intramuscularly. These routes, especially the intravenous infusion route, are often used in cases of DKA or coma associated with uncontrolled type 1 diabetes.

Regular insulin solution was actually the first medicinal insulin product developed. As noted earlier, it was originally isolated from bovine and porcine sources, but it is now made primarily from human insulin sources using recombinant DNA technology.

For clarity, some of the differences between regular insulin and the newer rapid-acting drugs should be noted. Both insulin lispro and insulin aspart are human insulin analogues. This means that they are insulin molecules with synthetic alterations to their chemical structures that alter their onset or duration of action. Both of these insulins have a faster onset of action and a shorter time to peak plasma level, but also a shorter duration of action, than does regular insulin.

PHARMACOKINETICS

Route	Onset of Action	Peak Plasma Concentration	Elimination Half-life	Duration of Action
Subcut	30-60 min	2.5 hr	Unknown	6-10 hr

INTERMEDIATE-ACTING INSULINS
insulin isophane suspension (NPH)
Insulin isophane suspension (also known as NPH insulin) is currently the only available intermediate-acting insulin product. NPH is an acronym for *neutral protamine Hagedorn* insulin, the original name of this type of insulin. NPH insulin is a sterile suspension of zinc insulin crystals and protamine sulfate in buffered water for injection. The suspension appears cloudy or opaque. NPH insulin has a slower onset of activity and longer duration of action than regular insulin, but not as long as those of the long-acting insulins. NPH insulin is often combined with regular insulin to reduce the number of insulin injections per day.

PHARMACOKINETICS

Route	Onset of Action	Peak Plasma Concentration	Elimination Half-life	Duration of Action
Subcut	1-2 hr	4-8 hr	Unknown	10-18 hr

LONG-ACTING INSULINS
◆ insulin glargine and insulin detemir
Two long-acting insulin products are now available: insulin glargine (Lantus) and insulin detemir (Levemir). Insulin glargine is normally a clear, colorless solution with a pH of 4.0. Once it is injected into subcutaneous tissue at physiologic pH, it forms microprecipitates that are slowly absorbed over the next 24 hours. It is a recombinant DNA–produced insulin analogue and is unique in that it provides a constant level of insulin in the body. This enhances its safety because blood levels do not rise and fall as with other insulins. Insulin glargine is usually dosed once daily, but the drug may be dosed every 12 hours, depending on the patient's glycemic response. Because insulin glargine provides a more prolonged, consistent blood glucose level, it is sometimes referred to as a *basal* insulin.

Often for those being switched from twice-daily NPH to insulin glargine, the initial daily glargine dose is reduced to 80% of the previous total NPH dose. Insulin detemir has a different mechanism of action from insulin glargine and the two insulins should not be considered interchangeable. The duration of action of insulin detemir is dose dependent, so that lower doses require twice-daily dosing and higher doses may be given once daily.

FIXED-COMBINATION INSULINS
Currently available fixed-combination insulin products include Humulin 70/30, Humulin 50/50, Novolin 70/30, Humalog Mix 75/25, Humalog 50/50, and NovoLog 70/30. Each of these products contains two different insulins, one intermediate-acting type and either one rapid-acting type (Humalog, NovoLog) or one short-acting type (Humulin), which work together in the body to optimize glycemic control. The numerical designations indicate the relative percentages of each of the two components in the product. Notice that in each case the numbers add up to 100 (percent). These products were developed to more closely simulate the varying levels of endogenous insulin that occur normally in nondiabetic people. To maintain constant blood glucose levels both after and between meals, insulin must be present. In most insulin regimens, patients take a combination of a rapid-acting insulin to deal with the surges in glucose that occur after meals and an intermediate or long-acting insulin for the period between meals when glucose levels are lower. However, this requires the mixing and administration of different types of insulins. Fixed-combination products were developed in an attempt to simplify the dosing process. The insulin lispro protamine component of Humalog Mix 75/25 is a modified insulin lispro molecule with a longer duration of action.

PHARMACOKINETICS

Route	Onset of Action	Peak Plasma Concentration	Elimination Half-life	Duration of Action
Subcut	1-2 hr	None	Unknown	24 hr

SLIDING-SCALE INSULIN DOSING

An important method for dosing insulin is referred to as the *sliding-scale method*. In this method, subcutaneous doses of rapid-acting (lispro or aspart) or short-acting (regular) insulin are adjusted according to blood glucose test results. This method is typically used in treating hospitalized diabetic patients whose insulin requirements may vary drastically because of stress (e.g., infections, surgery, acute illness), inactivity, or variable caloric intake, including receipt of *total parenteral nutrition (TPN)*. Sliding-scale insulin administration may also be used in type 1 patients receiving intensive insulin therapy. When an individual is on a sliding-scale insulin regimen, blood glucose concentrations are determined several times a day (e.g., before meals and at bedtime for patients on normal meal schedules, or every 4 to 6 hours around the clock for patients receiving TPN or enteral tube feedings. Subcutaneously administered regular insulin is then given in an amount that increases with the rise in blood glucose level. The disadvantage of sliding-scale dosing is that, because it delays insulin administration until hyperglycemia occurs, it does not meet basal insulin requirements and results in large swings in glucose control. Current research does not support the use of sliding scales, and many institutions are moving away from sliding-scale coverage and opting for insulin infusions until a stable state is reached and then appropriate insulin to cover the patient's metabolic needs. Nonetheless, sliding-scale dosing is still commonly used. The following is an example of a sliding dosing scale:

- No insulin for a blood glucose value of less than 140 mg/dL
- 2 units for a blood glucose value of 141 to 199 mg/dL
- 4 units for a blood glucose value of 200 to 249 mg/dL
- 6 units for a blood glucose value of 250 to 299 mg/dL
- 8 units for a blood glucose value of 300 mg/dL or higher

TRADITIONAL ORAL DRUGS FOR DIABETES

As previously described, type 2 diabetes is usually a very complex illness. Effective treatment involves several elements, including lifestyle modifications (e.g., diet control, exercise, smoking cessation), careful monitoring of blood glucose levels, and therapy with one or more drugs. In addition, the treatment of associated comorbid conditions is a necessity that serves to further complicate the entire process.

The latest consensus statement from the ADA and the European Association for the Study of Diabetes (EASD), recommends that new-onset type 2 diabetes be treated with both lifestyle interventions and the oral biguanide drug metformin, if there are no contraindications to the drug. This differs from past statements, which recommended lifestyle changes only as initial treatment. This latest consensus recognizes the reality that lifestyle changes, although essential, usually are not effective enough alone to lower blood glucose to the desired levels. If lifestyle modifications and the maximum tolerated metformin dose do not achieve the recommended A1C goals after 2 to 3 months, additional treatment with basal insulin or either a sulfonylurea or a thiazolidinedione is recommended. Studies have shown that metformin and the sulfonylureas (available in generic form) were either similar to or superior to the more expensive thiazolidinediones, glinides, and alpha-glucosidase inhibitors.

BIGUANIDE

Mechanism of Action and Drug Effects

Metformin is currently the only drug classified as a *biguanide*. It is considered a first-line drug and is the most commonly used oral drug for the treatment of type 2 diabetes. Metformin is believed to exert its beneficial effects in type 2 diabetes mellitus primarily by decreasing glucose production by the liver. It may also decrease intestinal absorption of glucose and improve insulin receptor sensitivity. This results in increased peripheral glucose uptake and use, and decreased hepatic production of triglycerides and cholesterol. Unlike sulfonylureas, metformin does not stimulate insulin secretion and therefore is not associated with hypoglycemia and weight gain.

Indications

As mentioned previously, the ADA-EASD guidelines now recommend metformin as the initial oral antidiabetic drug for treatment of newly diagnosed type 2 diabetes. Because it may also cause moderate weight loss, it is particularly useful for the many patients with type 2 diabetes who are overweight or obese. Metformin may be used as monotherapy or in combination with other oral antidiabetic drugs if single-drug therapy is unsuccessful. For this reason, it is available in combination products containing either sulfonylureas or thiazolidinediones. Metformin may also be combined with insulin.

Contraindications

Metformin is contraindicated in patients with renal disease or renal dysfunction (serum creatinine level higher than 1.5 mg/dL in males or higher than 1.4 mg/dL in females). Because metformin is primarily excreted by the kidneys, it can accumulate in these individuals, increasing the risk of development of lactic acidosis. Other contraindications include alcoholism, metabolic acidosis, hepatic disease, heart failure, and other conditions that predispose to tissue hypoxia and increase the risk of lactic acidosis.

Adverse Effects

The most common adverse effects of metformin are gastrointestinal. Metformin can cause abdominal bloating, nausea, cramping, a feeling of fullness, and diarrhea, especially at the start of therapy. These effects are all usually self-limiting and transient, and can be lessened by starting with low dosages, titrating up slowly, and taking the medication with food. Less common adverse effects with metformin are a metallic taste and a reduction in vitamin B_{12} levels after long-term use. Lactic acidosis is an extremely rare complication with metformin, but the risk increases with very high blood levels and/or clinical conditions predisposing to hypoxemia. Lactic acidosis is lethal in up to 50% of cases. Unlike sulfonylureas, metformin does not cause hypoglycemia.

Interactions

Metformin concentrations can be increased when the drug is given with cimetidine. Use of metformin with iodinated (iodine-containing) radiologic contrast media has been associated with both acute renal failure and lactic acidosis. For these reasons, metformin therapy should be discontinued the day of the test and for at least 48 hours after the patient undergoes any radiologic study that requires the use of such contrast media. Concurrent use of metformin with drugs that produce hypergly-

DOSAGES

Selected Oral Antidiabetic Drugs

Drug (Pregnancy Category)	Pharmacologic Class	Usual Dosage Range	Indications
acarbose (Precose) (B)	Alpha-glucosidase inhibitor	PO: 25-100 mg three times daily, taken with first bite of meal	
◆ glipizide (Glucotrol, Glucotrol XL) (C)	Second-generation sulfonylurea	PO: 5-10 mg daily (max daily dose 20 mg)	
◆ metformin (Glucophage, Glucophage XR) (B)	Biguanide	PO: 1000 mg twice daily or 850 mg twice daily; max daily dose 2550 mg for adults and 2000 mg for pediatric patients aged 10-16 yr	
◆ pioglitazone (Actos) (C)	Thiazolidinedione	PO: 15-45 mg once daily	
◆ repaglinide (Prandin) (C)	Meglitinide	PO: 0.5-4 mg three times daily; best taken 15 min before a meal	Diabetes mellitus type 2
Combination Oral Drugs			
glipizide/metformin (Metaglip) (C)	Combination sulfonylurea/ biguanide	PO: 1-2 tabs twice daily	
pioglitazone/metformin (ACTOplus Met) (C)	Combination thiazolidinedione/ biguanide	PO: 1 tab twice daily	
sitagliptin/metformin (Janumet) C	Combination incretin mimetic/ biguanide	PO: 1 tab twice daily	

PO, Oral.

cemia, such as diuretics and corticosteroids, may lead to loss of glucose control.

Dosages

For the recommended dosages of metformin, see the Dosages table above.

SULFONYLUREAS

Mechanism of Action and Drug Effects

The sulfonylureas are the oldest group of oral antidiabetic drugs. The drugs currently used are considered second-generation drugs with a better potency and adverse effect profile than first-generation drugs (such as acetazolamide and tolbutamide), which are no longer used clinically. Sulfonylureas bind to specific receptors on beta cells in the pancreas to stimulate the release of insulin. In addition, sulfonylureas appear to secondarily decrease the secretion of glucagon. For this class of drugs to be effective, the patient must still have functioning beta cells in the pancreas. Thus, these drugs work best during the early stages of the disease.

Indications

The ADA-EASD guidelines currently recommend sulfonylureas as second-step drugs for patients with type 2 diabetes whose A1C levels remain elevated when metformin is taken. Because they have different mechanisms of action, sulfonylureas can be used in conjunction with metformin and thiazolidinediones. Sulfonylureas should not be used in patients with advanced diabetes dependent on insulin administration, because the beta cells in such patients are no longer able to produce insulin.

Contraindications

Contraindications include hypoglycemia or conditions that can predispose to hypoglycemia, such as reduced caloric intake, ethanol use, or advanced age. There is a potential for cross allergy in

patients who are allergic to sulfonamide antibiotics. Although such an allergy is listed as a contraindication by the manufacturer, most clinicians will prescribe sulfonylureas for such patients. However, patients should be aware of the potential for cross allergy.

Adverse Effects

The most common adverse effect of the sulfonylureas is hypoglycemia, which depends on the dose, eating habits, and presence of hepatic or renal disease. Another predictable adverse effect is weight gain because of the stimulation of insulin secretion. Other adverse effects include skin rash, nausea, epigastric fullness, and heartburn.

Interactions

The hypoglycemic effect of second-generation sulfonylurea drugs may be enhanced when they are taken with alcohol, antacids, cimetidine, clofibrate, fluconazole, gemfibrozil, nonsteroidal antiinflammatory drugs, or sulfonamide antibiotics. Herbal supplements that are reported to increase the likelihood of hypoglycemia when given with sulfonylureas include garlic, ginger, and ginseng.

Drugs that are capable of reducing the hypoglycemic effect of sulfonylureas include carbamazepine, phenobarbital, phenytoin, cholestyramine, and rifampin.

Dosages

For the recommended dosages of sulfonylureas, see the Dosages table above.

GLINIDES

Mechanism of Action and Drug Effects

Repaglinide and nateglinide are currently the only two drugs in the glinide class. They are structurally different from the sulfonylureas but have a similar mechanism of action in that they also increase insulin secretion from the pancreas. However, they have a much shorter duration of action and must be given with each meal.

Indications

Like the sulfonylureas, the glinides are indicated for treatment of type 2 diabetes. They may be particularly useful for diabetic patients with high postprandial glucose levels. Glinides can be used along with metformin and thiazolidinediones, but should never be combined with sulfonylureas, because they share a similar mechanism of action.

Contraindications

Similar to those for the sulfonylureas.

Adverse Effects

The most commonly reported adverse effect of the glinides is hypoglycemia, which can occur particularly if food is not taken after a dose. Weight gain is also commonly reported.

Interactions

Drug interactions with the glinides are similar to those with the sulfonylureas.

Dosages

For the recommended dosages of the glinides, see the Dosages table on p. 498.

THIAZOLIDINEDIONES

Mechanism of Action and Drug Effects

The third major drug category to emerge for the oral treatment of type 2 diabetes mellitus besides the biguanides and the sulfonylureas is the thiazolidinediones or, simply, the *glitazones*. This class of drugs acts by regulating genes involved in glucose and lipid metabolism. The first drug in this class to be used in the United States was troglitazone (Rezulin). In 2000, it was removed from the market because of concerns about liver toxicity. However, two newer thiazolidinediones have taken its place: pioglitazone (Actos) and rosiglitazone (Avandia). They offer efficacy similar to that of troglitazone with less risk of hepatotoxicity. Thiazolidinediones are referred to as *insulin-sensitizing drugs*. They work to decrease insulin resistance by enhancing the sensitivity of insulin receptors. These drugs are also known to directly stimulate peripheral glucose uptake and storage, as well as to inhibit glucose and triglyceride production in the liver. Because glitazones affect gene regulation they have a slow onset of activity over several weeks, and maximal activity may not be evident for several months.

Indications

Thiazolidinediones are indicated for the management of type 2 diabetes. Because of their cost, adverse effect profile, and slow onset of action, they are usually reserved for those patients who cannot tolerate or cannot achieve glucose control with metformin or the sulfonylureas. Thiazolidinediones may also be combined with metformin or a sulfonylurea for synergistic effect. Only pioglitazone is approved for use with insulin.

Contraindications

Thiazolidinediones are contraindicated for use in patients with New York Heart Association class III or IV heart failure.

Adverse Effects

Rosiglitazone and pioglitazone both increase the risk of heart failure and are not recommended for use in patients with symptoms of heart failure. The glitazones also commonly cause peripheral edema and weight gain. The weight gain may be due to both water retention and an increase in adipose tissue. Glitazone use has also been associated with reduced bone mineral density and an increased risk of fractures, and rosiglitazone use may be associated with an increased risk of myocardial infarction. However, more definitive studies need to be completed to better define this risk.

Interactions

Clinically important interactions between rosiglitazone and other drugs have not been reported. Pioglitazone, on the other hand, is partly metabolized by cytochrome P-450 enzyme 3A4 (CYP3A4). Serum concentrations of pioglitazone may be increased if the drug is taken concurrently with a CYP3A4 inhibitor such as ketoconazole or erythromycin.

Dosages

For the recommended dosages of thiazolidinediones, see the Dosages table on p. 498.

ALPHA-GLUCOSIDASE INHIBITORS

Mechanism of Action and Drug Effects

Less commonly used oral drugs are the alpha-glucosidase inhibitors, acarbose (Precose) and miglitol (Glyset). As the name implies, these drugs work by reversibly inhibiting the enzyme alpha-glucosidase that is found in small intestine. This enzyme is responsible for the hydrolysis of oligosaccharides and disaccharides to glucose. When this enzyme is blocked, glucose absorption is delayed. The timing of administration of the alpha-glucosidase inhibitors is important, and they must be taken with food. When an alpha-glucosidase inhibitor is taken with a meal, excessive postprandial blood glucose elevation (a glucose "spike") can be prevented or reduced.

Indications

The alpha-glucosidase inhibitors are used to treat type 2 diabetes, usually in combination with another oral hypoglycemic drug. They may be particularly effective in controlling high postprandial glucose levels.

Contraindications

Because of their adverse gastrointestinal effects, alpha-glucosidase inhibitors are not recommended for use in patients with inflammatory bowel disease, malabsorption syndromes, or intestinal obstruction.

Adverse Effects

These drugs can cause a high incidence of flatulence, diarrhea, and abdominal pain. At high dosages they may also elevate levels of hepatic enzymes (transaminases). Unlike sulfonylureas, they do not cause hypoglycemia or weight gain.

Interactions

The bioavailability of digoxin, ranitidine, and propranolol may be reduced when they are taken with alpha-glucosidase inhibitors.

Dosages

For the recommended dosages of alpha-glucosidase inhibitors, see the Dosages table on p. 498.

DRUG PROFILES

acarbose

Acarbose (Precose) is one of the two currently available alpha-glucosidase inhibitors. The other drug in this drug category is miglitol (Glyset). As noted earlier, these drugs work by blunting the elevation of blood glucose levels after a meal. To work optimally they should be taken with the first bite of each meal. They also may be taken along with sulfonylurea drugs or with metformin. Acarbose use is contraindicated in patients with a hypersensitivity to alpha-glucosidase inhibitors, DKA, cirrhosis, inflammatory bowel disease, colonic ulceration, partial intestinal obstruction, or chronic intestinal disease.

PHARMACOKINETICS

Route	Onset of Action	Peak Plasma Concentration	Elimination Half-life	Duration of Action
PO	1-1.5 hr	2 hr	2-3 hr	Unknown

◆ glipizide

Glipizide (Glucotrol) is a second-generation sulfonylurea drug. In contrast to another second-generation sulfonylurea, glimepiride, glipizide has a very rapid onset and short duration of action, with no active metabolites. This confers many benefits. The rapid onset of action allows it to function much like the body normally does in response to meals when greater levels of insulin are required rapidly to deal with the increased glucose in the blood. When a patient with type 2 diabetes mellitus takes glipizide, it rapidly stimulates the pancreas to release insulin. This, in turn, facilitates the transport of excess glucose from the blood into the cells of the muscles, liver, and adipose tissues.

Glipizide use is contraindicated in cases of known drug allergy as well as in type 1 or brittle diabetes. Unlike most other oral antidiabetic drugs, it is not contraindicated in patients with severe renal failure. It works best if given 30 minutes before meals. This allows the timing of the insulin secretion induced by the glipizide to correspond with the elevation in blood glucose level induced by the meal in much the same way as endogenous insulin levels are raised in a person without diabetes. The extended-release dosage form of glipizide can be given once daily.

PHARMACOKINETICS

Route	Onset of Action	Peak Plasma Concentration	Elimination Half-life	Duration of Action
PO	1 hr	1-3 hr	2-5 hr	6-8 hr

◆ metformin

Metformin (Glucophage) is currently the only biguanide oral antidiabetic drug. It works primarily by inhibiting hepatic glucose production and increasing the sensitivity of peripheral tissue to insulin. Because its mechanism of action differs from that of sulfonylurea drugs, it may be given along with these drugs.

Metformin use is contraindicated in patients with a hypersensitivity to biguanides, hepatic or renal disease, alcoholism, or cardiopulmonary disease.

PHARMACOKINETICS

Route	Onset of Action	Peak Plasma Concentration	Elimination Half-life	Duration of Action
PO	Less than 1 hr	1-3 hr	1.5-5 hr	24 hr

◆ pioglitazone

Pioglitazone (Actos) is classified as a glitazone or thiazolidinedione derivative. It is marketed for the treatment of patients with type 2 diabetes. Pioglitazone and rosiglitazone (Avandia) are used alone or with a sulfonylurea, metformin, or insulin. Thiazolidinedione antidiabetic drugs work by decreasing insulin resistance. As noted earlier, the glitazones can worsen or precipitate heart failure and should be avoided in patients with cardiac disease. The safety of these drugs for use in pregnant women and children has not been established.

PHARMACOKINETICS

Route	Onset of Action	Peak Plasma Concentration	Elimination Half-life	Duration of Action
PO	Delayed	2 hr	3-7 hr	Unknown

◆ repaglinide

Repaglinide (Prandin) is one of two antidiabetic drugs classified as glinides, the other being nateglinide (Starlix). These drugs have a mechanism of action similar to that of the sulfonylureas in that they also stimulate the release of insulin from pancreatic beta cells. They are often especially helpful in the treatment of patients who have erratic eating habits, because the drug dose is skipped when a meal is missed. Contraindications include known drug allergy.

PHARMACOKINETICS

Route	Onset of Action	Peak Plasma Concentration	Elimination Half-life	Duration of Action
PO	15-60 min	1 hr	2-3 hr	4-6 hr

NEW ANTIDIABETIC DRUGS

AMYLIN MIMETICS

Amylin is a natural hormone secreted by the beta cells of the pancreas along with insulin in response to food. It functions to decrease postprandial plasma glucose levels, which it accomplishes in three ways:

1. It slows gastric emptying.
2. It suppresses glucagon secretion and hepatic glucose production.
3. It increases satiety (sense of having eaten enough).

Pramlintide (Symlin; pregnancy category C) was approved by the FDA in 2005 as the first *amylin mimetic* drug. It is available only as a subcutaneous injection and, when given before major meals, works by mimicking the action of the natural hormone amylin. The drug is indicated for use in patients with type 1 or type 2 diabetes receiving mealtime insulin who have failed to achieve optimal glucose control with insulin. In fact, it is the first drug approved for use in type 1 diabetes since insulin was discovered in the early twentieth century. Its use is contraindicated in patients with gastroparesis or those taking drugs that alter gastrointestinal motility. Adverse effects include nausea, vomiting, anorexia, and headache. The drug itself does not cause hypoglycemia, but if the patient is taking any prandial rapid- or short-acting insulin product, the insulin dose usually needs to be reduced by 50%. Pramlintide can delay the oral absorption of any drug taken at the same time and should be given at least 1 hour before other medications. Recommended dosage ranges are from 15 to 60 mcg for management of type 1 diabetes and 60 to 120 mcg for management of type 2 diabetes, taken before any major meal.

INCRETIN MIMETICS

Incretins are hormones released by the gastrointestinal tract in response to food. Incretins do the following:

1. Stimulate insulin secretion
2. Reduce postprandial glucagon production
3. Slow gastric emptying
4. Increase satiety

The most important incretin hormones that have been identified so far are glucagon-like peptide 1 (GLP-1) and gastric inhibitory peptide (GIP). These hormones are rapidly deactivated by the enzyme dipeptidyl peptidase IV (DPP-IV). Currently, there are two incretin mimetics, exenatide and sitagliptin.

Exenatide (Byetta; pregnancy category C) was approved by the FDA in 2005 as the first *incretin mimetic* drug. Exenatide is a long-acting analogue of GLP-1 that was initially derived from the salivary gland of the Gila monster. This drug is available only as a subcutaneous injection and is indicated only for patients with type 2 diabetes who have been unable to achieve blood glucose control with metformin, a sulfonylurea, and/or a glitazone. It cannot be used with insulin. It should be given 60 minutes before a meal. Adverse effects include nausea, vomiting, and diarrhea. Rare cases of hemorrhagic or necrotizing pancreatitis have also been reported. Patients may experience weight loss of 5 to 10 pounds. Like pramlintide, this drug can delay absorption of other orally administered drugs because of its slowing of gastric emptying. In patients taking sulfonylurea drugs, the dose may need to be reduced if hypoglycemia appears on initiation of exenatide therapy. The usual starting dosage is 5 mcg within 1 hour of both the morning and evening meals. If necessary, the dosage may be increased after 1 month to 10 mcg twice daily before meals. A new once weekly dosage form is currently under development.

DRUG PROFILE

♦ sitagliptin

Sitagliptin (Januvia) was approved by the FDA in 2006 as the second *incretin mimetic* drug but has an entirely different mechanism of action from exenatide. Sitagliptin is an oral drug that selectively inhibits the action of DPP-IV, thus increasing concentrations of the naturally occurring incretins GLP-1 and GIP. Sitagliptin is indicated for management of type 2 diabetes either as monotherapy or in combination with metformin, a sulfonylurea, or a glitazone, but not with insulin. Clinical trials have demonstrated A1C reductions of 0.6% to 0.8%, which is less than the reductions seen with traditional oral hypoglycemic drugs. Significant hypoglycemia may occur when the drug is combined with a sulfonylurea. There have been no significant adverse effects. However, in September 2009, the FDA received postmarketing cases of acute pancreatitis and advised that healthcare providers monitor patients closely for the development of pancreatitis after both initiation and dose increases. Sitagliptin is given once daily as a 100-mg tablet with or without food. Pregnancy category B.

PHARMACOKINETICS

Route	Onset of Action	Peak Plasma Concentration	Elimination Half-life	Duration of Action
PO	15-30 min	1 hr	12 hr	Unknown

HYPOGLYCEMIA

Hypoglycemia is an abnormally low blood glucose level (generally below 50 mg/dL). When the cause is organic and the effects are mild, treatment usually consists of dietary modifications, primarily a higher intake of protein and lower intake of carbohydrates, to prevent a rebound postprandial hypoglycemic effect. Hypoglycemia is also a common adverse effect of many antidiabetic drugs when their pharmacologic effects are greater than expected. Because the brain needs a constant amount of glucose to function, early symptoms of hypoglycemia include the central nervous system (CNS) manifestations of confusion, irritability, tremor, and sweating. Later symptoms include hypothermia and seizures. Without adequate restoration of normal blood and CNS glucose levels, coma and death will occur.

GLUCOSE-ELEVATING DRUGS

Oral forms of concentrated glucose are available for patients to use in the event of a hypoglycemic crisis. Dosage forms include rapidly dissolving buccal tablets and semisolid gel forms designed for oral use and rapid mucosal absorption. It should be pointed out that table sugar, which is sucrose, will not produce as rapid an effect as the glucose products intended for use by diabetic patients. This is because sucrose is a *disaccharide* (two-molecule) sugar that must first be digested in the body to yield glucose as a *monosaccharide* (one-molecule) by-product. In the hospital setting or when the patient is unconscious, intravenous glucose is an obvious option to treat hypoglycemia. Concentrations of up to 50% dextrose in water ($D_{50}W$) are most often used for this purpose.

In addition to oral and/or intravenous glucose, glucagon, a natural hormone secreted by the pancreas, is available as a subcutaneous injection to be given when a quick response to severe hypoglycemia is needed. Because glucagon injection may induce vomiting, an unconscious patient should be rolled onto his or her side before injection.

PHARMACOKINETIC BRIDGE
to Nursing Practice

Provision of insulin therapy by continuous subcutaneous insulin infusion (CSII) is becoming an option for selected diabetic patients in an attempt to minimize the risks and complications of the disease. One previously used option for achieving tight control of blood glucose levels was multiple daily injections of insulin (MDI). With CSII, normal serum glucose levels are maintained by the continuous delivery of basal insulin, and then with food intake—primarily carbohydrate consumption—bolus doses of insulin are given. Use of an insulin pump (i.e., CSII) leads to a more rapid, consistent absorption of the drug and reduction in the occurrence of hypoglycemia. Research has also shown that use of an insulin pump helps to decrease the occurrence of elevated prebreakfast serum glucose levels, often called the *dawn phenomenon* (referring to the dawn of the day). Because the insulin pump delivers insulin through the subcutaneous route and the infusion is a continuous one, fewer problems occur than with once- or twice-daily injections. Patients using CSII achieve mean serum glucose and A1C levels that remain somewhat lower than those associated with MDI, so that the risk for hypoglycemia is decreased. Understanding new and different drugs and their pharmacokinetic properties allows the nurse to help patients achieve better quality of life, minimize risks, and maximize wellness.

NURSING PROCESS

Assessment

Before administering any type of *antidiabetic* drug, the nurse must assess the patient's knowledge about the disease and recommended treatment. Head-to-toe physical assessment, medication history taking, and nursing assessment must be completed and documented. A medication history should include a list of the patient's current medications, including over-the-counter drugs, herbals, and supplements. Appropriate laboratory test results (e.g., fasting blood glucose level, A1C level) should be reviewed for any abnormalities compared with baseline levels. The prescriber's order for insulin must also be assessed, so that the correct drug, route, type of insulin (i.e., rapid acting, short acting, intermediate acting, short- and intermediate-acting mixtures, long acting), and dosage are implemented correctly. With assessment, it is important to keep in mind that allergic reactions are less likely to occur with *recombinant human insulins* because of their similarity with endogenous insulin; however, allergies may still occur and should be considered in the assessment. Contraindications, cautions, and drug interactions associated with the various forms of insulin have already been discussed and should be the focus of thorough assessment before any insulin is given. *Oral antidiabetic drugs* also require close assessment for contraindications, cautions, and drug interactions, and, for *sulfonylureas,* special attention to other drugs that have chemical or structural similarity (e.g., furosemide, sulfamethoxazole) because of the increased risk for cross allergy.

The nurse must also be aware that elderly or malnourished patients may react adversely to the *biguanides.* Contraindications, cautions, and interactions for this drug class have been previously discussed. Also important to remember is the interaction between metformin and the radiopaque dyes used for certain diagnostic purposes (e.g., computed tomography with contrast). The interaction is associated with an increased risk for renal dysfunction. With *thiazolidinediones,* another important caution to emphasize is the need to monitor liver function by reviewing ALT levels before drug therapy is initiated and periodically thereafter, such as every 3 months as ordered. Unstable serum glucose levels require immediate attention, so the patient should be assessed for any signs and symptoms of hypoglycemia (e.g., acute onset of nervousness, sweating, lethargy, weakness, cold and clammy skin, change in sensorium) or of hyperglycemia (e.g., tachycardia, blood glucose levels exceeding 150 mg/dL, and changes in respiration such as Kussmaul respiration). Assessment is even more critical for a diabetic patient who is also under stress, has an infection or is ill, is pregnant or lactating, or is experiencing trauma or any change in health status. With treatment, diabetic patients are at risk of hypoglycemia, with the potential danger of loss of consciousness; thus there is a need for constant assessment of serum glucose levels and neurologic status. Along with assessment of the therapeutic regimen and patient adherence to treatment, cultural factors, socioeconomic factors, and family support are also important to note and follow throughout therapy.

Nursing Diagnoses

- Risk for injury related to neurologic deficits (e.g., neuropathies) associated with diabetes mellitus
- Risk for infection related to the pathologic impact of diabetes on immune system function
- Imbalanced nutrition: less than body requirements related to the body's inability to use glucose (for Type 1)
- Imbalanced nutrition: more than body requirements related to excessive intake of nutrients (for Type 2)
- Deficient knowledge related to lack of information about diabetes mellitus, its management, and prevention of disease-related complications
- Ineffective therapeutic regimen management related to lack of experience with a significant daily treatment regimen

Planning

Goals

- Patient remains free of self-injury and complications of diabetes.
- Patient remains free of infection.
- Patient maintains adequate weight and dietary habits in the overall management of diabetes.
- Patient states the effects of diabetes on body function.
- Patient remains compliant with the medical regimen and adheres to treatment protocols.
- Patient states the importance of adherence to medication regimens, lifestyle changes, dietary restrictions, and avoidance of high-risk behaviors.
- Patient states the action and adverse effects of insulin or the oral hypoglycemic drugs.

Outcome Criteria

- Patient performs self-assessment and foot care as directed and as needed to maintain healthy skin.
- Patient immediately reports elevated temperature, difficult-to-heal lesions or sores, and any unusual redness of any area of the skin to the prescriber.
- Patient adheres to the diet recommended by the ADA or other dietary advisor per the orders of the prescriber or nutritional consultant.
- Patient eats a healthy diet, gets sufficient rest and relaxation, and notifies the prescriber should any unusual problems occur when customary activities are changed. Patient keeps all scheduled appointments with the prescriber to monitor therapeutic effectiveness and assess for complications of therapy.
- Patient takes medication as scheduled, monitors blood glucose levels, and watches for any signs and symptoms of hyperglycemia or hypoglycemia.

Implementation

With any patient who is taking *insulin* (or *oral antidiabetic drugs*), the nurse must always check serum glucose levels (and other related laboratory values, as ordered) before giving the drug so that accurate baseline glucose levels are obtained and documented. An additional check of the medication order and the prepared insulin dosage should be carried out with another registered nurse and charted, or performed per facility policy. NPH and premixed insulin mixtures should not be shaken but should be rolled between the hands before the prescribed dose is administered. The rolling helps to avoid air in the syringe and inaccurate dose administration. Insulins should also be administered at room temperature. Insulin may be stored at room temperature if used within 1 month; otherwise, refrigeration is needed. Refrigeration is also recommended in warm or hot climates and with

BOX 32-2   Administration, Handling, and Storage of Insulin

Dosages, Storage, Handling, and Mixing

1 Individualize insulin dosages (e.g., use sliding scale as ordered) and monitor closely for adequate control of hypoglycemia and hyperglycemia.
2 Adjust dosages, as ordered, to achieve fasting plasma glucose levels of between 100 mg/dL and 126 mg/dL in adults.
3 Store insulin for current use at room temperature. Avoid extreme temperatures and exposure to sunlight, because the insulin's protein structure will be permanently denatured. Extra vials not in use should be stored in the refrigerator. Vials being used in high environmental temperatures should also be stored in the refrigerator, but insulin should *never* be given cold. Never freeze insulin. To maintain drug stability, insulin should be stored for up to 1 month at room temperature and for up to 3 months in the refrigerator.
4 Discard unused vials if they have not been used for several weeks (or follow hospital policy). Do not use any insulin that does not have the proper clarity or color (e.g., clear for regular, cloudy for NPH).
5 Store prefilled insulin syringes in the refrigerator for up to 1 week. Store the syringe with the needle pointing upward to avoid clogging within the hub of the needle.

Administration

1 Administer insulin subcutaneously (see Chapter 10); however, regular insulin may be given intravenously in special situations (e.g., intravenous drip in patient with diabetic ketoacidosis; in postoperative patients), if ordered.
2 Roll the drug vial gently between the hands without shaking to avoid bubble formation in the vial, which may lead to inaccurate dosage withdrawal. Give mixed insulins within 5 minutes of mixing

to avoid binding of the solution and subsequent altered activity of the drugs.
3 Administer insulin at the recommended times, but always with meals or meal trays ready. Give insulin lispro and other rapid-acting insulins approximately 15 minutes before meals (it has a quicker onset of action) and only after monitoring the patient's fasting serum glucose level (as with all insulin administration). Give regular insulin (short-acting insulin) 30 minutes before meals, and NPH insulin 30 to 60 minutes before meals.
4 When giving regular and NPH insulin at the same time (if ordered), mix the two appropriately (see discussion of mixing insulins in the Implementation subsection under Nursing Process).
5 Administer insulin subcutaneously at a 90-degree angle. However, if the patient is emaciated, the injection may be given at a 45-degree angle. Insulin syringes should always be used (see text discussion and Chapter 10).
6 Instruct patients taking insulin injections to rotate sites within the same general location for about 1 week before moving to a new location (e.g., all injections for a week in the upper right thigh before moving a little lower on the right thigh). This technique allows for better insulin absorption. Each injection site should be at least $\frac{1}{2}$ to 1 inch away from the previous injection site. If this practice is followed, it will be approximately 6 weeks before the patient will have to rotate to a totally new area of the body. Note the following sites for subcutaneous insulin injections: thigh areas (front and back) and outer areas of the upper arm (middle third of the upper arm between the shoulder and the elbow).
7 Continuous subcutaneous insulin infusion and/or multiple daily injections may be ordered for tight glucose control.

any major changes in environmental temperatures from cold to hot. Expired or discolored insulin should not be used. For information about the handling, mixing, storage, and administration of insulin, see Box 32-2.

Insulin should be administered subcutaneously at a 90-degree angle unless the patient is emaciated, in which case it should be administered at a 45-degree angle. Only regular insulin may be administered intravenously; however, use of this route remains controversial because of absorption of the insulin into the intravenous bag and/or tubing. Only insulin syringes should be used. They are easy to identify because of their orange caps and calibration in units, not milliliters. These syringes have preattached needles that are 29 gauge and $\frac{1}{2}$ inch in length. When insulins are mixed (if ordered), the regular or rapid-acting insulin (unmodified and *clear*) should be withdrawn first, followed by withdrawal of the intermediate-acting or NPH insulin (modified and cloudy). This should be done *only* after the appropriate amount of air has been injected into the vials. The amount of air to be injected into the vials equals the prescribed number of units. Air should be injected into the intermediate-acting insulin vial first, followed by injection of air into the regular or rapid- or short-acting insulin vial. This helps prevent contamination of the rapid-acting insulin by the intermediate-acting insulin and modification of the unmodified (rapid-acting) insulin (see Table 32-4 and Chapter 10). Some fixed combinations of insulin products come prepared in premixed syringes.

Understanding of the action of the insulin and its related pharmacokinetics (e.g., onset, peak, duration) is critical for safe

care and patient education. For example, it is important to know that the rapid-acting insulins (insulin lispro, insulin aspart, and insulin glulisine) have an onset of action of about 15 minutes and must be given 15 minutes before meals, compared with 30 minutes before meals for regular insulin or a short-acting insulin. If lispro insulin is to be mixed with NPH (intermediate-acting) insulin, the combination should also be given 15 minutes before meals. The prescriber's orders should always be double-checked for clarification of the dosage and drug as well as of any change in dietary intake, such as a possible increase in carbohydrates and decrease in fat to avoid postprandial hypoglycemia.

Regardless of the specific type of recombinant human insulin used, understanding the peak, onset, and duration of action of the insulin to be used, such as rapid acting versus short acting versus intermediate acting versus long acting, will help the nurse determine when food or meals should be given. The intermediate-acting insulin (NPH) has an onset of action of 1-2 hours and so meals should be served at least 30 to 45 minutes prior to its administration. Many combination products of rapid- and short-acting with intermediate-acting insulin are available; these combination insulins should be given 15 to 30 minutes before meals. In the hospital setting, the nurse should be sure that meal trays have arrived on the unit before giving insulin to avoid time lapses and subsequent hypoglycemic episodes. The nurse must also be sure that other forms of allowed foods are available to the patient in case meals are delayed and insulin has already been administered.

Patients may require dosing by a sliding-scale method, which includes subcutaneous regular insulin doses adjusted according to serum glucose test results. Although controversial (see previous pharmacology discussion), sliding-scale dosing may be used for hospitalized diabetic patients experiencing drastic changes in serum glucose levels due to physical and/or emotional stress, infections, surgery, acute illness, inactivity, or variable caloric intake, as well as in patients needing intensive insulin therapy. When this insulin regimen is used, blood glucose levels are measured several times a day (e.g., every 4 hours, every 6 hours, or at specified times such as 7 AM, 11 AM, 4 PM, and midnight) to obtain fasting and/or premeal blood glucose values.

Oral antidiabetic drugs are usually given at least 30 minutes before meals, as ordered. Some of the sulfonylureas are to be taken with breakfast, the alpha-glucosidase inhibitors are always to be taken with the first bite of each main meal, and the thiazolidinediones are to be given once daily or in two divided doses. Exact timing of the dose should always be checked against the prescriber's order and with consideration of the drug's onset of action. With metformin (as with any antidiabetic drug or insulin), it is important for the nurse and/or patient to know what to do if symptoms of hypoglycemia occur—for example, the patient should take glucagon; eat glucose tablets or gel, corn syrup, or honey; drink fruit juice or a nondiet soft drink; or eat a small snack such as crackers or half a sandwich. If the patient receiving metformin is to undergo diagnostic studies with contrast dye, the prescriber will need to discontinue the drug prior to the procedure and restart it after the tests, but only after reevaluation of the

EVIDENCE-BASED PRACTICE

Tight Insulin Control

■ Review

Research has confirmed that intensive insulin therapy, although it carries many challenges, can help some patients with diabetes reduce complications and experience a better quality of life. More than 20 million Americans, or about 7% of the population, have diabetes mellitus, and serious complications and organ damage can result from the pathologic process. Heart disease, kidney disease, vascular disease, blindness, and amputations are the most common of the severely debilitating and/or fatal complications. Because of the mortality and morbidity rates associated with diabetes in the United Stats, tight control is seen as one way to possibly minimize risks and/or major complications as well as allow a more normal lifestyle. This is done through the use of continuous subcutaneous insulin infusions (CSII) via pump or by multiple daily injections (MDI).

■ Type of Evidence

The Diabetes Control and Complications Trial (DCCT) examined the use of intensive therapy versus conventional therapy in 1441 teenagers and young adults with type 1 diabetes. Intensive therapy involved hospitalization for stabilization of the disease and patient education, frequent dosing of insulin guided by the results of at least four serum glucose tests a day, four daily insulin injections or use of an insulin pump, monthly office visits, frequent telephone calls between the patients and nurse educators, dietary consultation, and exercise. Follow-up investigations occurred 4 years later.

■ Results of Study

The study found a 39% to 76% reduction in the incidence of various complications associated with diabetes in those receiving intensive therapy. Specifically, the findings of the DCCT showed that lowering blood glucose levels reduced the risk of eye disease by 75%, of kidney disease by 50%, and of nerve disease by 60%. DCCT participants were not expected to have many heart-related problems, because their average age was 27 years when the study was initiated; however, electrocardiography, blood pressure tests, and serum laboratory tests of lipid levels were performed for all participants to look for signs of cardiovascular disease. The study showed that the participants receiving intensive therapy had significantly lower risks of developing hyperlipidemia and subsequent cardiovascular or coronary heart disease. The risks of intensive therapy identified in the DCCT included hypoglycemia severe enough to require the assistance of another individual. Because of this

risk, researchers did not recommend intensive therapy for patients younger than 13 years of age, patients with heart disease or advanced complications, older adults, or patients with a history of frequent severe hypoglycemia.

A follow-up investigation conducted 4 years later (in 1997), known as the Epidemiology of Diabetes Interventions and Complications study, found that the original intensive therapy group continued to have a lower risk of eye, nerve, and kidney disease even though control had become less intensive. In 2003, some 6 years later, the patients still had reduced rates of nerve damage. Because of the long-term nature of the study and the moderately sized research sample, the results hold promise for the treatment of diabetes in those individuals willing to invest the required time, energy, and lifestyle changes.

■ Link of Evidence to Nursing Practice

The patients who are the best candidates for continuous subcutaneous insulin infusion are those who are diligent and committed to self-management of their diabetes, are willing to spend the time it takes to record serum glucose levels and insulin values in a journal four or more times a day, will make monthly or more frequent visits to their health care professionals, and are able to monitor carbohydrate intake closely. Individuals who have motor or cognitive impairments as well as those who are not committed to the intensive therapy may be unable to adhere to the strict regimen. The evidence strongly supports the value of tight control of glucose levels in helping to reduce long-term complications associated with diabetes. Not all patients are willing to spend the time and effort required to achieve tight glucose control, and the regimen is very stressful; however, every patient has the right to be informed of this option and its associated benefits and risks. This study produced ground-breaking results and has made an impact on the care of diabetic patients today. Many of the 1441 participants have been involved in the research for more than 20 years. To obtain more information for patients, contact the American Diabetes Association at 800-342-2383. In practicing evidence-based nursing, nurses look at new treatment approaches, such as the new therapy examined in this study, and their potential for improving patient care. Although the costs of intensive therapy are high, they are offset by the decrease in other medical expenses related to the complications of diabetes and by the improved quality of life.

Modified from National Institute of Diabetes and Digestive and Kidney Diseases: National diabetes statistics, 2004, available at *http:/diabetes.niddk.nih.gov/dm/pubs/statistics/index.htm;* Dow N: Tight insulin control: making it work, *RN* 68(7):44-52, 2005; National Institute of Diabetes and Digestive and Kidney Diseases: Diabetes Control and Complications Trial (DCCT), 2001, available at *http://diabetes.niddk.nih.gov/dm/pubs/control;* American Diabetes Association: Intensive diabetes control yields less nerve damage years later, 2004, available at *http://www.diabetes.org/for-media/2004-press-releases/neuropathy.jsp.*

patient's renal status. It is critical to the safe and efficient use of oral antidiabetics to be sure that food will be or is being tolerated before the dose is given. If the oral drug (and/or insulin) is taken and no meal is consumed or it is consumed at a later time than usual, hypoglycemia may be problematic and result in negative health consequences and even unconsciousness. Because the glitazones (e.g., rosiglitazone and pioglitazone) may both cause moderate weight gain and edema, it is important to weigh the patient daily at the same time every day and in the same amount of clothing. Several combination drug products are also available, including rosiglitazone plus metformin, glyburide plus metformin, and glipizide plus metformin. These should be given exactly as prescribed. Pramlintide should be given before any major meal. Exenatide is given by subcutaneous injection in patients with type 2 diabetes and cannot be used with insulin. Sitagliptin, a newer oral antidiabetic drug, is not to be used with insulin and may be taken with or without food.

In special situations, such as when the patient has been ordered to have nothing by mouth (NPO status) and is taking either an oral antidiabetic drug or insulin, it is crucial for the nurse to follow the prescriber's orders regarding drug administration. If there are no written orders about this situation, the prescriber should be contacted for further instructions. If a patient is on NPO status but is receiving an intravenous solution of dextrose, the prescriber may still order insulin, but this should always be clarified. The prescriber should also be contacted if a patient becomes ill and unable to take the usual dosage of an oral antidiabetic drug (or insulin). The patient should always wear a medical alert bracelet or necklace giving the diagnosis, list of medications, and emergency contact information.

It is also very important that the nurse stay informed and up to date about the latest research on diabetes and keep patients and family members well informed. For example, as previously discussed in the pharmacology section, macrovascular and microvascular problems are now being recognized to occur at FPG levels as low as 126 mg/dL. Also, the ADA, the National Institute of Diabetes and Digestive and Kidney Diseases, and the Centers for Disease Control and Prevention recommend that all adults 45 years of age and older be tested for elevated FPG levels every 3 years. See the Evidence-Based Practice box on p. 504 for more information on specific nursing research.

In summary, there are many nursing considerations related to drug therapy in patients with diabetes mellitus. Patient education is also very important and should begin the moment the patient has entered into the health care system or upon diagnosis. Instruction that is tailored to the patient's educational level and that uses appropriate teaching-learning concepts and teaching aids is important to patient adherence with the treatment regimen. In addition, the nurse should be sure that all necessary resources are made available to patients (e.g., financial assistance, visual assistance, dietary plans, daily menus, ADA information, transportation assistance, and Meals on Wheels and other community services). See the Patient Teaching Tips for more specific information.

Evaluation

It is important for the nurse to understand current therapeutic guidelines. The prevailing key diagnostic criterion for diabetes mellitus is hyperglycemia with a fasting blood glucose level of 126 mg/dL or higher or a nonfasting blood glucose level of 200 mg/dL or higher; however, the therapeutic response to insulin and any of the oral antidiabetic drugs is a decrease in blood glucose to the level prescribed by the prescriber or to near-normal levels. Most often, fasting blood glucose levels are used to measure the degree of glycemic control. To provide a picture of the patient's adherence to the therapy regimen for the previous several months, the level of A1C is measured. This value reflects how well the patient has been doing with diet and drug therapy. Patients with diabetes need to be monitored frequently by their prescribers (as well as at home) to make sure they are adhering to the therapy regimen as evidenced by normalization of blood test results. The patient should be monitored for indications of hypoglycemia or hyperglycemia and insulin allergy. With short-acting insulins such as lispro, because the onset of action is more rapid than with regular insulin and the duration of action is shorter, it is crucial for the nurse and the patient to monitor blood glucose levels very closely until the dosage is regulated and blood glucose is at the level the prescriber desires. Should a patient be switched from one insulin or oral antidiabetic drug to another, glucose levels must be monitored very closely at home or by the prescriber. The nurse must always evaluate whether identified goals and outcome criteria are being met and plan nursing care accordingly.

PATIENT TEACHING TIPS

- Patients should be encouraged to keep medical alert jewelry or a medical alert card on the person at all times and to keep medical information in clear view on the refrigerator at the patient's home.
- Instructions and demonstrations should be provided regarding the proper storage of insulin, the equipment needed for administration, the drawing up of insulin, the mixing of insulins (if ordered), the technique for insulin injections, rotation of subcutaneous insulin injection sites with provision of return demon-

strations from the patient (see Chapter 10 for more information about insulin injections). Other points to emphasize include that insulin may be stored at room temperature unless the heat is extreme or if the patient is traveling.. The patient should also receive instructions about how to rotate the subcutaneous insulin injection sites.
- A daily journal should be kept at all times.
- The patient should be educated about the need to have serum glucose levels monitored, as ordered and at the prescribed inter-

Continued

PATIENT TEACHING TIPS—cont'd

vals. Instructions that are specific to the patient's glucometer should also be emphasized. The patient should also receive thorough instructions about the importance of exercise, hygiene, foot care, the prescribed dietary plan, and weight control.

- Smoking and alcohol consumption should be avoided, and all dietary instructions should be followed. The patient also needs to understand the importance of avoiding skipping meals or skipping doses of insulin or oral antidiabetic drugs, and of contacting the prescriber for further instructions when needed.

- The difference between hypoglycemia and hyperglycemia should be explained (see earlier discussion for specific signs and symptoms) with emphasis on the treatment of each (e.g., having on hand quick sources of glucose, such as candy, sugar packets, over-the-counter glucose tablets, sugar cubes, honey, corn syrup, orange juice, or non-diet soda beverages for hypoglycemia, and having more insulin on hand for hyperglycemia, as ordered). The patient should be encouraged to keep quick dosage forms of glucose in possession at all times!

- Educate about situations or conditions that lead to altered serum glucose levels, such as fever, illness, stress, increased activity or exercise, surgery, emotional distress. Encourage contacting the prescriber for any questions or concerns about maintaining glucose control.

- Educate about the importance of knowing pre-meal serum glucose levels before taking insulin and the importance of timing meals as related to the type of insulin.

- The importance of having adequate supplies of insulin and equipment at all times and planning ahead for vacations should be emphasized. All medications and related equipment should be kept away from children. If needed, magnifying glass attachments are available for syringes and vials.

- Encourage any diabetic patient to report any yellow discoloration of the skin, dark urine, fever, sore throat, weakness, or unusual bleeding or easy bruising.

- The importance of A1C monitoring should be emphasized (e.g., at least two times a year for those with good glycemic control and quarterly for patients who are not at target values, have changed their therapy, or are not adhering to the therapy regimen) (Table 32-5). These recommendations apply to those taking oral antidiabetic drugs as well.

- Lifestyle modifications, including weight control, and glucose level maintenance with diet and exercise and/or drug therapy should be reviewed with the patient. Patients with type 2 diabetes have a greater therapeutic response to diet and exercise and glucose level control than patients with type 1 diabetes. ADA recommendations for fasting serum glucose level measurement should be followed. Educate about the importance of engaging in supervised exercise until the condition stabilizes. A nutritional consult with specific menu planning may help the patient with changes in intake (e.g., low-fat diet with 160 to 300 g of carbohydrates).

- The importance of the American Heart Association recommendations for diabetic patients should be emphasized including 30 minutes of exercise daily with use of a treadmill, prolonged walking, swimming or aquatic aerobics, bicycling, rowing, chair exercises, arm exercises, and non–weight-bearing exercises.

- Emphasize that therapy will be lifelong and that strict blood glucose control, drug therapy, and lifestyle changes is critical to reducing complications.

- The need for strict foot care should be emphasized to the patient and those involved in the patient's care, beginning with a basic assessment of the feet and toes every day to check for sores, lesions, cuts, bruises, ingrown toenails, and any other changes. Foot care is needed to enhance circulation and prevent infections and may include soaking the feet daily or as ordered in lukewarm water (the temperature of the water should be checked) and then adequately drying the feet and applying moisturizing lotion; checking the feet and legs for abnormal changes in color (e.g., purplish or reddish discoloration), cool temperature of the feet to the touch, swelling of the extremities or feet, and the appearance of any drainage; contacting the prescriber for further instructions if there is suspicion of any type of wound or alteration in skin integrity; and, having frequent pedicures and nail trimming by a podiatrist or other licensed, certified individual.

- Some of the oral antidiabetic drugs cause photosensitivity, so the patient should be instructed always to wear protective sunscreen and proper clothing when exposed to the sun and to wear protective eye goggles and sunscreen when using tanning beds.

Table 32-5 Diabetes Care: Correlation of Glycosylated Hemoglobin Levels with Mean Serum Glucose Levels

Hemoglobin A1C (%)	Mean Serum Glucose Level (mg/dL)	Mean Serum Glucose Level (mmol/L)
6	126	7.0
7	154	8.6
8	183	10.2
9	212	11.8
10	240	13.4
11	269	14.9
12	298	16.5

Data from American Diabetes Association. Available at *www.diabetes.org*.

- Insulin normally facilitates removal of glucose from the blood and its storage as glycogen in the liver.
- Type 1 diabetes mellitus was formerly known as *insulin-dependent diabetes* or *juvenile-onset diabetes*. Little or no endogenous insulin is produced by individuals with type 1 diabetes. It is much less common than type 2 diabetes and affects only about 10% of all diabetic patients. Patients with type 1 diabetes usually are not obese.
- The primary treatment for type 1 diabetes mellitus is insulin therapy. Patients with type 2 diabetes are managed with lifestyle changes (dietary changes, exercise, smoking cessation) and oral drug therapy (one or more drugs). If normal blood glucose levels are not achieved after 2-3 months of lifestyle chantes, treatment with oral antidiabetic drugs are often added to the regimen.
- Insulin was originally isolated from cattle and pigs, but bovine and porcine insulins are associated with a higher incidence of allergic reactions and insulin resistance than human insulin and are no longer available on the U.S. market.
- Complications associated with diabetes include retinopathy, neuropathy, nephropathy, hypertension, cardiovascular disease, and coronary artery disease.

- All rapid-acting, short-acting, and long-acting insulin preparations are clear solutions. Intermediate-acting insulins are cloudy solutions. Mixtures of short- and intermediate-acting insulin should look uniformly cloudy. The cloudy appearance of these mixtures is due to the presence of the intermediate-acting insulin. Vials of insulin should be rolled in the hands instead of shaken when used.
- Exact timing of the dose of insulin or oral antidiabetic drug should always be carefully checked against the prescriber's order and should take into consideration the drug's pharmacokinetics, including onset of action, peak, and duration of action.
- The techniques of CSII and MDI hold promise for patients by giving them tight control of serum glucose levels, which can help to decrease the complications of diabetes.
- Nursing care should be individualized with patient education focused on patient's needs and learning abilities. Information must be presented on all aspects of the disease process, drug therapy, and lifestyle modifications.

1 Which is most appropriate regarding the nurse's administration of a rapid-acting insulin to a hospitalized patient?
  a It should be given 15 minutes before the patient begins a meal.
  b It should be given half an hour before a meal.
  c It should be given an hour after a meal.
  d The timing of the insulin injection does not matter with insulin lispro.

2 Which statement would be appropriate for the nurse to include in patient teaching regarding type 2 diabetes?
  a "Insulin injections are never used with type 2 diabetes."
  b "Because you are not taking insulin injections, it is not necessary to measure your blood glucose levels."
  c "A person with type 2 diabetes still has functioning beta cells in his or her pancreas."
  d "Patients with type 2 diabetes usually have better control over their diabetes than those with type 1 diabetes."

3 The nurse monitoring for a therapeutic response to oral antidiabetic drugs will look for
  a fewer episodes of DKA.
  b weight loss of 5 pounds.
  c hemoglobin A1C levels of 6%.
  d glucose levels of 150 mg/dL.

4 A patient with type 2 diabetes is scheduled for magnetic resonance imaging (MRI) with contrast dye. The nurse reviews the orders and notices that the patient is receiving metformin (Glucophage). Which action by the nurse is appropriate?
  a Proceed with the MRI as scheduled
  b Notify the radiology department that the patient is receiving metformin

  c Expect to hold the metformin the day of the test and for 48 hours after the test is performed
  d Call the prescriber regarding holding the metformin for 2 days before the MRI is performed

5 A patient with type 2 diabetes has a new prescription for repaglinide (Prandin). After a week, she calls the office to ask what to do, because she keeps missing meals. "I work right through lunch sometimes, and I'm not sure if I should take it or not. What should I do?" What is the nurse's best response?
  a "You should try not to skip meals, but if that happens, you should also skip that dose of Prandin."
  b "We will probably need to change your prescription to insulin injections because you can't eat meals on a regular basis."
  c "Go ahead and take the pill when you first remember that you missed it."
  d "Take both pills with the next meal and try to eat a little extra to make up for what you missed at lunchtime."

6 A patient is taking metformin for new-onset type 2 diabetes mellitus. When reviewing potential adverse effects the nurse will include information about: (Select all that apply.)
  a Abdominal bloating
  b Nausea
  c Diarrhea
  d Hypoglycemia
  e Weight gain
  f Metallic taste

1. a, 2. c, 3. c, 4. c, 5. a, 6. a, b, c, f

CRITICAL THINKING ACTIVITIES: BEST ACTION

1 N.H. is a 25-year-old woman who has been diagnosed with type 1 diabetes mellitus. She has been placed on a 1500-calorie diabetic diet and is to be started on insulin glargine. N.H. has received teaching about her diet, about insulin injections, and about management of diabetes. She receives the first dose of insulin glargine at 9 PM; the next morning she complains of feeling "dizzy." She is diaphoretic, weak, and pale, with a heart rate of 110 beats/min. What should be the nurse's first action? What is the best explanation for these symptoms?

2 While making morning rounds, the nurse assesses a patient's ordered medications and finds that the patient is to be given NPH insulin each morning but is on orders to receive nothing by mouth because of a scheduled surgical procedure. What is the nurse's best action regarding the administration of the insulin?

3 A patient with type 2 diabetes comes to the emergency department with an acute asthma attack and pneumonia. Her condition is stabilized and she is admitted to the hospital to receive intravenous doses of antibiotics and corticosteroids. She says that, before this episode, she took oral drugs for diabetes and had her diabetes "under control," with fasting blood glucose levels ranging from 99 to 106 mg/dL on most mornings. However, the next morning, her fasting blood glucose level is 177 mg/dL, and her glucose levels remain elevated for the next few days. The patient is upset and declares, "I'm hardly eating anything extra. Why is my blood sugar so high?" What is the nurse's best answer?

For answers, see http://evolve.elsevier.com/Lilley.

CHAPTER 33

Adrenal Drugs

OBJECTIVES

When you reach the end of this chapter, you should be able to do the following:

1 Discuss the normal anatomy, physiology, and related functions of the adrenal glands, including specific hormones released from the glands.

2 Briefly compare the hormones secreted by the adrenal medulla with those secreted by the adrenal cortex.

3 Contrast Cushing's syndrome, Addison's disease, and addisonian crisis.

4 Compare the glucocorticoids and mineralocorticoids with regard to what roles they perform in normal bodily functions, what diseases alter them, and how they are used in pharmacotherapy.

5 Contrast the mechanisms of action, indications, dosages, routes of administration, cautions, contraindications, drug interactions, and adverse effects of glucocorticoids, mineralocorticoids, and antiadrenal drugs.

6 Develop a nursing care plan that includes all phases of the nursing process for patients taking adrenal and antiadrenal drugs.

e-Learning Activities

http://evolve.elsevier.com/Lilley

NCLEX Review Questions • Animations • Nursing Care Plans • Audio Glossary • Category Catchers • Medication Errors Checklists • IV Therapy Checklists • Calculators • Frequently Asked Questions • Content Updates • Supplemental Resources • Answers to Case Studies and Critical Thinking Activities

Drug Profiles

♦ aminoglutethimide, p. 514
♦ fludrocortisone, p. 513
  methylprednisolone, p. 514
♦ prednisone, p. 513

♦ *Key drug.*

Glossary

Addison's disease A potentially life-threatening condition caused by partial or complete failure of adrenocortical function with loss of the functions of the adrenal cortex and decrease in glucocorticoid, mineralocorticoid, and androgenic hormones. It is a chronic disease of hyposecretion of steroids. (p. 510)
Adrenal cortex The outer portion of the adrenal gland. (p. 509)
Adrenal crisis An acute, life-threatening state of profound adrenocortical insufficiency requiring immediate medical management. It is characterized by glucocorticoid deficiency, a drop in extracellular fluid volume, hyponatremia, and hyperkalemia. (p. 516)
Adrenal medulla The inner portion of the adrenal gland. (p. 509)
Aldosterone A mineralocorticoid hormone produced by the adrenal cortex that acts on the renal tubule to regulate sodium and potassium balance in the blood. (p. 510)
Cortex The general anatomic term for the outer layers of a body organ or other structure. (p. 509)
Corticosteroids Any of the natural or synthetic adrenocortical hormones; that is, those produced by the cortex of the adrenal gland (adrenocorticosteroids). (p. 510)

Cushing's syndrome A metabolic disorder characterized by abnormally increased secretion of the adrenocortical steroids. (p. 510)
Epinephrine An endogenous hormone secreted into the bloodstream by the adrenal medulla; also a synthetic drug that is an adrenergic vasoconstrictor and also increases cardiac output. (p. 510)
Glucocorticoids A major group of corticosteroid hormones that regulate carbohydrate, protein, and lipid metabolism and inhibit the release of adrenocorticotropic hormone (corticotropin). (p. 510)
Hypothalamic-pituitary-adrenal (HPA) axis A negative feedback system involved in regulating the release of corticotropin-releasing hormone by the hypothalamus, adrenocorticotropic hormone (corticotropin) by the pituitary gland, and corticosteroids by the adrenal glands. Suppression of the HPA may lead to Addison's disease and possible adrenal crisis or addisonian crisis. This suppression results from chronic disease or exogenous sources, such as long-term glucocorticoid therapy. (p. 510)
Medulla A general anatomic term for the most interior portions of an organ or structure. (p. 510)
Mineralocorticoids A major group of corticosteroid hormones that regulate electrolyte and water balance; in humans the primary mineralocorticoid is aldosterone. (p. 510)
Norepinephrine An adrenergic hormone, also secreted by the adrenal medulla, that increases blood pressure by causing vasoconstriction but does not appreciably affect cardiac output; it is the immediate metabolic precursor to epinephrine. (p. 510)

• • •

Anatomy, Physiology, and Disease Overview

ADRENAL SYSTEM

The adrenal gland is an endocrine organ that sits on top of the kidney like a cap. It is composed of two distinct parts called the **adrenal cortex** and the **adrenal medulla** that both structurally and functionally are very different from one another. In general, the term **cortex** refers to the outer layers of various organs (e.g., cerebral cortex), whereas the term **medulla** refers to the most internal layers. The adrenal cortex comprises roughly 80% to 90% of the entire adrenal gland; the remainder is the medulla. The adrenal cortex is made up of regular endocrine tissue (hormone driven), and the adrenal medulla is made up of neurosecretory endocrine tissue (driven by both hormones and peripheral autonomic nerve impulses). Therefore, the adrenal gland actually functions as two different endocrine glands, each secreting different hormones.

The adrenal medulla secretes two important hormones, both of which are catecholamines. These are **epinephrine,** or adrenaline, which accounts for about 80% of the secretion, and **norepinephrine,** or noradrenaline, which accounts for the other 20%. (Both of these hormones are discussed in Chapter 18 and are not described further in this chapter in any detail.) Some characteristics of the adrenal cortex and the adrenal medulla and the various hormones secreted by each are presented in Table 33-1.

The hormones secreted by the adrenal cortex, which are the focus of this chapter, are broadly referred to as **corticosteroids** because they arise from the cortex and they are made from the steroid known as cholesterol. There are two types of corticosteroids—**glucocorticoids** and **mineralocorticoids.** These are secreted by two different layers, or zones, of the cortex. The zona glomerulosa, which is the outer layer, secretes the mineralocorticoids, and the zona fasciculata, which lies under the zona glomerulosa, secretes the glucocorticoids. A third, inner layer, the zona reticularis, secretes small amounts of sex hormones. All the hormones secreted by the adrenal cortex are steroid hormones; that is, they have the steroid chemical structure.

The mineralocorticoids get their name from the fact that they play an important role in regulating mineral salts (electrolytes) in the body. In humans the only physiologically important mineralocorticoid is **aldosterone.** Its primary role is to maintain normal levels of sodium in the blood (sodium homeostasis) by causing sodium to be resorbed from the urine back into the blood in exchange for potassium and hydrogen ions. In this way aldosterone not only regulates blood sodium levels but also influences the potassium levels in the blood and blood pH.

Overall, the corticosteroids are necessary for many vital bodily functions. Some of the more important ones are listed in Box 33-1. Without these hormones, life-threatening consequences may arise.

Adrenal corticosteroids are synthesized as needed; the body does not store them as it does other hormones. The body levels of these hormones are regulated by the **hypothalamic-pituitary-adrenal (HPA) axis** in much the same way that the levels of hormones secreted by the endocrine glands discussed in previous chapters (pancreas, thyroid, and pituitary) are regulated. As the name implies, this axis consists of a very organized system of communications between the adrenal gland, the pituitary gland, and the hypothalamus. As is the case for the other endocrine glands, it uses hormones as the messengers and a negative feedback mechanism as the controller and maintainer of the process. This feedback mechanism operates as follows: When the level of a particular corticosteroid is low, corticotropin-releasing hormone is released from the hypothalamus into the bloodstream and travels to the anterior pituitary, where it triggers the release of adrenocorticotropic hormone (ACTH; also called *corticotro-*

TABLE 33-1 Adrenal Gland: Characteristics

Type of Tissue	Type of Hormone Secreted	Hormones Secreted and Related Drugs
Adrenal Cortex		
Endocrine	Glucocorticoids	adrenocorticotropic hormone, betamethasone, cortisone, dexamethasone, hydrocortisone, methylprednisolone, paramethasone, prednisolone, triamcinolone
	Mineralocorticoids	aldosterone, desoxycorticosterone, fludrocortisone
Adrenal Medulla		
Neuroendocrine	Catecholamines	epinephrine, norepinephrine

BOX 33-1 Adrenal Cortex Hormones: Biologic Functions

Glucocorticoids
Antiinflammatory actions
Carbohydrate and protein metabolism
Fat metabolism
Maintenance of normal blood pressure
Stress effects

Mineralocorticoids
Blood pressure control
Maintenance of serum potassium levels
Maintenance of pH levels in the blood
Sodium and water resorption

pin). The ACTH is transported in the blood to the adrenal cortex, where it stimulates the production of the corticosteroids. Corticosteroids are then released into the bloodstream. When they reach peak levels, a signal (negative feedback) is sent to the hypothalamus, and the HPA axis is inhibited until the level of the corticosteroids again falls below physiologic threshold, whereupon the axis is stimulated once again.

The oversecretion (hypersecretion) of adrenocortical hormones can lead to a group of signs and symptoms called **Cushing's syndrome.** The hypersecretion of glucocorticoids results in the redistribution of body fat from the arms and legs to the face, shoulders, trunk, and abdomen, which leads to the characteristic "moon face." Such a glucocorticoid excess can be due to any one of several causes, including ACTH-dependent adrenocortical hyperplasia or tumor, ectopic ACTH-secreting tumor, or excessive administration of steroids. The hypersecretion of aldosterone, or primary aldosteronism, leads to increased retention of water and sodium, which causes muscle weakness due to the potassium loss.

The undersecretion (hyposecretion) of adrenocortical hormones causes a condition known as **Addison's disease.** It is associated with decreased blood sodium and glucose levels, increased potassium levels, dehydration, and weight loss. The combination of a mineralocorticoid (fludrocortisone) and a glucocorticoid (prednisone or some other suitable drug) is used for treatment.

Pharmacology Overview

ADRENAL DRUGS

All the naturally occurring corticosteroids are also available as exogenous drugs, and there are also higher-potency synthetic analogues. The adrenal glucocorticoids are an extremely large group of steroids, and they are categorized in various ways. They can be classified by whether they are a natural or synthetic corticosteroid, by the method of administration (e.g., systemic, topical), by their salt and water retention potential (mineralocorticoid activity), by their duration of action (i.e., short, intermediate, or long acting), or by some combination of these methods. The only corticosteroid drug with exclusive mineralocorticoid activity is fludrocortisone. Its uses are much more specific than those of the glucocorticoids and are discussed in the drug profile for fludrocortisone. The currently available synthetic adrenal hormones and adrenal steroid inhibitors are listed in Table 33-2.

Mechanism of Action and Drug Effects

The action of the corticosteroids is related to their involvement in the synthesis of specific proteins. There are several steps to this process. Initially the steroid hormone binds to a receptor on the surface of a target cell to form a steroid-receptor complex, which is then transported through the cytoplasm to the nucleus of that target cell. Once inside the nucleus of the target cell, the complex stimulates the cell's deoxyribonucleic acid (DNA) to produce messenger ribonucleic acid (mRNA), which is then used as a template for the synthesis of a specific protein. It is these proteins that exert specific effects.

Most of the corticosteroids exert their effects by modifying enzyme activity; therefore, their role is more intermediary than direct. The naturally occurring mineralocorticoid aldosterone affects electrolyte and fluid balance by acting on the distal renal tubule to promote sodium resorption from the nephron into the blood, which pulls water and fluid along with it. In doing so it causes fluid and water retention, which leads to edema and hypertension. Aldosterone also promotes potassium and hydrogen excretion.

The glucocorticoid drugs hydrocortisone (called *cortisol* in its naturally occurring form) and cortisone have some mineralocorticoid activity and therefore have some of the same effects as aldosterone (i.e., fluid and water retention). Their other main effect is the inhibition of inflammatory and immune responses. Glucocorticoids primarily inhibit or help control the inflammatory response by stabilizing the cell membranes of inflammatory cells called *lysosomes,* decreasing the permeability of capillaries to the inflammatory cells, and decreasing the migration of white blood cells into already inflamed areas. They may lower fever by reducing the release of interleukin-1 from white blood cells. They also stimulate the *erythroid cells* that eventually become red blood cells. The glucocorticoids also promote the breakdown (catabolism) of protein, the production of glycogen in the liver (glycogenesis), and the redistribution of fat from peripheral to central areas of the body.

Indications

All of the systemically administered glucocorticoids have a similar clinical efficacy but differ in their potency and duration of action and in the extent to which they cause salt and water retention (Table 33-3). These drugs have broad indications, including the following:

- Adrenocortical deficiency
- Adrenogenital syndrome

TABLE 33-2 Available Synthetic Corticosteroids

Type of Hormone	Method of Administration	Individual Drugs
Adrenal steroid inhibitor	Systemic	aminoglutethimide
Glucocorticoid	Topical	alclometasone, betamethasone, clobetasol dexamethasone, fluocinolone, halobetasol hydrocortisone, mometasone, triamcinolone
	Systemic	betamethasone cortisone, dexamethasone, hydrocortisone, methylprednisolone, prednisolone, prednisone, triamcinolone
	Inhaled	beclomethasone, dexamethasone, flunisolide, triamcinolone fluticasone
	Nasal	beclomethasone, dexamethasone, flunisolide, triamcinolone
Mineralocorticoid	Systemic	fludrocortisone

TABLE 33-3 Systemic Glucocorticoids: A Comparison

Drug	Origin	Duration of Action	Equivalent Dose (mg)*	Salt and Water Retention Potential
betamethasone	Synthetic	Long	0.75	Very low
cortisone	Natural	Short	25	High
dexamethasone	Synthetic	Long	0.75	Very low
hydrocortisone	Natural	Short	20	High
methylprednisolone	Synthetic	Intermediate	4	Low
prednisolone	Synthetic	Intermediate	5	Low
prednisone	Synthetic	Intermediate	5	Low
triamcinolone	Synthetic	Intermediate	4	Very low

*Drugs with higher potency require smaller milligram doses than those with lower potency. This column lists the approximate dose equivalency between different drugs that is expected to achieve a comparable therapeutic effect.

- Bacterial meningitis (particularly in infants)
- Cerebral edema
- Collagen diseases (e.g., systemic lupus erythematosus)
- Dermatologic diseases (e.g., exfoliative dermatitis, pemphigus)
- Endocrine disorders (thyroiditis)
- Gastrointestinal (GI) diseases (e.g., ulcerative colitis, regional enteritis)
- Exacerbations of chronic respiratory illnesses such as asthma and chronic obstructive pulmonary disease
- Hematologic disorders (reduce bleeding tendencies)
- Ophthalmic disorders (e.g., nonpyogenic inflammations)
- Organ transplantation (decrease immune response to prevent organ rejection)
- Leukemias and lymphomas (palliative management)
- Nephrotic syndrome (remission of proteinuria)
- Spinal cord injury

Glucocorticoids are also administered by inhalation for the control of steroid-responsive bronchospastic states. However, glucocorticoid inhalers are not used as rescue inhalers for acute bronchospasm. Nasally administered glucocorticoids are used to manage rhinitis and to prevent the recurrence of polyps after surgical removal (see Chapter 36). The topical steroids are used in the management of inflammation of the eye, ear, and skin. Prednisone is the most commonly used oral drug, followed by dexamethasone. Methylprednisolone is the most commonly used injectable glucocorticoid, followed by hydrocortisone and dexamethasone. Betamethasone is the drug of choice for women in premature labor to accelerate fetal lung maturation.

Contraindications

Contraindications to the administration of glucocorticoids include drug allergy and may include cataracts, glaucoma, peptic ulcer disease, mental health problems, and diabetes mellitus. The adrenal drugs may intensify these diseases. For example, one common adverse effect seen in hospitalized patients is an increase in blood glucose levels, often requiring insulin. This is not to say that diabetic patients who require glucocorticoids should not receive them, but the clinician should be aware of the potential increases in blood glucose levels. Because of their immunosuppressant properties, glucocorticoids are often avoided in the presence of any serious infection, including septicemia, systemic fungal infections, and varicella. One exception to this rule is tuberculous meningitis, for which glucocorticoids may be used to prevent inflammatory central nervous system damage. Caution is emphasized in treating any patient with gastritis, reflux disease, or ulcer disease because of the potential of these drugs to cause gastric perforation, as well as any patient with cardiac, renal, and/or liver dysfunction because of the associated alterations in elimination.

Adverse Effects

The potent metabolic, physiologic, and pharmacologic effects of the corticosteroids can influence every body system, so these drugs can produce a wide variety of significant undesirable effects. The more common of these are summarized in Table 33-4. Moon facies is a very common adverse effect of long-term use. Two of the adverse effects most commonly seen in hospitalized patients are hyperglycemia and psychosis. The most serious ad-

TABLE 33-4 Corticosteroids: Common Adverse Effects

Body System	Adverse Effects
Cardiovascular	Heart failure, cardiac edema, hypertension—all due to electrolyte imbalances (e.g., hypokalemia, hypernatremia)
Central nervous	Convulsions, headache, vertigo, mood swings, psychic impairment, nervousness, insomnia
Endocrine	Growth suppression, Cushing's syndrome, menstrual irregularities, carbohydrate intolerance, hyperglycemia, hypothalamic-pituitary-adrenal axis suppression
Gastrointestinal	Peptic ulcers with possible perforation, pancreatitis, ulcerative esophagitis, abdominal distension
Integumentary	Fragile skin, petechiae, ecchymosis, facial erythema, poor wound healing, hirsutism, urticaria
Musculoskeletal	Muscle weakness, loss of muscle mass, osteoporosis
Ocular	Increased intraocular pressure, glaucoma, exophthalmos, cataracts
Other	Weight gain

verse effect of glucocorticoids is adrenal (or HPA) suppression, which is discussed in the drug profiles.

Interactions

Systemically administered corticosteroids can interact with many drugs:

- Their use with non–potassium-sparing diuretics (e.g., thiazides, loop diuretics) can lead to severe hypocalcemia and hypokalemia.
- Their use with aspirin, other nonsteroidal antiinflammatory drugs, and other ulcerogenic drugs produces additive GI effects and an increased chance of gastric ulcer development.
- Their use with anticholinesterase drugs produces weakness in patients with myasthenia gravis.
- Their use with immunizing biologicals inhibits the immune response to the biological.
- Their use with antidiabetic drugs may reduce the hypoglycemic effects of the latter and result in elevated blood glucose levels.

Many other drugs can interact with glucocorticoids; these include the following: thyroid hormones and antifungal drugs (such as fluconazole), which can decrease renal clearance of the adrenal drug; barbiturates and hydantoins, which can increase the metabolism of prednisone and similar drugs; oral anticoagulants, which interact with adrenal drugs in ways that can affect the international normalized ratio; and oral contraceptives, which can increase the half-life of adrenal drugs. Various other drug interactions may be possible between adrenal drugs and over-the-counter drugs and herbals.

Dosages

For information on the recommended dosages of adrenal drugs, see the Dosages table on p. 513.

DOSAGES

Selected Antiadrenal and Corticosteroid Drugs

Drug	Pharmacologic Class	Usual Dosage Range	Indications
◆ aminoglutethimide (Cytadren)	Adrenal corticosteroid inhibitor (antiadrenal drug)	**Adult** PO: 250 mg q6h; titrate in increments of 250 mg to a max daily dose of 2000 mg	Cushing's syndrome
◆ fludrocortisone (Florinef)	Synthetic mineralocorticoid	**Adult and pediatric (including infant)** PO: 0.05-0.2 mg q24h	Addison's disease; salt-losing adrenogenital syndrome
methylprednisolone (Solu-Medrol)	Systemic corticosteroid	**Adult** IV: 10-40 mg every 4 hr **Pediatric** IV: 0.5 mg/kg every 6 hr	Wide variety of endocrine disorders (including adrenocortical insufficiency) and rheumatic, collagen, dermatologic, allergic, ophthalmic, respiratory, hematologic, neoplastic, GI, and nervous system disorders; edematous states
◆ prednisone (Deltasone, Sterapred, Liquid Pred, others)	Synthetic intermediate-acting glucocorticoid	**Adult** PO: 5-60 mg/day **Pediatric** PO: 0.05-2 mg/kg/day divided daily-qid	Wide variety of endocrine disorders (including adrenocortical insufficiency) and rheumatic, collagen, dermatologic, allergic, ophthalmic, respiratory, hematologic, neoplastic, GI, and nervous system disorders; edematous states

GI, Gastrointestinal; *IV,* intravenous; *PO,* oral.

DRUG PROFILES

CORTICOSTEROIDS

The systemic corticosteroids consist of 13 chemically different but pharmacologically similar hormones. They all exert varying degrees of glucocorticoid and mineralocorticoid effects. Their differences are due to slight changes in their chemical structures.

Corticosteroid drugs can cross the placenta and produce fetal abnormalities. For this reason, they are classified as pregnancy category C drugs. They may also be secreted in breast milk and cause abnormalities in the nursing infant. Their use is contraindicated in patients who have exhibited hypersensitivity reactions to them in the past as well as in patients with fungal or bacterial infections. Short- or long-term use can lead to a condition known as *steroid psychosis.* One very important point about long-term use of steroids is that they must not be stopped abruptly. These drugs require a tapering of the daily dose, because the administration of these drugs causes the endogenous (body's own) production of the hormones to stop. This is referred to as *HPA or adrenal suppression.* This suppression can cause impaired stress response and place the patient at risk of developing hypoadrenal crisis (shock, circulatory collapse) in times of increased stress (i.e., surgery, trauma). Adrenal suppression can occur as early as 1 week after a corticosteroid is started. HPA suppression typically does not occur in patients taking prednisone 5 mg/day (or equivalent) or less. Tapering of daily doses allows the HPA axis the time to recover and to start stimulating the normal production of the endogenous hormones. Patients on long-term steroid therapy who are taking at least 10 mg/day (or equivalent) of prednisone and who undergo trauma or require surgery will need replacement doses of steroids (also known as *stress doses*).

◆ fludrocortisone

Fludrocortisone (Florinef) is the most commonly prescribed mineralocorticoid. It is used as partial replacement therapy for adrenocortical insufficiency in Addison's disease and in the treatment of salt-losing adrenogenital syndrome. It is contraindicated in cases of systemic fungal infection. Adverse effects generally relate to water retention and include heart failure, hypertension, and elevated intracerebral pressure (e.g., leading to seizures). Other potential adverse effects involve several body systems and include skin rash, menstrual irregularities, peptic ulcer, hyperglycemia, hypokalemia, potassium loss, muscle pain and weakness, compression bone fractures, glaucoma, and thrombophlebitis, among others. Drugs with which fludrocortisone interacts include anabolic steroids (increased edema); barbiturates, hydantoins, and rifamycins (increased fludrocortisone clearance); estrogens (reduced fludrocortisone clearance); amphotericin B and thiazide and loop diuretics (hypokalemia); anticoagulants (enhanced or reduced anticoagulant activity); antidiabetic drugs (reduced activity leading to hyperglycemia); digoxin (increased risk for dysrhythmias due to fludrocortisone-induced hypokalemia); salicylates (reduced efficacy); and vaccines (increased risk of neurologic complications). Fortunately, adverse effects and serious drug interactions secondary to fludrocortisone therapy are uncommon due to the relatively small dosages of the drug that are normally prescribed. This drug is available only in oral form as a 0.1-mg tablet. Pregnancy category C. Recommended dosages are given in the Dosages table above.

PHARMACOKINETICS

Route	Onset of Action	Peak Plasma Concentration	Elimination Half-life	Duration of Action
PO	10-20 min	1.7 hr	18-36 hr	Unknown

◆ prednisone

Prednisone (Deltasone) is one of the four intermediate-acting glucocorticoids; the others are methylprednisolone, prednisolone, and triamcinolone. These drugs have half-lives that are more than double those of the short-acting corticosteroids (2 to 5 hours), and therefore they have much longer durations of action. Prednisone is the preferred oral glucocorticoid for antiinflammatory or immunosuppressant purposes. Along with methylprednisolone and prednisolone, it is also used to treat exacerbations of chronic respiratory illnesses such as asthma and chronic bronchitis. This drug has only minimal mineralocorticoid properties and therefore alone is inadequate for the management of adrenocortical insufficiency (Addison's disease).

Prednisolone, a prednisone metabolite, is also the liquid drug form of prednisone. Prednisone itself comes in solid form. Pregnancy category C. Recommended dosages are given in the Dosages table on p. 513.

PHARMACOKINETICS

Route	Onset of Action	Peak Plasma Concentration	Elimination Half-life	Duration of Action
PO	Unknown	1-2 hr	18-36 hr	36 hr

methylprednisolone

Methylprednisolone (Solu-Medrol) is the most commonly used injectable glucocorticoid drug. It is used primarily as an antiinflammatory or immunosuppressant drug. It is usually given intravenously. It is available in a long-acting (depot) formulation as well. Like prednisone, it is a pregnancy category C drug. Most injectable formulations contain a preservative (benzyl alcohol) that cannot be given to children younger than 28 days of age.

PHARMACOKINETICS

Route	Onset of Action	Peak Plasma Concentration	Elimination Half-life	Duration of Action
IV	Immediate	30 min	3-4 hr	24-36 hr

ANTIADRENAL DRUG

Aminoglutethimide is an adrenal steroid inhibitor. Aminoglutethimide obstructs the normal actions or function of the adrenal cortex by inhibiting the conversion of cholesterol into adrenal corticosteroids. Aminoglutethimide is indicated for the treatment of Cushing syndrome, which results from an overproduction of corticosteroids by the adrenal gland. Use of antiadrenals is contraindicated in patients who have shown a previous hypersensitivity reaction to them. The most common adverse effects are nausea, anorexia, dizziness, and skin rash. Adverse effects for which to monitor include jaundice, skin lesions, hypotension, headache, lethargy, weakness, GI upset, and hepatotoxicity.

◆ aminoglutethimide

Aminoglutethimide (Cytadren) is used in the treatment of Cushing's syndrome, metastatic breast cancer, and adrenal cancer (see Chapters 47 and 48). It is available only in oral form. Pregnancy category D. Recommended dosages are given in the table on p. 513.

PHARMACOKINETICS

Route	Onset of Action	Peak Plasma Concentration	Elimination Half-life	Duration of Action
PO	Unknown	Unknown	9 hr	Unknown

NURSING PROCESS

Assessment

Before administering any of the *adrenal* or *antiadrenal drugs,* the nurse should perform a thorough physical assessment to determine the patient's nutritional and hydration status and immune status as well as to document baseline weight, intake and output,

---

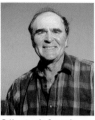
vital signs (especially blood pressure ranges), and the patient's skin condition. Important baseline laboratory values that may be assessed include serum sodium, serum potassium, blood urea nitrogen, serum glucose, and hemoglobin levels, and hematocrit. These specific laboratory tests are important because of the potential drug-related adverse effects. For instance, serum potassium levels usually decrease and blood glucose levels increase when a glucocorticoid (e.g., prednisone) is given. In addition, the patient's muscle strength and body stature should be assessed and documented. Hepatic function tests may also be ordered so that liver function can be assessed by examination of liver enzyme levels. Baseline data should be documented for comparison during and after drug therapy.

A thorough assessment should be performed to identify potential contraindications, cautions, and drug interactions (including interactions with prescription drugs, over-the-counter drugs, and herbals) associated with the adrenal and antiadrenal drugs (see previous discussion). Life span considerations associated with the administration of adrenal drugs include concerns about the use of these medications during pregnancy and lactation. Growth suppression may occur in children who are receiving long-term adrenal drug therapy (e.g., glucocorticoids) if the epiphyseal plates of the long bones have not closed. However, there may be situations in which the benefits to the therapy outweigh risks of the drug's adverse effects. The elderly are more prone to adrenal suppression with prolonged adrenal therapy and may require dosage alterations by the prescriber to minimize the impact of the drug on muscle mass, plasma volume, renal and hepatic function, blood pressure, and serum glucose and electrolyte levels. Adrenal drugs may exacerbate muscle weakness, produce fatigue, and worsen or precipitate osteoporosis. In addition, because the adrenal drugs are associated with the adverse effects of sodium retention, patients with edema and cardiac disease must be closely assessed for exacerbation of these conditions.

Nursing Diagnoses

- Imbalanced nutrition, more than body requirements, related to increased appetite resulting from glucocorticoid therapy
- Disturbed body image related to the physiologic effects of diseases of the adrenal gland on the body or the cushingoid appearance caused by drug therapy with glucocorticoids (e.g., prednisone)
- Excess fluid volume related to the fluid retention associated with glucocorticoid and mineralocorticoid use
- Risk for infection related to the antiinflammatory, immunosuppressive, metabolic, and dermatologic effects of long-term glucocorticoid therapy
- Impaired skin integrity related to the adverse effects of glucocorticoids
- Risk for injury related to the adverse effects of adrenal drug therapy, such as changes in sensorium and confusion

Planning
Goals

- Patient describes the healthy diet to follow during treatment.
- Patient experiences minimal body image disturbances.
- Patient exhibits minimal complications resulting from the fluid retention caused by mineralocorticoid therapy.
- Patient is free of infection during adrenal drug therapy.
- Patient's skin and mucous membranes remain intact during treatment.
- Patient maintains normal fluid and electrolyte levels.
- Patient remains free of changes in sensorium and possible confusion or dizziness from adrenal therapy.

Outcome Criteria

- Patient eats adequate food according to the food guide pyramid and maintains weight within the normal range with adequate menu planning.
- Patient openly verbalizes fears about body image disturbances and other changes to health care providers.

PREVENTING MEDICATION ERRORS

Look-Alike/Sound-Alike Drugs: Solu-Cortef and Solu-Medrol

Be careful about sound-alike, look-alike drugs! Medication errors often occur when drug names are similar.

Solu-Cortef is a trade name for hydrocortisone; Solu-Medrol is a trade name for methylprednisolone. Both are commonly used glucocorticoids and are given intravenously. However, 4 mg of Solu-Medrol is equivalent to 20 mg of Solu-Cortef; therefore, Solu-Medrol is five times stronger than Solu-Cortef. Despite the similar names, these drugs are not interchangeable!

- Patient experiences minimal problems with fluid volume excess and does not gain more than 2 pounds in 24 hours or 5 pounds or more in 1 week.
- Patient notifies the prescriber if the temperature is higher than 100° F (38° C).
- Patient performs frequent mouth and skin care to prevent infections and maintain intactness.
- Patient implements measures to minimize major electrolyte imbalances during adrenal drug therapy.
- Patient changes positions slowly and walks carefully to prevent injuries resulting from dizziness or syncope (caused by postural hypotension for which mineralocorticoids are taken).
- Patient identifies symptoms to report to the prescriber such as weight gain, shortness of breath, edema, dizziness, and/or syncope.
- Patient experiences minimal problems when being weaned off adrenal drugs.

Implementation

The nurse must understand how *glucocorticoids* work in the body so that the patient can be given proper explanations and education to maximize the drug's therapeutic effects and minimize adverse effects. Points to remember when giving these drugs include the following: (1) Hormone production by the adrenal gland is influenced by time of day and follows a diurnal (daily or 24-hour) pattern with peak levels occurring early in the morning between 6 AM and 8 AM, a decrease during the day, and a lower peak in the late afternoon between 4 PM and 6 PM. (2) Cortisol levels increase in response to both emotional and physiologic stress. (3) Cortisol levels also increase when endogenous levels decrease due to a physiologic negative feedback system. (4) When exogenous glucocorticoids are given, endogenous levels decrease; for endogenous production to resume, exogenous levels must be decreased gradually so that hormone output responds to the negative feedback system. (5) The best time to give exogenous glucocorticoids is early in the morning (6 AM to 9 AM), because this leads to the least amount of adrenal suppression.

Prednisone, an *adrenal drug*, may be given by the oral, intramuscular, and intravenous routes. All parenteral forms should be mixed per manufacturer guidelines, and intravenous doses should be given over the recommended time period and in the proper diluent. Intramuscular forms should always be administered into a large muscle mass such as the ventral gluteal site. If frequent injections are required, rotation of sites is needed to prevent tissue trauma and irritation. Oral dosage forms should be given with milk, food, or nonsystemic antacids (such as aluminum, calcium, or magnesium products), unless contraindicated, to minimize GI upset. Another option is for the prescriber to order an H_2-receptor antagonist or proton pump inhibitor to prevent ulcer formation, because glucocorticoids are often ulcerogenic. Patients should be encouraged to avoid alcohol as well as aspirin and other nonsteroidal antiinflammatory drugs to minimize gastric irritation and gastric bleeding. In long-term therapy, alternate-day dosing of glucocorticoids will help minimize the adrenal suppression. With oral and all other forms of glucocorticoids that are given short and/or long term, abrupt withdrawal must be avoided. Abrupt withdrawal of adrenal drugs (e.g., prednisone) may lead to a sudden decrease in or no production of endogenous glucocorticoids resulting in adrenal insufficiency. Signs and symptoms of partial or complete adrenal insufficiency or Addison's disease include fatigue, nausea, vomiting, and hypotension. If left untreated, this condition can lead to an **adrenal crisis** or a life-threatening state of profound adrenocortical insufficiency requiring immediate medical management. Signs and symptoms include a drop in extracellular fluid volume, hyponatremia, and hyperkalemia. This is also referred to as Addisonian crisis.

Other adrenal drug dosage forms include those for intraarticular, intrabursal, intradermal, intralesional, and intrasynovial administration. Intraarticular injections should not be overused, and if a joint is injected with medication, the patient should rest that area for up to 48 hours after the injection is given. Application of cold packs over the injected area may be indicated for up to the first 24 hours to help minimize the discomfort associated with intraarticular injections. Topical dosage forms (e.g., for skin, eye, or inhalation into the bronchial tree) are also available and should be given exactly as ordered. For dermatologic use, the skin should be clean and dry. Gloves should be worn and the medication applied with either a sterile tongue depressor or a cotton-tipped applicator. Sterile technique should be used if the skin is not intact. Nasally administered glucocorticoids (e.g., beclomethasone) should also be used exactly as ordered. Any written instructions that come with the product should be read and followed carefully. Before using the nasal sprays, the patient should first clear the nasal passages and then use the spray per instructions. After the nasal passages are cleared, the container is placed gently inside the nasal passage and the medication is released at the same time that the patient breathes in through the nose.

Glucocorticoid inhalers (e.g., beclomethasone, dexamethasone, flunisolide, triamcinolone, fluticasone) should be used strictly as ordered and the negative consequences of overuse should be explained to the patient. Use of these inhaled glucocorticoids may lead to fungal infections (candidiasis) of the oral mucosa and oral cavity, larynx, and pharynx. Therefore, the patient should rinse the mouth and oral mucous membranes with lukewarm water after each use to help prevent fungal overgrowth

and further complications. In addition to fungal infections, hoarseness, throat irritation, and dry mouth are also possible adverse effects associated with the use of inhaled glucocorticoids, and occurrence of any of these conditions should be reported to the prescriber immediately. See Chapter 10 and Patient Teaching Tips for more information on inhaled dosage forms.

If a patient is receiving long-term maintenance glucocorticoid therapy and requires surgery, the nurse should be sure that the patient's medical records are reviewed carefully. In addition, all nursing documentation and notes should be reviewed. If the preoperative orders do not include the maintenance dosage, the nurse should contact the surgeon and/or other prescriber and ensure that he or she is aware of the situation and the possible need for a rapid-acting corticosteroid. After surgery, the dosage of steroid may well be increased, with a gradual decrease in dosage over several days until the patient returns to baseline. In addition, the nurse should keep in mind that wound healing may be decreased if the patient has been on long-term therapy.

In summary, because of their suppressed immune systems, patients taking corticosteroids should avoid contact with people with known infections and report any fever, increased weakness and lethargy, or sore throat. Monitoring nutritional status, weight, fluid volume, electrolyte status, skin turgor, and glucose levels during therapy is very important to ensure safe and effective therapy. The prescriber should be notified if there is any weakness, joint pain, dyspnea, fever, dysrhythmias, depression, edema, or other unusual symptoms.

Evaluation

A therapeutic response to *glucocorticoids* includes a resolution of the underlying manifestations of the disease or pathology, such as a decrease in inflammation, increased feeling of well-being, less pain and discomfort in the joints, decrease in lymphocytes, or other improvement in the condition for which the medication was ordered. Adverse effects include weight gain; increased blood pressure; pulse irregularities; sodium increase and potassium loss; mental status changes such as aggression, depression, or psychosis; elevated glucose levels; decreased healing; GI upset; and ulcer-related symptoms. The systemic drugs may cause potassium depletion, which is manifested by fatigue, nausea, vomiting, muscle weakness, and dysrhythmias. Cushing's syndrome occurs with prolonged or frequent use of glucocorticoids and is characterized by moon face, obesity of the trunk area (often referred to as *belly fat*), increase in blood glucose and sodium levels, loss of serum potassium, wasting of muscle mass, buffalo hump, and other features previously discussed. Cataract formation and osteoporosis may also occur with long-term use. Rapid drops in cortisol levels (e.g., from abrupt withdrawal of medication) may lead to Addison's disease and addisonian crisis (see previous discussions). Therapeutic responses to aminoglutethimide include a decrease in the size of the tumor and a decrease in Cushing's syndrome. Adverse effects for which to monitor include nausea, anorexia, dizziness, and skin rash.

PATIENT TEACHING TIPS

- Medications (glucocorticoids) should be taken exactly as ordered and should never be abruptly discontinued. The prescriber should be contacted if there are situations that prevent proper dosing. Abrupt withdrawal may precipitate adrenal crisis or Addison's disease and possibly Addisonian crisis.

- If a once-a-day dose is missed with glucocorticoids, the patient should take the dose as soon as possible after remembering that the dose was missed. If the dose is *not* remembered until close to the time for the next dose, then the patient should skip the dose and resume the dosing on the next day without doubling up. If any questions arise, the patient should contact the prescriber. The patient should be educated about the adverse effects of long-term therapy, such as changes in body appearance including acne, buffalo hump, obesity of the trunk area, moon face, and thinning of the extremities, as well as cataract formation.

- With glucocorticoid therapy, education regarding bone health and ways to prevent falls should be emphasized due to the possibility of osteoporosis with long-term use. The prescriber may suggest a daily supplement of oral calcium and vitamin D.

- The prescriber should be contacted immediately if any signs and symptoms of acute adrenal insufficiency appear, such as anorexia, hypotension, hypoglycemia, weakness, nausea, psychologic changes, and restlessness. Any vomiting, diarrhea, acute illnesses, lower extremity edema, muscle weakness, and/or a severe, continual headache should also be reported.

- Fludrocortisone (a mineralocorticoid) should be taken with food or milk to minimize GI upset. With any of the adrenal drugs, weight gain of 2 pounds or more in 24 hours or 5 pounds or more in 1 week should be reported to the prescriber as soon as possible.

- The patient should be encouraged to keep a journal to document responses to treatment, blood pressure readings, daily weight measurements, and any adverse effects experienced.

- The patient should be encouraged to keep follow-up appointments with the prescriber so that electrolyte levels and adverse effects may be monitored. Also, the importance of maintaining a low-sodium and high-potassium diet, if ordered, should be emphasized.

- The patient should be encouraged to wear a medical identification bracelet or necklace with the diagnosis and a list of medications and allergies. A medical card with important relevant information should be on the person at all times and should be updated frequently.

POINTS TO REMEMBER

- The adrenal gland is an endocrine organ that is located on top of the kidney and is composed of two distinct tissues: the adrenal cortex and the adrenal medulla. The adrenal medulla secretes two important hormones: epinephrine and norepinephrine; the adrenal cortex secretes two classes of hormones known as *corticosteroids:* glucocorticoids and mineralocorticoids.

- The biologic functions of glucocorticoids include antiinflammatory actions; maintenance of normal blood pressure; carbohydrate, protein, and fat metabolism; and stress effects. The biologic functions of mineralocorticoids include sodium and water resorption, blood pressure control, and maintenance of potassium levels and pH of the blood.

- Patients taking adrenal drugs may receive them by various routes, such as orally, intramuscularly, intravenously, intranasally, intraarticularly, and by inhalation.

- Glucocorticoid inhaled dosage forms should be used only as prescribed and only after adequate patient education. Rinsing of the mouth after each use is needed to avoid oral fungal infections (oral candidiasis) and oral-pharyngeal irritation.

- Long-term or frequent glucocorticoid use produces increased levels of glucocorticoids, which can lead to Cushing's syndrome. Abrupt withdrawal of glucocorticoids leads to adrenal insufficiency and negative effects on the patient's homeostasis.

- With once-a-day dosing of these drugs, adrenal suppression from corticosteroid therapy can be minimized if the dose is given between 6 AM and 9 AM, but it should be given only as ordered.

NCLEX EXAMINATION REVIEW QUESTIONS

1 When monitoring for a therapeutic response to aminoglutethi-mide, the nurse will look for which potential outcomes?
   a Increase in Cushing's syndrome characteristics
   b Decrease in Cushing's syndrome characteristics
   c Increased lymphocyte levels
   d Growth suppression
2 The nurse has provided teaching about oral corticosteroid ther-apy to a patient. Which statement by the patient shows a poor understanding of the information about this therapy?
   a "I will report any fever or sore throat symptoms."
   b "I will stay away from anyone who has a cold or infection."
   c "I can stop this medication if I have severe adverse effects."
   d "I should take this drug with food or milk."
3 During long-term corticosteroid therapy, the nurse should moni-tor the patient for Cushing's syndrome, which is manifested by
   a weight loss.
   b moon face.
   c hypotension.
   d thickened hair growth.
4 When teaching a patient who has been prescribed a daily dose of prednisone, the nurse knows that the patient should be told to take the medication at which time of day to help reduce ad-renal suppression?

   a In the morning
   b At lunchtime
   c At dinnertime
   d At bedtime
5 Which teaching is appropriate for a patient who is taking an in-haled glucocorticoid for asthma?
   a "Exhale while pushing in on the canister of the inhaler."
   b "Blow your nose after taking the medication."
   c "Rinse the mouth thoroughly after taking the medication."
   d "Do not rinse the mouth after taking the medication."
6 During long-term corticosteroid therapy, the nurse should moni-tor the patient's laboratory results for adverse effects, such as: (Select all that apply.)
   a Increased serum potassium levels
   b Decreased serum potassium levels
   c Increased sodium levels
   d Decreased sodium levels
   e Hyperglycemia
   f Hypoglycemia

1. b, 2. c, 3. b, 4. a, 5. c, 6. b, c, e.

CRITICAL THINKING ACTIVITIES: BEST ACTION

1 A patient with type 2 diabetes mellitus will be receiving intrave-nous doses of methylprednisolone to prevent cerebral edema after a head injury. A new nurse is working with you as you prepare to give this medication. The nurse asks, "Isn't this drug going to cause problems for this patient? Should we be giving it?" What is your best answer?
2 A patient has been taking high doses of oral prednisone for a week due to an exacerbation of asthma symptoms. He is about to go home and is given a prescription for another week of prednisone therapy, but with doses tapering downward

before the medication is stopped. The patient asks, "Why should I bother with this drug if it's only for a week? Can't I just stop it now?" What is the nurse's best response to this question? Explain.
3 A patient has a new order for aminoglutethimide for treatment of Cushing's syndrome. While assessing the patient, the nurse reviews the patient's baseline laboratory results for abnormali-ties. Which laboratory results, if abnormal, would cause the nurse to clarify the order with the prescriber? Explain.

For answers, see *http://evolve.elsevier.com/Lilley*.

CHAPTER 34

Women's Health Drugs

OBJECTIVES

When you reach the end of this chapter, you should be able to do the following:

1 Discuss the normal anatomy and physiology of the female reproductive system.

2 Describe the normal hormonally mediated feedback system that regulates the female reproductive system.

3 Briefly describe the variety of disorders affecting women's health and the drugs used to treat them.

4 Discuss the rationale for use, indications, adverse effects, cautions, contraindications, drug interactions, dosages, and routes of administration for estrogen, progestins, uterine motility–altering drugs, and osteoporosis drugs.

5 Develop a nursing care plan that includes all phases of the nursing process for patients receiving any of the drugs related to women's health (e.g., estrogens, progestins, uterine mobility–altering drugs, and osteoporosis drugs).

e-Learning Activities

http://evolve.elsevier.com/Lilley

NCLEX Review Questions • Animations • Nursing Care Plans • Audio Glossary • Category Catchers • Medication Errors Checklists • IV Therapy Checklists • Calculators • Frequently Asked Questions • Content Updates • Supplemental Resources • Answers to Case Studies and Critical Thinking Activities

Drug Profiles

- ◆ alendronate, p. 528
  - calcitonin, p. 529
  - clomiphene, p. 530
  - contraceptive drugs, p. 527
- ◆ dinoprostone, p. 531
- ◆ estrogen, p. 523
- ◆ medroxyprogesterone, p. 525

  megestrol, p. 525
- ◆ methylergonovine, p. 532
- ◆ oxytocin, p. 532
  raloxifene, p. 529
  terbutaline, p. 533

◆ *Key drug.*

Glossary

Chloasma Hyperpigmentation from the hormone melanin in the skin, characterized by brownish macules on the cheeks, forehead, lips, and/or neck; a common dermatologic adverse effect of female hormonal medications (also called *melasma*). (p. 522)

Corpus luteum The structure that forms on the surface of the ovary after every ovulation and acts as a short-lived endocrine organ that secretes progesterone. (p. 520)

Endocrine glands Glands that secrete one or more hormones directly into the blood. (p. 520)

Estrogens The collective term for one of two major classes of female sex steroid hormones (the other is the *progestins*); of the estrogens, estradiol is responsible for most estrogenic physiologic activity. (p. 520)

Fallopian tubes The passages through which ova are carried from the ovary to the uterus. (p. 520)

Gonadotropin The hormone that stimulates the testes and ovaries. (p. 520)

Hormone replacement therapy (HRT) The term used to describe any replacement of natural body hormones with hormonal drug dosage forms. Most commonly, HRT refers to estrogen replacement therapy for treating symptoms associated with menopause-related estrogen deficiency. (p. 522)

Implantation The attachment to, penetration of, and embedding of the fertilized ovum in the lining of the uterine wall; it is one of the first stages of pregnancy. (Also called *nidation*, from the Latin word *nidus* meaning "nest.") (p. 520)

Menarche The first menses in a young woman's life and the beginning of cyclic menstrual function. (p. 520)

Menopause The cessation of menses that marks the end of a woman's childbearing capability. (p. 520)

Menses The normal flow of blood that occurs during menstruation. (p. 520)

Menstrual cycle The recurring cycle of changes in the endometrium in which the decidual layer is shed, regrows, proliferates, is maintained for several days, and is shed again at menstruation unless a pregnancy begins. (p. 520)

Nucleic acids Compounds involved in energy storage and release as well as in the determination and transmission of genetic characteristics. (p. 522)

Osteoporosis A condition characterized by the progressive loss of bone density and thinning of bone tissue; it is associated with increased risk of fractures. (p. 527)

Ova Female reproductive or germ cells (singular: *ovum;* also called *eggs*). (p. 520)

Ovarian follicles The location of egg production and ovulation in the ovary; the follicle is the precursor to the corpus luteum. (p. 520)

Ovaries The pair of female gonads located on each side of the lower abdomen beside the uterus. They store the *ova* (eggs) and release ova during the ovulation phase of the menstrual cycle. (p. 520)

Ovulation The rupture of the ovarian follicle, which results in the release of an unfertilized ovum into the peritoneal cavity, from which it normally enters the fallopian tube. (p. 520)

Progestins The collective term for one of the two major classes of female hormones (the other is the *estrogens*); of the progestins, progesterone is responsible for most progestational physiologic activity. (p. 520)

Puberty The period of life when the ability to reproduce begins. (p. 520)

Uterus The hollow, pear-shaped female organ in which the fertilized ovum is implanted (see *implantation*) and the fetus develops. (p. 520)

Vagina The part of the female genitalia that forms a canal from its external orifice through its vestibule to the uterine cervix. (p. 520)

• • •

Anatomy and Physiology Overview
FEMALE REPRODUCTIVE FUNCTIONS

The female reproductive system consists of the **ovaries, fallopian tubes, uterus, vagina,** and the external structure known as the *vulva.* The development of these primary sex structures, initiation of their subsequent reproductive functions (starting at **puberty**), and their maintenance are controlled by pituitary **gonadotropin** hormones and the female sex steroid hormones—the **estrogens** and **progestins.** Pituitary gonadotropins include follicle-stimulating hormone (FSH) and luteinizing hormone (LH). Both play a primary role in hormonal communication between the pituitary gland (see Chapter 30) and the ovaries in the continuous regulation of the **menstrual cycle** from month to month.

Estrogens are also responsible for stimulating the development of secondary female sex characteristics, including the characteristic breast, skin, and bone development and distribution of body fat and hair. Progestins help create optimal conditions for pregnancy in the endometrium just after **ovulation** and also promote the start of **menses** in the absence of a fertilized ovum.

The ovaries (female gonads) are paired glands located on each side of the uterus. They function both as **endocrine glands** and as reproductive glands. As reproductive glands, they produce mature **ova** within **ovarian follicles,** which are then ovulated—that is, released into the space in the peritoneal cavity between the ovary and the fallopian tube. Fingerlike projections known as *fimbriae* lie adjacent to each ovary and catch the released ovum and guide it into the fallopian tube. Once inside the fallopian tube the ovum is moved through its lumen to the uterus. This movement is accomplished through the muscular contractions of the tube walls and the actions of ciliated cells inside the lumen of the tube, which "beat" in the direction of the uterus. Fertilization of the ovum, when it occurs, often takes place in the fallopian tube.

As endocrine glands, the ovaries are responsible for producing the two major classes of sex steroid hormones, estrogens and progestins. Chemically speaking, each of these two major classes includes several distinct hormones. However, only two of these hormones occur in significant amounts, and these two have the greatest physiologic activity. These are the estrogen estradiol and the progestin progesterone. Estradiol is the principal secretory product of the ovary and has several estrogenic effects. One of these effects is the regulation of gonadotropin (FSH and LH) secretion via negative feedback to the pituitary gland. Others include promotion of the development of women's secondary sex characteristics, monthly endometrial growth, thickening of the vaginal mucosa, thinning of the cervical mucus, and growth of the ductal system of the breasts. Progesterone is the principle secretory product of the **corpus luteum** and has progestational effects. These include promotion of tissue growth and secretory activity in the endometrium following the estrogen-driven *proliferative phase* of the menstrual cycle. This important secretory process is required for endometrial egg **implantation** and maintenance of pregnancy. Other progestational effects include induction of menstruation when fertilization has not occurred and, during pregnancy, inhibition of uterine contractions, increase in the viscosity of cervical mucus (which protects the fetus from external contamination), and growth of the alveolar glands of the breasts.

TABLE 34-1 Phases of the Menstrual Cycle

Phase	Ovarian Follicle Activity	Endometrium Activity
Phase 1	Menstruation	Menstruation
Phase 2	Follicular phase (preovulatory)	Proliferative phase
Phase 3	Ovulation	Ovulation
Phase 4	Luteal phase (postovulatory)	Secretory phase

The uterus consists of three layers: the outer protective *perimetrium,* the muscular *myometrium,* and the inner mucosal layer known as the *endometrium.* The myometrium provides the powerful smooth muscle contractions needed for childbirth. The endometrium is the site of the following:

- Implantation of a fertilized ovum and subsequent development of the fetus
- Initiation of labor and birthing of the infant
- Menstruation

The vagina serves as a common passageway for birthing and menstrual flow. In addition, it is a receptacle for the penis during sexual intercourse and for the sperm after male ejaculation.

The menstrual cycle usually takes roughly 1 month to complete. Menstrual cycles begin during puberty with the first menses **(menarche)** and cease at **menopause,** which in most women occurs between 45 and 55 years of age. The hormonally controlled menstrual cycle consists of four distinct but interrelated phases that occur in overlapping sequence. Phase names correspond to activity in either the ovarian follicle or the endometrium (Table 34-1).

- **Phase 1:** the *menstruation phase,* which initiates the cycle and lasts from 5 to 7 days.
- **Phase 2:** the *follicular phase,* during which a mature ovum develops from an ovarian follicle. This phase is also called the *proliferative* or *preovulatory phase* and is characterized by rising estrogen secretion from the ovary and LH secretion from the pituitary gland. It terminates on or about day 14 of the cycle.
- **Phase 3:** the *ovulation phase,* which involves release of the unfertilized ovum from the ovary. This process occurs over a roughly 24- to 48-hour period starting at about day 14. Both estrogen and LH levels peak near this time.
- **Phase 4:** the final phase of the cycle, called the *luteal* or *postovulatory phase.* It is also known as the *secretory phase.* It occurs when the corpus luteum forms from the ruptured ovarian follicle. The corpus luteum is a mass of secretory cells on the surface of the ovary. Its primary function is to produce progesterone, which helps to optimize the endometrial mucosa for implantation of a fertilized ovum. The corpus luteum also serves as an initial source of the progesterone needed during early pregnancy. This function is later assumed by the developing placenta. If fertilization does not occur, the rising progesterone levels in the blood initiate the start of menstruation. The corpus luteum then degenerates, and the menstrual cycle begins again on or about day 28.

Figure 34-1 illustrates the sequence of hormone secretions and related events that take place during the menstrual cycle.

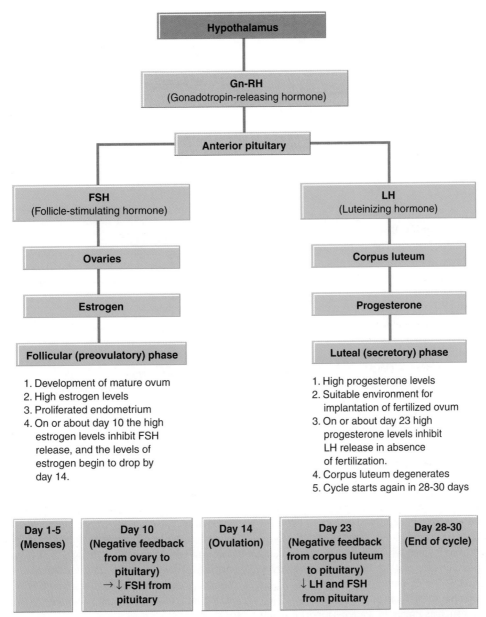

FIGURE 34-1   Hormonal activity during the monthly menstrual cycle. Gonadotropin-releasing hormone (Gn-RH) from the hypothalamus stimulates the pituitary gland, causing it to secrete follicle-stimulating hormone (FSH) early in the cycle (coinciding with the menses) and later luteinizing hormone (LH). FSH stimulates the ovaries to produce estrogen (primarily estradiol). Later in the cycle the combined surges in the levels of estrogen, Gn-RH, FSH, and LH stimulate ovulation. The corpus luteum then secretes estrogen and progesterone, which provide negative feedback to the hypothalamus and pituitary gland to reduce Gn-RH, FSH, and LH secretions. If the ovum (egg) is not fertilized by a spermatozoon, levels of estrogen and progesterone then fall to their monthly lows, Gn-RH and FSH rise again, and the onset of menses begins a new cycle.

▌Pharmacology Overview

FEMALE SEX HORMONES

ESTROGENS

There are three major endogenous estrogens: estradiol, estrone, and estriol. All are synthesized from cholesterol in the ovarian follicles and have the basic chemical structure of a steroid, known as the steroid nucleus. For this reason they are sometimes referred to as *steroid hormones*. Estradiol is the principal and most active of the three and represents the end product of estrogen synthesis.

The exogenous estrogenic drugs, those used as drug therapy, were developed because most of the endogenous estrogens are inactive when taken orally. These synthetic drugs fall into two categories, steroidal and nonsteroidal. Nonsteroidal estrogen products are no longer available in the United States because

---

BOX 34-1 Diethylstilbestrol

Between 1940 and 1971, an estimated 6 million mothers and their fetuses were exposed to diethylstilbestrol (DES). The drug was used to prevent reproductive problems such as miscarriage, premature delivery, intrauterine fetal death, and toxemia. This use resulted in significant complications of the reproductive system in both female and male offspring. Two large groups have been established to monitor these complications: the Registry for Research on Hormonal Transplacental Carcinogenesis and the National Cooperative Diethylstilbestrol Adenosis (DESAD) Project.

---

major adverse effects occurred when one of them, diethylstilbestrol (DES), was used in obstetrics. Box 34-1 describes this important episode in medical history. The estrogenic drugs currently in use are as follows:

- conjugated estrogens (Premarin)
- esterified estrogens (Estratab)
- estradiol transdermal (Estraderm, Climara, Vivelle)
- estradiol cypionate (Depo-Estradiol, DepoGen)
- estradiol valerate (Delestrogen)
- ethinyl estradiol (Estinyl)
- estradiol vaginal dosage forms (Vagifem, Estrace Vaginal Cream)
- estrone (Estrone Aqueous)
- estropipate (Ogen, Ortho-Est)

The most popular estrogen product in use today is an estrogen mixture known as *conjugated estrogens*. This mixture contains a combination of natural estrogen compounds equivalent to the average estrogen composition of the urine of pregnant mares, hence its brand name of Premarin. There is now a nonanimal source for this conjugated estrogen mixture. A product called Cenestin is composed of various conjugated estrogens obtained from soy and yam plants. This product was developed in response to consumer demand from women who wanted an alternative to an animal-derived product (see Herbal Therapies and Dietary Supplements box). Some women obtain other natural estrogen products from naturopathic prescribers and prefer these to standard prescription drugs such as Premarin. Patients report varying degrees of satisfaction with the numerous products available, and it can take both time and patience to find the best choice for a given individual. Ethinyl estradiol is one of the more potent estrogens and is most commonly found in oral contraceptive drugs. Another commonly used form of estrogen is the patch formulation. Several products exist, with the most commonly used called Climara (estradiol). Different patches are applied differently, thus patient education is necessary to ensure appropriate use.

Mechanism of Action and Drug Effects

The binding of estrogen to estrogen receptors stimulates the synthesis of **nucleic acids** (deoxyribonucleic acid [DNA] and ribonucleic acid [RNA]) and proteins, which are the building blocks for all living tissue. Estrogens are also required at puberty for the development and maintenance of the female reproductive system and the development of female secondary sex characteristics, a process known as *feminization*.

Estrogens produce their effects in estrogen-responsive tissues, which have a large number of estrogen receptors. These tissues

---

HERBAL THERAPIES AND DIETARY SUPPLEMENTS

Soy (Glycine max)

■ *Overview*

Soy is a bean commonly grown throughout the world. The isoflavones in soy are chemically similar to the female hormone estradiol. Some studies have shown soy to be useful in the prevention of menopausal symptoms in perimenopausal women. Estrasorb is a new form of estrogen therapy that is a soy-based emulsion applied like a lotion. Other studies have found that soy reduces both low-density lipoprotein and total cholesterol levels.

■ *Common Uses*

Reduction of cholesterol level, relief of menopause symptoms (alternative to hormonal therapy), osteoporosis prevention

■ *Adverse Effects*

Nausea, bloating, diarrhea, abdominal pain (ingested forms), and hypersensitivity reaction have been reported from soy. When Estrasorb is used, it has been found that estradiol is still present on the skin up to 8 hours after application and can transfer to men, which results in increased estradiol levels.

■ *Potential Drug Interactions*

Orally administered soy may interfere with thyroid hormone absorption (avoid concurrent use).

■ *Contraindications*

Allergy to soy products; Estrasorb shares the same contraindications as other estrogen products.

Follow manufacturer directions on label for use of specific preparations.

---

include the female genital organs, the breasts, the pituitary gland, and the hypothalamus. At the time of puberty the production of estrogen increases greatly. This causes initiation of the menses, breast development, redistribution of body fat, softening of the skin, and other feminizing changes. Estrogens play a role in the shaping of body contours and development of the skeleton. For instance, long bones are usually inhibited from growing, with the result that females are usually shorter than males.

Indications

Estrogens are used in the treatment or prevention of a variety of disorders that result primarily from estrogen deficiency. These conditions are listed in Box 34-2. **Hormone replacement therapy (HRT)** to counter such estrogen deficiency is most commonly known for its benefits in treating menopausal symptoms (e.g., hot flashes).

Contraindications

Contraindications for estrogen administration include known drug allergy, any estrogen-dependent cancer, undiagnosed abnormal vaginal bleeding, pregnancy, and active thromboembolic disorder (e.g., stroke, thrombophlebitis) or a history of such a disorder.

Adverse Effects

The most serious adverse effects of the estrogens are thromboembolic events. The most common undesirable effect of estrogen use is nausea. Photosensitivity also may occur with estrogen

BOX 34-2 Indications for Estrogen Therapy

- Atrophic vaginitis (shrinkage of the vagina and/or urethra)
- Hypogonadism
- Oral contraception (in combination with a progestin)
- Ovarian failure or castration
- Uterine bleeding
- Breast or prostate cancer (palliative treatment of advanced inoperable cases)
- Osteoporosis (treatment and prophylaxis)
- Vasomotor symptoms of menopause (e.g., hot flashes)

TABLE 34-2 Estrogens: Common Adverse Effects

Body System	Adverse Effects
Cardiovascular	Hypertension, thrombophlebitis, edema
Gastrointestinal	Nausea, vomiting, diarrhea, constipation, abdominal pain
Genitourinary	Amenorrhea, breakthrough uterine bleeding, enlarged uterine fibromyomas
Dermatologic	Chloasma (facial skin discoloration; also called *melasma*) hirsutism, alopecia
Other	Tender breasts, fluid retention, decreased carbohydrate tolerance, headaches

therapy. One common dermatologic effect of note is **chloasma.** This may be distressing to the patient in terms of body image. Chloasma consists of brownish, macular spots that often occur on the forehead, cheeks, lips, and neck. This and other adverse effects are listed in Table 34-2.

Interactions

Estrogens can decrease the activity of the oral anticoagulants, and the concurrent administration of rifampin and St. John's wort can decrease their estrogenic effect. Their use with tricyclic antidepressants may promote toxicity of the antidepressant. Smoking should be avoided during estrogen therapy, because this, too, can diminish the estrogenic effect and add to the risk for thrombosis.

Dosages

For the recommended dosages of some of the many available estrogen products, see the Dosages table on p. 524.

DRUG PROFILE

◆ estrogen

Estrogen is indicated for the treatment of many clinical conditions, primarily those resulting from estrogen deficiency (see Box 34-2). Many of these conditions occur around menopause, when the endogenous estradiol level is declining. Any estrogen capable of binding to the estrogen receptors in target organs can alleviate menopausal symptoms. As a general rule, the smallest dosage of estrogen that relieves the symptoms or prevents the condition is used. Although many women receive estrogen or estrogen-progestin therapy for many months or years, some clinicians (and patients) may prefer that the patient be weaned from such therapy in light of the known adverse effects.

Two studies that received media attention and were performed as part of the Women's Health Initiative (WHI), a large research program sponsored by the National Institutes of Health, demonstrated the possible detrimental effects of estrogen and estrogen-progestin therapy. Both studies attempted to determine the value of HRT, if any, in preventing diseases and conditions commonly affecting older women, including breast cancer, heart disease, stroke, and hip fracture. The WHI was launched in 1991 under the direction of the National Heart, Lung, and Blood Institute (NHLBI). In one of the WHI studies of HRT, research subjects who took a certain estrogen-progestin combination product were found to have an increased risk of breast cancer, heart disease, stroke, and blood clots, although their risk of hip fractures and colon cancer was reduced. These preliminary results were so alarming that this study of combined estrogen-progestin therapy was discontinued in 2002. A part of the WHI investigation focusing on cognitive function, the WHI Memory Study, also identified adverse cognitive effects in women receiving combination estrogen-progestin therapy. These patients showed an increased risk of developing dementia and demonstrated reduced performance on tests of cognitive function. A second HRT study was begun in which women who had undergone hysterectomy received estrogen alone without progestin. In March 2004, however, these participants were advised to stop taking their assigned medication, because the estrogen-only therapy appeared to be associated with an increased risk of stroke. The data also indicated that estrogen therapy had no effect on the rates of coronary heart disease or breast cancer but was associated with a reduced rate of hip fracture. Since publication of the WHI studies, much confusion and controversy has arisen. One of the biggest challenges of the WHI study is that the majority of the women studied were at least 10 years post-menopause. Recent data have suggested that the use of estrogen in women who are younger is beneficial. The North American Menopause Society released a position statement in July 2008 regarding estrogen use in perimenopausal and postmenopausal women. Recent data support the initiation of HRT around the time of menopause to treat menopause-related symptoms, to treat or reduce the risk of certain disorders such as osteoporosis or fractures in select postmenopausal women, or both. The benefit-risk ratio for menopausal HRT is favorable for women close to menopause but decreases with aging and with time since menopause in previously untreated women. Because this is a topic about which views are so rapidly changing, the reader is referred to the website of the North American Menopause Society at *http://www.menopause.org* for the latest position statements. Follow-up of the WHI study subjects is scheduled to continue until 2010.

The principal pharmacologic effects of all estrogens are similar because there are only slight differences in their chemical structures. These differences yield drugs of different potencies, which in turn makes them useful for a variety of indications. They also allow the drugs to be given by different routes of administration and at often highly customized dosages.

Many fixed estrogen-progestin combination products have been developed over the years. Their use is commonly referred to as *continuous combined hormone replacement therapy.* The rationale for the development of these drugs is that the use of estrogen therapy alone has been associated with an increased risk of endometrial hyperplasia, a possible precursor of endometrial cancer. The addition of continuously administered progestin to an estrogen regimen reduces the incidence of endometrial hyperplasia associated with unopposed estrogen therapy. Examples of these fixed combinations are conjugated estrogens with medroxyprogesterone, norethindrone acetate with ethinyl estradiol, and estradiol with norethindrone.

DOSAGES

Selected Estrogenic Drugs

Drug (Pregnancy Category)	Pharmacologic Class	Usual Dosage Range	Indications
◆ conjugated estrogens (Cenestin, Premarin) (X) and esterified estrogens (Estratab, Menest) (X)	Estrogenic hormone mixture	PO: 0.3-1.25 mg/day PO: 0.625-1.25 mg/day PO: 10 mg tid × 3 mo PO: 1.25 mg/day cyclically, 3 wk on, 1 wk off PO: 0.3-0.625 mg/day cyclically PO: 1.25-2.5 mg tid PO: 1.25 mg q4h × 24 hr, then 1.25 mg daily × 7-10 days	Atrophic vaginitis, kraurosis vulvae Vasomotor symptoms of menopause Breast cancer (palliative; male and female) Female castration, ovarian failure Female hypogonadism Prostate cancer Abnormal uterine bleeding
estradiol (Estrace) (X)	Estrogenic hormone	1-2 mg daily PO: 10 mg tid × 3 mo PO: 0.5 mg daily cyclically	Vasomotor symptoms of menopause, female castration, ovarian failure Breast cancer, prostate cancer Osteoporosis prophylaxis
estradiol transdermal (Estraderm, FemPatch, Vivelle, Climara, Menostar) (X)	Estrogenic hormone	Transdermal patch: 1 patch applied once or twice weekly to lower abdomen (not breast) ranging from 0.025 to 0.1 mg (instructions may vary by product)	Vasomotor symptoms of menopause

PO, Oral.

PROGESTINS

Available progestational medications, or progestins, include both natural and synthetic drugs. Progesterone is the most active natural progestational hormone and is the primary progestin component in most drug formulations. It is produced by the corpus luteum after each ovulation and during pregnancy by the placenta. In addition, there are two other major natural progestins. The first is 17-hydroxyprogesterone, an inactive metabolite of progesterone. The second is pregnenolone, a chemical precursor to all steroid hormones that is synthesized from cholesterol in the ovary as was described for the estrogens. Because orally administered progesterone is relatively inactive and parenterally administered progesterone causes local reactions and pain, chemical derivatives were developed that are effective orally and are also more potent. Their actions are also more specific and of longer duration. The following are some of the most commonly used progestins:

* hydroxyprogesterone (Hylutin)
* medroxyprogesterone (Amen, Provera, Depo-Provera)
* megestrol (Megace)
* norethindrone acetate (Aygestin)
* norgestrel (Ovrette, Ovral)
* progesterone (Prometrium)
* etonogestrel implant (Implanon)

Mechanism of Action and Drug Effects

All of the progestin products produce the same physiologic responses as those produced by progesterone itself. These responses include induction of secretory changes in the endometrium, including diminished endometrial tissue proliferation; an increase in the basal body temperature; thickening of the vaginal mucosa; relaxation of uterine smooth muscle; stimulation of mammary alveolar tissue growth; feedback inhibition (negative feedback) of the release of pituitary gonadotropins (FSH and LH); and alterations in menstrual blood flow, especially in the presence of estrogen.

Indications

Progestins are useful in the treatment of functional uterine bleeding caused by a hormonal imbalance, fibroids, or uterine cancer; in the treatment of primary and secondary amenorrhea; in the adjunctive and palliative treatment of some cancers and endometriosis; and, alone or in combination with estrogens, in the prevention of conception. They may also be helpful in preventing a threatened miscarriage and alleviating the symptoms of premenstrual syndrome. Medroxyprogesterone is the one most commonly used. Norethindrone and norgestrel are commonly used alone or in combination with estrogens as contraceptives. Megestrol is commonly used as adjunct therapy in the treatment of breast and endometrial cancers. When estrogen replacement therapy is initiated after menopause, progestins are often included to decrease the endometrial proliferation that can be caused by unopposed estrogen in women with an intact uterus. Formulations of progesterone itself are also used to treat female infertility (see Dosages table on p. 525).

Contraindications

Contraindications for progestin are similar to those for estrogens, as listed earlier.

Adverse Effects

The most serious undesirable effects of progestin use include liver dysfunction, commonly manifested as cholestatic jaundice; thrombophlebitis; and thromboembolic disorders such as pulmonary embolism. The more common adverse effects are listed in Table 34-3.

Interactions

There are reports of possible decreases in glucose tolerance when progestins are taken with antidiabetic drugs, and the dosage of the antidiabetic drug may need to be adjusted. The concurrent use of medroxyprogesterone or norethindrone and aminoglutethimide or rifampin induces increased metabolism of the progestin.

Dosages

For recommended dosages of the progestins, see the Dosages table below.

DRUG PROFILES

◆ medroxyprogesterone

Medroxyprogesterone (Amen, Provera, Depo-Provera) inhibits the secretion of pituitary gonadotropins, which prevents follicular maturation and ovulation, stimulates the growth of mammary tissue, and has an antineoplastic action against endometrial cancer. Medroxyprogesterone is used to treat uterine bleeding, secondary amenorrhea, endometrial cancer, and renal cancer and is also used as a contraceptive. Its most common use is to prevent endometrial cancer caused by estrogen replacement therapy. It is also sometimes used as adjunct therapy in certain types of cancer (see Chapter 48). Medroxyprogesterone is available in both oral and parenteral preparations. It is also available in a long-acting injection formulation called Depo-Provera. Depo-Provera is used for birth control, and one shot protects the woman for 3 months. There is concern about its use in women younger than 25 years of age and use for longer than 2 years due to the potential for bone density loss.

PHARMACOKINETICS

Route	Onset of Action	Peak Plasma Concentration	Elimination Half-life	Duration of Action
IM	Unknown	2-7 hr	14.5 hr	3 mo

megestrol

Megestrol (Megace) is a synthetic progestin that is structurally very similar to progesterone. Although megestrol shares the actions of the progestins, it is primarily used in the palliative management of recurrent, inoperable, or metastatic endometrial or breast cancer. It has also been used in the management of anorexia, cachexia, or unexplained substantial weight loss in patients with acquired immunodeficiency syndrome (AIDS). In addition, it may be used to stimulate appetite and promote weight gain in patients with cancer. It is available only for oral use.

PHARMACOKINETICS

Route	Onset of Action	Peak Plasma Concentration	Elimination Half-life	Duration of Action
PO	6-8 wk	1-3 hr	13-105 hr	4-10 mo

CONTRACEPTIVE DRUGS

Contraceptive drugs are medications used to prevent pregnancy. Contraceptive devices are nondrug methods of pregnancy prevention such as intrauterine devices, male and female condoms, cervical diaphragms, and others, which are beyond the scope of a pharmacology text. Patients must be informed, for their own safety, of the fact that contraceptive drug therapy serves only to prevent pregnancy and does not protect them from sexually transmitted diseases, including human immunodeficiency virus (HIV) infection/AIDS. This includes even spermicidal drugs such as the over-the-counter (OTC) foams for intravaginal use. These products most often contain the spermicide nonoxynol-9, which does kill sperm cells to prevent pregnancy but does not necessarily kill microbes capable of causing sexually transmitted diseases, including HIV infection.

Aside from sexual abstinence, oral contraceptives are the most effective form of birth control currently available. Estrogen-

TABLE 34-3 Progestins: Common Adverse Effects

Body System	Adverse Effects
Gastrointestinal	Nausea, vomiting
Genitourinary	Amenorrhea, spotting, changes in menstrual flow, changes in cervical erosion and secretions
Other	Edema, weight gain or loss, allergic rash, pyrexia, somnolence or insomnia, depression

DOSAGES

Selected Progestational Drugs

Drug (Pregnancy Category)	Pharmacologic Class	Usual Dosage Range	Indications
◆ medroxyprogesterone acetate (Provera, others) (X)	Progestin	PO: 2.5-10 mg/day for set number of days or cyclically (smaller doses may be given on a continuous daily basis)	Amenorrhea, uterine bleeding
		PO: 2.5-10 mg/day on last 10-13 days of each month to accompany estrogen dosing	Vasomotor symptoms of menopause
		PO: 400-1000 mg/wk	Metastatic endometrial or renal cancer
		400-800 mg/day	Severe weight loss in male and female patients with HIV/AIDS
megestrol (Megace) (X)		PO: 40 mg bid-qid	Uterine bleeding
		PO: 40-800 mg/day in divided doses	Breast or endometrial cancer

AIDS, Acquired immunodeficiency syndrome; *HIV*, human immunodeficiency virus (infection); *PO*, oral.

progestin combinations, often referred to as "the pill," are oral contraceptives that contain both estrogenic and progestational steroids. The most common estrogenic component is ethinyl estradiol, a semisynthetic steroidal estrogen. The most common progestin component is norethindrone.

The currently available oral contraceptives may be *biphasic, triphasic,* or *monophasic,* in terms of the doses taken at different times of the menstrual cycle. The newest are the extended-cycle oral contraceptives. The biphasic drugs contain a fixed estrogen dose combined with a low progestin dose for the first 10 days and a higher dose for the rest of the cycle and are available in 21- or 28-day dosage packages. The triphasic oral contraceptives contain three different estrogen-progestin dose ratios that are administered sequentially during the cycle and are provided in 21- or 28-day dosage packages. The triphasic products most closely duplicate the normal hormonal levels of the female cycle. These contraceptives also come in monophasic forms, in which the estrogen and progestin doses are the same throughout the cycle. There are also oral contraceptives that are progestin-only drugs. The monophasic and triphasic oral contraceptives are the most numerous on the market and the most widely prescribed. The extended-cycle oral contraceptives differ from the traditional 21 days on, 7 days off pills by decreasing or eliminating the hormone-free dosing interval. Consecutive days of hormonal therapy may extend to 84 to 365 days. Reasons for switching to an extended-cycle product include improved efficacy in women who forget to restart the pill and patient preference to decrease the frequency of menstrual bleeding. Some patients (e.g., those with menstrual irregularities) may require special assistance in selecting drug products with their prescribers. Three other important contraceptive medications are a long-acting injectable form of medroxyprogesterone, a transdermal contraceptive patch, and, most recently, an intravaginal contraceptive ring.

Mechanism of Action and Drug Effects

Contraceptive drugs prevent ovulation by inhibiting the release of gonadotropins and by increasing uterine mucous viscosity, which results in (1) decreased sperm movement and fertilization of the ovum, and (2) possible inhibition of implantation (nidation) of a fertilized egg (zygote) into the endometrial lining.

Oral contraceptives have many of the same hormonal effects as those normally produced by endogenous estrogens and progesterone. The contraceptive effect results mainly from the suppression of the hypothalamic-pituitary system that they induce, which in turn prevents ovulation. Other incidental benefits to their use are that they improve menstrual cycle regularity and decrease blood loss during menstruation. A decreased incidence of functional ovarian cysts and ectopic pregnancies has also been associated with their use.

Indications

Oral contraceptive drugs are primarily used to prevent pregnancy. In addition, they are used to treat endometriosis and hypermenorrhea and to produce cyclic withdrawal bleeding in patients with amenorrhea. Occasionally combination oral contraceptives are used to provide postcoital emergency contraception. Emergency contraception pills are not effective if the woman is already pregnant (i.e., egg implantation has occurred). They should therefore be taken within 72 hours of unprotected intercourse with a

TABLE 34-4 Oral Contraceptives: Common Adverse Effects

Body System	Adverse Effects
Cardiovascular	Hypertension, thrombophlebitis, edema, thromboembolism, pulmonary embolism, myocardial infarction
Central nervous	Dizziness, headache, migraines, depression, stroke
Gastrointestinal	Nausea, vomiting, diarrhea, anorexia, pancreatitis, cramps, constipation, increased appetite, increased weight, cholestatic jaundice
Genitourinary	Amenorrhea, cervical erosion, breakthrough bleeding, dysmenorrhea, breast changes

follow-up dose 12 hours after the first dose. They are intended to prevent pregnancy after known or suspected contraceptive failure or unprotected intercourse. Preven and Alesse are two ethinyl estradiol–levonorgestrel combination products that are commonly used for this indication. One new oral contraceptive of note is Seasonale (extended cycle), which includes both estrogen and progestin components. It is sold in packages containing 3 months' worth of medication, including 1 week's worth of nonhormonal tablets. This is because Seasonale reduces a woman's menstrual cycles to once every 3 months.

Contraindications

Contraindications to the use of oral contraceptives include known drug allergy to a specific product, pregnancy, and known high risk for or history of thromboembolic events such as myocardial infarction, venous thrombosis, pulmonary embolism, or stroke.

Adverse Effects

Common adverse effects associated with the use of oral contraceptives are listed in Table 34-4. These effects include hypertension, thromboembolism, alterations in carbohydrate and lipid metabolism, increases in serum hormone concentrations, and alterations in serum metal and plasma protein levels. It is the estrogen component that appears to be the source of most of these metabolic effects.

Interactions

Several drugs and drug classes can potentially reduce the effectiveness of oral contraceptives, which can possibly result in an unintended pregnancy. Patients must be educated about the need to use alternative birth control methods for at least 1 month during and after taking any of the following drugs: antibiotics (especially penicillins and cephalosporins), barbiturates, isoniazid, and rifampin. The effectiveness of other drugs, such as anticonvulsants, beta-blockers, hypnotics, antidiabetic drugs, warfarin, theophylline, tricyclic antidepressants, and vitamins, may be reduced when they are taken with oral contraceptives.

Dosages

For the recommended dosages of oral contraceptives, see the Dosages table on p. 527.

DOSAGES

Selected Contraceptive Drugs

Drug (Pregnancy Category)	Pharmacologic Class	Usual Dosage Range	Indications/Uses
Oral Contraceptives			
norethindrone and ethinyl estradiol (Ortho-Novum, Necon, Jenest, others) (X)	Biphasic: fixed estrogen–variable progestin 21- or 28-day products	For the most reliable contraceptive action, the patient should take all preparations according to instructions from prescriber or patient information product insert, at intervals not to exceed 24 hr	
norethindrone and ethinyl estradiol (Loestrin, Modicon, Necon, others) (X)	Monophasic: fixed estrogen-progestin combinations; 21- or 28-day products; 28-day products contain 7 inert tabs		
norethindrone and ethinyl estradiol (Ortho-Novum 7/7/7, Estrostep, Tri-Norinyl, others) (X)	Triphasic: 3 or 4 monthly phases of variable estrogen and progestin combinations; 21- or 28-day products; 28-day products contain 7 inert tabs		Prevention of pregnancy
levonorgestrel and ethinyl estradiol (Seasonale, Yaz, Lybrel, others)	Extended-cycle products		
Injectable Contraceptives (Depot)			
medroxyprogesterone (Depo-Provera) (X)	Progestin-only injectable contraceptive	IM: 150 mg q3mo	
Transdermal Contraceptives			
norelgestromin and ethinyl estradiol (X)	Fixed-combination estrogen-progestin transdermal contraceptive	Transdermal patch: 1 patch applied weekly × 3 wk each month, scheduled around menses in wk 4	
Intravaginal Contraceptives			
etonogestrel–ethinyl estradiol vaginal ring (NuvaRing) (X)	Fixed-combination estrogen-progestin intravaginal contraceptive	1 ring inserted into vagina by patient and left in place for 3 wk, followed by removal for 1 wk; new ring is then inserted	

IM, Intramuscular.

DRUG PROFILE

CONTRACEPTIVE DRUGS

The Dosages table above provides selected examples of the many contraceptive drugs available. All work in similar fashion to prevent pregnancy. If they are used during pregnancy, however, they can cause termination of pregnancy, and for this reason they are classified as pregnancy category X drugs by the U.S. Food and Drug Administration (FDA). Drugs that are *intended* for termination of pregnancy are known as *abortifacients* and are discussed later in this chapter.

DRUGS FOR OSTEOPOROSIS

Approximately 8 million women in the United States are currently affected by **osteoporosis,** or low bone mass with increased risk of fracture. Nearly 40% of U.S. women over 50 years of age will develop an osteoporotic fracture, and the annual costs to society equal nearly $11 billion. Risk factors for postmenopausal osteoporosis include white or Asian descent, slender body build, early estrogen deficiency, smoking, alcohol consumption, low-calcium diet, sedentary lifestyle, and family history of osteoporosis. Although osteoporosis is primarily a disorder that affects women, up to 20% of individuals with this condition are men.

Until recently, supplementation with calcium and vitamin D was strongly recommended for all women and men considered at risk for osteoporosis (e.g., those with a family history of the disorder). These supplements were thought to play a major role in the prevention of this common bone disorder. The current recommendation is that women, especially those older than age 60, *consider,* in discussions with their health care providers, taking calcium and vitamin D supplements for bone health.

Three major drug classes are currently the mainstays of treatment of existing osteoporosis: the bisphosphonates, the selective estrogen receptor modulators (SERMs), and the hormone calcitonin. Currently available bisphosphonates used for osteoporosis prevention and treatment include alendronate, ibandronate, risedronate, and the once-a-year injection zoledronic acid. Raloxifene and tamoxifen are the currently available SERMs. Tamoxifen is primarily used in oncology settings and is discussed further in Chapter 48. Raloxifene is indicated for use in the prevention and treatment of osteoporosis. A drug form of the hormone calcitonin is also commonly used. Teriparatide stimulates bone formation.

Mechanism of Action and Drug Effects
Bisphosphonates

The bisphosphonates work by inhibiting osteoclast-mediated bone resorption, which in turn indirectly enhances bone mineral density. *Osteoclasts* are bone cells that break down bone, causing calcium to be reabsorbed into the circulation; this resorption eventually leads to osteoporosis if not controlled or countered by adequate new bone formation. These drugs have become the primary drugs of choice for this condition, because their use is backed by the strongest clinical evidence to date indicating reversal of lost bone mass and reduction of fracture risk.

Selective Estrogen Receptor Modulators

Raloxifene helps prevent osteoporosis by stimulating estrogen receptors on bone and increasing bone density in a manner similar to that of the estrogens themselves.

Calcitonin

Like the natural thyroid hormone, calcitonin directly inhibits osteoclastic bone resorption.

Teriparatide

In contrast to the other therapies described thus far, which inhibit bone resorption, teriparatide is the first and currently the only drug available that acts by stimulating bone formation. It is a derivative of parathyroid hormone and works to treat osteoporosis by modulating the body's metabolism of calcium and phosphorus in a manner similar to that of the natural parathyroid hormone.

Indications

Raloxifene is primarily used for the prevention of postmenopausal osteoporosis. The bisphosphonates are used in both the prevention and treatment of osteoporosis. Teriparatide is used primarily for the subset of osteoporosis patients at highest risk of fracture (e.g., those with prior fracture) and calcitonin is used for treatment of osteoporosis.

Contraindications
Bisphosphonates

Contraindications to bisphosphonate use include drug allergy, hypocalcemia, esophageal dysfunction, and the inability to sit or stand upright for at least 30 minutes after taking the medication.

Selective Estrogen Receptor Modulators

The use of SERMs is contraindicated in women with a known allergy to these drugs, in women who are or may become pregnant, and in women with a venous thromboembolic disorder, including deep vein thrombosis, pulmonary embolism, and retinal vein thrombosis, or with a history of such a disorder.

Calcitonin

Contraindications to calcitonin use include drug allergy or allergy to salmon (the drug is salmon derived).

Teriparatide

Contraindications to the use of teriparatide include drug allergy.

Adverse Effects

The primary adverse effects of SERMs are hot flashes and leg cramps. Like estrogens they can increase the risk of venous thromboembolism and they are teratogenic. Leukopenia may also occur and predispose the patient to various infections. Postmenopausal women taking raloxifene were no more likely to develop breast, uterine, or ovarian cancer than were women taking a placebo. The most common adverse effects of bisphosphonates are headache, gastrointestinal (GI) upset, and joint pain. However, the bisphosphonates are usually well tolerated. There is a risk of esophageal burns with these medications if they become lodged in the esophagus before reaching the stomach. For this reason the patient should take these medications with a full glass of water and remain sitting upright or standing for at least 30 minutes afterward. Several case reports of osteonecrosis of the jaw in patients taking bisphosphonates have been released. In fact the FDA issued a public health advisory in January 2008 alerting practitioners to the possible association between bisphosphonate use and the development of severe (possibly incapacitating) bone, muscle, and/or joint pain, as well as low energy fractures when taking bisphosphates for long periods. Common adverse effects of calcitonin include flushing of the face, nausea, diarrhea, and reduced appetite. Common adverse effects of teriparatide include chest pain, dizziness, hypercalcemia, nausea, and arthralgia.

Interactions

Cholestyramine and ampicillin decrease the absorption of raloxifene, and raloxifene can decrease the effects of warfarin. Calcium supplements and antacids can interfere with the absorption of the bisphosphonates, and therefore these drugs should be spaced 1 to 2 hours apart to avoid this interaction. Calcium supplements, although often needed by patients with osteoporosis, are also more likely to cause hypercalcemia in patients receiving calcitonin. In addition, there have been case reports of teriparatide-associated hypercalcemia that has been implicated in digitalis toxicity. Aspirin and other nonsteroidal antiinflammatory drugs have the potential for additive GI irritation if taken with bisphosphonates.

Dosages

For the recommended dosages of osteoporosis drugs, see the Dosages table on p. 529.

DRUG PROFILES

◆ alendronate

Alendronate (Fosamax) is an oral bisphosphonate and the first nonestrogen nonhormonal option for preventing bone loss. This drug works by inhibiting and/or reversing osteoclast-mediated born resorption. Recall that *osteoclasts* are the bone cells that cause breakdown or *resorption* of bone tissue as part of their normal physiologic action. However, unchecked osteoclastic activity often leads to osteoporosis if not managed, so this drug class represents a major breakthrough in the treatment of osteoporosis. It is indicated for the prevention and treatment of osteoporosis in men and in postmenopausal women. It is also indicated for the treatment of glucocorticoid-induced osteoporosis in men and for the treatment of Paget disease in women.

Data show that alendronate therapy may reduce the risk of hip fracture by 51%, of spinal fracture by 47%, and of wrist fracture

DOSAGES

Selected Drugs Used Specifically for Osteoporosis

Drug (Pregnancy Category)	Pharmacologic Class	Usual Dosage Range	Indications/Uses
◆ alendronate (Fosamax) (C)	Bisphosphonate	PO: 5 mg/day or 35 mg/wk PO: 10 mg/day or 70 mg/wk	Osteoporosis prevention Osteoporosis treatment
calcitonin, salmon (Calcimar, Miacalcin, others) (C)	Calcitonin hormonal substitute derived from salmon	IM/subcut: 100 units/day Nasal spray: 200 units (1 spray)/day	Osteoporosis treatment
raloxifene (Evista) (X)	Selective estrogen receptor modulator	PO: 60 mg/day	Osteoporosis treatment

IM, Intramuscular; *PO,* oral; *subcut,* subcutaneous.

by 48%. Precautions should be taken in patients with dysphagia, esophagitis, esophageal ulcer, or gastric ulcer, because the drug can be very irritating. Case reports of esophageal erosions have been published. It is recommended that alendronate be taken with an 8-oz glass of water immediately upon arising in the morning and that the patient not lie down for at least 30 minutes after taking it. When patients whose condition has been stabilized on alendronate are hospitalized and cannot comply with these recommendations, the medication is often withheld. Alendronate has an extremely long terminal half-life, and going several days without taking a dose will do little to reduce the therapeutic efficacy of the drug.

Both alendronate and a similar drug, risedronate, are available only in tablet form for daily or weekly oral use. In 2005, the FDA also approved another bisphosphonate, ibandronate (Boniva), which is dosed orally once per month.

PHARMACOKINETICS

Route	Onset of Action	Peak Plasma Concentration	Elimination Half-life	Duration of Action
PO	3 wk	Unknown	Longer than 10 yr due to storage in bone tissue	Unknown

raloxifene

Raloxifene (Evista) is a SERM. It is used primarily for the prevention of postmenopausal osteoporosis. Interestingly, raloxifene has positive effects on cholesterol level, but it is not normally used specifically for this purpose. It may not be the best choice for women near menopause, because use of the drug is associated with the adverse effect of hot flashes. It is available only for oral use.

PHARMACOKINETICS

Route	Onset of Action	Peak Plasma Concentration	Elimination Half-life	Duration of Action
PO	8 wk	Unknown	28 hr	Unknown

calcitonin

Calcitonin, in its drug forms, is derived from salmon (fish) sources. Although it is available in both injectable form and nasal spray, the nasal spray (Miacalcin) is now more commonly used.

PHARMACOKINETICS

Route	Onset of Action	Peak Plasma Concentration	Elimination Half-life	Duration of Action
Inhalation (nasal spray)	Unknown	30-40 min	43 min	Unknown

DRUGS RELATED TO PREGNANCY, LABOR, DELIVERY, AND THE POSTPARTUM PERIOD

FERTILITY DRUGS

Infertility in women generally results from absence of ovulation (anovulation), which is normally due to various imbalances in female reproductive hormones. Such imbalances can occur at the level of the hypothalamus, the pituitary gland, the ovary, or any combination of these. Supplements of estrogens or progestins may be used to fortify the blood levels of these hormones when ovarian output is inadequate. The use of drug forms of these hormones was described earlier in this chapter.

Hormone deficiencies at the hypothalamic and pituitary levels are often treated with gonadotropin ovarian stimulants. These drugs stimulate increased secretion of gonadotropin-releasing hormone (Gn-RH) from the hypothalamus, which then results in increased secretion of FSH and LH from the pituitary gland. These hormones, in turn, stimulate the development of ovarian follicles and ovulation. They also stimulate ovarian secretion of the estrogens and progestins that are part of the normal ovulatory cycle. Proper selection and dosage adjustment of fertility drugs often requires the expertise of a fertility specialist. The various medical techniques used in the treatment of infertility, including drug therapy, are now collectively referred to as *assisted reproductive technology.* One particularly common specific technique is *in vitro fertilization,* which a woman's ovum is fertilized with her partner's sperm in a laboratory and the fertilized ovum is then medically implanted into the woman's uterus. Infants born through the use of this technique are commonly referred to as "test tube babies." The success of such fertilization techniques may be further aided with the use of medications such as those described earlier. Representative examples of ovulation stimulants include the drugs clomiphene, menotropins, and choriogonadotropin alfa.

Mechanism of Action and Drug Effects

Clomiphene is a nonsteroidal ovulation stimulant that works by blocking estrogen receptors in the uterus and brain. This results in a false signal of low estrogen levels to the brain. The hypothalamus and pituitary gland then increase their production of Gn-RH (from the hypothalamus) and FSH and LH (from the pituitary), which stimulates the maturation of ovarian follicles. Ideally this leads to ovulation and increases the likelihood of conception in a previously infertile woman.

Menotropins is the drug name for a standardized mixture of FSH and LH that is derived from the urine of postmenopausal women. The FSH component stimulates the development of ovarian follicles, which leads to ovulation. The LH component stimulates the development of the corpus luteum, which supplies female sex hormones (estrogens and progestins) during the first trimester of pregnancy. Choriogonadotropin alfa is a recombinant form (i.e., developed using recombinant DNA technology) of the hormone human chorionic gonadotropin. This hormone is naturally produced by the placenta during pregnancy and can be isolated from the urine of pregnant women. It is an analogue of LH and can provide a substitute for the natural LH surge that promotes ovulation. It does this by binding to LH receptors in the ovary and stimulating the rupture of mature ovarian follicles and the subsequent development of the corpus luteum. Human chorionic gonadotropin also maintains the viability of the corpus luteum during early pregnancy. This is critical, because the corpus luteum provides the supply of estrogens and progestins necessary to support the first trimester of pregnancy until the placenta assumes this role. Choriogonadotropin alfa is often given in a carefully timed fashion after FSH-active therapy such as menotropins or clomiphene therapy, when patient monitoring indicates sufficient maturation of ovarian follicles.

Indications

These drugs are used primarily for the promotion of ovulation in anovulatory female patients. They may also be used to promote spermatogenesis in infertile men. As was mentioned in the section on progestins, progesterone formulations are also used to treat female infertility.

Contraindications

Contraindications to the use of the ovarian stimulants include known drug allergy to a specific product and may also include primary ovarian failure, uncontrolled thyroid or adrenal dysfunction, liver disease, pituitary tumor, abnormal uterine bleeding, ovarian enlargement of uncertain cause, sex hormone–dependent tumors, and pregnancy.

Adverse Effects

The most common adverse effects of the ovulation stimulants are listed in Table 34-5.

Interactions

Few drugs interact with fertility drugs. The most notable are the tricyclic antidepressants, the butyrophenones (e.g., haloperidol), the phenothiazines (e.g., promethazine), and the antihypertensive drug methyldopa. When any of these drugs is taken with the fertility drugs, prolactin concentrations may be increased, which may impair fertility.

Dosages

For recommended dosages of clomiphene, see the Dosages table on p. 531.

TABLE 34-5 Fertility Drugs: Most Common Adverse Effects

Body System	Adverse Effects
Cardiovascular	Tachycardia, phlebitis, deep vein thrombosis, hypovolemia
Central nervous	Dizziness, headache, flushing, depression, restlessness, anxiety, nervousness, fatigue
Gastrointestinal	Nausea, bloating, constipation, abdominal pain, vomiting, anorexia
Other	Urticaria, ovarian hyperstimulation, multiple pregnancies, blurred vision, diplopia, photophobia, breast pain, fever

DRUG PROFILE

clomiphene

Clomiphene (Clomid) is primarily used to stimulate the production of pituitary gonadotropins, which in turn induces the maturation of the ovarian follicle and eventually ovulation. It is currently available only for oral use.

PHARMACOKINETICS

Route	Onset of Action	Peak Plasma Concentration	Elimination Half-life	Duration of Action
PO	4-12 days	Unknown	5 days	30 days

UTERINE STIMULANTS

A variety of medications are used to alter the dynamics of uterine contractions either to promote or to prevent the start or progression of labor. In the immediate postpartal period, medications may also be used to promote rapid shrinkage of the uterus to reduce the risk of postpartum hemorrhage.

Four types of drugs are used to stimulate uterine contractions: ergot derivatives, prostaglandins, the progesterone antagonist mifepristone (RU-486), and the hormone oxytocin. These drugs all act on the uterus, a highly muscular organ that has a complex network of smooth muscle fibers and a large blood supply. These drugs are often collectively referred to as *oxytocics,* after the naturally occurring hormone oxytocin, whose action they mimic. The uterus undergoes several changes during normal gestation and childbirth that at different times make it either resistant or susceptible to various hormones and drugs. Oxytocin is one of the two hormones secreted by the posterior lobe of the pituitary gland. The other is vasopressin, which is also known as *antidiuretic hormone* (see Chapter 30).

Mechanism of Action and Drug Effects

The uterus of a woman who is not pregnant is relatively insensitive to oxytocin, but during pregnancy the uterus becomes more sensitive to this hormone and is most sensitive at term (the end of gestation).

During childbirth, oxytocin stimulates uterine contraction, and during lactation it promotes the movement of milk from the mammary glands to the nipples. Another class of oxytocic drugs is the prostaglandins, natural hormones involved in regu-

DOSAGES

Selected Fertility Drugs

Drug (Pregnancy Category)	Pharmacologic Class	Usual Dosage Range	Indications
clomiphene (Clomid, Milophene, Serophene) (X)	Ovulation stimulant	PO: 50-100 mg daily × 5 days; repeatable cycle depending on response	Female infertility in selected patients

PO, Oral.

lating the network of smooth muscle fibers of the uterus. This network is known as the *myometrium.* The prostaglandins cause very potent contractions of the myometrium and may also play a role in the natural induction of labor. When the prostaglandin concentrations increase during the final few weeks of pregnancy, mild myometrial contractions, commonly known as *Braxton Hicks contractions,* are stimulated. The third major class of oxytocic drugs is the ergot alkaloids, which are also potent simulators of uterine muscle. These drugs increase the force and frequency of uterine contractions. One of the most politically charged prescription drug approvals ever made by the FDA was approval of the progesterone antagonist mifepristone (Mifeprex), also known as the "abortion pill." This drug also stimulates uterine contractions and is used to induce elective termination of pregnancy.

Indications

Oxytocin is available in a synthetic injectable form (e.g., Pitocin). This drug is used to induce labor at or near full-term gestation and to enhance labor when uterine contractions are weak and ineffective. Oxytocin is also used to prevent or control uterine bleeding after delivery, to induce completion of an incomplete abortion (including miscarriages), and to promote milk ejection during lactation.

The prostaglandins may be used therapeutically to induce labor by softening the cervix (cervical ripening) and enhancing uterine muscle tone. They may also be used to stimulate the myometrium to induce abortion during the second trimester when the uterus is resistant to oxytocin. Examples of these drugs are dinoprostone and misoprostol. Misoprostol is available as an oral tablet and is also used as a stomach protectant (see Chapter 45). For use in cervical ripening, it is administered intravaginally. It offers the great advantage of costing pennies as opposed to the hundreds of dollars paid for dinoprostone. Because of this, misoprostol is widely used in third-world countries as well as throughout the United States.

Ergot alkaloids are used after delivery of the infant and placenta to prevent postpartum uterine atony (lack of muscle tone) and hemorrhage.

Mifepristone is used to induce abortion and is often given with the synthetic prostaglandin drug misoprostol for this purpose.

Contraindications

Contraindications to the use of labor-inducing uterine stimulants include known drug allergy to a specific product and may include pelvic inflammatory disease, cervical stenosis, uterine

TABLE 34-6 Oxytocic Drugs: Most Common Adverse Effects

Body System	Adverse Effects
Cardiovascular	Hypotension or hypertension, chest pain
Central nervous	Headache, dizziness, fainting
Gastrointestinal	Nausea, vomiting, diarrhea
Genitourinary	Vaginitis, vaginal pain, cramping
Other	Leg cramps, joint swelling, chills, fever, weakness, blurred vision

fibrosis, high-risk intrauterine fetal positions before delivery, placenta previa, hypertonic uterus, uterine prolapse, or any condition in which vaginal delivery is contraindicated (e.g., increased bleeding risk). Contraindications to the use of abortifacients include known drug allergy as well as the presence of an intrauterine device, ectopic pregnancy, concurrent anticoagulant therapy or bleeding disorder, inadequate access to emergency health care, or the inability to understand or comply with follow-up instructions.

Adverse Effects

The most common undesirable effects of oxytocic drugs are listed in Table 34-6.

Interactions

Few clinically significant drug interactions occur with the oxytocic drugs. The most common and important of these involve sympathomimetic drugs. Combining drugs that produce vasoconstriction, such as sympathomimetics, with the oxytocic drugs can result in severe hypertension.

Dosages

For the recommended dosages of selected oxytocic drugs, see the Dosages table on p. 532.

DRUG PROFILES

◆ dinoprostone

Dinoprostone (Prostin E$_2$, Cervidil, Prepidil) is a synthetic derivative of the naturally occurring hormone prostaglandin E$_2$. It is used for the termination of pregnancy from the twelfth through the twentieth gestational weeks, for evacuation of the uterine contents in

DOSAGES

Selected Uterine Stimulants

Drug (Pregnancy Category)*	Pharmacologic Class	Usual Dosage Range	Indications/Uses
◆ dinoprostone (Prostin E₂, Prepidil, Cervidil) (X)	Prostaglandin E₂ abortifacient and cervical ripening drug	Vaginal suppository (Prostin E₂): 1 suppository (20 mg) into vagina at 3-5 hr intervals until uterine evacuation	Termination of pregnancy; uterine evacuation in cases of miscarriage or benign hydatidiform mole
		Cervical gel (Prepidil): 0.5 mg into cervical canal at 6-hr dosing intervals (max 1.5 mg/24 hr)	Cervical ripening for induction of labor
		Vaginal suppository (Cervidil): 10 mg into posterior vaginal fornix (space behind cervix) × 1 dose	Cervical ripening for induction of labor
◆ methylergonovine (Methergine) (X)	Oxytocic ergot alkaloid	IM/IV: 0.2 mg after delivery of placenta, repeatable at 2-4 hr intervals	Postpartum uterine atony and hemorrhage
		PO: 0.2 mg tid-qid for up to 7 days postpartum	
◆ oxytocin (Pitocin, Syntocinon) (X)	Oxytocic hypothalamic hormone	IV infusion: 0.5-20 milliunits/min, titrated to effect	Labor induction
		IV infusion: 10-40 units in 1 L of D₅LR titrated to effect	Postpartum uterine atony and hemorrhage
		IM: 10 units in a single dose after delivery of placenta	

D₅LR, Dextrose 5% in lactated Ringer's solution; *IM*, intramuscular; *IV*, intravenous; *PO*, oral.
*Use of these medications is contraindicated in pregnancy (pregnancy category X) unless needed for the indications listed.

the management of missed abortion or intrauterine fetal death up to 28 weeks of gestational age, for the management of nonmetastatic gestational trophoblastic disease, and for ripening of an unfavorable cervix in pregnant women at or near term when there is a medical or obstetric need for labor induction. It is available only for vaginal use in various dosage forms.

PHARMACOKINETICS

Route	Onset of Action	Peak Plasma Concentration	Elimination Half-life	Duration of Action
Topical gel	Rapid	30-45 min	Unknown	Not available

◆ methylergonovine

The ergot alkaloid methylergonovine (Methergine) is used primarily in the immediately postpartal period to enhance myometrial tone and reduce the likelihood of postpartum uterine hemorrhage. Its use is contraindicated in patients with a known hypersensitivity to ergot medications and in those with pelvic inflammatory disease. It also should not be used for augmentation of labor, before delivery of the placenta, or during a spontaneous abortion. Methylergonovine is available in both oral and injectable forms.

PHARMACOKINETICS

Route	Onset of Action	Peak Plasma Concentration	Elimination Half-life	Duration of Action
PO	5-15 min	30 min	2 hr	3 hr

◆ oxytocin

The drug oxytocin (Pitocin, Syntocinon) is the synthetic form of the endogenous hormone oxytocin and has all of its pharmacologic properties.

PHARMACOKINETICS

Route	Onset of Action	Peak Plasma Concentration	Elimination Half-life	Duration of Action
IV	Immediate	Immediate	3-5 min	1 hr

UTERINE RELAXANTS

When contractions of the uterus begin before term, it may be desirable to stop labor, because premature birth increases the risk of neonatal death. Postponing delivery by relaxing the uterine smooth muscles and helping to prevent contractions and the induction of labor increases the likelihood of the infant's survival. However, this measure is generally employed only after the twentieth week of gestation, because spontaneous labor occurring before the twentieth week is commonly associated with a nonviable fetus and thus is usually not interrupted. Only uterine contractions occurring between about 20 and 37 weeks of gestation are considered premature labor.

The nonpharmacologic treatment of premature labor includes bed rest, sedation, and hydration. Drugs given to inhibit labor and maintain the pregnancy are called *tocolytics*. Terbutaline is classified as a beta-adrenergic drug (see Chapter 18) and work by directly relaxing uterine smooth muscle. However, it should be noted that this use of terbutaline is "off label"; that is, the drug is not officially approved by the FDA for this purpose. Concentrated solutions of the electrolyte magnesium sulfate are also used intravenously for this purpose. Ritodrine is no longer available in the United States.

Mechanism of Action and Drug Effects

Tocolytics act by causing relaxation of uterine smooth muscle, thus stopping the uterus from contracting. They do so by stimulating beta-adrenergic receptors located on the bronchial tree, peripheral vasculature, and uterine smooth muscles. These are believed to be primarily beta$_2$-adrenergic receptors. The beta$_1$-adrenergic receptors are located in the heart and are not stimulated by terbutaline except at high dosages.

The drug effects of terbutaline are related to their beta-adrenergic effects. When the bronchial beta-adrenergic receptors are stimulated, the bronchi dilate and airway resistance decreases. When the beta-adrenergic receptors of the peripheral vasculature are stimulated, the blood vessels dilate and blood pressure decreases. Finally, when the beta-adrenergic receptors located on the uterine smooth muscle are stimulated by the beta agonist terbutaline, the uterine smooth muscle relaxes and premature contractions are thus halted.

Indications

Terbutaline is used to inhibit uterine contractions in preterm labor. Terbutaline was originally used as a bronchodilator in the symptomatic treatment of bronchial asthma and reversible bronchospasm (see Chapter 37).

Contraindications

Contraindications to the use of terbutaline include known drug allergy, cardiac dysrhythmia, pheochromocytoma (an adrenal tumor), pregnancy before the twentieth week of gestation, eclampsia, hypertension, thyrotoxicosis, antepartum hemorrhage, intrauterine fetal death, maternal cardiac disease, pulmonary hypertension, and uncontrolled diabetes.

TABLE 34-7 Tocolytic Drugs: Most Common Adverse Effects

Body System	Adverse Effects
Cardiovascular	Palpitations, tachycardia, hypertension, dysrhythmias, altered maternal and fetal heart rate and blood pressure, chest pain, pulmonary edema
Central nervous	Tremors, anxiety, insomnia, headache, dizziness, nervousness
Gastrointestinal	Nausea, vomiting, anorexia, bloating, constipation, diarrhea
Metabolic	Hyperglycemia, hypokalemia
Other	Rash, dyspnea, hyperventilation, glycosuria, lactic acidosis

Adverse Effects

The most common adverse effects of terbutaline are listed in Table 34-7. Terbutaline may cause pulmonary edema, which is associated with the following risk factors: excessive hydration, multiple gestation, and underlying cardiac disease. To reduce this risk, fluid intake should be limited to 2.5 to 3 L/day, sodium intake should be limited, and maternal pulse should be maintained at less than 130 beats/min.

Toxicity and Management of Overdose

The toxicity stemming from an overdose of a tocolytic and its management are similar to those for the other adrenergic drugs and are discussed in Chapter 18. For example, beta-blockers may be used to treat terbutaline overdose.

Interactions

Few drugs interact with uterine relaxants. The most notable are sympathomimetic drugs and beta-blockers. Sympathomimetic drugs may have additive cardiovascular effects when given with uterine relaxants, and beta-blockers may have antagonistic effects when combined with uterine relaxants.

Dosages

For the recommended dosages of terbutaline, see the Dosages table below.

DRUG PROFILE

terbutaline

Terbutaline (Brethine) is indicated for the prevention of preterm labor; it may also be used as a bronchodilator in the symptomatic treatment of asthma. As noted earlier, the preterm labor indication is actually "unlabeled," that is, the drug is not actually FDA approved for this use; the original indication for terbutaline was for respiratory problems. However, clinical obstetrical practice has demonstrated the usefulness of this drug in the management of preterm labor. Terbutaline is available in both oral and injectable forms. The injectable form is most commonly used for obstetrical purposes.

PHARMACOKINETICS

Route	Onset of Action	Peak Plasma Concentration	Elimination Half-life	Duration of Action
IV/subcut	5 min	30-60 min	20 hr	1.5-4 hr
PO	30-45 min	1-2 hr	20 hr	

DOSAGES

Selected Uterine Relaxants

Drug (Pregnancy Category)	Pharmacologic Class	Usual Dosage Range	Indications
terbutaline (Brethine) (B)	Beta$_2$-selective adrenergic agonist	IV infusion: 50-100 mcg/min, titrated to effect (max dose of 100 mcg) PO: 2.5-10 mg q4-6h as long as needed and tolerated by patient subcut: 0.25 mg every 0.5-3 hr	Preterm labor (unlabeled, non–FDA approved use)

FDA, Food and Drug Administration; *IV*, intravenous; *PO*, oral.

PHARMACOKINETIC BRIDGE
to Nursing Practice

Estrasorb is a new form of estrogen that is FDA approved to help ease the severity of postmenopausal hot flashes by increasing estrogen levels when these are found to be deficient in the patient. Estrasorb contains estradiol, which is identical to the estrogen produced in the woman's body. The absorption of the topical emulsion dosage form results in measurable levels of estradiol on the skin for up to 8 hours after application. It is important to fully understand this pharmacokinetic property, because the transfer of the drug to men may result. In fact, traces of Estrasorb have been found on males from such transfer for up to a 2-day period. This transfer of medication to other individuals may be reduced by allowing the dosage form to fully dry and then covering it with clothing before having contact with another individual. Although no specific investigation of the tissue distribution of the estradiol absorbed from Estrasorb in humans has been conducted, it is known that the distribution of exogenous estrogens is similar to that of endogenous estrogens. The metabolism of exogenous estrogens is also similar to that of endogenous estrogens, with biotransformation taking place mainly in the liver and excretion in the urine. The specific dosage form of an emulsion is desirable because it may be applied easily, once daily to the thighs and/or calves. One dose is contained in two separate foil pouches, and patients need to be fully aware of the application instructions. For example, sunscreen products should not be applied at the same time, because sunscreen reduces the absorption of Estrasorb.

Knowing the pharmacokinetic properties of Estrasorb is necessary for safe and efficient administration of the drug. It is also important to understand all the pharmacokinetic properties of this drug to be able to fully educate patients about the drug, its effect on the body, and the subsequent implications for its absorption, distribution, metabolism, and excretion.

NURSING PROCESS

Assessment

In this section, estrogen and progesterone drugs are discussed first, and then medroxyprogesterone, megestrol, menotropins, the gonadotropins, and clomiphene are covered. Next, information on uterine motility–altering drugs is provided, followed by a discussion of dinoprostone and, finally, consideration of the bisphosphonates and calcitonin. Before initiating therapy with any of the hormonal drugs (e.g., estrogens, progestins) or other women's health-related drugs, the patient's blood pressure, weight, blood glucose levels, and results of liver and renal function tests should be documented. Drug allergies, contraindications, cautions, and drug interactions should also be assessed for and documented. Patient assessment should also include obtaining a thorough medication history, medical history, and menstrual history as well as documenting vital signs, weight, and hormonal levels, if appropriate. Assessment of emotional stability is also important because of the potential for therapy-related depression. Results of the patient's last physical examination, clinician-performed breast examination, and gynecologic examination should be noted, as well.

Estrogen-only hormones should be given only after the following disorders and conditions have been ruled out: abnormal uterine bleeding, thromboembolic disorders, pregnancy, incomplete long-

bone growth, photosensitivity (a more common adverse effect with conjugated estrogens), estrogen receptor–positive breast cancer, personal history or family history of breast cancer, early menstruation, pregnancies late in life, endocrine disorders, renal and/or liver dysfunction, fluid retention disorders, and seizure activity. Assessment should also include questions about breast examination, breast self-examination practices, and dates of last complete physical examination and Papanicolaou (Pap) smear. The nurse must also assess the patient's knowledge about the use of hormones (e.g., estrogens and progestins), whether for contraception or replacement therapy. The patient's readiness to learn, educational level, and degree of adherence to other medication regimens must also be assessed. The success of treatment with oral contraceptives, hormone replacement medication, and other therapies depends heavily on the patient's understanding instructions.

With *oral contraceptive drugs* (e.g., combination estrogen-progestin drugs), the assessment should include a pregnancy test, assessment for cerebral and coronary vascular disease, jaundice, thromboembolic disorders, and malignancies of the reproductive tract or abnormal vaginal bleeding. There should also be close monitoring of patients with the following: uncontrolled hypertension, migraine headaches, visual disturbances, hyperlipidemia, asthma, blood dyscrasias, diabetes mellitus, heart failure, depression, and seizures. The concern is for exacerbation of these conditions and subsequent complications. Patients who smoke should also be closely monitored because of the increased risk of complications in smokers, especially those older than age 35 years. A smoking history should include documentation of the number of packs smoked per day and the number of years the patient has smoked. When combination oral contraceptives are used in emergency situations for postcoital conception, the same contraindications, cautions, and drug interactions apply, even if the drug is for one-time use. The indications for medroxyprogesterone and megestrol may be varied, for example, amenorrhea and abnormal uterine bleeding (for medroxyprogesterone) and palliative treatment of breast and endometrial cancers as well as promotion of increased appetite in patients with AIDS (for megestrol), but assessment is similar to that described earlier.

Use of *clomiphene* requires assessment of the patient's medical and medication history with attention to the patient's menstrual history. Medical history is critical, especially reproductive and uterine status, because use of the drug may result in multiple births and compromise maternal health status. Family stability and economic status must be assessed because of the risk of multiple births to make sure that as healthy a home as possible exists for everyone concerned. Cardiac, liver, and renal status must also be assessed, as ordered.

Terbutaline has the unlabeled use of inhibiting premature labor and should be used only in women in premature labor who are in the twentieth to thirty-seventh week of gestation. Women with other complications of pregnancy or with seizures, hypertension, diabetes, asthma, cardiac dysrhythmias, angina, or hypokalemia may receive this drug, but only if they are monitored very closely and if the benefits outweigh the risks. The contraindications, cautions, and drug interactions for terbutaline have been discussed previously; however, vital signs, with emphasis on maternal pulse rate and blood pressure and fetal heart rate, and a baseline electrocardiogram should be assessed and results available prior to use of the drug. It must be remembered that beta agonists or beta stimulants will decrease the therapeutic effects of terbutaline. The environment should be assessed as well. The setting should be a quiet one but should provide for constant maternal and fetal monitoring and the safe administration of the drug.

Before administering *uterine stimulants* (e.g., oxytocin or prostaglandins), the nurse should measure and document the patient's blood pressure, pulse, and respiration. Fetal heart rate and contraction-related fetal heart rates should also be determined and recorded. Because oxytocin therapy is associated with vasopressive and antidiuretic effects, it is even more important than normally to know fluid volume status. The nurse should know that when these drugs are administered, maternal blood pressure will decrease initially but will then rise (sometimes by up to 30%), and cardiac output and stroke volume will subsequently increase. Assessment for complications associated with the use of these drugs should include measurement of all vital signs, monitoring of intake and output, and observation for signs and symptoms of water intoxication (e.g., headache, fatigue, nausea, anorexia, lethargy, disorientation, seizures or coma, tachycardia, hypotension, and muscular cramps and weakness), which may even be fatal if not appropriately identified and treated. The mother and fetus should be assessed frequently for fetal distress and uterine contractions with either hypertonic or hypotonic patterns and the findings documented. For labor and delivery, the patient's cervix should be ready for induction (see a maternal and child health or obstetric nursing text for more information on the rating of the cervix). Constant monitoring of maternal blood pressure, pulse, contractions, and fluid status, as well as fetal heart rate monitoring, is needed. Oxytocin is *not* used during the first trimester except in some cases of spontaneous or induced abortion. The same considerations apply to the ergot alkaloids (e.g., methylergonovine), and the patient's vital signs and fetal heart rate should be assessed. A baseline neurologic assessment is important with attention to seizures. The nurse should continually assess for the signs of acute overdose, including nausea, vomiting, abdominal pain, numbness and tingling of the extremities, and hypertension. Contraindications, cautions, and drug interactions have been previously discussed for these drugs, as well as for the remaining women's health drugs.

The use of dinoprostone or other *prostaglandin E₂* drugs is indicated in specific situations requiring termination of pregnancy. The patient should be questioned about the presence of fibroids, pelvic inflammatory disease, pelvic stenosis, respiratory disease, and recent or past pelvic surgery and the answers documented.

With *osteoporosis drugs* (SERMs, biphosphonates), there are many contraindications, cautions, and drug interactions. Assessment for the following is also important to patient safety: premenopausal state; occurrence of thromboembolism, deep vein thrombosis, and/or pulmonary embolism; concurrent estrogen therapy; anticipated immobility or bed rest (SERMS should be discontinued 72 hours before the patient becomes immobile); aspiration risk; renal or liver dysfunction; high levels of calcium; the use of other drugs that are considered to be GI irritants; the presence of esophageal abnormalities or delayed esophageal emptying; and the inability to remain upright in either a sitting or standing position (remaining upright helps

CULTURAL IMPLICATIONS

Racial Disparities in the Survival of Women with Endometrial Cancers

The National Cancer Institute (NCI), part of the National Institutes of Health, has reported findings that suggest a biologic disparity in endometrial cancer between white and African American patients. Two separate studies performed in collaboration with the Walter Reed Army Medical Center and other institutions looked at patient outcomes in endometrial cancer clinical trials and at patterns of gene expression in endometrial tumors. Estimates were that in 2005 some 40,000 new cases of endometrial cancer would be diagnosed and some 7000 endometrial cancer–related deaths would occur. Research has shown that although the rate for new cancers is lower in African American women than in white women, African American women have a higher mortality rate from endometrial cancer than their white counterparts. In fact, an NCI review of research conducted from 1989 to 1994 reported that the 5-year survival rate for patients with endometrial cancer was 86% among whites but only 54% among African Americans. The cause of this disparity was believed to be multifactorial. One factor was cultural differences such as patterns of dealing with medical illness and inequality of access to appropriate cancer treatment. The disparity could also be related to biologic differences that lead to the occurrence of more aggressive tumors in African American females. Research evaluating global gene expression in endometrial cancer patients suggested that there are underlying molecular differences that may partially explain the differences in survival rates in whites and African Americans. The investigators noted that their research did not imply that African Americans and whites are genetically different but rather that there are multiple factors (e.g., environment and culture) that lead to differences in gene expression. Thus, there is a need to consider how racial differences may affect the way individuals respond to cancer treatment and to identify better therapies for high-risk minority groups.

Modified from Maxwell L: NCI studies examine racial disparity in survival among patients with endometrial cancer, NCI press release, March 21, 2005. Available at *http://www.cancer.gov.*

to prevent esophageal erosion and ulcers from reflux of the drug into the esophagus). Drug interactions have been discussed earlier in the chapter, but the nurse should note that any drugs that are associated with GI distress or ulcer formation (e.g., aspirin and nonsteroidal antiinflammatory drugs) should be avoided. Concerns about prolonged immobility should be addressed as well.

Nursing Diagnoses

- Risk for infection related to possible drop in white blood cell count due to the effects of SERMs
- Disturbed body image related to the effects of abnormal hormone levels, osteoporosis, or other female-related diseases or disorders
- Deficient knowledge related to lack of information about first-time drug therapy
- Acute pain related to a disorder of the female reproductive tract and related drug therapy
- Anxiety related to various female disorders and possible complications of the associated therapy
- Ineffective sexuality patterns related to abnormal levels of estrogen

- Decisional conflict related to the risks versus benefits of postmenopausal estrogen replacement therapy
- Risk for injury to the mother related to the adverse effects of uterine mobility–altering drugs
- Risk for injury to the infant related to premature labor and/or the adverse effects of tocolytics
- Excess fluid volume related to the adverse effect of retention associated with hormonal drugs and tocolytics

Planning
Goals

- Patient is free of body image disturbances.
- Patient states the rationale for hormonal replacement, combination oral contraceptives, osteoporosis drugs, uterine relaxants, or fertility drugs.
- Patient states the adverse effects of specific medications.
- Patient states the importance of compliance with hormonal therapy and other recommended pharmacologic and nonpharmacologic measures for the treatment of premature labor, preeclampsia, and/or fertility disorders.
- Patient openly states the need for improved sexual functioning and image before and during treatment.
- Patient verbalizes fears and concerns about the use of hormonal therapy.
- Patient verbalizes fears and concerns about pregnancy and its outcome.

Outcome Criteria

- Patient openly verbalizes concerns, fears, and anxieties about body image changes and the need for medication.
- Patient is compliant with the pharmacologic and nonpharmacologic therapy regimen and achieves successful management of osteoporosis, breast cancer, infertility, preeclampsia, or premature labor, or experiences effective birth control.
- Patient is free of complications and disturbing adverse effects associated with each group of drugs, such as chest pain, leg pain, blurred vision, thrombophlebitis, and leukopenia.
- Patient returns for regular follow-up visits with the prescriber for monitoring of the therapeutic and adverse effects of treatment.
- Patient has positive sexual patterns and habits while receiving hormonal therapy.
- Patient is free of complications associated with uterine mobility–altering drugs.

Implementation

Both *estrogens* and *progestins* should be administered in the lowest dosages possible and the dosages titrated as needed, but only as ordered. Intramuscular doses should be given deep in large muscle masses, and the injection sites should be rotated. Oral forms should be taken with food or milk to minimize GI upset. Progestin-only oral contraceptive pills are taken daily. It is important for the patient to take this oral contraceptive at the same time every day so that effective hormone serum levels are maintained. Because use of the progestin-only pill leads to a higher incidence of ovulatory cycles, there is an associated increased rate of contraceptive failure. The nurse should remember that this type of pill is usually prescribed for those women who cannot

CASE STUDY

Bisphosphonate Drug Therapy for Osteoporosis

© Martina Ebel

Mrs. S. is a relatively healthy 73-year-old retired clerk who has recently been diagnosed with postmenopausal osteoporosis. She has been prescribed treatment with ibandronate (Boniva), 150 mg each month. She has many questions, and you are reviewing the drug and its use with her.

1. Mrs. S. tells you that she likes to have breakfast, take her morning medicines, then lie down on the couch to read the morning newspaper. She asks whether the ibandronate will fit into her routine. What should you tell her?
2. Mrs. S. calls the clinic to ask what she should use for headaches. "I have several different types of headache pills, so aren't they all the same?" How should you respond?
3. A few months later, Mrs. S. comes in for a follow-up visit. She tells you that she is due for her next osteoporosis pill next week, but she has been having some jaw pains ever since she went to the dentist 2 weeks earlier to have a tooth pulled. She is worried that her osteoporosis has affected her jaw. What could be the reason for this pain? What do you think will be done about it?

For answers, see *http://evolve.elsevier.com/Lilley.*

tolerate estrogens or for whom estrogens are contraindicated. Often it is more effective in women who are older than 35 years of age. Combination estrogen-progestin pills contain low doses of drug. The low-dose monophasic and multiphasic types are provided as 21 days of pills followed by 7 days of placebo treatment, and the patient needs to understand how this treatment regimen works. The nurse should emphasize to the patient that the reduction in the level of estrogen has been associated with a decrease in adverse effects and a decrease in the risk for liver tumors, hypertension, and cardiovascular changes; however, more breakthrough bleeding will occur.

Medroxyprogesterone should be given as ordered. *Megestrol* is given orally and the patient should know whether the drug is being given to improve appetite so that appropriate dietary measures can be implemented. *Fertility drugs* (e.g., clomiphene) are often self-administered. The provision of specific instructions regarding how to administer the drug at home and how to monitor drug effectiveness is very important to improve the success of treatment. Journal tracking of the medication regimen is helpful to those involved in the care of the infertile patient or couple. See Patient Teaching Tips for more information.

Terbutaline use requires close and frequent monitoring of maternal blood pressure, pulse, temperature, and respirations. Terbutaline is usually given by intravenous pump with titration upward to the prescribed dose. Lactated Ringer's solution, dextrose 5% in water, or 0.9% (normal) saline should be used as ordered to help prevent fluid overload. Oral dosage forms are used for maintenance and can be administered at home, generally for long-term therapy. The patient should be positioned in the left lateral recumbent position to minimize hypotension, increase renal blood flow, and increase blood flow to the fetus. Frequent measurement of intake and output as well as maternal vital signs and fetal heart rate is critical to preventing complications of this therapy. Breath sounds should be auscultated for crackles or rhonchi as needed to help monitor fluid status due to the potential adverse reaction of pulmonary edema. The nurse should also check weight daily, monitor intake and output, and assess for pedal and/or dependent edema. The prescriber should be notified immediately if signs and symptoms of pulmonary edema or fluid overload are present. The rate of infusion or the dosage should be decreased, as ordered, if adverse effects such as tachycardia, hypertension, or nervousness develop. The antidote for terbutaline, if ordered, is the beta-blocker propranolol. The nurse must also be aware that these preterm labor patients should be monitored frequently for any increase in the intensity, duration, or frequency of contractions, as well as any palpitations, anxiety, shortness of breath, vomiting, dizziness, or tachycardia. In addition, any loss of fetal movement should be reported to the health care provider immediately. If the patient is diabetic, the health care provider will most likely order frequent measurement of serum glucose level. Due to the potential for hypokalemia with terbutaline, if any type of diuretic is administered, the patient should be closely monitored for any drop in potassium levels. Oral forms of terbutaline may be prescribed for home use while the patient is on bed rest to try to suppress premature onset of labor. The patient must be sure to keep all follow-up appointments.

Oxytocin should be administered only as ordered, and any instructions or protocols should be strictly followed. The cervix must be ripe (see earlier). *Prostaglandin E₂* may be instilled vaginally to help accomplish this if the mother's cervix is not ripe or at a Bishop score of 5 or higher. Because oxytocin has vasopressive and antidiuretic properties, the patient is at risk for hypertensive episodes as well as fluid retention, and constant monitoring of maternal blood pressure and pulse rate as well as fetal monitoring is required. The patient should report any of the following: strong contractions, edema, symptoms of water intoxication, palpitations, chest pain, and any changes in fetal movement. Intravenous infusions (via infusion pump) of oxytocin should be administered with the proper dilutional fluid and at the proper rate. To minimize the adverse effects of the drug, intravenous piggyback dosing is often ordered so that the diluted oxytocin solution can be discontinued immediately if maternal and/or fetal decline occurs while an intravenous line with hydration is maintained. Doses are generally titrated as ordered and are based on the progress of labor and degree of fetal tolerance of the drug. Should the labor progress at 1 cm/hr, oxytocin may no longer be needed. The decision is made by the prescriber and on an individual basis. Generally speaking, with oxytocin therapy, if there are hypertensive responses or major changes in the maternal vital signs *or* if the fetal heart rate decreases *or* if fetal movement stops, the prescriber should be contacted immediately. Hyperstimulation may also occur. If contractions are more frequent than every 2 minutes and last longer than 1 minute (and are accompanied by changes in other parameters), the infusion should be stopped and the prescriber contacted immediately. If this does occur, it is critical also to place the patient on the left side, maintain administration of intravenous fluids, and give oxygen as ordered (generally via tight face mask at 10 to 12 L/min). If there is concern about overstimulation, discuss concerns with the pre-

scriber and document actions thoroughly. Misoprostol may be used intravaginally for cervical ripening and should be given as ordered.

Dinoprostone is given by vaginal suppository to those who are 12 to 20 weeks pregnant and are seeking termination and/or to those patients in whom evacuation of the uterus is needed for the management of incomplete spontaneous abortion or intrauterine fetal death (up to 28 weeks). The drug should be given exactly as ordered, and the patient should be monitored closely.

The success of therapy with biphosphonates depends on providing thorough patient teaching and ensuring that the patient understands all aspects of the drug regimen. With oral biphosphonates, the nurse must emphasize the need to take the medication upon rising in the morning with a full glass (6 to 8 oz) of water at least 30 minutes before the intake of any food, other fluids, or other medication. In addition, the nurse must emphasize that the patient should remain upright in either a standing or sitting position for approximately 30 minutes after taking the drug to help prevent esophageal erosion or irritation. The patient taking the SERM raloxifene should be informed that the drug needs to be discontinued 72 hours before and during prolonged immobility. Therapy may be resumed once the patient becomes fully ambulatory and as ordered. Education about the best way to take these medications is important, as is education about the need to report any severe bone, muscle, and/or joint pain (see previous discussion about possible osteonecrosis of the jaw). See the Patient Teaching Tips.

Evaluation

Therapeutic responses to the various drugs discussed in this chapter should be measured by evaluating whether goals and outcome criteria have been met. Many drugs have been discussed, often with several indications for use; thus, the therapeutic response will be the occurrence of the indicated therapeutic effect, and the nurse will then also monitor for the associated adverse effects and/or toxicity. Therapeutic effects of *estrogens* may range from prevention of pregnancy to a decrease in menopausal symptoms to a reduction in the size of a tumor. Adverse effects of estrogens may include thromboembolism, edema, jaundice, abnormal vaginal bleeding, hyperglycemia, nausea, vomiting, increased appetite, and weight gain. Therapeutic responses to *progestins* include a decrease in abnormal uterine bleeding and the disappearance of menstrual disorders (e.g., amenorrhea). The adverse effects of progestins include edema, hypertension, cardiac symptoms, changes in mood and affect, and jaundice.

Therapeutic effects of oxytocin and other *uterine stimulants* include stimulation of labor and control of postpartum bleeding. Adverse effects may include drop in pulse rate, dysrhythmias, severe abdominal pain, and shocklike symptoms (e.g., decrease in blood pressure, increase in pulse rate). These adverse effects may indicate a dangerous complication and medical emergency. The primary therapeutic effect of *terbutaline* is the absence of preterm labor. Adverse maternal effects include palpitations, nausea, vomiting, headache, jitteriness, tremors, chest pain, and anxiety. Adverse neonatal effects include hypoglycemia, ileus, hypotension, and hypocalcemia.

The therapeutic effects of *fertility drugs* include successful fertilization. Adverse reactions include hot flashes, abdominal discomfort, blurred vision, GI upset, nervousness, depression, weight gain, and hair loss. Multiple births and birth defects are other possible consequences of therapy. The therapeutic effects of *dinoprostone* include therapeutic termination of pregnancy, and adverse effects include severe cramping and bleeding. Thera-

peutic effects of *osteoporosis drugs* include increased bone density and prevention or management of osteoporosis. Adverse effects are leukopenia, decreased platelet levels, thrombophlebitis, hot flashes, and leg cramps.

PATIENT TEACHING TIPS

- Hormonal drugs are usually tolerated better if taken with food or milk to minimize GI upset.
- With the use of oral contraceptives as well as any form of HRT with estrogens and/or progestins, the patient should be encouraged to openly discuss concerns about the medications. Assure the patient that, although risks may be associated with HRT, the prescriber will weigh each case individually and make a recommendation in each situation based on the benefits versus risks, but with the ultimate decision resting with the patient.
- With estrogens and progestins, the following should be reported to the prescriber immediately: chest pain, leg pain, blurred vision, headache, neck stiffness, neck pain, loss of vision, numbness of extremities, severe headache, edema, yellow discoloration of the skin or sclera, clay-colored stools, and abnormal vaginal bleeding.
- Patients should report a weight gain of 2 pounds or more in 24 hours or 5 pounds or more in 1 week, as well as any breakthrough bleeding, change in menstrual flow, or breast tenderness.
- Oral contraceptives should be taken exactly as ordered, and appointments for all follow-up examinations (e.g., a pelvic examination, Pap smear, and practitioner-performed breast examination) should be kept.
- Instruct on the importance of and technique for monthly breast self-examinations during the ideal time—that is, 7 to 10 days after the menses. The need for follow-up appointments and annual examinations by a health care provider must also be stressed.
- Hormones make the patient sensitive to sunlight and tanning beds, and so these should be avoided or the appropriate sun protection used.
- If the patient is using progesterone-only intravaginal gel with other gels, the patient should be sure to insert the other gels at least 6 hours before or after the progesterone-based product.
- Progesterone-filled intrauterine inserts are placed in the uterine cavity by a health care provider and their use should be accompanied by thorough education that the inserts are left in place for 1 year after insertion and then must be replaced. Abnormal uterine bleeding, cramping, abdominal pain, or amenorrhea should be reported immediately.
- The patient using an estrogen/progestin vaginal ring for contraception should be instructed on what to expect with its insertion. Use of this contraceptive device requires thorough teaching and follow-up, including instruction in insertion and removal techniques and a return demonstration before the patient leaves the prescriber's office. Inform patient that menstruation will follow in 2 to 3 days after the ring is removed and should be told to replace the used ring in its foil pouch and discard it in the trash, rather than flushing it down the commode.

- Oral contraceptive hormones should be taken at the same time every day. If one dose is missed, the patient should take the dose as soon as it is remembered and use a backup form of contraception. More specific instructions should be provided regarding the omission of more than one pill and/or 1 day's dose and should be specific to the prescribed oral contraceptive drug. It is important for patient safety and compliance to provide the patient with a phone number that can be called to obtain answers to questions about dosing, omissions, and so on.
- The importance of using condoms with oral contraception to prevent sexually transmitted diseases should be emphasized.
- It should be emphasized to the patient taking oral contraceptives that backup contraception (e.g., condom use) is needed when antibiotics, barbiturates, griseofulvin, isoniazid, or rifampin is taken. St. John's wort may also diminish the effectiveness of oral contraception.
- Estrasorb is generally applied once daily to the thighs and calves, as ordered, with one dose provided in two separate pouches. Sunscreen and other lotions should not be applied at the same time because they interfere with the drug. To reduce the chance of transfer of this medication to other individuals, the application areas should be allowed to dry completely before covering them with clothing. The drug contained in this dosage form, estradiol, has been found to be present on the skin up to 8 hours after application. The old dosage form should be removed and the area cleansed. Prior to applying a new dosage form, the site should be cleansed with soap and water.
- Bisphosphonates (e.g., alendronate) should be taken exactly as prescribed; that is, the drug should be taken at least 30 minutes before the first morning beverage, food, or other medication, and should be taken with at least 6 to 8 oz of water. The importance of remaining upright for at least 30 minutes after taking the medication to prevent esophageal and GI adverse effects should be emphasized. Esophageal irritation, dysphagia, severe heartburn, and retrosternal pain must be reported to the prescriber immediately to help prevent severe reactions.
- Patients taking bisphosphonates may also require supplemental calcium and vitamin D, as ordered by the prescriber.
- The patient should be educated about making lifestyle changes as recommended, such as engaging in weight-bearing exercise (e.g., walking), stopping smoking, and limiting or eliminating alcohol intake. These measures will help encourage fewer adverse effects of oral contraception and/or drug therapy with hormones.

POINTS TO REMEMBER

- Three major estrogens are synthesized in the ovaries: estradiol (the principal estrogen), progesterone, and estradiol. Exogenous estrogens can be classified into two main groups: steroidal estrogens (e.g., conjugated estrogens, esterified estrogens, estradiol) and nonsteroidal estrogens (e.g., chlorotrianisene, dienestrol, diethylstilbestrol).
- Progestins have a variety of uses, including treatment of uterine bleeding and amenorrhea, and adjunctive and palliative treatment of some cancers.
- Oral contraceptives containing a combination of estrogens and progestins are the most effective form of birth control currently available.

- Uterine stimulants (sometimes called *oxytocic drugs*) include ergot derivatives, prostaglandins, and oxytocin.
- Uterine relaxants (often called *tocolytic drugs*) are used to stop preterm labor and maintain pregnancy by halting uterine contractions. The most commonly used drug is terbutaline.
- A thorough nursing assessment is necessary to ensure the safe and effective use of female reproductive drugs. Information should be obtained on the patient's past medical problems, history of menses and problems with the menstrual cycle, medications taken (prescribed and OTC), number of pregnancies and miscarriages, last menstrual period, and any related surgical or medical treatments.

NCLEX EXAMINATION REVIEW QUESTIONS

1 The nurse is assessing a patient who is to receive dinoprostone. Which condition would be a contraindication to the use of this drug?
   a Pregnancy at 15 weeks' gestation
   b GI upset or ulcer disease
   c Ectopic pregnancy
   d Incomplete abortion
2 When teaching a patient who is taking oral contraceptive therapy for the first time, the nurse relates that adverse effects may include which of the following?
   a Dizziness
   b Nausea
   c Tingling in the extremities
   d Polyuria
3 The nurse is reviewing the use of obstetric drugs. Which situation is an indication for an oxytocin (Pitocin) infusion?
   a Termination of a pregnancy at 12 weeks
   b Hypertonic uterus
   c Cervical stenosis in a patient who is in labor
   d Induction of labor at full term
4 The nurse has provided patient education regarding therapy with the SERM raloxifene. Which statement from the patient reflects a good understanding of the instruction?
   a "When I take that long flight to Asia, I will need to stop taking this drug at least 3 days before I travel."

   b "I can continue this drug even when traveling as long as I take it with 8 oz of water each time."
   c "After I take this drug I must sit upright for at least 30 minutes."
   d "One advantage of this drug is that it will reduce my hot flashes."
5 The nurse is discussing therapy with clomiphene with a husband and wife who are considering trying this drug as part of treatment for infertility. It is important that they be informed of which possible effect of this drug?
   a Increased menstrual flow
   b Increased menstrual cramping
   c Multiple pregnancies
   d Sedation
6 A patient calls the clinic because she realized she missed one dose of an oral contraceptive. Which statement from the nurse is appropriate? (Select all that apply.)
   a "Go ahead and take the missed dose now, along with today's dose."
   b "Don't worry, you are still protected from pregnancy."
   c "Please come in to the clinic for a reevaluation of your therapy."
   d "Wait 7 days, then start a new pack of pills."
   e "You will need to use a backup form of contraception until the next cycle."

1. c, 2. b, 3. d, 4. a, 5. c, 6. a, e.

CRITICAL THINKING ACTIVITIES: BEST ACTION

1 A patient in her first pregnancy has spent 14 hours in labor and has made little progress. She is becoming exhausted, and the uterine contractions have decreased in strength. She is now receiving an oxytocin infusion. During this infusion, the nurse will perform many assessments. Which is most important?
2 The nurse is reviewing a cephalosporin prescription for a patient who has a severe sinus infection. The patient tells the nurse that she is taking a birth control pill and asks the nurse if there will

be any problems with the antibiotic. What is the nurse's best answer?
3 A woman comes into the emergency department. She says that she is pregnant but that she is having contractions every 3 minutes and she is "not due yet." She is very upset. While assessing her vital signs and fetal heart tones, what is the most important question the nurse should ask the patient?

For answers, see *http://evolve.elsevier.com/Lilly.*

CHAPTER 35

Men's Health Drugs

OBJECTIVES

When you reach the end of this chapter, you should be able to do the following:

1 Discuss the normal anatomy, physiology, and functions of the male reproductive system.
2 Compare the various men's health drugs, with discussion of their rationale for use, dosages, and dosage forms.
3 Describe the mechanisms of action, dosages, adverse effects, cautions, contraindications, drug interactions, and routes of administration for the various men's health drugs.
4 Develop a nursing care plan that includes all phases of the nursing process for patients receiving men's health drugs for treatment of benign prostatic hyperplasia, sexual dysfunction, hormone deficiency, or prostate cancer.

e-Learning Activities

Drug Profiles

finasteride, p. 544
◆ sildenafil, p. 544

◆ testosterone, p. 545

◆ *Key drug.*

Glossary

Anabolic activity Any metabolic activity that promotes the building up of body tissues, such as the activity produced by testosterone that causes the development of bone and muscle tissue; also called *anabolism.* (p. 540)

Androgenic activity The activity produced by testosterone that causes the development and maintenance of the male reproductive system and male secondary sex characteristics. (p. 540)

Androgens Male sex hormones responsible for mediating the development and maintenance of male sex characteristics. Chief among these are testosterone and its various biochemical precursors. (p. 540)

Benign prostatic hyperplasia (BPH) (also called hypertrophy) Nonmalignant (noncancerous) enlargement of the prostate gland. (p. 541)

Catabolism The opposite of anabolic activity; any metabolic activity that results in the breakdown of body tissues; also called *catabolism.* Examples of conditions in which catabolism occurs are debilitating illnesses such as end-stage cancer and starvation. (p. 540)

Erythropoietic effect The effect of stimulating the production of red blood cells (erythropoiesis). (p. 541)

Prostate cancer A malignant tumor within the prostate gland. (p. 542)

Testosterone The main androgenic hormone. (p. 540)

• • •

Anatomy and Physiology Overview

MALE REPRODUCTIVE SYSTEM

The male reproductive system consists of several structures, of which the testes and seminiferous tubules are the most important to the discussion in this chapter because they produce the primary male hormones. The testes, a pair of oval glands located in the scrotal sac, are the male gonads. The testes produce male sex hormones. The seminiferous tubules, which are channels in the testes, are the site of spermatogenesis, which is the process by which mature sperm cells are produced.

Androgens are the group of male sex hormones (primarily testosterone) that mediate the normal development and maintenance of the primary male sex characteristics as well as the secondary sex characteristics. Secondary male sex characteristics include advanced development of the prostate, seminal vesicles (two glands adjacent to the prostate), penis, and scrotum, as well as male hair distribution, laryngeal enlargement, and thickening of the vocal cords, and male body musculature and fat distribution. Androgens must be secreted in adequate amounts for these characteristics to appear. Probably the most important androgen is **testosterone,** which is produced from clusters of interstitial cells located between the seminiferous tubules. Besides having **androgenic activity,** testosterone is also involved in the development of bone and muscle tissue; inhibition of protein **catabolism** (metabolic breakdown); and retention of nitrogen, phosphorus, potassium, and sodium. These functions contribute to its **anabolic activity.** The hormone initiates the synthesis of specific proteins needed for androgenic and anabolic activity by binding to chromatin (strands of deoxyribonucleic acid [DNA]) in the nuclei of interstitial cells. In addition, testosterone appears to have an **erythropoietic effect** in that it stimulates the production of red blood cells (see Chapter 49).

Pharmacology Overview

ANDROGENS AND OTHER DRUGS PERTAINING TO MEN'S HEALTH

There are several synthetic derivatives of testosterone, and these were developed with the intention of improving the pharmacokinetic and pharmacodynamic characteristics of the naturally occurring hormone. One way that this was accomplished was by combining various esters with testosterone, which prolonged the duration of action of the hormone. For example, testosterone propionate is formulated as an oily solution, and its hormonal effects last for 2 to 3 days; the effects of testosterone cypionate and testosterone enanthate in oil last even longer. These drugs can be administered once every 2 to 4 weeks. Orally administered testosterone has very poor absorption, because most of the dose is metabolized and destroyed by the liver before it can reach the circulation (first-pass effect; see Chapter 2). To circumvent this problem, researchers developed methyltestosterone and fluoxymesterone. Both are synthetic dosage forms (tablets or capsules) designed to be effective following oral administration. Methyltestosterone is also available in a buccal tablet, which is dissolved in the buccal cavity (the space in the mouth between the cheek and teeth) and in an injectable form. Newer transdermal dosage forms for testosterone, including skin patches and a gel, have provided another way to circumvent the first-pass effect that occurs with oral administration of this hormone.

There are other chemical derivatives of naturally occurring testosterone known as *anabolic steroids.* These are synthetic drugs that closely resemble the natural hormone but possess high anabolic activity. Currently four anabolic steroid drug products are commercially available. These include oxymetholone (Anadrol-50), stanozolol (Winstrol), oxandrolone (Oxandrin), and nandrolone (Deca-Durabolin). These drugs are not commonly used, but U.S. Food and Drug Administration (FDA)–approved indications include anemia, hereditary angioedema, and metastatic breast cancer. Unlabeled (non–FDA-approved) uses for oxandrolone include treatment of human immunodeficiency virus (HIV)–associated wasting syndrome (debilitation related to disease-induced nutritional malabsorption) and alcoholic hepatitis. Anabolic steroids have a great potential for misuse by athletes, especially bodybuilders and weight lifters, because of their muscle-building properties. Improper use of these substances can have many serious consequences, such as sterility, cardiovascular diseases, and even liver cancer. For this reason anabolic steroids are currently classified as Schedule III controlled substances by the U.S. Drug Enforcement Administration. This classification implies that misuse of these drugs can lead to psychologic or physical dependence or both. Another synthetic androgen is danazol. Its labeled uses include treatment of hereditary angioedema, and, in women, endometriosis and fibrocystic breast disease.

Mechanism of Action and Drug Effects

The commercial forms of the natural and synthetic androgens and the synthetic anabolic steroids have effects similar to those of the endogenous androgens. These include stimulation of the normal growth and development of the male sex organs (primary sex characteristics) and development and maintenance of the secondary sex characteristics. One reason for the growth-promoting effects of androgens is that they stimulate the synthesis of ribonucleic acid (RNA) at the cellular level, thereby promoting cellular growth and reproduction. They also retard the breakdown of amino acids. These properties contribute to an increased synthesis of body proteins, which aids in the formation and maintenance of muscle tissue. Another potent anabolic effect of androgens is the retention of nitrogen, also essential for protein synthesis. Nitrogen also promotes the storage in the body of inorganic phosphorus, sulfate, sodium, and potassium, all of which have important metabolic roles, including protein synthesis, nerve impulse conduction, and muscular contractions. All of these effects result in weight gain and an increase in muscular strength. Finally, androgens also stimulate the production of erythropoietin by the kidney, which leads to enhanced erythropoiesis (red blood cell synthesis; see Chapter 49). However, the administration of exogenous androgens causes the release of endogenous testosterone to be inhibited as a result of the feedback inhibition of pituitary luteinizing hormone. Large doses of exogenous androgens may also suppress sperm production as a result of the feedback inhibition of pituitary follicle-stimulating hormone, which leads to infertility.

Androgen inhibitors are drugs that block the effects of naturally occurring (endogenous) androgens in the body. This is accomplished via inhibition of a specific enzyme, 5-alpha reductase. For this reason these drugs are also called 5-alpha reductase inhibitors. As previously mentioned, androgens maintain secondary sex characteristics, one of which is the growth and maintenance of the prostate. For unknown reasons, normal male physiology often results in an enlargement of the prostate known as **benign prostatic hyperplasia (BPH).** This process begins as early as 30 years of age and is present in at least 85% of men by the age of 80 years. The most troubling symptom is usually varying degrees of obstructed urinary outflow. Although surgical treatment by *transurethral resection of the prostate (TURP)* is a common strategy, BPH is also often amenable to treatment with a 5-alpha reductase inhibitor. There are currently two such drugs, finasteride and dutasteride. Finasteride, the prototypical drug for this class, works by inhibiting this enzyme, which normally converts testosterone to 5-alpha dihydrotestosterone (DHT). DHT is actually a somewhat more potent type of testosterone and is the principal androgen responsible for stimulating prostatic growth, as well as the expression of other male primary and secondary sex characteristics. Finasteride can dramatically lower the prostatic DHT concentrations, which helps to reduce the size of the prostate to ease the passage of urine. Fortunately, finasteride does not cause antiandrogen adverse effects that might be expected, such as loss of muscle strength, and fertility.

The drug effects of finasteride are limited primarily to the prostate, but this drug may also affect 5-alpha reductase–dependent processes elsewhere in the body, such as in the hair follicles, skin, and liver. For example, it has been noted that men taking finasteride experience increased hair growth. Therefore, finasteride is also

CULTURAL IMPLICATIONS

Men's Health Concerns: Prostate Cancer and Its Occurrence

Prostate cancer is the most common nonskin malignancy in men and is responsible for more deaths than any other cancer except lung cancer. However, microscopic evidence of prostate cancer is found at autopsy in many if not most men. The American Cancer Society estimated that about 218,890 new cases of prostate cancer were diagnosed in the United States during 2007. About 1 man in 6 will be diagnosed with prostate cancer during his lifetime, but only 1 man in 34 will die of it. A little over 1.8 million men in the United States are survivors of prostate cancer. The risk of developing and dying from prostate cancer is dramatically higher among blacks and of intermediate level among white males. The lowest occurrence is among the native Japanese. The following are some facts about the incidence, mortality, and racial-ethnic patterns of prostate cancer: (1) African American men are at highest risk of prostate cancer—it tends to start at a younger age in this group and grows faster than in men of other races. African American men have about a 60% higher incidence than white men. (2) White men are the group at next highest risk of prostate cancer, followed by Hispanic and Native American men. (3) African American men have twice the prostate cancer mortality rate of white men. (4) Prostate cancer mortality rates for whites and Hispanics have not decreased, whereas mortality rates for blacks and white non-Hispanics have declined.

From National Cancer Institute: Prostate cancer—step 1: find out about prostate cancer risk, available at *http://understandingrisk.cancer.gov/a_Prostate/01.cfm;* National Cancer Institute, Statistical Research and Applications Branch: DevCan—probability of developing or dying of cancer, software version 6.0, 2005, available at *http://srab.cancer.gov/devcan/.*

LIFE SPAN CONSIDERATIONS: The Elderly Patient

Sildenafil: Use and Concerns

- Over 10 million men experience erectile dysfunction (ED). The incidence of ED increases as age increases, and over 20% of patients with ED are 65 years of age or older.
- Sildenafil (Viagra) is a prescription medication that is commonly ordered to treat ED, but it is not without concerns and cautions for the patient. This is especially true for elderly patients, who generally have other medical conditions (e.g., renal disorders, hypertension, diabetes) and are usually taking more than one other prescribed medication.
- Liver function declines with age; therefore, drugs may not be metabolized as effectively in older adults as they are in younger adults. In addition, sildenafil is highly protein bound, which causes it to stay in the body longer and thus increases the possibility for drug interactions.
- A decreased dosage of sildenafil is generally indicated for patients over 65 years of age and for those with liver or renal impairment.
- Adverse effects to be concerned about in all patients, particularly older patients, include headache, flushing, urinary tract infection, diarrhea, rash, and dizziness.
- Sildenafil should be used cautiously in patients who have cardiac disease and angina, because these patients are at greater risk for complications, especially if they are taking nitrates for their cardiovascular disease.
- Discussing topics of a sexual nature may be comfortable for some patients but very anxiety producing for others. It is important for nurses to be aware of cultural and gender differences in how individuals perceive their own sexuality and how they generally deal with sexual performance issues. Nurses must be respectful of each individual's beliefs and feelings not only about his or her sexuality but also about other parts of the patient's whole self. This requires knowledge, sensitivity, and objectivity.

indicated for the treatment of male-pattern baldness. Research has demonstrated that the pharmacologic inhibition of 5-alpha reductase prevents the thinning of hair caused by increased levels of DHT. Finasteride is indicated for the treatment of baldness only in men, not in women. Finasteride can be teratogenic in pregnant women, but its use in women of any age (pregnant or not) still is not recommended by its manufacturer. Women should wear gloves when handling finasteride. However, another medication, minoxidil, can be used topically to treat baldness in both men and women. It is discussed in more detail in Chapter 56.

Another class of drugs that may be used to help alleviate the symptoms of obstruction due to BPH are the alpha$_1$-adrenergic blockers. These drugs are discussed in greater detail in Chapter 19. The alpha$_1$-adrenergic blockers that are most commonly used for symptomatic relief of obstruction secondary to BPH are terazosin (Hytrin), doxazosin (Cardura), tamsulosin (Flomax), and the newest such drug, alfuzosin (Uroxatral). Tamsulosin appears to have a greater specificity for the alpha$_1$-receptors in the prostate and thus may cause less hypotension.

There are also two other classes of androgen inhibitors. The first includes the androgen receptor blockers flutamide, nilutamide, and bicalutamide. These drugs work by blocking the activity of androgen hormones at the level of the receptors in target tissues (e.g., prostate). For this reason these drugs are used in the treatment of **prostate cancer** (see Chapter 48). The second class is the gonadotropin-releasing hormone (Gn-RH) analogues, including leuprolide, goserelin, and triptorelin. These drugs work

by inhibiting the secretion of pituitary gonadotropin, which eventually leads to a decrease in testosterone production. Both androgen receptor blockers and Gn-RH analogues are used most commonly to treat prostate cancer and are discussed in further detail in Chapter 48.

Sildenafil (Viagra) was the first oral drug approved for the treatment of erectile dysfunction. Sildenafil works by inhibiting the action of the enzyme phosphodiesterase. This in turn allows the buildup in the penis of the chemical cyclic guanosine monophosphate, which causes relaxation of the smooth muscle in the corpora cavernosa (erectile tubes) of the penis and permits the inflow of blood. Nitric oxide is also released inside the corpora cavernosa during sexual stimulation and contributes to the erectile effect. Two drugs that are similar but have a longer duration of action are vardenafil (Levitra) and tadalafil (Cialis). Collectively, these drugs are referred to as *erectile dysfunction drugs.* A second type of drug used to treat erectile dysfunction is the prostaglandin alprostadil. This drug must be given by injecting it directly into the erectile tissue of the penis or pushing a suppository form of the drug into the urethra.

A list of all of the men's health drugs mentioned in the chapter appears in Box 35-1. More information on selected drugs can be found in the Drug Profiles section. Antiandrogens and Gn-RH analogues are discussed in the antineoplastic drug chapters (see Chapter 48).

BOX 35-1 Currently Available Men's Health Drugs

Alpha₁-Adrenergic Blockers
doxazosin
tamsulosin
terazosin
alfuzosin

Anabolic Steroids
nandrolone
oxandrolone
oxymetholone
stanozolol

Other Androgens
danazol
fluoxymesterone
methyltestosterone
testosterone

Antiandrogens
bicalutamide
flutamide
nilutamide

5-Alpha Reductase Inhibitors
finasteride
dutasteride

Gonadotropin-Releasing Hormone Analogues
goserelin
leuprolide
triptorelin

Peripheral Vasodilator
minoxidil

Drugs for Erectile Dysfunction
sildenafil
tadalafil
vardenafil

TABLE 35-1 Men's Health Drugs: Indications

Drug	Indication
danazol	Endometriosis
	Fibrocystic breast disease
danazol and stanozolol	Hereditary angioedema
finasteride	Benign prostatic hyperplasia
	Male androgenetic alopecia
fluoxymesterone and methyltestosterone	Inoperable breast cancer
	Male hypogonadism
	Postpartum breast engorgement
methyltestosterone	Postpubertal cryptorchidism
minoxidil	Hypertension
	Female and male androgenetic alopecia
nandrolone	Metastatic breast cancer
oxymetholone	Various anemias
sildenafil, tadalafil, vardenafil	Erectile dysfunction
testosterone	Primary or secondary hypogonadism

Indications

The primary use for androgens is as hormone replacement therapy. Indications for other types of drugs discussed in this chapter are listed in Table 35-1.

Contraindications

Contraindications to the use of androgenic drugs include known androgen-responsive tumors. Use of sildenafil, vardenafil, and tadalafil is also contraindicated in men with major cardiovascular disorders, especially if they use nitrate medications such as nitroglycerin. Concurrent use of erectile dysfunction drugs and nitrates may cause severe hypotension, which may not respond to treatment. Use of finasteride is contraindicated in women (especially pregnant women) and children.

Adverse Effects

Although they are rare, some of the most devastating effects of androgenic steroids occur in the liver, where they cause the formation of blood-filled cavities, a condition known as *peliosis of the liver.* This condition is a possible consequence of the long-term administration of androgenic anabolic steroids and can be life threatening. Other serious hepatic effects are hepatic neoplasms (liver cancer), cholestatic hepatitis, jaundice, and abnormal liver

function. Fluid retention is another undesirable effect of androgens and may account for some of the weight gain seen in persons taking them. The serious adverse effects that can be caused by the androgens far outweigh the advantages to be gained from their use by those seeking improved athletic ability. Other less serious adverse effects of androgens are listed in Table 35-2.

Sildenafil, vardenafil, and tadalafil appear to have relatively favorable adverse effect profiles. In patients with preexisting cardiovascular disease, especially those taking nitrates (e.g., nitroglycerin, isosorbide mononitrate or dinitrate), these drugs can lower blood pressure substantially, potentially leading to more serious adverse events. Headache, flushing, and dyspepsia are the most common adverse effects reported. *Priapism* or abnormally prolonged penile erection is another relatively uncommon, but possible, adverse effect of both the erectile dysfunction drugs and the androgens. This condition is a medical emergency and warrants urgent medical attention. It is simply due to an excessive therapeutic drug response. As of this writing, the FDA is currently investigating unexplained case reports of visual losses in men using these drugs.

Finasteride has been reported to cause loss of libido, loss of erection, ejaculatory dysfunction, hypersensitivity reactions, gynecomastia, and severe myopathy. The drug has also caused a 50% decrease in prostate-specific antigen (PSA) concentrations. Pregnant women should not handle crushed or broken tablets on a regular basis because of the possibility of topical absorption, which can lead to teratogenic effects.

Interactions

Androgens, when used with oral anticoagulants, can significantly increase or decrease anticoagulant activity. They can also enhance the hypoglycemic effects of oral hypoglycemic (antidiabetic) drugs. Concurrent use of androgens with cyclosporine increases the risk of cyclosporine toxicity and is not recommended. Sildenafil, vardenafil, and tadalafil may cause severe hypotension when given together with nitrates such as nitroglycerin, isosorbide mononitrate, or isosorbide dinitrate. Alpha-blockers can cause additive hypotension when given with other drugs that lower blood pressure. Effects of tamsulosin may be increased

TABLE 35-2 Mens' Health Drugs: Selected Adverse Effects

Drug Class	Adverse Effects
Alpha₁-adrenergic blockers	Tachycardia, hypotension, chest pain, syncope, depression, dizziness, drowsiness, asthenia, rash, pruritus, impotence, urinary frequency, upper body muscular pain, dyspnea, flulike symptoms, visual changes, headache
Androgens (including anabolic steroids)	Headache, increased or reduced libido, anxiety, depression, acne, male pattern baldness, hirsutism, nausea, abnormal liver function test results, hepatic neoplasms, priapism, polycythemia, elevated cholesterol level, anaphylaxis (injection)
5-Alpha reductase inhibitors	Reduced libido, reduced semen volume, hypotension, dizziness, drowsiness
Peripheral vasodilator (topical minoxidil)	With topical route, usually limited to localized dermatologic reactions, including erythema, dermatitis, eczema, pruritus; possible systemic reactions theoretically include edema, chest pain, hypertension or hypotension, headache, dizziness, nausea, vomiting, diarrhea, sexual dysfunction, anemia, thrombocytopenia, muscular pain
Drugs for erectile dysfunction	Dizziness, headache, dyspepsia, nasal congestion, muscular pain, chest pain, hypertension or hypotension, rash, dermatitis, abnormal liver function test results, dry mouth, nausea, vomiting, diarrhea, gingivitis, priapism

DOSAGES

Selected Men's Health Drugs

Drug	Pharmacologic Class	Usual Dosage Range	Indications
finasteride (Propecia, Proscar)	5-Alpha reductase inhibitor	**Adult** PO: 1 mg daily (Propecia) PO: 5 mg daily (Proscar)	Androgenetic alopecia (baldness) (males only) Benign prostatic hyperplasia
◆ sildenafil (Viagra)	Phosphodiesterase inhibitor	**Adult (males only)** PO: 25-100 mg 1 hr before intercourse, no more than once daily	Erectile dysfunction
◆ testosterone cypionate (Depo-Testosterone)	Androgenic hormone	**Adult** IM: 200-400 mg q2-4wk **Adult and adolescent** IM: 50-400 mg q2-4wk	Inoperable breast cancer (in women) Delayed puberty or hypogonadism (in males)
◆ testosterone, transdermal (Testoderm, Androderm, AndroGel)	Androgenic hormone	**Adult and adolescent** Testoderm patch (applied only to scrotal skin): 4-6 mg/day Androderm patch (applied to skin of back, abdomen, upper arms, or thighs): 2.5-5 mg/day AndroGel (applied to shoulders, arms, or abdominal skin): 5 g daily (delivers 50 mg of testosterone)	Male hypogonadism

IM, Intramuscular; *PO,* oral.

when it is taken with azole antifungal drugs, erythromycin and clarithromycin, and cardiac drugs such as propranolol, verapamil, and protease inhibitors.

Dosages

For recommended dosages of the men's health drugs, see the Dosages table above.

■ DRUG PROFILES

finasteride

Finasteride (Proscar) use is contraindicated in patients who have shown a hypersensitivity to it and in pregnant women, and it is considered potentially dangerous for a pregnant woman even to handle crushed or broken tablets. The drug is currently available in two tablet forms of 1- and 5-mg strengths. The lower strength

is indicated for androgenetic alopecia in men. The higher strength is indicated for BPH, with clinical effects of prostate shrinkage in approximately 3 to 6 months of continual therapy. A similar but newer drug, dutasteride, is also indicated for BPH and is currently available in 0.5-mg capsule form. Both drugs are contraindicated in women and children. Pregnancy category X (for both). Refer to the table above for dosage information.

PHARMACOKINETICS

Route	Onset of Action	Peak Plasma Concentration	Elimination Half-life	Duration of Action
PO	3-12 mo	8 hr	4-15 hr	Unknown

◆ sildenafil

Sildenafil (Viagra) is approved by the FDA for the treatment of erectile dysfunction. Other erectile dysfunction drugs with longer durations of action include vardenafil and tadalafil. Sildenafil potentiates the physiologic sexual response, causing penile erection after sexual arousal by relaxing smooth muscle and increasing blood flow into the penis.

Sildenafil use is contraindicated in patients with a known hypersensitivity to it. Sildenafil can potentiate the hypotensive effects of nitrates, and its administration to patients who are using organic nitrates in any form, either regularly or intermittently, is therefore contraindicated. Dosage information for sildenafil appears in the table on p. 544.

PHARMACOKINETICS

Route	Onset of Action	Peak Plasma Concentration	Elimination Half-life	Duration of Action
PO	0.5-1 hr	1 hr	4 hr	4-6 hr

◆ testosterone

Testosterone (Androderm) is a naturally occurring anabolic steroid. It is used for primary and secondary hypogonadism but may also be used to treat oligospermia in men as well as inoperable breast cancer in women, where its purpose is to counteract tumor-enhancing estrogen activity. When it is used as hormone replacement therapy, a transdermal product is desirable. There are presently two transdermal patch formulations. They attempt to mimic the normal circadian variation in testosterone concentration seen in young healthy men, in whom the maximum testosterone levels occur in the early morning hours and the minimum concentrations occur in the evening. Of the two available transdermal delivery systems, Testoderm is always applied to the scrotal skin, whereas Androderm is always applied to skin elsewhere on the body and never to the scrotal skin. Patients should wash their hands and cover the area where testosterone is applied, as transfer to others can occur.

Testosterone use is contraindicated in patients with severe renal, cardiac, or hepatic disease; male breast cancer; prostate cancer; hypersensitivity; or genital bleeding, as well as in pregnant or lactating women. Testosterone is considered a Schedule III controlled substance under the Anabolic Steroids Control Act. It is available as intramuscular injections, transdermal gel, transdermal patches, and even implantable pellets. Pregnancy category X. Common dosages are listed in the table on p. 544.

PHARMACOKINETICS

Route	Onset of Action	Peak Plasma Concentration	Elimination Half-life	Duration of Action
Topical	1-2 hr	2-4 hr	10-100 min	2-4 wk

PHARMACOKINETIC BRIDGE
to Nursing Practice

Drugs used to manage erectile dysfunction (e.g., sildenafil) essentially work in the same way as the body to assist the male patient in achieving an erection. The related pharmacokinetics must be understood so that the drug is taken safely and effectively. Sildenafil is a rapidly absorbed drug with onset of action within 1 hour, peak plasma concentrations within 1 hour, and duration of action of up to 4 to 6 hours. If the drug is taken with a high-fat meal, absorption will be delayed, and it may take an additional 60 minutes for the drug to reach peak levels. This is yet another example of how specific drug pharmacokinetics may be affected by variables in a patient's everyday life, such as eating habits. Another pharmacokinetic consideration is that patients who are 65 years of age or older have reduced clearance of sildenafil and may experience increased plasma concentrations of free (or pharmacologically active) drug. This could possibly lead to drug accumulation and/or toxicity.

NURSING PROCESS

Assessment

Before any drug is given to a male patient for the treatment of benign or malignant diseases of the male reproductive tract, presenting symptoms should be thoroughly assessed and a complete history of past and present medical diseases or conditions obtained. In addition, assessment of the patient's urinary elimination patterns and any difficulties should be assessed and the findings documented. The health care provider usually performs a rectal examination to palpate for enlargement of the prostate or for other possible pathology. If enlargement exists, a serum PSA test will most likely be ordered, especially prior to any treatment, and the test may also be ordered during treatment. PSA levels may be increased in pathologic conditions such as prostate cancer, and levels should be documented and constantly monitored for baseline and comparative reasons. PSA levels should decrease with effective therapeutic regimens. More recent research encourages the use of a PSA value of less than 2.5 or 3 ng/mL as the criterion for normal levels, especially for younger patients.

With potentially teratogenic drugs such as *finasteride*, special handling precautions should be followed by health care personnel and any pregnant caregiver or partner. Gloves should be worn for protective reasons when these individuals handle the drug. Liver function should also be assessed to establish baseline liver function.

CASE STUDY

Erectile Dysfunction Drugs

© Olga OSA

Mr. S., a 63-year-old college professor, is in the office for a yearly checkup. He feels he is generally healthy, and he does not take any medications. He does say that he has one problem that he wants to discuss with the physician. During his physical examination, he tells the physician, "I have something embarrassing to ask. I want to try one of those drugs that can help my sex life." The physician reassures Mr. S. that there should be no embarrassment about this and asks several questions about Mr. S.'s sexual difficulties. At the end of the examination and assessment, Mr. S. is given a prescription for sildenafil (Viagra).

1. What teaching is important for Mr. S. before he starts this medication?
2. Eleven months later, Mr. S. is admitted to the emergency department with chest pains. After a thorough examination, including a cardiac catheterization, he is diagnosed with mild coronary artery disease and is started on isosorbide dinitrate, sustained release, 40 mg every 12 hours. He is given a follow-up appointment with his physician in 1 week. What is important to tell Mr. S. at this time?
3. Mr. S. comes to the office for the follow-up appointment and tells the nurse that he wants to try saw palmetto for his prostate health. He has a neighbor who takes it and has no problems with it, and he has noticed that he has had a slight increase in difficulty with urination. He is also upset about what he was told in the hospital about his medications. What should the nurse say to him at this time? What assessments should be done?

For answers, see *http://evolve.elsevier.com/Lilley.*

Drugs for erectile dysfunction should be given only after a physical examination has been performed by the prescriber. A thorough nursing assessment should be performed and medication history taken, if appropriate. These drugs are also associated with the adverse effects of hypotension, headache, and dyspepsia. Therefore, a cardiac history should be obtained and vital signs measured. A listing of all medications (prescription, over-the-counter, herbals) should be reviewed with special attention to the nitrates, which can lead to significant hypotension and possible negative consequences for the patient's cardiac status and health. Bowel sounds and bowel patterns should be assessed with notation of any dysphagia or gastrointestinal motility disorders. See pharmacology section for more information on adverse effects as well as contraindications, cautions, and drug interactions. With *testosterone* and related drugs, the patient should be assessed for cardiac disease because of the possible edema and subsequent added stress on the heart that can result with these drugs. Because androgenic anabolic steroids (e.g., testosterone) may increase weight, have a negative impact on bone growth, and elevate serum potassium, chloride, nitrogen, phosphorus, and cholesterol levels, the prescriber will generally order baseline laboratory testing. Renal function tests (e.g., BUN and serum creatinine levels), liver function tests (e.g., LDH, CPK, and bilirubin levels), cardiac enzyme assays, and PSA levels are generally ordered before the patient begins therapy with these drugs. The nurse should measure height and weight and assess for recent weight gain, bone disorders, and electrolyte imbalances before, during, and after therapy, as deemed appropriate. A history of male breast cancer, prostate cancer, and/or gynecomastia should also be ruled out before drug therapy is begun.

Nursing Diagnoses

- Disturbed body image related to sexual dysfunction and/or diseases of the male reproductive tract
- Fatigue related to the adverse effects of medications
- Excess fluid volume related to possible adverse effects of the medication (sodium retention)
- Impaired urinary elimination related to BPH and/or other male reproductive organ dysfunction or pathology
- Ineffective sexuality patterns related to the effects of treatment with testosterone and drugs used for erectile dysfunction
- Sexual dysfunction (male) related to inability to perform sexually due to erectile dysfunction
- Risk for injury related to the adverse effects (e.g., hypotension) of therapy with drugs used for erectile dysfunction
- Risk for situational low self-esteem related to sexual dysfunction secondary to medication use and/or disease states
- Deficient knowledge related to misinterpretation of information about self-medication

Planning
Goals

- Patient maintains a positive body image.
- Patient maintains normal activity levels during drug therapy with testosterone.
- Patient maintains normal sodium and fluid volume levels during drug therapy.
- Patient attains near-normal urinary elimination patterns.

- Patient experiences minimal alterations in sexual integrity and function during testosterone therapy.
- Patient remains compliant with the drug therapy regimen.
- Patient verbalizes feelings and concerns about actual or perceived changes in sexual patterns and functioning.

Outcome Criteria

- Patient verbalizes feelings, fears, and anxieties concerning potential for alteration in body image related to the disease process or the adverse effects of treatment with testosterone and related men's health drugs.
- Patient maintains healthy activity level during drug therapy and experiences minimal fatigue with gradual increase in performing activities of daily living.
- Patient states measures to be taken (such as dietary changes) to minimize edema related to sodium retention resulting from the use of large dosages of testosterone.
- Patient verbalizes feelings, anxieties, and fears of alteration in sexual patterns or functioning during drug therapy.
- Patient takes medications as prescribed and with appropriate follow-up.

Implementation

Finasteride may be given orally without regard to meals. The drug should be protected from exposure to light and heat. When used for treatment of the urinary symptoms of BPH, finasteride and related drugs may be ordered for approximately 6 months with a reevaluation of the condition at that time. Patients taking drugs for erectile dysfunction should be warned about potential adverse effects, such as dizziness, drop in blood pressure, and heartburn. In addition, the patient has the right to accurate and appropriate education about risk factors, adverse effects, and potential complications. See the Patient Teaching Tips for more information.

HERBAL THERAPIES AND DIETARY SUPPLEMENTS

Saw Palmetto (*Serenoa repens, Sabal serrulata*)

■ **Overview**
Saw palmetto comes from a tree that is also known as the American dwarf palm. The therapeutically active part of the tree is its ripe fruit. Saw palmetto is believed to inhibit dihydrotestosterone and 5-alpha reductase. A prostatic-specific antigen test and digital rectal examination should be performed before initiation of treatment with saw palmetto for benign prostatic hyperplasia.

■ **Common Uses**
Diuretic, urinary antiseptic, treatment of benign prostatic hyperplasia, treatment of alopecia

■ **Adverse Effects**
Gastrointestinal upset, headache, back pain, dysuria

■ **Potential Drug Interactions**
Nonsteroidal antiinflammatory drugs, hormones such as estrogen replacement therapy and oral contraceptives, immunostimulants

■ **Contraindications**
None

The therapeutic effects of *testosterone* are maximized when the drug is taken as ordered and at regular intervals so that steady levels are maintained. If the drug is being used for hypogonadism or induction of puberty, dosages may be managed differently, so that at the end of the growth spurt the patient is placed on maintenance dosages. Testoderm transdermal patches should be placed on clean, dry scrotal skin that has been shaved for optimal skin contact and should be replaced every 22 to 24 hours or as ordered. Androderm patches should be placed on clean, dry skin on the back, abdomen, upper arms, or thighs; the scrotum and bony areas (shoulder, hip) should be avoided. These patches are often ordered to be changed every 7 days. Because various types of transdermal patch are available, the nurse should be sure the patient understands which type of patch is to be used, and where and how it is to be applied. If the drug is given intramuscularly, the vial of medication should be mixed thoroughly by agitating it before withdrawing the prescribed amount of medication. See the Herbal Therapies and Dietary Supplements box for a description of saw palmetto, an herbal supplement that is often taken to relieve symptoms of an enlarged prostate.

Evaluation

The therapeutic effects of drugs related to the male reproductive tract include improvement of the condition and/or signs and symptoms for which the patient is being treated, such as hypogonadism, sexual dysfunction, erectile dysfunction, and urinary elimination problems caused by BPH. The therapeutic effects of some drugs (e.g., finasteride) may not be seen for 6 to 12 months, so it is important for the nurse to observe and monitor the patient for the intended effects of the drugs. In addition, the nurse should evaluate for the adverse effects of these medications (see the pharmacology section for specific adverse effects). Goals and outcome criteria should always be evaluated to see if the patient's needs have been met.

PATIENT TEACHING TIPS

- With finasteride, education about the drug's therapeutic effects as well as adverse effects should be provided at the patient's educational level (see pharmacology discussion for more information). Female family members, significant others, and caregivers who are pregnant or of childbearing age should be educated about the need to avoid exposure during handling of this drug, including *not* touching any broken or crushed tablets, which could result in exposure to the drug and the risk of teratogenic effects. Wearing of gloves is recommended.
- Finasteride may be given orally without regard to meals. It should be protected from exposure to light and heat.
- Sildenafil should be taken about 1 hour before sexual activity. This drug, and other drugs for erectile dysfunction, should not be taken with nitrates because it may lead to significant hypotensive consequences that could be life threatening.
- Inform the patient that drug therapy for erectile dysfunction is not effective without sexual stimulation and arousal.

- With testosterone, educate about all therapeutic and adverse effects. It should be emphasized to the patient that follow-up appointments are an important aspect of effective therapy with testosterone (as well as with any drugs discussed in this chapter).
- Instruct the patient that used or unwrapped transdermal dosage forms should be discarded by flushing in the commode to keep any possible accidental application or ingestion by children (or anyone else).
- Any swelling of the extremities, jaundice, or prolonged painful erections should be reported immediately to the prescriber. Prolonged erection (i.e., longer than 4 hours) is considered a medical emergency.
- Testosterone should not be withdrawn abruptly except under the supervision of the prescriber. Weaning is usually done over several weeks.

POINTS TO REMEMBER

- The most commonly used drugs related to male health and the male reproductive tract are finasteride, sildenafil, and testosterone. The nurse needs to know the way these drugs work and their adverse effects, contraindications, cautions, and drug interactions to ensure their safe and effective use.
- Testosterone is responsible for the development and maintenance of the male reproductive system and secondary sex characteristics. Oral testosterone has very poor pharmacokinetic and pharmacodynamic characteristics, and therefore it is recommended that testosterone be administered via injection (parenteral route) or a transdermal patch.

- Methyltestosterone was developed to circumvent the problems associated with the oral administration of testosterone.
- Finasteride is usually indicated to stop growth of the prostate in men with BPH and to treat men with androgenic alopecia.
- Patients taking drugs for erectile dysfunction (e.g., sildenafil) should be warned about potential adverse effects, such as hypotension, headache, and heartburn.
- There are major concerns about heart-related deaths associated with concurrent use of nitrates and drugs used for erectile dysfunction. Patient education should focus on the prevention of drug interactions and related adverse effects and complications.

NCLEX EXAMINATION REVIEW QUESTIONS

1 A patient has been taking finasteride (Proscar) for almost a year. The nurse knows that which is most important to evaluate at this time?
   a Complete blood count
   b PSA levels
   c Blood pressure
   d Fluid retention

2 The nurse is performing an assessment of a patient who is asking for a prescription for sildenafil (Viagra). Which finding would be a contraindication to its use?
   a Age of 65 years
   b History of hypertension
   c Medication list that includes nitrates
   d Medication list that includes saw palmetto

3 During a counseling session for a group of teenage athletes, the use of androgenic steroids is discussed. The nurse will explain that which problem is a rare but devastating effect of androgenic steroid use?
   a Peliosis of the liver
   b Bradycardia
   c Kidney failure
   d Tachydysrhythmias

4 The nurse is teaching a patient about the possible adverse effects of erectile dysfunction drugs. The patient should know that if he experiences priapism, or an erection that lasts longer than 4 hours, the most important action is to
   a stay in bed until the erection ceases.
   b apply an ice pack for 30 minutes.
   c turn on his left side and rest.
   d seek medical attention immediately.

5 A patient is asking about the use of saw palmetto for prostate health. The nurse tells him that drugs that interact with saw palmetto include:
   a Acetaminophen (Tylenol)
   b Nitrates
   c Nonsteroidal antiinflammatory drugs
   d Antihypertensive drugs

6 When the Testoderm form of testosterone is ordered to treat hypogonadism in a teenaged boy, which instructions by the nurse are correct? (Select all that apply.)
   a Place the patch on clean, dry skin on the back, upper arms, abdomen, or thighs.
   b Place the patch on clean, dry scrotal skin that has been shaved.
   c Place the patch on clean, dry scrotal skin, but do not shave the skin first.
   d Replace the patch every 7 days.
   e Replace the patch every 22 to 24 hours.

1. b, 2. c, 3. a, 4. d, 5. c, 6. b, e.

CRITICAL THINKING ACTIVITIES: BEST ACTION

1 During morning medication rounds, you are about to give a dose of finasteride when the patient asks you to crush the pill, which is not enteric coated. What is your best action at this time?

2 A male patient calls the office to ask about topical testosterone gel. This morning, he applied the daily dose to his upper arms and, without thinking, picked up his young granddaughter soon afterward. He wants to know if the medication can cause a problem in his granddaughter. What is your best answer?

3 During an office checkup, a patient tells you, "Ever since I started that pill for my prostate gland I'm having trouble with sex. I just don't have the interest anymore. Could it be the pill?" When you check his medical record, you see that he started taking dutasteride, a 5-alpha reductase inhibitor, 3 months ago. What is your best answer?

For answers, see *http://evolve.elsevier.com/Lilley*.

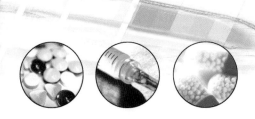
Drugs Affecting the Respiratory System

STUDY SKILLS TIPS

Study on the Run, PURR

STUDY ON THE RUN, PURR

The basic approach in applying Study on the Run (SOTR) is to make use of small blocks of time that are otherwise nonproductive. Plan, Rehearse, and Review do not require that the entire chapter be covered in one study session. These steps produce their benefits by promoting repetition of learning.

Where Is the Time?

SOTR time is everywhere. In the course of a single day you might have an hour or more that can be used for SOTR activities. It is just a matter of becoming aware of little bits and pieces of your day that can ordinarily slip away without being productive. Small blocks of time are everywhere in your day; it just takes a little creativity on your part to become aware of them. Finishing an examination early, standing in the checkout line, waiting for the teakettle to boil, or even waiting for the washing machine to finish the last spin before you change loads can be time used for SOTR. Get creative and be flexible. Remember, every minute of time you use this way is a minute of time you will not have to find later.

SOTR and Plan

Remember the importance of questioning as an essential component in Plan. Look at the chapter objectives for Chapter 37. There are five objectives presented for this chapter. Work on the questions for as many of these objectives as can be covered in the time you have. If you complete questions for only two objectives, do not look upon it as failure to complete something. Instead, learn to view what you have done as that much less to do later. The time you spend now frees up that much more time during your large blocks of study time for intense study reading.

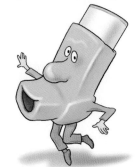

Will you forget the questions you generated in this session before you have the opportunity to read the chapter? If you make it a habit to ask questions as a continuing part of all study, you will find that you remember the focus questions very well. If you have trouble remembering your own questions, write the questions in the margins of the text. Gradually you will find that questioning becomes such an automatic procedure that you will be able to dispense with writing questions. You will remember them.

SOTR and Vocabulary

One of the most challenging aspects of a course like this is the almost overwhelming vocabulary load. If the new vocabulary load were not enough, there is also the need to keep reviewing previous parts and chapters because some term that was introduced three chapters ago has reappeared and you do not remember it clearly. Creating your own vocabulary cards is a perfect SOTR activity.

The basic card model is simple. The word, common form, prefix, or suffix appears on the card front. The back of the card may have just a little information (the minimum being a definition of what is on the front) or may contain considerable information. I recommend that you include part, chapter, and page number on the back so that you can locate the term quickly if the need arises. In addition, you may want to add a specific example from the text or of your own creation to help clarify the term. Put as much information on the back as you find useful.

Creating Vocabulary Cards with SOTR

Use the time between classes to create several personal vocabulary cards. Grab your text and your blank note cards. Open to the next chapter you will be studying. Flip over to the glossary pages. Write the first word from the glossary on the front of a blank note card. Turn the card over. Write the part and chapter numbers and the page number for the glossary on the card. Pick a standard location for this. Put these numbers in a top or bottom corner, but make sure you put them in the same corner every time. Eventually this becomes a habit and makes the preparation process faster. It also helps when you are making use of the cards, because you will know exactly what information you put on the card and where you put it. Put this card aside and repeat the process with the next term in the glossary. In those few minutes before you go to class you can have completed the basic preparation for a full set of cards covering, for example, the 17 terms in the Chapter 36 glossary.

Notice that all I proposed was that you copy the term and the location information. I did not tell you to copy the definition in the glossary at this time. The term used in the context of a sentence and a paragraph may be much easier to understand. If, as you read the chapter, you feel that the glossary definition is also useful to have on this card, you can always flip back by using the location information you put on the card.

SOTR and Vocabulary Review

Your vocabulary cards are ideal for SOTR action. Carry a pack of cards with you at all times. Whenever you have even a minute or two, you can pull out a stack of cards from previous chapters or the current chapter. Use the oral ask-and-answer method discussed in the *Study Guide.* For instance, the first term in the glossary for Chapter 37 is *allergen.* Ask yourself aloud, "What is an allergen?" Then try to answer the question aloud. Answer: "An allergen is a substance that produces an allergic reaction." It is not necessary to recall the exact answer presented in the glossary and/or chapter. What is important is that you respond with a clear and meaningful answer. The answer given earlier is not exactly the same as that stated in the glossary, but the general concept is the same. Once you have stated your answer, turn the card over and check to make sure that you were correct. Each time you do this with a term, you are strengthening your long-term memory, and you will find that it takes less and less time to recall the terms you need.

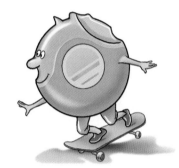

Vocabulary cards can also be used with your study group. You may want to give oral quizzes to each other. This is one sure way to check that your answer is stated clearly.

SOTR and Chapter Review

Chapter review can be overwhelming if you think that review means rereading the material and that you therefore need large blocks of uninterrupted time. There is a much more efficient way to review, and it works well in short time blocks, which makes it a perfect technique for SOTR.

Look at the first page of Chapter 36. You should instantly see a number of visible structures that make it easy to review key terms and concepts without rereading the entire block of material. First, there is the chapter title: Antihistamines, Decongestants, Antitussives, and Expectorants. What are antihistamines? This is a question you would have generated when you were engaged in the Plan step of PURR. Now that you have read the chapter, repeat the question and answer it aloud. Answer aloud because you will hear what you say and will either know the material or need to mark it to come back and reread. Now ask a more complex question: "What is the role of antihistamines? What do they do?" Now try to answer these questions. If you can, then you do not need to reread to find out what antihistamines are. Next, looking at p. 552, you will notice some terms in **bold print.** Apply the same process. Using the boldface words and phrases as stimuli, ask questions and try to answer them to your own satisfaction. If you cannot develop a satisfactory answer, then you know that some rereading is needed. However, it is very focused. You are not trying to reread everything on the page, only the material right there that is associated with the term.

At the top of the first column on p. 553 you will see a list. Look at the sentence preceding the list: "This explains why the release of excessive amounts of histamine can lead to anaphylaxis and severe allergic symptoms and may result in any or all of the following physiologic changes . . ." Ask questions. If you can answer them, no reading is necessary. If you cannot answer, you know that the answers are found immediately after this sentence in the indented list. Use the structures in the chapter to accomplish focused review. Comprehension is improved and long-term memory is strengthened, and your test grades will reflect this.

The benefits of SOTR are enormous. There are no drawbacks. You are using time that otherwise would be "wasted," and this time now becomes productive study time. The more active you become in looking for SOTR opportunities, the more you will find. The more SOTR time you spend, the better student you will become.

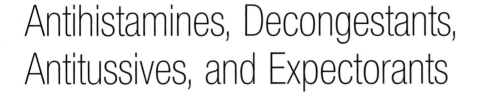
Antihistamines, Decongestants, Antitussives, and Expectorants

OBJECTIVES

When you reach the end of this chapter, you should be able to do the following:

1 Provide specific examples of the drugs categorized as antihistamines (both sedating and nonsedating), decongestants, antitussives, and expectorants.

2 Discuss the mechanisms of action, indications, contraindications, cautions, drug interactions, adverse effects, dosages, and route of administration for antihistamines, decongestants, antitussives, and expectorants.

3 Develop a nursing care plan that includes all phases of the nursing process for patients taking any of the antihistamines, decongestants, antitussives, and/or expectorants.

e-Learning Activities

http://evolve.elsevier.com/Lilley

NCLEX Review Questions • Animations • Nursing Care Plans • Audio Glossary • Category Catchers • Medication Errors Checklists • IV Therapy Checklists • Calculators • Frequently Asked Questions • Content Updates • Supplemental Resources • Answers to Case Studies and Critical Thinking Activities

Drug Profiles

benzonatate, p. 559
codeine, p. 559
◆ dextromethorphan, p. 559
◆ diphenhydramine, p. 556
◆ guaifenesin, p. 560
◆ loratadine, p. 555
naphazoline, p. 557

◆ *Key drug.*

Glossary

Adrenergics (sympathomimetics) Drugs that stimulate the sympathetic nerve fibers of the autonomic nervous system which use epinephrine or epinephrine-like substances as neurotransmitters. (p. 556)

Antagonists Drugs that exert an action opposite to that of another drug or compete for the same receptor sites. (p. 553)

Anticholinergics (parasympatholytics) Drugs that block the action of acetylcholine and similar substances at acetylcholine receptors, which results in inhibition of the transmission of parasympathetic nerve impulses. (p. 556)

Antigens Substances that, upon entering to the body, are capable of inducing specific immune responses and in turn reacting with the specific products of such responses, such as certain antibodies and specifically sensitized T lymphocytes. Antigens can be soluble (e.g., a foreign protein) or particulate or insoluble (e.g., a bacterial cell). (p. 553)

Antihistamines Substances capable of reducing the physiologic and pharmacologic effects of histamine, including a wide variety of drugs that block histamine receptors. (p. 553)

Antitussive A drug that reduces coughing, often by inhibiting neural activity in the cough center of the central nervous system. (p. 558)

Corticosteroids Any of the hormones produced by the adrenal cortex, either in natural or synthetic drug form. They influence or control many key processes in the body, such as carbohydrate and protein metabolism, the maintenance of serum glucose levels, electrolyte and water balance, and the functions of the cardiovascular system, skeletal muscle, kidneys, and other organs. (p. 556)

Decongestants Drugs that reduce congestion or swelling, especially of the upper or lower respiratory tract. (p. 556)

Empiric therapy A method of treating disease based on observations and experience without a knowledge of the precise cause of or mechanism responsible for the disorder or the way in which the therapeutic drug or procedure produces improvement or cure. (p. 552)

Expectorants Drugs that increase the flow of fluid in the respiratory tract, usually by reducing the viscosity of bronchial and tracheal secretions, and facilitate their removal by coughing and ciliary action. (p. 559)

Histamine antagonists Drugs that compete with histamine for binding sites on histamine receptors. (p. 553)

Influenza A highly contagious infection of the respiratory tract caused by a myxovirus and transmitted by airborne droplets. (p. 552)

Nonsedating antihistamines Newer medications that work peripherally to block the actions of histamine and therefore do not have the central nervous system effects of many of the older antihistamines; also called *second-generation antihistamines* and *peripherally acting antihistamines*. (p. 555)

Reflex stimulation An irritation of the respiratory tract occurring in response to an irritation of the gastrointestinal tract. (p. 558)

Rhinovirus Any of about 100 serologically distinct ribonucleic acid (RNA) viruses that cause about 40% of acute respiratory illnesses. (p. 552)

Sympathomimetic drugs A class of drugs whose effects mimic those resulting from the stimulation of organs and structures by the sympathetic nervous system. They do this by occupying adrenergic receptor sites and acting as agonists or by increasing the release of norepinephrine at postganglionic nerve endings. (p. 557)

Upper respiratory tract infection (URI) Any infectious disease of the upper respiratory tract, including the common cold, laryngitis, pharyngitis, rhinitis, sinusitis, and tonsillitis. (p. 552)

● ● ●

Anatomy, Physiology, and Disease Overview

Most common colds result from a viral infection, most often infection with a **rhinovirus** or an **influenza** virus. These viruses normally invade the tissues (mucosa) of the upper respiratory tract (nose, pharynx, and larynx) to cause an **upper respiratory tract infection (URI).** The inflammatory response elicited by these invading viruses stimulates excessive mucus production. This fluid drips behind the nose, down the pharynx, and into the esophagus and lower respiratory tract, which leads to symptoms typical of a cold: sore throat, coughing, and upset stomach. The irritation of the nasal mucosa often triggers the sneeze reflex and also causes the release of several inflammatory and vasoactive substances, which results in the dilation of the small blood vessels in the nasal sinuses and leads to nasal congestion. The treatment of the common symptoms of URI involves the combined use of antihistamines, nasal decongestants, antitussives, and expectorants. Many of these drugs are available without prescription. However, these drugs can only relieve the symptoms of a URI. They can do nothing to eliminate the causative pathogen. In 2008, the U.S. Food and Drug Administration (FDA) issued recommendations that over-the-counter (OTC) cough and cold products not be given to children younger than 2 years of age. This followed numerous case reports of symptoms such as oversedation, seizures, tachycardia, and even death in toddlers medicated with such products. There is also evidence that such medications are simply not effective in small children, and parents are advised to consult their pediatrician on the best ways to manage these illnesses. Antiviral drugs are currently the only drugs that are effective, but treatment with these mediations is often hampered by the fact that the viral cause cannot be readily identified. Because of this, the treatment rendered can only be based on what is believed to be the most likely cause, given the presenting clinical symptoms. Such treatment is called **empiric therapy.** Some patients seem to gain benefit from the use of herbal products and other supplements, such as vitamin C, to prevent the onset of cold signs and symptoms or at least to decrease their severity. Herbal products commonly used for colds are echinacea and goldenseal (see Herbal Therapies and Dietary Supplements boxes on this page). The practitioner should recognize, however, that there are limited controlled research data regarding the efficacy of herbal products and also that some of them can have significant drug-drug or drug-disease interactions.

Pharmacology Overview

ANTIHISTAMINES

Histamine is a bodily substance that performs many functions. It is involved in nerve impulse transmission in the central nervous system (CNS), dilation of capillaries, contraction of smooth muscles, stimulation of gastric secretion, and acceleration of the heart rate. There are two types of cellular receptors for histamine.

HERBAL THERAPIES AND DIETARY SUPPLEMENTS

Echinacea *(Echinacea)*

■ *Overview*
The three species of echinacea used medicinally are *Echinacea angustifolia, Echinacea pallida,* and *Echinacea purpurea.* Echinacea has been shown in clinical trials to reduce cold symptoms and recovery time when taken early in the illness. This is believed to be due to its immunostimulant effects. At this time there is no strong research evidence to warrant recommending the herb for urinary tract infections, wound healing, or prevention of colds; further study is needed to provide evidence of its therapeutic effects and indications.

■ *Common Uses*
Stimulation of the immune system, antisepsis, treatment of viral infections and influenza-like respiratory tract infections, promotion of healing of wounds and chronic ulcerations

■ *Adverse Effects*
Dermatitis, upset stomach or vomiting, dizziness, headache, unpleasant taste

■ *Potential Drug Interactions*
Amiodarone, cyclosporine, phenytoin, methotrexate, ketoconazole, barbiturates; tolerance likely to develop if used for more than 8 weeks. Because some preparations have a high alcohol content, they may cause acetaldehyde syndrome in patients taking disulfiram (Antabuse) to prevent alcohol abuse (see Chapter 9).

■ *Contraindications*
Contraindicated for patients with acquired immunodeficiency syndrome, tuberculosis, connective tissue diseases, multiple sclerosis

---

HERBAL THERAPIES AND DIETARY SUPPLEMENTS

Goldenseal *(Hydrastis canadensis)*

■ *Overview*
Goldenseal is found in wooded areas from the northeastern to midwestern United States. It is the dried root of the plant that is most commonly used for its various biologically active alkaloids. These components have been shown to have antibacterial, antifungal, and antiprotozoal activity. The alkaloid berberine has both anticholinergic and antihistaminic activity.

■ *Common Uses*
Treatment of upper respiratory tract infections, allergies, nasal congestion, and numerous genitourinary, skin, ophthalmic, and otic conditions

■ *Adverse Effects*
Gastrointestinal (GI) distress, emotional instability, mucosal ulceration (e.g., when used as a vaginal douche)

■ *Potential Drug Interactions*
Gastric acid suppressors (including antacids, histamine H_2 blockers [e.g., ranitidine], proton pump inhibitors [e.g., omeprazole]): theoretically reduced effectiveness due to acid-promoting effect of herb
Antihypertensives: theoretically reduced effectiveness due to vasoconstrictive activity of herb

■ *Contraindications*
Acute or chronic GI disorders; pregnancy (has uterine stimulant properties); should be used with caution by those with cardiovascular disease

---

Data from Jellin J et al: *Natural medicines comprehensive database,* ed 6, Stockton, Calif, 2004, Therapeutic Research Faculty; Skidmore-Roth L: *Mosby's handbook of herbs and natural supplements,* ed 2, St Louis, 2004, Mosby.

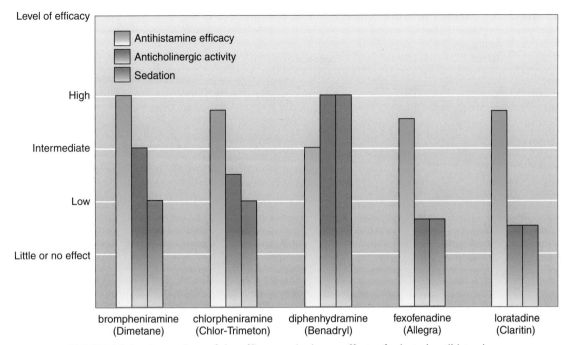

FIGURE 36-1   Comparison of the efficacy and adverse effects of selected antihistamines.

Histamine 1 (H$_1$) receptors mediate smooth muscle contraction and dilation of capillaries, and histamine 2 (H$_2$) receptors mediate acceleration of the heart rate and gastric acid secretion. This explains why the release of excessive amounts of histamine can lead to anaphylaxis and severe allergic symptoms and may result in any or all of the following physiologic changes:

- Constriction of smooth muscle, especially in the stomach and lungs
- Increase in body secretions
- Vasodilatation and increased capillary permeability, which results in the movement of fluid out of the blood vessels and into the tissues and thus causes a drop in blood pressure and edema

Antihistamines are drugs that directly compete with histamine for specific receptor sites. For this reason, they are also called **histamine antagonists.** Antihistamines that compete with histamine for the H$_2$ receptors are called H$_2$ **antagonists** or *H$_2$ blockers* and include such drugs as cimetidine, ranitidine, and famotidine. Because they act on the gastrointestinal (GI) system, they are discussed in detail in Chapter 50. This chapter focuses on the H$_1$ antagonists (also called *H$_1$ blockers*); these are the drugs more commonly known by the name *antihistamines.* They are very useful drugs, because approximately 10% to 20% of the general population is sensitive to various environmental allergens. Histamine is a major inflammatory mediator in many allergic disorders, such as allergic rhinitis (e.g., hay fever and mold, dust allergies), anaphylaxis, angioedema, drug fevers, insect bite reactions, and urticaria (itching).

H$_1$ antagonists include drugs such as diphenhydramine, chlorpheniramine, fexofenadine, loratadine, and cetirizine. They are of greatest value in the treatment of nasal allergies, particularly seasonal hay fever. They are also given to relieve the symptoms of the common cold, such as sneezing and runny nose. In this regard they are palliative, not curative; that is, they can help al-

leviate the symptoms of a cold but can do nothing to destroy the virus causing it.

The clinical efficacy of the more than one dozen different antihistamines is very similar, although they have varying degrees of antihistaminic, anticholinergic, and sedating properties. The particular actions of, and hence the indications for, a particular antihistamine are determined by its specific chemical makeup. All antihistamines compete with histamine for the H$_1$ receptors in areas such as the smooth muscle surrounding blood vessels and bronchioles. They also affect the secretions of the lacrimal, salivary, and respiratory mucosal glands, which are the primary anticholinergic actions of antihistamines. Because of their antihistaminic properties, they are indicated for the treatment of allergies. These drugs also differ from each other in their potency and their adverse effects, especially in the degree of drowsiness they produce. The antihistaminic, anticholinergic, and sedative properties of some of the more commonly used antihistamines are summarized in Figure 36-1. These effects make them useful for the treatment of problems such as vertigo, motion sickness, insomnia, and cough. Several classes of antihistamines are listed in Table 36-1, along with their various anticholinergic and sedative effects.

Mechanism of Action and Drug Effects

During allergic reactions, histamine and other substances are released from mast cells, basophils, and other cells in response to **antigens** circulating in the blood. The histamine molecules then bind to and activate other cells in the nose, eyes, respiratory tract, GI tract, and skin, producing the characteristic allergic signs and symptoms. For example, in the respiratory tract histamine causes extravascular smooth muscle (e.g., in the bronchial tree) to contract, whereas antihistamines cause it to relax. Also, histamine causes pruritus by stimulating nerve endings. Antihistamines can prevent or alleviate this itching.

TABLE 36-1 Effects of Various Antihistamines

Chemical Class	Anticholinergic Effects	Sedative Effects	Comments
Alkylamines			
brompheniramine	Moderate	Low	Cause less drowsiness and more CNS stimulation; suitable for daytime use.
chlorpheniramine	Moderate	Low	
dexchlorpheniramine	Moderate	Low	
Ethanolamines			
clemastine	High	Moderate	Substantial anticholinergic effects; commonly cause sedation; at usual dosages, drowsiness occurs in about 50% of patients; diphenhydramine and dimenhydrinate also used as antiemetics.
diphenhydramine	High	High	
dimenhydrinate	High	High	
Ethylenediamines			
pyrilamine	Low to none	Low	Weak sedative effects, but adverse GI effects are common.
Phenothiazine			
promethazine	High	High	Drugs in this class are principally used as antipsychotics; some are useful as antihistamines, antipruritics, and antiemetics.
Piperidines			
azatadine	Moderate	Moderate	Commonly used in the treatment of motion sickness; hydroxyzine is used as a tranquilizer, sedative, antipruritic, and antiemetic.
cyproheptadine	Moderate	Low	
hydroxyzine	Moderate	Moderate	
phenindamine	Moderate	Low to none	
Miscellaneous			
fexofenadine	Low to none	Low to none	Very few adverse anticholinergic or sedative effects; almost exclusively antihistaminic effects; can be taken during the day because no sedative effects occur; in general they are longer acting and have fewer adverse effects than other classes.
loratadine	Low to none	Low to none	

CNS, Central nervous system; *GI,* gastrointestinal.

TABLE 36-2 Antihistamines: Drug Effects

Body System	Histamine Effects	Antihistamine Effects
Cardiovascular (small blood vessels)	Dilates blood vessels, increases blood vessel permeability (allows substances to leak into tissues)	Reduces dilation of blood vessels and increased permeability
Immune (release of various substances commonly associated with allergic reactions)	Released from mast cells along with several other substances, which results in allergic reactions	Does not stabilize mast cells or prevent the release of histamine and other substances, but does bind to histamine receptors and prevent the actions of histamine
Smooth muscle (on exocrine glands)	Stimulates salivary, gastric, lacrimal, and bronchial secretions	Reduces salivary, gastric, lacrimal, and bronchial secretions

Circulating histamine molecules normally bind to histamine receptors on basophils and mast cells. This stimulates further release of histamine stored within these cells. Antihistamine drugs work by blocking the histamine receptors on the surfaces of basophils and mast cells, thereby preventing the release and actions of histamine stored within these cells. They do not push off histamine that is already bound to a cell surface receptor but compete with histamine for unoccupied receptors. Therefore, these drugs are most beneficial when given early in a histamine-mediated reaction, before all of the free histamine molecules bind to cell membrane receptors. The binding of H$_1$ blockers to these receptors prevents the adverse consequences of histamine binding: vasodilation; increased GI, respiratory, salivary, and lacrimal secretions; and increased capillary permeability with resultant edema. The various drug effects of antihistamines are listed in Table 36-2.

Indications

Antihistamines are most beneficial in the management of nasal allergies, seasonal or perennial allergic rhinitis (e.g., hay fever), and some of the typical symptoms of the common cold. They are also useful in the treatment of allergic reactions, motion sickness, Parkinson's disease (due to their anticholinergic effects), and vertigo. In addition, they are sometimes used as a sleep aid.

Contraindications

Use of antihistamines is generally contraindicated in cases of known drug allergy. They should also not be used as the sole drug therapy during acute asthmatic attacks. In such cases a rapidly acting bronchodilator such as albuterol, or in extreme cases epinephrine, is generally the most urgently needed medication. Other contraindications may include narrow-angle glaucoma, cardiac disease, kidney disease, hypertension, bronchial asthma, chronic obstructive pulmonary disease, peptic ulcer disease, seizure disorders, benign prostatic hyperplasia, and pregnancy. Fexofenadine is not recommended for children younger than 6 years of age or those with renal impairment. Desloratadine is not recommended for pediatric patients. Loratadine is not recommended for children younger than 2 years of age. Antihistamines should generally be used with caution in patients with impaired liver function or renal insufficiency, as well as in lactating mothers.

Adverse Effects

Drowsiness is usually the chief complaint of people who take antihistamines, but the sedative effects vary from class to class (see Table 36-1). Fortunately, sedative effects are much less common, although still possible, with the newer "nonsedating" drugs. The anticholinergic (drying) effects of antihistamines can cause adverse effects such as dry mouth, changes in vision, difficulty urinating, and constipation. Reported adverse effects of the antihistamines are listed in Table 36-3.

Interactions

When fexofenadine is given with erythromycin, increased fexofenadine concentrations can result. Ketoconazole, cimetidine, and erythromycin may increase concentrations of loratadine. Alcohol, monoamine oxidase inhibitors (MAOIs), and CNS depressants may increase the CNS depressant effects of diphenhydramine and cetirizine. Concurrent use of anticholinergic drugs may also lead to more anticholinergic adverse effects such as dry mouth and constipation. Antihistamine effects may be potentiated excessively by interactions with apple, grapefruit and orange juice as well as with St. John's wort. Rifampin reduces the absorption of fexofenadine. An allergist will usually recommend discontinuation of antihistamine drug therapy at least 4 days prior to allergy testing.

Dosages

For the recommended dosages of selected antihistamines, see the Dosages table on p. 556.

DRUG PROFILES

Although some antihistamines are prescription drugs, most are available OTC. Antihistamines are available in many dosage forms to be administered orally, intramuscularly, intravenously, or topically.

NONSEDATING ANTIHISTAMINE

A major advance in antihistamine therapy occurred with the development of the **nonsedating antihistamines** loratadine, cetirizine, and fexofenadine. These drugs were developed in part to eliminate many of the unwanted adverse effects (mainly sedation) of the older antihistamines. These drugs work peripherally to

TABLE 36-3 Antihistamines: Reported Adverse Effects

Body System	Adverse Effects
Cardiovascular	Local anesthetic (quinidine-like) effect on the cardiac conduction system, which can result in dysrhythmias, arrest, hypotension, palpitations, syncope, dizziness
Central nervous	Sedation (mild drowsiness to deep sleep), dizziness, muscular weakness, paradoxical excitement, restlessness, insomnia, nervousness, seizures
Gastrointestinal	Anorexia, nausea, vomiting, diarrhea or constipation, hepatitis, jaundice
Other	Dryness of mouth, nose, and throat; urinary retention; impotence; vertigo; visual disturbances; blurred vision; tinnitus; headache; rarely agranulocytosis, hemolytic anemia, leukopenia, thrombocytopenia, pancytopenia

block the actions of histamine and therefore do not have the CNS effects that many older antihistamines do. For this reason these drugs are also called *peripherally acting antihistamines* because they tend not to cross the blood-brain barrier, unlike their traditional counterparts. Another advantage of these drugs over the older antihistamines is that they have longer durations of action, which allows some of them to be taken only once a day. This further increases patient adherence to therapy. These three drugs replace the two original nonsedating antihistamines terfenadine and astemizole, which were withdrawn from the U.S. market in the 1990s following the occurrence of several cases of fatal drug-induced cardiac dysrhythmias. Fexofenadine is actually the active metabolite of terfenadine but is not associated with such severe cardiac effects, nor are loratadine or cetirizine.

◆ loratadine

Loratadine (Claritin) is a nonsedating antihistamine. It needs to be taken only once a day. Structurally it is similar to cyproheptadine and azatadine, but unlike these drugs it cannot distribute into the CNS, which alleviates the sedative effects associated with traditional antihistamines. Loratadine is used to relieve the symptoms of seasonal allergic rhinitis (e.g., hay fever) as well as chronic urticaria. Loratadine has recently been converted to OTC status. However, a drug containing its primary active metabolite, desloratadine, has recently come on the U.S. market and is currently available by only by prescription.

Drug allergy is the only contraindication to the use of loratadine. The drug is available in oral form as a 10-mg tablet, as a 1-mg/mL syrup, as a 10-mg rapidly disintegrating tablet, and in a combination tablet with the decongestant pseudoephedrine. Pregnancy category B. See the Dosages table on p. 556 for dosage information.

PHARMACOKINETICS

Route	Onset of Action	Peak Plasma Concentration	Elimination Half-life	Duration of Action
PO	1-3 hr	8-12 hr	8-24 hr	24 hr

TRADITIONAL ANTIHISTAMINE

The traditional antihistamines are the older drugs that work both peripherally and centrally. They also have anticholinergic effects, which in some cases make them more effective than nonsedat-

DOSAGES

Selected Antihistamines

Drug (Pregnancy Category)	Pharmacologic Class	Usual Dosage Range	Indications
Nonsedating Antihistamine			
◆ loratadine (Claritin) (B)	H₁ antihistamine	**Adult and pediatric 6 yr and older** PO: 10 mg once daily **Pediatric 2-5 yr** PO: 5 mg once daily	Allergic rhinitis, chronic urticaria
Traditional Antihistamine (More Commonly Associated with Sedation)			
◆ diphenhydramine (Benadryl) (B)	H₁ antihistamine	**Pediatric more than 10 kg** PO/IM/IV: 12.5-25 mg tid-qid	Allergic disorders, nighttime insomnia, motion sickness
		Adult and pediatric 12 yr and older PO: 25-50 mg at bedtime	Nighttime insomnia
		Adult only PO/IM/IV: 25-50 mg tid-qid	Allergic disorders, PD symptoms
		Adult only PO: 25-50 mg tid-qid	Motion sickness

IM, Intramuscular; *IV,* intravenous; *PD,* Parkinson's disease; *PO,* oral.

ing antihistamines. Some of these commonly used older drugs are diphenhydramine, brompheniramine, chlorpheniramine, dimenhydrinate, meclizine, and promethazine. These drugs are used either alone or in combination with other drugs in the symptomatic relief of many disorders ranging from insomnia to motion sickness. Many patients respond to and tolerate the older drugs quite well, and because many are generically available, they are much less expensive. These drugs are available both OTC and by prescription.

◆ diphenhydramine

Diphenhydramine (Benadryl) is an older, traditional antihistamine that works both peripherally and centrally. It also has potent anticholinergic and sedative effects. In fact, it is still often used as a hypnotic drug because of its sedating effects. This use is not generally advised in elderly patients, however, because of the "hangover" effect and increased potential for falls. Diphenhydramine is one of the most commonly used antihistamines, in part because of its excellent safety profile and efficacy. It has the greatest range of therapeutic indications of any antihistamine available. It is used for the relief or prevention of histamine-mediated allergies and motion sickness, the treatment of Parkinson's disease (due to its anticholinergic effects; see Chapter 16), and the promotion of sleep (see Chapter 13). It is also used in conjunction with epinephrine in the management of anaphylaxis and in the treatment of acute dystonic reactions.

Diphenhydramine is classified as a pregnancy category B drug, and its use is contraindicated in patients with a known hypersensitivity to it, nursing mothers, neonates, and patients with lower respiratory tract symptoms. It is available in oral, parenteral, and topical preparations. In oral form, diphenhydramine is available as capsules, tablets, and liquid, as well as in several combination products that contain other cough and cold medications. In parenteral form, diphenhydramine is available as an injection. In topical form, diphenhydramine is available as a cream, gel, and spray. It also is available in combination with several other drugs that are commonly given topically, such as calamine, camphor, and zinc oxide. These combination preparations come in the form of aerosols, creams, gels, and lotions. The recommended dosages

for the oral and injectable forms are given in the Dosages table above.

PHARMACOKINETICS

Route	Onset of Action	Peak Plasma Concentration	Elimination Half-life	Duration of Action
PO	15-30 min	2-4 hr	2-7 hr	4 hr

DECONGESTANTS

Nasal congestion is due to excessive nasal secretions and inflamed and swollen nasal mucosa. The primary causes of nasal congestion are allergies and URIs, especially the common cold. There are three separate groups of nasal **decongestants: adrenergics (sympathomimetics),** which are the largest group; **anticholinergics (parasympatholytics),** which are somewhat less commonly used; and selected topical **corticosteroids** (intranasal steroids).

Decongestants can be taken orally to produce a systemic effect, can be inhaled, or can be administered topically to the nose. Each method of administration has its advantages and disadvantages. Decongestants administered by the oral route include pseudoephedrine, which is available OTC. A commonly used nasal decongestant spray is phenylephrine, which is also OTC.

Drugs administered by the oral route produce prolonged decongestant effects, but the onset of action is more delayed and the effect less potent than for decongestants applied topically. However, the clinical problem of rebound congestion associated with topically administered drugs is almost nonexistent with oral dosage forms. Rebound congestion occurs because of the very rapid absorption of drug through mucous membranes and delivery to adrenergic receptors within respiratory tissues, followed by a more rapid decline in therapeutic activity. This is in contrast to oral dosage forms, which provide a more gradual increase and decline in pharmacologic activity due to the time required for GI absorption. Decongestants suitable for nasal inhalation include ephedrine, oxymetazoline, phenylephrine, and tetrahydrozoline.

Inhaled intranasal steroids and anticholinergic drugs are not generally associated with rebound congestion and are often used prophylactically to prevent nasal congestion in patients with chronic upper respiratory tract symptoms. Commonly used intranasal steroids include the following:

- beclomethasone dipropionate (Beconase)
- budesonide (Rhinocort)
- flunisolide (Nasalide)
- fluticasone (Flonase)
- triamcinolone (Nasacort)

The only intranasal anticholinergic drug in common use at this time is ipratropium nasal spray (Atrovent).

Mechanism of Action and Drug Effects

Nasal decongestants are most commonly used for their ability to shrink engorged nasal mucous membranes and relieve nasal stuffiness. Adrenergic drugs (e.g., ephedrine, oxymetazoline) accomplish this by constricting the small arterioles that supply the structures of the upper respiratory tract, primarily the blood vessels surrounding the nasal sinuses. When these blood vessels are stimulated by alpha-adrenergic drugs, they constrict. Because sympathetic nervous system stimulation produces the same effect, these drugs are sometimes referred to as *sympathomimetics*. Once these blood vessels shrink, the nasal secretions in the swollen mucous membranes are better able to drain, either externally through the nostrils or internally through reabsorption into the bloodstream or lymphatic circulation.

Nasal steroids are aimed at the inflammatory response elicited by invading organisms (viruses and bacteria) or other antigens (e.g., allergens). The body responds to these antigens by producing inflammation in an effort to isolate or wall off the area and by attracting various cells of the immune system to consume and destroy the offending antigens. Steroids exert their antiinflammatory effect by causing these cells to be turned off or rendered unresponsive. It should be kept in mind, however, that the goal is *not* complete immunosuppression of the respiratory tract but rather the modulation of inflammatory symptoms to improve patient comfort and air exchange. The drug effects of intranasal steroids are discussed in more detail in Chapter 33.

Indications

Nasal decongestants reduce the nasal congestion associated with acute or chronic rhinitis, the common cold, sinusitis, and hay fever or other allergies. They may also be used to reduce swelling of the nasal passages and to facilitate visualization of the nasal and pharyngeal membranes before surgery or diagnostic procedures.

Contraindications

Contraindications to the use of decongestants include drug allergy and, in the case of adrenergic drugs, narrow-angle glaucoma, uncontrolled cardiovascular disease, hypertension, diabetes, hyperthyroidism, and prostatitis. The drugs may also be contraindicated in situations in which the patient is unable to close his or her eyes (such as after a cerebrovascular accident), as well as in patients with a history of cerebrovascular accident or transient ischemic attacks, cerebral arteriosclerosis, long-standing asthma, benign prostatic hyperplasia, or diabetes.

Adverse Effects

Adrenergic drugs are usually well tolerated. Possible adverse effects of these drugs include nervousness, insomnia, palpitations, and tremor. The most common adverse effects of intranasal steroids are localized and include mucosal irritation and dryness.

Although a topically applied adrenergic nasal decongestant can be absorbed into the bloodstream, the amount absorbed is usually too small to cause systemic effects at normal dosages. Excessive dosages of these medications, however, are more likely to cause systemic effects elsewhere in the body. These may include cardiovascular effects such as hypertension and palpitations and CNS effects such as headache, nervousness, and dizziness. These systemic effects are the result of alpha-adrenergic stimulation of the heart, blood vessels, and CNS.

Interactions

There are few significant drug interactions with nasal decongestants. Systemic **sympathomimetic drugs** and sympathomimetic nasal decongestants are more likely to cause drug toxicity when given together. MAOIs may result in additive pressor effects (e.g., raising of the blood pressure) when given with sympathomimetic nasal decongestants. Other interacting drugs include methyldopa and urinary acidifiers and alkalinizers.

Dosages

For the recommended dosages of naphazoline, the only nasal decongestant profiled, see the Dosages table on p. 558.

DRUG PROFILE

Many of the decongestants are OTC drugs, but the more potent drugs that can cause serious adverse effects are available only by prescription. Use of adrenergic drugs is usually contraindicated in patients with diabetes, hypertension, cardiac disease, thyroid dysfunction, prostatitis, or a known hypersensitivity to these drugs. Although nasal steroids are relatively safe, their use is also contraindicated in some circumstances, including in patients with nasal mucosal infections (because of their ability to depress the body's immune response as part of their antiinflammatory effect) or known drug allergy.

Many inhaled corticosteroids (e.g., beclomethasone, dexamethasone, flunisolide) are discussed in greater detail in Chapter 33. The adrenergic drugs (e.g., naphazoline) are discussed in this chapter. Both of these drug categories are generally first-line drugs for the treatment of chronic nasal congestion.

naphazoline

Naphazoline (Privine) is chemically and pharmacologically very similar to the other sympathomimetic drugs oxymetazoline, tetrahydrozoline, and xylometazoline. When these drugs are administered intranasally they cause dilated arterioles to constrict, which reduces nasal blood flow and congestion. During a cold the blood vessels that surround the nasal sinus are usually dilated and engorged with plasma, white blood cells, mast cells, histamines, and many other blood components that are involved in fighting infections of the respiratory tract. This swelling, or dilation, blocks the nasal passages, which results in nasal congestion. Naphazoline and its chemically related cousins are classified as pregnancy category C drugs and have the same contraindications as the other nasal decongestants. Naphazoline for nasal administration is available as a 0.05% solution and

DOSAGES

Selected Decongestant, Expectorant, and Antitussive Drugs

Drug (Pregnancy Category)	Pharmacologic Class	Usual Dosage Range	Indications
benzonatate (Tessalon Perles) (C)	Nonopioid antitussive	**Adult and pediatric older than 10 yr** PO: 100-200 mg tid	Cough
codeine (as part of a combination product such as Dimetane-DC, Tussar SF, Novahistine DH, Robitussin A-C, others) (C)	Opioid antitussive	**Adult and pediatric older than 12 yr** PO: 10-20 mg q4-6h, max 120 mg/24 hr **Pediatric 6-12 yr** PO: 5-10 mg q4-6h, max 60 mg/24 hr **Pediatric 2-5 yr** PO: 2.5-5 mg q4-6h, max 30 mg/24 hr	
◆ dextromethorphan (as part of a combination product such as Vicks Formula 44, Robitussin DM, others) (C)	Nonopioid antitussive	**Adult and pediatric older than 12 yr** PO: 10-30 mg q4-8h, max 120 mg/24 hr **Pediatric 6-12 yr** PO: 5-10 mg q4h or 15 mg q6-8h, max 60 mg/24 hr **Pediatric 2-6 yr** PO: 2.5-7.5 mg q4-8h, max 30 mg/24 hr	
◆ guaifenesin (glyceryl guaiacolate) (Guiatuss, Humibid, Robitussin, Mucinex, others) (C)	Expectorant	**Adult and pediatric 12 yr and older** PO: 100-400 mg q4h, max 2400 mg/24 hr **Pediatric 6-12 yr** PO: 100-200 mg q4h, max 1200 mg/24 hr **Pediatric 2-6 yr** PO: 50-100 mg q4h, max 600 mg/24 hr	Respiratory congestion, cough
naphazoline (Privine) (C)	Alpha-adrenergic vasoconstrictor	**Adult and pediatric 12 yr and older** 0.05%, 1 or 2 drops or sprays in each nostril q6h prn, usually for no more than 3-5 days	Nasal congestion

is meant to be instilled into each nostril. Common dosages for this drug are given in the Dosages table above.

PHARMACOKINETICS

Route	Onset of Action	Peak Plasma Concentration	Elimination Half-life	Duration of Action
Intranasal	5-10 min	Unknown	Unknown	2-6 hr

ANTITUSSIVES

Coughing is a normal physiologic function and serves the purpose of removing potentially harmful foreign substances and excessive secretions from the respiratory tract. The cough reflex is stimulated when receptors in the bronchi, alveoli, and pleura (lining of the lungs) are stretched. This causes a signal to be sent to the cough center in the medulla of the brain, which in turn stimulates the cough. Although most of the time coughing is a beneficial response, there are times when it is not useful and may even be harmful (e.g., after a surgical procedure such as hernia repair or in cases of nonproductive or "dry" cough). In these situations it may enhance patient comfort and reduce respiratory distress to inhibit this otherwise normal response through the use of an **antitussive** drug. There are two main categories of antitussive drugs: opioid and nonopioid.

Although all opioid drugs have antitussive effects, only codeine and its semisynthetic derivative hydrocodone are used as antitussives. Both drugs are effective in suppressing the cough reflex, and if they are taken in the prescribed manner, their use should not lead to dependency. These two drugs are usually in-

corporated into various combination formulations with other respiratory drugs and are rarely used alone for the purpose of cough suppression.

Nonopioid antitussive drugs are less effective than opioid drugs and are available either alone or in combination with other drugs in an array of OTC cold and cough preparations. Dextromethorphan is the most widely used of the nonopioid antitussive drugs and is a derivative of the synthetic opioid levorphanol. Benzonatate is another nonopioid drug.

Mechanism of Action and Drug Effects

The opioid antitussives codeine and hydrocodone suppress the cough reflex through direct action on the cough center in the CNS (medulla). Opioid antitussives also provide analgesia and have a drying effect on the mucosa of the respiratory tract, which increases the viscosity of respiratory secretions. This helps to reduce symptoms such as runny nose and postnasal drip. The nonopioid cough suppressant dextromethorphan works in the same way. Because it is not an opioid, however, it does not have analgesic properties, nor does it cause addiction or CNS depression. Another nonopioid antitussive is benzonatate. Its mechanism of action is entirely different from that of the other drugs. Benzonatate suppresses the cough reflex by anesthetizing (numbing) the stretch receptor cells in the respiratory tract, which prevents **reflex stimulation** of the medullary cough center.

Indications

Although they have other properties, such as analgesic effects for the opioid drugs, antitussives are used primarily to stop the cough reflex when the cough is nonproductive and/or harmful.

Contraindications

The only absolute contraindication to the antitussives is drug allergy. Relative contraindications include opioid dependency (for opioid antitussives) and high risk for respiratory depression (e.g., in frail elderly patients). Patients with these conditions are often able to tolerate lower medication dosages and still experience some symptom relief.

Additional contraindications and cautions include the following:

- *benzonatate:* no known contraindications but cautious use in those with productive cough
- *dextromethorphan:* contraindications of hyperthyroidism, advanced cardiac and vessel disease, hypertension, glaucoma and use of MAOIs within the past 14 days
- *diphenhydramine:* see antihistamines
- *codeine and hydrocodone:* contraindicated with alcohol use; extremely cautious use required with CNS depression, anoxia, high serum levels of carbon dioxide (hypercapnia), and respiratory depression; cautious use required with increased intracranial pressure, impaired renal function, liver diseases, benign prostatic hyperplasia, Addison's disease, and chronic obstructive pulmonary disease

Adverse Effects

The following are the common adverse effects of selected antitussive drugs:

- *benzonatate:* dizziness, headache, sedation, nausea, constipation, pruritus, and nasal congestion
- *codeine:* sedation, nausea, vomiting, lightheadedness, and constipation
- *dextromethorphan:* dizziness, drowsiness, and nausea
- *diphenhydramine:* sedation, dry mouth, and other anticholinergic effects
- *hydrocodone:* sedation, nausea, vomiting, lightheadedness, and constipation

Interactions

Very few drug interactions occur with benzonatate, although some are associated with the use of opioid antitussives and dextromethorphan. Opioid antitussives (codeine and hydrocodone) may potentiate the effects of other opioids, general anesthetics, tranquilizers, sedatives and hypnotics, tricyclic antidepressants, alcohol, and other CNS depressants.

Dosages

For the recommended dosages of selected antitussive drugs, see the Dosages table on p. 558.

DRUG PROFILES

Antitussives come in many oral dosage forms and are available both with and without a prescription. Most of the opioid antitussives are available only by prescription because of the associated abuse potential. Dextromethorphan is the most popular nonnarcotic antitussive available OTC.

benzonatate

Benzonatate (Tessalon Perles) is a nonopioid antitussive drug that, as mentioned earlier, is thought to work by anesthetizing or numbing the cough receptors. It is available only in oral form as a 100-mg capsule. Its use is contraindicated in patients with a known hypersensitivity to it. Pregnancy category C. Common dosages are listed in the Dosages table on p. 558.

PHARMACOKINETICS

Route	Onset of Action	Peak Plasma Concentration	Elimination Half-life	Duration of Action
PO	15-20 min	Unknown	Unknown	3-8 hr

codeine

Codeine (Dimetane-DC) is a very popular opioid antitussive drug. It is used in combination with many other respiratory medications to control coughs. Because it is an opioid, it is potentially addictive and can depress respirations as part of its CNS depressant effects. For this reason codeine-containing cough suppressants are more tightly controlled substances. Although most states allow OTC purchase of at least one oral liquid combination product, the purchaser usually must be at least 18 years of age and be willing to sign a log book kept at the pharmacy. More commonly the patient has obtained a prescription for such products. Codeine alone, without being combined with other drugs, is a Schedule II drug. Codeine-containing cough suppressants are available in many oral dosage forms: solutions, tablets, capsules, and suspensions. Their use is contraindicated in patients with a known hypersensitivity to opiates and in those who have respiratory depression, increased intracranial pressure, seizure disorders, or severe respiratory disorders. Pregnancy category C. Common dosages are listed in the table on p. 558.

PHARMACOKINETICS

Route	Onset of Action	Peak Plasma Concentration	Elimination Half-life	Duration of Action
PO	15-30 min	34-45 min	2.5-4 hr	4-6 hr

◆ dextromethorphan

Dextromethorphan is a nonopioid antitussive that is available alone or in combination with many other cough and cold preparations. It is widely used because it is safe and nonaddicting and does not cause respiratory or CNS depression, when used in recommended dosages. Dextromethorphan has become a popular drug of abuse and is discussed in detail in Chapter 9. Its use is contraindicated in cases of drug allergy, asthma or emphysema, or persistent headache. Dextromethorphan is available as lozenges, solution, liquid-filled capsules, granules, tablets (chewable, extended release, and film coated), and extended-release suspension. Pregnancy category C. Common dosages are listed in the Dosages table on p. 558.

PHARMACOKINETICS

Route	Onset of Action	Peak Plasma Concentration	Elimination Half-life	Duration of Action
PO	15-30 min	2.5 hr	Unknown	3-6 hr

EXPECTORANTS

Expectorants aid in the expectoration (i.e., coughing up and spitting out) of excessive mucus that has accumulated in the respiratory tract by breaking down and thinning out the secretions. They are administered orally either as single drugs or in combination with other drugs to facilitate the flow of respiratory secretions by reducing the viscosity of tenacious secretions. The actual clinical effectiveness of expectorants is somewhat questionable, however. Placebo-controlled clinical evaluations have failed to strongly confirm that expectorants reduce the viscosity of sputum. Despite this, expectorants are popular drugs, are contained in most OTC cold and cough preparations, and provide symptom relief for many users. The most common expectorant in OTC products is guaifenesin (formerly known as glyceryl guaiacolate).

Mechanism of Action and Drug Effects

Expectorants have one of two different mechanisms of action, depending on the drug. The first is reflex stimulation, in which loosening and thinning of respiratory tract secretions occurs in response to an irritation of the GI tract produced by the drug. Guaifenesin is the only such drug currently available. The second mechanism of action is direct stimulation of the secretory glands in the respiratory tract.

Indications

Expectorants are used for the relief of productive cough commonly associated with the common cold, bronchitis, laryngitis, pharyngitis, pertussis, influenza, and measles. They may also be used for the suppression of coughs caused by chronic paranasal sinusitis. By loosening and thinning sputum and the bronchial secretions, they may also indirectly diminish the tendency to cough.

Contraindications

Guaifenesin is contraindicated if drug allergy is present.

Adverse Effects

The adverse effects of expectorants are minimal. Guaifenesin may cause nausea, vomiting, and gastric irritation.

Interactions

There are no known significant interactions involving guaifenesin.

Dosages

The recommended dosages of guaifenesin, the only expectorant profiled, are given in the Dosages table on p. 558.

DRUG PROFILE

◆ guaifenesin

Guaifenesin (Mucinex) is a very commonly used expectorant that is available in several different oral dosage forms: capsules, tablets, solutions, and granules. It is used in the symptomatic management of coughs of varying origin. It is beneficial in the treatment of productive coughs because it thins mucus in the respiratory tract that is difficult to cough up. There are few published pharmacokinetic data on guaifenesin, but its half-life is estimated to be approximately 1 hour. This short half-life helps to explain why it is usually dosed several times throughout the day. Although this drug remains popular, however, there is some evidence in the literature to suggest that it has no greater therapeutic activity than water in terms of loosening respiratory tract secretions. Pregnancy category C. See the Dosages table on p. 558 for the common dosages.

NURSING PROCESS

Assessment

When the patient is to be given drugs to treat symptoms related to the respiratory tract, the nurse should begin the assessment by gathering data about the condition and determining whether

symptoms are caused by an allergic reaction. Obtaining the patient's medical history and medication profile, completing a thorough head-to-toe physical assessment, and taking a nursing history are critical to understanding possible causes, risks, or links to diseases or conditions such as allergy, a cold, and/or flu. For example, if an allergic reaction to a drug, food, or substance has occurred, the patient may be experiencing signs and symptoms such as hives, wheezing or bronchospasm, tachycardia, and/or hypotension that may require immediate medical treatment. However, if the cause is a cold or flu, the symptoms will be different and will be treated completely differently in most cases. The drug of choice is then selected based on the severity of the symptoms.

Most *nonsedating antihistamines* (e.g., fexofenadine, loratadine, desloratadine, cetirizine) are not to be used in patients younger than 6 years of age. Allergies and other contraindications, cautions, and drug interactions should be assessed prior to use. It is important to remember with the traditional and nontraditional antihistamines that if allergy testing is to be performed, these medications should be discontinued at least 4 days before the testing, but only on a prescriber's order.

Before administering the *traditional antihistamines* such as diphenhydramine, chlorpheniramine, or brompheniramine, the nurse must ensure that the patient has no allergies to this group of medications, even though these drugs are used for allergic reactions. Contraindications, cautions, and drug interactions need to be assessed with these and all other drugs. Use of these antihistamines is of concern in patients who are experiencing an acute asthma attack and in those who have lower respiratory tract disease or are at risk for pneumonia. The rationale for not using these drugs in these situations is that antihistamines dry up secretions; if the patient cannot expectorate the secretions, the secretions may become viscous (thick), occlude airways, and lead to atelectasis or further infection or occlusion of the bronchioles. It is also important to know that these drugs may lead to paradoxical reactions in the elderly, with subsequent irritability as well as dizziness, confusion, sedation, and hypotension.

With *antitussive* therapy, assessment is tailored to the patient and the specific drug. Most of these drugs result in sedation, dizziness, and drowsiness, so assessment of the patient's safety is very important. An assessment for allergies, contraindications, cautions, and drug interactions should be completed and the findings documented. Respiratory assessment (as for all of the drugs in this chapter) should include rate, rhythm and depth, as well as breath sounds, presence of cough, and description of cough and sputum if present. For individuals with chronic respiratory disease, the prescriber may order serum measurements of carbon dioxide, partial pressure of arterial oxygen, and other blood gas analyses (e.g., blood pH). Pulse oximetry readings with measurement of vital signs may be used to provide more information.

Use of *decongestants* requires assessment of contraindications, cautions, and drug interactions. Because decongestants are available in oral, nasal drop and spray, and eyedrop dosage forms, any condition that could affect the functional structures of the eye or nose may be a possible caution or contraindication. Decongestants may increase blood pressure and heart rate, so assessment and documentation of the patient's blood pressure, pulse, and other vital parameters should be carried out. Because so many of these drugs are found in OTC cough and cold products and have been associated with numerous cases of oversedation, seizures,

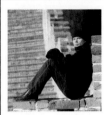
tachycardia, and even in death in children younger than 2 years of age, the FDA has issued warnings that these drugs are not to be used in this patient group. Assessment of age thus becomes very important in these situations, and medical attention should be sought as needed.

Inhaled intranasal steroids and *anticholinergic drugs* are not generally associated with rebound congestion but may be used prophylactically to prevent nasal congestion in patients with chronic upper respiratory tract symptoms. A thorough assessment for contraindications, cautions, and drug interactions needs to be performed prior to use of these drugs (as for all the drugs in this chapter). For patients who have a cough and need to bring up secretions more easily, *expectorants* are often recommended or prescribed. In addition to assessing all the parameters identified previously, the nurse should assess cough and sputum, if present.

Nursing Diagnoses

- Impaired gas exchange related to the disorder, condition, or disease affecting the respiratory system and various respiratory-related signs and symptoms
- Deficient knowledge related to the effective use of cold medications and other related products due to lack of information and patient teaching
- Ineffective airway clearance related to diminished ability to cough and/or a suppressed cough reflex (with antitussives)
- Risk for injury or falls related to the sedating adverse effects of many of these drugs
- Risk for injury related to sensory-perceptual alterations from drug-induced drowsiness and/or sedation

Planning
Goals

- Patient states rationale for the use of antihistamine, expectorant, antitussive, or decongestant.
- Patient states the adverse effects of medication.
- Patient states the importance of compliance with the therapy regimen.
- Patient identifies symptoms to report to the prescriber.

- Patient states the importance of scheduling and keeping follow-up appointments with the prescriber.
- Patient indicates relief of symptoms with treatment.
- Patient regains near-normal or normal (baseline) respiratory patterns and function.
- Patient remains free of excessive drowsiness or sedation.

Outcome Criteria

- Patient remains compliant with the antihistamine, antitussive, decongestant, or expectorant medication regimen until symptoms are resolved or the prescriber orders discontinuation.
- Patient takes medications exactly as prescribed to avoid complications of therapy, achieve maximal effectiveness, and minimize adverse effects.
- Patient reports any of the following symptoms to the prescriber immediately: increase in cough, congestion, shortness of breath, chest pain, fever (a temperature above 100.4° F or 38° C), or any change in sputum production or color (i.e., if not clear or if a change from baseline).
- Patient identifies specific safety precautions to help prevent injury related to drug-induced CNS depressant adverse effects, such as moving purposefully and slowly, asking for assistance as needed, minimizing use of other CNS depressant drugs, and, if elderly or at high risk for injury, obtaining assistance with activities of daily living and with mobility.
- Patient reports resolution of symptoms and an improved health status, such as return of temperature to baseline, return of secretions or sputum to clear color and normal consistency, return to normal breathing rate and patterns, and clearing of breath sounds.

Implementation

If patients are receiving any of the newer *nonsedating antihistamines,* the drugs should be taken very carefully and as directed. Reduced dosages may be needed for patients who are elderly or have decreased renal function. These newer H_1 receptor antagonist drugs do not cross the blood-brain barrier as readily as do older antihistamines and are therefore less likely to cause sedation. They are generally very well tolerated with minimal adverse effects.

Patients taking *traditional antihistamines* (e.g., diphenhydramine) should take the medications as prescribed. Most of these medications, including the OTC antihistamines, are best tolerated when taken with meals. Although food may slightly decrease absorption of these drugs, it has the benefit of minimizing the GI upset these drugs may cause. Patients who experience dry mouth should be encouraged to chew or suck on candy (sugar-free if needed) or OTC throat, cough, or cold lozenges, or to chew gum, as well as to perform frequent mouth care to ease the dryness and related discomfort. Other OTC or prescribed cold or cough medications should not be taken with antihistamines unless they were previously approved or ordered by the prescriber because of the potential for serious drug interactions. Dosage amounts and routes may vary depending on whether the patient is elderly, adult aged, or younger than 12 years, so proper dosing and usage should be encouraged. Blood pressure and other vital signs should be monitored as needed. The elderly and children should be monitored for any paradoxical reactions, which are common with these drugs.

With *antitussives,* chewable or lozenge forms of the drugs should be used exactly as ordered. Drowsiness or dizziness may occur with the use of antitussives; therefore, patients should be cautioned against driving a car or engaging in other activities that requires mental alertness until they feel back to normal. If the antitussive contains codeine, the CNS depressant effects of the narcotic opiate may further depress breathing and respiratory effort. Other antitussives, such as dextromethorphan, as well as the codeine-containing drugs should be given at evenly spaced intervals so that the drug reaches a steady state.

Patients taking *decongestants,* such as pseudoephedrine or phenylephrine, are generally using the drugs for nasal decongestion. These drugs come in oral dosage forms, including sustained-release and chewable forms. With any of the drugs discussed in this chapter and the disorders or diseases for which they are being taken, it is also important to encourage fluid intake of up to 3000 mL a day, unless contraindicated. The fluid helps to liquefy secretions, assists in breaking up thick secretions, and makes it easier to cough up secretions. Patient teaching tips for these drugs are presented below.

Evaluation

A therapeutic response to drugs given to treat respiratory conditions, such as *antihistamines, antitussives, decongestants,* and *expectorants,* includes resolution of the symptoms for which the drugs were originally prescribed or taken. These symptoms may include cough; nasal, sinus, or chest congestion; nasal, salivary, and lacrimal gland hypersecretion; motion sickness; sneezing; watery, red, or itchy eyes; itchy nose; allergic rhinitis; and allergic symptoms. Some of the antihistamines, such as diphenhydramine, are also helpful as sleep aids, and a therapeutic response when taken for this purpose would be the successful induction of sleep. Adverse effects for which to monitor in patients using any of these drugs include excessively dry mouth, drowsiness, oversedation, dizziness (lightheadedness), paradoxical excitement, nervousness, dysrhythmias, palpitations, GI upset, urinary retention, fever, dyspnea, chest pain, headache, and insomnia, depending on the drug prescribed.

PATIENT TEACHING TIPS

- The patient should be educated about the possibility of tolerance to the sedating effects of traditional antihistamines. The patient should be instructed to avoid activities that require alertness until tolerance to sedation occurs or until the patient accurately judges the fact that the drug has no impact on motor skills or responses to motor activities. Another element to include in patient education is a list of drugs the patient should avoid, including alcohol and CNS depressants.
- With traditional and nonsedating antihistamines, a humidifier may be needed to help liquefy sections making expectoration of sputum easier. Intake of fluids should always be encouraged, unless contraindicated.
- Patients with upper or lower respiratory symptoms or disease processes should know to avoid dry air, smoke-filled environments, and allergens.
- The patient should be encouraged *always* to check for possible drug interactions because of the many OTC and prescription drugs that could lead to adverse effects if taken concurrently.
- The patient should be educated about taking the medication with food to help avoid GI upset.
- Any difficulty breathing, palpitations, hallucinations, or tremors should be reported to the prescriber immediately.
- Antitussives should be taken with caution, and the patient must be fully aware that any fever, chest tightness, change in sputum from clear to colored, difficult or noisy breathing, activity intolerance, or weakness should be reported.
- The patient should be instructed to use decongestants only as ordered and to adhere to instructions regarding dose and frequency. It should be emphasized to the patient that frequent, long-term, or excessive use of decongestants (whether oral forms or nasal inhaled forms) may lead to rebound congestion in which the nasal passages become more congested as the effects of the drug wear off; when this occurs, the patient generally uses more of the drug, precipitating a vicious cycle with more congestion. The patient should be instructed to report excessive dizziness, heart palpitations, weakness, sedation, and/or excessive irritability to the prescriber.
- Patients taking expectorants should avoid alcohol and products containing alcohol, and they should not use these medications for longer than 1 week. If cough or symptoms continue, they should know to contact their prescriber. Intake of fluids should be encouraged (unless contraindicated) to help thin secretions for easier expectoration.
- Decongestants and expectorants are recommended to treat cold symptoms, but the patient should be encouraged to report to the prescriber a fever of higher than 100.4° F (38° C), cough, or other symptoms lasting longer than 4 days when decongestants or any of the other drugs presented in this chapter are used.

POINTS TO REMEMBER

- There are two types of histamine blockers: H_1 blockers and H_2 blockers. H_1 blockers are the drugs to which most people are referring when they use the term *antihistamine*. H_1 blockers prevent the harmful effects of histamine and are used to treat seasonal allergic rhinitis, anaphylaxis, reactions to insect bites, and so forth. H_2 blockers are used to treat gastric acid disorders, such as hyperacidity or ulcer disease.
- Educate about the purposes of the medication regimen, the expected adverse effects, and any drug interactions. A list of all medications (prescription, over-the-counter, and herbal) should be provided to all health care providers.

- Decongestants work by causing constriction of the engorged and swollen blood vessels in the sinuses, which decreases pressure and allows mucous membranes to drain. Nurses must understand the action of these drugs and know other important information such as significant adverse effects, including cardiac and CNS-stimulating effects.
- Nonopioid antitussive drugs may also cause sedation, drowsiness, or dizziness. Patients should not drive a car or engage in other activities that require mental alertness if these adverse effects occur. Codeine-containing antitussives may lead to CNS depression; they should be used cautiously and should not be mixed with anything containing alcohol.

NCLEX EXAMINATION REVIEW QUESTIONS

1 When assessing a patient who is to receive a decongestant, the nurse will recognize that a potential contraindication to this drug would be
   a glaucoma.
   b fever.
   c ulcer disease.
   d allergic rhinitis.
2 When giving decongestants, the nurse must remember that these drugs have alpha-adrenergic–stimulating effects that may result in
   a fever.
   b bradycardia.
   c hypertension.
   d CNS depression.
3 The nurse is reviewing a patient's medication orders for prn (as necessary) medications that can be given to a patient who has bronchitis with a productive cough. Which drug should the nurse choose?
   a An antitussive
   b An expectorant
   c An antihistamine
   d A decongestant

4 The nurse knows that an antitussive cough medication would be the best choice for which patient?
   a A patient with a productive cough
   b A patient with chronic paranasal sinusitis
   c A patient who has had recent abdominal surgery
   d A patient who has influenza
5 A patient is taking a decongestant to help reduce symptoms of a cold. The nurse should instruct the patient to observe for which possible symptom, which may indicate an adverse effect of this drug?
   a Increased cough
   b Dry mouth
   c Slower heart rate
   d Heart palpitations
6 The nurse is giving an antihistamine and will observe the patient for which side effects? (Select all that apply.)
   a Hypertension
   b Dizziness
   c "Hangover" effect
   d Drowsiness
   e Tachycardia
   f Dry mouth

1 a, 2 c, 3 b, 4 c, 5 d, 6 b, c, d, f

CRITICAL THINKING ACTIVITIES: BEST ACTION

1 A patient calls the clinic to ask the nurse about taking an antihistamine for a "terrible cold." She says she is so tired of sneezing and blowing her nose. The nurse asks about the patient's history and finds out that the patient has a history of asthma. What is the nurse's best answer regarding this patient's use of an antihistamine?
2 An elderly patient is discussing the use of guaifenesin with the nurse. He asks, "What else can I do to fight this terrible cold? I don't want to just take a pill." What is the nurse's best answer?

3 A patient is recovering from an emergency exploratory laparotomy. He had a cold before his surgery and is now coughing up large amounts of whitish yellow sputum. He is receiving intravenous fluids and antibiotics. He asks the nurse for something to make him stop coughing. The nurse reviews the medication sheet and sees both an expectorant and an antitussive ordered. Which medication would be the best choice at this time? Explain.

For answers, see *http://evolve.elsevier.com/Lilley*.

CHAPTER 37

Bronchodilators and Other Respiratory Drugs

OBJECTIVES

When you reach the end of this chapter, you should be able to do the following:

1 Describe the anatomy and physiology of the respiratory system.
2 Discuss the impact of respiratory drugs on various lower and upper respiratory tract diseases and conditions.
3 List the classifications of drugs used to treat diseases and conditions of the respiratory system and provide specific examples.
4 Discuss the mechanisms of action, indications, contraindications, cautions, drug interactions, dosages, routes of administration, adverse effects, and toxic effects of the bronchodilators and other respiratory drugs.
5 Develop a nursing care plan that includes all phases of the nursing process for patients who use bronchodilators and other respiratory drugs.

http://evolve.elsevier.com/Lilley

NCLEX Review Questions • Animations • Nursing Care Plans • Audio Glossary • Category Catchers • Medication Errors Checklists • IV Therapy Checklists • Calculators • Frequently Asked Questions • Content Updates • Supplemental Resources • Answers to Case Studies and Critical Thinking Activities

Drug Profiles

◆ albuterol, p. 569
fluticasone propionate, p. 575
ipratropium, p. 570
methylprednisolone, p. 575

◆ montelukast, p. 572
◆ salmeterol, p. 569
theophylline, p. 571

◆ *Key drug.*

Glossary

Allergen Any substance that evokes an allergic response. (p. 565)
Allergic asthma Bronchial asthma caused by hypersensitivity to an allergen or allergens. (p. 565)
Alveoli Microscopic sacs in the lungs where oxygen is exchanged for carbon dioxide; also called *air sacs.* (p. 565)
Antibodies Immunoglobulins produced by lymphocytes in response to bacteria, viruses, or other antigenic substances. (p. 565)
Antigen A substance (usually a protein) that causes the formation of an antibody and reacts specifically with that antibody. (p. 565)
Asthma attack The onset of wheezing together with difficulty breathing. (p. 565)
Bronchial asthma The general term for recurrent and reversible shortness of breath resulting from narrowing of the bronchi and bronchioles; it is often referred to simply as *asthma.* (p. 565)

Bronchodilators Medications that improve airflow by relaxing bronchial smooth muscle cells (e.g., xanthines, adrenergic agonists). (p. 566)
Chronic bronchitis Chronic inflammation of the bronchi. (p. 565)
Emphysema A condition of the lungs characterized by enlargement of the air spaces distal to the bronchioles. (p. 565)
Immunoglobulins Proteins belonging to any of five structurally and antigenically distinct classes of antibodies present in the serum and external secretions of the body; they play a major role in immune responses; *immunoglobulin* is often abbreviated *Ig.* (p. 565)
Lower respiratory tract (LRT) The division of the respiratory system composed of organs located almost entirely within the chest. (p. 564)
Status asthmaticus A prolonged asthma attack. (p. 565)
Upper respiratory tract (URT) The division of the respiratory system composed of organs located outside the chest cavity (thorax). (p. 564)

• • •

Anatomy, Physiology, and Disease Overview

The main function of the respiratory system is to deliver oxygen to, and remove carbon dioxide from, the cells of the body. To perform this deceptively simple task requires a very intricate system of tissues, muscles, and organs called the *respiratory system.* It consists of two divisions or tracts: the upper and lower respiratory tracts. The **upper respiratory tract (URT)** is composed of the structures that are located outside of the chest cavity or *thorax.* These are the nose, nasopharynx, oropharynx, laryngopharynx, and larynx. The **lower respiratory tract (LRT)** is located almost entirely within the thorax and is composed of the trachea, all segments of the bronchial tree, and the lungs. The

URT and LRT have four main accessory structures that aid in their overall function. These are the oral cavity (mouth), the rib cage, the muscles of the rib cage (intercostal muscles), and the diaphragm. The upper and lower respiratory tracts together with the accessory structures make up the respiratory system, and the elements of this system are in constant communication with each other as they perform the vital function of respiration and the exchange of oxygen for carbon dioxide.

The air we breathe is a mixture of many gases. During inhalation, oxygen molecules from the air diffuse across the semipermeable membranes of the **alveoli,** where they are exchanged for carbon dioxide molecules, which are then exhaled. The lungs also filter, warm, and humidify the air we breathe. The oxygen is then delivered to the cells by the blood vessels of the circulatory system, where the respiratory system then transfers the oxygen it has extracted from inhaled air to the hemoglobin protein molecules contained within red blood cells. Also within the circulatory system, the cellular metabolic waste product carbon dioxide is collected from the tissues by the red blood cells. This waste is then transported back to the lungs via the circulatory system, where it diffuses back across the alveolar membranes and is then exhaled into the air. The respiratory system also plays a central role in speech, smell, and regulation of pH (acid-base balance).

DISEASES OF THE RESPIRATORY SYSTEM

Several diseases impair the function of the respiratory system. Those that affect the URT include colds, rhinitis, and hay fever. These conditions and the drugs used to treat them are discussed in Chapter 36. The major diseases that impair the function of the LRT include asthma, **emphysema,** and **chronic bronchitis.** The one feature these diseases have in common is that they all involve the obstruction of airflow through the airways. Chronic obstructive pulmonary disease (COPD) is the name applied collectively to emphysema and chronic bronchitis, because the obstruction is relatively constant. Asthma that is persistent and present most of the time despite treatment is also considered a COPD. Cystic fibrosis and infant respiratory distress syndrome are other disorders that affect the LRT, but because the treatment for them places more emphasis on nonpharmacologic than on pharmacologic measures, they are not a focus of the discussion in this chapter.

Asthma

Bronchial asthma is defined as a recurrent and reversible shortness of breath and occurs when the airways of the lung (bronchi and bronchioles) become narrow as a result of bronchospasm, inflammation and edema of the bronchial mucosa, and the production of viscous (sticky) mucus. The alveolar ducts and alveoli distal to the bronchioles remain open, but the obstruction to the airflow in the airways prevents carbon dioxide from getting out of the air spaces and oxygen from getting into them. Wheezing and difficulty breathing are the symptoms. When an episode has a sudden and dramatic onset, it is referred to as an **asthma attack.** Most asthma attacks are short, and normal breathing is subsequently recovered. However, an asthma attack may be prolonged for several minutes to hours and may not respond to typical drug therapy. This is a condition known as **status asthmaticus** and often requires hospitalization. The onset of asthma

---

BOX 37-1 Steps Involved in an Attack of Allergic Asthma

1. The offending allergen provokes the production of hypersensitive antibodies (most commonly immunoglobulin E [IgE]) that are specific to the allergen. This immunologic response initiates patient sensitivity.
2. The IgE antibodies are homocytotropic and collect on the surface of mast cells, thus sensitizing the patient to the allergen.
3. Subsequent allergen contact provokes the antigen-antibody reaction on the surface of mast cells.
4. Mast cell integrity is then violated, and these cells release chemical mediators stored in the cell. They also synthesize and then release other chemical mediators. These mediators include bradykinin, eosinophil chemotactic factor of anaphylaxis, histamine, prostaglandins, and slow-reacting substance of anaphylaxis (SRS-A).
5. The released chemical mediators, especially histamine and SRS-A, trigger bronchial constriction and an asthma attack.

---

occurs before 10 years of age in 50% of patients and before 40 years of age in about 80% of patients.

There are three categories of asthma: allergic, idiopathic, and mixed allergic-idiopathic asthma. Approximately 2% of the general population is affected by one of these three types. Allergic asthma accounts for approximately 30% to 35% of the cases of asthma, idiopathic asthma for about 35% to 50%, and the mixed form for the remaining cases.

Allergic asthma is caused by a hypersensitivity to an allergen or allergens in the environment. An **allergen** is any substance that elicits an allergic reaction. In patients with seasonal asthma the allergen is a substance such as pollen or mold, which is present only periodically (seasonally). The offending allergens in patients with nonseasonal asthma are substances such as dust, mold, and animal danders, which are present in the environment throughout the year. Cigarette smoke, from either smoking or exposure to secondhand smoke, is another common allergen. Examples of common food allergens include nuts, eggs, and corn. Exposure to the offending allergen in a patient with either type of allergic asthma causes an immediate allergic reaction in the form of an asthma attack. This attack is mediated by antibodies already present in the patient's body that chemically recognize the allergen to be a foreign substance, or **antigen.** These **antibodies** are specialized immune system proteins known as **immunoglobulins.** The antibody in individuals with asthma is usually immunoglobulin E (IgE), which is one of the five types of antibodies in the body (the others are IgG, IgA, IgM, and IgD). On exposure to the allergen, the patient's body responds by mounting an immediate and potent antigen-antibody reaction *(immune response).* This reaction occurs on the surfaces of cells such as *mast cells* that are rich in *histamines, leukotrienes,* and other substances involved in the immune response. These substances are collectively known as *inflammatory mediators,* and they are released from the mast cells as part of the immune response. This in turn, as described in Chapter 36, triggers the mucosal swelling and bronchoconstriction that are characteristic of an allergic asthma attack. The sequence of events that occurs in a patient with allergic asthma is shown in Box 37-1.

The specific cause of idiopathic, or intrinsic, asthma is unknown. It is not mediated by IgE, and there is often no family

---

BOX 37-2 Classifications of Drugs Used to Treat Asthma

Long-Term Control
Leukotriene receptor antagonists
cromolyn
Inhaled steroids
ipratropium
Long-acting beta$_2$ agonists
nedocromil
theophylline

Quick Relief
Intravenous systemic corticosteroids
Short-acting inhaled beta$_2$ agonists

TABLE 37-1 Stepwise Therapy for the Management of Asthma

Step	Drug Classification
Step 1	Short-acting inhaled beta$_2$ agonists as needed
Step 2	Preferred: low-dose inhaled corticosteroid (ICS)
	Alternative: cromolyn, nedocromil, leukotriene receptor antagonist (LTRA), or theophylline
Step 3	Preferred: low-dose ICS and long-acting beta$_2$ agonist (LABA) or medium-dose ICS
	Alternative: low-dose ICS and either LTRA, theophylline, or zileuton
Step 4	Preferred: medium-dose ICS plus LABA
	Alternative: medium-dose ICS plus either LTRA, theophylline, or zileuton
Step 5	High-dose ICS and LABA and consider omalizumab for patients with allergies
Step 6	High-dose ICS and LABA and oral corticosteroid and consider omalizumab for patients with allergies

---

history of allergies in affected patients. However, certain factors have been noted to precipitate asthma attacks in these patients, including respiratory infections, stress, cold weather, and strenuous work or exercise. As the name implies, mixed allergic-idiopathic asthma results from a combination of allergic and idiopathic factors. Patients with any type of asthma who know their suspected "triggers," whether an allergen, the weather, or another factor, are advised to avoid these triggers as much as is feasible as part of managing their disease. When it is not feasible or advisable to avoid a certain trigger (e.g., exercise), patients should work with their prescribers to mitigate the response to these triggers through appropriate drug therapy (e.g., use of a bronchodilator inhaler before exercise or other strenuous activity).

The National Asthma Education and Prevention Panel (NAEPP) of the National Heart, Lung, and Blood Institute has maintained ongoing guidelines for the diagnosis and management of asthma since 1989. The current guideline revision was published in 2007. In general, these guidelines classify asthma medications as either for long-term symptom control or rapid symptom relief. The specific drugs in each classification are listed in Box 37-2. The guidelines advocate the use of a stepwise approach in the treatment of asthma. The particular steps and recommended drug classifications for treatment at each step are listed in Table 37-1.

Chronic Bronchitis

Chronic bronchitis is a continuous inflammation of the bronchi. The inflammation in the associated bronchioles (smaller bronchi) is responsible for most of the airflow obstruction. Chronic bronchitis involves the excessive secretion of mucus and certain pathologic changes in the bronchial structure. The disease can arise as a result of repeated episodes of acute bronchitis or in the context of chronic generalized diseases. It is usually precipitated by prolonged exposure to bronchial irritants. One of the most common is cigarette smoke. Some patients acquire the disease because of other predisposing factors such as viral or bacterial pulmonary infections during childhood. Others may have mild impairment of the ability to inactivate *proteolytic* (protein-destroying) enzymes, which then damage the airway mucosal tissues. Unknown genetic characteristics may be responsible as well.

Emphysema

Emphysema is a condition in which the air spaces enlarge as a result of the destruction of the alveolar walls. This appears to be caused by the effect of proteolytic enzymes released from leukocytes in response to alveolar inflammation. Because the alveolar walls are partially destroyed, the surface area available for oxygen and carbon dioxide exchange is reduced, which impairs effective respiration. As with chronic bronchitis, cigarette smoke appears to be the primary irritant responsible for precipitating the underlying inflammation that leads to the development of emphysema. There is also an associated genetic deficiency in some people of the enzyme alpha$_1$-antitrypsin.

TREATMENT OF DISEASES OF THE LOWER RESPIRATORY TRACT

In the past the treatment of asthma and other COPDs focused primarily on the use of drugs that cause the airways to dilate. Now there is a greater understanding of the pathophysiology of asthma. The emphasis of research has shifted from the bronchoconstriction component of the disease to the inflammatory component. This is also reflected in the various medication classes used to treat COPDs, although bronchodilators still play an important role. A synopsis of the mechanisms of action of the various classes of antiasthmatic drugs is provided in Table 37-2. Figure 37-1 gives an overview of the various drugs used in asthma.

Pharmacology Overview

BRONCHODILATORS

Bronchodilators are an important part of the pharmacotherapy for all COPDs. These drugs are able to relax bronchial smooth muscle bands to dilate the bronchi and bronchioles that are narrowed as a result of the disease process. There are three classes of such drugs: beta agonists, anticholinergics, and xanthine derivatives.

TABLE **37-2** Mechanisms of Antiasthmatic Drug Action

Antiasthmatic	Mechanism in Asthma Relief
Anticholinergics	Block cholinergic receptors, thus preventing the binding of cholinergic substances that cause constriction and increase secretions
Leukotriene receptor antagonists	Modify or inhibit the activity of leukotrienes, which decreases arachidonic acid–induced inflammation and allergen-induced bronchoconstriction
Beta agonists and xanthine derivatives	Raise intracellular levels of cyclic adenosine monophosphate, which in turn produces smooth muscle relaxation and dilates the constricted bronchi and bronchioles
Corticosteroids	Prevent the inflammation commonly provoked by the substances released from mast cells
Mast cell stabilizers (cromolyn and nedocromil)	Stabilize the cell membranes of the mast cells in which the antigen-antibody reactions take place, thereby preventing the release of substances such as histamine that cause constriction

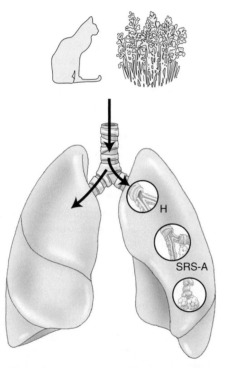

ALLERGENS such as dust, wool blankets, feather pillows, pollen, etc., in hypersensitive persons with IgE antibodies stimulate mast cells in lungs to release histamine (H) and slow-reacting substance of anaphylaxis (SRS-A).

HISTAMINE stimulates larger bronchi to cause smooth muscle spasms, inflammation, and edema.

SRS-A stimulates small bronchi to cause smooth muscle swelling.

Result is spasms of smooth bronchial muscle, increased mucus secretions, swollen mucosa, hyperinflation of alveoli eventually leading to loss of elasticity and collapsed alveoli.

H

SRS-A

LEUKOTRIENE ANTAGONISTS block the release of leukotrienes in the lungs. Inflammation causes an increase in leukotrienes, substances that constitute the slow-reacting substance of anaphylaxis (SRS-A).

THEOPHYLLINE increases cyclic AMP to inhibit breakdown of sensitized mast cells that stimulate the release of histamine, serotonin, and SRS-A.

MAST CELL STABILIZERS inhibit the release of histamine from mast cells to reduce allergic effects.

SYMPATHETIC AGONISTS stimulate sympathetic systems to decrease mucus secretions and relax bronchial muscle spasms.

CORTICOSTEROIDS produce an antiinflammatory effect and reduce mucus secretions and tissue histamine.

FIGURE 37-1 Overview of the effects of various antiasthmatic medications. (From McKenry LM, Tessier E, Hogan M: *Mosby's pharmacology in nursing,* ed 22, St Louis, 2006, Mosby.)

BETA-ADRENERGIC AGONISTS

The beta agonists are a large group of drugs that are commonly used during the acute phase of an asthmatic attack to quickly reduce airway constriction and restore airflow to normal. They are agonists or stimulators of the adrenergic receptors in the sympathetic nervous system. The beta and alpha adrenergic receptors are discussed in Chapters 18 and 19. The beta agonists imitate the effects of norepinephrine on these receptors. For this reason they are also called *sympathomimetic bronchodilators.* Available asthma-related drugs in this class include albuterol (e.g., Ventolin), formoterol (Foradil) epinephrine, metaproterenol (Alupent), and salmeterol (Serevent). Salmeterol is a long acting drug which should never be used for acute treatment.

Mechanism of Action and Drug Effects

The beta agonists dilate airways by stimulating the beta$_2$-adrenergic receptors located throughout the lungs.

There are three subtypes of these drugs, based on their selectivity for beta$_2$ receptors:

1. Nonselective adrenergic drugs, which stimulate the beta, beta$_1$ (cardiac), and beta$_2$ (respiratory) receptors. Example: epinephrine.
2. Nonselective beta-adrenergic drugs, which stimulate both beta$_1$ and beta$_2$ receptors. Example: metaproterenol.
3. Selective beta$_2$ drugs, which primarily stimulate the beta$_2$ receptors. Example: albuterol.

These drugs can also be categorized according to their routes of administration as oral, injectable, or inhaled. The various beta agonist bronchodilators are listed in Table 37-3.

The bronchioles are surrounded by smooth muscle. If this smooth muscle contracts, the airways are narrowed and the amount of oxygen and carbon dioxide exchanged is reduced. The action of beta agonist bronchodilators begins at the specific receptor stimulated and ends with the dilation of the airways. However, many reactions must take place at the cellular level for this bronchodilation to occur. When a beta$_2$-adrenergic receptor is stimulated by a beta agonist, adenylate cyclase, which is an enzyme needed to make cyclic adenosine monophosphate (cAMP), is activated and produces more cAMP. The increased levels of cAMP made available by adenylate cyclase cause bronchial smooth muscles to relax, which results in bronchial dilation and increased airflow into and out of the lungs.

Nonselective adrenergic agonist drugs such as epinephrine also stimulate beta-adrenergic receptors, causing constriction within the blood vessels. This vasoconstriction reduces the amount of edema or swelling in the mucous membranes and limits the quantity of secretions normally produced by these membranes. In addition, these drugs stimulate beta$_1$ receptors, which results in cardiovascular adverse effects such as an increase in heart rate, force of contraction, and blood pressure, as well as central nervous system (CNS) effects such as nervousness and tremor.

Drugs such as albuterol that predominantly stimulate the beta$_2$ receptors have more specific drug effects. By primarily stimulating the beta$_2$-adrenergic receptors of the bronchial and vascular smooth muscles, they cause bronchodilation and may also have a dilating effect on the peripheral vasculature, which results in a decrease in diastolic blood pressure.

TABLE 37-3 Beta Agonist Bronchodilators

Drug	Type	Trade Names	Administration
albuterol	Beta$_2$	Proventil, Ventolin	PO, inhalation
ephedrine	Alpha/beta	None (various generic)	IM, IV, subcut
epinephrine	Alpha/beta	Adrenalin	Subcut, IM,
formoterol	Beta$_2$	Foradil, Perforomist	Inhalation
metaproterenol	Beta$_1$/beta$_2$	Alupent	PO, inhalation
levalbuterol	Beta$_2$	Xopenex	Inhalation
metaproterenol	Beta$_1$/beta$_2$	Alupent, Metaprel	PO, inhalation
pirbuterol	Beta$_2$	Maxair	Inhalation
salmeterol	Beta$_2$	Serevent, Serevent Diskus	Inhalation
terbutaline	Beta$_2$	Brethine	PO, subcut, inhalation

IM, Intramuscular; *IV,* intravenous; *PO,* oral; *subcut,* subcutaneous.

Indications

The primary respiratory therapeutic effect of the beta agonists is the relief of bronchospasm related to bronchial asthma, bronchitis, and other pulmonary diseases. However, they are also used for beneficial therapeutic effects outside the respiratory system. Because some of these drugs have the ability to stimulate both beta$_1$- and alpha-adrenergic receptors, they may be used to treat hypotension and shock (see Chapter 18) or to produce uterine relaxation (see Chapter 34).

Contraindications

Contraindications include drug allergy, uncontrolled cardiac dysrhythmias, and high risk of stroke (because of the vasoconstrictive drug actions).

Adverse Effects

Mixed alpha/beta agonists produce the greatest array of undesirable effects. These include insomnia, restlessness, anorexia, cardiac stimulation, hyperglycemia, tremor, and vascular headache. The adverse effects of the nonselective beta agonists are limited to beta-adrenergic effects, including cardiac stimulation, tremor, anginal pain, and vascular headache. The beta$_2$ drugs can cause both hypertension and hypotension, vascular headaches, and tremor. Overdose management may include careful administration of a beta-blocker while the patient is under close observation. Because the half-life of most adrenergic agonists is relatively short, however, the patient may just be observed while the body eliminates the medication.

Interactions

When nonselective beta-blockers are used with the beta agonist bronchodilators, the bronchodilation from the beta agonist is diminished. The use of beta agonists with monoamine oxidase inhibitors and other sympathomimetics is best avoided, because of the enhanced risk for hypertension. Patients with diabetes may require an adjustment in the dosage of their hypoglycemic drugs,

DOSAGES

Bronchodilators

Drug (Pregnancy Category)	Pharmacologic Class	Usual Dosage Range	Indications
◆ albuterol (Proventil, Proventil Repetabs, Ventolin, others) (C)	Beta₂ agonist	**Pediatric 2-6 yr** PO: 0.1-0.2 mg/kg 3 times daily **Pediatric 7-11 yr** PO: 2 mg 3-4 times daily **Adult and pediatric 12 yr and older** PO: 2-4 mg 3-4 times daily Inhalation solution: 2.5 mg 3-4 times daily **Adult and pediatric 4 yr and older** MDI: 2 puffs q4-6h Allergic and nonallergic rhinorrhea	Asthma, bronchospasm
ipratropium (Atrovent) (B)	Anticholinergic	**Adult and pediatric 12 yr and older** MDI: 2 puffs 4 times daily Nasal spray, 0.03%: 2 sprays 2-3 times daily Nasal spray, 0.06%: 2 sprays 3-4 times daily Inhalation solution: 500 mcg 3-4 times daily	

IM, Intramuscular; *IV*, intravenous; *MDI*, metered-dose inhaler; *PO*, oral.

especially patients receiving epinephrine, because of the increase in blood glucose levels that can occur.

Dosages

For recommended dosages of selected beta agonists, see the Dosages table above.

DRUG PROFILES

◆ albuterol

Albuterol (Proventil) is one of six beta₂-specific bronchodilating beta agonists. Other similar drugs include bitolterol (Tornalate), levalbuterol (Xopenex), pirbuterol (Maxair), salmeterol (Serevent Diskus), and terbutaline (Brethine). Although albuterol is the most commonly used drug in this class, salmeterol has a unique 12-hour duration of action, which makes it an attractive alternative. If albuterol is used too frequently, dose-related adverse effects may be seen, because albuterol loses its beta₂-specific actions, especially at larger dosages. As a consequence, the beta₁ receptors are stimulated, which causes nausea, increased anxiety, palpitations, tremors, and an increased heart rate.

Albuterol is available for both oral and inhalational use. Inhalational dosage forms include metered-dose inhalers (MDIs) as well as solutions for inhalation. The levorotatory isomeric form of albuterol, levalbuterol, is strictly for inhalational use and is sometimes prescribed as an albuterol alternative for patients with certain risk factors (e.g., tachycardia, including tachycardia associated with albuterol treatment).

PHARMACOKINETICS

Route	Onset of Action	Peak Plasma Concentration	Elimination Half-life	Duration of Action
Inhalation	Immediate	10-25 min	3-4 hr	3-4 hr

◆ salmeterol

Salmeterol (Serevent) is a long acting beta₂ agonist bronchodilator. It is used for the maintenance treatment of asthma and COPD. Because it is a long-acting drug, it should never be used for acute treatment. It is given twice daily for maintenance treatment only.

In 2006, a large randomized clinical trial showed that use of salmeterol was associated with an increase in asthma-related deaths (when added to usual asthma therapy). The risk appears to be higher in African American patients than in whites. Adverse effects include immediate hypersensitivity reactions, headache, hypertension, and neuromuscular and skeletal pain. Salmeterol should never be given more than twice daily nor should the maximum daily dose (one puff twice daily) be exceeded. It is available as a powder for inhalation either alone (Serevent Diskus) or combined with a corticosteroid (ADVAIR Diskus).

PHARMACOKINETICS

Route	Onset of Action	Peak Plasma Concentration	Elimination Half-life	Duration of Action
Inhalation	Asthma: 30-48 min COPD: 2 hr	Asthma: 2-4 hr COPD: 3-4.5 hr	5.5 hr	12 hr

ANTICHOLINERGICS

Currently there are two anticholinergic drugs used in the treatment of COPD: ipratropium and tiotropium.

Mechanism of Action and Drug Effects

On the surface of the bronchial tree are receptors for acetylcholine (ACh), the neurotransmitter for the parasympathetic nervous system. When the parasympathetic nervous system releases ACh from its nerve endings, it binds to the ACh receptors on the surface of the bronchial tree, which results in bronchial constriction and narrowing of the airways. Anticholinergic drugs block these ACh receptors to prevent bronchoconstriction. This indirectly causes airway dilation.

Indications

Because their actions are slow and prolonged, anticholinergics are used for prevention of the bronchospasm associated with chronic bronchitis or emphysema and not for the management of acute symptoms.

Contraindications

The only usual contraindication to the use of bronchial anticholinergic drugs is drug allergy, including allergy to atropine or to soy lecithin (found in some of the inhalational formulations), or allergy to related food products such as peanut oils, peanuts, soybeans, and other legumes (beans). There have been reported cases of severe anaphylactic reactions to ipratropium inhalers in patients with peanut allergy, and such use should be avoided.

Adverse Effects

The most commonly reported adverse effects of ipratropium and tiotropium therapy are related to the drugs' anticholinergic effects and include dry mouth or throat, nasal congestion, heart palpitations, gastrointestinal (GI) distress, urinary retention, increased intraocular pressure, headache, coughing, and anxiety. Ipratropium is classified as a pregnancy category B drug; tiotropium is a category C.

Drug Interactions

Possible additive toxicity may occur when anticholinergic bronchodilators are taken with other anticholinergic drugs.

Dosages

See the Dosages table on p. 569.

DRUG PROFILE

ipratropium

Ipratropium (Atrovent) is the oldest and most commonly used anticholinergic bronchodilator. It is pharmacologically very similar to atropine (see Chapter 21). It is available both as a liquid aerosol for inhalation and as a multidose inhaler; both form are usually dosed twice daily. A newer but similar drug is tiotropium (Spiriva), which is formulated for once-daily dosing. Many patients also benefit from taking both a beta₂ agonist and an anticholinergic drug, with the most popular combination being albuterol and ipratropium. Although many patients receive the two drugs separately, two combination products are available containing both of these drugs: Combivent (an MDI) and DuoNeb (an inhalation solution).

PHARMACOKINETICS

Route	Onset of Action	Peak Plasma Concentration	Elimination Half-life	Duration of Action
Inhalation	5-15 min	1-2 hr	1.6 hr	4-5 hr

XANTHINE DERIVATIVES

The natural xanthines consist of the plant alkaloids caffeine, theobromine, and theophylline, but only theophylline and caffeine are currently used clinically. Synthetic xanthines include aminophylline and dyphylline. Caffeine, which is actually a metabolite of theophylline, has other uses described later.

Mechanism of Action and Drug Effects

Xanthines cause bronchodilation by increasing the levels of the energy-producing substance cAMP. They do this by competitively inhibiting phosphodiesterase, the enzyme responsible for breaking down cAMP. In patients with COPD, cAMP plays an

integral role in the maintenance of open airways. Higher intracellular levels of cAMP contribute to smooth muscle relaxation and also inhibit IgE-induced release of the chemical mediators that drive allergic reactions (histamine, slow-reacting substance of anaphylaxis, and others).

Theophylline is metabolized to caffeine in the body, whereas aminophylline is metabolized to theophylline. Theophylline and other xanthines also stimulate the CNS, but to a lesser degree than caffeine. This stimulation of the CNS has the beneficial effect of acting directly on the medullary respiratory center to enhance respiratory drive. In large doses, theophylline may stimulate the cardiovascular system, which results in both an increased force of contraction (positive inotropy) and an increased heart rate (positive chronotropy). The increased force of contraction raises cardiac output and hence blood flow to the kidneys. This, in combination with the ability of the xanthines to dilate blood vessels in and around the kidney, increases the glomerular filtration rate, which produces a diuretic effect.

Indications

Xanthines are used to dilate the airways in patients with asthma, chronic bronchitis, or emphysema. They may be used in mild to moderate cases of acute asthma and as an adjunct drug in the management of COPD. However, xanthines are now deemphasized as

DOSAGES

Theophylline Salts

Drug (Pregnancy Category)	Pharmacologic Class	Usual Dosage Range	Indication
theophylline (Elixophyllin, Theo-Dur, Uniphyl, others) (C)	Xanthine-derived bronchodilator	**Adult** PO: 400-600 mg/day in 1-4 divided doses	Asthma

treatment for milder asthma because of their greater potential for drug interactions and the greater interpatient variability in therapeutic drug levels in the blood. Because of their relatively slow onset of action, xanthines are more often used for the prevention of asthmatic symptoms than for the relief of acute asthma attacks. However, they are often preferred as adjunct bronchodilators for patients with chronic bronchitis or emphysema.

Caffeine is primarily used without prescription as a CNS stimulant, or analeptic (see Chapter 14), to promote alertness (e.g., for long-duration driving or studying). It is also used as a cardiac stimulant in infants with bradycardia and for enhancement of respiratory drive in infants in neonatal intensive care units. It is not normally used clinically in adults for these purposes, although theoretically it would have similar effects.

Contraindications

Contraindications to therapy with xanthine derivatives include drug allergy, uncontrolled cardiac dysrhythmias, seizure disorders, hyperthyroidism, and peptic ulcers.

Adverse Effects

The common adverse effects of the xanthine derivatives include nausea, vomiting, and anorexia. In addition, gastroesophageal reflux has been observed to occur during sleep in patients taking these drugs. Cardiac adverse effects include sinus tachycardia, extrasystole, palpitations, and ventricular dysrhythmias. Transient increased urination and hyperglycemia are other possible adverse effects. Overdose and other toxicity of xanthine derivatives are usually treated by the repeated administration of doses of activated charcoal.

Interactions

The use of xanthine derivatives with any of the following drugs causes the serum level of the xanthine derivative to be increased: allopurinol, cimetidine, macrolide antibiotics (e.g., erythromycin), quinolones (e.g., ciprofloxacin), influenza vaccine, and oral contraceptives. Their use with sympathomimetics, or even caffeine, can produce additive cardiac and CNS stimulation. Rifampin increases the metabolism of theophylline, which results in decreased theophylline levels. A reported herbal interaction is the tendency of St. John's wort (Hypericum perforatum) to enhance the rate of xanthine drug metabolism; thus, higher dosages of theophylline and other xanthine derivatives may be needed in patients using this popular herbal preparation. Cigarette smoking has a similar effect because of the enzyme-inducing effect of nicotine. Interacting foods include charcoal-broiled, high-protein, and low-carbohydrate foods. These foods may reduce serum levels of xanthines through various metabolic mechanisms.

Dosages

For the recommended dosages of selected theophylline salts, see the Dosages table above.

DRUG PROFILE

theophylline

Theophylline (Elixophyllin) is the most commonly used xanthine derivative. It is available in oral, rectal, injectable (as aminophylline), and topical dosage forms. Besides theophylline, which occurs in various salt forms, the other xanthine bronchodilators used clinically for the treatment of bronchoconstriction are aminophylline and dyphylline. These drugs are prodrugs of theophylline; they are metabolized to theophylline in the body. Aminophylline is the most commonly used of these prodrugs and is sometimes given intravenously to patients with status asthmaticus who have not responded to fast-acting beta agonists such as epinephrine.

The beneficial effects of theophylline can be maximized by maintaining levels in the blood within a certain target range. If these levels become too high, many unwanted adverse effects can occur. If the levels become too low, the patient receives little therapeutic benefit. Although the optimal level may vary from patient to patient, most standard references have suggested that the therapeutic range for theophylline blood level is 10 to 20 mcg/mL. However, most clinicians now advise levels between 5 and 15 mcg/mL. Laboratory monitoring of drug blood levels is common to ensure adequate dosage, especially in the hospital setting.

PHARMACOKINETICS

Route	Onset of Action	Peak Plasma Concentration	Elimination Half-life	Duration of Action
PO	Unknown	1-2 hr	7-9 hr	12 hr

NONBRONCHODILATING RESPIRATORY DRUGS

Bronchodilators are just one type of drug used to treat asthma, chronic bronchitis, and emphysema; as discussed earlier, these drugs include beta-adrenergic agonists and xanthines. There are also other drugs that are effective in suppressing various underlying causes of some of these respiratory illnesses. These include leukotriene receptor antagonists (montelukast, zafirlukast, and zileuton), and corticosteroids (beclomethasone, budesonide, dexamethasone, flunisolide, fluticasone, and triamcinolone). Another drug class known as *mast cell stabilizers* is now rarely used. However, these drugs are still listed in the national guidelines as *alternative* therapy and include cromolyn and nedocromil. As their class name implies, they work by stabilizing the cell membranes of mast cells to prevent the release of inflammatory mediators such as histamine.

LEUKOTRIENE RECEPTOR ANTAGONISTS

A newer class of asthma medications are the *leukotriene receptor antagonists (LTRAs)*. LTRAs became the first new class of asthma medications to be introduced in the United States in more than 20 years when the first of these was made available in the 1990s.

Before the development of LTRAs, most asthma treatments focused on relaxing the contraction of bronchial muscles with bronchodilators. More recently, researchers have begun to understand how asthma symptoms are caused by the immune system at the cellular level. A chain reaction starts when a trigger allergen, such as cat hair or dust, initiates a series of chemical reactions in the body. Several substances are produced, including a family of molecules known as *leukotrienes*. In people with asthma, leukotrienes cause inflammation, bronchoconstriction, and mucus production. This in turn leads to coughing, wheezing, and shortness of breath. As their name implies, LTRAs prevent leukotrienes from attaching to receptors located on circulating immune cells (e.g., lymphocytes in the blood) as well as local immune cells within the lungs (e.g., alveolar macrophages). This alleviates asthma symptoms in the lungs by reducing inflammation.

Mechanism of Action and Drug Effects

Currently two subclasses of LTRAs are available. These subclasses differ in the mechanism by which they block the inflammatory process in asthma. The first subclass of LTRAs acts by an indirect mechanism and inhibits the enzyme 5-lipoxygenase, which is necessary for leukotriene synthesis. Zileuton (Zyflo) is the only drug of this type currently available. Drugs in the second subclass of LTRAs act more directly by binding to the D_4 leukotriene receptor subtype in respiratory tract tissues and organs. These drugs include montelukast (Singulair) and zafirlukast (Accolate).

The drug effects of LTRAs are primarily limited to the lungs. Through their reduction of leukotriene synthesis or action, they prevent smooth muscle contraction of the bronchial airways, decrease mucus secretion, and reduce vascular permeability (which reduces edema). Other antileukotriene effects of these drugs include prevention of the mobilization and migration of such cells as neutrophils and lymphocytes into the lungs. This also serves to reduce airway inflammation.

Indications

The LTRAs montelukast, zafirlukast, and zileuton are used for the prophylaxis and long-term treatment of asthma in adults and children 12 years of age and older. Montelukast is the most widely used of these drugs and has also been approved for treatment of allergic rhinitis, a condition discussed in Chapter 36. These drugs are not meant for the management of acute asthmatic attacks. Improvement with their use is typically seen in about 1 week.

Contraindications

Drug allergy or other previous adverse drug reaction is the primary contraindication to the use of these drugs. Allergy to povidone, lactose, titanium dioxide, or cellulose derivatives is also

important to note, because these are inactive ingredients in these drugs.

Adverse Effects

The adverse effects of LTRAs differ depending on the specific drug. The most commonly reported adverse effects of zileuton, after headaches, are dyspepsia, nausea, dizziness, and insomnia. The most common adverse effects of zafirlukast, after headaches, are nausea and diarrhea. Both drugs may also lead to liver dysfunction. For this reason, liver enzyme levels should be monitored regularly in patients taking these drugs, especially early in the course of therapy.

Interactions

Montelukast has fewer drug interactions than zafirlukast or zileuton. It does not interact with theophylline, warfarin, digoxin, prednisone, or either the estrogen or progestin components of combination oral contraceptives. Phenobarbital decreases montelukast concentrations. For information on the drugs that interact with zafirlukast and zileuton, see Table 37-4.

Dosages

For recommended dosages of montelukast, see the Dosages table on p. 573.

DRUG PROFILE

LTRAs are a new class of asthma medications. The three drugs currently available are zileuton, zafirlukast, and montelukast. They are used primarily for oral prophylaxis and long-term treatment of asthma. These drugs are not recommended for treatment of acute asthma attacks.

◆ montelukast

Montelukast (Singulair) belongs to the same subcategory of LTRAs as zafirlukast. Montelukast and zafirlukast work by blocking leukotriene D_4 receptors to augment the inflammatory response. Montelukast offers the advantage of being U.S. Food and Drug Administration approved for use in children 2 years of age and older. It also has fewer adverse effects and drug interactions than zafirlukast. Use of montelukast is contraindicated in patients with a known hypersensitivity to it. It is available only for oral use. Pregnancy category B. Common dosages are given in the table on p. 573.

PHARMACOKINETICS

Route	Onset of Action	Peak Plasma Concentration	Elimination Half-life	Duration of Action
PO	30 min	3-4 hr	2.7-5 hr	24 hr

CORTICOSTEROIDS

Corticosteroids, also known as *glucocorticoids,* are either naturally occurring or synthetic drugs used in the treatment of pulmonary diseases for their antiinflammatory effects. All have actions similar to those of the natural steroid hormone cortisol, which is chemically the same as the drug hydrocortisone. Synthetic steroids are now more commonly used in drug therapy. They can be given by inhalation, orally, or even intravenously in severe cases of asthma. Corticosteroids administered by in-

TABLE 37-4 Drug Interactions: Leukotriene Receptor Antagonists

Drug	Interacting Drugs	Mechanism	Result
montelukast (Singulair)	phenobarbital, rifampin	Increased metabolism	Decreased montelukast levels
zafirlukast (Accolate)	aspirin	Decreased clearance	Increased zafirlukast levels
	erythromycin	Decreased bioavailability	Decreased zafirlukast levels
	tolbutamide, phenytoin, carbamazepine	Inhibited metabolism	Increased tolbutamide, phenytoin, and carbamazepine levels
	warfarin	Decreased clearance	Increased warfarin levels
zileuton (Zyflo)	propranolol	Decreased clearance	Increased propranolol levels
	theophylline	Decreased clearance	Increased theophylline levels
	warfarin	Decreased clearance	Increased warfarin levels

DOSAGES

Selected Antileukotriene Drug

Drug (Pregnancy Category)	Pharmacologic Class	Usual Dosage Range	Indications
◆ montelukast (Singulair) (B)	Leukotriene receptor antagonist	**Pediatric 2-5 yr** 4 mg daily in evening **Pediatric 6-14 yr** 5 mg daily in evening **Adult and pediatric 15 yr and older** 10 mg daily in evening	Asthma (prophylaxis and maintenance treatment)

halation have an advantage over orally administered corticosteroids in that their action is limited to the topical site in the lungs. This generally prevents systemic effects. The chemical structures of the corticosteroids given by inhalation have also been slightly altered to limit their systemic absorption from the respiratory tract. The corticosteroids administered by inhalation include the following:

- beclomethasone dipropionate (Beclovent)
- budesonide (Pulmicort Turbuhaler)
- dexamethasone sodium phosphate (Decadron Phosphate Respihaler)
- flunisolide (AeroBid)
- fluticasone (Flonase)
- triamcinolone acetonide (Azmacort)

The systemic use of corticosteroids was described in Chapter 33. The systemic corticosteroids most commonly used for respiratory illness include the following:

- prednisone (oral)
- methylprednisolone (intravenous or oral)

Mechanism of Action and Drug Effects

Although the exact mechanism of action of the corticosteroids has not been determined, it is conjectured that they have the dual effect of both reducing inflammation and enhancing the activity of beta agonists. The corticosteroids previously mentioned produce their antiinflammatory effects through a complex sequence of actions. The overall effect is to prevent various nonspecific inflammatory processes. These include the accumulation of inflammatory mediators as well as altered vascular permeability (which causes edema).

They essentially work by stabilizing the membranes of cells that normally release very harmful bronchoconstricting substances. These cells include *leukocytes,* which is another name for white blood cells (WBCs). There are five different types of WBC, each with its own specific characteristics. The five types of WBC, their role in the inflammatory process, and the way in which corticosteroids inhibit their normal action, combat inflammation, and produce bronchodilation are summarized in Table 37-5. In particular, inflammatory mediators are primarily released by *lymphocytes* in the circulation as well as by *mast cells* and *alveolar macrophages.* These latter two cell types are stationary (noncirculating) inflammatory cells that remain localized in the various tissues and organs of the respiratory tract.

Corticosteroids have also been shown to restore or increase the responsiveness of bronchial smooth muscle to beta-adrenergic receptor stimulation, which results in more pronounced stimulation of the beta$_2$ receptors by beta agonist drugs such as albuterol. It may take several weeks of continuous therapy before the full therapeutic effects of the corticosteroids are realized.

Indications

Inhaled corticosteroids are now used for the primary treatment of bronchospastic disorders to control the inflammatory responses that are believed to be the cause of these disorders. They are often used concurrently with bronchodilators, primarily beta-adrenergic agonists. In respiratory illnesses, systemic corticosteroids are generally used only to treat acute exacerbations, or severe asthma. Their long-term use is associated with adverse effects (see later). The NAEPP recommends long-term use in cases of truly disabling illness (Step 6 of the recom-

TABLE 37-5 White Blood Cells (Leukocytes)

WBC Type*	Role in Inflammation	Corticosteroid Effect
Granulocytes		
Neutrophils (65%)	Contain powerful lysosomes (very small bodies that hold cellular digestive enzymes); release chemicals that destroy invading organisms and also attack other WBCs	Stabilize cell membranes so that inflammation-causing substances are not released
Eosinophils (2%-5%)	Function mainly in allergic reactions and protect against parasitic infections; ingest inflammatory chemicals and antigen-antibody complexes	Little if any effect
Basophils (0.5%-1%)	Contain histamine, an inflammation-causing substance, and heparin, an anticoagulant	Stabilize cell membranes so that histamine is not released
Agranulocytes		
Lymphocytes (25%)	Two types: T lymphocytes and B lymphocytes; T cells attack infecting microbial or cancerous cells; B cells produce antibodies against specific antigens	Decrease activity of the lymphocytes
Monocytes (3%-5%)	Produce macrophages, which can migrate out of the bloodstream to such places as mucous membranes, where they are capable of engulfing large bacteria or virus-infected cells	Inhibit macrophage accumulation in already inflamed areas, thus preventing more inflammation

WBC, White blood cell.
*Value in parentheses is the percentage of all leukocytes represented by the given type.

mended therapeutic approach) in which the benefits of this drug therapy arguably outweigh the adverse effects. When a more pronounced antiinflammatory effect is needed, however, as in an acute exacerbation of asthma or other chronic obstructive pulmonary disease, intravenous corticosteroids (e.g., methylprednisolone) are often used.

Contraindications

Drug allergy is the primary contraindication. It should also be emphasized that these drugs are not intended as sole therapy for acute asthma attacks. Inhaled corticosteroids are contraindicated in patients who are hypersensitive to glucocorticoids, in patients whose sputum tests positive for *Candida* organisms, and in patients with systemic fungal infection.

Adverse Effects

The main undesirable local effects of typical doses of inhaled corticosteroids in the respiratory system include pharyngeal irritation, coughing, dry mouth, and oral fungal infections. Patients should be instructed to rinse the mouth after use of an inhaled corticosteroid. Most of the drug effects of inhaled corticosteroids are limited to their topical site of action in the lungs. Because of the chemical structure of these inhaled dosage forms, there is relatively little systemic absorption of the drugs when they are administered by inhalation at normal therapeutic dosages. However, the degree of systemic absorption is more likely to be increased in patients who require higher inhaled dosages. When there is significant systemic absorption, which is most likely with high-dose intravenous or oral administration, corticosteroids can affect any of the organ systems in the body. Some of these systemic drug effects include adrenocortical insufficiency, increased susceptibility to infection, fluid and electrolyte disturbances, endocrine effects, CNS effects (insomnia, nervousness, seizures), and dermatologic and connective tissue effects, including brittle skin, bone loss, and osteoporosis.

One important point to remember pertains to patients who are switched to inhaled corticosteroids after receiving systemic corticosteroids, especially at high dosages for an extended period. Patient deaths have been reported due to adrenal gland failure in such cases when the switch to inhaled corticosteroids is made quickly and the dosage of systemic corticosteroids is not reduced gradually. Prevention of this occurrence requires careful clinical monitoring with slow tapering of systemic drug dosages. The patient dependent on systemic corticosteroids may need up to 1 year of recovery time after discontinuation of systemic therapy. There is evidence that bone growth is suppressed in children and adolescents taking corticosteroids. This suppression is more apparent in children receiving larger systemic (versus inhaled) dosages over longer treatment durations. Growth should be tracked (e.g., with standardized charts), and medications should be reevaluated should growth suppression become evident. In some cases, supplemental growth hormone may be prescribed.

Interactions

Drug interactions are more likely to occur with systemic (versus inhaled) corticosteroids. These drugs may increase serum glucose levels, possibly requiring adjustments in dosages of antidiabetic drugs. Because of interactions related to metabolizing enzymes, they may also raise the blood levels of the immunosuppressants cyclosporine and tacrolimus. Likewise, the antifungal drug itraconazole may reduce clearance of the steroids, whereas phenytoin, phenobarbital, and rifampin may enhance it. There is also greater risk for hypokalemia with concurrent use of potassium-depleting diuretics such as hydrochlorothiazide and furosemide.

Dosages

For recommended dosages of selected corticosteroids, see the Dosages table on p. 575.

DOSAGES

Selected Corticosteroids

Drug (Pregnancy Category)	Pharmacologic Class	Usual Dosage Range	Indications
fluticasone propionate (Flovent, Flonase) (C)	Synthetic glucocorticoid	**Adult and pediatric 12 yr and older** Flovent MDI, 3 strengths available: 88-880 mcg twice daily **Pediatric 4-11 yr** Flovent inhalation powder, 3 strengths available: 50-100 mcg twice daily **Adult and pediatric 12 yr and older** Flovent inhalation powder, 3 strengths available: 100-1000 mcg twice daily	Asthma (prophylaxis and maintenance treatment); seasonal allergic rhinitis
methylprednisolone (Solu-Medrol injection, Medrol tablets) (C)	Synthetic glucocorticoid	Dosage varies as above, but usually 40-125 mg IV, 1-3 times daily, usually tapered down Oral taper: usually from 24 to 2 mg daily	Exacerbations of asthma or COPD

COPD, Chronic obstructive pulmonary disease; *IV,* intravenous; *MDI,* metered-dose inhaler.

■ DRUG PROFILES

fluticasone propionate

Fluticasone is administered intranasally (Flonase) (one inhalation in each nostril daily) and by oral inhalation (Flovent) (usually one inhalation by mouth twice daily). Recently fluticasone became available in a combination formulation with the bronchodilator salmeterol (ADVAIR Diskus).

PHARMACOKINETICS

Route	Onset of Action	Peak Plasma Concentration	Elimination Half-life	Duration of Action
Inhalation	Unknown	Unknown	3 hr	Up to 24 hr

methylprednisolone

Methylprednisolone is a systemic corticosteroid available in both oral (Medrol) and injectable (Solu-Medrol) forms.

PHARMACOKINETICS

Route	Onset of Action	Peak Plasma Concentration	Elimination Half-life	Duration of Action
IV	Immediate	30 min	3-4 hr	24-36 hr

MONOCLONAL ANTIBODY ANTIASTHMATIC

Omalizumab (Xolair) is the newest antiasthmatic medication to become available. It is a monoclonal antibody that selectively binds to the immunoglobulin IgE, which in turn limits the release of mediators of the allergic response. Omalizumab is given by injection and has the potential for producing anaphylaxis. Patients receiving omalizumab must be monitored closely for hypersensitivity reactions.

NURSING PROCESS

Assessment

The net drug effect of beta agonists, xanthine derivatives, anticholinergics, LTRAs, and corticosteroids is improved airflow in airway passages and increased oxygen supply. Cautions, contra-

indications, and drug interactions (discussed previously) should be assessed before these drugs are administered. In a thorough assessment of patients receiving any of the respiratory drugs, the patient's skin color, temperature, respiration rate (which should be more than 12 and less than 24 breaths/min), respiration depth and rhythm, breath sounds, blood pressure, and pulse should be monitored as needed. The nurse should also determine if the patient is having problems with cough, dyspnea, orthopnea, or hypoxia, or has other signs or symptoms of respiratory distress. The patient should also be assessed for the presence of any of the following: sternal retractions, cyanosis, restlessness, activity intolerance, cardiac irregularities, palpitations, hypertension, tachycardia, and use of accessory muscles to breathe. The anterior-posterior diameter of the thorax should be determined and pulse oximetry reading noted to determine oxygen saturation levels. The patient should be assessed for a history of allergies, and any specific allergens (e.g., dust, pollen, mold, mildew, nuts, or other foods) should be noted. If a cough is present, its character, frequency, and presence or absence of sputum should be noted. The color of the sputum should also be noted. A complete medication history should be obtained that includes information about prescription and over-the-counter (OTC) drugs, herbal products, alternative therapies, use of nebulizers and/or humidifiers, use of a home air conditioner, and intactness of the heating and air conditioning system. The characteristics of any respiratory symptoms (e.g., seasonally induced, exercise or stress induced) and any family history of respiratory diseases should be noted. Any environmental exposures as well as precipitating and alleviating factors for any respiratory symptoms and/or disease processes should be identified. An excellent resource for the assessment of asthma can be found online at *http://www.asthma.com/asthma_control_test.html.* Smoking habits should also be assessed, because smoking exacerbates respiratory symptoms and nicotine interacts with many respiratory drugs.

Cardiac status may be compromised due to respiratory distress; thus the patient's blood pressure, pulse rate, heart sounds, and electrocardiogram, if ordered, need to be assessed closely. Blood gas analysis may be indicated with attention to the patient's pH, oxygen, carbon dioxide, and serum bicarbonate levels. The nail beds should be assessed for abnormalities (e.g., clubbing, cyanosis), and the area around the lips should be examined for cyanotic changes. Restlessness is often the first sign of hypoxia, so assessing for this as needed is critical, and it should be reported to the prescriber if present. If chest radiographs, scans, or magnetic resonance images have been ordered, the findings should be reviewed. Along with a physical assessment, a psychosocial and emotional assessment is needed, because anxiety, stress, and fear may only further compromise the patient's respiratory status and oxygen levels. The nurse should be sure to note the age of the patient, because drug sensitivity is increased in elderly and pediatric patients.

For the *beta agonists,* cautions, contraindications, and drug interactions associated with these drugs have been discussed previously, and a general overview of the required respiratory assessment has been provided; however, the need to assess for allergies to the fluorocarbon propellant in inhaled dosage forms should also be emphasized. The patient's intake of caffeine (e.g., chocolate, tea, coffee, candy, and sodas) and use of OTC medications containing caffeine (e.g., appetite suppressants, pain relievers) should be assessed. The intake of caffeine is important to determine, because of its sympathomimetic effects and possible potentiation of adverse effects associated with albuterol and other beta agonists (e.g., tachycardia and hypertension from cardiac stimulation, vascular headache and tremors from CNS stimulation). Educational level and readiness to learn should also be assessed to aid in preparing patient education, such as instructions about the use of MDIs, nebulizers, and other dosage forms.

Respiratory *anticholinergic drugs* and their cautions, contraindications, and drug interactions have been discussed previously. Assessments for patients taking these drugs should include those mentioned earlier as well as assessment for any history of GI disorders, heart palpitations, benign prostatic hyperplasia (because of drug-induced urinary retention), or glaucoma (because of drug-induced increase in intraocular pressure). Patients with an allergy to soy lecithin, peanut oils, peanuts, soybeans, or other legumes have shown a higher risk of allergy to the anticholinergics, and the patient should be assessed for such allergies before these drugs are given. Ipratropium and its aerosol forms have been associated with bronchospasms, and thus the patient should be assessed for any preexisting problems with the use of MDIs. If a combination product containing both ipratropium and albuterol is prescribed, the patient needs assessment appropriate to the use of both of these drugs.

Assessment for patients prescribed *xanthine derivatives* (e.g., theophylline) should include identification of any contraindications, cautions, and drug interactions (see previous discussion). Cardiovascular and CNS stimulation may occur with these drugs, thus careful cardiac and neurologic assessment is required. GI reflux may also occur with these drugs, so an assessment for bowel patterns and preexisting disease, such as gastroesophageal reflux and/or ulcers, is also important. Results of renal and liver function tests should also be assessed if these are ordered. Baseline urinary patterns must be assessed due to possible transient urinary frequency. A dietary assessment should include questions about consumption of a low-carbohydrate, high-protein diet and intake of charcoal-broiled meat. These dietary practices may lead

---

> **LIFE SPAN CONSIDERATIONS: The Elderly Patient**
>
> ### Xanthine Derivatives
>
> - Xanthine derivatives should be administered cautiously with careful monitoring in the elderly because sensitivity to these drugs is increased in this patient population due to decreased drug metabolism.
> - Elderly patients should be assessed for signs and symptoms of xanthine toxicity, which include nausea, vomiting, restlessness, insomnia, irritability, and tremors. Discriminating the cause of restlessness (e.g., hypoxia versus drug toxicity) is important to patient safety.
> - Elderly patients should never chew or crush sustained-released dosage forms and remain aware of drug interactions, especially interactions with other asthma-related drugs/bronchodilators. Advise the elderly to avoid omitting and/or doubling up on doses. If a dose is missed, the prescriber should be contacted for further instructions.
> - Monitoring of serum levels during follow-up visits is important to avoid possible toxicity and ensure therapeutic blood levels.
> - Lower dosages may be necessary initially in the elderly, not only because of their increased sensitivity to the drug but also because of the possibility of decreased liver and renal functioning. Close monitoring for adverse effects and toxicity should be part of everyday therapy, and palpitations and increased blood pressure (from cardiovascular and central nervous system stimulation) should be noted and reported.

---

to increased theophylline elimination and possibly decreased therapeutic levels of the drugs, whereas a high-carbohydrate, low-protein diet may decrease excretion of the drug and lead to theophylline toxicity. Caffeine-containing foods, beverages, prescription drugs, OTC drugs, and herbals should be noted because of possible cardiovascular and CNS stimulation. It is important to remember that many OTC and prescription antimigraine preparations contain caffeine.

With *corticosteroids* (also known as *glucocorticoids*), baseline assessment of vital signs, breath sounds, and heart sounds should be performed. Assessment for underlying adrenal disorders is important because of the adrenal suppression that occurs with the use of these medications. Age should be noted, because corticosteroids may be problematic for the pediatric patient if long-term therapy and/or high dosage amounts are used. The systemic impact on the pediatric patient is suppressed growth (see pharmacology section for further discussion). As with the other drugs in this chapter, awareness of basic information about these drugs, especially their action, is very important for safe use and prevention of medication errors. For example, glucocorticoids are used for their antiinflammatory effects, beta agonists and xanthines for their bronchodilating effects, and anticholinergics for their blockage of cholinergic receptors. Knowing what drugs do and why they are used helps to prevent or decrease medication errors and adverse effects. See Chapter 33 for more information on these antiinflammatory adrenal drugs.

With *LTRAs,* it is important to assess for contraindications, cautions, and drug interactions. Liver functioning should be determined because of specific concerns about the use of these drugs in patients with altered hepatic function. As with other

PREVENTING MEDICATION ERRORS

Oral Ingestion of Capsules for Inhalation Devices

Some inhalation products use capsules and a device that pierces the capsules to allow the powdered medication to be inhaled with a special inhaler. Two products, Foradil Aerolizer (formoterol fumarate inhalation powder) and Spiriva HandiHaler (tiotropium bromide inhalation powder) contain such capsules. Even though these capsules are packaged with inhaler devices, they closely resemble oral capsules. The U.S. Food and Drug Administration (FDA) has received reports that the capsules have been taken orally by patients, which can potentially result in adverse effects. If the capsules are swallowed instead of taken using the inhalation device, the medication's onset of action may be delayed, the efficacy is reduced, and as a result the patient receives inadequate drug delivery. The FDA has taken steps to work with the drug manufacturers to mark the packaging clearly. Nurses need to be certain to instruct patients on the proper use and correct route of administration for these inhaled drugs to prevent their confusion with oral products.

medications, the elderly are more sensitive to these drugs. The type of asthma attack is also important to note, because these drugs are used more for prevention and long-term treatment.

Omalizumab, a *monoclonal antibody antiasthmatic drug*, requires additional assessment of known risks associated with certain malignancies. Taking a thorough nursing history will help identify any of these risks, and the information obtained should be documented.

Nursing Diagnoses

- Impaired gas exchange related to pathophysiologic changes caused by respiratory disease
- Fatigue related to the disease process
- Risk for injury related to bronchospasms caused by the disease and to the adverse effects of various respiratory medications
- Anxiety related to the "unknowns" associated with respiratory disease and to the adverse effects of drug therapy
- Disturbed sensory perception related to the CNS stimulation caused by bronchodilators
- Deficient knowledge related to unfamiliarity with the medication treatment regimen and the disease process
- Risk for ineffective peripheral tissue perfusion related to adverse effects of beta agonists.
- Noncompliance with the medication regimen related to undesirable adverse effects of drug therapy

Planning
Goals

- Patient experiences minimal exacerbations of the disease while compliant with the medication regimen.
- Patient states the importance of rest to recovery.
- Patient is free of self-injury related to the disease or to the adverse effects of the medication.
- Patient remains compliant with the medication regimen and with the nonpharmacologic therapies.
- Patient follows up with health care providers as instructed by the prescriber.

- Patient does not increase or decrease the dosage or stop taking the medication without the approval of the prescriber.
- Patient's respiratory status improves because of compliance with the medication therapy.
- Patient's circulation remains intact and strong during therapy.

Outcome Criteria

- Patient briefly describes the disease process, its signs and symptoms, and the precipitating factors.
- Patient states measures to take to prevent self-injury resulting from the disease or the adverse effects of the medication, such as taking medications as prescribed.
- Patient is well rested, with plans to rest during periods of disease exacerbation.
- Patient states the expected adverse effects of the drug being taken, such as palpitations, nervousness, mood changes, and insomnia.
- Patient contacts the prescriber if increased dyspnea, shortness of breath, increased cough, or fever occurs.
- Patient states the importance of taking the medication as prescribed, the reasons for not increasing or decreasing the dosage of the drug, and the importance of not stopping the drug therapy to prevent complications and exacerbations related to the disease or the adverse effects of medications.
- Patient states situations to report to the prescriber that are indicative of poor perfusion/circulation, such as palpitations, chest pain, swelling of the feet, bluish discoloration of the nail beds and/or lips, and coolness of the extremities.

Implementation

Nursing interventions that apply to patients with respiratory disease processes (e.g., COPD, asthma, other upper and lower respiratory tract disorders) include patient education and an emphasis on compliance and prevention, in addition to the specific actions related to the prescribed drug therapy. Measures to implement to prevent, relieve, or decrease the manifestations of the disease should be emphasized to the patient at all times, and the patient's awareness of specific precipitating and relieving factors should be increased. *Bronchodilators* and other respiratory drugs should be given exactly as prescribed and by the prescribed route (e.g., parenterally, orally, by intermittent positive pressure breathing, or by inhalation). The proper method for administering the inhaled forms of these drugs should be demonstrated to the patient, who should provide a return demonstration. The patient should also be strongly discouraged from taking more than the prescribed dose of the *beta agonists, xanthines, and other respiratory drugs* because of the excessive cardiac demands related to adverse effects of cardiac and CNS stimulation (hypertension and tachycardia) that may occur. The use of MDIs requires coordination to inhale the medication correctly and to obtain approximately 10% of drug delivery to the lungs. If a second puff of the same drug is ordered, wait 1 to 2 minutes between puffs. If a second type of inhaled drug is ordered, wait 2 to 5 minutes between the medications, or take as prescribed. Use of a spacer may be indicated to increase the amount of drug delivered. See the Legal and Ethical Principles box for information concerning the environmental hazards associated with MDIs. Dry powder inhalers are small hand-held devices that deliver a specific amount of dry micronized power with each inhaled breath. Their use does not require the same degree of coordination as do MDIs, they deliver about 20% of the drug to the lung, and they have no propellants and as such do not pose problems for the environment. One to two minutes should also be allowed between each puff. A nebulizer dosage form delivers small amounts of misted droplets of the drug to the lungs through a small mouthpiece or mask. Although a nebulizer may take a longer time to deliver the drug to the lungs than the inhalers, the nebulizer dosage form may be more effective for some patients. See Chapter 10 for more information.

Beta agonists should be taken exactly as prescribed. Overdosage may be life-threatening, and so the patient must receive adequate education that emphasizes the need for the proper dosage and frequency. Oral sustained-released tablets should not be crushed or chewed and should be taken with food to decrease GI upset. Instructions for inhaled dosage forms are presented in Patient Teaching Tips. Before, during, and after therapy with these drugs, it is important to reassess the respiratory status and breath sounds. *Anticholinergic drugs* used for respiratory diseases (e.g., ipratropium), should be taken daily as ordered and with appropriate use of the MDI. See Patient Teaching Tips for more information on the administration of these drugs. It is important to wait from 1 to 2 minutes (or as prescribed) before inhaling the second dose of the drug to allow for maximal lung penetration. Exact instructions should be included in the prescriber's order for the medication and may vary. Rinsing the mouth with water immediately after use of any inhaled or nebulized drug may help to prevent mucosal irritation and dryness.

Xanthine derivatives should also be given exactly as prescribed. If they are to be administered parenterally, the nurse should always determine the correct diluent and rate of administration. Intravenous infusion pumps should be used to ensure dosage accuracy and help prevent toxicity. Too rapid an infusion may lead to profound hypotension with possible syncope, tachycardia, seizures, and even cardiac arrest. To prevent a sudden increase in drug release and irritating effects on the gastric mucosa, timed-release preparations should not be crushed or chewed. Oral forms should be taken with food to decrease GI upset. Suppository forms of the drug should be refrigerated, and patients should notify the prescriber if rectal burning, itching, or irritation occurs. The patient should continue to be monitored for respiratory status and improvement in baseline condition during drug therapy.

Inhaled *corticosteroids* (glucocorticoids) should also be used exactly as prescribed, and the patient should be cautioned about overuse. The medication should be taken as ordered every day, regardless of whether the patient is feeling better or not. Often these drugs (e.g., flunisolide) are used as maintenance drugs and are taken twice daily for maximal response. An inhaled $beta_2$ agonist may be used before the inhaled corticosteroid to provide bronchodilation before administration of the antiinflammatory drug. The bronchodilator inhaled drug is generally taken 2 to 5 minutes (or as ordered) before the corticosteroid aerosol. All equipment (inhalers or nebulizers) should be kept clean, with filters cleaned and changed (nebulizers), and maintained in good working condition. Use of a spacer may be indicated, especially if success with inhalation is limited. Rinsing of the mouth immediately after use of the inhaler or nebulizer dosage forms of corticosteroids is recommended to help prevent overgrowth of oral fungi and subsequent development of oral candidiasis

LEGAL AND ETHICAL PRINCIPLES

Chlorofluorocarbons and the Environment

The U.S. Food and Drug Administration (FDA) issued a final rule on albuterol metered-dose inhalers (MDIs) that use chlorofluorocarbon (CFC) propellants and their effect on the environment. The concern was that the CFCs that propel the medicine into the lungs via the inhaler harm the ozone layer. Under the FDA final rule, which was published in the March 31, 2005, issue of the *Federal Register* and reported in a talk paper released on the same date, these inhalers were no longer to be produced, marketed, or sold in the United States after December 31, 2008. The Department of Health and Human Services (DHHS) said that sufficient supplies of two FDA-approved and environmentally friendly albuterol inhalers would be available by that date. This would allow a phasing out of other similar inhalers that are not environmentally friendly. The FDA and DHHS are encouraged that drug manufacturers are proactively implementing programs to help patients afford the the non-CFC albuterol MDIs, which are more expensive than the CFC devices. CFC-containing MDIs used to treat respiratory diseases were previously exempted from a general ban on CFC production and importation under an international agreement established through the Montreal Protocol on Substances that Deplete the Ozone Layer and the U.S. Clean Air Act. The FDA final rule also created the basis for the phase-out of CFC-containing albuterol products by withdrawing their "essential use" status as of December 31, 2008.

In January 2006, the FDA also recommended a ban on some of the nonprescription inhalers containing propellants that are known to harm the ozone layer. An FDA advisory panel voted to support the removal of essential use status for these over-the-counter inhalers (e.g., Primatene Mist), and the agency may opt to begin a rule-making process that would include public comment. The American Lung Association agreed with the recommendations of the FDA. The association also expressed concern for the many individuals who use over-the-counter asthma inhalers because they lack insurance that covers prescription drug costs or have no medical insurance at all. This concern echoes the need for adequate access to health care by all Americans.

Modified from U.S. Food and Drug Administration: FDA talk paper: FDA publishes final rule on chlorofluorocarbons in metered dose inhalers, March 31, 2005, available at *http://www.fda.gov/cder/mdi/default.htm;* further information may be obtained at *http://www.WebMD.com* and 888-INFO-FDA; Edelman NH, American Lung Association: Statement on FDA's recommendation to ban CFC inhalers, January 25, 2006, available at *http://www.lungusa.org.*

(thrush). Pediatric patients may need a prescriber's order to have these medications on hand at school and during athletic events or physical education. Peak flow meter use is also encouraged to help patients of all ages better regulate their disease. Journaling to record peak flow levels, signs and symptoms of the disease, any improvement, and any adverse effects associated with therapy may be helpful. For pediatric patients, use of systemic forms of corticosteroids is a concern. Specifically, in children the use of systemic forms of these drugs may lead to suppression of the hypothalamic-pituitary-adrenal axis and subsequent growth stunting. However, the benefits are considerable when compared to the risks. Inhaled forms are often combined with short-term systemic therapy in pediatric patients. The nurse should continue to monitor the patient's condition during therapy with a focus on the respiratory, cardiac, and central nervous systems.

The *LTRAs,* specifically zileuton, montelukast, and zafirlukast, are given orally. Of most concern are the montelukast chewable tablets, which contain aspartame and approximately 0.842 mg of phenylamine per 5-mg tablet. Some patients may need to avoid these substances. Patient education should also emphasize that these drugs are indicated for treatment of chronic, not acute, asthma. These drugs should be taken as ordered and on a continuous schedule, even if symptoms improve. Fluid intake should increase, as with all the respiratory drugs, to help decrease the viscosity of secretions.

The *monoclonal antibody antiasthmatic drug* omalizumab should be taken exactly as ordered. It is given as a subcutaneous injection and requires either instruction in self-injection or frequent visits to the prescriber, nurse, or other health care provider to receive the injection. This drug is usually given every 2 to 4 weeks. Omalizumab is not indicated for acute asthma attacks and it may be used in conjunction with other acute-acting asthma medications.

Evaluation

The therapeutic effects of any of the drugs used to improve the control of acute or chronic respiratory diseases and to treat or help prevent respiratory symptoms including the following: a decrease in dyspnea, wheezing, restlessness, and anxiety; improved respiratory patterns with return to normal rate and quality; improved activity tolerance and arterial blood gas levels; improved quality of life; and decreased severity and incidence of respiratory symptoms. The therapeutic effects of bronchodilators (e.g., xanthines, beta agonists) include decreased symptoms and increased ease of breathing. Blood levels of theophylline should be between 5 and 15 mcg/mL and should be frequently monitored. Peak flow meters are easy to use and help reveal early decreases in peak flow caused by bronchospasms. They also aid in monitoring treatment effectiveness. Other respiratory drugs should produce the therapeutic effects related to the specific drug. Adverse effects for which to monitor during therapy include the following: *beta agonists* and *anticholinergics*—nausea, vomiting, anorexia, urinary retention, and increased intraocular pressure; *xanthenes*—nausea, vomiting, anorexia, dyspepsia, and cardiac and CNS stimulation; *corticosteroids*—adrenocortical insufficiency, increased susceptibility to infection, fluid and electrolyte disturbances, endocrine effects, insomnia, nervousness, seizures, and dermatologic and connective tissue effects, including brittle skin, bone loss, and osteoporosis; *LTRAs*—dyspepsia, headaches, nausea, dizziness, and insomnia; *monoclonal antibody antiasthmatic drugs*—fatigue, joint pain, and pain, swelling, redness, and/or increased warmth at the injection site.

PATIENT TEACHING TIPS

Beta Agonists
- Educate about maintaining healthy living habits (e.g., regular health checkups, forcing fluids, eating three balanced meals daily, engaging in consistent exercise as tolerated and as ordered).
- Instruct about any potential drug interactions.
- Patients with asthma, bronchitis, or COPD, should be encouraged to avoid precipitating events such as exposure to conditions or situations that may lead to bronchoconstriction and/or worsening of the disorder (e.g., allergens, stress, smoking, and/or air pollutants).
- Instructions should be given about the proper use and care of MDIs, dry powder inhalers, and other such devices. (For example, 1 to 2 minutes [or as ordered] should lapse before a second puff.) See Chapter 10 for more specific information.

Xanthines
- Educate about the interaction between smoking and xanthines, e.g., smoking decreases the blood concentrations of aminophylline and theophylline. Xanthines also interact with charcoal-broiled foods causing decreased serum xanthine drugs.
- Instruct patient about food and beverage items that contain caffeine (e.g., chocolate, coffee, cola, cocoa, tea), because their consumption can exacerbate CNS stimulation.
- Encourage the patient that he or she needs to take medications around the clock to maintain steady-state drug levels. Extended-released dosage forms and other oral dosage forms should not be crushed or chewed. Any worsening of adverse effects, such as epigastric pain, nausea, vomiting, tremors, and headache should be reported immediately.

- The patient should be encouraged to keep follow-up appointments because of their importance in monitoring therapeutic levels of medications and therapeutic effectiveness.

Anticholinergics
- The patient should be educated that ipratropium is used prophylactically to decrease the frequency and severity of asthma and must be taken as ordered and generally year round for therapeutic effectiveness. This drug should not be given if there is an existing allergy to soybeans, peanuts, or other legumes.
- Forcing fluids should be encouraged, unless contraindicated, to decrease the viscosity of secretions and increase the expectoration of sputum.
- When inhaled forms of these drugs (and other respiratory drugs) are used, the patient should be instructed to take the prescribed number of puffs of the inhaler and no more than two puffs with one dosing or as ordered. The patient should be educated about how to properly use an MDI with or without a spacer, how to use a dry powder inhaler, and how to properly clean and store the equipment (see Chapter 10). Patients should wait 2 to 5 minutes (or as prescribed) before the use of additional, different inhaled medications.

Corticosteroids (Glucocorticoids)
- In addition to adhering to the specified dose and frequency of these drugs, if inhaled forms are used, the patient should practice good oral hygiene (e.g., rinsing of the mouth) after the last inhalation. Rinsing the mouth with water is appropriate and necessary to prevent oral fungal infections. The patient should be

Continued

PATIENT TEACHING TIPS—cont'd

given instructions about keeping the inhaler clean, including weekly removing the canister from the plastic casing and washing the casing in warm, soapy water. Once the casing is dry, the canister and mouthpiece may be put back together and the cap applied. The glucocorticoid may predispose patient to oral fungal overgrowth; thus the need for implicit instructions for cleaning of inhaled devices.

- Instruct patient to keep track of the doses left in the MDI as follows: The number of doses in the canister should be noted and the number of days the doses will last should be calculated. For example, assume that two puffs are taken four times a day, and the inhaler has a capacity of 200 inhalations. Two puffs four times a day equals eight inhalations per day. Eight divided into 200 yields 25; that is, the inhaler will last approximately 25 days. The MDI should be marked with the date it will be empty and a refill obtained a few days before that date. Note that using extra doses will alter the refill date. Expiration dates should always be checked.
- Journaling is important and include notation of how the patient feels, medications being taken, adverse effects, and precipitators/alleviators/symptoms of the asthma/illness.
- A medical alert bracelet or necklace should be worn at all times and medical card with the diagnoses and list of medications and allergies kept on the person at all times. Emergency contact persons and phone numbers should also be listed.
- With intranasal dosage forms, nasal passages should be cleared before administration. The head should be tilted slightly forward and the spray tip inserted into one nostril and pointed toward the inflamed nasal turbinates. The medication should be pumped into the nasal passage as the patient sniffs inward while holding the other nostril closed. This procedure should then be repeated in the other nostril. Any unused portion should be discarded after 3 months or by the expiration date.

- Educate about the fact that excess levels of systemic corticosteroids may lead to Cushing's syndrome with symptoms such as moon face, acne, an increase in fat pads, and swelling. Although use of inhaled forms helps to minimize this problem, education about it remains important to patient safety. As noted previously, the risk of occurrence of these signs and symptoms is higher when these drugs are given systemically (e.g., oral or parenteral dosage forms).
- Educate about the possibility of Addisonian crisis which may occur if a systemic corticosteroid is abruptly discontinued. These drugs require weaning prior to discontinuation of the medication. Addisonian crisis may be manifested by nausea, shortness of breath, joint pain, weakness, and fatigue and the prescriber should be contacted immediately should these occur.
- Educate about the importance of reporting to the prescriber any weight gain of 2 pounds or more in 24 hours or 5 pounds or more in 1 week.

Leukotriene Receptor Antagonists

- The patient should be educated about the action and purpose of LTRAs and told that they work differently by preventing leukotriene formation and thus preventing/decreasing inflammation, bronchoconstriction, and mucus production. Emphasize that these drugs are indicated for prevention, not treatment, of acute asthmatic attacks.

Monoclonal Antibody Antiasthmatic Drugs

- Omalizumab is used for the treatment of moderate to severe asthma and not for aborting acute asthma attacks. The patient should provide return demonstrations of subcutaneous injection techniques. The patient should be instructed to keep medications and needles, syringes, and other equipment out of the reach of children and to use puncture-proof needle waste containers. Each needle is used for only one injection.

POINTS TO REMEMBER

- The beta agonists stimulate beta$_1$ and beta$_2$ receptors. The beta$_2$ agonists are the most specific for the lungs.
- Xanthines such as theophylline help to relax the smooth muscles of the bronchioles by inhibiting phosphodiesterase. Phosphodiesterase breaks down cAMP, which is needed to relax smooth muscles.
- Anticholinergic drugs are used for maintenance and not for relief of acute bronchospasms and work by blocking the bronchoconstrictive effects of ACh.

- Corticosteroids (e.g., beclomethasone, dexamethasone, flunisolide, triamcinolone) have many indications and work by stabilizing the membranes of cells that release harmful bronchoconstricting substances.
- The LTRAs, such as zileuton and zafirlukast, are given orally. Adverse effects include headache, dizziness, insomnia, and dyspepsia.
- Omalizumab, a monoclonal antibody antiasthmatic drug, works by preventing the release of mediators that lead to allergic responses. It is given for preventative purposes.

NCLEX EXAMINATION REVIEW QUESTIONS

1 A patient who has a history of asthma is experiencing an acute episode of shortness of breath and needs to take a medication for immediate relief. Which medication will the nurse choose for this situation?

a A beta agonist, such as albuterol

b An antileukotriene, such as montelukast

c A corticosteroid, such as fluticasone

d An anticholinergic, such as ipratropium

2 After a nebulizer treatment with the beta agonist albuterol, the patient complains of feeling a little "shaky," with slight tremors of the hands. His heart rate is 98 beats/min, increased from the pretreatment rate of 88 beats/min. The nurse knows that this reaction is an

a expected adverse effect of the medication.

b allergic reaction to the medication.

c indication that he has received an overdose of the medication.

d idiosyncratic reaction to the medication.

3 A patient has been receiving an aminophylline (xanthine derivative) infusion for 24 hours. The nurse will expect to see which adverse effect when assessing the patient during the infusion?

a CNS depression

b Sinus tachycardia

c Increased appetite

d Temporary urinary retention

4 During a teaching session for a patient who will be receiving a new prescription for the LTRA montelukast (Singulair), the nurse should tell the patient that the drug has which therapeutic effect?

a Improves the respiratory drive

b Loosens and removes thickened secretions

c Reduces inflammation in the airway

d Stimulates immediate bronchodilation

5 After the patient takes a dose of an inhaled corticosteroid, such as fluticasone, what is the most important action the patient should do next?

a Hold the breath for 60 seconds

b Rinse out the mouth with water

c Follow the corticosteroid with a bronchodilator inhaler, if ordered

d Repeat the dose in 15 minutes if the patient feels short of breath

6 A patient has been given an MDI of albuterol and is instructed to take two puffs three times a day, with doses 6 hours apart. The inhaler contains 200 actuations. Calculate how many days the inhaler will deliver this ordered dose.

1. a, 2. a, 3. b, 4. c, 5. b, 6. approximately 33 days (6 puffs per day divided into 200).

CRITICAL THINKING ACTIVITIES: BEST ACTION

1 A patient is taking a xanthine derivative and asks the nurse about drinking coffee with the medication. What would be the nurse's best answer?

2 A patient has a new prescription for an LTRA. He asks the nurse, "So, will this new medicine help me when I have an asthma attack?" What would be the nurse's best answer?

3 A 13-year-old is taken to the school clinic because he started to have an asthma attack while running outside in the cold air. The school nurse has two inhalers on file for him: fluticasone and albuterol. Which inhaler is the best choice at this time? Explain.

For answers, see *http://evolve.elsevier.com/Lilley.*

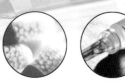

PART 7

Antiinfective and Antiinflammatory Drugs

STUDY SKILLS TIPS

Nursing Process • Assessment
Nursing Diagnoses • Evaluation

NURSING PROCESS

This study model focuses on the Nursing Process section in Chapter 38. Since there is a Nursing Process section at the end of each chapter, the discussion of the example in Chapter 38 is applicable to all chapters.

ASSESSMENT

What is the purpose of this section? Each time you begin to read the Nursing Process section of a chapter, you need to ask this question. What are you supposed to learn? What are you supposed to know? What are you supposed to be able to do? All these questions relate to your role as a nurse. Consider the following sentence from this section in Chapter 38.

> In general, <u>before the administration of any antibiotic</u>, it is <u>crucial to gather data regarding a history of or symptoms indicative of hypersensitivity or allergic reactions (from mild reactions with rash, pruritus, or hives to severe reactions with laryngeal edema, bronchospasms, hypotension, and possible cardiac arrest).</u>

Assessment clearly has to do with patient care. You are assessing the patient in relation to the pharmacologic interventions that this chapter discusses. Some underlining has been done in this section to bring into sharper focus some of the things that you must be very aware of as you study.

First, notice the use of the word *crucial* in the first line. Something is so important at this point that it cannot be ignored. Immediately the questioning process should be activated. What is crucial? The answer follows immediately in the sentence. You must assess for history of or symptoms indicative of hypersensitivity or allergic reactions. The sentence goes on

to identify the kind of data that should be available, and the sentence makes it clear that these data must be obtained *before the administration* of any drug. Each of the data factors is important, and each relates to other parts and chapters in this text. The next item to notice is hypersensitivities. Some individuals are *allergic* to certain antibiotics. It would be dangerous and possibly fatal, however, to administer an antibiotic to a patient if he or she is *hypersensitive.*

Another data item specifies rash, pruritus, or hives and laryngeal edema, bronchospasms, hypotension, and possible cardiac arrest. As you read this, you should instantly think of the reactions to which they refer. Then you should try to recall information from this chapter that related the specific antibiotics to these reactions. Learning is cumulative. The Nursing Process section assumes you have read and understood what was presented earlier in the chapter.

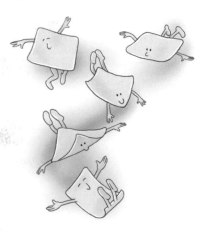

Often you will encounter standard medical abbreviations. As you read on in the Assessment section, you find this sentence:

> Further assessment should include determination of the patient's age, weight, baseline vital sign values with body temperature, and examination of the results of any laboratory tests that have been ordered, such as liver function studies (AST and ALT levels), kidney function studies

(usually blood urea nitrogen and creatinine levels), cardiac function studies (pertinent laboratory tests, electrocardiogram), ultrasonography (if indicated), culture and sensitivity tests, complete blood count (CBC), hemoglobin (Hgb) level and hematocrit (Hct), and platelet and clotting tests.

In earlier Study Skills Tips, it has been suggested that you prepare vocabulary cards for these abbreviations to help you in a situation such as this. You need to know what *AST, ALT, BUN, CBC, Hgb,* and *Hct* mean, what they measure, and how they relate to appropriate and effective administration of antibiotics. If these letters are not meaningful to you, then you will not be able to link what you know about the antibiotics with what you must know about administering them as a nurse. Many test questions on nursing examinations use the standard abbreviations, and you must know them instantly and be able to relate them to the situation covered. As you look at antibiotic administration and *CBC, Hgb,* and *Hct,* think what a test question might ask about these data elements in a real application in patient care. This is what the nursing process is all about.

NURSING DIAGNOSES

The same first question applies here as in every other section. What am I supposed to learn? Since the focus is on administration of antibiotics, the expectation you should bring to this is an awareness of your role in diagnosis. What should you look for in working with patients that affects the administration of antibiotics?

This same procedure should be applied to the Planning, Goals, Outcome Criteria, and Implementation sections. Consider what each of these headings suggests about the nursing process, and read and evaluate the information, relating it to what you have already learned. Also consider the implications of the information as possible 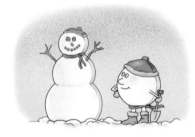 test questions that may ask you to do more than recall specific facts. As an example, consider the following case:

> Patient A, age 23, has a fever of 100.8° F (38.2 ° C). She was admitted yesterday and delivered a healthy infant 8 hours ago. She is breast-feeding the newborn. What antibiotics might be administered for the fever? What specific antibiotics should be used with caution or eliminated from consideration?

This case demonstrates the need to read and think critically. Not only do you need to remember the specific facts from the chapter, but you should also be able to take a case study example and apply those facts to that specific situation.

EVALUATION

Evaluation is the final section under Nursing Process. What are you supposed to evaluate?

> Evaluation should include monitoring of goals, outcome criteria, and therapeutic effects and adverse effects. Therapeutic effects of antibiotics include a decrease in the signs and symptoms of the infection; a return to normal vital signs, including temperature, and negative results on culture and sensitivity tests; normal results for CBC; and improved appetite, energy level, and sense of well-being. Evaluation for adverse effects includes monitoring for specific drug-related adverse effects (see each drug profile).

First you should look for the positive responses (therapeutic effects) set forth in the preceding text sample that indicate the patient is responding favorably to the treatment. However, then you read, "Evaluation for adverse effects includes…." This says that part of your role in evaluation is to monitor the patient for negative responses and be prepared to educate the patient about the effects he or she is experiencing and possible steps to help alleviate the symptoms.

The Nursing Process section in each chapter should be read carefully and thoughtfully, because it is in this section where you begin to see how the complex pharmacologic material presented earlier in the chapter fits into your role as a nurse. This material should be read with the same concern and care that you have given to the highly complex material earlier in the chapter, because this is the section in which you must think about *application* of all you have learned. Your thinking process may be stimulated when you review this section with your study group. Each person brings his or her understanding and experience to the discussion. The insights can be richer and the learning more complete as you exchange ideas. Apply the PURR model with a study group or alone and be an active questioner and reader, and you will be successful in working with the Nursing Process section in each chapter.

CHAPTER 38

Antibiotics Part 1

OBJECTIVES

When you reach the end of this chapter, you should be able to do the following:

1 Discuss the general principles of antibiotic therapy.
2 Explain how antibiotics work to rid the body of infection.
3 Briefly compare the characteristics and uses of antiseptics and disinfectants.
4 List the most commonly used antiseptics and disinfectants.
5 Discuss nursing considerations associated with the use of antiseptics and disinfectants.
6 Discuss the pros and cons of antibiotic use with attention to the overuse or abuse of antibiotics and development of drug resistance.
7 Classify the various antibiotics by general category, including sulfonamides, penicillins, cephalosporins, macrolides, and tetracyclines.
8 Discuss the mechanisms of action, indications, cautions, contraindications, routes of administration, and drug interactions for the sulfonamides, penicillins, cephalosporins, macrolides, and tetracyclines.
9 Identify drug-specific adverse effects and toxic effects of each of the antibiotic classes listed earlier and cite measures to decrease their occurrence.
10 Briefly discuss superinfection, including its etiology and prevention.
11 Develop a nursing care plan that includes all phases of the nursing process for patients receiving drugs in each of the following classes of antibiotic: sulfonamides, penicillins, cephalosporins, macrolides, and tetracyclines.

e-Learning Activities

http://evolve.elsevier.com/Lilley
NCLEX Review Questions • Animations • Nursing Care Plans • Audio Glossary • Category Catchers • Medication Errors Checklists • IV Therapy Checklists • Calculators • Frequently Asked Questions • Content Updates • Supplemental Resources • Answers to Case Studies and Critical Thinking Activities

Drug Profiles

◆ amoxicillin, p. 594
   ampicillin, p. 594
◆ azithromycin and clarithromycin, p. 600
   aztreonam, p. 598
◆ cefazolin, p. 595
   cefepime, p. 597
◆ cefoxitin, p. 596
   ceftazidime, p. 597
◆ ceftriaxone, p. 597
   cefuroxime, p. 596

◆ cephalexin, p. 595
   demeclocycline, p. 601
◆ doxycycline, p. 601
◆ erythromycin, p. 599
◆ imipenem/cilastatin, p. 597
   nafcillin, p. 593
◆ penicillin G and penicillin V potassium, p. 592
   sulfamethoxazole/trimethoprim (co-trimoxazole), p. 590
   tigecycline, p. 601

◆ *Key drug.*

Glossary

Antibiotic Having or pertaining to the ability to destroy or interfere with the development of a living organism. The term is used most commonly to refer to antibacterial drugs. (p. 585)
Antiseptic One of two types of *topical antimicrobial agent;* a chemical that inhibits the growth and reproduction of microorganisms without necessarily killing them. Antiseptics are also called *static agents.* (p. 586)
Bactericidal antibiotics Antibiotics that kill bacteria. (p. 591)
Bacteriostatic antibiotics Antibiotics that do not actually kill bacteria but rather inhibit their growth. (p. 589)
Beta-lactam The designation for a broad, major class of antibiotics that includes four subclasses: penicillins, cephalosporins, carbapenems, and monobactams; so named because of the beta-lactam ring that is part of the chemical structure of all drugs in this class. (p. 590)
Beta-lactamase Any of a group of enzymes produced by bacteria that catalyze the chemical opening of the crucial beta-lactam ring structures in beta-lactam antibiotics. (p. 590)
Beta-lactamase inhibitors Medications combined with certain penicillin drugs to block the effect of beta-lactamase enzymes. (p. 590)
Colonization The establishment and growth of microorganisms on the skin, open wounds, or mucous membranes, or in secretions without causing adverse clinical signs or symptoms. (p. 586)
Community-associated infection An infection that is acquired by persons who have not been hospitalized or had a medical procedure recently (within the past year). (p. 586)
Definitive therapy The administration of antibiotics based on known results of culture and sensitivity testing identifying the pathogen causing infection. (p. 587)

584

Disinfectant One of two types of *topical antimicrobial agent;* a chemical applied to nonliving objects to kill microorganisms. Also called *cidal agents.* (p. 586)

Empiric therapy The administration of antibiotics based on the practitioner's judgment of the pathogens most likely to be causing an apparent infection; it involves the presumptive treatment of an infection to avoid treatment delay before specific culture information has been obtained. (p. 587)

Glucose-6-phosphate dehydrogenase (G6PD) deficiency An inherited disorder in which the red blood cells are partially or completely deficient in glucose-6-phosphate dehydrogenase, a critical enzyme in the metabolism of glucose. Certain medications can cause hemolytic anemia in patients with this disorder. This is an example of a *host factor* related to drug therapy. (p. 588)

Health care–associated infection An infection that is acquired during the course of receiving treatment for another condition in a health care facility. The infection is not present or incubating at the time of admission. (p. 586)

Host factors Factors that are unique to the body of a particular patient that affect the patient's susceptibility to infection and response to various antibiotic drugs. (p. 588)

Infections Invasions and multiplications of microorganisms in body tissues. (p. 585)

Microorganisms Microscopic living organisms (also called *microbes*). (p. 585)

Prophylactic antibiotic therapy Antibiotics taken before anticipated exposure to an infectious organism in an effort to prevent the development of infection. (p. 587)

Pseudomembranous colitis A necrotizing inflammatory bowel condition that is often associated with antibiotic therapy. A more general term that is also used is *antibiotic-associated colitis.* (p. 587)

Slow acetylation A common genetic host factor in which the rate of metabolism of certain drugs is reduced. (p. 588)

Subtherapeutic Referring to antibiotic treatment that is ineffective in treating a given infection. Possible causes include inappropriate drug therapy, insufficient drug dosing, and bacterial drug resistance. (p. 587)

Superinfection (1) An infection occurring during antimicrobial treatment for another infection, resulting from overgrowth of an organism not susceptible to the antibiotic used. (2) A secondary microbial infection that occurs in addition to an earlier primary infection, often due to weakening of the patient's immune system function by the first infection. (p. 587)

Teratogens Substances that can interfere with normal prenatal development and cause one or more developmental abnormalities in the fetus. (p. 588)

Therapeutic Referring to antibiotic therapy that results in sufficient concentrations of the drug in the blood or other tissues to render it effective against specific bacterial pathogens. (p. 587)

• • •

Anatomy, Physiology, and Disease Overview

MICROBIAL INFECTION

A person is normally able to remain healthy and resistant to infectious **microorganisms** because of the existence of certain host defenses. These defenses take various forms, including actual physical barriers such as intact skin or the ciliated respiratory mucosa, or physiologic defenses such as the gastric acid in the stomach and immune factors such as antibodies. Other defenses are the phagocytic cells (macrophages and polymorphonuclear neutrophils) that are part of the reticuloendothelial system.

Microorganisms are everywhere in both the external environment and many parts of the internal environment of our bodies. They can be harmful to humans or they can be beneficial under normal circumstances but become harmful when conditions are altered in some way. Every known major class of microbes contains organisms that can infect humans. This includes bacteria, viruses, fungi, and protozoans. The focus of this chapter is common bacterial **infections.**

Recall from microbiology that bacteria may take a number of different shapes. This property of bacteria is called their *morphology* (Figure 38-1), and they are often group based on this property. Bacteria may also be grouped according to other common recognizable characteristics. One of the most important ways of categorizing different bacteria is on the basis of their response to the *Gram stain* procedure. Bacterial species that stain purple with Gram staining are classified as gram-positive organisms. Bacteria that stain red are classified as gram-negative organisms. This seemingly simple difference proves to be very significant in guiding the choice of **antibiotic** therapy.

Gram-positive organisms have very thick cell wall, known as peptidoglycan, and they also have a thick outer capsule. Gram-negative organisms have a cell wall structure that is more complex, with a smaller outer capsule and peptidoglycan layer and two cell membranes: an outer and an inner membrane (Figure 38-2). These differences usually make gram-negative bacterial infections more difficult to treat, because the drug molecules have a harder time penetrating the more complex cell walls of gram-negative organisms.

When a person's normal host defenses are somehow compromised, that person becomes susceptible to infection. The microorganisms invade and multiply in the body tissues, and if the infective process overwhelms the body's own defense system, the infection becomes clinically apparent. The patient then usually manifests some of the following classic signs and symptoms of infection: fever, chills, sweats, redness, pain and swelling, fatigue, weight loss, increased white blood cell (WBC) count, and the formation of pus. Not all patients will exhibit signs of the infection. This is especially true in elderly and immunocompromised patients.

To help the body and its normal host defenses combat an infection, antibiotic therapy is often required. Antibiotics are most effective when their actions are combined with functioning bodily defense mechanisms. Often patients will become colo-

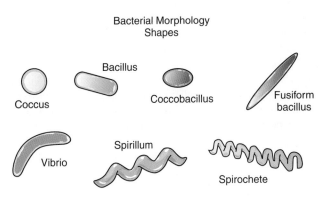

Bacterial Morphology Shapes

Coccus   Bacillus   Coccobacillus   Fusiform bacillus

Vibrio   Spirillum   Spirochete

FIGURE 38-1 General morphology of bacteria. (From Murray PR et al: *Medical microbiology,* ed 6, St Louis, 2009, Mosby.)

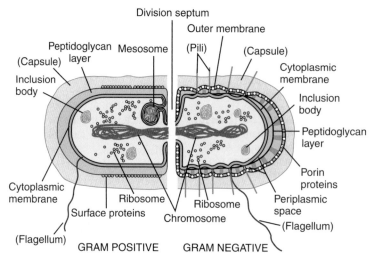

FIGURE 38-2 Gram-positive and gram-negative bacteria. A gram-positive bacterium has a thick layer of peptidoglycan *(left)*. A gram-negative bacterium has a thin peptidoglycan layer and an outer membrane *(right)*. Structures in parentheses are not found in all bacteria. (From Murray PR et al: *Medical microbiology,* ed 6, St Louis, 2009, Mosby.)

nized with bacteria. Although bacteria are present in open wounds, in secretions, on mucous membranes, or on the skin, these patients do not have any overt signs of infection. **Colonization** does not require antibiotic treatment. However, it is not uncommon for these colonizations to be treated, which can cause problems with the development of resistant organisms.

A **community-associated infection** is defined as an infection that is acquired by a person who has not recently (within the past year) been hospitalized or had a medical procedure (such as dialysis, surgery, catheterization). A **health care–associated infection,** previously known as a *nosocomial infection,* is defined as an infection that a patient acquires during the course of receiving treatment for another condition in a health care facility. The infection was not present or incubating at the time of admission. Heath care–associated infections are one of the top ten leading causes of death in the United States. They tend to be more difficult to treat, primarily because the causative microorganisms have been exposed to strong antibiotics in the past and are the most drug resistant and the most virulent. The particular organisms that cause hospital-associated infections have changed over time, with methicillin-resistant *Staphylococcus aureus* (MRSA) now being the most common. Other serious pathogens include *Enterococcus, Klebsiella, Acinetobacter,* and *Pseudomonas aeruginosa.* Most of these microorganisms are now resistant to many of the commonly used antibiotics.

Health care–associated infections develop in approximately 10% of hospitalized patients, and the cost of treating these infections amounts to $4 to $11 billion annually. Most of these infections (70% or more) are either urinary tract infections (UTIs) or postoperative wound infections. Often they are acquired from various devices, such as mechanical ventilators, intravenous (IV) infusion lines, catheters, and dialysis equipment. Areas of the hospital where the risk for acquiring a hospital-associated infection is particularly high are the critical care, dialysis, oncology, transplant, and burn units. This is because the host defenses of the patients in these areas are typically compromised, which makes them more vulnerable to infection. Over 70% of hospital-

TABLE 38-1 Antiseptics Versus Disinfectants

	Antiseptics	Disinfectants
Where used	Living tissue	Nonliving objects
Toxic?	No	Yes
Potency	Lower	Higher
Activity against organisms	Primarily inhibits growth (bacteriostatic)	Kills (bactericidal)

associated infections are preventable. The most common mode of transmitting hospital-associated infections is by direct contact. The most important thing health care professionals can do to prevent the spread of these potentially deadly infections is to wash their hands. In fact, the Joint Commission has made the prevention of infection a primary focus, and it is a 2009 national patient safety goal.

Other methods of reducing hospital-associated infections include the use of disinfectants and antiseptics. A **disinfectant** is able to kill organisms and is used only on nonliving objects to destroy organisms that may be present on them. Disinfectants are sometimes called *cidal agents.* An **antiseptic** generally only inhibits the growth of microorganisms but does not necessarily kill them and is applied exclusively to living tissue. Antiseptics are also called *static agents.* The differences between disinfectants and antiseptics in a clinical sense are summarized in Table 38-1. Topical antimicrobial drugs are discussed further in Chapter 56.

Pharmacology Overview

The selection of antimicrobial drugs requires clinical judgment and detailed knowledge of pharmacologic and microbiologic factors. Antibiotics have three general uses: empiric therapy, definitive therapy, and prophylactic or preventative therapy. Antibiotic drug therapy should begin with a clinical assessment of the patient to determine whether he or she has the common signs and symptoms of infection previously mentioned. The patient should also be assessed during and after antibiotic therapy to evaluate the effectiveness of the drug therapy, monitor for adverse drug effects, and make sure the infection is not recurring.

Often the signs and symptoms of an infection appear long before a causative organism can be identified. When this happens and the risk of life-threatening or severe complications is high (e.g., suspected acute meningitis), an antibiotic is given to the patient immediately. The antibiotic selected is one that can best kill the microorganisms known to be the most common causes of the infection. This is called **empiric therapy.** Before the start of empiric antibiotic therapy, specimens should be obtained from suspected areas of infection to be cultured in an attempt to identify a causative organism. It must be emphasized that culture specimens should be obtained before drug therapy is initiated whenever possible. Otherwise, the presence of antibiotics in the tissues may result in misleading culture results. However, sometimes it is not possible to obtain a sample (especially sputum) in a reasonable amount of time, and antibiotic therapy should be begun without a sample in that situation. If an organism is identified in the laboratory, it is then tested for susceptibility to various antibiotics. The results of these tests can confirm whether the empiric therapy chosen is appropriate for eradicating the organism identified. If not, therapy can be adjusted to optimize its efficacy against the specific infectious organism(s). Once the results of culture and sensitivity testing are available (usually in 48 to 72 hours), the antibiotic therapy is then tailored to treat the identified organism by using the most narrow-spectrum, least toxic drug based on sensitivity results. This is known as **definitive therapy.** Broad-spectrum antibiotics are those that are active against numerous organisms (gram positive, gram negative, and anaerobic). Narrow-spectrum antibiotics are effective against only a few organisms. Once the results of culture and sensitivity testing are available, it is always better to use an antibiotic that targets the specific organism identified (i.e., a narrow-spectrum antibiotic). Overuse of broad-spectrum antibiotics contributes to resistance. It should always be the goal of therapy to use the most narrow-spectrum drug when possible based on sensitivity results.

Antibiotics are also given for prophylaxis. This is often the case, for example, when patients are scheduled to undergo a procedure (i.e., surgery) in which the likelihood of dangerous microbial contamination is high during or after the procedure. **Prophylactic antibiotic therapy** is used to prevent an infection. The risk of infection varies depending on the procedure being performed. For example, the risk of infection in a patient undergoing coronary artery bypass surgery (with standard preoperative cleansing of the body) is relatively low compared with that in a person undergoing intraabdominal surgery for the treatment of injuries sustained in a motor vehicle accident. In the latter case, contamination with bacteria from the gastrointestinal (GI) tract is more likely to be present in the abdominal cavity. This would constitute a contaminated or "dirty" surgical field, and therefore the likelihood of clinically serious infection would be much higher. Antibiotic therapy would likely be required for a longer period after the procedure. To be effective, prophylactic antibiotics need to be given before the procedure, generally 30 minutes before to ensure adequate tissue penetration. The Surgical Care Improvement Project (SCIP) is a national performance improvement project that provides hospitals with evidence-based recommendations on the administration of prophylactic antibiotics. More information can be found at *http://www.jointcommission.org/PerformanceMeasurement/PerformanceMeasurement/SCIP.*

To optimize antibiotic therapy, the patient should be continuously monitored for both **therapeutic** efficacy and adverse drug effects. A therapeutic response to antibiotics is one in which there is a decrease in the specific signs and symptoms of infection compared with the baseline findings (e.g., fever, elevated WBC count, redness, inflammation, drainage, pain). Antibiotic therapy is said to be **subtherapeutic** when these signs and symptoms do not improve. This can result from use of an incorrect route of drug administration, inadequate drainage of an abscess, poor drug penetration to the infected area, insufficient serum levels of the drug, or bacterial resistance to the drug. Antibiotic therapy is considered toxic when the serum levels of the antibiotic are too high or when the patient has an allergic or other major adverse reaction to the drug. These reactions include rash, itching, hives, fever, chills, joint pain, difficulty breathing, or wheezing. Relatively minor adverse drug reactions such as GI discomfort and diarrhea are quite common with antibiotic therapy and are usually not severe enough to require drug discontinuation.

Superinfection can occur when antibiotics reduce or completely eliminate the normal bacterial flora, which consists of certain bacteria and fungi that are needed to maintain normal function in various organs. When these bacteria or fungi are killed by antibiotics, other bacteria or fungi are permitted to take over and cause infection. An example of a superinfection caused by antibiotics is the development of a vaginal yeast infection when the normal vaginal bacterial flora is reduced by antibiotic therapy and yeast growth is no longer kept in balance. Antibiotic use is strongly associated with the potential for the development of diarrhea. As noted earlier, antibiotic-associated diarrhea is a common adverse effect of antibiotics. However, it becomes a serious superinfection when it causes antibiotic-associated colitis, also known as **pseudomembranous colitis.** This happens because antibiotics disrupt the normal gut flora and can cause an overgrowth of *Clostridium difficile.* The most common symptom of *C. difficile* colitis is watery diarrhea, abdominal pain, and fever. Whenever a person who was previously treated with antibiotics develops watery diarrhea, the person should be tested for *C. difficile* infection. If the results are positive, the patient will need to be treated for this serious superinfection.

Another type of superinfection occurs when a second infection closely follows the initial primary infection and comes from an external source (as opposed to normal body flora). A common example is a case in which a patient who already has a viral respiratory infection develops a secondary bacterial infection. This is likely due to weakening of the patient's immune system function by the primary viral infection. Although the viral infection will not respond to antibiotic therapy, antibiotics may be needed to treat the secondary bacterial infection. This situation calls for some diagnostic finesse on the part of the prescriber, who should avoid prescribing unnecessary antibiotics for a viral infection. The presence of colored sputum (e.g., green or yellow) may be a sign of a bacterial superinfection during a viral respiratory illness. Patients will often expect to receive an antibiotic prescription even when they show no signs of a bacterial superinfection. From their perspective, they know they are "sick" and want "some medicine" to expedite their recovery from illness. This can create both diagnostic confusion and an emotional dilemma for the prescriber. Over the decades many very treatable bacterial infections have become increasingly resistant to antibiotic therapy. One major cause of this phenomenon is considered to be the overprescribing of antibiotics, often in the clinical situations described earlier. Antibiotic resistance is now considered one of the world's most pressing public health problems. Another factor that contributes to this problem is the tendency of many patients not to complete their antibiotic regimen. Patients should be counseled to take the entire course of prescribed antibiotic drugs, even if they feel that they are no longer ill.

Food-drug and drug-drug interactions are common problems when antibiotics are taken. One of the more common food-drug interactions is that between milk or cheese and tetracycline, which results in decreased GI absorption of tetracycline. An example of a drug-drug interaction is that between quinolone antibiotics and antacids or multivitamins with iron, which leads to decreased absorption of quinolones. This is especially important, as will be discussed later, because quinolone antibiotics are used orally to treat serious infections. If they are not absorbed, treatment failure is likely to ensue.

Other important factors that must be understood to use antibiotics appropriately are host-specific factors, or **host factors.** These are factors that pertain specifically to a given patient, and they can have an important bearing on the success or failure of antibiotic therapy. Some of these host factors are age, allergy history, kidney and liver function, pregnancy status, genetic characteristics, site of infection, and host defenses.

Age-related host factors are those that apply to patients at either end of the age spectrum. For example, infants and children may not be able to take certain antibiotics such as tetracyclines, which affect developing teeth or bones; quinolones, which may affect bone or cartilage development in children; and sulfonamides, which may displace bilirubin from albumin and precipitate kernicterus (hyperbilirubinemia) in neonates. The aging process affects the function of various organ systems. As people age there is a gradual decline in the function of the kidneys and liver, the organs primarily responsible for metabolizing and eliminating antibiotics. Therefore, depending on the level of kidney or liver function of a given older adult, dosage adjustments may be necessary. Pharmacists often play a role in evaluating the dosages of antibiotics and other medications to ensure optimal dosing for a given patient's level of organ function.

A patient history of allergic reaction to an antibiotic plays an important role in the selection of the most appropriate antibiotic for that patient. Penicillins and sulfonamides are two broad classes of antibiotic to which many people have allergic anaphylactic reactions. Symptoms of anaphylaxis include flushing, itching, hives, anxiety, fast irregular pulse, and throat and tongue swelling. The most dangerous such reaction is anaphylactic shock, in which a patient can suffocate from drug-induced respiratory arrest. Although this outcome is the most extreme, the potential for it does underscore the importance of consistently assessing patients for drug allergies and documenting any known allergies clearly in the medical record. All reported drug allergies should be taken seriously and investigated further before a final decision is made about whether to administer a given drug. Many patients will say that they are "allergic" to a medication when in fact what they experienced was a common mild adverse effect such as stomach upset or nausea. Patients who report drug allergies should be asked open-ended questions to elicit descriptions of prior allergic reactions so that the actual severity of the reaction can be assessed. The most common severe reactions to any medication that need to be noted in the patient's chart are any difficulty breathing; significant rash, hives, or other skin reaction; and severe GI intolerance. Although some antibiotics are ideally taken on an empty stomach, eating a small amount of food with the medication may be sufficient to help the patient tolerate it and realize its therapeutic benefits.

Pregnancy-related host factors are also important to the selection of appropriate antibiotics, because several antibiotics can pass through the placenta and cause harm to the developing fetus. Drugs that cause development abnormalities in the fetus are called **teratogens.** Their use by pregnant women can result in birth defects.

Some patients also have certain genetic abnormalities that result in various enzyme deficiencies. These conditions can adversely affect drug actions in the body. Two of the most common examples of such genetic host factors are **glucose-6-phosphate dehydrogenase (G6PD) deficiency** and **slow acetylation.** The administration of antibiotics such as sulfonamides, nitrofurantoin, and dapsone to a person with G6PD deficiency may result in the hemolysis, or destruction, of red blood cells. Patients who are slow acetylators have a physiologic makeup that causes certain drugs to be metabolized more slowly than usual in a chemical step known as *acetylation.* This can lead to toxicity from drug accumulation. (See Chapter 4.)

The anatomic site of the infection is another important host factor to consider when deciding not only which antibiotic to use but also the dosage, route of administration, and duration of therapy. Some antibiotics do not penetrate into the site of infection, such as the lung or bone or abscesses, which can lead to treatment failures.

Consideration of these host factors helps prescribers and pharmacists to ensure optimal drug selection for each individual patient. Continued patient assessment and proper monitoring of antibiotic therapy increase the likelihood that this therapy will be safe and effective.

ANTIBIOTICS

Antibiotics are classified into many broad categories based on their chemical structure. Some of the more common of these categories are sulfonamides, penicillins, cephalosporins, macrolides, quinolones, aminoglycosides, and tetracyclines. In addition to chemical structure, other characteristics that distinguish one class of drugs from the next include antibacterial spectrum, mechanism of action, potency, toxicity, and pharmacokinetic properties. The four most common mechanisms of antibiotic action are: (1) interference with bacterial cell wall synthesis, (2) interference with protein synthesis, (3) interference with replication of nucleic acids (deoxyribonucleic acid [DNA] and ribonucleic acid [RNA]), and (4) antimetabolite action that disrupts critical metabolic reactions inside the bacterial cell. Figure 38-3 portrays these mechanisms of action in combating bacterial infections and indicates which mechanism is used by several

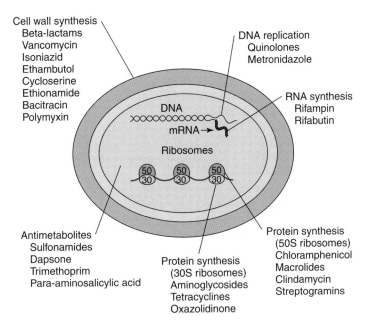

FIGURE 38-3 Basic sites of antibiotic activity. *DNA,* Deoxyribonucleic acid; *mRNA,* messenger ribonucleic acid; *RNA,* ribonucleic acid. (From Murray PR et al: *Medical microbiology,* ed 6, St Louis, 2009, Mosby.)

major antibiotic classes. Perhaps the greatest challenge in understanding antimicrobial therapy is remembering the types and species of microorganisms against which a given drug can act. The list of individual microorganisms against which a given drug has activity can be quite extensive and can seem daunting to the inexperienced practitioner. Most antimicrobials have activity against only one *type* of microbe (e.g., bacteria, viruses, fungi, protozoans). However, a few drugs do have activity against more than one class of organisms. The reader should recognize that his or her understanding of antimicrobial therapy will deepen with clinical experience. The field of infectious disease treatment is continually evolving, largely because of the continual emergence of resistant bacterial strains. For this reason, drug indications change frequently, often from year to year, as various bacterial species become resistant to previously effective antiinfective therapy. It is always appropriate to check the most current reference materials or consult with colleagues (e.g., nurses, pharmacists, prescribers) when questions remain. Pharmacists are excellent resources regarding antibiotics. Many hospitals now have pharmacists who are specially trained in treatment of infectious disease.

SULFONAMIDES

Sulfonamides were one of the first groups of drugs used as antibiotics. Although there are many compounds in the sulfonamide family, only sulfamethoxazole combined with trimethoprim (a nonsulfonamide antibiotic), known as Bactrim, Septra, or co-trimoxazole and often abbreviated as SMX-TMP, is used commonly in clinical practice. Sulfisoxazole combined with erythromycin (a macrolide antibiotic) is occasionally used in pediatrics. Sulfasalazine, another sulfonamide, is used to treat ulcerative colitis and rheumatoid arthritis and is not used as an antibiotic.

Mechanism of Action and Drug Effects

Sulfonamides do not actually destroy bacteria but inhibit their growth. For this reason they are considered **bacteriostatic antibiotics.** They inhibit the growth of susceptible bacteria by preventing bacterial synthesis of folic acid, a B-complex vitamin that is required for the proper synthesis of *purines,* one of the chemical components of nucleic acids (DNA and RNA). Chemical components of folic acid include paraaminobenzoic acid (PABA), pteridine, and glutamic acid. Specifically, in a process known as competitive inhibition, sulfonamides compete with PABA for the bacterial enzyme *tetrahydropteroic acid synthetase,* which incorporates PABA into the folic acid molecule during biosynthesis. Because sulfonamides are capable of blocking a specific step in a biosynthetic pathway, they are also considered antimetabolites. However, microorganisms that require exogenous folic acid (not synthesized by the bacterium itself) are not affected by sulfonamide antibiotics. Therefore, these drugs do not affect folic acid metabolism in human cells. Trimethoprim, although not a sulfonamide, works via a similar mechanism, inhibiting dihydrofolic acid reduction to tetrahydrofolate, which results in inhibition of the enzymes of the folic acid pathway.

Indications

Sulfonamides have a broad spectrum of antibacterial activity, including activity against both gram-positive and gram-negative organisms. These antibiotics achieve very high concentrations in the kidneys, through which they are eliminated. Therefore, sulfamethoxazole/trimethoprim is often used in the treatment of UTIs. The combination of these two drugs allows for an additive antibacterial effect. Commonly susceptible organisms include strains of *Enterobacter* species (spp.), *Escherichia coli, Klebsiella* spp., *Proteus mirabilis, Proteus vulgaris,* and *S. aureus.* Unfortunately, however, resistant bacterial strains are a growing problem, as is the case with other antibiotic classes. Results of culture and sensitivity testing help to optimize drug selection in individual cases. This combination drug is also used for respiratory tract infections. However, it is now less effective against streptococci infecting the upper respiratory tract and pharynx. Another specific use for sulfamethoxazole/trimethoprim is prophylaxis and treatment of opportunistic infections in patients with human immunodeficiency virus (HIV) infection, especially infection by *Pneumocystis jirovecii*, a common cause of HIV-associated pneumonia. Sulfamethoxazole/trimethoprim is also a drug of choice for infection caused by the bacterium *Stenotrophomonas maltophilia*. Although an uncommon infection, it is associated with prolonged hospitalization. Sulfamethoxazole/trimethoprim has become common treatment for outpatient *Staphylococcus* infections, due to the high rate of methicillin-resistant *S. aureus* (MRSA) infections. MRSA and other resistant organism are discussed in Chapter 39.

Contraindications

Use of sulfonamides is contraindicated in cases of known drug allergy to sulfonamides. Chemically related drugs such as the sulfonylureas (used to treat diabetes; see Chapter 32), thiazide and loop diuretics (see Chapter 26), and carbonic anhydrase inhibitors (see Chapter 26) are generally considered relatively safe in a patient who has a sulfonamide allergy. However, the cyclooxygenase-2 inhibitor celecoxib (Celebrex) should not be used (see Chapter 44). It is important to differentiate between sulfites and sulfonamides. Sulfites are commonly used as preservatives in everything from wine to food to injectable drugs. A person allergic to sulfonamide drugs may or may not also be allergic to sulfite preservatives. The use of sulfonamides is also contraindicated in pregnant women at term and in infants younger than 2 months of age.

Adverse Effects

Sulfonamide drugs are a common cause of allergic reaction. Patients will sometimes refer to this as "sulfa allergy" or even "sulfur allergy." Although immediate reactions can occur, sulfonamides typically cause delayed cutaneous reactions. These reactions frequently begin with fever followed by a rash (morbilliform eruptions, erythema multiforme, or toxic epidermal necrolysis). Photosensitivity reactions are another type of skin reaction that is induced by exposure to sunlight during sulfonamide drug therapy. In some cases, such reactions can result in severe sunburn. Such reactions are also common with the *tetracycline* class of antibiotics discussed later in this chapter, as well as with various other drug classes (see Index) and may occur immediately or have a delayed onset. Other reactions to sulfonamides include mucocutaneous, GI, hepatic, renal, and hematologic complications, all of which may be fatal in severe cases. It is believed that sulfonamide reactions are immune mediated and involve the production of reactive drug metabolites in the body. Reported adverse effects of the sulfonamides are listed in Table 38-2.

Interactions

Sulfonamides can have clinically significant interactions with a number of other medications. Sulfonamides may potentiate the hypoglycemic effects of sulfonylureas in diabetes treatment, the

TABLE 38-2 Sulfonamides: Reported Adverse Effects

Body System	Adverse Effects
Blood	Agranulocytosis, aplastic anemia, hemolytic anemia, thrombocytopenia
Gastrointestinal	Nausea, vomiting, diarrhea, pancreatitis, hepatotoxicity
Integumentary	Epidermal necrolysis, exfoliative dermatitis, Stevens-Johnson syndrome, photosensitivity
Other	Convulsions, crystalluria, toxic nephrosis, headache, peripheral neuritis, urticaria, cough, pulmonary infiltrates

toxic effects of phenytoin, and the anticoagulant effects of warfarin, which can lead to hemorrhage. Sulfonamides may increase the likelihood of cyclosporine-induced nephrotoxicity. Patients receiving any of the above drug combinations may require more frequent monitoring. Sulfonamides may also reduce the efficacy of oral contraceptives. Patients taking the drugs should be advised to use additional contraceptive methods.

Dosages

For recommended dosages of selected sulfonamides, see the Dosages table on p. 591.

DRUG PROFILE

Sulfonamides work by interfering with bacterial synthesis of the essential nutrient *folic acid*. Most sulfonamide therapy today uses the combination drug sulfamethoxazole/trimethoprim.

sulfamethoxazole/trimethoprim (co-trimoxazole)
Co-trimoxazole (Bactrim) is a fixed-combination drug product containing a 5:1 ratio of sulfamethoxazole to trimethoprim. It is available in both oral and injectable dosage forms.

PHARMACOKINETICS

Route	Onset of Action	Peak Plasma Concentration	Elimination Half-life	Duration of Action
PO	Variable	2-4 hr	7-12 hr	12 hr

BETA-LACTAM ANTIBIOTICS

The **beta-lactam** antibiotics are very commonly used drugs, so named because of the beta-lactam ring that is part of their chemical structure (Figure 38-4). This broad group of drugs includes four major subclasses: penicillins, cephalosporins, carbapenems, and monobactams. They share a common structure and mechanism of action. They inhibit the synthesis of the bacterial peptidoglycan cell wall. Some bacterial strains produce the enzyme **beta-lactamase**. This enzyme provides a mechanism for bacterial resistance to these antibiotics. The enzyme can break the chemical bond between the carbon (C) and nitrogen (N) atoms in the structure of the beta-lactam ring. When this happens, all beta-lactam drugs lose their antibacterial efficacy. Because of this, additional drugs known as **beta-lactamase inhibitors** are added to the dosage forms of several

DOSAGES

Selected Sulfonamide Combination Drug Product

Drug (Pregnancy Category)	Pharmacologic Class	Usual Dosage Range*	Indications
sulfamethoxazole/trimethoprim (co-trimoxazole, SMX-TMP, SMZ-TMP) (Bactrim, Septra) (C)	Sulfonamide and folate antimetabolite	**Adult and pediatric** IV/PO: 8-20 mg/kg/day divided twice a day (dose is in terms of trimethoprim component) **Adult** PO: 160 mg TMP/800 mg SMX twice daily (every 12 hr) **Pediatric** PO: 150 mg/m^2 TMP/750 mg/m^2 SMX daily × 3 consecutive days/wk	UTI, shigellosis enteritis; higher doses for nocardiosis and *Pneumocystis jirovecii* infection *P. jirovecii* prophylaxis, otitis media, acute exacerbation of chronic bronchitis

IV, Intravenous; *PO,* oral; *UTI,* urinary tract infection.
*Dosage ranges are typical but are not necessarily exhaustive due to space limitations. Clinical variations may occur. Check current drug handbook for exact dosages for specific indications.

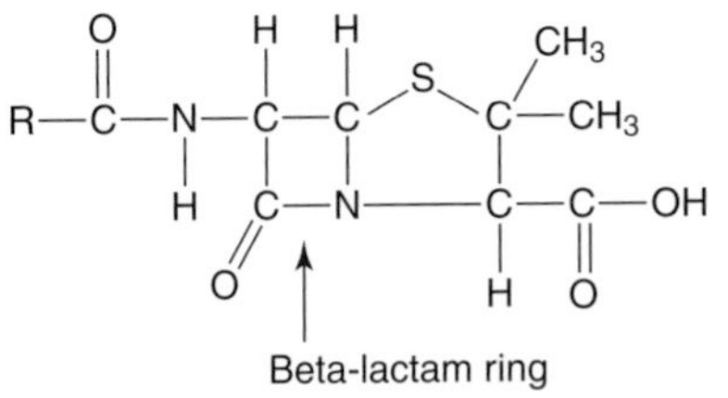

FIGURE 38-4   Chemical structure of penicillins showing the beta-lactam ring. *R,* Variable portion of drug chemical structure.

of the penicillin antibiotics to make the drug more powerful against beta-lactamase–producing bacterial strains. Each of the four classes of beta-lactam antibiotics is examined in detail in the following sections.

PENICILLINS

The penicillins are a very large group of chemically related antibiotics that were first derived from a mold (fungus) often seen on bread or fruit. The penicillins can be divided into four subgroups based on their structure and the spectrum of bacteria that they can kill: natural penicillins, penicillinase-resistant penicillins, aminopenicillins, and extended-spectrum penicillins. Examples of antibiotics in each subgroup and a brief description of their characteristics are given in Table 38-3.

Penicillins are **bactericidal antibiotics,** meaning they kill a wide variety of gram-positive and some gram-negative bacteria. However, some bacteria have acquired the capacity to produce enzymes capable of destroying penicillins. As noted earlier, these enzymes are called *beta-lactamases,* and they can inactivate the penicillin molecules by opening the beta-lactam ring. The beta-lactamases that specifically inactivate penicillin molecules are called *penicillinases.* Bacterial strains that produce these drug-inactivating enzymes were a therapeutic obstacle until drugs were synthesized that inhibit these enzymes. Three of these beta-lactamase inhibitors are clavulanic acid (also called *clavulanate*), tazobactam, and sulbactam. These drugs bind with the beta-lactamase enzyme itself to prevent the en-

zyme from breaking down the penicillin molecule, although they are not always effective. The following are examples of currently available combinations of a penicillin and a beta-lactamase inhibitor:

- ampicillin/sulbactam (Unasyn)
- amoxicillin/clavulanic acid (Augmentin)
- ticarcillin/clavulanic acid (Timentin)
- piperacillin/tazobactam (Zosyn)

Mechanism of Action and Drug Effects

The mechanism of action of penicillins involves the inhibition of bacterial cell wall synthesis. Once distributed by the patient's bloodstream to infected areas, penicillin molecules slide through bacterial cell walls to get to their site of action. Some penicillins, however, are too large to pass through the openings in the cell walls, and because they cannot get to their site of action they cannot kill the bacteria. Some bacteria make the openings in their cell walls small so that the penicillin cannot get through to kill them. The penicillin molecules that do gain entry into the bacterium must then find the appropriate binding sites. These are known as *penicillin-binding proteins.* By binding to these proteins, the penicillin molecules interfere with normal cell wall synthesis, causing the formation of defective cell walls that are unstable and easily broken down (see Figure 38-3). Bacterial death usually results from lysis (rupture) of the bacterial cells due to this drug-induced disruption of cell wall structure.

Indications

Penicillins are indicated for the prevention and treatment of infections caused by susceptible bacteria. The microorganisms most commonly destroyed by penicillins are gram-positive bacteria, including *Streptococcus* spp., *Enterococcus* spp., and *Staphylococcus* spp. Most natural penicillins have little if any ability to kill gram-negative bacteria. However, the extended-spectrum penicillins (i.e., piperacillin/tazobactam [Zosyn]) have excellent gram-positive, gram-negative, and anaerobic coverage. Because of this, the extended-spectrum penicillins are used to treat many hospital-associated infections, including pneumonia, intraabdominal infections, and sepsis.

TABLE 38-3 Classification of Penicillins

Subclass	Generic Drug Names	Description
Natural penicillins	penicillin G, penicillin V	Although many modifications of the original natural (mold-produced) structure have been made, these are the only two in current clinical use. Penicillin G is the injectable form for IV or IM use; penicillin V is a PO dosage form (tablet and liquid).
Penicillinase-resistant drugs	cloxacillin, dicloxacillin, nafcillin, oxacillin	Stable against hydrolysis by most staphylococcal penicillinases (enzymes that normally break down the natural penicillins).
Aminopenicillins	amoxicillin, ampicillin	Have an amino group attached to the basic penicillin structure that enhances their activity against gram-negative bacteria compared with natural penicillins.
Extended-spectrum drugs	piperacillin, ticarcillin, carbenicillin, piperacillin/tazobactam	Have wider spectra of activity than do all other penicillins.

IM, Intramuscular; *IV,* intravenous; *PO,* oral.

Contraindications

Penicillins are usually safe and well-tolerated medications. The only usual contraindication is known drug allergy. It is very important for nurses to obtain an accurate history regarding the type of reaction that occurs in patients who state they are allergic to penicillins. It is also important to note that often drugs are referred to by their trade names, and these don't always end in "cillin" (e.g., Zosyn, Augmentin). Many medication errors have occurred when a penicillin drug called by its trade name is given to a patient with a penicillin allergy. When these errors are analyzed, the common reason is that the person administering the drug didn't realize that the drug with the non-"cillin" name was a penicillin.

Adverse Effects

Allergic reactions to the penicillins occur in 0.7% to 4% of treatment courses. The most common reactions are urticaria, pruritus, and angioedema. A wide variety of idiosyncratic (unpredictable) drug reactions can occur, such as maculopapular eruptions, eosinophilia, Stevens-Johnson syndrome, and exfoliative dermatitis. Maculopapular rash occurs in about 2% of treatment courses with natural penicillin and 5.2% to 9.5% of those with ampicillin. Anaphylactic reactions are much less common, occurring in 0.004% to 0.015% of patients. Severe reactions are much more common with injected than with orally administered penicillin, as is the case with most antibiotics. A common clinical scenario is that in which a prescriber wants to administer a cephalosporin to a patient reporting a penicillin allergy. Patients who are allergic to penicillins have an increased risk of allergy to other beta-lactam antibiotics. The incidence of cross-reactivity between cephalosporins and penicillins is reported to be between 1% and 4%. Patients reporting penicillin allergy should be asked to describe their prior allergic reaction. It is very important for the nurse to document the type of reaction The decision to continue with cephalosporin therapy in such cases is often a matter of clinical judgment, based on the severity of reported prior reactions to penicillin drugs, the nature of the infection, the drug susceptibility of the infective organism if known, and the availability and patient tolerance of other alternative antibiotics. Generally speaking, only those patients with a history of throat swelling or hives should not receive cephalosporins. Some patients may require skin testing and desensitization.

TABLE 38-4 Penicillins: Reported Adverse Effects

Body System	Adverse Effects
Central nervous	Lethargy, hallucinations, anxiety, depression, twitching, coma, seizures
Gastrointestinal	Nausea, vomiting, diarrhea, transient increases of AST and ALT levels, abdominal pain, colitis, taste alterations, oral candidiasis
Hematologic	Anemia, increased bleeding time, bone marrow depression, granulocytopenia
Metabolic	Hyperkalemia, hypokalemia, alkalosis
Skin	Pruritus, hives, rash

ALT, Alanine aminotransferase; *AST,* aspartate aminotransferase.

Penicillins are generally well tolerated and associated with very few adverse effects. As with many drugs, the most common adverse effects involve the GI system. The most common adverse effects of the penicillins are listed in Table 38-4.

Interactions

Many drugs interact with penicillins; some have positive effects, and others have harmful effects. The most common and clinically significant drug interactions associated with penicillin use are listed in Table 38-5.

Dosages

For dosage information for selected penicillins, see the Dosages table on p. 593.

DRUG PROFILES

Penicillins are classified as pregnancy category B drugs. They are very safe antibiotics. Their use is contraindicated in patients with a hypersensitivity to them, but because of their relatively good adverse effects profile, there are otherwise very few contraindications to their use.

NATURAL PENICILLINS
◆ penicillin G and penicillin V potassium

Penicillin G has three salt forms: benzathine, procaine, and potassium. All of these forms are given by injection, either intravenously (IV) or intramuscularly (IM). The benzathine and procaine salts are

TABLE 38-5 Penicillins: Drug Interactions

Drug Interacting with Penicillins	Mechanism	Result
Aminoglycosides (IV) and clavulanic acid	Additivity	More effective killing of bacteria
methotrexate	Decreased renal elimination of methotrexate	Increased methotrexate levels
neomycin (an oral aminoglycoside)	Reduced absorption of penicillin in GI tract when both drugs are given orally	Reduced penicillin efficacy; avoid concurrent use or consider injectable penicillin instead
Potassium supplements, table salt	penicillin G potassium has 1.7 mEq of potassium ion per million units; penicillin G sodium has 2 mEq of sodium ion per million units	Effects unlikely for most patients but may precipitate or worsen hyperkalemia and hypernatremia; monitor sodium and/or potassium levels as needed in patients at risk and choose alternative drugs if indicated
NSAIDs	Compete for protein binding	More free and active penicillin (may be beneficial)
Oral contraceptives	Uncertain	May decrease efficacy of the contraceptive
probenecid	Competes for elimination	Prolongs the effects of penicillins
rifampin	Inhibition	May inhibit the killing activity of penicillins
warfarin	Reduced vitamin K from gut flora	Enhanced anticoagulant effect of warfarin

GI, Gastrointestinal; *IV,* intravenous; *NSAIDs,* nonsteroidal antiinflammatory drugs.

DOSAGES

Selected Penicillins

Drug (Pregnancy Category)	Pharmacologic Class	Usual Dosage Range	Indications
◆ amoxicillin (Amoxil) (B)	Aminopenicillin	**Pediatric** PO: 40-90 mg/kg/day divided q8-12h **Adult** PO: 250-500 mg q8h	Otitis media; sinusitis; various susceptible respiratory, skin, and urinary tract infections; dental prophylaxis for bacterial endocarditis; *Helicobacter pylori* infection
Ampicillin (generic only) (B)	Aminopenicillin	**Adult** PO/IV/IM: 1-12 g/day divided q4-6h **Pediatric** 50-400 mg/kg/day divided q4-6h	Primarily infection with gram-negative organisms such as *Shigella, Salmonella, Escherichia, Haemophilus, Proteus,* and *Neisseria* spp.; infection with some gram-positive organisms
nafcillin (generic only) (B)	Penicillinase-resistant penicillin	**Adult** IV/IM: 500-1000 mg q4-6h **Pediatric** IV/IM: 50-200 mg/kg/day divided q4-6h	Infection with penicillinase-producing staphylococci
◆ penicillin V potassium (Pen-Vee K) (B)	Natural penicillin	**Adult and pediatric** PO: 125-500 mg q6-8h **Adult and pediatric** IV: 150-300 mg/kg/day divided q4-6h	Primarily infection with gram-positive organisms such as *Streptococcus* (including *Streptococcus pneumoniae*) and *Staphylococcus* spp.

IM, Intramuscular; *IV,* intravenous; *PO,* oral; *spp.,* species.

used as longer-acting IM injections. They are formulated into a thick, white, pastelike material that is designed for prolonged dissolution and absorption from the IM site of injection. These preparations should *never* be given IV, however, because their consistency is too thick for IV administration, and such use can be fatal. The IM formulations can be especially helpful for treating the sexually transmitted disease syphilis, because often only one injection is needed, and therefore it can be given one time at a clinic that treats sexually transmitted diseases. Penicillin G potassium is formulated for IV use. Penicillin V potassium is available only for oral use.

PHARMACOKINETICS

Route	Onset of Action	Peak Plasma Concentration	Elimination Half-life	Duration of Action
PO	Variable	30-60 min	30 min	4-6 hr
IV	Variable	30 min	24-54 min	4-6 hr

PENICILLINASE-RESISTANT PENICILLINS
nafcillin

Nafcillin is one of the four currently available penicillinase-resistant penicillins; the other three are cloxacillin, dicloxacillin, and oxacillin. Nafcillin is available only in injectable form, whereas cloxacillin and dicloxacillin are available only in oral form. Oxacillin is available in both oral and injectable forms. The penicillinase-resistant penicillins are able to resist breakdown by the penicillin-destroying enzyme (penicillinase) commonly produced by bacteria such as staphylococci. For this reason they may also be referred to as *antistaphylococcal penicillins*. The chemical structure of these drugs features a large, bulky side chain near the beta-lactam ring. This side chain serves as a barrier to the penicillinase enzyme, preventing it from breaking the beta-lactam ring, which would inactivate the drug. There are, however, certain strains of staphylococci, specifically *S. aureus,* that are resistant to these drugs. Such bacteria therefore require alternative antibiotic regimens.

PHARMACOKINETICS

Route	Onset of Action	Peak Plasma Concentration	Elimination Half-life	Duration of Action
IV	Variable	15-30 min	30-60 min	6 hr

AMINOPENICILLINS

There are two aminopenicillins: amoxicillin and ampicillin. They are so named because of the presence of a free amino group (⁻NH$_2$) in their chemical structure. This structural feature gives aminopenicillins enhanced activity against gram-negative bacteria against which the natural and penicillinase-resistant penicillins are relatively ineffective. The aminopenicillins are also effective against many gram-positive organisms. Amoxicillin is an analogue of ampicillin.

◆ amoxicillin

Amoxicillin is a very commonly prescribed aminopenicillin. Amoxicillin is used to treat infections caused by susceptible organisms in the ears, nose, throat, genitourinary tract, skin, and skin structures. Pediatric dosages are sometimes higher than in the past because of the development of increasingly resistant *Streptococcus pneumoniae* organisms. The drug is available only for oral use and can be given with or without food.

PHARMACOKINETICS

Route	Onset of Action	Peak Plasma Concentration	Elimination Half-life	Duration of Action
PO	0.5-1 hr	1-2 hr	1-1.5 hr	6-8 hr

ampicillin

Ampicillin is available in three different salt forms: anhydrous, trihydrate, and sodium. The different salt forms are administered by different routes. Ampicillin anhydrous and trihydrate are both administered orally, whereas ampicillin sodium is given parenterally. This drug is still currently available, although it is now used less frequently than before because of resistance.

PHARMACOKINETICS

Route	Onset of Action	Peak Plasma Concentration	Elimination Half-life	Duration of Action
PO	Variable	1-2 hr	1-1.5 hr	4-6 hr
IV	Variable	5 min	1-1.8 hr	6-8 hr

EXTENDED-SPECTRUM PENICILLINS

By making a few changes in the basic penicillin structure, drug developers produced another generation of penicillins that have a wider spectrum of activity than that possessed by either of the other two classes of semisynthetic penicillins (penicillinase-resistant penicillins and aminopenicillins) or by the natural penicillins. Currently three extended-spectrum penicillins are available: carbenicillin, piperacillin, and ticarcillin, however they are rarely used by themselves. Both ticarcillin and piperacillin are available in fixed-combina-

tion products that include beta-lactamase inhibitors. The ticarcillin fixed-combination product (Timentin) includes clavulanate potassium. Piperacillin is available in combination with tazobactam (a combination called Zosyn). These beta-lactamase–inhibiting products allow for enhanced multiorganism coverage, especially against anaerobic organisms that are common in intestinal infections and *Pseudomonas* spp., which are common in hospital-acquired infections. Zosyn is commonly used in hospitalized patients with suspected or documented serious infections. Because of its broad spectrum of activity (gram positive, gram negative and anaerobic), it is often used as empiric therapy. Zosyn and Timentin are available only by injection.

CEPHALOSPORINS

Cephalosporins are semisynthetic antibiotics widely used in clinical practice. They are structurally and pharmacologically related to the penicillins. Like penicillins, cephalosporins are bactericidal and work by interfering with bacterial cell wall synthesis. They also bind to the same penicillin-binding proteins inside bacteria that were described earlier for the penicillins. Although there are a variety of such proteins, they are collectively referred to as *penicillin binding* regardless of the type of beta-lactam drug involved.

Cephalosporins can destroy a broad spectrum of bacteria, and this ability is directly related to the chemical changes that have been made to their basic cephalosporin structure. Modifications to this chemical structure by pharmaceutical scientists have given rise to four generations of cephalosporins, with a fifth generation currently awaiting approval from the U.S. Food and Drug Administration. Depending on the generation, these drugs may be active against gram-positive, gram-negative, or anaerobic bacteria. They are not active against fungi and viruses. The different drugs of each generation have certain chemical similarities, and thus they can kill similar spectra of bacteria. In general, the level of gram-negative coverage increases with each successive generation. The first-generation drugs have the most gram-positive coverage, and the later generations have the most gram-negative coverage. Anaerobic coverage is found only with the second-generation drugs. Cefepime, cefdinir, and cefditoren pivoxil are the oral third-generation cephalosporins. Ceftobiprole, the newest cephalosporin, often referred as the fifth generation, has a broad spectrum and covers gram-positive (including MRSA) and gram-negative organisms. The currently available parenteral and oral cephalosporin antibiotics are listed in Table 38-6. As is often the case, injectable drugs produce higher serum concentrations than drugs administered by the oral route and thus are used to treat more serious infections.

The safety profiles, contraindications, and pregnancy ratings of the cephalosporins are very similar to those of the penicillins. The most commonly reported adverse effects are mild diarrhea, abdominal cramps, rash, pruritus, redness, and edema. Because cephalosporins are chemically very similar to penicillins, a person who has had an allergic reaction to penicillin may also have an allergic reaction to a cephalosporin. This is referred to as *cross-sensitivity*. Various investigators have observed that the incidence of cross-sensitivity between penicillins and cephalosporins is between 1% and 4%. However, only those patients who have had a serious anaphylactic reaction to penicillin should

TABLE **38-6** Cephalosporins: Parenteral and Oral Preparations

First Generation		Second Generation		Third Generation		Fourth Generation	Fifth Generation
IV	PO	IV	PO	IV	PO	IV	IV
cefazolin	cefadroxil	cefoxitin	cefaclor	cefoperazone	cefpodoxime	cefepime	ceftobiprole†
cephradine	cephalexin	cefuroxime	cefuroxime	cefotaxime	proxetil*		
	cephradine	cefotetan	axetil*	ceftizoxime	ceftibuten		
		loracarbef	cefprozil	ceftriaxone	cefdinir		
				ceftazidime			

IV, Intravenous; *PO,* oral.
*Prodrug salts that aid in drug delivery into gastrointestinal tract.
†Not yet marketed at time of publication.

TABLE **38-7** Cephalosporins: Drug Interactions

Interacting Drug	Mechanism	Result
ethanol (alcohol)	Accumulation of acetaldehyde metabolite of ethanol	Acute alcohol intolerance (disulfiram-like reaction) after drinking alcoholic beverages within 72 hr of taking cefotetan. Symptoms include stomach cramps, nausea, vomiting, diaphoresis, pruritus, headache, and hypotension.
Antacids, iron	Decreased absorption of certain oral cephalosporins (cefdinir, cefditoren)	Decreased effectiveness of drug
probenecid	Decreased renal excretion	Increased cephalosporin levels
Oral contraceptives (OCs)	Enhanced OC metabolism	Increased risk for unintended pregnancy

definitely not be given cephalosporins. As a class the cephalosporins are very safe and effective antibiotics, and they should not be unnecessarily avoided because of overcautiousness about possible cross-sensitivity.

Penicillins and cephalosporins are practically identical in their mechanism of action, drug effects, therapeutic effects, and adverse effects. For that reason, this information is not repeated for the cephalosporins, and the reader is referred to the pertinent discussions in the section on the penicillin drugs. Cephalosporins of all generations are very safe drugs that are categorized as pregnancy category B drugs. Their use is contraindicated in patients who have shown a hypersensitivity to them and in any patient with a history of life-threatening allergic reaction to penicillins. Drug interactions are listed in Table 38-7.

Dosages

For the recommended dosages of selected cephalosporins, see the Dosages table on p. 596.

DRUG PROFILES

FIRST-GENERATION CEPHALOSPORINS
First-generation cephalosporins are usually active against gram-positive bacteria and have limited activity against gram-negative bacteria. They are available in both parenteral and oral forms. Currently available first-generation cephalosporins include cefadroxil, cefazolin, cephalexin, and cephradine.

◆ cefazolin
Cefazolin (Ancef) is a prototypical first-generation cephalosporin. As with all first-generation cephalosporins, it provides excellent coverage against gram-positive bacteria but limited coverage against gram-negative bacteria. It is available only for parenteral use. It is used commonly for surgical prophylaxis and for susceptible staphylococcal infections.

PHARMACOKINETICS

Route	Onset of Action	Peak Plasma Concentration	Elimination Half-life	Duration of Action
IV	Variable	5 min	1.2-2.5 hr	8 hr

◆ cephalexin
Cephalexin (Keflex) is a prototypical oral first-generation cephalosporin. It also provides excellent coverage against gram-positive bacteria but limited coverage against gram-negative bacteria. It is available only for oral use. Cephradine is another oral first-generation cephalosporin.

PHARMACOKINETICS

Route	Onset of Action	Peak Plasma Concentration	Elimination Half-life	Duration of Action
PO	Variable	1 hr	0.6-2 hr	6-12 hr

SECOND-GENERATION CEPHALOSPORINS
Second-generation cephalosporins have coverage against gram-positive organisms similar to that of the first-generation cephalosporins but have enhanced coverage against gram-negative bacteria. Both parenteral and oral formulations are available. Currently available second-generation cephalosporins include cefaclor, cefoxitin, cefuroxime, cefotetan, cefprozil, and loracarbef. These drugs differ

DOSAGES

Selected Cephalosporins

Drug (Pregnancy Category)	Pharmacologic Class	Usual Dosage Range	Indications
◆ cefazolin (Kefzol, Ancef) (B)	First-generation cephalosporin	**Adult** IV/IM: 500-1000 mg q6-8h **Pediatric** IV/IM: 25-50 mg/kg/day divided q6-8h	Infections: due to gram positive organisms, some penicillinase-producing organisms, and some gram-negative organisms; preop and postop surgical prophylaxis
◆ cefoxitin (Mefoxin) (B)	Second-generation cephalosporin	**Adult** IV/IM: 3-12 g/day divided q6-8h **Pediatric** IV/IM: 80-160 mg/kg/day divided q4-6h, not to exceed 12 g/day	Infections; less coverage of gram-positive organisms, greater coverage of gram-negative and anaerobic organisms
cefuroxime (Kefurox, Zinacef); cefuroxime axetil* (Ceftin, tablet form) (B)	Second-generation cephalosporin	**Adult** PO (tabs): 125-500 mg bid **Pediatric** PO tabs: 125-250 mg bid **Pediatric** PO oral suspension: 20-30 mg/kg/day divided bid **Adult** IV/IM: 750-1500 mg q8h **Pediatric** IV/IM: 50-240 mg/kg/day, divided q6-8h	Comparable to those for cefazolin and provides more coverage of gram-negative organisms
ceftazidime (Fortaz, Tazidime) (B)	Third-generation cephalosporin	**Adult** IV/IM: 250-2000 mg q6-12h **Pediatric** IV/IM: 30-50 mg/kg/day divided q8-12h	Infections; more extensive coverage of gram-negative organisms, including *Pseudomonas* spp.
◆ ceftriaxone (Rocephin) (B)	Third-generation cephalosporin	**Adult** IV/IM: 1-2 g given once daily except for meningitis, for which it is twice daily **Pediatric** IV/IM: 50-100 mg/kg/day divided daily-bid (as above)	Comparable to those for ceftazidime; also preop surgical prophylaxis
cefepime (Maxipime) (B)	Fourth-generation cephalosporin	**Adult** IV/IM: 250-2000 mg daily-bid **Pediatric** IV/IM: 50 mg/kg q12h	Infections; provides more extensive coverage of gram-negative organisms and better gram-positive coverage than third generation, including organisms causing intraabdominal infections

IM, Intramuscular; *IV*, intravenous; *PO*, oral; *preop*, preoperative; *postop*, postoperative; *spp.*, species.
*Cefuroxime axetil and cefditoren pivoxil are both prodrugs for PO use that are hydrolyzed into the active ingredient in the fluids of the gastrointestinal tract.

slightly with regard to their antibacterial coverage. Cefoxitin and cefotetan are often referred to as *cephamycins* and have better coverage against various anaerobic bacteria such as *Bacteroides fragilis, Peptostreptococcus* spp., and *Clostridium* spp. than the other drugs in this class.

◆ cefoxitin

Cefoxitin (Mefoxin) is a parenteral second-generation cephalosporin. It provides excellent gram-positive coverage and better gram-negative coverage than the first-generation drugs. Cefoxitin has been used extensively as a prophylactic antibiotic in patients undergoing abdominal surgery because it can effectively kill intestinal bacteria, including anaerobes. Normal intestinal flora include gram-positive, gram-negative, and anaerobic bacteria.

PHARMACOKINETICS

Route	Onset of Action	Peak Plasma Concentration	Elimination Half-life	Duration of Action
IV	Variable	0.5 hr	1 hr	8 hr

cefuroxime

Cefuroxime sodium (Zinacef) is the parenteral form of this second-generation cephalosporin. The oral form is a different salt, cefuroxime axetil (Ceftin). Cefuroxime is a very versatile second-generation cephalosporin. It has more activity against gram-negative bacteria than first-generation cephalosporins but a narrower spectrum of activity against gram-negative bacteria than third-generation cephalosporins. It differs from the cephamycins such as cefoxitin in that it does not kill anaerobic bacteria. Cefuroxime axetil is a prodrug. It has little antibacterial activity until it is hydrolyzed in the liver to its active cefuroxime form. It is available only for oral use. Cefuroxime sodium is available only in injectable form.

PHARMACOKINETICS

Route	Onset of Action	Peak Plasma Concentration	Elimination Half-life	Duration of Action
PO	Variable	2-3 hr	1.3 hr	6-8 hr
IV	Variable	30 min	1-2 hr	6-8 hr

THIRD-GENERATION CEPHALOSPORINS

The available third-generation cephalosporins include cefotaxime, cefpodoxime, ceftazidime, ceftibuten, cefdinir, ceftizoxime, and ceftriaxone. These are the most potent of the first three generations of cephalosporins in fighting gram-negative bacteria, but they generally have less activity than first- and second-generation drugs against gram-positive organisms.

Because of specific changes in the basic cephalosporin structure, ceftazidime has significant activity against *Pseudomonas* spp. However resistance is beginning to limit its usefulness. Cefpodoxime, cefdinir, cefditoren pivoxil, and ceftibuten are currently the only third-generation cephalosporins available for oral use. All the other third-generation drugs are available only in parenteral forms.

◆ ceftriaxone

Ceftriaxone (Rocephin) is an extremely long-acting third-generation drug that can be given only once a day for the treatment of most infections. It also has the unique characteristic of being able to pass easily through the blood-brain barrier. For this reason it is one of the few cephalosporins that is indicated for the treatment of meningitis, an infection of the meninges of the brain. The spectrum of activity of ceftriaxone is similar to that of the other third-generation drugs cefotaxime and ceftizoxime. It can be given both IV and IM. In some cases of infection, one IM injection can eradicate the infection. Ceftriaxone is 93% to 96% bound to plasma protein, a proportion higher than that of many of the other cephalosporins. This drug is also unique in that it is metabolized in the intestine after biliary excretion. It should not be given to hyperbilirubinemic neonates or to patients with severe liver dysfunction. It should not be administered with calcium infusions. This drug is available only for injection.

PHARMACOKINETICS

Route	Onset of Action	Peak Plasma Concentration	Elimination Half-life	Duration of Action
IV	Variable	1.5-4 hr	4.3-8.7 hr	24 hr

ceftazidime

Ceftazidime (Ceptaz, Fortaz, Tazidime) is a parenterally administered third-generation cephalosporin with excellent activity against difficult-to-treat infections with gram-negative bacteria such as *Pseudomonas* spp. It is the third-generation cephalosporin of choice for many indications because of its excellent spectrum of activity and safety profile; however, resistance is beginning to limit its usefulness, and it is generally given in combination with an aminoglycoside (discussed in Chapter 39). It is available only in injectable form.

PHARMACOKINETICS

Route	Onset of Action	Peak Plasma Concentration	Elimination Half-life	Duration of Action
IV/IM	Variable	1 hr	2 hr	8-12 hr

FOURTH-GENERATION CEPHALOSPORINS
cefepime

Cefepime (Maxipime) is the prototypical fourth-generation cephalosporin. Cefepime is a broad-spectrum cephalosporin that most closely resembles ceftazidime in its spectrum of activity. It differs from ceftazidime in that it has increased activity against many *Enterobacter* spp. (gram negative) as well as gram-positive organisms. Cefepime is indicated for the treatment of uncomplicated and complicated UTIs, uncomplicated skin and skin structure infections, and pneumonia. It is available only in injectable form.

PHARMACOKINETICS

Route	Onset of Action	Peak Plasma Concentration	Elimination Half-life	Duration of Action
IV	0.5 hr	0.5-1.5 hr	2 hr	8-12 hr

FIFTH-GENERATION CEPHALOSPORINS

Ceftobiprole is the newest cephalosporin. It has a broader spectrum of activity than the current cephalosporins. It is effective against a wide variety of organisms, including MRSA and *Pseudomonas* spp. It is available only in injectable form. At the time of publication, it has not yet been marketed.

CARBAPENEMS

Carbapenems have among the broadest antibacterial action of any antibiotics to date. They are bactericidal and inhibit cell wall synthesis. Because of this, they are often reserved for complicated body cavity and connective tissue infections in acutely ill hospitalized patients. They are also effective against many gram-positive organisms. One hazard of carbapenem use is drug-induced seizure activity, which occurs in a relatively small percentage of patients but is obviously undesirable. However, the risk of seizures can be reduced by proper dosage adjustment in truly impaired patients. There is a small risk of cross allergenicity in patients with penicillin allergies. Only those patients with anaphylactic-type reactions to penicillins should not receive a carbapenem. Currently available carbapenems include imipenem/cilastatin, meropenem, ertapenem, and doripenem. Carbapenems must be infused over 60 minutes.

DRUG PROFILE

◆ imipenem/cilastatin

Imipenem/cilastatin (Primaxin) is a fixed combination of imipenem, which is a semisynthetic carbapenem antibiotic similar to beta-lactam antibiotics, and cilastatin, an inhibitor of an enzyme that breaks down imipenem. Imipenem has a wide spectrum of activity against gram-positive and gram-negative aerobic and anaerobic bacteria. Cilastatin is a unique drug in that it inhibits an enzyme in the kidneys called *dehydropeptidase*, which would otherwise quickly break down the imipenem. Cilastatin also blocks the renal tubular secretion of imipenem, which prevents imipenem from being excreted by the kidneys, the primary route of elimination of the drug.

Imipenem/cilastatin exerts its antibacterial effect by binding to penicillin-binding proteins inside bacteria, which in turn inhibits bacterial cell wall synthesis. Unlike many of the penicillins and cephalosporins, imipenem/cilastatin is very resistant to the antibiotic-inhibiting actions of beta-lactamases. Drugs with which it potentially interacts include cyclosporine, ganciclovir, and probenecid, all of which may potentiate the central nervous system (CNS) adverse effects (including seizures) of imipenem. Concurrent use with these drugs should be avoided whenever clinically feasible. The most serious adverse effect associated with imipenem/cilastatin therapy is seizures, which have been reported in up to 1.5% of patients receiving less than 500 mg every 6 hours. In patients receiving high dosages of the drug (more than 500 mg every 6 hours), however, there is about a 10% incidence of seizures. Seizures are more likely in elderly and renally impaired patients. Seizures have been associated with all of the carbapenems, but the data suggests that they are most likely to occur with imipenem/cilastatin.

DOSAGES

Selected Carbapenem and Monobactam

Drug (Pregnancy Category)	Pharmacologic Class	Usual Dosage Range		Indications
aztreonam (Azactam) (B)	Monobactam	**Adult** IV/IM: 500-1000 mg q6-12h IV: 2 g q12h **Pediatric** IV/IM: 30 mg/kg every 6-8 hr		Primarily UTI caused by gram-negative organisms, severe systemic infections
◆ imipenem/cilastatin (Primaxin) (C)	Carbapenem	**Adult** IV: 250-500 mg q6-8h IM: 500-750 mg q12h **Pediatric** 15-25 mg/kg every 6 hr		Infection with gram-positive, gram-negative, and aerobic bacteria, including *Pseudomonas aeruginosa;* includes infections of bone, joint, skin, or soft tissue and endocarditis, pneumonia, UTI, intraabdominal and pelvic infections, and septicemia

IM, Intramuscular; *IV,* intravenous; *UTI,* urinary tract infection.

Imipenem/cilastatin is indicated for the treatment of bone, joint, skin, and soft tissue infections; bacterial endocarditis caused by *S. aureus;* intraabdominal bacterial infections; pneumonia; UTIs and pelvic infections; and bacterial septicemia caused by susceptible bacterial organisms. The IM form of imipenem/cilastatin contains lidocaine, and its use is therefore contraindicated in patients with a known drug allergy to lidocaine or related local anesthetics. All dosage forms contain the same number of milligrams of both imipenem and cilastatin.

Meropenem (Merrem) is the second drug in the carbapenem class of antibiotics. Compared with imipenem/cilastatin, meropenem appears to be somewhat less active against gram-positive organisms, more active against Enterobacteriaceae, and equally active against *P. aeruginosa.* However, meropenem is the only carbapenem currently indicated for treatment of bacterial meningitis. Ertapenem (Invanz) has a spectrum of activity comparable to that of imipenem/cilastatin, although it is not active against *Enterococcal* or *Pseudomonas* spp. Doripenem (Doribax) is the newest carbapenem. It has less seizure potential than imipenem/cilastatin. It is indicated for intraabdominal infections, pyelonephritis, UTIs, and pneumonia. For recommended dosages of imipenem/cilastatin, see the Dosages table on page 000.

PHARMACOKINETICS

Route	Onset of Action	Peak Plasma Concentration	Elimination Half-life	Duration of Action
IV	Variable	2 hr	2-3 hr	6-8 hr

MONOBACTAMS

DRUG PROFILE

aztreonam

Aztreonam (Azactam) is the only monobactam antibiotic to be developed thus far. It is a synthetic beta-lactam antibiotic that is primarily active against aerobic gram-negative bacteria, including *E. coli, Klebsiella* spp., and *Pseudomonas* spp. Aztreonam is a bactericidal antibiotic. It destroys bacteria by inhibiting bacterial cell wall synthesis, which results in lysis. Aztreonam is indicated for the treatment of moderately severe systemic infections and UTIs. It is often combined with other antibiotics for the treatment of intraabdominal and gynecologic infections. It has the theoretical therapeutic advantage of preserving normal gram-positive and anaerobic flora, unlike many other beta-lactam antibiotics. Aztreonam is available only in injectable form. Its use is contraindicated in patients with a known drug allergy, although it is believed to have less allergic cross-reactivity with other beta-lactam antibiotics. Common adverse effects include rash, nausea, vomiting, and diarrhea. For dosage information on this monobactam, see the Dosages table above.

PHARMACOKINETICS

Route	Onset of Action	Peak Plasma Concentration	Elimination Half-life	Duration of Action
IV/IM	Variable	1 hr	1.5-2.1 hr	6-12 hr

MACROLIDES

The macrolides are a large group of antibiotics that first became available in the early 1950s with the introduction of erythromycin. Macrolides are considered bacteriostatic; however, in high enough concentrations they may be bactericidal to some susceptible bacteria. There are four main macrolide antibiotics: azithromycin, clarithromycin, dirithromycin, and erythromycin. Azithromycin and clarithromycin are two of the newer drugs in the class, and together with the original drug, erythromycin, are currently the most widely used of the macrolides. Although the spectra of antibacterial activity of both azithromycin and clarithromycin are similar to that of erythromycin, the former have longer durations of action than erythromycin, which allows them to be given less often. They produce fewer and milder GI tract adverse effects than erythromycin, and azithromycin is usually dosed over a shorter length of time than many of the erythromycin products. Azithromycin and clarithromycin also exhibit better efficacy in eradicating various bacteria and are capable of better tissue penetration. Because erythromycin has a bitter taste and is quickly degraded by the acidity of the stomach, several salt forms and many dosage formulations were developed to circumvent these problems.

Mechanism of Action and Drug Effects

Macrolide antibiotics are bacteriostatic drugs that inhibit protein synthesis by binding reversibly to the 50S ribosomal subunits of susceptible microorganisms.

Macrolides are effective in the treatment of a wide range of infections. These include various infections of the upper and lower respiratory tract, skin, and soft tissue caused by some strains of *Streptococcus* and *Haemophilus;* spirochetal infections such as syphilis and Lyme disease; gonorrhea; and *Chlamydia, Mycoplasma,* and *Corynebacterium* infections. Gonorrheal infections have become increasingly difficult to treat with macrolide monotherapy, so these drugs are sometimes used in combination with other antibiotics such as cephalosporins. Macrolides are also somewhat unique among antibiotics in that they are especially effective against several bacterial species that often reproduce inside host cells instead of just in the bloodstream or interstitial spaces. Common examples of such bacteria, some of which were previously listed, are *Listeria, Chlamydia, Legionella* (one species of which causes legionnaires disease), *Neisseria* (one species of which causes gonorrhea), and *Campylobacter.*

Indications

Infections caused by *Streptococcus pyogenes* (group A beta-hemolytic streptococci) are inhibited by macrolides, as are mild to moderate upper and lower respiratory tract infections caused by *Haemophilus influenzae.* Spirochetal infections that are treated with erythromycin and other macrolides are syphilis and Lyme disease. Various forms of gonorrhea and *Chlamydia* and *Mycoplasma* infections are also susceptible to the effects of macrolides.

A therapeutic effect of erythromycin outside its antibiotic actions is its ability to irritate the GI tract, which stimulates smooth muscle and GI motility. This may be of benefit to patients who have decreased GI motility, such as delayed gastric emptying in diabetic patients (known as *diabetic gastroparesis*). It has also been shown to be helpful in facilitating the passage of feeding tubes from the stomach into the small bowel. Azithromycin and clarithromycin are approved for the prevention and treatment of *Mycobacterium avium-intracellulare* complex infections. This is a common *opportunistic infection* often associated with HIV infection/acquired immunodeficiency syndrome (AIDS) (see Chapter 40). Clarithromycin also has been approved for use in combination with omeprazole for the treatment of patients with active ulcer associated with *Helicobacter pylori* infection.

Contraindications

The only usual contraindication to macrolide use is known drug allergy. In fact, as indicated earlier, macrolides are often used as alternative drugs for patients with allergies to beta-lactam antibiotics.

TABLE 38-8   Macrolides: Reported Adverse Effects

Body System	Adverse Effects
Cardiovascular	Palpitations, chest pain, QTc prolongation (rare)
Central nervous	Headache, dizziness, vertigo
Gastrointestinal	Nausea, hepatotoxicity, heartburn, vomiting, diarrhea, stomatitis, flatulence, cholestatic jaundice, anorexia, abnormal taste
Integumentary	Rash, pruritus, urticaria, thrombophlebitis at intravenous site
Other	Hearing loss, tinnitus

Adverse Effects

The older macrolide products, primarily erythromycin formulations, have many adverse effects. Most affect the GI tract, although the two newest macrolides, azithromycin and clarithromycin, seem to be associated with a lower incidence of these GI tract complications. Reported adverse effects are listed in Table 38-8.

Interactions

There are a number of potential drug interactions with the macrolides. Two properties of macrolides that are the source of many of these interactions are that they are highly protein bound and they are metabolized in the liver. For drugs metabolized in the liver drug, interactions commonly arise from competition between the different drugs for metabolic enzymes, specifically the enzymes known as the *cytochrome P-450 complex.* Such enzymatic effects generally lead to more pronounced drug interactions than does competition for protein binding. The result is a delay in the metabolic clearance of one or more interacting drugs and thus a prolonged and possibly toxic drug effect. Examples of some especially common drugs that compete for hepatic metabolism with the macrolides are carbamazepine, cyclosporine, digoxin, theophylline, and warfarin. When macrolides are given with these drugs the results are enhanced effects and possible toxicity of the latter drugs. Such drug combinations should be avoided when possible. When a macrolide is given together with any of these drugs, the patient should be observed for signs of drug toxicity, and appropriate laboratory measurements (e.g., blood drug levels) should be obtained. Macrolides can also reduce the efficacy of oral contraceptives. Clarithromycin and erythromycin should not be used with moxifloxacin, pimozide, thioridazine, or other drugs that prolong the QTc interval, because malignant dysrhythmias can occur. Concurrent use of simvastatin or lovastatin with clarithromycin or erythromycin is not recommended. Azithromycin is not as prone to such interactions as are the other macrolides, because of its minimal effects on the cytochrome P-450 enzymes.

Dosages

For recommended dosages of selected macrolide antibiotics, see the Dosages table on p. 600.

DRUG PROFILES

Macrolide antibiotics are used to treat a variety of infections. Of the four macrolide drugs currently available, erythromycin has been available the longest and has been the mainstay of treatment for various infections for more than four decades. Azithromycin and clarithromycin have fewer adverse effects and a better pharmacokinetics profile than older drugs. Dirithromycin is less commonly used.

Macrolide use is contraindicated in patients with known drug allergy. Because these drugs are significantly protein bound and are metabolized in the liver, they may interact with other drugs that are also highly protein bound or hepatically metabolized.

◆ erythromycin

Erythromycin, which goes by many product names, was for many years the most commonly prescribed macrolide antibiotic. However, other macrolides are now more commonly used. The drug is available in several different salt and dosage forms for oral use that were developed to circumvent some of the drawbacks it has chemically. An injectable form is also available for IV use. Erythromycin is also

DOSAGES

Selected Macrolides

Drug (Pregnancy Category)	Pharmacologic Class	Usual Dosage Range	Indications
◆ azithromycin (Zithromax) (B)	Semisynthetic macrolide	**Adult** PO: 500 mg × 1 dose, then 250 mg daily × 4 days IV: 250-500 mg × 1 dose, then PO: 250-500 mg × 3-7 days depending on the infection **Pediatric** PO: 5-12 mg/kg once a day × 4 days or as 30 mg/kg single dose (max dose 500 mg) IV: 10 mg/kg × 1 day then 5 mg/kg/day × 4 days	Comparable to those for erythromycin, but especially GU and respiratory tract infections, including MAC infections
◆ clarithromycin (Biaxin) (C)	Semisynthetic macrolide	**Adult** PO: 500 mg twice daily **Pediatric** PO: 7.5 mg/kg twice daily (max 500 mg/dose)	Comparable to those for erythromycin, but especially GU and respiratory tract infections, including MAC infections
◆ erythromycin (E-mycin, EryPed, Eryc, E.E.S., many others) (B)	Natural macrolide	**Adult*** PO: 250-500 mg qid **Pediatric*** 30-100 mg/kg/day divided qid	Infections of respiratory and GI tracts and skin caused by various gram-positive, gram-negative, and miscellaneous organisms

GI, Gastrointestinal; *GU,* genitourinary; *IV,* intravenous; *MAC, Mycobacterium avium-intracellulare* complex; PO, oral.
*There are many dosage forms, and dosages may vary from those listed.

available in topical forms for dermatologic use (see Chapter 56) and in ophthalmic dosage forms (see Chapter 57). The absorption of oral erythromycin is enhanced if it is taken on an empty stomach, but because of the high incidence of stomach irritation associated with its use, many of these drugs are taken with a meal or snack.

◆ azithromycin and clarithromycin

Azithromycin (Zithromax) and clarithromycin (Biaxin) are semisynthetic macrolide antibiotics that differ structurally from erythromycin and as a result have advantages over it. These include better adverse effect profiles, including less GI tract irritation, and more favorable pharmacokinetic properties. Both have very similar spectra of activity that differ only slightly from that of erythromycin. The two drugs are used for the treatment of both upper and lower respiratory tract and skin structure infections.

Azithromycin has excellent tissue penetration, so that it can reach high concentrations in infected tissues. It also has a long duration of action, which allows it to be dosed once daily. It is usually given in a regimen of 500 mg on day 1 and then 250 mg daily for four days. Taking the drug with food decreases both the rate and extent of GI absorption. The drug is available in oral and injectable forms.

Clarithromycin is given orally twice daily in adults and children older than 6 months of age. It can be given with or without food. The extended-release preparation should not be crushed.

PHARMACOKINETICS (AZITHROMYCIN)

Route	Onset of Action	Peak Plasma Concentration	Elimination Half-life	Duration of Action
PO	Variable	2.5-4 hr	60-70 hr	Up to 24 hr

PHARMACOKINETICS (CLARITHROMYCIN)

Route	Onset of Action	Peak Plasma Concentration	Elimination Half-life	Duration of Action
PO	Variable	2-4 hr	3-7 hr	Up to 12 hr

KETOLIDES

Telithromycin (Ketek) is currently the only drug in a new class known as *ketolides*. It is derived from erythromycin A and has better acid stability and better antibacterial coverage than the macrolides. Its mechanism of action is also similar to that of the macrolides. However, telithromycin has been associated with severe liver damage, and its use is very limited.

TETRACYCLINES

The tetracyclines are bacteriostatic drugs that inhibit bacterial protein synthesis by binding to the 30S bacterial ribosome. The three naturally occurring tetracyclines are demeclocycline, oxytetracycline, and tetracycline. The two semisynthetic tetracyclines are doxycycline and minocycline. The newest tetracycline antibiotic is tigecycline (Tygacil). Tigecycline is indicated for skin and soft tissue infections, intraabdominal infections, and pneumonia. It is effective against many resistant bacteria. The available tetracycline antibiotics are listed in Box 38-1.

Tetracyclines are chemically and pharmacologically similar to one another. The most significant chemical characteristic of these drugs is their ability to bind to (chelate) divalent (Ca^{++}, Mg^{++}) and trivalent (Al^{+++}) metallic ions to form insoluble complexes. Therefore, their coadministration with milk, antacids, or iron salts causes a considerable reduction in the oral absorption of the tetracycline. In addition, their strong affinity for calcium usually precludes their use in pediatric patients younger than 8 years of age, because it can result in significant tooth discoloration. These drugs should also be avoided in pregnant women and nursing mothers. The drugs do pass into breast milk, and this can be another route of exposure leading to tooth discoloration in nursing children.

Tetracyclines primarily differ from one another in the following ways:

- *Oral absorption:* All except tigecycline are adequately absorbed, but doxycycline and minocycline have the best absorption.
- *Body tissue penetration:* Doxycycline and minocycline possess the best penetration potential (brain and cerebrospinal fluid).
- *Half-life and resulting dosage schedule:* See the Dosages table on p. 602 and pharmacokinetics information in the Drug Profiles section.

Mechanism of Action and Drug Effects

Tetracyclines work by inhibiting protein synthesis in susceptible bacteria. They inhibit the growth of and kill a very wide range of *Rickettsia, Chlamydia,* and *Mycoplasma* organisms, as well as a variety of gram-negative and gram-positive bacteria. They are also useful in the treatment of spirochetal infections, such as syphilis and Lyme disease, and pelvic inflammatory disease. Demeclocycline possesses a unique drug effect in that it inhibits the action of antidiuretic hormone, which makes it useful in the treatment of the syndrome of inappropriate secretion of antidiuretic hormone (SIADH).

Indications

Tetracyclines have a wide range of activity, and all drugs in this class are effective against essentially the same spectrum of microbes. They inhibit the growth of many gram-negative and gram-positive organisms and even of some protozoans. Traditionally used to treat acne in adolescents and adults, they are also considered the drugs of choice for the treatment of the following infections caused by susceptible organisms:

- *Chlamydia:* lymphogranuloma venereum, psittacosis, and nonspecific endocervical, rectal, and urethral infections
- *Mycoplasma: Mycoplasma* pneumonia
- *Rickettsia:* Q fever, rickettsial pox, Rocky Mountain spotted fever, and typhus
- *Other bacteria:* acne, brucellosis, chancroid, cholera, granuloma inguinale, shigellosis, spirochetal relapsing fever, Lyme disease, *H. pylori* infections associated with peptic ulcer disease (used as part of the treatment regimen), syphilis (used as an alternative drug to treat patients with penicillin allergy); tetracyclines are now unreliable in treating gonorrhea due to the development of resistant bacterial strains
- *Protozoa:* balantidiasis

Contraindications

The only usual contraindication is known drug allergy. However, tetracyclines should be avoided in pregnant and nursing women and should not be given to children younger than 8 years of age.

Adverse Effects

All tetracyclines cause similar adverse effects. They can cause discoloration of the permanent teeth and tooth enamel hypoplasia in both fetuses and children and possibly retard fetal skeletal development if taken during pregnancy. Other clinically significant undesirable effects include photosensitivity, which is most frequent in patients taking demeclocycline; alteration of the intestinal and vaginal flora, which can result in diarrhea or vaginal candidiasis; reversible bulging fontanelles in neonates; thrombocytopenia, possible coagulation irregularities, and hemolytic anemia; and exacerbation of systemic lupus erythematosus. Other effects include gastric upset, enterocolitis, and maculopapular rash.

Interactions

There are several significant drug interactions associated with the use of tetracyclines. When tetracyclines are taken with antacids, antidiarrheal drugs, dairy products, calcium, enteral feedings, or iron preparations, the oral absorption of the tetracycline is reduced. Tetracyclines can potentiate the effects of oral anticoagulants, which necessitates more frequent monitoring of anticoagulant effect and possible dosage adjustment. They can also antagonize the effects of bactericidal antibiotics and oral contraceptives. In addition, depending on the dosage, they can cause blood urea nitrogen levels to be increased.

Dosages

For dosage information for selected tetracyclines, see the Dosages table on p. 602.

DRUG PROFILES

Tetracyclines were one of the first classes of antibiotic capable of providing coverage against a broad spectrum of microorganisms. Their use is contraindicated in patients who have had hypersensitivity reactions to them in the past and in lactating women. Resistance to one tetracycline implies resistance to all tetracyclines.

demeclocycline

Demeclocycline (Declomycin) is a naturally occurring tetracycline antibiotic that is derived from strains of *Streptomyces.* It is used both for its antibacterial action and for its ability to inhibit the action of antidiuretic hormone in SIADH. Demeclocycline has all the characteristics of this class of tetracyclines. It is available only for oral use.

◆ doxycycline

Doxycycline (Doryx) is a semisynthetic tetracycline antibiotic. It is useful in the treatment of rickettsial infections such as Rocky Mountain spotted fever, chlamydial and mycoplasmal infections, spirochetal infections, and many infections with gram-negative organisms. It can also be used for the prevention and treatment of anthrax and malaria. Doxycycline may also be used in the treatment of acne. It is available in both oral and injectable forms.

PHARMACOKINETICS

Route	Onset of Action	Peak Plasma Concentration	Elimination Half-life	Duration of Action
PO	Variable	1.5-4 hr	14-24 hr	Up to 10-12 hr

tigecycline

Tigecycline (Tygacil) is the newest tetracycline, referred to as a *glycylcycline.* It differs from other tetracyclines in that it is effective against many organisms resistant to others in its class. It is indi-

DOSAGES

Selected Tetracyclines

Drug (Pregnancy Category)	Pharmacologic Class	Usual Dosage Range	Indications
demeclocycline (Declomycin) (D)	Tetracycline	**Adult** PO: 150 mg qid or 300 mg bid **Pediatric older than 8 yr*** 7-13 mg/kg divided bid-qid	Infections; provides broad antibacterial coverage, including treatment of skin infections and respiratory, GI, and GU tract infections
♦ doxycycline (Vibramycin, others) (D)	Tetracycline	**Adult** PO: 100 mg bid first day, then 100 mg daily thereafter **Pediatric older than 8 yr*** PO/IV: 2.5 mg/kg/day in 1-2 divided doses, not to exceed 200 mg/day	Comparable to those for demeclocycline
tigecycline (Tygacil) (D)	Glycylcycline	**Adult** IV: 100 mg × 1 then 50 mg q12h	Skin and skin structure infections, MRSA infections, intraabdominal infections

GI, Gastrointestinal; *GU,* genitourinary; *IV,* intravenous; *MRSA,* methicillin-resistant *Staphylococcus aureus; PO,* oral.
*Use of tetracyclines is contraindicated in children younger than 8 yr and in pregnant women because of the risk of significant tooth discoloration in children.

cated for the treatment of complicated skin and skin structure infections caused by susceptible organisms, including MRSA and vancomycin-sensitive *Enterococcus faecalis,* and for the treatment of complicated intraabdominal infections. Tigecycline is given by injection only. Nausea and vomiting are the most common adverse effects, occurring in 20% to 30% of patients.

PHARMACOKINETICS

Route	Onset of Action	Peak Plasma Concentration	Elimination Half-life	Duration of Action
IV	Immediate	Immediate after infusion	27 hr	12 hr

The remaining antibiotic classes are discussed in Chapter 39.

NURSING PROCESS

Assessment

In general, before the administration of any *antibiotic,* it is crucial to gather data regarding a history of or symptoms indicative of hypersensitivity or allergic reactions (from mild reactions with rash, pruritus, or hives to severe reactions with laryngeal edema, bronchospasms, hypotension, and possible cardiac arrest). Further assessment should include determination of the patient's age, weight, baseline vital signs with body temperature, and examination of the results of any laboratory tests that have been ordered, such as liver function studies (AST and ALT levels), kidney function studies (usually BUN and creatinine levels), cardiac function studies (pertinent laboratory tests, electrocardiogram), ultrasonography (if indicated), culture and sensitivity tests, complete blood count (CBC), and platelet and clotting tests. Intake and output measurements should be noted, if appropriate (e.g., more than 30 mL/hr or 600 mL/day). Baseline neurologic assessment findings are important to note because of the possibility of CNS adverse effects. Bowel sounds and patterns should be assessed because of potential antibiotic-related GI tract adverse effects. An assessment for contraindica-

tions, cautions, and drug interactions should also be carried out, and a complete list of all medications, including over-the-counter drugs, herbals, and dietary supplements, should be obtained. Cultural assessment is also important because of the well-documented variations in responses among different racial and ethnic groups as well as some patients' use of folk remedies or alternative therapies to try to alleviate infections. Learning preparedness, willingness to learn, and educational level should be assessed because of the importance of patient education to safe medication administration. Baseline findings from assessment of the oral mucosa, respiratory tract, GI tract, and genitourinary tract should be noted, because of the risk of superinfection in these areas. Superinfections are often evidenced by fever, lethargy, mouth sores, perineal itching, and other system-related symptoms (see earlier discussion). Because antibiotic resistance is so prevalent, questions about long-term use, overuse, or abuse of antibiotics should be posed to the patient or caregiver. Assessment information related to each group of antibiotics is presented in the following paragraphs.

For patients taking *sulfonamides,* a careful assessment for drug allergies to sulfa-type drugs, such as oral sulfonylureas (antidiabetic drugs) and thiazide diuretics, is critical to patient safety. A thorough skin assessment during drug therapy is also important because of the potential for occurrence of the adverse effect of Stevens-Johnson syndrome. Red blood cell counts are usually assessed before beginning sulfonamide therapy because of the possibility of drug-related anemias. Renal function should also be determined because of the potential for drug-related crystalluria.

With *penicillins,* because of the high incidence of hypersensitivity, drug allergies should be determined before initiation of therapy. In addition, the patient should be assessed for a history of asthma, sensitivity to multiple allergens, aspirin allergy, and sensitivity to cephalosporins, because these are associated with a higher risk for penicillin allergy. If procaine penicillin is to be given, also assess for procaine hypersensitivity. Hepatic and renal functioning should also be assessed. Results of culture and sen-

CASE STUDY

Antibiotic Therapy

© Arvind Balaraman

Mr. G. has been a resident of an assisted care facility since experiencing a left-sided stroke 5 years ago. Presently his cardiovascular status and cerebrovascular status are stable. However, he has had a productive cough and a low-grade fever for 2 days. After physical assessment and chest radiographic examination, the prescriber diagnoses pneumonia of the left lower lobe of the lung. The prescriber instructs that a sputum specimen be obtained and orders intravenous piperacillin/tazobactam (Zosyn) 2.25 g every 8 hours and oral theophylline (Theo-Dur) 300 mg every 12 hours. Mr. G. also takes warfarin (Coumadin) 2 mg every evening. Maalox 30 mL has been ordered as needed for gastrointestinal upset, and oral ibuprofen 400 mg can be given as needed for pain. The prescriber also asks the nurse to start the antibiotic "as soon as possible."

1. Explain the rationale behind the use of tazobactam with piperacillin in the Zosyn.
2. Which order should the nurse execute first? Explain.
3. What concerns or drug interactions should the nurse be aware of with the use of Zosyn and the other medications ordered for Mr. G.?
4. What parameters should be monitored to determine whether the Zosyn is working? Explain your answer.

For answers, see *http://evolve.elsevier.com/Lilley.*

sitivity testing should be noted as soon as they are available. Because of possible CNS and/or GI adverse effects, a thorough neurologic, abdominal, and bowel assessment should be completed. Especially important for patients with electrolyte disturbances, cardiac disease, and/or renal disease would be assessment of serum sodium and potassium levels, primarily because of the high sodium and potassium ion concentrations in some penicillin preparations. For example, penicillin G contains 1.7 mEq of potassium ion per million units and 2 mEq of sodium ion per million units (see Table 38-5). With these particular preparations, if a patient has heart failure, fluid overload, or cardiac dysrhythmias, then a high sodium or potassium level (hypernatremia or hyperkalemia) can lead to exacerbation of these problems. With any dosage form of the penicillins, it is important to patient safety to assess for the possibility of an immediate, accelerated, or delayed allergic reaction. The nurse must also remember that a small percentage of patients taking penicillins may develop serious superinfections as well as colitis; therefore, thorough bowel and GI tract assessment for this potential complication should be ongoing.

Carbapenems are similar to penicillins, and thus assessment for allergy to the penicillin group (see previous discussion on penicillins) is needed. Assessment for neurologic functioning and the presence of any seizure disorders is needed because of the possibility of CNS adverse effects such as tremors and seizures. A thorough assessment of the abdomen and GI tract functioning is required because of potential drug-related exacerbation of diarrhea, nausea, and vomiting.

With *cephalosporins,* thorough assessment of allergies, including allergy to penicillins, is required because of possible cross-sensitivity. Baseline vital sign values, CBC, bleeding and clotting times, as well as results of renal and hepatic function tests should be assessed and monitored, as ordered. Assessment for severe diarrhea, bloody stools, and abdominal pain is needed in patients taking this group of drugs due to adverse effects. It is also important to obtain information about the specific drug and to note the generation of cephalosporins to which it belongs, because each of the five drug generations has distinctive adverse effects and/or complications in addition to commonalities with the other groups.

With *tetracyclines,* culture and sensitivity reports should be assessed carefully, as appropriate. In patients with preexisting kidney or liver disease, results of renal and liver function tests are needed. There is also concern regarding the use of these drugs in patients younger than 8 years of age because of the problem of permanent mottling and discoloration of the teeth. Use of these drugs in pregnancy may also pose problems for the fetus. Assessment for any whitish sore patches on the oral mucosa (due to candidiasis or yeast infection) as well as any vaginal itching, pain, and/or cottage cheese–like discharge (due to vaginal candidiasis) is important for early identification and early treatment of superinfections (see previous discussion).

With *macrolides,* assessment of baseline cardiac function (because of the risk of exacerbation of heart disease) and a thorough assessment of renal and liver function may help to identify adverse effects early in therapy. Drug interactions have been discussed previously, but special consideration should be given to concurrent use of a macrolide and warfarin. These drugs, when given together, may alter clotting ability, so platelet counts and results of clotting studies (e.g., international normalized ratio, prothrombin time, partial thromboplastin time) must be examined. In addition, the use of antibiotics with oral contraceptives is always a concern, because it may lead to contraceptive failure.

Antiseptics and disinfectants have been put in this chapter because they are appropriate given the chapter content. See Box 38-2 for a brief summary of nursing-related considerations for these agents.

Nursing Diagnoses

- Risk for infection related to the patient's compromised immune status before treatment due to bacterial invasion
- Risk for injury (compromised organ function) related to the adverse effects of medications (e.g., anemias, hepatic and renal toxicity) and the weakened physical state
- Acute pain related to infection and adverse reaction to medications
- Deficient knowledge related to lack of information about the disease process and the medication regimen
- Noncompliance with the treatment regimen related to lack of information and/or inability to pay for and obtain the necessary medication

Planning
Goals

- Patient remains free of the signs and symptoms of infection once therapy is completed.
- Patient experiences minimal adverse effects as well as full therapeutic effects of antibiotic therapy.

- Patient remains compliant with the antibiotic therapy regimen for the full duration of treatment.
- Patient experiences improvement in any discomfort or pain related to the infection.
- Patient remains informed about the drug therapy as well as about other treatment modalities and/or alternative therapies.
- Patient returns to the prescriber for follow-up visits as recommended.

Outcome Criteria

- Patient states the signs and symptoms of an infection or its worsening, such as fever, pain, malaise, chills, joint pain, and increase in site-related symptoms.
- Patient describes improvement in the body's response to a resolving infection with subsequent increase in energy level and ability to carry out the activities of daily living.
- Patient states the adverse effects of antibiotic therapy, such as GI upset, nausea, and diarrhea (specific to each class) and indicates which adverse effects to report to the prescriber, such as severe GI symptoms, jaundice (yellowish discoloration of skin and sclera), and severe skin rashes.
- Patient implements actions to minimize the GI distress and other adverse effects associated with antibiotic therapy, such as forcing fluids and eating dairy products like yogurt and buttermilk, as appropriate.

- Patient experiences increased periods of comfort related to a resolving infectious process.
- Patient keeps all follow-up appointments and takes appropriate measures after completing antibiotic therapy, as explained by the prescriber.

Implementation

General nursing interventions that apply to antibiotics include the following: (1) Giving oral antibiotics within the recommended time frames and fluids/foods as indicated. (2) All medication should be taken as ordered and in full and around the clock to maintain effective blood levels unless otherwise instructed by the prescriber. (3) Doses should not be omitted or doubled up. (4) Oral antibiotics should not be given at the same time as antacids, calcium supplements, iron products, laxatives containing magnesium, or some of the antilipemic drugs (see pharmacology listing of drug interactions). (5) Herbal products and dietary supplements should be used only if they do not interact with the antibiotic. (6) Continual monitoring for hypersensitivity reactions past the initial assessment phase because immediate reactions may not occur for up to 30 minutes; accelerated reactions may occur within 1 to 72 hours, and delayed responses may occur after 72 hours. These are characterized by wheezing; shortness of breath; swelling of the face, tongue, or hands; itching; or rash. (7) If there are signs of a possible hypersensitivity reaction, the first thing the nurse should do is stop the dosage form immediately (if IV, stop the infusion), contact the prescriber, and monitor the patient closely.

Sulfonamides should always be taken as directed and with forcing of fluids (2000 to 3000 mL/24 hr) to prevent drug-related crystalluria. Oral dosage forms should be taken with food to minimize GI upset. It is also important to encourage patients to immediately report the following to the prescriber: worsening abdominal cramps, stomach pain, diarrhea, blood in the urine, severe or worsening rash, shortness of breath, and fever.

With *penicillins,* as with other antibiotics, the natural flora in the GI tract may be killed off by the antibiotic. Unaffected GI bacteria such as *C. difficile* may overgrow (see pharmacology discussion for more information). This process may be prevented by the consumption of probiotics, such as products containing lactobacillus, supplements, or cultured dairy products like yogurt, buttermilk, and kefir. Kefir is prepared using milk from sheep, goats, and cows. Soy milk kefirs are now also commercially available. The following are important when various penicillin formulations are given: (1) Take oral penicillins with at least 6 oz of water (not juices); No juices because acidic fluids nullify the drug's antibacterial action. (2) Penicillin V, amoxicillin, and amoxicillin/clavulanate should be taken with water 1 hour before or 2 hours to maximize absorption; however, because of GI upset, it may need to be taken with a snack or meals. (3) Procaine and benzathine salt penicillins are thick solutions that should be administered as ordered; they should be given IM using at least a 21-gauge needle and into a large muscle mass with rotation of sites as needed. (4) IM imipenem/cilastatin should be reconstituted in sterile saline, with plain lidocaine—as ordered and if the patient has no allergy to it—and given into a large muscle mass. (5) With IV penicillins (e.g., ampicillin), as with any IV therapy, the proper diluent should be used and the medication infused over the recommended time. The IV rate and site should be checked (check site for swelling, tendernesss, heat, redness, and pain) and changed, as appropriate. (6) Check for compatabilities of IV fluids and drugs prior to infusion. (7) Should the patient experience an anaphylactic reaction to a penicillin, epinephrine and other emergency drugs should be given as ordered and supportive treatment (e.g., oxygen) available at all times.

Orally administered *cephalosporins* should be given with food to decrease GI upset. Alcohol and alcohol-containing products should be avoided due to the potentiation of a disulfiram-like reaction with some of the cephalosporins. With the newer cephalosporins, as with many drug groups, the nurse must check the drug names carefully to ensure patient safety, because many drug names sound alike, and this can lead to medication errors. Cephalosporin use may also predispose the patient to colitis, especially if preexisting GI disease is documented.

Tetracyclines cause photosensitivity, so precautions should be taken to avoid sun exposure and tanning bed use. Oral doses should be given with at least 8 oz of fluids and food to minimize GI upset. However, tetracyclines should *not* be given with dairy products, antacids, sodium bicarbonate, kaolin or pectin, or iron, because these chelate or bind with the antibiotic and decrease the antibiotic effect. These interacting foods and drugs may be given 2 hours before or 3 hours after the tetracycline to avoid this inter-

action. IV doxycycline is very irritating to the veins, and the IV infusion site should be checked frequently. Patients should be encouraged to report abdominal pain, nausea, vomiting, visual changes, and/or jaundice.

Macrolides should be administered with the same precautions as other antibiotics. Macrolides should *not* be given with or immediately before or after fruit juices to avoid interaction with the drug. The patient should be informed about the many drug interactions (discussed in the pharmacology section of this chapter), including those with over-the-counter drugs, herbal products, and dietary supplements. Patients should report severe rash, itching, hives, difficulty swallowing, jaundice, dark urine, and/or pale stools to their prescriber immediately.

Evaluation

Evaluation should include monitoring of goals, outcome criteria, and therapeutic effects and adverse effects. Therapeutic effects of *antibiotics* include a decrease in the signs and symptoms of the infection; a return to normal vital signs, including temperature, and negative results on culture and sensitivity tests; normal results for CBC; and improved appetite, energy level, and sense of well-being. Evaluation for adverse effects includes monitoring for specific drug-related adverse effects (see each drug profile).

PATIENT TEACHING TIPS

- Provide patient with a list of foods and beverages that may interact negatively with antibiotics, such as alcohol, acidic fruit juices, and dairy products.
- Advise patient to report severe adverse effects to the prescriber and to keep any follow-up visits so that the effectiveness of therapy monitored. Laboratory tests (e.g., CBC) may also be performed at these visits. Foods that may help prevent superinfections (e.g., vaginal yeast infections) include yogurt, buttermilk, and kefir (see earlier discussion). New yogurts, termed *probiotics*, are available for re-establishing the natural flora of the GI tract.
- Educate patients who are taking oral contraceptives for birth control, about the interactions between them and certain antibiotics. This is because effectiveness of oral contraceptives may be decreased with certain antibiotics. Back-up methods of contraception are encouraged.
- A medical alert bracelet or necklace should be worn at all times providing access to a list of medications, drug allergies, and medical diagnoses. This information should also be kept on a written card carried on the patient's person at all times.
- For *sulfonamides,* the medication should be taken with plenty of fluids (2000 to 3000 mL/24 hr) to prevent drug-related crystalluria or precipitate formation in the kidneys. These drugs should also be taken with food to decrease GI adverse effects. Worsening abdominal cramps, stomach pain, diarrhea, blood in the urine, severe or worsening rash, shortness of breath, or fever should be reported to the prescriber immediately.

- For *penicillins,* medication should be taken exactly as prescribed and for the full duration indicated (as for all antibiotics), with doses spaced at regularly scheduled intervals. Oral dosage forms are to be taken with water, and the following beverages should be avoided: caffeine-containing beverages, citrus fruit, cola beverages, fruit juices, and tomato juice (decrease effectiveness of the antibiotic). If the patient must take a penicillin drug four times a day, the patient should set up a reminder system (with cell phone alarms or a watch) so that blood levels remain steady. For *cephalosporins,* the patient should be told to report diarrhea, flulike symptoms, blistering or peeling of the skin, hearing loss, breathing difficulty, or seizures to the prescriber immediately. Foul-smelling, loose, frequent, and/or bloody stools should also be reported.
- For *tetracyclines,* advise patients to avoid exposure to tanning beds and direct sunlight or to use sunscreen and/or wear protective clothing because of drug-related photosensitivity. These photosensitive effects may be noticed within a few minutes to hours after taking the drug and may last up to several days after the drug has been discontinued.
- For *macrolides,* the patient should take the drug as directed and should check for interactions with other drugs being taken at the same time, especially interactions between erythromycin and other medications. For some drugs in this class (e.g., azithromycin), newer dosage forms are available in 3-day and even 1-day dose packs rather than the 5-day dose pack. The nurse should always be sure that the patient knows the proper dosage and instructions for the drug the patient is taking.

- Antibiotics are either bacteriostatic or bactericidal. Bacteriostatic antibiotics inhibit the growth of bacteria but do not directly kill them. Bactericidal antibiotics directly kill the bacteria.
- Most antibiotics work by inhibiting bacterial cell wall synthesis in some way. Bacteria have survived over the ages because they can adapt to their surroundings. If a bacterium's environment includes an antibiotic, over time it can mutate in such a way that it can survive an attack by the antibiotic. The production of beta-lactamases is one way in which bacteria can fend off the effects of antibiotics.
- Nurses need to be aware of the most common adverse effects of antibiotics, which include nausea, vomiting, and diarrhea. Nurses

should inform patients that antibiotics should be taken for the prescribed length of time.
- Each class of antibiotics is associated with specific cautions, contraindications, drug interactions, and adverse effects that must be carefully assessed for and monitored by the nurse.
- Because normally occurring bacteria are killed during antibiotic therapy, superinfections may arise during treatment. These may be manifested by the following signs and symptoms: fever, perineal itching, oral lesions, vaginal irritation and discharge, cough, and lethargy.

NCLEX EXAMINATION REVIEW QUESTIONS

1 A patient is scheduled for colorectal surgery tomorrow. He does not have sepsis, his WBC count is normal, he has no fever, and he is otherwise in good health. However, there is an order to administer an antibiotic on call before he goes to surgery. The nurse knows that the rationale for this antibiotic order is to
   a provide empiric therapy.
   b provide prophylactic therapy.
   c treat for a superinfection.
   d reduce the number of resistant organisms.
2 A teenaged patient is taking a tetracycline drug as part of treatment for severe acne. When the nurse teaches this patient about drug-related precautions, which is the most important information to convey?
   a When the acne clears up, the medication may be discontinued.
   b This medication should be taken with antacids to reduce GI upset.
   c The patient should use sunscreen or avoid exposure to sunlight, because this drug may cause photosensitivity.
   d The teeth should be observed closely for signs of mottling or other color changes.
3 A newly admitted patient reports a penicillin allergy. The prescriber has ordered a second-generation cephalosporin as part of the therapy. Which of the nursing actions below is appropriate?
   a Call the prescriber to clarify the order because of the patient's allergy.
   b Give the medication and monitor for adverse effects.
   c Ask the pharmacy to change the order to a first-generation cephalosporin.
   d Administer the drug with an nonsteroidal antiinflammatory to reduce adverse effects.

4 During patient education regarding an oral macrolide such as erythromycin, the nurse should include which information?
   a If GI upset occurs, the drug will have to be stopped.
   b The drug should be taken with an antacid to avoid GI problems.
   c The patient should take each dose with a sip of water.
   d The patient may take the drug with a small snack to reduce GI irritation.
5 A woman who has been taking an antibiotic for a UTI calls the nurse practitioner to complain of severe vaginal itching. She has also noticed a thick, whitish vaginal discharge. The nurse practitioner suspects that
   a this is an expected response to antibiotic therapy.
   b the UTI has become worse instead of better.
   c a superinfection has developed.
   d the UTI is resistant to the antibiotic.
6 The nurse is reviewing the orders for wound care, which include use of an antiseptic. Which statements best describe the use of antiseptics? (Select all that apply.)
   a Antiseptics are appropriate for use on living tissue.
   b Antiseptics work by sterilizing the surface of the wound.
   c Antiseptics are applied to nonliving objects to kill microorganisms.
   d The patient's allergies should be assessed before using the antiseptic.
   e Antiseptics are used to inhibit the growth of microorganisms on the wound surface.

1. b, 2. c, 3. a, 4. d, 5. c, 6. a, d, e.

CRITICAL THINKING ACTIVITIES: BEST ACTION

1 The nurse is reviewing the medications that are due this morning for a patient and notes the following orders:
   doxycycline, 200 mg, by mouth (PO) every morning
   Multivitamin with iron, 1 tablet, PO every morning
   Mylanta, 30 mL, twice a day PO
   What is the nurse's best action regarding how these medications are given?
2 The nurse is reviewing the orders for a patient who has been admitted for treatment of pneumonia. The antibiotic orders include an order for penicillin. However, when the patient is asked

about his allergies, he lists "penicillin" as one of his allergies. What should be the next action of the nurse?
3 A 79-year-old patient has been admitted for treatment of osteomyelitis. His orders include IV imipenem/cilastatin, oral lisinopril, oral phenytoin, and a prn order for acetaminophen for a temperature over 101° F (38.3° C) or for pain. The nurse is reviewing the patient's history and new orders. After reviewing the orders, what is the first action the nurse should take?

For answers, see *http://evolve.elsevier.com/Lilley*.

CHAPTER 39

Antibiotics Part 2

OBJECTIVES

When you reach the end of this chapter, you should be able to do the following:

1. Review the general principles of antibiotic therapy and review all of the antibiotics covered previously in Chapter 38 in preparation for discussion of the following antibiotics or antibiotic classes: aminoglycosides, quinolones, clindamycin, metronidazole, nitrofurantoin, vancomycin, and several other miscellaneous antibiotics.

2. Describe the advantages and disadvantages associated with the use of antibiotics, including overuse and abuse of antibiotics, development of drug resistance, superinfections, and antibiotic-associated colitis.

3. Discuss the indications, cautions, contraindications, mechanisms of action, adverse effects, toxic effects, routes of administration, and drug interactions for the aminoglycosides, fluoroquinolones, clindamycin, metronidazole, nitrofurantoin, vancomycin, and miscellaneous antibiotics.

4. Develop a nursing care plan that includes all phases of the nursing process for the patient receiving antibiotics.

---

e-Learning Activities

NCLEX Review Questions • Animations • Nursing Care Plans • Audio Glossary • Category Catchers • Medication Errors Checklists • IV Therapy Checklists • Calculators • Frequently Asked Questions • Content Updates • Supplemental Resources • Answers to Case Studies and Critical Thinking Activities

Drug Profiles

amikacin, p. 610
♦ ciprofloxacin, p. 613
♦ clindamycin, p. 613
colistimethate, p. 616
daptomycin, p. 616
♦ gentamicin, p. 610
levofloxacin, p. 613

linezolid, p. 614
♦ metronidazole, p. 615
neomycin, p. 611
nitrofurantoin, p. 615
quinupristin/dalfopristin, p. 615
tobramycin, p. 611
♦ vancomycin, p. 615

♦ *Key drug.*

Glossary

Concentration-dependent killing A property of some antibiotics, especially aminoglycosides, whereby achieving a relatively high plasma drug concentration, even if briefly, results in the most effective bacterial kill (compare *time-dependent killing*). (p. 608)

Extended-spectrum beta-lactamases (ESBLs) A group of beta-lactamase enzymes produced by some organisms that makes the organism resistant to all beta-lactam antibiotics (penicillins and cephalosporins) and aztreonam. Patients infected by such organisms must be in contact isolation, and proper hand washing is key to preventing the spread of the infections. (p. 608)

***Klebsiella pneumoniae* carbapenemase (KPC)** An enzyme first found in isolates of the bacterium *Klebsiella pneumoniae* that renders the organism resistant to all carbapenem antibiotics as well as beta-lactam antibiotics and monobactams. Such organisms produce a very serious resistant infection. (p. 608)

Methicillin-resistant *Staphylococcus aureus* (MRSA) A strain of *Staphylococcus aureus* that is resistant to the beta-lactamase penicillin known as methicillin. Originally, the abbreviation *MRSA* referred exclusively to methicillin-resistant *S. aureus*. It is now used more commonly to refer to strains of *S. aureus* that are resistant to several drug classes, and therefore, depending on the context or health facility, it may also stand for "multidrug-resistant *S. aureus*." (p. 608)

Microgram One millionth of a gram. Be careful not to confuse with milligram (one thousandth of a gram), which is a thousand times greater than 1 microgram. Confusion of these two units sometimes results in drug dosage errors. (p. 609)

Minimum inhibitory concentration (MIC) A laboratory measure of the lowest concentration of a drug needed to kill a certain standardized amount of bacteria. (p. 609)

Multidrug-resistant organisms Bacteria that are resistant to one or more classes of antimicrobial drugs. These include multidrug-resistant *Staphylococcus aureus*, extended-spectrum beta-lactamase–producing organisms, and *Klebsiella pneumoniae* carbapenemase–producing organisms. All are discussed in this chapter. (p. 608)

Nephrotoxicity Toxicity to the kidneys, often drug induced and manifesting as compromised renal function. (p. 609)

Ototoxicity Toxicity to the ears, often drug induced and manifesting as varying degrees of hearing loss that is more likely to be permanent than the impaired renal function resulting from nephrotoxicity. (p. 609)

Postantibiotic effect A period of continued bacterial suppression that occurs after brief exposure to certain antibiotic drug classes, especially aminoglycosides and carbapenems (see Chapter 38). The mechanism of this effect is uncertain. (p. 609)

Pseudomembranous colitis A necrotizing inflammatory bowel condition that is often associated with antibiotic therapy. Some antibiotics (e.g., clindamycin) are more likely to produce it than others. A more general term that is also used is *antibiotic-associated colitis*. (p. 614)

Synergistic effect Drug interaction in which the bacterial killing effect of two antibiotics given together is greater than the sum of the individual effects of the same drugs given alone. (p. 609)

Therapeutic drug monitoring Ongoing monitoring of plasma drug concentrations and dosage adjustment based on these values as well as other laboratory indicators such as kidney and liver function test results; it is often carried out by a pharmacist in collaboration with medical, nursing, and laboratory staff. (p. 608)

Time-dependent killing A property of most antibiotic classes whereby prolonged high plasma drug concentrations are required for effective bacterial kill (compare *concentration-dependent killing*). (p. 608)

Vancomycin-resistant *Enterococcus* (VRE) *Enterococcus* species that are resistant to beta-lactam antibiotics and vancomycin. Most commonly refers to *Enterococcus faecium*. (p. 608)

• • •

This chapter is a continuation of Chapter 38 and focuses on additional classes of antibiotics. Chapter 39 describes the various antibiotics that are used for more serious and harder-to-treat infections. Many of the drugs discussed in this chapter are given by the *parenteral* (injection) route only, a route generally reserved for treating more clinically serious infections in the hospital setting. Also included are miscellaneous drugs that are unique in their class, as well as newer drugs and drug classes. This chapter also focuses on multidrug-resistant organisms, specifically **methicillin-resistant** *Staphylococcus aureus* (MRSA), **vancomycin-resistant** *Enterococcus* (VRE), organisms producing **extended-spectrum beta-lactamases (ESBLs),** and organisms producing *Klebsiella pneumoniae* **carbapenemase (KPC).**

MULTIDRUG RESISTANCE

Organisms that are resistant to one or more classes of antimicrobial drugs are referred to as **multidrug-resistant organisms.** These include MRSA, VRE, and ESBL- and KPC-producing organisms. MRSA has been around for many years, and new antibiotics have been developed to treat MRSA. However, the threat that MRSA will become resistant to all antibiotics currently available is all too real. MRSA is no longer seen just in hospitals; it has spread to the community setting, and approximately 50% of staphylococcal infections contracted in the community involve MRSA, depending on location. Local community and hospital MRSA strains vary. VRE is usually seen in urinary tract infections. Some newer antibiotics have been developed to successfully treat VRE, as well as MRSA. ESBL- and KPC-producing bacteria are the newest players in this saga. Organisms that produce ESBL are resistant to all beta-lactam antibiotics and aztreonam, and can be treated only with carbapenems or sometimes quinolones. In the noble effort to treat infection with ESBL-producing organisms, the use of carbapenems increased, and unfortunately in response bacteria created a new means of resistance, namely, the ability to produce KPC. When patients become infected with KPC-producing bacteria, there are only two known antibiotics that can be used, tigecycline and colistimethate. Reports of resistance to these antibiotics have been reported, which leaves the patient untreatable. Multidrug-resistant organisms are one of the world's top health problems. When patients become infected with such an organism, they must be placed in contact isolation. Many hospitals are placing all patients infected with KPC-producing bacteria in one area, and some hospitals have been shut down due to this organism. Proper hand washing is of the utmost importance. These organisms are spread by contact, so all health care professionals must wash their hands before and after all patient contact.

Pharmacology Overview

AMINOGLYCOSIDES

The aminoglycosides are a group of natural and semisynthetic antibiotics that are classified as *bactericidal* drugs (see Chapter 38). They are potent antibiotics, which makes aminoglycosides the drugs of choice for the treatment of particularly virulent infections. The aminoglycoside antibiotics available for clinical use are listed in Table 39-1. These drugs can be given by several different routes, but they are not given orally because of their poor oral absorption. An exception to this is neomycin (see Drug Profiles). The three aminoglycosides most commonly used for the treatment of systemic infections are amikacin, gentamicin, and tobramycin. Serum levels of these drugs are routinely monitored in patients' blood samples. Dosages are then adjusted to maintain known optimal levels that maximize drug efficacy and minimize the risk for toxicity. This process is known as **therapeutic drug monitoring.** Aminoglycoside therapy is commonly monitored in this way due to the nephrotoxicity and ototoxicity associated with these drugs. Most commonly, dosing is adjusted to the patient's level of renal function, based on estimates of creatinine clearance calculated from serum creatinine values. This task is often carried out by a hospital pharmacist, consulting for the prescriber. Not only are serum levels measured to prevent toxicity, but it has been shown that for the aminoglycosides to be effective, the serum level should be at least eight times higher than the **minimum inhibitory concentration (MIC).** The MIC for any antibiotic is a measure of the lowest concentration of drug needed to kill a certain standard amount of bacteria. This value is determined *in vitro* (in the laboratory) for each drug. It has been shown that other classes of antibiotics, such as beta-lactams, act through **time-dependent killing,** that is, the amount of time the drug is above the MIC is critical for maximal bacterial kill. However, aminoglycosides work primarily through **concentration-dependent killing;** that is, achieving a drug plasma concentration that is a certain level above the MIC, even for a brief period of time, results in the most effective bacterial kill. For this reason, although these drugs were originally given in three daily intravenous doses, the current predominant practice is *once-daily aminoglycoside dosing.* Dosages of 5 to 7 mg/kg/day are used. Several clinical studies have shown that once-daily dosing provides a sufficient plasma drug concentration for bacterial kill, along with equal or lower risk for toxicity compared with multiple daily dosing regimens. Use of a once-daily regimen instead of the traditional three-times-daily regimen also reduces the nursing care time required and often allows for outpatient or even home-based aminoglycoside drug therapy.

Peak (highest) drug levels for once-daily regimens are usually not measured it is assumed that the peak level for a single daily dose will be short lived and will drop within a reasonable time frame. However, *trough* (lowest) levels are routinely measured to ensure adequate renal clearance of the drug and avoid toxicity. Dosage information for selected aminoglycosides appears in the Dosages table on p. 611. Dosage regimens and ranges for serum levels may vary for different institutions.

With once-daily dosing, the blood sample for trough measurement should be drawn at least 12 hours after completion of dose administration and closer to 18 hours afterward for renally im-

TABLE 39-1 Aminoglycoside Antibiotics

Serum Drug Levels	Peak		Trough	
	Multiple Daily Dosing*	**Once-Daily Dosing**	**Multiple Daily Dosing**	**Once-Daily Dosing**
amikacin	15-30 mcg/mL†	Usually not measured	5-10 mcg/mL	Less than 10 mcg/mL
gentamicin and tobramycin	4-10 mcg/mL	Usually not measured	1-2 mcg/mL	Less than 1 mcg/mL

*q8h or q12h.

†mcg = **microgram;** note that 1 microgram = $\frac{1}{1000}$ (one thousandth of a) milligram or $\frac{1}{1,000,000}$ (one millionth of a) gram. Also note that microgram is abbreviated *mcg*, while milligram is abbreviated *mg.*

paired patients. The therapeutic goal is a trough concentration at or below 1 mcg/mL (which is considered undetectable). The reason is that trough levels above 2 mcg/mL are associated with greater risk for both **ototoxicity** and **nephrotoxicity.** Ototoxicity (toxicity to the ears) often manifests as some degree of temporary or permanent hearing loss. Nephrotoxicity (toxicity to the kidneys) manifests as varying degrees of reduced renal function. This is generally indicated by results on laboratory tests such as serum creatinine level. A rising serum creatinine level suggests reduced creatinine clearance by the kidneys and is indicative of declining renal function. Trough levels are normally monitored initially then once every 5 to 7 days until the drug therapy is discontinued. The patient's serum creatinine level should also be measured at least every 3 days as an index of renal function, and drug dosages should be adjusted as needed for any changes in renal function.

Traditional dosing of aminoglycosides (i.e., three times a day) can still be used. When an aminoglycoside is given in this manner, both peak and trough levels are measured. Samples for measurement of peak levels are drawn 30 minutes after a 30-minute infusion, and samples for measurement of trough levels are drawn just before the next dose. Pharmacists can adjust the dose based on a pharmacokinetic evaluation of these levels. When the drug is given in the traditional manner, the desired peak levels vary depending on the type of organism and the site of infection. Higher levels are needed when treating pneumonia, as opposed to treating a urinary tract infection. Because the aminoglycosides are eliminated by the kidney, the drug concentrates in the urine, so lower dosages can be used to treat urinary tract infections. Regardless of the infection being treated, however, it is desirable to keep the trough levels below 2 mcg/mL. Table 39-1 lists the *traditional* desired drug levels for these drugs.

Mechanism of Action and Drug Effects

Aminoglycosides work in a way that is similar to that of the tetracyclines in that they also bind to ribosomes, specifically the 30S ribosome, and thereby prevent protein synthesis in bacteria (see Figure 38-3). Often aminoglycosides are used in combination with other antibiotics such as beta-lactams or vancomycin in the treatment of various infections, because the combined effect of the two antibiotics is greater than the sum of the effects of each drug acting separately. This is known as a **synergistic effect.** When aminoglycosides are used in combination with beta-lactam antibiotics (i.e., penicillins, cephalosporins, monobactams [see Chapter 38]), the beta-lactam antibiotic should be given first. This is because the beta-lactams break down the cell wall of the bacteria and allow the aminoglycoside to gain access to the ribosomes where they work. Aminoglycosides also have a property known as the **postantibiotic**

effect. This is a period of continued bacterial growth suppression that occurs *after* short-term antibiotic exposure, as in once-daily aminoglycoside dosing (see earlier). Carbapenems are another antibiotic class with a postantibiotic effect. The postantibiotic effect is enhanced with higher peak drug concentrations and concurrent use of beta-lactam antibiotics.

As is the case with most antibiotic drug classes, various bacterial mechanisms of resistance to aminoglycosides have emerged among both gram-positive and gram-negative species previously more susceptible to these drugs. The prevalence and strength of such resistance varies for different drugs, organisms, patient populations, disease states, and geographic prescribing patterns.

Indications

The toxicity associated with aminoglycosides normally limits their use to treatment of serious gram-negative infections and specific conditions involving gram-positive cocci, in which case gentamicin is usually given in combination with a penicillin. Gram-negative infections commonly treated with aminoglycosides include those caused by *Pseudomonas* species (spp.) and several organisms belonging to the Enterobacteriaceae family (facultatively anaerobic gram-negative rods), including *Escherichia coli, Proteus* spp., *Klebsiella* spp., and *Serratia* spp. Such infections are often treated with a suitable aminoglycoside and an extended-spectrum penicillin, third-generation cephalosporin, or carbapenem. Gram-positive infections treated with aminoglycosides may include infections due to *Enterococcus* spp. and *S. aureus,* and bacterial endocarditis, which is usually streptococcal in origin. A regimen of three daily doses is more common when treating gram-positive infections, because this often enhances synergy with other antibiotics that are used. Aminoglycosides are never used alone to treat gram-positive infections. Aminoglycosides are also used for prophylaxis in procedures involving the gastrointestinal or genitourinary tract, because such procedures carry high risk for enterococcal bacteremia. They are also commonly given in combination with either ampicillin or vancomycin (for penicillin-allergic patients) to surgical patients with a history of valvular heart disease, because diseased heart valves are also more prone to enterococcal infection.

Aminoglycosides should be administered with caution in premature and full-term neonates. Because of the renal immaturity of these patients, prolonged actions of the aminoglycosides and a greater risk for toxicities may result. Serious pediatric infections for which aminoglycosides are commonly used include pneumonia, meningitis, and urinary tract infections. Drug selection for both pediatric and adult patients is based on the susceptibility of the causative organism. Refer to Table 39-2 for more information

TABLE 39-2 Aminoglycosides: Comparative Spectra of Antimicrobial Activity

Aminoglycoside	Spectrum of Activity
amikacin	*Acinetobacter* spp., *Enterobacter aerogenes*, *Escherichia coli*, *Klebsiella pneumoniae*, *Proteus* spp., *Providencia* spp., *Pseudomonas* spp., *Serratia* spp., *Staphylococcus*
gentamicin	*E. aerogenes*, *E. coli*, *K. pneumoniae*, *Proteus* spp., *Pseudomonas* spp., *Salmonella* spp., *Serratia* spp. (nonpigmented), *Shigella* spp.
neomycin	Toxicity limits use to gastrointestinal tract (hepatic coma, *E. coli* diarrhea, and antisepsis) and as a topical antibacterial
streptomycin	*Klebsiella granulomatis* (granuloma inguinale), *Yersinia pestis* (plague), *Francisella tularensis* (tularemia), *Mycobacterium tuberculosis* (tuberculosis), *Streptococcus* spp. (nonhemolytic endocarditis)
tobramycin	*Citrobacter* spp., *Enterobacter* spp., *E. coli*, *Klebsiella* spp., *Proteus* spp., *Providencia* spp., *P. aeruginosa*, *Serratia* spp.

spp., Species.

on the antibacterial spectra of specific aminoglycosides. A few aminoglycosides have even more specific indications. Streptomycin is active against *Mycobacterium* spp. (see Chapter 41), whereas paromomycin is used to treat amebic dysentery, a protozoal intestinal disease (see Chapter 43). Aminoglycosides are relatively inactive against fungi, viruses, and most anaerobic bacteria.

Contraindications

The only usual contraindication is known drug allergy. The pregnancy categories of these drugs range from C to D. Aminoglycosides have been shown to cross the placenta and cause fetal harm when administered to pregnant women. There have been several case reports of total irreversible bilateral congenital deafness in the children of women receiving aminoglycosides during pregnancy. Therefore, aminoglycosides should be used in pregnant women only in the event of life-threatening infections against which safer drugs are ineffective. These drugs are also distributed in breast milk. Their use should be avoided in lactating women to avoid risk of drug toxicity in nursing infants.

Adverse Effects

Aminoglycosides are very potent antibiotics and are capable of potentially serious toxicities, especially to the kidneys *(nephrotoxicity)* and to the ears *(ototoxicity)*, in which they can affect hearing and balance functions. Duration of drug therapy should be as short as possible, based on sound clinical judgment and monitoring of the patient's progress. Nephrotoxicity typically occurs in 5% to 25% of patients and is usually manifested by urinary casts (visible remnants of destroyed renal cells), proteinuria, and increased blood urea nitrogen (BUN) and serum creatinine levels. It is usually reversible, but the patient's renal function test results should be monitored throughout therapy. In contrast, ototoxicity is less common, occurring in 3% to 14% of patients, and often is not reversible. It can result in varying degrees of perma-

nent hearing loss, depending on the dosage and duration of drug therapy. It is believed to result from injury to the eighth cranial nerve (CN VIII, also called the *cochleovestibular nerve* or *auditory nerve*) and involves both cochlear damage (hearing loss) and vestibular damage (disrupted sense of balance). Symptoms include dizziness, tinnitus, a sense of fullness in the ears, and hearing loss. Other less common effects include headache, paresthesia, vertigo, skin rash, fever, overgrowth of nonsusceptible organisms, and neuromuscular paralysis (very rare and reversible). The risk for these toxicities is greatest in patients with preexisting renal impairment, patients already receiving other renally toxic drugs, and patients receiving high-dose or prolonged aminoglycoside therapy.

Interactions

The risk for nephrotoxicity can be increased with concurrent use of other nephrotoxic drugs such as vancomycin, cyclosporine, and amphotericin B. Concurrent use with loop diuretics increases the risk for ototoxicity. In addition, because aminoglycosides, like many other antibiotics, kill intestinal bacterial flora, they also reduce the amount of vitamin K produced by these gut bacteria. These normal flora normally serve to balance the effects of oral anticoagulants such as warfarin (Coumadin). Therefore, aminoglycosides can potentiate warfarin toxicity. Concurrent use with neuromuscular blocking drugs may prolong the duration of action of the neuromuscular blockade.

Dosages

For recommended dosages of selected aminoglycosides, see the Dosages table on p. 611.

DRUG PROFILES

Historically, the aminoglycoside antibiotics were used primarily to treat gram-negative infections. However, they are now used as a synergistic drug in the treatment of gram-positive infections as well. They are normally given intravenously or intramuscularly, but neomycin is administered only orally, rectally, or topically. Topical dosage forms of both gentamicin and tobramycin are also available for dermatologic (see Chapter 56) and ophthalmic (see Chapter 57) use. Currently available aminoglycosides include amikacin, gentamicin, kanamycin, neomycin, streptomycin, and tobramycin. Dosage and other information appear in the Dosages table on p. 611.

amikacin

Amikacin (Amikin) is a semisynthetic aminoglycoside antibiotic that is often used to treat infections that are resistant to gentamicin or tobramycin. It is available only in injectable form.

PHARMACOKINETICS

Route	Onset of Action	Peak Plasma Concentration	Elimination Half-life	Duration of Action
IV	Variable	1 hr	2-3 hr	8-12 hr
IM	Variable	30 min-2 hr	2-3 hr	8-12 hr

♦ gentamicin

Gentamicin (Garamycin) is one of the most commonly used aminoglycosides in clinical practice today. It can be given either intravenously or intramuscularly, and the dosage is the same for both routes. It is indicated for the treatment of infection with several susceptible gram-positive and gram-negative bacteria. Gentamicin

DOSAGES

Selected Aminoglycosides

Drug (Pregnancy Category)	Usual Dosage Range	Indications/Uses
amikacin (Amikin) (D)	**Adult and pediatric** IV: 15 mg/kg/day divided 2-3 times daily or 15-20 mg/kg once daily **Neonatal*** IV: 10 mg/kg load, then 7.5 mg/kg q12h	Primarily infection with gentamicin- and tobramycin-resistant gram-negative organisms along with severe staphylococcal infections
◆ gentamicin (Garamycin) (C)	**Adult** IV/IM: 2-6 mg/kg/day divided 1-4 times daily or 5-7 mg/kg once daily **Pediatric and neonatal** IV/IM: 2-2.5 mg/kg q8h	Primarily gram-negative infections along with severe staphylococcal infections
neomycin (Neo-Fradin) (C)	**Adult** PO/PR: 3000-9000 mg divided between 3-9 doses **Pediatric†** PO/PR: 90 mg/kg/day q4h × 2 days	Preoperative bowel cleansing (also used with different dosage regimens for hepatic encephalopathy)
tobramycin (Nebcin, TOBI) (D)	**Adult** IV/IM: 3-6 mg/kg/day divided 1-3 times daily or 5-7 mg/kg once daily **Pediatric** IV/IM: 6-7.5 mg/kg/day divided 3-4 times daily **Neonatal*** IV/IM: 3 mg/kg q24h or 2 mg/kg q12h	Primarily gram-negative infections along with severe staphylococcal infections

IM, Intramuscular; *IV*, intravenous; *PO*, oral; *PR*, rectal.
*Dosing and frequency vary depending on age.
†Safe and effective use has not been established by the manufacturer.

is available in several dosage forms, including injections, topical ointments, and ophthalmic drops and ointments.

PHARMACOKINETICS

Route	Onset of Action	Peak Plasma Concentration	Elimination Half-life	Duration of Action
IV	Variable	30 min	2-3 hr	Up to 24 hr
IM	Variable	30-90 min	2-3 hr	Up to 24 hr

tobramycin

Tobramycin (Nebcin) has dosages, routes of administration, and indications that are comparable to those for gentamicin for generalized infections. In addition, it is commonly used to treat recurrent pulmonary infections in patients with cystic fibrosis by both injectable and inhaled dosing. It is also available in topical and ophthalmic dosage forms.

PHARMACOKINETICS

Route	Onset of Action	Peak Plasma Concentration	Elimination Half-life	Duration of Action
IV	Variable	30 min	2-3 hr	Up to 24 hr
IM	Variable	30-90 min	2-3 hr	Up to 24 hr

neomycin

Neomycin (Neo-Fradin) is most commonly used for bacterial decontamination of the gastrointestinal tract before surgical procedures, and it is given both orally and rectally (as an enema) for this purpose. Other uses include topical application for skin infections, bladder irrigation, and treatment of *E. coli* diarrhea, hepatic encephalopathy, and eye infections. In hepatic encephalopathy, the drug helps reduce the number of ammonia-producing bacteria in the gastrointestinal tract. The subsequent reduced blood ammonia levels sometimes result in improvement of neurologic symp-

toms of the hepatic illness. This drug is not available in injectable form but instead is available in tablets, solutions, and powders for oral, topical, or irrigation administration.

PHARMACOKINETICS

Route	Onset of Action	Peak Plasma Concentration	Elimination Half-life	Duration of Action
PO	Variable	1-4 hr	3 hr	Up to 24 hr

QUINOLONES

Quinolones, sometimes referred to as *fluoroquinolones*, are very potent bactericidal broad-spectrum antibiotics. Currently available quinolone antibiotics include norfloxacin, ciprofloxacin, levofloxacin, and moxifloxacin. With the exception of norfloxacin, these antibiotics have excellent oral absorption. In many cases, the extent of oral absorption is comparable to that of intravenous injection.

Mechanism of Action and Drug Effects

Quinolone antibiotics destroy bacteria by altering their deoxyribonucleic acid (DNA) (see Figure 38-3). They accomplish this by interfering with the bacterial enzymes DNA gyrase and topoisomerase IV. Quinolones do not seem to affect the corresponding mammalian enzymes and therefore do not inhibit the production of human DNA.

These drugs kill susceptible strains of mostly gram-negative and some gram-positive organisms. Some quinolones are also believed to diffuse into and concentrate themselves in human neutrophils, killing bacteria such as *S. aureus, Serratia marcescens,* and *Mycobacterium fortuitum* that sometimes accumulate in these cells. Nonetheless, bacterial resistance to quinolone antibiotics has been identified among several bacterial species, including *Pseudomonas aeruginosa, S. aureus, Pneumococcus* spp., *Enterococcus* spp., and the broad Enterobacteriaceae family that includes *E. coli.*

Indications

Quinolones are active against a wide variety of gram-negative and selected gram-positive bacteria. Most are excreted primarily by the kidneys, which contain a high percentage of unchanged drug. This characteristic, together with the fact that they have extensive gram-negative coverage, makes them suitable for treating complicated urinary tract infections. They are also commonly used to treat respiratory, skin, gastrointestinal, bone, and joint infections, and sexually transmitted diseases.

Ciprofloxacin (Cipro) was the first quinolone to enjoy widespread use. Resistance was soon seen in *Pseudomonas* and some *Streptococcus* spp. Ciprofloxacin is available both orally and by injection and is currently the only quinolone available as a generic, which means that it costs significantly less than the other quinolones. Levofloxacin (Levaquin) is somewhat more active than ciprofloxacin against gram-positive organisms such as *Streptococcus pneumoniae,* including penicillin-resistant strains, as well as *Enterococcus* and *S. aureus.* Moxifloxacin is also effective against *S. pneumoniae* as well as some strains of *S. aureus* and entero-

cocci. However, MRSA and VRE are generally also resistant to moxifloxacin. The activity of moxifloxacin against many enteric gram-negative bacteria and *P. aeruginosa* is similar to that of levofloxacin and less than that of ciprofloxacin. Moxifloxacin often has stronger anaerobic bacterial coverage. Norfloxacin has limited oral absorption but is available only in oral form, so its use is limited to genitourinary tract infections. Quinolones are often combined with aminoglycosides to treat *P. aeruginosa* infections. Moxifloxacin also has some *in vitro* activity against anaerobes.

The use of quinolones in prepubescent children is not generally recommended, because these drugs have been shown to affect cartilage development in laboratory animals. However, more recent evidence suggests that judicious use in children might be less of a risk than previously thought, and in fact these drugs are used commonly in children with cystic fibrosis. Box 39-1 lists selected microbes commonly susceptible to quinolone therapy in general, but there is some variation in spectra among drugs. Table 39-3 gives common indications for individual drugs.

Contraindications

The only true contraindication is known drug allergy.

Adverse Effects

Quinolones are capable of causing a variety of adverse effects, the most common of which are listed in Table 39-4. Bacterial overgrowth is another possible complication of quinolone therapy, but this is more commonly associated with long-term use. More worrisome is a cardiac effect that involves prolongation of the QT interval on the electrocardiogram (ECG). Dangerous cardiac dysrhythmias are more likely to occur when quinolones are taken by patients receiving class Ia and class III antidysrhythmic drugs such as disopyramide and amiodarone. For this reason, such drug combinations should be avoided. There is some debate regarding this effect, but cases are still reported. A black box warning is required by the U.S. Food and Drug Administration for all quinolones because of the increased risk of tendonitis and tendon rupture with use of the drugs. This effect is more common in elderly patients, patients with renal failure, and those receiving concurrent glucocorticoid therapy (e.g., prednisone). Central nervous system stimulation (i.e., seizures) has been reported. Quinolones must be infused over 1 to 1.5 hours.

BOX 39-1 Overview of Quinolone-Susceptible Organisms

- Gram-positive: *Streptococcus* (including *Streptococcus pneumoniae*), *Staphylococcus, Enterococcus, Listeria monocytogenes*
- Gram-negative: *Neisseria gonorrhea, Neisseria meningitidis, Haemophilus influenzae, Haemophilus parainfluenzae,* Enterobacteriaceae (including *Escherichia coli, Enterobacter, Klebsiella, Proteus mirabilis, Salmonella, Shigella), Acinetobacter, Pseudomonas aeruginosa, Pasteurella multocida, Legionella, Mycoplasma pneumoniae, Chlamydia*
- Anaerobes: *Bacteroides fragilis, Peptococcus, Peptostreptococcus* (moxifloxacin strongest)
- Other: *Rickettsia* (ciprofloxacin only)

TABLE 39-3 Quinolones: Common Indications for Specific Drugs

Generic Name (Trade Name, Year of FDA Approval)	Antibacterial Spectrum	Common Indications
norfloxacin (Noroxin, 1986)	Extensive gram-negative and selected gram-positive coverage	Urinary tract infections, prostatitis, STDs
ciprofloxacin (Cipro, 1987)	Comparable to that of norfloxacin	Anthrax (inhalational, postexposure); respiratory, skin, urinary tract, prostate, intraabdominal, gastrointestinal, bone, and joint infections; typhoid fever; STDs; selected nosocomial pneumonias
levofloxacin (Levaquin, 1996)	Comparable to that of norfloxacin	Respiratory and urinary tract infections; prophylaxis in various transrectal and transurethral prostate surgical procedures
moxifloxacin (Avelox, 1999)	Comparable to that of norfloxacin	Respiratory and skin infections; CAP caused by PRSP; anaerobic infections

CAP, Community-acquired pneumonia; *FDA,* U.S. Food and Drug Administration; *PRSP,* penicillin-resistant streptococcal pneumonia; *STD,* sexually transmitted disease.

Interactions

There are several drugs that interact with quinolones. Concurrent use of the quinolones with antacids, iron, zinc preparations, or sucralfate causes the oral absorption of the quinolone to be greatly reduced. Patients should take calcium and magnesium supplements at least 1 hour before or after taking quinolones. Tube feedings can also reduce the absorption of quinolones. Probenecid can reduce the renal excretion of quinolones, and the use of some quinolones with theophylline or caffeine may increase their effects. Nitrofurantoin, discussed later in this chapter, can antagonize the antibacterial activity of the quinolones, and oral anticoagulants should be used with caution in patients receiving quinolones because of the antibiotic-induced alteration of the intestinal flora, which affects vitamin K synthesis.

Dosages

For recommended dosages of selected quinolones, see the Dosages table below.

DRUG PROFILES

◆ ciprofloxacin

Ciprofloxacin (Cipro) was one of the first of the newer broad-coverage, potent quinolones to become available. It was first marketed in an oral form but is also available in injectable, ophthalmic (see Chapter 57), and otic (see Chapter 58) formulations. Because of its excellent bioavailability, it can work as well as many intravenous antibiotics. It is also capable of killing a wide range of gram-negative bacteria and is even effective against traditionally difficult-to-kill gram-negative bacteria such as *Pseudomonas*. Some anaerobic bacteria as well as atypical organisms such as *Chlamydia*, *Mycoplasma*, and *Mycobacterium* can also be killed by ciprofloxacin. It is also a drug of choice for anthrax (infection with *Bacillus anthracis*).

PHARMACOKINETICS

Route	Onset of Action	Peak Plasma Concentration	Elimination Half-life	Duration of Action
IV	30 min	1 hr	3-4.8 hr	Up to 12 hr
PO	Variable	1-2 hr	3-4.8 hr	Up to 12 hr

levofloxacin

Levofloxacin (Levaquin) is one of the most widely used quinolones. It has a broad spectrum of activity similar to that of ciprofloxacin, but it has the advantage of once-daily dosing. Levofloxacin is available in both oral and injectable forms.

PHARMACOKINETICS

Route	Onset of Action	Peak Plasma Concentration	Elimination Half-life	Duration of Action
IV	Variable	1-2 hr	6-8 hr	Up to 24 hr
PO	Variable	2 hr	6-8 hr	Up to 24 hr

MISCELLANEOUS ANTIBIOTICS

There are a number of antibiotics that do not fit into any of the previously described broad categories. Most have somewhat unique indications or are especially preferred for a particular type of infection. Although they may not be used as commonly as drugs from the other major classes, they are still of clinical importance. Several of these drugs are described individually in the following drug profiles. See the Dosages table on page 000 for dosing information for these drugs.

DRUG PROFILES

◆ clindamycin

Clindamycin (Cleocin) is a semisynthetic antibiotic. Clindamycin can be either bactericidal or bacteriostatic (see Chapter 38), depending on the concentration of the drug at the site of infection and on the infecting bacteria. It inhibits protein synthesis in bacteria (see Figure 38-3). It is indicated for the treatment of chronic bone infections, genitourinary tract infections, intraabdominal infections, anaerobic pneumonia, septicemia caused by streptococci and staphylococci, and serious skin and soft tissue infections caused by susceptible bacteria. Most gram-positive bacteria, in-

---

TABLE 39-4   Quinolones: Reported Adverse Effects

Body System	Adverse Effects
Central nervous	Headache, dizziness, fatigue, insomnia, depression, restlessness, convulsions
Gastrointestinal	Nausea, constipation, increased AST and ALT levels, flatulence, heartburn, vomiting, diarrhea, oral candidiasis, dysphagia, pseudomembranous colitis
Integumentary	Rash, pruritus, urticaria, photosensitivity (with lomefloxacin), flushing
Other	Ruptured tendons and tendonitis (black box warning added 2008), fever, chills, blurred vision, tinnitus

ALT, Alanine aminotransferase; *AST,* aspartate aminotransferase.

DOSAGES

Selected Quinolones

Drug	Pharmacologic Class	Usual Dosage Range	Indication/Uses
◆ ciprofloxacin (Cipro) (C)	Fluoroquinolone	**Adult*** IV: 200-400 mg q12h PO: 250-750 mg q8-12h	Broad gram-positive and gram-negative coverage for infections throughout the body
levofloxacin (Levaquin) (C)		**Adult only** IV/PO: 250-750 mg once daily	Various susceptible bacterial infections

IV, Intravenous; *PO,* oral.

*Not normally recommended for children younger than 18 yr due to finding of adverse musculoskeletal effects in studies of immature animals.

Dosages

Selected Miscellaneous Antibiotics

Drug (Pregnancy Category)	Pharmacologic Class	Usual Dosage Range	Indications
◆ clindamycin (Cleocin) (B)	Lincosamide	**Adult** IV/PO: 300-900 mg bid-qid **Pediatric** IV/PO: 8-25 mg/kg/day divided tid-qid	Anaerobic infections; streptococcal and staphylococcal infections of bone, skin, respiratory, and GU tract
colistimethate (Colisitin) (C)	Polypeptide	2.5-5 mg/kg/day; infuse over 3-5 min	Treatment of KPC-producing organisms; renal and neurotoxicity common
daptomycin (Cubicin) (B)	Lipopeptide	**Adult only** IV: 4 mg/kg once daily × 7-14 days	Complicated skin and soft tissue infections
linezolid (Zyvox) (C)	Oxazolidinone	**Adult only** IV/PO: 400-600 mg q12h	VRE infections; skin and respiratory infections caused by various *Staphylococcus* and *Streptococcus* spp.
◆ metronidazole (Flagyl) (B)	Nitroimidazole	**Adult*** IV/PO: 250-500 mg q6-12h	Primarily anaerobic and gram-negative infections of abdominal cavity, skin, bone, and respiratory and GU tracts
nitrofurantoin (Macrodantin, Furadantin) (B)	Nitrofuran	**Adult** PO: 50-100 mg qid **Pediatric** PO: 5-7 mg/kg/day divided qid	Primarily UTIs caused by gram-negative organisms and *Staphylococcus aureus*
quinupristin/dalfopristin (Synercid) (B)	Streptogramins	**Adult and pediatric** IV: 7.5 mg/kg q8-12h	VRE infections; skin infections caused by streptococcal and staphylococcal infections
vancomycin (Vancocin, Vancoled) (B, oral; C injection)	Tricyclic glycopeptide	**Adult** IV/PO: 1 g q12h (IV) or 500 mg q6h (PO) **Pediatric†** IV/PO: 10 mg/kg q6h	Severe staphylococcal infections, including MRSA infections; other serious gram-positive infections, including streptococcal infections

GU, Genitourinary; *IV,* intravenous; *KPC, Klebsiella pneumoniae* carbapenemase; *MRSA,* methicillin-resistant *Staphylococcus aureus; PO,* oral; *spp.,* species; *UTIs,* urinary tract infections; *VRE,* vancomycin-resistant *Enterococcus.*
*Not normally used in children except to treat amebiasis.
†Dose variable depending on age of patient.

cluding staphylococci, streptococci, and pneumococci, are susceptible to clindamycin's actions. It also has the special advantage of being active against several anaerobic organisms and is most often used for this purpose. However, resistant strains of gram-positive, gram-negative, and anaerobic organisms do exist. Also, all Enterobacteriaceae are resistant to clindamycin.

Clindamycin is contraindicated in patients with a known hypersensitivity to it, those with ulcerative colitis or enteritis, and infants younger than 1 month of age. Gastrointestinal tract adverse effects are the most common and include nausea, vomiting, abdominal pain, diarrhea, pseudomembranous colitis, and anorexia. **Pseudomembranous colitis,** also known as *antibiotic-associated colitis,* is a necrotizing inflammatory bowel condition that is often associated with antibiotic therapy, especially clindamycin therapy. Clindamycin is available in oral, injectable, and topical (see Chapter 56) forms.

Clindamycin is also known to have some neuromuscular blocking properties that may enhance the actions of neuromuscular drugs used in perioperative and intensive care settings, such as vecuronium (see Chapter 12). Patients receiving both drugs should be monitored for excessive neuromuscular blockade and respiratory paralysis, and appropriate ventilatory support provided as needed.

PHARMACOKINETICS

Route	Onset of Action	Peak Plasma Concentration	Elimination Half-life	Duration of Action
PO	30 min	45 min	2-3 hr	6 hr
IM/IV	Variable	IM: 3 hr	2-3 hr	IM: 8-12 hr

linezolid

Linezolid (Zyvox) is the first antibacterial drug in a new class of antibiotics known as *oxazolidinones.* This drug works by inhibiting bacterial protein synthesis. Linezolid was originally developed to treat infections associated with vancomycin-resistant *Enterococcus faecium,* more commonly referred to as VRE. VRE infection is notoriously difficult to treat and often occurs as a *nosocomial* (hospital-acquired) infection. Linezolid is commonly used to treat hospital-acquired pneumonia; complicated skin and skin structure infections, including cases caused by MRSA; and gram-positive infections in infants and children. MRSA is a virulent organism and, as noted earlier, stands for "methicillin-resistant *S. aureus.*" However, methicillin, a penicillinase-resistant penicillin, has recently been removed from the U.S. market. Nonetheless, *MRSA* is still the term used, although oxacillin is now the test drug for this organism. To confuse things even further, oxacillin is rarely used for therapy, and nafcillin is the most commonly used drug for methicillin-susceptible *S. aureus.* MRSA is notorious for causing serious infections, especially in the hospital setting. Linezolid is also approved for treatment of community-acquired pneumonia and uncomplicated skin and skin structure infections.

The most commonly reported adverse effects attributed to linezolid are headache, nausea, diarrhea, and vomiting. It has also been shown to decrease platelet count. Linezolid is contraindicated in patients with a known hypersensitivity to it. It is available in oral and injectable forms. It has excellent oral absorption, which allows patients to continue oral therapy at home for serious infections that would otherwise require hospitalization. With regard to drug interactions, linezolid has the potential to strengthen the vasopressor (prohypertensive) effects of various vasopressive drugs (see Chapter 18) such as dopamine by an unclear mechanism. Also, there have been postmarketing case reports of this drug causing *serotonin syndrome* when used concurrently with serotonergic drugs such as the selective serotonin reuptake inhibitor (SSRI) antidepressants (see Chapter 17). It is recommended that the SSRI be stopped while the patient is receiving linezolid therapy; however, often this is not realistic. Finally, tyramine-containing foods such as aged cheese or wine, soy sauce, smoked meats or fish, and sauerkraut can interact with linezolid to raise blood pressure.

PHARMACOKINETICS

Route	Onset of Action	Peak Plasma Concentration	Elimination Half-life	Duration of Action
PO	Variable	1-2 hr	5 hr	12 hr
IV	Variable	Immediate	6-7 hr	8-12 hr

◆ metronidazole

Metronidazole (Flagyl) is an antimicrobial drug of the class *nitroimidazole*. It has especially good activity against anaerobic organisms and is widely used to treat intraabdominal and gynecologic infections that are caused by such organisms. Examples of the *anaerobes* against which it is active are *Peptostreptococcus* spp., *Eubacterium* spp., *Bacteroides* spp., and *Clostridium* spp. The drug is also indicated for treatment of protozoal infections such as amebiasis and trichomoniasis (see Chapter 43). It works by interfering with microbial DNA synthesis, and in this regard is similar to the quinolones (see Figure 38-3). It is used orally to treat antibiotic-associated colitis; however, resistance is being noted. Metronidazole is contraindicated in cases of drug allergy. It is available in both oral and injectable forms. It is classified as a pregnancy category B drug, although it is not recommended for use during the first trimester of pregnancy. Adverse effects include dizziness, headache, gastrointestinal discomfort, nasal congestion, and reversible neutropenia and thrombocytopenia. Drug interactions include acute alcohol intolerance when it is taken with alcoholic beverages, due to the accumulation of acetaldehyde, the principal alcohol metabolite. Patients should avoid alcohol for 24 hours before initiation of therapy and for at least 36 hours after the last dose of metronidazole. Metronidazole may also increase the toxicity of lithium, the benzodiazepines, cyclosporine, calcium channel blockers, various antidepressants (e.g., venlafaxine), warfarin, and other drugs. In contrast, phenytoin and phenobarbital may reduce the effects of metronidazole. These interactions occur because of various enzymatic effects involving the cytochrome P-450 liver enzymes that result in altered drug metabolism when these drugs are taken concurrently with metronidazole.

PHARMACOKINETICS

Route	Onset of Action	Peak Plasma Concentration	Elimination Half-life	Duration of Action
PO	Variable	1-2 hr	8 hr	Unknown
IV	Variable	1 hr	8 hr	Unknown

nitrofurantoin

Nitrofurantoin (Macrodantin) is an antibiotic drug of the class *nitrofuran*. It is indicated primarily for urinary tract infections caused by *E. coli*, *S. aureus*, *Klebsiella* spp., and *Enterobacter* spp. The drug is believed to work by interfering with the activity of enzymes that regulate bacterial carbohydrate metabolism and also by disrupting bacterial cell wall formation. It is contraindicated in cases of drug allergy and also in cases of significant renal function impairment, because the drug concentrates in the urine. The drug is available only for oral use. Adverse effects include gastrointestinal discomfort, dizziness, headache, skin reactions (mild to severe reported), blood dyscrasias, ECG changes, possibly irreversible peripheral neuropathy, and hepatotoxicity. Although hepatotoxicity is rare, it is often fatal. Interacting drugs are few and include probenecid, which can reduce renal excretion of nitrofurantoin, and antacids, which can reduce the extent of its gastrointestinal absorption.

PHARMACOKINETICS

Route	Onset of Action	Peak Plasma Concentration	Elimination Half-life	Duration of Action
PO	2.5-4.5 hr	30 min	0.5-1 hr	5-8 hr

quinupristin/dalfopristin

Quinupristin and dalfopristin (Synercid) are two streptogramin antibacterials marketed in a 30:70 fixed combination. The combination drug is approved for intravenous treatment of bacteremia and life-threatening infection caused by VRE and for treatment of complicated skin and skin structure infections caused by *S. pyogenes* and *S. aureus*, including MRSA.

Common adverse effects are arthralgias and myalgias, which may become severe. Adverse effects related to the infusion site, including pain, inflammation, edema, and thrombophlebitis, have developed in approximately 75% of patients treated through a peripheral intravenous line. The drug is contraindicated in patients with a known hypersensitivity to it. It is available only in injectable form. Drug interactions are limited, the most serious being potential increase in levels of cyclosporine, which can be addressed by laboratory monitoring and dosage adjustment of cyclosporine. Quinupristin/dalfopristin must be infused with 5% dextrose in water (D$_5$W) only and cannot be mixed with saline or heparin, including heparinized flushes.

PHARMACOKINETICS

Route	Onset of Action	Peak Plasma Concentration	Elimination Half-life	Duration of Action
IV	1-2 hr	3-4 hr	1-3 hr	8-12 hr

◆ vancomycin

Vancomycin (Vancocin) is a natural bactericidal antibiotic structurally unrelated to any other commercially available antibiotics. It destroys bacteria by binding to the bacterial cell wall, producing immediate inhibition of cell wall synthesis and death (see Figure 38-3). This mechanism differs from that of beta-lactam antibiotics.

Vancomycin is the antibiotic of choice for the treatment of MRSA infection and infections caused by many other gram-positive bacteria. It is not active against gram-negative bacteria, fungi, or yeast. Oral vancomycin is indicated for the treatment of antibiotic-induced pseudomembranous colitis *(Clostridium difficile)* and for the treatment of staphylococcal enterocolitis. Because the oral formulation is poorly absorbed from the gastrointestinal tract, it is used for its local effects on the surface of the gastrointestinal tract. The parenteral form is indicated for the treatment of bone and joint infections and bacterial bloodstream infections caused by *Staphylococcus* spp. Resistance to vancomycin has been noted with increasing frequency in patients with infections caused by *Enterococcus* organisms. These strains have been isolated most often from gastrointestinal tract infections but have also been isolated from skin, soft tissue, and bloodstream infections. Resistance to MRSA has been rarely reported to occur with vancomycin.

Vancomycin is contraindicated in patients with a known hypersensitivity to it. It should be used with caution in those with preexisting renal dysfunction or hearing loss, as well as in elderly patients and neonates. Vancomycin is similar to the aminoglycosides in that there are very specific drug levels in the blood that are safe. If the levels are too low (less than 5 mcg/mL), the dosage may be subtherapeutic with reduced antibacterial efficacy. If the blood levels are too high (over 50 mcg/mL), toxicities may result, the two most severe of which are ototoxicity (hearing loss) and nephrotoxicity (kidney damage). Nephrotoxicity is more likely to occur with concurrent therapy with other nephrotoxic drugs such as aminoglycosides and cyclosporine. Vancomycin can also cause additive neuromuscular blocking effects with patients receiving neuromuscular blockers. Another common adverse effect that is bothersome but usually not harmful is known as *red man syndrome*. This syndrome is characterized by flushing and/or itching of the head, face, neck, and upper trunk area. It is most commonly seen when the drug is infused too rapidly. It can usually be alleviated by slowing the rate of infusion of the dose to at least 1 hour. Rapid infusions may also cause hypotension. Optimal blood levels of vancomycin are a peak level of 18 to 50 mcg/mL and a trough level of 10 to 20 mcg/mL. Measurement of peak levels is no longer routinely recommended, and only trough levels are commonly monitored. Blood samples for measurement of trough levels should be drawn immediately before administration of the next dose. Because of the increase in resistant organisms, many clinicians use a trough level of 15 to 20 mcg/mL as their goal.

PHARMACOKINETICS

Route	Onset of Action	Peak Plasma Concentration	Elimination Half-life	Duration of Action
IV	Variable	1 hr	4-6 hr	Up to 24 hr Longer in renal dysfunction

daptomycin

Daptomycin (Cubicin) is currently the only drug of the new class known as *lipopeptides*. Its mechanism of action is not completely known, but it binds to gram-positive cells in a calcium-dependent process and disrupts the cell membrane potential. It is used to treat complicated skin and soft tissue infections caused by susceptible gram-positive bacteria, including MRSA and VRE. This drug is contraindicated in cases of drug allergy. It is available only in injectable form. Adverse reactions include hypotension or hypertension (low incidence for both), headache, dizziness, rash, gastrointestinal discomfort, elevated liver enzyme levels, local injection site reaction, renal failure, dyspnea, and fungal infection. The precise mechanisms for these reactions are uncertain, but all occur in a relatively small percentage of patients (fewer than 5%). Major drug interactions have yet to be identified; however, there is a theoretical risk of increased myopathy when daptomycin is given in conjunction with hydroxymethylglutaryl–coenzyme A (HMG-COA) reductase inhibitors, commonly referred to as *statins*.

PHARMACOKINETICS

Route	Onset of Action	Peak Plasma Concentration	Elimination Half-life	Duration of Action
IV	Unknown	30 min	8-9 hr	Unknown

colistimethate

Colistimethate (Coly-Mycin) is a polypeptide antibiotic that penetrates and disrupts the bacterial membrane of susceptible strains of gram-negative bacteria. It is commonly referred to as colistin. It is an old drug that fell out of clinical use when newer, less toxic drugs became available. Unfortunately, due to the emergence of infections with KPC-producing organisms, it is now being used

again, often as one of the only drugs available to treat KPC. Colistin is available for intravenous, intramuscular, and inhalational administration. It has serious adverse effects, including renal failure and neurotoxic effects such as paresthesia, numbness, tingling, vertigo, dizziness, and impairment of speech. It can cause acute respiratory failure when administered by inhalation. Colistin crosses the placenta and should be used with caution in pregnant women. Colistin is infused over 3 to 5 minutes.

PHARMACOKINETICS

Route	Onset of Action	Peak Plasma Concentration	Elimination Half-life	Duration of Action
IV	Unknown	5 min	2-3 hr	8-12 hr

NURSING PROCESS

Assessment

Many of the antibiotics discussed in this chapter, in contrast to those in Chapter 38, are the types of drugs that are often reserved for treatment of more potent infections and are mainly administered by parenteral routes; thus, they demand more skillful and thorough assessment of the patient and specific drug. These antibiotics all require a critical assessment for any history of or current symptoms indicative of hypersensitivity or allergic reactions (from mild reactions with rash, pruritus, or hives to severe reactions with laryngeal edema, bronchospasms, hypotension, and possible cardiac arrest). Further assessment associated with these groups of antibiotics in general should include conducting a nursing physical examination and recording age, weight, and baseline vital sign values, including body temperature. Diagnostic and laboratory studies that may be ordered include the following: (1) for assessing liver function—AST and ALT levels; (2) for assessing renal function—urinalysis, BUN level, and serum creatinine level; (3) for assessing cardiac function—ECG, echocardiography, ultrasonography, and/or cardiac enzyme levels; (4) for assessing sensitivity of the bacteria to the antibiotic—culture and sensitivity testing of infected tissue or blood samples; (5) for baseline blood values—white blood cell (WBC) count, hemoglobin level, hematocrit, red blood cell (RBC) count, and platelet and clotting values. A baseline neurologic assessment should include assessment for baseline sensory and motor intactness and/or assessment of any alterations in neurologic functioning—for example, altered sensorium and level of consciousness—because of the potential for central nervous system adverse effects. Baseline abdominal and gastrointestinal assessments are important, with a focus on bowel patterns and bowel sounds because of the possibility of gastrointestinal adverse effects. Contraindications, cautions, and drug interactions should also be noted, and a complete list of the patient's medications, including over-the-counter drugs, herbals, and dietary supplements should be obtained. A cultural assessment is important because of the various responses of certain racial and ethnic groups to specific drugs as well as the potential use of alternative healing practices.

With any antibiotic, it is important for the nurse to assess for *superinfection* or a secondary infection that occurs with the destruction of normal flora during antibiotic therapy (see Chapter 38). Fungal superinfections are evidenced by fever, lethargy, perineal itching, and other anatomically related symptoms. The status of the patient's immune system and overall condition is

Vancomycin

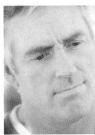

Mr. M., a 45-year-old quadriplegic, is being treated for an infected stage IV sacral pressure ulcer. The wound cultures have indicated the presence of multidrug-resistant *Staphylococcus aureus* (MRSA). The physician has ordered intravenous vancomycin to be given every 12 hours, application of wet-to-dry dressings (twice a day) as part of the treatment, as well as a referral to the enterostomal therapist. In addition, Mr. M. is placed on contact precautions because of the MRSA.

© Monkey Business Images

1. What should you assess before starting the vancomycin infusion?
2. Two days later, Mr. M. complains of feeling "hot" in his face and neck, and itching in those same areas. His face and neck are flushed. What do you suspect is happening?
3. What can you do to minimize complications during vancomycin infusions?
4. The physician orders measurement of vancomycin blood levels. What is the therapeutic goal when vancomycin levels are monitored?
5. What is the single best action you can take to prevent the spread of Mr. M.'s MRSA infection?

For answers, see *http://evolve.elsevier.com/Lilley.*

important to assess, because if there is a deficiency (e.g., in patients with cancer, autoimmune disorders such as lupus, acquired immunodeficiency syndromes, and any chronic illness) the patient's ability to physically resist infection may be diminished. Antibiotic resistance is a continual concern with antibiotic drug therapy, especially in pediatrics and in large health care institutions and long-term care facilities. This possibility of resistance to certain antibiotics should be considered when assessing patients for symptoms of infection and superinfection. Once a thorough assessment has been performed and follow-up to therapy considered, the nurse should share information about prevention of antibiotic resistance (see Implementation).

With *aminoglycosides,* the nurse should assess for hypersensitivity and preexisting conditions, and obtain a list of all medications the patient is taking, because of the many cautions, contraindications, and drug interactions associated with these drugs. The aminoglycosides are known for their ototoxicity and nephrotoxicity; therefore, baseline hearing tests with audiometry and assessment of vestibular function as well as renal function studies (BUN level, urinalysis, serum and urine creatinine levels) should be performed and all results documented. If renal baseline functioning is decreased or abnormal, dosage amounts may need to be adjusted by the prescriber because of the nephrotoxicity. A thorough neuromuscular assessment should be performed, because of the potential for drug-related neurotoxicity and higher risk for complications in those with impaired neurologic functioning; for example, patients with myasthenia gravis or Parkinson's disease may experience worsening of muscle weakness because of the drug's neuromuscular blockade. Neonates (because of the immaturity of the nervous and renal systems) and the elderly (because of decreased neurologic and renal functioning) are at highest risk for nephrotoxicity, neurotoxicity, and ototoxic-

ity and require careful assessment before and during drug therapy. Hydration status should also be assessed.

Quinolones, such as ciprofloxacin, require careful assessment for drug allergies. Preexisting central nervous system conditions (e.g., seizure or stroke disorders) may be exacerbated by the concurrent use of these drugs, and therefore careful history taking is needed before drugs in this group are administered. Assessment of bowel activity is required, as well as assessment of neuromuscular functioning because of the potential for dizziness, headache, and visual changes. The timing of medication doses should also be reviewed and other drugs the patient is receiving assessed, because of the interaction of these drugs with antacids (see previous discussion of drug interactions) and the preferred dosing time of 2 hours after meals. It is important to remember that many drugs interact with these antibiotics, including iron, multivitamin products, and zinc. The latter drugs may be used but should not be given within 2 hours of the quinolones, because they decrease absorption of the quinolones. Blood glucose levels and results of renal and liver function tests should also be assessed and documented. Intake and output amounts should also be assessed and documented.

The patient should be assessed for hypersensitivity to either *clindamycin* or related compounds, and this sensitivity as well as any allergy to aspirin should be documented. Although drug interactions have been discussed previously, it is important to emphasize that clindamycin should never be given at the same time as neuromuscular blocking drugs. In addition, because of the risk for antibiotic-associated colitis, blood dyscrasias, and nephrotoxicity, it is critical (to patient safety) to assess gastrointestinal patterns, presence of abdominal pain, frequency and consistency of stools, WBC counts, platelet count, and BUN and serum creatinine levels.

Linezolid is used to treat diabetic foot infections, community-acquired infections, VRE infections, nosocomial pneumonias, and other severe infections. A discerning and careful assessment of the patient's underlying immune status and renal, liver, gastrointestinal, and hematologic functioning is critical to patient safety and to early identification of adverse and toxic effects. A systems-related nursing assessment would focus on the patient's history of infections, response to infections, and overall immune status, as well as intake and output, bladder functioning, any presence of jaundice or liver enlargement (noted on abdominal palpation or percussion), bowel sounds, bowel patterns, and any complaints of gastrointestinal symptoms (e.g., nausea, vomiting, diarrhea, abdominal pain). Related laboratory or diagnostic testing might include immunoglobulin levels, WBC count, RBC count, platelet count, hemoglobin level, hematocrit, BUN level, creatinine level, urinalysis, and levels of ALT, AST, ALP, and GGT. These assessments are all very important for safe use and for the prevention of possible adverse and toxic effects, as well as for the patient's overall well-being. Should the patient be immune compromised and have renal or liver dysfunction, adverse effects may be exacerbated, leading to complications and/or toxicity.

Patients taking *metronidazole* need to be assessed for allergy to the drug and to other nitroimidazole derivatives. As with all medications, contraindications, cautions, and drug interactions should be assessed for and the findings documented (see pharmacology discussion). Culture and sensitivity reports should be reviewed before therapy is started, and baseline assessments of the neurologic system (dizziness, numbness, tingling, and other sensory and motor abnormalities), gastrointestinal system (bowel sounds, bowel problems and patterns), and genitourinary system (urinary patterns, color of urine, and intake and output) should be carried out. The nurse should inquire about alcohol intake, because of the interaction of alcohol with the drug. A disulfiram-like reaction may occur, characterized by flushing of the face, tachycardia, palpitations, nausea, and vomiting.

Assessment of allergies and any history of asthma (which puts the patient at risk for drug allergy) are important with *nitrofurantoin*. Renal and liver function should be assessed. A history of glucose-6-phosphate dehydrogenase deficiency (see Chapters 2 and 38) is of concern, because patients with this disorder have a greater risk for hemolytic anemia. Patients who are debilitated are at greater risk for peripheral neuropathies. Other medications that are neurotoxic should be avoided, because their use increases the risk for neurologic adverse effects (e.g., irreversible peripheral neuropathy). The nurse should take note of the patient's skin, including color, turgor, and intactness, because of the possibility of drug-related risk Stevens-Johnson syndrome. Assessment should also include description of respiratory patterns and breath sounds, and notation of cough if present. With *quinupristin/dalfopristin,* vital signs as well as the results of baseline liver and renal function tests and complete blood count should be assessed so that baseline levels related to the infection will be available. An assessment of gastrointestinal functioning is also important, with a focus on bowel patterns, bowel sounds, and abdominal pain, because of the potential for antibiotic-associated colitis.

With *vancomycin,* the patient assessment should include questioning about other medications the patient is taking, especially drugs that are nephrotoxic or ototoxic. Vital signs should be assessed with close attention to blood pressure during infusion of the drug. Bowel patterns and sounds should be assessed because of the risk for gastrointestinal adverse effects. Baseline hearing status should be assessed due to the risk for ototoxicity, as should urinary patterns due to risk for nephrotoxicity. As previously discussed, trough drug levels must be monitored during therapy. The color of the patient's skin should be noted because of the risk for red man syndrome. Because of multiple drug and diluent incompatibilities, as with several of the other parenteral antibiotics mentioned previously in this chapter, the nurse must always stop and assess for potential fluid and medication interactions.

With the emergence of multidrug-resistant organisms (e.g., MRSA, VRE, and ESBL- and KPC-producing organisms), it is important to ensure that proper hand-washing techniques are used by health care providers and caregivers. All antibiotics with which the patient has been treated are also important to document.

Nursing Diagnoses

- Risk for infection related to the patient's compromised immune status before and during treatment
- Risk for injury to self (compromised organ function) related to adverse effects of medications (e.g., ototoxicity and nephrotoxicity) and weakened physical state
- Acute pain related to infection and/or adverse reaction to medications
- Deficient knowledge related to lack of information and experience with the medication regimen

- Ineffective therapeutic regimen management related to lack of information about the proper use of antibiotics and the lack of patient's experience with the therapy

Planning
Goals

- Patient is free of the signs and symptoms of infection once therapy is completed.
- Patient experiences minimal adverse effects of antibiotic therapy.
- Patient remains compliant with antibiotic therapy regimen.
- Patient experiences improvement in discomfort or pain associated with the infection.
- Patient returns for follow-up visits as recommended.
- Patient completes entire course of antibiotics as ordered.

Outcome Criteria

- Patient experiences an increased sense of well-being related to the resolving of the infection.
- Patient states the signs and symptoms of an infection (e.g., fever, pain, malaise) and reports them if they occur while taking antibiotics.
- Patient is able to identify the adverse effects of antibiotic therapy, such as gastrointestinal upset, nausea, and diarrhea (specific to each drug class).
- Patient experiences increased periods of comfort and improved energy levels related to the resolving of the infectious process and minimal adverse effects of therapy.
- Patient states the reasons for compliance with therapy (i.e., to adequately eradicate bacteria).
- Patient states the measures to take to minimize the gastrointestinal distress associated with antibiotic therapy, such as taking the medication with yogurt or other foods, as appropriate.
- Patient keeps follow-up appointments to be evaluated for therapeutic effects and complications of therapy.

Implementation

Aminoglycosides should be given exactly as ordered and with adequate hydration. Fluid intake of up to 3000 mL/day should be encouraged unless contraindicated, especially with oral dosage forms. Parenteral dosage forms are the most commonly used. Neomycin is the only oral dosage form available. Because of the potential for nephrotoxicity and ototoxicity, the patient's renal function is determined and monitored during therapy. Dosing is adjusted based on estimates of creatinine clearance calculated from the patient's serum creatinine level. This assists in keeping a close watch on the patient's renal function and thus helps to prevent toxicity. Alteration in auditory, vestibular, and/or renal function may indicate the need for possible dosage adjustment or withdrawal of the drug. Consumption of yogurt or buttermilk may help prevent antibiotic-induced superinfections (see Chapter 38). The patient should be instructed to report to the prescriber any changes in hearing, ringing in the ears (tinnitus), or a full feeling in the ears. Nausea, vomiting with motion, ataxia, nystagmus, and dizziness should also be reported immediately. Redness, burning, and itching of the eyes may indicate an adverse reaction to ophthalmic forms, and redness over the skin area may indicate an adverse reaction to topical forms. Intramuscular administration sites should be checked for induration. If noted, it should be reported immediately to the prescriber, and the site should not be reused. Intravenous sites should be checked for heat, swelling, redness, pain, or red streaking over the vein (phlebitis) as per institutional protocol or policy.

Gentamicin sulfate comes in intrathecal, ophthalmic, topical, and parenteral dosage forms. Special considerations for each of these routes include the following: (1) Intramuscular: Give deeply and slowly to minimize discomfort. (2) Intravenous: Check for incompatibilities with other drugs and give only clear or very slightly yellow solutions that have been diluted with either normal saline (NS) or D_5W, infusing as prescribed. (3) Intrathecal: This dosage form should be preservative free and, as a point of information, mixed with an estimated 10% cerebrospinal fluid or NS and given over a period of 3 to 5 minutes. (4) Ophthalmic: Refer to Chapter 10 for specific instructions on administering eyedrops and ointments. Serum drug peak and trough levels are usually measured with multiple daily dosing, whereas only trough levels are generally monitored with once-daily dosing. Refer to Table 39-1 for more information on peak and trough levels of aminoglycosides.

As noted earlier, neomycin, another aminoglycoside, is the only drug in this class that is given orally and is also available topically as an over-the-counter drug. Oral neomycin is generally used in special situations such as for preoperative bowel preparation, treatment of diarrhea caused by *E. coli,* and treatment of hepatic encephalopathy, and should be given exactly as ordered. Another important nursing consideration for neomycin—as well as other aminoglycosides—is to monitor respiratory status constantly if the drug is used in a patient with neuromuscular disease. All dosage amounts are generally based on body weight. Nursing considerations associated with the use of tobramycin sulfate are similar to those discussed for parenteral, ophthalmic, and topical dosage forms of gentamicin.

Quinolones should be taken exactly as prescribed and for the full course of treatment. The patient should not take antacids at the same time as oral quinolones to prevent inactivation of the antibiotic. It is recommended that the oral quinolone be given 2 hours before antacids or ferrous sulfate to avoid alteration in the antibiotic's absorption. Calcium, magnesium, zinc, and copper should also be avoided. Alkaline foods and fluids, such as dairy products, peanuts, and sodium bicarbonate, may lead to a higher incidence of crystalluria due to a more alkaline urinary pH and should be avoided. Forcing of fluids and increased intake of fluids and foods high in ascorbic acid (e.g., cranberry juice and citrus fruits) is recommended, however, to prevent crystalluria. Patients should restrict coffee intake to avoid nervousness, insomnia, anxiety, and tachycardia. See Patient Teaching Tips for more information.

Clindamycin should be administered as ordered, whether by oral, topical, intravaginal, intravenous, or intramuscular route. Oral forms should be taken with 8 oz of water or other fluid and dosed evenly over 24 hours, as with other dosage forms. Oral solutions should *never* be refrigerated after they are reconstituted because of thickening of the solution. With topical forms, it is important to avoid simultaneous use of peeling or abrasive acne products, soaps, or alcohol-containing cosmetics to prevent cumulative effects. Topical forms should be applied in a thin layer to the affected area. Intravaginal doses are usually given by applicator—for example, one full applicator at bedtime for 3 to 7 days, or one suppository at bedtime for 3 days. Bedtime use is recommended for comfort reasons. Perineal pads may be worn to catch any leakage of the medicine from the vagina. Intravenous dosage forms should be infused by piggyback technique and as ordered. Most references state *never* to give these drugs via parenteral intravenous push. Doses of the drug should be diluted and infused per manufacturer guidelines and as ordered. Too rapid intravenous infusion can lead to severe hypotension and possible cardiac arrest. Intramuscular dosage forms should be given deep into the muscle.

Linezolid is generally given orally or intravenously. Oral doses should be evenly spaced and given with food or milk to decrease the possibility of gastrointestinal upset. Oral suspension forms should be given within 21 days of reconstitution. Intravenous doses should be protected from light and infused over 30 to 120 minutes, and should not be mixed with any other medication. Because of the risk for antibiotic-associated colitis, superinfections, and myelosuppression, the nurse must be constantly alert for the occurrence of frequent, loose, and foul-smelling stools; severe genital and/or anal pruritus; and severe mouth soreness. In addition, complete blood counts should be monitored closely (e.g., weekly) during therapy.

Oral forms of *metronidazole* should be given with food or meals to help decrease gastrointestinal upset. Extended-release dosage forms should not be chewed and should be taken on an empty stomach. Intravaginal doses are recommended to be administered at bedtime, and topical creams, ointments, or lotions are to be applied thinly to the affected area. An applicator should be used for intravaginal dosages. Generally speaking, gloves are worn to protect from undue exposure to medication, and the nurse should always wear gloves as a part of Standard Precautions. Topical forms should not be applied close to the eyes to avoid irritation. Intravenous dosage forms should be stored at room temperature and are supplied in a ready-to-use infusion bag.

Nitrofurantoin is available in oral forms and should be given with plenty of fluids, food, or milk to decrease gastrointestinal upset. Crushing of tablets should be avoided to help prevent tooth staining and gastrointestinal upset. Because of the risk for superinfection, hepatotoxicity, and peripheral neuropathy (which may be irreversible), the nurse should document the findings from constant monitoring for the signs and symptoms of these adverse effects. Superinfection has been discussed previously. The nurse should be aware that jaundice, itching, rash, and liver enlargement may indicate toxic effects to the liver, whereas numbness and tingling may occur with peripheral neuropathy. In addition, constant monitoring of breath sounds and breathing patterns, and observation for any cough are important because of the risk for permanent impairment of lung function.

For *quinupristin/dalfopristin,* only intravenous dosage forms are available, and these are stable for only 1 hour at room temperature. The drug should be reconstituted using only D_5W or sterile water for injection, and a gentle swirling action instead of shaking should be used to mix the drug (to help minimize foaming). A diluted infusion bag of the drug is stable for up to 6 hours, or 54 hours if refrigerated. These characteristics are important to know to help prevent untoward complications. Infusions are generally given over at least 60 minutes. It should also be noted that NS and lactated Ringer's solution are incompatible solutions. The same measures as with other antibiotics should be implemented to monitor for superinfection, hepatotoxicity, and antibiotic-associated colitis. It is very important to report any of the following to the prescriber should they occur: diarrhea with fever, abdominal pain, mucus or blood in the stools, and swollen face or tongue. If these symptoms occur, the patient should be monitored and the drug withheld until further orders are received from the prescriber.

Vancomycin may be used orally but is poorly absorbed by this route; this is the reason that more use of parenteral dosage forms is seen. A reconstituted powder dose form may be administered via nasogastric tube, and oral solutions are stable for 2 weeks if refrigerated. Note that powder forms for oral dosing are not to be used for intravenous administration. Intravenous dosage forms should be reconstituted as recommended (e.g., with either D_5W or NS) and should be infused over at least 60 minutes. Too rapid an infusion of vancomycin or administration by intravenous push may lead to severe hypotension and red man syndrome. Red man syndrome is characterized by flushing of the neck and face and a decrease in blood pressure. Extravasation may cause local skin irritation and damage, so frequent monitoring of the infusion, and in particular the intravenous site, is needed. Constant monitoring for drug-related neurotoxicity, nephrotoxicity, ototoxicity, and superinfection remain critical to patient safety. In addition, adequate hydration (at least 2 L of fluids every 24 hours unless contraindicated) is most important to prevent nephrotoxicity. Optimal peak blood levels of vancomycin range from 18 to 50 mcg/mL with a trough level of 10 to 20 mcg/mL (see pharmacology discussion for further information).

Because of the significant issue of multidrug-resistant organisms, it is important to encourage patients and family members not to abuse or overuse antibiotics and always to report immediately to the prescriber any signs and symptoms of an infection that is not resolving or responding to antibiotic therapy. *Colistin* and *tigecycline* may be prescribed, and it is important to give these medications exactly as prescribed and with close monitoring to track the patient's overall status and improvement in the underlying infection. Regardless of drug management, in today's health care settings (acute and long-term facilities, medical offices, urgent care centers, emergency departments) as well as in the home setting and abroad, proper and thorough hand-washing technique must be taught and demonstrated. Hand washing should be performed often, especially during cold and flu season, before and after preparing food, and after engaging in any of the following activities: going to the bathroom or changing diapers; touching bare human body parts; coughing, sneezing, or using a handkerchief or disposable tissue; eating or drinking; using tobacco; using the telephone; shaking hands; and playing with pets. The Centers for Disease Control and Prevention recommend the following as the proper hand-washing technique: Wash hands with warm running water and soap; lather well by rubbing hands vigorously for at least 15 to 20 seconds; pay attention to the wrist area, backs of the hands, areas between the fingers, and under the fingernails; and rinse well. Allow the water to run while drying hands with a paper towel and then use a dry paper towel as a barrier between the faucet and clean hands while turning off the water. If soap and water are not available and hands are not visibly soiled, gel hand sanitizers or alcohol-based hand wipes containing at least 60% ethyl alcohol or isopropanol may be used. Once the gel is applied and all surfaces covered, rub hands until gel is dry.

Evaluation

Evaluation focused on goals, outcome criteria, therapeutic effects, and adverse effects should be ongoing once antibiotic therapy has been initiated. Patients should report a decrease in symptoms (e.g., infection) as well as absence of injury to self and a decrease in pain. Therapeutic goals include all those previously mentioned as well as a return to normal of all blood counts and vital sign values, negative results on culture and sensitivity testing, as well as improved appetite, energy level, and sense of well-being. Signs and symptoms of the infection should also resolve. Another aspect of evaluation is monitoring for adverse effects of therapy such as superinfections, antibiotic-associated colitis, nephrotoxicity, ototoxicity, neurotoxicity, hepatotoxicity, and other drug-specific adverse effects.

PATIENT TEACHING TIPS

Aminoglycosides
- The patient should be educated about the drug, its purpose, and adverse effects, including the risk of hearing loss, which may occur even after therapy has been completed. Any change in hearing should be reported immediately to the prescriber.
- Forcing fluids up to 3000 mL/day, unless contraindicated, is important with any medication but especially with antibiotics to maximize absorption of oral doses and minimize some of the adverse effects.
- Any persistent headache, nausea, or vertigo should be reported to the prescriber. Educate about the signs and symptoms of superinfection, such as diarrhea; vaginal discharge; stomatitis; glottitis; black, hairy tongue; loose and foul-smelling stools; and cough.

Quinolones
- Exposure to the sun and tanning beds should be avoided. Use of sunglasses and sunscreen protection is recommended.
- Patients should report dizziness, restlessness, stomach distress, diarrhea, headache, inflammation of the tendons, confusion, and an irregular or rapid heartbeat to the prescriber.
- Drug interactions occurring between these antibiotics and oral anticoagulants (e.g., warfarin [Coumadin]) should be part of patient teaching. Frequent coagulation studies (measurement of international normalized ratio) should be done so that clotting ability is monitored and appropriate action taken as needed.

PATIENT TEACHING TIPS—cont'd

Clindamycin

- The patient should be instructed not to use topical forms near the eyes or near any abraded areas to avoid irritation.
- When vaginal dosage forms are used, the patient should be instructed not to engage in sexual intercourse for the duration of therapy, and to administer the entire course of antibiotics as ordered to obtain maximal therapeutic benefit.
- Should cream dosage forms get into the eyes accidentally, the eyes should be rinsed immediately with copious amounts of cool tap water.

Vancomycin

- The patient should be instructed to report any changes in hearing such as ringing in the ears or a feeling of fullness in the ears. Any nausea, vomiting, unsteady gait, dizziness, generalized tingling (usually after intravenous dosing), chills, fever, rash, and/or hives should also be reported.
- Therapeutic serum levels will be monitored throughout therapy; this monitoring is key to prevention of toxicity. The patient should be told that follow-up appointments are important for monitoring serum drug levels and identifying possible toxic effects.

Linezolid

- Therapy must be continued for the full prescribed length of treatment (as with all antibiotics).

- The patient should be educated to avoiding tyramine-containing foods (e.g., red wine, aged cheeses) while taking the drug.
- Severe abdominal pain, fever, severe diarrhea, and/or worsening of signs and symptoms of infection should be reported to the prescriber immediately.

Metronidazole

- Warn the patient that the urine may turn red-brown or a darker color. Caution patients to avoid alcohol and any alcohol-containing products (e.g., cough preparations and elixirs) while taking the drug because of the risk for a disulfiram-like reaction (e.g., severe vomiting).
- The patient should be educated about the purpose of the drug, such as its use as either an antibacterial or an antifungal medication, because this knowledge is crucial to achieving therapeutic effects and preventing adverse effects.

Nitrofurantoin

- The patient should be warned that the urine may become dark yellow or brown during drug therapy.
- Cough, fever, chest pain, difficulty breathing, numbness or tingling of extremities, and alopecia should be reported to the prescriber.

POINTS TO REMEMBER

- Over the years, bacteria have developed enzymes and mechanisms to interact with antibiotics and render the antibiotic ineffective. Multidrug resistance is a significant health issue, and such resistant organisms include ESBL- and KPC-producing bacteria, MRSA, and VRE.
- The aminoglycosides are a group of natural and semisynthetic antibiotics that are classified as *bactericidal* drugs, are very potent, and are capable of potentially serious toxicities (e.g., nephrotoxicity, ototoxicity).
- Quinolones are very potent, bactericidal, broad-spectrum antibiotics and include norfloxacin, ciprofloxacin, levofloxacin, moxifloxacin, gatifloxacin, and gemifloxacin.
- Clindamycin is a semisynthetic derivative of lincomycin, an older antibiotic.
- Linezolid is an antibacterial drug used to treat infections associated with vancomycin-resistant *Enterococcus faecium*, more commonly referred to as VRE. VRE is a difficult infection to treat and often occurs as a *nosocomial* (hospital-acquired) infection.
- Metronidazole (Flagyl) is an antimicrobial drug of the class nitroimidazole, has good activity against anaerobic organisms, and is widely used for intraabdominal and gynecologic infections; it is also used to treat protozoal infections (e.g., amebiasis, trichomoniasis).

- Nitrofurantoin (Macrodantin, Furadantin) is an antibiotic drug of the class *nitrofuran*. It is indicated primarily for urinary tract infections caused by *E. coli, S. aureus, Klebsiella* spp., and *Enterobacter* spp.
- Quinupristin and dalfopristin (Synercid) are two streptogramin antibacterials approved for intravenous treatment of bacteremia and life-threatening infection caused by VRE and for treatment of complicated skin and skin structure infections caused by *S. aureus* and *S. pyogenes.*
- Daptomycin (Cubicin) is used to treat complicated skin and soft tissue infections.
- Use of these antibiotics requires a critical assessment for any history or current symptoms indicative of hypersensitivity or allergic reactions (from mild reactions with rash, pruritus, and hives to severe reactions with laryngeal edema, bronchospasms, hypotension, and possibly cardiac arrest).
- With use of any antibiotic, it is important for the nurse to assess for *superinfection*, or a secondary infection that occurs because of the destruction of normal flora during antibiotic therapy. Superinfections may occur in the mouth, respiratory tract, gastrointestinal and genitourinary tracts, and on the skin. Fungal infections are evidenced by fever, lethargy, perineal itching, and other anatomically related symptoms.

NCLEX EXAMINATION REVIEW QUESTIONS

1 While assessing a woman who is receiving an antibiotic for community acquired pneumonia, the nurse notes that the patient has a thick, white vaginal discharge. The patient is also complaining about perineal itching. The nurse suspects that the patient has
  a resistance to the antibiotic.
  b an adverse effect of the antibiotic.
  c a superinfection.
  d an allergic reaction.

2 A patient has been admitted for treatment of an infected leg ulcer and will be started on intravenous linezolid. The nurse is reviewing the list of the patient's current medications. Which type of medication, if listed, would be of most concern if taken with the linezolid?
  a Beta-blocker
  b Oral anticoagulant
  c Selective serotonin reuptake inhibitor antidepressant
  d Thyroid replacement hormone

3 When administering vancomycin, the nurse knows that which of the following is the most important thing to assess before giving a dose?
  a Renal function
  b WBC count
  c Liver function
  d Platelet count

4 During therapy with an intravenous aminoglycoside, the patient calls the nurse and says, "I'm hearing some odd sounds, like ringing, in my ears." Which is the best action of the nurse at this time?
  a Reassure the patient that these are expected adverse effects
  b Reduce the rate of the intravenous infusion
  c Increase the rate of the intravenous infusion
  d Stop the infusion immediately and notify the prescriber

5 When giving intravenous quinolones, the nurse needs to keep in mind that these drugs may have serious interactions with which drugs?
  a Selective serotonin reuptake inhibitor antidepressants
  b Nonsteroidal antiinflammatory drugs
  c Oral anticoagulants
  d Antihypertensives

6 The nurse is administering an intravenous aminoglycoside to a patient who has had gastrointestinal surgery. Which nursing measures are appropriate? (Select all that apply.)
  a Report a trough drug level of 0.8 mcg/mL and hold the drug
  b Enforce a strict fluid restriction
  c Monitor serum creatinine levels
  d Instruct the patient to report dizziness or a feeling of fullness in the ears
  e Warn the patient that the urine may turn darker in color

1. c, 2. c, 3. a, 4. d, 5. c, 6. c, d.

CRITICAL THINKING ACTIVITIES: BEST ACTION

1 A patient who has been receiving intravenous doses of metronidazole has been discharged and will continue therapy with oral doses of this medication. The patient remarks, "I'm so glad to be going home. Our annual office party is tomorrow night, and I've been looking forward to it all year long." What is the nurse's best response to the patient?

2 A patient has been receiving therapy with the aminoglycoside tobramycin, and the nurse notes that the patient's latest trough drug level was 3 mcg/mL. This drug is given daily, and the next dose is due in 1 hour. Based on this trough drug level, what is the nurse's best action? Explain.

3 A patient has a urinary tract infection caused by *Pseudomonas* spp. Two antibiotics have been ordered, both due at 0900:
gentamicin, 300 mg, intravenously, daily (due at 0900), infuse over 60 minutes
ceftazidime, 500 mg intravenously, every 12 hours (due at 0900 and 2100), infuse over 30 minutes
Which antibiotic should the nurse infuse first? Explain.

For answers, see *http://evolve.elsevier.com/Lilley.*

CHAPTER 40

Antiviral Drugs

OBJECTIVES

When you reach the end of this chapter, you should be able to do the following:

1 Discuss the effects of the immune system with attention to the various types of immunity.
2 Describe the effects of viruses in the human body.
3 List specific drugs categorized as non–human immunodeficiency virus (HIV) antivirals and HIV antivirals or antiretrovirals.
4 Discuss the process of immunosuppression in patients with viral infections, specifically those with HIV infection.
5 Describe the stages of acquired immunodeficiency syndrome (AIDS) and various drugs used to manage the illness.
6 Discuss the mechanism of action, indications, contraindications, cautions, routes, adverse effects, and toxic effects of the various non-HIV antiviral and HIV antiviral drugs.
7 Develop a nursing care plan that includes all phases of the nursing process for patients receiving non-HIV and HIV antiviral drugs.

e-Learning Activities

http://evolve.elsevier.com/Lilley

NCLEX Review Questions • Animations • Nursing Care Plans • Audio Glossary • Category Catchers • Medication Errors Checklists • IV Therapy Checklists • Calculators • Frequently Asked Questions • Content Updates • Supplemental Resources • Answers to Case Studies and Critical Thinking Activities

Drug Profiles

◆ acyclovir, p. 630
amantadine and rimantadine, p. 628
enfuvirtide, p. 637
◆ ganciclovir, p. 630
◆ indinavir, p. 637
◆ nevirapine, p. 638

maraviroc, p. 637
oseltamivir and zanamivir, p. 631
raltegravir, p. 638
ribavirin, p. 631
tenofovir, p. 638
◆ zidovudine, p. 639

◆ *Key drug.*

Glossary

Acquired immunodeficiency syndrome (AIDS) Infection caused by the *human immunodeficiency virus (HIV),* which weakens the host's immune system, giving rise to *opportunistic infections* by pathogens that normally coexist in the body with minimal health affects. (p. 624)

Antibodies Immunoglobulin molecules that have an antigen-specific amino acid sequence and are synthesized by the humoral immune system (antibodies produced from B lymphocytes) in response to exposure to a specific antigen, the purpose of which is to attack and destroy molecules of this antigen. (p. 625)

Antigen A substance, usually a protein, that is foreign to a host (e.g., human) and causes the formation of an antibody and reacts specifically with that antibody. Examples of antigens include bacterial exotoxins, viruses, and allergens. An allergen (e.g., dust, pollen, mold) is a specific type of antigen that causes allergic reactions (see Chapter 36). (p. 625)

Antiretroviral drugs A specific term for antiviral drugs that work against *retroviruses* such as HIV. (p. 626)

Antiviral drugs A general term for drugs that destroy viruses, either directly or indirectly by suppressing their replication. (p. 625)

Cell-mediated immunity One of two major parts of the immune system. It consists of *nonspecific* immune responses mediated primarily by T lymphocytes (T cells) and other immune system cells (e.g., monocytes, macrophages, neutrophils) but not by antibody-producing cells (B lymphocytes). (p. 625)

Deoxyribonucleic acid (DNA) A *nucleic acid* composed of *nucleotide* units that contain molecules of the sugar deoxyribose, phosphate groups, and purine and pyrimidine bases. DNA molecules transmit genetic information and are found primarily in the nuclei of cells. (Compare with *ribonucleic acid [RNA]*.) (p. 624)

Fusion The process by which viruses attach themselves to, or fuse with, the cell membranes of host cells, in preparation for infecting the cell for purposes of viral *replication*. (p. 624)

Genome The complete set of genetic material of any organism; it may consist of multiple chromosomes (groups of DNA or RNA molecules) in higher organisms; a single chromosome, as in bacteria; or one or two DNA or RNA molecules, as in viruses. (p. 624)

Herpesviruses Several different types of viruses belonging to the family Herpesviridae that cause various forms of herpes infection. (p. 625)

Host Any organism (human, animal, or plant) that is infected with a microorganism, such as bacteria or viruses. (p. 624)

Human immunodeficiency virus (HIV) The *retrovirus* that causes AIDS. (p. 624)

Humoral immunity One of two major parts of the immune system. It consists of *specific* immune responses in the form of antigen-specific antibodies produced from B lymphocytes. (p. 625)

Immunoglobulins Synonymous with immune globulins. Glycoproteins (sugar proteins) synthesized and used by the humoral immune system to attack and kill any substance (antigen) that is foreign to the body. An immunoglobulin with an antigen-specific amino acid sequence is called an *antibody* and is able to recognize and inactivate molecules of a specific *antigen*. (p. 625)

Influenza viruses The viruses that causes influenza, an acute viral infection of the respiratory tract. There are three types of influenza virus: A, B, and C. Currently, medications are available only to treat types A and B. (p. 626)

Nucleic acids A general term referring to DNA and RNA. These complex biomolecules contain the genetic material of all living organisms, which is passed to future generations during reproduction. (p. 624)

Nucleoside A structural component of nucleic acid molecules (DNA or RNA) that consists of a purine or pyrimidine base attached to a sugar molecule. (p. 626)

Nucleotide A nucleoside that is attached to a phosphate unit, which makes up the side chain "backbone" of a DNA or an RNA molecule. (p. 626)

Opportunistic infections Infections caused by any type of microorganism that occur in an immunocompromised host but normally would not occur in an immunocompetent host. (p. 626)

Protease An enzyme that breaks down the amino acid structure of protein molecules by chemically cleaving the peptide bonds that link together the individual amino acids. (p. 632)

Replication Any process of duplication or reproduction, such as that involved in the duplication of nucleic acid molecules (DNA or RNA) during the reproduction processes of all living organisms. This is also the term used most often to describe the entire process of viral reproduction, which occurs only inside the cells of an infected host organism. (p. 624)

Retroviruses Viruses belonging to the family Retroviridae. These viruses contain RNA (as opposed to DNA) as their *genome* and replicate using the enzyme *reverse transcriptase*. Currently the most clinically significant retrovirus is HIV. (p. 625)

Reverse transcriptase An RNA-directed DNA polymerase enzyme. Such an enzyme promotes the synthesis of a DNA molecule from an RNA molecule, which is the reverse of the usual process. HIV replicates in this manner. (p. 632)

Ribonucleic acid (RNA) A nucleic acid composed of *nucleotide* units that contain molecules of the sugar ribose, phosphate groups, and purine and pyrimidine bases. RNA molecules transmit genetic information and are found in both the nuclei and cytoplasm of cells. (Compare with *deoxyribonucleic acid [DNA]*.) (p. 624)

Virion A mature virus particle. (p. 624)

Viruses The smallest known class of microorganisms; viruses can only replicate inside host cells. (p. 624)

• • •

Anatomy, Physiology, and Disease Overview

GENERAL PRINCIPLES OF VIROLOGY

Viruses are very small microorganisms, usually many times smaller than bacteria. For this reason, they are usually seen only with the strongest microscopes, such as electron microscopes. Unlike bacteria, viruses can reproduce, or replicate, only inside the cells of their **host,** which can be a human, animal, plant, or other type of microorganism (e.g., bacterium, protozoan). In this respect, all viruses are obligate intracellular parasites. It must be emphasized that viruses are not cells, per se, but instead are particles that infect and replicate inside of cells. A mature virus particle is known as a **virion.** Compared with other organisms, virions have a relatively simple structure that consists of the *genome,* the *capsid,* and the *envelope.* The **genome** is the inner core of the virion, which is composed of single- or double-stranded **deoxyribonucleic acid (DNA)** or **ribonucleic acid (RNA)** molecules, but not both. Viruses are the simplest of all organisms, because the cells of more complex organisms have either much larger nucleic acid strands or multiple strands, which make up

chromosomes. The latter is the case with higher organisms, including humans. The viral capsid is a protein coat that surrounds and protects the genome. It also plays a role in the process of **fusion** between the virions and the host cells. Fusion occurs when virions attach themselves to host cells in preparation for infecting the cells. The envelope is the outermost layer of the virion and is present in some, but not all, viruses. It has a lipoprotein (lipid and protein) structure containing viral antigens that are often chemically specific for various proteins on the surface of the host cell membranes *(cell surface proteins)*. This biochemical specificity, when present, also facilitates the fusion process. The **human immunodeficiency virus (HIV),** which causes **acquired immune deficiency syndrome (AIDS),** functions in this manner.

Viruses can enter the body through at least four routes: inhalation through the respiratory tract, ingestion via the gastrointestinal tract, transplacentally via mother to infant, and inoculation via skin or mucous membranes. The inoculation route can take several forms, including sexual contact, blood transfusions, sharing of syringes or needles (as in injection drug use), organ transplantation, and animal bites (including human, animal, insect, spider, and others). As mentioned earlier, once inside the body the virus particles, or virions, begin to attach themselves to the outer membranes of host cells *(cell membranes or plasma membranes)* as illustrated in Figure 40-1.

The viral genome then passes through the plasma membrane into the cytoplasm of the host cell. It later enters the cell *nucleus,* where the **replication** process begins. The virion may use its own or host enzymes (or both) to direct the replication process. In the host cell nucleus, the viral genome uses the cell's own genetic material, the **nucleic acids** RNA and DNA, to synthesize viral nucleic acids and proteins. These are then used to construct complete new virions. These new virions then exit the infected host cell by budding through the plasma membrane and go on to infect other host cells, where the replication process continues. The degenerative changes in the cell associated with viral replication are known as the *cytopathic effect* and usually result in the destruction of the host cell. Repeated over time, cumulative host cell destruction gives rise to the pathologic effects of the virus, which can eventually impair or even kill the host organism.

Although this cytopathic effect is the most common outcome, there are other possible outcomes of viral infection. One is *viral transformation,* which involves mutation of the host cell DNA or RNA and can result in malignant (cancerous) host cells. Viruses that can induce cancer in this way are known as *oncogenic* viruses. More common than viral transformation is *latent,* or dormant, infection in which the virions remain inside host cells but do not actively replicate to any significant degree. For example, HIV infection may have a lengthy dormant phase of 10 years or longer before giving rise to AIDS in an infected person. HIV infection is discussed in greater detail later in this chapter in the section on retroviruses.

Viruses are ubiquitous (widespread) in the environment, and most viral infections may not even be noticed before they are eliminated by the host's immune system. These are referred to as "silent" viral infections. Although the host's immune system acts to neutralize viral infection, it can become overwhelmed, depending on how strong, or *virulent,* the virus is and how rapidly it replicates inside host cells. In most cases, however, a person's

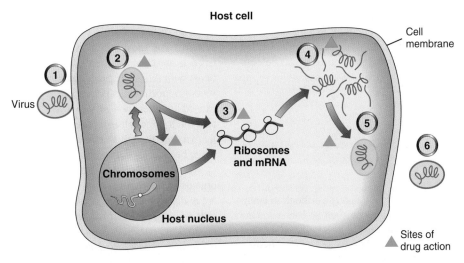

1. Attachment to host cell
2. Uncoating of virus, and entry of viral nucleic acid into host cell nucleus
3. Control of DNA, RNA, and/or protein production
4. Production of viral subunits
5. Assembly of virions
6. Release of virions

FIGURE 40-1   Virus replication. Some viruses integrate into host chromosome and enter a period of latency. *mRNA,* Messenger RNA. (Modified from Brody TM, Larner J, Minneman KP: *Human pharmacology: molecular to clinical,* ed 3, St Louis, 1998, Mosby.)

immune system is able to arrest and eliminate the virus. Host immune responses to viral infections are classified as either *nonspecific* or *specific.* Nonspecific immune responses include *phagocytosis* (eating) of viral particles by leukocytes (white blood cells) such as neutrophils, macrophages, monocytes, and T lymphocytes (T cells). Another important nonspecific immune response is the release of *cytokines* from these leukocytes. Cytokines are biochemical substances (e.g., histamine, tumor necrosis factor) that stimulate other protective immune functions. In addition, these *activated* immune system cells may also phagocytize infected host cells to curb the growth and spread of infection. These types of immune responses are collectively referred to as **cell-mediated immunity.** Cell-mediated immunity is nonspecific in the sense that it does not involve **antibodies** that are specific for a given **antigen.** In contrast, *specific* immune responses include the production of antibodies from B lymphocytes (B cells). These are immune-system proteins (immunoglobulins) that are chemically specific for viral antigens. This type of immune response is also called **humoral immunity.** Immune system function is discussed in further detail in Chapters 45 and 47.

OVERVIEW OF VIRAL ILLNESSES AND THEIR TREATMENT

There are at least 6 classes of DNA viruses and at least 14 classes of RNA viruses that are known to infect humans. Some of the more prominent viral illnesses include smallpox (poxviruses), sore throat and conjunctivitis (adenoviruses), warts (papovaviruses), influenza (orthomyxoviruses), respiratory infections (coronaviruses, rhinoviruses), gastroenteritis (rotaviruses, Norwalk-like viruses), HIV/AIDS **(retroviruses),** herpes **(herpesviruses),** and hepatitis (hepadnaviruses). Effective drug therapy is currently available only for a relatively small number of active viral infections. The drug therapy for hepatitis is discussed further in Chapter 49 on biologic response–modifying drugs. HIV belongs to the relatively unique viral class known as *retroviruses* and is discussed in greater detail in a separate section of this chapter.

Fortunately, many viral illnesses are survivable (e.g., chickenpox), even if bothersome and uncomfortable. The incidence of some of these illnesses has been reduced by the development of effective vaccines (e.g., vaccines for polio, smallpox, measles, chickenpox). Vaccines are discussed in more detail in Chapter 46. However, many other viral illnesses are either fatal or have much more severe long-term outcomes (e.g., hepatitis, HIV infection).

Antiviral drugs are chemicals that kill or suppress viruses by either destroying virions or inhibiting their ability to replicate. Even the best medications currently available probably never fully eradicate a virus completely from its host. However, the body's immune system has a better chance of controlling or eliminating a viral infection when the ability of the virus to replicate itself is suppressed. Drugs that actually destroy virions include various disinfectants and immunoglobulins. Disinfectants such as povidone-iodine (Betadine) are *virucides* and are commonly used to disinfect medical equipment as well as various parts of the body during invasive procedures. Such drugs are discussed further in Chapter 38.

Immunoglobulins are concentrated antibodies that can attack and destroy viruses. They are isolated and pooled from human or animal blood. In their activity they may be either nonspecific (e.g., human gamma globulin) or specific (e.g., rabies immunoglobulin, varicella-zoster immunoglobulin). Although such substances can technically be considered as antiviral drugs, they are more commonly thought of as immunizing drugs and are therefore discussed in further detail in Chapter 46. A few antiviral drugs, such as the interferons, stimulate the body's immune system to kill the virions directly. These drugs are discussed in Chapter 49.

The current antiviral drugs are all synthetic compounds that work indirectly by inhibiting viral replication as opposed to directly by destroying mature virions themselves. As noted earlier, only relatively few of the numerous known viruses can be controlled by current drug therapy. Some of the viruses in this group are the following

- Cytomegalovirus (CMV)
- Hepatitis viruses
- Herpesviruses
- HIV
- **Influenza viruses** ("flu" viruses)
- Respiratory syncytial virus

Active viral infections are usually much more difficult to eradicate than those caused by other microbes such as bacteria. One reason is that viruses replicate only inside host cells rather than replicating independently in the bloodstream or in other tissues. Most antiviral drugs must therefore enter these cells to disrupt viral replication. The need to develop antiviral drugs that are not overly toxic to host cells is one reason that there are relatively few effective antiviral medications on the market. However, the HIV/AIDS epidemic that began in the early 1980s strongly boosted antiviral drug research. This has increased the number of available antiviral drugs to treat HIV and other viral infections such as influenza, CMV infection, and varicella-zoster virus (VZV) infection. Many drugs for the treatment of HIV are approved by the U.S. Food and Drug Administration (FDA) via an accelerated process, which means that they are approved faster than other drugs, because of the nature of the illness. Because of the rapid addition of HIV drugs to the market, it is beyond the scope of this book to list every available drug. The reader is referred to the FDA website on approved AIDS drugs at *http://www.fda.gov/oashi/aids/virals.html* for the most recently approved AIDS drugs.

Another major reason viral illnesses are difficult to treat is that the virus has often replicated itself many thousands or even millions of times before symptoms of illness appear. Therefore, one goal in the field of infectious disease treatment is to be able to diagnose viral illnesses before an infecting virus has undergone widespread replication in a human host. This would theoretically allow the dual benefit of both early drug therapy and easier elimination of the virus by the host's immune system. This has happened to some degree with HIV infection, with relatively early diagnosis made possible by blood tests to screen for HIV antibodies. Of course, the patient must also be alerted of the need to seek medical care before serious illness develops.

Recall that for a virus to replicate, virions must first attach themselves to host cell membranes in a process known as *fusion.* Once inside the cell, the viral genome makes nucleic acids and proteins, which are then used to build new viral particles, or virions (see Figure 40-1). All virions contain a genome that consists of either DNA or RNA, but not both. Antiviral drugs inhibit this replication process in various ways. Most antiviral drugs enter the same cells that the viruses enter. Once inside, these antiviral drugs interfere with viral nucleic acid synthesis. Other antiviral drugs work by preventing the fusion process itself.

The best responses to antiviral drug therapy are usually seen in patients with competent immune systems. The immune system can work synergistically with the drug to eliminate or suppress viral activity. Patients who are *immunocompromised* (have weakened immune systems) are at greater risk for **opportunistic infections,** infections caused by organisms that would not normally harm an *immunocompetent* person (one with a healthy immune system). The most common examples of immunocompromised patients are cancer patients, organ transplant recipients, and patients with AIDS. These patients are prone to frequent and often severe opportunistic infections of many types, including those caused by other (non-HIV) viruses, bacteria, fungi, and protozoans. Such infections often require long-term prophylactic antiinfective drug therapy to control the infection and prevent its recurrence because of compromised host immune functions.

Recall that there are two types of nucleic acid found in living organisms: DNA and RNA. There are also five organic bases that are major structural components of these nucleic acids. DNA consists of long chains of *deoxyribose* sugar molecules, phosphate groups, and *purine* (*adenine* or *guanine*) and *pyrimidine* (*cytosine* or *thymine*) bases. *RNA* consists of long chains of *ribose* sugar molecules linked to phosphate groups, together with *purine* (*adenine* or *guanine*) and *pyrimidine* (*cytosine* or *uracil*) bases. A **nucleoside** is a single unit consisting of a base and its attached sugar molecule. Nucleosides have names similar to their bases with minor spelling modifications (e.g., adenosine, guanosine, cytidine, thymidine). A **nucleotide** is a nucleoside plus its attached phosphate molecule. Most antiviral drugs are synthetic *purine* or *pyrimidine* nucleoside or nucleotide analogues. Some pharmacology texts categorize the antiviral drugs based on their nucleoside-nucleotide activity. However, for ease of learning, this book divides antiviral drugs into drugs that treat HIV infections and those that treat non-HIV viral infections. **Antiretroviral drugs** are indicated specifically for the treatment of infections caused by HIV, the virus that causes AIDS. The effectiveness of antiviral drugs varies widely among patients and even over time in the same patient.

HERPES SIMPLEX VIRUS AND VARICELLA-ZOSTER VIRUS INFECTIONS

The family of viruses known as *Herpesviridae* includes those viruses that cause all kinds of herpes infection. There are several specific *types* of such viruses. *Herpes simplex virus type 1 (HSV-1)* causes *mucocutaneous herpes*—usually in the form of perioral blisters ("fever blisters" or "cold sores"). *Herpes simplex virus type 2 (HSV-2)* causes genital herpes. *Human herpesvirus 3 (HHV-3)* causes both chickenpox and shingles. This virus is more commonly known as *herpes zoster virus* or *varicella-zoster virus (VZV). Human herpesvirus 4 (HHV-4),* more frequently known as *Epstein-Barr virus,* is associated with illnesses such as infectious mononucleosis ("mono") and chronic fatigue syndrome. *Human herpesvirus 5 (HHV-5)* is more commonly known as *cytomegalovirus (CMV)* and is the cause of CMV retinitis (a serious viral infection of the eye) and CMV disease, which is most commonly seen in immunocompromised patients. *Human herpesviruses 6 and 7* are not especially clinically significant, and infection with these viruses may be more likely to occur in immunocompromised patients. *Human herpesvirus 8,* also known as *Kaposi's sarcoma herpesvirus,* is an *oncogenic* (cancer-inducing) virus believed to cause Kaposi's sarcoma, an AIDS-associated cancer. All of these viruses occur, often asymptomatically, in varying percentages of the population. Types 3 through 7 normally do not cause diseases that require medication, except in the case of immunocompromised patients. However, the HSVs (types 1 and 2) and VZV

(HHV-3) commonly cause illnesses that are now routinely treated with prescription medications.

Herpes Simplex Viruses

Although there can be anatomic overlap between the two types of HSV, HSV-1 infection is most commonly associated with perioral blisters and is therefore often thought of as "oral herpes." In contrast, HSV-2 infection is most commonly associated with blisters on both male and female genitalia and is therefore commonly referred to as "genital herpes." Although they usually do not cause serious or life-threatening illness, both infections are annoying and highly transmissible through close physical contact (e.g., kissing, sexual intercourse). Outbreaks of painful skin lesions occur *intermittently* (come and go), with periods of *latency* (no sores or other symptoms) occurring between acute outbreaks. Although antiviral medications are not always clinically required and are *not* curative, they can speed up the process of remission and reduce the duration of painful symptoms. This is especially true if the medications are started early in a given outbreak. Patients may also be prescribed an ongoing lower dose of antiviral drug for *prophylaxis* (prevention) of outbreaks. Situations in which HSV infections can become especially serious, even life-threatening, are those involving immunocompromised patients and virus transmission to a newborn infant. *Neonatal herpes* is often a life-threatening infection, and babies with this disease are often treated in neonatal intensive care units with intravenous antiviral drugs. However, these treatments fail in many cases, with infant death and/or permanent disability common. Therefore, the best strategy is to *prevent* transmission to the newborn infant. For this reason, obstetricians will usually recommend delivery by cesarean section ("C-section") for any mother with active genital herpes lesions.

Varicella-Zoster Virus

VZV is a type of herpesvirus (HHV-3) that most commonly causes *chickenpox (varicella)* in childhood, remains dormant for many years, and can then reemerge in later adulthood as painful *herpes zoster* lesions known as *shingles.*

Chickenpox is usually an uncomfortable but self-limiting disease of childhood. However, it is highly contagious and easily spread by either direct contact with weeping lesions or via droplet inhalation. It may also lead to significant scarring. The serious condition known as *Reye's syndrome* (fatty liver damage with encephalopathy) may also complicate varicella, as can other viral infections such as influenza. Herpes zoster, more commonly known as *shingles,* is caused by the reactivation of VZV from its dormant state, often decades after a case of childhood chickenpox. It is also referred to simply as *zoster.* Its most common manifestation is in the form of skin lesions that follow nerve tracts, known as *dermatomes,* along the skin surface. The most common site of these lesions is around the side of the trunk, although they can appear in other areas (e.g., along trigeminal nerve dermatomes of the face). Zoster lesions are often quite painful, and some patients even require opioids for pain control. In addition, postherpetic neuralgias (long-term nerve pain) remain following shingles outbreaks in up to 50% of elderly patients. Early administration of antiviral drugs such as acyclovir may speed recovery, but this effect is usually not dramatic. The best results are generally seen when the antiviral drug is started within 72 hours of symptom onset.

Active childhood varicella (chickenpox) infections are usually self-limiting and are not normally treated with antiviral drugs, except in high-risk (e.g., immunocompromised) pediatric patients. The varicella virus vaccine was approved in 1995 and is now routinely recommended for healthy children older than 1 year of age who have not had chickenpox. It has been shown effective in producing VZV immunity in HIV-positive children who are reasonably healthy. A new vaccine, Zostavax, is available for prevention of herpes shingles in patients 60 years or older.

In a small percentage of shingles cases, skin lesions may progress beyond the usual dermatome regions, and the virus can cause solid organ infections such as pneumonitis, hepatitis, encephalitis, and optic neuritis (infection of the optic nerve). Such infections are uncommon, and elderly and immunocompromised patients are the most vulnerable. Rarely, these serious infections can also be due to first-time exposure to varicella (chickenpox). In general, these more serious infections require intravenous antiviral drugs, especially in high-risk patients. Intravenous acyclovir is the most commonly used drug, and it can sometimes prevent fatalities or disability. Less serious infections are usually treated orally with acyclovir, valacyclovir, or famciclovir. Topical dosage forms of some of these drugs are also available and are discussed further in Chapter 56. Although VZV reactivation is comparable in pathology to that of HSV (e.g., oral or genital herpes lesions), VZV reactivation occurs much less regularly than does HSV reactivation because of a lack of reactivation genes. Secondary bacterial infections (e.g., group A *Streptococcus* skin infection) are common with VZV exacerbations, so antibiotics may also be needed. This is especially true in cases of ophthalmic involvement.

Pharmacology Overview of Antivirals (non-HIV)

The drugs discussed in this section include those used to treat non-HIV viral infections such as those caused by influenza viruses, HSV, VZV, and CMV. There are also antiviral drugs used to treat infections with hepatitis A, B, and C viruses. However, hepatitis treatment is covered in detail in Chapter 49 because it involves some additional unique drug therapy.

Mechanism of Action and Drug Effects

Most of the current antiviral drugs work by blocking the activity of a polymerase enzyme that normally stimulates the synthesis of new viral genomes. The result is impaired viral replication, which ideally results in viral concentrations low enough to allow elimination of the virus by the patient's immune system. If this does not occur, the virus may either enter a dormant state or remain at a low level of replication with continuous drug therapy.

Indications

The antivirals discussed in this section are those used to treat HSV, VZV and CMV infections and are listed in Table 40-1.

Contraindications

Most of the antiviral drugs used to treat non-HIV viral infections are surprisingly well tolerated. The only usual contraindication for most of these drugs is known severe drug allergy. However, a small number of contraindications are listed for a few of the antiviral drugs. Amantadine is contraindicated in lactating women, children younger than 12 months of age, and patients with an eczematous rash. Famciclovir is contraindicated in cases of allergy to the drug itself or to a similar drug called penciclovir, which is used topically to treat *herpes labialis* (perioral sores). Because cidofovir has such a strong propensity for renal toxicity, it is contraindicated in patients who already have severely compromised renal function as well as those receiving concurrent drug therapy with other highly nephrotoxic drugs. It is also contraindicated in cases of allergy to probenecid, because probenecid is recommended as concurrent drug therapy with cidofovir to help alleviate its nephrotoxicity. Ribavirin also has additional specific contraindications besides drug allergy. Because of the drug's teratogenic potential, it is also contraindicated in pregnant women and even in their male sexual partners. The aerosol form also should not be used by pregnant women or by women who may become pregnant during exposure to the drug. This includes health care providers administering the drug in aerosol form, because of the potential for second-hand inhalation on the part of the health care provider.

TABLE 40-1 Examples of Antiviral Drugs (Non-HIV)

Drug	Indications
Drugs to Treat Herpesviruses	
acyclovir, valacyclovir	Herpes simplex types 1 and 2, herpes zoster, chickenpox
trifluridine	Herpes simplex keratitis
Drugs to Treat Influenza Viruses	
amantadine	Influenza A
rimantadine	Influenza A
zanamivir, oseltamivir	Influenza A and B
Miscellaneous Antivirals	
ribavirin	Respiratory syncytial virus infection
cidofovir	Cytomegalovirus infection
foscarnet	Cytomegalovirus infection, acyclovir herpes simplex infections

HIV, Human immunodeficiency virus.

Adverse Effects

The adverse effects of the antiviral drugs are as different as the drugs themselves. Each has its own specific adverse effect profile. Because viruses reproduce in human cells, selective killing is difficult, and consequently many healthy human cells, in addition to virally infected cells, may be killed in the process, which results in more serious toxicities for these drugs. However, this effect is usually not as pronounced as in cancer chemotherapy, which often kills many more healthy cells. The more serious adverse effects are listed by drug in Table 40-2.

Interactions

The significant drug interactions that occur with the antiviral drugs arise most often when they are administered via systemic routes such as intravenously and orally. Many of these drugs are also applied topically to the eye or body, however, and the incidence of drug interactions associated with these routes of administration is much lower. Selected common drug interactions for both antiviral and antiretroviral drugs are listed in Table 40-3.

Dosages

For recommended dosages of some of the commonly used antiviral drugs, see the Dosages table on p. 630.

DRUG PROFILES

amantadine and rimantadine

Amantadine (Symmetrel), one of the earliest antiviral drugs, has a narrow antiviral spectrum in that it is active only against influenza A viruses. It has been used both prophylactically and therapeutically. However, the 2008 guidelines of the Centers for Disease Control and Prevention (CDC) did not recommend the use of amantadine or rimantadine to prevent or treat the flu. The recommendations on the use of amantadine change yearly based on the type of influenza that is prevalent. The reader is referred to *http://www.cdc.gov/flu/professionals/treatment* for the latest recommendations.

Rimantadine is a structural analogue of amantadine that has the same spectrum of activity, mechanism of action, and clinical indications. However, it differs from amantadine in that it has a longer half-life and causes fewer central nervous system adverse effects

TABLE 40-2 Selected Antiviral Drugs: Adverse Effects

Drug	Adverse Effects
acyclovir	Nausea, vomiting, diarrhea, headache, transient burning when topically applied
amantadine, rimantadine	Insomnia, nervousness, lightheadedness, anorexia, nausea, anticholinergic effects, orthostatic hypertension
didanosine	Pancreatitis, peripheral neuropathies, seizures
foscarnet	Headache, seizures, hypocalcemia, hypophosphatemia, hyperphosphatemia, hypokalemia, acute renal failure, bone marrow suppression, nausea, vomiting, diarrhea
ganciclovir	Bone marrow toxicity, nausea, anorexia, vomiting, headache, seizures
indinavir	Nausea, abdominal pain, headache, diarrhea, vomiting, weakness or fatigue, insomnia, flank pain, taste changes, acid regurgitation, back pain, indirect hyperbilirubinemia, nephrolithiasis
nevirapine	Rash, fever, nausea, headache, elevation in liver enzyme levels
ribavirin	Rash, conjunctivitis, anemia, mild bronchospasm
trifluridine	Ophthalmic effects: burning, swelling, stinging, photophobia, pain
vidarabine	Ophthalmic effects: burning, lacrimation, keratitis, foreign body sensation, pain, photophobia, uveitis, stromal edema
zalcitabine	Peripheral neuropathy, rash, ulcers
zidovudine	Bone marrow suppression, nausea, headache

TABLE 40-3 Selected Antiviral Drugs: Interactions

Drug	Interacting Drugs	Interaction
Non-HIV Drugs		
Acyclovir	interferon	Additive antiviral effects
	probenecid	Increased acyclovir levels due to decreasing renal clearance
	zidovudine	Increased risk for neurotoxicity
Amantadine	Anticholinergic drugs	Increased adverse anticholinergic effects
	CNS stimulants	Additive CNS stimulant effects
Ganciclovir	foscarnet	Additive or synergistic effect against cytomegalovirus and herpes simplex virus type 2
	imipenem	Increased risk for seizures
	zidovudine	Increased risk for hematologic toxicity (i.e., bone marrow suppression)
Ribavirin	Nucleoside reverse transcriptase inhibitors	Increase risk of hepatotoxicity and lactic acidosis
HIV Drugs		
Indinavir	Drugs metabolized by the CYP3A4 hepatic microsomal enzyme system (astemizole, cisapride, triazolam, and midazolam)	Competition for metabolism resulting in elevated blood levels and potential toxicity
	ketoconazole	Increased plasma concentrations of ganciclovir
	rifabutin and ketoconazole	Increased plasma concentrations of rifabutin and ketoconazole
	rifampin	Increased metabolism of indinavir
Nevirapine	Drugs metabolized by the CYP3A4 hepatic microsomal enzyme system	Increased metabolism of these drugs
	Oral contraceptives	Decreased plasma concentrations of oral contraceptives
	Protease inhibitors	Decreased plasma concentrations of protease inhibitors
	rifampin and rifabutin	Decreased nevirapine serum concentration
Tenofovir	acyclovir, cidofovir, ganciclovir, valacyclovir	May increase serum concentrations of tenofovir
	Protease inhibitors	Increase serum concentrations of tenofovir
Maraviroc	CYP3A4 inhibitors (azole antifungals, clarithromycin, doxycycline, erythromycin, isoniazid, nefazodone, nicardipine, protease inhibitors, quinidine, telithromycin, and verapamil)	May increase maraviroc toxicity
	CYP3A4 inducers (phenytoin, carbamazepine, rifampin)	May decrease the effects of maraviroc
	St. John's wort	May decrease the effects of maraviroc
Raltegravir	atazanavir (with or without ritonavir)	May increase effects of raltegravir
	rifampin	May decrease effects of raltegravir
Zidovudine	acyclovir	Increased neurotoxicity
	interferon beta	Increased serum levels of zidovudine
	Cytotoxic drugs	Increased risk for hematologic toxicity
	didanosine and zalcitabine	Additive or synergistic effect against HIV
	ganciclovir and ribavirin	Antagonize the antiviral action of zidovudine

CNS, Central nervous system; *CYP3A4,* cytochrome P-450 enzyme 3A4; *HIV,* human immunodeficiency virus.

such as dizziness and blurred vision. Rimantadine has gastrointestinal adverse effects similar to those of amantadine. Both medications may be used in children. Both drugs are available only for oral use.

PHARMACOKINETICS

Route	Onset of Action	Peak Plasma Concentration	Elimination Half-life	Duration of Action
PO	Within 48 hr	1-4 hr	17 hr	12-24 hr

◆ acyclovir

Acyclovir (Zovirax) is a synthetic nucleoside analogue that is used mainly to suppress the replication of HSV-1, HSV-2, and VZV. Acyclovir is considered the drug of choice for the treatment of both initial and recurrent episodes of these viral infections.

Acyclovir is available in oral, topical, and injectable formulations. Its topical use is discussed in Chapter 56. Other similar antiviral drugs include valacyclovir and famciclovir. However, these

latter two drugs are currently available only for oral use and are indicated for the treatment of less serious infections. Note the slight inconsistencies in the spelling of these drug names. Valacyclovir is a prodrug that is metabolized to acyclovir in the body. It has the advantage of greater oral bioavailability and less frequent dosing (three times daily versus five times daily for acyclovir). It may also provide more effective relief of pain from zoster lesions.

PHARMACOKINETICS

Route	Onset of Action	Peak Plasma Concentration	Elimination Half-life	Duration of Action
PO	1.5-2 hr	1.5-2 hr	2-3 hr	10-15 hr
IV	Variable	1 hr	3 hr	8 hr

◆ ganciclovir

Like acyclovir, ganciclovir (Cytovene) is a synthetic nucleoside analogue of guanosine, but it has a much different spectrum of anti-

DOSAGES

Antiviral Drugs (Non-HIV)

Drug (Pregnancy Category)	Pharmacologic Class	Usual Dosage Range	Indications
◆ acyclovir (Zovirax) (B)	Antiherpesvirus	**Pediatric younger than 12 yr** IV: 10-20 mg/kg q8h × 7-10 days **Pediatric 12 yr to adult** IV: 5-10 mg/kg q8h × 7-10 days PO: 200-800 mg q4h 5 times daily × 7-10 days, or PO: 20 mg/kg (max 800 mg/dose) 5 times daily × 5 days	HSV-1 and HSV-2 infection, including genital herpes, mucocutaneous herpes, herpes encephalitis; herpes zoster (shingles); higher-dose therapy for acute episodes; lower-dose therapy for viral suppression Chickenpox (varicella)
amantadine (Symmetrel) (C)	Antiinfluenza	**Pediatric 1-9 yr** 4.4-8.8 mg/kg/day divided once or twice daily **Pediatric 9-12 yr** 100 mg twice daily **Adolescent and adult 13-64 yr** 200 mg/day or divided bid **Adult older than 65 yr** 100 mg daily	Influenza A
oseltamivir (Tamiflu) (C)	Antiinfluenza	**Pediatric 1-12 yr* or less than 15 kg** 30 mg twice daily **15-22 kg** 45 mg twice daily **23-40 kg** 60 mg twice daily **More than 40 kg or 13 yr to adult** 75 mg twice daily	Influenza A or B
ribavirin (Virazole) (X)	Anti-RSV	**Pediatric** Aerosol: 6 g reconstituted to 20 mg/mL via continuous aerosol 12-18 hr/day for 3-7 days	Severe RSV infection in hospitalized infants and toddlers
zanamivir (Relenza) (C)	Antiinfluenza	**Pediatric 7 yr to adult** Inhalation*: 10 mg (two 5-mg powder doses) twice daily; first day's doses must be at least 2 hr apart and q12h thereafter	Influenza A or B

NOTE: When pediatric dosages are not provided, dosing guidelines for pediatric patients are not firmly established for the drug in question and should be based on the careful clinical judgment of a qualified prescriber.
HIV, Human immunodeficiency virus; *HSV-1, HSV-2,* herpes simplex virus types 1 and 2; *IV,* intravenous; *PO,* oral; *RSV,* respiratory syncytial virus.
*Use bronchodilator inhaler first if applicable.

viral activity. It is indicated for the treatment of infections caused by CMV. CMV is carried by up to 50% of the adult population and normally causes no harm. However, in immunocompromised patients (including premature infants), it can cause life-threatening or disabling opportunistic infections. Valganciclovir (Valcyte), foscarnet (Foscavir), and cidofovir (Vistide) are three other antiviral drugs that are used in the treatment of CMV infection. Of these three antiviral drugs, ganciclovir is the one most often used for this purpose. A common site of CMV infections in the immunocompromised patient is the eye, and the result is CMV retinitis, a devastating viral infection that can lead to blindness. Ganciclovir is most commonly administered intravenously or orally. However, there is also an ophthalmic form (Vitrasert) for treating active CMV retinitis, which must be surgically inserted. Ganciclovir is also administered to *prevent* CMV *disease* (generalized infection) in high-risk patients, such as those receiving organ transplants.

The dose-limiting toxicity of ganciclovir treatment is bone marrow suppression, whereas that of foscarnet and cidofovir is renal toxicity. These toxicities should be kept in mind when deciding which drug is more appropriate in a particular patient. For example, a heart transplant recipient who contracts CMV retinitis is immunocompromised because of immunosuppressant drug therapy and is most likely taking cyclosporine, which is nephrotoxic. Therefore, using foscarnet in this patient may be more dangerous than using ganciclovir. On the other hand, a patient who contracts a CMV infection and is immunocompromised because of a bone marrow transplant might be better treated using foscarnet.

Valganciclovir is a prodrug of ganciclovir, formulated for oral use, that is metabolized to ganciclovir in the body. As is the case described previously for valacyclovir and acyclovir, the prodrug provides greater oral bioavailability and allows less frequent daily dosing. Cidofovir and foscarnet are available only in injectable form.

PHARMACOKINETICS

Route	Onset of Action	Peak Plasma Concentration	Elimination Half-life	Duration of Action
PO	Unknown	24 hr	4.8 hr	Variable

oseltamivir and zanamivir

Oseltamivir (Tamiflu) and zanamivir (Relenza) belong to one of the newest classes of antiviral drugs known as *neuraminidase inhibitors*. These drugs are active against influenza virus types A and B. They are indicated for the treatment of uncomplicated acute illness caused by influenza infection in adults. They have been shown to reduce the duration of influenza infection by several days. The neuraminidase enzyme enables budding virions to escape from infected cells and spread throughout the body. Neuraminidase inhibitors are designed to stop this process in the body, speeding recovery from infection.

The most commonly reported adverse events with oseltamivir are nausea and vomiting; those with zanamivir are diarrhea, nausea, and sinusitis. Oseltamivir is available only for oral use. The drug is indicated for prophylaxis and treatment of influenza infection. Zanamivir is available in blister packets of dry powder for inhalation. It is currently indicated only for treatment of active influenza illness. Treatment with oseltamivir and zanamivir ideally should begin within 2 days of symptom onset.

PHARMACOKINETICS (OSELTAMIVIR)

Route	Onset of Action	Peak Plasma Concentration	Elimination Half-life	Duration of Action
PO	Unknown	1-2 hr	1-3 hr	5-15 hr

PHARMACOKINETICS (ZANAMIVIR)

Route	Onset of Action	Peak Plasma Concentration	Elimination Half-life	Duration of Action
PO	Unknown	1-2 hr	2-5 hr	10-24 hr

ribavirin

Ribavirin (Virazole) is a synthetic nucleoside analogue of guanosine, as are many of the other antiviral drugs, but it has a spectrum of antiviral activity that is broader than that of other currently available antiviral drugs. It interferes with both RNA and DNA synthesis and as a result inhibits both protein synthesis and viral replication overall.

The inhalational form (Virazole) is used primarily in the treatment of hospitalized infants with severe lower respiratory tract infections caused by respiratory syncytial virus. This drug was first available only in inhalational form. More recently oral dosage forms have become available for use in the treatment of hepatitis C; these are discussed in Chapter 49.

PHARMACOKINETICS

Route	Onset of Action	Peak Plasma Concentration	Elimination Half-life	Duration of Action
Inhalation	Unknown	End of inhalation	1.4-2.5 hr	Variable
PO	Unknown	2-3 hr	120-170 hr	Unknown

Disease Overview of HIV Infection and AIDS

The first U.S. cases of acquired immune deficiency syndrome (AIDS) were recognized in 1981 in 31 previously healthy homosexual men in Los Angeles and New York City. These first patients mysteriously developed *Pneumocystis carinii* pneumonia (PCP) or Kaposi's sarcoma, both normally extremely rare illnesses. (PCP is now known as *Pneumocystis jirovecii* pneumonia). Within months, similar disease patterns were recognized in intravenous drug users

and in hemophiliac patients who had been transfused with blood-derived clotting factors. Other cases began to occur in hospitalized patients transfused with a variety of blood-derived products. In 1983 human T-cell lymphotropic virus type 3 (HTLV-3) was isolated from a patient with lymphadenopathy (swollen lymph nodes), and in 1984 this virus was demonstrated to be the cause of AIDS. The virus was later renamed *human immunodeficiency virus (HIV)*, a member of the retrovirus family. There are two recognized types of HIV: human immunodeficiency virus type 1 (HIV-1) and human immunodeficiency virus type 2 (HIV-2). Both cause AIDS, but HIV-2 is primarily localized in western Africa, with HIV-1 causing the majority of the HIV pandemic in the rest of the world. By 1985, a laboratory technique known as *enzyme-linked immunosorbent assay* (ELISA) was developed. This technique allowed the detection of HIV exposure based on the presence of human antibodies to the virus in blood samples. This diagnostic breakthrough led to an appreciation of the enormity of HIV prevalence both in U.S. high-risk groups and as an emerging world pandemic, especially in developing countries. This laboratory screening technique also helped to restore the safety of the transfusion blood supply, although it is not 100% reliable.

The retrovirus family got its name upon discovery of a unique feature of its replication process. Retroviruses are all RNA viruses and are unique in their use of the enzyme **reverse transcriptase** during their replication process. This enzyme promotes the synthesis of complementary (mirror image) DNA molecules from the viral RNA genome. A second enzyme, *integrase*, promotes the integration of this viral DNA into the host cell DNA. This hybrid DNA complex is known as a *provirus*. It produces new viral RNA genomes and proteins, which in turn combine to make mature HIV virions that infect other host cells. Another important enzyme is

protease, which serves to chemically separate the new viral RNA from viral protein molecules. These components are initially synthesized into one large macromolecular strand, and the protease enzyme carefully breaks up this strand into its key components. Figure 40-2 shows the major structural features of the HIV virion, and Figure 40-3 illustrates the steps in its replication process. Reverse transcriptase is not normally found in host cells—both reverse transcriptase and integrase are carried by the virus itself. "Reversal" of the usual replication processes led to the name *re-*

verse transcriptase for this enzyme and also to the name *retrovirus* for this family of viruses. Furthermore, the fact that retroviruses synthesize DNA from viral RNA molecules is also a reversal of the norm, because in most other organisms, RNA molecules are synthesized *from* DNA molecules as part of the reproductive process. Reverse transcriptase has a high rate of errors when stringing together the purine and pyrimidine bases during transcription of the viral RNA genome into a DNA molecule in the replication process. This allows more frequent genetic mutations among HIV virions and often results in viral strains that are resistant to both medications and the patient's immune system. Such mutations also hamper the development of an effective vaccine against the virus. Drugs used to treat HIV are called *antiretrovirals.*

The most common routes of transmission of HIV are sexual activity, intravenous drug use, and perinatal transfer from mother to child. According to CDC data, an estimated 56,300 people became newly infected with HIV in 2006. Transmission was most common in homosexual or bisexual men (53% of cases). High-risk heterosexual intercourse accounted for 31% of cases and intravenous drug use for 12% of cases. African American males and females had a rate of HIV infection seven times higher than that seen in white Americans. Cases of sexual transmission via oral mucosa have also been documented. However, it should be emphasized that no solid evidence to date confirms transmission of HIV by more casual contact, including hugging, kissing, coughing, sneezing, swimming in pools, and sharing of food, water, eating utensils, or toilet facilities. HIV also is not transmitted by insect bites, unlike some other viral illnesses. Although HIV can be isolated from almost any body

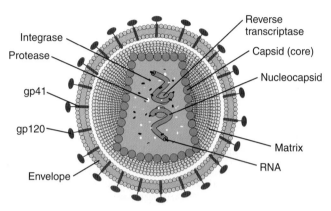

FIGURE 40-2 Human immunodeficiency virus. Within the core capsid, the diploid, single-stranded, positive-sense RNA is complexed to nucleoprotein. *gp,* Glycoprotein. (From *Dorland's illustrated medical dictionary,* ed 31, Philadelphia, 2007, Saunders.)

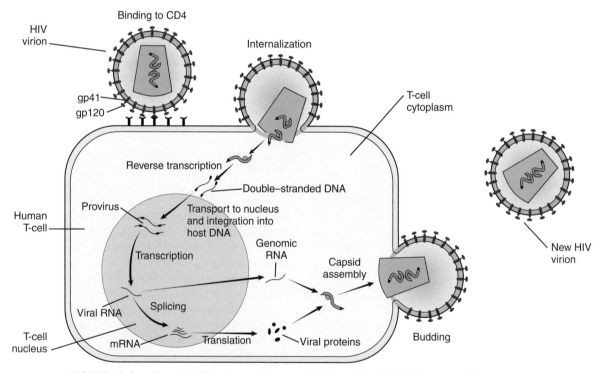

FIGURE 40-3 Life cycle of the human immunodeficiency virus (HIV). The extracellular envelope protein gp120 binds to CD4 on the surface of T lymphocytes or mononuclear phagocytes, while the transmembrane protein gp41 mediates the fusion of the viral envelope with the cell membrane. *gp,* Glycoprotein; *mRNA,* messenger RNA. (From *Dorland's illustrated medical dictionary,* ed 31, Philadelphia, 2007, Saunders.)

fluid, including tears, sweat, saliva, and urine, its concentrations in these fluids are much lower than those in blood and genital secretions. In approximately 6% of cases, specific risk factors cannot be determined. The risk for transmission to health care workers via percutaneous (needlestick) injuries is currently calculated at approximately 0.3%. Observing Standard Precautions to avoid contact with all body fluids during patient care dramatically reduces the risk for caregiver infection (see Box 10-1).

The rate of new infections is rising more rapidly in minority populations, especially among African Americans and Hispanics. Worldwide, there are now more than 40 million cases of HIV/AIDS, with more than 80% occurring in developing countries. Patients in these countries often lack access to adequate drug therapy. Untreated HIV-infected pregnant women transmit the virus to their infants in 15% to 30% of pregnancies. This can occur transplacentally, causing infection in utero, or during birth. When the first antiretroviral drugs were developed in the 1980s, it was feared that they would be too toxic and even teratogenic if given to pregnant women. However, prophylactic antiretroviral treatment of infected mothers has been shown to reduce infant infection by at least two thirds and is not normally harmful to either mother or infant. Medication may also be given prophylactically to the newborn infant, typically for the first 6 weeks of life. Of course, infants and children with established HIV infection must usually continue taking medication indefinitely. Breast milk can transmit the virus to the infant in 10% to 20% of cases, and therefore breast-feeding is contraindicated in more developed countries. In developing countries, however, breast-feeding may be the only available source of nutrition for the infant and therefore worth the risk. Box 40-1 summarizes key epidemiologic concepts related to HIV/AIDS.

HIV infection that is untreated or treatment resistant eventually leads to severe immune system failure, with death occurring secondary to opportunistic infections. AIDS often progresses over a period of several years. Various health organizations, including the CDC and the World Health Organization (WHO), have published classification systems describing various "stages" of this infection. The most recent WHO model lists four stages as follows:

- Stage 1: asymptomatic infection
- Stage 2: early, general symptoms of disease
- Stage 3: moderate symptoms
- Stage 4: severe symptoms, often leading to death

Stage 1 refers to the first few weeks or months after initial exposure to the virus. Patients may be asymptomatic but may show signs of *persistent generalized lymphadenopathy* or swollen lymph nodes ("swollen glands"). Persistent generalized lymphadenopathy is more specifically defined as inflammation of the lymph nodes in at least two sites outside the inguinal (groin) area that lasts for some months. During this time, the virus is present in the blood at low levels and has a low rate of replication. An important measure of immune function, the *CD4 count,* is usually still within normal limits at 350 cells/mm³ of blood. *CD4* refers to the protein on the cell surface of helper T lymphocytes, to which HIV virions attach themselves. Helper T cells normally function by releasing *cytokines.* Cytokines are chemicals that activate and modulate *cell-mediated immunity,* which, as noted earlier, is a general term for all immune system actions other than those involving antibodies. Immune system function is

described further in Chapter 49. Helper T cells circulate in the blood and are the primary target cells for HIV. It is ultimately through widespread destruction of these helper T cells in the blood that HIV infection weakens the patient's immune system.

Stage 2 involves continued lymphadenopathy along with other symptoms, including fever, rash, sore throat, night sweats, malaise, diarrhea, idiopathic thrombocytopenia, oral candidiasis, and herpes zoster (shingles). In the early years of the epidemic (early 1980s), this stage was also known as *AIDS-related complex* or *ARC.* These symptoms may actually resolve spontaneously about the time of seroconversion, which is when the patient's own antibodies to the virus (HIV antibodies) begin to appear in blood samples. Seroconversion usually occurs 3 weeks to 3 months after exposure. At this point, the patient is said to be *HIV positive.* However, the patient may not have further progression of symptoms for 1 to 10 years. During this stage, the CD4 T-cell count begins to drop, and HIV antibody levels rise as part of an attempt by the patient's own immune system to neutralize the virus. The virus begins to multiply in the body but does not necessarily produce disabling symptoms. This stage is often the first presenting sign of HIV infection, and stage 1 may not have been noticed or reported by the patient.

During *stage 3,* the infection progresses to a moderately symptomatic state. Weight loss, chronic diarrhea, and fever continue, and CD4 counts continue to drop. Opportunistic infections begin, including severe bacterial pneumonias, and pulmonary tuberculosis (TB). Pulmonary TB is usually more severe in persons with AIDS and is currently the leading cause of death worldwide for HIV-infected patients. Opportunistic infections

---

BOX 40-1 Epidemiology of HIV Infection

Disease Viral Factors
- Developed virus is easily inactivated and must be transmitted in body fluids
- Disease has a long prodromal or incubation period
- Virus can be shed before development of identifiable symptoms

Transmission
- Virus is present in blood, semen, and vaginal secretions

Groups at Risk
- Intravenous drug abusers; sexually active people with many partners (homosexual and heterosexual); prostitutes; newborns of HIV-positive mothers
- Blood and organ transplant recipients and hemophiliacs: before 1985 (before screening programs)

Geographic Factors
- Continuously expanding epidemic worldwide
- No particular seasonal pattern of infection (i.e., unlike influenza)

Modes of Control
- Antiviral drugs limit progression of disease.
- Vaccines for prevention and treatment are in trials.
- Monogamous sex using safe sexual practices helps limit spread.
- Sterile injection needles should be used.
- Large-scale screening programs have been developed to test blood for transfusions, organs for transplantation, and clotting factors given to hemophiliacs.

Data from U.S. Department of Health and Human Services: AIDSinfo (AIDS information website), available at *http://www.aidsinfo.nih.gov.*
HIV, Human immunodeficiency virus.

are so named because the destruction by HIV of the patient's immune system gives the "opportunity" for normally harmless microorganisms in the body to proliferate to cause serious infections. These infections may become life-threatening or produce significant disability (e.g., blindness from CMV retinitis).

In *stage 4* (formerly called *full-blown AIDS*), viral replication rises dramatically, which results in increasing destruction of helper T cells and a corresponding decrease in CD4 counts. At this point, there is a major decline in immune system function, and the illness begins to seriously affect the entire body. When the CD4 count drops below 200 cells/mm^3, fever, night sweats, and malaise resume and are now accompanied by increasingly severe *opportunistic infections,* such as *Mycobacterium avium-intracellulare* complex infection and *Pneumocystis jirovecii* pneumonia. Other common opportunistic infections include parasitic infections such as cryptosporidial diarrhea and toxoplasmosis encephalitis; viral infections such as HSV mouth ulcers, disseminated extrapulmonary tuberculosis, esophagitis, pneumonitis, CMV pneumonia, and CMV retinitis; and fungal infections, such as candidiasis of the gastrointestinal and respiratory tracts, and invasive aspergillosis of the lungs. Similarly opportunistic disorders are HIV-associated neoplasms. The most common of these are Kaposi's sarcoma and various types of lymphoma. There is also some evidence that cervical cancer is more likely to be diagnosed in advanced stages in HIV-infected women. *HIV wasting syndrome* is yet another defining condition of the disease and involves major weight loss, chronic diarrhea, more frequent or even constant fever, and chronic fatigue. In addition to attacking helper T cells and macrophages, the HIV virus can also cause pathologic changes in organs such as the brain (HIV-induced encephalopathy and dementia), bone marrow, lungs (recurrent pneumonia), and skin. Death is most likely when the CD4 count falls below 50 cells/mm^3. The viral load, which is measured as the number of viral RNA copies per milliliter of blood, also continues to rise uncontrollably. If this condition persists, death often ensues. All of these manifestations are said to be the *defining conditions* of AIDS. Box 40-2 lists several such conditions.

Figure 40-4 illustrates events that roughly correlate with these four stages of HIV infection. This figure shows the hypothetical natural course of the disease through the previously described stages in patients *without* treatment. Patients who are effectively treated with drug therapy usually do not progress through all of these stages, or at least such progression is slowed considerably (by years). In fact, advances in antiretroviral drug therapy have given rise to increasingly greater numbers of long-term survivors of HIV infection. *Highly active antiretroviral therapy (HAART)* refers to combinations of antiretroviral drugs ("cocktails") that are now standard for treating HIV-infected patients. This combination therapy (HAART) is normally begun immediately upon confirmation of HIV infection. Opportunistic infections are treated with infection-specific antimicrobial drugs (see corresponding chapters) as they arise. Prophylactic treatment for opportunistic infections is also common and is most frequently given when a patient's CD4 count falls below 200 cells/mm^3. Opportunistic malignancies, such as Kaposi's sarcoma and lymphomas, are also treated with specific antineoplastic medications, which are discussed in Chapters 47 and 48, as well as with radiation and/or surgery as indicated. *Long-term survival* is defined as

---

BOX 40-2 Indicator Diseases of AIDS

Opportunistic Infections
Protozoal
- Toxoplasmosis of the brain
- Cryptosporidiosis with diarrhea
- Isosporiasis with diarrhea

Fungal
- Candidiasis of the esophagus, trachea, and lungs
- *Pneumocystis jirovecii* pneumonia
- Cryptococcosis (extrapulmonary)
- Histoplasmosis (disseminated)
- Coccidioidomycosis (disseminated)

Viral
- Cytomegalovirus disease
- Herpes simplex virus infection (persistent or disseminated)
- Progressive multifocal leukoencephalopathy
- Hairy leukoplakia caused by Epstein-Barr virus

Bacterial
- *Mycobacterium avium-intracellulare* complex infection (disseminated)
- Any atypical mycobacterial disease
- Extrapulmonary tuberculosis
- *Salmonella* septicemia (recurrent)
- Pyogenic bacterial infections (multiple or recurrent)

Opportunistic Neoplasias
- Kaposi's sarcoma
- Primary lymphoma of the brain
- Other non-Hodgkin's lymphomas

Others
- HIV wasting syndrome
- HIV encephalopathy
- Lymphoid interstitial pneumonia

From Mandell GL et al: *Principles and practices of infectious diseases,* ed 6, Philadelphia, 2005, Churchill Livingstone.
AIDS, Acquired immunodeficiency syndrome; *HIV,* human immunodeficiency virus.

---

living with HIV infection for at least 10 to 15 years after infection. Some particularly remarkable patients have lived for several years with CD4 counts remaining at levels considered fatal. Improved drug therapy against both HIV and opportunistic infections is believed to play an important role in these unusual cases. Other remarkable patients are the long-term nonprogressors. These are long-term survivors who have maintained normal CD4 counts and low HIV viral loads despite not receiving *any* anti-HIV drug treatment. These patients are usually able to mount especially strong cell-mediated and humoral immune responses that prevent progression of the viral infection. They are also the subject of much research to identify the mechanisms of their survival and hopefully to find ways to share these advantages with other patients. Research attempts to develop an effective anti-HIV vaccine are also underway throughout the world. Several *preclinical* (animal) studies using monkeys have been carried out. Human clinical trials have been conducted since 1990, primarily in non–HIV-infected research volunteers. However, vaccines are also being studied in HIV-positive patients. Despite encouraging data regarding potential benefits, the design of an effective HIV vaccine continues to remain elusive.

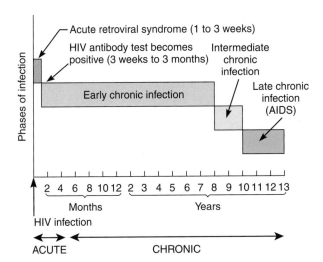

FIGURE 40-4 Timeline for the spectrum of untreated HIV infection. The timeline represents the course of untreated illness from the time of infection to clinical manifestations of disease. (From Lewis SM et al: *Medical-surgical nursing: assessment and management of clinical problems,* ed 7, St Louis, 2007, Mosby.)

Pharmacology Overview of Drugs Used to Treat HIV Infection

Much has happened in medical science since the AIDS virus was first identified in the early 1980s. The increasing urgency and public awareness of the HIV epidemic have stimulated much research in the fields of immunology and pharmacology. This has resulted in the development of several increasingly effective antiretroviral drugs, as well as of antiviral drugs in general. Although new drug combinations have definitely prolonged lives and offered hope to many people, these medications often carry significant toxicities. Furthermore, HIV/AIDS is still not considered to be a curable disease, although there have been some remarkable recoveries and apparent cures in a small number of individuals. There are currently five classes of antiretroviral drugs, including the *reverse transcriptase inhibitors,* the *protease inhibitors,* the *fusion inhibitors,* and the newest classes, the *entry inhibitor–CCR5 coreceptor antagonists* and the *HIV integrase strand transfer inhibitors.* There are currently two subclasses of reverse transcriptase inhibitors: nucleoside reverse transcriptase inhibitors (NRTIs) and the nonnucleoside reverse transcriptase inhibitors (NNRTIs). Drugs from many of these drug classes are combined together into a single drug dosage form for ease of use. See Table 40-4 for lists of drugs and their respective classes. As stated earlier, HIV drug therapy is rapidly changing, and the reader is referred to various websites including the FDA's site at *http://www.fda.gov/oashi/aids/virals. html* for the most up-to-date listing.

Mechanism of Action and Drug Effects

Although HIV/AIDS is a very complex illness, the mechanisms of action of the various drug classes are fortunately straightforward and distinct. The name of each class of medication provides a reminder of its role in suppressing the viral replication process.

TABLE **40-4** **Examples of Antiretrovirals Used to Treat HIV**

Generic Name	Trade Name
Nucleoside Reverse Transcriptase Inhibitors	
abacavir	Ziagen
abacavir/lamivudine	Epzicom
abacavir/zidovudine/lamivudine	Trizivir
didanosine (enteric coated)	Videx EC
didanosine (dideoxyinosine)	Videx
emtricitabine	Emtriva
lamivudine	Epivir
stavudine (d4T)	Zerit
tenofovir	Viread
tenofovir/emtricitabine	Truvada
zalcitabine	Hivid
zidovudine	Retrovir
Nonnucleoside Reverse Transcriptase Inhibitors	
delavirdine	Rescriptor
efavirenz	Sustiva
etravirine	Intelence
nevirapine	Viramune
Protease Inhibitors	
amprenavir	Agenerase
atazanavir	Reyataz
darunavir	Prezista
fosamprenavir	Lexiva
indinavir	Crixivan
lopinavir/ritonavir	Kaletra
nelfinavir	Viracept
ritonavir	Norvir
saquinavir mesylate	Invirase
tipranavir	Aptivus
Fusion Inhibitor	
enfuvirtide	Fuzeon
Entry Inhibitor–CCR5 Coreceptor Antagonist (also known as CCR5 antagonist)	
maraviroc	Selzentry
HIV Integrase Strand Transfer Inhibitor (also known as integrase inhibitor)	
raltegravir	Isentress
Mulitclass Combination Products	
efavirenz/emtricitabine/tenofovir	Atripla
abacavir/lamivudine/zidovudine	Trizivir
lamivudine/zidovudine	Combivir
lopinavir/ritonavir	Kaletra

CCR5, Chemokine receptor 5; *HIV,* human immunodeficiency virus.

Thus, reverse transcriptase inhibitors work by blocking activity of the enzyme reverse transcriptase. Reverse transcriptase promotes the synthesis of new viral DNA molecules from the RNA genome of the parent virion. The protease inhibitors work by inhibiting the protease retroviral enzyme. This enzyme promotes the breakup of chains of protein molecules at designated points, a process necessary for viral replication. There is also one combination protease inhibitor that includes both lopinavir and ritonavir. Both medications are protease inhibitors. The ritonavir component also serves to inhibit *cytochrome P-450*–mediated

TABLE **40-5** Recommendations for Occupational HIV Exposure Chemoprophylaxis

Type of Exposure	Source	Prophylaxis?	Therapy
Percutaneous	Blood	Recommended	zidovudine + lamivudine + indinavir; OR
	Fluid containing visible blood or other potentially infectious fluid or tissue		zidovudine + lamivudine ± indinavir
Mucous membrane	Blood	Offer	zidovudine + lamivudine
	Fluid containing visible blood or other potentially infectious fluid or tissue	Offer	zidovudine + lamivudine ± indinavir; OR zidovudine ± lamivudine
Skin (i.e., prolonged contact, extensive area, area without skin integrity)	Blood	Offer	zidovudine + lamivudine ± indinavir

HIV, Human immunodeficiency virus.

enzymatic metabolism of the lopinavir component. There is currently only one fusion inhibitor. This compound works by inhibiting viral fusion. This is the process by which an HIV virion attaches to (fuses with) the membrane of a host cell (T lymphocyte) before infecting it in preparation for viral replication. The entry inhibitors–CCR5 coreceptor antagonists, or CCR5 antagonists (maraviroc), work by selectively and reversibly binding to the type 5 chemokine coreceptors located on the CD4 cells that are used by the HIV virion to gain entry to the cells. The integrase strand transfer inhibitors, also referred to as integrase inhibitors (raltegravir), work by inhibiting the catalytic activity of the enzyme integrase thus preventing integration of the proviral gene into human DNA.

Single-drug therapy was most common in the early years of the HIV epidemic, partly due to a lack of treatment options. However, both the development of multiple antiretroviral drugs and the emergence of resistant viral strains have given rise to combination drug therapy as the current standard of care. This is the most effective treatment to date and, as noted earlier, is referred to as *highly active antiretroviral therapy* (HAART). HAART usually includes at least three medications. The most commonly recommended drug combinations include two or three NRTIs; two NRTIs plus one or two protease inhibitors; or an NRTI plus an NNRTI with one or two protease inhibitors. Despite the effectiveness of HAART, prescribers may still need to alter a given patient's drug regimen in cases of major drug intolerance (see Adverse Effects) or drug resistance. A given patient's HIV strain can still evolve and mutate over time, which allows it to become resistant to any drug therapy, especially when that therapy is used for a prolonged period of time. Evidence of drug resistance includes a falling CD4 count and/or increased viral load in a patient in whom a given drug regimen previously kept those parameters under control.

All antiretroviral drugs have similar therapeutic effects, to varying degrees. They reduce the viral load, which is the number of viral RNA copies per milliliter of blood. A viral load of less than 50 copies/mL is considered to be an undetectable viral load and is a primary goal of antiretroviral therapy. HIV-infected patients should ideally be followed by practitioners with extensive training and specialization in drug therapy for infectious diseases. These practitioners must often make careful choices and changes in drug

therapy over time, based on a given patient's clinical response and severity of any drug-related toxicities. When effective, treatment leads to a significant reduction in mortality and incidence of opportunistic infections, improves patient's physical performance, and significantly increases T-cell counts.

Indications

The only usual indication for all of the current antiretroviral drugs is active HIV infection. Prophylactic therapy is also given to individuals such health care workers and high-risk infants with known potential exposure to HIV (e.g., via needlestick injuries in hospitals [Table 40-5]).

Contraindications

Because of the potentially fatal outcome of HIV infection, the only usual contraindication to a given medication is known severe drug allergy or other intolerable toxicity. Most of the current antiretroviral drug classes have several alternative drugs to choose from, should a patient be especially intolerant of a given drug.

Adverse Effects

Common adverse effects of selected antiretroviral drugs are listed in Table 40-2. A few key adverse effects are discussed in more detail later. The need to modify drug therapy because of adverse effects is not uncommon. The goal is to find the regimen that will best control a given patient's infection and that has as tolerable an adverse effect profile as possible. Different patients vary widely in their drug tolerance, and their tolerance may change over time. Thus, medication regimens often must be strategically individualized and evolve with the course of the patient's illness. Approximately 25% of HIV-infected patients in the United States are also infected with hepatitis C virus (HCV), which tends to cause more severe disease in HIV patients. Hepatitis C is the most important cause of chronic liver disease in the United States and is the most common reason for liver transplantation. Unfortunately, HAART is strongly correlated with increased mortality from HCV-induced liver disease, because the anti-HIV drugs produce strain on the liver. A major adverse effect of protease inhibitors is lipid abnormalities, including *lipodystrophy,* or redistribution of fat stores under the skin. This condition often results in cosmetically undesirable outcomes for the patient, such as a "hump" at the posterior base of the neck and also a *skeletonized* (bony) appearance of the face. In addition, dyslipidemias such as hypertriglyceridemia can occur, and insulin resistance and type 2 diabetes symptoms can result. It is reported that in these cases, switching a patient from a protease inhibitor to an NNRTI may help to reduce such symptoms without decreasing antiretroviral efficacy. The increase in long-term antiretroviral drug therapy due to prolonged disease survival has led to the emergence of another long-term adverse effect associated with these medications—bone demineralization and possible osteoporosis. When this condition occurs, it may require treatment with standard medications for osteoporosis, such as calcium, vitamin D, and bisphosphonates (see Chapter 34).

Interactions

Common selected drug interactions involving both antiretrovirals and other antivirals are listed in Table 40-3.

Dosages

Because of rapidly changing antiviral drug therapy and the complexity of dosing and the disease state, only selected dosages are listed in this book (see Dosages table on p. 638). The reader is referred to an up-to-date drug information handbook for specifics on dosing.

DRUG PROFILES

enfuvirtide

Enfuvirtide (Fuzeon) is the only medication in one of the newest classes of antiretroviral drugs, called *fusion inhibitors.* It works by suppressing the fusion process whereby a virion is attached to the outer membrane of a host T cell before entry into the cell and subsequent viral replication. This mechanism of action serves as yet another example of how antiretroviral drugs are strategically designed to interfere with specific steps of the viral replication process. As mentioned previously, the use of combinations of drugs that work by different mechanisms improves a patient's chances for continued survival by reducing the likelihood of viral resistance to the drug therapy regimen. Enfuvirtide is indicated for treatment of HIV infection in combination with other antiretroviral drugs. Adult and pediatric patients have shown comparable tolerance of the drug in clinical trials thus far. Use of this drug in combination with other standard antiretroviral drugs has been associated with markedly reduced viral loads, compared with drug regimens that did not include this drug. The drug is currently available only in injectable form.

PHARMACOKINETICS

Route	Onset of Action	Peak Plasma Concentration	Elimination Half-life	Duration of Action
Subcut	Unknown	4-8 hr	4 hr	Unknown

◆ indinavir

Indinavir (Crixivan) belongs to the *protease inhibitor* class of antiretroviral drugs. Others include ritonavir (Norvir), nelfinavir (Viracept), amprenavir (Agenerase), fosamprenavir (Lexiva), atazanavir (Reyataz), tipranavir (Aptivus), ritonavir (Norvir), darunavir (Prezista), and the combination product lopinavir/ritonavir (Kaletra). Indinavir can be taken in combination with other anti-HIV therapies or alone. This drug is best dissolved and absorbed in an acidic gastric environment, and the presence of high-protein and high-fat foods reduces its absorption. Therefore, it is recommended that it be administered in a fasting state. Indinavir therapy produces increases in CD4 cell counts and significant reductions in viral load. Protease inhibitors are commonly given in combination with two reverse transcriptase inhibitors to maximize efficacy and decrease the likelihood of viral drug resistance. Indinavir is relatively well tolerated in most patients. Nephrolithiasis (kidney stones) occur in approximately 4% of patients. Patients who take indinavir are encouraged to drink at least 48 oz of liquids every day to maintain hydration and help avoid nephrolithiasis. Indinavir and all other protease inhibitors are available only for oral use.

PHARMACOKINETICS

Route	Onset of Action	Peak Plasma Concentration	Elimination Half-life	Duration of Action
PO	2 wk to therapeutic effect	0.5-1 hr	1.5-2.5 hr	6 mo

maraviroc

Maraviroc (Selzentry) is the only drug available in a new class of antiretrovirals called *CCR5 antagonists.* Maraviroc works by selectively and reversibly binding to the chemokine coreceptors located on the CD4 cells. It is used in treatment-experienced patients with evidence of viral replication and HIV-1 strains resistant to multiple antiretroviral therapy. Patients must receive an FDA-approved medication guide before this drug is dispensed. Hepatotoxicity with allergic-type features has been reported. Drug interactions of significance include interactions with cytochrome P-450 3A4 (CYP3A4) inhibitors (azole antifungals, clarithromycin, doxycycline, erythromycin, isoniazid, nefazodone, nicardipine, protease inhibitors, quinidine, telithromycin, and verapamil), which may increase maraviroc toxicity. CYP3A4 inducers, including phenytoin, carbamazepine, nafcillin, and rifampin, may decrease maraviroc's effects. Maraviroc is available only for oral use.

PHARMACOKINETICS

Route	Onset of Action	Peak Plasma Concentration	Elimination Half-life	Duration of Action
PO	Unknown	0.5-4 hr	14-18 hr	Unknown

◆ nevirapine

Nevirapine (Viramune) is an *NNRTI.* This is the second class of antiviral drugs indicated for the treatment of HIV infection. Other currently available NNRTIs include delavirdine (Rescriptor), efavirenz (Sustiva), and etravirine (Intelence). These drugs are often used in combination with *NRTIs.*

Nevirapine is well tolerated compared with other therapies for HIV. The most common adverse events associated with nevirapine therapy are rash, fever, nausea, headache, and abnormal liver function test results. Nevirapine and the other NNRTIs are available only for oral use.

PHARMACOKINETICS

Route	Onset of Action	Peak Plasma Concentration	Elimination Half-life	Duration of Action
PO	2 hr	2-4 hr	25-30 hr	24 hr

raltegravir

Raltegravir (Isentress) is the only drug in the new class called *integrase inhibitors.* Raltegravir works by inhibiting the activity of the integrase enzyme, thus preventing integration of the proviral gene into human DNA. Raltegravir is used in treatment-experienced

DOSAGES

HIV/AIDS Drugs

Drug (Pregnancy Category)	Pharmacologic Class	Usual Dosage Range
enfuvirtide (Fuzeon) (B)	Fusion inhibitor	**Pediatric 6-16 yr** Subcut: 2 mg/kg twice daily (max 90 mg/dose) **17 yr to adult** Subcut: 90 mg twice daily
◆ indinavir (Crixivan) (C)	Protease inhibitor	**Adult** PO: 800 mg q8h
maraviroc (Selzentry) (B)	CCR5 antagonist	**Adults and children older than 16 yr** 300 mg twice daily
◆ nevirapine (NVP) (Viramune) (C)	Nonnucleoside reverse transcriptase inhibitor	**Pediatric 2 mo-8 yr** PO: 4 mg/kg daily × 14 days, then 7 mg/kg twice daily **8 yr to adult** PO: 4 mg/kg daily × 14 days, then 4 mg/kg twice daily **Adult** PO: 200 mg daily × 14 days, then twice daily
raltegravir (Isentress) (C)	Integrase Inhibitor	**Adults and children older than 16 yr** 400 mg twice daily
tenofovir (Viread) (B)	Nucleotide reverse transcriptase inhibitor	**Adult** PO: 300 mg once daily
◆ zidovudine (AZT, ZDV) (Retrovir) (C)	Nucleoside reverse transcriptase inhibitor	**Pediatric 0-3 mo*** PO: 2 mg/kg q6h starting within 12 hr after birth and through 6 wk of age IV: 1.5 mg/kg q6h **Pediatric 6 wk-12 yr** PO: 160 mg/m² q8h (max 200 mg/dose) **Adult** PO: 100 mg q4h around the clock if symptomatic; q4h while awake if asymptomatic IV: 1 mg/kg over 1 hr; 5-6 times daily **Pregnant women** PO: 100 mg 5 times daily during pregnancy until start of labor, then give IV bolus dose of 2 mg/kg over 1 hr followed by an IV infusion of 1 mg/kg/hr until the umbilical cord is clamped

NOTE: Where pediatric doses are not provided, dosing guidelines for pediatric patients are not firmly established for the drug in question and should be based on the careful clinical judgment of a qualified prescriber.

AIDS, Acquired immunodeficiency syndrome; *CCR5,* chemokine receptor 5; *HIV,* human immunodeficiency virus; *IV,* intravenous; *PO,* oral; *subcut,* subcutaneous.
*Drug should be continued either IV or PO through at least 6 wk of age.

patients with virus that shows multidrug resistance and active replication. Myopathy and rhabdomyolysis have been reported, as well as an immune reconstitution syndrome, which may result in an inflammatory response to a residual opportunistic infection. Raltegravir does not interact with CYP3A4 inducers or inhibitors (as do many other AIDS drugs).

PHARMACOKINETICS

Route	Onset of Action	Peak Plasma Concentration	Elimination Half-life	Duration of Action
PO	Unknown	3 hr	9 hr	Unknown

tenofovir

Tenofovir (Viread) is one of many *NRTIs*. Others in this class include emtricitabine (Emtriva), lamivudine (Epivir), stavudine (Zerit), and abacavir (Ziagen), as well as many combination products. Lactic acidosis and severe hepatomegaly have been reported with this drug and others in its class. This drug is indicated for use against HIV infection in combination with other antiretroviral drugs. It is currently available only for oral use.

PHARMACOKINETICS

Route	Onset of Action	Peak Plasma Concentration	Elimination Half-life	Duration of Action
PO	4-8 days for therapeutic effect	1 hr	10-14 hr	7 days

◆ zidovudine

Zidovudine (Retrovir), also known as azidothymidine or AZT, is a synthetic nucleoside analogue of thymidine that has had an enormous impact on the treatment and quality of life of patients infected with HIV who have AIDS. It was the very first, and for a long time the only, anti-HIV medication that offered patients with AIDS any hope in the early years of the epidemic. Zidovudine, along with various other antiretroviral drugs, is given to HIV-infected pregnant women and even to newborn babies to prevent maternal transmission of the virus to the infant.

The major dose-limiting adverse effect of zidovudine is bone marrow suppression, and this is often the reason a patient with an HIV infection must be switched to another anti-HIV drug such as zalcitabine or didanosine. Some patients may receive a combination of two of these drugs, in lower dosages, to maximize their combined actions. This strategy may reduce the likelihood of toxicity. Zidovudine is available in both oral and injectable formulations.

PHARMACOKINETICS

Route	Onset of Action	Peak Plasma Concentration	Elimination Half-life	Duration of Action
PO	At least 6 mo for therapeutic effect	0.4-1.5 hr	0.8-2 hr	3-5 hr

Disease Overview of Other Viral Infections

There are numerous other viral infections; however, four of recent special significance are avian flu, West Nile virus (WNV) infection, severe acute respiratory syndrome (SARS), and the novel influenza virus (H1N1). All of these viral infections have resulted in significant morbidity and mortality, sometimes requiring aggressive supportive care in an intensive care unit setting.

In 1999, the first North American cases of *WNV infection* occurred in New York City. WNV is a member of the arbovirus family and is transmitted to humans by mosquitoes. It also infects animals, primarily birds, and has been detected in horses and cows. In humans, WNV infection can lead to meningitis and encephalitis. In 2001, an epidemic occurred with more than 4000 documented human cases, including 284 deaths. Organ transplant patients constituted one of the key groups infected. The virus can also be transmitted through blood transfusions and has been detected in breast milk. It is currently being investigated to determine whether maternal-fetal transmission can occur during pregnancy. In July 2003, national blood banks began screening blood donations for WNV using newly developed laboratory techniques. There are currently no specific antiviral medications or vaccines available for treatment of human WNV infection. Prevention focuses on reducing mosquito reproduction by eliminating unneeded pools of water near residential environments.

November 2002 marked the emergence of a new, serious viral illness known as *severe acute respiratory syndrome,* or *SARS.* A large outbreak later occurred in Singapore in March 2003. This outbreak was eventually traced to a traveler returning from Hong Kong. Cases later appeared in Europe and North America. SARS can range from a mild to a life-threatening respiratory illness. The disease usually resolves on its own within 3 to 4 weeks. However, 10% to 20% of patients required mechanical ventilation and intensive care support, and the overall fatality rate is 3%. Although standard antiviral drugs, including oseltamivir, have been used to treat SARS, no specific drug therapy has proved to be definitively helpful. The cause of SARS has been determined to be a coronavirus, which was named the *SARS coronavirus.* Coronaviruses commonly cause mild to moderate upper respiratory tract illnesses in humans, including the common cold.

Avian influenza or "bird flu" is an influenza virus infection that has been shown to infect birds in Europe and both birds and humans in Asia. This disease is caused by an influenza A virus known as *avian influenza A, subtype H5N1.* The virus is carried in the intestines of many wild birds worldwide, often without causing any serious illness. However, more serious infections can be fatal and spread rapidly among an entire flock of birds. Usually, these viruses do not infect humans. However, since 1997, there have been cases of human infection, mostly following contact with infected birds or their secretions or excrement (e.g., in poultry workers). Most of these cases have occurred in Europe and Asia. There have also been one documented case in New York and one in Virginia of infection with H7N2 virus, another avian influenza virus subtype. Human to human transmission has been especially rare. Symptoms in humans have ranged from typical flulike symptoms such as fever, cough, sore throat, and muscle aches to eye infections and acute respiratory illness, sometimes with life-threatening complications. This virus is resistant to amantadine and rimantadine, although it is believed (but remains to be confirmed) that zanamivir and oseltamivir would likely offer some therapeutic benefit for this condition.

Many health experts fear a flu pandemic caused by this virus, should it mutate to a more easily transmissible form. This occurs frequently with influenza viruses in general, which is why a new seasonal flu vaccine must be developed each year. Although no one can predict if and when such a pandemic might occur with this virus, WHO and other health agencies, including the CDC, are continuously monitoring activity patterns as well as the virus's resistance to other antiviral drugs. Some countries, including the United States, have also implemented a ban on the import of birds from countries where avian influenza has been shown to be prevalent.

In 2009, the World Health Organization signaled that a pandemic was underway with the new influenza virus H1N1 (originally called *swine flu*). The H1N1 virus spreads person to person, much the same way the regular seasonal influenza virus spreads. Symptoms include fever, cough, sore throat, body aches, chills, and fatigue. Severe illness and death have occurred with H1N1. A vaccine was developed and made available in October 2009. Antiviral medications such as oseltamivir or zanamivir are recommended for all patients with suspected or confirmed influenza requiring hospitalization. Prophylactic treatment should be considered for patients at high risk of complications.

NURSING PROCESS

Assessment

Before administering an antiviral drug, the nurse should perform a thorough medical and physical assessment and take a medication history. This is important to ensure safe medication use. Any known allergies to the medication should be noted. It is important for the nurse to also assess the patient's nutritional status and baseline vital signs because of the profound effects of viral illnesses, especially if the patient is immune compromised. Contraindications, cautions, and drug interactions associated with all of the antiviral drugs have been discussed previously.

Assessment related to the use of *non-HIV antivirals* includes inquiry about the patient's allergy to medications as well as a listing of any prescription and over-the-counter drugs, herbals, and dietary supplements. Energy levels, any weight loss, vital signs, and the characteristics of any visible lesions should be assessed and the findings documented for baseline comparison before initiation of therapy. Age is also important, because the safety and efficacy of these drugs have not been proven in children younger than 2 years of age. Rimantadine and amantadine are the drugs that may be used in children, but assessment for allergies, cautions, contraindications, and drug interactions as well as any underlying gastrointestinal symptoms and/or diseases is still required. Elderly patients may require dosage adjustments because of altered renal and hepatic functioning. There should be further concern if the patient is taking other medications that are nephrotoxic or if the patient has underlying dehydration or mineral and electrolyte imbalances. These conditions need to be identified and managed before initiation of therapy to prevent drug-related complications. Results of any HIV testing should be assessed to determine baseline values. Other laboratory tests that will most likely be ordered include white blood cell count, red blood cell (RBC) count, blood urea nitrogen (BUN) level, creatinine clearance, and liver function studies. If amantadine is being used as an antiviral for treatment of influenza, caution should be taken if there is a history of hypotension because of the potential for further hypotension and possible falls. Close attention should be given to the patient's pulse rate and blood pressure. Postural blood pressures may be needed. Specimens from blood, feces, throat, and urine may also be ordered before drug therapy for further assessment when antivirals are given.

With ribavirin, analysis of respiratory secretions via sputum specimen will most likely be ordered for diagnostic purposes prior to initiation of drug therapy. In addition, baseline renal, hepatic, cardiac, and pulmonary functioning should be assessed carefully. With respiratory illness, breath sounds, respiratory rate and patterns, cough, sputum production, and vital signs including temperature should also be assessed and documented. Ribavirin is also associated with the potential for teratogenic effects and should not be given during pregnancy or handled by health care personnel who are or might be pregnant. A dose-limiting toxicity of ganciclovir treatment is bone marrow suppression, and thus close review of blood cell counts, including complete blood count (CBC), RBC count, and platelet count, is needed. With foscarnet and cidofovir, renal function must be assessed because of the potential for renal toxicity. Before giving acyclovir, the nurse not only should carry out the usual vital sign measurement and history taking but should also be sure to assess the drug order closely. Other antiviral drugs with names similar to acyclovir are valacyclovir and famciclovir, so the nurse must be careful that the right drug is being given to avoid a medication error. Famciclovir also requires assessment of allergies, especially allergy to probenecid, because of the possibility of cross allergy. Oseltamivir and zanamivir, useful against influenza virus types A and B, must be given as ordered; close assessment of the drug, the patient, and the drug's indication is needed, because treatment with these drugs should begin within 2 days of the onset of flu symptoms.

Use of *HIV antivirals* or *antiretrovirals* requires close assessment of allergies, cautions, contraindications, and drug interactions. Use of protease inhibitors require assessment of the patient's medical history, vital signs, baseline weight, allergies, medication history, and results of baseline laboratory tests, such as CBC, RBC count, and renal and liver function studies. These laboratory tests

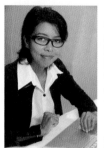
are also generally ordered during the different phases of treatment, and results should be documented appropriately. Age is an important assessment factor, because many of the drugs (e.g., abacavir) cannot be used safely in pediatric patients between the ages of 3 months and 13 years. In the elderly, dosages of many of these drugs may need to be reduced by the prescriber.

The antiretroviral drug maraviroc requires assessment of allergies and liver function as well as review of the list of medications the patient is taking because of the lengthy list of interacting drugs (see previous discussion). Raltegravir, a newer drug, is associated with myopathies and breakdown of muscle cells, and thus baseline notation of skeletal muscle functioning and pain level is crucial to patient safety. Baseline measurement and frequent monitoring of vital signs, including temperature, are important due to the possibility of opportunistic infections. The prescriber may also order CBCs and other laboratory studies before, during, and after therapy (as with many of these drugs). Bone marrow suppression is a dose-limiting adverse effect of zidovudine, and so blood cell counts and results of clotting studies need to be reviewed before and during therapy. Other drugs may need to be used should such suppression occur.

With any of the drugs presented in this chapter, especially those used for management of HIV infection, assessment of the patient's knowledge about the illness and the need for long-term and often lifelong therapy is crucial. In addition, a knowledge of the patient's educational level, reading level, the way in which the patient learns best, and familiarity with community resources is important to implement patient education effectively. Assessment of mental status and emotional state is important because of the psychologic impact of chronic illness. Value systems, social patterns, hobbies, support systems, and spiritual beliefs should also be noted and documented. For patients with chronic illnesses, the synthesis of this information will help ensure the development of a nursing care plan that is complete and holistic.

Nursing Diagnoses

- Acute pain related to the signs and symptoms associated with non-HIV viral infections, HIV infection, and HIV-related illnesses
- Risk for injury related to falls due to the adverse effects of non-HIV antiviral and antiretroviral (HIV antiviral) medications
- Risk for injury related to the immunosuppressive effects of viral disease processes and their treatment
- Deficient knowledge related to the lack of information about and experience with long-term medication therapy and lack of information about the viral infection, its transmission, and its treatment
- Activity intolerance related to weakness secondary to decreased energy from pathology of viral infections
- Risk for impaired tissue integrity from a break in the skin due to viral lesions and other skin-related problems

Planning

Goals

- Patient is free of symptoms of viral infection once therapy is completed.
- Patient adheres to the prescribed therapy regimen.
- Patient experiences improved energy and appetite and improved ability to engage in activities of daily living for the duration of therapy.
- Patient states the rationale for treatment of self and for treatment of any of the patient's active sexual partners if diagnosed with genital herpes or other viral sexually transmitted diseases.
- Patient experiences minimal adverse effects of non-HIV antivirals and HIV antivirals (antiretrovirals).
- Patient reports diminished signs and symptoms of viral infection with drug therapy.
- Patient reports healing of lesions and restoration of intact skin integrity.

Outcome Criteria

- Patient experiences increased periods of comfort as a result of successful treatment of viral infection.
- Patient states the physical impact of a viral infection on the patient's overall state of health (e.g., compromised immune system) and the effect of appropriate therapy with either non-HIV antivirals and/or HIV antivirals (antiretrovirals).
- Patient states the rationale for the treatment regimen as well as the need for treatment of any partners with whom the patient has been sexually active to prevent worsening of symptoms and to decrease the severity of disease-related episodes and other viral diseases.
- Patient identifies the possible adverse effects of the non-HIV antivirals, such as diarrhea, headache, nausea, and insomnia.
- Patient identifies the possible adverse effects of the HIV antivirals (antiretrovirals), such as gastrointestinal upset, immunosuppression, malaise, loss of energy, and loss of strength.
- Patient states the adverse effects to report (see earlier) as well as measures to take to help minimize the severity of the adverse effects of the HIV antiviral drugs, such as conservation of energy, consumption of well-balanced meals, administration of prescribed medications as ordered, and use of holistic measures, including imagery, relaxation, meditation, yoga, and other related health-preserving interventions.
- Patient states the appropriate and recommended measures to take to prevent the spread of viral infection as well as the means of containing, preventing the spread, and promoting the healing of lesions during and after antiviral or antiretroviral therapy.

Implementation

Nursing interventions pertinent to patients receiving *non-HIV antivirals* include use of the appropriate technique when applying or administering ointments, aerosol powders, or intravenous or oral forms of medication (see Box 10-1). Wearing gloves and washing hands thoroughly before and after the administration of medication are necessary to prevent contamination of the site and spread of infection. The nurse must remember that strict adherence to Standard Precautions is important to the safety of both the patient and the nurse. Also see Chapter 39 for a brief discussion of proper hand washing for patients. The use of non-HIV antivirals as well as HIV antivirals or antiretrovirals may lead to superimposed infection or superinfection, and the nurse must constantly monitored for such infections as well as implement measures for their prevention (see Chapters 38 and 39).

Oral antivirals should be given with meals to help minimize gastrointestinal upset. Capsules should be stored at room temperature, and they should not be crushed or broken. Topical dosage forms (e.g., acyclovir) should be applied using a finger cot or rubber glove to prevent autoinoculation. Eye contact should be avoided. Intravenous acyclovir is stable for 12 hours at room temperature and will often precipitate when refrigerated. Intravenous infusions should be diluted as recommended (e.g., with 5% dextrose in water or normal saline) and infused with caution. Infusion over longer than 1 hour is suggested to avoid the renal tubular damage seen with more rapid infusions. Adequate hydration should be encouraged during the infusion and for several hours afterward to prevent drug-related crystalluria. The intravenous site should be continually assessed. Any redness, heat, pain, swelling, or red streaks indicate possible phlebitis. The characteristics of any lesions should be documented. Appropriate isolation should be implemented for individuals with chickenpox or herpes zoster, and analgesics should be given for comfort. Laboratory testing to assess renal and hepatic functioning, as well as monitoring of the patient's CBC, should be ongoing with the use of antivirals. Monitoring of vital signs, with special attention to blood pressure, should be conducted throughout therapy with these medications, especially acyclovir and amantadine, because of the potential for drug-related orthostatic hypotension.

Amantadine, and other antivirals, should be taken for the entire course of therapy, and if a dose is missed the patient should take the dose as soon as it is remembered or contact the prescriber for further instructions. Should dry mouth occur, sucking on sugarless candy or chewing gum might be helpful. Daily mouth care, including the use of dental floss, and regular dental preventive visits are encouraged. Saliva substitutes may be needed, and if dry mouth continues for longer than 2 weeks, the prescriber should be contacted for further management measures. Livedo reticularis, a red-blue network-like mottling of the skin caused by congestion of the superficial capillaries, may occur, and patient education about this is important. Discontinuation of amantadine will reverse this discoloration. It is often recommended that the second dose of the drug be given several hours before bedtime to prevent insomnia. Famciclovir should be taken for the full course of therapy, and for patients who have genital herpes, the directions are usually to provide evenly spaced doses around the clock. Ganciclovir, if given intravenously, should be diluted with 5% dextrose in water or normal saline to a concentration and in a time frame indicated by the prescriber and authoritative sources. Administration into large veins is recommended to provide the dilution needed to minimize the risk for vein irritation. When the solution of ganciclovir is being handled, exposure of the eyes, mucous membranes, and skin to the drug should be avoided, and the use of latex gloves and safety glasses is recommended for handling and preparation. Should the drug come in contact with these areas, the eyes should be flushed with plain water and other affected areas should be washed thoroughly with soap and water. Ribavirin may be given by nasal or oral inhalation, but the drug should not be administered to pregnant women or handled by a health care provider who is (or may be) pregnant. When certain antivirals are given, the order should be checked closely against the drug being administered, because other drugs are spelled similarly or sound alike. For example, acyclovir may be mistaken for valacyclovir and famciclovir. When the patient is taking oseltamivir and other non-HIV antivirals for influenza, it is important to remember that this medication should be prescribed and is most effective if started within 2 days of the onset of flu symptoms.

Aerosol generators are available from the drug manufacturer. Reservoir solutions should be discarded if levels are low or empty and should be changed every 24 hours. Patients taking ribavirin and similar drugs for treatment of respiratory syncytial virus via a small particle aerosol generator (SPAG) device should be taught how to properly mix and administer the drug. The drug (e.g., ribavirin powder) should be reconstituted as instructed in the manufacturer guidelines. Old solutions left in the equipment should be discarded before adding fresh medication. Drugs given using SPAG equipment are usually administered 12 to 18 hours daily for up to 7 days, beginning within 3 days of the onset of symptoms. Much controversy exists about the use of this drug in patients on ventilators, and only health care providers who are specially trained in this drug and its use should administer it in such cases. Any "rain out" in the tubing of the ventilator should be emptied frequently, and the nurse should always monitor breath sounds in patients receiving inhaled forms of this drug, whether they are receiving artificial ventilation or not. Zanamivir is administered by inhalation using a Diskhaler device. It is important to be sure that the patient exhales completely first; then, while holding the mouthpiece between their teeth with lips snug around it and tongue down and out of the way. The patient should then inhale deeply through the mouth and then hold the breath as long as possible before exhaling the drug and the breath. The mouth should be rinsed with water to prevent irritation and dryness and the patient should never exhale into the diskhaler. In addition, during treatment with any of the antivirals, blood counts, including platelet, neutrophil, and thrombocyte counts, should be performed periodically.

HIV antivirals, or *antiretrovirals,* include numerous drugs, and general types of nursing actions are reviewed and specific drug-related information is presented, as appropriate. With regard to dosage forms, there are special administration and handling guidelines for some of the antiretroviral drugs. With zidovudine, the nurse must monitor for the adverse effects of abdominal pain, elevated serum amylase or triglyceride levels, nausea, and vomiting, and report these to the prescriber immediately, because they may indicate pancreatitis. If the patient experiences signs and symptoms of an opportunistic infection (e.g., respiratory signs and symptoms, fever, changes in oral mucosa), the prescriber should be contacted immediately. Patients should be weighed, or encouraged to weigh themselves, at least two times a week, and a gain of 2 pounds or more in 24 hours or 5 pounds or more in 1 week should be reported. Headaches may occur with some of these drugs, and therefore analgesia should be provided, as ordered.

With some antiretrovirals, avoidance of high-fat meals and an altered dosage amount for elderly patients are recommended, but only as ordered. Film-coated oral dosage forms should not be altered in any way. The taste of ritonavir may be improved by mixing it with chocolate milk or a nutritional beverage within 1 hour of its dosing. Ritonavir's dosage form should be protected from light. Absorption of oral dosage forms of zidovudine is not impeded by taking the drug with food or milk, but the patient should be kept upright while the medication is administered and for up to 30 minutes afterward to prevent esophageal ulceration. Intravenous doses should be given only if the solution is clear and does not contain any particulate matter, and the appropriate dosage, diluents, and infusion time should be used. Because these drugs often come in oral dosage forms, it is usually recommended that they be given with food. Zidovudine and other antiretrovirals are generally administered at evenly spaced intervals around the clock—as ordered—to ensure steady-state levels. With all oral and parenteral dosage forms of antiretrovirals, the patient should be observed for nausea and vomiting as well as any changes in weight, anorexia, or changes in bowel activity and patterns. Maraviroc and tenofovir are available for oral dosing and should be given as prescribed. Throughout therapy, it must always be remembered that the goal of treatment is to find the regimen that provides the best control of the individual patient's infection with the most tolerable adverse effects possible. Because patients vary greatly in their drug tolerance, medication regimens must be carefully individualized. Therefore, nursing assessment, documentation, nursing interventions, and evaluation are all very crucial to the success of a therapeutic regimen. Other nursing interventions associated with these drugs include: (1) Monitoring continually for adverse effects throughout therapy with a focus on the various organ systems, such as gastrointestinal, neurologic, renal, and hepatic. (2) With oral forms of indinavir and nevirapine, encourage forcing of fluids (unless contraindicated) of at least 6 to 8 glasses of water daily to maintain adequate hydration and help prevent nephrolithiasis. (3) Nevirapine, zidovudine, and similar drugs may be associated with a rash; however, if the rash is accompanied by blistering, fever, malaise, myalgias, oral lesions, swelling or edema, and conjunctivitis, the prescriber should be contacted immediately. (4) If drug therapy results in worsening of signs and symptoms, the prescriber should be contacted immediately and the drug may be discontinued. (5) Continually monitoring laboratory testing (e.g., CBC, RBC count, hemoglobin level, hematocrit, platelet count, renal/liver function studies, HIV RNA levels), with abnormalities reported to the prescriber. See Patient Teaching Tips for more information.

Evaluation

The therapeutic effects of *non-HIV antivirals* and *HIV antivirals* or *antiretrovirals* include elimination of the virus or a decrease in the symptoms of the viral infection. There may be a delayed progression of HIV infection and AIDS as well as a decrease in flulike symptoms and/or the frequency of herpetic flare-ups and other lesion breakouts. Herpetic lesions should crust over, and the frequency of recurrence should decrease. In addition, there should be constant evaluation for the occurrence of adverse effects and toxicity associated specific antiviral and antiretroviral drugs. These specific adverse effects are listed in Table 40-2. The nursing care plan should always be reevaluated to ensure that the goals and outcome criteria have been met. It is also the nurse's responsibility to remain constantly attentive in reviewing reports from the CDC, other federal and state health care agencies, and public health care organizations regarding new strains of viruses and flu syndromes (see earlier discussion).

PATIENT TEACHING TIPS

- Alert patient to the adverse effect of dizziness and instruct for them to use caution while driving or participating in activities requiring alertness while taking antiviral drugs. All medications should be taken exactly as prescribed and for the full course of therapy.
- Instruct patient on all possible drug interactions including over-the-counter medications.
- Immunocompromised patients should avoid crowds and persons with infections.
- Standard precautions and safe sex practices should be advocated for patients with sexually transmitted viral diseases, such as HIV-positive individuals. Condom use is a necessity for prevention of these viral infections and other sexually transmitted diseases; however, presence of genital herpes requires sexual abstinence.
- Female patients with genital herpes should have a Papanicolaou smear test (Pap test) performed every 6 months or as ordered by the prescriber to monitor the virus and the effectiveness of therapy.
- Gingival hyperplasia may occur with some antivirals and with long-term use, so the patient should be educated about the need for frequent oral hygiene.
- The patient should be told to report the following adverse reactions to the prescriber: decrease in urinary output, changes in sensorium, dizziness, confusion, syncope, nausea, vomiting, and diarrhea.
- Provide patient with adequate demonstrations, teaching aids and instructions for special application procedures (e.g., instillation of ophthalmic drops, use of finger cots or gloves when applying medication to lesions; use of respiratory inhalation forms).

- Explain that gloves or finger cots are needed for mediation application and cleansing to prevent the spread of lesions.
- Encourage forcing fluids up to 3000 mL/24 hr unless contraindicated.
- The patient should be educated that antiviral drugs provide suppression of the virus but are not a cure.
- The patient should be told to start therapy with drugs such as valacyclovir (or other antivirals) at the first sign of a recurrent episode of genital herpes or herpes zoster. In addition, it should be explained that early treatment within 24 to 48 hours of symptom onset is needed to achieve full therapeutic results.
- Any difficulty breathing; drastic changes in blood pressure; bleeding; new symptoms; worsening of infection, fever, or chills; or other unusual problems should be reported to the prescriber immediately.
- Emphasize the importance of follow-up appointments.
- The patient should be given appropriate drug-specific instructions (e.g., with didanosine, the patient should avoid alcohol, which will lead to a disulfiram-like reaction; the patient should take indinavir with water only and without food for optimal effects, although taking the drug with a light meal, skim milk, tea, or juice is acceptable and will help decrease gastrointestinal adverse effects; stavudine is associated with adverse effects such as abdominal discomfort, fatigue, dyspnea, numbness, nausea, tingling, vomiting, and weakness; with zidovudine, the patient should report any bleeding from the gums, nose, or rectum and should notify the prescriber if there is any difficulty breathing, headache, insomnia, muscle weakness, or worsening of infection).

POINTS TO REMEMBER

- Viruses are difficult to kill and to treat because they live inside human cells, and most antiviral drugs work by inhibiting replication of the virus. In this chapter, antiviral drugs are categorized as either non-HIV antivirals or HIV antivirals (antiretrovirals).
- Non-HIV antivirals include amantadine, rimantadine, acyclovir, ganciclovir, oseltamivir, zanamivir, and ribavirin. HIV antivirals include enfuvirtide, indinavir, maraviroc, nevirapine, raltegravir, tenofovir, and zidovudine.
- Antiretroviral drugs should be administered only after the prescriber's orders are read and understood and after a thor-

ough nursing assessment is performed that includes a review of the patient's nutritional status, weight, baseline vital sign values, and renal and hepatic functioning as well as an assessment of heart sounds, neurologic status, and gastrointestinal tract functioning.
- Comfort measures and supportive nursing care should accompany drug therapy. Patients should be encouraged to drink plenty of fluids and to space medications around the clock, as ordered, to maintain steady blood levels of the drug.

NCLEX EXAMINATION REVIEW QUESTIONS

1 During treatment with zidovudine, the nurse needs to monitor for which potential adverse effect?
  a Retinitis
  b Deep vein thromboses
  c Kaposi's sarcoma
  d Bone marrow suppression

2 After giving an injection to a patient with HIV infection, the nurse accidentally receives a needlestick from a too-full needle disposal box. Recommendations for occupational HIV exposure may include the use of which drug(s)?
  a Didanosine
  b Lamivudine and enfuvirtide
  c Zidovudine, lamivudine, and indinavir
  d Acyclovir

3 When the nurse is teaching a patient who is taking acyclovir for genital herpes, which statement by the nurse is accurate?
  a "This drug will help the lesions to dry and crust over."
  b "Acyclovir will eradicate the herpes virus."
  c "This drug will prevent the spread of this virus to others."
  d "Be sure to give this drug to your partner, too."

4 A patient who has been newly diagnosed with HIV has many questions about the effectiveness of drug therapy. After a teaching session, which statement by the patient reflects a need for more education?
  a "I will be monitored for adverse effects and improvements while I'm taking this medicine."
  b "These drugs do not eliminate the HIV, but hopefully the amount of virus in my body will be reduced."

  c "There is no cure for HIV."
  d "These drugs will eventually eliminate the virus from my body."

5 After surgery for organ transplantation, a patient is receiving ganciclovir, even though he does not have a viral infection. Which statement best explains the rationale for this medication therapy?
  a Ganciclovir is used to prevent potential exposure to the HIV virus.
  b This medication is given prophylactically to prevent influenza A infection.
  c Ganciclovir is given to prevent CMV infection.
  d The drug works synergistically with antibiotics to prevent superinfections.

6 The nurse is reviewing the use of multidrug therapy for HIV with a patient. Which statements are correct regarding the reason for using multiple drugs to treat HIV? (Select all that apply.)
  a The combination of drugs has fewer associated toxicities.
  b The use of multiple drugs is more effective against resistant strains of HIV.
  c Effective treatment results in reduced T-cell counts.
  d The goal of this treatment is to reduce the viral load.
  e This type of therapy reduces the incidence of opportunistic infections.

1. d, 2. c, 3. a, 4. d, 5. c, 6. b, d, e.

CRITICAL THINKING ACTIVITIES: BEST ACTION

1 A 19-year-old male transfer college student who came from Europe to the United States was diagnosed with HIV approximately 7 months ago. He has been going through several treatment regimens, but the infectious disease physician is planning to change his medication. He has been taking several anti-HIV drugs and is now being treated with didanosine. He has experienced some bone marrow depression off and on during the last few months. The student asks you, "Why is the doctor changing to didanosine therapy? Am I okay? What side effects does this new medicine have?" What are your best answers to his questions?

2 A young adult female patient underwent bone marrow transplantation and less than a year later she contracted a CMV infection. She is concerned about the medications and asks, "Are antiviral drugs going to be a problem? What if I get pregnant?" What is the nurse's best response? Explain your answer.

3 A college student has had the symptoms of the flu since Friday, but she does not go to the student health office until the following Tuesday. She tells the nurse that she is "miserable" and that she heard about Tamiflu on the Internet. She wants to take it to "keep the flu from getting worse." What is the nurse's best response to the student's request?

For answers, see *http://evolve.elsevier.com/Lilley.*

CHAPTER 41

Antitubercular Drugs

OBJECTIVES

When you reach the end of this chapter, you should be able to do the following:

1   Identify the various first-line and second-line drugs indicated for the treatment of tuberculosis.

2   Discuss the mechanisms of action, dosages, adverse effects, routes of administration, special dosing considerations, cautions, contraindications, and drug interactions of the various antitubercular drugs.

3   Develop a nursing care plan that includes all phases of the nursing process for patients receiving antitubercular drugs.

4   Develop a comprehensive teaching guide for patients and families impacted by the diagnosis and treatment of antitubercular drugs.

e-Learning Activities

http://evolve.elsevier.com/Lilley

NCLEX Review Questions • Animations • Nursing Care Plans • Audio Glossary • Category Catchers • Medication Errors Checklists • IV Therapy Checklists • Calculators • Frequently Asked Questions • Content Updates • Supplemental Resources • Answers to Case Studies and Critical Thinking Activities

Drug Profiles

ethambutol, p. 649
◆ isoniazid, p. 649
pyrazinamide, p. 650
rifabutin, p. 650

rifampin, p. 651
rifapentine, p. 651
streptomycin, p. 651

◆ *Key drug.*

Glossary

Aerobic Requiring oxygen for the maintenance of life. (p. 645)

Antitubercular drugs Drugs used to treat infections caused by *Mycobacterium* bacterial species. (p. 647)

Bacillus A rod-shaped bacterium. (p. 645)

Granulomas Small nodular aggregations of inflammatory cells (e.g., macrophages, lymphocytes); usually characterized by clearly delimited boundaries, as found in *tuberculosis.* (p. 645)

Isoniazid The primary and most commonly prescribed tuberculostatic drug. (p. 649)

Multidrug-resistant tuberculosis (MDR-TB) Tuberculosis that demonstrates resistance to two or more drugs. (p. 646)

Slow acetylator An individual with a genetic defect that causes a deficiency in the enzyme needed to metabolize isoniazid, the most widely used tuberculosis drug. (p. 650)

Tubercle The characteristic lesion of *tuberculosis;* a small round gray translucent granulomatous lesion, usually with a *caseated* (cheesy) consistency in its interior. (See *granuloma.*) (p. 645)

Tubercle bacilli Another common name for rod-shaped tuberculosis bacteria; essentially synonymous with *Mycobacterium tuberculosis.* (p. 645)

Tuberculosis (TB) Any infectious disease caused by species of *Mycobacterium,* usually *Mycobacterium tuberculosis* (adjectives: *tuberculous, tubercular*). (p. 645)

• • •

Anatomy, Physiology, and Disease Overview

TUBERCULOSIS

Tuberculosis (TB) is the medical diagnosis of any infectious disease caused by a bacterial species known as *Mycobacterium.* TB is most commonly characterized by **granulomas** in the lungs. These are nodular accumulations of inflammatory cells (e.g., macrophages, lymphocytes) that are *delimited* ("walled off" with clear boundaries) and have a center that has a cheesy or *caseated* consistency. *Casein* is the name of a protein that is prevalent in cheese and milk. Although there are technically two mycobacterial species that can cause TB, *Mycobacterium tuberculosis* and *Mycobacterium bovis,* infections caused by *M. tuberculosis* (abbreviated MTB) are far more common. There are also several other mycobacterial species, including *Mycobacterium leprae,* which causes leprosy, and *Mycobacterium avium-intracellulare* complex, which causes a disease that is similar to TB but often has gastrointestinal symptoms, both of which have varying susceptibility to different drugs used for TB. Infections with these bacteria are much less of a public health problem and hence are not the focus of this chapter. MTB is an aerobic bacillus, which means that it is a rod-shaped microorganism (**bacillus**) that requires a large supply of oxygen to grow and flourish (**aerobic**). This bacterium's need for a highly oxygenated body site explains why *Mycobacterium* infections most commonly affect the lungs. However, other common sites of infection are the growing ends of bones and the brain (cerebral cortex). Less common sites of infection include the kidney, liver, and genitourinary tract, as well as virtually every other tissue and organ in the body.

These **tubercle bacilli** (a common synonym for MTB) are transmitted from one of three sources: humans, cattle (adjective: bovine, hence the species name *M. bovis*), or birds (adjective: avian), although bovine and avian transmission are much less common than human transmission. **Tubercle** bacilli are conveyed in droplets expelled by infected people or animals during coughing or sneezing and then inhaled by the new host. After these infectious droplets are inhaled, the infection spreads to the susceptible organ sites by means of the blood and lymphatic sys-

645

tem. MTB is a very slow-growing organism, which makes it more difficult to treat than most other bacterial infections. Many of the antibiotics used to treat TB work by inhibiting growth rather than by directly killing the organism. The reason is that microorganisms that grow more slowly are more difficult to kill, because their cells are not as metabolically active as those of faster-growing organisms. Most bactericidal (cell-killing) drugs work by disrupting critical cellular metabolic processes in the organism. Therefore, the most drug-susceptible organisms are those with faster (not slower) metabolic activity.

At the other end of the TB patient spectrum are infected persons whose host defenses have been broken down as the result of immunosuppressive drug therapy, chemotherapy for cancer, or an immunosuppressive disease such as acquired immunodeficiency syndrome (AIDS). In these individuals, the disease can inflict devastating and irreversible damage. The first infectious episode is considered the *primary* TB infection; *reinfection* represents the more chronic form of the disease. However, TB does not develop in all people who are exposed to the bacteria. In some cases, the bacteria become dormant and walled off by calcified or fibrous tissues. These patients may test positive for exposure but are not necessarily infectious because of this dormancy process. The steps for diagnosis of TB are listed in Box 41-1.

TB cases have been reported on a national level in the United States beginning in 1953. Since that time, the TB incidence decreased in most years until about 1985. At that point, the epidemic of human immunodeficiency virus (HIV) infection was growing strongly, and the TB incidence began to rise for the first time in 20 years because of the development of TB in patients coinfected with HIV. Many cities were unprepared to handle this reemergence of TB. After an 18% increase in TB incidence between 1985 and 1991, a 50% decline was recorded from 1992 through 2002, and a 3.2% decline was seen from 2005 to 2006. In 2006, 13,767 new cases were reported in the United States. The rate in 2006 represented the lowest recorded number of cases since 1953. This is attributed to intensified public health efforts aimed at preventing, diagnosing, and treating TB as well as HIV infection, including more effective antiretroviral drug therapy (see Chapter 40). However, the *rate* of decline has now slowed, primarily due to one contributing factor: the number of **multidrug-resistant tuberculosis (MDR-TB)** cases. An upward trend in drug resistance, especially to isoniazid (abbreviated INH) and rifampin, has been observed since the 1970s. As recently as the 1990s, one third of TB cases in New York City were resistant to at least one drug, and 20% to both isoniazid and rifampin. Fortunately, these numbers have since declined, which has been attributed to stronger TB-related public health efforts. Nonetheless, the prevalence and growth of TB continues to be greater in the larger global community, and TB infects one third of the world's population. It is currently second only to HIV infection in the number of deaths caused by a single infectious organism. MDR-TB is defined as TB that is resistant to both isoniazid and rifampin, according to the World Health Organization. Close contacts of patients with MDR-TB need to be treated as well. Extensively drug-resistant tuberculosis (XDR-TB) is a relatively rare type of MDR-TB. It is resistant to almost all drugs used to treat TB, including the two best first-line drugs, isoniazid and rifampin. It also resistant to the best second-line medications. Because XDR-TB is resistant to the most powerful first-

---

BOX 41-1 Diagnosis of Tuberculosis

Step 1: Tuberculin skin test (Mantoux test)
Step 2: If skin test results are positive, then chest radiograph
Step 3: If chest radiograph shows signs of tuberculosis, then culture of sputum* or stomach secretions

*The acid-fast bacillus smear test is performed on sputum as a quick method of determining whether tuberculosis treatment and precautions are needed until a more definite diagnosis is made.

---

line and second-line drugs, patients are left with treatment options that are much less effective and often have worse treatment outcomes. XDR-TB is of special concern for patients who have AIDS or are otherwise immunocompromised. Not only are these patients more likely to contract TB, they are also more likely to die of it. At this point, XDR-TB is rare.

Several factors have contributed to this health care crisis, but one very important source of the problem is the increasing numbers of people in groups that are particularly susceptible to the infection—the homeless, undernourished or malnourished individuals, HIV-infected persons, drug abusers, cancer patients, those taking immunosuppressant drugs, and those who live in crowded and poorly sanitized housing facilities. All of these circumstances also favor the acquisition of a drug-resistant infection. Members of racial and ethnic minority groups are at greater risk than white populations and account for two thirds of new cases. Asian and Hispanic immigrants are at particularly high risk, accounting for more than half of all U.S. cases of foreign-acquired TB. Also in 2006, more U.S. cases were reported in Hispanics than in any other ethnic group.

Pharmacology Overview

ANTITUBERCULAR DRUGS

The drugs used to treat infections caused by all forms of *Mycobacterium* are called *antitubercular drugs,* and these drugs fall into two categories: *primary* or *first-line* and *secondary* or *second-line* drugs. As these designations imply, primary drugs are those tried first, whereas secondary drugs are reserved for more complicated cases, such as those resistant to primary drugs. The antimycobacterial activity, efficacy, and potential adverse and toxic effects of the various drugs determine the class to which they belong. Isoniazid is a primary antitubercular drug and is the most widely used. It can be administered either as the sole drug in the prophylaxis of TB or in combination with other antitubercular drugs in the treatment of TB. The various first- and second-line antibiotic drugs are listed in Box 41-2. There are also two miscellaneous TB-related injections—one diagnostic, the other a vaccine. These are described in Box 41-3.

An important consideration during drug selection is the relative likelihood of drug-resistant organisms and drug toxicity. Following are other key elements that are important in the planning and implementation of effective therapy:

- Drug-susceptibility tests should be performed on the first *Mycobacterium* species that is isolated from a patient specimen (to prevent the development of MDR-TB).

BOX 41-2 First- and Second-Line Antitubercular Drugs

First-Line Drugs
ethambutol
isoniazid (INH)
pyrazinamide (PZA)
rifabutin
rifampin
rifapentine
streptomycin

Second-Line Drugs
amikacin
capreomycin
cycloserine
ethionamide
kanamycin
levofloxacin
ofloxacin
para-aminosalicylic acid (PAS)

BOX 41-3 Miscellaneous Tuberculosis-Related Injections

Purified protein derivative (PPD): A diagnostic injection given intradermally in doses of 5 tuberculin units (0.1 mL) to detect exposure to the tuberculosis (TB) organism. It is composed of a protein precipitate derived from TB bacteria. A positive result is indicated by induration (not erythema) at the site of injection and is known as the *Mantoux* reaction, named for the physician who described it.

Bacille Calmette-Guérin (BCG): A vaccine injection derived from an inactivated strain of *Mycobacterium bovis*. Although it is not normally administered in the United States because the risk is not as high, it is used in much of the world to vaccinate young children against tuberculosis. Although it does not prevent infection, evidence indicates that it reduces active tuberculosis by 60% to 80% and is even more effective at preventing more severe cases involving dissemination of infection throughout the body.

- Before the results of the susceptibility tests are known, the patient should be started on a four-drug regimen consisting of isoniazid, rifampin, pyrazinamide (PZA), and ethambutol or streptomycin, which together are 95% effective in combating the infection. The use of multiple medications reduces the possibility of the organism's becoming drug resistant.
- Once drug susceptibility results are available, the regimen should be adjusted accordingly.
- Patient adherence to the prescribed drug regimen and any adverse effects of therapy should be monitored closely, because the incidence of both patient noncompliance and adverse effects is high.
- Despite the availability of many drugs to combat TB and the efforts mounted to detect and treat victims of the disease, treatment has been made difficult by two problems previously mentioned: patient nonadherence with therapy and the growing incidence of drug-resistant organisms.

Mechanism of Action and Drug Effects

The mechanisms of action of the various antitubercular drugs vary depending on the drug. These drugs act on MTB by inhibiting protein synthesis, inhibiting cell wall synthesis, or various other mechanisms. The **antitubercular drugs** are listed in Table 41-1 by their mechanism of action. The major effects of drug therapy include reduction of cough and, therefore, reduction of the infectiousness of the patient. This normally occurs within 2 weeks of the initiation of drug therapy, assuming that the patient's TB strain is drug sensitive.

Indications

Antitubercular medications are indicated for the treatment of TB infections, including both pulmonary and extrapulmonary TB. Most antitubercular drugs have not been fully tested for their effects in pregnant women. However, the combination of isoniazid and ethambutol has been used to treat pregnant women with clinically apparent TB without teratogenic complications. Rifampin is another drug that is usually safe during pregnancy and is a more likely choice for more advanced disease.

Besides being used for the initial treatment of TB, antitubercular drugs have also proved effective in the management of treatment failures and relapses. Infection with species of *Mycobacterium* other than *M. tuberculosis* and atypical mycobacterial infections have also been successfully treated with these drugs. Nontuberculous *Mycobacteria* may also be susceptible to antitubercular drugs. However, in general, antitubercular drugs are not as effective against other species of *Mycobacterium* as they are against MTB. Some of these other species that may be of particular concern in immunocompromised patients such as AIDS patients are *M. avium-intracellulare* complex, *Mycobacterium flavescens*, *Mycobacterium marinum*, and *Mycobacterium kansasii*. Additional *Mycobacterium* infections that may respond to antitubercular drugs are those caused by *Mycobacterium fortuitum*, *Mycobacterium chelonae*, *Mycobacterium smegmatis*, *Mycobacterium xenopi*, and *Mycobacterium scrofulaceum*. Treatment regimens for these non-TB mycobacterial infections often include the macrolide antibiotics clarithromycin or azithromycin (see Chapter 38), either alone or in combination with one or more antitubercular drugs.

In summary, antitubercular drugs are primarily used for the prophylaxis or treatment of TB. The effectiveness of these drugs depends on the type of infection, adequate dosing, sufficient duration of treatment, adherence to the drug regimen, and selection of an effective drug combination. The indications of the different antitubercular drugs are listed in Table 41-2.

Contraindications

Contraindications to the use of various antitubercular drugs include severe drug allergy and major renal or liver dysfunction. However, it must be recognized that the urgency of treating a potentially fatal infection may have to be balanced against any prevailing contraindications. In extreme cases, patients are sometimes given a drug to which they have some degree of allergy with supportive care that enables them at least to tolerate the medication. Examples of such supportive care are treatment with antipyretics (e.g., acetaminophen), antihistamines (e.g., diphenhydramine), or even corticosteroids (e.g., prednisone, methylprednisolone).

Reported contraindications that are specific to cycloserine include epilepsy and significant mental illness. One relative con-

TABLE 41-1 Antitubercular Drugs: Mechanisms of Action

Drugs	Description
Inhibit Protein Synthesis	
amikacin, kanamycin, capreomycin, rifabutin, rifampin, rifapentine, streptomycin	Streptomycin and kanamycin work by interfering with normal protein synthesis and causing the production of faulty proteins. Rifampin and capreomycin act at different points in the protein synthesis pathway from streptomycin and kanamycin. Rifampin inhibits RNA synthesis and may also inhibit DNA synthesis. Human cells are not as sensitive as the mycobacterial cells and are not affected by rifampin except at high drug concentrations. Capreomycin inhibits protein synthesis by preventing translocation on ribosomes.
Inhibit Cell Wall Synthesis	
cycloserine, ethionamide, isoniazid	Cycloserine acts by inhibiting the amino acid (d-alanine) involved in the synthesis of cell walls. Isoniazid and ethionamide also act at least partly to inhibit the synthesis of wall components, but the mechanisms of these two drugs are still not clearly understood.
Other Mechanisms	
ethambutol, ethionamide, isoniazid, para-aminosalicylic acid, pyrazinamide	Other proposed mechanisms of action for isoniazid exist. Isoniazid is taken up by mycobacterial cells and undergoes hydrolysis to isonicotinic acid, which reacts with cofactor NAD to form a defective NAD that is no longer active as a coenzyme for certain life-sustaining reactions in the *Mycobacterium tuberculosis* organism. Ethionamide directly inhibits mycolic acid synthesis, which eventually has the same deleterious effects on the TB organism as isoniazid. Ethambutol affects lipid synthesis, which results in the inhibition of mycolic acid incorporation into the cell wall and thus inhibits protein synthesis. Para-aminosalicylic acid acts as a competitive inhibitor of para-aminobenzoic acid in the synthesis of folate. The mechanism of action of pyrazinamide in the inhibition of TB is unknown. It can be either bacteriostatic or bactericidal, depending on the susceptibility of the particular *Mycobacterium* organism and the concentration of the drug attained at the site of infection.

NAD, Nicotinamide adenine; *TB,* tuberculosis.

TABLE 41-2 Antitubercular Drugs: Clinical Uses

Drug	Clinical Uses
amikacin, kanamycin	Used in combination with other antitubercular drugs in the treatment of clinical TB. Not intended for long-term use.
capreomycin	Used with other antitubercular drugs for the treatment of pulmonary TB caused by *Mycobacterium tuberculosis* after first-line drugs fail, drug resistance appears, or drug toxicity occurs.
cycloserine	Used with other antitubercular drugs for treatment of active pulmonary and extrapulmonary TB after failure of first-line drugs.
ethambutol	Indicated as a first-line drug for treatment of TB.
ethionamide	Used with other antitubercular drugs in treatment of clinical TB after failure of first-line drugs and for treatment of other types of mycobacterial infections.
isoniazid	Used alone or in combination with other antitubercular drugs in treatment and prevention of clinical TB.
para-aminosalicylic acid	Used in combination with other antitubercular drugs for treatment of pulmonary and extrapulmonary *M. tuberculosis* infection after failure of first-line drugs.
pyrazinamide	Used with other antitubercular drugs in treatment of clinical TB.
rifabutin	Used to prevent or delay development of *Mycobacterium avium-intracellulare* bacteremia and disseminated infections in patients with advanced HIV infection.
rifampin	Used with other antitubercular drugs in treatment of clinical TB.
	Used in treatment of diseases caused by mycobacteria other than *M. tuberculosis.*
	Used for preventive therapy in patients exposed to isoniazid-resistant *M. tuberculosis.*
	Used to eliminate meningococci from the nasopharynx of asymptomatic *Neisseria meningitidis* carriers when risk for meningococcal meningitis is high.
	Used for chemoprophylaxis in contacts of patients with HiB infection.
	Used with at least one other antiinfective drug in the treatment of leprosy.
	Used in the treatment of endocarditis caused by methicillin-resistant staphylococci, chronic staphylococcal prostatitis, and multiple-antiinfective–resistant pneumococci.
rifapentine	Used with other antitubercular drugs in the treatment of clinical TB.
streptomycin	Used in combination with other antitubercular drugs in the treatment of clinical TB and other mycobacterial diseases.

HiB, Haemophilus influenzae type b; *HIV,* human immunodeficiency virus; *TB,* tuberculosis.

traindication to ethambutol is optic neuritis. Chronic alcohol use, especially when associated with major liver damage, may also be a contraindication to therapy with any antitubercular drug, with the cautions mentioned earlier kept in mind. Other contraindications for specific drugs, if any, can be found in the drug profiles presented later.

Adverse Effects

Antitubercular drugs are fairly well tolerated. Isoniazid, one of the mainstays of treatment, is noted for causing pyridoxine deficiency and liver toxicity. For this reason, supplements of pyridox-ine (vitamin B_6; see Chapter 54) are often given concurrently with isoniazid, with a common oral dose of 50 mg daily. The most problematic drugs and their associated adverse effects are listed in Table 41-3.

Interactions

The drugs that can interact with antitubercular drugs can cause significant effects. See Table 41-4 for a listing of selected interactions. Besides these drug interactions, isoniazid can cause false-positive readings on urine glucose tests (e.g., Clinitest) and an increase in the serum levels of the liver function enzymes alanine aminotransferase and aspartate aminotransferase.

Dosages

For the recommended dosages of selected antitubercular drugs, see the Dosages table on p. 650.

TABLE 41-3 Antitubercular Drugs: Common Adverse Effects

Drug	Adverse Effects
amikacin, kanamycin	Ototoxicity, nephrotoxicity
capreomycin	Ototoxicity, nephrotoxicity
cycloserine	Psychotic behavior, seizures
ethambutol	Retrobulbar neuritis, blindness
ethionamide	GI tract disturbances, hepatotoxicity
isoniazid	Peripheral neuropathy, hepatotoxicity, optic neuritis and visual disturbances, hyperglycemia
levofloxacin, ofloxacin	Dizziness, headache, GI disturbances, visual disturbances, insomnia
para-aminosalicylic acid	GI tract disturbances, hepatotoxicity
pyrazinamide	Hepatotoxicity, hyperuricemia
rifabutin	GI tract disturbances; rash; neutropenia; red-orange-brown discoloration of urine, feces, saliva, sputum, sweat, tears, skin
rifampin	Hepatitis; hematologic disorders; red-orange-brown discoloration of urine, tears, sweat, sputum
rifapentine	GI upset; red-orange-brown discoloration of tears, sweat, skin, teeth, tongue, sputum, saliva, urine, feces, CSF
streptomycin	Ototoxicity, nephrotoxicity, blood dyscrasias

CSF, Cerebrospinal fluid; *GI,* gastrointestinal.

DRUG PROFILES

ethambutol

Ethambutol (Myambutol) is a first-line bacteriostatic drug used in the treatment of TB that is believed to work by diffusing into the myco-bacteria and suppressing ribonucleic acid (RNA) synthesis, which thereby inhibits protein synthesis. Ethambutol is included with iso-niazid, streptomycin, and rifampin in many TB combination-drug therapies. It may also be used to treat other mycobacterial diseases. It is contraindicated in patients with known optic neuritis, because it can both exacerbate and cause this condition, which can result in varying degrees of vision loss. It is also contraindicated in children younger than 13 years of age. It is available only in oral form.

PHARMACOKINETICS

Route	Onset of Action	Peak Plasma Concentration	Elimination Half-life	Duration of Action
PO	Variable	2-4 hr	3.3 hr	24 hr

◆ isoniazid

Isoniazid (also called INH) is not only the mainstay in the treatment of TB but also the most widely used antitubercular drug. It may be given either as a single drug for prophylaxis or in combina-

---

TABLE 41-4 Antitubercular Drugs: Drug Interactions

Drug	Interacting Drugs	Mechanism	Results
Aminosalicylate	probenecid	Reduces excretion	Increased aminosalicylate levels
	Salicylates	Has additive effects	Aminosalicylate toxicity
Isoniazid	Antacids	Reduces absorption	Decreased isoniazid levels
	cycloserine, ethionamide, rifampin	Has additive effects	Increased central nervous system and hepatic toxicity
	phenytoin + carbamazepine	Decreases metabolism	Increased phenytoin and carbamazepine effects
Streptomycin	Nephrotoxic and neurotoxic drugs		Increased toxicity
	Oral anticoagulants	Alter intestinal flora	Increased bleeding tendencies
Rifampin	Beta-blockers		
	Benzodiazepines		
	cyclosporine, oral anticoagulants, oral antidiabetics, oral contraceptives, phenytoin, quinidine, sirolimus, theophylline	Increase metabolism	Decreased therapeutic effects of these drugs

DOSAGES

Selected Antitubercular Drugs

Drug (Pregnancy Category)	Pharmacologic Class	Usual Dosage Range	Indications
ethambutol (Myambutol) (B)	Synthetic first-line antimycobacterial	**Adult and pediatric** PO: 15-25 mg/kg/day; may also be divided in 2×/wk and 3×/wk dosage regimens with higher doses; no maximum dose listed	
◆ isoniazid (INH), generic only (C)	Synthetic first-line antimycobacterial	**Adult** PO: 5 mg/kg daily (max 300 mg) or 15 mg/kg 1-3×/wk (max 900 mg/dose) **Pediatric** PO: 10-20 mg/kg/day (max 300 mg) or 20-40 mg/kg 2-3×/wk (max 900 mg/dose)	
pyrazinamide (generic only) (C)	Synthetic first-line antimycobacterial	**Adult and pediatric** PO: 15-30 mg/kg/day (max 2 g) or 50-70 mg/kg 2-3×/wk (max 3-4 g/dose)	
rifabutin (Mycobutin) (B)	Semisynthetic first-line antimycobacterial antibiotic	**Adult only** PO: 150-300 mg once daily	Active TB
rifampin (Rifadin, Rimactane) (C)	Semisynthetic first-line antimycobacterial antibiotic	**Adult** PO/IV: 10 mg/kg up to 600 mg once daily **Pediatric** PO/IV*: 10-20 mg/kg/day or 2-3×/wk (max 600 mg/dose for all regimens)	
rifapentine (Priftin) (C)	Semisynthetic first-line antimycobacterial antibiotic	**Adult only** PO: 600 mg 2×/wk for first 2 mo; then 1×/wk for 4 mo	
streptomycin (generic only) (D)	Antimycobacterial aminoglycoside antibiotic	**Adult and pediatric** IM/IV:15-40 mg/kg 1-3×/wk (max 1-1.5 g/dose)	

IM, Intramuscular; *IV,* intravenous; *PO,* oral; *TB,* tuberculosis.
*Use of intramuscular and subcutaneous injections is contraindicated due to soft tissue toxicity.

tion with other antitubercular drugs for the treatment of active TB. It is a bactericidal drug that kills the mycobacteria by disrupting cell wall synthesis and essential cellular functions. Isoniazid is metabolized in the liver through a process called *acetylation,* which requires a certain enzymatic pathway to break down the drug. However, some people have a genetic deficiency of the liver enzymes needed for this to occur. Such people are called **slow acetylators.** When isoniazid is taken by slow acetylators, the isoniazid accumulates, because there is not enough of the enzymes to break down the isoniazid. Therefore, the dosages of isoniazid may need to be adjusted downward in these patients.

Isoniazid is most commonly used in oral form, although an injection is available. There is also a combination oral formulation containing both isoniazid and rifampin (Rifamate). Another combination drug product, Rifater, contains rifampin, isoniazid, and pyrazinamide. Isoniazid is contraindicated in those with previous isoniazid-associated hepatic injury or any acute liver disease.

PHARMACOKINETICS

Route	Onset of Action	Peak Plasma Concentration	Elimination Half-life	Duration of Action
PO	Variable	1-2 hr	1-4 hr	24 hr

pyrazinamide

Pyrazinamide is an antitubercular drug that can be either bacteriostatic or bactericidal, depending on its concentration at the site of infection and the particular susceptibility of the mycobacteria. It is commonly used in combination with other antitubercular drugs

for the treatment of TB. Its mechanism of action is unknown, but it is believed to work by inhibiting lipid and nucleic acid synthesis in the mycobacteria. Pyrazinamide is available only in generic oral form. It is contraindicated in patients with severe hepatic disease or acute gout. It is also not normally used in pregnant patients in the United States, due to a lack of teratogenicity data, although it is often used in pregnant patients in other countries.

PHARMACOKINETICS

Route	Onset of Action	Peak Plasma Concentration	Elimination Half-life	Duration of Action
PO	Variable	2 hr	9-10 hr	24 hr

rifabutin

Rifabutin is the second of three currently available *rifamycin* antibiotics, following rifampin. Although it is considered a first-line TB drug by some clinicians, it is more commonly used to treat infections caused by *M. avium-intracellulare* complex, which includes several non-TB mycobacterial species. This is also the case with the two other rifamycin-derived drugs, rifampin and rifapentine. A notable adverse effect of rifabutin, as well as rifampin (see later), is that it can turn urine, feces, saliva, skin, sputum, sweat, and tears a red-orange-brown color. Rifabutin is currently available only for oral use.

PHARMACOKINETICS

Route	Onset of Action	Peak Plasma Concentration	Elimination Half-life	Duration of Action
PO	Variable	2-4 hr	16-69 hr	1 to several days

rifampin

Rifampin (Rifadin) is the first of the rifamycin class of synthetic macrocyclic antibiotics, which also includes rifabutin and rifapentine. The term *macrocyclic* connotes the very large and complex hydrocarbon ring structure included in all three of the rifamycin compounds. Rifampin has activity against many *Mycobacterium* species, as well as against *Meningococcus, Haemophilus influenzae* type b, and *M. leprae*. It is a broad-spectrum bactericidal drug that kills the offending organism by inhibiting protein synthesis. Rifampin is used either alone in the prevention of TB or in combination with other antitubercular drugs in its treatment. Rifampin is available in both oral and parenteral formulations and, as previously mentioned, in combination with isoniazid (Rifamate). Rifampin is available in both oral and injectable forms. Rifampin is contraindicated in patients with known drug allergy to it or to any other rifamycin (i.e., rifabutin, rifapentine).

PHARMACOKINETICS

Route	Onset of Action	Peak Plasma Concentration	Elimination Half-life	Duration of Action
PO	Variable	2-4 hr	3 hr	Up to 24 hr

rifapentine

Rifapentine (Priftin) is a derivative of rifampin. It offers advantages over rifampin in that it has a much longer duration of action and possibly better efficacy. It has been shown to have greater antimycobacterial efficacy and macrophage penetration. Its accumulation into tissue macrophages allows it to work synergistically against bacterial cells that are ingested by the macrophage during phagocytosis ("cell eating"). Rifapentine is available only for oral use.

PHARMACOKINETICS

Route	Onset of Action	Peak Plasma Concentration	Elimination Half-life	Duration of Action
PO	Unknown	5-6 hr	14-17 hr	1 to several days

streptomycin

Streptomycin is an aminoglycoside antibiotic currently available only in generic form. Introduced in 1944, it was the very first drug available that could effectively treat TB. Because of its toxicities it is used most commonly today in combination drug regimens for the treatment of MDR-TB infections. Streptomycin is currently available only in injectable form. It is usually not given to pregnant patients due to risk of fetal harm.

PHARMACOKINETICS

Route	Onset of Action	Peak Plasma Concentration	Elimination Half-life	Duration of Action
IM	Variable	1-2 hr	2-3 hr	Up to 24 hr

NURSING PROCESS

Assessment

Before administering any of the *antitubercular drugs*, and to ensure the safe and effective use of these medications, the nurse should obtain a thorough medical history, medication profile, and nursing history for the patient as well as perform a complete head-to-toe physical assessment. Any specific history of diagnoses or symptoms of TB, as well as the results of the patient's last purified protein derivative or tuberculin skin test and the reaction at the site of the intradermal injection, should be noted. The most recent chest radiograph and results should also be reviewed. Results of liver function studies (e.g., bilirubin level, liver enzyme levels) need to be assessed, because, as noted earlier, severe liver dysfunction is a contraindication. Not only are these values important for assessing liver function, but they also provide comparative baseline data throughout therapy. Because some drugs can lead to peripheral neuropathies, baseline neurologic functioning should also be noted prior to therapy. Hearing status should be assessed, especially when streptomycin is to be used, because of its drug-related ototoxicity.

Assessment of age is also important, because the likelihood of adverse reactions and toxicity is increased in the elderly due to age-related liver dysfunction, and the safety of these drugs in children 13 years of age and younger has not been established. The nurse should also check the patient's complete blood count before administering isoniazid because of the potential for drug-related hematologic disorders. Renal studies, such as serum creatinine level, blood urea nitrogen level, and urinalysis, should be performed at the start of antituberculin therapy as well as throughout therapy, as ordered. Uric acid baseline levels should be noted, because these values may increase and precipitate gout. Analysis of sputum specimens is usually ordered as well, to aid in determining the appropriate drug regimen. An eye examination should be performed and baseline eye function assessed before therapy with isoniazid or ethambutol. Pyrazinamide use requires careful assessment of allergic reactions to other antitubercular drugs because of high cross-sensitivity. Contraindications, cautions, and drug interactions have been discussed previously.

Nursing Diagnoses

- Risk for injury related to neurologic adverse effects of antitubercular drugs, noncompliance with the drug therapy regimen, and an overall poor health status
- Ineffective therapeutic regimen management related to poor compliance with antitubercular drug therapy and lack of knowledge about long-term therapies
- Ineffective family therapeutic regimen management related to poor compliance and poor housing and living conditions
- Deficient knowledge related to the disease process and treatment protocol

Planning
Goals

- Patient experiences minimal adverse effects of drug therapy for tuberculosis.
- Patient takes medication regularly and for the length of time prescribed.
- Patient remains free of injury related to adverse effects (e.g., peripheral neuropathies) and drug interactions with the antitubercular drugs.
- Patient remains free of drug-related toxic effects and states the importance of reporting any symptoms of toxic effects to the prescriber immediately.
- Patient remains compliant with the drug therapy.

Outcome Criteria

- Patient reports therapeutic effects (improved signs and symptoms) and possible adverse effects (neuropathies, gastrointestinal upset) of the drug regimen.

- Patient takes medication as ordered and regularly, with acknowledgement of more effective therapy and prevention of complications, relapses, or recurrences.
- Patient states the drugs that interact with antitubercular drug such as salicylates, antacids, and anticoagulants and maintains drug safety.
- Patient reports toxic effects such as jaundice, renal problems, hearing loss, severe neuropathies, and/or blindness to the prescriber should they occur.
- Patient shows improvement of disease state with adherence to the drug regimen including a decrease in cough, fever, and sputum production, and laboratory values return to normal.

Implementation

Because drug therapy is the mainstay of treatment for TB and often lasts for up to 24 months, patient education is critical, with a special emphasis on adherence to the drug regimen. Simple, clear, and concise instructions should be given to the patient, with appropriate use of audiovisuals and take-home information. This education should include the fact that multiple drugs are often used to improve cure rates. All antitubercular drugs should be taken exactly as ordered and at the same time every day. Consistent use and dosing around the clock are critical to maintaining steady blood levels and minimizing the chances of resistance to the drug therapy. Instructions to the patient should always emphasize the need for strict adherence to the therapeutic regimen.

Although many drugs should be given without food for maximum absorption, antitubercular drugs may need to be taken with food to minimize gastrointestinal upset. There should be constant monitoring for any signs and symptoms of liver dysfunction such as fatigue, jaundice, nausea, vomiting, dark urine, and anorexia, and any of these should be reported to the prescriber. If vision changes occur (e.g., altered color perception, changes in visual acuity), in particular with ethambutol use, these changes should be reported immediately to the prescriber. Uric acid levels should be monitored during therapy, and the patient should be observed for symptoms of gout such as hot, painful, or swollen joints of the big toe, knee, or ankle. In addition, the prescriber should be notified if there are signs and symptoms of peripheral neuropathy (e.g., numbness, burning, and tingling of extremities). Pyridoxine (vitamin B₆) may be beneficial for isoniazid-induced peripheral neuropathy. If the prescriber has ordered collection of a sputum specimen to test for acid-fast bacilli, it is best to obtain the sample early in the morning. The most common order is for three consecutive morning specimens, with a repeat specimen several weeks later. All drugs should be taken as ordered and without any omission of doses for maximal therapeutic results.

Follow-up visits to the prescriber are important for monitoring therapeutic effects and watching for adverse effects and toxicity. If intravenous dosing of an antitubercular drug is ordered, the nurse should be sure to use the appropriate diluent and to infuse over the recommended time. The intravenous site should be monitored every hour during the infusion for extravasation with possible tissue inflammation (e.g., redness, heat, and swelling at the intravenous site). See Patient Teaching Tips for more information on antitubercular drugs.

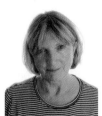
Cultural considerations associated with these drugs include the fact that when patients have active TB thorough patient teaching of all family members is required, and some family members may need prophylactic therapy for up to 1 full year. Because some cultural practices include living in close-knit communities or close living quarters, this teaching is critical to make sure the spread of this highly communicable disease is adequately prevented. All family members or those in close contact with the patient must receive the same thorough instructions about maintaining health while taking their medications appropriately, with emphasis on adherence.

Evaluation

The nurse should always document patient responses, or lack of them, to therapy. A therapeutic response to antitubercular therapy is manifested by a decrease in the symptoms of TB, such as cough and fever, and by weight gain. The results of laboratory studies (culture and sensitivity tests) and the chest radiographic findings should confirm the clinical findings of resolution of the infection. Meeting of goals and outcome criteria should also be evaluated to confirm that the infection is being adequately treated and that the drug therapy is providing therapeutic relief without complications or toxicity and with minimal adverse effects. Patients also need to be monitored for the occurrence of adverse reactions to antitubercular drugs, such as fatigue; nausea; vomiting; fever; loss of appetite; depression; jaundice; numbness, tingling, or burning of the extremities; abdominal pain; changes in vision; and easy bruising. Because of the need for long-term therapy and possible treatment of family or those in close contact, further evaluation of the home setting is also needed.

PATIENT TEACHING TIPS

- Medications should be taken exactly as ordered by the prescriber with attention to long-term therapy and strict adherence to the drug regimen. Treatment may be ineffective if drugs are taken intermittently or stopped once the patient begins to feel better.
- Follow-up appointments with the prescriber or health clinic should be kept so that the infection and therapeutic effectiveness may be closely monitored.
- The patient should avoid alcohol while taking antitubercular drugs. The patient should check with the prescriber before taking any other type of medication.
- Pyridoxine (vitamin B$_6$) may be indicated to prevent isoniazid-precipitated peripheral neuropathies and numbness, tingling, or burning of the extremities.
- A patient taking isoniazid or rifampin should be educated to report occurrence of the following adverse effects to the prescriber immediately: fever, nausea, vomiting, loss of appetite, unusual bleeding, or numbness or tingling of the extremities.
- Sunscreen and protective clothing should be worn to avoid ultraviolet light exposure. Drug-related photosensitivity reactions may be avoided by preventing exposure to the sun.
- The patient should report flulike symptoms, gastrointestinal upset, and rash to the prescriber immediately.

- Women taking oral contraceptives who are prescribed rifampin must be switched to another form of birth control, because oral contraceptives become ineffective when given with this drug.
- During initial periods of the illness, every effort should be made to wash the hands and cover the mouth when coughing or sneezing. Methods of proper disposal of secretions should be emphasized.
- The importance of proper rest, good sleep habits, adequate nutrition, and maintenance of general health should be emphasized. Antitubercular drugs and other medications should be kept out of the reach of children.
- A medical alert tag or bracelet with a list of allergies, prescription drugs, and medical conditions should be worn at all times. Written medical information should also be kept on the patient's person.
- Any increase in fatigue, cough, or sputum production; bloody sputum; chest pain; unusual bleeding; or yellow skin and/or eyes should be reported to the prescriber immediately.
- Patients taking rifampin, rifabutin, or rifapentine may experience red-orange-brown discoloration of the skin, sweat, tears, urine, feces, sputum, saliva, cerebrospinal fluid, and tongue as an adverse effect of the drug. The discoloration reverses with discontinuation of the drug; however, contact lenses may be permanently stained.

POINTS TO REMEMBER

- All antitubercular drugs should be taken exactly as prescribed, with emphasis on adherence to the therapeutic regimen and long-term dosing combined with healthy living practices.
- Therapeutic effects include resolution of pulmonary and extrapulmonary MTB infections.
- Vitamin B$_6$ is needed to combat the peripheral neuropathy associated with isoniazid.
- Women taking oral contraceptive therapy who are prescribed rifampin should be counseled on other forms of birth control

because of the ineffectiveness of oral contraception when rifampin is taken.
- Patients should be educated about the importance of strict adherence to the drug regimen for improvement or cure of the condition. Instructions about drug interactions and the need to avoid alcohol while taking any of these medications should be provided in written and oral formats.

NCLEX EXAMINATION REVIEW QUESTIONS

1 The nurse is teaching a patient who is starting antitubercular therapy with rifampin. Which adverse effects would the nurse expect to see?
  a Headache and neck pain
  b Glaucoma and gynecomastia
  c Reddish brown urine
  d Numbness or tingling of extremities

2 During antitubercular therapy with isoniazid, the patient received another prescription for pyridoxine. Which statement by the nurse best explains the rationale for this second medication?
  a "This vitamin will help to improve your energy levels."
  b "This helps to prevent neurologic adverse effects."
  c "It works to protect your heart from toxic effects."
  d "This drug works to reduce gastrointestinal adverse effects."

3 When the nurse is counseling a woman who is beginning antitubercular therapy with rifampin, which statement by the nurse is most important regarding potential drug interactions?
  a "If you are taking birth control pills, you will need to switch to another form of birth control."
  b "Your birth control pills will remain effective while you are taking rifampin."
  c "You will need to switch to a stronger form of oral contraceptive while taking rifampin."
  d "You can take the birth control pills with the rifampin without problems, but it may cause your urine to turn reddish orange."

4 When counseling a patient who has been newly diagnosed with TB, the nurse should make sure that the patient realizes that he or she is contagious
  a during all phases of the illness.
  b any time up to 18 months after therapy begins.
  c during the postictal phase of TB.
  d during the initial period of the illness and its diagnosis.

5 While monitoring a patient, the nurse knows that a therapeutic response to antitubercular drugs would be:
  a The patient states that he or she is feeling much better.
  b The patient's laboratory test results show a lower white blood cell count.
  c The patient reports a decrease in cough and night sweats.
  d There is a decrease in symptoms, along with improved chest radiograph and sputum culture results.

6 The nurse is monitoring for liver toxicity in a patient who has been receiving long-term isoniazid therapy. Manifestations of liver toxicity include: (Select all that apply.)
  a Orange discoloration of sweat and tears
  b Darkened urine
  c Dizziness
  d Fatigue
  e Visual disturbances
  f Jaundice

1. c, 2. b, 3. a, 4. d, 5. d, 6. b, d, f.

CRITICAL THINKING ACTIVITIES: BEST ACTION

1 The nurse is reviewing medication therapy with a patient who has been newly diagnosed with TB. The patient asks, "How will the doctors know when I'm better? Will I have this disease forever?" What is the nurse's best answer?

2 A 28-year-old health care worker has been diagnosed with active TB. She will be taking rifampin and is reviewing her current list of medications with the office nurse and asks, "I use birth control because we really don't want children right now. Can I still use 'the pill'?" What is the nurse's best answer?

3 P.T., a 48-year-old businessman, has been taking rifapentine as part of therapy for TB. He has been told that his bodily secretions will turn a reddish orange-brown color, and he asks, "What about my contact lenses? I can still wear them, right?" What is the nurse's best answer?

For answers, see *http://evolve.elsevier.com/Lilley*.

CHAPTER 42

Antifungal Drugs

OBJECTIVES

When you reach the end of this chapter, you should be able to do the following:

1 Identify the various antifungal drugs.
2 Describe the mechanisms of action, indications, contraindications, routes of administration, adverse and toxic effects, and drug interactions of the various antifungal drugs.
3 Develop a nursing care plan that includes all phases of the nursing process for patients receiving antifungal drugs.

e-Learning Activities

http://evolve.elsevier.com/Lilley

NCLEX Review Questions • Animations • Nursing Care Plans • Audio Glossary • Category Catchers • Medication Errors Checklists • IV Therapy Checklists • Calculators • Frequently Asked Questions • Content Updates • Supplemental Resources • Answers to Case Studies and Critical Thinking Activities

Drug Profiles

- ◆ amphotericin B, p. 659
- caspofungin, p. 659
- ◆ fluconazole, p. 659

- nystatin, p. 659
- terbinafine, p. 659
- voriconazole, p. 661

◆ *Key drug.*

Glossary

Antimetabolite A drug or other substance that is a either a receptor antagonist or that resembles a normal human metabolite and interferes with its function in the body, usually by competing for the metabolite's usual receptors or enzymes. (p. 656)

Dermatophyte One of several fungi, often found in soil, that infect skin, nails, or hair of humans. (p. 655)

Ergosterol An unsaturated hydrocarbon of the vitamin D group isolated from yeast, mushrooms, ergot, and other fungi; the main sterol in fungal membranes. (p. 657)

Fungi A very large, diverse group of eukaryotic microorganisms that require an external carbon source and that form a plant structure known as a *thallus*. Fungi consist of yeasts and molds. (p. 655)

Molds Multicellular fungi characterized by long, branching filaments called *hyphae*, which entwine to form a complex branched structure known as a *mycelium*. (p. 655)

Mycosis The general term for any fungal infection. (p. 655)

Pathologic fungi Fungi that cause mycoses. (p. 655)

Sterols Substances in the cell membranes of fungi to which polyene antifungal drugs bind. (p. 657)

Yeasts Single-celled fungi that reproduce by budding. (p. 655)

• • •

Anatomy, Physiology, and Disease Overview

FUNGAL INFECTIONS

Fungi are a very large and diverse group of microorganisms that include all yeasts and molds. **Yeasts** are single-celled fungi that reproduce by *budding* (in which a daughter cell forms by pouching out of and breaking off from a mother cell). These organisms have common practical uses in the baking of breads and the preparation of alcoholic beverages. **Molds** are multicellular and are characterized by long, branching filaments called *hyphae,* which entwine to form a mat called a *mycelium.* Some fungi are part of the normal flora of the skin, mouth, intestines, and vagina.

The infection caused by a fungus is called a **mycosis.** A variety of fungi can cause clinically significant infections or *mycoses.* These are called **pathologic fungi,** and the infections they cause range in severity from mild infections with annoying symptoms (e.g., athlete's foot) to systemic mycoses that can become life threatening. These infections are acquired by various routes: the fungi can be ingested orally; they can grow on or in the skin, hair, or nails; and, if the fungal spores are airborne, they can be inhaled. There are four general types of mycotic infection: *systemic, cutaneous, subcutaneous,* and *superficial.* The latter three are infections of various layers of the *integumentary* system (skin, hair, or nails). Fungi that cause integumentary infections are known as **dermatophytes,** and such infections are known as *dermatomycoses.* The most severe systemic fungal infections generally affect people whose host immune defenses are compromised. Commonly, these are patients who have received organ transplants and are taking immunosuppressive drug therapy, cancer patients who are immunocompromised as a result of their chemotherapy, and patients with acquired immunodeficiency syndrome (AIDS). In addition, the use of antibiotics, antineoplastics, or immunosuppressants such as corticosteroids may result in colonization of *Candida albicans,* followed by the development of a systemic infection. When the infection affects the mouth, it is referred to as *oral candidiasis,* or *thrush.* It is common in newborns and immunocompromised patients. Vaginal

TABLE **42-1** **Mycotic Infections**

Mycosis	Fungus	Endemic Location	Reservoir	Transmission	Primary Tissue Affected
Systemic Infections					
Aspergillosis	*Aspergillus* spp.	Universal	Soil	Inhalation	Lungs
Blastomycosis	*Blastomyces dermatitidis*	North America	Soil, animal droppings	Inhalation	Lungs
Candidiasis	*Candida albicans, glabrata, krusei, tropicalisis, parapsilosis*	Universal	Humans	Direct contact, overgrowth in response to treatment with antibiotic to which it is nonsusceptible	Blood, lungs
Coccidioidomycosis	*Coccidioides immitis*	Southwestern United States	Soil, dust	Inhalation	Lungs
Cryptococcosis	*Cryptococcus neoformans*	Universal	Soil, bird and chicken droppings	Inhalation	Lungs, meninges of brain
Histoplasmosis	*Histoplasma capsulatum*	Universal		Inhalation	Lungs
Superficial/Topical Infections					
Candidiasis	*Candida albicans*	Universal	Humans	Direct contact, overgrowth in response to treatment with antibiotic to which it is nonsusceptible	Mucous membrane, skin; disseminated (may be systemic)
Dermatophytosis, tinea	*Epidermophyton* spp. *Microsporum* spp. *Trichophyton* spp.	Universal	Humans	Direct and indirect contact with infected persons	Scalp, skin (e.g., groin, feet)
Tinea versicolor	*Malassezia furfur*	Universal	Humans	Unknown*	Skin

spp., Species.
**Malassezia* spp. are a usual part of the normal human flora and appear to cause infection in only select individuals.

candidiasis, commonly called a *yeast infection*, often affects pregnant women, women with diabetes mellitus, women taking antibiotics, and women taking oral contraceptives. The characteristics of some of the systemic, cutaneous, and superficial mycotic infections are summarized in Table 42-1.

▎Pharmacology Overview
ANTIFUNGAL DRUGS

The drugs used to treat fungal infections are called *antifungal drugs.* Systemic mycotic infections and some cutaneous or subcutaneous mycoses are treated with oral or parenteral drugs, but these constitute a fairly small group of drugs, only three or four of which are commonly used. There are few such drugs because the fungi that cause these infections have proved to be very difficult to kill, and research into new and improved drugs has occurred at a slow pace, with relatively few important advances made so far. One difficulty that has slowed the development of new drugs is that often the chemical concentrations required for experimental drugs to be effective cannot be tolerated by human beings. Those drugs that proved successful in the treatment of systemic mycoses as well as severe dermatomycoses include amphotericin B, caspofungin, fluconazole, flucytosine, griseofulvin, itraconazole, ketoconazole, micafungin, nystatin, terbinafine, posaconazole, anidulafungin, and voriconazole. These drugs are the focus of this chapter.

Topical antifungal drugs are by far the most commonly used drugs in this class and are most often administered without pre-

scription for the treatment of dermatomycoses as well as oral and vaginal mycoses. Although topical drug therapy is usually sufficient for these conditions, systemic oral medications are also sometimes used, especially for more severe or recurrent cases. Antifungal drugs available for topical use are discussed further in Chapter 56. There is also a single antifungal drug (natamycin) for ophthalmic use (see Chapter 57).

Two antifungal drugs, flucytosine and griseofulvin, are individually listed and are not specifically classified according to their chemical structures. The remaining drugs currently include four specific chemical classes: *polyenes* (amphotericin B and nystatin), *imidazoles* (ketoconazole), *triazoles* (fluconazole, itraconazole, voriconazole, and posaconazole), and the *echinocandins* (caspofungin, micafungin, and anidulafungin). The imidazoles and triazoles are sometimes referred to by the more general term *azole antifungals.* Also included in some of these classes are drugs for topical use, which again are described further in Chapter 56.

Mechanism of Action and Drug Effects

The mechanisms of action of the various antifungal drugs differ for different drug subclasses. Flucytosine, also known as *5-fluorocytosine* (5-FC), acts in much the same way as the antiviral drugs. It is an **antimetabolite,** which is a drug that disrupts critical cellular metabolic pathways of the fungal cell. Once inside a susceptible fungal cell, the drug is deaminated by the enzyme *cytosine deaminase* to 5-fluorouracil (5-FU). Because human cells do not have this enzyme, they are not harmed by this antimetabolite. Once the 5-FU is generated inside the fungal cell, it interferes with fungal deoxyribonucleic acid (DNA) synthesis, which results in both inhibition of cell growth and reproduction, and cell death. 5-FU is also available as an antineoplastic (anticancer) drug and is discussed in more detail in Chapter 47.

Griseofulvin, like flucytosine, is one of the older types of antifungal drugs. It works by preventing susceptible fungi from reproducing. It enters the fungal cell through an energy-dependent transport system and inhibits fungal mitosis (cell division) by binding to key structures known as *microtubules*. It has also been proposed that griseofulvin causes the production of defective DNA, which is then unable to replicate. Although both griseofulvin and flucytosine are still currently available on the U.S. market, in clinical use they have been largely replaced by the newer antifungal drug classes.

The polyenes act by binding to **sterols** in the cell membranes of fungi. The main sterol in fungal membranes is **ergosterol.** Human cell membranes have cholesterol instead of ergosterol. Because polyene antifungals have a strong chemical affinity for ergosterol instead of cholesterol, they do not bind to human cell membranes and therefore do not kill human cells. Once the polyene drug molecule binds to the ergosterol, a channel forms in the fungal cell membrane that allows potassium and magnesium ions to leak out of the fungal cell. This loss of ions causes fungal cellular metabolism to be altered, which leads to death of the cell.

Imidazoles and triazoles act as either fungistatic or fungicidal drugs, depending on their concentration in the fungus. They are most effective in combating rapidly growing fungi and work by inhibiting fungal cell cytochrome P-450 enzymes. These enzymes are needed to produce ergosterol. The allylamine terbinafine is believed to act by a similar mechanism. When the production of ergosterol is inhibited, other sterols called *methylsterols* are produced instead. This results in a defect similar to that caused by the polyene antifungals, namely, a leaky cell membrane that allows needed electrolytes to escape. The fungal cells die because they cannot carry on cellular metabolism.

The echinocandins caspofungin, micafungin, and anidulafungin act by preventing the synthesis of *glucans,* essential components of fungal cell walls that are not present in mammalian cells. This also contributes to fungal cell death. Some of the fungi that are susceptible to these drugs are the pathogens involved in the various mycoses listed in Box 42-1.

Indications

Indications for the use of the various antifungal drugs are specific to the drug. The adverse effects of the newer antifungals are fewer and less serious than those of the older drugs. However, the drug of choice for the treatment of many severe systemic fungal infections remains one of the oldest antifungals, amphotericin B, which does have major adverse effects. Amphotericin B is effective against a wide range of fungi. It is sometimes given with flucytosine in the treatment of *Candida* and cryptococcal infections because of the synergy of the two drugs. Amphotericin B is also effective for treating aspergillosis, blastomycosis, candidiasis, coccidioidomycosis, cryptococcosis, fungal endocarditis, histoplasmosis, zygomycosis, fungal septicemia, and many other systemic fungal infections. The activity of nystatin is similar to that of amphotericin B, but its usefulness is limited because of its toxic effects when given in the dosages required to accomplish

---

BOX 42-1 Fungal Species Susceptible to Current Antifungal Drugs

Superficial/Topical Mycoses
Epidermophyton spp.
Malassezia furfur (causes tinea versicolor)
Microsporum spp.
Sporothrix spp.
Trichophyton spp.

Systemic Mycoses
Absidia spp.
Aspergillus spp.
Basidiobolus spp.
Blastomyces dermatitidis
Candida spp.
Coccidioides immitis
Conidiobolus spp.
Cryptococcus neoformans
Histoplasma capsulatum
Mucor spp.
Rhizopus spp.
Scedosporium apiospermum

Spp., Species.

---

the same antifungal actions as amphotericin B. It is also not available in parenteral form. Nystatin is most commonly used to treat oropharyngeal candidiasis, commonly referred to as *thrush.*

Fluconazole and itraconazole are synthetic azole antifungals. Fluconazole can pass into the cerebrospinal fluid (CSF) and inhibit the growth of cryptococcal fungi. This makes it effective in the treatment of cryptococcal meningitis. Both drugs are active against oropharyngeal and esophageal *Candida* infections. Itraconazole is capable of only poor CSF penetration but can be widely distributed throughout other areas of the body. It is indicated for the treatment of fungal infections in immunocompromised and nonimmunocompromised patients with disseminated candidiasis, histoplasmosis, blastomycosis, and aspergillosis. Ketoconazole, a systemic imidazole, inhibits many dermatophytes and fungi that cause systemic mycoses, but it is not active against *Aspergillus* organisms or *Phycomycetes* (common molds) such as *Mucor* species (spp.). Fortunately the newest triazole antifungal drug, voriconazole, does have activity against some of these more tenacious fungi, including *Aspergillus* spp. causing invasive infection, *Scedosporium* spp., and *Fusarium* spp.

Of the azole antifungals, fluconazole is the most effective for combating infections with *Candida, Cryptococcus, Blastomyces,* and *Histoplasma* organisms. Fluconazole is very effective against vaginal candidiasis. One dose of 150 mg of fluconazole can cure many vaginal candidal infections.

Flucytosine inhibits *Cryptococcus neoformans, C. albicans,* and many *Cladosporium* and *Phialophora* spp. It does not inhibit *Aspergillus, Sporothrix, Blastomyces,* or *Histoplasma* spp. or *Coccidioides immitis.*

Griseofulvin inhibits dermatophytes of *Microsporum, Trichophyton,* and *Epidermophyton* spp. It has no effect on filamentous fungi such as *Aspergillus,* yeasts such as *Candida* spp., or dimorphic species such as *Histoplasma.* Terbinafine is a synthetic allylamine derivative used in a systemic oral form for treatment of

TABLE 42-2 Selected Antifungal Drugs: Common Adverse Effects and Cautions

Body System	Adverse Effects	Cautions
amphotericin B (Sy)		
Cardiovascular	Cardiac dysrhythmias	Recheck dosage and type of amphotericin B being administered
Central nervous	Neurotoxicity; tinnitus; visual disturbances; hand or feet numbness, tingling, or pain; convulsions	
Renal	Renal toxicity, potassium loss, hypomagnesemia	
Pulmonary	Pulmonary infiltrates, other respiratory difficulties	
Other (infusion related)	Fever, chills, headache, malaise, nausea, occasionally hypotension, gastrointestinal upset, anemia	
fluconazole (Sy)		
Gastrointestinal	Nausea, vomiting, diarrhea, stomach pain	Use with caution in patients with renal or hepatic dysfunction
Other	Increased liver enzyme levels, dizziness	
caspofungin (Sy)		
Central nervous	Fever, chills, headache	
Cardiovascular	Hypotension, peripheral edema, tachycardia	
Gastrointestinal	Nausea, vomiting, diarrhea, hepatotoxicity	
Hematologic	Decreased hemoglobin and hematocrit, leukopenia, anemia	
Integumentary	Rash, facial edema, itching	
voriconazole (Sy)		
Central nervous	Hallucinations	
Gastrointestinal	Nausea, vomiting	
Hepatic	Increase liver enzyme levels	
Integumentary	Rash	
Other	Photophobia, hypokalemia	
nystatin (T)		
Gastrointestinal	Nausea, vomiting, anorexia, diarrhea, cramps	Local irritation may occur
Integumentary	Rash, urticaria	
terbinafine (Sy, T)		
Central nervous	Headache, dizziness	Rarely causes irritation
Gastrointestinal	Nausea, vomiting, diarrhea	
Integumentary	Rash, pruritus	
Other	Alopecia, fatigue	

Sy, Systemic; *T,* topical.

onychomycoses—fungal infections of the fingernails or toenails. Topical forms of terbinafine are also used for various skin infections (see Chapter 56).

Contraindications

Drug allergy, liver failure, kidney failure, and porphyria (for griseofulvin) are the most common contraindications for antifungal drugs. Itraconazole should not be used to treat onychomycoses in patients with severe cardiac problems. Voriconazole can cause fetal harm in pregnant women.

Adverse Effects

The major adverse effects and clinical problems caused by antifungal drugs are encountered most commonly in conjunction with amphotericin B treatment. Drug interactions and hepatotoxicity are the primary concerns in patients receiving other antifungal drugs, but the intravenous administration of amphotericin B is associated with a multitude of adverse effects. The most common and problematic of the adverse effects of the various anti-

fungal drugs are listed in Table 42-2. With amphotericin B treatment in particular, prescribers commonly order various premedications (including antiemetics, antihistamines, antipyretics, and corticosteroids) to prevent or minimize infusion-related reactions. The likelihood of such reactions can also be reduced by using longer-than-average drug infusion times (i.e., 2 to 6 hours) for this particular drug.

Interactions

There are many important drug interactions associated antifungal drugs, some of which can be life threatening. A common underlying source of the problem is that many of the antifungal drugs, as well as other drugs, are metabolized by a frequently used enzyme system in the liver called the *cytochrome P-450 system.* The result of the coadministration of two drugs that are both broken down by this system is that they compete for the limited amount of enzymes, and one of the drugs ends up accumulating. Key drug interactions for the systemic antifungal drugs are summarized in Table 42-3.

TABLE 42-3 Antifungal Drugs: Drug Interactions

Drug	Possible Effects
amphotericin B	
Digitalis glycosides	amphotericin B–induced hypokalemia may increase the potential for digitalis toxicity
Nephrotoxic drug	Additive nephrotoxicity
Thiazide diuretics	Severe hypokalemia or decreased adrenal cortex response to corticotrophin
fluconazole, itraconazole	
cyclosporine, phenytoin, sirolimus	Increased plasma concentrations of both drugs
Oral anticoagulants	Increased effects of anticoagulants seen as increases in PT
Oral hypoglycemics	Reduced metabolism of hypoglycemic drugs
Griseofulvin	
Oral anticoagulants	Decreased effects of anticoagulants seen as decreases in PT
Oral contraceptives, estrogen-containing products	Decreased effectiveness of these drugs
voriconazole	
quinidine	Prolongation of QT interval on electrocardiogram

PT, Prothrombin time.

Dosages

For the recommended dosages of selected antifungal drugs, see the Dosages table on p. 660.

DRUG PROFILES

◆ amphotericin B

As previously mentioned, amphotericin B (Fungizone) remains the drug of choice for the treatment of severe systemic mycoses. The main drawback of amphotericin B therapy is that the drug causes many adverse effects. Almost all patients given the drug intravenously experience fever, chills, hypotension, tachycardia, malaise, muscle and joint pain, anorexia, nausea and vomiting, and headache. For this reason, as noted earlier, pretreatment with an antipyretic (acetaminophen), antihistamines, and antiemetics may be conducted to decrease the severity of the infusion-related reaction.

Lipid formulations of amphotericin B have been developed in an attempt to decrease the incidence of its adverse effects and increase its efficacy. There are currently three lipid preparations of amphotericin B: amphotericin B lipid complex (Abelcet), amphotericin B cholesteryl complex (Amphotec), and liposomal amphotericin B (AmBisome). These lipid dosage forms have a much higher cost than conventional amphotericin B and for this reason are often used only when patients are intolerant of or have an infection refractory to nonlipid amphotericin B.

Amphotericin B is contraindicated in patients who have shown hypersensitivity reactions to it and in those with severe bone marrow suppression or renal impairment. However, patients who have life-threatening fungal infections may still be treated with this drug if culture results indicate that no other drug will kill the caus-

ative organism. The drug is available in injectable, oral, and topical preparations. Often a 1-mg test dose is given over 20 to 30 minutes to see if the patient will tolerate the amphotericin. The drug has been used as a local irrigant (in bladder irrigation) for the treatment of candidal cystitis and has been used intrapleurally and intraperitoneally for the treatment of fungal infections in those body cavities.

PHARMACOKINETICS

Route	Onset of Action	Peak Plasma Concentration	Elimination Half-life	Duration of Action
IV	Variable	1 hr	1-15 days	18-24 hr

caspofungin

Caspofungin (Cancidas) was the first echinocandin antifungal drug, approved in 2001. It is used for treatment of severe *Aspergillus* infection (invasive aspergillosis) in patients who are intolerant of or have infections refractory to other drugs. Caspofungin doses should be reduced in patients with impaired liver function. The drug is available only in injectable form. In 2005, a second echinocandin known as micafungin (Mycamine) was approved, and in 2007, a third, anidulafungin (Eraxis), was approved.

PHARMACOKINETICS

Route	Onset of Action	Peak Plasma Concentration	Elimination Half-life	Duration of Action
IV	Unknown	1 hr	9-50 hr	Unknown

◆ fluconazole

Fluconazole (Diflucan) has proved to be a significant improvement in the area of antifungal treatment. It has a much better adverse effect profile than that of amphotericin B, and it also has excellent coverage against many fungi. In fact, it is often preferred to amphotericin B because of these qualities. Oral fluconazole has excellent bioavailability, which means that almost the entire dose administered is absorbed into the circulation. Fluconazole is available in both oral and injectable forms.

PHARMACOKINETICS

Route	Onset of Action	Peak Plasma Concentration	Elimination Half-life	Duration of Action
PO	1 hr	1-2 hr	22-30 hr	Variable

nystatin

Nystatin (Mycostatin) is a polyene antifungal drug that is often applied topically for the treatment of candidal diaper rash, taken orally as prophylaxis against candidal infections during periods of neutropenia in patients receiving immunosuppressive therapy, and used for the treatment of oral and vaginal candidiasis. It is not available in a parenteral form but does come in several oral and topical formulations.

PHARMACOKINETICS

Route	Onset of Action	Peak Plasma Concentration	Elimination Half-life	Duration of Action
PO	24 hr	2 hr	Unknown	Unknown

terbinafine

Terbinafine (Lamisil) is classified as an allylamine antifungal drug and is currently the only drug in its class. It is available in a topical cream, gel, and spray for treating superficial dermatologic infections, including tinea pedis (athlete's foot), tinea cruris (jock itch), and tinea corporis (ringworm). A tablet form is also available for

DOSAGES

Selected Antifungal Drugs

Drug (Pregnancy Category)	Pharmacologic Class	Usual Dosage Range	Indications
◆ amphotericin B (Amphocin, Fungizone) (B)	Polyene antifungal	IV: Initial daily dose, 0.25 mg/kg; titrate up to 0.5-1.5 mg/kg/day Topical: apply cream or lotion 2-4 times daily	Systemic infections with broad spectrum of fungi Topical candidiasis
amphotericin B lipid complex; dosages vary with product as follows:	Polyene antifungal	**Adult and pediatric**	Systemic fungal infections
Abelcet (B)		IV: 5 mg/kg once daily, infused at 2.5 mg/kg/hr	
Amphotec (B)		IV: 3-4 mg/kg/day, infused at 1 mg/kg/hr	
AmBisome (B)		IV: 3-5 mg/kg/day, infused over 1-2 hr	
caspofungin (Cancidas) (C)	Echinocandin antifungal	**Adult only** IV: 70 mg loading dose on day 1, followed by 50 mg/day thereafter; infuse doses over 1 hr	Invasive aspergillosis in patients who do not tolerate or respond to other drugs
◆ fluconazole (Diflucan) (C)	Synthetic triazole antifungal	**Adult** PO: 150 mg in a single dose	Vaginal candidiasis
		Adult IV/PO: 100-400 mg/day × 2-5 wk (dose and duration dependent on severity of infection) **Pediatric** IV/PO: 3-12 mg/kg, same guidelines as for adult	Oropharyngeal and esophageal candidiasis, systemic candidiasis
		Adult IV/PO: 200-400 mg/day × 10-12 wk after negative CSF culture results **Pediatric** IV/PO: 3-12 mg/kg ×10-12 wk after negative CSF culture results	Cryptococcal meningitis
nystatin (Nilstat, Mycostatin, Nystex) (C)	Polyene antifungal	**Infant** PO: 200,000 units (2 mL) oral suspension in oral cavity 4 times daily	Oral candidiasis
		Adult and pediatric PO: 400,000-600,000 units (4-6 mL) oral suspension in oral cavity 4 times daily	
		Adult and pediatric PO (troche): 200,000-400,000 units (1-2 troches dissolved in mouth) 4-5 times daily	
		Adult only PO (tab): 500,000-1,000,000 units (1-2 tabs) 3 times daily	Intestinal candidiasis
		Topical (cream, lotion, or powder): apply 2-3 times daily	Topical candidiasis
terbinafine (Lamisil) (B)	Synthetic allylamine antifungal	**Adult only** PO: 250 mg/day × 6 wk (fingernail) or × 12 wk (toenail)	Onychomycosis (fungal infection of fingernail or toenail)
		Topical cream or solution: apply twice daily to affected area × 1-4 wk	Athlete's foot (tinea pedis), jock itch (tinea cruris), or ringworm (tinea corporis)
voriconazole (Vfend) (D)	Synthetic triazole antifungal	**Adult only** PO: 200 mg q12h IV: 6 mg/kg q12h × 2 doses followed by 4 mg/kg q12h	Invasive aspergillosis; other major fungal infections in patients who do not tolerate or respond to other antifungal drugs

CSF, Cerebrospinal fluid; *IV,* intravenous; *PO,* oral.

systemic use and is used primarily to treat onychomycoses of the fingernails or toenails.

PHARMACOKINETICS

Route	Onset of Action	Peak Plasma Concentration	Elimination Half-life	Duration of Action
PO	Unknown	1-2 hr	22-26 hr	Unknown

voriconazole

Voriconazole (Vfend) is also a newer antifungal drug, approved by the U.S. Food and Drug Administration in 2002. It is used for treating severe fungal infections caused by *Aspergillus* spp. (invasive aspergillosis). It is also used for a variety of other severe fungal infections, such as those caused by *Scedosporium* and *Fusarium* spp. Voriconazole is contraindicated in patients who have a known drug allergy to it and in patients who are taking certain other drugs metabolized by the cytochrome P-450 enzyme 3A4 (e.g., quinidine) because of the risk for induction of serious cardiac dysrhythmias. It is also the only antifungal drug contraindicated in pregnancy. The drug is available in oral and injectable forms.

PHARMACOKINETICS

Route	Onset of Action	Peak Plasma Concentration	Elimination Half-life	Duration of Action
PO	Unknown	1-2 hr	Variable	Unknown

NURSING PROCESS

Assessment

Although topical dosage forms are discussed in detail in Chapter 56, it is still important to discuss these forms and related nursing process issues here. Vital signs, weight, hemoglobin level, hematocrit, red blood cell counts (RBCs), complete blood counts (CBCs) with differential, liver and renal function test results, and culture and sensitivity test results should all be assessed and the findings documented before initiation of antifungal therapy. Before administering amphotericin B (or any other antifungal drug), the nurse should identify any contraindications, cautions, and drug interactions, which have been discussed previously. Allergy to amphotericin B and/or sulfites should be noted and considered a contraindication. Any other nephrotoxic drugs need to be avoided, if at all possible. Baseline renal function studies would be warranted in this situation. There is a risk for severe adverse reactions with intravenous antifungal administration (e.g., amphotericin B), so assessment of any special premedication orders for antiemetics, antihistamines, antipyretics, and/or antiinflammatory drugs, should be completed. Caspofungin and other antifungals require recording of baseline vital signs, liver function test results, and CBCs. Patients receiving griseofulvin should be assessed thoroughly for allergy to penicillin because of the possibly higher risk for allergic reactions to the antifungal in patients with penicillin allergy. Miconazole use is associated with adverse cardiovascular effects; therefore, pulse rate, blood pressure, and electrocardiogram findings should be noted, as should any history of cardiac disease. Use of nystatin lozenges should be avoided in children younger than 5 years of age. Terbinafine requires close monitoring of liver function test results, especially in patients receiving treatment for longer than 6 weeks. Voriconazole should be given only after baseline liver and kidney function test results have been noted.

Amphotericin B

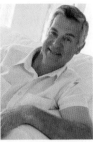

© Monkey Business Images

A.B., a 63-year-old retired delivery driver, has been hospitalized for pneumonia. Since his admission, he has been diagnosed with a severe systemic fungal infection, and an amphotericin B infusion will be started. Before beginning this medication, the nurse assesses the results of his renal and liver function laboratory studies, as well as his complete blood count. The patency of the intravenous line is verified, and the nurse gives A.B. a dose of acetaminophen (Tylenol) as well as an antihistamine before starting the infusion.

1. What is the purpose of the acetaminophen and antihistamine?
2. The nurse stays with the patient for the first 15 minutes of the infusion and monitors A.B.'s vital signs. Explain the rationale for these nursing actions.
3. One hour after the infusion is completed, A.B. calls the nurse and says that he feels as if he may vomit and has chills, yet feels hot at the same time. What should the nurse do?
4. A.B. continues to feel "terrible" the rest of the night, and the next morning his physician, Dr. F., changes the order to liposomal amphotericin B (AmBisome). Why did the physician continue an antifungal medication? What is the rationale behind this order change?

For answers, see *http://evolve.elsevier.com/Lilley*.

See pharmacology discussion for cautions, contraindications, and drug interactions for all antifungals.

Nursing Diagnoses

- Acute pain related to symptoms of the infectious process
- Deficient knowledge related to lack of information and experience with the antifungal drug therapy
- Risk for injury related to adverse effects of the medication treatment regimen

Planning
Goals

- Patient states the rationale for adherence to the antifungal therapy regimen.
- Patient states the common adverse effects of antifungal drug therapy and ways to prevent injury to self.
- Patient exhibits relief of the symptoms previously associated with the fungal infection.
- Patient states the importance of making and keeping follow-up appointments with the prescriber.

Outcome Criteria

- Patient is free of drug-induced complications or experiences minimal adverse effects of the antifungal drug therapy (e.g., nausea, vomiting, gastrointestinal upset) for the duration of treatment.
- Patient remains compliant with the medication regimen without skipping doses and experiences relief of infection with a return to normal vital signs and negative findings on culture and sensitivity tests after the full course of therapy.

- Patient experiences improved appetite, energy level, and physical strength and stamina after taking the antifungal drugs for the prescribed period.
- Patient returns to the prescriber regularly as recommended by the prescriber for constant monitoring of the infection and of drug therapy with various blood tests (e.g., CBC with differential, RBC count, hemoglobin level, hematocrit, renal and liver function tests).

Implementation

The nursing interventions appropriate for patients receiving antifungal drugs vary depending on the particular drug. It is often necessary for the nurse to check the vital signs of patients receiving any of the antifungals at least every 15 to 30 minutes during an intravenous infusion, or as needed. The nurse should monitor all laboratory values (see earlier) during therapy. Weight should also be documented frequently, as indicated, with long-term or at-home therapy, because a gain of 2 pounds or more in a 24-hour period or 5 pounds or more in 1 week may indicate possible medication-induced renal damage, and the need for prompt medical attention. The nurse should follow manufacturer guidelines and the prescriber's order for specific solutions and rates of intravenous administration. With intravenous amphotericin B, solutions that are cloudy or have precipitates should not be administered. Use of an intravenous infusion pump is recommended. Once the intravenous infusion has begun, vital signs should be monitored every 15 minutes or as needed to assess for adverse reactions such as cardiac dysrhythmias, visual disturbances, paresthesias (numbness or tingling of the hands or feet), respiratory difficulty, pain, fever, chills, and nausea. Should these adverse effects or a severe reaction occur, the infusion should be discontinued (while the patient is closely monitored) and the prescriber contacted. The intravenous site should be monitored for signs of phlebitis (e.g., heat, pain, and redness over the vein), as per hospital policy. See Patient Teaching Tips for further information.

Only clear solutions of caspofungin should be used, and doses should be diluted with the recommended amount of normal saline.

Liver toxicity may occur, and thus liver function should be monitored during therapy. In addition, the patient should be monitored for the occurrence of tachycardia, hypotension, fever, chills, or headache. Hemoglobin level and hematocrit should be measured frequently as well, because of the possibility of drug-induced anemias. Fluconazole may be given either orally or intravenously, with intravenous dosage forms used if there is a specific indication or if the oral dosage forms are poorly tolerated. Intravenous dosage forms should be administered only if clear, and no other medication should be added to the solution. The occurrence of itching or a rash should be reported immediately, and the patient's temperature, bowel activity, and stool consistency should also be monitored. Nystatin may be given orally in the form of lozenges or troches, which should be slowly and completely dissolved in the mouth for optimal effects; these should not be chewed or swallowed whole. If a suspension is used, the patient should swish the medication solution thoroughly in the mouth for as long as possible before swallowing. Terbinafine may be given orally or topically. Local skin reactions that need to be reported include blistering, itching, oozing, redness, and swelling. Oral doses of voriconazole should be given 1 hour before or 1 hour after a meal, and intravenous doses may be diluted with 5% dextrose in water or normal saline and the accurate dose infused over the recommended time period. Visual acuity must be monitored when this drug is given (especially if ordered for longer than 28 days) and any changes reported to the prescriber.

Evaluation

The therapeutic effects of antifungals include improvement and eventual resolution of the signs and symptoms of the fungal infection if the patient has remained totally adherent to the therapy regimen. Improved energy levels and improvement in overall sense of well-being with a normal temperature and other vital sign values also indicate a therapeutic response. Specific adverse effects for which to monitor in patients receiving these drugs are listed in Table 42-2. Goals and outcome criteria should be evaluated in the context of the nursing care plan.

PATIENT TEACHING TIPS

- Female patients taking antifungal medications for the treatment of vaginal infections should abstain from sexual intercourse until the treatment is completed and the infection is resolved and should be told to continue to take the medication even if they are actively menstruating. Patients should notify the prescriber if symptoms persist after treatment is completed.
- Some patients receiving amphotericin B may need long-term treatment (i.e., over weeks to months). If so, possible adverse effects include tinnitus, blurred vision, burning and itching at the infusion site, headache, rash, fever, chills, hypokalemia, gastrointestinal upset, and various anemias. Patients should weigh themselves daily and notify the prescriber if they gain more than 2 pounds in a 24-hour period or 5 pounds or more in 1 week. Muscle weakness may occur due to hypokalemia, so serum potassium levels should be monitored.
- When taking caspofungin, any problems with shortness of breath, itching, facial swelling, and/or a rash must be reported immediately to the prescriber.

- Fluconazole may cause dizziness, and therefore the patient should not drive until adverse effects are resolved. Good hygiene should be recommended.
- The patient should be given proper dosing instructions for nystatin (e.g., swish and swallow). The patient should be fully informed about how to apply the drug. If vaginal troches are prescribed, the appropriate applicator should be used with a gloved hand and inserted high into the vagina; then hand washing should follow.
- The patient should be encouraged to keep affected body areas clean and dry and to wear light and cool clothing. Contact of the topical dosage form with the eyes, mouth, nose, or other mucous membranes should be avoided. The patient should be instructed to report any adverse effects such as skin irritation and diarrhea.
- Voriconazole should be taken 1 hour before or 1 hour after meals. The patient should be encouraged to avoid driving at night because of possible visual changes, such as blurred vision and/or photophobia. The patient should be encouraged to avoid direct sunlight and to use effective contraception.

POINTS TO REMEMBER

- Fungi are a very large and diverse group of microorganisms and consist of yeasts and molds. Yeasts are single-celled fungi that may be harmful (e.g., causing infections) or helpful (e.g., aiding in baking or brewing beer). Molds are multicellular and are characterized by long, branching filaments called *hyphae*.
- Candidiasis is an opportunistic fungal infection caused by *C. albicans* and occurs in patients taking broad-spectrum antibiotics, antineoplastics, or immunosuppressants, as well as in immunocompromised persons. When candidiasis occurs in the mouth, it is commonly called *oral candidiasis* or *thrush*. Oral candidiasis is more commonly seen in newborns or immunocompromised persons.
- Vaginal candidiasis is a yeast infection and occurs most commonly in individuals with diabetes mellitus, women taking oral contraceptives, and pregnant women.

- Antifungals may be administered either systemically or topically. Some of the most common systemic antifungals are amphotericin B and fluconazole; an example of a topical antifungal is nystatin.
- Before administering antifungals, the nurse must thoroughly assess for allergies as well as interactions with other drugs patients are taking, including prescription drugs, over-the-counter drugs, and herbals.
- Amphotericin B must be properly diluted according to manufacturer guidelines and administered using an intravenous infusion pump. Tissue extravasation of fluconazole at the intravenous infusion site leads to tissue necrosis; therefore, the site should be checked hourly and the assessment documented.

NCLEX EXAMINATION REVIEW QUESTIONS

1 The nurse is assessing a patient who is about to receive antifungal drug therapy. Which problem would be of most concern?
  a Endocrine disease
  b Hepatic disease
  c Cardiac disease
  d Pulmonary disease
2 While monitoring a patient who is receiving intravenous amphotericin B, the nurse expects to see which adverse effect(s)?
  a Hypertension
  b Bradycardia
  c Fever and chills
  d Diarrhea and stomach cramps
3 When administering antifungal drug therapy, the nurse knows that a problem that contributes to many of the drug interactions with antifungals is
  a polyuria.
  b gallbladder metabolism.
  c bone distribution.
  d cytochrome P-450 enzyme system.
4 During an infusion of amphotericin B, the nurse knows that which administration technique may be used to minimize infusion-related adverse effects?

  a Forcing of fluids during the infusion
  b Infusing the medication quickly
  c Infusing the medication over a longer period of time
  d Stopping the infusion for 2 hours after half of the bag has infused, then resuming 1 hour later
5 When the nurse is teaching a patient who is taking nystatin lozenges for oral candidiasis, which instruction by the nurse is correct?
  a "Chew the lozenge carefully before swallowing."
  b "Dissolve the lozenge slowly and completely in your mouth."
  c "Dissolve the lozenge until it is half the original size, then swallow it."
  d "These lozenges should be swallowed whole with a glass of water."
6 When monitoring a patient who is receiving caspofungin, the nurse should look for which serious adverse effects? (Select all that apply.)
  a Blood dyscrasias
  b Hypotension
  c Cardiac palpitations
  d Tinnitus
  e Hepatotoxicity

1. b, 2. c, 3. d, 4. c, 5. b, 6. a, b, e.

CRITICAL THINKING ACTIVITIES: BEST ACTION

1 The nurse is reviewing newly written orders for a patient who has a vaginal yeast infection. One order reads, "Fluconazole, 150 mg, one tablet by mouth now for vaginal yeast infection." The unit secretary sees the order and asks, "Is that a mistake? How can one pill help that problem?" What is the nurse's best answer?
2 A patient has a severe respiratory aspergillosis and has not responded to antifungal therapy after 4 days. There is a new order

for caspofungin (Cancidas). What is the most important assessment action by the nurse before administering this drug?
3 When the nurse is administering medications, the patient takes the oral nystatin suspension and says, "I know how to take this." He then swallows the liquid medication all at once. What is the nurse's best action at this time?

For answers, see *http://evolve.elsevier.com/Lilley*.

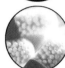

CHAPTER *43*

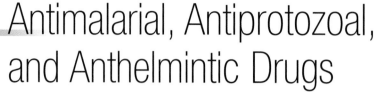

Antimalarial, Antiprotozoal, and Anthelmintic Drugs

OBJECTIVES

When you reach the end of this chapter, you should be able to do the following:

1. Briefly discuss the infectious process associated with malaria, other protozoal infections, and helminth infections.

2. Compare the signs and symptoms of malarial, other protozoal, and helminthic infection processes.

3. Identify the more commonly used antimalarial, antiprotozoal, and anthelmintic drugs.

4. Discuss the mechanisms of action, indications, cautions, contraindications, adverse effects, dosages, drug interactions and routes of administration of the antimalarial, antiprotozoal, and anthelmintic drugs.

5. Develop a nursing care plan that includes all phases of the nursing process for patients receiving antimalarial, antiprotozoal, or anthelmintic drugs.

e-Learning Activities

http://evolve.elsevier.com/Lilley

NCLEX Review Questions • Animations • Nursing Care Plans • Audio Glossary • Category Catchers • Medication Errors Checklists • IV Therapy Checklists • Calculators • Frequently Asked Questions • Content Updates • Supplemental Resources • Answers to Case Studies and Critical Thinking Activities

Drug Profiles

atovaquone, p. 671
◆ chloroquine and
  hydroxychloroquine, p. 668
◆ mebendazole, p. 674
  mefloquine, p. 668
◆ metronidazole, p. 671

pentamidine, p. 671
praziquantel, p. 674
◆ primaquine, p. 668
  pyrantel, p. 674
  pyrimethamine, p. 668

───────────
◆ *Key drug.*

Glossary

Anthelmintic A drug that destroys or prevents the development of parasitic worm (helminthic) infections. Also called *antihelmintic* or *vermicide;* notice that the terms for the drug categories are spelled with only one *h*, which appears in the second syllable of the term, whereas the term for worm infection *(helminthic)* is spelled with two *h*'s, appearing in both the second and third syllables of the term. (p. 671)

Antimalarial drugs Drugs that destroy or prevent the development of the malaria parasite (*Plasmodium* sp.) in human hosts. Antimalarial drugs are a subset of the broader category of antiprotozoal drugs. (p. 665)

Antiprotozoal A drug that destroys or prevents the development of protozoans in human hosts. (p. 668)

Helminthic infections Parasitic worm infections. (p. 671)

Malaria A widespread protozoal infectious disease caused by four species of the genus *Plasmodium*. (p. 664)

Parasite Any organism that feeds on another living organism (known as a *host*) in a way that results in varying degrees of harm to the host organism. (p. 665)

Parasitic protozoans Harmful protozoans that live on or in human beings or animals and cause disease in the process. (p. 664)

Protozoans Single-celled organisms that are the smallest and simplest members of the animal kingdom. (p. 664)

• • •

Anatomy, Physiology, and Disease Overview

There are more than 28,000 known types of **protozoans,** which are single-celled organisms. Those that live on or in humans are called **parasitic protozoans.** Billions of people worldwide are infected with these organisms, and, as a result, these infections are considered a serious public health problem. Some of the more common protozoal infections are malaria, leishmaniasis, trypanosomiasis, amebiasis, giardiasis, and trichomoniasis. They are relatively uncommon in the United States but are becoming increasingly prevalent in immunocompromised individuals, including those with acquired immunodeficiency syndrome (AIDS). Protozoal diseases are especially prevalent among people living in tropical climates because it is easier for protozoans to survive and be transmitted in environments that are warm and humid year round. Although the population of the United States is relatively free of many of these protozoal infections, international travel and the immigration of people from other countries where such infections are endemic are providing opportunities for increased exposure.

MALARIA

The most significant protozoal disease in terms of morbidity and mortality is **malaria.** Worldwide, it is estimated that 350 to 500 million people are infected, with an annual death rate of 1 million to 2 million people. In Africa alone, malaria accounts for more than 1 million infant deaths a year. The geographic areas with the highest prevalence are sub-Saharan Africa, Southeast Asia, and Latin America. In 2006, the United States had 1564 cases of malaria. Malaria is caused by a particular genus of protozoans called *Plasmodium,* and there are four species of organisms in this genus, each with its own characteristics and its own ability to resist being killed by antimalarial drugs. These four species are *Plasmodium vivax, Plasmodium falciparum, Plasmodium malariae, and Plasmodium ovale.* Although *P. vivax* is the most widespread of the four, *P. falciparum* is nearly as widespread and causes greater problems with drug resistance. The two remaining species are much less common and more geographically limited in their occurrence, but they can still cause serious malarial infections. Most commonly, malaria is transmitted by the bite of an infected female *anopheline* mosquito. This type of mosquito is endemic to many tropical regions of the earth. Malaria can also be transmitted by blood transfusions, congenitally from mother to infant via an infected placenta, or through the use of contaminated needles by drug abusers. Despite the combined efforts of many countries to eradicate malaria, it remains one of the most devastating infectious diseases in the world. As is also the case with tuberculosis (see Chapter 41) and AIDS (see Chapter 40), many lives are lost to malaria, and the cost of treating and preventing the disease imposes a tremendous economic burden on the often poor countries where the disease is prevalent.

The *Plasmodium* life cycle is quite complex and involves many stages. The organism has two interdependent life cycles: the *sexual cycle,* which takes place inside the mosquito, and the *asexual cycle,* which occurs in the human host (Figure 43-1). In addition, the asexual cycle of the **parasite** consists of a phase outside the erythrocyte (primarily in liver tissues) called the *exoerythrocytic phase* (or the *tissue phase*) and a phase inside the erythrocyte called the *erythrocytic phase* (or the *blood phase*). The malarial parasite undergoes many changes during these two phases (Figure 43-2). Malaria signs and symptoms are often described in terms of the *classic malaria paroxysm*. A paroxysm is a sudden recurrence or intensification of symptoms. Symptoms include chills and rigors, followed by fevers of up to 104° F (40° C) and diaphoresis, frequently leading to extreme fatigue and prolonged sleep. This syndrome often repeats itself periodically in 48- to 72-hour cycles. Other common symptoms include headache, nausea, and joint pain.

Pharmacology Overview
ANTIMALARIAL DRUGS

Treatment for malaria should not be initiated until the diagnosis has been confirmed by laboratory investigations. Once the diagnosis of malaria has been confirmed, appropriate antimalarial treatment must be initiated immediately. Treatment should be guided by three main factors: the infecting *Plasmodium* species, the clinical status of the patient, and the drug susceptibility of the infecting parasites as determined by the geographic area where the infection was acquired. Because the resistance patterns are constantly changing, depending on geographic location, the reader is referred to the website of the Centers for Disease Control and Prevention (CDC) at *http://www.cdc.gov/malaria/diagnosis_treatment/clinicians2.htm* for the most up-to-date information. People traveling to different parts of the world may require antimalarial prophylaxis and should check with their prescribers and/or the CDC website just mentioned for specific drug therapy.

Antimalarial drugs administered to humans cannot affect the parasite during its sexual cycle when it resides in the mosquito. Instead, these drugs work against the parasite during its asexual cycle, which takes place within the human body. Often these drugs are given in various combinations to achieve an additive or synergistic antimalarial effect. One example is the combination of the two antiprotozoal drugs atovaquone and proguanil

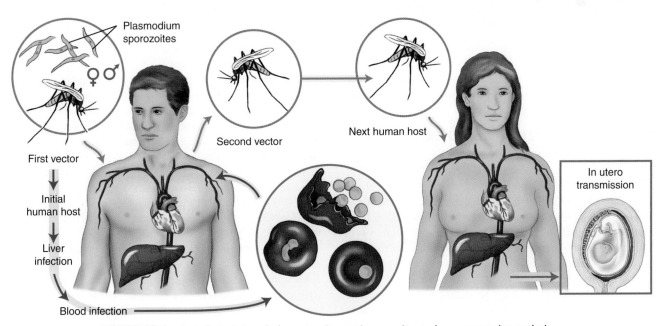

FIGURE 43-1 An infected *Anopheles* mosquito carries parasites to humans, causing malaria. These parasites mature in the liver before entering the bloodstream and rupturing red blood cells. A pregnant woman infected with malaria may transmit the disease to her unborn child.

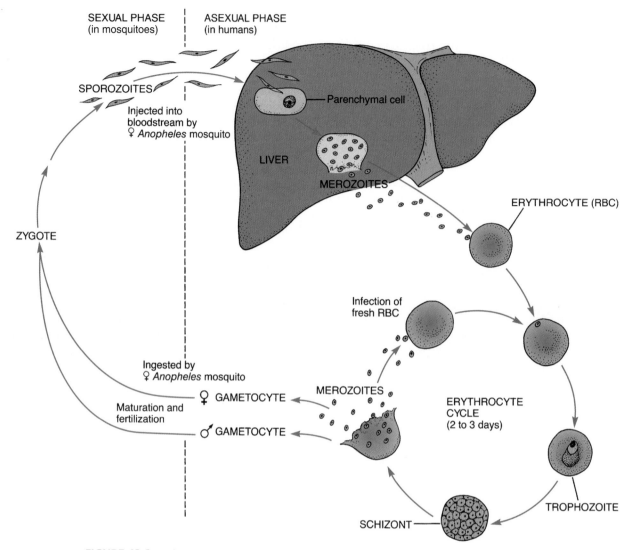

FIGURE 43-2   Life cycle of the malarial parasite. (From Lehne RA: *Pharmacology for nursing care,* ed 7, St Louis, 2010, Saunders.)

(Malarone). The antibiotic combination of pyrimethamine and sulfadoxine (Fansidar) is also commonly used, especially in cases caused by drug-resistant organisms.

Mechanism of Action and Drug Effects

The mechanisms of action of the various antimalarial drugs differ depending on the chemical family to which they belong. The *4-aminoquinoline derivatives* (chloroquine and hydroxychloroquine) work by inhibiting deoxyribonucleic acid (DNA) and ribonucleic acid (RNA) polymerase, enzymes essential to DNA and RNA synthesis by the parasite cells. Parasite protein synthesis is also disrupted, because protein synthesis is dependent on proper nucleic acid (DNA and RNA) function. These drugs are also believed to raise the pH within the parasite, which interferes with the parasite's ability to metabolize and use erythrocyte hemoglobin and is one reason these drugs are ineffective during the exoerythrocytic phase (tissue phase) of infection. All of these actions contribute to the destruction of the parasite. Quinine, quinidine, and mefloquine are thought to be similar to

the 4-aminoquinoline derivatives in their actions in that all are also believed to raise the pH within the parasite.

The *diaminopyrimidines* (pyrimethamine and trimethoprim [see Chapter 38]) work by inhibiting dihydrofolate reductase, an enzyme that is needed for the production of certain vital substances in malarial parasites. Specifically, inhibiting this enzyme blocks the synthesis of tetrahydrofolate, which is a precursor of purines and pyrimidines (nucleic acid components) and certain amino acids (protein components) that are essential for the growth and survival of plasmodia parasites. These two drugs are effective only during the erythrocytic phase. Pyrimethamine and trimethoprim are often used with a sulfonamide (sulfadoxine or dapsone) because of the resulting synergistic effects exerted by such drug combinations. Tetracyclines such as doxycycline (see Chapter 38) and lincomycins such as clindamycin (see Chapter 39) may also be used in combination with some of the other antimalarial drugs because of the synergistic effects resulting from these drug combinations.

Primaquine, an *8-aminoquinoline* that is structurally similar to the 4-aminoquinolines mentioned earlier, has the ability to

TABLE 43-1 Antimalarial Drugs: Common Adverse Effects

Body System	Adverse Effects
chloroquine and hydroxychloroquine	
Gastrointestinal	Diarrhea, anorexia, nausea, vomiting, abdominal distress
Central nervous	Dizziness, anxiety, headache, reduced seizure threshold
Other	Alopecia, rash, pruritus
mefloquine	
Central nervous	Headache, dizziness, insomnia, visual disturbances, increased anxiety, convulsions, depression, psychosis
Gastrointestinal	Stomach pain, anorexia, nausea, vomiting
primaquine	
Gastrointestinal	Nausea, vomiting, abdominal distress
Other	Headaches, pruritus, dark discoloration of urine, hemolytic anemia due to G6PD deficiency
pyrimethamine	
Gastrointestinal	Anorexia; vomiting; taste disturbances; soreness, redness, swelling, or burning of tongue; diarrhea; throat pain; swallowing difficulties; sores, ulcerations, or white spots in mouth; sore throat
Other	Fever, increased bleeding, increased weakness, rash, hemolytic anemia resulting from G6PD deficiency, severe hypersensitivity reactions
quinine	
Central nervous	Visual disturbances, dizziness, severe headaches, tinnitus, hearing loss
Gastrointestinal	Diarrhea, nausea, vomiting, abdominal pain or discomfort
Other	Rash, pruritus, hives, respiratory difficulties, wheezing

G6PD, Glucose-6-phosphate dehydrogenase.

TABLE 43-2 Antimalarial Drugs: Drug Interactions

Drug	Mechanism	Result
chloroquine		
divalproex, valproic acid	Decreased serum levels of valproic acid	Loss of seizure control
mefloquine		
Beta-blockers, calcium channel blockers quinidine, quinine	Unknown	Increased risk of dysrhythmia, cardiac arrest, seizures
primaquine		
Other hemolytic drugs	Unknown	Increased risk for myelotoxic effects (monitor for muscle weakness)

bind to and alter parasitic DNA and is one of the few drugs that is effective in the exoerythrocytic phase. Atovaquone/proguanil also works by interference with nucleic acid synthesis.

The drug effects of the antimalarial drugs are mostly limited to their ability to kill parasitic organisms, most of which are *Plasmodium* species (spp.). However, some of these drugs have other effects and therapeutic uses. Hydroxychloroquine also has antiinflammatory effects and is sometimes used in the treatment of rheumatoid arthritis and systemic lupus erythematosus. Quinine and quinidine can also decrease the excitability of both cardiac and skeletal muscles. Quinidine is still currently used to treat certain types of cardiac dysrhythmias (see Chapter 23).

Indications

Antimalarial drugs are used to kill *Plasmodium* organisms, the parasites that cause malaria. As discussed earlier, different antimalarial drugs work during different phases of the parasite's growth inside the human. The antimalarials that exert the greatest effect on all four *Plasmodium* organisms during the erythrocytic or blood phase are chloroquine, hydroxychloroquine, and pyrimethamine. Other drugs that are known to work during the blood phase are

quinine, quinidine, and mefloquine. Because these drugs are ineffective during the exoerythrocytic phase, however, they cannot *prevent* infection. The most effective antimalarial drug for eradicating the parasite during the exoerythrocytic or tissue phase is primaquine, which actually works during both phases. Primaquine is indicated specifically for infection with *P. vivax*. Chloroquine and hydroxychloroquine (4-aminoquinolines) are the drugs of choice for the treatment of susceptible strains of malarial parasites. They are highly toxic to all *Plasmodium* spp., except resistant strains of *P. falciparum.*

Quinine is indicated for infection with chloroquine-resistant *P. falciparum,* which can cause a type of malaria that affects the brain. Quinine can be used alone but is more commonly given in combination with pyrimethamine, a sulfonamide, or a tetracycline (such as doxycycline). Pyrimethamine is another antimalarial antibiotic that is commonly used in combination with the sulfonamide antibiotic sulfadoxine (Fansidar) for prophylaxis against chloroquine-resistant *P. falciparum* and *P. vivax.* However, drug resistance in most locations has reduced its use for this purpose. Other antimalarial drugs are generally preferred for the treatment of active disease. Mefloquine is a newer antimalarial drug that may also be used for both prophylaxis and treatment of malaria caused by *P. falciparum* or *P. vivax.* The drug combination atovaquone and proguanil (Malarone) is also used for prevention and treatment of *P. falciparum* infection.

Contraindications

Contraindications to various antimalarial drugs include drug allergy, tinnitus (ear ringing), and pregnancy (quinine). Severe renal, hepatic, or hematologic dysfunction may also be a contraindication to the use of antimalarial drugs. Other drug-specific contraindications are noted in the drug profiles that follow.

Adverse Effects

Antimalarial drugs cause diverse adverse effects, and these are listed for each drug in Table 43-1.

Interactions

Some common drug interactions associated with antimalarial drugs are listed in Table 43-2.

Dosages

For the recommended dosages of selected antimalarial drugs, see the Dosages table on p. 669.

DRUG PROFILES

The dosing instructions for several of the antimalarial drugs can be confusing, because tablet strengths listed on the medication packaging often indicate the strength of the tablet in terms of the entire salt form of the drug, not just the active ingredient itself, which is referred to as the *base ingredient.* However, dosing guidelines often list recommended dosages in terms of the base ingredient and not the entire salt. For example, as described later in the drug profile for chloroquine, the tablets come in 250- and 500-mg strengths of the salt form of the drug, but these tablets actually only have 150 and 300 mg, respectively, of the active ingredient or base. The reader is advised to be mindful of these distinctions.

◆ chloroquine and hydroxychloroquine

Chloroquine (Aralen) is a synthetic antimalarial drug that is chemically classified as a 4-aminoquinoline derivative. In addition to malaria, it is also indicated for treatment of other parasitic infections, such as amebiasis. Hydroxychloroquine is another synthetic 4-aminoquinoline derivative that differs from chloroquine by only one hydroxyl group (⁻OH). Its efficacy in treating malaria is comparable to that of quinine. Both medications also possess antiinflammatory actions and have been used to treat rheumatoid arthritis and systemic lupus erythematosus since the 1950s. However, only hydroxychloroquine is now used for those indications.

Contraindications include visual field changes, optic neuritis, and psoriasis, but it should be kept in mind that the use of the medication may still be warranted in urgent clinical situations, based on sound clinical judgment.

Chloroquine and hydroxychloroquine are available only for oral use. Both drugs are classified as pregnancy category C drugs, but it is recommended that they be used in pregnant women only in truly urgent clinical situations. These drugs are also distributed into breast milk.

PHARMACOKINETICS (CHLOROQUINE)

Route	Onset of Action	Peak Plasma Concentration	Elimination Half-life	Duration of Action
PO	8-10 hr	2 hr	3-5 days	Variable

PHARMACOKINETICS (HYDROXYCHLOROQUINE)

Route	Onset of Action	Peak Plasma Concentration	Elimination Half-life	Duration of Action
PO	4 hr	2-3 hr	32-50 days	Variable

mefloquine

Mefloquine (Lariam) is an analogue of quinine that is indicated for the management of mild to moderate acute malaria and for the prevention and treatment of malaria caused by chloroquine-resistant organisms. It is also used to treat multidrug-resistant strains of *P. falciparum,* which, as already noted, is a very difficult species of *Plasmodium* to kill. The drug is commonly used prophylactically by travelers to prevent malarial infection while visiting malaria-endemic areas. The tetracycline antibiotic doxycycline (see Chapter 38) is also commonly used for this purpose. Mefloquine is available only for oral use.

PHARMACOKINETICS

Route	Onset of Action	Peak Plasma Concentration	Elimination Half-life	Duration of Action
PO	Less than 24 hr	7-24 hr	21-22 days	Variable

◆ primaquine

Primaquine is similar in chemical structure and antimalarial activity to the 4-aminoquinolines, but it is classified as an 8-aminoquinoline. As previously noted, however, it is one of the few antimalarial drugs that can destroy the malarial parasites while they are in their exoerythrocytic phase (tissue phase). It is indicated for curative therapy in acute cases of *P. vivax, P. ovale,* and to a lesser degree, *P. falciparum* infection.

Primaquine is contraindicated in patients with allergy or any disease states that may cause granulocytopenia (rheumatoid arthritis, systemic lupus erythematosus). Primaquine should be used with caution in patients with methemoglobinemia, porphyria, methemoglobin reductase deficiency, and glucose-6-phosphate dehydrogenase (G6PD) deficiency. It is available only for oral use.

PHARMACOKINETICS

Route	Onset of Action	Peak Plasma Concentration	Elimination Half-life	Duration of Action
PO	2 hr	1-3 hr	4-10 hr	24 hr

pyrimethamine

Pyrimethamine (Daraprim) is a synthetic antimalarial drug that is structurally related to trimethoprim (see Chapter 38). Both drugs are chemically subclassified as *diaminopyrimidines.* Fansidar is a commonly used fixed-combination drug product that contains 500 mg of sulfadoxine and 25 mg of pyrimethamine. Pyrimethamine is contraindicated in patients with megaloblastic anemia caused by folate deficiency. It is available only for oral use.

PHARMACOKINETICS

Route	Onset of Action	Peak Plasma Concentration	Elimination Half-life	Duration of Action
PO	6 hr	2-6 hr	4 days	Up to 2 wk

OTHER PROTOZOAL INFECTIONS

There are several other common protozoal infections. These include amebiasis (caused by *Entamoeba histolytica*), giardiasis (caused by *Giardia lamblia*), pneumocystosis caused by *Pneumocystis jirovecii* (formerly *Pneumocystis carinii*), toxoplasmosis (caused by *Toxoplasma gondii*), and trichomoniasis, (caused by *Trichomonas vaginalis*). Like malaria, these diseases are also more prevalent in tropical regions.

These protozoal infections can be transmitted in a number of ways: from person to person (e.g., via sexual contact), through the ingestion of contaminated water or food, through direct contact with the parasite, or by the bite of an insect (mosquito or tick). These infections can be systemic and occur throughout the body or they can be localized to a specific region. For example, amebiasis most commonly affects the gastrointestinal tract (e.g., amebic dysentery), whereas pneumocystosis is predominantly a pulmonary infection.

The more common protozoal infections are described briefly in Table 43-3, and the **antiprotozoal** drugs commonly used in their treatment are listed. Only selected drugs are discussed here. Patients whose immune systems are compromised are at particular risk for acquiring a protozoal infection. Often such infections are fatal in these patients.

DOSAGES

Selected Antimalarial Drugs

Drug (Pregnancy Category)	Pharmacologic Class	Usual Dosage Range	Indications/Uses
◆ chloroquine (Aralen) (C)	Synthetic antimalarial and antiamebic	**Adult*** PO: 300 mg base weekly, beginning 1-2 wk before and continuing for 4 wk after visiting endemic area	Malaria prophylaxis
		PO: 600 mg base on day 1, followed by 300 mg 6 hr later and on days 2 and 3	Malaria treatment
◆ hydroxychloroquine (Plaquenil) (C)	Synthetic antimalarial	**Adult*** PO: 310 mg base weekly, beginning 1-2 wk before and continuing through 4 wk after visiting endemic area	Malaria prophylaxis
		PO: 620 mg base on day 1, followed by 310 mg 6 hr later and once daily on days 2 and 3	Malaria treatment
mefloquine (Lariam) (C)	Synthetic antimalarial	**Adult** PO: 250 mg weekly beginning 1-2 wk before travel and continuing until 4 wk after visiting endemic area **Pediatric** PO: Weekly dosing as above based on weight as follows: 10-19 kg: ¼ tab 20-30 kg: ½ tab 31-45 kg: ¾ tab More than 45 kg: 1 tab (250 mg)	Malaria prophylaxis
		Adult PO: 1250 mg (5 tabs) in a single dose **Pediatric** PO: 15-25 mg/kg in a single dose, not to exceed 1250 mg	Malaria treatment
◆ primaquine (generic only) (C)	Synthetic antimalarial	**Adult** PO: 30 mg base daily × 14 days **Pediatric** PO: 0.5 mg base/kg/day daily × 14 days	For cure or prevention of relapse of malarial infection with *Plasmodium vivax;* may also be used for *P. vivax* malaria in patients intolerant of chloroquine or if chloroquine is not available
pyrimethamine (Daraprim) (C)	Folic acid antagonist, antimalarial, antitoxoplasmotic drug	**Adult and pediatric older than 10 yr** PO: 25 mg weekly **Pediatric 4-10 yr** PO: 12.5 mg weekly **Pediatric infant to 3 yr** PO: 6.25 mg weekly	Malaria prophylaxis
		Adult and pediatric older than 10 yr PO: 50 mg daily × 2 days **Pediatric 4-10 yr** PO: 25 mg daily × 2 days	Malaria treatment

ASAP, As soon as possible; *IM,* intramuscular; *PO,* oral.
*Only adult dosages are given. Pediatric dosages range from 5-10 mg/kg but should not exceed adult dosages.

ANTIPROTOZOAL DRUGS

Several drugs used to treat malaria are also used to treat nonmalarial protozoal infections, including chloroquine, primaquine, pyrimethamine, and atovaquone. Other antiprotozoal drugs normally used against nonmalarial parasites include iodoquinol, metronidazole, paromomycin, and pentamidine.

Mechanism of Action and Drug Effects

Antiprotozoal drugs work by several different mechanisms. The most commonly used of these drugs, together with brief descriptions of their mechanisms of action, are given in Table 43-4. Pyrimethamine and chloroquine were discussed earlier in this chapter in the section on malaria. The drug effects of antiproto-

TABLE 43-3 Types of Protozoal Infections and Common Drug Therapy

Infection	Description	Antiprotozoal Drug
Amebiasis	Caused by the protozoal parasite *Entamoeba histolytica*. Infection mainly resides in the large intestine but can also migrate to other parts of the body, such as the liver. Usually transmitted in contaminated food or water.	chloroquine, metronidazole, paromomycin, iodoquinol
Giardiasis	Caused by *Giardia lamblia*. The most common intestinal protozoal infection, usually residing in the intestinal mucosa (most commonly the duodenum). May cause diarrhea, bloating, and foul-smelling stools. Transmitted in contaminated food or water or by contact with stool from infected persons.	metronidazole, nitazoxanide, quinacrine, furazolidone, albendazole, paromomycin
Pneumocystosis	Pneumonia caused by *Pneumocystis jirovecii* that occurs exclusively in immunocompromised individuals. Always fatal if left untreated.	trimethoprim/sulfamethoxazole, dapsone, atovaquone, primaquine, pentamidine, clindamycin
Toxoplasmosis	Caused by *Toxoplasma gondii*. Can produce systemic infection in both immunocompetent and immunocompromised hosts. Domesticated animals, usually cats, serve as intermediate host for parasites, passing infective oocysts in their feces.	sulfonamides with pyrimethamine, clindamycin, metronidazole
Trichomoniasis	Sexually transmitted disease caused by *Trichomonas vaginalis*.	metronidazole

TABLE 43-4 Selected Antiprotozoal Drugs: Mechanisms of Action

Drug	Mechanism of Action
atovaquone	Atovaquone selectively inhibits mitochondrial electron transport, reducing synthesis of adenosine triphosphate (required for cellular energy). Also inhibits nucleic acid synthesis.
metronidazole	Interfers with DNA, resulting in inhibition of protein synthesis and cell death in susceptible organisms.
pentamidine	Inhibits production of much-needed substances such as DNA and RNA. Can bind to and aggregate ribosomes. Is directly lethal to *Pneumocystis jirovecii* by inhibiting glucose metabolism, protein and RNA synthesis, and intracellular amino acid transport.

TABLE 43-5 Selected Antiprotozoal Drugs: Indications

Drug	Indications
atovaquone	Indicated for treatment of acute mild to moderately severe *Pneumocystis jirovecii* pneumonia in patients who cannot tolerate co-trimoxazole
iodoquinol	Indicated for treatment of intestinal amebiasis in asymptomatic carriers of *Entamoeba histolytica*; also has been used for treatment of *Giardia lamblia* and *Trichomonas vaginalis* infections
metronidazole	Indicated for treatment of bacterial (including anaerobic), protozoal, and helminthic infections
pentamidine	Indicated for treatment of *P. jirovecii* pneumonia

zoal drugs are primarily limited to their ability to kill various forms of protozoal parasites.

Indications

Antiprotozoal drugs are used to treat various protozoal infections, ranging from intestinal amebiasis to pneumocystosis. Indications for selected drugs are summarized in Table 43-5. Atovaquone and pentamidine are used for the treatment of *P. jirovecii* infection. Iodoquinol, metronidazole, and paromomycin are all used to treat intestinal amebiasis. Metronidazole is effective against several forms of bacteria, including anaerobic bacteria (see Chapter 39), as well as against protozoans and helminths (parasitic worms). Worm infection (helminthiasis) is discussed later in the chapter.

Contraindications

Contraindications to the use of antiprotozoal drugs include known drug allergy. Additional contraindications may include serious renal, liver, or other illnesses, with the seriousness of the infection weighed against the patient's overall condition.

Adverse Effects

The adverse effects of antiprotozoal drugs vary greatly depending on the drug and are listed in Table 43-6.

Interactions

The common drug and laboratory test interactions associated with the use of antiprotozoal drugs are listed in Table 43-7. Some of these interactions can result in severe toxicities, and it is therefore important to know of them and to understand the mechanism involved.

Dosages

For dosage information for selected antiprotozoal drugs, see the Dosages table on p. 672.

DRUG PROFILES

atovaquone

Atovaquone (Mepron) is a synthetic antiprotozoal drug indicated for the treatment of mild to moderate *P. jirovecii* pneumonia in patients who cannot tolerate co-trimoxazole (trimethoprim/sulfamethoxazole [see Chapter 38]). It is available only for oral use.

PHARMACOKINETICS

Route	Onset of Action	Peak Plasma Concentration	Elimination Half-life	Duration of Action
PO	8-24 hr	24-96 hr	2-3 days	Unknown

◆ metronidazole

Metronidazole (Flagyl) is an antiprotozoal drug that also has fairly broad antibacterial activity as well as **anthelmintic** activity. The therapeutic uses of metronidazole are many and range from the treatment of trichomoniasis, amebiasis, and giardiasis to the treatment of anaerobic bacterial infections and antibiotic-induced

---

TABLE 43-6 Selected Antiprotozoal Drugs: Adverse Effects

Body System	Adverse Effects
atovaquone	
Cardiovascular	Hypotension
Hematologic	Anemia
Integumentary	Pruritus, urticaria, rash, oral candidiasis
Gastrointestinal	Anorexia, increased liver enzyme levels, acute pancreatitis, nausea, vomiting, diarrhea, constipation, abdominal pain
Central nervous	Dizziness, headache, anxiety
Metabolic	Hyperkalemia, hyperglycemia, hyponatremia
Other	Sweating, cough
iodoquinol	
Hematologic	Agranulocytosis
Integumentary	Rash; pruritus; discolored skin, hair, nails
Central nervous	Headache, agitation, peripheral neuropathy
Eyes, ears, nose, and throat	Blurred vision, sore throat, optic neuritis
Gastrointestinal	Anorexia, gastritis, abdominal cramps, nausea, vomiting, diarrhea
Other	Fever, chills, vertigo, weakness, dysesthesia
metronidazole	
Central nervous	Headache, dizziness, confusion, fatigue, convulsions, peripheral neuropathy
Eyes, ears, nose, and throat	Blurred vision, sore throat, dry mouth, metallic taste, glossitis
Gastrointestinal	Abdominal cramps, nausea, vomiting, diarrhea
Genitourinary	Darkened urine, dysuria
Hematologic	Leukopenia, bone marrow depression
Integumentary	Rash, pruritus, urticaria, flushing
paromomycin	
Gastrointestinal	Stomach cramps, nausea, vomiting, diarrhea
Central nervous	Hearing loss, dizziness, tinnitus
pentamidine	
Cardiovascular	Hypotension, dysrhythmias
Hematologic	Anemia, leukopenia, thrombocytopenia
Integumentary	Pain at injection site, pruritus, urticaria, rash
Genitourinary	Acute renal failure
Gastrointestinal	Increased liver enzyme levels, acute pancreatitis, metallic taste, nausea, vomiting, diarrhea
Central nervous	Disorientation, hallucinations, dizziness, confusion
Respiratory	Cough, shortness of breath, bronchospasm
Metabolic	Hyperkalemia, hypocalcemia, hypoglycemia followed by hyperglycemia
Other	Fatigue, chills, night sweats

---

pseudomembranous colitis (see Chapters 38 and 39). Metronidazole is believed to directly kill protozoans by causing free-radical reactions that damage their DNA and other vital biomolecules. Tinidazole (Tindamax) is a newer, similar drug that is available in Canada.

Metronidazole is contraindicated during the first trimester of pregnancy. It is available in both oral and injectable form.

PHARMACOKINETICS

Route	Onset of Action	Peak Plasma Concentration	Elimination Half-life	Duration of Action
PO	1 hr	1-2 hr	8 hr	Variable

pentamidine

Pentamidine (NebuPent, Pentam 300) is an antiprotozoal drug that is used mainly for the management of *P. jirovecii* pneumonia, although it is sometimes used to treat various other protozoal infections. It works by inhibiting protein and nucleic acid synthesis. It is used for the treatment of active pneumocystosis and for prophylaxis of *P. jirovecii* pneumonia in patients at high risk for initial or recurrent *Pneumocystis* infection, such as patients with human immunodeficiency virus (HIV) infection and AIDS.

The only contraindication to pentamidine is hypersensitivity to the drug. Hypersensitivity is more common when the drug is administered by inhalation. An allergic reaction to the inhalational form does not preclude its administration by either the intramuscular or intravenous route, due to the seriousness of the *Pneumocystis* infection. The drug should also be used with caution in patients with blood dyscrasias, hepatic or renal disease, diabetes mellitus, cardiac disease, hypocalcemia, or hypertension. Pentamidine is available as an oral inhalational solution and also in injectable form.

PHARMACOKINETICS

Route	Onset of Action	Peak Plasma Concentration	Elimination Half-life	Duration of Action
Inhalation	0.5-1 hr	Less than 1 hr	6-9 hr	Variable

HELMINTHIC INFECTIONS

Parasitic **helminthic infections** (worm infections) are a worldwide problem. It has been estimated that one third of the world's population is infected with these parasites, but persons living in undeveloped countries where sanitary conditions are often poor are by far the most common victims. The incidence of worm infection in developed countries where sewage treatment is adequate is much lower, and usually only a few select helminthic diseases are the source of the problem. The most prevalent helminthic infection in the United States is enterobiasis, caused by one genus of roundworm, *Enterobius*.

Helminths that are parasitic in humans are classified in the following way:

- Platyhelminthes (flatworms)
- Cestodes (tapeworms)
- Trematodes (flukes)
- Nematodes (roundworms)

The characteristics of a few of the most common of the many helminthic infections are summarized in Table 43-8. These usually first infect the intestines of their host and reside there but can sometimes also migrate to other tissues.

TABLE 43-7 Antiprotozoal Drugs: Drug and Laboratory Test Interactions

Drug	Mechanism	Result
atovaquone	Competition for binding on protein, resulting in free, active atovaquone	Highly protein-bound drugs (e.g., warfarin, phenytoin) may increase atovaquone drug concentrations and risk of adverse reactions
iodoquinol	Increase in protein-bound serum iodine concentrations, reflecting a decrease in iodine 131 uptake	May interfere with certain thyroid function test results
metronidazole	Decreased absorption of vitamin K from the intestines due to elimination of the bacteria needed to absorb vitamin K, leading to increased plasma acetaldehyde concentration after ingestion of alcohol	Alcohol causes a disulfiram-like reaction; action of warfarin may be increased (increased bleeding risk)
pentamidine	Additive nephrotoxic effects	Use with an aminoglycoside, amphotericin B, colistin, cisplatin, methoxyflurane, polymyxin B, or vancomycin may result in nephrotoxicity

DOSAGES

Selected Antiprotozoal Drugs

Drug (Pregnancy Category)	Pharmacologic Class	Usual Dosage Range	Indications/Uses
Atovaquone* (Mepron) (C)	Synthetic anti-*Pneumocystis* drug	**Adult and adolescent 13-16 yr** PO: 750 mg twice daily with meal × 21 days	Prophylaxis of PJP; treatment of active PJP
◆ metronidazole (Flagyl) (X, first trimester; B, 2nd and 3rd trimesters)	Amebicide, antibacterial, trichomonacide	**Adult** PO: 500-750 mg 3 times daily × 5-10 days **Pediatric** PO: 35-50 mg/kg (max 750 mg/dose) 3 times daily × 5-10 days	Amebiasis, including amebic liver abscess
		Adult 7-day treatment PO: 250 mg 3 times daily × 7 days **Pediatric 7-day treatment** PO: 5 mg/kg 3 times daily × 7 days	Trichomoniasis, giardiasis
pentamidine (NebuPent, Pentam 300) (C)	Synthetic anti-*Pneumocystis* drug	**Adult and pediatric** Inhalation aerosol: 300 mg q4wk IV/IM: 4 mg/kg daily × 14-21 days	Prophylaxis of PJP; treatment of active PJP

IM, Intramuscular; *IV*, intravenous; *PO*, oral; *PJP, Pneumocystis jirovecii* pneumonia.
*Note: A combination product containing atovaquone and the drug proguanil is also used against malaria.

ANTHELMINTIC DRUGS

Unlike protozoans, which are the single-celled members of the animal kingdom, helminths are larger and have complex multicellular structures. Anthelmintic drugs (also spelled *antihelmintic*) work to destroy these organisms by disrupting their structures. The currently available anthelmintic drugs are very specific with regard to the worms they can kill. For this reason, the causative worm in an infected host should be accurately identified before treatment is started. This can usually be done by analyzing samples of feces, urine, blood, sputum, or tissue from the infected host for the presence of ova or larvae of the particular parasite.

Several anthelmintics are commercially available in the United States. These include the following:
- albendazole (Albenza)
- ivermectin (Stromectol)
- mebendazole (Vermox)
- praziquantel (Biltricide)
- pyrantel (Antiminth)
- thiabendazole (Mintezol)

Other drugs, such as niclosamide and piperazine, may be available either in other countries or by special request from the CDC. As previously mentioned, anthelmintics are very specific in their actions. Albendazole and mebendazole can be used to treat both tapeworms and roundworms. Praziquantel is a drug that can kill flukes (trematodes). The most commonly used anthelmintics and the specific class of worms they can effectively kill are summarized in Table 43-9.

Mechanism of Action and Drug Effects

The mechanisms of action of the various anthelmintics vary greatly from drug to drug, although there are some similarities among the drugs used to kill similar types of worms. The various anthelmintic drugs and their respective mechanisms of action are listed in Table 43-10. The drug effects of the anthelmin-

TABLE 43-8 Helminthic Infections

Infection	Organism and Other Facts
Nematodes (Various Intestinal and Tissue Roundworms)	
Ascariasis	Caused by *Ascaris lumbricoides* (giant roundworm); worm resides in small intestine; treated with pyrantel, mebendazole, or albendazole
Enterobiasis	Caused by *Enterobius vermicularis* (pinworm); worm resides in large intestine; treated with pyrantel, mebendazole, or albendazole
Platyhelminthes (Intestinal Tapeworms or Flatworms)	
Diphyllobothriasis	Caused by *Diphyllobothrium latum* (fish worm); acquired from fish; treated with paromomycin, praziquantel, or albendazole
Hymenolepiasis	Caused by *Hymenolepis nana* (dwarf tapeworm); treated with niclosamide, paromomycin, praziquantel, or albendazole
Taeniasis	Caused by *Taenia saginata* (beef tapeworm); acquired from beef; treated with paromomycin, praziquantel, or albendazole
	Caused by *Taenia solium* (pork tapeworm); acquired from pork; treated with paromomycin, praziquantel, or albendazole

TABLE 43-9 Anthelmintics: Class of Worms Killed

Anthelmintic Drug	Cestodes	Nematodes	Trematodes
albendazole	Yes	Yes	Yes
ivermectin	No	Yes	No
mebendazole	Yes	Yes	No
piperazine and pyrantel	No	Yes (giant worm and pinworm)	No
praziquantel	Yes	No	Yes

tic drugs are limited to their ability to kill various forms of worms and flukes.

Indications

Anthelmintic drugs are used to treat roundworm, tapeworm, and fluke infections. Specific drugs are used to treat specific helminthic infections.

Contraindications

The only usual contraindication to a specific anthelmintic drug product is known drug allergy. Pyrantel is contraindicated in patients with liver disease. Praziquantel is also contraindicated in patients with *ocular cysticercosis* (tapeworm infection of the eye).

Adverse Effects

The anthelmintic drugs show a remarkable diversity in their drug-specific adverse effects. Common adverse effects are listed in Table 43-11.

Interactions

The concurrent use of pyrantel with piperazine is not recommended, and pyrantel should be used cautiously in patients with hepatic impairment. Pyrantel has also been shown to raise blood levels of theophylline in pediatric patients. The anticonvulsants carbamazepine and phenytoin (see Chapter 15) may reduce the blood levels of mebendazole. Thiabendazole may raise the blood levels of xanthines such as theophylline. Albendazole blood levels may be raised by dexamethasone and cimetidine, as well as the anthelmintic praziquantel. Histamine H_2 antagonists (e.g., cimetidine, ranitidine) may also raise blood levels of praziquantel.

Dosages

For dosage information for selected anthelmintic drugs, see the Dosages table on p. 674.

TABLE 43-10 Anthelmintics: Mechanisms of Action

Drug	Mechanism of Action	Indication
albendazole	Cells of intestinal and tissue-dwelling larvae are selectively destroyed by degenerating cytoplasmic microtubules. This in turn causes secretory substances to accumulate intracellularly, which leads to impaired cholinesterase secretion and glucose. Glycogen becomes depleted, which leads to decreased ATP production and energy depletion, which immobilizes and kills the worm.	Neurocysticercosis, hydatid disease
ivermectin	Potentiates inhibitory signals in the CNS of nematodes, which leads to their paralysis.	Nondisseminated intestinal infection with *Strongyloides* (threadworms)
mebendazole	Selectively and irreversibly inhibits the uptake of glucose and other nutrients. Results in the depletion of endogenous glycogen stores, with eventual autolysis of the parasitic worm and death.	Trichuriasis (whipworm infection), enterobiasis, ascariasis, *Ancylostoma* (common hookworm) infection, *Necator* (American hookworm) infection
praziquantel	Increases permeability of the cell membrane of susceptible worms to calcium, which results in the influx of calcium. This causes the worms to be dislodged from their usual site of residence in the mesenteric veins to the liver; they are then killed by host tissue reactions.	Schistosomiasis, opisthorchiasis (liver fluke infection), clonorchiasis (infection with Chinese or Oriental liver fluke), diphyllobothriasis (fish worm infection), hymenolepiasis (dwarf tapeworm infection), neurocysticercosis
pyrantel	Blocks ACh at the neuromuscular junction, which results in paralysis of the worm. Paralyzed worm is then expelled from the GI tract by normal peristalsis.	Ascariasis, enterobiasis, other helminthic infections
thiabendazole	Inhibits the helminth-specific enzyme fumarate reductase.	Cutaneous larva migrans (creeping eruption), strongyloidiasis, trichinosis

ACh, Acetylcholine; *ATP*, adenosine triphosphate; *CNS*, central nervous system; *GI*, gastrointestinal.

DRUG PROFILES

Anthelmintics are available only as oral preparations and, with the exception of pyrantel, all require a prescription. Different drugs are selected to treat infection with different helminthic species.

◆ mebendazole

Mebendazole (Vermox) is a synthetic anthelmintic drug that may be used in the treatment of many types of roundworm and a few types of tapeworm infections. It is available only for oral use.

PHARMACOKINETICS

Route	Onset of Action	Peak Plasma Concentration	Elimination Half-life	Duration of Action
PO	Less than 2 hr	2-4 hr	6-12 hr	Variable

praziquantel

Praziquantel (Biltricide) is one of the primary anthelmintic drugs used for the treatment of various fluke infections. It is also useful against many species of tapeworm. It is contraindicated in pa-

tients with ocular worm infestation (*ocular cysticercosis*). It is available only for oral use.

PHARMACOKINETICS

Route	Onset of Action	Peak Plasma Concentration	Elimination Half-life	Duration of Action
PO	1 hr	1-3 hr	4-5 hr	Variable

pyrantel

Pyrantel (Antiminth, Reese's Pinworm) is a pyrimidine-derived anthelmintic drug that is indicated for the treatment of infection with intestinal roundworms, including ascariasis, enterobiasis, and other helminthic infections. It is the only anthelmintic available in the United States without a prescription. It is available only for oral use.

PHARMACOKINETICS

Route	Onset of Action	Peak Plasma Concentration	Elimination Half-life	Duration of Action
PO	1 hr	1-3 hr	Unknown	Unknown

TABLE 43-11 Anthelmintics: Common Adverse Effects

Body System	Adverse Effects
mebendazole	
Gastrointestinal	Diarrhea, abdominal pain
Hematologic	Myelosuppression
primaquine	
Gastrointestinal	Nausea, vomiting, abdominal distress
Other	Headaches, pruritus, dark discoloration of urine, hemolytic anemia due to glucose-6-phosphate dehydrogenase deficiency
pyrantel	
Central nervous system	Headache, dizziness, insomnia
Dermatologic	Skin rash
Gastrointestinal	Anorexia, abdominal cramps, diarrhea, nausea, vomiting
praziquantel	
Central nervous system	Dizziness, headache, drowsiness
Gastrointestinal	Abdominal pain, nausea
Other	Malaise

NURSING PROCESS

Assessment

Before beginning treatment with an *antimalarial drug,* the nurse should obtain a thorough medication history, perform a head-to-toe physical assessment, and measure vital signs. The nurse should give special attention to, and document, any of the manifestations of malaria such as chills, profound sweating, headache, nausea, joint aching, fatigue, or exhaustion. Other signs and symptoms include periodic diaphoresis and a remittent fever as high as 104° to 105° F (40° to 40.5° C). Baseline visual acuity, renal function test results, gastrointestinal status, and electrocardiogram findings are also important to assess and document because of the possible drug-related adverse effects of cranial nerve VIII involvement (quinine and chloroquine), renal impairment (quinine), and cardiovascular problems (quinine). Contraindications, cautions, and drug interactions should be assessed for and noted before administration of any of the antimalarials, antiprotozoals, or anthelmintics.

Antiprotozoal drugs and their contraindications, cautions, and drug interactions have been previously discussed, and in addition to these, the patient should be assessed for renal, cardiac, and liver

---

DOSAGES

Selected Anthelmintic Drugs

Drug (Pregnancy Category)	Pharmacologic Class	Usual Dosage Range	Indications
◆ mebendazole (Vermox) (C)	General anthelmintic	**Adult and pediatric** PO: 100 mg twice daily × 3 days PO: 100 mg in a single dose	Variety of worm infections *Enterobius* spp.
praziquantel (Biltricide) (B)	Trematode anthelmintic	**Adult and pediatric** PO: approx 20-25 mg/kg 3 times daily × 1 day	Fluke infections
pyrantel (Antiminth, Reese's Pinworm, Pin-Rid, Pin-X) (C)	Nematode anthelmintic	**Adult and pediatric** PO: 11 mg/kg in a single dose (max dose 1 g)	Roundworm infections

PO, oral.

dysfunction, as well as thyroid disease. The patient's baseline visual acuity should be determined and documented prior to initiation of therapy. Metronidazole should be given only after the patient has been assessed for allergy to any of the nitroimidazole derivatives, and to parabens for the topical dosage forms. Appropriate specimens for analysis should be obtained before treatment. Patients with blood dyscrasias, central nervous system disorders, or liver dysfunction require thorough assessment prior to use of these drugs. Atovaquone requires careful assessment for gastrointestinal problems, including nausea and vomiting; skin assessment; documentation of predrug hemoglobin levels; and assessment of the results of renal and/or liver function studies.

With any of the *anthelmintic drugs,* a thorough history of the foods eaten, especially meat and fish, and their means of preparation should be obtained. Other individuals in the family household should also be assessed for helminth infection. Obtaining stool specimens is also indicated. The patient's energy level, ability to perform the activities of daily living, weight, appetite, and any other symptoms should also be assessed and the findings documented. The nurse should assess not only for contraindications and cautions, but also for possible drug interactions (see previous pharmacology discussion).

Nursing Diagnoses

- Risk for injury related to adverse effects of the medication
- Risk for impaired tissue integrity related to lesions caused by the infestation
- Risk for infection related to a break in skin integrity associated with infestation-related lesions
- Imbalanced nutrition, less than body requirements, related to the disease process and adverse effects of medication
- Deficient knowledge related to the infection and its drug treatment
- Ineffective therapeutic regimen management related to poor compliance with treatment and lack of knowledge about the infection and its treatment

Planning

Goals

- Patient is free of self-injury related to the adverse effects of medication.
- Patient remains free of infection during duration of therapy.
- Patient remains injury free throughout the prescribed drug regimen.
- Patient maintains normal body weight during drug therapy.
- Patient remains compliant with drug therapy regimen for the prescribed length of time.
- Patient experiences minimal body image changes related to the disease.
- Patient states the adverse effects of medication, as well as symptoms or adverse reactions to report to the prescriber.

Outcome Criteria

- Patient states measures to take to minimize self-injury related to the adverse effects of medication, such as following instructions regarding medication dose and time of administration and avoiding drug interactions.
- Patient states various measures to prevent worsening of lesions and minimize tissue injury, such as washing hands

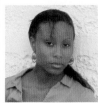

CASE STUDY

Metronidazole

© Matt Antonino

T.J., a 28-year-old graduate student, just returned from an archeology internship in a third-world country. She has had severe diarrhea for several days and has been diagnosed with intestinal amebiasis. She will receive fluids for rehydration and metronidazole (Flagyl) as part of her treatment.

1. What is one specific laboratory test that should be ordered before initiation of the metronidazole therapy?

2. T.J. is started on the intravenous piggyback infusions, and after a day she reports that her diarrhea has decreased and that she feels a little better. During afternoon rounds, she tells the nurse that she feels dizzy and tired, and has some nausea. She asks, "Is this because of my infection?" How should the nurse respond?

3. T.J. is discharged to home with a prescription to take the metronidazole for 2 more weeks. The nurse knows that one serious adverse effect is leukopenia. What symptoms should the nurse tell T.J. to report?

4. A week later, T.J. calls to tell the nurse that she went out to a bar with some friends and became very ill after having a drink. Explain what happened.

For answers, see *http://evolve.elsevier.com/Lilley.*

thoroughly; reporting worsening of lesions and/or drainage, fever, or joint pain; and taking medication as prescribed.
- Patient lists foods to be included in his or her diet to improve overall health based on the U.S. Department of Agriculture food pyramid guidance system.
- Patient states the symptoms of the infection, such as fever, lethargy, and loss of appetite.
- Patient understands the rationale for treatment for the prescribed length of time.
- Patient states the symptoms to report to the prescriber, such as worsening of infection, anorexia, and fever.
- Patient verbalizes feelings about altered body image openly with a health care professional.
- Patient states the importance of complying with therapy and returning for follow-up visits to the prescriber to monitor progress and check for adverse reactions.

Implementation

With *antimalarials,* the nurse should monitor—or have the patient monitor—urinary output (which should be more than 600 mL/day). At least 6 to 8 oz of water or other fluid should be taken with each dosage, with forcing of fluids unless contraindicated. Because antimalarials concentrate in the liver first, it is important for the patient to recognize the importance of follow-up visits to the prescriber so that liver function can be monitored during therapy. This is especially true if the patient has a history of alcohol abuse or drinks a considerable amount of alcohol. Chloroquine and hydroxychloroquine are administered orally and should be given exactly as prescribed. Dosing should be followed as prescribed, with specific attention to the loading doses, subsequent doses, prophylactic dosing, cautions, contraindications, and drug interactions (see previous information in the pharmacology section of this chapter). See Patient Teaching Tips for further information.

Most of the *antiprotozoal drugs* (e.g., atovaquone, metronidazole) should be given with food when taken orally. Quinine sulfate, an antiprotozoal, must be administered intact because it is very irritating to the gastrointestinal mucosa. Oral dosage forms of metronidazole should be given with food to decrease gastrointestinal upset. Intravenous doses should infuse over more than 30 to 60 minutes and should never be given as an intravenous bolus. During use of this drug, changes in neurologic status should be reported to the prescriber. All anthelmintic drugs should be administered as ordered and for the prescribed length of time. Patients should be warned that thiabendazole, an anthelmintic, may give the urine an asparagus-like odor or the skin an unusual odor. Any syrup forms of these drugs should be stored in tight and closed containers to prevent chemical changes in the drug. Collection of stool specimens, if indicated with the anthelmintics or other antiparasitic drugs, should be performed using a clean container, and the stool should not be in contact with water, urine, or chemicals because of the risk of destroying the parasitic worms. See Patient Teaching Tips for more information on these drugs.

Evaluation

The nurse should monitor the patient for the therapeutic effects of the antimalarials, antiprotozoals, and anthelmintic drugs such as improved energy levels and decrease in and/or eventual resolution of all symptoms. Evaluation of proper hygiene and prevention of the spread of the infestation or infection is also important. With these three groups of drugs, it is important also to evaluate for the adverse effects associated with each type of drug: gastrointestinal upset, liver problems, anemias, thrombocytopenia, cardiac irregularities, and visual changes, including those indicating a risk for retinal damage, which may be irreversible. The *antimalarial drugs* may precipitate hemolysis in patients with G6PD deficiency (mostly African American patients and those of Mediterranean ancestry); therefore, such patients should be closely monitored for this complication during the treatment protocol. See Chapter 2 for further discussion of G6PD deficiency. With *antiprotozoal drugs*, the patient should be monitored for visual disturbances, gastrointestinal distress, blurred vision, and altered hearing. Patients being treated with *anthelmintics* should be evaluated for adverse effects such as pallor, anorexia, and sudden decrease in red blood cells (RBCs), white blood cells (WBCs), and hemoglobin level.

PATIENT TEACHING TIPS

- Antimalarials are known to cause gastrointestinal upset; however, this may be decreased if the medication is taken with food. The patient should be told to contact the prescriber if there is nausea, vomiting, profuse diarrhea, or abdominal pain and to report immediately any visual disturbances, dizziness, jaundice or yellowing of the skin or sclera of the eye, or pruritus.
- The patient should be educated about the need for prophylactic doses of antimalarials, as prescribed, before visiting malaria-infested countries as well as the need to obtain appropriate treatment upon return.
- Alcohol should not be consumed while taking antimalarials.
- Antimalarials, like all other medications, should be kept out of the reach of children.
- The patient should be informed about the adverse effects associated with quinine-containing drugs, such as dizziness, visual blurring, and yellow discoloration of the skin (often referred to as *cinchonism*). The entire course of medication should be taken as directed.
- Antiprotozoals should be taken exactly as prescribed, and the importance of adherence to the drug regimen should be emphasized, as for any of the three groups of drugs.
- Metronidazole should be taken with food. Alcohol, including cough syrups and elixirs (which contain alcohol), should be avoided when taking this drug.
- The patient should be told to avoid activities that require mental alertness or quick motor responses while taking this drug until

the patient's neurologic responses have been determined to be back within normal limits.
- A patient taking metronidazole for a sexually transmitted disease should avoid sexual intercourse until the prescriber states otherwise.
- When the patient is taking metronidazole for amebiasis, instructions should include how to check stool samples correctly and safely, and how to dispose of samples properly.
- Topical forms of the drug should be applied with a finger cot or gloved hand, and the patient should be cautioned to avoid contact of the drug with the eyes. The patient should be told that makeup or other cosmetics may be applied after topical drug application.
- Metronidazole may precipitate dizziness, so the patient should be encouraged to be cautious in all activities until a response to the drug is noted and is consistent.
- Anthelmintics should be taken exactly as prescribed, and the importance of compliance with the drug regimen should be emphasized. The patient should also be encouraged to notify the prescriber immediately if the patient experiences fatigue, fever, pallor, anorexia, darkened urine, or abdominal, leg, or back pain, which could indicate a sudden decrease in RBCs, hemoglobin level, or WBCs.

POINTS TO REMEMBER

- Malaria is caused by *Plasmodium*, a particular genus of protozoans, and is transmitted by the bite of an infected female mosquito. The drug primaquine attacks the parasite when it is outside the RBC (exoerythrocytic phase).
- Other common protozoal infections are amebiasis, giardiasis, pneumocystosis, toxoplasmosis, and trichomoniasis. Protozoans are parasites that are transmitted by person-to-person contact, ingestion of contaminated water or food, direct contact with the parasite, and the bite of an insect (mosquito or tick).
- Antiprotozoals include atovaquone and pentamidine. Metronidazole is an antibacterial, antiprotozoal, and anthelmintic. The drugs iodoquinol and paromomycin directly kill protozoans such as *Entamoeba histolytica*.

- Anthelmintics are drugs used to treat parasitic worm infections caused by cestodes (tapeworms), nematodes (roundworms), and trematodes (flukes).
- Nursing considerations with the use of any of the antimalarials, antiprotozoals, and anthelmintics include assessment for contraindications, cautions, and drug interactions. Contraindications to the use of antimalarials include pregnancy, G6PD deficiency, and a history of drug allergy. Contraindications to the use of antiprotozoals include hypersensitivity; underlying renal, cardiac, thyroid, or liver disease; and pregnancy. Contraindications to the use of anthelmintics include a history of hypertension, hypersensitivity, visual difficulty, and severe hepatic, renal, or cardiac disease.

NCLEX EXAMINATION REVIEW QUESTIONS

1 The nurse is reviewing the medication history of a patient who is taking hydroxychloroquine. However, the patient's chart does not reveal a history of malaria or travel out of the country. The patient is most likely taking this medication for
   a *Plasmodium*.
   b thyroid disorders.
   c roundworms.
   d rheumatoid arthritis.
2 Which teaching point would be appropriate to include when the nurse is informing patients about the adverse effects of antimalarials?
   a The skin may turn blotchy while these medications are taken.
   b These medications may cause anorexia and abdominal distress.
   c These drugs may cause increased urinary output.
   d The patient may experience periods of diaphoresis and chills.
3 When teaching a patient about the potential drug interactions with antiprotozoal drugs, the nurse should include information about
   a acetaminophen.
   b warfarin.
   c decongestants.
   d antibiotics.

4 Before administering antiprotozoal drugs, the nurse should review which baseline assessment?
   a Prothrombin time
   b Serum magnesium level
   c Hemoglobin level
   d Arterial blood gas concentrations
5 The nurse knows that antimalarial drugs are used to treat patients with infections caused by which protozoans?
   a *Plasmodium* spp.
   b *Candida albicans*
   c *Pneumocystis jirovecii*
   d *Mycobacterium tuberculosis*
6 When giving metronidazole, the nurse implements appropriate administration techniques, including: (Select all that apply.)
   a Giving oral forms with food
   b Giving oral forms on an empty stomach with a full glass of water
   c Infusing intravenous doses over 30 to 60 minutes
   d Administering intravenous doses by bolus over 5 minutes
   e Obtaining ordered specimens before starting the medication

1. d, 2. b, 3. b, 4. c, 5. a, 6. a, c, e.

CRITICAL THINKING ACTIVITIES: BEST ACTION

1 You are preparing to give mebendazole to a patient who has an infection with *Necator* (American hookworm). The patient is very worried about this infection and its treatment, and asks you, "What will this drug do to me? Does it have bad side effects? I'm already sick enough!" What is your best answer?
2 Your roommate is traveling to a country where there is high risk for malaria infection. She asks you what you think the nurse

practitioner will order for her, if anything at all. What is your best response to her question?
3 A patient with a history of AIDS has severe *Pneumocystis jirovecii* pneumonia. As you prepare the ordered dose of pentamidine inhalation, the patient asks you, "What are you doing? Can't you give that to me in a pill?" What is your best response?

For answers, see *http://evolve.elsevier.com/Lilley.*

CHAPTER 44

Antiinflammatory and Antigout Drugs

OBJECTIVES

When you reach the end of this chapter, you should be able to do the following:

1. Discuss the inflammatory response and the part it plays in the generation of pain.
2. Compare the disease processes or pathologies that are inflammatory in nature with those of gout.
3. Discuss the mechanisms of action, indications, adverse effects, dosage ranges, routes of administration, cautions, contraindications, drug interactions, and toxicities of the various antiinflammatory and antigout drugs.
4. Develop a nursing care plan that includes all phases of the nursing process for patients receiving antiinflammatory and/or antigout drugs.

e-Learning Activities

http://evolve.elsevier.com/Lilley

NCLEX Review Questions • Animations • Nursing Care Plans • Audio Glossary • Category Catchers • Medication Errors Checklists • IV Therapy Checklists • Calculators • Frequently Asked Questions • Content Updates • Supplemental Resources • Answers to Case Studies and Critical Thinking Activities

Drug Profiles

- ◆ allopurinol, p. 686
- ◆ aspirin, p. 684
- ◆ celecoxib, p. 685
  colchicine, p. 686
- ◆ ibuprofen, p. 685
- ◆ indomethacin, p. 685
- ◆ ketorolac, p. 685
  probenecid, p. 686
  sulfinpyrazone, p. 687

  ◆ *Key drug.*

Glossary

Done nomogram A standard data graph, originally published in 1960 in the journal *Pediatrics*, for rating the severity of aspirin toxicity following overdose. Serum salicylate levels are plotted against time elapsed since ingestion. (p. 682)

Gout Hyperuricemia (elevated blood uric acid level); the arthritis caused by tissue buildup of uric acid crystals. (p. 685)

Inflammation A localized protective response stimulated by injury to tissues that serves to destroy, dilute, or wall off (sequester) both the injurious agent and the injured tissue. (p. 678)

Nonsteroidal antiinflammatory drugs (NSAIDs) A large and chemically diverse group of drugs that possess analgesic, antiinflammatory, antirheumatic, and antipyretic (fever-reducing) activity. (p. 679)

Salicylism The syndrome of salicylate toxicity, including symptoms such as tinnitus (ringing sound in the ears), nausea, and vomiting. (p. 682)

• • •

Anatomy, Physiology, and Disease Overview

Inflammation is defined as a localized protective response stimulated by injury to tissues, which serves to destroy, dilute, or wall off (sequester) both the injurious agent and the injured tissue. Classic signs and symptoms of inflammation include pain, fever, loss of function, redness, and swelling. These symptoms result from arterial, venous, and capillary dilation; enhanced blood flow and vascular permeability; exudation of fluids, including plasma proteins; and leukocyte migration into the inflammatory focus. The inflammatory response is mediated by a host of endogenous compounds, including proteins of the complement system, histamine, serotonin, bradykinin, leukotrienes, and prostaglandins, the latter two being major contributors to the symptoms of inflammation.

Arachidonic acid is released from phospholipids in cell membranes in response to a triggering event (e.g., an injury). It is metabolized in either the *prostaglandin* pathway or the *leukotriene pathway,* both of which are branches of the arachidonic acid pathway, as shown in Figure 44-1. Both of these pathways lead to inflammation, edema, headache, and other pain characteristic of the body's response to injury or inflammatory illnesses such as arthritis.

In the prostaglandin pathway, arachidonic acid is converted by the enzyme *cyclooxygenase* into various prostaglandins. Prostaglandins mediate inflammation by inducing vasodilation and enhancing vasopermeability. These effects in turn potentiate the action of proinflammatory substances such as histamine and bradykinin in the production of edema and pain. These symptoms arise as a result of prostaglandin-induced hyperalgesia (excessive sensitivity). In this situation, stimuli that normally would not be painful, such as simply moving a joint through its natural range of motion, become painful because of the inflammatory process at work. Fever results when prostaglandin E_2 is synthesized in the

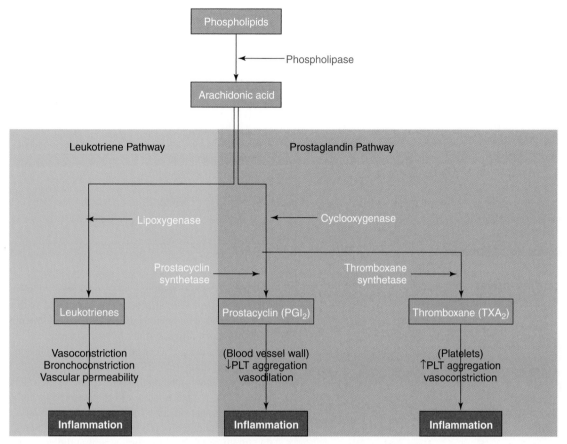

FIGURE 44-1 Arachidonic acid pathway. *PGI₂,* Prostaglandin I₂; *PLT,* platelet; *TXA₂,* thromboxane A₂.

preoptic hypothalamic region, the area of the brain that regulates temperature.

The leukotriene pathway utilizes lipoxygenases to metabolize the arachidonic acid and convert it into various leukotrienes. Although leukotrienes are more newly discovered than prostaglandins and not as well studied, they are also mediators of inflammation, promoting vasoconstriction, bronchospasms, and increased vascular permeability with resultant edema. (See Chapter 37.)

Pharmacology Overview

NONSTEROIDAL ANTIINFLAMMATORY DRUGS

Nonsteroidal antiinflammatory drugs (NSAIDs) are among the most commonly prescribed drugs. Every year, over 70 million prescriptions are written for these drugs. This represents more than 5% of all prescriptions. Currently more than 23 different NSAIDs are available in the United States. Some of these are used much more commonly than others. A given patient may respond better to one NSAID than to others, in terms of both symptom relief and adverse effects.

NSAIDs comprise a large and chemically diverse group of drugs that possess analgesic, antiinflammatory, and antipyretic (antifever) activity. They are also used for the relief of mild to moderate headaches, myalgia, neuralgia, and arthralgia; alleviation of postoperative pain; relief of the pain associated with ar-

thritic disorders such as rheumatoid arthritis, juvenile arthritis, ankylosing spondylitis, and osteoarthritis; and treatment of *gout* and *hyperuricemia* (discussed later in this chapter). Aspirin is used for its effect in inhibiting platelet aggregation, which has been shown to have protective qualities against certain cardiovascular events such as myocardial infarction and stroke. Steroidal antiinflammatory drugs (e.g., prednisone, dexamethasone) are also used for similar purposes and were discussed in Chapter 33. NSAIDs have a generally more favorable adverse effect profile than steroidal antiinflammatory drugs.

In 1899, acetylsalicylic acid (ASA; aspirin) was marketed and rapidly became the most widely used drug in the world. The success of aspirin established the importance of drugs with antipyretic, analgesic, and antiinflammatory properties—the properties that all NSAIDs share. The widespread use of aspirin also yielded evidence of its potential for causing major adverse effects. Gastrointestinal intolerance, bleeding, and renal impairment became major factors limiting its long-term administration. As a result, efforts were mounted to develop drugs that did not have the adverse effects of aspirin. This led to the discovery of other NSAIDs, which in general are associated with a lower incidence of and less serious adverse effects and are often better tolerated than aspirin in patients with chronic diseases. If aspirin were to be a newly discovered drug today, it would require a prescription.

As a single class, NSAIDs constitute an exceptional variety of drugs, and they are used for an equally wide range of indications. Box 44-1 categorizes these drugs into a number of distinct

---

BOX 44-1 Chemical Categories of NSAIDs

Salicylates
aspirin
diflunisal (Dolobid)
salsalate (Salistab)
choline salicylate (Arthropan)

Acetic Acid Derivatives
diclofenac sodium (Voltaren)
indomethacin (Indocin)
sulindac (Clinoril)
tolmetin (Tolectin)
etodolac (Lodine)
ketorolac (Toradol)
meclofenamate (generic only)
mefenamic acid (Ponstel)

Cyclooxygenase-2 Inhibitors
celecoxib (Celebrex)

Enolic Acid Derivatives
nabumetone (Relafen)
meloxicam (Mobic)
piroxicam (Feldene)

Propionic Acid Derivatives
fenoprofen (Nalfon)
flurbiprofen (Ansaid)
ibuprofen (Motrin, Advil, others)
ketoprofen (Orudis KT)
naproxen (Naprosyn, Aleve)
oxaprozin (Daypro)

NSAID, Nonsteroidal antiinflammatory drug.

BOX 44-2 NSAIDs: FDA-Approved Indications

Acute gout
Acute gouty arthritis
Ankylosing spondylitis
Bursitis
Fever
Juvenile rheumatoid arthritis
Mild to moderate pain
Osteoarthritis
Primary dysmenorrhea
Rheumatoid arthritis
Tendinitis
Various ophthalmic uses

FDA, Food and Drug Administration; *NSAID,* nonsteroidal antiinflammatory drug.

---

chemical classes. The NSAIDs have been approved for a variety of indications and are considered the drug of choice for most of the conditions listed in Box 44-2. Almost all NSAIDs are used for the treatment of rheumatoid arthritis (see Chapter 49) and degenerative joint disease (osteoarthritis). Several of these drugs are available in sustained-release formulations. This allows once- or twice-daily dosing, which is known to improve patients' adherence to prescribed drug therapy regimens.

Mechanism of Action and Drug Effects

The NSAIDs work through inhibition of the leukotriene pathway, the prostaglandin pathway, or both. More specifically, NSAIDs relieve pain, headache, and inflammation by blocking the chemical activity of the enzyme called *cyclooxygenase (COX)*. It is now recognized that there are at least two types of cyclooxygenase. Cyclooxygenase-1 (COX-1) is the isoform of the enzyme that promotes the synthesis of prostaglandins, which have primarily beneficial effects on various body functions. One example is their role in maintaining an intact gastrointestinal mucosa. In contrast, the cyclooxygenase-2 (COX-2) isoform promotes the synthesis of prostaglandins that are involved in inflammatory processes. In 1998, the newest class of NSAIDs, the COX-2 inhibitors, were approved. These drugs work by specifically inhibiting the COX-2 isoform of cyclooxygenase and theoretically have limited or no effects on COX-1. Previous NSAIDs nonspecifically inhibited both COX-1 and COX-2 activity. This greater enzyme specificity of the COX-2 inhibitors allows for the beneficial antiinflamma-

tory effects while reducing the prevalence of adverse effects, such as gastrointestinal ulceration, associated with the nonspecific NSAIDs. The leukotriene pathway is inhibited by some antiinflammatory drugs, but not by salicylates.

The main drug effects of NSAIDs are analgesic, antiinflammatory, and antipyretic effects. All NSAIDs can be ulcerogenic and induce gastrointestinal bleeding due to their activity against tissue COX-1. One notable effect of aspirin is its inhibition of platelet aggregation, also known as its *antiplatelet activity*. Aspirin has the unique property among NSAIDs of being an irreversible inhibitor of COX-1 receptors within the platelets themselves. This in turn results in reduced formation of thromboxane A_2, a substance that normally promotes platelet aggregation. This antiplatelet action has made aspirin, along with thrombolytic drugs (see Chapter 28), a primary drug in the treatment of acute myocardial infarction and many other thromboembolic disorders. Other NSAIDs generally lack these antiplatelet effects.

Indications

Some of the therapeutic uses of this broad class of drugs are listed in Table 44-1; however, NSAIDs are primarily used for their analgesic, antiinflammatory, and antipyretic effects, and for platelet inhibition. NSAIDs are also widely used for the treatment of rheumatoid arthritis (see Chapter 49) and osteoarthritis, as well as other inflammatory conditions, rheumatic fever, mild to moderate pain, and acute gout. They also have proved beneficial as adjunctive pain relief medications in patients with chronic pain syndromes, such as pain from bone cancer and chronic back pain. For the relief of pain they are sometimes combined with an opioid (see Chapter 11). They tend to have an opioid-sparing effect when given together with opioids, because the drugs attack pain using two different mechanisms. This often allows less opioids to be used. Unlike opioids, NSAIDs show a ceiling effect that limits their effectiveness; that is, any further increase in the dosage beyond a certain level increases the risk for adverse effects without a corresponding increase in the therapeutic effect. In contrast, opioid dosages may be titrated almost indefinitely to increasingly higher levels, especially in terminally ill patients with severe pain.

The appropriate selection of an NSAID is a clinical judgment based on consideration of the patient's history, including any previous medical conditions; the intended use of the drug; the

TABLE 44-1 Suggested NSAIDs for Patients with Various Medical Conditions

Medical Condition	Recommended NSAID
Ankylosing spondylitis	indomethacin, diclofenac
Diabetic neuropathy	Sulindac
Dysmenorrhea	Fenamates, naproxen, ibuprofen
Gout	indomethacin, naproxen, sulindac
Headaches	aspirin, naproxen. Ibuprofen
Hepatotoxicity	tolmetin, naproxen, ibuprofen, piroxicam, fenamates
History of aspirin or NSAID allergy	Avoid if possible; if deemed necessary, consider a nonacetylated salicylate
Hypertension	sulindac, nonacetylated salicylate, ibuprofen, etodolac
Osteoarthritis	diclofenac, oxaprozin, indomethacin
Risk for gastrointestinal toxicity	COX-2 inhibitors (celecoxib), nonacetylated salicylate, enteric-coated aspirin, diclofenac, nabumetone, etodolac, ibuprofen, oxaprozin
Risk for nephrotoxicity	sulindac, nonacetylated salicylate, nabumetone, etodolac, diclofenac, oxaprozin
Warfarin therapy	sulindac, tolmetin, naproxen, ibuprofen, oxaprozin

COX, Cyclooxygenase; *NSAID,* nonsteroidal antiinflammatory drug.

TABLE 44-2 NSAIDs: Adverse Effects

Body System	Adverse Effects
Cardiovascular	Moderate to severe noncardiogenic pulmonary edema
Gastrointestinal	Most frequent: dyspepsia, heartburn, epigastric distress, nausea; less frequent: vomiting, anorexia, abdominal pain, gastrointestinal bleeding, mucosal lesions (erosions or ulcerations)
Hematologic	Altered hemostasis through effects on platelet function
Hepatic	Acute reversible hepatotoxicity
Renal	Reduction in creatinine clearance, acute tubular necrosis with renal failure
Other	Skin eruption, sensitivity reactions, tinnitus, hearing loss

NSAID, Nonsteroidal antiinflammatory drug.

BOX 44-3 FDA Required Warnings on All NSAIDs

The following black box warning must now be included in the packaging for all NSAIDs:

Cardiovascular Risk

- NSAIDs may cause an increased risk of serious cardiovascular thrombotic events, myocardial infarction, and stroke, which can be fatal. This risk may increase with duration of use. Patients with cardiovascular disease or risk factors for cardiovascular disease may be at greater risk.
- NSAIDs are contraindicated for the treatment of perioperative pain in the setting of coronary artery bypass graft surgery.

Gastrointestinal Risk

- NSAIDs cause an increased risk of serious gastrointestinal adverse events, including bleeding, ulceration, and perforation of the stomach or intestines, which can be fatal. These events can occur at any time during use and without warning symptoms. Elderly patients are at greater risk for serious gastrointestinal events.

See Chapter 4 for more information on black box warnings.
FDA, Food and Drug Administration; *NSAID,* nonsteroidal antiinflammatory drug.

---

patient's previous experience with NSAIDs; the patient's preference; and the cost.

Contraindications

Contraindications to NSAIDs include known drug allergy and conditions that place the patient at risk for bleeding, such as rhinitis (risk for epistaxis [nosebleed]), vitamin K deficiency, and peptic ulcer disease. Patients with documented aspirin allergy should not receive NSAIDs. Other common contraindications are those that apply to most drugs and include severe renal or hepatic disease. NSAIDs are generally rated as pregnancy category C drugs for use during the first two trimesters of pregnancy but are rated as pregnancy category D (not recommended) for use during the third trimester. This is because NSAID use has been associated with both excessive maternal bleeding and neonatal toxicity during the perinatal period. These drugs also are not recommended for nursing mothers, because they are known to be excreted into human milk. Because of the potential of NSAIDs to increase bleeding, patients undergoing elective surgery should stop taking NSAIDs at least 1 week prior to surgery.

Adverse Effects

Although NSAIDs are the most widely used class of drugs, and some are available without prescription, their potential for serious adverse events has been underemphasized. Over 100,000 hospitalizations occur each year due to NSAID use, with over 16,000 deaths reported annually. One of the more common and potentially serious adverse effects of the NSAIDs is their effect on the gastrointestinal tract. Symptoms can range from mild symptoms such as heartburn to the most severe gastrointestinal complication, gastrointestinal bleeding. Most fatalities associated with NSAID use are related to gastrointestinal bleeding. In addition, acute renal failure is quite common with NSAID use,

especially if the patient is dehydrated. The potential adverse effects of NSAIDs are listed in Table 44-2. It should be noted that not all adverse effects necessarily apply to all drugs, but many do. In fact, in 2006 the U.S. Food and Drug Administration (FDA) began requiring a black box warning on all of the NSAIDs (see Box 44-3 on the black box warning for NSAIDs as well as Chapter 4).

As stated earlier, many of the adverse effects of NSAIDs are secondary to their inactivation of protective prostaglandins that help maintain the normal integrity of the stomach lining. However, the drug misoprostol (Cytotec) has proved successful in preventing the gastric ulcers and hence gastrointestinal bleeding that can occur in patients receiving NSAIDs. Misoprostol is a synthetic prostaglandin E_1 analogue that inhibits gastric acid secretion and also has a cytoprotective component, although the mechanism responsible for this action is unclear. This drug also has abortifacient properties, which were discussed in Chapter 34.

TABLE 44-3 Acute or Chronic Salicylate Intoxication: Signs and Symptoms

Body System	Signs and Symptoms
Cardiovascular	Increased heart rate
Central nervous	Tinnitus, hearing loss, dimness of vision, headache, dizziness, mental confusion, lassitude, drowsiness
Gastrointestinal	Nausea, vomiting, diarrhea
Metabolic	Sweating, thirst, hyperventilation, hypoglycemia or hyperglycemia

TABLE 44-4 Acute Salicylate Intoxication: Treatment

Severity	Treatment
Mild	1. Dosage reduction or discontinuation of salicylates 2. Symptomatic and supportive therapy
Severe	1. Discontinuation of salicylates 2. Intensive symptomatic and supportive therapy 3. Dialysis if: high salicylate levels, unresponsive acidosis (pH less than 7.1), impaired renal function or renal failure, pulmonary edema, persistent CNS symptoms (e.g., seizures, coma), progressive deterioration despite appropriate therapy

CNS, Central nervous system.

Renal function depends partly on prostaglandins. Disruption of prostaglandin function by NSAIDs is sometimes strong enough to precipitate acute or chronic renal failure, depending on the patient's current level of renal function. The use of NSAIDs can compromise existing renal function. Renal toxicity can occur in patients who are dehydrated, those with heart failure or liver dysfunction, and those taking diuretics or angiotensin-converting enzyme inhibitors.

Toxicity and Management of Overdose

Salicylate toxicity is not as common as it used to be; however, there are both chronic and acute manifestations of salicylate toxicity. *Chronic salicylate intoxication* is also known as **salicylism** and results from either short-term administration of high dosages or prolonged therapy with high or even lower dosages. The most common signs and symptoms of acute or chronic salicylate intoxication are listed in Table 44-3.

The most common manifestations of chronic intoxication in adults are tinnitus and hearing loss. Those in children are hyperventilation and central nervous system (CNS) effects such as dizziness, drowsiness, and behavioral changes. Metabolic complications such as metabolic acidosis and respiratory alkalosis often occur to varying degrees in cases of chronic salicylate intoxication. Metabolic acidosis can also occur with acute intoxication, but it is usually less severe than that in patients with chronic intoxication. Hypoglycemia may also arise and can be life threatening. The treatment of chronic intoxication is based on the presenting symptoms.

The signs and symptoms of *acute salicylate toxicity* are similar to those of chronic intoxication, but the effects are often more pronounced and occur more quickly. Acute salicylate overdose usually results from the ingestion of a single toxic dose, and its severity can be judged based on the estimated amount ingested (in milligrams per kilogram of body weight), as follows:
- Little or no toxicity: less than 150 mg/kg
- Mild to moderate toxicity: 150 to 300 mg/kg
- Severe toxicity: 300 to 500 mg/kg
- Life-threatening toxicity: over 500 mg/kg

It should be noted, however, that even doses lower than 150 mg/kg have resulted in fatal toxicity. A serum salicylate concentration measured 6 hours or longer after the ingestion may be used in conjunction with the **Done nomogram** to estimate the severity of intoxication and help guide treatment. The Done nomogram is a graphic plot of serum salicylate level as a function of time since salicylate ingestion. It was first published in a 1960 issue of the journal *Pediatrics* and is still used today for gauging salicylate toxicity. This nomogram is intended for estimating only the severity of acute intoxications and not the severity of chronic salicylate intoxication. Table 44-4 describes, in general terms, the treatment for cases of varying severity. Treatment goals include removing salicylate from the gastrointestinal tract and/or preventing its further absorption; correcting fluid, electrolyte, and acid-base disturbances; and implementing measures to enhance salicylate elimination, including hemodialysis.

An acute overdose of nonsalicylate NSAIDs (e.g., ibuprofen) causes effects similar to those of salicylate overdose, but they are generally not as extensive or as dangerous. Symptoms include CNS toxicities such as drowsiness, lethargy, mental confusion, paresthesias (abnormal touch sensations), numbness, aggressive behavior, disorientation, and seizures, and gastrointestinal toxicities such as nausea, vomiting, and gastrointestinal bleeding. Intense headache, dizziness, cerebral edema, cardiac arrest, and death have also been known to occur in extreme cases. Treatment consists of the immediate removal of the ingested drug by inducing emesis with gastric lavage. This is followed by the administration of activated charcoal, with supportive and symptomatic treatment initiated thereafter. Unlike in the case of salicylates, hemodialysis appears to be of no value in enhancing the elimination of nonsalicylate NSAIDs.

Interactions

Drug interactions associated with the use of salicylates and other NSAIDs can result in significant complications and morbidity. Some of the more common of these are listed in Table 44-5.

NSAIDs can also interfere with laboratory test results. Specifically, salicylates can cause what are usually minor and transient elevations in the levels of liver enzymes (alanine aminotransferase, aspartate aminotransferase), but unlike with acetaminophen (see Chapter 11) cases of severe hepatotoxicity are rare. Hematocrit, hemoglobin level, and red blood cell (RBC) count can drop if any drug-induced gastrointestinal bleeding does occur, and bleeding time may be prolonged. NSAID-induced hyperkalemia or hyponatremia can also occur.

Dosages

For the recommended dosages of various NSAIDs, see the Dosages table on p. 683.

TABLE 44-5 Salicylates and Other NSAIDs: Drug Interactions

Interacting Drug	Mechanism	Result
Alcohol	Additive effect	Increased gastrointestinal bleeding
Anticoagulants	Platelet inhibition, hypoprothrombinemia	Increased bleeding tendencies
aspirin and other salicylates with other NSAIDs	Reduction of NSAID absorption, additive gastrointestinal toxicities	Increased gastrointestinal toxicity with no therapeutic advantage
Corticosteroids and other ulcerogenic drugs	Additive toxicities	Increased ulcerogenic effects
cyclosporine	Inhibition of renal prostaglandin synthesis	May increase the nephrotoxic effects of cyclosporine
Diuretics and ACE inhibitors	Inhibition of prostaglandin synthesis	Reduced hypotensive and diuretic effects
Protein-bound drugs	Competition for binding	More pronounced drug actions
Uricosurics	Antagonism	Decreased uric acid excretion
Herbals: feverfew, garlic, ginger, gingko	Interference with platelet function	Increased risk of bleeding

ACE, Angiotensin-converting enzyme; *NSAID,* nonsteroidal antiinflammatory drug.

DOSAGES

Most Commonly Used NSAIDs

Drug (Pregnancy Category*)	Pharmacologic Class	Usual Dosage Range	Indications
◆ aspirin (ASA; many product names) (C/D)	Salicylate	**Adult** PO/PR: 325-650 mg 4-6 times daily (max 4 g/day)	Fever, pain
		PO/PR: 3.2-6 g/day divided q4-6h	Arthritis
		PO: 81-325 mg once daily	Thromboprevention
		Pediatric PO/PR: 10-15 mg/kg q4-6h	Fever, pain
		PO/PR: 80-100 mg/kg/day	Inflammation
◆ celecoxib (Celebrex) (C/D)	COX-2 inhibitor	**Adult and adolescent older than 15 yr** PO: 100-200 mg/day given in 1 or 2 doses	Arthritis, acute pain, primary dysmenorrhea
		PO: 400 mg twice daily	FAP (to reduce number of heredity colon polyps)
		Pediatric Less than 25 kg: 50 mg twice daily More than 25 kg: 100 mg twice daily	Juvenile rheumatoid arthritis
◆ ibuprofen (Motrin, Advil, others) (C/D)	Propionic acid derivative	**Adult** 1200-3200 mg/day divided 3-4 times daily **Pediatric** 20-40 mg/kg/day divided 3-4 times daily	Arthritis, fever, pain, dysmenorrhea
◆ indomethacin (Indocin, Indocin SR) (C/D)	Acetic acid derivative	**Adult** PO/PR: 25-50 mg 2-3 times daily (max 200 mg/day) **Pediatric** PO/PR: 1-2 mg/kg/day divided 2-4 times daily (max 200 mg/day)	Arthritis, including acute gouty arthritis, acute painful shoulder due to bursitis or tendonitis
◆ ketorolac (Toradol) (C/D)	Acetic acid derivative	**Adult†** PO‡: 10 mg q4-6h (max 40 mg/day) IV/IM: 15-60 mg q6-12h (max 120 mg/day if younger than 65 yr; max 60 mg/day if 65 yr or older) Maximum treatment 5 days	Acute painful conditions that would otherwise require opioid-level analgesia

ASA, Acetylsalicylic acid; *COX,* cyclooxygenase; *FAP,* familial adenomatous polyposis; *IM,* intramuscular; *IV,* intravenous; *NSAID,* nonsteroidal antiinflammatory drug; *PO,* oral; *PR,* rectal; *SR,* sustained release.

*Pregnancy category C/D = C, first trimester; D, third trimester.

†Pediatric dosing guidelines are not as well established, but the recommended range for IV, IM, or PO use is 0.4-1 mg/kg as a single dose for acute conditions (e.g., sports injury).

‡PO form is recommended only when transitioning from injectable form to oral form of ketorolac.

DRUG PROFILES

SALICYLATES

Aspirin is the most commonly used of all salicylates. Although aspirin is available over the counter, many of the other salicylate drugs do require a prescription. These include diflunisal (Dolobid), choline magnesium trisalicylate (Trilisate), and salsalate (Salsitab). Salicylates are most commonly used in solid oral dosage forms (i.e., tablets, capsules). Other available dosage forms include a topical cream (Aspercreme), rectal suppositories, and oral liquids. Aspirin is also contained in many combination products, including aspirin/acetaminophen/caffeine combinations such as Excedrin and aspirin/antacid combinations (e.g., Bufferin). Aspirin also is available in special dosage forms, such as enteric-coated aspirin (Ecotrin), designed to protect the stomach mucosa by dissolving in the duodenum.

◆ aspirin

Aspirin is known chemically as acetylsalicylic acid (ASA). It is the prototype salicylate and NSAID and is the most widely used drug in the world. A daily aspirin tablet (81 mg or 325 mg) is now routinely recommended as prophylactic therapy for adults who have strong risk factors for developing coronary artery disease or stroke, even if they have no previous history of such an event. The 81-mg strength (which is traditionally thought of as "children's" aspirin) and the 325-mg strength appear to be equally beneficial for the prevention of thrombotic events. For this reason, the lower strength is often chosen for patients who have any elevated risk for bleeding, such as those with previous stroke history or history of peptic ulcer disease and those taking the anticoagulant warfarin (Coumadin). Aspirin is also often used to treat the pain associated with headache, neuralgia, myalgia, and arthralgia, as well as other pain syndromes resulting from inflammation. These include arthritis, pleurisy, and pericarditis. Patients with systemic lupus erythematosus may also benefit from aspirin therapy because of its antirheumatic effects. Aspirin is also used for its antipyretic action.

Aspirin and other salicylates all have one very specific contraindication. This drug class is contraindicated in children with flulike symptoms, because the use of these drugs has been strongly associated with Reye's syndrome. This is an acute and potentially life-threatening condition involving progressive neurologic deficits that can lead to coma and may also involve liver damage. It is believed to be triggered by viral illnesses such as influenza as well as by salicylate therapy itself, in the presence of a viral illness. Survivors of this condition may or may not suffer permanent neurologic damage.

PHARMACOKINETICS

Route	Onset of Action	Peak Plasma Concentration	Elimination Half-life	Duration of Action
PO	15-30 min	1-2 hr	5-9 hr	4-6 hr

LIFE SPAN CONSIDERATIONS: The Pediatric Patient

Reye's Syndrome

Reye's syndrome is associated with the administration of aspirin to children and teenagers and is a potentially life-threatening illness. Encephalopathy and liver damage are two of the serious complications resulting from Reye's syndrome, which usually occurs after a viral infection such as chickenpox or influenza B, during which time aspirin is often given to decrease fever. To reduce the risk for Reye's syndrome, aspirin or medications that contain aspirin should not be given to children or teenagers to treat viral illnesses or fever. Other names for aspirin include acetylsalicylic acid, acetylsalicylate, salicylic acid, and salicylate. Other drugs that can be used instead of aspirin to reduce fever and relieve pain include acetaminophen and ibuprofen. Check the label on any medication that is to be given to a child, because aspirin is contained in many over-the-counter drugs, for example, Alka-Seltzer, some Excedrin products, and Pepto-Bismol.

Signs and Symptoms of Reye's Syndrome

- Altered liver function
- Encephalopathy and fatty degeneration of the viscera, primarily in children and teenagers
- Changes in level of consciousness
- Coma, flaccid paralysis, loss of deep tendon reflexes
- Hypoglycemia
- Seizures
- Vomiting

Medical Management

- Provide supportive treatment in intensive care unit
- Maintain life functions, restore metabolic balance, and control cerebral edema
- Administer intravenous glucose (10% or higher) for treatment of hypoglycemia

- Monitor blood glucose level; insulin may be needed
- Administer vitamin K for clotting problems
- Give fresh frozen plasma if needed for significant bleeding
- Provide prophylactic antiepileptic drugs
- Monitor intracranial pressure
- Initiate cautious fluid administration
- Administer osmotic diuretics with steroids if needed to treat cerebral edema

Nursing Management

- Critical care setting often indicated for care of these patients
- Assess neurologic status, vital signs, and arterial and central venous pressures
- Monitor blood gas concentrations and intracranial pressure as ordered
- Control temperature to prevent elevations and increased O_2 demands
- Elevate the head of the bed
- Monitor intake and output
- Initiate hyperventilation (if patient is intubated and if ordered) to reduce intracranial pressure by lowering CO_2 levels and increasing O_2 levels
- Provide a quiet environment
- Handle gently
- Monitor for seizure activity
- Provide family support during critical phase of the illness
- Provide physical and emotional support for the child and family with recovery
- Ensure appropriate spiritual care
- Educate the public about Reye's syndrome and its life-threatening complications

Modified from Mayo Foundation for Medical Education and Research, November 17, 2005, No. DS00142. Available at http://www.mayoclinic.com/health/reyes-syndrome/DS00142.

ACETIC ACID DERIVATIVES

There are several acetic acid derivatives, and they are listed in Table 44-1. Indomethacin and ketorolac are the most commonly used.

◆ indomethacin

Like the other NSAIDs, indomethacin (Indocin) has analgesic, antiinflammatory, antirheumatic, and antipyretic properties. Its therapeutic actions are of particular use in the treatment of rheumatoid arthritis, osteoarthritis, acute bursitis or tendonitis, ankylosing spondylitis, and acute gouty arthritis. The drug is available for both oral and rectal use. An injectable form of the drug is also used intravenously (IV) to promote closure of patent ductus arteriosus, a heart defect that sometimes occurs in premature infants.

PHARMACOKINETICS

Route	Onset of Action	Peak Plasma Concentration	Elimination Half-life	Duration of Action
PO	30 min	2 hr	4.5 hr	4-6 hr

◆ ketorolac

Ketorolac (Toradol) is somewhat unique in that, although it does have some antiinflammatory activity, it is used primarily for its powerful analgesic effects. Its analgesic effects are comparable to those of narcotic drugs such as morphine, which can make it a desirable choice for opiate-addicted patients who have acute pain control needs, because ketorolac lacks the addictive properties of the opioids. Ketorolac is indicated for the treatment of moderate to severe acute pain such as that resulting from orthopedic injuries or surgery. Ketorolac is the only NSAID that can be given orally or by injection, and there is also a dosage form for ophthalmic use (see Chapter 57). It is available only by prescription. It is indicated for short-term use (up to 5 days) to manage moderate to severe acute pain. It is not indicated for treatment of minor pain or chronic pain. The main adverse effects of ketorolac include renal impairment, edema, gastrointestinal pain, dyspepsia, and nausea. It is important to note that the drug can only be used for 5 days, because of its potential adverse effects on the kidney and gastrointestinal tract.

PHARMACOKINETICS

Route	Onset of Action	Peak Plasma Concentration	Elimination Half-life	Duration of Action
IV/IM	0.5 hr	1-2 hr	5-7 hr	4-6 hr

PROPIONIC ACID DERIVATIVES
◆ ibuprofen

Ibuprofen (Motrin, Advil) is the prototype NSAID in the propionic acid category, which also includes fenoprofen, flurbiprofen, ketoprofen, naproxen, and oxaprozin. Ibuprofen is the most commonly used of the propionic acid drugs because of the numerous indications for its use and because of its relatively safe adverse effect profile. It is often used for its analgesic effects in the management of rheumatoid arthritis, osteoarthritis, primary dysmenorrhea, gout, dental pain, and musculoskeletal disorders; in addition, it is used for its antipyretic actions. Naproxen is the second most commonly used NSAID, with a reportedly somewhat better adverse effect profile than ibuprofen, as well as fewer drug interactions with angiotensin-converting enzyme inhibitors given for hypertension. Both drugs are available only for oral use in both over-the-counter and prescription strengths.

PHARMACOKINETICS

Route	Onset of Action	Peak Plasma Concentration	Elimination Half-life	Duration of Action
PO	30-60 min (analgesic) 7 days (antiinflammatory)	1-2 hr	2-4 hr	4-6 hr

CYCLOOXYGENASE-2 INHIBITORS

The COX-2 inhibitors were developed primarily to decrease the gastrointestinal adverse effects characteristic of other NSAIDs because of their COX-2 selectivity. However, they are not totally devoid of gastrointestinal toxicity. Gastritis and upper gastrointestinal bleeding have been reported with their use, although much less frequently than with the older NSAIDs. Originally there were three COX-2 inhibitors; however, because the use of rofecoxib (Vioxx) and valdecoxib (Bextra) was found to be associated with an increased risk for adverse cardiovascular events, including myocardial infarction, stroke, and death, these two were removed from the U.S. market.

◆ celecoxib

Celecoxib (Celebrex) was the first COX-2 inhibitor and is the only one remaining on the market. It is indicated for the treatment of osteoarthritis, rheumatoid arthritis, acute pain symptoms, ankylosing spondylitis, and primary dysmenorrhea. More recently, this drug has also been approved for reduction of colon polyps in patients with an inherited condition known as *familial adenomatous polyposis*. It is available only for oral use. There is evidence that celecoxib may pose a risk of cardiovascular events similar to that associated with rofecoxib and valdecoxib. However there is inconsistency in the literature regarding the true potential for these effects. Celecoxib currently remains on the U.S. market, although its use is now being monitored more closely by the FDA. Other adverse effects associated with celecoxib include headache, sinus irritation, diarrhea, fatigue, dizziness, lower extremity edema, and hypertension. COX-2 inhibitors have little effect on platelet function. Celecoxib should not be used in patients with known sulfa allergy.

PHARMACOKINETICS

Route	Onset of Action	Peak Plasma Concentration	Elimination Half-life	Duration of Action
PO	1 hr	3 hr	11 hr	4-8 hr

ENOLIC ACID DERIVATIVES

The enolic acid derivatives include piroxicam, meloxicam, and nabumetone. Piroxicam and meloxicam are very potent drugs that are commonly used in the treatment of mild to moderate osteoarthritis, rheumatoid arthritis, and gouty arthritis. Both are available only in oral dosage formulations and have contraindications similar to those of the other NSAIDs.

Nabumetone (Relafen) is a relatively newer NSAID that is better tolerated than some of the others in terms of gastrointestinal adverse effects. It is relatively nonacidic compared with most of the other NSAIDs, which may account for its improved gastrointestinal tolerance. Currently it is indicated only for the treatment of osteoarthritis and rheumatoid arthritis.

ANTIGOUT DRUGS

Gout is caused by the overproduction of uric acid or decreased uric acid excretion, or both. This overproduction and/or decreased excretion can often result in hyperuricemia (too much uric acid in the blood). Persons with gout either overproduce or underexcrete uric acid. When the body contains too much uric acid, deposits of uric acid crystals collect in tissues and joints. This causes an inflammatory response and extreme pain, because these crystals are like small needles that jab and stick into sensitive tissues and joints, which is an end product of purine metabolism. Purines are part of the normal dietary intake and are used

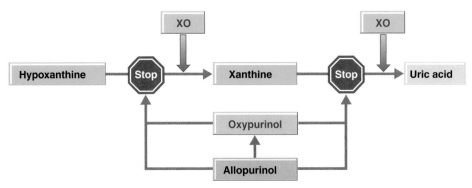

FIGURE 44-2   Uric acid production. *XO,* Xanthine oxidase.

to make the essential structural units of deoxyribonucleic acid (DNA) and ribonucleic acid (RNA). During purine metabolism, they are converted from hypoxanthine to xanthine and eventually to uric acid. The normal pathway for purine metabolism is depicted in Figure 44-2. This pathway is overactive in patients with gout and is reduced by antigout drug therapy. The goals of gout treatment are to decrease the symptoms of an acute attack and to prevent recurrent attacks.

DRUG PROFILES

Although specific antigout drugs are available, the NSAIDs (described earlier) are considered first-line therapy for most patients with gout. The specific antigout drugs—allopurinol (Zyloprim), colchicine, probenecid (Benemid), and sulfinpyrazone (Anturane)—are targeted at the underlying defect in uric acid metabolism, which causes either overproduction or underexcretion of uric acid (see Figure 44-2). Both of these pathologic processes lead to tissue accumulations of uric acid crystalline deposits *(gouty deposits)* and symptoms of gout. Not all gouty deposits occur within joints. Gouty arthritis is the condition in which one or more joints are inflamed due to the collection of gouty deposits inside the joint anatomy. This is also called *articular gout,* whereas gout that occurs in tissues outside of the joints is called *abarticular gout.*

◆ allopurinol

The beneficial effect of allopurinol (Zyloprim) in the relief of gout is the inhibition of the enzyme xanthine oxidase, which thereby prevents uric acid production. Allopurinol is indicated for patients whose gout is caused by the excess production of uric acid (hyperuricemia). Oxypurinol, a metabolite of allopurinol, also prevents uric acid production. Oxypurinol is available as an orphan drug for patients with hyperuricemia who are intolerant of allopurinol therapy. Allopurinol is also used to prevent acute tumor lysis syndrome (see Chapter 47).

Allopurinol is contraindicated in patients with a hypersensitivity to it. Significant adverse effects of the drug include agranulocytosis, aplastic anemia, and serious and potentially fatal skin conditions such as exfoliative dermatitis, Stevens-Johnson syndrome, and toxic epidermal necrolysis. Azathioprine and mercaptopurine both significantly interact with allopurinol, and as a result, their dosages may have to be adjusted. Allopurinol is available only for oral use. The usual recommended adult dosage is 200 to 600 mg/day, and the maximum dosage is 800 mg/day. Pregnancy category C.

PHARMACOKINETICS

Route	Onset of Action	Peak Plasma Concentration	Elimination Half-life	Duration of Action
PO	1-2 wk	30-120 min	18-30 hr	Unknown

colchicine

Colchicine is the oldest available therapy for acute gout and is considered second-line therapy, after the NSAIDs. Colchicine appears to be effective in the treatment of gout by reducing the inflammatory response to the deposits of urate crystals in joint tissue. Its mechanism of action is not clearly defined, but it is thought to inhibit the metabolism, mobility, and *chemotaxis* of polymorphonuclear leukocytes. Chemotaxis is the chemical attraction of leukocytes to the site of inflammation, which worsens an inflammatory response.

Colchicine is a powerful inhibitor of cell mitosis and can cause short-term leukopenia. For this reason it is generally used for the short-term treatment of acute attacks of gout. Its more severe adverse effects can include bleeding into the gastrointestinal or urinary tracts, and the drug should be stopped should such effects appear. Colchicine is contraindicated in patients with hypersensitivity to it and in those with severe renal, gastrointestinal, hepatic, or cardiac disorders, and blood dyscrasias. There is no specific antidote for colchicine poisoning. The drug is available in oral forms only. Until 2008, it was also available in injectable form, but at that time the FDA asked that it no longer be manufactured in or shipped to the United States, because of the potential for life-threatening adverse effects.

For acute gout, colchicine is given in an initial dose of 0.6 to 1.2 mg, followed by 0.6 mg/hr until either pain is relieved, the patient develops severe nausea and diarrhea, or a total of 6 mg has been administered. Some clinicians choose to limit the cumulative dose to 3 mg. When colchicine is used for treatment of acute gout, 3 days must pass before a second course of therapy is initiated. Colchicine is also used for prophylaxis of acute attacks in dosages of 0.6 mg once or twice a day. Colchicine dosage must be reduced with renal impairment. Pregnancy category D.

PHARMACOKINETICS

Route	Onset of Action	Peak Plasma Concentration	Elimination Half-life	Duration of Action
PO	12 hr	0.5-2 hr	12-30 min	12 hr

probenecid

Probenecid (Benemid) inhibits the reabsorption of uric acid in the kidney and thus increases the excretion of uric acid. Drugs that promote uric acid excretion are known as *uricosurics*. In some patients, gout is due to the underexcretion of uric acid. Probenecid works by binding to the special transporter protein in the proximal convoluted renal tubule that takes uric acid from the urine and places it back into the blood. The probenecid is then reabsorbed back into the bloodstream while the uric acid remains in the urine and is excreted. Besides being used to treat the hyperuricemia associated with gout and gouty arthritis, it also has the ability to delay the renal excretion of penicillin, which increases the serum levels of penicillin and prolongs its effect (see Chapter 38). Probenecid is available as a 500-mg oral tablet. The usual adult dosage is 250 mg twice a day with food, milk, or antacids for 1 week, followed by 500 mg twice daily thereafter. This dosage may be adjusted as needed to maintain desirable serum uric acid levels. Contraindications include peptic ulcer disease and blood dyscrasias. Probenecid is ineffective and should not be used in patients with renal impairment. Pregnancy category B.

PHARMACOKINETICS

Route	Onset of Action	Peak Plasma Concentration	Elimination Half-life	Duration of Action
PO	1 hr	3 hr	3-17 hr	8 hr

sulfinpyrazone

Sulfinpyrazone (Anturane) is also a uricosuric drug and works similarly to probenecid. Despite its generic name, it is not a sulfonamide drug per se but is chemically related to phenylbutazone, an early NSAID, which is no longer available on the U.S. market. Like other NSAIDs, however, sulfinpyrazone can be ulcerogenic and is therefore contraindicated in patients with peptic ulcer disease and in patients with underlying blood dyscrasias. It may cause bone marrow suppression, and blood cell counts should be monitored periodically during prolonged therapy. Sulfinpyrazone is available only for oral use. The usual initial adult dosage is 100 to 200 mg twice a day for 1 week. The subsequent adjusted maintenance dosage can range from 200 to 800 mg daily. Pregnancy category C (category D during the third trimester).

PHARMACOKINETICS

Route	Onset of Action	Peak Plasma Concentration	Elimination Half-life	Duration of Action
PO	2 hr	1-2 hr	3 hr	4-10 hr

NURSING PROCESS

Assessment

Before administering any of the antiinflammatory, antigout, and/or related drugs, it is critical to patient safety and drug effectiveness to assess for drug allergies, contraindications, cautions, and drug interactions associated with each drug in these major groups of drugs. This specific information has been discussed previously in the pharmacology section of this chapter as well as in various tables and drug profiles. Each of the major drug categories is discussed in this nursing process section, with attention to specific drugs as deemed appropriate. Before administering any antiinflammatory drug, the nurse should perform a thorough head-to-toe physical assessment, measure vital signs, perform a nursing assessment, and take a thorough medication history with notation of any prescription, over-the-counter, herbal, and/or alternative drugs the patient is taking. Results of laboratory tests reflecting hematologic, renal, and hepatic functioning should be analyzed before initiation of therapy as ordered. These tests will

---

HERBAL THERAPIES AND DIETARY SUPPLEMENTS

Glucosamine and Chondroitin

■ *Overview*

Glucosamine is chemically derived from glucose. Its chemical name is 2-amino-2-deoxyglucose sulfate.

Chondroitin is a protein usually isolated from bovine (cow) cartilage. To date, there are no reports of any type of disease transmission from cows to humans with chondroitin.

■ *Common Uses*

These two supplements are often used in combination, and sometimes individually, to treat pain from osteoarthritis. Although they are most commonly taken orally, injectable forms are commercially available (e.g., for administration by naturopathic prescribers).

■ *Adverse Effects*

Glucosamine: Usually mild adverse effects that are comparable to those of placebo in clinical studies, including gastrointestinal discomfort, drowsiness, headache, and skin reactions.

Chondroitin: No major ill effects in studies lasting from 2 months to 6 years. Gastrointestinal discomfort is the most common adverse effect but is usually well tolerated.

■ *Potential Drug Interactions*

Both supplements: May enhance the anticoagulant effects of warfarin. The patient's international normalized ratio should be measured more frequently during glucosamine/chondroitin therapy, and the warfarin dosage adjusted if indicated.

Glucosamine: May cause an increase in insulin resistance, necessitating the need for higher dosages of oral hypoglycemics or insulin.

■ *Contraindications*

Both supplements: No specific contraindications listed, but avoidance during pregnancy is recommended due to lack of firm safety data.

---

most likely include RBC count, hemoglobin level, hematocrit, white blood cell count, platelet count, BUN level, and liver enzyme levels such as ALP, AST, and LDH. If NSAIDs are used short term for other conditions (e.g., fever, acute pain), laboratory studies are not usually indicated since these drugs are available over the counter.

With aspirin, NSAIDs, other antiinflammatory drugs and antigout drugs, it is important to assess and document the duration, onset, location, and type of inflammation and/or pain the patient is experiencing as well as any precipitating, exacerbating, or relieving factors. Interference of the symptoms with the patient's ability to perform the activities of daily living (ADLs) should also be noted. All joints should be inspected with attention to deformities, immobility or limitations in mobility, overlying skin condition, and presence of any heat or swelling over the joint. Age is important to assess as well, because aspirin and many of the other NSAIDs are not to be used in children and teenagers due to the increased risk for Reye's syndrome (see the Life Span Considerations box on p. 684). These drugs should also be used very cautiously in the elderly. Assessing the odor of aspirin is also important, because a vinegary odor is associated with a chemical breakdown of the drug. With aspirin, the patient should be assessed for a history of asthma, wheezing, or other respiratory problems because of the increased incidence of allergic reactions to aspirin in these individuals. Also with aspirin, it

---

LIFE SPAN CONSIDERATIONS: The Elderly Patient

NSAIDs

It is anticipated that by 2030 there will be more than 60 million Americans aged 65 years and older, exceeding 20% of the population. It is also anticipated that the use of over-the-counter NSAIDs will be widespread and increasing in this population and will require special attention and education to prevent and/or minimize adverse effects. Understanding the physiologic changes of the elderly patient will help ensure safe and effective use of these medications.

The underlying pharmacokinetic characteristics and physical and biologic changes in the elderly must be understood. Even if older patients have normal kidney and liver function, these patients have a reduced rate of drug metabolism and drug elimination compared with younger adults.

Patients 65 years and older do not have to be ill for NSAIDs to adversely affect them because of normal age-related physiologic changes. The presence of chronic or multiple illnesses will result in increased incidence of adverse reactions.

Some changes noted in the elderly that effect drug treatment include changes in renal elimination, protein binding, body composition, drug distribution, drug clearance, and sensitivity to drugs, as well as an increased incidence of adverse reactions to all sorts of medications.

Older patients at risk for renal insufficiency because of natural physiologic changes may experience changes in fluid balance as well as changes in drug reabsorption, excretion, and filtration processes. This may lead to drug toxicity.

Cardiac output drops by 25% between the ages of 25 and 65, which results in decreased blood flow to the kidneys and, consequently, reduced glomerular filtration rate. There is also an overall decline in circulating blood volume, which may affect overall pharmacokinetics and lead to decreased drug absorption, distribution, metabolism, and excretion.

Many individuals older than 65 years of age become slow metabolizers of medications, which affects the way NSAIDs are handled by the liver. In addition, the liver decreases in size and weight with advancing age, and liver blood flow decreases. Drug metabolism is affected by these changes, which results in the need to possibly decrease drug dosages and/or monitor very closely for toxicity.

Gastrointestinal functioning is impacted by aging, with a more acidic content of gastric juice and decreased gastric motility. This may lead to slower emptying of the stomach and result in decreased intestinal absorption and drug absorption. Serum levels of drugs, including NSAIDs, may be higher due to these changes, and the overall drug dosage may need to be decreased. It has also been documented that the elderly may be at increased risk for developing NSAID-related gastrointestinal problems.

Interventions to help decrease NSAID-related adverse reactions include asking questions, listing all drugs, teaching about all medications, and assessing the patient's gastrointestinal, cardiovascular, and neurologic systems, depending on patient complaints.

For more information, see Durrance S: Older adults and NSAIDs: avoiding adverse reactions, 2004, available at *http://www.medscape.com/viewarticle/466796*. *NSAID,* Nonsteroidal antiinflammatory drug.

---

is important to identify patients who have been diagnosed with what is called the *aspirin triad,* which includes asthma, nasal polyps, and rhinitis. These conditions are considered to put the patient at risk for reactions to aspirin. Other contraindications, cautions, and drug interactions for aspirin and other NSAIDs have been discussed previously. The nurse must remember that salicylic acid or aspirin and other NSAIDs have antiinflammatory, antipyretic, analgesic, and antiplatelet activity but also carry a risk for ulcerogenic and bleeding adverse effects. Use of NSAIDs requires close assessment not only for gastrointestinal upset but also for any preexisting peripheral edema. Baseline CBC, results of blood chemistry analysis with electrolyte levels, BUN level, creatinine level, liver function test results, and bleeding/clotting times should also be noted prior to initiation of drug therapy. Ketorolac use requires assessment of the drug order as well, because it is important to be sure the drug has been ordered for a short term (e.g., no more than 5 days) and for patients experiencing moderate to severe acute pain. The patient should be assessed for underlying signs of infection before the use of any NSAID or other antiinflammatory drug, because these drugs can mask symptoms. With use of celecoxib, assessment should also include documentation of any gastrointestinal disorders such as bleeding and ulcers.

With *antigout* drugs, the patient should be assessed for any history of gastrointestinal distress, ulcers, or cardiac, renal, or liver disease, and baseline hydration status should be determined. Serum uric acid levels are generally measured before initiation of therapy for baseline comparisons, as ordered. Urinary output should also be closely assessed prior to and during the drug therapy to ensure an output of at least 30 to 60 mL/hr. Levels of BUN,

serum creatinine, ALP, AST, ALT, and LDH are some of the more common blood tests performed before therapy to obtain baseline values for comparison. Also worthy of mentioning for *antigout drugs* (e.g., allopurinol, colchicine, probenecid) is that these drugs may be used for either their short-term or long-term effects. Therefore, the nurse must assess the order and indication for the antigout drug to ensure that the patient is receiving the appropriate treatment. The nurse should also assess for all contraindications, cautions, and drug interactions (see earlier discussion).

Nursing Diagnoses

- Acute pain related to the disease process or injury to joints and other disease-affected areas
- Activity intolerance related to the condition or disease process causing the pain
- Risk for injury to self related to the effects of the disease and even its treatment on mobility and performance of ADLs
- Ineffective health maintenance related to lack of knowledge about pharmacologic and nonpharmacologic treatment measures
- Deficient knowledge related to first-time drug therapy for treatment of a disease process

Planning
Goals

- Patient is able to describe the use of the medication as it relates to the relief of inflammation and pain.
- Patient experiences pain relief or relief of symptoms within the expected time frame.

- Patient uses nonpharmacologic measures to enhance drug therapy to decrease inflammation so that he or she can increase performance of ADLs, including walking.
- Patient reports adverse effects to the prescriber as indicated.
- Patient remains compliant with the medication therapy regimen.

Outcome Criteria

- Patient states that pain and changes in joints and mobility are characteristic of inflammation, injury, or related disease processes and will decrease with effective therapy.
- Patient identifies factors that aggravate or alleviate pain, such as movement, activity, exercise, change in weather or atmosphere, etc.
- Patient states nonpharmacologic measures to use to promote comfort, increase joint function and mobility, and increase performance of ADLs (e.g., biofeedback, imagery, massage, application of hot or cold packs, physical therapy, and relaxation therapy).
- Patient states adverse effects associated with the specific group of drugs.
- Patient lists symptoms to report to the prescriber immediately.
- Patient states the importance of correct dosing and consistency in the self-administration of medication.
- Patient returns for follow-up visits with the prescriber and states the importance of returning for evaluating the success of treatment and/or monitoring for adverse or toxic effects.

Implementation

If *aspirin* is used, the oral dosage forms should be given with food, milk, or meals. Sustained-release or enteric-coated tablets should not be crushed or broken. Serum levels of aspirin should be monitored if aspirin therapy is used for its antiarthritic effect. Measurement of serum aspirin levels is also important for distinguishing among mild, moderate, and severe toxicity. Although aspirin therapy is not generally recommended or commonly used because of its toxicity, the nurse should remain current about the drug (see pharmacology discussion). The nurse should be alert to signs of toxicity such as gastric ulcers, gastric bleeding, and other bleeding and report these to the prescriber for immediate treatment. If aspirin is used as an antipyretic, the patient's temperature should begin to decrease within 1 hour. For more information on the safe use of aspirin, see Patient Teaching Tips.

Non-aspirin NSAIDs may also come in enteric-coated or sustained-release preparations, and these should not be crushed or chewed. Oral dosage forms of these drugs—including ketorolac—may be taken with antacids or food to decrease gastrointestinal upset or irritation. Moderate to severe gastrointestinal upset, dyspepsia with nausea, vomiting, abdominal pain, and blood in the stool or vomitus should be reported to the prescriber immediately. Other ulcerogenic substances (e.g., alcohol, prednisone, aspirin-containing products, other NSAIDs) should be avoided to help minimize risk of gastrointestinal mucosal breakdown. During therapy with NSAIDs, the patient should be monitored constantly for bowel patterns, stool consistency, and any occurrence of gastrointestinal symptoms and/or dizziness and the findings documented. Laboratory tests whose results may need monitoring with high-dose or long-term treatment include CBC; BUN levels; platelet counts; and serum bilirubin, ALP, AST, and ALT levels. Safe ambulation should always be emphasized with

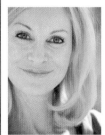
NSAID use as well as with the use of any other antiinflammatory drugs and/or analgesics. With ketorolac, it is also important to understand that dosing should not exceed a 5-day time period for either the oral, intramuscular, or IV dosage forms. Intramuscular injections should be administered slowly into a large muscle mass, and IV dosage forms are recommended to be administered over a period of no less than 15 seconds. Celecoxib should be administered only as ordered and, as with the other NSAIDs, alcohol, aspirin, salicylates, and over-the-counter drugs containing any of these should be avoided. Celecoxib may be taken without regard to meals; however, taking the drug with food and fluids may decrease any gastrointestinal upset. Any stomach or abdominal pain, gastrointestinal problems, unusual bleeding, blood in the stool or vomitus, chest pain, edema, and/or palpitations should be reported immediately to the prescriber.

The *antigout drugs* are somewhat different from the NSAIDs, with different mechanisms of action and also very different nursing considerations. Colchicine should be taken on an empty stomach for more complete absorption; therefore, it should be taken at least 1 hour before or 2 hours after meals. IV colchicine, if prescribed, should be administered as recommended per manufacturer guidelines and over the recommended time period. Regardless of dosage form, the patient should always increase fluid intake to up to 3 liters per day, unless contraindicated. Alcohol and any over-the-counter cold relief products that contain alcohol should be avoided while this medication is being taken. In addition, patients with gout must be instructed that adherence to the complete medical regimen—both pharmacologic and nonpharmacologic—is critical to successful treatment. If allopurinol is prescribed, it should be given with meals to minimize the occurrence of gastrointestinal symptoms such as nausea, vomiting, and anorexia. If allopurinol is to be administered in conjunction with chemotherapy (in an attempt to decrease hyperuricemia associated with malignancy and cell death from successful treatment), it is recommended that it be given a few days before the antineoplastic therapy. Patients taking allopurinol should be instructed to increase fluid intake to 3 L/day, to avoid hazardous activities if dizziness or drowsiness occurs with the medication, and to avoid the use of alcohol and caffeine because these drugs will increase uric acid levels and decrease the level of allopurinol.

Evaluation

Aspirin and *NSAIDs* may vary in their potency and antiinflammatory and analgesic effects. Therapeutic responses to NSAIDs include the following: decrease in acute pain; decrease in swelling, pain, stiffness, and tenderness of a joint or muscle area; improved ability to perform ADLs; improved muscle grip and strength; reduction in fever; return to normal laboratory values for CBC, RBC count, hemoglobin level, hematocrit, and sedimentation rate; and return to a less inflamed state as evidenced by improved sedimentation rates, radiographic examination, computed tomographic scan, or magnetic resonance imaging. Use of *COX-II inhibitors* should also result in improved joint function and fewer inflammation-based signs and symptoms. Patients should begin to show improvement in mobility and the ability to perform ADLs with any of these drugs, but within a time frame that may be up to 2 to 3 months, depending on the drug. Monitoring for the occurrence of adverse effects and toxicity is essential to the safe and effective use of aspirin, COX-II inhibitors, other NSAIDs, and *antigout drugs* (see Table 44-2).

Therapeutic responses to the *antigout* drug colchicine include decreased pain in the affected joints and increased sense of well-being. The patient should be monitored closely for or should report to the prescriber any increased pain, blood in the urine, excessive fatigue and lethargy, or chills or fever. A therapeutic response to allopurinol, another antigout drug, includes a decrease in pain in the joints, a decrease in uric acid levels, and a decrease in stone formation in the kidneys.

PATIENT TEACHING TIPS

- These drugs—if in sustained-release or enteric-coated dosage forms—should not be crushed/chewed. Ringing in the ears, any persistent gastrointestinal or abdominal pain, and easy bruising or bleeding should be reported to the prescriber immediately.
- Educate that the full antiinflammatory effect of the drug may not be apparent immediately, depending on the specific drug. For example, onset of full therapeutic antiinflammatory action may take 7 days for ibuprofen or 30 to 60 minutes for its analgesic effects.
- A list of all medications should be shared with all health care professionals/dentists especially if the patient is taking high dosages of aspirin or has been taking aspirin or other NSAIDs for prolonged periods. Aspirin and other NSAIDs should also be discontinued 1 week before any type of surgery, including oral or dental surgery, per the prescriber's or surgeon's orders.
- Aspirin and other drugs should be kept out of the reach of children. If a child (or adult) has consumed large or unknown quantities of aspirin or other NSAIDs, a poison control center should be contacted and/or emergency medical attention sought immediately. Children and teenagers should not take aspirin because of the risk of Reye's syndrome. Acetaminophen in the recommended dosage range is usually preferred.
- The patient should be educated about the adverse effects of aspirin, such as gastrointestinal upset, nausea, vomiting, diarrhea, dizziness, and tinnitus. Table 44-3 discusses signs and symptoms of acute or chronic salicylate intoxication. Any black or tarry stools, bleeding around the gums, petechiae (very small red-brown spots), ecchymosis (easy bruising), and purpura (large red spots) should be reported to the prescriber immediately.
- Educate about the most common adverse effects of the NSAIDs (see Table 44-2). Instruct that NSAIDs should be taken with food, milk, or antacids to help minimize gastrointestinal distress. Other problems about which to alert patients include the possible risk of stomatitis and ulcers of the oral mucosa.
- Education should be included about the many drug interactions with aspirin, other NSAIDs, and antigout drugs (see pharmacology discussion for a complete listing).
- The patient should be alerted to look-alike sound-alike drugs, especially Celebrex (celecoxib), which may be confused with Celexa (citalopram) or Cerebyx (fosphenytoin).

POINTS TO REMEMBER

- NSAIDs are one of the most commonly prescribed categories of drugs.
- The first drug in this category to be synthesized was salicylic acid or aspirin. Aspirin is often identified as and included in discussion of antiinflammatory drugs. NSAIDs have analgesic, antiinflammatory, and antipyretic activity; aspirin also has antiplatelet activity. NSAIDs are often used in the treatment of gout, osteoarthritis, juvenile arthritis, rheumatoid arthritis, dysmenorrhea, and musculoskeletal injuries such as strains and sprains.
- The three main adverse effects of NSAIDs are gastrointestinal intolerance, bleeding (often gastrointestinal bleeding), and renal impairment. Misoprostol (Cytotec) may be given to prevent gastrointestinal intolerance and ulcers resulting from NSAID use. It is classified as a prostaglandin analogue. There are also many con-

traindications to the use of NSAIDs, such as gastrointestinal tract lesions, peptic ulcers, and bleeding disorders.
- Most oral NSAIDs are better tolerated if taken with food to minimize gastrointestinal upset.
- Patients taking NSAIDs should be closely monitored for the occurrence of bleeding, such as blood in the stools or vomitus. When NSAIDs are used to decrease joint inflammation in arthritis patients, full therapeutic effects may not be experienced for a week or longer.
- Antigout drugs are indicated for either acute or chronic gout or gout prophylaxis. Diarrhea and abdominal pain are common adverse effects. Antigout drugs are often given to patients during cancer chemotherapy that causes cell death to avoid goutlike syndromes and pain.

NCLEX EXAMINATION REVIEW QUESTIONS

1 When a patient is receiving long-term NSAID therapy, which drug may be given to prevent the serious gastrointestinal adverse effects of NSAIDs?
  a misoprostol (Cytotec)
  b metoprolol (Lopressor)
  c metoclopramide (Reglan)
  d magnesium sulfate

2 The nurse recognizes that manifestations of NSAID toxicity include:
  a Constipation
  b Nausea and vomiting
  c Tremors
  d Urinary retention

3 During a teaching session about antigout drugs, the nurse would tell the patient that antigout drugs work by which mechanism?
  a Increasing blood oxygen levels
  b Decreasing leukocytes and platelets
  c Increasing protein and rheumatoid factors
  d Decreasing serum uric acid levels

4 When the nurse is teaching about antigout drugs, which statement by the nurse is accurate?
  a "Drink only limited amounts of fluids with the drug."
  b "This drug may cause limited movements of your joints."

  c "There are very few drug interactions with these medications."
  d "Colchicine is best taken on an empty stomach."

5 A mother calls the clinic to ask what medication to give her 5-year-old child for a fever during a bout of chickenpox. The nurse's best response would be:
  a "Your child is 5 years old, so it would be okay to use children's aspirin to treat his fever."
  b "Start with acetaminophen or ibuprofen, but if those do not work, then you can try aspirin."
  c "You can use children's dosages of acetaminophen or ibuprofen, but aspirin is not recommended."
  d "It is best to wait to let the fever break on its own without medication."

6 A 49-year-old patient has been admitted with possible chronic salicylate intoxication after self-treatment for arthritis pain. The nurse will assess for which symptoms of salicylate intoxication?
  a Tinnitus
  b Headache
  c Constipation
  d Nausea
  e Bradycardia

1. a, 2. b, 3. d, 4. d, 5. c, 6. a, b, d.

CRITICAL THINKING ACTIVITIES: BEST ACTION

1 P.T., age 68, is instructed to take aspirin, 81 mg every morning with breakfast, as part of treatment after having a myocardial infarction. When discussing the aspirin therapy, he asks you, "Will this also help my arthritis?" What is your best answer?

2 H.M. has been taking ibuprofen (Motrin), 800 mg three times a day, for treatment of arthritis. She is scheduled for a laparoscopy. She asks you, "I hope I can continue the Motrin, because I really

ache if I don't take it. It's just minor surgery, right?" What is your best answer?

3 Henry has been diagnosed with gout and will be taking colchicine. When reviewing the instructions for the medication, he asks, "I like to take my pills with breakfast." What is your best response to Henry?

For answers, see *http://evolve.elsevier.com/Lilley.*

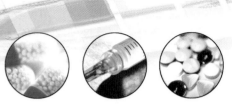

Immune and Biologic Modifiers and Chemotherapeutic Drugs

STUDY SKILLS TIPS

Manage Time • Evaluate Prior Performance

Anticipate the Test • Plan for Distributed Study

MANAGE TIME

The first step in preparing for a chapter or part exam is to plan for the time needed. Let us begin by assuming that the next test you have will cover the chapters in Part 8. First examine the material to determine just how much there is to cover. Look at the objectives, the glossary, and the number of pages of text in each chapter. This will help you determine just how big a task you face. As you are doing this, also consider how much study time you have been devoting to these chapters in the days before the exam. If you have been doing regular study with frequent review sessions, then the demand on your time in the day or two just before the exam will be less than if you have to do a major "cram" session to try to catch up on study that has been put off. The basic question to answer here is a simple one: "How much time do I need to schedule for exam preparation?" The answer varies with each student. Some will need 6, 8, or more hours of preparation time in the 2 to 3 days before the exam. Others will find that 3, 4, or 5 hours will be adequate. You must assess your own learning and prior success to determine what time is necessary for you, but you must set time aside and use it effectively.

There is one thing that should play a major role in helping you determine how much time you will need to set aside. Evaluate your performance on prior exams. How have you been doing? How much time have you been spending to achieve that level? If you are not achieving according to your capabilities, then you should certainly consider spending more time preparing for the next exam. If you are achieving at a satisfactory level, then plan on devoting about the same amount of time to test preparation as you have devoted before.

The next step in preparing for an exam is to organize the time. Write down what you are going to study and when, as well as

how much time you will spend. Consider the following example based on the materials in Chapters 47 and 49:

1. Review Chapter 47 objectives. Monday, 4:00 to 4:30 PM. Note objectives that are unclear for further review.
2. Question and answer review. Monday, 4:30 to 5:15 PM.
3. Self-test, Chapter 47 glossary. Monday, 6:30 to 7:00 PM. Note terms that need further review for mastery.
4. Review Chapter 49 objectives. Monday, 7:00 to 7:30 PM.
5. Question and answer review. Monday, 7:30 to 8:00 PM.
6. Self-test, Chapter 49 glossary. Monday, 8:00 to 8:30 PM.

The advantage to this test preparation model is that you now know where you must focus in the days before the exam.

EVALUATE PRIOR PERFORMANCE

As you begin preparing to review for any exam, take some time to look back at previous exams. Evaluate your performance and use that evaluation to improve on subsequent tests. As you look at prior tests, consider the following factors.

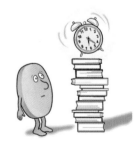

What Type of Errors Did I Make?

As students we often find that there are certain question types or forms that are missed consistently. Assess your errors and try to pinpoint any recurring patterns in your mistakes. Did you miss questions that contained an exemption in the multiple-choice stem? Question stems that state, "All of the following except" and "Which of the following would not be …" are exemption questions. Questions like this are often missed because they contain too many apparently correct responses. Remember that an exemption stem means you are looking for the one response choice that is *wrong*. The stem asks you to identify the inappropriate response, and it is the best choice.

Did I Have Trouble with Questions That Required Mastery of Terminology?

As part of the evaluation of prior tests, also look at questions that demanded mastery of the terms from the chapters. If you missed more than one or two questions of that type, then you know you need to spend more time reviewing terminology.

Did I Miss Concept Questions?

If the question asked you to apply a principle, evaluate a drug response, or in some other way apply knowledge from the course, you are dealing with concepts rather than facts. If you missed a number of concept questions, then you should spend more of your review time studying applications and principles than memorizing facts and terms. Working with a study group may help you to improve your responses to concept questions.

Did I Make Errors Because I Did Not Know the Material?

This question focuses on the quality of your learning. If you miss one or two questions on an exam because you did not learn (or did not remember) the material, it is not a major problem. There will almost always be one or two questions that one does not remember. If you are analyzing past performance and find that there are several questions on which you guessed because you did not recall any information that seemed relevant to the question, it may be necessary to put more time into review. This may involve doing more oral rehearsal so that the material is stored in long-term memory. Whatever the cause, it is essential that you acknowledge to yourself that you have missed questions because you did not know the material. Once you have acknowledged the problem, take steps to correct it.

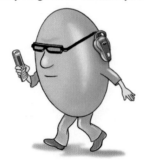

ANTICIPATE THE TEST

Do not wait until exam time to find out what you should know. As you do your review, try to think like the instructor. Generate questions that you think might be a part of the test. This does not mean you need to try to write multiple-choice stems and choices, but you should be trying to focus your review in a way that will facilitate learning and long-term memory. The process of working with a study group to anticipate test questions and to quiz each other can help move concepts from short-term memory to long-term memory.

Here are some examples of questioning that you might use based on material found in Chapter 49.

1. What are biologic response modifiers?
2. What is the role of biologic response modifiers in the care of patients with cancer?
3. What is the role of the immune system in treating cancer?

These sample questions were drawn from just the first few pages of the chapter. Some questions may focus on literal comprehension and are relatively easy to generate. Being able to answer them is important, but if all of your questions are literal, it may be difficult to answer questions that require application of principles and concepts. For that reason, it is essential that some questions require analysis, synthesis, and/or evaluation of the material. A study group is helpful in creating this more complicated type of question. The process of discussion can generate ideas you may not develop on your own. Answers to these questions require the learner to put together the literal information and relate the terms to the concepts being explained.

PLAN FOR DISTRIBUTED STUDY

One of the major problems that many students encounter when trying to review for a test is waiting too long to begin the review, which forces them into a review pattern of long hours of intensive study all packed into the last day or two before the exam. This is known as "cramming," and although cramming does work to some degree, it is not the most effective way to learn. A better model is to distribute the review over a period of several days with short study sessions of 30 minutes to 1 hour several times each day. Distributing practice in this way allows time for you to think about what you have been learning, and it fosters long-term memory. Studying with a group adds variety to your study time and provides another method of receiving and processing information.

One important consideration is spending more of the review time doing oral rehearsal ("ask and answer" sessions) and not simply rereading material. Oral rehearsal encourages active learning, which enhances your ability to concentrate, improves comprehension and memory, and thus improves test performance. Oral rehearsals work well in study groups, but if you are satisfied with the test results you get by reviewing alone, keep doing what works for you.

CHAPTER 45

Immunosuppressant Drugs

OBJECTIVES

When you reach the end of this chapter, you should be able to do the following:

1 Discuss the role of immunosuppressive therapy in organ transplantation and in the treatment of autoimmune diseases.

2 Discuss the mechanisms of action, contraindications, cautions, adverse effects, routes of administration, drug interactions, and toxicity of the most commonly used immunosuppressants.

3 Develop a nursing care plan that includes all phases of the nursing process for patients receiving immunosuppressants after organ transplantation or for the treatment of autoimmune disease.

e-Learning Activities

Drug Profiles

◆ azathioprine and mycophenolate mofetil, p. 699
   basiliximab and daclizumab, p. 699

◆ cyclosporine, p. 699
   glatiramer acetate, p. 699
◆ muromonab-CD3, p. 699
   sirolimus and tacrolimus, p. 699

◆ *Key drug.*

Glossary

Autoimmune diseases A large group of diseases characterized by the subversion or alteration of the function of the immune system so that the immune response is directed against normal tissue(s) of the body, which results in pathologic conditions. (p. 694)

Grafts The term used for transplanted tissues or organs. (p. 699)

Immune-mediated diseases A large group of diseases that result when the cells of the immune system react to a variety of situations, such as transplanted organ tissue or drug-altered cells. (p. 694)

Immunosuppressants Drugs that decrease or prevent an immune response. (p. 694)

Immunosuppressive therapy A drug treatment used to suppress the immune system. (p. 694)

• • •

Anatomy, Physiology, and Disease Overview

IMMUNE SYSTEM

The purpose of the *immune system* is to distinguish self from nonself and to protect the body from foreign material (antigens). There are three layers of barriers to protect the body (Figure 45-1). There are two types of immunity: humoral immunity, which is mediated by B lymphocytes, and cellular immunity, which is mediated by T lymphocytes. This chapter focuses on drugs that suppress the T lymphocytes. The immune system defends the body against invading pathogens, foreign antigens, and its own cells that become cancerous, or neoplastic. Besides performing this beneficial function, however, it can also sometimes attack itself and cause what are known as **autoimmune diseases** or **immune-mediated diseases.** It also participates in hypersensitivity, or anaphylactic, reactions, which can be life threatening. The rejection of kidney, liver, and heart (whole organ) transplants is directed by the immune system as well.

Drugs that decrease or prevent an immune response, and hence suppress the immune system, are known as **immunosuppressants.** Treatment with such drugs is referred to as **immunosuppressive therapy,** and it is used to selectively eradicate certain cell lines that play a major role in the rejection of a transplanted organ. These cell lines must be targeted and selectively altered or suppressed, or organ rejection will occur. The primary immunosuppressant drugs are the corticosteroids (see Chapter 33), cyclophosphamide (see Chapter 47), azathioprine, cyclosporine, muromonab-CD3, tacrolimus, glatiramer acetate, daclizumab, basiliximab, and sirolimus.

Pharmacology Overview

IMMUNOSUPPRESSANT DRUGS

Mechanism of Action and Drug Effects

All immunosuppressants have similar mechanisms of action in that they all selectively suppress certain T-lymphocyte cell lines. By suppressing the T-lymphocyte cell lines, these drugs prevent their involvement in the immune response. This results in a pharmacologically immunocompromised state similar to that in a cancer patient whose bone marrow and immune cells have been destroyed as a result of chemotherapy or that in a patient with acquired immunodeficiency syndrome (AIDS) whose immune cells have been destroyed by the human immunodeficiency virus (HIV). Each drug differs in the exact way in which it suppresses certain cell lines involved in an immune response. Table 45-1 gives the mechanisms of action and indications of the available immunosuppressant drugs.

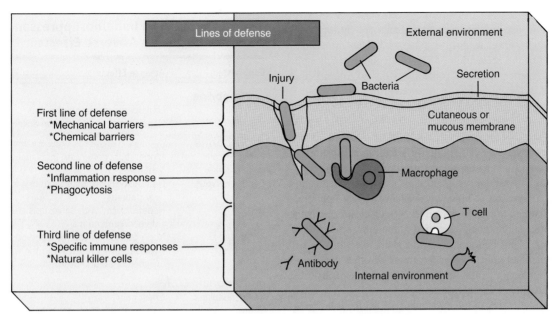

FIGURE 45-1   A simplified depiction of the complicated immune system. (From Thibodeau GA, Patton KT: *Anatomy and physiology,* ed 6, St Louis, 2006, Mosby.)

TABLE 45-1 Available Immunosuppressant Drugs: Mechanisms of Action and Indications

Drug Name, Year of FDA Approval	Mechanism of Action	Indications/Uses
azathioprine (Imuran), 1980	Blocks metabolism of purines, inhibiting the synthesis of T-cell DNA, RNA, and proteins and thereby blocking immune response	Organ rejection prevention in kidney transplantation; treatment of rheumatoid arthritis
basiliximab* (Simulect), 1998	Suppresses T-cell activity by blocking the binding of the cytokine mediator IL-2 to a specific receptor	Organ rejection prevention in kidney transplantation
cyclosporine (Sandimmune, Neoral, Gengraf), 1983	Inhibits activation of T cells by blocking the production and release of the cytokine mediator IL-2	Organ rejection prevention in kidney, liver, and heart transplantation; treatment of rheumatoid arthritis and psoriasis. Unlabeled uses† include rejection prevention in pancreas, bone marrow, and heart/lung transplantation.
daclizumab* (Zenapax), 1997	Suppresses T-cell activity by blocking the binding of the cytokine mediator IL-2 to a specific receptor	Organ rejection prevention in kidney transplantation
glatiramer acetate (Copaxone), 1996	Precise mechanism unknown; believed to somehow modify immune system processes that are associated with MS symptoms	Reduction of relapse frequency in patients with RRMS
muromonab-CD3* (Orthoclone OKT3), 1986	Binds to CD3 glycoprotein on T-cell receptors, which blocks antigen recognition and reverses graft rejection that is already in progress	Treatment of acute organ rejection in kidney, liver, and heart transplantation
mycophenolate mofetil (CellCept), 1995	Prevents proliferation of T cells by inhibiting intracellular purine synthesis	Organ rejection prevention in kidney, liver, and heart transplantation
sirolimus (Rapamune), 1999	Inhibits T-cell activation by binding to an intracellular protein known as FKBP-12 that subsequently prevents cellular proliferation	Organ rejection prevention in kidney transplantation
tacrolimus (Prograf), 1994	Inhibits T-cell activation, possibly by binding to an intracellular protein known as FKBP-12	Organ rejection prevention in liver, kidney, or heart transplantation. Unlabeled uses† include rejection prevention in bone marrow, pancreas, pancreatic islet cell, and small intestine transplantation; treatment of autoimmune diseases and severe psoriasis.

FDA, Food and Drug Administration; *FKBP-12,* FK-binding protein 12; *IL-2,* interleukin-2; *MS,* multiple sclerosis; *RRMS,* relapsing-remitting multiple sclerosis.
*Note that "ab" in any drug name usually indicates that it is a monoclonal antibody synthesized using recombinant DNA technology.
†Non-FDA approved but under investigation.

Indications

The therapeutic uses of immunosuppressants are multiple and vary from drug to drug, as noted in Table 45-1. They are primarily indicated for the prevention of organ rejection, which is the focus of this chapter. However, some are also used to treat other immunologic illnesses, such as rheumatoid arthritis (see Chapter 49) and multiple sclerosis. Only muromonab-CD3 is indicated for treatment of organ rejection once rejection of the transplanted organ has begun. The four newer drugs (basiliximab, daclizumab, sirolimus, and mycophenolate mofetil), are all immunosuppressants used in transplant patients and are indicated for organ rejection prophylaxis. Azathioprine is used as an adjunct medication to prevent the rejection of kidney transplants and to ameliorate severe rheumatoid arthritis (see Chapter 49). Cyclosporine is the primary immunosuppressant drug used in the prevention of kidney, liver, heart, and bone marrow transplant rejection. It may also have beneficial effects in the treatment of other conditions with an immunologic cause, such as certain types of arthritis, psoriasis, and irritable bowel disease.

Tacrolimus has many of the same therapeutic effects as cyclosporine and is indicated for the prevention of heart, kidney, or liver transplant rejection. Glatiramer acetate is the only immunosuppressant currently indicated for treatment of multiple sclerosis. Specifically, it is indicated for reduction of the frequency of relapses (exacerbations) in a type of multiple sclerosis known as *relapsing-remitting multiple sclerosis*. This is currently its sole indication.

Contraindications

The main contraindication for all immunosuppressants is known drug allergy. Relative contraindications, depending on the patient's condition, may include renal or hepatic failure, hypertension, and concurrent radiation therapy. Pregnancy is not necessarily a contraindication to the use of these drugs, but immunosuppressants should be given to pregnant women only in clinically urgent situations.

Adverse Effects

Many of the adverse effects of the immunosuppressants can be devastating, especially to a transplant patient. Although not strictly an adverse effect, a heightened susceptibility to opportunistic infections is a major risk factor in immunosuppressed patients. Other adverse effects are limited to the particular drug. Some of the most common of these are listed in Table 45-2.

Interactions

Immunosuppressant drugs have many drug interactions and are listed in Table 45-3. Cyclosporine, tacrolimus, and sirolimus are capable of many drug interactions, several of which can be very harmful and result in toxicity or in organ rejection. All immunosuppressant drugs can reduce the effectiveness of vaccines. Grapefruit can inhibit metabolizing enzymes and thus can increase the activity of cyclosporine, tacrolimus, and sirolimus. Patients who eat grapefruit or drink grapefruit juice need not avoid it entirely but are advised to maintain a steady consumption of this fruit. They are also advised to notify their prescriber if their grapefruit consumption levels change, because this may require either an increase or decrease in the dosage of the immunosuppressant. Grapefruit juice may increase the bioavailability of cyclosporine by 20% to 200%. Cyclosporine may sometimes be administered with grapefruit juice intentionally to achieve therapeutic blood levels of cyclosporine with decreased dosages. The manufacturer of cyclosporine does not endorse this practice.

Because the antibodies basiliximab, daclizumab, and muromonab-CD3 are generally given in a relatively short single course of therapy, they have few recognized drug interactions. However, cases of encephalopathy have occurred in patients in whom the antiinflammatory drug indomethacin (see Chapter 44) was used concurrently with muromonab-CD3.

The potential for interactions between immunosuppressant drugs and herbal preparations also should not be overlooked. For example, the enzyme-inducing properties of St. John's wort have been demonstrated to reduce the therapeutic levels of cyclosporine and cause organ rejection. The immunostimulant properties of cat's claw and echinacea may be similarly undesirable in transplant recipients, because they have effects that are opposite those of the immunosuppressants.

Dosages

For the recommended dosages of selected immunosuppressant drugs, see the Dosages table on p. 698.

TABLE 45-2 Selected Immunosuppressant Drugs: Common Adverse Effects

Body System	Adverse Effects
azathioprine	
Hematologic	Leukopenia, thrombocytopenia
Hepatic	Hepatotoxicity is a common adverse effect
cyclosporine	
Cardiovascular	Moderate hypertension in as many as 50% of patients
Central nervous	Neurotoxicity, including tremors, in about 20% of patients
Hepatic	Hepatotoxicity with cholestasis and hyperbilirubinemia
Renal	Nephrotoxicity is common and dose limiting
Other	Hypersensitivity reactions to the vehicle, gingival hyperplasia, and hirsutism
muromonab-CD3	
Cardiovascular	Chest pain
Central nervous	Pyrexia (fever), chills, tremors
Gastrointestinal	Vomiting, nausea, diarrhea
Respiratory	Dyspnea, wheezing, pulmonary edema
Other	Flulike symptoms, fluid retention
tacrolimus	
Central nervous	Agitation, anxiety, confusion, hallucinations, neuropathy
Renal	Albuminuria, dysuria, acute renal failure, renal tubular necrosis
Antibody Immunosuppressants	
(basiliximab, daclizumab, and muromonab-CD3)	Cytokine release syndrome, which includes such immune-mediated symptoms as fever, dyspnea, tachycardia, sweating, chills, headache, nausea, vomiting, diarrhea, muscle and joint pain, and general malaise

TABLE 45-3 Immunosuppressant Drugs: Selected Drug Interactions

Drug	Mechanism	Result
cyclosporine		
clarithromycin fluconazole amiodarone Estrogens verapamil allopurinol cimetidine diltiazem Protease inhibitors	Inhibit metabolism of cyclosporine	Increased cyclosporine levels and toxicity
phenytoin phenobarbital carbamazepine rifampin St. John's wort	Induce metabolism of cyclosporine	Decreased cyclosporine levels and reduce effect
gentamicin tobramycin ciprofloxacin NSAIDs vancomycin	Enhance nephrotoxicity of cyclosporine	Kidney failure
Grapefruit juice	Increases absorption of cyclosporine	Cyclosporine toxicity
sirolimus		
cyclosporine	Unknown	Increased sirolimus concentrations
fluconazole ketoconazole clarithromycin erythromycin Protease inhibitors verapamil diltiazem Grapefruit juice	Inhibit metabolism of sirolimus	Increased sirolimus concentration and effect
rifampin phenytoin phenobarbital carbamazepine St. John's wort	Induce metabolism of sirolimus	Decreased sirolimus concentration and effect
tacrolimus		
amphotericin gentamicin tobramycin	Increase nephrotoxicity of tacrolimus	Renal failure
clarithromycin fluconazole ketoconazole voriconazole Protease inhibitors verapamil diltiazem Grapefruit juice	Inhibit metabolism of tacrolimus	Increased effect of tacrolimus
rifampin phenytoin phenobarbital carbamazepine St. John's wort	Induce metabolism of tacrolimus	Decreased effect of tacrolimus

ACE, Angiotensin-converting enzyme; *NSAIDs,* nonsteroidal antiinflammatory drugs.

Continued

TABLE 45-3 Immunosuppressant Drugs: Selected Drug Interactions—cont'd

Drug	Mechanism	Result
mycophenolate mofetil		
Antacids		
iron	Reduce absorption of mycophenolate	Decreased effect of mycophenolate
cholestyramine		
Oral contraceptives	Mycophenolate decreases progesterone levels	Possible pregnancy
rifampin	Induces metabolism of mycophenolate	Decreased effect of mycophenolate
azathioprine		
ACE inhibitors	Have additive effects	Leukopenia
allopurinol	Decreases metabolism of azathioprine	Bone marrow depression
warfarin	Unknown	Decreased effect of warfarin

DOSAGES

Selected Immunosuppressant Drugs

Drug (Pregnancy Category)	Pharmacologic Class	Usual Dosage Range	Indications/Uses
◆ azathioprine (Imuran) (D)	Purine antagonist	**Adult and pediatric** IV/PO: 2-5 mg/kg/day to start, then 1-3 mg/kg/day maintenance	Prevention of rejection of kidney transplants
		Adult PO: 1 mg/kg/day as a single or divided dose for 6-8 wk, then may increase prn by 0.5 mg/kg/day q4wk to a maximum of 2.5 mg/kg/day	Treatment of rheumatoid arthritis
basiliximab (Simulect) (B)	Monoclonal antibody	**Pediatric 2-15 yr, less than 35 kg** IV: 10 mg within 2 hr of transplant surgery, then 4 days afterward	Prevention of rejection of kidney transplants
		Adult and pediatric 35 kg or more Use 20-mg doses in same regimen	
◆ cyclosporine (Sandimmune, Neoral) (C)	Polypeptide antibiotic	**Adult and pediatric** PO: 15 mg/kg as a single dose 4-12 hr preop; continue same dose daily postop for 1-2 wk, then reduce by 5%/wk to a maintenance dose of 5-10 mg/kg/day IV: 5-6 mg/kg as a single dose 4-12 hr preop and continued daily postop until patient can be switched to PO dosing	Prevention of rejection of kidney, liver, heart transplants
daclizumab (Zenapax) (C)	Monoclonal antibody	**Adult and pediatric** IV: Bolus injection of 1 mg/kg 24 hr preop and for 4 additional postop doses, spaced 14 days apart	Prevention of rejection of kidney transplants
glatiramer acetate (Copaxone) (B)	Miscellaneous biologic	**Adult only** Subcut: 20 mg once daily	RRMS
◆ muromonab-CD3 (Orthoclone OKT3) (C)	Monoclonal antibody	**Adult and pediatric** IV: 2.5-5 mg/day as a single bolus injection for 10-14 days (pediatric patients often started with 2.5 mg/day)	Treatment of active rejection of kidney transplants; treatment of active rejection of liver, heart, pancreas, and bone marrow transplants that are resistant to conventional treatment
mycophenolate mofetil (CellCept, Myfortic) (C)	Miscellaneous	**Adult** IV/PO: 1 g twice daily (delayed-release formulation) **Pediatric** IV/PO: 600 mg/m^2 twice daily (maximum daily dose: 400 mg or 720 mg twice daily)	Prevention of rejection of kidney transplants
sirolimus (Rapamune) (C)	Fungus derived	**Adult and pediatric** IV/PO: 6-mg loading dose on day 1, followed by maintenance dose of 2 mg/day	Prevention of rejection of kidney transplants
tacrolimus (Prograf) (C)	Fungus derived	**Adult and pediatric** IV: 0.03-0.05 mg/kg/day as continuous IV infusion; then PO: 0.1-0.2 mg/kg/day divided q12h	Prevention of rejection of liver and kidney transplants

IV, Intravenous; *PO,* oral; *postop,* postoperatively; *preop,* preoperatively; *RRMS,* relapsing-remitting multiple sclerosis; *subcut,* subcutaneous.

As previously stated, the primary use for the immunosuppressant drugs discussed in this chapter is the prevention of organ rejection. Other immunologic disorders, such as rheumatoid arthritis and multiple sclerosis, may also be treated with these drugs. Selected immunosuppressants are described further in the drug profiles that follow.

◆ azathioprine and mycophenolate mofetil

Azathioprine (Imuran) is a chemical analogue of the physiologic purines, such as adenine and guanine. It blocks T-cell proliferation by inhibiting purine synthesis, which in turn prevents synthesis of deoxyribonucleic acid (DNA). Mycophenolate mofetil (CellCept) is another immunosuppressant drug whose mechanism of action is similar to that of azathioprine. Both are used for prophylaxis of organ rejection concurrently with other immunosuppressant drugs, such as cyclosporine and corticosteroids. Both drugs are available in both oral and injectable forms.

PHARMACOKINETICS (AZATHIOPRINE)

Route	Onset of Action	Peak Plasma Concentration	Elimination Half-life	Duration of Action
PO	2-4 days*	1-2 hr	5 hr	Unknown

*6-8 wk for rheumatoid arthritis.

PHARMACOKINETICS (MYCOPHENOLATE MOFETIL)

Route	Onset of Action	Peak Plasma Concentration	Elimination Half-life	Duration of Action
PO	4 wk	0.8-1.8 hr	8-16 hr	Unknown

basiliximab and daclizumab

Basiliximab (Simulect) and daclizumab (Zenapax) are both monoclonal antibodies that work by inhibiting the binding of the cytokine mediator interleukin-2 (IL-2) to the high-affinity IL-2 receptor. These drugs are used to prevent rejection of transplanted kidneys **(grafts)** and are generally used as part of a multidrug immunosuppressive regimen that includes cyclosporine and corticosteroids. Both basiliximab and daclizumab have a tendency to cause the allergy-like reaction known as *cytokine release syndrome*, which can be severe and even involve anaphylaxis. Patients are often premedicated with corticosteroids (e.g., intravenous methylprednisolone) in an effort to avoid or alleviate this problem. Both basiliximab and daclizumab are available only in injectable form.

PHARMACOKINETICS (BASILIXIMAB)

Route	Onset of Action	Peak Plasma Concentration	Elimination Half-life	Duration of Action
IV	1 day	3-4 days	7-9 days	Unknown

PHARMACOKINETICS (DACLIZUMAB)

Route	Onset of Action	Peak Plasma Concentration	Elimination Half-life	Duration of Action
IV	1 day	3-5 days	20 days	Unknown

◆ cyclosporine

Cyclosporine (Sandimmune, Neoral, Gengraf) is an immunosuppressant drug that is indicated for the prevention of organ rejection. It is a very potent immunosuppressant and the principal drug in many immunosuppressive drug regimens. It works by inhibiting the production and release of IL-2. Like azathioprine, it may also be used for the treatment of other immunologic disorders, such as various forms of arthritis, psoriasis, and irritable bowel disease.

Cyclosporine is available in both oral and injectable forms, under the three brand names noted earlier. Although these three products contain the same active ingredient (cyclosporine), they cannot be used interchangeably. When a change is made from Neoral or Gengraf to Sandimmune, the starting dose should be a 1:1 mg amount, but dosage adjustments may be necessary to compensate for the greater bioavailability of Neoral and Gengraf. It is recommended that cyclosporine blood concentration be monitored in patients changing from one product to another. Cyclosporine has a narrow therapeutic range, and for this reason laboratory monitoring of drug levels may be used to ensure therapeutic plasma concentrations and avoid toxicity.

PHARMACOKINETICS

Route	Onset of Action	Peak Plasma Concentration	Elimination Half-life	Duration of Action
PO	1-3 hr	3.5 hr	1-2 hr (parent compound) 10-27 hr (metabolites)	Unknown

glatiramer acetate

Glatiramer acetate (Copaxone) is a mixture of random polymers of four different amino acids. This mixture results in a compound that is antigenically similar to myelin basic protein. This is a protein that is found on the myelin sheaths of nerves. The drug is believed to work by blocking T-cell autoimmune activity against this protein, which reduces the frequency of the neuromuscular exacerbations associated with multiple sclerosis. This drug is mixed in the sugar known as mannitol; therefore, it is contraindicated in patients who are allergic to that component. It is available only in injectable form.

◆ muromonab-CD3

Muromonab-CD3 (Orthoclone OKT3) is the only drug indicated for the reversal (not just the prevention) of graft rejection. It is a monoclonal antibody, synthesized using recombinant DNA technology, and it is very similar to the antibodies produced naturally by the body (immunoglobulins G, M, D, A, and E). It specifically targets the binding sites on the T cells that recognize foreign invaders, such as a transplanted organ. It differs from human antibodies in that it comes from mice. As described previously, other monoclonal antibodies used for the prevention of organ rejection are basiliximab and daclizumab. Muromonab-CD3, often called OKT3, is contraindicated in patients with a hypersensitivity to murine products and in those who are experiencing fluid overload. Muromonab-CD3 can cause cytokine release syndrome, and patients are often pretreated with a corticosteroid as described previously for basiliximab and daclizumab. This drug is available only in injectable form.

PHARMACOKINETICS

Route	Onset of Action	Peak Plasma Concentration	Elimination Half-life	Duration of Action
IV	Rapid	3 days	Unknown	Unknown

sirolimus and tacrolimus

Sirolimus (Rapamune) is another immunosuppressant drug, similar in structure to tacrolimus (Prograf). Sirolimus is a macrocyclic immunosuppressive, antifungal, and antitumor drug. It works by inhibiting T-lymphocyte activation in response to antigenic stimulation and inhibits antibody production, which in turn suppresses cytokine mediated T-cell proliferation. Sirolimus and tacrolimus are structurally related and act through similar mechanisms. Sirolimus is available only for oral use, whereas tacrolimus is available in both oral and injectable forms.

PHARMACOKINETICS (SIROLIMUS)

Route	Onset of Action	Peak Plasma Concentration	Elimination Half-life	Duration of Action
PO	Rapid	1-3 hr	60-80 hr	Unknown

PHARMACOKINETICS (TACROLIMUS)

Route	Onset of Action	Peak Plasma Concentration	Elimination Half-life	Duration of Action
PO	Variable	0.5-4 hr	21-61 hr	Unknown

NURSING PROCESS

Assessment

Before administering any of the *immunosuppressants,* the nurse should perform a thorough patient assessment with baseline measurement of vital signs and weight. A thorough history of past and present medical conditions should be obtained, and the following systems assessment information should be documented: (1) preexisting diseases that impact the patient's immune status, such as diabetes, hypertension, and cancer; (2) urinary functioning and patterns; (3) presence of jaundice, edema, and/or ascites; (4) history of cardiac disease and/or dysrhythmias, chest pain, or heart failure; (5) level of central nervous system functioning, with attention to any seizure disorders, alteration of motor or sensory function, paresthesias, or changing levels of consciousness; (6) respiratory status and baseline respiratory functioning, breath sounds, and presence of asthma, pulmonary diseases, wheezing, cough, activity intolerance, dyspnea, or sputum production; (7) gastrointestinal functioning and patterns, with notation of bowel patterns and bowel disease; (8) musculoskeletal intactness, with attention to ability to perform the activities of daily living, range of motion, and appearance of joints and any deformities; and (9) presence and location of any inflammatory reactions as well as any pain, redness, and/or drainage. In addition, the following laboratory and diagnostic tests may be ordered, and the results should be analyzed: renal function tests with blood urea nitrogen (BUN) and creatinine levels; hepatic function tests with ALP, AST, ALT, and bilirubin levels; and cardiovascular function with baseline electrocardiogram. See Table 45-2 for information on other systems affected by the immunosuppressant drugs. All cautions, contraindications, and drug interactions should be assessed for and noted (see previous pharmacology discussion).

Azathioprine requires assessment of white blood cell and platelet counts with notation of any signs and symptoms of infection as well as any bleeding tendencies due to the potential for drug-related leukopenia and thrombocytopenia. For cyclosporine, related contraindications, cautions, and drug interactions have been discussed previously, but specific assessment of the functional level of all organs as well as assessment for any underlying cardiovascular, central nervous system, hepatic, and/or renal disease are needed because of potential drug related toxicities involving these systems and the physiologic impact of the organ transplant process. A baseline oral assessment is needed, because gingival hyperplasia is a known adverse effect. Measurement of serum potassium

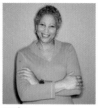
and uric acid levels will most likely be ordered and these indicators assessed frequently to monitor for increased or toxic levels. Generally speaking, with most organ transplants, mild nephrotoxicity may occur within 2 to 3 months, whereas severe toxicity occurs closer to the time of the actual transplantation.

Daclizumab requires assessment of baseline vital signs with specific attention to blood pressure and pulse rate. Any immune-compromising disorders or infectious disease processes should also be noted. Laboratory studies (e.g., hemoglobin level, hematocrit, white blood cell and platelet counts) should be performed and the results documented before, during (monthly), and after therapy. If the leukocyte count drops below 3000 cells/mm^3, the drug should be discontinued, but only after the prescriber is contacted. Muromonab-CD3 should be given only after documentation of baseline weight and thorough assessment of all vital parameters (e.g., vital signs). This is important because of possible drug-related edema, fluid retention, and fever. A chest radiograph is usually ordered within 24 hours of beginning the drug to be sure that baseline lung fields are clear and without fluid.

Tacrolimus requires obtaining a thorough patient history with attention to medication use and performing a physical assessment with close attention to renal functioning through monitoring of BUN, serum creatinine and serum electrolyte levels. When the drug is administered, the patient requires very close assessment for the first 30 minutes with the first dose of the medication. Concern for anaphylactic reaction also continues past this first 30 minutes and first dose, and it is usually important to confirm that resuscitative equipment is accessible and functioning, and that appropriate doses of epinephrine and oxygen are also readily available. With basiliximab, daclizumab, and muromonab-CD3 (antibody immunosuppressants), thorough documentation of baseline vital signs and other presenting complaints is necessary because of the possible occurrence of cytokine release syndrome. This is manifested by the immune-mediated symptoms listed in Table 45-2.

Nursing Diagnoses

- Risk for injury to self related to the physiologic effects of the disease, overall weakness, and the adverse effects of immunosuppressants
- Risk for injury related to allergic reaction and subsequent systemic responses involving hypersensitivity reactions to immunosuppressants
- Risk for infection related to altered immune status caused by chronic disease, treatment with immunosuppressants, and the transplantation process
- Acute pain (e.g., joint and muscle aches and pain and flulike symptoms) related to adverse effects of immunosuppressant medications
- Noncompliance related to undesired adverse effects of drug treatment and lack of knowledge

Planning

▍Goals

- Patient experiences minimal complications and injuries during drug therapy.
- Patient experiences maximal comfort during drug therapy.
- Patient remains compliant with drug therapy and comes in for follow-up visits with the prescriber.
- Patient states symptoms of adverse reactions to therapy and exacerbation of illness that should be reported to the prescriber.
- Patient states the importance of reporting any signs and symptoms of allergic reactions to the nurse, prescriber, or other health care provider.

▍Outcome Criteria

- Patient states measures to help minimize unpleasant adverse effects of drug therapy, such as taking acetaminophen for fever and joint pain, reporting unusually high blood pressure readings, and engaging in relaxation therapy, massage, and biofeedback.
- Patient reports an improvement in energy levels, decrease in disease-related symptoms, increased ability to carry out activities of daily living, and overall mental status improvement.
- Patient adheres to the schedule of follow-up visits with the prescriber and other health care professionals to monitor for the therapeutic effects of immunosuppressant therapy (e.g., decreased symptomatology) as well as for any adverse effects and/or toxic reactions to the medication (e.g., myalgias, arthralgias).
- Patient notifies the prescriber immediately if fever, rash, sore throat, fatigue, or other unusual problems or symptoms develop.
- Patient states measures to implement to enhance comfort while taking immunosuppressant therapy (e.g., use of non-

aspirin analgesics, rest, biofeedback, therapeutic touch or massage, imagery, diversional activities, hypnosis).
- Patient notifies the appropriate health care personnel—or emergency medical services (EMS) personnel if in a home setting—if the patient experiences difficulty breathing, shortness of breath, flushing of the face, urticaria, rash or welts, dizziness, or syncope.
- Patient states appropriate measures to take—after contacting the prescriber and/or EMS personnel—to help alleviate the risk for further systemic symptoms of hypersensitivity, such as taking diphenhydramine or related drugs to alter allergic reaction, as ordered.

Implementation

Oral *immunosuppressants* should be taken with food to minimize gastrointestinal upset. It is also important, because of the immunosuppressed state of patients receiving immunosuppressants, that oral forms of the drugs be used whenever possible to decrease the risk for infection associated with parenteral injections and subsequent injury to the first line of defense (skin). An oral antifungal medication may be ordered to treat the oral candidiasis that may occur in these patients as a consequence of the treatment and the disease process; however, significant drug interactions may occur between the immunosuppressant and the antifungal drug, so the nurse must always check for such drug interactions. It is very important with the use of any of the immunosuppressants to be sure that supportive treatment equipment and related drugs are available in case of an anaphylactic or allergic reaction. The nurse should be aware of the high risk for such an occurrence and be constantly prepared. The use of premedication protocols involving various antihistamines and/or antiinflammatory drugs is also common.

Cyclosporine is now available in several oral formulations, but these are not to be used interchangeably. Oral solutions should not be refrigerated. Oral liquid dosage forms should be administered using a calibrated liquid measuring device. Oral solutions may be mixed in a glass container with chocolate milk, milk, or orange juice and served at room temperature. Once the solution is mixed, the nurse must make sure the patient drinks it immediately. Styrofoam containers or cups should be avoided, because the drug has been found to adhere to the inside wall of such containers.

When administered intravenously, cyclosporine should be diluted as recommended by the manufacturer and given according to standards of care and institutional policy. Cyclosporine is usually diluted with normal saline or 5% dextrose in water and infused using an intravenous infusion pump. It should be infused over the recommended time period. The patient should be monitored closely during the infusion, especially during the first 30 minutes, for any allergic reactions, as manifested by facial flushing, urticaria, wheezing, dyspnea, and rash. Vital sign values should also be recorded frequently. It is also important to monitor the patient's levels of BUN, lactate dehydrogenase, AST, and ALT closely during therapy, as ordered, to detect possible renal and hepatic impairment. Oral hygiene should be performed frequently to prevent gum problems. The prescriber will also order blood testing to confirm therapeutic serum levels of cyclosporine, and these serum drug levels should be closely monitored. Intravenously administered muromonab-CD3 is usually infused over 1 minute. When the dose is prepared, the medication must be withdrawn from the ampule through a low protein-binding 0.22-micron filter, and the filter must be detached and a new sterile needle applied after the medication is withdrawn. A premedication protocol is generally followed (see previous discussion) to help minimize reactions. Both sirolimus and tacrolimus have long half-lives, so toxicity is an added concern because of possible cumulative effects. Basiliximab and daclizumab are administered parenterally. Manufacturer guidelines regarding the type and amount of dilutional solution should be followed, and the intravenous drip should be closely monitored. Use of an intravenous infusion pump may help to ensure that the proper dose is administered. Sirolimus and tacrolimus should be administered as ordered by either the intravenous or oral route. If intravenous tacrolimus is to be discontinued and maintenance dosing needed, oral tacrolimus is usually ordered to be given 8 to 12 hours after the discontinuation of the intravenous drug. Intravenous solution should not be stored in polyvinyl chloride containers and should be administered in an appropriately designed container and tubing. Oral doses of tacrolimus should be given on an empty stomach and put in a glass container. As with cyclo-sporine, the drug should not be put in Styrofoam containers, and the patient should consume no grapefruit within 2 hours of taking the drug. Complete blood counts, liver enzyme levels, and serum potassium levels need to be monitored for the duration of therapy with these drugs as well.

Evaluation

There should be continual evaluation and reevaluation of patient goals and outcome criteria related to the nursing process and administration of *immunosuppressants*. In addition, therapeutic responses to immunosuppressants should be evaluated and may include acceptance of the transplanted organ or graft in transplant patients and improved symptoms in those with autoimmune disorders. Complete blood count; erythrocyte sedimentation rate; C-reactive protein level; liver, kidney, and cardiac function tests; pulmonary function tests; chest radiography; and analysis of T-lymphocyte surface phenotype are a few of the tests for which results may be evaluated during and after drug therapy. Evaluation for drug-specific adverse effects and toxicity (see Table 45-2) and specific therapeutic drug levels (as prescribed) should be ongoing.

PATIENT TEACHING TIPS

• Patients should understand the importance of avoiding situations that pose an increased risk of exposure to infection, such as being in crowds, malls, or movie theaters. They should also understand the importance of reporting any fever, sore throat, chills, joint pain, or fatigue to the prescriber as these may indicate infection and require immediate medical attention.
• Female patients receiving immunosuppressants should be educated about the need to use some form of contraception during treatment and for up to 12 weeks after therapy ends.
• Patients taking cyclosporine should be told to take the drug at the same time every day (as with most immunosuppressants) and, if a dose is omitted, to contact the prescriber for further instructions.
• Follow-up appointments are important because of the need to monitor patient's status through examinations and blood testing.
• Educate about the adverse effects of cyclosporine (e.g., headache, tremor) and told to avoid consumption of grapefruit or grapefruit juice because of the potential for an increase in the blood concentration of cyclosporine.
• Gelcaps should be stored in a cool, dry environment and should not be exposed to light. The dosage form should be kept in its original packaging. Also, patients should avoid prolonged exposure to the sun and should be encouraged to wear sunscreen and protective clothing when outdoors.
• Patients who are to undergo transplant surgery and who are receiving cyclosporine should know that several days before surgery they may be told to take the cyclosporine with corticosteroids, and they may also be given an oral antifungal as prophylaxis for *Candida* infections
• Patients taking oral forms of cyclosporine should be told to take the medication with meals or mixed with milk to minimize gastrointestinal upset.
• Patients taking azathioprine or muromonab-CD3 should be informed that several days before transplant surgery they should take all their medication by the oral route if possible and avoid intramuscular injection, which carries the risk for infection.
• All immunosuppressants taken at home should be taken exactly as ordered and at the same time every day. Patients should be educated about the adverse effects of the medication and should be instructed to report problems of particular concern, such as fever, chest pain, dizziness, headache, problems with urination, rash, and respiratory and/or other infections.

POINTS TO REMEMBER

• Immunosuppressants decrease or prevent the body's immune response.
• Some of the clinical uses for immunosuppressants are suppression of immune-mediated disorders, malignancies and improvement of short-term and long-term allograft survival.
• Nursing considerations include the possible need to administer oral antifungals, which are generally given with immunosuppressant medications to treat the oral candidiasis that occurs as a result of immunosuppression and fungal overgrowth. The nurse should inspect the oral cavity as often as necessary (at least once every shift) for any white patches on the tongue, mucous membranes, and/or oral pharynx. These patches may indicate oral candidiasis.
• Another nursing consideration with the immunosuppressants is the need to monitor the results of prescriber-ordered laboratory studies such as hemoglobin level, hematocrit, and white blood cell and platelet counts. Should the values drop below normal ranges, the prescriber should be notified.

NCLEX EXAMINATION REVIEW QUESTIONS

1 A patient has a new order for glatiramer acetate. The patient has not had an organ transplant. The nurse knows that the patient must be receiving this drug for which condition?
   a Rheumatoid arthritis
   b Psoriasis
   c Irritable bowel syndrome
   d Relapse-remitting multiple sclerosis
2 While assessing a patient who is to receive muromonab-CD3, the nurse knows that which condition would be a contraindication for this drug?
   a Acute myalgia
   b Fluid overload
   c Polycythemia
   d Diabetes mellitus
3 During therapy with azathioprine (Imuran), the nurse must monitor for which common adverse effect?
   a Bradycardia
   b Diarrhea
   c Thrombocytopenia
   d Vomiting
4 During a teaching session for a patient receiving an immunosuppressant drug, the nurse should include which statement?
   a "It is better to use oral forms of these drugs to prevent the occurrence of thrush."

   b "You will remain on antibiotics to prevent infections."
   c "It is important to use some form of contraception during treatment and for up to 12 weeks after the end of therapy."
   d "Be sure to take your medications with grapefruit juice to enhance its effects."
5 During drug therapy with basiliximab, the nurse monitors for signs of cytokine release syndrome, which results in
   a fever, dyspnea, and general malaise.
   b neurotoxicity and peripheral neuropathy.
   c thrombocytopenia with increased bleeding tendencies.
   d hepatotoxicity with jaundice.
6 When assessing a patient who is to begin therapy with an immunosuppressant drug, the nurse recognizes that such drugs should be used cautiously in patients with which condition(s)? (Select all that apply.)
   a Renal dysfunction
   b Glaucoma
   c Anemia
   d Hepatic dysfunction
   e Pregnancy
   f Myalgia

1. d, 2. b, 3. c, 4. c, 5. a, 6. a, d, e.

CRITICAL THINKING ACTIVITIES: BEST ACTION

1 The nurse is explaining the purpose of cyclosporine to R.S., a 58-year-old who has had a heart transplant. R.S. asks, "How does this keep my immune system from attacking my new heart?" What would be the nurse's best answer?
2 A patient is about to receive muromonab-CD3 as part of post-transplant drug therapy. As the nurse prepares to administer the drug, the physician walks in and says, "You gave the premedica-

tion, right?" The nurse knows that the most appropriate pre-medication would have been what drug, and why?
3 T.T. is on call for lung transplant surgery—she has been told the procedure could occur within the next 4 days. The surgeon writes an order that says, "Avoid injections as much as possible." A new nurse questions this order, asking, "What does Dr. S. mean by that?" What would be the nurse's best answer?

For answers, see *http://evolve.elsevier.com/Lilley.*

CHAPTER 46

Immunizing Drugs and Biochemical Terrorism

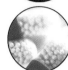

OBJECTIVES

When you reach the end of this chapter, you should be able to do the following:

1 Discuss the importance of immunity as it relates to the various immunizing drugs and their use in patients of all ages.

2 Identify the diseases that are treated or prevented with toxoids or vaccines.

3 Compare the mechanisms of action, indications, cautions, contraindications, adverse effects, toxicity, drug interactions, and routes of administration of various toxoids and vaccines.

4 Develop a nursing care plan that includes all phases of the nursing process related to the administration of immunizing drugs across the life span.

5 Develop a nursing care plan covering aspects of the nursing process related to bioterrorism, with emphasis on the nurse's role.

e-Learning Activities

http://evolve.elsevier.com/Lilley

NCLEX Review Questions • Animations • Nursing Care Plans • Audio Glossary • Category Catchers • Medication Errors Checklists • IV Therapy Checklists • Calculators • Frequently Asked Questions • Content Updates • Supplemental Resources • Answers to Case Studies and Critical Thinking Activities

Drug Profiles

- ◆ diphtheria and tetanus toxoids, and acellular pertussis vaccine tetanus (adsorbed), p. 709
  Haemophilus influenzae type b conjugate vaccine, p. 713
- ◆ hepatitis B immunoglobulin, p. 715
- ◆ hepatitis B virus vaccine (inactivated), p. 713
  herpes zoster vaccine, p. 714
  human papillomavirus vaccine, p. 714
- ◆ immunoglobulin, p. 715
- ◆ influenza virus vaccine, p. 713

- ◆ measles, mumps, and rubella virus vaccine (live), p. 713
- ◆ pneumococcal vaccine, polyvalent and seven valent, p. 714
- ◆ poliovirus vaccine (inactivated), p. 714
  rabies immunoglobulin, p. 715
  rabies virus vaccine, p. 714
  $Rh_0(D)$ immunoglobulin, p. 715
  tetanus immunoglobulin, p. 715
- ◆ varicella virus vaccine, p. 714
  varicella-zoster immunoglobulin, p. 715

◆ *Key drug.*

Glossary

Active immunization A type of immunization that causes development of a complete and long-lasting immunity to a certain infection through exposure of the body to the associated disease antigen; it can be natural active immunization (i.e., having the disease) or artificial active immunization (i.e., receiving a vaccine or toxoid). (p. 705)

Active immunizing drugs Toxoids or vaccines that are administered to a host (human or animal) to stimulate host production of antibodies. (p. 708)

Antibodies Immunoglobulin molecules that have an antigen-specific amino acid sequence and are synthesized by the humoral immune system (B cells) in response to exposure to a specific antigen (foreign substance). Their purpose is to attack and destroy molecules of this antigen. (p. 705)

Antibody titer The amount of an antibody needed to react with and neutralize a given volume or amount of a specific antigen. (p. 708)

Antigens Substances, usually proteins and foreign to a host (human or animal), that stimulate the host to produce antibodies and that react specifically with those antibodies. Examples of antigens include bacterial exotoxins and viruses. An allergen (e.g., dust, pollen, mold) is an antigen that can produce an immediate-type hypersensitivity reaction or allergy. (p. 705)

Antiserum A serum that contains antibodies. It is usually obtained from an animal that has been immunized against a specific antigen, either by injection with the antigen or by infection with specific microorganisms that produce the antigen. (p. 708)

Antitoxin An antiserum against a toxin (or toxoid). It is most often a purified antiserum obtained from animals (usually horses) by injection of a toxin or toxoid so that antibodies to the toxin (i.e., antitoxin) can be collected from the animals and used to provide artificial passive immunity to humans exposed to a given toxin (e.g., tetanus immunoglobulin). (p. 708)

Antivenin An antiserum against a venom (poison produced by an animal) used to treat humans or other animals that have been envenomed (e.g., by snakebite, spider bite, or scorpion sting). (p. 708)

Biologic antimicrobial drugs Substances of biologic origin used to prevent, treat, or cure infectious diseases (e.g., vaccines, toxoids, immunoglobulins). These drugs are often simply referred to as *biologics*. However, *biologics* also refers to drugs of bioterrorism (e.g., anthrax spores, smallpox virus), depending on the context. (p. 706)

Bioterrorism The use of infectious biologic or chemical agents as weapons for human destruction. (p. 716)

Booster shot A repeat dose of an antigen, such as a vaccine or toxoid, which is usually administered in an amount smaller than that used in the original immunization. It is given to maintain the immune response of a previously immunized patient at, or return the response to, a clinically effective level. (p. 708)

Cell-mediated immune system The immune response that is mediated by T cells (as opposed to B cells, which produce antibodies). T cells mount their immune response through activities such as the release of cytokines (chemicals that stimulate other protective immune functions; e.g., production of nasal secretions to help eliminate pathogens via the nose) as well as through direct cytotoxicity (e.g., phagocytosis of an antigen). (p. 705)

Herd immunity Resistance to a disease on the part of an entire community or population because a large proportion of its members are immune to the disease. (p. 708)

Immune response A cascade of biochemical events that occurs in response to entry into the body of an antigen (foreign substance); key processes of the immune response include phagocytosis (literally "eating of cells") of foreign microorganisms and synthesis of antibodies that react with (by chemically binding to) molecules of specific antigens to inactivate them. Immune response centers around the blood but may also involve the lymphatic system and the *reticuloendothelial system* (see later). (p. 705)

Immunization The induction of immunity by administration of a vaccine or toxoid (active immunization) or antiserum (passive immunization). (p. 706)

Immunizing biologics Toxoids, vaccines, or immunoglobulins that are targeted against specific infectious microorganisms or toxins. (p. 706)

Immunoglobulins Glycoproteins synthesized and used by the humoral immune system (B cells) to attack and kill all substances foreign to the body. The term is synonymous with *immune globulins.* (p. 705)

Passive immunization A type of immunization in which immunity to infection is conferred by bypassing the host's immune system and injecting a person with antiserum or concentrated antibodies obtained from other humans or animals that directly give the host the means to fight off an invading microorganism (artificial passive immunization). The host's immune system therefore does not have to manufacture these antibodies. This process also occurs when antibodies pass from mother to infant during breast-feeding or through the placenta during pregnancy (natural passive immunization). (p. 705)

Passive immunizing drugs Drugs containing antibodies or antitoxins that can kill or inactivate pathogens by binding to the associated antigens. These are directly injected into a person (host) and provide that person with the means to fend off infection, bypassing the host's own immune system. (p. 707)

Recombinant Relating to or containing a combination of genetic material from two or more organisms. Such genetic recombination is one of the key methods of biotechnology and is often used to manufacture immunizing drugs and various other medications. (p. 708)

Reticuloendothelial system Specialized cells located in the liver, spleen, lymphatics, and bone marrow that remove miscellaneous particles from the circulation, such as aging antibody molecules. (p. 708)

Toxin Any poison produced by a plant, animal, or microorganism that is highly toxic to other living organisms. (p. 706)

Toxoids Bacterial exotoxins that are modified or inactivated (by chemicals or heat) so that they are no longer toxic but can still bind to host B cells to stimulate the formation of antitoxin; toxoids are often used in the same manner as vaccines to promote artificial active immunity in humans. They are one type of active immunizing drug (e.g., tetanus toxoid). (p. 706)

Vaccines Suspensions of live, attenuated, or killed microorganisms that can promote an artificially induced active immunity against a particular microorganism. They are another type of active immunizing drug (e.g., tetanus vaccine). (p. 706)

Venom A poison that is secreted by an animal (e.g., snake, insect, or spider). (p. 708)

· · ·

Anatomy, Physiology, and Disease Overview

IMMUNITY AND IMMUNIZATION

Centuries ago it was noticed that people who contracted certain diseases acquired an immune tolerance to the disease so that, when exposed to it again, they did not experience a second bout of illness. This basic observation prompted scientists to investigate ways of artificially producing this tolerance. Along with this came an understanding of the way in which the normal immune system functions, knowledge important to an understanding of how immunizing drugs work. Briefly, when the body first comes into contact with **antigens** (foreign proteins) from an invading organism, specific information is imprinted into a cellular "memory bank" of the immune system. The body can then effectively fight any future invasion by that same organism by mounting an **immune response.** This cellular memory bank consists of specialized immune cells known as *memory cells.* When an antigen presents itself to a person's humoral immune system (B cells, or B lymphocytes) by binding to B cells, the B cells differentiate into two other types of cells. One type is the memory cells. The second type is known as *plasma cells,* the role of which is to produce large volumes of antibodies against the antigen in question. **Antibodies** are immunoglobulin molecules that have antigen-specific amino acid sequences. **Immunoglobulins,** or *immune globulins,* are glycoprotein molecules synthesized by the humoral immune system for the purpose of destroying all substances that the body recognizes as foreign. Immunoglobulins can be general or specific. A general immunoglobulin lacks a specific amino acid sequence that allows it to recognize a specific antigen. An immunoglobulin with such a specific amino acid sequence is known as an *antibody.* It is because of this process that people rarely suffer twice from certain diseases such as mumps, chickenpox, and measles. Instead they have a complete and long-lasting immunity to those infections.

In contrast to the humoral immune system, which is the focus of this chapter, the **cell-mediated immune system** is the branch of the immune system that does not synthesize antibodies. Instead, it is driven by T cells (T lymphocytes) and works by the release of *cytokines* (chemicals that promote other immune system functions such as inflammatory responses, runny nose, etc.) and by *phagocytosis* (engulfing and destruction of the antigens by the T cells). The cell-mediated immune system is discussed in Chapter 45, because it is the target of immunosuppressant drugs. To varying degrees, these two immune system branches work simultaneously or even interdependently. The humoral immune system is also activated and/or driven partly by cytokines from the cell-mediated immune system.

There are two ways of obtaining immunity to certain infections: **active immunization** and **passive immunization.** Each can be an artificial or natural process. In artificial active immunization, the body is clinically exposed to a relatively harmless form of an antigen that does not cause an actual infection. Information about the antigen is then imprinted into the memory of the immune system as described earlier, and the body's defenses are stimulated to resist any subsequent exposure (by producing antibodies). In contrast, natural active immunization occurs when a person acquires immunity by surviving the disease itself and

TABLE 46-1 Active Versus Passive Immunization

Characteristic	Active	Passive
Artificial		
Type of immunizing drug	Toxoid or vaccine	Immunoglobulin or antitoxin
Mechanism of action	Results from an antigen-antibody response similar to that after antigen exposure in natural disease process	Results from direct administration of exogenous antibodies; antibody concentration will decrease over time, so if reexposure is expected, it is wise to continue passive immunizations.
Use	To prevent development of active disease in the event of exposure to a given antigen in people who have at least a partially functioning immune system	To provide temporary protection against disease in people who are immunodeficient, those for whom active immunization is contraindicated, and those who have been exposed to or anticipate exposure to the organism or toxin; an antibody response is not stimulated in the host.
Natural		
Mechanism of action	Production of one's own antibodies during actual infection	Transmission of antibodies from mother to infant through placenta or during breast-feeding

producing antibodies to the disease-causing organism. Artificial passive immunization involves clinical administration of serum or concentrated immunoglobulins obtained from humans or animals, which directly gives the inoculated individual the substance needed to fight off the invading microorganism. This type of **immunization** bypasses the host's immune system. Finally, natural passive immunization occurs when antibodies are transferred from the mother to her infant in breast milk or through the bloodstream via the placenta during pregnancy. The major differences between active and passive immunization are summarized in Table 46-1 and are discussed in greater depth in the following sections.

Active Immunization

In general, **biologic antimicrobial drugs** (also referred to simply as *biologics*) are substances such as antitoxins, antisera, toxoids, and vaccines that are used to prevent, treat, or cure infectious diseases. Toxoids and vaccines are known as **immunizing biologics,** and they target a particular infectious microorganism.

Toxoids

Toxoids are substances that contain antigens, most often in the form of bacterial (usually gram-positive bacterial) exotoxins. These substances have been detoxified or weakened (attenuated) with chemicals or heat, which renders them nontoxic and unable to revert back to a toxic form. Nonetheless, they remain highly antigenic and can stimulate an artificial active immune response (production of antitoxin antibodies) when injected into a host patient. These antibodies can then neutralize the same exotoxin upon any future exposure. Toxoids were first developed in 1923 at the Pasteur Institute by Gaston Ramon and his associates, and modern versions are effective against diseases such as diphtheria and tetanus caused by **toxin**-producing bacteria.

Vaccines

Vaccines are suspensions of live, attenuated (weakened), or killed (inactivated) microorganisms that can stimulate production of antibodies against the particular organism. As with toxoids, these slight alterations in the bacteria and viruses prevent the person injected with the vaccine from contracting the disease but

are still able to promote active immunization against the organism, including an antibody response. People vaccinated with live bacteria or viruses (as well as those who recover from an actual infection) enjoy lifelong immunity against that particular disease. However, only partial immunity is conferred on those vaccinated with killed bacteria or viruses, and for this reason they must be given periodic booster shots to maintain immune system protection against infection with the given organism. One exception to this is the smallpox vaccine, because it uses live cowpox virus (vaccinia virus) instead of the more virulent smallpox virus.

Edward Jenner, an English physician born in 1749, noticed that milkmaids who had contracted cowpox infections were rarely victims of smallpox and was the first to study the relationship of cowpox to smallpox immunity. His observation led to the development of the smallpox vaccine. In 1796, Jenner successfully immunized a young boy against smallpox by vaccinating him with cowpox virus obtained from a cowpox vesicle on an infected cow. With the help of the modern version of this vaccine, smallpox was considered to be eradicated as of 1980. However, following the terrorist attacks in the United States on September 11, 2001, fears arose of a large-scale bioterrorism attack using the smallpox virus. By 2003, these fears had subsided somewhat, and the Centers for Disease Control and Prevention (CDC) released guidelines recommending routine early detection surveillance activities on the part of all public health agencies. These guidelines also included a plan for rapid vaccination of local populations in the event of a suspected smallpox outbreak and listed several high-priority high-risk groups, including direct health care personnel, who should be vaccinated first if a suspected outbreak occurs.

Today there are more than 20 infectious diseases for which vaccines are available. New vaccines appear periodically but not with the rapidity of other types of drugs, because of the complexities of developing a safe and effective vaccine. Most modern vaccines are produced in a laboratory by genetic engineering methods and contain some extract of the pathogen, or a synthetic extract, rather than the microbe itself. Some vaccines, such as influenza vaccine, may contain actual whole or split virus particles. Most, however, contain a smaller fraction of the organism, such as the bacterial capsular polysaccharides that are used to make pneumococcal vaccine. The attenuating or killing agent is usually a chemical such as formaldehyde or a physical mechanism such as heat. Attenuation may also be accomplished by repeated passage of the microbe through some medium such as a fertile hen egg or a special tissue culture. The search for new and better drugs will never end. Current goals include finding vaccines against human immunodeficiency virus infection/acquired immunodeficiency syndrome (HIV/AIDS) and malaria; the ultimate goal is to develop an effective vaccine against all infectious diseases. The currently available immunizing vaccines are listed in Box 46-1. Note that the drug given to prevent respiratory syncytial virus (RSV) infection is not an immunizing drug per se but is a specialized antiviral drug. It is discussed in Chapter 40. The RSV immunoglobulin is listed in Box 46-1. People who travel to different parts of the world may require specific vaccines. This information can be found on the CDC website at *http://www.cdc. gov/travel/contentVaccinations.aspx.*

The current childhood immunization schedule published by the CDC is available at *http://www.cdc.gov/vaccines.* This advisory is published annually as a joint effort of the American Academy of Pediatrics, the CDC's Advisory Committee on Immunization Practices, and the American Academy of Family Physicians. The CDC also posts on its website a catch-up schedule for children who may have missed scheduled immunizations. The CDC's current adult immunization schedule can be found online at *http://www.cdc.gov/nip/recs/adult-schedule.pdf.*

Passive Immunization

In passive immunization, the host's immune system is bypassed, and the person is inoculated with serum containing immunoglobulins obtained from other humans or animals. These substances give the person the means to fight off the invading organism. This is known as *artificially acquired passive immunity* and it confers temporary immunity against a particular antigen following exposure to the antigen. It differs from active immunization in that it produces a transitory (short-lived) immune state and the antibodies are already prepared for the host—the host's immune system does not have to synthesize its own antibodies. This allows for more rapid prevention or treatment of disease. Important examples include immunization with tetanus immunoglobulin, hepatitis immunoglobulin, rabies immunoglobulin, and snakebite antivenin.

Passive immunization occurs naturally between a mother and the fetus or the nursing infant when the mother passes maternal antibodies directly, either through the placenta to the fetus or through breast milk to the nursing infant. This is called *naturally acquired passive immunity.*

There are specific populations that can benefit from passive immunization but not from active immunization (Table 46-1). These are people who have been rendered immunodeficient for one reason or another (e.g., by drugs or disease) and who therefore cannot mount an immune response to a toxoid or vaccine injection because their immune system is suppressed. **Passive immunizing drugs** are also used in people who already have the given disease, especially those with diseases that are rapidly harmful or fatal, such as rabies, tetanus, and hepatitis. Because these diseases can progress rapidly, the body does not have time to mount an adequate immune defense against them before death

---

BOX 46-1   Available Immunizing Drugs

Passive Immunizing Drugs
antivenin, pit viper (Crotalidae), polyvalent
Crotalidae polyvalent immune Fab (for pit viper snakebite;
    e.g., rattlesnake, water moccasin)
antivenin, *Latrodectus mactans* (black widow spider)
antivenin, *Micrurus fulvius* (coral snake)
botulism immunoglobulin
cytomegalovirus immunoglobulin (human)
digoxin immune Fab
hepatitis B immunoglobulin
immunoglobulin, intramuscular
immunoglobulin, intravenous
lymphocyte immunoglobulin, antithymocyte globulin
rabies immunoglobulin (human)
respiratory syncytial virus immunoglobulin, intravenous (human)
$Rh_0(D)$ immunoglobulin
tetanus immunoglobulin
vaccinia immunoglobulin
varicella-zoster immunoglobulin (chickenpox/shingles)

Active Immunizing Drugs
BCG (bacille Calmette-Guérin) vaccine (tuberculosis)
diphtheria and tetanus toxoids (adsorbed)
diphtheria and tetanus toxoids, and acellular pertussis vaccine
    (adsorbed)
diphtheria and tetanus toxoids, acellular pertussis, and *Haemophilus*
    influenzae type b conjugate vaccines
diphtheria and tetanus toxoids, acellular pertussis (adsorbed),
    hepatitis B (recombinant), and inactivated poliovirus vaccine
    combined
H. influenzae type b conjugate vaccine
H. influenzae type b conjugate vaccine with hepatitis B vaccine
hepatitis A virus vaccine (inactivated)
hepatitis B virus vaccine (recombinant)
hepatitis A virus vaccine (inactivated) and hepatitis B virus vaccine
    (recombinant)
herpes zoster virus vaccine (live, attenuated)
human papillomavirus vaccine (attenuated)
influenza virus vaccine
Japanese encephalitis virus vaccine
measles virus* vaccine (live, attenuated)
measles, mumps, and rubella virus vaccine (live)
meningococcal bacterial vaccine
mumps virus vaccine (live)
pneumococcal bacterial vaccine, polyvalent
pneumococcal seven-valent conjugate vaccine
poliovirus vaccine (inactivated)
rabies virus vaccine
rubella virus vaccine (live)
rubella and mumps virus vaccine (live)
rubella, measles, and mumps virus vaccine (live)
Smallpox virus vaccine†
tetanus toxoid (fluid)
tetanus toxoid (adsorbed)
typhoid bacterial vaccine
varicella virus vaccine
yellow fever virus vaccine

*Also known as rubeola virus.
†Not currently on the U.S. market but according to the Centers for Disease Control and Prevention website may be reintroduced because of current bioterrorism threats.

occurs. The passive immunization of such individuals confers a temporary protection that is usually sufficient to keep the invading organisms from killing them, even though it does not stimulate an antibody response.

The passive immunizing drugs are divided into three groups: antitoxins, immunoglobulins, and snake and spider antivenins. An **antitoxin** is a purified **antiserum** that is usually obtained from horses inoculated with the toxin. An immunoglobulin is a concentrated preparation containing predominantly immunoglobulin G and is harvested from a large pool of blood donors. An **antivenin,** often referred to as *antivenom*, is an antiserum containing antibodies against a **venom,** which is a poison secreted by an animal such as a reptile, insect, or other arthropod (e.g., spider). Most antivenins are obtained from animals (usually horses) that have been injected with the particular venom; however, the newer ones are produced by **recombinant** technology. The serum contains immunoglobulins that can neutralize the toxic effects of the venom.

Pharmacology Overview
IMMUNIZING DRUGS

Mechanism of Action and Drug Effects

Active immunizing drugs consist of vaccines and toxoids that may be administered either orally or intramuscularly and work by stimulating the humoral immune system. This system synthesizes substances called *immunoglobulins,* of which there are five distinct types, designated as M, G, A, E, and D. These immunoglobulins attack and kill the foreign substances that invade the body. In this case these foreign substances are called *antigens,* and the immunoglobulins are called *antibodies.*

Vaccines contain substances that trigger the formation of these antibodies against specific pathogens. Sometimes these substances are the actual live or attenuated (weakened) pathogen or a killed pathogen. The amount of antibodies they cause to be produced can be measured in the blood. The **antibody titer** is a measure of how many antibodies to a given antigen are present in the blood and is used to assess whether enough antibodies are present to protect the body effectively against the particular pathogen. Sometimes the antibody levels decline over time. When this happens, another dose of the vaccine is given to restore the antibody titers to a level that can protect the person against the infection. This repeat dose is referred to as a **booster shot.** Toxoids are altered forms of bacterial toxins that stimulate the production of antibodies in the same way as vaccines.

Because both toxoids and vaccines rely on the immunized host to mount an immune response, the host's immune system must be intact. Therefore, patients who are immunocompromised (i.e., who cannot mount an immune response), such as those undergoing immunosuppressive cancer chemotherapy, those receiving immunosuppressive therapy to prevent the rejection of transplanted organs, and those with immunosuppressive diseases such as AIDS, may not benefit from receiving vaccines or toxoids. Instead, their clinical situations may warrant giving them passive immunizing drugs such as immunoglobulins.

Passive immunizing drugs are the actual antibodies (immunoglobulins) that can kill or inactivate the pathogen. The process is called *passive* because the person's immune system does not participate in the synthesis of antibodies; instead, the antibodies are provided by the immunizing drug. As noted earlier, immunity acquired in this way generally lasts for a much shorter time than that produced by active immunization. Passive immunization lasts only until the injected immunoglobulins are removed from the person's immune system by the **reticuloendothelial system.** The reticuloendothelial system is composed of specialized cells in the liver, spleen, lymphatics, and bone marrow.

Indications

Vaccines and toxoids are active immunizing drugs that have been developed for the prevention of many illnesses caused by bacteria and their toxins, as well as those caused by various viruses. Antivenins, antitoxins, and immunoglobulins are passive immunizing drugs. Such drugs can inactivate spider and snake venom, bacterial toxins (exotoxins), and potentially lethal viruses. Box 46-1 lists the currently available immunizing drugs. The successful immunization of 95% or more of a population confers protection on the entire population. This is called **herd immunity.**

Antivenins, also known as *antisera,* are used to prevent or minimize the effects of poisoning by the venoms of crotalids (rattlesnakes, copperheads, cottonmouths, water moccasins), black widow spiders, and coral snakes, some of which can be lethal. Most healthy adults do not die from the bites of spiders or snakes if they receive prompt and appropriate treatment (i.e., administration of the appropriate antivenin). However, very young children and older persons with health problems are particularly susceptible to the effects of the venom of some of these animals. In either situation, an antivenin is needed to neutralize the venom.

Contraindications

Contraindications to the administration of immunizing drugs include allergy to the immunization itself or allergy to any of its components, such as eggs or yeast. In the case of a potentially fatal illness such as rabies, the drug may still need to be given and any allergic reaction controlled with other medications. Administration of some immunizing drugs is best deferred until after recovery from a febrile illness or temporary immunocompromised state (e.g., following cancer chemotherapy), if possible. However, this is often a matter of clinical judgment, and the individual patient's condition and risk factors for serious illness may be arguments for or against administration of a given immunizing drug at a given time.

Adverse Effects

The undesirable effects of the various immunizing drugs can range from mild and transient to serious and even life threatening. These are listed in Table 46-2. Minor reactions can be treated with acetaminophen and rest. More severe reactions, such as fever higher than 103° F (39.4° C), should be treated with acetaminophen and sponge baths. Serum sickness sometimes occurs after repeated injections of equine (horse)–derived immunizing drugs. The signs and symptoms consist of edema of the face, tongue, and throat; rash; urticaria; arthritis; adenopathy; fever; flushing; itching; cough; dyspnea; cyanosis; vomiting; and cardiovascular collapse. Serum sickness is best treated with analgesics, antihistamines, epinephrine, and/or corticosteroids. In these cases hospitalization may be required.

TABLE 46-2 Immunizing Drugs: Minor and Severe Adverse Effects

Body System	Adverse Effects
Minor Effects	
Central nervous	Fever, adenopathy
Integumentary	Minor rash, soreness at injection site, urticaria, arthritis
Severe Effects	
Central nervous	Fever higher than 103° F (39.4° C), encephalitis, convulsions, peripheral neuropathy, anaphylactic reaction, shock, unconsciousness
Integumentary	Urticaria, rash
Respiratory	Dyspnea
Other	Cyanosis

Any serious or unusual reactions to immunizing drugs should be reported to the Vaccine Adverse Event Reporting System (VAERS). This is a national vaccine safety surveillance program that is cosponsored by the Food and Drug Administration (FDA) and the CDC. A report can be submitted via the toll-free telephone number 800-822-7967. Alternatively, a reporting form can be printed from the website of either the FDA *(http://www.fda.gov)* or the CDC *(http://www.cdc.gov)*. These websites have extensive information describing this reporting system and the data collected by it. Such data are used to improve the quality of immunizing drugs and can even be grounds for an FDA recall of biologic drugs whose adverse effects exceed acceptable safety thresholds.

In the early 1980s, in response to vaccine-related injuries, many parents became reluctant to immunize their children against common, and even potentially fatal, childhood illnesses. Increasing numbers of legal actions were also brought by parents of injured children. In 1986, the U.S. Congress passed the Childhood Vaccine Injury Act, which in turn established the National Vaccine Injury Compensation Program (VICP). The purpose was to create a no-fault alternative to the civil tort system, which had driven many vaccine manufacturers out of the field. Serious adverse events following vaccination are very uncommon. The Vaccine Injury Table published in 2005 by the Health Resources and Services Administration itemizes serious adverse events reported for vaccines that are covered under the VICP, as well as the expected time frame for such events to occur. The first symptom must appear within the listed time frame (Table 46-3) for it to be presumed to be caused by the vaccine. This table was updated in 2007. For more information, the reader is referred to *http://www.hrsa.gov/Vaccinecompensation/table.htm.* There continues to be controversy in the national news pertaining to the link between immunizations and autism in children. It is thought that thimerosal (a mercury-containing preservative used in vaccines) may have been a causative link, so since 2001 thimerosal has no longer been used in the preparation of vaccines.

Interactions

Drug interactions are not generally a problem with the majority of immunizing drugs, because they are normally given in a single dose or a relatively small number of doses. One drug class of note that can potentially reduce the efficacy of immunizing drugs is immunosuppressive drugs, including corticosteroids (see Chapter 33), transplant antirejection drugs (see Chapter 45), and cancer chemotherapy drugs (see Chapters 47 and 48). All of these drugs can, to varying degrees, hinder the generation of the active immunity that would normally occur following vaccine or toxoid administration. The bacille Calmette-Guérin vaccine for tuberculosis (used mostly outside the United States in developing countries) can cause false-positive results on the tuberculin skin test (see Chapter 41). Some vaccines should not be given close in time to one other. For example, the meningococcal vaccine, whole-cell pertussis vaccine, and typhoid vaccine together have an undesirably large bacterial endotoxin content and should not be administered simultaneously. The effectiveness of measles, mumps, and rubella vaccines may be reduced by concurrent interferon therapy (see Chapter 49). Influenza vaccine may also theoretically lose efficacy if given while antiviral influenza drugs are being taken (see Chapter 40). Recommendations are to give the influenza vaccine at least 48 hours after stopping such antiviral drug therapy. In general, immunizations requiring intramuscular injection should be given with particular caution (and with appropriate monitoring) to patients receiving anticoagulant drugs such as warfarin (see Chapter 28). The nurse should review the package insert for any immunizing drugs given to obtain the latest information and identify other specific drug interactions that may occur. Hepatitis B immunoglobulin interacts with live vaccines; administration of such vaccines should be deferred until 3 months after the dose of immunoglobulin is given.

Dosages

For the recommended dosages of selected immunizing drugs, see the Dosages table on p. 711.

DRUG PROFILES

Some of the more commonly used vaccines, toxoids, and immunoglobulins are described in the following sections. The immunizing drugs currently available commercially in the United States, including several combination vaccines for prevention of more than one disease, are listed in Box 46-1. Combination vaccines obviously reduce the number of injections that the patient receives, and thus their use is desirable when possible, especially in children.

ACTIVE IMMUNIZING DRUGS
diphtheria and tetanus toxoids, and acellular pertussis vaccine (adsorbed)

The active immunizing drugs include diphtheria and tetanus toxoids and the acellular pertussis vaccine (adsorbed) (Tripedia, Daptacel, Infanrix). *Adsorption* refers to the laboratory techniques used to make most vaccines and toxoids. The biologic materials (i.e., virus or toxin particles) are adsorbed (separated out of solution and dried) onto carrier media such as alum, from which they are later removed for packaging into final dosage forms. Diphtheria, tetanus, and pertussis are very different disorders, but an injection that combines all three vaccines (DTP; also commonly called DPT) was been routinely given to children since the 1940s. In 1996, a new vaccine combination called *diphtheria and tetanus toxoids with acellular* pertussis vaccine (adsorbed) (DTaP) was approved for the full childhood immunization series and has replaced DPT. It uses a different form of the pertussis component, known as *acellular pertussis.* Acellular pertussis consists of only a

TABLE 46-3 U.S. Department of Health and Human Services Vaccine Injury Table

Vaccine	Adverse Event	Time Interval
Tetanus toxoid–containing vaccines (e.g., DTaP, Tdap, DTP-Hib, DT, Td, TT)	Anaphylaxis or anaphylactic shock	0-4 hr
	Brachial neuritis	2-28 days
	Any acute complication or sequela (including death) of above events	NA
Pertussis antigen–containing vaccines (e.g., DTaP, Tdap, DTP, P, DTP-Hib)	Anaphylaxis or anaphylactic shock	0-4 hr
	Encephalopathy (or encephalitis)	0-72 hr
	Any acute complication or sequela (including death) of above events	NA
Measles, mumps, and rubella virus–containing vaccines in any combination (e.g., MMR, MR, M, R)	Anaphylaxis or anaphylactic shock	0-4 hr
	Encephalopathy (or encephalitis)	5-15 days
	Any acute complication or sequela (including death) of above events	NA
Rubella virus–containing vaccines (e.g., MMR, MR, R)	Chronic arthritis	7-42 days
	Any acute complication or sequela (including death) of above event	NA
Measles virus–containing vaccines (e.g., MMR, MR, M)	Thrombocytopenic purpura	7-30 days
	Vaccine-strain measles viral infection in an immunodeficient recipient	0-6 mo
	Any acute complication or sequela (including death) of above events	NA
Polio live virus–containing vaccines (OPV)	Paralytic polio	
	In a nonimmunodeficient recipient	0-30 days
	In an immunodeficient recipient	0-6 mo
	In a vaccine-associated community case	NA
	Vaccine-strain polio viral infection	
	In a nonimmunodeficient recipient	0-30 days
	In an immunodeficient recipient	0-6 mo
	In a vaccine-associated community case	NA
	Any acute complication or sequela (including death) of above events	NA
Polio inactivated virus–containing vaccines (e.g., IPV)	Anaphylaxis or anaphylactic shock	0-4 hr
	Any acute complication or sequela (including death) of above event	NA
Hepatitis B antigen–containing vaccines	Anaphylaxis or anaphylactic shock	0-4 hr
	Any acute complication or sequela (including death) of above event	NA
Haemophilus influenzae type b polysaccharide conjugate vaccines	No condition specified for compensation	NA
Varicella vaccine	No condition specified for compensation	NA
Rotavirus vaccine	No condition specified for compensation	NA
Vaccines containing live, oral, rhesus-based rotavirus	Intussusception	0-30 days
	Any acute complication or sequela (including death) of above event	NA
Pneumococcal conjugate vaccines	No condition specified for compensation	NA
Any new vaccine recommended by the Centers for Disease Control and Prevention for routine administration to children, after publication by the Secretary of DHHS of a notice of coverage*	No condition specified for compensation	NA

From Health Resources and Services Administration: *National vaccine injury compensation program fact sheet*, Atlanta, 2005, The Administration.
DHHS, Department of Health and Human Services; *DT*, diphtheria and tetanus vaccine; *DTaP*, diphtheria, tetanus, and acellular pertussis vaccine; *DTP*, diphtheria, tetanus, and pertussis vaccine; *Hib, Haemophilus influenzae* type b conjugate vaccine; *IPV*, inactivated poliovirus; *M*, measles vaccine; *MMR*, measles, mumps, and rubella vaccine; *MR*, measles and rubella vaccine; *NA*, not applicable; *OPV*, oral polio vaccine; *P*, pertussis vaccine; *R*, rubella vaccine; *Td*, tetanus and diphtheria toxoids; *Tdap*, tetanus and diphtheria toxoids and acellular pertussis vaccine; *TT*, tetanus toxoid.
*As of December 1, 2004, hepatitis A vaccines have been added to the Vaccine Injury Table under this category. As of July 1, 2005, *trivalent* influenza vaccines have been added to the table under this category. Trivalent influenza vaccines are given annually during the flu season either by needle and syringe or in a nasal spray. All influenza vaccines routinely administered in the United States are trivalent vaccines covered under this category. See "News" on the National Vaccine Injury Compensation Program website *(http://www.hrsa.gov/vaccinecompensation)* for more information.

DOSAGES

Selected Immunizing Drugs

Drug (Pregnancy Category)	Pharmacologic Class	Usual Dosage Range*	Indications/Uses
Active Immunizing Drugs			
diphtheria, tetanus, and acellular pertussis vaccine (DTaP) only) (Adacel)	Mixed toxoid/vaccine	**Pediatric only** IM: Series of three 0.5-mL injections; age of first injection 6 wk-7 yr; give second and third doses at 4-8 wk intervals	Prophylaxis against diphtheria, tetanus, and pertussis
Haemophilus influenzae type b conjugate vaccine (HibTITER) (C)	Bacterial capsular antigenic extract vaccine	**Pediatric** **Infant 2-6 mo** Give three IM injections (0.5 mL each) about 2 mo apart **Previously unvaccinated child 7-11 mo** Give two IM injections about 2 mo apart **Previously unvaccinated child 12-14 mo** Give only one IM injection	*H. influenzae* type b prophylaxis
◆ hepatitis B virus vaccine, inactivated (Recombivax HB) (C)	Viral surface antigen vaccine	**Pediatric to age 10 yr** IM: 5 mcg (0.5 mL) at birth, then again at 1 mo and 6 mo **Adult** IM: Three 10-mcg (1-mL) doses: day 0, 1 mo, and 6 mo	Hepatitis B virus prophylaxis
◆ influenza virus vaccine (Fluzone, FluShield, Fluvirin) (C)	Viral surface antigen vaccine	**Pediatric 6 mo-9 yr** IM: Single yearly dose (two doses of 0.25 mL at least 1 mo apart if receiving influenza vaccine for first time) **Adult** IM: Single yearly dose (0.5 mL)	Influenza prophylaxis
◆ measles, mumps, and rubella virus vaccine, live (M-M-R II)	Live, attenuated viral vaccine	**Adult and pediatric older than 12 mo** Subcut: 0.5-mL single dose; booster recommended for children entering middle or high school	Prophylaxis against measles, mumps, and rubella
◆ pneumococcal vaccine, polyvalent (Pneumovax 23) (C)	Bacterial capsular antigenic extract vaccine	**Adult and pediatric 2 yr and older** Subcut: 0.5 mL × 1	*Streptococcus pneumoniae* prophylaxis
◆ poliovirus vaccine, inactivated (IPOL) (C)	Inactivated viral vaccine	**Pediatric (infant)** Subcut: Three 0.5-mL doses: 4-8 wk, 2-4 mo, and 6-12 mo **Adult** Subcut: Two 0.5-mL doses 1-2 mo apart, then a third dose 6-12 mo later	Polio prophylaxis
rabies virus vaccine (Imovax, RabAvert) (C)	Inactivated viral vaccine	**Adult and pediatric** *Postexposure prophylaxis* IM: 1 mL on days 0, 3, 7, 14, and 28 (with one dose of rabies immunoglobulin [see later] within 8 days of first vaccine dose) *Preexposure prophylaxis for those at high risk for rabies exposure (e.g., veterinarians)* IM/ID: 1 mL IM or 0.1 mL ID on days 0, 7, and once between days 21 and 28, for a total of three doses; then q2-5yr, depending on antibody titers	Rabies prophylaxis

ID, Intradermal; *IM,* intramuscular; *subcut,* subcutaneous.
*Note: Dosages given are only for brands listed. Dosing amounts and regimens may vary for different brands. The user should always follow manufacturer's current dosing directions.

Continued

DOSAGES

Selected Immunizing Drugs—cont'd

Drug (Pregnancy Category)	Pharmacologic Class	Usual Dosage Range*	Indications/Uses
tetanus and diphtheria toxoids, adsorbed (Td), (Decavac) (C)	Mixed toxoid	**Adult and unvaccinated pediatric older than 7 yr** IM: 0.5 mL on day 0; second dose 4-8 wk later; third dose 6-12 mo later	Prophylaxis against diphtheria and tetanus
◆ varicella virus vaccine (Varivax) (C)	Live, attenuated viral vaccine	**Adult and pediatric older than 12 yr** Subcut: Two 0.5-mL doses given 4-8 wk apart **Pediatric 1-12 yr** Subcut: One 0.5-mL dose	Prophylaxis against varicella virus (causes chickenpox and shingles)
Passive Immunizing Drugs			
◆ hepatitis B immunoglobulin (BayHep B, Nabi-HB) (C)	Pooled human immunoglobulin	**Infant (of mother known to be hepatitis B positive)** IM: 0.5 mL within 12 hr after birth **Adult** IM: 0.06 mg/kg after exposure and 30 days later	Passive hepatitis B prophylaxis
◆ immunoglobulin intravenous (Gammar-P IV, Panglobulin NF, others) (C)	Pooled human immunoglobulin	Dosages vary widely; refer to manufacturer's current dosage information for specific indications	Therapy for many disorders, including primary immune deficiency syndrome, pediatric AIDS, idiopathic thrombocytopenic purpura, B-cell lymphocytic leukemia
rabies immunoglobulin (Imogam, Rabies-HT, BayRab) (C)	Pooled human immunoglobulin	**Adult and pediatric** Single dose of 20 IU/kg; infiltrate as much of dose as possible into bite wound area and give remainder IM in gluteal region; do not give into same site as rabies vaccine	Rabies prophylaxis
Rh₀(D) immunoglobulin (RhoGAM, MICRhoGAM) (C)	Immunosuppressant globulin	**Adult female** IM (full dose): Inject total contents of a single vial within 72 hr after delivery IM (microdose): Inject full contents of a single vial after spontaneous or elective abortion of pregnancy of 12 wk gestation or less	Postpartum antibody suppression to prevent hemolytic disease of future newborns
tetanus immunoglobulin (BayTet) (C)	Pooled human immunoglobulin	**Adult and pediatric** IM: 250 units as a single dose IM: 3000-6000 units as a single dose	Postexposure tetanus prophylaxis Tetanus treatment

AIDS, Acquired immunodeficiency syndrome.

single weakened toxoid, whereas previous pertussis vaccines contained multiple toxoids; this may reduce the number of adverse effects seen from DTP. Currently DTaP is the preferred preparation for primary and booster immunization against these diseases in children from 6 weeks to 6 years of age, unless use of the pertussis component is contraindicated.

Tetanus, diphtheria, and pertussis are prevalent in the populations of many developing countries throughout the world. Full immunization against these diseases with DTP or DTaP is recommended for travelers to these areas and as well as for their inhabitants. A combination product containing only tetanus and diphtheria toxoids (Td) is administered to persons 7 years of age and older who require a primary or booster immunization against teta-

nus for routine wound management. Booster doses should be given approximately every 10 years. Emergency booster doses of Td (for adult use) are unnecessary when the wound is clean and minor (not tetanus prone), provided that the patient has received a primary or booster immunization against tetanus within the previous 10 years.

Pertussis (whooping cough) is much less common in children older than 7 years of age and in adults. The Td combination (adsorbed) is generally given to children 7 years of age and older and to adults with functioning immune systems. However, there is recent evidence that pertussis is actually recurring among adults (whose previous vaccine-induced immunity has waned), who in turn are passing it on to their children. Cases of pertussis tripled between 2001 and 2004. It is recommended that patients between the ages of 11 and 64 get booster doses, especially if they are in regular contact with newborns.

These toxoids (DTP, DTaP, and Td) are available only as parenteral preparations to be given as deep intramuscular injections. Their use is contraindicated in persons who have had a prior systemic hypersensitivity reaction or a neurologic reaction to one of the ingredients. Some manufacturers state that use is contraindicated in cases of concurrent acute or active infections but not in cases of minor illness. Although there have been very few studies, if any, documenting the safety of their use in pregnant women, it is generally considered safe to give diphtheria, tetanus, and pertussis toxoids after the first trimester.

Haemophilus Influenzae type b conjugate vaccine
Haemophilus influenzae type b (Hib) (HibTITER, ActHIB, Liquid PedvaxHIB) vaccine is a noninfectious, bacteria-derived vaccine. It is made by extracting *H. influenzae* particles that are antigenic and chemically attaching these particles to a protein carrier medium for use in injections. The vaccine is given by injection to adults and children considered at high risk for acquiring *H. influenzae* infection. Conditions that may predispose an individual to Hib infection are septicemia, pneumonia, cellulitis, arthritis, osteomyelitis, pericarditis, sickle cell anemia, an immunodeficiency syndrome, and Hodgkin's disease. Before this vaccine was developed, infections caused by Hib were the leading cause of bacterial meningitis in children 3 months to 5 years of age. This form of bacterial meningitis has a mortality rate of 5% to 10%. Of those who survive, 20% to 45% suffer serious morbidity in the form of neurologic deficits. All Hib vaccine products are parenteral formulations that are administered intramuscularly.

◆ hepatitis B virus vaccine (inactivated)
Hepatitis B virus vaccine (inactivated) (Recombivax HB, Engerix-B) is a noninfectious viral vaccine containing hepatitis B surface antigen (HBsAg). It is made from viral particles and yeast using recombinant DNA technology. In this technique, DNA from two or more organisms is combined. Yeast cells then produces this viral antigenic substance in mass quantities. The substance is then attached to a carrier medium (alum) and made into a vaccine injection preparation. This antigenic HBsAg is used to promote active immunity to hepatitis B infection in persons considered at high risk for potential exposure to the hepatitis B virus or HBsAg-positive materials (e.g., blood, plasma, serum). Health care workers, for example, are persons considered at high risk, and many hospitals require this vaccination.

Use of the vaccine is contraindicated in persons who are hypersensitive to yeast. Pregnancy is not considered a contraindication to use. The vaccine is administered by intramuscular injection and is given as a series of three injections. There are three main formulations designed for three different populations: a pediatric formulation for neonates, infants, children, and adolescents; an adult formulation for persons older than 20 years of age; and a dialysis formulation for predialysis and dialysis patients and for other immunocompromised individuals.

◆ influenza virus vaccine
The influenza virus vaccine (Fluzone, Fluvirin, FluMist) is the vaccine used to prevent influenza. Each year before the influenza season begins this vaccine should be administered to persons at high risk of contracting influenza. Such inoculation is the single most important influenza control measure. FluMist is given intranasally, whereas the others are given intramuscularly.

Each year a new influenza vaccine is developed by virology researchers. It usually contains three different influenza virus strains (usually two type A and one type B strain). These strains are chosen from among the hundreds of influenza virus strains in the environment based on the latest epidemiologic data indicating which influenza viruses will most likely circulate in North America in the upcoming winter. The vaccine is made from highly purified, egg-grown viruses that have been rendered noninfectious (inactivated). Influenza is characterized by abrupt onset of fever, myalgia, sore throat, and nonproductive cough. Severe malaise may last several days. More severe illness can occur in certain populations. Older individuals, children, and adults with underlying serious health problems (e.g., HIV infection, asthma, cardiopulmonary disease, cancer, diabetes) are at increased risk for complications from influenza infection. Health care personnel are also considered a high-risk group. Increased mortality results not only from influenza and pneumonia but also from cardiopulmonary and other chronic diseases that can be exacerbated by influenza. More than 90% of the deaths attributed to pneumonia and influenza occur among persons 65 years of age or older. Another fairly unusual but important risk group is children and teenagers who are receiving long-term aspirin therapy (e.g., for juvenile arthritis) and who therefore might be at risk for developing Reye's syndrome after influenza (see Chapter 44).

The effectiveness of influenza vaccine in preventing illness varies. Factors that may alter its effectiveness are the age and immunocompetence of the vaccine recipient and the degree of similarity between the virus strains included in the vaccine and those that actually predominate during a given influenza season. Healthy persons younger than 65 years of age have a 70% chance of avoiding illness caused by influenza virus when there is a good match between the vaccine and the circulating viruses.

Older persons, especially those residing in nursing homes, can avoid severe illness, secondary complications, and death by taking the influenza vaccine. In frail older persons, the vaccine can prevent hospitalization and pneumonia up to 50% to 60% of the time and death up to 80% of the time. Achieving a high rate of vaccination among nursing home residents can reduce the spread of infection in a facility, thus preventing disease through herd immunity. The CDC now recommends that children aged 5 to 18 years, as well as all children at high risk (i.e., immunosuppressed children) receive the influenza vaccine.

◆ measles, mumps, and rubella virus vaccine (live)
The measles, mumps, and rubella vaccine (M-M-R II) is a virus preparation consisting of live measles, mumps, and rubella viruses that are weakened (attenuated). The vaccine promotes active immunity to these diseases by inducing the production of virus-specific immunoglobulin G and immunoglobulin M antibodies. The antibody response to initial vaccination resembles that caused by primary natural infection.

Administration of the measles vaccine or any of the combination products that includes the measles virus is contraindicated in persons with a history of anaphylactic or anaphylactoid reaction, or some other immediate reaction to egg ingestion. Use of these products is also contraindicated in persons who have had an anaphylactic reaction to topically or systemically administered neomycin, because this antibiotic is used as a preservative in some of the vaccine preparations. These vaccines should not be administered to pregnant women, and pregnancy should be avoided for 3 months after measles virus vaccination and 30 days after vaccination with a rubella-containing (measles-rubella or measles-mumps-rubella [MMR]) measles virus vaccine. This precaution is based on the theoretic risk that the live virus vaccine may cause a fetal infection.

◆ pneumococcal vaccine, polyvalent and seven valent

Two forms of vaccine against pneumococcal pneumonia are available that also protect against any illness caused by *Streptococcus pneumoniae. Pneumococcus* is the common name for the bacterium *S. pneumoniae,* the causative organism of this common bacterial infection. The polyvalent type of vaccine (Pneumovax 23) is used primarily in adults. (The term *polyvalent* refers to the fact that the vaccine is designed to be effective against the 23 strains of pneumococcus most commonly implicated in adult cases of pneumonia.) This vaccine also may sometimes be recommended for pediatric patients at higher risk for pneumonia as a result of serious chronic illnesses, especially those who are immunocompromised. However, the seven-valent vaccine is the pneumococcal vaccine that is routinely recommended for children. Its official full name is *seven-valent conjugate vaccine* (diphtheria CRM197 protein, or Prevnar). The name *seven-valent* refers to the fact that the vaccine is designed to immunize against the top seven pneumococcal strains found in pediatric pneumonia cases. In 2008, the CDC recommended that all smokers aged 19 to 64 years receive the pneumococcal vaccine. Contraindications to the use of either vaccine include known drug allergy to components of the vaccine itself, as well as the presence of current significant febrile illness or immunosuppressed state as a result of drug therapy (e.g., cancer chemotherapy). The vaccine may sometimes still be given in such cases, if it is felt that withholding the vaccine poses an even greater risk to the patient.

◆ poliovirus vaccine (inactivated)

The use of live oral polio vaccine (OPV) is no longer routine in the United States, due to case reports of vaccine-acquired polio. Since 1979 the only indigenous cases of poliomyelitis reported in the United States (44 cases) have been associated with use of the live OPV. Injected doses of inactivated polio vaccine (brand name, IPOL) are instead recommended for routine use. The use of OPV should be reserved for the following groups: populations that are the target of mass vaccination campaigns to control outbreaks of paralytic polio, unvaccinated children who will be traveling in fewer than 4 weeks to areas in which polio is endemic, and children of parents who object to the recommended number of IPV injections.

rabies virus vaccine

Although vaccination against the rabies virus is not normally a routine immunization, situations requiring it occur periodically in many practice settings. Rabies virus vaccine (Imovax, RabAvert) is produced using laboratory techniques involving infected human cell cultures and selected antimicrobial drugs. Rabies is a virus that can infect a variety of mammals, including skunks, foxes, raccoons, bats, dogs, and cats. The virus is usually transferred to humans by an animal bite and almost universally causes fatal brain tissue destruction if the patient is not treated with rabies vaccine and immunoglobulin (discussed later). Current recommendations call for a total of five intramuscular injections on days 0, 3, 7, 14, and 28 following an animal bite that raises concern for rabies transmission. This includes a bite by any animal whose rabies immunization status is unknown or which escapes and cannot be observed for signs of rabies. This type of treatment is known as *postexposure prophylaxis. Preexposure prophylaxis* is recommended for persons at high risk for exposure to the rabies virus (e.g., veterinarians). The preexposure course consists of only three injections on day 0, day 7, and sometime between days 21 and 28. Periodic booster shots are also recommended for such individuals approximately every 2 to 5 years, or based on the levels of the patient's rabies virus antibody titers. Patients who have been previously immunized who have a new bite may need only two booster shots on days 0 and 3. Contraindications to the administration of rabies vaccine include a history of allergic reaction to the vaccine itself or to the drugs neomycin, gentamicin, or amphotericin B. However, given the life-threatening nature of rabies infection, treatment may still be required, with supportive therapy (e.g., epinephrine, diphenhydramine, corticosteroids) provided to minimize allergic reactions. Patients with any kind of febrile illness should delay occupational preexposure prophylaxis treatment until the illness has subsided.

human papillomavirus vaccine

The papillomavirus vaccine (Gardasil) is the first and only vaccine known to prevent cancer. Human Papillomavirus Virus (HPV) is a common cause of genital warts and cervical cancer. The vaccine is recommended for all girls aged 11 and 12 and for women aged 13 to 26 years who have not yet been vaccinated. Genital HPV is a common virus that is transmitted through genital contact, most often during sex. Most sexually active people will get HPV at some time in their lives, although most will never even know it. It is most common in people in their late teens and early twenties. Every year, about 12,000 women are diagnosed with cervical cancer and almost 4000 women die from this disease in the United States.

HPV vaccine protects against four types of HPV: two types known to cause 70% of reported cervical cancers and two types known to cause 90% of genital warts. The vaccine is given in three injections—the first dose, then two more doses 2 months and 6 months later. It is contraindicated in patients who show hypersensitivity to yeast or to their first injection of the vaccine. The HPV vaccine is not recommended for pregnant patients, because appropriate studies have not been completed. Pain on injection is common.

herpes zoster vaccine

Zoster vaccine (Zostavax) is a newly released vaccine (first available in 2008) for the prevention of herpes zoster. Herpes zoster, also known as *shingles,* is an extremely painful condition caused by the varicella-zoster virus that also causes chickenpox. The vaccine is recommended for patients 60 years or older to prevent reactivation of the zoster virus that causes shingles. It is a one-time vaccine. The vaccine does not prevent postherpetic neuralgia. It can be given to patients who have already had shingles. Herpes zoster virus vaccine is a live attenuated vaccine. Its use is contraindicated in patients with hypersensitivity to neomycin, gelatin, or any component of the vaccine. It is also contraindicated in immunosuppressed patients or those receiving immunosuppressant therapy, as well as in pregnant women. Because it is a live vaccine, there is a risk of transmission of the virus from the person who is vaccinated to other people. The vaccine is not to be used for the prevention of chickenpox and should not be given to children. The drug must be stored in the freezer.

◆ varicella virus vaccine

The live attenuated varicella virus vaccine (Varivax) is used to prevent varicella (chickenpox). Varicella primarily occurs in children younger than 8 years of age or in individuals with compromised immune systems such as the elderly or HIV-infected patients. It is estimated that only 10% of children older than 12 years of age are still susceptible to varicella. Only 2% of adults develop varicella-zoster virus infections. However, 50% of the deaths associated with varicella are in adults. Half of these are in immunocompromised patients.

The virus in varicella vaccine is attenuated by the passage of virus particles through human and embryonic guinea pig cell cultures. Varicella vaccine must be stored in a freezer. It should not be given to immunodeficient patients or to patients who have received high doses of systemic steroids in the previous month. It is also recommended that salicylates be avoided for 6 weeks after administration of varicella vaccine because of the possibility of Reye's syndrome (see Chapter 44). The varicella vaccine should be given at 12 months of age and then a second dose should be given at age 4 to 6 years. All patients need to receive a second dose.

PASSIVE IMMUNIZING DRUGS
The currently available antivenins, antitoxins, and immunoglobulins that comprise the passive immunizing drugs are listed in Box 46-1. Those that are more commonly used are described in the following profiles.

◆ hepatitis B immunoglobulin
Hepatitis B immunoglobulin (BayHep B, Nabi-HB) is used to provide passive immunity against hepatitis B infection in the postexposure prophylaxis and treatment of persons exposed to hepatitis B virus or HBsAg-positive materials (e.g., blood, plasma, serum). It is prepared from the plasma of human donors with high titers of antibodies to HBsAg. All donors are tested for HIV antibodies to prevent HIV transmission.

Because of the possible devastating consequences of hepatitis B infection, pregnancy is not considered a contraindication to the use of hepatitis B immunoglobulin when there is a clear need for it.

◆ immunoglobulin
Immunoglobulin (BayGam, Octagam) is available in both intramuscular and intravenous dosage forms. It provides passive immunity by increasing antibody titer and antigen-antibody reaction potential. Immunoglobulins are given to help prevent certain infectious diseases in susceptible persons or to ameliorate the diseases in those already infected. Immunoglobulins are pooled from the blood of at least 1000 human donors. This plasma is prepared by cold alcohol fractionation and usually washed with a detergent to destroy any harmful viruses, such as hepatitis virus or HIV. There are many FDA-approved and non–FDA-approved uses for immunoglobulins; the approved uses are listed in Box 46-2. In recent years there has been a shortage of immunoglobulin products. The supply of these drugs is dependent on donors. Because of fluctuations in supply and the unfavorable risk/benefit ratio of using products derived from human donors, product insurers have restricted reimbursement to force practitioners to administer the drugs for FDA-approved indications only. "Off-label" or non–FDA-approved uses have been severely curtailed because of such restrictions as well as because of product shortages.

BOX 46-2   Current FDA-Approved Indications for Immunoglobulins*

Pediatric HIV infection
B-cell chronic lymphocytic leukemia
Bone marrow transplantation
Hepatitis A
Idiopathic thrombocytopenic purpura
Kawasaki disease
Immunoglobulin deficiencies
Measles
Primary immunodeficiency diseases
Rubella
Varicella

FDA, Food and Drug Administration; *HIV,* human immunodeficiency virus.
*Approved routes of administration are intramuscular and intravenous.

Rh₀(D) immunoglobulin
Rh$_0$(D) immunoglobulin (RhoGAM, WinRho) is used to suppress the active antibody response and the formation of anti-Rh$_0$(D) antibodies in an Rh$_0$(D)-negative person exposed to Rh-positive blood. Because an Rh$_0$(D)-negative person reacts to Rh-positive blood as if it were a foreign, "nonself" substance, an immune response develops against it and an antigen-antibody reaction occurs. This reaction can be fatal. The administration of this immunoglobulin helps to prevent the reaction. The most common use of this product is in cases of maternal-fetal Rh incompatibility (postpartum). Only the mother is normally dosed, and the treatment objective is to prevent a harmful maternal immune response to a fetus during a future pregnancy should an Rh-negative mother become pregnant with an Rh-positive child.

Rh$_0$(D) immunoglobulin is prepared from the plasma or serum of adults with a high titer of anti-Rh$_0$(D) antibody to the red blood cell antigen Rh$_0$(D). Administration of this immunoglobulin is contraindicated in persons who have been previously immunized with this drug and in Rh$_0$(D)-positive/Du-positive patients. It is normally given postpartum but is rated as a pregnancy category C drug.

rabies immunoglobulin
Rabies immunoglobulin (BayRab, Imogam Rabies-HT) is a passive immunizing drug that is administered concurrently with rabies virus vaccine following suspected exposure to the rabies virus. In humans this usually occurs after an animal bite. Rabies immunoglobulin is derived from human cells that are harvested from persons who have been immunized with rabies vaccine. The only contraindication to its use is drug allergy, although an allergic patient may still need to be dosed rather than face infection with the almost universally fatal rabies virus. The decision to dose a patient in such a case is based on the probability of rabies infection given the particular circumstances surrounding the animal bite.

tetanus immunoglobulin
Tetanus immunoglobulin (BayTet) is a passive immunizing drug effective against tetanus. It contains tetanus antitoxin antibodies that neutralize the bacterial exotoxin produced by *Clostridium tetani*, the bacterium that causes tetanus. Tetanus immunoglobulin is prepared from the plasma of adults hyperimmunized with the tetanus toxoid and is given as prophylaxis to persons with tetanus-prone wounds. It may also be used to treat active tetanus.

varicella-zoster immunoglobulin
Varicella-zoster immunoglobulin (VZIG; available only in generic form from the American Red Cross) can be used to modify or prevent chickenpox in susceptible individuals who have had recent significant exposure to the disease. VZIG should be administered within 96 hours of exposure. Candidates for therapy with VZIG are those at high risk of serious disease or complications if they become infected with the varicella-zoster virus. Two examples are newborn children, including premature infants with significant exposure, and immunocompromised adults. If the infection manifests in a pregnant woman within 5 days of delivery, a dose of VZIG is recommended for the infant. It may also be beneficial to both mother and infant when given to the mother during pregnancy, preferably as soon as possible after diagnosis of infection. Healthy adults, including pregnant women, should be evaluated on a case-by-case basis. The duration of protection against infection provided by VZIG is at least 3 weeks. VZIG is prepared from the plasma of normal blood donors with high antibody titers to varicella-zoster virus.

TABLE 46-4 Illnesses Caused by CDC Category "A" Possible Bioterrorism Agents*

Name of Illness	Causative Organism	Clinical Presentation	Prevention/Treatment
Anthrax	Bacterium: *Bacillus anthracis*	Inhalational form most severe and can lead to potentially fatal bacteremia	Vaccine available; treatable with antibiotics such as ciprofloxacin and dicloxacillin
Smallpox	Virus: vaccinia	Flulike symptoms followed by total-body disfiguring rash	Vaccine available and may be effective for up to 3 days after exposure; antiviral drug cidofovir possibly effective
Botulism	Bacterium: *Clostridium botulinum*	Visual changes; dry mouth; muscle weakness; progressive downward paralysis, including paralysis of diaphragm	Vaccine available only for highly exposed persons; antitoxin effective if given early in disease; immunoglobulin also now available; antibiotics of no benefit
Tularemia	Bacterium: *Francisella tularensis*	Severe, potentially life-threatening respiratory illness	Vaccine still under review by FDA; treatable with antibiotics such as tetracycline and ciprofloxacin
Viral hemorrhagic fever	Viruses: several viral causes, including Ebola, Marburg, and Lassa viruses, yellow fever virus, Argentine hemorrhagic fever virus	Bleeding from body orifices and in internal organs in severe cases; possible renal failure and coma	No vaccines except for yellow fever virus and Argentine hemorrhagic fever virus; no current treatment other than supportive care; prevention focuses on rodent control
Plague	Bacterium: *Yersinia pestis*	Can occur in lungs (pneumonic plague), skin (bubonic plague—most common), or blood (septicemic plague); death possible from respiratory failure and shock	No vaccine currently available in U.S.; antibiotics best if given within 24 hr and include gentamicin and tetracycline

Data from U.S. Centers of Disease Control and Prevention. Available at *http://emergency.cdc.gov/bioterrorism/.*
CDC, Centers for Disease Control and Prevention; *FDA,* Food and Drug Administration.
*Classified as "high-priority" biologic diseases by the CDC.

Biologic and Chemical Terrorism

Because of the terrible tragedy that happened on September 11, 2001, there is heightened concern regarding the potential use of infectious or otherwise toxic agents as weapons against human populations. A terrorist attack involving the use of pathogenic microorganisms or other biologic agents is referred to as **bioterrorism,** whereas an attack in which harmful chemical agents are used is called *chemical terrorism.* In June 2002, President George W. Bush signed into law the Public Health Security and Bioterrorism Preparedness and Response Act (the Bioterrorism Act). This legislation marked the official beginning of the President's Countering Bioterrorism Initiative, which attempts to address this issue proactively as a matter of public health. The Center for Biologics Evaluation and Research (CBER), a branch of the FDA, is an important participant in this public health initiative. Recent CBER activities include the funding of rapid development by private industry of new vaccines for the prevention of anthrax and smallpox as well as vaccinia immunoglobulin, to prepare for possible bioterrorist attack using these infectious organisms. Although smallpox vaccine is no longer routinely administered in the United States, supplies are maintained by the CDC in the event of a smallpox bioterrorist attack. The Department of Defense currently owns all lots of anthrax vaccine produced in the United States. Although the CDC does not currently recommend public inoculation with the anthrax vaccine, it is administered prophylactically to military personnel considered to be at higher risk of anthrax exposure because of the location and

nature of their assigned duties. The Environmental Health Laboratory of the CDC's Division of Laboratory Sciences oversees planned responses to chemical terrorist attacks. One of its newest developments is the Rapid Toxic Screen. This laboratory test is able to analyze the blood and/or urine of multiple patients to detect 150 chemicals that could potentially be used in a terrorist attack to confirm exposure and direct treatment decisions. Tables 46-4 and 46-5 provide examples of microorganisms and chemical agents, respectively, believed potentially likely to be used in a terrorist attack. The chemical agents listed all have a history of prior military use. Because a small-scale attack with anthrax has already occurred in the United States, this disease is also discussed in more detail in the following section.

ANTHRAX

In October 2001, the month following the September 11 terrorist attacks, six U.S. Postal Service workers were infected with anthrax via contaminated mail. Two of them did not survive. Anthrax is a bacterial infectious disease caused by spores of the bacterium *Bacillus anthracis.* In humans, infection can occur via three routes of exposure: skin (20% mortality), gastrointestinal tract (25% to 75% mortality), and inhalation (80% or higher mortality). Antibiotics such as the fluoroquinolone ciprofloxacin are used to treat more severe cases (i.e., the inhalational form). Milder cases (i.e., cutaneous and gastrointestinal forms) are often treated with the tetracycline antibiotic doxycycline. The vaccine is produced from an attenuated strain of *B. anthracis.* It has a calculated efficacy level of

TABLE 46-5 Possible Chemical Terrorism Agents

Agent (Classification)	Effects	Treatment
Sarin (nerve gas)	Headache, runny nose, difficulty breathing, seizures	Remove from area; provide supportive care (e.g., mechanical ventilation). Specific antidote drugs include atropine, pralidoxime, and pyridostigmine. FDA approved special pediatric atropine dosage forms in 2003.
Mustard (blistering agent)	Skin burns, pulmonary edema, ocular damage	Rinse copiously with water; remove contaminated clothing; provide airway support as needed. FDA approved special skin lotion in 2003.
Cyanide (blood agent)	Seizures, gastrointestinal hemorrhage, respiratory arrest	Remove from area; provide airway support. Specific antidote drug therapy includes the chemicals amyl nitrite (by inhalation), and sodium nitrite and sodium thiosulfate (both by injection).
Chlorine (choking agent)	Eye and respiratory irritation; pulmonary edema	Remove from area; remove contaminated clothing; provide airway support.
Radioactive elements	DNA mutations, tissue fibrosis, vascular insufficiency, bone marrow toxicity, organ failure, pneumonitis, enteritis	Several chelating drugs are used to facilitate bodily excretion of various radioactive elements. For example, in 2004, FDA approved two new drugs (pentetate calcium trisodium and pentetate zinc trisodium) for internal decontamination of various radioactive elements (plutonium, americium, curium).
Ricin (by-product of processing of castor beans for production of castor oil)	Respiratory failure, seizures, fever, cough, diarrhea	Remove from exposure; remove and dispose of contaminated clothing; provide supportive care as needed (e.g., mechanical ventilation, intravenous hydration).

FDA, Food and Drug Administration.

92.5% for protection against anthrax infection. Anthrax vaccination is recommended not only for selected military personnel, as mentioned earlier, but also for others considered to be at higher than average risk for exposure to the bacterium. Included are veterinarians and others who handle potentially infected animals as well as workers who process imported animal hair, which is used to manufacture various commercial products.

NURSING PROCESS

Assessment

Before administering a toxoid or vaccine, the nurse should gather complete information about the patient's health history, including a list of medications taken (prescription, over-the-counter, and herbal), reactions to drugs, present and past health status, previous allergy test results, use of any immunosuppressants, presence of autoimmune or immunosuppressive diseases or infections, pregnancy and lactation status, and any unusual reaction to any substance. When pediatric patients are to receive a vaccine or toxoid, the prescribed immunization schedule and dose must be followed. The Department of Health and Human Services, and specifically the CDC, provides the latest recommendations for adult and pediatric immunizations in the United States. These recommendations are easily accessible on the Internet at *http://www.cdc.gov* and should be referred to and kept close at hand in any facility that administers these drugs. It is crucial for the nurse to stay current regarding immunization cautions and contraindications. This website and other

published materials from the CDC on immunization are an important source of information.

Because *passive immunizing drugs* may precipitate serum sickness, elderly patients and those who have chronic illnesses or are debilitated must be assessed very carefully before treatment. This may include measuring vital signs, completing the nursing assessment, and obtaining the medication history as well as examining the results of any laboratory testing ordered by the prescriber. The patient's general health status should be documented with attention to any illness and overall well-being. See the pharmacology discussion on passive vaccines as well as Box 46-1 and Table 46-1 for further information.

For the various *active immunizing drugs,* the pharmacology section and Tables 46-1, 46-2, and 46-3, as well as the Dosages table, provides more specific insight and information including contraindications, cautions, and drug interactions. It is also important to note that use of these drugs in the following patient groups should be considered carefully: pregnant patients; those with active infections (especially those caused by the same pathogen or organism producing the same toxin); patients with severe febrile illnesses excluding minor illnesses such as a cold, mild infection, ear infection, or low-grade fever; and patients with a history of reactions or serious adverse effects to the drug. In addition, research has shown that patients who are already immunosuppressed (e.g., those with AIDS, elderly patients, those with chronic diseases or cancer, neonates) are at increased risk for serious adverse effects to toxoids or vaccines; therefore, these drugs should be used cautiously or not at all in such patients. Many adults assume that the vaccines they received as children will protect them for a lifetime. This is usually the case. However, some adults were never vaccinated as children, or newer vaccines were not available at the time they were vaccinated. In addition, immunity may fade over time, and as individuals age they may become more susceptible to serious diseases caused by common infections, such as *Pneumococcus* infections.

Tetanus, diphtheria, and pertussis vaccines are to be used in patients aged 6 weeks to 6 years and are contraindicated in those with previous vaccine reactions. In addition, their use is contraindicated in patients with any type of neurologic reactions to the vaccine. The *H. influenzae* type b vaccine is administered to adults and children considered at high risk for acquiring *H. influenzae* infection, such as individuals with septicemia, pneumonia, cellulitis, arthritis, osteomyelitis, pericarditis, sickle cell anemia, an immunodeficiency syndrome, or Hodgkin's disease. Hepatitis B virus vaccines are indicated for those at high risk for exposure to the hepatitis B virus or HBsAg-positive materials (e.g., blood, plasma, serum), such as health care workers. This vaccine is contraindicated in those allergic to yeast. It is also important to assess the need of the patient receiving the vaccine, because there are different formulations for pediatric patients, adults over the age of 20 years, and individuals receiving dialysis or other immunocompromised patients. The influenza virus vaccine is contraindicated in those with previous hypersensitivity. The MMR vaccine is contraindicated in pregnant women and in those with an anaphylactic reaction to topically or systemically administered neomycin.

Pneumococcal vaccine is contraindicated in those with known allergy to the drug or its components or in those patients with significant febrile illness or immunosuppressed state as a result of drug therapy (e.g., chemotherapy). Contraindications to the administration of rabies vaccine include a history of allergic reaction to the vaccine itself or to the drugs neomycin, gentamicin, or amphotericin B. However, the risk/benefit ratio must be considered, and if treatment is required, then pretreatment with other drugs may be ordered (see pharmacology discussion).

The HPV vaccine should not be given to patients with allergies to yeast or patients who have a documented allergic reaction to the first injection of HPV vaccine. This vaccine is also contraindicated in pregnancy. The herpes zoster virus vaccine should not be administered to patients allergic to neomycin or gelatin, or to pregnant patients.

Bioterrorism and *chemical terrorism* are unfortunately a reality in today's society. The nurse's role may range from contributing significantly during preparations for a biologic terrorist attack after a warning has been issued or performing triage and carrying out the nursing process during such an attack. The nurse's role may also include assessing individuals, groups, and communities and providing related education to help people understand the benefits of being informed, making plans, and maintaining a state of preparedness at all times insofar as is possible. Cultural background, level of knowledge and education, age, motor skills, cognitive abilities, awareness of extended family members and their level of preparedness, and ability to manage stress and to think during a crisis are just a few of the areas worthy of assessment in relation to bioterrorism. Nurses also have a responsibility to ensure that, regardless of the situation, they maintain a calm, reassuring, compassionate, caring, and empathic manner during the assessment phase (and all other phases of the nursing process) in the care of those in need and avoid excessively anxiety-provoking comments or actions. Just discussing the topic of terrorism or bioterrorism can

---

CASE STUDY

Varicella Vaccination

© Monkey Business Images

Mrs. T. has taken her daughter, 12-month-old, Jamie, for her well-baby checkup. Jamie has been healthy overall and is due for the varicella virus vaccination. The nurse reviews the vaccination process with Mrs. T. and gives her information about what to expect after the vaccination.

1. Mrs. T. looks at the information sheet and then asks, "This is just one shot, right? After this she'll be immune to chickenpox. What a relief that will be!" How should the nurse respond?
2. The nurse reviews the information with Mrs. T. and tells her that a slight fever may develop. She asks Mrs. T. what she has at home to give to Jamie if a fever or discomfort at the injection site develops. Mrs. T. replies, "Oh, I have children's aspirin." What instructions should the nurse give regarding this?
3. The next morning, the skin around Jamie's injection site is slightly swollen, red, and warm to the touch. Mrs. T. calls the office to "make sure everything is all right." What further assessment questions should the nurse ask Mrs. T.?
4. Mrs. T.'s grandmother, who is 65 years old, is visiting and tells Mrs. T., "Oh, I had that same vaccine 2 months ago! I don't ever want to get shingles." Is she correct? Did she receive the same vaccine that Jamie did?

For answers, see *http://evolve.elsevier.com/Lilley.*

---

evoke fear and other emotions in individuals, and so questioning and assessment must be conducted in a way that is calming and provides a sense of control.

Nursing Diagnoses

- Risk for injury related to possible adverse effects of or allergic reactions to an immunizing drug
- Acute pain related to local and/or systemic effects of the injection of a toxoid, vaccine, or passive immunizing drug
- Deficient knowledge related to the use of toxoids, vaccines, or passive immunizing drugs
- Anxiety related to suspected risk of bioterrorism

Planning
Goals

- Patient states the adverse effects of the medication.
- Patient experiences minimal discomfort stemming from the administration of a toxoid, vaccine, or passive immunizing drug.
- Patient remains compliant with the therapeutic regimen.
- Patient returns for follow-up injections and booster injections and for follow-up visits with the prescriber.
- Patient states the importance of proactive behavior and education related to the risk of bioterrorism.

Outcome Criteria

- Patient experiences minimal adverse effects of or allergic reactions to the immunizing drug, such as fever, chills, myalgias, and bronchospasms, and is able to manage these effects with the use of acetaminophen and diphenhydramine if ordered.
- Patient uses measures such as the application of warm packs to the site of injection, as indicated and as ordered by the

prescriber, to help relieve localized discomfort or alleviate any localized reactions.

- Patient remains compliant with the therapeutic regimen for the prevention of illness or disease through follow-up visits with the prescriber.
- Patient states any problems or concerns to report immediately to the prescriber, such as fever higher than 101° F (38.3° C), infection, wheezing, increasing weakness, or any other unusual reaction.
- Patient states methods of remaining well informed about the possibility of bioterrorism and specific actions for self-protection, including reading reliable sources, staying abreast of local and national news, and even keeping special kits in the home containing items useful in a disaster, such as hurricane preparedness kits and, even more importantly, Homeland Security bioterrorism kits.

Implementation

When any *immunizing drug* is administered, it is crucial to patient safety always to check and then recheck the specific protocols and schedules of administration. It is also important to follow the manufacturer's recommendations concerning storage and administration of the drug, routes and site of administration, dosage, precautions pertaining to the drug's use, and contraindications to its use. Parents of young children must be encouraged and taught how to maintain an accurate journal of the child's immunization status, including dates of immunization and the reaction(s), if any. If the patient experiences discomfort at the injection site, application of warm compresses or administration of acetaminophen may help. With regard to the possibility of *bioterrorism,* patients need to be kept well informed, but the nurse must be constantly aware of the need to minimize anxiety. See *http://evolve.elsevier.com/Lilley* for more information on specific federal agencies, centers, initiatives, and online resources related to bioterrorism and homeland security. Also see Patient Teaching Tips for more specific information.

Evaluation

The therapeutic response in patients receiving *immunizing drugs* is the prevention or amelioration of the specific disease being targeted. Adverse reactions for which to monitor in patients receiving immunizing drugs are specific to the drug, but there may be a localized reaction including swelling, redness, discomfort, and heat at the site of injection or a more serious reaction that should be reported immediately to the prescriber (e.g., high fever, lymphadenopathy, rash, itching, joint pain, severe flulike symptoms, decreased level of consciousness, and/or shortness of breath). For a complete list of expected reactions or adverse effects, including minor and severe, see Table 46-2. As immunizing drugs improve and newer ones are developed, it is hoped that fewer adverse effects will occur and fewer adverse drug events and complications will be seen.

PATIENT TEACHING TIPS

- A localized reaction to the injection sometimes occurs when toxoids and vaccines are administered. The patient should be told that the discomfort can be relieved by placing warm compresses on the injection site, resting, and taking acetaminophen and/or diphenhydramine, as directed by the prescriber. Instructions for the care of infants or children experiencing such reactions are generally given by the child's prescriber when the immunizing drug is administered.

- The patient or parent/caregiver should notify the prescriber if high or prolonged fever, rash, itching, or shortness of breath occurs after the vaccination.
- The patient or parent/caregiver should always keep a double record (two copies stored in separate places) of all of the medications being taken, especially all vaccinations received.
- A vaccine adverse event reporting system is available through the FDA by calling 800-822-7967.

POINTS TO REMEMBER

- A foreign substance in the body is termed an *antigen;* the body creates a substance called an *antibody* specifically to bind to it.
- B lymphocytes (B cells), when stimulated by the binding of an antigen molecule, begin to differentiate into memory cells and plasma cells.
- Memory cells remember what that particular antigen looks like in case the body is exposed to the same antigen again in the future. Plasma cells manufacture the antibodies and will mass-produce clones of the antibodies upon reexposure to a particular antigen.
- The two types of immunity are active and passive immunity. Different types of drugs are used to induce each, and these drugs are indicated for different populations, as follows:
  - Active immunization involves administration of a toxoid or a vaccine that exposes the body to a relatively harmless form of the antigen (foreign invader) to imprint cellular memory and stimulate the body's defenses to fight any subsequent exposure. It provides long-lasting or permanent immunity. The recipient must have an active, functioning immune system to benefit.

- Passive immunization involves the administration of immunoglobulins, antitoxins, or antivenins. Serum or concentrated immunoglobulins are obtained from humans or animals and, after screening and testing, are injected into the patient, directly giving the individual the ability to fight off an invading microorganism or inactivate a toxin. Passive immunization provides temporary protection and does not stimulate an antibody response in the host. It is used in patients who are immunocompromised or who have been exposed to, or anticipate exposure to, an organism or toxin.
- Patients who should not receive immunizing drugs include those with active infections, febrile illnesses, or a history of a previous reaction to the drug. Use of these drugs in pregnant women is also usually contraindicated.
- Patients who are immunocompromised are at greater risk of experiencing serious adverse effects from immunizing drugs.
- Parents should keep updated records of their children's and their own immunizations with any toxoids or vaccines.

NCLEX EXAMINATION REVIEW QUESTIONS

1 When assessing a patient who will be receiving an immunizing drug, the nurse will consider which condition to be a possible contraindication?
  a Anemia
  b Pregnancy
  c Ear infection
  d Common cold

2 When giving a vaccination to an infant, the nurse should tell the mother to expect which adverse effect?
  a Fever over 103° F (39.4° C)
  b Rash
  c Soreness at the injection site
  d Chills

3 In the emergency department, several patients have possibly been exposed to anthrax. The nurse will prepare to administer prophylactic doses of
  a ciprofloxacin.
  b cidofovir.
  c immunoglobulin.
  d antitoxin.

4 During a routine checkup, a 72-year-old patient is advised to receive an influenza vaccine injection. He questions this, saying, "I had one last year. Why do I need another one?" What is an appropriate response from the nurse?
  a "The effectiveness of the vaccine wears off after 6 months."
  b "Each year a new vaccine is developed based on the flu strains that are likely to be in circulation."

  c "When you reach age 65, you need boosters on an annual basis."
  d "Taking the flu vaccine each year allows you to build your immunity to a higher level each time."

5 A patient is in the urgent care center after stepping on a rusty tent nail. The nurse evaluates the patient's immunity status and knows that a tetanus booster is necessary if it has been how long since the patient's last booster shot?
  a 1 year
  b 2 years
  c 5 years
  d 10 years

6 The nurse is providing teaching after an adult receives a booster immunization. Which adverse reactions should be reported immediately to the health care provider?
  a Swelling and redness at the injection site
  b Fever of 100° F (37.8° C)
  c Joint pain
  d Heat over the site of injection
  e Rash
  f Shortness of breath

CRITICAL THINKING ACTIVITIES: BEST ACTION

1 R.T. is in the emergency department after receiving a bite from a black widow spider *(Latrodectus mactans)*. As you administer the antivenin for the black widow spider bite, he asks you, "Now will I be immune to black widow spiders after this shot? That's good, because we have a lot of them around the barn." What is the best response to his question? Explain.

2 Within 2 hours after the patient receives a tetanus booster vaccination, his wife calls the clinic. "He says that he is feeling weird

and a little short of breath. You said to call if he is having a reaction, but it's hard to tell what is happening." What is the first instruction the nurse should give to this patient's wife?

3 You are working as a staff nurse on a medical-surgical unit in a suburban area. A co-worker asks you, "What are we supposed to do if this area has a terrorist attack, such as an anthrax exposure?" What is your best answer?

For answers, see *http://evolve.elsevier.com/Lilley.*

CHAPTER 47

Antineoplastic Drugs Part 1: Cancer Overview and Cell Cycle–Specific Drugs

Timothy R. McGuire

OBJECTIVES

When you reach the end of this chapter, you should be able to do the following:

1 Briefly describe the concepts related to carcinogenesis.

2 Define the different types of malignancy.

3 Discuss the purpose and role of the various treatment modalities in the management of cancer.

4 Define *antineoplastic*.

5 Discuss the role of antineoplastic therapy in the treatment of cancer.

6 Contrast the cell cycle of normal cells and malignant cells with regard to growth, function, and response of the cell to chemotherapeutic drugs and other treatment modalities.

7 Compare the characteristics of highly proliferating normal cells (including cells of the hair follicles, gastrointestinal tract, and bone marrow) with the characteristics of highly proliferating cancerous cells.

8 Briefly describe the specific differences between cell cycle–specific and cell cycle–nonspecific antineoplastic drugs (cell cycle–nonspecific drugs and miscellaneous other antineoplastics are discussed in Chapter 48).

9 Identify the drugs that are categorized as cell cycle specific, including mitotic inhibitors, topoisomerase inhibitors, and antineoplastic enzymes.

10 Describe the common adverse effects and toxic reactions associated with the various antineoplastic drugs, including the causes for their occurrence and methods of treatment, such as antidotes for toxicity.

11 Discuss the mechanisms of action, indications, dosages, routes of administration, cautions, contraindications, and drug interactions of cell cycle–specific drugs, including mitotic inhibitors, topoisomerase inhibitors, and antineoplastic enzymes.

12 Apply knowledge about the various antineoplastic drugs to the development of a comprehensive nursing care plan for patients receiving cell cycle–specific drugs, including mitotic inhibitors, topoisomerase inhibitors, and antineoplastic enzymes.

e-Learning Activities

http://evolve.elsevier.com/Lilley

NCLEX Review Questions • Animations • Nursing Care Plans • Audio Glossary • Category Catchers • Medication Errors Checklists • IV Therapy Checklists • Calculators • Frequently Asked Questions • Content Updates • Supplemental Resources • Answers to Case Studies and Critical Thinking Activities

Drug Profiles

♦ asparaginase, p. 737
capecitabine, p. 733
cladribine, p. 732
♦ cytarabine, p. 733
♦ etoposide, p. 735
fludarabine, p. 732
fluorouracil, p. 733

gemcitabine, p. 733
irinotecan, p. 737
♦ methotrexate, p. 732
♦ paclitaxel, p. 735
pegaspargase, p. 737
topotecan, p. 737
♦ vincristine, p. 736

♦ *Key drug.*

Glossary

Analogue A chemical compound with a structure similar to that of another compound but differing from it with respect to some component. (p. 730)

Anaplasia The absence of the cellular differentiation that is part of the normal cellular growth process (see *differentiation;* adjective: *anaplastic*). (p. 726)

Antineoplastic drugs Drugs used to treat cancer. Also called *cancer drugs, anticancer drugs, cancer chemotherapy,* and *chemotherapy.* (p. 726)

Benign Denoting a neoplasm that is noncancerous and therefore not an immediate threat to life. (p. 722)

Cancer A malignant neoplastic disease, the natural course of which is fatal (see *neoplasm*). (p. 722)

Carcinogen Any cancer-producing substance or organism. (p. 725)

Carcinomas Malignant epithelial neoplasms that tend to invade surrounding tissue and metastasize to distant regions of the body. (p. 722)

Cell cycle–nonspecific Denoting antineoplastic drugs that are cytotoxic in any phase of the cellular growth cycle. (p. 727)

Cell cycle–specific Denoting antineoplastic drugs that are cytotoxic during a specific phase of the cellular growth cycle. (p. 727)

Clone A cell or group of cells that is genetically identical to a given parent cell. (p. 722)

Differentiation An important part of normal cellular growth in which immature cells mature into specialized cells. (p. 722)

Dose-limiting adverse effects Adverse effects that prevent an antineoplastic drug from being given in higher dosages, often restricting the effectiveness of the drug. (p. 729)

Emetic potential The potential of a drug to cause nausea and vomiting. (p. 729)

Extravasation The leakage of any intravenously or intraarterially administered medication into the tissue space surrounding the vein or artery. Such an event can cause serious tissue injury, especially with antineoplastic drugs. (p. 730)

Growth fraction The percentage of cells in mitosis at any given time. (p. 725)

Intrathecal A route of drug injection through the theca of the spinal cord and into the subarachnoid space. This route is used to deliver certain chemotherapy medications to kill cancer cells in the central nervous system. (p. 732)

Leukemias Malignant neoplasms of blood-forming tissues characterized by the replacement of normal bone marrow cells with leukemic blasts resulting in abnormal numbers and forms of immature white blood cells in the circulation. (p. 723)

Lymphomas Malignant neoplasms of lymphoid tissue. (p. 723)

Malignant Tending to worsen and cause death; anaplastic, invasive, and metastatic. (p. 722)

Metastasis The process by which a cancer spreads from the original site of growth to a new and remote part of the body (adjective: *metastatic*). (p. 722)

Mitosis The process of cell reproduction occurring in somatic (nonsexual) cells and resulting in the formation of two genetically identical daughter cells containing the diploid (complete) number of chromosomes characteristic of the species. (p. 725)

Mitotic index The number of cells per unit (usually 1000 cells) undergoing mitosis during a given time. (p. 725)

Mutagen A chemical or physical agent that induces or increases genetic mutations by causing changes in deoxyribonucleic acid (DNA). (p. 725)

Mutation A permanent change in DNA that is transmissible to future cellular generations. Mutations can transform normal cells into cancer cells. (p. 722)

Myelosuppression Suppression of bone marrow function, which can result in dangerously reduced numbers of red and white blood cells and platelets. (p. 729)

Nadir Lowest point in any fluctuating value over time; for example, the lowest white blood cell count measured after the count has been depressed by chemotherapy. (p. 730)

Neoplasm Any new and abnormal growth, specifically growth that is uncontrolled and progressive; a synonym for *tumor*. A *malignant* neoplasm or tumor is synonymous with *cancer*. (p. 722)

Nucleic acids Molecules of DNA and ribonucleic acid (RNA) in the nucleus of every cell (hence the name *nucleic acid*). Chromosomes are made up of DNA and encode all of the genes necessary for cellular structure and function. (p. 725)

Oncogenic Cancer producing, often applied to tumor-inducing viruses. (p. 724)

Paraneoplastic syndromes Symptom complexes arising in patients with cancer that cannot be explained by local or distant spread of their tumors. (p. 723)

Primary lesion The original site of growth of a tumor. (p. 722)

Sarcomas Malignant neoplasms of the connective tissues arising in bone, fibrous, fatty, muscular, synovial, vascular, or neural tissue, often first presenting as painless swellings. (p. 723)

Tumor A new growth of tissue characterized by a progressive, uncontrolled proliferation of cells. Tumors can be solid (e.g., brain tumor) or circulating (e.g., leukemia or lymphoma), and *benign* (noncancer-

ous) or *malignant* (cancerous). Circulating tumors are more precisely called *hematologic tumors* or *hematologic malignancies*. A tumor is also called a *neoplasm*. (p. 722)

Tumor lysis syndrome A common metabolic complication of chemotherapy for rapidly growing tumors. It is characterized by the presence of excessive cellular waste products and electrolytes, including uric acid, phosphate, and potassium, and by reduced serum calcium levels. (p. 731)

· · ·

Anatomy, Physiology, and Disease Overview

Cancer is a broad term encompassing a group of diseases that are characterized by cellular transformation (e.g., by genetic **mutation**), uncontrolled cellular growth, and possible invasion into surrounding tissue and metastasis to other tissues or organs distant from the original body site. This cellular growth differs from normal cellular growth in that cancerous cells do not possess a growth control mechanism. Lack of cellular **differentiation** or maturation into specialized, productive cells is also a common characteristic of cancer cells. Figure 47-1 illustrates the multiple steps involved in the development of cancer. Cancerous cells will continue to grow and invade adjacent structures, and they may break away from the original tumor mass and travel by means of the blood or lymphatic system to establish a new clone of cancer cells and create a metastatic growth elsewhere in the body. A **clone** is a cell or group of cells that is genetically identical to a given parent cell. For the remainder of this and the next chapter, the term *cancer* will generally be used to refer to any type of malignant neoplasm.

Metastasis refers to the spreading of a cancer from the original site of growth **(primary lesion)** to a new and remote part of the body (*secondary* or *metastatic lesion*). The terms *malignancy, neoplasm,* and *tumor* are often used as synonyms for cancer. A **neoplasm** ("new tissue") is a mass of new cells. It is another term for **tumor.** There are two types of tumors: benign and malignant. A **benign** tumor is of a uniform size and shape and displays no invasiveness (in terms of infiltrating other tissues) or metastatic properties. The terms *nonmalignant* and *benign* suggest that tumors may be harmless, which is true in most cases. However, a benign tumor can be lethal if it grows large enough to mechanically interrupt the normal function of a critical tissue or organ. **Malignant** neoplasms consist of cancer cells that invade (infiltrate) surrounding tissues and metastasize to other tissues and organs. Some of the various characteristics of benign and malignant neoplasms are listed in Table 47-1.

Over 100 types of cancer affect humans. Various tumor types based on tissue categories include sarcomas, carcinomas, lymphomas, leukemias, and tumors of nervous tissue origin. Examples of these common types of malignant tumors are presented in Table 47-2. It is important to know the tissue of origin, because this determines the type of treatment used, the likely response to therapy, and the prognosis.

Carcinomas arise from epithelial tissue, which is located throughout the body. This tissue covers or lines all body surfaces, both inside and outside the body. Examples are the skin, the mucosal lining of the entire gastrointestinal (GI) tract, and the lining

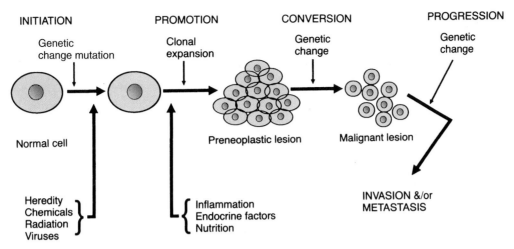

FIGURE 47-1 Schematic model of multistep carcinogenesis. *Genetic change* refers to events such as the activation of protooncogenes or drug resistance genes or the inactivation of tumor suppressor genes, antimetastasis genes, or apoptosis (normal cell death). Genetic change may be relatively minimal, as with the translocations seen in various leukemias, or it may involve multiple sequential genetic alterations, as exemplified by the development of colon cancer. (From Haskell CM: *Cancer treatment,* ed 5, Philadelphia, 2001, Saunders.)

TABLE 47-1 Tumor Characteristics: Benign and Malignant

Characteristic	Benign	Malignant
Potential to metastasize	No	Yes
Encapsulated	Yes	No
Similar to tissue of origin	Yes	No
Rate of growth	Slow	Unpredictable and unrestrained
Recurrence after surgical removal	Rare	Common

TABLE 47-2 Tumor Classification Based on Specific Tissue of Origin

Tissue of Origin	Malignant Tissue
Epithelial = Carcinomas	
Glands or ducts	Adenocarcinomas
Respiratory tract	Small and large cell carcinomas
Kidney	Renal cell carcinoma
Skin	Squamous cell, epidermoid, and basal cell carcinoma; melanoma
Connective = Sarcomas	
Fibrous tissue	Fibrosarcoma
Cartilage	Chondrosarcoma
Bone	Osteogenic sarcoma (Ewing's tumor)
Blood vessels	Kaposi's sarcoma
Synovia	Synoviosarcoma
Mesothelium	Mesothelioma
Lymphatic = Lymphomas	
Lymph tissue	Lymphomas (e.g., Hodgkin's, non-Hodgkin's)
Nerve	
Glia	Glioma
Adrenal medulla nerves	Pheochromocytoma
Blood and Bone Marrow	
White blood cells	Leukemia
Bone marrow	Multiple myeloma

of the bronchial tree (lungs). The purpose of these epithelial tissues is to protect the body's vital organs.

Sarcomas are malignant tumors that arise primarily from connective tissues, but some sarcomas are tumors of epithelial cell origin. Connective tissue is the most abundant and widely distributed of all tissues and includes bone, cartilage, muscle, and lymphatic and vascular structures. Its purpose is to support and protect other tissues.

Lymphomas are cancers within the lymphatic tissues. **Leukemias** arise from the bone marrow and are cancers of blood and bone marrow. Leukemias differ from carcinomas and sarcomas in that the cancerous cells do not form solid tumors but are interspersed throughout the lymphatic or circulatory system and interfere with the normal functioning of these systems. For this reason, they are sometimes referred to as *circulating tumors,* although *hematologic malignancy* is a more precise term. Lymphomas can be quite bulky and are usually classified as solid tumors.

Cancer patients may also experience various groups of symptoms that cannot be directly attributed to the spread of a cancerous tumor. Such symptom complexes are referred to as **paraneoplastic syndromes.** They are estimated to occur in up to 15% of patients with cancer and may even be the first sign of malignancy. *Cachexia* (general ill health and malnutrition) is the most com-

mon such symptom complex. Examples of other common paraneoplastic syndromes are given in Table 47-3. These syndromes are believed to result from the effects of biologically or immunologically active substances, such as hormones and antibodies, secreted by the tumor cells. Many patients also exhibit more generalized symptoms, such as anorexia, weight loss, fatigue, and fever.

TABLE 47-3 Paraneoplastic Syndromes Associated with Some Cancers

Paraneoplastic Syndrome	Associated Cancer
Hypercalcemia, sensory neuropathies, SIADH	Lung
Disseminated intravascular coagulation	Leukemia
Cushing's syndrome	Lung, thyroid, testes, adrenal
Addison's syndrome	Adrenal, lymphoma

SIADH, Syndrome of inappropriate secretion of antidiuretic hormone.

ETIOLOGY OF CANCER

The etiology of cancer remains a mystery for the most part, and cancer researchers have made slow progress toward identifying possible causes. In recent years, certain etiologic factors have come to light, however, and some of these and the cancers with which they are causally associated are listed in Table 47-4. Radiation, oncogenic viruses, and immunologic, ethnic, genetic, age-related, and sex-related characteristics are among the causative factors identified.

Age- and Sex-Related Differences

The probability that a neoplastic disease will develop generally increases with advancing age. However, a number of rare cancers, such as acute lymphocytic leukemia and Wilms tumor, occur predominantly in pediatric patients.

With the exception of cancers affecting the reproductive system, few cancers exhibit a sex-related difference in incidence. Lung and urinary cancers are more common in men than in women, but this may have more to do with exogenous factors such as smoking patterns and occupational exposure to environmental toxins than to sex-related characteristics. The incidence of colon, rectal, pancreatic, and skin cancers are comparable in men and women. A number of hematologic cancers have a slight male predominance.

Genetic and Ethnic Factors

Few cancers have been confirmed to have a hereditary basis (some types of breast, colon, and stomach cancer are exceptions). However, the understanding of tumor biology has helped guide therapy tremendously. Two such advances are determination of hormone receptor status and identification of specific gene expression in various types of tumor cells. For example, some tumor cells have been shown to express on their cell membrane surfaces either estrogen receptors or progesterone receptors, and some tumor cells express specific genes such as the HER2/neu gene. Because these indicators aid in classification of a patient's tumor, they also help in choosing appropriate drug therapy, predicting response to therapy, and anticipating prognosis. Discovery of the *BRCA1* and *BRCA2* genes has allowed identification of women who are at risk of breast cancer because they have a certain alteration in one of these BRCA genes. Many women with a family history of breast cancer choose to be tested for the presence of a BRCA gene mutation, and the discovery of such a cancer-associated mutation has led some women to undergo pro-

TABLE 47-4 Cancer: Proposed Etiologic Factors

Risk Factor	Associated Cancer
Environment	
Radiation (ionizing)	Leukemia, breast, thyroid, lung
Radiation (ultraviolet)	Skin, melanoma
Viruses	Leukemia, lymphoma, nasopharyngeal
Food	
Aflatoxin	Liver
Dietary factors	Colon, breast, endometrial, gallbladder
Lifestyle	
Alcohol	Esophageal, liver, stomach, laryngeal, breast
Tobacco	Lung, oral, esophageal, laryngeal, bladder
Medical Drugs	
Diethylstilbestrol (DES)	Vaginal in offspring, breast, testicular, ovarian
Estrogens	Endometrial, breast
Alkylating drugs	Leukemia, bladder
Occupational	
Asbestos	Lung, mesothelioma
Aniline dye	Bladder
Benzene	Leukemia
Vinyl chloride	Liver
Reproductive History	
Late first pregnancy, early menses	Breast
No children	Ovarian
Multiple sexual partners	Cervical, uterine

phylactic breast removal. Tumors with identifiable gene expression patterns can show a familial pattern of inheritance. For example, Burkitt's lymphoma is more common in young African children and children of African descent. Another example of an ethnic predisposition is the high incidence of nasopharyngeal cancer in persons of Chinese descent. These associations with race are complicated by a well-recognized viral pathogenesis for both diseases.

Oncogenic Viruses

Extensive research has indicated that there are cancer-causing **(oncogenic)** viruses that can affect most mammalian species. Examples include human papillomavirus, the various cat leukemia viruses, the Rous* sarcoma virus in chickens, and the Shope* papillomavirus in rabbits.

The herpesviruses are common examples of oncogenic viruses. Epstein-Barr virus is a type of herpesvirus. It is most commonly recognized as the cause of infectious mononucleosis (commonly referred to as "mono" or the "kissing disease"). However, it is also associated with the development of Burkitt's lymphoma and nasopharyngeal cancer as discussed earlier. Infection with human papillomavirus (often abbreviated as HPV) has been linked to both cervical and anal cancer.

*Drs. P. Rous and R. Shope were early investigators of oncogenic viruses.

Occupational and Environmental Carcinogens

A **carcinogen** is any substance that can cause cancer. In the nucleus of every cell are found molecules of **nucleic acids,** so named because of their location in the cell nucleus. The two types of nucleic acids are *deoxyribonucleic acid (DNA)* and *ribonucleic acid (RNA)*. DNA molecules are the master molecules of genetic material within cells and contain the approximately 30,000 genes of the human genome. Genes are transcribed into messenger RNA molecules, which in turn are translated into protein molecules necessary for cellular structure and function. This process is discussed further in the section on alkylating drugs in Chapter 48. A **mutagen** is any substance or physical agent (e.g., radiation) that induces changes in DNA molecules. Mutations often *transform* normal cells into cancer cells. Thus, *mutagenicity* is associated with and often (but not always) leads to carcinogenicity. The U.S. Food and Drug Administration (FDA) regulations mandate that carcinogenic studies be performed before any new drug is approved for use. However, no amount of clinical testing can fully reveal all of a drug's possible carcinogenic effects, because testing methods are not always satisfactory and some cancers may be species related. Carcinogenic effects may not be observed in the laboratory animals on which the drug has been tested but may be reported when the drugs are used in human subjects. Given the relatively small numbers of patients tested in clinical research trials, the carcinogenic potential of a given drug may not be observed until after the drug is marketed for use in the general population. If patterns of carcinogenicity begin to emerge during this period of postmarketing surveillance (or postmarketing studies), the drug may be recalled from the market.

Radiation

Radiation is a well-known and potent carcinogenic agent. There are two basic types of radiation: (1) *ionizing,* or high-energy, radiation, and (2) *nonionizing,* or low-energy, radiation. Both types can be carcinogenic. Ionizing radiation is very potent and can penetrate deeply into the body. It is called *ionizing* because it causes the formation of ions within living cells. This type of radiation (e.g., that used in x-ray studies) is also used to treat (irradiate) cancerous tumors (e.g., radium implants). Nonionizing radiation is much less potent and cannot penetrate deeply into the body. Ultraviolet light is an example of this type of radiation and is the cause of skin cancer. In contrast to chemotherapy, radiation therapy is considered to be a locoregional and not a systemic cancer treatment. Adverse effects of radiation therapy (e.g., radiation burns; nausea with GI tract irradiation) tend to be more localized to the site of treatment as well. Scientific specialists known as *radiation oncologists* are involved in the planning of radiation treatments, including calculation of the appropriate dose *(dosimetry)*.

Immunologic Factors

The immune system plays an important role in the body in terms of cancer surveillance and the elimination of neoplastic cells. Neoplastic cells are believed to develop routinely in everyone, but in healthy persons the immune system recognizes them as abnormal and eliminates them by means of cell-mediated immunity (cytotoxic T lymphocytes; see Chapter 49). It has also been shown that the incidence of cancer is much higher in immunocompromised individuals. Examples are patients undergoing cancer chemotherapy, organ transplant patients receiving immunosuppressive therapy, and patients with immunologic impairment or immunologic disease, including acquired immunodeficiency syndrome (AIDS). The relationship between cancer and a suppressed immune system has also been noted in cancer patients being treated with immunosuppressive drugs after organ transplantation. The higher rates of cancers such as skin cancer and lymphoma in transplant patients is a result of this aggressive use of drugs to prevent organ rejection.

Cell Growth Cycle

Normal cells in the body divide *(proliferate)* in a controlled and organized fashion, and this growth is regulated by various mechanisms. In contrast, cancer cells lack such regulatory mechanisms and divide uncontrollably, although some modification of cancer cell division may occur if blood flow to the cancer is disrupted. Often the growth of cancer cells is more constant or continuous than that of nonmalignant cells. Thus, one important growth index for malignant tumors is the time it takes for the tumor to double in size. This *doubling time* varies greatly for various types of cancers and is directly related to and important in determining the prognosis for a particular patient. Cancer treatment that cannot destroy every neoplastic cell does not prevent the regrowth of the tumor. The time it takes for regrowth to occur depends on the doubling time of the particular cancer. For instance, Burkitt's lymphoma has an extremely short doubling time. This shorter doubling time is associated with a tumor that, although it may be chemosensitive, is often difficult to cure due to rapid regrowth.

The cell growth characteristics of normal and neoplastic cells are similar. Both types of cells pass through five distinct gap phases: G_0, the *resting* phase, in which the cell is considered out of the cell cycle; G_1, the first gap phase; S, the *synthesis* phase; G_2, the second gap phase; and M, the **mitosis** phase. During mitosis, one cell divides into two identical *daughter* cells. Mitosis is further subdivided into four distinct subphases related to the time periods before and during the alignment and separation of the chromosomes (DNA strands): *prophase, metaphase, anaphase,* and *telophase*. A complete cell cycle from one mitosis to the next is called the *generation time* and it is different for all tumors, ranging from hours to days. The cell growth cycle and the events that occur in the various phases are summarized in Table 47-5. Figure 47-2 shows where in the general phases of the cell cycle the various cell cycle–specific chemotherapeutic drugs show their greatest activity.

The growth activity in a mass of tumor cells can also be characterized, and it has an important bearing on the killing power of chemotherapeutic drugs. The *percentage* of cells undergoing mitosis at any given time is called the **growth fraction** of the tumor. The *actual number* of cells that are in the M phase of the cell cycle is called the **mitotic index.** Chemotherapy is most effective when used in a rapidly dividing or *highly proliferative* tumor.

Cells in the bone marrow that have the capacity for self-renewal and repopulation of the different types of blood and bone marrow cells are known as hematopoietic *stem cells*. In the bone marrow, the hematopoietic stem cell divides asynchronously, regenerating itself while producing a cell that will go through a

TABLE 47-5 Cell Cycle Phases

Phase	Description
G_0: Resting phase	Most normal human cells exist predominantly in this phase. Cancer cells in this phase are not susceptible to the toxic effects of cell cycle–specific drugs.
G_1: First gap phase or *postmitotic* phase	Enzymes necessary for DNA synthesis are produced.
S: DNA synthesis phase	DNA synthesis takes place, from DNA strand separation to replication of each strand to create duplicate DNA molecules.
G_2: Second gap phase or *premitotic* phase	RNA and specialized proteins are made.
M: Mitosis phase	Divided into four subphases: prophase, metaphase, anaphase, and telophase; cell divides (reproduces) into two *daughter* cells.

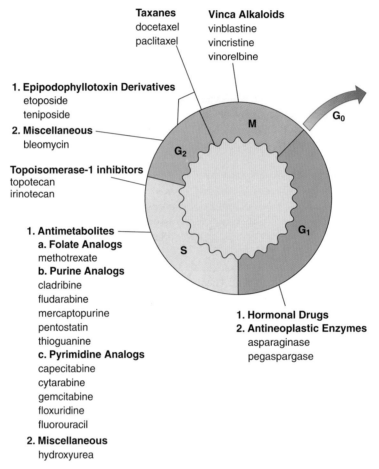

FIGURE 47-2 General phase of the cell cycle in which the various cell cycle–specific chemotherapeutic drugs have their greatest proportionate kill of cancer cells.

series of cell divisions to produce mature blood cells. Tumors in the bone marrow that affect a cell close to the stem cell are unable to mature and are considered poorly differentiated. The level of differentiation within a tumor, whether solid or circulating, becomes especially important in the treatment of neoplasms. This is because more highly differentiated tumors generally have a better therapeutic response (tumor shrinkage) to treatments such as chemotherapy and radiation. In contrast, some cancers, such as leukemia, involve proliferation of immature white blood cells (WBCs) known as *blast cells*. Cancers with a larger proportion of such *undifferentiated* cells are often less responsive to chemo-

therapy or radiation and therefore are more difficult to treat. Lack of normal cellular differentiation is known as **anaplasia,** and such undifferentiated cells are said to be *anaplastic* cells.

Pharmacology Overview

CANCER DRUG NOMENCLATURE

The more technical term for cancer is *malignant neoplasm*. Drugs used to treat cancer are therefore known as **antineoplastic drugs** but are also called *cancer drugs, anticancer drugs,* and, most commonly, *cytotoxic chemotherapy* or just *chemotherapy.* The nomenclature (naming system) of cancer drugs can be somewhat more complex and confusing than that for other drug classes. Cancer treatment is an intensively researched area in health care with many active research protocols. Multiple names are often used for the same drug, depending on its stage of development.

Recall from earlier chapters that medications have a chemical name, a generic name, and a trade name. This section introduces yet another name for medications, especially cancer drugs, that is often encountered in clinical practice: the *investigational* or *protocol* name. A drug's chemical name is used by the chemists who first discover and work with the drug. This is generally the first name used to identify a particular chemical compound, often before it is classified as a "drug" with known therapeutic properties. The chemical name is based on the standard chemical nomenclature recommended by the International Union of Pure and Applied Chemists (IUPAC). For this reason, it is also often known as the *IUPAC name*. The generic name is frequently first assigned to a chemical compound after a pharmaceutical manufacturer has determined that it is worthy of continued clinical research. It is often at this point that the chemical compound becomes an investigational drug.

Generic names are usually shorter and less complex than chemical names, and their spelling is often at least loosely based on the chemical characteristics of the drug. The trade name is a marketing name used by the manufacturer of a given drug primarily to market the drug. The trade name is frequently strategically chosen to be shorter and easier to pronounce and remember than the chemical, protocol, or generic name.

During the time before marketing and while a given medication is undergoing clinical research, it is frequently referred to by its protocol name. The protocol name is often a code name that consists of a combination of letters and numbers separated by one or more dashes. Although investigational drugs for all disease classes usually have some kind of protocol name, protocol names tend to be used more commonly in patient care settings for cancer drugs than for other drug classes. Here are two typical examples that illustrate these concepts:

Other Name	Generic Name	Trade Name
STI-571 (protocol name)	Imatinib	Gleevec
5-fluorouracil* (chemical name)	fluorouracil	Adrucil

*The "5" refers to the position of a fluorine atom in the cyclic ring structure of the uracil molecule.

DRUG THERAPY

Cancer is normally treated using one or more of three major medical approaches: surgery, radiation therapy, and chemotherapy. The term *chemotherapy* is a general term that technically can refer to chemical (drug) therapy for any kind of illness. In practice, however, this term usually refers to the pharmacologic treatment of cancer.

Normal cells in the body divide (proliferate) in a controlled and organized fashion, and this growth is regulated by means of various mechanisms. In contrast, cancer cells lack regulatory mechanisms, and they proliferate uncontrollably. Figure 47-3 shows what is termed the *Gompertzian tumor growth curve,* which illustrates the effects on patient clinical status of tumor

growth over time. Figure 47-4 shows how various combinations of cancer treatment may succeed, or fail, over time.

Cancer chemotherapy drugs can be subdivided into two main groups based on where in the cell cycle they have their effects. Antineoplastic drugs that are cytotoxic (cell killing) in any phase of the cycle are called **cell cycle–nonspecific** drugs. Those drugs that are cytotoxic during a specific cell cycle phase are called **cell cycle–specific** drugs. It should be noted, however, that these are broad categories that describe the *predominant* activity of a drug with regard to cell cycle. Individual drugs may have actions that fall into both of these categories. Regardless of the cell cycle characteristics of a drug, it is more effective on rapidly growing tumors. This chapter has described the various individual phases of the cell cycle and discusses the corresponding cell cycle–specific drugs. Chapter 48 focuses on cell cycle–nonspecific drugs as well as various miscellaneous antineoplastic drugs.

The ultimate goal of any anticancer regimen is to kill every neoplastic cell and produce a cure, but this goal is not achieved in most cases. Fortunately some patients' immune systems may be able to clear the remaining tumor. Factors that affect the chances of cure and the length of patient survival include the cancer stage at the time of diagnosis, the type of cancer and its doubling time, the efficacy of the cancer treatment, the development of drug resistance, and the general health of the patient. When total cure is not possible, the primary goal of therapy is to control the growth of the cancer while maintaining the best quality of life for the patient with the least possible level of discomfort, least compromise in performing the activities of daily living, and fewest treatment adverse effects.

It must be strongly emphasized that cancer care and treatment involve many rapidly evolving medical sciences. Cancer is an intensively researched area, with the ultimate goals being to prevent cancer and to prevent premature death in those diagnosed with it. Chemotherapy medications are often dosed as part of complex, specific treatment protocols that are subject to frequent revision by oncology clinicians and researchers. For these reasons the reader must recognize that the drug dosing information provided in this chapter is intended only to be representative of current cancer treatment and is not absolute or comprehensive. Oncology nursing is a highly specialized area of practice with focused ongoing continuing education requirements that may vary among state jurisdictions. Furthermore, the indications that are listed for each specific drug are the primary FDA-approved indications that are current at the time of this writing. These, too, may change unpredictably with time as a given drug is determined to be more (or less) effective for treating certain types of cancer. Also, in clinical practice, patients are often treated with one or more antineoplastic medications in "off-label" uses; that is, the drug is not currently approved for those particular uses by the FDA. As noted earlier, however, only the current FDA-approved indications are generally mentioned in this chapter.

No antineoplastic drug is effective against all types of cancer. Most cancer drugs have a low therapeutic index, which means that a fine line exists between therapeutic and toxic levels. Clinical experience has shown that a combination of drugs is usually more effective than single-drug therapy. Because drug-resistant cells often develop, exposure to multiple drugs with multiple

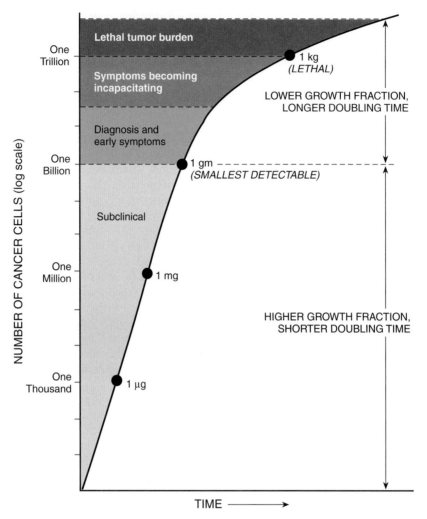

FIGURE 47-3   Gompertzian tumor growth curve showing the relationship between tumor size and clinical status. (From Lehne RA: *Pharmacology for nursing care,* ed 6, St Louis, 2007, Saunders.)

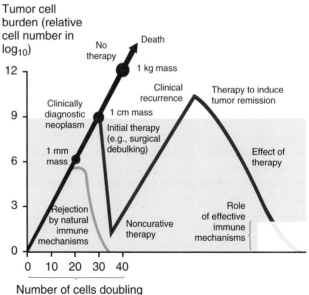

FIGURE 47-4   Relationship between tumor cell burden and phases of cancer treatment. (From McCance KL: *Pathophysiology: The biologic basis for disease in adults and children,* ed 5, St Louis, 2006, Mosby.)

BOX 47-1 Relative Emetic Potential of Selected Antineoplastic Drugs*

Low (Less Than 10% to 30%)
asparaginase
bleomycin
busulfan
capecitabine
chlorambucil
cladribine
cytarabine (less than 1000 mg/m^2)
daunorubicin, liposomal
docetaxel
doxorubicin (less than 20 mg/m^2)
doxorubicin, liposomal
estramustine
etoposide
floxuridine
fludarabine
fluorouracil (less than 1000 mg/m^2)
gefitinib
gemcitabine
hydroxyurea
imatinib
melphalan
mercaptopurine
methotrexate (less than 250 mg/m^2)
mitomycin
paclitaxel
pegaspargase
pentostatin
rituximab
teniposide
thioguanine
thiotepa
topotecan
trastuzumab
tretinoin

vinblastine
vincristine
vinorelbine

Moderate (30% to 60%)
altretamine
cyclophosphamide (less than 750 mg/m^2)
dactinomycin
daunorubicin (50 mg/m^2 or less)
doxorubicin (20 to 60 mg/m^2)
epirubicin (less than 90 mg/m^2)
idarubicin
ifosfamide (1500 mg/m^2 or less)
irinotecan
methotrexate (250 to 1000 mg/m^2)
mitoxantrone (15 mg/m^2 or less)
temozolomide

High (60% to More Than 90%)
carboplatin
carmustine
cisplatin
cyclophosphamide (750 to more than 1500 mg/m^2)
cytarabine (more than 1000 mg/m^2)
dacarbazine
dactinomycin
daunorubicin (more than 50 mg/m^2)
doxorubicin (more than 60 mg/m^2)
ifosfamide (more than 1500 mg/m^2)
lomustine
mechlorethamine
methotrexate (more than 1000 mg/m^2)
mitoxantrone (more than 15 mg/m^2)
oxaliplatin
procarbazine
streptozocin

*Drugs in this list not covered in this chapter are described in Chapter 48.

---

mechanisms and sites of action will destroy more subpopulations of cells. The delayed onset of resistance to a particular antineoplastic drug is thus one benefit of combination drug therapy. To be most effective, however, the drugs used in such a combination regimen should possess the following characteristics:

- Some efficacy even as single drugs in the treatment of the particular type of cancer
- Different mechanisms of action so that the cytotoxic effect is maximized; this includes differences in cell cycle specificity
- No or minimal overlapping toxicities

One major drawback to the use of antineoplastic drugs is that nearly all of them cause adverse effects. These toxicities generally stem from the fact that chemotherapy drugs affect rapidly dividing cells—both harmful cancer cells and healthy, normal cells. Three types of rapidly dividing human cells are the cells of hair follicles, GI tract cells, and bone marrow cells. Because most of today's antineoplastic drugs cannot differentiate between cancer cells and healthy cells, the healthy cells are also destroyed, so hair loss, nausea and vomiting, and bone marrow toxicity are the undesirable consequences. Effects on the GI tract and bone marrow are often **dose-limiting adverse effects;** that is, the patient can no longer tolerate an increase in dosage that may be necessary to adequately treat the cancer and achieve good disease response.

As noted, hair follicle cells are rapidly dividing cells. Cancer drugs that affect these cells often cause the adverse effect known as *alopecia,* or hair loss. Many patients, especially women, choose to wear wigs, hats, or scarves to disguise this adverse effect. Some antineoplastic drugs are more harmful to the epithelial cells of the stomach and intestinal tract, which often leads to diarrhea and mucositis, and may also increase the risk of nausea and vomiting. The likelihood that a given drug will produce vomiting is known as its **emetic potential.** Anticancer drugs cause nausea and vomiting by stimulating the cells of the *chemoreceptor trigger zone.* Several antiemetic drugs are used to prevent these symptoms. These are described in Chapter 52. Box 47-1 lists the relative emetic potential of selected chemotherapy drugs.

Myelosuppression, also known as *bone marrow suppression* or *bone marrow depression*, is another unwanted adverse effect of certain antineoplastics. It commonly results from drug- or radiation-induced destruction of certain rapidly dividing cells in the bone marrow, primarily the cellular precursors of WBCs, red blood cells (RBCs), and platelets. This can also occur secondary to the disease processes of the cancer itself. Myelosuppression, in turn, leads to leukopenia, anemia, and thrombocytopenia. The cancer patient is often at greater risk for infection because of *leukopenia* (reduced WBC count) secondary to chemotherapy. Patients often need antibiotics intravenously (IV), either to prevent or to treat bacterial infections. Such patients are referred to as being *neutropenic.* Drug-induced *anemia* (reduced RBC count) often leads to hypoxia and fatigue, whereas *thrombocytopenia* (reduced platelet count) makes the patient more susceptible to bleeding. The lowest level of WBCs in the blood following chemotherapy (or radiation) treatment is called the **nadir.** The time until the nadir is reached in a given patient may become shorter and the recovery time for the bone marrow may become longer with multiple courses of antineoplastic treatment. The nadir normally occurs roughly 10 to 28 days after dosing, depending on the particular cancer drug or combination of drugs that is used to treat the patient. Anticipation of this nadir based on known cancer drug data can be used to guide the timing of prophylactic (preventative) administration of antibiotics and blood stimulants known as *hematopoietic growth factors* (see Chapter 49).

Common indications for various antineoplastic drugs are listed in the Dosages tables. Also provided in various locations in this and the next chapter are tables and boxes (Tables 47-8 and 48-2 and Boxes 48-1 and 48-2) containing drug-specific guidelines for the treatment of **extravasation**—unintended leakage of a chemotherapy drug (with vesicant potential) into the surrounding tissues outside of the IV line.

Because of the often severe toxicity of cancer medications, a current major focus of cancer drug research is the development of *targeted* drug therapy. Targeted drug therapy utilizes drugs that recognize a specific molecule involved in cancer cells growth, while mostly sparing healthy cells. One example of such targeted therapy is the newer class of cancer drugs known as *monoclonal antibodies* (see Chapter 49).

Pharmacokinetic data for antineoplastic medications is seldom used to guide dosing. Assay complexity coupled with a poor correlation between blood concentration and toxicity and efficacy limits its value. Only a handful of anticancer drugs benefit from therapeutic drug monitoring. For these reasons pharmacokinetic data are not included with the drug profiles in this chapter.

In spite of their notorious toxicity, given the often fatal outcome of neoplastic diseases, most cancer drugs are only rarely considered to be absolutely contraindicated for a given patient. Even if a patient has a known allergic reaction to an antineoplastic medication, the urgency of treating the patient's cancer necessitates administering the medication and treating any allergic symptoms with premedications such as antihistamines, corticosteroids, and acetaminophen. For these reasons, no specific contraindications are listed for any of the drugs in this chapter.

Common relative contraindications for cancer drugs include weakened status of the patient as manifested by indicators such as very low WBC count, ongoing infectious process, severe compromise in nutritional and hydration status, reduced kidney or liver function, or a decline in organ function in any system that may be further affected by the toxic effect of the drug being administered. These are situations in which chemotherapy treatment is commonly delayed until the patient's status improves. In general, most chemotherapy is held when the WBC count is less than 500 cells/mm^3. Alternatively, dosages are often reduced for frail elderly patients or others with significantly compromised organ system function, depending on the drugs used.

Reduction in fertility is often a major concern in postpubertal patients. Cancer also complicates 1 in 1000 pregnancies. Both radiation and chemotherapy treatments can cause significant permanent fetal harm or death. The greatest risk is during the first trimester. Chemotherapy treatment during the second or third trimester is more likely to improve maternal outcome without significant fetal risk. However, radiation treatment poses great risk to the fetus throughout pregnancy and should be reserved for the postpartum period if possible. Prepubertal patients are more resilient, however, and can have normal puberty and fertility.

In the elderly, *frailty* refers to loss of most of the patient's functional reserve and limited ability to tolerate even minimal physiologic stress (e.g., chemotherapy treatment). More robust elderly patients are certainly better candidates for cancer treatment, although frail patients often benefit as well, especially in terms of *palliative* (noncurative) symptom control.

CELL CYCLE–SPECIFIC ANTINEOPLASTIC DRUGS

Cell cycle–specific drug classes include antimetabolites, mitotic inhibitors, alkaloid topoisomerase II inhibitors, topoisomerase I inhibitors, and antineoplastic enzymes. These drugs are collectively used to treat a variety of solid and/or circulating tumors, although some drugs have much more specific indications than others.

ANTIMETABOLITES

A compound that is structurally similar to a normal cellular metabolite is known as an **analogue** of that metabolite. Analogues may have agonist or antagonist activity relative to the corresponding cellular compounds. An antagonist analogue is also known as an *antimetabolite.*

Mechanism of Action and Drug Effects

Antineoplastic antimetabolites are cell cycle–specific analogues that work by antagonizing the actions of key cellular metabolites. More specifically, antimetabolites inhibit cellular growth by interfering with the synthesis or actions of three classes of compounds critical to cellular reproduction: the vitamin *folic acid* and *purines* and *pyrimidines,* the two classes of compounds that make up the bases contained in *nucleic acid* molecules (DNA and RNA). These drugs work via two mechanisms: (1) by falsely substituting for purines, pyrimidines, or folic acid; and (2) by inhibiting critical enzymes involved in the synthesis or function of these compounds. Thus, they ultimately inhibit the synthesis of DNA, RNA, and proteins, all of which are necessary for cell survival. Antimetabolites work primarily in the S phase of the cell cycle, during which DNA synthesis is most active. The available antimetabolites and the metabolites they antagonize are as follows:

Folate antagonists
- methotrexate (MTX)
- pemetrexed

Purine antagonists
- cladribine
- fludarabine (F-AMP)
- mercaptopurine (6-MP)
- pentostatin
- thioguanine (6-TG)

Pyrimidine antagonists
- capecitabine

- cytarabine (ara-C)
- floxuridine (FUDR)
- fluorouracil (5-FU)
- gemcitabine

Folic Acid Antagonism

The antimetabolite methotrexate is an analogue of folic acid and inhibits the action of dihydrofolate reductase, an enzyme responsible for converting folic acid to a chemically reduced form that is used in the biosynthesis of other molecules. This inhibition prevents the formation of the folate, the reduced or anionic form of folic acid, that is needed for the synthesis of DNA. The result is that DNA is not produced and the cell dies. In practice, the terms *folic acid* and *folate* are often used interchangeably. Pemetrexed is the name of a newer folate antagonist with a mechanism of action similar to that of methotrexate.

Purine Antagonism

The purine bases present in DNA and RNA are adenine and guanine (see the discussion in Chapter 48), and they are required for the synthesis of the purine nucleotides that are incorporated into the nucleic acid molecules. Mercaptopurine and fludarabine are synthetic analogues of adenine, and thioguanine is a synthetic analogue of guanine. Cladribine is a more general purine antagonist, whereas pentostatin inhibits the action of the critical enzyme *adenosine deaminase*. Cladribine is unique in that it actually lacks cell cycle specificity relative to other drugs in its class. However, it is included in this section because of its similar pharmacology and mechanism of action. All of these drugs work by ultimately interrupting the synthesis of both DNA and RNA.

Although allopurinol is chemically similar to purines, it does not disrupt DNA synthesis. Instead, it inhibits xanthine oxidase, which reduces serum and/or urinary levels of *uric acid*. Rasburicase is an enzyme that degrades uric acid to more soluble end products. Uric acid is a common waste product that often accumulates in the blood following lysis of tumor cells, part of a condition known as **tumor lysis syndrome** (see Adverse Effects).

Pyrimidine Antagonism

Of the pyrimidine bases, cytosine and thymine occur in the structure of DNA molecules, and cytosine and uracil are part of the structure of RNA molecules. These bases are essential for DNA and RNA synthesis. Floxuridine and fluorouracil are synthetic analogues of uracil, and cytarabine is a synthetic analogue of cytosine. Capecitabine is actually a prodrug of fluorouracil and is converted to that drug in the liver and other body tissues. Because of its prodrug form it can be given orally. Gemcitabine inhibits the action of two essential enzymes, *DNA polymerase* and *ribonucleotide reductase*. Overall, these drugs act in a way that is very similar to that of the purine antagonists, incorporating themselves into the metabolic pathway for the synthesis of DNA and RNA and thereby interrupting the synthesis of both of these nucleic acids.

Indications

Antimetabolite antineoplastic drugs are used for the treatment of a variety of solid tumors and some hematologic cancers. They may also be used in combination chemotherapy regimens to enhance the overall cytotoxic effect. Methotrexate is also used to treat severe cases of psoriasis (a skin condition) as well as rheumatoid arthritis

(see Chapter 49). Because some of these drugs are available in both oral and topical preparations, they are sometimes used for low-dose maintenance and palliative (noncurative) cancer therapy.

Allopurinol and rasburicase are both indicated for the hyperuricemia associated with tumor lysis syndrome and are usually given in anticipation of this condition during various chemotherapy regimens associated with this syndrome. Allopurinol is also used commonly in oral form to treat gout (see Chapter 44). Rasburicase is used primarily in pediatric patients, and there is little published information to date regarding its use in adults. The commonly used drugs and their common specific therapeutic uses are listed in the Dosages table on p. 734.

Adverse Effects

Like most antineoplastic drugs, antimetabolites can cause hair loss, nausea, vomiting, diarrhea, and myelosuppression. The relative emetic potentials for some of these drugs are listed in Box 47-1. In addition, these and other antineoplastic drug classes are associated with other major types of toxicity including neurologic, cardiovascular, pulmonary, hepatobiliary, GI, genitourinary, dermatologic, ocular, otic, and metabolic toxicity. Common manifestations of these various toxicities are listed in Table 47-6, roughly in order of increasing severity. Note that a single drug may not cause all of the specific symptoms that are listed for each toxicity category, and actual symptoms may vary widely in severity among patients. The most common general symptoms are fever and malaise. Metabolic toxicity also includes tumor lysis syndrome, a common postchemotherapy condition. This syndrome is often associated with *induction* (initial) chemotherapy for rapidly growing hematologic malignancies. It may include hyperphosphatemia, hyperkalemia, and hypocalcemia. These electrolyte abnormalities are often treated with diuretics such as mannitol, IV calcium supplementation, oral or rectal potassium exchange resin and oral aluminum hydroxide. Hyperuricemia can lead to nephropathy, and hemodialysis may be required in severe cases of tumor lysis syndrome.

A severe, but usually reversible, form of dermatologic toxicity is known as *palmar-plantar dysesthesia* or paresthesia (also called *hand-foot syndrome*). It can range from mild symptoms such as painless swelling and erythema to painful blistering of the patient's palms and soles. Other severe, but fortunately uncommon, dermatologic syndromes that can similarly affect the skin in more generalized regions include *Stevens-Johnson syndrome* and *toxic epidermal necrolysis.*

Interactions

As is true for cancer drugs in general, the administration of one antimetabolite drug with another that causes similar toxicities may result in additive toxicities. Therefore, the respective risks and benefits should be weighed carefully before therapy is initiated with either another antimetabolite or any other drug possessing a similar toxicity profile. Table 47-7 lists some known common examples of drugs that cause interactions with antimetabolites.

Dosages

For information on the dosages of selected antimetabolite chemotherapeutic drugs, see the Dosages table on p. 734. It is important to note that dosages of antineoplastics are highly variable based on type of cancer, prior therapy, and planned coadministration of other agents.

TABLE 47-6 Common Manifestations of Antineoplastic Toxicity

Type of Toxicity	Common Manifestations
Neurologic	Fatigue, weakness, depression, agitation, euphoria, insomnia, sedation, headache, reduced libido, confusion, amnesia, hallucinations (visual and auditory), dizziness, loss of taste or altered taste sensations, dysarthria (joint pain), polyneuropathy (e.g., numbness in extremities), neuritis, paresthesia (abnormal touch sensations), facial paralysis, migraine, tremor, hemiplegia, loss of consciousness, seizures, ataxia, stroke, encephalopathy
Cardiovascular	Hot flushes, edema, thrombophlebitis and bleeding (e.g., near infusion site), chest pain, tachycardia, bradycardia, other dysrhythmias, angina, venous or arterial thrombosis, transient ischemic attacks, heart failure, myocardial ischemia, pericarditis, pericardial effusion, pulmonary embolism, aneurysm, cardiomyopathy, myocardial infarction, stroke, cardiac arrest, sudden cardiac death
Pulmonary-respiratory	Cough, rhinorrhea (runny nose), sore throat, sinusitis, bronchitis, pharyngitis, laryngitis, epistaxis (nosebleed), abnormal breath sounds, asthma, bronchospasms, atelectasis, pleural effusion, hemoptysis, hypoxia, respiratory distress, pneumothorax, diffuse interstitial pneumonitis, fibrosis, hemorrhage, anaphylaxis and generalized allergic reactions
Hepatobiliary	Increased bilirubin and liver enzyme levels, jaundice, cholestasis, acalculic cholecystitis (inflamed gallbladder without stones), hepatitis, sclerosis, fibrosis, fatty liver changes, venoocclusive hepatic disease, cirrhosis, hepatic coma
Gastrointestinal (GI)	Dyspepsia (heartburn), hiccups, gingivitis (inflamed gums), glossitis (inflamed tongue), abdominal pain, nausea, vomiting, diarrhea, constipation, gastroenteritis, stomatitis (painful mouth sores), oral candidiasis (thrush), ulcers, proctalgia (rectal pain), hematemesis, GI hemorrhage, melena (blood in stool), toxic intestinal dilation, ileus (bowel paralysis), ascites, necrotizing enterocolitis
Genitourinary	Oliguria, nocturia, dysuria, proteinuria, crystalluria, hematuria, urinary retention, abnormal renal function test results, hemorrhagic cystitis, renal failure
Dermatologic	Rash, erythema, pruritus, ecchymosis, dryness, edema, photosensitivity, sweating, discoloration (pigmentation changes), freckling, petechiae, purpura, numbness, tingling, hypersensitivity, fissuring, scaling, seborrhea, acne, eczema, psoriasis, skin hypertrophy, subcutaneous nodules, alopecia, nail disorder including onycholysis (loss of nails), dermatitis, cellulitis, excoriation, maceration, ulceration, urticaria, abscesses, benign skin neoplasm, hemorrhage (at injection site), palmar-plantar dysesthesia-paresthesia, toxic epidermal necrolysis, Stevens-Johnson syndrome
Ocular	Eye irritation, increased lacrimation, nystagmus, photophobia, visual changes, conjunctivitis, keratitis, dacryostenosis (narrowing of lacrimal duct)
Otic	Hearing loss
Metabolic	Weight loss or gain, anorexia, dehydration, hypokalemia, hypocalcemia, hypomagnesemia, hypertriglyceridemia, hyperglycemia, syndrome of inappropriate secretion of antidiuretic hormone, hypoadrenalism, protein-losing enteropathy, hyperuricemia, tumor lysis syndrome
Musculoskeletal	Back pain, limb pain, bone pain, myalgia, joint stiffness, arthralgia, muscle weakness, fibromyositis

DRUG PROFILES

FOLATE ANTAGONIST

◆ methotrexate

Methotrexate is the prototypical antimetabolite antineoplastic of the folate antagonist group and is currently one of only two antineoplastic folate antagonists used clinically. It has proved useful for the treatment of solid tumors such as breast, head and neck, and lung cancers and for the management of acute lymphocytic leukemia and non-Hodgkin's lymphomas. Methotrexate also has immunosuppressive activity, because it can inhibit lymphocyte multiplication. For this reason it may be useful in the treatment of rheumatoid arthritis (see Chapter 49). Its combined immunosuppressant and antiinflammatory properties also make it useful for the treatment of psoriasis.

High-dose methotrexate is associated with bone marrow suppression, and it is always given in conjunction with the "rescue" drug *leucovorin*. Leucovorin is an antidote for folic acid antagonists. Basically leucovorin rescues the healthy cells from methotrexate. Methotrexate is available in both injectable and oral (tablet) form. A preservative-free injectable formulation is required for **intrathecal** (spinal) administration, used in treatment of some cancers. Currently the only other folate antagonist is a newer drug called pemetrexed, which has an action similar to that of methotrexate. However, it is much less widely used because of its limited indications for treatment of certain types of lung cancer.

PURINE ANTAGONISTS

The currently available purine antagonists are cladribine, fludarabine, mercaptopurine, pentostatin, and thioguanine. Mercaptopurine and thioguanine are administered orally, whereas the other three are available only in injectable form. These drugs are used largely in the treatment of leukemia and lymphoma.

cladribine

Cladribine (Leustatin) is indicated specifically for the treatment of a certain type of leukemia known as hairy cell leukemia, so named because of the appearance of its cancerous cells under the microscope.

fludarabine

Fludarabine (Fludara), like cladribine, also has a very specific single indication—in this case, chronic lymphocytic leukemia. It is also commonly used in the treatment of follicular lymphoma and as part of salvage therapy in acute myelogenous leukemia.

pyrimidine antagonists

The currently available pyrimidine antagonists are capecitabine, cytarabine, floxuridine, fluorouracil, and gemcitabine. These drugs are used more commonly than the purine antagonists. They are available only in parenteral formulations except for capecitabine, which is currently available only in tablet form. Dosage and other information appear in the Dosages table on p. 734.

TABLE 47-7 Selected Antimetabolites: Common Drug Interactions

Antimetabolite	Interacting Drug	Observed and Reported Effects*
capecitabine	warfarin	Altered coagulation test results with potential for fatal bleeding
	phenytoin	Reduced phenytoin clearance and toxicity
	leucovorin	Potentiation of capecitabine with possible toxicity
cladribine	None listed	None listed
cytarabine	digoxin	Reduced absorption likely due to cytarabine-induced damage to intestinal mucosa; elixir form may be better absorbed
	Aminoglycoside antibiotics	Reduced antibiotic efficacy against *Klebsiella pneumoniae* infections
floxuridine	None listed	None listed
fludarabine	cytarabine	Increased antitumor activity of cytarabine
	pentostatin	Potentially fatal pulmonary toxicity; do not use together
fluorouracil	warfarin	Enhanced anticoagulant effects
	leucovorin	Same as for capecitabine
	cimetidine	Increases toxicity of fluorouracil
gemcitabine	None listed	None listed
mercaptopurine (6-MP)	allopurinol	Inhibition of 6-MP metabolism by inhibition of xanthine oxidase enzyme, with possible enhanced 6-MP toxicity; reduce dose to one third to one fourth
	warfarin	6-MP reported to both enhance and inhibit its effects
	Hepatotoxic drugs	Increased risk of liver toxicity
methotrexate (MTX)	Protein-bound drugs and weak organic acids (e.g., salicylates, sulfonamides, sulfonylureas, phenytoin, tetracyclines)	Possible displacement of MTX from protein-binding sites, enhancing its toxicity
	penicillins, NSAIDs	Possible reduced renal elimination of MTX with potentially fatal hematologic and GI toxicity
	Live virus vaccines	Viral infection (true for any immunosuppressive drug)
	folic acid	Reduced MTX efficacy (theoretical only)
	theophylline	Reduced theophylline clearance
	Hepatotoxic drugs	Increased risk of liver toxicity
pentostatin	fludarabine	Potentially fatal pulmonary toxicity
thioguanine	busulfan	Reports of hepatotoxicity, esophageal varices, and portal hypertension
	Other cytotoxic drugs in general	Reports of hepatotoxicity

GI, Gastrointestinal; *NSAIDs,* nonsteroidal antiinflammatory drugs.
*Note that not all mechanisms for these drug interactions have been clearly identified. The information in this table is based on reported clinical observations, with mention of known or theorized mechanisms when available.

capecitabine

Capecitabine (Xeloda) is indicated primarily for the treatment of metastatic breast cancer.

◆ cytarabine

Cytarabine (ara-C) (Cytosar) is used primarily for the treatment of leukemias (acute myelocytic and lymphocytic leukemia and meningeal leukemia) and non-Hodgkin's lymphomas. As previously noted, it is available only in injectable form and may be given IV, subcutaneously, or intrathecally. It is also now available in a special encapsulated liposomal form for intrathecal use only in treating meningeal leukemia.

fluorouracil

Fluorouracil (5-FU) (Efudex) is used in a variety of treatment regimens, including the palliative treatment of cancers of the colon, rectum, stomach, breast, and pancreas. It also is used in the adjuvant setting in the treatment of breast and colorectal cancer.

gemcitabine

Gemcitabine (Gemzar) is an antineoplastic drug structurally related to cytarabine. Gemcitabine is believed to have antitumor activity superior to that of cytarabine. It is used as first-line therapy for locally advanced or metastatic cancer of the pancreas and for the treatment of non–small cell lung cancer. It is increasingly used to treat other solid tumors, including breast cancer.

MITOTIC INHIBITORS

Mitotic inhibitors include natural products obtained from the periwinkle plant and semisynthetic drugs obtained from the mandrake plant (also known as the "may apple"). The periwinkle plant contains antineoplastic alkaloids. These vinca alkaloids include vinblastine, vincristine, and vinorelbine. Two newer plant-derived drugs are the taxanes. These include paclitaxel, once derived from the bark of the slow-growing Western (Pacific) yew tree, and docetaxel, a semisynthetic taxane produced from the needles of the European yew tree. The current process of isolating the starting material for paclitaxel from the needles has made the drug supply more abundant. Docetaxel is pharmacologically similar to paclitaxel. Dosage and other information appears in the Dosages table on p. 735.

Mechanism of Action and Drug Effects

Depending on the particular drug, these plant-derived compounds can work in various phases of the cell cycle (late S phase, throughout G_2 phase, and M phase), but they all work shortly before or during mitosis and thus retard cell division. Each different subclass inhibits mitosis in a unique way.

The vinca alkaloids (vincristine, vinblastine, and vinorelbine) bind to the protein *tubulin* during the metaphase of mitosis (M phase). This prevents the assembly of key structures called

DOSAGES

Selected Antimetabolites

Drug (Pregnancy Category)	Pharmacologic Class	Usual Dosage Range*	Indications
capecitabine (Xeloda) (D)	Pyrimidine antagonist (analogue)	PO: 1250 mg/m² bid for 2 wk, followed by 1-wk rest period; this 3-wk cycle repeatable as ordered	Metastatic colorectal and breast cancer
cladribine (Leustatin) (D)	Purine antagonist (analogue)	IV: 0.09 mg/kg/day by continuous infusion for 7 consecutive days	Hairy cell leukemia
◆ cytarabine (Cytosar-U) (D)	Pyrimidine antagonist (analogue)	IV: 100 mg/m²/day by continuous infusion for 7 days (other regimens as well)	Leukemias (several varieties), NHL
fludarabine (Fludara) (D)	Purine antagonist (analogue)	IV: 25 mg/m²/day for 5 consecutive days; repeatable q28d	Various acute and chronic leukemias, NHL
fluorouracil (Adrucil) (D)	Pyrimidine antagonist (analogue)	IV: short infusion: 400 mg/m²; continuous infusion: 2400 mg/m² over 46 hr; dosage varies afterward depending on patient response	Colon, rectal, breast, esophageal, head and neck, cervical, and renal cancer
gemcitabine (Gemzar) (D)	Pyrimidine antagonist (analogue)	IV: 1000 mg/m² once weekly or as protocol dictates; cycle may be repeated or modified according to patient tolerance	Pancreatic, non–small cell lung, and bladder cancer
◆ methotrexate (Trexall, tablet form; otherwise generic) (X)	Folate antagonist (analogue)	IV: 30-40 mg/m²/wk PO: 15-30 mg/day for 5 days, repeated q7d for 3-5 courses	Acute lymphocytic† leukemia; gestational choriocarcinoma; breast, head and neck, and many other cancers

IV, Intravenous; *NHL,* non-Hodgkin's lymphoma; *PO,* oral.
*Note: Dosages are highly variable.
†The term *lymphocytic* is synonymous in the literature with the term *lymphoblastic.*

---

microtubules. This, in turn, results in the dissolution of other important structures known as *mitotic spindles.* Without these mitotic spindles, cells cannot reproduce properly. This results in inhibition of cell division and cell death.

The yew tree derivatives (taxanes) paclitaxel and docetaxel both act in the late G_2 phase and M phase of the cell cycle. They work by causing the formation of nonfunctional microtubules, which halts mitosis during metaphase.

Indications

Mitotic inhibitors are used to treat a variety of solid tumors and some hematologic malignancies. They are often used in combination chemotherapy regimens to enhance the overall cytotoxic effect. Selected drugs and some of their specific therapeutic uses are listed in the Dosages table on p. 735.

Adverse Effects

Like many of the antineoplastic drugs, mitotic inhibitor antineoplastic drugs can cause hair loss, nausea and vomiting, and myelosuppression (see Table 47-6). The emetic potential of some of these drugs is given in Box 47-1.

Toxicity and Management of Extravasation

Most of the mitotic inhibitor antineoplastics are administered IV, and extravasation of these drugs is potentially serious. Specific antidotes and additional measures to be taken for the treatment of extravasation of the mitotic inhibitors are given in Table 47-8.

TABLE 47-8 Mitotic Inhibitor and Etoposide Extravasation: Listed Specific Antidote

Drug	Antidote Preparation	Method
etoposide teniposide vinblastine vincristine	hyaluronidase (Wydase) 150 units/mL: add 1 mL NaCl (150 units/mL)	1. Inject 1-6 mL into the extravasated site with multiple subcut injections. 2. Repeat subcut dosing over the next few hours. 3. Apply warm compresses.* No total dose established.

Subcut, Subcutaneous.
*Important: Administration of corticosteroids and topical cooling appear to worsen toxicity.

Interactions

A variety of drug interactions are possible with most antineoplastic drugs, some more significant than others. A few basic principles should be kept in mind that apply to all antineoplastic drug classes. Any drug that reduces the clearance of an anticancer drug also increases the risk of toxicity, whereas a drug that increases the elimination of an anticancer drug reduces its efficacy. The use of multiple antineoplastic drugs can cause severe neutropenia and infection, due to additive bone marrow suppression. Patients should be monitored and treated accordingly for hematologic toxicity and infections. Observed drug interactions specific for mitotic inhibitors are summarized in Table 47-9.

TABLE 47-9 Selected Mitotic Inhibitors and Etoposide: Common Drug Interactions

Drug	Interacting Drug/Observed and Reported Effects*
etoposide	warfarin: enhanced anticoagulation cyclosporine: reduced etoposide clearance
docetaxel	CYP3A4 inhibitors (azole antifungals, ciprofloxacin, clarithromycin, imatinib, verapamil, many others): enhanced docetaxel effect (possible toxicity) CYP3A4 inducers (e.g., carbamazepine, rifampin, phenytoin): reduced docetaxel effect
paclitaxel	doxorubicin: increased cardiotoxicity CYP3A4 inhibitors and inducers: same as for docetaxel
vincristine	phenytoin: reduced phenytoin concentrations with consequent enhanced seizure risk asparaginase: reduced vincristine clearance and increased neurotoxicity (give vincristine 12-24 hr before asparaginase) mitomycin: increased risk of pulmonary toxicity CYP3A4 inhibitors and inducers: same as for docetaxel

CYP3A4, Cytochrome P-450 liver enzyme 3A4.
*Note that not all mechanisms for these drug interactions have been clearly identified. The information in this table is based on reported clinical observations, with mention of known or theorized mechanisms when available.

Dosages

For information on the dosages of selected mitotic inhibitors and alkaloid topoisomerase II inhibitors, see the Dosages table on this page.

ALKALOID TOPOISOMERASE II INHIBITORS

Etoposide and teniposide are semisynthetic derivatives of *epipodophyllotoxin*, which is obtained from the resinous extract of the mandrake plant. Whereas podophyllotoxin inhibits mitosis, the epipodophyllotoxin derivatives (etoposide and teniposide)

exert their cytotoxic effects by inhibiting the enzyme *topoisomerase II*, which causes breaks in DNA strands. These drugs work during the late S phase and the G_2 phase of the cell cycle.

Dosages

For information on the dosages of selected mitotic inhibitors and alkaloid topoisomerase II inhibitors, see the Dosages table on this page.

▌ DRUG PROFILES

SELECTED MITOTIC INHIBITORS AND ETOPOSIDE
◆ etoposide

Etoposide (VP-16) (VePesid) is a semisynthetic epipodophyllotoxin derivative with topoisomerase II inhibiting activity. Its structure, mechanism of action, and adverse effect profile are similar to those of teniposide. As previously noted, it is believed to kill cancer cells in the late S phase and the G_2 phase of the cell cycle. It is indicated for the treatment of small cell lung cancer and testicular cancer. It is available in both oral and injectable forms; however, the oral form is poorly absorbed and has fallen out of favor because it produces significant toxicities without therapeutic benefit. The IV drug is formulated in a hydroalcoholic diluent, which can cause toxicity (hypotension) if administered in too high a concentration. A water-soluble form of the drug (Etopophos) can eliminate these administration issues, but it is very expensive compared with the standard preparation.

◆ paclitaxel

Paclitaxel (Taxol) is a natural mitotic inhibitor that was originally isolated from the bark of the Pacific yew tree. The European yew tree is the source for another mitotic inhibitor known as docetaxel (Taxotere). Paclitaxel is currently approved for the treatment of ovarian cancer, breast cancer, non–small cell lung cancer, and Kaposi's sarcoma, among other cancers. Paclitaxel is water insoluble (hydrophobic), and for this reason it is put into a solution containing oil rather than water. The particular oil used is a type of castor oil called Cremophor EL, the same oil with which cyclosporine is formulated. Many patients tolerate it poorly and show hypersensitivity associated with infusion. For this reason, before

DOSAGES

Selected Mitotic Inhibitors and Etoposide

Drug (Pregnancy Category)	Pharmacologic Class	Usual Dosage Range*	Indications
Epipodophyllotoxin Derivative			
◆ etoposide (VePesid, Toposar, Etopophos) (D)	Topoisomerase II inhibitor	IV: 50-160 mg/m²/day for 4-5 days, then repeated cycles and dosage based on type of cancer	Testicular and small cell lung cancer
Taxane			
◆ paclitaxel (Taxol, Onxol) (D)	Inhibitor of tubulin depolymerization	IV: 135-250 mg/m² q3wk	Ovarian, breast, esophageal, bladder, head and neck, cervical cancer; non–small cell and small cell lung cancer; Kaposi's sarcoma
Vinca Alkaloid			
◆ vincristine (Oncovin, Vincasar PFS) (D)	Inhibitor of tubulin polymerization	IV: 1.4 mg/m² q1wk; usual max dose 2 mg; fatal if given intrathecally	ALL, AML, HL, NHL, rhabdomyosarcoma, neuroblastoma, Wilms tumor, brain tumors, small cell lung cancer, Kaposi's sarcoma

ALL, Acute lymphocytic leukemia; *AML,* acute myelocytic leukemia; *HL,* Hodgkin's lymphoma; *IV,* intravenous; *NHL,* non-Hodgkin's lymphoma.
*Note that dosages may vary widely among treatment protocols.

patients receive paclitaxel they are premedicated with a steroid (dexamethasone), H_1 receptor antagonist (diphenhydramine), and H_2 receptor antagonist (ranitidine). Paclitaxel is available only in injectable form. There is an albumin-bound form of the drug (Abraxane) that is not associated with severe infusion reactions.

◆ vincristine

Vincristine is an alkaloid isolated from the periwinkle plant that is indicated for the treatment of acute lymphocytic leukemia and other cancers. It is available only in injectable form. It is an M phase–specific drug that inhibits mitotic spindle formation. Vincristine is the most significant neurotoxin of the cytotoxic drug class, but it continues to be used in part because of its relative lack of bone marrow suppression. Special care must be taken not to inadvertently give vincristine via the intrathecal route. Several deaths have been reported due to this error. The World Health Organization and the Institute for Safe Medication Practices suggest that vincristine be diluted in 25 mL of fluid and never dispensed via a syringe to prevent this lethal error from occurring. A special warning is required for all vincristine products dispensed that states "Lethal if given intrathecally, for IV use only." (See the Preventing Medication Errors box on this page.)

TOPOISOMERASE I INHIBITORS

Topoisomerase I inhibitors are a relatively new class of chemotherapy drugs. The two drugs currently available in this class are topotecan and irinotecan. Both are semisynthetic analogues of the compound camptothecin, which was originally isolated in the 1960s from *Camptotheca acuminata,* a Chinese shrub. For this reason, these drugs are also referred to as *camptothecins.*

Mechanism of Action and Drug Effects

The Chinese shrub–derived camptothecins inhibit proper DNA function in the S phase by binding to the DNA–topoisomerase I complex. This complex normally allows DNA strands to be temporarily cleaved and then reattached in a critical step known as *religation.* The binding of the camptothecin drugs to this complex retards this religation process, which results DNA strand break.

Indications

The two currently available topoisomerase I inhibitors are used primarily to treat ovarian and colorectal cancer. Topotecan has been shown to be effective even in cases of metastatic ovarian cancer that has failed to respond to platinum-containing regimens (e.g., cisplatin, carboplatin) and paclitaxel. Topotecan is also used to treat small cell lung cancer. Irinotecan is currently approved for the treatment of metastatic colorectal cancer, small cell lung cancer, and cervical cancer.

Adverse Effects

As with many cancer chemotherapeutic drugs, the main adverse effect of topotecan is bone marrow suppression. Topotecan should not be given to patients with baseline neutrophil counts of less than 1500 cells/mm³. Other adverse effects are relatively minor compared with those of the other antineoplastic drug classes. These include mild to moderate nausea, vomiting, and diarrhea; headache; rash; muscle weakness; and cough.

PREVENTING MEDICATION ERRORS

Vincristine: Right Route Is Essential

For several years, the Institute for Safe Medication Practices has recommended changes in procedures to ensure that vincristine and other vinca alkaloids are not given intrathecally (via the spinal route). Administering these drugs via the spinal route is almost always fatal, and the death is slow and excruciating. Mistakes occur when the drug is drawn up in a syringe for intravenous administration and then is inadvertently given via the intrathecal route. These errors are preventable. The World Health Organization has suggested that pharmacies prepare vincristine in a diluted volume, such as in a 50-mL minibag of normal saline, to deter practitioners from giving the drug intrathecally. Drugs given intrathecally are not normally dispensed in a minibag. The nurse, who may be assisting the health care practitioner with intrathecal procedures, needs to be aware of the potential fatal error that may occur if vincristine is given via the wrong route. For more information, go to *http://www.ismp.org.*

Irinotecan causes more severe adverse effects than topotecan. In addition to producing similar hematologic adverse effects, it has been associated with severe diarrhea known as *cholinergic diarrhea* that may occur during irinotecan infusion. It is recommended that this condition be treated with atropine unless use of that drug is strongly contraindicated. Delayed diarrhea may occur 2 to 10 days after infusion of irinotecan. This diarrhea can be severe and even life threatening. Delayed diarrhea should be treated aggressively with loperamide. There is a well-recognized polymorphism in the irinotecan-metabolizing enzymes that, when present, may reduce drug elimination and therefore increase the severity of bone marrow suppression and diarrhea. There is a moderate risk of nausea and vomiting with irinotecan, which requires appropriate supportive care such as IV rehydration and antiemetic drug therapy.

Interactions

Topotecan has a unique drug interaction involving the *granulocyte colony-stimulating factor* filgrastim (see Chapter 49). Filgrastim is commonly used to enhance WBC recovery after chemotherapy. When topotecan is given along with filgrastim, myelosuppression has actually been shown to be worsened. It is recommended that filgrastim be administered 24 hours after completion of the topotecan infusion. Laxatives and diuretics should not be given with irinotecan, because of the potential to worsen the dehydration resulting from the severe diarrhea that this drug can produce. Severe cardiovascular toxicity, including thrombosis, pulmonary embolism, stroke, and acute fatal myocardial infarction, have been reported when irinotecan is given with fluorouracil and leucovorin. The role of irinotecan in this toxicity syndrome is unclear, because fluorouracil is a well-recognized cause of myocardial ischemia, including myocardial infarction and sudden death. Such drug combinations should be given with careful monitoring. Several additional recognized drug interactions occur with irinotecan, which are summarized in Table 47-10.

Dosages

For recommended dosages of selected topoisomerase I inhibitors, see the Dosages table on p. 737.

DOSAGES

Selected Topoisomerase I Inhibitors

Drug (Pregnancy Category)	Pharmacologic Class	Usual Dosage Range*	Indications
irinotecan (Camptosar) (D)	Synthetic camptothecin	IV: 125-350 mg/m² on various days depending on protocol	Metastatic colorectal cancer, small cell lung cancer, cervical cancer
topotecan (Hycamtin) (D)	Semisynthetic camptothecin	IV: 1.5 mg/m² once daily for 5 consecutive days on a repeatable 21-day course	Ovarian and small cell lung cancer

IV, Intravenous.
*Note: Dosages are highly variable.

TABLE 47-10 Irinotecan: Common Drug Interactions

Interacting Drug	Observed and Reported Effects*
CYP2B6 inhibitors (e.g., paroxetine, sertraline)	Increased effects and toxicity of irinotecan
CYP3A4 inhibitors (e.g., azole antifungals, ciprofloxacin, clarithromycin, imatinib, isoniazid, verapamil)	Increased effects and toxicity of irinotecan; concurrent use not recommended
CYP2B6 inducers (e.g., carbamazepine, phenytoin, nevirapine)	Reduced effects of irinotecan
CYP3A4 inducers (e.g., aminoglutethimide, carbamazepine, rifampin, nevirapine, phenytoin)	Reduced effects of irinotecan
St. John's wort (CYP3A4 inducer)	Reduced effects of irinotecan; stop St. John's wort 2 wk before initiating irinotecan therapy

CYP2B6, Cytochrome P-450 liver enzyme 2B6; *CYP3A4,* cytochrome P-450 liver enzyme 3A4.
*Note that not all mechanisms for these drug interactions have been clearly identified. The information in this table is based on reported clinical observations, with mention of known or theorized mechanisms when available.

DRUG PROFILES

irinotecan
Irinotecan (Camptosar) is often given with both fluorouracil and leucovorin. It is available only in injectable form.

topotecan
After initial therapy with other antineoplastics, cancer cells commonly become resistant to their effects. The use of topotecan (Hycamtin) to treat ovarian cancer and small cell lung cancer has been studied extensively. As noted earlier, it produces therapeutic responses even in cases in which powerful drugs such as cisplatin and paclitaxel have failed. It is available only in injectable form.

ANTINEOPLASTIC ENZYMES

Two antineoplastic enzymes are commercially available: asparaginase and pegaspargase. A third, *Erwinia* asparaginase, is available only by special request from the National Cancer Institute for patients who have developed allergic reactions to *Escherichia coli*–based asparaginase. All three drugs are synthesized from cultures of certain bacteria using recombinant DNA technology.

Indications
The antineoplastic enzymes are currently approved exclusively for the treatment of acute lymphocytic leukemia.

Adverse Effects
Of particular note for the antineoplastic enzymes is a fairly unique adverse effect of impaired pancreatic function. This can lead to hyperglycemia and severe or fatal pancreatitis. Other types of adverse effects associated with these drugs are dermatologic, hepatic, genitourinary, neurologic, musculoskeletal, GI, and cardiovascular effects.

Interactions
Commonly reported drug interactions involving the antineoplastic enzymes are summarized in Table 47-11.

Dosages
Dosages for the antineoplastic enzymes are given in the Dosages table on p. 738.

DRUG PROFILES

◆ asparaginase
Asparaginase (Elspar) is used for the treatment of acute lymphocytic leukemia. Its mechanism of action is slightly different from that of traditional antineoplastic drugs in that it is an enzyme that catalyzes the conversion of the amino acid asparagine to aspartic acid and ammonia. Leukemic cells are then unable to synthesize the asparagine required for the synthesis of DNA and proteins needed for cell survival.

The only commercially available asparaginase product in the United States is the Elspar product manufactured by Merck, Inc. This product is derived from the *E. coli* bacterium, and it is common for patients to develop allergic reactions to it. When this happens, one alternative is to switch to a product synthesized from an *Erwinia* bacteria. As noted earlier, this product is not sold commercially in the United States but is available by special request from the National Cancer Institute. Another treatment alternative is to use the commercially available pegaspargase product described in the following drug profile. All antineoplastic enzymes are available only in injectable form.

pegaspargase
Pegaspargase (Oncaspar) has a mechanism of action, indications, and contraindications similar to those of asparaginase. It is essentially the same enzyme that has been formulated so as to reduce its allergenic potential. This process involves chemical conjugation of the enzyme with units of a relatively inert compound known as

DOSAGES

Selected Antineoplastic Enzymes

Drug (Pregnancy Category)	Pharmacologic Class	Usual Dosage Range*	Indications
◆ asparaginase (Elspar) (C)	*Escherichia coli*–derived L-asparagine amidohydrolase enzyme	IV/IM: 200 units/kg/day to 40,000 units per dose depending on protocol	Acute lymphocytic leukemia
pegaspargase (Oncaspar) (C)	Pegylated version of asparaginase	IV/IM: 2500 IU/m² q14d (smaller pediatric dosages)	Acute lymphocytic leukemia (usually in patients who have developed an allergy to asparaginase)

IM, Intramuscular; *IV,* intravenous.
*Note: Dosages are highly variable.

TABLE 47-11 Selected Antineoplastic Enzymes: Common Drug Interactions

Enzyme	Interacting Drug/Observed and Reported Effects*
asparaginase	cyclophosphamide, mercaptopurine, vincristine: interference with efficacy or clearance of asparaginase
	mercaptopurine, methotrexate, prednisone: enhanced liver toxicity of asparaginase
	methotrexate: reduced antineoplastic effect when given concurrently, but possibly enhanced antineoplastic effect when given 9-10 days before or shortly after methotrexate
	prednisone: hyperglycemia (give asparaginase after prednisone)
	vincristine: neuropathy (give asparaginase after vincristine)
	aspirin, NSAIDs, dipyridamole, heparin, warfarin: use with caution due to possible coagulation abnormalities

NSAIDs, Nonsteroidal antiinflammatory drugs.
*Note that not all mechanisms for these drug interactions have been clearly identified. The information in this table is based on reported clinical observations, with mention of known or theorized mechanisms when available.

monomethoxypolyethylene glycol. Because polyethylene glycol is abbreviated PEG, this process is known as *pegylation.* It is a process that is increasingly used in formulating various drugs, some of which are described in other chapters (e.g., see Chapter 49). These drugs are recognized by the prefix *peg* in their generic names. Pegaspargase is usually prescribed for patients who have developed an allergy to asparaginase—a common occurrence, as mentioned earlier, especially with repeated treatment.

NURSING PROCESS

Assessment

Antineoplastic therapy requires the following aspects of a thorough physical assessment: a nursing history; past and present medical history; family history; a medication profile with a notation of allergies as well as a listing of all prescription drugs, over-the-counter drugs, and herbals; height, weight, and vital signs; and baseline hearing and vision testing (as ordered). Bowel and bladder patterns, neurologic status, heart sounds, heart rhythm, breath sounds, and lung function should also be assessed. The skin and mucosa should be examined and turgor, hydration, color, and temperature noted. Any signs and symptoms of fear and anxiety should be assessed, with attention to complaints of insomnia, irritability, shakiness, restlessness, and/or palpitations, any unusual problems that could be attributed to stress and anxiety. An assessment of cultural, emotional, spiritual, sexual, and financial influences, concerns, and issues should also be completed. The patient's ability to perform activities of daily living and the patient's mobility status and gait also should be noted. Assessing for pain is also an important part of the care of these patients. The patient should be assessed for oral, pharyngeal, esophageal, and/or abdominal pain; painful swallowing; epigastric or gastric pain, especially after eating spicy or acidic foods; achiness in joints or lower extremities; and numbness, tingling, and any burning or sharp pain that is general or localized. Pain should be assessed using an intensity rating scale (e.g., 0 to 10, where 0 = no pain and 10 = worse pain ever). The pattern of pain should also be noted, with a focus on the location, quality, onset, duration, and precipitating or alleviating factors. The patient should also be asked about past experiences with pain and about any drug, nondrug, or alternative therapies used and successes or failures in its treatment. Cultural beliefs and background as they relate to pain are important to assess, because the individual's culture may affect how pain is perceived, verbalized, and treated (see Chapter 11).

Contraindications, cautions, drug interactions, and drug allergies should also be assessed and documented prior to the use of these drugs. Laboratory tests that are usually ordered include levels of electrolytes and minerals, uric acid levels, complete blood count, platelet count, bleeding time, tests of renal and hepatic function, and cardiac enzyme levels (see Laboratory Values Related to Drug Therapy box). Assays of tumor markers may also be ordered to establish baseline levels and determine the impact of the disease and subsequent therapy on the patient. For more information about the specific adverse effects associated with the destruction of various populations of normal cells due to chemotherapy, see Box 47-2. Specific areas of assessment related to the more common adverse effects of chemotherapy on normal, rapidly dividing cells include the following:

- For *altered nutritional status* and *impaired oral mucosa:* Assess signs and symptoms of altered nutrition with a focus on weight loss, abnormal serum protein-albumin and blood urea

LABORATORY VALUES RELATED TO DRUG THERAPY

Rationales for Assessment and Monitoring of Blood Cell Counts with Antineoplastics

Antineoplastic drugs kill both normal and abnormal cells that are rapidly dividing, and thus the bone marrow and its rapidly dividing cellular constituents are negatively impacted. Because of this characteristic of chemotherapeutic drugs, red blood cells (RBCs), white blood cells (WBCs), and platelets are suppressed and therefore their levels require frequent monitoring. This box presents information specifically on RBCs and hemoglobin (Hgb) and hematocrit (Hct) levels as well as platelet levels. Chapter 48 presents more information on WBCs with neutrophil counts and nadir levels.

Laboratory Test	Normal Ranges	Rationale for Assessment
RBC count	M: 4.6-6.2 million cells/mm^3 F: 4.2-5.4 million cells/mm^3	Bone marrow suppression from antineoplastics affects RBC values, leading to severe anemia. RBCs carry oxygen—attached to the hemoglobin—from the lungs to the rest of the body. RBCs also help carry carbon dioxide back to the lungs for exhalation. Therefore, if RBC counts are low (e.g., with anemia), the body does not get the oxygen it needs, which leads to lack of energy, fatigue, intolerance of activity, shortness of breath, and hypoxemia. For the cancer patient who may already be experiencing the effects of bone marrow suppression from the disease and then from the treatment, this loss of oxygen saturation will be exacerbated resulting in a lesser ability to get up and about and perform activities of daily living.
Hct	M: 40%-54% F: 37%-47%	Hct measures the amount of space or volume of RBCs in the blood, so if the RBC value is low the Hct is also low. The impact of this low value is discussed above under RBCs.
Hgb level	M: 14-18 g/dL F: 12-16 g/dL	Hgb is the major substance in RBCs. It carries oxygen and is responsible for the red color of the blood cell. With low levels of Hgb, the consequence to the patient is as noted with RBCs.
Platelet count	150,000-140,000 platelets/mm^3	Platelets are the smallest type of blood cell and play a large role in the process of blood clotting. When bleeding occurs, the platelets swell, clump, and form a plug that helps stop the bleeding. Therefore, if platelet levels are lower than 100,000 platelets/mm^3, the patient is at high risk for uncontrolled bleeding and/or hemorrhage. Some guidelines may use a platelet count of 50,000 platelets/mm^3 and above as the criterion. Seek out further information in policies and procedures or contact the prescriber.

F, Female; *M,* male.

---

nitrogen (BUN) levels (a negative nitrogen status due to low protein levels would be indicated by a decreasing BUN level), weakness, fatigue, lethargy, poor skin turgor, and pale conjunctiva. Assess oral mucosa for any signs and symptoms of *stomatitis,* such as pain or burning in the mouth, difficulty swallowing, taste changes, viscous saliva, dryness, cracking, and/or fissures with or without bleeding of the mucosa.

- For *effects on the GI mucosa:* Assess bowel sounds (hyperactive or hypoactive vs. normoactive) and assess for signs and symptoms of *diarrhea,* such as frequent, loose stools (more than three stools per day), urgency, and abdominal cramping, and obtain information about the presence of blood in the stool as well as consistency, color, odor, and amount. Assess for *nausea and vomiting* and determine whether symptoms are acute, delayed, or anticipatory; if vomiting occurs, determine the color, amount, consistency, frequency, and odor, and whether blood is present. The severity of nausea and vomiting may be rated using a scale of 1 to 10 (where 10 is the worst symptoms) or using the terms *mild, moderate,* and *severe.*
- For *alopecia:* Assess the patient's views, concerns, and emotions about potential hair loss. Assess the patient's need to prepare for hair loss, either by leaving the hair as it is and allowing it to fall out on its own; having the hair cut short; or wearing a scarf, hat, bandana, or hair wrap and/or purchasing a wig before the hair is actually lost. Purchasing a wig prior to chemotherapy will allow for a closer match to a patient's pre-chemotherapy hairstyle.

- For *bone marrow suppression:* Assess for signs and symptoms of *anemia,* or the decrease in RBCs, hemoglobin level, and hematocrit (e.g., pallor of the skin, oral mucous membranes, and conjunctiva; fatigue; lethargy; loss of interest in activities; shortness of breath; and inability to concentrate). Assess for signs and symptoms of *leukopenia* or *neutropenia* (decrease in WBCs [usually less than 2000 cells/mm^3] and/or in absolute neutrophil count [below 500 cells/mm^3]), including fever; chills; tachycardia; abnormal breath sounds; productive cough with purulent, green, or rust-colored sputum; change in the color of the urine; lethargy, fatigue; and/or acute confusion. Assess for signs and symptoms of *thrombocytopenia* (decrease in thrombocytes [usually less than 100,000] and platelet clotting factors), including indications of unusual bleeding such as petechiae; purpura; ecchymosis; gingival (gum) bleeding; excessive or prolonged bleeding from puncture sites (e.g., intramuscular or IV administration sites or blood draw sites); unusual joint pain; blood in the stool, urine, or vomitus; and a decrease in blood pressure with elevated pulse rate (see the Laboratory Values Related to Drug Therapy box in this chapter as well as Chapters 28 and 29; also see Box 47-2). Always check normal range values.
- For possible *sterility, teratogenesis,* damage to ovaries with *amenorrhea:* In adult male patients, assess baseline reproductive history with attention to sexual functioning, fathering of children, and/or past or current reproductive or sexual problems or concerns. In female adult patients, in addition to the relevant aspects already mentioned, inquire about fertility,

menstrual and childbearing history, menstrual irregularities, and age at onset of menses and menopause, if applicable.

With *cell cycle–specific drugs*, all allergies, cautions, contraindications, and drug interactions should be documented. Most *antimetabolite drugs* do not produce severe emesis (i.e., in fewer than 10% of cases); however, pentostatin and some of the pyrimidine analogues have emetic potential and require assessment of baseline GI functioning. In addition, the folate antagonists are not as likely to cause emesis but may be associated with GI abnormalities, such as ulcers and stomatitis. Because these drugs are generally administered parenterally (IV), assessing peripheral access areas or central venous sites is critical to prevent risk of damage to surrounding tissue, joints, and tendons. IV sites should be assessed every hour or as needed for redness, swelling, heat, and pain. One specific assessment consideration associated with the use of the antimetabolite cytarabine is monitoring for the occurrence of *cytarabine syndrome*. This syndrome usually occurs within 6 to 12 hours after drug administration and is characterized by fever, myalgia, bone pain, nausea, vomiting, occasional chest pain, and rash.

In patients receiving *mitotic inhibitors* (e.g., vinblastine, vincristine) and *alkaloid topoisomerase II inhibitors* (e.g., etoposide) baseline hepatic and renal function tests should be performed, and serum uric acid levels also should be measured because the levels rise with increased cell death. The increase in uric acid may precipitate or exacerbate gout. Other mitotic inhibitors, docetaxel and

paclitaxel, are associated with severe neutropenia and a decrease in platelet counts (see the Laboratory Values Related to Drug Therapy box and Chapter 49); thus, blood counts must be performed before, during, and after drug therapy. The patient should be constantly assessed for severe hypersensitivity reactions, characterized by dyspnea, severe hypotension, angioedema, and generalized urticaria during treatments. Drops in blood cell counts may even occur before any clinical evidence is present. Baseline neurologic functioning as well as the presence of any peripheral neuropathies should be noted. Because these drugs have multiple incompatibilities and are either irritants (irritating the IV site and vein) or vesicants (causing cell death with extravasation and necrosis with ulcerations), the nurse should know all potential solution and drug interactions and should document initial and follow-up assessments of the IV site.

Topoisomerase I inhibitors are associated with hematologic adverse effects, and thus baseline WBC counts are needed. Bone marrow suppression is predictable, noncumulative, reversible, and manageable, and therefore drugs such as topotecan should not be given to patients with baseline neutrophil counts of fewer than 1500 cells/mm³. Irinotecan causes more severe adverse effects than topotecan, and thus related systems should be assessed and the findings noted. The potential for irinotecan-related *cholinergic diarrhea* requires continual assessment of the GI tract. Diarrhea may appear 2 to 10 days after the irinotecan infusion, and further medical treatment may be required if severe forms of diarrhea occur. Severe cardiovascular toxicity, including thrombosis, pulmonary embolism, stroke, and acute fatal myocardial infarction, are related adverse effects and require cautious and skillful assessment of related systems. These adverse effects have been seen when irinotecan is given with IV fluorouracil and leucovorin. These drug combinations should be given with careful monitoring. Severe nausea and vomiting may also occur.

The use of *natural enzyme* drugs (e.g., asparaginase, pegaspargase) requires documentation of any history of chickenpox. Any current outbreak of chickenpox or herpes zoster should be reported to the prescriber, because the virus may create problems for the patient. Any recent cytotoxic treatment or radiation therapy should also be noted because of the potential for worsening of adverse effects and toxicity. Any history of seizures; the presence of numbness or tingling in the extremities, nervousness, irritability, or confusion; and the level of mobility, muscle strength, and gait should be documented. Because of the risk of pancreatitis, the patient should be assessed for moderate to severe abdominal pain (upper left quadrant) and for nausea and vomiting. Coagulopathies may occur, so baseline blood cell counts are also important to assess and document (see the Laboratory Values Related to Drug Therapy box in this chapter and Chapter 28). It is also important to assess for high serum ammonia levels and complaints of headache.

Genetic considerations are an additional area of importance in the treatment of cancer with antineoplastics, as well as with all drug therapy. Individuals should be assessed for the presence of the following characteristics before chemotherapy is initiated: (1) genetic markers for oral cancers, (2) genetic determinants of testosterone or estrogen metabolism, and (3) genetically linked enzyme system abnormalities such as those involving specific cytochrome P-450 enzymes that metabolically convert nicotine to a carcinogenic substance. These genetic factors are very complex; nevertheless, the nurse should be aware of the possible influence of genetic differences and should look to those involved in drug research and administration for additional information. See Chapter 5 for more information on Genetics as related to drug therapy and the nursing process.

Nursing Diagnoses

- Activity intolerance related to drug-induced anemia with fatigue and lethargy caused by antineoplastic drugs
- Anxiety related to the unknowns of therapy, illness, and the fear of death
- Disturbed body image related to drug-induced alopecia, darkening of the skin, and sexual dysfunctioning
- Constipation related to the adverse effects of antineoplastic drugs
- Ineffective coping related to fears about cancer, its treatment, and dying
- Diarrhea related to the adverse effects of antineoplastic drugs
- Risk for infection related to drug-induced bone marrow suppression with possible leukopenia and neutropenia
- Imbalanced nutrition, less than body requirements, related to loss of appetite, nausea, vomiting, stomatitis, and changes in taste as a result of antineoplastic therapy
- Impaired oral mucous membrane related to the adverse effects of stomatitis, leukopenia, and neutropenia
- Nausea (and vomiting) related to the adverse effects of antineoplastic therapy
- Acute pain related to the disease process and drug-induced joint pain, stomatitis, nausea and vomiting, and other discomforts associated with antineoplastic cell cycle–specific therapy (e.g., neuropathies)
- Impaired physical mobility related to drug-induced anemia and fatigue
- Situational low self-esteem related to the physiologic impact of cancer and related treatment

Planning
Goals

- Patient maintains levels of activity and mobility, as tolerated and without major muscle mass loss, during drug treatment.
- Patient remains calm and comfortable without moderate or severe anxiety during therapy.
- Patient maintains an intact and healthy body image and effective coping mechanisms while experiencing alopecia, skin changes, and sexual dysfunction associated with antineoplastic drugs.
- Patient experiences minimal problems due to oral and GI adverse effects—specifically stomatitis, constipation, diarrhea, nausea, and vomiting—while taking antineoplastic drugs.
- Patient experiences minimal risks for infection as well as minimal breaks in the integrity of the skin and oral mucous membranes (possibly due to the occurrence of stomatitis) while receiving antineoplastic drugs.
- Patient remains safe and free from injury with minimal neurologic, sensory, and motor deficits due to the adverse effects of antineoplastic drugs.
- Patient's nutritional status returns to normal during the recovery period and after completion of the antineoplastic protocol.

- Patient regains normal urinary patterns during and after antineoplastic therapy.

Outcome Criteria

- Patient states measures to maximize activity levels and mobility, such as conserving energy by planning activities, seeking assistance, and maintaining range of motion daily.
- Patient uses nonpharmacologic, complementary, and alternative therapies (e.g., relaxation, music therapy, pet therapy, biofeedback, massage, therapeutic touch, diversion) as well as prescribed drug therapy to control pain and discomfort related to the adverse effects of antineoplastic drugs or the disease process itself.
- Patient states measures to enhance levels of comfort during drug therapy, such as managing pain (see earlier); taking antiemetics as prescribed; keeping skin clean, dry, and moist; and maintaining range of motion daily.
- Patient openly verbalizes any anxieties, fears, concerns, or feelings of upset or depression about changes in body image and self-concept to help in coping.
- Patient states measures to assist in maintaining healthy breathing and respiratory patterns as well as measures to prevent respiratory infections, such as performance of deep breathing exercises, frequent hand washing, forcing of fluids, consumption of a well-balanced diet, avoidance of malls and other crowded places, and avoidance of persons with colds, flu, or communicable respiratory illnesses while undergoing chemotherapy.
- Patient states and demonstrates ways to minimize oral mucosal breakdown, such as performing frequent mouth care and dental hygiene measures using mild toothpaste, gentle sponge-type toothettes, and non–alcohol-based mouthwash, and taking fluid frequently while undergoing drug therapy.
- Patient demonstrates the use of various measures to enhance skin integrity while undergoing antineoplastic therapy, such as keeping skin clean, dry, and lubricated.
- Patient understands the importance of daily measures to help minimize the risk of self-injury related to the adverse effects of bone marrow suppression, such as avoiding crowds, monitoring temperature daily or as needed, not using straight razors, and avoiding venipuncture and injections if possible.
- Patient uses nonpharmacologic methods (e.g., consumption of a well-balanced diet with fiber and roughage as allotted, intake of fluids, exercise) and pharmacologic methods (e.g., use of stool softeners or bulk-forming laxatives) to regain and/or maintain normal or prechemotherapy bowel elimination patterns.
- Patient states ways to minimize risk for injury from neurologic adverse effects of chemotherapy by establishing a safety plan that includes removing throw rugs or furniture that may lead to falls, using assistive devices such as a walker or cane, having a bedside commode, using night lights, and instituting other measures to ease mobility.
- Patient adheres to daily regimen for increasing urinary health, such as forcing fluids, consuming fluids that minimize urinary infections (e.g., cranberry juice), and maintaining daily hydration while undergoing antineoplastic therapy.

(Note that the nursing diagnoses, goals, and outcome criteria presented here are appropriate to treatment with many antineoplastic drugs as well as the particular cell cycle–specific and other drugs discussed in this chapter.)

Implementation

Antineoplastic drugs are some of the most toxic medications given to patients because they cause the death of normal cells along with the death of cancer cells. The high potency of these drugs also places the patient at higher risk for toxicity, serious complications, and adverse effects. The possibility of such adverse effects and toxicities requires skillful nursing care based on cautious and thorough assessment and subsequent critical thinking. General considerations in nursing implementation applicable to most antineoplastic drugs as well as some specific aspects of implementation related to cell cycle–specific drugs are discussed in the following paragraphs. Other nursing process information related to cell cycle–nonspecific drugs is presented in Chapter 48.

For antineoplastic therapy in general, nursing considerations related to *reducing fear and anxiety* include establishing a therapeutic relationship beginning with trust and empathy. In addition, the nurse should always approach the patient in a warm, empathic, and supportive manner while projecting confidence in providing nursing care. Explanations and teaching about the patient's illness, care, and treatments should be individualized and appropriate to the patient's educational level. Collaboration with all members of the health care team is needed. Patients should be encouraged to consider relaxation techniques such as listening to music, performing yoga, and engaging in guided imagery. It may be necessary to call on all potential sources of support, including social services, counseling services, financial assistance services, Meals on Wheels, and religious-spiritual or belief systems while respecting the patient's holistic needs. Appropriate consults may also be necessary with other practitioners such as a licensed clinical social worker, discharge planner, clinical psychiatrist, mental health nurse, nurse practitioner, and oncology nurse specialist, as well as with support groups for the patient, family, and/or significant others.

A variety of interventions that may be indicated for the management of *stomatitis* or excessive oral mucosa dryness and irritation include the following: (1) Oral hygiene should be performed before and after eating or as needed to provide cleanliness and comfort. Lemon, glycerin, undiluted peroxide, or alcohol-containing products should be avoided because of their drying and irritating effects. (2) Use of a soft-bristle toothbrush or soft-tipped toothette or swab with solutions of diluted warm saline is recommended. Chlorhexidine gluconate (Peridex) may also be useful. (3) If dentures are worn, they should be removed and cleaned frequently and, if stomatitis is severe, inserted only at mealtimes. (4) Using over-the-counter saliva substitutes, keeping the lips moist, and using sugarless candy or gum to stimulate saliva flow may be helpful. (5) Spicy, acidic, or hot foods; alcohol; and tobacco should be avoided. (6) Oral antifungal suspensions (e.g., nystatin) may be ordered if white patches are noted on the oral mucosa, and analgesic solutions (e.g., lidocaine swish and swallow) may be used to help manage discomfort. Other regimens may be prescribed, as needed.

Nausea and vomiting occur commonly with antineoplastic drugs. Emetic potential varies depending on the drug and treatment protocol (see earlier discussion and Box 47-1). Measures to enhance comfort during times of nausea and vomiting include restricting oral intake; removing noxious odors or sights to avoid stimulating the vomiting center; performing oral hygiene as needed; promoting relaxation through slow, deep breathing and other techniques; consuming small, frequent meals and eating slowly; and consuming clear liquids and a bland diet. Use of IV fluids may be indicated if nausea and vomiting are severe. Antiemetics are also a vital part of antineoplastic therapy (see Chapter 52 for more specific drug-related information). Premedication with antiemetics 30 to 60 minutes before administration of the antineoplastic(s) is the preferred treatment protocol to help reduce nausea and vomiting, prevent dehydration and malnutrition, and promote comfort. Combination antiemetic drug therapy may be more effective than single-drug therapy. IV hydration may also be helpful in preventing complications.

Diarrhea is also a common adverse effect of antineoplastic therapy. The following nursing interventions have proved to be helpful: (1) Oral intake of irritating, spicy, and gas-producing foods; caffeine; high-fiber foods; alcohol; very hot or cold foods or beverages; and lactose-containing foods and beverages should be limited. (2) Appropriate personnel should be consulted, as ordered, to help the patient and family plan meals and arrange ways to meet the patient's dietary and bowel elimination needs. (3) Opioids (e.g., paregoric) or synthetic opioids (e.g., loperamide, diphenoxylate hydrochloride) may be ordered as antidiarrheals. Adsorbents-protectants and antisecretory drugs may also help reduce GI upset and diarrhea (see Chapter 52).

To address *nutritional concerns*, the following measures may prove beneficial in improving oral intake and nutritional status: (1) Perform a 24-hour recall of food intake and report the typical week's diet for the patient. (2) Antiemetic therapy, pain management, mouth care, and hydration may reduce the adverse effects of therapy and improve appetite. (3) Taste alterations may be eased through consumption of mild-tasting foods and the use of cold chicken, turkey, or cheese for protein sources. (4) Plastic rather than metal utensils can be used if the patient complains of a metallic taste. (5) Encourage eating foods that are easy to swallow, such as custards; gelatins; puddings; milkshakes; eggnog; commercially prepared high-protein, high-calorie supplemental shakes; mashed white or sweet potatoes; blended drinks with crushed ice, fruit, and yogurt; nutritional supplement drinks and snacks; frozen popsicles; and lactose-free ice cream. (6) Sticky or dry foods should be avoided, and the patient should eat small, frequent meals in an environment that is conducive to eating (e.g., free of odors and excess noise). (7) Appetite stimulants such as megestrol acetate or dronabinol should be used, as ordered. (8) Energy conservation should be practiced, with frequent rest periods before and after meals.

Alopecia is a common adverse effect of antineoplastics and is very disturbing regardless of age or gender. The patient and family should be warned about the possibility of hair loss and told when it will occur (usually 7 to 10 days after treatment begins) and that it is reversible. Patients should know that new hair growth is often a different color and/or texture from the hair lost. Information should be provided about the options of acquiring a wig or hairpiece, or wearing scarves or hats, before the actual hair loss, and the patient should be told that the American Cancer Society may be a resource for these items and possibly for financial assistance.

Antineoplastic-induced bone marrow suppression leads to *anemias, leukopenia, neutropenia,* and *thrombocytopenia* (see previous discussion and Laboratory Values Related to Drug Therapy boxes in this chapter and Chapter 48). Anemias result in fatigue and loss of energy and are common adverse effects of therapy and the disease process. Anemias may require blood transfusions, peripheral blood stem cell treatment, or treatment with prescribed medications such as iron preparations, folic acid, or erythropoietic growth factors (e.g., epoetin or darbepoetin alfa). These injections may be given at home and may be administered at the first sign of a decrease in RBC counts.

Risk of infection from leukopenia or neutropenia and/or immunosuppression is one of the more significant adverse effects that deserves close attention. The patient and family and/or caregivers need to understand that when WBC counts are low, the patient is at high risk for infection and that defenses remain low until the counts recover. Following Standard Precautions and using good hand-washing technique are most important in preventing transmission of infection in the hospital and home settings. Because fever is a principal early sign of infection, oral or axillary temperature should be taken at least every 4 hours during periods in which the patient is at risk. Taking the temperature rectally should be avoided to minimize tissue trauma, breaks in skin integrity, and thus loss of the first line of defense. Temperature elevations to 101° F (38.3° C) or above should be reported immediately to the prescriber so that appropriate treatment can be initiated and complications avoided.

If needed, and as ordered, administration of colony-stimulating factors may be beneficial. Filgrastim, pegfilgrastim, and sargramostim are examples of drugs given to accelerate WBC recovery during antineoplastic drug therapy. These drugs may be used to minimize neutropenia. These medications act on the bone marrow to enhance neutrophil production and help decrease the incidence, severity, and duration of neutropenia. These drugs must be administered within a certain time frame (see Chapter 49). Patients with *immune suppression* should be encouraged to be aware of environments and persons to avoid, such as individuals who have recently been vaccinated (who may have a subclinical infection) or who have a cold or flu or other symptoms of an infection. Maintaining a "low-microbe" diet by washing fresh fruits and vegetables and making sure foods are well cooked is also recommended. Patients should perform oral care frequently (see discussion of stomatitis) and turn, cough, and deep breathe to help prevent stasis of respiratory secretions.

Thrombocytopenia is also an adverse effect of antineoplastic therapy and puts the patient at risk for bleeding. Platelet counts, coagulation studies, RBC counts, hemoglobin levels, and hematocrit values should be monitored and any decreases reported (see the Laboratory Values Related to Drug Therapy box). Injections should be avoided if possible, and alternative routes of administration sought. If injections or venipunctures are absolutely necessary, the nurse should use the smallest gauge needle possible and apply gentle, prolonged pressure to the site afterward. Patients undergoing bone marrow aspiration should be monitored closely after the procedure for bleeding at the aspiration site. Blood pressure monitoring should be performed only as needed and should be done quickly without overinflation of the cuff to avoid bruising. The nurse should monitor the patient for bleeding from the mouth, gums, and nose and for bleeding after teeth brushing and should report excessive bleeding to the prescriber.

The patient should be aware that antineoplastics may also have a *negative impact on the reproductive tract,* causing de-

struction of the germinal epithelium of the testes and damage to the ovaries and to a fetus (teratogenesis). Other problems may include sterility; amenorrhea; premature menopausal symptoms of hot flashes, decreased vaginal secretions, and mood changes or irritability; and decreased libido or sexual dysfunction. Male patients should be counseled about the risk of sterility, which is often irreversible. The option of sperm banking before chemotherapy should be discussed with male patients, if appropriate. Female patients of childbearing age who are sexually active should protect themselves against pregnancy because of the risk of embryonic death. Contraceptive measures are encouraged during chemotherapy and for up to 8 weeks after discontinuation of therapy; however, some antineoplastic drugs require use of contraception for up to 2 years after completion of treatment because of the long-term risk for genetic abnormalities.

With *antimetabolites,* the prescriber's orders should always be followed regarding premedication with antiemetics and/or antianxiety drugs. Orders or protocol for the use of other symptom-control medications should be followed, as prescribed. GI adverse effects are common with antimetabolites and usually occur on about the fourth day, which may require preplanning for special pharmacologic interventions (e.g., antiemetics, antispasmodics, analgesics) and nonpharmacologic measures (dietary changes, oral care). Antibiotic therapy may also be ordered prophylactically. See earlier discussion of nursing considerations associated with stomatitis, loss of appetite, diarrhea, nausea, nutrition, hydration, vomiting, and anemias. For further discussion of the handling of antimetabolites and other IV antineoplastic drugs, see Box 47-3.

Cytarabine should be used with extreme caution in handling and administration by the various routes (IV, subcutaneous, or intrathecal). Other major concerns with cytarabine therapy are bone marrow suppression (see earlier discussion) and cytarabine syndrome (see assessment section). If high dosages are used, cytarabine may also cause central nervous system, GI, and/or pulmonary toxicity, so close monitoring of these systems is important to patient safety and comfort. For intrathecal administration, the drug may be reconstituted with sodium chloride, or the prescriber may use the patient's spinal fluid. Fluorouracil should not be added to any other IV infusions and should be administered by itself in the appropriate diluent. When an infusion port is not used, IV sites should not be over joints, tendons, or small veins, or in extremities that are edematous. IV dosages should be given exactly as ordered with constant monitoring of the IV site, infusion port, and/or infusion solution and equipment. If IV infiltration occurs, the protocol for management of infiltration should be followed and the prescriber contacted. All hospital or infusion protocols should be followed without exception, because treatment of extravasation is handled differently depending on the specific drug. If extravasation of a vesicant occurs, the drug is usually discontinued immediately, leaving the IV cannula in place (for possible use of antidotes through cannula to access affected area) and following facility protocol. Antidotes and use of other drugs, as well as use of hot or cold packs, is usually outlined in the protocol for managing extravasation (see Box 48-1). For a more in-depth discussion of IV antineoplastic vesicants and their basic management, see *http://evolve. elsevier.com/Lilley*. If topical forms of the drug are used, the patient should be told to apply the drug exactly as ordered and to the affected area only. Gloves or finger cots should be used to apply the topical dosage form.

Gemcitabine, an antimetabolite, is dosed based on absolute granulocyte counts and platelet nadirs and is given if the counts exceed 1500×10^6 cells/L and $100,000 \times 10^6$ platelets/L, respectively. IV solutions should be kept at room temperature to avoid crystallization and used within 24 hours. Infusions are to be given as ordered. Antiemetics and antidiarrheals may be needed. Mercaptopurine comes in oral dosage forms and should be given as ordered. Finally, the antimetabolite methotrexate has numerous toxicities and adverse effects that may be minimized by appropriate medical treatment. For example, there may be orders for boosting the immune status and blood cell counts before aggressive therapy is initiated. Cytoprotective drugs are used. Continue to monitor creatinine clearance, as ordered, to detect any nephrotoxicity. Nutritional status may be enhanced by the intake of foods high in folic acid, including bran, dried beans, nuts, fruits, asparagus, and other fresh vegetables, if tolerated. Consumption of these foods is yet another measure to help minimize the possibility of methotrexate toxicity. Should GI upset and/or stomatitis occur, the patient may need to decrease any sources of irritation (e.g., high-fiber food) (see previous discussion). Methotrexate is usually given orally or IV. The nurse should wear gloves when giving the drug, and if any of the powder comes in contact with the skin, the area should be washed immediately and thoroughly with soap and water. (See Box 48-3 for discussion of concerns in the handling and administration of vesicant drugs.)

For the *mitotic inhibitors,* specifically the taxane family of drugs and docetaxel in particular, premedication protocols are usually specified and include administration of oral corticosteroids (e.g., dexamethasone) beginning several days before day 1 of therapy to help decrease the risk of hypersensitivity. Vital signs should be measured frequently during the infusion, especially in the first hour of the infusion. Closely monitor the patient for the sudden onset of bronchospasms, flushing of the face, and localized skin reactions; these may indicate a hypersensitivity response requiring immediate treatment. The prescriber should be contacted immediately. These symptoms may occur within just a few minutes of beginning the infusion. In addition, any dyspnea, abdominal distension, crackles in the lungs, or dependent edema during therapy should be tended to immediately by medical personnel. Cutaneous reactions may also appear during therapy and include rash on the hands and feet; these also need immediate attention and treatment. With paclitaxel, the patient may also be premedicated with diphenhydramine, corticosteroids, and H_2 antagonist drugs. All measures should be taken to minimize tissue trauma (e.g., avoidance of intramuscular injections and rectal temperature taking, if possible) to promote comfort and prevent bleeding and infection.

With the *topoisomerase I inhibitors* irinotecan and topotecan, blood counts should be monitored closely with every treatment. A drop in blood counts and/or diarrhea (see previous discussion) may cause a temporary postponement of therapy. Extravasation of the solution should be treated immediately and protocol followed. Ensuring that IV sites remain patent is critical to the prevention of tissue damage secondary to extravasation of antineoplastic drugs considered to be irritants and/or vesicants. Nausea

CASE STUDY

Facing Chemotherapy

©Monkey Business Images

Mrs. D., a 48-year-old married mother of two teenaged daughters, has been diagnosed with breast cancer. She has undergone lumpectomy to remove the tumor and is about to start adjuvant chemotherapy. She states that she has "faced the facts" about her disease and the threat to her life but says, "I know this is silly, but I hate the thought of losing my hair to this disease."

1. What measures can be taken to help her deal with her hair loss?
2. Ten days after the chemotherapy, her neutrophil count drops to 2000 cells/mm³. She has been hospitalized because she has developed a cough, and several of her friends have come in to visit her. What actions should be taken to protect her from infection?
3. During rounds, the nurse finds Mrs. D. curled up in the bed and sobbing. Mrs. D. says that she feels "so afraid" and is worried about who will care for her family if she dies. What should the nurse do?

For answers, see *http://evolve.elsevier.com/Lilley.*

and vomiting may lead to dehydration and electrolyte disturbances, so patients should be aware of the need to report these symptoms immediately before negative consequences occur (see previous discussion for specific interventions). IV incompatibilities are numerous for both these drugs and should be an area of constant concern. With topotecan, IV extravasation is usually accompanied by only a mild local reaction such as erythema or bruising and, if noted, should be managed immediately to avoid further trauma and/or risk for loss of skin integrity (the first line of defense against infection). Headaches and difficulty breathing may be more common with topotecan; therefore, the patient should be monitored closely for these symptoms with every administration.

The *enzyme antineoplastics* asparaginase and pegaspargase should be handled with extreme caution and care. An intradermal test dose of asparaginase may be given before therapy begins or when a week or longer has passed between doses. With asparaginase and pegaspargase, if the solution comes in contact with the skin, thorough washing/rinsing of the area should occur with copious amounts of water for a minimum of 15 minutes. During therapy, if there are signs and symptoms of oliguria, anuria (renal failure), or pancreatitis, the drug will most likely be discontinued. The intramuscular route of administration is usually preferred because it carries a lower risk of causing clotting abnormalities, GI disorders, and renal and hepatic toxicity. If solutions are cloudy, they should not be used. If more than 2 mL is required for a dose, two injections should be given. Pancreatitis is problematic with these drugs and can be serious, so close attention should be given to symptoms such as severe abdominal pain with nausea and vomiting. Serum lipase and amylase levels should be constantly monitored. If any signs or symptoms of pancreatitis occur, these drugs are usually discontinued immediately. Use of cytoprotective drugs has been briefly discussed in the pharmacology section of this chapter, and further discussion is provided in Chapter 49.

Evaluation

Evaluation of nursing care should focus on reviewing whether goals and outcomes are being met as well as monitoring for therapeutic responses and adverse and toxic effects of the antineoplastic therapy. Therapeutic responses may manifest as clinical improvement, decrease in tumor size, and decrease in metastatic spread. Evaluation of nursing care with reference to goals and outcomes may reveal improvements related to a decrease in adverse effects and a decrease in the impact of cancer on the patient's well-being, with increases in comfort, nutrition, hydration, energy levels, ability to carry out the activities of daily living, and quality of life. Goals and outcomes should be revisited to identify more specific areas to monitor. In addition, certain laboratory studies such as tumor marker levels, levels of carcinoembryonic antigens, RBC and WBC counts, and platelet counts may be performed to aid in determining how well the treatment protocol has worked. Also, if neutrophils drop below 500 cells/mm^3, chemotherapy may be discontinued but then reinitiated when the level is back at 1500. Other blood counts are considered too. As part of the evaluation, prescribers may also order additional radiographs, computed tomographic scans, magnetic resonance images, tissue analysis, or other studies appropriate to the diagnosis both during and after antineoplastic therapy has been completed, at time intervals related to the anticipated tumor response.

PATIENT TEACHING TIPS

- GI adverse effects and irritation to the oral and GI mucosa may be decreased by avoiding intake of alcohol, tobacco, spicy and high-fiber foods, citrus fruit juices or foods, and foods that are too hot or cold or have a rough texture.
- Daily mouth care is needed. Mouth sores, pain, or white patches should be reported to the prescriber immediately. Headache, fatigue, faintness, shortness of breath (possibly indicative of anemia), bleeding, easy bruising (possibly indicative of a drop in platelet count), sore throat, and fever (possibly indicative of infection) should be reported immediately to the appropriate prescriber. Fever and/or chills may be the first sign of an oncoming infection.
- Contraception, sperm banking, and other reproductive issues (see previous discussion) should be discussed with male patients and women of childbearing age.
- Information about over-the-counter medications to avoid (e.g., aspirin, ibuprofen, and any combination products containing these over-the-counter drugs), should be emphasized to the patient while the patient is receiving antineoplastic drugs.
- Antineoplastics may cause alopecia (hair loss). Before therapy, the patient should have the opportunity to discuss options for hair and scalp care. These options may include, but are not limited to, having the hair cut short before treatment; selecting, purchasing, or renting a wig or hairpiece comparable to the patient's existing hair in color, texture, length, and style; or having bandanas, scarves, or hats on hand before the hair is actually lost. Although hair loss is temporary, patients need to be informed that it will occur. The American Cancer Society may be a resource for wigs and hairpieces.
- The following websites are helpful online resources for the patient and significant others: *http://www.fda.gov, http://www.fda.gov/oc/oha, http://www.nih.gov, http://www.healthfinder.gov, http://www.who.int/en,* and *http://www.oncolink.upenn.edu.*

- With *cytarabine,* the patient should be encouraged to increase fluid intake to help decrease the risk of dehydration and/or hyperuricemia.
- With *fluorouracil* and *gemcitabine,* frequent oral hygiene should be encouraged, and the patient should report bleeding, bruising, chest pain, diarrhea, nausea, vomiting, heart palpitations, infection, and changes in vision to the prescriber immediately. Sun protection is needed with fluorouracil, including avoidance of overexposure to sun or ultraviolet light and the use of protective clothing, sunscreen, and sunglasses.
- With *mercaptopurine,* alcohol should be avoided to help minimize drug toxicity.
- With *methotrexate,* the patient should be told to notify the prescriber if nausea and vomiting are problematic or uncontrollable, or if fever, sore throat, muscle aches and pains, or unusual bleeding occurs. Alcohol, salicylates, nonsteroidal antiinflammatory drugs, and exposure to sunlight or ultraviolet light should be avoided. Both male and female patients should use contraceptive measures for up to 3 months or longer, if appropriate.
- With *taxanes,* specifically paclitaxel, the patient should report any signs or symptoms of neuropathy (e.g., numbness or tingling of the extremities) to the prescriber immediately.
- With *etoposide* and *teniposide* as with other antineoplastics, if white blood cell counts are low, patients should be cautioned to avoid individuals who are ill. Additionally, any easy bleeding, bruising, difficulty breathing, fever, sore throat, or chills should be reported immediately to the prescriber.
- With *asparaginase* and *pegaspargase,* the patient should be encouraged to force fluids and should be instructed to report any severe nausea or vomiting, bleeding, excessive fatigue, or fever or other signs or symptoms of infection.

POINTS TO REMEMBER

- Cancers are diseases that are characterized by uncontrolled cellular growth.
- *Malignancy* refers specifically to a neoplasm that is anaplastic, invasive, and metastatic, as opposed to benign.
- Tumors are generally classified by tissue of origin, as follows: epithelial (carcinoma), connective (sarcoma), lymphatic (lymphoma), and leukocytes (leukemia).
- Antineoplastics are drugs that are used to treat malignancies. They may be either cell cycle–specific or cell cycle–nonspecific drugs or may have miscellaneous actions.
- Cell cycle–specific drugs kill cancer cells during specific phases of the cell growth cycle. Cell cycle–nonspecific drugs kill cancer cells during any phase of the cell growth cycle.
- Chemotherapy, or antineoplastic drug therapy, requires very skillful and perceptive nursing care, and the nurse must act prudently and make critical decisions about the nursing care of patients receiving these drugs.

- Cell cycle–specific drug classes include antimetabolites, mitotic inhibitors, alkaloid topoisomerase II inhibitors, topoisomerase I inhibitors, and antineoplastic enzymes.
- Antineoplastic antimetabolites are cell cycle–specific antagonistic analogues that work by inhibiting the actions of key cellular metabolites.
- Two plant-derived antineoplastic drugs are the taxanes paclitaxel, derived from the bark of the slow-growing Western (Pacific) yew tree, and docetaxel, a semisynthetic taxoid produced from the needles of the European yew tree. Docetaxel is pharmacologically similar to paclitaxel.
- The topoisomerase I inhibitors topotecan and irinotecan comprise a relatively new class of chemotherapy drugs.
- Antineoplastic enzymes include asparaginase and pegaspargase.
- Several drugs are available that are classified as cytoprotective and help reduce the toxicity of various antineoplastics.

NCLEX EXAMINATION REVIEW QUESTIONS

1 A patient is experiencing stomatitis after a round of chemotherapy. Which intervention by the nurse is correct?
   a Clean the mouth with a soft-bristle toothbrush and warm saline solution.
   b Rinse the mouth with commercial mouthwash twice a day.
   c Use lemon-glycerin swabs to keep the mouth moist.
   d Keep dentures in the mouth between meals.
2 The nurse is caring for a patient who becomes severely nauseated during chemotherapy. Which intervention is most appropriate?
   a Encourage light activity during chemotherapy as a distraction
   b Provide antiemetic medications 30 to 60 minutes before chemotherapy begins
   c Provide antiemetic medications only upon the request of the patient
   d Hold fluids during chemotherapy to avoid vomiting
3 The nurse monitors a patient who is experiencing thrombocytopenia from severe bone marrow suppression by looking for
   a severe weakness and fatigue.
   b elevated body temperature.
   c decreased skin turgor.
   d excessive bleeding and bruising.

4 A patient receiving chemotherapy is experiencing severe bone marrow suppression. Which nursing diagnosis is most appropriate at this time?
   a Activity intolerance
   b Risk for infection
   c Disturbed body image
   d Impaired physical mobility
5 If extravasation of an antineoplastic medication occurs, which intervention should the nurse perform first?
   a Apply cold compresses to the site while elevating the arm
   b Inject subcutaneous doses of epinephrine around the IV site every 2 hours
   c Stop the infusion immediately while leaving the catheter in place
   d Inject the appropriate antidote through the IV catheter
6 The nurse is assessing a patient who has experienced severe neutropenia after chemotherapy and will monitor for which possible signs of infection in this patient? (Select all that apply.)
   a Elevated WBC count
   b Fever
   c Nausea
   d Sore throat
   e Chills

1. a, 2. b, 3. d, 4. b, 5. c, 6. b, d, e.

CRITICAL THINKING ACTIVITIES: BEST ACTION

1 A patient who has undergone three chemotherapy sessions is now experiencing stomatitis, and his wife exclaims, "He won't eat! What kinds of food can I give him? I'm concerned because he has no appetite and now he has these mouth sores." What is the nurse's best response? Explain.
2 A patient is receiving irinotecan as part of his chemotherapy regimen. He will be receiving the dose shortly and will then be sent home. The nurse is providing patient teaching before giving him the medication. What is one of the most important problems for which he will need to be ready once he is home? Explain the nurse's best action.

3 A patient is receiving chemotherapy that includes the antimetabolite cytarabine. Several hours after the treatment, the patient begins to complain of shortness of breath. The nurse examines the patient and finds that his pulse rate is 118 beats/min, he has slight edema in his lower extremities, and crackles are audible over the bases of the lungs. In addition, his pulse oximetry reading is 92% (previously it was 99%) on room air. What action should the nurse take next?

For answers, see *http://evolve.elsevier.com/Lilley*.

CHAPTER 48

Antineoplastic Drugs Part 2: Cell Cycle–Nonspecific and Miscellaneous Drugs

Timothy R. McGuire

OBJECTIVES

When you reach the end of this chapter, you should be able to do the following:

1 Review the concepts related to carcinogenesis, the types of malignancies and related terminology, and the different treatment modalities, including the use of cell cycle–nonspecific and miscellaneous antineoplastic drugs (see Chapter 47).

2 Identify the various drugs that are classified as cell cycle nonspecific or hormonal, or that are considered miscellaneous drugs.

3 Discuss the common adverse effects and toxic effects of the cell cycle–nonspecific and miscellaneous antineoplastic drugs, including the reasons for their occurrence and methods of treatment, such as any antidotes.

4 Describe the mechanisms of action, indications, dosages, routes of administration, cautions, contraindications, and drug interactions of the cell cycle–nonspecific drugs, hormonal drugs, and miscellaneous antineoplastic drugs.

5 Apply knowledge about the cell cycle–nonspecific, hormonal agonist-antagonist, and other miscellaneous antineoplastic drugs and their characteristics in the development of a comprehensive nursing care plan for patients with cancer who are receiving these drugs.

6 Briefly describe extravasation and other major adverse effects associated with the antineoplastics discussed in this chapter, including discussion of protocols and antidotes.

---

e-Learning Activities

http://evolve.elsevier.com/Lilley

NCLEX Review Questions • Animations • Nursing Care Plans • Audio Glossary • Category Catchers • Medication Errors Checklists • IV Therapy Checklists • Calculators • Frequently Asked Questions • Content Updates • Supplemental Resources • Answers to Case Studies and Critical Thinking Activities

Drug Profiles

bevacizumab, p. 753
◆ cisplatin, p. 750
◆ cyclophosphamide, p. 750
◆ doxorubicin, p. 752
hydroxyurea, p. 753

imatinib, p. 753
◆ mechlorethamine, p. 750
mitotane, p. 753
mitoxantrone, p. 752
octreotide, p. 754

◆ *Key drug.*

Glossary

Alkylation A chemical reaction in which an alkyl group is transferred from one molecule to another. In chemotherapy, alkylation leads to damage of the cancer cell deoxyribonucleic acid (DNA) and cell death. (p. 748)

Bifunctional Referring to those alkylating drugs composed of molecules that have two reactive alkyl groups and that are therefore able to alkylate at two sites on the DNA molecule. (p. 748)

Extravasation The leakage of any intravenously or intraarterially administered medication into the tissue space surrounding the vein or artery. Such an event can cause serious tissue injury, especially with antineoplastic drugs. (p. 748)

Mitosis The process of cell reproduction occurring in somatic (non-sexual) cells and resulting in the formation of two genetically identical daughter cells, each containing the diploid (complete) number of chromosomes characteristic of the species. (p. 748)

Polyfunctional Referring to the action of alkylating drugs that can engage in several alkylation reactions with cancer cell DNA molecules per single molecule of drug. (p. 748)

• • •

This chapter is a continuation of Chapter 47 and focuses on additional classes of antineoplastic drugs. Chapter 47 describes the various antineoplastic drugs that are effective against cancer cells during specific phases in the *cell growth cycle*. In contrast, this chapter focuses on drugs that have antineoplastic activity regardless of the phase of the cell cycle. Also discussed in this chapter are drugs that are classified as *miscellaneous* antineoplastics either because of their lack of clear cell cycle specificity or their unique or *novel* (new) mechanisms of action. For a description of the cell growth cycle, see Chapter 47.

Pharmacology Overview

CELL CYCLE–NONSPECIFIC ANTINEOPLASTIC DRUGS

There are currently two broad classes of cell cycle–nonspecific cancer drugs: alkylating drugs and cytotoxic antibiotics.

ALKYLATING DRUGS

Records of the use of drugs to treat cancer date back several centuries. However, truly successful systemic cancer chemotherapy treatments are not documented until the 1940s. At this time, the first alkylating drugs were developed from mustard gas agents that were used for chemical warfare before and during World War I. The first drug to be developed was mechlorethamine, which is also known as *nitrogen mustard.* It is the prototypical drug of this class and is still used today for cancer treatment. Since its antineoplastic activity was discovered in the mid-twentieth century, many analogues have been synthesized for use in the treatment of cancer, and they are collectively referred to as *nitrogen mustards* also.

The alkylating drugs commonly used in clinical practice in the United States today fall into three categories: *classic alkylators* (the *nitrogen mustards*); *nitrosoureas,* which have a different chemical structure than the nitrogen mustards but also work by **alkylation;** and *miscellaneous alkylators,* which also have a different chemical structure than the nitrogen mustards but are known to work at least partially by alkylation. These drugs are used to treat a wide spectrum of malignancies. The drugs in each category are as follows:

Classic alkylators (nitrogen mustards)
- chlorambucil
- cyclophosphamide
- ifosfamide
- mechlorethamine
- melphalan

Nitrosoureas
- carmustine
- lomustine
- streptozocin

Miscellaneous alkylators
- altretamine
- busulfan
- carboplatin
- cisplatin
- dacarbazine
- oxaliplatin
- procarbazine
- temozolomide
- thiotepa

Mechanism of Action and Drug Effects

The alkylating drugs work by preventing cancer cells from reproducing. Specifically, they alter the chemical structure of the cells' deoxyribonucleic acid (DNA), which is essential to the reproduction of any cell. DNA molecules consist of two adjacent strands, each consisting of alternating sequences of phosphate and sugar molecules (Figure 48-1). These components make up what is called the "backbone" of the DNA strands. These two strands are chemically linked to each other by the third DNA structural element: nitrogen-containing bases (adenine, guanine, thymine, and cytosine, abbreviated A, G, T, and C, respectively). These bases are bound to the sugar molecules of the DNA backbone, and two bases, linked to each other by hydrogen bonds, form the molecular bridges between the two DNA strands that bring them into the double helix structure. A *nucleotide,* which consists of one molecule each of base, sugar, and phosphate that are bound together, is the structural unit of the molecules of both DNA and ribonucleic acid (RNA), another nucleic acid that is important in cellular reproduction. Messenger RNA (mRNA) molecules are produced by DNA molecules during the complex process of transcription. These mRNA molecules differ from DNA molecules in at least three ways: they are single stranded (instead of double stranded), the thymine base is replaced by another base known as *uracil (U),* and the sugar molecule is *ribose,* which has a slightly different structure from that of the *deoxyribose* molecules of DNA.

During the normal process of reproduction, the double helix uncoils, and its two strands separate. A strand of RNA is then assembled next to each single DNA strand in a process known as *transcription.* RNA strands, in turn, are involved in both protein synthesis *(translation)* and replication of the original DNA structure before cell division, or **mitosis.** These processes ultimately result in the creation of a new cell with the same DNA sequence, and thus the same characteristics, as its parent cell.

Alkyl groups that are part of the chemical structure of antineoplastic alkylating drugs attach to DNA molecules by forming covalent bonds with the bases described earlier. As a result, abnormal chemical bonds form between the adjacent DNA strands, which leads to the formation of defective nucleic acids that are then unable to perform the normal cellular reproductive functions mentioned previously. This leads to cell death.

Alkylating drugs can also be characterized by the number of alkylation reactions in which they can participate. **Bifunctional** alkylating drugs have two reactive alkyl groups that are able to alkylate two sites on the DNA molecule. **Polyfunctional** alkylating drugs can participate in several alkylation reactions. Figure 48-2 shows the location along the DNA double helix where the alkylating drugs work.

Indications

The most commonly used alkylating drugs today are effective against a wide spectrum of malignancies, including both solid and hematologic tumors. Common examples of the various types of cancer that different alkylating drugs are used to treat are listed in the Dosages table on p. 751.

Adverse Effects

Alkylating drugs are capable of causing all of the dose-limiting adverse effects described in Chapter 47. Other adverse effects are described in Table 48-1. The relative emetic potential of the various alkylating drugs is given in Box 47-1. The adverse effects of these drugs are important because of their severity, but they can often be prevented or minimized by prophylactic measures. For instance, nephrotoxicity from cisplatin can often be prevented by adequately hydrating the patient with intravenous fluids. Drug **extravasation** (Box 48-1) occurs when an intravenous catheter punctures the vein and medication leaks (infil-

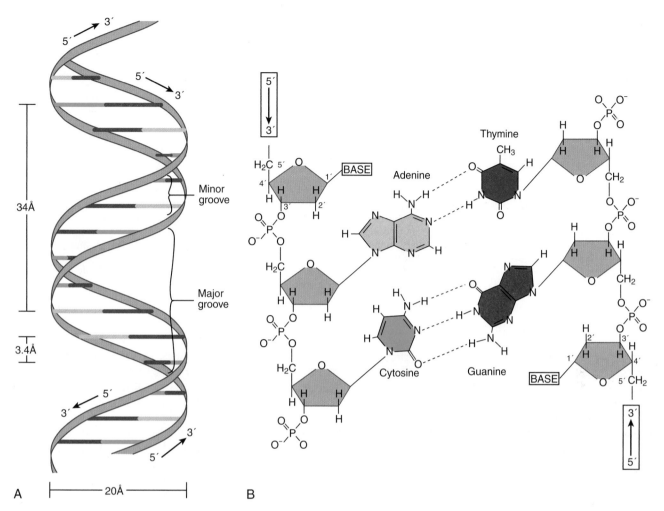

FIGURE 48-1   Deoxyribonucleic acid (DNA) double helix. **A,** Diagrammatic model of the helical structure, showing its dimensions, the major and minor grooves, the periodicity of the bases, and the antiparallel orientation of the backbone chains (represented by ribbons). The base pairs (represented by rods) are perpendicular to the axis and lie stacked one on another. **B,** The chemical structure of the backbone and bases of DNA, showing the sugar-phosphate linkages of the backbone and the hydrogen bonding between the base pairs. There are two hydrogen bonds between adenine and thymine, and three between cytosine and guanine. (From *Dorland's illustrated medical dictionary,* ed 31, Philadelphia, 2007, Saunders.)

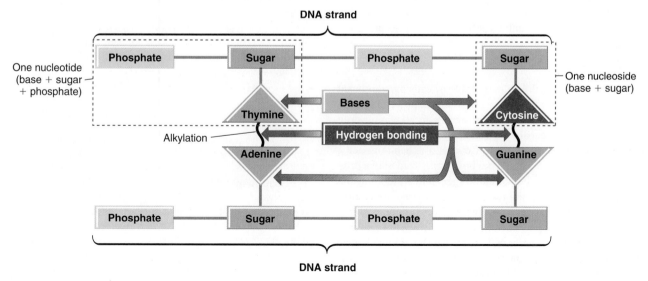

FIGURE 48-2   Organization of deoxyribonucleic acid (DNA) and site of action of alkylating drugs.

BOX 48-1 Extravasation of Antineoplastics

Extravasation is one of the more devastating complications of antineoplastic therapy and may lead to extensive tissue damage, the need for skin grafting, other problems in the surrounding areas, and even loss of limb. Because many cell cycle–specific and cell cycle–nonspecific drugs are given intravenously, there is a constant danger of extravasation of vesicants and subsequent injury, including permanent damage to nerves, tendons, and muscles. However, skillful and perceptive nursing care may help to prevent extravasation or to identify it early if it does occur, which can reduce the severity of tissue damage. There are important reasons for the placement of central venous intravenous catheters rather than peripheral catheters when long-term treatment is anticipated. Infiltration may occur with any intravenous catheter; it is the specific drug and its characteristics, such as irritant (irritating the IV site or vein) or vesicant (causing cell death with extravasation and necrosis with ulcerations) properties, that poses the concern. Because peripheral veins are small and offer minimal dilution of the intravenous drug with blood, there is a greater risk of severe and irreversible damage if a substance infil-

trates and spreads to surrounding tissues, including muscles, tendons, and ligaments. If the drug is a vesicant, extravasation may lead to massive tissue injury, whereas extravasation of an irritant results in significantly less damage. Central venous access is needed for administration of vesicants to avoid the problems associated with extravasation. Should extravasation of a vesicant be suspected, immediate action should be taken, and the antidote, if known, should be given following strict procedures. Steps to help manage extravasation include the following: (1) Stop the infusion immediately and contact the prescriber, but leave the intravenous catheter in place. (2) Usually, aspiration of any residual drug and/or blood from the catheter is performed next. (3) Consult institutional policy or guidelines or the pharmacist regarding the use of antidotes, application of hot or cold packs and/or sterile occlusive dressings, and elevation and rest of the affected limb. The extravasation incident must be thoroughly documented with attention to all phases of the nursing process related to the problem. Remember to always consult facility protocol and guidelines.

Data from National Cancer Institute website, *http://www.nci.hih.gov; http://dcb.nci.nih.gov/thinktank/Executive_Summary_of_Inflammation_and_Cancer_Think_Tank. doc*; United States Pharmacopeial Convention: *USP DI volume 1: drug information for the health care professional,* Greenwood Village, Colo, 2005, Micromedex. Internet resources for additional information: *http://www.americancancersociety.com, http://www.OncoLink.com, http://www.hospicenet.org, http://www.acponline.org/ public/hcare.*

TABLE 48-1 Commonly Used Alkylating Drugs: Severe Adverse Effects

Drug	Adverse Effects
busulfan	Pulmonary fibrosis
carboplatin	Less nephrotoxicity and neurotoxicity but more bone marrow suppression than cisplatin
cisplatin	Nephrotoxicity, peripheral neuropathy, ototoxicity
cyclophosphamide	Hemorrhagic cystitis

trates) into the surrounding tissues. With cancer chemotherapeutic drugs, in particular doxorubicin (a cytotoxic antibiotic), extravasation can cause severe tissue damage and *necrosis* (tissue death). Extravasation antidotes for selected drugs are listed in Table 48-2.

Interactions

Only a few alkylating drugs are capable of causing significant drug interactions. The most important rule for preventing such drug interactions is to avoid administering an alkylating drug with any other drug capable of causing similar toxicities. For example, a major adverse effect of cisplatin is nephrotoxicity. Therefore, if possible, it should not be administered with a drug such as an aminoglycoside antibiotic (gentamicin, tobramycin, or amikacin) because of the resulting additive nephrotoxic effects and hence the increased likelihood of renal failure. Mechlorethamine and cyclophosphamide, both of which have significant bone marrow–suppressing effects, ideally should not be administered with radiation therapy or with other drugs that suppress the bone marrow. In general, the nurse should work with available pharmacy and oncology staff to proactively an-

ticipate (and avoid, if possible) undesirable drug and treatment interactions.

Dosages

For the recommended dosages of selected alkylating drugs, see the Dosages table on p. 751. It is important to note that dosages are highly variable based on type of cancer, previous drugs used, and concurrent drug administration.

DRUG PROFILES

The most widely used alkylating drugs, based on standard treatment protocols, are profiled here. Information for these drugs also appears in the Dosages table on p. 751.

◆ cisplatin

Cisplatin (Platinol) is an antineoplastic drug that contains platinum in its chemical structure. It is classified as a probable alkylating drug because it is believed to destroy cancer cells in the same way as the classic alkylating drugs—by forming cross-links with DNA and thereby preventing its replication. It is also considered a bifunctional alkylating drug.

Cisplatin is used for the treatment of many solid tumors, such as bladder, lung, testicular, and ovarian tumors. It is available only in injectable form. Medication errors, resulting in deaths, have occurred when cisplatin was confused for carboplatin. The best practice is to use both trade name and generic name when dealing with chemotherapy drugs.

◆ cyclophosphamide

Cyclophosphamide (Cytoxan) is a nitrogen mustard derivative that was discovered during the course of research to improve mechlorethamine. It is a polyfunctional alkylating drug and is a prodrug requiring *in vivo* activation. It is used in the treatment of cancers of the bone and lymph, as well as other solid tumors. Cyclophosphamide is also used in the treatment of leukemias and multiple myeloma. It is available in both oral and injectable dosage forms.

TABLE 48-2 Alkylating Drug Extravasation: Specific Antidotes

Drug	Antidote Preparation	Method
carmustine	Mix equal parts 1 mEq/mL sodium bicarbonate (premixed) with sterile NS (1:1 solution); resulting solution is 0.5 mEq/mL.	1. Inject 2-6 mL IV through the existing line along with multiple subcut injections into the extravasated site. 2. Apply cold compresses. 3. Total dose should not exceed 10 mL of 0.5-mEq/mL solution.
mechlorethamine	Mix 4 mL 10% sodium thiosulfate with 6 mL sterile water for injection.	1. Inject 5-6 mL IV through the existing line with multiple subcut injections into the extravasated site. 2. Repeat subcut injections over the next few hours. 3. Apply cold compresses. 4. No total dose has been established.

IV, Intravenous; *NS,* normal saline; *subcut,* subcutaneous.

DOSAGES

Selected Alkylating Drugs

Drug (Pregnancy Category)	Pharmacologic Subclass	Usual Dosage Range*	Indications
◆ cisplatin (Platinol-AQ) (D)	Platinum coordination complex	IV: 50-100 mg/m² q4wk	Metastatic testicular, ovarian, and bladder cancer; brain tumors; esophageal, head, neck, lung, and cervical cancer
◆ cyclophosphamide (Cytoxan, Neosar) (D)	Classic alkylator	IV: 3-5 mg/kg 2×/wk **(many other regimens as well)**	HL, NHL, leukemia; breast, ovarian, and testicular cancer; retinoblastoma; almost every solid tumor
◆ mechlorethamine (Mustargen) (D)	Classic alkylator	IV: 6 mg/m² day 1 and day 28 q4wk	HL, NHL, leukemia, bronchogenic carcinoma, others

HL, Hodgkin's lymphoma; *IV,* intravenous; *NHL,* non-Hodgkin's lymphoma.
*Note: Dosages are highly variable.

◆ mechlorethamine

Mechlorethamine (nitrogen mustard) (Mustine) is the prototypical alkylating drug. It is a nitrogen analogue of sulfur mustard (mustard gas) that was used for chemical warfare in World War I. As noted earlier, mechlorethamine was the very first alkylating antineoplastic drug discovered, and its beneficial effects in the treatment of various cancers were identified after the war. Although its use has declined with the development of newer and better drugs, it continues to be administered occasionally in the treatment of Hodgkin and Non-Hodgkin lymphoma.

Mechlorethamine is a bifunctional alkylating drug capable of forming cross-links between two DNA nucleotides, which interferes with RNA transcription and prevents cell division and protein synthesis. It is available in a parenteral form only, for administration intravenously or by an intracavitary route, such as intrapleurally or intraperitoneally. It can also be used topically for treatment of cutaneous T-cell lymphoma.

CYTOTOXIC ANTIBIOTICS

The cytotoxic antibiotics consist of natural substances produced by the mold *Streptomyces* as well as semisynthetic substances in which chemical changes are made in the natural molecule. Cytotoxic antibiotics have bone marrow suppression as a common toxicity. The one exception is bleomycin, which instead causes pulmonary toxicity (pulmonary fibrosis and pneumonitis). Other severe toxicities associated with the use of cytotoxic antibiotics

PREVENTING MEDICATION ERRORS

Sound-Alike Drugs: "Rubicins"

The anthracycline chemotherapy drugs have the same sound-alike suffix and are often nicknamed the "rubicins." These drugs include daunorubicin, doxorubicin, epirubicin, idarubicin, and valrubicin. Even though these drugs are in the same class, their use and drug effects are different. Medication errors have occurred because one "rubicin" has been mistaken for another. It is important to refer to these drugs by both trade and generic names rather than as a "rubicin."

are heart failure (daunorubicin) and in rare cases acute left ventricular failure (doxorubicin). The available cytotoxic antibiotics, categorized according to the specific subclass to which they belong, are as follows:

Anthracyclines
* daunorubicin
* doxorubicin
* epirubicin
* idarubicin
* valrubicin

Other cytotoxic antibiotics
* bleomycin (which is actually a cell cycle–specific drug)
* dactinomycin
* mitomycin
* mitoxantrone

TABLE 48-3 Cytotoxic Antibiotics: Severe Adverse Effects

Drug	Adverse Effects
bleomycin	Pulmonary fibrosis, pneumonitis
dactinomycin, daunorubicin	Liver toxicity, tissue damage in the event of extravasation, heart failure
doxorubicin, idarubicin	Liver and cardiovascular toxicities
mitomycin	Liver, kidney, and lung toxicities
mitoxantrone	Cardiovascular toxicity
plicamycin	Tissue damage secondary to extravasation

BOX 48-2 Treatment of Doxorubicin Extravasation

1. Cool the site to patient tolerance for 24 hours.
2. Elevate and rest the extremity for 24 to 48 hours, then have the patient resume normal activity as tolerated.
3. If pain, erythema, or swelling persists beyond 48 hours, discuss with the prescriber the need for surgical intervention or other treatment options.

Data from National Cancer Institute website, *http://www.nci.hih.gov;* United States Pharmacopeial Convention: *USP DI volume 1: drug information for the health care professional,* Greenwood Village, Colo, 2005, Micromedex; Internet resources for additional information: *http://www.americancancersociety.com; http://www.OncoLink.com; http://www.hospicenet.org; http://www.acponline.org/public/hcare; http://www.acponline.org/public*

Mechanism of Action and Drug Effects

Cytotoxic antibiotic antineoplastic drugs are cell cycle–nonspecific drugs. They interact with DNA through a process called *intercalation,* in which the drug molecule is inserted between the two strands of a DNA molecule, ultimately blocking DNA synthesis. These drugs inhibit the enzyme *topoisomerase II,* which leads to DNA strand breaks. Many of these drugs are able to generate free radicals, which also leads to DNA strand breaks and programmed cell death.

Indications

Cytotoxic antibiotics are used to treat a variety of solid tumors and some hematologic malignancies as well. Commonly used examples of these drugs and the malignancies they are used to treat are presented in the Dosages table on p. 753.

Adverse Effects

As with all of the antineoplastic drugs, cytotoxic antibiotics have the undesirable effects of hair loss, nausea and vomiting, and myelosuppression. The emetic potential of the various drugs in this category is given in Box 47-1. Major adverse effects specific to the cytotoxic antibiotics are listed in Table 48-3.

Toxicity and Management of Overdose

Severe cases of cardiomyopathy are associated with large cumulative doses of doxorubicin. Routine monitoring of cardiac ejection fraction with multiple-gated acquisition (MUGA) scans, cumulative dose limitations, and the use of cytoprotective drugs such as dexrazoxane can decrease the incidence of this devastating toxicity. Box 48-2 outlines the management of doxorubicin extravasation.

Interactions

The cytotoxic antibiotics that are used in chemotherapy interact with many drugs. They all tend to produce increased toxicities when used in combination with other chemotherapeutic drugs or with radiation therapy. Some drugs, most notably bleomycin and doxorubicin, have been known to cause serum digoxin levels to increase. Patients receiving one of these drugs along with digoxin should be observed for signs of digoxin toxicity. Dosage reduction or elimination of digoxin therapy may be indicated (see Chapter 22).

Dosages

For recommended dosages of selected cytotoxic antibiotic drugs, see the Dosages table on p. 753.

DRUG PROFILES

◆ doxorubicin

Doxorubicin (Adriamycin) is used in many combination chemotherapy regimens. The drug is contraindicated in patients with a known hypersensitivity to it, patients with severe myelosuppression, and patients who are at risk for severe cardiac toxicity because they have already received a large cumulative dose of any of the anthracycline antineoplastics. It is available only in injectable form. Doxorubicin is also now available in a liposomal drug delivery system (Doxil). In this dosage formulation the drug is encapsulated in a lipid molecule bilayer called a *liposome.* The advantages of liposomal encapsulation are reduced systemic toxicity and increased duration of action. Liposomal encapsulation extends the biologic half-life of doxorubicin to 50 to 60 hours and increases its affinity for cancer cells. The liposomal dosage formulation is currently indicated for the treatment of Kaposi's sarcoma, which primarily affects individuals infected with the human immunodeficiency virus (HIV) that causes acquired immunodeficiency syndrome (AIDS).

mitoxantrone

Mitoxantrone (Novantrone) is indicated for the treatment of acute nonlymphocytic leukemia and prostate cancer as well as the neurologic disorder multiple sclerosis. It is available only in injectable form.

MISCELLANEOUS ANTINEOPLASTICS

The miscellaneous antineoplastic drugs are those that, because of their unique structure and mechanism of action, cannot be classified into the previously described categories. However, some drugs that are originally classified as miscellaneous drugs are later reclassified as more is learned about their mechanisms of action and other characteristics. Drugs currently in the miscellaneous category include bevacizumab, hydroxyurea, imatinib, mitotane, hormonal drugs, and radioactive and related antineoplastic drugs. Selected miscellaneous drugs are profiled in the following sections.

DRUG PROFILES

The various drugs in the miscellaneous category of antineoplastics are used to treat a wide range of neoplasms. Hydroxyurea and imatinib are administered orally. Bevacizumab and mitotane are available only in injectable form.

DOSAGES

Selected Cytotoxic Antibiotics

Drug (Pregnancy Category)	Pharmacologic Subclass	Usual Dosage Range*	Indications
Anthracycline Antibiotics			
◆ doxorubicin, conventional (Adriamycin, Rubex) (D)	Anthracycline	IV: 30-75 mg/m² q7-28d (depending on type of cancer)	Multiple cancers, including breast, bone, and ovarian cancer, and leukemia, neuroblastoma, HL, NHL
◆ doxorubicin, liposomal (Doxil) (D)	Anthracycline	IV: 20-50 mg/m² q3-4wk for as long as tolerated and tumor is responsive to treatment	AIDS-related Kaposi's sarcoma when other chemotherapy drugs have failed or patient is intolerant of them; recurrent metastatic ovarian cancer
Anthracenedione Antibiotic			
mitoxantrone (Novantrone) (D)	Anthracenedione	IV: 12 mg/m² q3wk (prostate cancer) **(many other regimens as well)**	Prostate cancer, acute myelocytic leukemia

AIDS, Acquired immunodeficiency syndrome; *HL,* Hodgkin's lymphoma; *IV,* intravenous; *NHL,* non-Hodgkin's lymphoma.
*Note: Dosages are highly variable.

bevacizumab

Bevacizumab (Avastin) is the first, and currently the only, approved antineoplastic drug in a new category—*angiogenesis inhibitors. Angiogenesis* is the creation of new blood vessels that supply oxygen and other blood nutrients to growing tissues. In the case of malignant tumors, angiogenesis that occurs within the tumor mass promotes continued tumor growth. As a tumor enlarges, its central tissues gradually die off *(necrosis).* However, its outer portion continues to grow, often to fatal proportions, with blood supplied through angiogenesis. Thus, inhibiting this process offers a promising new mechanism for antineoplastic drug action. Bevacizumab is a recombinant "humanized" monoclonal immunoglobulin G1 antibody derived from mouse antibodies. The scientific name for any compound derived from mouse tissue is *murine. Humanization* refers to the use of recombinant DNA techniques to make animal-derived antibody proteins more genetically similar to those of humans. Immunoglobulin G1 is a subtype of *immunoglobulin G,* the principal class of antibodies produced by mammalian immune systems (see Chapter 46). This drug works by binding to and inhibiting the biologic activity of human *vascular endothelial growth factor (VEGF).* VEGF is an endogenous protein that normally promotes angiogenesis in the body. Bevacizumab is available only in injectable form. The only recognized contraindication is severe drug allergy or allergy to other murine products.

Adverse reactions include those affecting the cardiovascular system (hypertension or hypotension, thrombosis), central nervous system (CNS) (pain, headache, dizziness), skin (alopecia, dry skin), metabolism (weight loss, hypokalemia), gastrointestinal (GI) tract (nausea, vomiting, diarrhea), kidneys (nephrotoxicity with proteinuria), and respiratory tract (infection). More severe effects can occur in any of these systems but are much less common than those listed. Drug interactions reported to date are limited but include potentiation of the cardiotoxic affects of the anthracycline antibiotics such as doxorubicin.

hydroxyurea

Hydroxyurea (Hydrea) is an antimetabolite that interferes with the synthesis of DNA by inhibiting the incorporation of thymidine into DNA. More specifically, it inhibits ribonucleotide reductase, which is involved in conversion of ribonucleotides to deoxyribonucleotides. It works primarily in the S and G₁ phases of the cell cycle, which makes it a cell cycle–specific drug like all other antimetabolites. It is used in the treatment of squamous cell carcinoma in concert with radiation to take advantage of its radiosensitizing activity. It is also used in the treatment of various types of leukemia. The drug is available only in oral form. Adverse reactions include edema, drowsiness, headache, rash, hyperuricemia, nausea, vomiting, dysuria, myelosuppression, elevated liver enzyme levels, muscular weakness, peripheral neuropathy, nephrotoxicity, dyspnea, and pulmonary fibrosis. Drugs with which it interacts include the anti-HIV drugs zidovudine, zalcitabine, and didanosine (see Chapter 40), all of which can actually have a synergistic effect with hydroxyurea. Concurrent use with fluorouracil increases the risk of neurotoxic symptoms. Because hydroxyurea can reduce the clearance of cytarabine, dosage reduction of cytarabine is recommended when the two are used concurrently.

imatinib

Imatinib (Gleevec) is the standard of care for the treatment of chronic myeloid leukemia (CML). It works by inhibiting the action of a key enzyme (bcr-abl tyrosine kinase) responsible for causing CML. Although its name sounds similar to those of various monoclonal antibody drugs, imatinib is not a monoclonal antibody but rather a targeted therapy. It is available only in oral form. Common adverse reactions include fatigue, headache, rash, fluid retention, GI and hematologic effects, musculoskeletal pain, cough, and dyspnea. Potential drug interactions are numerous and involve other drugs metabolized by the cytochrome P-450 hepatic enzymes. Examples include amiodarone, verapamil, warfarin, azole antifungals, antidepressants, and antibiotics. A pharmacist may be needed to review the patient's medication regimen and adjust dosages or delete medications accordingly, in collaboration with the patient's prescriber.

mitotane

Mitotane (Lysodren) is an adrenal cytotoxic drug that is indicated specifically for the treatment of inoperable adrenal corticoid carcinoma. It is available only in oral form. Adverse reactions include CNS depression, rash, nausea, vomiting, muscle weakness, and headache. Reported drug interactions include enhanced CNS depressive effects when taken concurrently with other CNS depressants (e.g., benzodiazepines). Mitotane may also increase the clearance of both warfarin and phenytoin, reducing their effects.

TABLE 48-4 Hormonal Antineoplastics: Adverse Effects

Class	Drug	Adverse Effects
Aromatase inhibitors	anastrozole, aminoglutethimide	Vasodilation, hypertension, hot flashes, mood disorders, weakness, arthritis
Selective estrogen receptor modulators	tamoxifen, toremifene	Flushing, hypertension, peripheral edema, mood disorders, depression, hot flashes, nausea, weakness
Progestins	megestrol, medroxyprogesterone	Hypertension, chest pain, headache, weight gain, hepatotoxicity, dizziness, abdominal pain
Androgens	fluoxymesterone, testolactone	Menstrual irregularities, virilization of female, gynecomastia, hirsutism, acne, anxiety, headache, nausea
Estrogen receptor antagonists	fulvestrant	Vasodilation, pain, headache, hot flushes, nausea, vomiting, pharyngitis
Antiandrogens	bicalutamide, flutamide, nilutamide	Peripheral edema, pain, hot flushes, gynecomastia, anemia, nausea, diarrhea
Gonadotropin-releasing hormone agonists	leuprolide, goserelin	Rash, pain on injection, alopecia, body odor
Antineoplastic hormone	estramustine	Edema, dyspnea, leg cramps, breast tenderness, nausea, anorexia, diarrhea

Finally, the potassium-sparing diuretic spironolactone may negate the effects of mitotane.

octreotide
Octreotide (Sandostatin) (see Chapter 30) is a unique medication used for management of a cancer-related condition called *carcinoid crisis* and treatment of the diarrhea caused by vasoactive intestinal peptide–secreting tumors (VIPomas).

HORMONAL ANTINEOPLASTICS

Hormonal drugs are used in the treatment of a variety of neoplasms in both males and females. The rationale is that sex hormones act to accelerate the growth of some common types of malignant tumors, especially certain types of breast and prostate cancer. Therefore, therapy may involve administration of hormones with opposing effects (i.e., male vs. female hormones) or drugs that block the body's sex hormone receptors. These drugs are used most commonly as palliative and adjuvant therapy. For certain types of cancer they may also be used as drugs of first choice. Some of the more commonly used hormonal drugs for female-specific neoplasms such as breast cancer are the aromatase inhibitors anastrazole and aminoglutethimide, the selective estrogen receptor modulators tamoxifen and toremifene, the progestins megestrol and medroxyprogesterone, the androgens fluoxymesterone and testolactone, and the estrogen receptor antagonist fulvestrant. For male-specific neoplasms such as prostate cancer, the following drugs are used: the antiandrogens bicalutamide, flutamide, and nilutamide; and the antineoplastic hormone estramustine. The most common adverse effects of these drugs used to treat female and male cancers are listed in Table 48-4.

RADIOPHARMACEUTICALS AND RELATED ANTINEOPLASTICS

Antineoplastic drugs that are usually administered by prescribers include porfimer sodium and various radioactive pharmaceuticals (radiopharmaceuticals). Porfimer sodium is used to

BOX 48-3 Concerns in the Handling and Administration of Vesicant Drugs

The handling and administration of antineoplastic drugs is very controversial, because the nurse mixing and giving the drug may experience negative consequences. In most institutions, the pharmacy department is responsible for mixing these drugs, and preparation is carried out carefully in an appropriate environment with use of a laminar airflow hood and personal protective equipment (mask, gown, gloves). Many facilities recommend taking special precautions during the care of a patient who is receiving chemotherapy, such as double-flushing the patient's bodily secretions in the commode and using special hampers for the disposal of all items that come into contact with the patient, including used personal protective equipment. Special spill kits are employed to clean up even the smallest chemotherapy spills. These precautions are necessary to protect the health care provider from the cytotoxic effects of these drugs. In addition, proper and up-to-date knowledge about these drugs is important to safe and appropriate nursing care. All nurses giving these drugs must be certified to administer chemotherapy and must remain current in their level of practice and competencies related to this treatment modality. All equipment and containers should be handled appropriately once the infusion is completed, and the hands and any exposed areas must be washed to ensure the safety of the health care provider. The Centers for Disease Control and Prevention and the Oncology Nursing Society offer exceptional resources for individuals involved in the care of patients receiving chemotherapy.

treat esophageal or bronchial tumors that are present on the surface mucosa. The medication is given intravenously, and administration is followed by one or more sessions of laser light therapy to the esophageal or bronchial mucosa for direct tumor lysis and manual débridement. Radiopharmaceuticals are used to treat a variety of cancers or symptoms caused by cancers. Five commonly used radioisotopes are chromic phosphate P 32 (for cancer-induced peritoneal or pleural effusions), samarium SM 153 lexidronam (for bone cancer pain), sodium iodide I 131 (for thyroid cancer and hyperthyroidism), sodium phosphate P 32 (for various leukemias and palliative treatment of bone

LABORATORY VALUES RELATED TO DRUG THERAPY

Rationales for Assessment and Monitoring of Blood Cell Counts with Antineoplastics

Laboratory Test	Normal Ranges	Rationale for Assessment
Leukocytes (WBCs)	5000-10,000 cells/mm³	WBCs protect against infection, and when an infection develops, the WBCs attack and destroy the causative bacteria, virus, or other organism. In response to the infection, WBCs increase in number dramatically. If WBC levels are decreased from antineoplastic treatment and subsequent bone marrow suppression, and should they decrease to levels less than 2000 cells/mm³ (leukopenia), there is a high risk for severe infection and immunosuppression.
WBC components:		The major types of WBCs are neutrophils, lymphocytes, monocytes, eosinophils, and
Neutrophils	47%-77% or above 2000/mm³	basophils. Immature neutrophils are called *band neutrophils* and their number, along with neutrophil counts, provides a picture of the patient's immune system. If neutrophils are
Band neutrophils	0%-3%	decreased to levels of less than 500 cells/mm³ (neutropenia), then there is risk for severe infection. If band neutrophils are included in the WBC differential count, then an abnormally low value reinforces the risk for severe infection (see Chapter 47).
Nadir	See normal range of each blood cell	*Nadir* refers to the lowest levels of bone marrow cells that are reached. The time to reach this nadir may become shorter and the recovery time longer with successive courses of antineoplastic treatment. A general estimate of the time to nadir is 10-28 days. Anticipation of the nadir allows the oncologist and health care team to develop a preventative treatment plan, which may include use of biologic response modifiers and antibiotics.

NOTE: Similar information on red blood cell and platelet counts is presented in Chapter 47. Also note that chemotherapy may be discontinued with anemia, leukopenia, neutropenia, and/or thrombocytopenia. Once counts recover (sometimes more quickly with certain drugs), treatment is often reinitiated.
WBCs, White blood cells.

metastases), and strontium Sr 89 chloride (for bone cancer pain). Two drugs used in the treatment of various forms of non-Hodgkin's lymphoma are iodine I 131 tositumomab (Bexxar) and yttrium Y 90 ibritumomab tiuxetan (yttrium 90–labeled CD20 antibody; Zevalin). These medications are usually administered by nuclear medicine specialists.

CYTOPROTECTIVE DRUGS AND MISCELLANEOUS TOXICITY INHIBITORS

Several drugs are available that are classified as cytoprotective drugs. These medications help to reduce the toxicity of various antineoplastics. The decision about whether to use them is often very patient specific, as is the case with chemotherapy regimens. Such decisions are generally made by patients' oncologists. All of these drugs are normally administered intravenously with the exception of allopurinol, which may also be given orally. Extravasation of irritants and vesicants was discussed in Table 47-8. For more information related to extravasation and the handling and administration of antineoplastics, see Boxes 48-1, 48-2, and 48-3. Also see the Laboratory Values Related to Drug Therapy box on p. 755.

NURSING PROCESS

Antineoplastics are some of the most toxic drugs given to patients (see Chapter 47), and because of these toxicities, serious complications and adverse effects may occur. Nursing care must be based on a thorough knowledge of cancer, its treatment, and the subsequent effects of different treatment modalities. This chapter presents information about cell cycle–nonspecific, hormonal, and miscellaneous antineoplastic drugs, whereas Chapter 47 covers cell cycle–specific antineoplastic drugs.

Assessment

The overall assessment of patients taking any of these drugs should begin with a thorough nursing history, medication profile, and past and present medical history. Vital signs should be measured and recorded, and the presence of conditions that represent cautions or contraindications as well as potential drug interactions should be documented. A head-to-toe physical assessment should be performed that includes attention to the following: skin turgor and level of moisture, and integrity of the skin and oral mucosa; baseline level of neurologic functioning including level of consciousness, alertness, motor and sensory intactness, reflexes, and presence of any abnormal sensations; bowel sounds, bowel patterns, and inquiry into any problems such as diarrhea, constipation, nausea, vomiting, or reflux; color, amount, and odor of urine; breath sounds as well as respiratory rate, rhythm, and depth; and heart sounds. Laboratory tests that may be ordered include fluid and electrolyte levels (sodium, potassium, chloride, magnesium, calcium), red blood and white blood cell count, hemoglobin, hematocrit, renal and hepatic function tests, and serum protein-albumin levels.

For patients receiving *alkylating drugs,* such as cisplatin and cyclophosphamide, bone marrow suppression, pulmonary fibrosis, nephrotoxicity and/or neurotoxicity may occur; thus an appropriate and thorough nursing assessment is needed (see Assessment in Chapter 47). Deep tendon reflexes and baseline hearing level should also be assessed and documented. Use of busulfan may result in pulmonary fibrosis, so baseline pulmonary function testing and a thorough respiratory assessment are needed. High-dose cyclophosphamide may lead to hemorrhagic cystitis, so urinary patterns and any abnormal symptoms need to be documented. Level of hydration should also be noted before cyclophosphamide is administered.

One of the major adverse effects associated with the use of *cytotoxic antibiotics* (e.g., bleomycin) is pulmonary fibrosis, and therefore medical testing (e.g., radiographs, computed tomographic [CT] scans, magnetic resonance imaging scans, arterial blood gas levels, and partial pressures of CO_2 and O_2) may be ordered. When doxorubicin is given intravenously, it is generally administered via a central line indwelling catheter device (e.g., Port-A-Cath or MediPort), because if it is given by peripheral intravenous line and extravasation occurs, there is a risk for necrosis with tissue sloughing that may erode through the layers of skin and underlying supportive structures (e.g., muscles, ligaments). See pharmacology discussion of extravasation as well as Table 48-2 and Box 48-3. In addition, in patients with documented cardiac disease or a history of thoracic irradiation doxorubicin must be administered with extreme caution. CT scans and ultrasound studies may be needed before and during treatment to assess cardiac ejection fraction because of the risk of cardiomyopathy, which is often associated with cumulative doses. These tests may also aid in evaluating the effectiveness of the cytoprotective drug dexrazoxane, which is used to help decrease the risk of life-threatening cardiac toxicities.

Use of *hormonal antineoplastic drugs* requires that a thorough medical, nursing, and medication history be obtained. Many of the drugs included in this category are presented in depth in Chapters 34 and 35 which also discuss aspects of the nursing process related to their use, and additional information is available online at *http://evolve.elsevier.com/Lilley.* Assessment associated with the use of *estrogen antagonists* such as fulvestrant, tamoxifen, raloxifene, and toremifene citrates often begins with a review of the results of any tumor estrogen receptor assays, computed tomographic scans, radiographs, and other diagnostic testing. Complete blood cell counts, clotting studies, liver function studies, lipid profiles, and serum cholesterol and calcium levels should be measured before and during drug therapy and the results noted, so that drug-related changes can be identified early and appropriate actions taken. A neurologic and cardiac assessment should be performed (see previous discussion and Chapter 47) with attention to baseline complaints of any pain, abnormal sensations, or headaches. Any menopausal symptoms should be noted upon assessment because of the possible adverse effect of vasodilation and hot flushes. In addition, these drugs may cause nausea and vomiting, and so a thorough GI assessment should be completed.

Blood cell counts, hemoglobin level, hematocrit, blood pressure, and weight should be measured before and during the use of *androgens* (e.g., testosterone). For female patients, a thorough gynecologic history should be completed with attention to any menstrual issues or problems because of the adverse effect of menstrual irregularities. Results of liver function studies should be noted as well. It is also important to assess the patient's body image and feelings of self-esteem because of the possible adverse effects of hirsutism and virilization in female patients. See Chapter 35 and *http://evolve.elsevier.com/Lilley* for more information on these side effects (of androgens).

Flutamide and leuprolide are *antiandrogens.* In rare cases flutamide may cause liver failure; thus some level of assessment should be performed for jaundice or yellowish discoloration of the skin and eyes, dark yellow urine, flulike symptoms, abdominal pain, extreme fatigue, and loss of appetite. Urinary patterns and sexual functioning are also important to assess with attention to any existing problems or difficulties. A nursing assessment

should establish baseline cardiac functioning and document any existing cardiac disease states because of the potential adverse effects of edema and anemia, which may further compromise the patient's health status. A thorough GI and gynecologic assessment should be performed because of the possibility for nausea, diarrhea, and hot flushes. Documentation of the use of a reliable form of birth control is important because of teratogenic effects. Male sperm production may be affected (see Chapter 47), and a decline in sexual functioning and/or desire may occur.

With use of *gonadotropin-releasing hormone agonists*, such as leuprolide and goserelin, the patient must be assessed for allergies to the drugs. Contraceptive history is important, because women who are taking these drugs must use a nonhormonal contraceptive. Often the prescriber will order laboratory tests for serum testosterone level and prostatic acid phosphatase level for male patients before and during therapy; an increase will be noted during the initial week of therapy and then levels will return to baseline by 4 weeks. Assessment of the cardiac system should include evaluation of heart sounds, pulse rate and rhythm, blood pressure, and weight, and examination for the presence of edema.

For patients taking *antiadrenal drugs* (e.g., mitotane), in addition to performing a basic assessment, the nurse should inquire about any GI disturbances and appetite, and assess emotional status because of the common adverse effects of diarrhea, loss of appetite, mental depression, sedation, nausea, and vomiting. The miscellaneous drugs glucocorticoids and mineralocorticoids may be given to prevent adrenal insufficiency and may also play a part in the therapeutic regimen, and so an understanding of baseline functioning through examination of laboratory test results (see previous discussion of laboratory testing) is also important. Forcing fluids, monitoring blood counts, preventing infection, treating nausea and vomiting, checking for abnormal peripheral sensations, and maximizing energy levels are all important with the use of hydroxyurea because of its adverse effects (see earlier discussion).

Nursing Diagnoses

- Activity intolerance related to drug-induced anemia with fatigue and lethargy
- Anxiety related to the unknowns of therapy and illness
- Disturbed body image related to drug-induced alopecia, darkening of the skin, and sexual dysfunction (such as is seen with cyclophosphamide, nitrosoureas, and other alkylating drugs)
- Decreased cardiac output related to the adverse effect of cardiotoxicity associated with cytotoxic antibiotics
- Diarrhea related to the adverse effects of antineoplastic drugs
- Disturbed sensory perception (hearing loss, optic neuritis) related to ototoxicity associated with cisplatin
- Imbalanced nutrition, less than body requirements, related to loss of appetite, nausea, vomiting, stomatitis, and changes in taste as a result of antineoplastic therapy
- Impaired urinary elimination related to the adverse effects of cyclophosphamide (hemorrhagic cystitis and nephrotoxicity)
- Ineffective breathing pattern related to the adverse effect of pulmonary toxicity associated with some antineoplastic drugs
- Risk for injury related to loss of reflexes, numbness of the hands and feet, and ataxia caused by cisplatin-related neurotoxicity

Planning

Goals

- Patient maintains as healthy a diet as possible with adequate intake of protein, vitamins, and other nutrients to increase energy and stamina and allow continued performance of the activities of daily living during antineoplastic treatment.
- Patient maintains an intact and healthy body image and effective coping mechanisms while experiencing alopecia, skin changes, and sexual dysfunction associated with antineoplastic therapy.
- Patient verbalizes concerns, fears, and anxieties associated with changes in body image.
- Patient's cardiac output remains within normal limits while the patient is taking antineoplastics.
- Patient states foods and fluids that should be avoided to prevent further GI irritation and is able to identify foods that help bulk up stool and minimize problems from diarrhea.
- Patient remains safe and free from injury with minimal neurologic, sensory, and motor deficits from the adverse effects of antineoplastic therapy.
- Patient receives consultation regarding appropriate dietary intake and fluid and electrolyte needs, help with meal planning, grocery shopping tips, and information on the consumption of various food groups and use of medications, as ordered, to prevent problems of nutritional imbalance.
- Patient regains normal urinary patterns during and after antineoplastic therapy.

Outcome Criteria

- Patient openly verbalizes any anxieties, fears, concerns, or feelings of being upset or depressed about changes in body image and self-concept and seeks out appropriate resources for help in coping, such as spiritual support, therapeutic touch, counseling, and talking with family, friends, and other individuals with cancer who have been trained to visit cancer patients. (Such individuals can be located through the American Cancer Society and community support groups.)
- Patient adheres to a daily "heart-healthy" regimen of conserving energy, planning activities, and consistently monitoring pulse rate and blood pressure and asks for assistance with care and activities as needed.
- Patient adheres to a daily regimen for increasing urinary health, such as forcing fluids, consuming fluids that minimize urinary infections (e.g., cranberry juice), and maintaining daily hydration while receiving antineoplastic therapy.
- Patient states measures to follow for pulmonary health, including avoiding individuals with influenza, colds, fever, or other illnesses; avoiding smoking and exposure to second-hand smoke; coughing and performing deep breathing frequently during waking hours; forcing fluids; and taking prophylactic antibiotic therapy, if ordered.
- Patient states ways to minimize risk for injury (from neurologic adverse effects) by development of a safety plan that includes ridding the home of throw rugs and furniture that may lead to falls, using assistive devices such as a walker or cane, having a bedside commode available, installing night lights, and instituting other measures to aid mobility. (See Chapter 47 for additional nursing diagnoses, goals, and outcome criteria that may be relevant to the discussion here.)

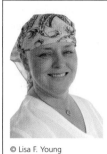

CASE STUDY

Chemotherapy with Alkylating Drugs

W.S. is receiving cisplatin as part of treatment for ovarian cancer. She is receiving her third treatment today and has just arrived at the cancer treatment center for her outpatient infusion. W.S. says that she has felt "okay" during the time between the last treatment and today but dreads how she will feel after today.

© Lisa F. Young

1. While the nurse prepares to start the infusion, what is important for the nurse to assess before beginning the chemotherapy?
2. What will the nurse do before the infusion to help reduce or prevent adverse effects?
3. During the infusion, W.S. mentions that she is hearing a slight "roaring" sound and that she feels a bit dizzy. What should the nurse do?
4. After stopping the infusion, the nurse spills some of the chemotherapy solution on her arm and the floor. What should the nurse do?

For answers, see *http://evolve.elsevier.com/Lilley.*

Implementation

Before initiating drug therapy with the cell cycle-nonspecific drugs, hormonal antineoplastics and miscellaneous drugs, the nurse must be completely knowledgeable about the drug, its use, and its impact on all rapidly dividing cells, whether normal or malignant (see Chapters 34, 35, and 47 for additional information).

With *alkylating drugs,* the patient will more than likely experience problems related to bone marrow suppression, such as anemia, leukopenia, and thrombocytopenia (see Chapter 47 for specific interventions). Other nursing considerations for alkylating drugs include measuring vital signs every 1 to 2 hours, or as needed, during infusion of these drugs; forcing fluids; monitoring intake and output; following orders for intravenous therapy for hydration; and monitoring any vomiting and reporting to the prescriber if vomiting is uncontrolled. The patient should be monitored constantly for abnormal peripheral sensations. Any numbness or tingling should be reported to the prescriber. Ringing or roaring in the ears or hearing loss should also be reported. Because hemorrhagic cystitis is associated with cyclophosphamide use, hydration must be maintained to minimize this adverse effect. These and all other antineoplastics should be handled with caution because of their possible carcinogenic, mutagenic, and teratogenic properties (see Box 48-3).

Another commonly used alkylating drug, cisplatin, is nephrotoxic, and renal function test results must be monitored frequently during therapy. Intravenous hydration is often required at a rate of 100 to 200 mL/hr starting before cisplatin administration with a total of 2000 to 3000 mL/day, depending on the dose of cisplatin and if not contraindicated. Aluminum needles or administration sets should not be used with many of these drugs because aluminum can degrade the platinum compounds in them, and the nurse must ensure that the proper infusion equipment is used. Drug-induced neuropathies may occur, so the patient should be encouraged to avoid extremely cold temperatures or the handling of cold objects during the infusion, because this may exacerbate the toxicity. Other drugs in this group may be given by various routes, such as intrapericardial, intratumoral, and intravesical, so appropriate interventions will need to be performed per the manufacturer's guidelines or hospital policy. Pulmonary toxicity may occur with some of the alkylating drugs, particularly busulfan and carmustine, so the nurse should be alert to cough, shortness of breath, and abnormal breath sounds. These adverse effects should be reported immediately to the prescriber. Reconstitution of the parenteral formulations any of these drugs should be performed according to the manufacturer's guidelines and suggestions, because not all diluents are compatible.

Patients receiving *cytotoxic antibiotics* such as bleomycin may require more frequent monitoring of pulmonary function, and baseline chest radiographs may be obtained for comparison with subsequent radiographs if pneumonitis occurs at a later point. Results of liver and renal function tests should be monitored throughout therapy as well. Hyperuricemia may occur, so provision of fluids and hydration are important to minimize this adverse effect. With doxorubicin, the urine may turn a reddish color for a few days after the treatment, and the patient should be warned about this effect to ease any fears or anxieties associated with this change. Stomatitis may be more severe with ulceration of the mucous membranes during the first week. Bone marrow suppression, alopecia, vomiting, diarrhea, and nausea are also problematic with these drugs (see Chapter 47). Cardiac toxicity may occur; therefore, heart and breath sounds should be checked frequently and the patient weighed daily. An increase of 2 pounds or more in 24 hours or 5 pounds or more in 1 week should be reported.

Use of *hormone antagonists* in the treatment of various neoplasms is common, particularly with breast and prostate cancer. Associated nursing interventions and patient education for the use of these hormone antagonists are discussed in depth in Chapters 34 and 35. Corticosteroid therapy and related nursing considerations are presented in Chapter 33. Further information and discussion regarding the use of hormones and hormone antagonists in the treatment of patients with various types of cancer can also be found online at *http://evolve.elsevier.com/Lilley.*

Hydroxyurea is used sparingly in a couple of treatment protocols. This drug is given orally. Monitoring of platelet and leukocyte counts is important to avoid harm to the patient. Monitoring should be ongoing during therapy. If platelet count falls below 100,000 platelets/mm³ or leukocyte count falls below 2000 cells/mm³, therapy may need to be temporarily halted until counts rise toward the normal values. See earlier discussion in Chapter 47 about nursing considerations associated with anemias, fatigue, weakness, bleeding tendencies, and infection.

In addition to the nursing interventions discussed earlier and in Chapter 47, keeping epinephrine, antihistamines, and antiinflammatories available in case of an allergic or anaphylactic reaction is highly recommended. Each antineoplastic drug has its own peculiarities and its own set of cautions, contraindications, nursing implementations, and toxicities. *Cytoprotective drugs* are useful in

---

BOX 48-4 Indications of an Oncologic Emergency

Fever and/or chills with a temperature higher than 100° F (37.8° C)
New sores or white patches in the mouth or throat
Swollen tongue with or without cracks and bleeding
Bleeding gums
Dry, burning, "scratchy," or "swollen" throat
A cough that is new and persistent
Changes in bladder function or patterns
Blood in the urine
Changes in gastrointestinal or bowel patterns, including "heartburn" or nausea, vomiting, constipation, or diarrhea lasting longer than 2 or 3 days
Blood in the stools

NOTE: The patient should contact the prescriber immediately if any of the listed signs or symptoms occurs. If the prescriber is not available, the patient should seek medical treatment at the closest emergency department.

---

reducing certain toxicities. For example, use of intravenous amifostine may help to reduce the renal toxicity associated with cisplatin; intravenous or oral allopurinol may be given to reduce hyperuricemia (see Table 47-6 and Box 47-2). Other major concerns related to the care of patients receiving chemotherapy are the oncologic emergencies that arise because of damage occurring to rapidly dividing normal cells as well as rapidly dividing cancerous cells. Some of the complications that are potential emergencies include infections, infusion reactions and allergy, stomatitis with severe ulceration, bleeding, metabolic aberrations, severe diarrhea, renal failure, liver failure, and cardiac toxicity, including dysrhythmia or heart failure (Box 48-4). See *http://evolve.elsevier.com/Lilley* for information on resources for patients with cancer.

Evaluation

Evaluation of nursing care should center on determining whether goals and outcomes have been met, as well as on monitoring for therapeutic responses and adverse and toxic effects of antineoplastic therapy. Therapeutic responses may manifest as clinical improvement, decrease in tumor size, and decrease in metastatic spread. Evaluation of nursing care with reference to goals and outcomes may reveal improvements related to a decrease in adverse effects; a decrease in the impact of cancer on the patient's well-being; an increase in comfort, nutrition, and hydration; improved energy levels and ability to carry out the activities of daily living; and improved quality of life. The goals and outcomes can be revisited to identify more specific areas to monitor. In addition, certain laboratory studies such as measurement of tumor marker levels, levels of carcinoembryonic antigens, and red blood cell, white blood cell, and platelet counts may also be used to determine how well the goals and outcomes have been met. As part of the evaluation, prescribers may also order additional radiographs, computed tomographic scans, magnetic resonance images, tissue analyses, and other studies appropriate to the diagnosis during and after antineoplastic therapy, at time intervals related to anticipated tumor response.

PATIENT TEACHING TIPS

- Aspirin, ibuprofen, and products containing these drugs should be avoided to help prevent excessive bleeding.
- Be open with discussion about the risk of alopecia (a complete discussion is presented in Chapter 47).
- Encourage forcing of fluids up to 3000 mL/day, if not contraindicated, to prevent dehydration and further weakening and, in the case of cyclophosphamide therapy, to prevent or help manage hemorrhagic cystitis.
- Constipation and diarrhea may be problematic and so educate about ways to help manage these alterations in bowel status that may be due to the antineoplastic or due to narcotics used for pain management. To help avoid constipation, forcing of

fluids and consumption of a balanced diet are important; however, the oncologist generally orders either a stool softener or a mild noncramping laxative to prevent the problem. Diarrhea is generally treated by dietary restrictions and use of antidiarrheals as ordered.

- The following are helpful online resources for the patient and significant others: *http://www.fda.gov*, *http://www.fda.gov/oc/oha*, *http://www.nih.gov*, *http://www.healthfinder.gov*, *http://www.who.int/en*, and *http://www.oncolink.upenn.edu*.
- Follow protocols and facility guidelines regarding extravasation, including the stopping of the infusion.

POINTS TO REMEMBER

- Antineoplastics are drugs that are used to treat malignancies and are classified as cell cycle–specific drugs, cell cycle–nonspecific drugs, miscellaneous antineoplastics, and hormonal drugs.
- Cell cycle–specific drugs kill cancer cells during specific phases of the cell growth cycle, whereas the cell cycle–nonspecific drugs discussed in this chapter kill cancer cells during any phase of the growth cycle.
- Chemotherapy, or antineoplastic drug therapy, requires very skillful and perceptive nursing care, and the nurse must act prudently and make critical decisions about the nursing care of patients receiving these drugs.
- Knowledge is important to ensure patient safety and also to protect the nurse from the adverse effects of antineoplastics.

- Extreme caution must be exercised in the handling and administration of cell cycle–nonspecific (as well as cell cycle–specific) drugs.
- Hormonal drugs, both agonists and antagonists, and female and male hormones, are used to treat a variety of malignancies.
- Extravasation of strong vesicants (doxorubicin) may lead to severe tissue injury with complications such as permanent damage to muscles, tendons, and ligaments, and possible loss of limb.
- Oncologic emergencies occur as a consequence of cell death and may be life threatening. Skillful assessment and immediate intervention may help to decrease the severity of the problem or even reduce the occurrence of such emergencies.

NCLEX EXAMINATION REVIEW QUESTIONS

1 A patient who is receiving chemotherapy with cisplatin has developed pneumonia. The nurse would be concerned about nephrotoxicity if which type of antibiotic was ordered as treatment for the pneumonia at this time?
  a Penicillin
  b Sulfa drug
  c Fluoroquinolone
  d Aminoglycoside

2 During treatment with doxorubicin, the nurse must monitor closely for which potentially life-threatening adverse effect?
  a Nephrotoxicity
  b Peripheral neuritis
  c Cardiomyopathy
  d Ototoxicity

3 While teaching a patient who is about to receive cyclophosphamide chemotherapy, the nurse should instruct the patient to watch for potential adverse effects, such as:
  a Cholinergic diarrhea
  b Hemorrhagic cystitis
  c Peripheral neuropathy
  d Ototoxicity

4 When chemotherapy with alkylating drugs is planned, the nurse expects to implement which intervention to prevent nephrotoxicity?
  a Hydrating the patient with intravenous fluids before chemotherapy
  b Limiting fluids before chemotherapy
  c Monitoring drug levels during chemotherapy
  d Assessing creatinine clearance during chemotherapy

5 During therapy with the cytotoxic antibiotic bleomycin, the nurse will assess for a potentially serious adverse effect by monitoring
  a blood urea nitrogen and creatinine levels.
  b cardiac ejection fraction.
  c respiratory function.
  d cranial nerve function.

6 While administering bevacizumab (Avastin), what will the nurse assess to look for drug-related toxicities? (Select all that apply.)
  a Blood pressure
  b Color of the skin and sclera of the eye (for jaundice)
  c Blood glucose level
  d Urine protein level
  e Hearing

CRITICAL THINKING ACTIVITIES: BEST ACTION

1 During an infusion of carmustine, the patient dislodges the intravenous catheter, and infiltration of the medication occurs. What is the nurse's best action?

2 A patient has been receiving bleomycin irrigations through a chest tube for 3 days. Today he begins to have an irregular and slow heart rhythm, complains of nausea, and says, "I'm seeing yellow hazy circles around the lights." He thinks the chemo-therapy is causing these problems. What is the nurse's best action? Explain.

3 During a prechemotherapy teaching session, the patient hears that she will be receiving a cytotoxic antibiotic as part of the medication regimen. The patient asks, "How can this drug help cancer? It's an antibiotic!" What is the nurse's best answer?

For answers, see *http://evolve.elsevier.com/Lilley.*

CHAPTER 49

Biologic Response–Modifying and Antirheumatoid Drugs

OBJECTIVES

When you reach the end of this chapter, you should be able to do the following:

1 Describe the basic anatomy, physiology, and functions of the immune system.

2 Compare the two major classes of biologic response–modifying drugs: hematopoietic drugs and immunomodulating drugs.

3 Discuss the mechanisms of action, indications, dosages, routes of administration, adverse effects, cautions, contraindications, and drug interactions of the different biologic response–modifying drugs.

4 Describe the pathology associated with rheumatoid arthritis.

5 Discuss the mechanisms of action, indications, dosages, routes of administration, adverse effects, cautions, contraindications, and drug interactions of the different antirheumatoid drugs.

6 Develop a nursing care plan that includes all phases of the nursing process for patients receiving biologic response–modifying drugs and for those receiving antirheumatoid drugs.

e-Learning Activities

http://evolve.elsevier.com/Lilley

NCLEX Review Questions • Animations • Nursing Care Plans • Audio Glossary • Category Catchers • Medication Errors Checklists • IV Therapy Checklists • Calculators • Frequently Asked Questions • Content Updates • Supplemental Resources • Answers to Case Studies and Critical Thinking Activities

Drug Profiles

abatacept, p. 776
adalimumab, p. 771
◆ aldesleukin, p. 774
alemtuzumab, p. 771
anakinra, p. 774
bevacizumab, p. 772
cetuximab, p. 772
denileukin diftitox, p. 774
◆ epoetin alfa, p. 766
etanercept, p. 776
◆ filgrastim, p. 767
gemtuzumab ozogamicin, p. 772
ibritumomab tiuxetan, p. 772
infliximab, p. 772
◆ interferon alfa-2a, interferon alfa-2b, interferon alfa-n3, inter-

feron alfacon-1, peginterferon alfa-2a, and peginterferon alfa-2b, p. 768
◆ interferon beta-1a, interferon beta-1b p. 769
interferon gamma-1b, p. 769
leflunomide, p. 776
methotrexate, p. 776
natalizumab, p. 772
◆ oprelvekin, p. 767
◆ rituximab, p. 772
◆ sargramostim, p. 767
tositumomab and iodine I 131 tositumomab, p. 772
trastuzumab, p. 772

◆ *Key drug.*

Glossary

Adjuvant A nonspecific *immunostimulant;* that is, an immunostimulant that somehow enhances overall immune function, rather than stimulating the function of a specific immune system cell or cytokine through specific chemical reactions. An example is bacille Calmette-Guérin vaccine. (p. 774)

Antibodies Immunoglobulin molecules (see Chapter 46) that have the ability to bind to and inactivate antigen molecules through formation of an antigen-antibody complex. This process ideally serves to inactivate foreign antigens that enter the body and are capable of causing disease. (p. 763)

Antigen A biologic or chemical substance that is recognized as foreign by the body's immune system. (p. 763)

Arthritis Inflammation of one or more joints. (p. 775)

Autoimmune disorder A disorder that occurs when the body's tissues are attacked by its own immune system. (p. 774)

B lymphocytes (B cells) Leukocytes of the humoral immune system that develop into plasma cells, which produce the antibodies that bind to and inactivate antigens. B cells are one of the two principal types of lymphocytes; *T lymphocytes* are the other. (p. 763)

Biologic response–modifying drugs A broad class of drugs that includes hematopoietic drugs and immunomodulating drugs. Often referred to as *biologic response modifiers (BRMs)*, these drugs alter the body's response to diseases such as cancer as well as autoimmune, inflammatory, and infectious diseases. Examples are cytokines (e.g., interleukin, interferons), monoclonal antibodies, and vaccines. Also called *biomodulators* or *immunomodulating drugs*. *Biologic response–modifying drugs* may be *adjuvants, immunostimulants,* or *immunosuppressants.* (p. 762)

Cell-mediated immunity The collective term for all immune responses that are mediated by T lymphocytes (T cells). Also called *cellular immunity.* Cell-mediated immunity acts in collaboration with *humoral immunity.* (p. 763)

Colony-stimulating factors Cytokines that regulate the growth, differentiation, and function of bone marrow stem cells. (p. 764)

Complement The collective term for about 20 different proteins normally present in plasma that assist other immune system components (e.g., B cells and T cells) in mounting an immune response. (p. 772)

Cytokines The generic term for nonantibody proteins released by specific cell populations (e.g., activated T cells) on contact with antigens. Cytokines act as intercellular mediators of an immune response. Although no cytokines are antibodies, all cytokines are proteins. (p. 763)

Cytotoxic T cells Differentiated T cells that can recognize and lyse (rupture) target cells that bear foreign antigens on their surfaces. These antigens are recognized by the corresponding specific antigen receptors that are expressed (displayed) on the cytotoxic T-cell surface. Also called *natural killer cells*. (p. 763)

Differentiation The process of cellular development from a simplified into a more complex and specialized cellular structure. In hematopoiesis, it refers to the multistep processes involved in the maturation of blood cells, in which generalized pluripotent stem cells in the bone marrow develop along different cellular paths to yield mature, specialized blood components such as erythrocytes, leukocytes, and platelets. (p. 764)

Disease-modifying antirheumatic drugs (DMARDs) Medications used in the treatment of rheumatic diseases that have the potential to arrest or slow the actual disease process instead of providing only antiinflammatory and analgesic effects (like the nonsteroidal antiinflammatory drugs). (p. 775)

Hematopoiesis The collective term for all of the body's processes originating in the bone marrow that result in the formation of various types of blood components (adjective: *hematopoietic*). It includes the three main processes of *differentiation* (see earlier): erythropoiesis (formation of red blood cells, or erythrocytes), leukopoiesis (formation of white blood cells, or leukocytes), and thrombopoiesis (formation of platelets, or thrombocytes). (p. 762)

Humoral immunity The collective term for all immune responses that are mediated by B cells, which ultimately work through the production of antibodies against specific antigens. Humoral immunity acts in collaboration with *cell-mediated immunity*. (p. 763)

Immunoglobulins Complex immune system glycoproteins that bind to and inactivate foreign antigens. The term is synonymous with *immune globulins*. (p. 763)

Immunomodulating drugs Collective term for various subclasses of biologic response–modifying drugs that specifically or nonspecifically enhance or reduce immune responses. The three major types of immunomodulators, based on mechanism of action, are adjuvants, immunostimulants, and immunosuppressants (see Chapter 45). (p. 762)

Immunostimulant A drug that enhances immune response through specific chemical interactions with particular immune system components. An example is interleukin-2. (p. 774)

Immunosuppressant A drug that reduces immune response through specific chemical interactions with particular immune system components. An example is cyclosporine (see Chapter 45). (p. 768)

Interferons One type of cytokine that promotes resistance to viral infection in uninfected cells and can also strengthen the body's immune response to cancer cells. (p. 767)

Leukocytes The collective term for all subtypes of white blood cells. Leukocytes include the granulocytes (neutrophils, eosinophils, and basophils), monocytes, and lymphocytes (B cells and T cells). Some monocytes also develop into tissue macrophages. (p. 763)

Lymphokine-activated killer (LAK) cell *Cytotoxic T cells* that have been further activated by interleukin-2 and therefore have a stronger and more specific response against cancer cells. (p. 773)

Lymphokines Cytokines that are produced by sensitized T lymphocytes on contact with antigen particles. (p. 763)

Memory cells Cells involved in the humoral immune system that remember the exact characteristics of a particular foreign invader or antigen for the purpose of expediting immune response in the event of future exposure to this antigen. (p. 763)

Monoclonal Denoting a group of identical cells or organisms derived from a single cell. (p. 763)

Plasma cells Cells derived from B cells that are found in the bone marrow, connective tissue, and blood. They produce antibodies. (p. 763)

Rheumatism General term for any of several disorders characterized by inflammation, degeneration, or metabolic derangement of connective tissue structures, especially joints and related structures. (p. 774)

T helper cells Cells that promote and direct the actions of various other cells of the immune system. (p. 763)

T lymphocytes (T cells) Leukocytes of the cell-mediated immune system. Unlike B cells, they are not involved in the production of antibodies but instead occur in various cell subtypes (e.g., T helper cells, T suppressor cells, and cytotoxic T cells) that act through direct cell-to-cell contact or through production of cytokines that guide the functions of other immune system components (e.g., B cells, antibodies). (p. 763)

T suppressor cells Cells that regulate and limit the immune response, balancing the effects of T helper cells. (p. 763)

Tumor antigens Chemical compounds expressed on the surfaces of tumor cells. They signal to the immune system that these cells do not belong in the body, labeling the tumor cells as foreign. (p. 763)

• • •

Anatomy, Physiology, and Disease Overview

OVERVIEW OF IMMUNOMODULATORS

Over the last two decades medical technology has developed a group of drugs whose primary site of action is the immune system. This has resulted in some new additions to the class of drugs known as **biologic response–modifying drugs,** or *biologic response modifiers(s)*. These drugs alter the body's response to diseases such as cancer and autoimmune, inflammatory, and infectious diseases. These drugs can enhance or restrict the patient's immune response to disease, can stimulate a patient's *hematopoietic* (blood-forming) function, and can even prevent disease. **Hematopoiesis** is the collective term for all of the blood component–forming processes of the bone marrow. Two broad classes of biologic response–modifying drugs are *hematopoietic drugs* and **immunomodulating drugs.** Subclasses of immunomodulating drugs include *interferons, monoclonal antibodies, interleukin receptor agonists and antagonists, and miscellaneous drugs. Disease-modifying antirheumatic drugs* are drugs that are used to treat rheumatoid arthritis, which is discussed later in this chapter.

Immunomodulating drugs are defined as medications that therapeutically alter a patient's immune response. In cancer treatment, they make up the fourth type of cancer therapy, along with surgery, chemotherapy, and radiation. The human immune system is most commonly viewed as the body's natural defense against primarily pathogenic bacteria and viruses. However, it also has effective antitumor capabilities. An intact immune system can identify cells as malignant and destroy them. In contrast to chemotherapeutic drugs, a healthy immune system can distinguish between tumor cells and normal body tissues. Normal cells are recognized as "self" and are not damaged, whereas tumor cells are recognized as "foreign" and are destroyed. It is known that people routinely develop cancerous cells in their bodies on a regular basis. Normally the immune system is able to eliminate these cells before they multiply to uncontrollable levels. It is only when the natural immune responses fail to keep pace with these initially microscopic cancer cell growths that a person develops a true "cancer" requiring clinical intervention.

With regard to action against cancer cells in particular, there are three common mechanisms by which current biologic response–modifying drugs work. The first mechanism is enhancement or restoration of the host's immune system defenses against the tumor. The second is a direct toxic effect of the molecules of a particular drug on the tumor cells, which causes them to *lyse,* or rupture. The third mechanism is adverse modification of the tumor's biology, which makes it harder for the tumor cells to survive and reproduce.

Some immunomodulating drugs are used to treat autoimmune, inflammatory, and infectious diseases. In these instances, the drug functions either to reduce the patient's inappropriate immune response (in the case of inflammatory and autoimmune diseases such as rheumatoid arthritis) or to strengthen the patient's immune response against microorganisms (especially viruses) and cancer cells. To better understand these complex drugs, a review of immune system physiology is beneficial.

IMMUNE SYSTEM

The immune system is an intricate biologic defense network of cells that are capable of distinguishing an unlimited variety of substances as either foreign ("nonself") or a natural part of the host's body ("self"). When a foreign substance such as a bacteria or virus enters the body, the immune system recognizes it as being nonself and mounts an immune response to eliminate or neutralize the invader. Tumors are not truly foreign substances because they arise from cells of normal tissues whose genetic material (deoxyribonucleic acid [DNA] and ribonucleic acid [RNA]) has somehow mutated, causing uncontrolled cell growth. Tumor cells express chemical compounds on their surfaces that signal the immune system that these cells are a threat. These chemical markers are called **tumor antigens** or *tumor markers,* and they label the tumor cells as abnormal cells. An **antigen** is any substance that the body's immune system recognizes as foreign. Recognition of antigens varies among individuals, which is why some people are more prone than others to immune-related diseases such as allergies, inflammatory diseases, and cancer.

The two major components of the body's immune system are **humoral immunity,** mediated by B-cell functions (primarily *antibody* production; see later), and **cell-mediated immunity,** which is mediated by T-cell functions. These two systems act together to recognize and destroy foreign particles and cells in the blood or other body tissues. Communication between these two divisions is vital to the success of the immune system as a whole. Attack against tumor cells by antibodies produced by the **B lymphocytes (B cells)** of the humoral immune system prepares those tumor cells for destruction by the **T lymphocytes (T cells)** of the cell-mediated immune system. This is just one example of the effective way that the two divisions of the immune system communicate with each other for a collaborative immune response.

Humoral Immune System

The primary functional cells of the humoral immune system are the B lymphocytes. They are also called *B cells* because they originate in the bone marrow. Antigens that enter the body send a biochemical signal to B lymphocytes when the antigen molecules bind to antigen receptors that are located on the B cells. The B cells that are capable of generating a particular antibody normally re-

main dormant until the corresponding antigen is detected. These B cells then mature or *differentiate* into **plasma cells,** which in turn produce antibodies. **Antibodies** are **immunoglobulins** (large glycoprotein molecules; glyco = sugar; protein = amino acid chain) that bind to specific antigens, forming an *antigen-antibody complex* that inactivates disease-causing antigens.

The immune system in a healthy individual is genetically preprogrammed to be able to mount an antibody response against literally millions of different antigens. This ability results from the individual's lifetime antigen exposure and is further developed through exposure to new antigens and passed down through many generations. Antibodies that a single plasma cell makes are all identical. They are therefore called **monoclonal** antibodies, and they are active against the single specific antigen that was originally recognized by their ancestor B cell as foreign. Since the 1980s, monoclonal antibodies have also been prepared synthetically using recombinant DNA technology, which has resulted in newer drug therapies.

There are five major types of naturally occurring immunoglobulins in the body: immunoglobulins A, D, E, G, and M. These unique types have different structures and functions and are found in various areas of the body. During an immune response, when B lymphocytes differentiate into plasma cells, some of these B cells become **memory cells** instead. Memory cells "remember" the exact characteristics of a particular foreign invader or antigen, which allows a stronger and faster immune response in the event of reexposure to the same antigen. The cells of the humoral immune system are shown in Figure 49-1.

Cell-Mediated Immune System

The primary functional cells of the cell-mediated (as opposed to antibody-mediated) immune system are the T lymphocytes. They are also referred to as *T cells* because, although they originate in the bone marrow like their B-cell counterparts, they mature in a mediastinal gland known as the *thymus.* There are three distinct populations of T cells: cytotoxic T cells, T helper cells, and T suppressor cells. They are distinguished by the different functions that they perform. **Cytotoxic T cells** directly kill their targets by causing cell lysis or rupture. **T helper cells** are considered the master controllers of the immune system. They direct the actions of many other immune components, such as lymphokines and cytotoxic T cells. **Lymphokines** are a subset of a broader category of blood proteins known as *cytokines.* **Cytokines** are nonantibody proteins that serve as chemical mediators of a variety of physiologic functions. Lymphokines are those cytokines that are released by T lymphocytes upon contact with antigens and serve as chemical mediators of the immune response. **T suppressor cells** have an effect on the immune system that is opposite to that of T helper cells and serve to limit or control the immune response. A healthy immune system has about twice as many T helper cells as T suppressor cells at any given time.

The major cells involved in the destruction of cancer cells are believed to be part of the cell-mediated immune system. The cancer-killing cells of the cellular immune system include macrophages (derived from monocytes), natural killer (NK) cells (another type of lymphocyte), and polymorphonuclear **leukocytes** (not lymphocytes), which are also called *neutrophils.* In contrast, T suppressor cells have the most important negative influence on antitumor actions of the immune system. Overactive

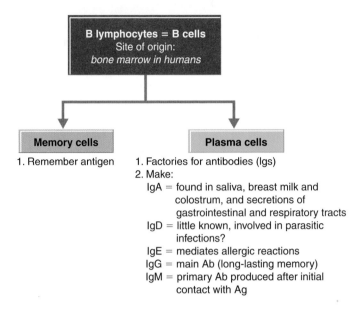

FIGURE 49-1   Cells of the humoral (antibody-mediated) immune system. *Ig,* Immunoglobulin.

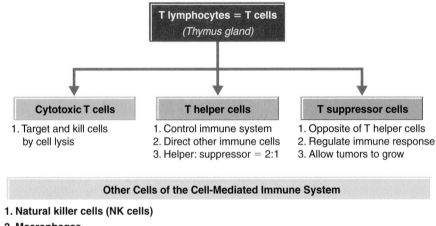

FIGURE 49-2   Cells of the cellular immune system.

T suppressor cells may be responsible for clinically significant cancer cases by permitting tumor growth beyond immune system's control. Figure 49-2 shows the components of the cellular immune system.

Pharmacology Overview

Therapy with biologic response–modifying drugs combines the knowledge of several disciplines, including general biology, genetics, immunology, pharmacology, medicine, and nursing. The general therapeutic effects of these drugs are as follows:

- Enhancement of hematopoietic function
- Regulation or augmentation (enhancement) of the immune response, including cytotoxic or cytostatic activity against cancer cells
- Inhibition of metastases, prevention of cell division, or inhibition of cell maturation

Box 49-1 lists the currently available biologic response–modifying drugs used in the treatment of cancer and other illnesses that have varying levels of immune system–related pathophysiology. The drugs are classified according to their biologic effects.

HEMATOPOIETIC DRUGS

Hematopoietic drugs include several newer medications developed over the past 10 to 15 years. Falling into this category are two erythropoietic drugs (epoetin alfa and darbepoetin alfa), three **colony-stimulating factors** (filgrastim, pegfilgrastim, and sargramostim), and one platelet-promoting drug (oprelvekin). All of these drugs promote the synthesis of various types of major blood components by promoting the growth, **differentiation,** and function of their corresponding precursor cells in the bone marrow.

BOX 49-1 Biologic–Response Modifying Drugs

Hematopoietic Drugs
Colony-Stimulating Factors
filgrastim (G-CSF)
pegfilgrastim
sargramostim (GM-CSF)

Other
darbepoetin alfa
epoetin alfa
oprelvekin (IL-11)

Immunomodulating Drugs
Interferons
interferon alfa-2a
interferon alfa-2b*
peginterferon alfa-2a
peginterferon alfa-2b
interferon alfacon-1
interferon alfa-n3
interferon beta-1a
interferon beta-1b
interferon gamma-1b

Monoclonal Antibodies
alemtuzumab
gemtuzumab ozogamicin
ibritumomab tiuxetan
rituximab
trastuzumab

Interleukin Receptor Agonists and Antagonists
Agonist
aldesleukin (IL-2)

Antagonists
anakinra
denileukin diftitox

Miscellaneous Immunomodulators
Tumor Necrosis Factor Receptor Antagonist
etanercept

Enzymes
pegademase bovine

Retinoid Receptor Agonists
tretinoin
bexarotene

Adjuvants (Nonspecific Immunostimulants)
bacille Calmette-Guérin vaccine
leflunomide
levamisole
mitoxantrone
thalidomide
abatacept

G-CSF, Granulocyte colony-stimulating factor; *GM-CSF,* granulocyte-macrophage colony-stimulating factor; *IL,* interleukin.
*Also available in combination with the antiviral drug ribavirin.

Mechanism of Action and Drug Effects

Although the hematopoietic drugs are not toxic to cancer cells, they do have beneficial effects in the treatment of cancer. All hematopoietic drugs have the same basic mechanism of action. They decrease the duration of chemotherapy-induced anemia, neutropenia, and thrombocytopenia and enable higher dosages of chemotherapy to be given; decrease bone marrow recovery time

after bone marrow transplantation or irradiation; and stimulate other cells in the immune system to destroy or inhibit the growth of cancer cells, as well as virus- or fungus-infected cells.

All of these drugs are produced by recombinant DNA technology, which allows them to be essentially identical to their endogenously produced counterparts. These substances work by binding to receptors on the surfaces of specialized *progenitor cells* in the bone marrow. These cells are responsible for the production of three particular cell lines: red blood cells (RBCs), white blood cells (WBCs), and platelets. When a hematopoietic drug binds to a progenitor cell surface, the immature progenitor cell is stimulated to mature, proliferate (reproduce itself), differentiate (transform into its respective type of specialized blood component), and become functionally active. Hematopoietic drugs may enhance certain functions of mature cell lines as well.

Epoetin alfa is a synthetic derivative of the human hormone *erythropoietin,* which is produced primarily by the kidney. It promotes the synthesis of erythrocytes (RBCs) by stimulating RBC progenitor cells in the bone marrow. It is also called *EPO.* Darbepoetin alfa, a newer drug, is a longer-acting form of epoetin alfa. Filgrastim is a colony-stimulating factor that stimulates progenitor cells for the subset of WBCs (leukocytes) known as *granulocytes* (including basophils, eosinophils, and neutrophils). For this reason it is also commonly called *granulocyte colony-stimulating factor* (G-CSF). Pegfilgrastim is a newer, longer-acting form of filgrastim. Sargramostim is also a CSF that works by stimulating the bone marrow precursor cells that synthesize both granulocytes and the phagocytic (cell-eating) cells known as *monocytes,* some of which become *macrophages.* For this reason it is also called *granulocyte-macrophage colony-stimulating factor* (GM-CSF). Oprelvekin, the newest drug, is also classified as an *interleukin,* namely, interleukin-11 (IL-11). Other interleukins are discussed later in this chapter. Oprelvekin stimulates the bone marrow cells, specifically megakaryocytes, that eventually give rise to platelets.

Indications

Hematopoietic drugs have many specific therapeutic uses. Neutrophils are the most important granulocytes for fighting infection. Because administration of colony-stimulating factors reduces the duration of low neutrophil counts, these drugs reduce the incidence and duration of infections. Infections normally appear in patients who have experienced destruction of bone marrow cells as a result of chemotherapy. Colony-stimulating factors stimulate these cells to grow and mature and thus directly oppose the detrimental bone marrow actions of chemotherapeutic drugs (see Interactions later). Colony-stimulating factors also enhance the functioning of mature cells of the immune system, such as macrophages and granulocytes. This increases the ability of the body's immune system to kill cancer cells, as well as virus- and fungus-infected cells. Ultimately these properties allow patients to receive higher dosages of chemotherapy. Similar benefits occur with epoetin alfa and oprelvekin with regard to RBC and platelet counts, respectively.

The effect of hematopoietic drugs on the bone marrow cells also reduces the recovery time after bone marrow transplantation and radiation therapy. Dosages of chemotherapy used in bone marrow transplantation are often much higher than those used in conventional chemotherapy. Both the chemotherapy and radiation therapy are toxic to the bone marrow. When one or more colony-stimulating factors are administered as part of the drug therapy for bone marrow transplantation, bone marrow cell counts return to normal in a drastically shortened time. This helps to increase the likelihood of a successful bone marrow transplantation and therefore patient survival. Specific drug indications are listed in the Dosages table on this page.

Contraindications

Contraindications for all these drugs include drug allergy. Use of epoetin and darbepoetin is contraindicated in cases of uncontrolled hypertension and when hemoglobin levels are above certain levels (see drug profile). Use of filgrastim, sargramostim, and pegfilgrastim is contraindicated in the presence of more than 10% myeloid blasts (immature tumor cells in the bone marrow), because colony-stimulating factors may stimulate malignant growth of these myeloid tumor cells.

Adverse Effects

Adverse effects associated with the use of hematopoietic drugs are mild. The most common are fever, muscle aches, bone pain, and flushing. Table 49-1 lists additional adverse effects. However, the U.S. Food and Drug Administration (FDA) published a public health advisory in 2006 when it was discovered that use of epoetin by patients with higher than recommended hemoglobin levels was associated with increased adverse effects such as heart attack, heart failure, stroke, and death.

TABLE 49-1 Hematopoietic Drugs: Common Adverse Effects

Body System	Adverse Effects
Cardiovascular	Hypertension (epoetin alfa), edema
Gastrointestinal	Anorexia, nausea, vomiting, diarrhea
Integumentary	Alopecia, rash
Respiratory	Cough, dyspnea, sore throat
Other	Fever, blood dyscrasias, headache, bone pain

Interactions

Filgrastim and sargramostim have significant drug interactions when these two drugs are given with *myelosuppressive* (bone marrow depressant) antineoplastic drugs. Remember that these two drugs are administered to enhance the production of bone marrow cells; therefore, when myelosuppressive antineoplastics are given with them, the drugs directly antagonize each other. Typically filgrastim and sargramostim are not given within 24 hours of administration of myelosuppressive antineoplastics. However, they are often given soon after this time to help prevent the WBC nadir from dropping to dangerous levels and also to speed WBC recovery. It is also recommended that these drugs be used with caution or not be given with other medications that can potentiate their *myeloproliferative* (bone marrow–stimulating) effects. Two examples are lithium and corticosteroids.

Dosages

For the recommended dosages of hematopoietic drugs see the Dosages table on this page.

DRUG PROFILES

◆ epoetin alfa

Epoetin alfa (Epogen) is a biosynthetic form of the natural hormone erythropoietin, which is normally secreted by the kidneys in response to a decrease in RBCs. Epoetin alfa is used to treat anemia that is associated with end-stage renal disease, human immunodeficiency virus (HIV) infection, and cancer. Epoetin causes the progenitor cells in the bone marrow to manufacture large numbers of immature RBCs and to greatly speed up their maturation. This medication is ineffective without adequate body iron stores. Most patients receiving epoetin alfa should also receive an oral iron preparation. A newer, longer-acting form of epoetin called *darbepoetin* is available that reduces the required number of injections, although one cost study found that there is no significant difference in overall cost between the two. Both drugs are available for injection only and can be given intravenously or subcutaneously. When the drugs are given by the subcutaneous route, the onset of action is slower, and lower dosages can be used.

In 2006, the FDA issued a public health advisory regarding the overzealous use of epoetin. It was found that when hemoglobin

DOSAGES

Hematopoietic Drugs

Drug (Pregnancy Category)	Pharmacologic Class	Usual Dosage Range	Indications
◆ epoetin alfa (Epogen, Procrit) (C)	Human recombinant hormone (erythropoietin) analogue	IV/subcut: 2000-40,000 units 1-3 times per week, depending on weight and indication	Chemotherapy-induced anemia; anemia associated with chronic renal failure, zidovudine therapy (for HIV infection); reduction of need for blood transfusions in surgical patients
◆ filgrastim (Neupogen) (C)	Colony-stimulating factor	IV/subcut: 5-10 mcg/kg/day	Chemotherapy-induced leukopenia
◆ oprelvekin (IL-11) (Neumega) (C)	Synthetic human interleukin analogue	**Adult only** Subcut: 50 mcg/kg daily for up to 21 days	Chemotherapy-induced thrombocytopenia
◆ sargramostim (Leukine) (C)	Colony-stimulating factor	IV: 250 mcg/m²/day	Chemotherapy-induced leukopenia

HIV, Human immunodeficiency virus; *IL,* interleukin; *IV,* intravenous; *subcut,* subcutaneous.

levels are above 12 gm/dL and the drug is continued, patients experienced serious adverse events, including heart attack, stroke, and death. Because of these findings, epoetin should not be given to renal patients unless their hemoglobin level is less than 12 gm/dL; for cancer patients, the hemoglobin level should be less than 10 gm/dL.

PHARMACOKINETICS

Route	Onset of Action	Peak Plasma Concentration	Elimination Half-life	Duration of Action
Subcut or IV	7-10 days	5-24 hr	4-13 hr	Variable

◆ filgrastim

Filgrastim (Neupogen) is a synthetic analogue of human granulocyte colony-stimulating factor and is commonly referred to as *G-CSF. Filgrastim* promotes the proliferation, differentiation, and activation of the cells that make granulocytes. Granulocytes are the body's primary defense against bacterial and fungal infections. Filgrastim has the same pharmacologic effects as endogenous human G-CSF, which is normally secreted by specialized leukocytes known as *monocytes, macrophages,* and mature *neutrophils.* Filgrastim is indicated to prevent or treat febrile neutropenia in patients receiving myelosuppressive antineoplastics for nonmyeloid (non–bone marrow) malignancies. It should be given *before* a patient develops an infection, but not within 24 hours before or after myelosuppressive chemotherapeutic drugs. Pegfilgrastim (Neulasta) is a long-acting form of filgrastim that reduces the number of injections required. Both drugs are available for injection only. These drugs are usually discontinued when a patient's absolute neutrophil count (ANC) is above 1000 cells/mm³. A normal ANC is 1500 cells/mm³, and less than 500 cells/mm³ is considered neutropenia.

PHARMACOKINETICS

Route	Onset of Action	Peak Plasma Concentration	Elimination Half-life	Duration of Action
Subcut or IV	1 hr	2-6 hr	3-5 hr	12-24 hr

◆ sargramostim

Sargramostim (Leukine) is a synthetic analogue of human granulocyte-macrophage colony-stimulating factor and is commonly referred to as *GM-CSF.* There are three major subsets of leukocytes: granulocytes, monocytes, and lymphocytes (B cells and T cells). As noted earlier, granulocytes are further subdivided into basophils, eosinophils, and neutrophils, with neutrophils the most important in fighting infection. Macrophages are tissue-based (as opposed to circulating) cells that are derived from monocytes, which circulate in the blood. Neutrophils, monocytes, and macrophages make up the three main categories of phagocytic (cell-eating) blood cells, and they literally ingest foreign cells and other antigens as part of their immune system function. Sargramostim has the same pharmacologic effects as endogenous human GM-CSF. It stimulates the proliferation, differentiation, and activation of the cells in the bone marrow that eventually become granulocytes, monocytes, and macrophages.

Sargramostim is indicated for promoting bone marrow recovery after autologous (own marrow) or allogenic (donor marrow) bone marrow transplantation in patients with various types of leukemia and lymphoma. This drug is available for injection only.

PHARMACOKINETICS

Route	Onset of Action	Peak Plasma Concentration	Elimination Half-life	Duration of Action
Subcut or IV	4 hr	2 hr	2 hr	10 days

◆ oprelvekin

Oprelvekin (Neumega) is both a hematopoietic drug and one of the three currently available interleukins. However, its function is similar to that of the colony-stimulating factors (filgrastim and sargramostim) in that it enhances synthesis of a specific blood component—in this case, the platelets. It is indicated for the prevention of chemotherapy-induced severe thrombocytopenia and avoidance of the need for platelet transfusions. Its use is contraindicated in cases of drug allergy. It is available for injection only.

PHARMACOKINETICS

Route	Onset of Action	Peak Plasma Concentration	Elimination Half-life	Duration of Action
Subcut	5-9 days*	3 hr	7 hr	14 days

*Platelet counts begin to increase.

INTERFERONS

Interferons are proteins that have three basic properties: they are antiviral, antitumor, and immunomodulating. Chemically they are glycoproteins. There are three different groups of interferon drugs—the alpha, beta, and gamma interferons—each with its own antigenic and biologic activity. Interferons are most commonly used in the treatment of certain viral infections and certain types of cancer.

Mechanism of Action and Drug Effects

Interferons are recombinantly manufactured substances that are identical to the interferon cytokines that are naturally present in the human body. Therefore, they have the same properties. In the body, interferons are naturally produced by activated T cells and by other cells in response to viral infection. Interferons protect human cells from virus attack by enabling the human cells to produce enzymes that stop viral replication and prevent viruses from penetrating into healthy cells. Interferons prevent cancer cells from dividing and replicating and also increase the activity of other cells in the immune system, such as macrophages, neutrophils, and natural killer cells. Their effect on cancer cells is believed to be caused by a combination of direct inhibition of DNA and protein synthesis within cancer cells (antitumor effects) and multiple immunomodulatory effects on the host's immune system. Interferons increase the cytotoxic activity of natural killer cells and the phagocytic ability of macrophages. Interferons are also believed to increase the expression of cancer cell antigens on the cell surface, which enables the immune system to recognize cancer cells more easily, specifically marking them for destruction.

Overall, interferons have three different effects on the immune system. They can (1) restore its function if it is impaired, (2) augment (amplify) the immune system's ability to function as the body's defense, and (3) inhibit the immune system from working. This latter function may be especially useful when the immune system has become dysfunctional, causing an *autoimmune* disease. This is believed to be the case in multiple sclerosis. Two interferons (interferon beta-1a and interferon beta-1b) are specifically indicated for treatment of multiple sclerosis. Inhibiting the dysfunctional immune system prevents further damage to the body from the disease process.

Indications

The beneficial actions of interferons (antiviral, antineoplastic, and immunomodulatory) make them excellent drugs for the treatment of viral infections, various cancers, and some autoimmune disorders. Currently accepted indications for interferons are listed in the Dosages table.

Contraindications

Contraindications to the use of interferons include known drug allergy and may include autoimmune disorders, hepatitis or liver failure, concurrent use of **immunosuppressant** drugs, Kaposi's sarcoma related to acquired immunodeficiency syndrome (AIDS), and severe liver disease.

Adverse Effects

The most common adverse effects can be broadly described as flulike symptoms: fever, chills, headache, malaise, myalgia, and fatigue. The major dose-limiting adverse effect of interferons is fatigue. Patients taking high dosages become so exhausted that they are often confined to bed. Other adverse effects of interferons are listed in Table 49-2.

Interactions

Drug interactions are seen with both interferon alfa-2a and interferon alfa-2b when they are used with drugs that are metabolized in the liver via the cytochrome P-450 enzyme system. The combination results in decreased metabolism and increased accumulation of these drugs, which leads to drug toxicity. There is also some evidence that using interferons together with antiviral drugs such as zidovudine enhances the activity of both drugs but may lead to toxic levels of zidovudine. Interferons can also interact with angiotensin-converting enzyme inhibitors to produce blood abnormalities such as anemia and diminished WBC and platelet counts. Interferon beta products can enhance the anticoagulant effects of warfarin, which may place the patient at greater risk for bleeding. Additive toxic effects to the bone marrow can occur when interferon gamma products are used with other myelosuppressive drugs.

Dosages

For the recommended dosages of interferons see the Dosages table on p. 769.

TABLE 49-2 Interferons: Adverse Effects

Body System	Adverse Effects
General	Flulike syndrome, fatigue
Cardiovascular	Tachycardia, cyanosis, ECG changes, MI (rare), orthostatic hypotension
Central nervous	Mild confusion, somnolence, irritability, poor concentration, seizures, hallucinations, paranoid psychoses
Gastrointestinal	Nausea, diarrhea, vomiting, anorexia, taste alterations, dry mouth
Hematologic	Neutropenia, thrombocytopenia
Renal and hepatic	Increased BUN and creatinine levels, proteinuria, abnormal liver function test results (transaminases)

BUN, Blood urea nitrogen; *ECG,* electrocardiogram; *MI,* myocardial infarction.

The three major classes of interferon drugs are alfa, beta, and gamma, which are sometimes also written using the lowercase Greek letters α, β, and γ, respectively. The "alfa" designation is synonymous with the Greek letter "alpha," but "alfa" is now more commonly used clinically. The interferons vary in their antigenic makeup, biologic actions, and pharmacologic properties. The best known interferon class is interferon alfa. Interferon products are biologic response–modifying drugs that can be broadly classified as cytokines. Cytokines are immune system proteins that serve two essential functions: they direct the actions and communication between the cell-mediated and humoral divisions of the immune system, and they augment or enhance the immune response. Other cytokines include tumor necrosis factor (TNF), interleukins, and colony-stimulating factors. Interferons were first found to have antiviral activity in 1957. Their beneficial effects in treating cancer were discovered much later.

INTERFERON ALFA PRODUCTS
♦ **interferon alfa-2a, interferon alfa-2b, interferon alfa-n3, interferon alfacon-1, peginterferon alfa-2a, peginterferon alfa-2b**

The most commonly used interferon products are in the alfa class. They are also referred to as *leukocyte interferons* because they are produced from human leukocytes. Two newer types of interferon alfa include peginterferon alfa-2a and peginterferon alfa-2b. The *peg* refers to the attachment of a polymer chain of the hydrocarbon polyethylene glycol (PEG). This "pegylation" process increases the size of the interferon molecule. This increased size delays drug absorption, increases half-life, and decreases plasma clearance rate, which prolongs the drug's therapeutic effects. In addition, pegylation is believed to reduce the immunogenicity of the interferon and thus delay its recognition and destruction by the immune system. Similarly, pegfilgrastim, mentioned previously in this chapter, is a pegylated form of filgrastim and is also longer acting. The alfa-2a and alfa-2b interferons share the following indications: chronic hepatitis C, hairy cell leukemia, and AIDS-related Kaposi's sarcoma. Interferon alfa-2a (only) is also indicated for the treatment of chronic myelogenous leukemia. Additional indications unique to interferon alfa-2b are chronic hepatitis B, malignant melanoma (an often fatal form of skin cancer), follicular lymphoma (so named because its malignant cells gather in clumps called *follicles*—not to be confused with hair follicles), and condylomata acuminata (virally induced genital or venereal warts). Peginterferon alfa-2a and peginterferon alfa-2b are currently indicated only for treatment of chronic hepatitis C.

Interferon alfa-n3 is a polyclonal mixture of all interferon alfa subtypes. It is the product of pooled human leukocytes. Its only current indication is condylomata acuminata. Interferon alfacon-1 is a purely synthetic (i.e., non–naturally occurring) recombinant product that is currently indicated only for treatment of hepatitis C.

All interferons are most commonly given by either intramuscular or subcutaneous injection. However, some have been given by intravenous and intraperitoneal routes as well. It is important to note that some interferons are commonly dosed in millions of units, and these doses may be abbreviated "MU." However, MU is an unacceptable abbreviation. The nurse should always double-check to make sure that this is the correct dose, because the prescriber's writing of "MU" can sometimes be mistaken for "mg" or "mcg." If there is any question in the nurse's mind about the dose of any medication, the nurse should double-check with the prescriber, pharmacist, or other experienced colleague before administering the medication to the patient. Although this is true for all medications, it is a special consideration for interferons and

DOSAGES

Interferons

Drug (Pregnancy Category)	Pharmacologic Class	Usual Dosage Range	Indications
◆ interferon alfa-2a (Roferon-A) (C)	Immunomodulator, antiviral, antineoplastic	IM/subcut: 3 million units 3 times per week, depending on indication	Chronic hepatitis C, hairy cell leukemia, AIDS-related Kaposi's sarcoma, chronic myelogenous leukemia
◆ interferon alfa-2b (Intron-A) (C)	Immunomodulator, antiviral, antineoplastic	IM/subcut: 1-30 million units 3 times per week*	Hairy cell leukemia, malignant melanoma, follicular lymphoma, condylomata acuminata (venereal-genital warts), AIDS-related Kaposi's sarcoma, chronic hepatitis C, chronic hepatitis B
◆ peginterferon alfa-2a (Pegasys) (C)	Immunomodulator, antiviral	Subcut: 180 mcg weekly for 48 wk	Chronic hepatitis C
◆ peginterferon alfa-2b (PEG-Intron) (C)	Immunomodulator, antiviral	Subcut: 1 mcg/kg/wk for 1 yr†	Chronic hepatitis C
◆ interferon alfa-n3 (Alferon-N) (C)	Immunomodulator, antiviral	Intralesional: 250,000 units (0.05 mL) into the base of each wart 2 times per week for up to 8 wk	Condylomata acuminata
◆ interferon alfacon-1 (Infergen) (C)	Immunomodulator, antiviral	Subcut: 9 mcg 3 times per week for 24 wk	Chronic hepatitis C
◆ interferon beta-1a (Avonex, Rebif) (C)	Immunomodulator	IM (Avonex): 30 mcg 1 time per week Subcut (Rebif): 44 mcg 3 times per week	Multiple sclerosis
interferon gamma-1b (Actimmune) (C)	Immunomodulator	**BSA more than 0.5 m^2** Subcut: 50 mcg/m^2 3 times per week **BSA less than 0.5 m^2** Subcut: 1.5 mcg/kg 3 times per week	Chronic granulomatous disease, osteopetrosis

AIDS, Acquired immunodeficiency syndrome; *BSA,* body surface area; *IM,* intramuscular; *subcut,* subcutaneous.
*May also be given by intravenous infusion for melanoma. Route and dose vary depending on indication.
†Dose is 1.5 mcg/kg/wk if given with ribavirin capsules (see Chapter 40).

other biologic response–modifying drugs, because of both their potency and their dosage variability.

INTERFERON BETA PRODUCTS
◆ interferon beta-1a, interferon beta-1b
Interferon beta-1a and interferon beta-1b are the two currently available beta products. They interact with specific cell receptors found on the surfaces of human cells and possess antiviral and immunomodulatory activity. Both are produced by recombinant DNA techniques and are indicated for the treatment of relapsing multiple sclerosis to slow the progression of physical disability and decrease the frequency of clinical exacerbations. Drug allergy, including allergy to human albumin, is currently the only contraindication. Both drugs are available for injection only.

INTERFERON GAMMA PRODUCT
interferon gamma-1b
Interferon gamma-1b (Actimmune) is another type of synthetic product produced by recombinant DNA technology. It is indicated for the treatment of serious infections associated with chronic granulomatous disease, a genetic immunodeficiency, and osteopetrosis, a genetic bone disease characterized by abnormally dense bone, anemia, and frequent fractures. The drug is available for injection only.

MONOCLONAL ANTIBODIES

Monoclonal antibodies are quickly becoming standards of therapy in many areas of medicine, including treatment of cancer, rheumatoid arthritis and other inflammatory diseases, multiple sclerosis, and organ transplantation. In cancer treatment they have advantages over traditional antineoplastics in that they can specifically target cancer cells and have minimal effect on healthy cells. This reduces many of the adverse effects traditionally associated with antineoplastic drugs. There are currently 10 commercially available monoclonal antibodies used to treat cancer and rheumatoid arthritis. These are listed in the Dosages table. Another drug, muromonab, is used in kidney transplantation and was discussed in Chapter 45. The *mab* suffix in a drug name is usually an abbreviation for "monoclonal antibody."

Mechanism of Action, Drug Effects, and Indications

Because these drugs are so diverse, specific information for each appears in the individual drug profiles provided later in this chapter.

TABLE 49-3 Selected Immunomodulating Drugs: Common Adverse Effects

Drug	Adverse Effects
adalimumab	Localized inflammatory reaction at the injection site, infectious processes such as upper respiratory tract and urinary tract infections, and higher rates of various malignancies. Although such effects are likely related to the immunosuppressive properties of this drug, rheumatoid arthritis patients, especially those with more severe disease, are also known to experience higher rates of cancer.
alemtuzumab	Rash, pruritus (itching), nausea, vomiting, diarrhea, dyspnea, cough, rigors (muscle spasms), fever, fatigue, pain (especially skeletal pain), myelosuppression
bevacizumab	Deep vein thrombosis, hypertension, diarrhea, abdominal pain, constipation, vomiting, GI hemorrhage, leukopenia, asthenia (muscular fatigue and weakness), headache, dizziness, dry skin, proteinuria, hypokalemia, epistaxis, weight loss
cetuximab	Headache, insomnia, skin rash, conjunctivitis, GI discomfort, anemia, leukopenia, dehydration, edema, weight loss, dyspnea, asthenia, back pain, fever
gemtuzumab ozogamicin	Rash, herpes simplex outbreak of the skin, anorexia, constipation, diarrhea, nausea, vomiting, hypokalemia, cough, dyspnea, epistaxis (nosebleed), abdominal pain, asthenia, chills, fever, headache, infection
ibritumomab tiuxetan	Nausea, myelosuppression, asthenia, infection, chills
infliximab	Headache, rash, GI discomfort, dyspnea, upper and lower respiratory tract infection
natalizumab	Depression, fatigue, headache, GI discomfort, urinary tract infection, lower respiratory tract infection, joint pain. Of even greater concern are four case reports from 2005 and 2006 of a rare and potentially fatal brain disorder known as *progressive multifocal leukoencephalopathy*. At the time of this writing, the drug remains on the U.S. market but is under scrutiny by the FDA.
rituximab	Fever, chills, headache. Potentially fatal infusion-related events can also occur with rituximab, including severe bronchospasm, dyspnea, hypoxia, pulmonary infiltrates, adult respiratory distress syndrome, hypotension, and angioedema. *Tumor lysis syndrome* (see Chapter 47) with acute renal failure has also been reported. Because of these potentially fatal adverse effects, this drug should be used only after consideration of other treatment options. The drug should be stopped immediately if such a reaction appears imminent, and indicated supportive care provided.
tositumomab and iodine I 131 tositumomab	Headache, rash, GI discomfort, muscle pains, dyspnea, pharyngitis, asthenia, fever, chills, infection
trastuzumab	Fever, chills, headache, infection, nausea, vomiting, diarrhea, dizziness, headache, insomnia, rash, GI discomfort, edema, dyspnea, rhinitis, asthenia, back pain, fever, chills, infection

FDA, Food and Drug Administration; *GI,* gastrointestinal.

Contraindications

The only clear contraindication to the use of monoclonal antibodies reported thus far is drug allergy to a specific product. Their use is also usually contraindicated in patients with known active infectious processes due to their immunosuppressive qualities. Although known drug allergy is a contraindication, depending on the urgency of the clinical situation, a given monoclonal antibody may be the only viable treatment option for a seriously ill patient. In such situations, allergic symptoms may be controlled with supportive medications such as diphenhydramine and acetaminophen (for fever control). Infliximab has been shown to worsen severe cases of heart failure and should be dosed at no more than 5 mg/kg and only after considering other treatment options for its indications. Use of alemtuzumab is also contraindicated in patients with active systemic infections and immunodeficiency conditions, including AIDS.

Adverse Effects

Many, if not most, patients receiving these very potent drugs manifest acute symptoms that are comparable to classic allergy or flulike symptoms, such as fever, dyspnea, and chills. The primary objective is to administer the medication and control such symptoms as well as possible. Because the mechanisms of action of these drugs is to work through augmentation (or inhibition) of the human immune response, they can have a variety of adverse effects, some mild, some severe, that affect several body systems. Drug-specific adverse effects with the highest reported incidence (10% to 50% or more) are listed in Table 49-3. Again, the risk of such adverse effects must be weighed against the severity of the patient's underlying illness. It should be noted that many of these adverse effects may also be associated with the patient's disease process (e.g., infections) and even with life in general (e.g., headache, depression). This is especially true for the milder effects.

Interactions

Drug interactions associated with monoclonal antibodies are relatively few, and no major food interactions are listed. Administration of adalimumab with the anti–rheumatoid arthritis drug anakinra (an interleukin) may increase the risk of serious infections secondary to neutropenia. The clearance of natalizumab may be reduced by concurrent administration of interferon beta-1a (both used for multiple sclerosis). Coadministration of anti-TNF drugs (e.g., etanercept, anakinra) with infliximab may also increase the risk of neutropenia and infections. Etanercept should also not be given concurrently with varicella-zoster immune globulin (VZIG) because of undesirable drug interactions. However, etanercept may be resumed after completion of VZIG therapy. Bevacizumab is associated with increased risk of severe diarrhea and neutropenia when given concurrently with another anti–colorectal cancer drug, irinotecan (see Chapter 47). Pacli-

DOSAGES

Monoclonal Antibodies

Drug (Pregnancy Category)	Pharmacologic Class	Usual Dosage Range	Indications
adalimumab (Humira) (B)	Anti–TNF-alpha monoclonal antibody	**Adult only** Subcut: 40 mg every other week; may advance to 40 mg weekly if indicated	Severe, progressive RA for which other RA therapies have failed
alemtuzumab (Campath) (C)	Anti–glycoprotein CD52	IV: 3-10 mg daily to maximum tolerated dose, then 30 mg 3 times per week (alternate days) for up to 12 wk	B-cell chronic lymphocytic leukemia
bevacizumab (Avastin) (C)	Anti–human vascular endothelial growth factor	IV: 5-10 mg/kg every 14 days	Metastatic colorectal cancer
cetuximab (Erbitux) (C)	Anti–human epidermal growth factor	IV: 400 mg/m^2 loading dose, then 250 mg/m^2 weekly	Metastatic colorectal cancer
gemtuzumab ozogamicin (Mylotarg) (D)	Conjugate with cytotoxic antibiotic	IV: 9 mg/m^2 × 2 doses 14 days apart	Acute myeloid leukemia
ibritumomab tiuxetan (Zevalin) (D)	Chelator immunoconjugate	IV: 250 mg/m^2 × 2 doses 7 to 9 days apart	Non-Hodgkin's lymphoma
infliximab (Remicade) (B)	Anti–TNF-alpha	IV: 3-5 mg/kg at 0, 2, and 6 wk, then every 6 wk	Ankylosing spondylitis, Crohn disease, RA
natalizumab (Tysabri) (C)	Anti–alpha$_4$ integrin subunit	IV: 300 mg every 4 wk	Multiple sclerosis
◆ rituximab (Rituxan) (C)	Anti–CD20 surface antigen	IV: 375 mg/m^2 1 time per week × 4 doses	Non-Hodgkin's lymphoma
tositumomab and iodine I 131 tositumomab (Bexxar) (X)	Radioactive MAB	IV: Complex dosing regimen involving both drug components—follow instructions in package insert as ordered	Non-Hodgkin's lymphoma
trastuzumab (Herceptin) (B)	Anti–HER2 protein MAB	IV: Loading dose, 4 mg/kg IV: Maintenance dose, 2 mg/kg/wk	Breast cancer

IV, Intravenous; *MAB,* monoclonal antibody; *RA,* rheumatoid arthritis; *subcut,* subcutaneous; *TNF,* tumor necrosis factor.

taxel (see Chapter 47) has been shown to reduce the clearance of trastuzumab when the two are administered concurrently to treat breast cancer.

Dosages

For the recommended dosages of the monoclonal antibodies see the Dosages table on p. 771.

DRUG PROFILES

All of the monoclonal antibodies are synthesized using recombinant DNA technology. Because of the complexities of this technology, these drugs tend to be much more expensive than most other medications, with prices in the hundreds or thousands of dollars per single dose. Because of their cost, insurance companies may require that other less costly medications be tried first and be found ineffective. The majority of monoclonal antibodies are used to treat various forms of cancer. Their advantage is that they offer greater cell-killing specificity aimed at cancer cells instead of all body cells. Nonetheless, these drugs are associated with significant adverse effects and therefore with risk, which must be weighed against the benefit using expert clinical judgment. Severe allergic inflammatory-type infusion reactions can occur, Patients may therefore be premedicated with acetaminophen or diphenhydramine to reduce the occurrence of such reactions. If reactions do occur, they may be treated with diphenhydramine and other drugs such as epinephrine and corticosteroids. Conventional phar-

macokinetic data are not listed for the majority of these drugs because they do not follow standard pharmacokinetic models owing to their unique behavior in the body. It is known, however, that they may remain in the affected tissues for many weeks or months. The elimination half-life is given in the following profiles when known.

adalimumab

Adalimumab (Humira) works through its specificity for human *TNF-alpha*. TNF-alpha is a naturally occurring cytokine that is involved in normal inflammatory and immune responses. Adalimumab is indicated for the treatment of severe cases of rheumatoid arthritis that have failed to respond to other medications, including methotrexate. It can be used either alone or concurrently with such medications. In patients with rheumatoid arthritis, elevated levels of TNF are found in the synovial fluid in the spaces of affected joints. In addition to preventing TNF-alpha molecules from binding to TNF cell surface receptors adalimumab also modulates the inflammatory biologic responses that are induced or regulated by TNF. Use of adalimumab is contraindicated in patients with any active infectious process, whether localized or systemic, acute or chronic.

alemtuzumab

Alemtuzumab (Campath) was approved by the FDA in 2001 to treat B cell–mediated chronic lymphocytic leukemia. It is classified as a recombinant humanized antibody that is directed against the *CD52 glycoprotein* that appears on the surfaces of virtually all B and

T lymphocytes. *Humanization* involves the insertion of human DNA sequences during drug production to make the drug better tolerated by human patients. It is used specifically in patients for whom other first-line chemotherapy treatments, including treatment with alkylating drugs and the antimetabolite fludarabine (see Chapter 47), have failed. Its contraindications are drug allergy, active systemic infection, and documented immunodeficiency disease such as HIV-positive status. Half-life is 10 hours to 30 days.

bevacizumab

Bevacizumab (Avastin) was approved in 2004 for the treatment of metastatic colon or rectal cancer in combination with the first-line antineoplastic drug 5-fluorouracil (see Chapter 47). It is unique in that it binds to and inhibits vascular endothelial growth factor, a protein that promotes development of new blood vessels in tumors (as well as in normal body tissues). It has no listed contraindications but may complicate surgical wound healing because of its antivascular effects. Half-life is 11 to 50 days.

cetuximab

Cetuximab (Erbitux) was also approved in 2004 for the treatment of metastatic colorectal cancer. It is a recombinant monoclonal antibody made from both human and mouse *(murine)* genetic material and is designed for concurrent use with the second-line antineoplastic drug irinotecan (see Chapter 47). It binds to *epidermal growth factor* on the surface of tumor cells, where it hinders cell growth through interference with cell metabolism. It is used either in combination with irinotecan or alone in patients who are intolerant of the latter drug. It has no listed contraindications but is known to cause severe infusion reactions in up to 3% of patients receiving it. Half-life is 97 to 114 hours.

gemtuzumab ozogamicin

Gemtuzumab ozogamicin (Mylotarg) was approved by the FDA in 2000 as the first monoclonal antibody indicated for treatment of leukemia. It is designed to treat acute myelocytic leukemia (also called *acute myelogenous* or *myeloid leukemia*). This drug is unique in that it consists of a recombinant humanized antibody that is linked ("conjugated") to a cytotoxic antineoplastic antibiotic, ozogamicin. This type of drug complex is known as an *immunoconjugate*. This particular complex binds to the CD33 cell surface antigen, which is expressed on the surface of leukemia blasts (malignant immature WBCs) in more than 80% of patients with acute myelocytic leukemia. The binding of the antibody portion of the drug to this receptor leads to internalization of the drug complex by the leukemic blast. At this point the ozogamicin component is released inside the lysosomes (called *suicide sacs* in biology) of the malignant cell, which leads to DNA damage and cell death. Half-life is 40 to 100 hours.

ibritumomab tiuxetan

Ibritumomab tiuxetan (Zevalin) was approved in 2002 for treating B-cell non-Hodgkin's lymphoma. This drug is another immunoconjugate, consisting of ibritumomab conjugated with the metal chelator tiuxetan. This drug comes in kits that also include one of two radioactive metal isotopes (radioisotopes). The antibody binds to the CD20 antigen that occurs on the surfaces of both normal and malignant B lymphocytes. Once the complex is bound to the cells, the tiuxetan component binds the radioisotope, which is administered as another part of the anticancer therapy. Radioactive beta emission from the bound radioisotope, a unique feature of this drug, induces free radical formation and cell damage in both the cell containing the drug complex and neighboring cells.

infliximab

Infliximab (Remicade) is one of the earliest monoclonal antibodies, approved in 1998. It works through an anti–TNF-alpha action, similar to adalimumab. It is approved for the treatment of ankylosing spondylitis, Crohn disease, and rheumatoid arthritis. It has the special contraindication of severe heart failure (class III or IV on the New York Heart Association scale), because it may worsen this condition. It also carries an FDA black box warning reporting cases of fatal tuberculosis and/or fungal infections associated with the use of this drug. It is recommended that patients be tested for latent tuberculosis before it is administered. Half-life is 8 to 9 days.

natalizumab

Natalizumab (Tysabri) was approved in late 2004 for the treatment of multiple sclerosis. It is a humanized monoclonal antibody derived from murine myeloma cells. Natalizumab works by binding to the alpha$_4$ subunits of *integrins*, proteins found on the surfaces of leukocytes (with the exception of neutrophils). These proteins are implicated in the multiple sclerosis disease process, but the exact mechanism by which this drug exerts its therapeutic effects has not been determined. However, the drug is known to inhibit the leukocyte adhesion that is mediated by these alpha$_4$ protein subunits and that is also believed to be part of the disease process. Natalizumab has no listed contraindications. Half-life is 11 days. Natalizumab was pulled from the market only 1 year after it was approved due to reports of patients' developing multifocal leukoencephalopathy, a rare and serious viral infection of the brain. In 2006, the FDA allowed the marketing of natalizumab to resume under a special distribution program. Only patients who are enrolled in the program are allowed to receive the drug.

◆ rituximab

Rituximab (Rituxan) specifically binds to antigen CD20. This antigen is a protein on the membranes of both normal and malignant B cells found in patients with non-Hodgkin's lymphoma. Antigen CD20 is expressed in more than 90% of B-cell non-Hodgkin's lymphomas. Once rituximab binds to these B cells, a host immune response causes lysis of the cells. Rituximab has become a standard drug for the treatment of patients with follicular low-grade non-Hodgkin's lymphoma for whom previous therapy has failed. It is recommended that patients be premedicated with acetaminophen and diphenhydramine before each infusion of the drug to reduce its well-known infusion-related adverse effects.

tositumomab and iodine I 131 tositumomab

Tositumomab and iodine I 131 tositumomab (Bexxar) were approved by the FDA in 2003 for the treatment of non-Hodgkin's lymphoma. This drug is a murine monoclonal antibody with a dual radioactive and nonradioactive component. Both components bind to the CD20 antigen, a transmembrane protein that, as noted earlier, is expressed on the cell membranes of more than 90% of B-cell non-Hodgkin's lymphoma cells. Theoretical mechanisms of action include induction of *apoptosis* (programmed cell death), *complement-dependent* cytotoxicity, or antibody-dependent cytotoxicity mediated by the drug itself. **Complement** is a collective term for about 20 different proteins normally present in plasma that aid other immune system components (e.g., B cells and T cells) in mounting an immune response.

trastuzumab

Trastuzumab (Herceptin) kills tumor cells by mediating antibody-dependent cellular cytotoxicity. It accomplishes this by inhibiting proliferation of human tumor cells that overexpress the HER2 protein. The HER2 protein is overexpressed in 25% to 30% of primary malignant breast tumors and has been established as an adverse prognostic factor for early-stage breast cancer. Because of the relatively selective expression of HER2 on cancer cells, it has been an appealing target for antineoplastic therapy. The combination of trastuzumab and paclitaxel (see Chapter 47) has produced encouraging results. Trastuzumab has a special black box warning from the FDA reporting cases of ventricular dysfunction and heart failure associated with this drug. Patients should be monitored for signs and symptoms of heart failure and ventricular dysfunction before and during treatment. In addition, fatal hypersensitivity reactions, infusion reactions, and pulmonary events have occurred in association with its use; therefore, careful clinical judgment, risk evaluation, and informed patient consent are called for in its use. Half-life is 10 to 30 days.

BOX 49-2 Interleukin-2: Drug Effects

Modulating Effects
Proliferation of T cells
Synthesis and secretion of cytokines
Increased production of B cells (antibodies)
Proliferation and activation of NK cells
Proliferation and activation of LAK cells

Enhancing Effects
Enhancement of killer T cell activity
Amplification of the effects of cytokines
Enhancement of the cytotoxic actions of NK cells and LAK cells

---

LAK, Lymphokine-activated killer; *NK*, natural killer.

INTERLEUKINS AND RELATED DRUGS

Interleukins are a natural part of the immune system and are classified as *lymphokines*. Lymphokines are soluble proteins that are released from activated lymphocytes such as natural killer cells. There are several known interleukins in the body (IL-2, IL-3, IL-4, IL-5, IL-6, and IL-11), and more are being identified as knowledge of the immune system increases.

The pharmaceutical interleukin receptor agonists currently available are aldesleukin (IL-2), oprelvekin (IL-11), denileukin diftitox, and anakinra. Oprelvekin was mentioned with the hematopoietic drugs earlier in this chapter and is used to help patients produce platelets. It has a dual classification as both an interleukin and hematologic drug. Both aldesleukin and oprelvekin are synthesized using recombinant DNA technology and are patterned after corresponding natural interleukins in the body. Denileukin diftitox is also recombinant DNA derived, but it contains fragments of both diphtheria toxin and aldesleukin. A fourth drug, anakinra, is actually an IL-1 receptor antagonist. It is also a recombinant product that is patterned after its natural counterpart in the body.

Mechanism of Action and Drug Effects

Interleukins cause multiple effects in the immune system, one of which is antitumor action. IL-2 is produced by activated T cells in response to macrophage-"processed" antigens and secreted interleukin (IL-1). It was formerly called *T-cell growth factor* because, among other actions, it aids in the growth and differentiation of T lymphocytes. The IL-2 derivative aldesleukin acts indirectly to stimulate or restore immune response. Aldesleukin binds to receptor sites on T cells, which stimulates the T cells to multiply. One type of cell that results from this multiplication is the **lymphokine-activated killer (LAK) cell.** These LAK cells recognize and destroy only cancer cells and ignore normal cells. Aldesleukin is currently the most widely used of the interleukin drugs. A detailed list of its specific immunomodulating effects appears in Box 49-2.

Denileukin diftitox consists of one segment (denileukin) that is patterned after natural human IL-2 and a second segment (diftitox) that is patterned after diphtheria toxin. It is an IL-2 receptor antagonist and binds to cell surface IL-2 receptors that are expressed on both normal and certain malignant cells. It causes cell death upon binding to these receptors through the cytocidal activity of diphtheria toxin, which inhibits intracellular protein synthesis.

Anakinra is a recombinant form of the natural human IL-1 receptor antagonist. It competitively inhibits the binding of IL-1 to its corresponding receptor sites, which are expressed in many different tissues and organs.

Indications

Aldesleukin was previously indicated only for the treatment of metastatic renal cell carcinoma, a malignancy that originates in the kidney tissues. It is now also approved for the treatment of metastatic melanoma. Denileukin diftitox is currently indicated only as therapy for a skin-based lymphoma known as *cutaneous T-cell lymphoma*, which often metastasizes to other areas of the body. Anakinra is indicated for symptom control in patients with rheumatoid arthritis for whom other therapy has failed.

Contraindications

Contraindications to the administration of aldesleukin include drug allergy, organ transplantation, and abnormal results on thallium cardiac stress tests or pulmonary function tests. For denileukin diftitox, the only usual contraindication is drug allergy, as is also the case for anakinra.

Adverse Effects

Unfortunately, therapy with aldesleukin is commonly complicated by severe toxicity. A syndrome known as *capillary leak syndrome* is responsible for the severe toxicities of aldesleukin. As the name implies, capillary leak syndrome refers to a condition induced by interleukin therapy in which the capillaries lose their ability to retain vital colloids such as albumin, protein, and other essential components of blood. Because the capillaries are "leaky," these substances migrate into the surrounding tissues. This results in massive fluid retention (20 to 30 pounds), which can lead to the life-threatening problems of respiratory distress, heart failure, dysrhythmias, and myocardial infarction. Fortunately, these are all reversible after discontinuation of the interleukin therapy. Close patient monitoring and vigorous supportive care are essential in the patient receiving aldesleukin therapy. Other adverse effects that may be associated with aldesleukin therapy are fever, chills, rash, fatigue, hepatotoxicity, myalgias, headaches, and eosinophilia.

DOSAGES

Interleukins and Related Drugs

Drug (Pregnancy Category)	Pharmacologic Class	Usual Dosage Range	Indications
◆ aldesleukin [IL-2] (Proleukin) (C)	Human recombinant IL-2 analogue	IV: 600,000 IU/kg (0.037 mg/kg) q8h (14 doses)	Metastatic renal cell carcinoma or melanoma
anakinra (Kineret) (B)	IL-1 receptor antagonist	Subcut: 100 mg/day	Rheumatoid arthritis
denileukin diftitox (Ontak) (C)	Recombinant IL-2 and diphtheria toxin protein	IV: 9 or 18 mcg/kg/day for 5 consecutive days every 21 days	Cutaneous T-cell lymphoma

IL, Interleukin; *IV,* intravenous; *subcut,* subcutaneous.

The most common adverse effects associated with denileukin diftitox administration are nausea, vomiting, anorexia, diarrhea, hypoalbuminemia, elevated liver enzyme levels, edema, dyspnea, cough, fever, chills, asthenia, generalized pain, chest pain, infection, and headache. Anakinra has a much milder adverse effect profile that includes local reactions at the injection site, various respiratory tract infections, and headache.

Interactions

Aldesleukin, when given with antihypertensives, can produce additive hypotensive effects. Coadministration of corticosteroids with aldesleukin can reduce its antitumor effectiveness. The toxic effects of aldesleukin are increased when it is administered with aminoglycosteroids, indomethacin, cytotoxic chemotherapeutic drugs, methotrexate, asparaginase, and doxorubicin. No particular drug interactions have been reported to date for denileukin diftitox. Anakinra should not be used (or used cautiously) with adalimumab, etanercept, and infliximab due to increased risk of serious infections.

Dosages

For the recommended dosages of the interleukin agonists and antagonists, see the Dosages table on p. 774.

DRUG PROFILES

The interleukins are a group of naturally occurring cytokines in the body that originally were believed to be produced by and to act primarily on leukocytes (WBCs). They are now recognized as multifunctional cytokines that are produced by a variety of cells but act at least partly within the lymphatic system.

◆ aldesleukin

Aldesleukin (Proleukin) is a human IL-2 derivative that is manufactured using recombinant DNA technology. It is a cytokine that is produced by lymphocytes and is therefore classified as a lymphokine. Aldesleukin is currently approved only for the treatment of metastatic renal cell carcinoma and metastatic melanoma, despite its activity against other cancers. Off-label uses include HIV infection and AIDS, and non-Hodgkin's lymphoma. Aldesleukin is contraindicated in patients with drug allergy, abnormal thallium stress test or pulmonary function tests (due to potential drug effects on cardiopulmonary function), and organ transplants (due to the immunostimulating qualities of the drug, which may cause organ rejection). The drug is available only for injection.

denileukin diftitox

Denileukin diftitox (Ontak) is an IL-2 receptor antagonist that is produced using recombinant DNA technology. It is used to treat cutaneous T-cell lymphoma. Its only current contraindication is drug allergy. It is available for injection only.

anakinra

Anakinra (Kineret) is an IL-1 receptor antagonist that is also recombinant DNA synthesized. It is used to help control symptoms of rheumatoid arthritis. Its only current contraindication is drug allergy. It is available for injection only.

MISCELLANEOUS IMMUNOMODULATING DRUGS

In addition to the drugs in the major classes discussed thus far, there are several additional medications that can be broadly classified as miscellaneous immunomodulating drugs. They work by various specific and nonspecific mechanisms. A special term used for **immunostimulant** drugs that work by a nonspecific mechanism is **adjuvant**. These miscellaneous medications, including some that are classified as adjuvants, are listed in Table 49-4.

Rheumatoid Arthritis

Rheumatism is a general term for any of several disorders characterized by inflammation, degeneration, or metabolic derangement of connective tissue structures, especially joints and related structures such as muscles, tendons, bursae, fibrous tissue, and ligaments. Rheumatoid arthritis is a chronic **autoimmune disorder** that commonly causes inflammation and tissue damage in joints. It can also cause anemia and diffuse inflammation in the lungs, eyes, and pericardium of the heart, and subcutaneous nodules under the skin (Figure 49-3). It is a painful and oftentimes disabling disease. It is diagnosed primarily based on symptoms and the results of a blood test for rheumatoid factor. Symptoms include pain, stiffness, and reduced range of motion. Treatment encompasses both pharmacologic and nonpharmacologic modalities, including physical and occupational therapy. There is no known cure for rheumatoid arthritis, and the goal of therapy is to alleviate current symptoms and to prevent further damage of the joints. Rheumatoid arthritis affects over 2 million people in the United States and usually appears between the ages of 25 and 50. Women are two to three times more likely than men to have rheu-

TABLE 49-4 Miscellaneous Immunomodulating Drugs

Drug (Trade and Other Names)	Classification	Indications	Mechanism of Action
abatacept (Orencia)	Selective costimulation modulator	RA	Inhibits T-cell activation
bexarotene (Targretin)	Retinoid receptor agonist	Cutaneous T-cell lymphoma	Exact mechanism unknown; binds to and activates retinoid X receptor subtypes; this regulates the expression of genes that control cellular differentiation
BCG vaccine (Pacis, TICE BCG, TheraCys)	Live virus vaccine, adjuvant	Localized bladder cancer	Promotes local inflammation and immune response in bladder mucosa
etanercept (Enbrel)	TNF receptor antagonist	RA (including juvenile) and psoriatic arthritis	Blocks effects of TNF, a major inflammatory mediator in RA
leflunomide (Arava)	Antimetabolite	RA	Exerts antiinflammatory effects via inhibition of cellular DNA synthesis
levamisole (Ergamisol)	Immunostimulant, adjuvant	Dukes stage C colon cancer (given with fluorouracil)	Exact mechanism unclear, but may enhance the therapeutic effects of fluorouracil and have its own immunostimulatory effects
mitoxantrone (Novantrone)	Anthracycline antibiotic (also an antineoplastic drug)	MS (secondary chronic type)	Inhibits cellular DNA synthesis, which reduces neurologic disability in MS (exact mechanism unclear)
pegademase bovine (Adagen)	Immunostimulant	SCID	Modified enzyme that compensates for deficiency of the enzyme adenosine deaminase, which is associated with SCID
thalidomide (Thalomid)	Immunostimulant	Erythremia nodosum*	Exact mechanism unclear, but may have anti-TNF properties, which counter the disease process
tretinoin (Vesanoid)	Retinoid receptor agonist	Acute promyelocytic leukemia	Induces differentiation and maturation of leukemic cells, reducing proliferation of immature, disease-causing cells

BCG, Bacille Calmette-Guérin; *MS,* multiple sclerosis; *RA,* rheumatoid arthritis; *SCID,* severe combined immunodeficiency disease; *TNF,* tumor necrosis factor.
*An inflammatory reaction in the subcutaneous fat, often following a bacterial infection or in reaction to drugs such as oral contraceptives or sulfonamides.

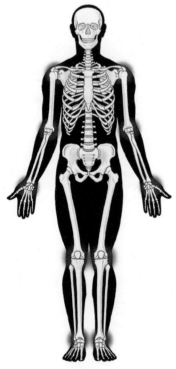

FIGURE 49-3   Areas of the body affected by rheumatoid arthritis. Rheumatoid arthritis is most frequently seen in the shoulders, elbows, wrists, knees, and ankles, and it often affects the joints on both sides of the body equally.

matoid arthritis. Smokers and those with a family history are also at risk. Osteoarthritis is another type of **arthritis** that tends to be an age-related degeneration of joint tissues resulting in pain and reduced function. This section focuses on rheumatoid arthritis.

Because rheumatoid arthritis is a disease characterized by inflammation, the nonsteroidal antiinflammatory drugs (NSAIDs) are the most commonly used (see Chapter 44). Full dosages of NSAIDs are tried in the early stages of rheumatoid arthritis. Corticosteroids, also potent antiinflammatory drugs (see Chapter 33) are also used to prevent inflammatory symptoms. These drugs, although they are effective in reducing inflammation, do not actually affect the disease itself. **Disease-modifying antirheumatic drugs (DMARDs)** not only provide antiinflammatory and analgesic effects but they can arrest or slow the disease processes associated with arthritis.

DISEASE-MODIFYING ANTIRHEUMATOID ARTHRITIS DRUGS

DMARDs are drugs that modify the disease of rheumatoid arthritis. They exhibit antiinflammatory, antiarthritic, and immunomodulating effects and work by inhibiting the movement of various cells into an inflamed, damaged area, such as a joint. These cells (neutrophils, monocytes, and macrophages) are responsible for causing many of the deleterious effects of chronic rheumatoid arthritis. By preventing the accumulation of these inflammatory cells in the area of the diseased joint, antiarthritic drugs prevent progression of the disease. DMARDs often have a slow onset of action of several weeks, versus minutes to hours for NSAIDs. For this reason, DMARDs are sometimes also referred to as *slow-acting antirheumatic drugs (SAARDs)*. They used to be thought of as second-line drugs for the treatment of arthritis because they can have much more toxic adverse effects than do the NSAIDs. However, the American College of Rheumatology updated its treatment guidelines in 2008 and now recommends the use of DMARDs as first-line therapy in many patients. The guidelines differentiate the DMARDs into nonbiologic and biologic DMARDs. Nonbiologic DMARDs include methotrexate, leflunomide, hydroxychloroquine (see Chapter 43), and sulfasalazine (see Chapter 38). The guidelines recommend starting with methotrexate or leflunomide in most patients. Use of the other drugs, including the biologic DMARDs, is generally reserved for those patients who do not respond to methotrexate or leflunomide. The biologic DMARDs include etanercept, infliximab, adalimumab, abatacept, and rituximab. Box 49-3 lists the DMARDs. Etanercept and abatacept are discussed in this section; infliximab, adalimumab, and rituximab were discussed in the section of the chapter on monoclonal antibodies.

Mechanism of Action, Indications, and Adverse Effects

The mechanism of action and adverse effects of the different DMARDs vary. The individual drug profiles provide information on mechanism of action and adverse effects. All of these drugs are indicated for the treatment of rheumatoid arthritis, and some have other uses as previously mentioned.

Contraindications

DMARDs should not be used in patients with active bacterial infections, active herpes zoster, active or latent tuberculosis, or acute or chronic hepatitis B or C. Etanercept, infliximab, and adalimumab should not be used in patients with heart failure, lymphoma, or multiple sclerosis. Methotrexate and leflunomide should be avoided during pregnancy and lactation.

DRUG PROFILES

methotrexate

Methotrexate is an anticancer drug that is commonly used for treatment of rheumatoid arthritis in much lower dosages than those used for cancer. It is usually started at dosages of 7.5 to

10 mg/wk but can be increased to 25 mg/wk. It is very important to note that the drug is given once per week, not once per day. Serious medication errors, including deaths, have occurred when an order is mistranscribed and the drug is given daily instead of once a week. It is usually given orally for rheumatoid arthritis, but it can also be given by injection. Bone marrow suppression is the main adverse effect of methotrexate. The onset of antirheumatic action is 3 to 6 weeks. The half-life of the drug is 3 to 10 hours.

leflunomide

Leflunomide (Arava) is indicated for the treatment of active rheumatoid arthritis. It modulates or alters the response of the immune system to rheumatoid arthritis. It has antiproliferative, antiinflammatory, and immunosuppressive activity. Its most common adverse effects are diarrhea, respiratory tract infection, alopecia, elevated liver enzyme levels, and rash. It is contraindicated in women who are or may become pregnant and should not be used by nursing mothers or those with a hypersensitivity to it. It is a pregnancy category X drug. Aspirin, other NSAIDs, and/or low-dose corticosteroids may be continued during leflunomide therapy. The drug is available only for oral use. The half-life is 14 to 15 days.

etanercept

Etanercept (Enbrel) is a recombinant DNA–derived TNF-blocking drug. It binds TNF and blocks its interaction with cell surface receptors. It is indicated for the treatment of rheumatoid arthritis (including juvenile rheumatoid arthritis) and moderate to severe chronic plaque psoriasis. It is contraindicated in patients with hypersensitivity to it and in those with sepsis and active infections (including chronic or local infections). It should be used with caution in patients with preexisting demyelinating central nervous system disorders, heart failure, or significant hematologic abnormalities. Some dosage forms may contain latex, so patients should be screened for latex allergy. Reactivation of hepatitis and tuberculosis have been reported. Live vaccines should not be given with etanercept. Common adverse effects include headache, injection site reaction, upper respiratory tract infection, dizziness, and weakness. The drug is administered subcutaneously. Drugs with which it interacts include anakinra, which may increase the risk of infection and cyclophosphamide, which may increase the risk of malignancy. It is a pregnancy category B drug. It is not known if the drug is excreted in breast milk, and its use is not recommended in lactating women. The onset of action is 1 to 2 weeks and the half-life is 72 to 132 hours.

abatacept

Abatacept (Orencia) is a selective costimulation modulator; it inhibits T-cell activation. Abatacept is indicated for the treatment of rheumatoid arthritis. It is contraindicated in patients with hypersensitivity to it or any of its components. Caution should be used in patients with a history of recurrent infections or chronic obstructive pulmonary disease. Patients should be brought up to date with all current immunizations before starting abatacept therapy. Adverse effects include headache, upper respiratory tract infections, and hypertension. Abatacept may increase the risk of infections associated with live vaccines and may decrease response to dead and/or live vaccines. It should not be given with anakinra or TNF-blocking drugs because of the risk of serious infections. It should not be given with the herb echinacea, which has immunostimulant properties. Abatacept is dosed according to body weight and is given at 4-week intervals. It is administered intravenously, and a filter should be used. The half-life is 8 to 25 days.

NURSING PROCESS

Assessment

Before administering any of the *biologic response–modifying drug* and other drugs included in this chapter, the nurse must assess his or her own knowledge about these medications with attention to their action and pharmacokinetic properties, as well as associated cautions, contraindications, drug interactions, adverse effects, and toxicities. The patient must then be assessed for the presence of any conditions that represent contraindications or cautions to their administration, for the use of other potentially interacting drugs, and for hypersensitivity to the drug, egg proteins, or immunoglobulin G. Further assessment should include a head-to-toe examination that covers the following: (1) respiratory system with attention to respiratory rate, rhythm, and depth as well as breath sounds with listening for any adventitious (abnormal) sounds; (2) cardiac system with attention to vital signs, heart sounds, heart rate and rhythm, and oxygen saturation levels, as well as assessment for edema and/or shortness of breath, presence of cyanotic discoloration around the mouth or nail beds, and any chest pain; (3) central nervous system with a focus on baseline mental status and assessment for any seizure-like activity or central nervous system abnormalities; and (4) immune system with notation of any history of chronic illnesses, ability to fight off infections, and history of suppressed immunity. Nutritional status, height, and weight should be noted as well as results of any prescribed laboratory tests, such as complete blood count (CBC) and especially hemoglobin level and hematocrit, serum protein and albumin levels, and immunoglobin levels (see Nursing Process in Chapters 47 and 48). Presence or absence of underlying diseases, symptoms, and success or failure of medication regimens in the past should also be documented, as with all drug regimens. Assessment should also include gathering data about the patient's ability to carry out the activities of daily living, emotional and socioeconomic status, educational level, learning needs, desire and ability to learn, past coping strategies, support systems, and self-care abilities.

For *hematopoietic biologic response–modifying drugs,* the following assessments should be performed in addition to the aforementioned. (1) For *erythropoietin* and similar drugs: The patient should be assessed for a history of hypertension, seizure activity, thrombosis, and chest pain, because these conditions may be exacerbated by the drug. Renal function should be evaluated, because patients with chronic renal failure who receive these drugs may experience transient rises in blood pressure. Iron stores should be assessed by measuring transferrin saturation, which must be at least 20%, and ferritin level, which should be at 100 ng/mL. These levels allow appropriate erythropoietin stimulation. Possible subcutaneous and/or intravenous sites should be assessed and blood pressure measured before initiation of therapy and early in treatment. For further discussion of the use of epoetin and the FDA's public health advisory statement calling for administration of the drug only to those with hemoglobin levels of less than 10 gm/dL, see the pharmacology section. (2) For *colony-stimulating factors:* CBC results should be assessed; for example, with filgrastim and sargramostim, counts should be determined before and throughout therapy to monitor

for problems with leukocytosis and thrombocytosis. Hepatic functioning should be assessed by determining levels of liver enzymes (as ordered). Potential intravenous and subcutaneous sites should be assessed, and, if appropriate, chemotherapy-induced absolute neutrophil nadir (low point) should be noted, because timing of the dose is critical in helping to boost blood cell counts. For example, with filgrastim, the drug should *not* be given within 24 hours before or after the chemotherapy. In addition, any existing pain, especially joint or bone pain, is important to document because of the possible adverse effect of mild, moderate, or severe bone pain with filgrastim.

Before *interferons* (e.g., interferon alfa-2a or alfa-2b; interferon gamma-1b) are given, the patient's CBC should be documented because long-term therapy with these drugs may lead to bone marrow suppression. Other serum laboratory values such as platelet counts, blood urea nitrogen and creatinine levels, and ALP and AST levels should be checked before treatment and twice weekly during therapy or as ordered. A urinalysis is also part of laboratory testing. Before aldesleukin is used, it is important for the nurse to document baseline vital sign measurements, neurologic functioning, bowel status, and results of liver and renal studies. These laboratory and baseline assessments are important because of possible drug-related impaired renal and liver functioning. Capillary leak syndrome is also associated with the use of interleukin drugs, so it is important to document any edema and to assess baseline vital signs and baseline cardiac, respiratory, renal, and liver status. The symptoms of this potentially fatal syndrome include hypotension, reduced organ perfusion, extravasation of plasma proteins and fluid, and symptoms of heart failure, cardiac irregularities, and respiratory distress. (See the Pharmacology section for further discussion.) Because of these concerns, the interleukins may not be administered to patients with cardiac diseases or symptoms (e.g., hypotension, hypertension, angina). Any allergy to proteins of *Escherichia coli* should be noted because of cross-sensitivity to interferon.

With the use of all *monoclonal antibody drugs* (e.g., alemtuzumab, rituximab, trastuzumab), blood pressure should be monitored and the patient should be observed for any gastrointestinal signs and symptoms, fatigue, weakness, or malaise. The medication order should also be examined for timing of the dose, because different protocols are used. Intravenous sites should be assessed, and with rituximab, withholding antihypertensives for 12 hours before infusion may be considered, as ordered, to avoid any transient hypotensive episodes. Hepatic, renal, and cardiac function tests should be assessed with the use of trastuzumab.

With *DMARDs* close assessment of any past or present medical conditions as well a thorough assessment of allergies is required, and a medication profile should be compiled listing prescription drugs, herbals, and over-the-counter drugs. Because bone marrow suppression is the main adverse effect, baseline blood cell and platelet counts need to be assessed and these counts monitored before, during, and after therapy. Another important area for assessment is the medication order by the prescriber, because serious medication errors have occurred when the order for this drug has been transcribed incorrectly and the drug has been given daily instead of in the recommended once-weekly dosing. Documentation of the findings of a baseline head-to-toe physical assessment as well as notation of musculoskeletal changes due to the pathology of arthritis and related changes in activities of daily living and other basic activities is needed before drug therapy is initiated as well as throughout the therapeutic regimen.

Before initiation of therapy with leflunomide, a complete assessment of hepatic and renal functioning as well as baseline blood cell counts is necessary. Because of the possible adverse effects of diarrhea and respiratory infections, gastrointestinal functioning and bowel patterns should be assessed and a complete history of gastrointestinal disorders obtained prior to beginning therapy with the drug. Respiratory assessment should include obtaining a history of past and present disorders and infections as well as noting breath sounds, presence of sputum, and baseline respiratory rate, rhythm, and depth. Etanercept and similar drugs should be given only after documentation of any current, active infections and testing for tuberculosis and hepatitis. For children diagnosed with juvenile rheumatoid arthritis, it is recommended that all childhood immunizations be completed before therapy if at all possible.

Nursing Diagnoses

- Acute pain related to the adverse effects of biologic response–modifying drugs
- Altered nutrition, less than body requirements, related to the adverse effects of biologic response-modifying drugs
- Impaired skin integrity (rash) related to the adverse effects of biologic response–modifying drugs
- Risk for falls related to weakness and fatigue from the disease process as well as from drug effects
- Impaired gas exchange related to the adverse effects of the various biologic response–modifying drugs

Planning
Goals

- Patient experiences adequate control of pain during drug treatment.
- Patient regains prechemotherapy (and as near normal as possible) nutritional status.

- Patient experiences minimal weight loss during therapy.
- Patient maintains or regains normal bowel and bladder patterns.
- Patient's mucous membranes maintain and/or regain intactness during therapy.
- Patient is free of self-injury related to drug therapy.

Outcome Criteria

- Patient describes nutritional needs and daily meal planning reflecting dietary needs, such as consumption of a high-calorie, low-residue, high-protein diet, high energy foods from protein and complex carbohydrates and forcing of fluids.
- Patient states measures to minimize gastrointestinal adverse effects, such as eating small, frequent meals and avoiding spicy foods.
- Patient forces fluids up to 3000 mL/day, unless contraindicated, using creative means such as consumption of flavored water, decaffeinated iced tea, lemonade, sugar-free juices (if appropriate), and cranberry juice, with adequate urinary output noted.
- Patient's skin and mucous membranes remain intact and clean through daily bathing, skin care with moisturizing products, and daily oral hygiene with flossing as well as follow-up care with a dental professional.
- Patient states ways to minimize self-injury related to weakness and fatigue from the disease process and related treatment with biologic response–modifying drugs, such as by using assistive devices and grab bars or rails; removing rugs, mats, or other obstacles in the bedroom, bathroom, and other parts of the house; maintaining muscle mass and energy; and obtaining assistance in performing the activities of daily living, if needed.

Implementation

Generally speaking, *biologic response–modifying drugs* should be given exactly as prescribed and in keeping with manufacturer guidelines to minimize all expected and untoward adverse effects. Vital signs, with special attention to temperature, should also be measured throughout drug therapy. Premedication with acetaminophen and diphenhydramine may be deemed necessary when any of the biologic response–modifying drugs are administered. With some of the biologic response–modifying drugs, treatment with opioids, antihistamines, and/or antiinflammatory drugs may be required for the management of bone pain and chills should treatment with acetaminophen or diphenhydramine not be successful. Antiemetics may also be needed for any drug-related nausea or vomiting and may be administered before the specific biologic response–modifying drug is taken. Antiemetics may even need to be dosed around the clock if nausea and vomiting are problematic. The patient should be encouraged to rest when tired, not to overdo it during therapy, and to contact the prescriber if profound fatigue or loss of appetite is experienced. The patient should force fluids up to 3000 mL/day (unless contraindicated) to promote excretion of the by-products of cellular breakdown. Consultation with a dietitian or nutritionist may be helpful for the patient to learn about a nourishing diet to promote health and wellness (e.g., foods high in protein, complex carbohydrates, and necessary minerals, vitamins, and/or herbals). Menu planning and grocery shopping may also be discussed, with specific suggestions provided in each individual patient care situation. Nowadays, many grocery stores support Internet food shopping with car pickup at the store on the same day, and many stores also deliver at no or minimal cost to the patient. Patients should be informed about community resources (e.g., Meals on Wheels, respite care organizations, physical and occupational therapists) as needed. A social services agency should be contacted if the patient needs assistance in covering the cost of treatments or other services.

Another nursing intervention is to give the drug at night or at bedtime to decrease daytime fatigue. *Interferons* are administered parenterally by either the subcutaneous, intravenous, or intramuscular route, depending on the drug. For example, interferon alfa-2a is given subcutaneously or intramuscularly. Epoetin alfa may be given intravenously or subcutaneously, and the dosage may change depending on hematocrit values. If there is no response to the drug, the patient should undergo a workup (as ordered) for iron deficiency; underlying infection, inflammation, or malignancies; occult blood loss; hematologic disease; hemolysis; folic acid or vitamin B_{12} deficiency; and aluminum intoxication. Recommendations for the administration of epoetin alfa are to give the drug without shaking the vial and with only one use per vial; to use the smallest possible amount per injection (e.g., 1 mL or less per injection)—but always as ordered; to change the needle once the medication has been withdrawn from the vial; and to apply ice to numb the injection site. With sargramostim, only one dose should be withdrawn per vial, and as with all vials and packages, expiration dates should be checked. Vials should not be shaken but should be rolled between the hands. Filgrastim drug vials contain single-dose-only portions and should be stored in the refrigerator. Oprelvekin should not be used if any discoloration or particulate matter is noted in the vial. Treatment may be ordered to begin within 6 to 24 hours after completion of antineoplastic therapy. Daily subcutaneous dosing for 14 days has been found to produce dose-dependent platelet elevations, with counts increasing within 5 to 9 days of starting injections. Once oprelvekin is discontinued, counts remain increased for about 7 days and return to baseline within 14 days. Subcutaneous sites for oprelvekin administration include the thigh, abdomen, hip, and upper arm. When drugs are given subcutaneously, injection sites should be rotated. See Patient Teaching Tips for more information.

Patients requiring treatment with methotrexate should receive a test dose, and the importance of once-weekly dosing should be noted. Etanercept should be injected subcutaneously into the thigh, abdomen, or upper arm with rotation of injection sites. Leflunomide is given very cautiously and while liver and renal functioning are monitored; it should be administered orally with meals or food to minimize gastrointestinal upset.

CASE STUDY

Hematopoietic Biologic Response Modifiers

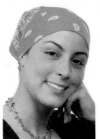

© Brian Chase

J.T., a 37-year-old homemaker, is receiving a second round of chemotherapy as part of treatment for ovarian cancer. Chemotherapeutic drugs may lead to the adverse effect of bone marrow suppression of various blood cell components.

1. What symptoms would the nurse expect to see if J.T. had diminished production of platelets? Red blood cells? White blood cells? Explain your answers.

Two weeks after this round of chemotherapy, J.T.'s hemoglobin level is 7.9 g/dL (pretherapy value was 11 g/dL) and the hematocrit is 28.5% (pretherapy value was 34%). The following orders are received: epoetin alfa (Epogen) 150 units/kg subcutaneously three times a week; ferrous sulfate, 300 mg by mouth daily.

2. What is the purpose of the order for ferrous sulfate?
3. For what conditions should the nurse assess before beginning the epoetin therapy?
4. The nurse should monitor J.T. closely. What assessment findings would be of the most concern during this therapy?
5. After 5 weeks, J.T.'s hemoglobin level is 11.4 g/dL and her hematocrit is 33%. The next dose of epoetin is due today. What action should the nurse take?

For answers, see *http://evolve.elsevier.com/Lilley*

Evaluation

Therapeutic responses to *biologic response–modifying drugs* include a decrease in the growth of the lesion or mass, decreased tumor size, and an easing of symptoms related to the tumor or disease process. Other therapeutic effects are an improvement in WBC, RBC, and platelet counts and/or a return to normal levels, and absence of infection, anemias, and hemorrhage. Journaling may help provide health care providers with more data from which to evaluate the patient's response during and after therapy. Possible adverse effects for which to evaluate are presented in Tables 49-1 and 49-2. Use of *DMARDs* should produce therapeutic results within the documented time frame (often weeks) with the patient experiencing increased ability to move joints, less discomfort, and an overall increased sense of improvement and well-being. Toxicity of these drugs may be manifested by liver, renal, and respiratory dysfunction and, for methotrexate, bone marrow suppression.

PATIENT TEACHING TIPS

- The patient should avoid hazardous tasks because of the central nervous system changes noted with several *biologic response–modifying drugs*. Fatigue is also a common adverse effect, and excessive fatigue should be reported.
- Signs of infection, such as sore throat, diarrhea, vomiting, and/or a fever of 100° F (37.8° C) or higher should be reported to the prescriber immediately. Excessive fatigue, loss of appetite, edema and bleeding should also be reported.
- Pregnancy is discouraged while the patient is taking a *biologic response–modifying drug*, so education should include information about contraceptive choices and the need to use contraception for up to 2 years after completion of therapy.
- Inform patient that adverse effects associated with *biologic response–modifying drug* usually disappear within 72 to 96 hours after therapy has been discontinued.

- Interleukins may be self-administered; therefore, the patient should learn self-injection technique and proper disposal of equipment (e.g., needles, syringes). A corresponding written instruction sheet should be provided for the patient, and the patient should keep a daily journal to record the site of injection and an overall rating of how the patient feels.
- Bone pain and flulike symptoms often occur with some of the *biologic response–modifying drugs*, and the use of non-opioid or, in some cases, opioid analgesics may be required. Some patients may find relief with ibuprofen.
- With DMARDs, patients should express improved joint function and decreased pain. Encourage reporting of any bleeding, excess fatigue, fever, and respiratory symptoms.

POINTS TO REMEMBER

- Cancer treatment has traditionally involved surgery, radiation, and chemotherapy. Surgery and radiation are usually local or regional therapies. Chemotherapy is generally systemic, but it often does not completely eliminate all of the cancer cells in the body. Adjuvant therapy is frequently used to destroy undetected distant micrometastases.
- The humoral and cellular immune systems act together to recognize and destroy foreign particles and cells. The humoral immune system is composed of lymphocytes that are known as B cells until they are transformed into plasma cells when they come in contact with an antigen (foreign substance). The plasma cells then manufacture antibodies to that antigen.
- *Biologic response–modifying drugs* provide another treatment option for patients who have malignancies and/or those who are receiving chemotherapy and have a need to boost blood cell counts. *Biologic response–modifying drugs* include hematopoietics and immunomodulating drugs. Interferons, interleukins, monoclonal antibodies, and miscellaneous drugs are the catego-

ries of immunomodulating drugs. Use of these drugs may augment, restore, or modify host defenses against the tumor.
- Nursing management associated with the administration of *biologic response–modifying drugs* focuses on the use of careful aseptic technique and other measures to prevent infection, proper nutrition, oral hygiene, monitoring of blood counts, and management of the adverse effects, including joint/bone pain and flu-like symptoms.
- The recommend therapy with nonbiologic DMARDs usually begins with methotrexate or leflunomide for most patients. Biologic DMARDs are generally reserved for those patients whose disease does not respond to methotrexate or leflunomide. The biologic DMARDs include etanercept, infliximab, adalimumab, abatacept, and rituximab.
- Filgrastim and sargramostim are not administered within 24 hours of a myelosuppressive antineoplastic, and the timeframe for their use should be followed (as prescribed), whether in an inpatient or home setting.

NCLEX EXAMINATION REVIEW QUESTIONS

1 The nurse is conducting a class on drugs for malignant tumors for a group of new oncology staff members. Which best describes the action of interferons in the management of malignant tumors?
  a Interferons increase the production of specific anticancer enzymes.
  b Interferons have antiviral and antitumor properties and strengthen the immune system.
  c Interferons stimulate the production and activation of T lymphocytes and cytotoxic T cells.
  d Interferons help improve the cell killing action of T cells because they are retrieved from healthy donors.

2 When planning care for a patient who is receiving interferon therapy, the nurse must keep in mind that the major dose-limiting factor is
  a fatigue.
  b bone marrow suppression.
  c fever.
  d nausea and vomiting.

3 The nurse is administering methotrexate as part of the treatment for rheumatoid arthritis and will monitor for signs of bone marrow suppression, such as:
  a Edema
  b Tinnitus
  c Increased bleeding tendencies
  d Tingling in the extremities

4 In caring for a patient receiving therapy with a myelosuppressive antineoplastic drug, the nurse notes an order to begin filgrastim after the chemotherapy is completed. Which of the following statements correctly describes when the nurse should begin the filgrastim therapy?
  a It can be started during the chemotherapy.
  b It should begin immediately after the chemotherapy is completed.
  c It should not be initiated until 24 hours after the chemotherapy is completed.
  d It should not be started until at least 72 hours after the chemotherapy is completed.

5 A patient with renal failure has severe anemia, and there is an order for darbepoetin. As the nurse assesses the patient, which condition listed should the nurse consider a contraindication to use of this medication?
  a Uncontrolled hypertension
  b Diabetes mellitus
  c Hypothyroidism
  d Angina

6 A patient is to receive filgrastim (Neupogen) after therapy with carmustine and radiation therapy for treatment of a brain tumor. The patient weighs 132 pounds. The protocol that the oncologist has written states that the filgrastim should be dosed at 5 mcg/kg. Filgrastim comes in a 300-mcg/mL vial. What dose should the patient receive? How many milliliters will the patient be given?

1. b, 2. a, 3. c, 4. c, 5. a, 6. 300 mcg; 1 mL.

CRITICAL THINKING ACTIVITIES: BEST ACTION

1 A patient who has been receiving an alkylating chemotherapeutic drug is to receive the colony-stimulating factor pegfilgrastim (Neulasta). A new nurse is preparing to start the pegfilgrastim as soon as the chemotherapy is completed, and the charge nurse is reviewing the orders. What is the best action of the charge nurse at this time? Explain.

2 The nurse is monitoring a patient who is receiving the interleukin drug aldesleukin (Proleukin). The patient is experiencing fever, chills, fatigue, dyspnea, slight crackles, ankle edema rated as 2+, and headache. Which of these assessment findings should cause the most concern, and what is the nurse's best action at this time?

3 The nurse is preparing to administer etanercept (Enbrel) to a patient with severe rheumatoid arthritis. During the assessment, the nurse notes that the patient has a history of moderate psoriasis, type 2 diabetes mellitus, and allergies to penicillin and latex. What is the nurse's best action at this time?

For answers, see *http://evolve.elsevier.com/Lilly.*

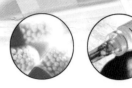
Drugs Affecting the Gastrointestinal System and Nutrition

STUDY SKILLS TIPS

Active Questioning • What Are the Right Questions?

Kinds of Questions • Questioning Application

ACTIVE QUESTIONING

There is one technique for study that cannot be overemphasized: active questioning. In the PURR study model, it is critical to be able to generate questions in the Plan, Rehearsal, and Review steps. The questions you generate when applying the PURR method are essential in helping you maintain concentration as you study, improving your comprehension as you read assigned material, and developing your long-term memory. Active questioning is a strategy that you must practice continuously. It is a strategy that develops with practice.

WHAT ARE THE RIGHT QUESTIONS?

Some questions generated during the Plan step will be useful and will focus on exactly the right issues for maximum learning. On the other hand, sometimes the questions generated by looking at the chapter outline or accented material in the body of the text will be inappropriate. These questions seem logical and important when you are working with the limited amount of information available in the Plan step, but as you read the chapter you will find that they miss the mark. Do not

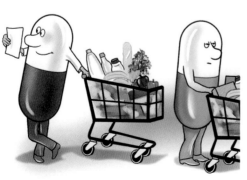

worry about whether each question you ask is perfectly focused. As you read, rehearse, and review the material, you can and should revise questions based on your growing understanding of the material. The important point is to ask many questions to help you maintain active involvement in the learning process and anticipate questions that will appear on exams. The more questions you ask, the more effective you will become, both as an active questioner and as an active learner.

KINDS OF QUESTIONS

First, you must realize that there is more than one kind of question to be asked. Over the years, many questioning hierarchies have been proposed by educators and scholars. The different kinds of questions identified vary from three or four to as many as seven or eight. The following is a simple approach that focuses on two types of questions.

Literal Questions

Literal questions are those that are answered directly and specifically by the text. When you were reading a story in elementary school and the teacher asked, "What did Sally do when she lost her movie money?" you were able to answer easily because the question asked for specific information that was stated clearly and directly in the story. If you were reading an American history text and found a topic heading for "The First President," an obvious question would be, "Who was the first president?" The answer is one that would be stated clearly and directly in the body of this topic. These are examples of literal questions. A literal question usually has a single correct response. The answer is stated directly in the text, and every reader will find that same information.

Interpretive Questions

Interpretive questions are more challenging questions that require the reader to interpret, synthesize, evaluate, and analyze the material. Interpretive questions require knowing the literal information in addition to understanding the reading material well enough to be able to select several different pieces or bits of data and put them together to formulate a response that demonstrates your understanding. In the American history example about the first president, an interpretive question might be, "Why was George Washington considered to be such an exemplary model as the first president of the new nation?" This question requires not only that you know the literal facts about Washington, but also that you be able to evaluate and judge those facts to reach a conclusion that could be supported by the literal information. Even though a question is interpretive, it is possible that there is only one correct response. However, it is equally possible that there is more than one correct response to an interpretive question. The literal information can be evaluated in a number of different ways in responding to the question, and the answers derived by different readers will vary. This is why it is a good choice to work with a study group when reviewing for interpretive questions. A study group can develop a variety of responses that result in a more comprehensive understanding of the course material. This depth of learning is what is necessary to pass not only your course test but also the NCLEX examination, as well as to become a competent nurse. Both literal and interpretive questions are essential in the learning process.

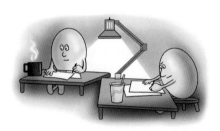

Questioning Application

Italicization is used to gain the reader's attention and to indicate that the italicized material is especially noteworthy. Accented material should always be considered as a potential source of

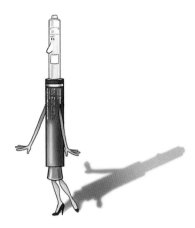

questions. Again, the questioning can begin with simple, literal questions, but it is essential that interpretive questions also be asked. Your questions should require that you read for broader general understanding and not just focus on "the facts."

At the end of each chapter there is a section entitled Critical Thinking Activities: Best Action. Even though this information is often stated in question form, you should consider generating additional questions of your own. The first question in Chapter 53 is, "The nurse is about to administer calcium supplemental therapy to a patient with a history of cardiac disease. What is the most important assessment that is needed before the nurse gives the drug?" In answering this question, some additional questions will help you focus your learning. What is calcium supplemental therapy? How does calcium affect cardiac patients? Why? Is calcium supplemental therapy inappropriate for all cardiac patients? If not, what are the circumstances that might rule out supplemental calcium? Of what signs and symptoms should the caregiver be aware if calcium supplemental therapy is being administered to a cardiac patient?

The more active you become as a questioner, the easier it will become to ask the kinds of questions that are necessary for your own learning.

CHAPTER 50

Acid-Controlling Drugs

OBJECTIVES

When you reach the end of this chapter, you should be able to do the following:

1 Discuss the physiologic influence of various pathologies, such as peptic ulcer disease, gastritis, spastic colon, gastroesophageal reflux disease, and hyperacidic states, on the health of patients and their gastrointestinal tracts.

2 Describe the mechanisms of action, indications, cautions, contraindications, drug interactions, adverse effects, dosages, and routes of administration for the following classes of acid-controlling drugs: antacids, histamine 2 (H_2)–blocking drugs (H_2 receptor antagonists), proton pump inhibitors, and acid suppressants.

3 Develop a nursing care plan that includes all phases of the nursing process for patients receiving acid-controlling drugs.

-Learning Activities

http://evolve.elsevier.com/Lilley

NCLEX Review Questions • Animations • Nursing Care Plans • Audio Glossary • Category Catchers • Medication Errors Checklists • IV Therapy Checklists • Calculators • Frequently Asked Questions • Content Updates • Supplemental Resources • Answers to Case Studies and Critical Thinking Activities

Drug Profiles

antacids, general, p. 788
♦ cimetidine, p. 790
♦ famotidine, p. 791
lansoprazole, p. 792
misoprostol, p. 792

omeprazole, p. 791
pantoprazole, p. 792
ranitidine, p. 790
simethicone, p. 793
♦ sucralfate, p. 792

♦ *Key drug.*

Glossary

Antacids Basic compounds composed of different combinations of acid-neutralizing ionic salts. (p. 787)
Chief cells Cells in the stomach that secrete the gastric enzyme pepsinogen (a precursor to *pepsin*). (p. 785)
Gastric glands Secretory glands in the stomach containing the following cell types: parietal, chief, mucous, endocrine, and enterochromaffin. (p. 785)
Gastric hyperacidity The overproduction of stomach acid. (p. 784)
Hydrochloric acid (HCl) An acid secreted by the *parietal cells* in the lining of the stomach that maintains the environment of the stomach at a pH of 1 to 4. (p. 785)
Mucous cells Cells whose function in the stomach is to secrete mucus that serves as a protective mucous coat against the digestive properties of HCl. Also called *surface epithelial cells.* (p. 785)
Parietal cells Cells in the stomach that produce and secrete HCl. These cells are the primary site of action for many of the drugs used to treat acid-related disorders. (p. 785)
Pepsin An enzyme in the stomach that breaks down proteins. (p. 785)

One of the conditions of the stomach requiring drug therapy is hyperacidity, or excessive acid production. Left untreated, hyperacidity can lead to serious conditions such as acid reflux, ulcer disease, esophageal damage, and even esophageal cancer. Overproduction of stomach acid is also referred to as **gastric hyperacidity.**

Anatomy, Physiology, and Disease Overview

ACID-RELATED PATHOPHYSIOLOGY

The stomach secretes several substances with various physiologic functions, including the following:

- Hydrochloric acid, an acid that aids digestion and also serves as a barrier to infection
- Bicarbonate, a base that is a natural mechanism to prevent hyperacidity
- Pepsinogen, an enzymatic precursor to pepsin, an enzyme that digests dietary proteins
- Intrinsic factor, a glycoprotein that facilitates gastric absorption of vitamin B_{12}
- Mucus, which protects the stomach lining from both hydrochloric acid and digestive enzymes
- Prostaglandins, which have a variety of antiinflammatory and protective functions (see Chapter 44)

The stomach, although one structure, can be divided into three functional areas. Each area is associated with specific glands. These glands are composed of different cells, and these cells secrete different substances. Figure 50-1 shows the three functional areas of the stomach and the distribution of the associated types of stomach glands.

The three primary types of glands in the stomach are the cardiac, pyloric, and gastric glands. These glands are named for their positions in the stomach. The cardiac glands are located around the cardiac sphincter (also known as the *gastroesophageal sphincter*); the gastric glands are in the fundus, also known as the *greater part of the body of the stomach;* and the pyloric

784

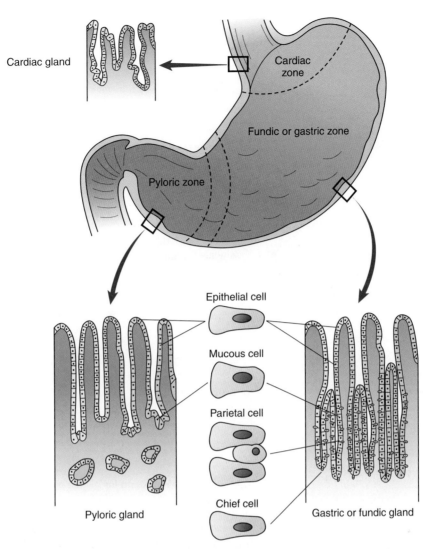

FIGURE 50-1   The three zones of the stomach and the associated glands.

glands are in the pyloric region and in the transitional area between the pyloric and the fundic zones. The gastric glands are the most numerous and are of primary importance to the discussion of acid-related disorders and drug therapy.

The **gastric glands** are highly specialized secretory glands composed of several different types of cells: parietal, chief, mucous, endocrine, and enterochromaffin. Each cell secretes a specific substance. The three most important cell types are parietal cells, chief cells, and mucous cells. These cells are depicted in Figure 50-1.

Parietal cells produce and secrete **hydrochloric acid (HCl).** They are the primary site of action for many of the drugs used to treat acid-related disorders. **Chief cells** secrete *pepsinogen.* Pepsinogen is a *proenzyme* (enzyme precursor) that becomes **pepsin** when activated by exposure to acid. Pepsin breaks down proteins and is therefore referred to as a *proteolytic* enzyme. **Mucous cells** are mucus-secreting cells that are also called *surface epithelial cells.* The secreted mucus serves as a protective coating against the digestive action of hydrochloric acid and digestive enzymes.

These three cell types play an important role in the digestive process. When the balance of these cells and their secretions is impaired, acid-related diseases can occur. The most harmful of these involve *hypersecretion* of acid and include *peptic ulcer disease* and *esophageal cancer.* However, the most common condition is mild to moderate hyperacidity. Many lay terms (e.g., indigestion, sour stomach, heartburn, acid stomach) have been used to describe this condition of overproduction of hydrochloric acid by the parietal cells. Hyperacidity is often associated with *gastroesophageal reflux disease (GERD).* This is the tendency of excessive and acidic stomach contents to back up, or *reflux,* into the lower (and even upper) esophagus. Over time this condition can lead to more serious disorders such as *erosive esophagitis* and *Barrett esophagus,* a precancerous condition. Therefore, to prevent serious disorders from occurring and to promote patient comfort, GERD is aggressively treated with one or more of the medications described in this section.

Hydrochloric acid, as noted earlier, is an acid that is secreted by the parietal cells in the lining of the stomach. It is the primary substance secreted in the stomach that maintains the environment of the stomach at a pH of 1 to 4. This acidity aids in the proper digestion of food and also serves as one of the body's defenses against microbial infection via the gastrointestinal (GI) tract. Several substances stimulate hydrochloric acid secretion by the

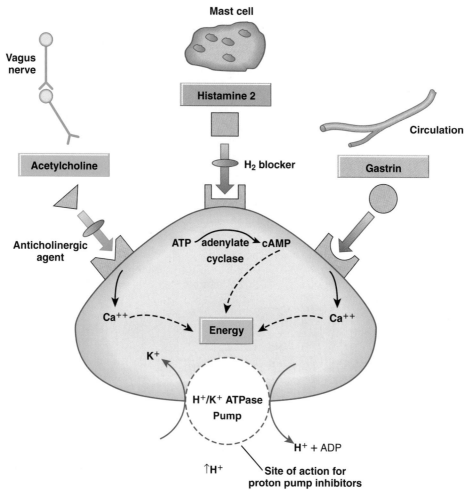

FIGURE 50-2 Parietal cell stimulation and secretion. *ADP,* Adenosine diphosphate; *ATP,* adenosine triphosphate; *ATPase,* adenosine triphosphatase; *cAMP,* cyclic adenosine monophosphate.

parietal cells, such as food, caffeine, chocolate, and alcohol. In moderation, any of these is usually not problematic. However, excessive consumption of large, fatty meals or alcohol, as well as emotional stress, may result in hyperproduction of hydrochloric acid from the parietal cells and lead to hypersecretory disorders such as peptic ulcer disease.

The parietal cell is the source of hydrochloric acid production, and it is the primary target for many of the most effective drugs for the treatment of acid-related disorders. A closer look at how the parietal cell receives signals to produce and secrete hydrochloric acid will enhance the understanding of the mechanism of action of many of the drugs used to treat acid-related disorders.

The wall of the parietal cell contains three types of receptors: acetylcholine (ACh), histamine, and gastrin. When any one of these is occupied by its corresponding chemical stimulant (ACh, histamine, or gastrin, which can all be considered *first messengers*), the parietal cell will produce and secrete hydrochloric acid. Figure 50-2 shows the parietal cell with its three receptors. Once these receptors have become occupied, a *second messenger* is sent inside the cell. In the case of histamine receptors, occupation results in the production of adenylate cyclase. Adenylate cyclase converts adenosine triphosphate

(ATP) to cyclic adenosine monophosphate (cAMP), which provides energy for the *proton pump.* The proton pump—or, more precisely, the hydrogen–potassium–adenosine triphosphatase (ATPase) pump—is a pump for the transport of hydrogen ions and is located in the parietal cells. The pump requires energy to work. If energy is present, the proton pump will be activated, and the pump will be able to transport hydrogen ions needed for the production of hydrochloric acid.

In the case of both ACh and gastrin receptors, the second messenger that drives the proton pump is not cAMP but is instead calcium ions. Anticholinergic drugs (see Chapter 21) such as atropine block ACh receptors, which also results in decreased hydrogen ion secretion from the parietal cells. However, these drugs are no longer used for this purpose and have been superseded by other drug classes discussed in this chapter. There is currently no drug to block the binding of the hormone gastrin to its corresponding receptor on the parietal cell surface.

Peptic ulcer disease is a general term for gastric or duodenal ulcers that involve digestion of the GI mucosa by the enzyme pepsin. Pepsin normally breaks down only food proteins and is the activated form of pepsinogen. Pepsinogen is produced by the chief cells of the stomach in response to hydrochloric acid released from the parietal cells. The sight, smell, and taste of food and its presence in the stomach are the primary stimulus for the release of hydrochloric acid from the parietal cells. Because the process of ulceration is driven by the proteolytic (protein breakdown) actions of pepsin together with the caustic effects of hydrochloric acid, peptic ulcer disease and related problems are also referred to by the more general term *acid-peptic disorders.*

In 1983, a gram-negative spiral bacterium, *Campylobacter pylori,* was isolated from several patients with gastritis. Over the next few years this bacterium was studied further, and it became implicated in the pathophysiology of peptic ulcer disease. The official name of the bacterium was changed to *Helicobacter pylori* because it was felt to have more characteristics of the *Helicobacter* genus. The prevalence of *H. pylori* as measured by serum antibody tests is approximately 40% to 60% for patients older than 60 years of age but only 10% for those younger than 30 years of age. The bacterium is found in the GI tracts of roughly 90% of patients with duodenal ulcers and 70% of those with gastric ulcers. However, this bacterium is also found in many patients who do not have peptic ulcer disease, and its presence is not associated with acute, perforating ulcers. These latter observations suggest that more than one factor is involved in ulceration. The American College of Gastroenterologists published treatment guidelines in 2007 for *H. pylori* infections. First-line therapy includes a 10- to 14-day course of a proton pump inhibitor (discussed later in this chapter) and the antibiotics clarithromycin and either amoxicillin or metronidazole (see Chapters 38 and 39) or a combination of a proton pump inhibitor, bismuth subsalicylate (see Chapter 51), and the antibiotics tetracycline and metronidazole (see Chapters 38 and 39). Many different combinations are used, but all incorporate the aforementioned key drugs.

Stress-related mucosal damage is an important issue for critically ill patients. Stress ulcer prophylaxis (or therapy to prevent severe GI damage) is undertaken in almost every critically ill patient in an intensive care unit (ICU). GI lesions are a common finding in ICU patients, especially within the first 24 hours after admission. The etiology and pathophysiology of stress-related mucosal damage is multifactorial and is not fully understood. Factors include decreased blood flow, mucosal ischemia, hypoperfusion, and reperfusion injury. Procedures performed commonly in critically ill patients, such as passing nasogastric (NG) tubes, placing patients on ventilators, and others, predispose patients to bleeding of the GI tract. Coagulopathy, a history of peptic ulcer or GI bleed, sepsis, use of steroids, ICU stay of longer than 1 week, and occult bleeding are considered to indicate high risk of GI lesions. Guidelines suggest that all such patients receive either a histamine receptor–blocking drug or a proton pump inhibitor, both of which are discussed in detail in this chapter.

Pharmacology Overview

ANTACIDS

Antacids are basic compounds used to neutralize stomach acid. Most commonly they are nonprescription salts of aluminum, magnesium, calcium, and/or sodium. They have been used for centuries in the treatment of patients with acid-related disorders. The ancient Greeks used crushed coral (calcium carbonate) in the

first century AD to treat patients with dyspepsia. Antacids were the principal antiulcer treatment, along with anticholinergic drugs, until the introduction of the *histamine 2 (H_2) receptor antagonists* in the late 1970s. The use of anticholinergic drugs has fallen out of favor; however, the antacids, especially the over-the-counter (OTC) formulations, are still used extensively. They are available in a variety of dosage forms, some including more than one antacid salt. In addition, many antacid preparations also contain the *antiflatulent* (antigas) drug simethicone (see the section on miscellaneous acid-controlling drugs), which reduces gas and bloating.

Many aluminum- and calcium-based formulations also include magnesium, which not only contributes to the acid-neutralizing capacity but also counteracts the constipating effects of aluminum and calcium. There are multiple salts of calcium, with calcium carbonate being used most often. However, calcium antacids may lead to the development of kidney stones and increased gastric acid secretion, so they are not used as frequently as other antacids. Antacids containing magnesium should be avoided in patients with renal failure. Sodium bicarbonate is a highly soluble antacid form with a quick onset but short duration of action.

Mechanism of Action and Drug Effects

Antacids work primarily by neutralizing gastric acidity. They do not prevent the overproduction of acid but instead help to neutralize acid secretions. It is also believed that antacids promote gastric mucosal defensive mechanisms, especially at lower dosages. They do this by stimulating the secretion of mucus, prostaglandins, and bicarbonate from the cells inside the gastric glands. Mucus serves as a protective barrier against the destructive actions of hydrochloric acid. Bicarbonate helps buffer the acidity of hydrochloric acid. Prostaglandins prevent histamine from binding to its corresponding parietal cell receptors, which inhibits the production of adenylate cyclase. Without adenylate cyclase, no cAMP can be formed and no second messenger is available to activate the proton pump (see Figure 50-2).

The primary drug effect of antacids is the reduction of the symptoms associated with various acid-related disorders, such as pain and reflux ("heartburn"). A dose of antacid that raises the gastric pH from 1.3 to 1.6 (only 0.3 point) reduces gastric acidity by 50%, whereas acidity is reduced by 90% if the pH is raised an entire point (e.g., 1.3 to 2.3). Antacid-associated pain reduction is thought to be a result of base-mediated inhibition of the protein-digesting ability of pepsin, increase in the resistance of the stomach lining to irritation, and increase in the tone of the cardiac sphincter, which reduces reflux from the stomach.

Indications

Antacids are indicated for the acute relief of symptoms associated with peptic ulcer, gastritis, gastric hyperacidity, and heartburn.

Contraindications

The only usual contraindication to antacid use is known allergy to a specific drug product. Other contraindications may include severe renal failure or electrolyte disturbances (because of the potential toxic accumulation of electrolytes in the antacids themselves) and GI obstruction (antacids may stimulate GI motility when it is undesirable because of the presence of an obstructive process requiring surgical intervention).

BOX 50-1 Nursing Concerns for Patients Taking Antacids

Aluminum, used to reduce gastric acid, binds to phosphate and may lead to hypercalcemia. Early hypercalcemia is characterized by constipation, headache, increased thirst, dry mouth, decreased appetite, irritability, and a metallic taste in the mouth. Later signs and symptoms of hypercalcemia include confusion, drowsiness, increase in blood pressure, irregular heart rate, nausea, vomiting, and increased urination. Use of aluminum-based antacids may also produce hypophosphatemia, which is characterized by loss of appetite, malaise, muscle weakness, and/or bone pain. The use of calcium-containing antacids (e.g., calcium carbonate) may lead to *milk-alkali syndrome,* which is associated with headache, anorexia, nausea, vomiting, and unusual tiredness. Use of sodium bicarbonate may lead to metabolic alkalosis if the drug is abused or used over the long term. Alkalosis is manifested by irritability, muscle twitching, numbness and tingling, cyanosis, slow and shallow respirations, headache, thirst, and nausea. Acid rebound occurs with the discontinuation of antacids that have high acid-neutralizing capacity and with overuse or misuse of antacid therapy. If acid neutralization is sudden and high, the result is an immediate elevation in pH to alkalinity and just as rapid a decline in pH to a more acidic state in the gut.

Adverse Effects

The adverse effects of the antacids are limited. The magnesium preparations, especially milk of magnesia, can cause diarrhea. Both the aluminum- and calcium-containing formulations can result in constipation. Calcium products can also cause kidney stones. Excessive use of any antacid can theoretically result in systemic alkalosis. This is more common with sodium bicarbonate. Another adverse effect that is more common with the calcium-containing products is rebound hyperacidity, or acid rebound, in which the patient experiences hyperacidity when antacid use is discontinued. Long-term self-medication with antacids may mask symptoms of serious underlying disease such as bleeding ulcer or malignancy. Patients with ongoing symptoms should undergo regular medical evaluations, because additional medications or other interventions may be needed. Box 50-1 lists several specific nursing concerns for patients taking antacids.

Interactions

Antacids are capable of causing several interactions when administered with other drugs. There are four basic mechanisms by which antacids cause interactions:

- *Adsorption* of other drugs to antacids, which reduces the ability of the other drug to be absorbed into the body
- *Chelation,* which is the chemical inactivation of other drugs that produces insoluble complexes
- *Increased stomach pH,* which increases the absorption of basic drugs and decreases the absorption of acidic drugs
- *Increased urinary pH,* which increases the excretion of acidic drugs and decreases the excretion of basic drugs

Most drugs are either weak acids or weak bases. Therefore, pH conditions in both the GI and urinary tracts will affect the extent to which drug molecules are absorbed. Common examples of drugs whose effects may be chemically enhanced by the presence of antacids (due to pH effects) are benzodiazepines, sulfonylureas (effects may also be reduced, depending on the drugs involved), sympathomimetics, and valproic acid. More commonly, the pres-

ence of antacids reduces the efficacy of interacting drugs by interfering with their GI absorption. Such drugs include allopurinol, tetracycline, thyroid hormones, captopril, corticosteroids, digoxin R, histamine antagonists, phenytoin, isoniazid, ketoconazole, methotrexate, nitrofurantoin, phenothiazines, salicylates, and quinolone antibiotics. Patients are advised to dose any interacting drugs at least 1 to 2 hours before or after antacids are taken. Significant patient harm may ensue when the quinolone antibiotics (ciprofloxacin, levofloxacin) are given with antacids. These antibiotics are administered orally to treat serious infections. Antacids can reduce their absorption by over 50%. Thus, antacids must be given either 2 hours before or 2 hours after the dose of a quinolone antibiotic.

Dosages

For information on dosages for selected antacid drugs, see the Dosages table on p. 789.

DRUG PROFILES

antacids, general

Some of the available aluminum, magnesium, calcium, and sodium salts that are used in many of the antacid formulations are listed in Box 50-2. There are far too many individual antacid products on the market to mention all formulations. Briefly, OTC antacid formulations are available as capsules, chewable tablets, effervescent granules and tablets, powders, suspensions, and plain tablets. This allows patients a variety of options for self-medication. Pharmacokinetic parameters are not normally listed for antacids, but these drugs are generally excreted quickly through the GI tract and/or the electrolyte homeostatic mechanisms of the kidneys. Antacids are generally considered safe for use during pregnancy if prolonged administration and high dosages are avoided. However, it is recommended that pregnant women consult their health care providers before taking an antacid. Aluminum- and sodium-based antacids are often recommended for patients with renal compromise because they are more easily excreted than antacids in other categories. Calcium-containing antacids are currently advertised as an extra source of calcium. Calcium carbonate neutralization will produce gas and possibly belching. For this reason, it may be combined with an antiflatulent drug such as simethicone (see section on miscellaneous acid-controlling drugs). Magnesium-containing antacids commonly have a laxative effect, and frequent administration of these antacids alone often cannot be tolerated. Both calcium- and magnesium-based antacids are more likely to accumulate to toxic levels in patients with renal disease and are often avoided in this patient group.

H₂ RECEPTOR ANTAGONISTS

H₂ receptor antagonists, commonly abbreviated as H2RAs and also called *H₂ receptor blockers,* are the prototypical acid-secretion antagonists. These drugs reduce but do not completely abolish acid secretion. They have become the most popular drugs for the treatment of many acid-related disorders, including peptic ulcer disease. This can be attributed to their efficacy, patient acceptance, and excellent safety profile. These drugs include cimetidine, ranitidine, famotidine, and nizatidine. There is little difference among the four available H₂ receptor antagonists from the standpoint of efficacy. All are available OTC.

DOSAGES

Selected Antacid Drugs*

Drug (Pregnancy Category)	Pharmacologic Class	Usual Dosage Range	Indications
aluminum hydroxide (Amphojel) (A)	Aluminum-containing antacid	**Adult** PO: 600-1500 mg 3-6 times per day	Hyperacidity
aluminum hydroxide and magnesium hydroxide (Maalox, Mylanta) (A)	Combination antacid	**Adult** 400-2400 mg 3-6 times per day	Hyperacidity
calcium carbonate (Tums) (A)	Calcium-containing antacid	**Adult** PO: 0.5-1.5 g prn	Hyperacidity
magnesium hydroxide (milk of magnesia) (A)	Magnesium-containing antacid	**Adult** PO: 0.65-1.3 g prn, up to 4 times per day	Hyperacidity (more commonly used as a laxative)

PO, Oral.

*Many more antacid products are available on the market than appear in this table. Dosages given are approximate dosages of active ingredients; there may be variations among different products and different dosage forms of the same product.

BOX 50-2 Antacids

Antacids: Salt Content

Magnesium Salts	Aluminum Salts	Calcium Salts	Sodium Salts
carbonate hydroxide oxide trisilicate	carbonate hydroxide	carbonate	bicarbonate citrate

Commonly Available Antacid Products
Magnesium-Containing Antacids
Carbonate salt: Gaviscon Liquid, Gaviscon Extra Strength Relief Formula Tablets
Hydroxide salt: milk of magnesia
Oxide salt: Mag-Ox (included for information only; used primarily as a magnesium supplement)
Trisilicate salt: Gaviscon Tablets

Aluminum-Containing Antacids
Carbonate salt: Basaljel
Hydroxide salt: ALternaGEL, Amphojel
Combination products: Gaviscon, Maalox, Mylanta, Di-Gel

Calcium-Containing Antacids
Carbonate salt: Tums, Maalox Antacid Caplets, Extra Strength Alkets Antacid

Sodium-Containing Antacids
Bicarbonate salt: Alka-Seltzer
Citrate salt: Citra pH

Mechanism of Action and Drug Effects

H_2 receptor antagonists competitively block the H_2 receptor of acid-producing parietal cells. This makes the parietal cell less responsive not only to histamine but also to the stimulation of ACh and gastrin. This is shown in Figure 50-2. Up to 90% inhibition of vagal- and gastrin-stimulated acid secretion occurs when histamine is blocked. However, complete inhibition has not been shown. The effect of these drugs is reduced hydrogen ion secretion from the parietal cells, which results in an increase in the pH of the stomach and relief of many of the symptoms associated with hyperacidity-related conditions.

Indications

H_2 receptor antagonists have several therapeutic uses, including treatment of GERD, peptic ulcer disease, and erosive esophagitis; adjunct therapy in the control of upper GI tract bleeding; and treatment of pathologic gastric hypersecretory conditions such as *Zollinger-Ellison syndrome.* The latter is one form of *hyperchlorhydria,* or excessive gastric acidity. H_2 receptor antagonists are commonly used for stress ulcer prophylaxis in critically ill patients.

Contraindications

The only usual contraindication to the use of H_2 receptor antagonists is a known drug allergy. Liver and/or kidney dysfunction are relative contraindications that may warrant dosage adjustment.

Adverse Effects

The H_2 receptor antagonists have a remarkably low incidence of adverse effects (fewer than 3% of cases). The four available H_2 receptor antagonists are similar in many respects but have some differences in adverse effect profiles. Table 50-1 lists the adverse effects associated with these drugs. Central nervous system adverse effects occur in fewer than 1% of patients taking these drugs but are sometimes seen in the elderly. These adverse effects include confusion and disorientation. The nurse should be alert for mental status changes when giving these drugs, especially if they are new to the patient. Cimetidine may induce impotence and gynecomastia. This is the result of cimetidine's inhibition of estradiol metabolism and displacement of dihydrotestosterone from peripheral androgen-binding sites. All four H_2 receptor antagonists may increase the secretion of prolactin from the anterior pituitary. Thrombocytopenia has been reported with ranitidine and famotidine.

Interactions

Cimetidine carries a higher risk of drug interactions than the other three drugs, especially in the elderly. These interactions may be of clinical importance. Cimetidine binds enzymes of the hepatic cytochrome P-450 microsomal oxidase system. This is a

TABLE 50-1 H₂ Receptor Antagonists: Adverse Effects

Body System	Adverse Effects
Cardiovascular	Hypotension (monitor for this effect with intravenous administration)
Central nervous	Headache, lethargy, confusion, depression, hallucinations, slurred speech, agitation
Endocrine	Increased prolactin secretion, gynecomastia (with cimetidine)
Gastrointestinal	Diarrhea, nausea, abdominal cramps
Genitourinary	Impotence, increased blood urea nitrogen, creatinine levels
Hepatobiliary	Elevated liver enzyme levels, jaundice
Hematologic	Agranulocytosis, thrombocytopenia, neutropenia, aplastic anemia
Integumentary	Urticaria, rash, alopecia, sweating, flushing, exfoliative dermatitis

group of enzymes in the liver that metabolize many different drugs. By inhibiting the metabolism of drugs metabolized via this pathway, cimetidine may raise the blood concentrations of certain drugs. Ranitidine has only 10% to 20% of the binding action of cimetidine on the P-450 system, and nizatidine and famotidine have essentially no effect. This interaction has little clinical significance for most drugs; however, significant interactions are more likely to arise with medications having a narrow therapeutic range, such as theophylline, warfarin, lidocaine, and phenytoin. All H₂ receptor antagonists may inhibit the absorption of certain drugs, such as ketoconazole, that require an acidic GI environment for gastric absorption. Smoking has also been shown to decrease the effectiveness of H₂ antagonists. For optimal results, H₂ receptor antagonists should be taken 1 to 2 hours before antacids.

Dosages

For dosage information for the H₂ antagonists, see the Dosages table on p. 790.

DRUG PROFILES

H₂ receptor antagonists are the prototypical acid-secretion antagonists. These drugs reduce acid secretion. They are among the most commonly used drugs in the world, due to their efficacy, OTC availability, and overall excellent safety profile. However, this drug class has been partially replaced by proton pump inhibitors (see the next section).

◆ cimetidine

In 1977, cimetidine (Tagamet) became the first drug in this class to be released on the market. It is the prototypical H₂ receptor antagonist and was the first major prescription drug to go OTC. Because of its potential to cause drug interactions, its use has been largely replaced by ranitidine and famotidine. Cimetidine is still used to treat certain allergic reactions.

PHARMACOKINETICS

Route	Onset of Action	Peak Plasma Concentration	Elimination Half-life	Duration of Action
PO	15-60 min	1-2 hr	2 hr	4-5 hr

ranitidine

Ranitidine (Zantac) was the second H₂ receptor antagonists introduced. It does not carry the concerns over drug interactions that cimetidine has and has become the most widely used H₂ receptor antagonist. It is available in oral and intravenous forms. Dosing is different for the different forms: oral ranitidine is dosed as 150 mg twice a day or 300 mg at bedtime, whereas the intravenous form is dosed at 50 mg every 8 hours.

PHARMACOKINETICS

Route	Onset of Action	Peak Plasma Concentration	Elimination Half-life	Duration of Action
PO	1 hr	2-4 hr	2-3 hr	4-12 hr
IV	30 min	1 hr	2-3 hr	4-12 hr

DOSAGES

Selected H₂ Receptor Antagonists

Drug (Pregnancy Category)	Usual Dosage Range	Indications
◆ cimetidine (Tagamet, Tagamet HB) (B)	**Adult** PO: 200 mg bid	Dyspepsia, heartburn
	PO: 300 mg qid or 400 mg bid and at bedtime or 800 mg at bedtime	Ulcers
	PO: 1600 mg/day divided in 2 to 4 doses	GERD
	PO/IM/IV: 300 mg tid and at bedtime; do not exceed 2400 mg/day	Pathologic hypersecretion
◆ famotidine (Pepcid, Pepcid AC) (B)	**Adult** PO: 10 mg daily-bid	Dyspepsia, heartburn
	PO: 40 mg daily at bedtime or 20 mg bid	Ulcers
	PO: 20-160 mg q6h	Pathologic hypersecretion
	IV: 20 mg q12h	GERD
	PO: 20 mg bid	
ranitidine (Zantac) (B)	**Adult** PO: 75 mg bid	Dyspepsia, heartburn
	PO: 150 mg daily-bid or 300 mg at bedtime	Ulcers
	PO: 150 mg bid	Pathologic hypersecretion, GERD
	PO: 150 mg qid	Erosive esophagitis

GERD, Gastroesophageal reflux disease; *IM,* intramuscular; *IV,* intravenous; *PO,* oral.

◆ **famotidine**

Famotidine (Pepcid) was the last H$_2$ receptor antagonist introduced and, like ranitidine, has no drug interaction concerns. It is available in oral and injectable forms. The dosing is the same for both forms.

PHARMACOKINETICS

Route	Onset of Action	Peak Plasma Concentration	Elimination Half-life	Duration of Action
PO	1.4 hr	3 hr	2.6-4 hr	9-12 hr
IV	Immediate	1.5 hr	2.6-4 hr	9-12 hr

PROTON PUMP INHIBITORS

The newest drugs introduced for the treatment of acid-related disorders are the *proton pump inhibitors (PPIs)*. These include lansoprazole (Prevacid), omeprazole (Prilosec), rabeprazole (AcipHex), pantoprazole (Protonix), and esomeprazole (Nexium). These drugs are even more powerful than the H$_2$ receptor antagonists. The PPIs bind directly to the hydrogen-potassium-ATPase pump mechanism and irreversibly inhibit the action of this enzyme, which results in a total blockage of hydrogen ion secretion from the parietal cells.

Mechanism of Action and Drug Effects

The action of the hydrogen-potassium-ATPase pump is the final step in the acid-secretory process of the parietal cell (see Figure 50-2). If chemical energy is present to run the pump, the pump will transport hydrogen ions out of the parietal cell, which increases the acid content of the surrounding gastric lumen and lowers the pH. Because hydrogen ions are *protons* (positively charged atoms), this ion pump is also called the *proton pump*. PPIs bind irreversibly to the proton pump. This inhibition prevents the movement of hydrogen ions out of the parietal cell into the stomach and thereby blocks all gastric acid secretion. The PPIs stop over 90% of acid secretion over 24 hours, which makes most patients temporarily *achlorhydric* (without acid). However, food absorption is not affected. For acid secretion to return to normal after a PPI has been stopped, the parietal cell must synthesize new hydrogen-potassium-ATPase. Although there are other proton pumps in the body, hydrogen-potassium-ATPase is structurally and mechanically distinct from other hydrogen-transporting enzymes and appears to exist only in the parietal cells. Thus, the action of PPIs is limited to its effects on gastric acid secretion.

Indications

PPIs are currently indicated as first-line therapy for erosive esophagitis, symptomatic GERD that is poorly responsive to other medical treatment such as therapy with H$_2$ receptor antagonists, short-term treatment of active duodenal ulcers and active benign gastric ulcers, gastric hypersecretory conditions (e.g., Zollinger-Ellison syndrome), and nonsteroidal antiinflammatory drug (NSAID)–induced ulcers, and for stress ulcer prophylaxis. Long-term therapeutic uses include maintenance of healing of erosive esophagitis and pathologic hypersecretory conditions, including both GERD and Zollinger-Ellison syndrome. All of the PPIs can be used in combination with antibiotics to treat patients with *H. pylori* infections. The PPIs can be given orally or through an NG or percutaneous enterogastric tube. For example, esomeprazole capsules may be opened, the granules dissolved in 50 mL of water, and the solution given through the tube. Similar tubal

administration is also listed by the manufacturer for lansoprazole capsules and omeprazole powder for oral suspension. The drug packaging should be consulted for drug-specific instructions. The nurse must be aware of the particle size of the drug once it is in solution and the tube size being used. For example, pantoprazole granules are to be used with NG tubes that are larger than 16 gauge and may clog the tube if used with small tubes. Several of the PPIs are now also available for intravenous use.

Contraindications

The only usual contraindication to use of the PPIs is known drug allergy.

Adverse Effects

PPIs are generally well tolerated. The frequency of adverse effects has been similar to that for placebo or H$_2$ receptor antagonists. There was some early concern that long-term use of PPIs might promote malignant gastric tumors. This has not proved to be the case, however, and this initial concern has subsided. There are some concerns that these drugs may be overprescribed and may predispose patients to GI tract infections because of the reduction of the normal acid-mediated antimicrobial protection. New concerns have arisen over the potential for long-term users of PPIs to develop osteoporosis. This is thought to be due to the inhibition of stomach acid, and it is speculated that PPIs speed up bone mineral loss.

Interactions

Few drug interactions occur with the PPIs; however, they may increase serum levels of diazepam and phenytoin. There may be an increased chance of bleeding in patients who are taking both a PPI and warfarin. Other possible interactions include interference with the absorption of ketoconazole, ampicillin, iron salts, and digoxin. When given with clopidogrel, there is some concern of an increased risk of death if the patient has acute coronary syndrome. Sucralfate may delay the absorption of PPIs. Food may decrease absorption of the PPIs, and it is recommended that they be taken on an empty stomach.

Dosages

For recommended dosages of selected PPIs, see the Dosages table on p. 792.

DRUG PROFILES

omeprazole

Omeprazole (Prilosec) was the first drug in this breakthrough class of antisecretory drugs. Omeprazole and rabeprazole are not available in injectable form. Other PPIs include lansoprazole (Prevacid), esomeprazole (Nexium), and pantoprazole (Protonix). Orally administered PPIs (and H$_2$ receptor antagonists) often work best when taken 30 to 60 minutes before meals. Omeprazole was the first PPI to become available generically, and many insurance companies dictate its use as a first-line drug unless there is a documented treatment failure. As more of the PPIs become available in generic form, this will become a nonissue.

PHARMACOKINETICS

Route	Onset of Action	Peak Plasma Concentration	Elimination Half-life	Duration of Action
PO	2 hr	5 days	0.5-1 hr	1-5 days

DOSAGES

Selected Proton Pump Inhibitors

Drug (Pregnancy Category)	Usual Dosage Range	Indications
lansoprazole (Prevacid) (B)	**Adult** PO: 30 mg daily	GERD, ulcer, erosive esophagitis
omeprazole (Prilosec) (C)	**Adult** PO: 20 mg/day for 4-8 wk PO: 60 mg PO once daily initially, then titrated and given in single or multiple daily doses, with dosage titration up to a maximum of 120 mg PO tid	Esophagitis, duodenal ulcer Hypersecretory conditions
pantoprazole (Protonix) (B)	**Adult** PO/IV: 20-80 mg/day depending on indication	GERD, ulcer, stress ulcer prophylaxis

GERD, Gastroesophageal reflux disease; *IV*, intravenous; *PO*, oral.

lansoprazole

Lansoprazole (Prevacid) is available in a delayed-release capsule, granules for oral suspension, and orally disintegrating tablets (Prevacid SoluTab). The capsules can be opened and mixed (not crushed) with apple juice for administration via NG tube, or the Solu-tab can be dissolved in water. Lansoprazole drug is also available as Prevpac, a combination product for the treatment of *H. Pylori* infection.

PHARMACOKINETICS

Route	Onset of Action	Peak Plasma Concentration	Elimination Half-life	Duration of Action
PO	1.7 hr	4 wk	1-2 hr	24 hr

pantoprazole

Pantoprazole (Protonix) was the first PPI available for intravenous use. It was also the first drug to be used as a continuous infusion for the treatment of GI bleeding. It is available as an oral tablet and as delayed-release granules for NG administration. However, the granules are large, and the NG tube must be at least size 16, or the granules may clog the tube.

PHARMACOKINETICS

Route	Onset of Action	Peak Plasma Concentration	Elimination Half-life	Duration of Action
PO	2.5 hr	2-2.5 hr	1 hr	7 days
IV	End of infusion	End of infusion	1 hr	7 days

MISCELLANEOUS ACID-CONTROLLING DRUGS

There are a few other acid-controlling drugs that are unique in terms of their mechanisms and other features. These include sucralfate, misoprostol, and simethicone. They are profiled individually in the following paragraphs. Other drugs are bismuth subsalicylate (Pepto-Bismol; see Chapter 51) and metoclopramide (see Chapter 52).

DRUG PROFILES

◆ sucralfate

Sucralfate (Carafate) is a drug used as a mucosal protectant in the treatment of active stress ulcerations and in long-term therapy for peptic ulcer disease. Sucralfate acts locally, not systemically, binding directly to the surface of an ulcer. Sucralfate has as its basic structure a sugar, sucrose. Sulfate and aluminum hydroxide groups are attached to this sugar in the places where there are normally hydroxyl groups. Once sucralfate comes into contact with the acid of the stomach, it begins to dissociate into aluminum hydroxide (an antacid) and sulfate anions. The aluminum salt stimulates secretion of both mucus and bicarbonate base. The sulfated sucrose molecules of sucralfate are attracted to and bind to positively charge tissue proteins at the bases of ulcers and erosions, forming a protective barrier that can be thought of as a liquid bandage. By binding to the exposed proteins of ulcers and erosions, sucralfate also limits the access of pepsin. As noted earlier, pepsin is an enzyme that normally breaks down proteins in food but can have the same effect on GI epithelial tissue, either causing ulcers or making them worse. Sucralfate also binds and concentrates *epidermal growth factor*, present in the gastric tissues, which promotes ulcer healing. In addition, the drug stimulates the gastric secretion of prostaglandin molecules, which serve a mucoprotective function. Despite its many beneficial actions, sucralfate has fallen out of common use because its effects are transient and multiple daily dosing (up to four times daily) is therefore needed. It is indicated for stress ulcers, esophageal erosions, and peptic ulcer disease. The only usual contraindication to sucralfate use is drug allergy. Adverse effects are uncommon but include nausea, constipation, and dry mouth. Only minimal systemic absorption occurs, and the drug is virtually inert. Drug interactions mainly involve physical interference with the absorption of other drugs. This can be alleviated by taking other drugs at least 2 hours ahead of sucralfate. Sucralfate is also best given 1 hour before meals and at bedtime. It is a pregnancy category B drug that is normally dosed at 1 g orally four times daily.

PHARMACOKINETICS

Route	Onset of Action	Peak Plasma Concentration	Elimination Half-life	Duration of Action
PO	1 hr	2-4 hr	6-20 hr	3-6 hr

misoprostol

Misoprostol (Cytotec), a prostaglandin E analogue, has been shown to effectively reduce the incidence of gastric ulcers in patients taking NSAIDs (see Chapter 44). Prostaglandins have a wide variety of biologic activities. They are thought to inhibit gastric acid secretion. They are also believed to protect the gastric mucosa from injury (*cytoprotective* function), possibly by enhancing the local production of mucus or bicarbonate, by promoting local cell regeneration, and by helping to maintain mucosal blood flow. Use of misoprostol is contraindicated in patients with known drug allergy and in pregnant women (see later). Adverse effects include headache, GI distress, and vaginal bleeding. There are no major drug interactions, although antacids may reduce drug absorption.

Although some studies show that synthetic analogues of prostaglandins promote the healing of duodenal ulcers, the drugs must be used in dosages that usually produce disturbing adverse effects, such as abdominal cramps and diarrhea. Thus, they are not believed to be as effective as H_2 receptor antagonists and PPIs for this indication. Misoprostol is also used for its abortifacient properties as discussed in Chapter 34. For this reason, it is a pregnancy category X drug. The usual dosage is 200 mcg four times daily with meals for the duration of NSAID therapy in patients at high risk for ulceration.

PHARMACOKINETICS

Route	Onset of Action	Peak Plasma Concentration	Elimination Half-life	Duration of Action
PO	2 days	12 min	20-40 min	1-2 days

simethicone

Simethicone (Mylicon) is used to reduce the discomforts of gastric or intestinal gas (flatulence) and aid in its release via the mouth or rectum. It is therefore classified as an *antiflatulent* drug. Gas commonly appears in the GI tract as a consequence of the swallowing of air as well as normal digestive processes. Gas in the upper GI tract is composed of swallowed air and thus consists largely of nitrogen. It is usually expelled from the body by belching. The composition of flatus, however, is determined largely by the dietary intake of carbohydrates and the metabolic activity of the bacteria in the intestines.

Some foods, including legumes (beans) and cruciferous vegetables (e.g., cauliflower, broccoli), are well known for their gas-producing ability. Gas can also result from disorders such as diverticulitis, dyspepsia (heartburn), peptic ulcers, and spastic or irritable colon, and gaseous distention can occur postoperatively. Simethicone works by altering the elasticity of mucus-coated gas bubbles, which causes them to break into smaller ones. This reduces gas pain and facilitates the expulsion of gas via the mouth or rectum. Simethicone has no listed adverse effects, drug interactions, or pharmacokinetic parameters. It is available only for oral use. The usual simethicone dosage is 1 to 2 tablets four to six times daily as needed. A variety of different simethicone products are available for OTC use.

NURSING PROCESS

Assessment

Before an *acid-controlling drug* is given, a thorough patient assessment should be performed with attention to past and present medical history and special focus on GI tract–related disorders and signs and symptoms of ulcer disease and GERD. Current bowel patterns, any change in bowel patterns or GI tract functioning, and GI tract–related pain should also be assessed and documented. Results of baseline serum chemistry laboratory tests, as ordered, should be assessed with specific attention to hepatic function (e.g., serum ALP, ALT, AST levels) and renal function (serum creatinine level). Contraindications, cautions, and drug interactions have already been discussed, and a thorough assessment for these should be completed. The knowledge that acid-controlling drugs have many interactions should spark close attention to all medications the patient is taking, which underscores the importance of obtaining a medication history that includes information about prescription drugs, OTCs, and herbals. Other components of assessment include performing a physical examination and taking a thorough cardiac history with close attention

to a history of heart failure, hypertension, and/or other cardiac diseases, and the presence of edema, fluid and electrolyte imbalances, or renal disease. One reason it is important to assess for these conditions is that the high sodium content of various antacids may lead to exacerbation of cardiac problems, renal dysfunction, and fluid-electrolyte problems.

When *antacids* containing aluminum and/or magnesium are used, all other medications the patient is taking should be identified, and information about cautions and contraindications should be noted (see pharmacology discussion). It is important to note that combination products containing both magnesium and aluminum may have fewer adverse effects than either type of antacid by itself. For example, aluminum-containing antacids are associated with constipation, whereas magnesium-containing antacids may lead to diarrhea. The net effect of a combination of these antacids is a balancing out of both adverse effects and fewer problems with altered bowel patterns. Calcium-based antacids may also be used, especially as a source of calcium; however, they carry the risks of rebound hyperacidity, milk-alkali syndrome, and changes in systemic pH, especially if the patient has abnormal renal functioning (see Box 50-1). Sodium bicarbonate is generally not recommended as an antacid because of the high risk for systemic electrolyte disturbances and alkalosis. The sodium content of sodium bicarbonate is also high, and this is very problematic for patients who have hypertension, heart failure, or renal insufficiency.

For patients using *H_2 receptor antagonist drugs*, renal and liver function as well as level of consciousness should be assessed because of possible drug-related adverse effects. The elderly are known to react to these drugs with more disorientation and confusion. Drugs such as cimetidine and famotidine should not be administered simultaneously with antacids. These drugs may be spaced 1 hour apart if both drugs need to be given. Patients taking nizatidine or ranitidine require assessment of baseline blood chemistry results with attention to levels of BUN, creatinine, bilirubin, and ALP, AST, and ALT to document renal and hepatic functioning before treatment is initiated.

For *PPIs* (e.g., lansoprazole, omeprazole, and pantoprazole), assessment of swallowing capacity is required because of the size of some of the oral capsules. Assessment of renal and liver function and a complete blood count may be recommended prior to beginning therapy with these medications. Drug interactions have been discussed previously in the pharmacology section, and the patient's medication list should always be checked before this or any other type of medication is given.

Other drugs used by patients with GI disorders include sucralfate and simethicone. The use of simethicone (an antiflatulent) and sucralfate (an ulcer adherent) requires assessment of the patient's bowel patterns and bowel sounds, and evaluation for abdominal distention and rigidity. Treatment of peptic ulcer disease has become focused on the use of antibiotics (to attack the *H. pylori* bacteria) with frequent dosing of other drugs. The GI tract should be assessed, and signs and symptoms should be noted. With misoprostol, pregnancy should be ruled out prior to use.

Nursing Diagnoses

- Acute pain related to gastric hyperacidity and other GI disorders such as ulcer disease
- Constipation related to the adverse effects of aluminum-containing antacids and other drugs used to treat hyperacidity

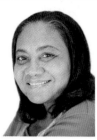

CASE STUDY

Proton Pump Inhibitors

A 50-year-old attorney has self-treated for heartburn for years by drinking large amounts of antacids. She finally made an appointment with her family practice physician, who referred her to a gastroenterologist. Her family practice physician instructed her to stop taking the antacids.

1. Why did the physician ask her to stop taking the antacids?

In a few weeks, the attorney had an endoscopy, and it was discovered that she had gastroesophageal reflux disease (GERD) and gastritis secondary to stress-induced hyperacidity. The physician has prescribed the proton pump inhibitor (PPI) omeprazole (Prilosec) 20 mg once a day.

2. What other conditions will the gastroenterologist test for during this diagnostic stage?
3. What is the rationale for the use of PPIs to treat GERD?
4. What patient teaching is important regarding the PPI?

© Rob Marmion

For answers, see *http://evolve.elsevier.com/Lilley*.

- Diarrhea related to the adverse effects of magnesium-containing antacids and other drugs used to treat hyperacidity
- Deficient knowledge related to lack of information about antacids, H₂ receptor antagonists, or PPIs, including their use and potential adverse effects

Planning

Goals

- Patient has minimal to no pain during therapy with antacids or other acid-controlling drugs.
- Patient experiences minimal adverse effects while using antacids or other acid-controlling drugs.
- Patient remains compliant with the therapeutic regimen.

Outcome Criteria

- Patient experiences increased comfort related to the use of acid-controlling drugs, abdominal massage, application of heat if appropriate, and frequent repositioning.
- Patient states adverse effects of antacids, H₂ receptor antagonists, and PPIs, including constipation, diarrhea, headache, and confusion, and seeks advice from the prescriber if adverse effects worsen or are not relieved after several days.
- Patient states the importance of compliance with the drug regimen and strict adherence to medication instructions regarding the use of acid-controlling drugs to adequately resolve symptoms of the hyperacidity or other GI disorder.

Implementation

When giving acid-controlling drugs, the nurse should always be sure that chewable tablets are chewed thoroughly by the patient and that liquid forms are thoroughly shaken before they are taken. *Antacids* should be given with at least 8 oz of water to enhance absorption of the antacid in the stomach, except for newer forms that are rapidly dissolving drugs. Should constipation or diarrhea occur with single-component drugs, the nurse

should suggest a combination aluminum- and magnesium-based product to the prescriber and educate the patient about the adverse effects of aluminum-only or magnesium-only products. It is also recommended that antacids be given as ordered but not within 1 to 2 hours of other medications because of the effect of antacids on the absorption of oral medications. This dosing schedule can be implemented safely by the nurse without interrupting safe dosing of other medications. The dosing will differ if the prescriber has ordered the drug to be given with antacids. Antacid overuse or misuse, or the rapid discontinuation of antacids with high acid-neutralizing capacity, may lead to acid rebound. Therefore, antacids should be used only as prescribed and/or as directed.

Because so many *H₂ receptor antagonists* and other acid-controlling drugs are now available OTC, it is important to instruct the patient about proper use (see Patient Teaching Tips). For example, cimetidine should be taken with meals, and antacids, if also used, should be taken 1 hour before or after the cimetidine. Intravenous dosing and related mixing and infusing for intravenous cimetidine are similar to those described later for intravenous famotidine. Famotidine may be given orally in tablet or suspension form and without regard to meals or food. Rapid release forms of famotidine dissolve quickly under the patient's tongue and can be taken without water. Ranitidine should be given as ordered and, if administered with antacids, should be given 1 hour before or after the antacid. Intravenous forms of famotidine or ranitidine should be diluted with appropriate solutions and given within the documented time frame. With intravenous ranitidine, cardiac irregularities and hypotension may occur with rapid infusion. The nurse should refer to appropriate sources for information on other specific drugs and their intravenous administration. For all these H₂ receptor antagonists, blood pressure readings should be monitored as needed during intravenous infusion because of the risk of hypotension. The patient should continue to be monitored for GI tract bleeding with the diagnosis of ulcers or GI irritation. Blood in the stools or the occurrence of black, tarry stools or hematemesis should be reported. The nurse should also listen to bowel sounds and examine the abdomen to monitor for possible complications.

With *PPIs*, lansoprazole oral dosage forms should be given as ordered and with fluids. If the patient has difficulty swallowing these capsules, a capsule may be opened and the granules sprinkled over at least a tablespoon of applesauce, which should be swallowed immediately. The nurse should be sure to monitor for abdominal pain, distention, and abnormal bowel sounds. Omeprazole should be administered before meals, and the capsule should be taken whole and not crushed, opened, or chewed. Omeprazole may also be given with antacids if ordered. The nurse should always double-check the names and dosages of these drugs to ensure that they are not confused with similarly named drugs. Pantoprazole may be given orally without crushing or splitting of the tablet form. Intravenous pantoprazole should be given exactly as ordered using the correct dilutional fluids and infusion over the recommended time period.

Other drugs such as simethicone may also be added to the oral medication protocol with PPIs. Simethicone is usually well tolerated. It is to be taken *after* meals and at bedtime. Tablets should be chewed thoroughly and suspensions shaken well before use. Sucralfate is usually given 1 hour before meals and at bedtime. Tablets may be crushed or dissolved in water, if needed. Antacids should be avoided for 30 minutes before or after administration of sucralfate. Misoprostol should be given with food and is usually ordered to be taken with meals and at bedtime. Suggestions for patient education for these drugs are presented in Patient Teaching Tips.

Evaluation

Therapeutic response to the administration of *antacids, H₂ receptor antagonists, PPIs,* and *other related drugs* includes the relief of symptoms associated with peptic ulcer, gastritis, esophagitis, gastric hyperacidity, or hiatal hernia (i.e., decrease in epigastric pain, fullness, and abdominal swelling). Adverse effects for which to monitor include all of those listed for each of the drug categories and range from constipation or diarrhea to nausea, vomiting, abdominal pain, hypotension, and cardiac irregularities. Milk-alkali syndrome, acid rebound, hypercalcemia, and metabolic alkalosis are known complications associated with the various antacids; the patient must also be evaluated for these adverse effects and measures taken to prevent or resolve them. Therapeutic response to all of the drugs in the various categories discussed in this chapter is also measured by evaluating whether the identified goals and outcome criteria have been met.

PATIENT TEACHING TIPS

- Medications should not be taken, unless prescribed, within 1 to 2 hours of taking an antacid because of their impact on the absorption of many medications in the stomach.
- The prescriber should be contacted immediately if the patient experiences severe or prolonged constipation and/or diarrhea; increase in abdominal pain; abdominal distension; nausea; vomiting; hematemesis; or black, tarry stools (a sign of possible GI tract bleeding).
- If the patient is taking enteric-coated medications, the patient should know that the use of antacids may promote premature dissolution of the enteric coating. Enteric coatings are used to diminish the stomach upset caused by irritating medications, and if the coating is destroyed early in the stomach, gastric upset may occur.
- Encourage patient to take H₂ receptor antagonists exactly as prescribed. Inform patient about how smoking decreases the drug's effectiveness. H₂ receptor antagonists should not be taken within 1 hour of antacids, and the patient should be told that occurrence of a prolonged headache with therapy should be reported to the prescriber immediately. A patient requiring treatment with these drugs should also be encouraged to avoid aspirin, other NSAIDs, alcohol, and/or caffeine because of their ulcerogenic or irritating effects on the GI tract.
- Omeprazole and other PPIs should be taken before meals, and the patient should be told that if lansoprazole is being used, the granules may be sprinkled from the capsule into a tablespoon of applesauce if needed. If lansoprazole is taken with sucralfate, it should be taken 30 minutes before the latter drug.
- The patient should follow the manufacturer's directions when taking simethicone. Chewable forms must always be chewed thoroughly; liquid preparations should be shaken thoroughly before administration. A patient with a gas problem or flatulence should be encouraged to avoid problematic foods (e.g., spicy, gas-producing foods) and carbonated beverages.
- Sucralfate should be taken on an empty stomach, and antacids should be avoided or, if indicated, taken 2 hours before or 1 hour after sucralfate administration. Taking sips of tepid water, keeping fluids nearby, and using sugarless or sour hard candy may help relieve dry mouth.
- For a patient taking the drug regimen for the treatment of *H. pylori* infection–peptic ulcer disease, it is important to emphasize the need to take each drug, including the antibiotics, exactly as prescribed and without fail to guarantee success in the treatment. If treatment protocols are not followed appropriately, the condition may likely reoccur.

POINTS TO REMEMBER

- The stomach secretes many substances (hydrochloric acid, pepsinogen, mucus, bicarbonate, intrinsic factor, and prostaglandins).
- The parietal cell is responsible for the production of acid.
- In acid-related disorders there is an impairment of the balance among the substances secreted by the stomach.
- H₂ receptor antagonists are H₂ blockers that bind to and block histamine receptors located on parietal cells. This blockade renders these cells less responsive to stimuli and thus decreases their acid secretion. Up to 90% inhibition of acid secretion can be achieved with the H₂ receptor antagonists.
- PPIs block the final step in the acid production pathway, the hydrogen-potassium-ATPase pump, and they block all acid secretion.
- Sucralfate is used for the treatment of peptic ulcer disease and stress-related ulcers. It binds to tissue proteins in the eroded area and prevents exposure of the ulcerated area to stomach acid.
- Misoprostol is a synthetic prostaglandin analogue that inhibits gastric acid secretion and is used to prevent NSAID-related ulcers.
- Cautious use of antacids is recommended in patients who have heart failure, hypertension, or other cardiac diseases or who require sodium restriction, especially if the antacid is high in sodium.
- Many drug interactions occur with the acid-controlling drugs due to alteration of oral dosage forms, and so other medications should not be taken within 1 to 2 hours of taking an antacid. Antacids are sometimes to be avoided when other acid-controlling drugs are taken.
- Magnesium-aluminum combination antacids are used to prevent the adverse effects of constipation and diarrhea. Some of the more serious concerns with antacids include acid rebound, hypercalcemia, milk-alkali syndrome, and metabolic alkalosis.

NCLEX EXAMINATION REVIEW QUESTIONS

1 A 30-year-old business executive is taking simethicone for excessive flatus associated with diverticulitis. During a patient teaching session, the nurse explains the mechanism of action of simethicone by saying:
   a "It neutralizes gastric pH, thereby preventing gas."
   b "It buffers the effects of pepsin on the gastric wall."
   c "It decreases gastric acid secretion and thereby minimizes flatus."
   d "It causes mucus-coated gas bubbles to break into smaller ones."

2 When evaluating the medication list of a patient who will be starting therapy with an H₂ receptor antagonist, the nurse is aware that which drug may interact with it?
   a Codeine
   b Penicillin
   c Ketoconazole
   d Acetaminophen

3 When administering sucralfate, which action by the nurse is most correct?
   a Giving the drug with meals
   b Giving the drug on an empty stomach
   c Instructing the patient to restrict fluids
   d Waiting 30 minutes before administering other drugs

4 A patient with a history of renal problems is asking for advice about which antacid he should use. What should the nurse recommend?

   a Antacids should not be used by patients who have renal problems.
   b The patient should choose antacids that are aluminum based.
   c The patient should choose antacids that are calcium based.
   d The patient should choose antacids that are magnesium based.

5 A patient who is taking oral tetracycline complains of heartburn and requests an antacid. The nurse should
   a give the tetracycline, but delay the antacid for 1 to 2 hours.
   b give the antacid, but delay the tetracycline for at least 4 hours.
   c administer both medications together.
   d explain that the antacid cannot be given while the patient is taking the tetracycline.

6 When the nurse is administering a PPI, which actions by the nurse are most correct? (Select all that apply.)
   a Giving the PPI on an empty stomach
   b Giving the PPI with meals
   c Making sure the patient does not crush or chew the capsules
   d Instructing the patient to open the capsule and chew the contents for best absorption
   e Administering the PPI only when the patient complains of heartburn

1. d, 2. c, 3. b, 4. b, 5. a, 6. a, c.

CRITICAL THINKING ACTIVITIES: BEST ACTION

1 A father brings his 2-month-old infant to the pediatric clinic and says, "He seems to have so much gas! Is there anything that can help?" The pediatrician suggests an infant formulation of simethicone. The father asks, "What does this drug do?" What is the nurse's best answer?

2 A patient wants to use an antacid, but he has been told that he has decreased renal function. What is the nurse's best answer when he asks, "What antacids can I use?" Explain your answer.

3 A patient tells the nurse, "I like taking antacids because they coat my stomach and protect my ulcer." What is the nurse's best response to this statement?

For answers, see *http://evolve.elsevier.com/Lilley*.

CHAPTER 51

Bowel Disorder Drugs

OBJECTIVES

When you reach the end of this chapter, you should be able to do the following:

1 Discuss the anatomy and physiology of the gastrointestinal tract, including the process of peristalsis.

2 Identify the various factors affecting bowel elimination and/or bowel patterns.

3 List the various groups of drugs used to treat alterations in bowel elimination, specifically diarrhea, constipation, and irritable bowel syndrome (IBS).

4 Discuss the mechanisms of action, indications, cautions, contraindications, drug interactions, dosages, routes of administration, and adverse effects of the various antidiarrheals, laxatives, and IBS drugs.

5 Develop a nursing care plan that includes all phases of the nursing process for patients taking antidiarrheals, laxatives, and IBS drugs.

e-Learning Activities

http://evolve.elsevier.com/Lilley

NCLEX Review Questions • Animations • Nursing Care Plans • Audio Glossary • Category Catchers • Medication Errors Checklists • IV Therapy Checklists • Calculators • Frequently Asked Questions • Content Updates • Supplemental Resources • Answers to Case Studies and Critical Thinking Activities

Drug Profiles

belladonna alkaloid combinations, p. 800
bisacodyl, p. 805
bismuth subsalicylate, p. 799
◆ diphenoxylate with atropine, p. 800
◆ docusate salts, p. 803
◆ glycerin, p. 803
Lactobacillus, p. 800

◆ lactulose, p. 805
◆ loperamide, p. 800
magnesium salts, p. 805
methylcellulose, p. 803
mineral oil, p. 803
polyethylene glycol 3350, p. 805
◆ psyllium, p. 803
◆ senna, p. 806

◆ *Key drug.*

Glossary

Antidiarrheal drugs Drugs that counter or combat diarrhea. (p. 797)
Constipation A condition of abnormally infrequent and difficult passage of feces through the lower gastrointestinal tract. (p. 800)
Diarrhea The abnormally frequent passage of loose stools. (p. 797)
Irritable bowel syndrome (IBS) A recurring condition of the intestinal tract characterized by bloating, flatulence, and often periods of diarrhea that alternate with periods of constipation. (p. 806)
Laxatives Drugs that promote bowel evacuation, such as by increasing the bulk of the feces, softening the stool, or lubricating the intestinal wall. (p. 800)

• • •

Anatomy, Physiology, and Disease Overview

Diarrhea and the diseases associated with it account for 5 to 8 million deaths per year in infants and small children and are among the leading causes of death and morbidity in underdeveloped nations. The key symptoms of gastrointestinal (GI) disease are abdominal pain, nausea and/or vomiting, and diarrhea. **Diarrhea** is defined as the passage of stools with abnormally increased frequency, fluidity, and weight, or increased stool water excretion. *Acute diarrhea* refers to diarrhea of sudden onset in a previously healthy individual. It lasts from 3 days to 2 weeks and is self-limiting, resolving without sequelae. *Chronic diarrhea* lasts for longer than 3 to 4 weeks and is associated with recurrent passage of diarrheal stools, possible fever, loss of appetite, nausea, vomiting, weight reduction, and chronic weakness.

The probable cause of diarrhea should be taken into consideration when designing a drug regimen to treat it. Causes of acute diarrhea include drugs, bacteria, viruses, nutritional factors, and protozoa. Causes of chronic diarrhea include tumors, acquired immunodeficiency syndrome (AIDS), diabetes mellitus, hyperthyroidism, Addison's disease, and irritable bowel syndrome. Treatment is directed at the cessation of the increased stool frequency associated with diarrhea, alleviation of abdominal cramps, fluid resuscitation and electrolyte replacement, and prevention of weight loss and nutritional deficits from malabsorption. Often, replacement of fluids is the only treatment needed. Patients with diarrhea associated with a bacterial or parasite infection should not use antidiarrheal drugs, because this will cause the organism to stay in the body longer and will prolong recovery.

Pharmacology Overview

ANTIDIARRHEALS

Drugs used to treat diarrhea are called **antidiarrheal drugs.** They are divided into different groups based on the specific mechanism of action: *adsorbents, antimotility drugs* (anticholinergics and opi-

TABLE 51-1 Antidiarrheals: Drug Categories and Selected Drugs

Category	Antidiarrheal Drugs
Adsorbents	activated charcoal, aluminum hydroxide, bismuth subsalicylate, cholestyramine, polycarbophil
Anticholinergics	atropine, hyoscyamine
Opiates	opium tincture, paregoric, codeine, diphenoxylate, loperamide
Intestinal flora modifiers	*Lactobacillus acidophilus, Lactobacillus GG*

TABLE 51-2 Selected Antidiarrheals: Adverse Effects

Drug	Adverse Effects
bismuth subsalicylate	Increased bleeding time, constipation, dark stools, confusion, tinnitus, metallic taste, blue gums
atropine, hyoscyamine	Urinary retention and hesitancy, impotence, headache, dizziness, anxiety, drowsiness, confusion, bradycardia, hypotension, dry skin, flushing, blurred vision, increased pressure in eyes
codeine, diphenoxylate	Drowsiness, sedation, dizziness, lethargy, nausea, vomiting, constipation, hypotension, urinary retention, flushing, respiratory depression

ates), and *intestinal flora modifiers* (also known as *probiotics* and *bacterial replacement drugs*). The specific classes and the drugs in each are listed in Table 51-1. Please note that antidiarrheal and laxative drugs do not have the classic pharmacokinetics of other drugs, and thus pharmacokinetics tables such as those presented throughout the book are not included in this chapter.

Mechanism of Action and Drug Effects

Antidiarrheal drugs have varying mechanisms of action. *Adsorbents* act by coating the walls of the GI tract. They bind the causative bacteria or toxin to their adsorbent surface for elimination from the body through the stool. *Adsorption* is similar to absorption but differs in that it involves the chemical binding of substances (e.g., ions, bacterial toxins) onto the *surface* of an adsorbent. In contrast, *absorption* generally refers to the penetration of a substance into the *interior* structure of the adsorbant or the uptake of a substance across a surface (e.g., the absorption of dietary nutrients into the intestinal villi). The adsorbent bismuth subsalicylate is a form of aspirin, or acetylsalicylic acid, and therefore it also has many of the same drug effects as aspirin (see Chapter 44). Activated charcoal not only is helpful in coating the walls of the GI tract and adsorbing bacteria but also is useful in cases of overdose because of its drug-binding properties. The antilipemic drugs colestipol and cholestyramine (see Chapter 29) are anion exchange resins that are sometimes prescribed as antidiarrheal adsorbents and lipid-lowering drugs. Besides binding to diarrhea-causing toxins, they have the additional benefit of decreasing cholesterol levels.

Anticholinergic drugs work to slow peristalsis by reducing the rhythmic contractions and smooth muscle tone of the GI tract. They are used in combination with adsorbents and opiates (see later). Anticholinergics are discussed in detail in Chapter 21.

Intestinal flora modifiers are products obtained from bacterial cultures, most commonly *Lactobacillus* organisms, which make up the majority of the body's normal bacterial flora. These organisms are commonly destroyed by antibiotics. Intestinal flora modifiers work by replenishing these bacteria, which helps to restore the balance of normal flora and suppress the growth of diarrhea-causing bacteria.

The primary action of *opiates* (see Chapter 11) in diarrhea treatment is to reduce bowel motility. A secondary effect that make opiates beneficial in the treatment of diarrhea is reduction of the pain associated with diarrhea by relief of rectal spasms. Because they decrease the transit time of food through the GI tract, they permit longer contact of the intestinal contents with the absorptive surface of the bowel, which increases the absorp-

tion of water, electrolytes, and other nutrients from the bowel and reduces stool frequency and net volume.

Indications

Antidiarrheal drugs are indicated for the treatment of diarrhea of various types and levels of severity. Adsorbents are more likely to be used in milder cases, whereas anticholinergics and opiates tend to be used in more severe cases. Intestinal flora modifiers are often helpful in patients with antibiotic-induced diarrhea.

Contraindications

Contraindications to the use of antidiarrheals include known drug allergy and any major acute GI condition, such as intestinal obstruction or colitis, unless the drug is ordered by the patient's prescriber after careful consideration of the specific case.

Adverse Effects

The adverse effects of the antidiarrheals are specific to each drug family. Most of these potential effects are minor and are not life threatening. The major adverse effects of specific drugs in each drug class are listed in Table 51-2. Intestinal flora modifiers do not have any listed adverse effects.

Interactions

Many drugs are absorbed from the intestines into the bloodstream, where they are delivered to their respective sites of action. A number of the antidiarrheals have the potential to alter this normal process, by either increasing or decreasing the absorption of these other drugs.

The adsorbents can decrease the effectiveness of many drugs primarily by decreasing the absorption of certain drugs. Examples include digoxin, clindamycin, quinidine, probenecid, and hypoglycemic drugs. The oral anticoagulant warfarin (see Chapter 28) is more likely to cause increased bleeding times or bruising when coadministered with adsorbents. This is thought to be because the adsorbents bind to vitamin K, which is needed to make certain clotting factors. Vitamin K is synthesized by the normal bacterial flora in the bowel. The toxic effects of methotrexate are more likely to occur when it is given with adsorbents.

The therapeutic effects of the anticholinergic antidiarrheals can be decreased by coadministration with antacids. Amanta-

DOSAGES

Selected Antidiarrheal Drugs

Drug (Pregnancy Category)	Pharmacologic Class/Indication	Usual Dosage Range	Onset of Action
belladonna alkaloids/phenobarbital combinations (Donnatal Elixir, Donnatal capsules and tablets, Donnatal Extentabs) (C to X)	Fixed-combination anticholinergic/diarrhea	**Adult** PO: Donnatal Elixir, 5-10 mL tid-qid Donnatal capsules and tablets, 1-2 caps or tabs tid-qid PO: Donnatal Extentabs, 1 tab q8-12h	1-2 hr
bismuth subsalicylate (Pepto-Bismol) (D)	Antimicrobial, antidiarrheal/diarrhea	Doses repeated q30-60 min, not to exceed 8 per day; all doses PO **Pediatric 3-5 yr** 5 mL or ⅓ tab **Pediatric 6-12 yr** 10 mL or ⅔ tab **Adult** 30 mL or 2 tab	0.5-2 hr
◆ diphenoxylate with atropine (Lomotil) (C)	Opioid with anticholinergic/diarrhea	**Pediatric 2-12 yr** 0.3-0.4 mg/kg/day in 4 divided doses; use with caution in young children due to variable response **Adult** 2 tabs qid (max of 8 tabs/day)	40-60 min
Lactobacillus acidophilus (Bacid, Lactinex) (A)	Intestinal flora modifier/dietary supplementation,* diarrhea, need for bacterial replacement	**Adult** PO (Bacid): 2 caps bid-qid PO (Lactinex): 1 packet granules with liquid or food tid-qid; 4 tabs tid-qid with liquid or food	Unknown
◆ loperamide (Imodium A-D, Pepto Diarrhea Control) (B)	Opiate antidiarrheal/diarrhea	**Pediatric 2-5 yr** PO: 1 mg tid (liquid only) **Pediatric 6-8 yr (21.8-26.8 kg)** PO: 2 mg after the first unformed stool, followed by 1 mg PO after each subsequent unformed stool; not to exceed 4 mg/day for 2 days **Pediatric 9-12 yr (27.3-43.2 kg)** PO: 2 mg after the first unformed stool, followed by 1 mg PO after each subsequent unformed stool; not to exceed 6 mg/day for 2 days **Adult** PO: 4 mg followed by 2 mg after each BM (not to exceed 16 mg/day)	1-3 hr

BM, Bowel movement; *PO,* oral.

*Often used to treat uncomplicated diarrhea, although this is an off-label (non–U.S. Food and Drug Administration approved) use.

dine, tricyclic antidepressants, monoamine oxidase inhibitors, opiates, and antihistamines, when given with anticholinergics, can result in increased anticholinergic effects. The opiate antidiarrheals have additive central nervous system (CNS) depressant effects if they are given with CNS depressants, alcohol, narcotics, sedatives-hypnotics, antipsychotics, or skeletal muscle relaxants.

Bismuth subsalicylate can lead to increased bleeding times and bruising when administered with warfarin as well as aspirin and other nonsteroidal antiinflammatory drugs. It can also cause confusion in the elderly. Cholestyramine, when administered with glipizide, can result in decreased hypoglycemic effects. Cholestyramine also decreases the absorption of any drug that is given within 2 hours of it. It is important for the nurse not to give any drug within 2 hours before or 2 hours after cholestyramine.

Dosages

For the recommended dosages of antidiarrheal drugs, see the Dosages table on p. 799.

DRUG PROFILES

Drug therapy for diarrhea depends on the specific cause of the diarrhea (if known). All antidiarrheals are orally administered drugs available as suspensions, tablets, or capsules. Some antidiarrheals are over-the-counter (OTC) medications, whereas others require a prescription.

ADSORBENTS
bismuth subsalicylate
Bismuth subsalicylate (Pepto-Bismol) is a salicylate by chemical structure; therefore, it should be used with caution in children and teenagers who have or are recovering from chickenpox or influenza because of the risk of Reye's syndrome (see Life Span Considerations: The Pediatric Patient box). It can also cause all of the adverse effects that are associated with an aspirin-based product (see Chapter 44). Two alarming but harmless adverse effects are temporary darkening of the tongue and the stool. Bismuth subsalicylate is available OTC for oral use.

ANTICHOLINERGICS
The anticholinergics atropine and hyoscyamine are used either alone or in combination with other antidiarrheals because they

Antidiarrheal Preparations

- If diarrhea is accompanied by fever, malaise, or abdominal pain, contact the prescriber immediately because of the possibility of excessive fluid and electrolyte loss. Dehydration and electrolyte loss occur very rapidly in the pediatric patient because of the patient's size and sensitivity to loss of fluid volume and electrolytes through the stool.
- Always contact the prescriber or pharmacist for the proper dosage of antidiarrheals if the child is 6 years of age or younger or if there is any doubt as to proper dosing. Never hesitate to contact the prescriber with any concern or question regarding any medication recommended for the pediatric patient.
- Bismuth subsalicylate is a salicylate by chemical structure; therefore, it should be used with caution in children and teenagers because of the risk of Reye's syndrome (see p. 799).
- Immediately report to the prescriber any abdominal distention, firm abdomen, painful abdomen, or worsening of or lack of improvement in diarrhea 24 to 48 hours after medication administration. Measurement of the amount of diarrhea by the number of soiled diapers or number of stools per day provides important information.
- Antidiarrheal preparations should always be given cautiously to the pediatric patient. If symptoms persist or dehydration occurs (e.g., no tears and decreased urine output in the child), contact the prescriber.
- If the patient is sluggish, lethargic, or confused or the diarrhea is bloody, contact the prescriber immediately or go to the closest emergency facility.

slow GI tract motility. These drugs are referred to as *belladonna alkaloids* and are discussed in Chapter 21. Their safety margin is not as wide as that of many of the other antidiarrheals, because they can cause serious adverse effects if used inappropriately. For this reason they are available only by prescription.

belladonna alkaloid combinations

Belladonna alkaloids can be used to treat many GI disorders, including diarrhea; however, their use is limited. Donnatal is the most commonly used drug in this class. Use of the belladonna alkaloid preparations is contraindicated in patients who have shown a hypersensitivity to anticholinergics and in patients with narrow-angle glaucoma, GI obstruction, myasthenia gravis, paralytic ileus, and toxic megacolon. Donnatal tablets contain a combination of four different alkaloids: atropine, hyoscyamine, phenobarbital, and scopolamine. Available dosage forms of this combination include elixir, tablets, and extended-release tablets. Donnatal Extentabs contain increased amounts of the aforementioned ingredients. Pregnancy category C to X, depending on the ingredients of the specific product.

OPIATES

There are five opiate-related antidiarrheal drugs: codeine, diphenoxylate with atropine, loperamide, paregoric, and tincture of opium. The only opiate-related antidiarrheal that is available as an OTC medication is loperamide; all others are prescription-only drugs because of the risks of respiratory depression and dependency associated with opiate use. Numerous medication errors and deaths have been reported with paregoric and tincture of opium. For those reasons, their use is very limited.

◆ diphenoxylate with atropine

Diphenoxylate (Lomotil, Lonox) is a synthetic opiate agonist that is structurally related to meperidine. It acts on smooth muscle of the intestinal tract, inhibiting GI motility and excessive GI propulsion.

It has little or no analgesic activity; however, because it is an opioid, abuse and physical dependence may occur. Diphenoxylate is combined with subtherapeutic quantities of atropine to discourage its use as a recreational opiate drug. The amount of atropine present in the combination is too small to interfere with the conjugated diphenoxylate. When taken in large dosages, however, the combination results in extreme anticholinergic effects (e.g., dry mouth, abdominal pain, tachycardia, blurred vision).

Use of the combination of diphenoxylate and atropine is contraindicated in patients experiencing diarrhea associated with pseudomembranous colitis or toxigenic bacteria, because the drug's anticholinergic effects might be problematic in such conditions. This drug product is available only for oral use.

◆ loperamide

Loperamide (Imodium A-D) is a synthetic antidiarrheal that is similar to diphenoxylate. It inhibits both peristalsis in the intestinal wall and intestinal secretion, thereby decreasing the number of stools and their water content. Although the drug exhibits many characteristics of the opiate class, physical dependence on loperamide has not been reported. Because of its safety profile it is the only opiate antidiarrheal drug that is available as an OTC medication. Loperamide use is contraindicated in patients with severe ulcerative colitis, pseudomembranous colitis, and acute diarrhea associated with *Escherichia coli*.

INTESTINAL FLORA MODIFIERS

Intestinal flora modifiers suppress the growth of diarrhea-causing bacteria and reestablish the flora that normally reside in the intestine. They are bacterial cultures of *Lactobacillus* organisms.

Lactobacillus

Lactobacillus acidophilus (Bacid) and *Lactobacillus GG* (Culturelle) are acid-producing bacteria prepared in a concentrated, dried culture for oral administration. They are a normal inhabitant of the GI tract where, through the fermentation of carbohydrates (which produces lactic acid), they create an unfavorable environment for the overgrowth of harmful fungi and bacteria. *L. acidophilus* has been used for more than 75 years for the treatment of uncomplicated diarrhea, particularly that caused by antibiotic therapy that destroys normal intestinal flora.

LAXATIVES

Laxatives are used for the treatment of **constipation,** which is defined as the abnormally infrequent and difficult passage of feces through the lower GI tract. Constipation is a symptom, not a disease; it is a disorder of movement through the colon and/or rectum that can be caused by a variety of diseases or drugs. Some of the more common causes of constipation are listed in Table 51-3.

The GI tract is responsible for the digestive process, which involves (1) ingestion of dietary intake, (2) digestion of dietary intake into basic nutrients, (3) absorption of basic nutrients, and (4) storage and removal of fecal material via defecation (Figure 51-1).

Ingestion → digestion → absorption → storage and removal

The usual time span between ingestion and defecation is 24 to 36 hours. The last segment of the GI tract, the large intestine (colon), is responsible for (1) forming the stool by removing excess water from the fecal material, (2) temporarily storing the stool until defecation, and (3) extracting essential vitamins from the intestinal bacteria (especially vitamin K). The colon is 120 to 150 cm long and is separated from the small intestine by the ileocecal valve. The colon extends into the rectum, which terminates at the anus. The rectum is the temporary storage site for the stool, which is composed of water and unabsorbed and indigestible material. Evacuation of the rectal contents is accomplished by bowel movements.

A bowel movement (defecation) is a reflex act that involves both smooth and skeletal muscles. The entry of feces into the rectum stimulates mass peristaltic movement that results in a bowel movement. However, voluntary initiation or inhibition of defecation is also possible via skeletal muscle pathways.

TABLE 51-3 Causes of Constipation

Cause	Examples
Adverse drug effects	Analgesics, anticholinergics, iron supplements, aluminum antacids, calcium antacids, opiates, calcium channel blockers
Lifestyle	Poor bowel movement habits: voluntary refusal to defecate resulting in constipation
	Diet: poor fluid intake and/or low-residue (low-roughage) diet or excessive consumption of dairy products
	Physical inactivity: lack of proper exercise, especially in elderly individuals
	Psychologic factors: anxiety, stress, hypochondria
Metabolic and endocrine disorders	Diabetes mellitus, hypothyroidism, pregnancy, hypercalcemia, hypokalemia
Neurogenic disorders	Autonomic neuropathy, intestinal pseudo-obstruction, multiple sclerosis, spinal cord lesions, Parkinson's disease, stroke

Treatment of constipation should be individualized, with consideration of the patient's age, concerns, and expectations; duration and severity of constipation; and potential contributing factors. Treatment can be either surgical (in extreme cases) or nonsurgical. Nonsurgical treatments can be separated into three broad approaches: dietary (e.g., fiber supplementation), behavioral (e.g., increased physical activity), and pharmacologic. The focus in this chapter is on pharmacologic treatment.

Laxatives are among the most misused OTC medications. Long-term and often inappropriate use of laxatives may result in laxative dependence, produce damage to the bowel, or lead to previously nonexistent intestinal problems. With the exception of the bulk-forming type, laxatives should not be used for long periods. Laxatives are divided into five major groups based on their mechanism of action: bulk forming, emollient, hyperosmotic, saline, and stimulant laxatives. Table 51-4 lists the currently available laxative drugs categorized by drug family. The onset of action of laxatives is the most important pharmacokinetic feature of these drugs and is listed in the Dosage table on p. 804.

Mechanism of Action and Drug Effects

All laxatives promote bowel movements, but each class of laxative has a different mechanism of action. Laxatives may act by (1) affecting fecal consistency, (2) increasing fecal movement through the colon, and/or (3) facilitating defecation through the rectum. *Bulk-forming laxatives* act in a manner similar to that of the fiber naturally contained in the diet. They absorb water into the intestine, which increases bulk and distends the bowel to initiate reflex bowel activity, thus promoting a bowel movement.

Emollient laxatives are also referred to as *stool softeners* (docusate salts) and *lubricant laxatives* (mineral oil). Fecal soft-

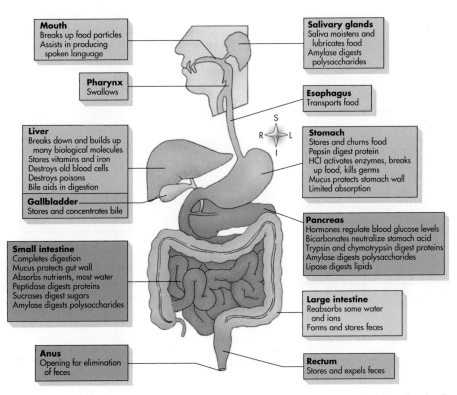

FIGURE 51-1 The digestive system. (From Patton KT, Thibodeau GA: *Mosby's handbook of anatomy and physiology*, St Louis, 2000, Mosby.)

eners work by lowering the surface tension of GI fluids, so that more water and fat are absorbed into the stool and the intestines. The lubricant type of emollient laxatives works by lubricating the fecal material and the intestinal wall and preventing absorption of water from the intestines. Instead of being absorbed, this water in the bowel softens and expands the stool. This promotes bowel distension and reflex peristaltic actions, which ultimately lead to defecation.

Hyperosmotic laxatives work by increasing fecal water content, which results in distention, increased peristalsis, and evacuation. Their site of action is limited to the large intestine. *Saline laxatives* increase osmotic pressure in the small intestine by inhibiting water absorption and increasing both water and electrolyte (salt) secretions from the bowel wall into the bowel lumen. This results in a watery stool. The increased distention promotes peristalsis and evacuation. Rectal enemas of sodium phosphate, a saline laxative, produce defecation 2 to 5 minutes after administration.

As the name implies, *stimulant laxatives* stimulate the nerves that innervate the intestines, which results in increased peristalsis. They also increase fluid in the colon, which increases bulk and softens the stool. Table 51-5 summarizes the specific drug effects of the different classes of laxatives.

In 2008, a new class of drugs was approved for the treatment of very specific types of constipation related to opioid use and bowel resection surgery. These peripherally acting opioid antagonists include methylnaltrexone (Relistor) and alvimopan (Entereg). These drugs block the entrance of an opioid drug into the bowel cells, thus allowing bowels to function normally, even with continued opioid use. Methylnaltrexone is approved only for terminally ill (hospice) patients who have opioid-induced constipation. It is available as an injection only and is given once a day. Alvimopan is indicated to accelerate GI recovery time following partial large or small bowel resection surgery. Patients must be hospitalized and registered to receive Alvimopan.

Indications

The following are some of the more common uses of laxatives:
- Facilitation of bowel movements in patients with inactive colon or anorectal disorders
- Reduction of ammonia absorption in hepatic encephalopathy (lactulose only)
- Treatment of drug-induced constipation
- Treatment of constipation associated with pregnancy and/or postobstetric period
- Treatment of constipation caused by reduced physical activity or poor dietary habits
- Removal of toxic substances from the body
- Facilitation of defecation in megacolon
- Preparation for colonic diagnostic procedures or surgery

See Table 51-6 for specific therapeutic indications for each laxative drug class.

Contraindications

All categories of laxatives share the same general contraindications and precautions, including avoidance in cases of drug allergy and the need for cautious use in the presence of the following: acute surgical abdomen; appendicitis symptoms such as abdominal pain, nausea, and vomiting; fecal impaction (mineral oil enemas excepted); intestinal obstruction; and undiagnosed abdominal pain.

Adverse Effects

The adverse effects of the various drugs are specific to the laxative group. Most of the adverse effects from laxatives are confined to the intestine; however, the overuse and misuse of laxatives lead to many unwanted effects that are not expected or

---

TABLE 51-4 Laxatives: Drug Categories and Selected Drugs

Category	Laxative Drugs
Bulk forming	psyllium, methylcellulose
Emollient	docusate salts, mineral oil
Hyperosmotic	polyethylene glycol, lactulose, sorbitol, glycerin
Saline	magnesium hydroxide, magnesium sulfate, magnesium citrate
Stimulant	senna, bisacodyl

TABLE 51-6 Laxatives: Indications

Category	Indication
Bulk forming	Acute and chronic constipation, irritable bowel syndrome, diverticulosis
Emollient	Acute and chronic constipation, fecal impaction, anorectal conditions requiring facilitation of bowel movements
Hyperosmotic	Chronic constipation, bowel preparation for diagnostic and surgical procedures
Saline	Constipation, bowel preparation for diagnostic and surgical procedures
Stimulant	Acute constipation, bowel preparation for diagnostic and surgical procedures

---

TABLE 51-5 Laxatives: Drug Effects

Drug Effect	Bulk	Emollient	Hyperosmotic	Saline	Stimulant
Increases peristalsis	Yes	Yes	Yes	Yes	Yes
Causes increased secretion of water and electrolytes in small bowel	Yes	Yes	No	Yes	Yes
Inhibits absorption of water in small bowel	Yes	Yes	No	Yes	Yes
Increases wall permeability in small bowel	No	Yes	No	No	Yes
Acts only in large bowel	No	No	Yes	No	No
Increases water in fecal mass	Yes	Yes	Yes	Yes	Yes
Softens fecal mass	Yes	Yes	Yes	Yes	Yes

TABLE 51-7 Laxatives: Adverse Effects

Category	Adverse Effects
Bulk forming	Impaction above strictures, fluid disturbances, electrolyte imbalances, gas formation, esophageal blockage, allergic reaction
Emollient	Skin rashes, decreased absorption of vitamins, lipid pneumonia, electrolyte imbalances
Hyperosmotic	Abdominal bloating, rectal irritation, electrolyte imbalances
Saline	Magnesium toxicity (with renal insufficiency), electrolyte imbalances, cramping, diarrhea, increased thirst
Stimulant	Nutrient malabsorption, skin rashes, gastric irritation, electrolyte imbalances, discolored urine, rectal irritation

designed to occur with appropriate use. The major adverse effects of the laxative drugs are listed in Table 51-7.

Interactions

Laxatives alter intestinal function; therefore, they can interact with other drugs, because many drugs are absorbed in the intestines. Bulk-forming laxatives can decrease the absorption of antibiotics, digoxin, nitrofurantoin, salicylates, tetracyclines, and warfarin. Mineral oil can decrease the absorption of fat-soluble vitamins (A, D, E, and K). Hyperosmotic laxatives can cause increased CNS depression if they are given with barbiturates, general anesthetics, opioids, or antipsychotics. Oral antibiotics can decrease the effects of lactulose. Stimulant laxatives decrease the absorption of antibiotics, digoxin, nitrofurantoin, salicylates, tetracyclines, and oral anticoagulants.

Dosages

For the recommended dosages of selected laxatives, see the Dosages table on p. 804.

DRUG PROFILES

Laxatives are used for the treatment of constipation. Such treatment must involve an understanding of the whole patient. Many drugs in the five major groups of laxatives are available as OTC medications, whereas others require a prescription for use. The following profiles describe the prototypical drugs in each of the laxative groups.

BULK-FORMING LAXATIVES
Bulk-forming laxatives are composed of water-retaining (hydrophilic) natural and synthetic cellulose derivatives. Psyllium is an example of a natural bulk-forming laxative, and methylcellulose is an example of a synthetic cellulose derivative. Bulk-forming drugs increase water absorption, which results in greater total volume (bulk) of the intestinal contents. Bulk-forming laxatives tend to produce normal, formed stools. Their action is limited to the GI tract, so there are few, if any, systemic effects. However, they should be taken with liberal amounts of water to prevent esophageal obstruction and/or fecal impaction. The bulk-forming laxatives are all obtainable OTC, are among the safest laxatives available, and are the only ones that are recommended for long-term use.

methylcellulose
Methylcellulose (Citrucel) is a synthetic bulk-forming laxative that attracts water into the intestine and absorbs excess water into the stool, stimulating the intestines and increasing peristalsis. Specific contraindications include GI obstruction and hepatitis. Methylcellulose is an oral drug available in powdered form that provides approximately 2 g of fiber per heaping tablespoon.

◆ psyllium
Psyllium (Metamucil) is a natural bulk-forming laxative obtained from the dried seed of the *Plantago psyllium* plant. It has many of the characteristics of methylcellulose. Psyllium use is contraindicated in patients with intestinal obstruction or fecal impaction. Its use is also contraindicated in patients experiencing abdominal pain and/or nausea and vomiting. Psyllium is available for oral use in wafer and powder form.

EMOLLIENT LAXATIVES
Emollient laxatives either directly lubricate the stool and the intestines, as with mineral oil, or act as fecal softeners. By lubricating the fecal material and the intestinal walls, lubricant emollient laxatives prevent water from moving out of the intestines, which softens and expands the stool. Stool softeners (docusate salts) work by lowering the surface tension of fluids, which allows more water and fat to be absorbed into the stool and the intestines.

◆ docusate salts
Docusate salts (calcium and sodium) (Colace) are stool-softening emollient laxatives that facilitate the passage of water and lipids (fats) into the fecal mass, which softens the stool. These drugs are used to treat constipation, soften fecal impactions, and facilitate bowel movements in patients with hemorrhoids and other painful anorectal conditions. They do not cause patients to defecate, they simply soften the stool to ease its passage. In addition to the docusate salt formulations, combination products are also available. Docusate use is contraindicated in patients with intestinal obstruction, fecal impaction, or nausea and vomiting.

mineral oil
Mineral oil (Kondremul Plain) eases the passage of stool by lubricating the intestines and preventing water from escaping the stool. Mineral oil is the only lubricant laxative in the emollient category. It is a mixture of liquid hydrocarbons derived from petroleum and is most commonly used to treat constipation associated with hard stools or fecal impaction.

Mineral oil use is contraindicated in patients with intestinal obstruction, abdominal pain, or nausea and vomiting. Mineral oil drugs are available as enemas and in products for oral use. There are also combination products that contain mineral oil, such as Haley's M-O, which includes both mineral oil and milk of magnesia (magnesium hydroxide).

HYPEROSMOTIC LAXATIVES
The hyperosmotic laxatives glycerin, lactulose, sorbitol, and polyethylene glycol (PEG) relieve constipation by increasing the water content of the feces, which results in distention, peristalsis, and evacuation. They are most commonly used to treat constipation and to evacuate the bowels before diagnostic and surgical procedures.

◆ glycerin
Glycerin (Fleet Babylax) promotes bowel movement by increasing osmotic pressure in the intestine, which draws fluid into the colon. Because it is a very mild laxative, it is often used in children. Glycerin has properties similar to those of sorbitol, another hyperosmotic laxative. Glycerin use is contraindicated in patients who

DOSAGES

Selected Laxatives

Drug (Pregnancy Category)	Pharmacologic Class	Usual Dosage Range	Onset of Action
bisacodyl (Dulcolax)	Stimulant laxative	**Pediatric younger than 2 yr** 5-mg suppository **Pediatric older than 2 yr** 10-mg suppository **Pediatric older than 6 yr** PO: 0.3 mg/kg **Adult** 5-15 mg oral or 10 mg-suppository	Oral: 6-12 hr Rectal: 15-60 minutes
◆ docusate sodium (Colace, others) and docusate calcium (Surfak, others) (C)	Fecal softener, emollient laxative	**Pediatric 2-11 yr*** PO: 33-120 mg/day divided daily-tid **Pediatric 12 yr and older, and adult*** PO: 50-300 mg/day divided daily-qid	1-3 days
◆ glycerin (Sani-Supp, Colace, Fleet Babylax) (C)	Hyperosmotic laxative	**Adult and pediatric** Rectal only: Insert one adult, child, or infant suppository PR daily-bid prn; attempt to retain 15-30 min; suppository does not have to melt to induce BM	16-36 min
◆ lactulose (Enulose, Chronulac, others) (B)	Disaccharide, hyperosmotic laxative	**Pediatric, infant†** PO: 2.5-10 mL/day divided bid-qid **Child and adolescent†** PO: 40-90 mL/day divided bid-qid **Adult†** PO: 30-45 mL tid-qid	24 hr
magnesium citrate (generic only), magnesium sulfate (Epsom salts by various manufacturers) (B)	Saline laxative	***Citrate, PO*** **Pediatric younger than 6 yr** 0.5 mL/kg (max 200 mL); may repeat q4-6h until stools clear **Pediatric 6-11 yr** 100-150 mL × 1 dose **Adult** 120-300 mL × 1 dose	0.5-3 hr
methylcellulose (Citrucel, others) (B)	Bulk-forming laxative	**Pediatric 6-11 yr** ½ dose for pediatric 12 yr and older and adult **Pediatric 12 yr and older, and adult** PO: 1 heaping tbsp in 8 oz cold water daily-tid	12-24 hr
mineral oil (Kondremul Plain, Fleet Oil-Retention Enema) (B)	Emollient laxative	***PO*** **Pediatric 6-11 yr** 5-15 mL oil or 10-25 mL Kondremul Plain emulsion **Pediatric 12 yr and older, and adult** 15-45 mL oil or 30-75 mL Kondremul Plain emulsion taken at bedtime ***Rectal enema*** **Pediatric 2-11 yr** PR: 59 mL × 1 **Pediatric 12 yr and older, and adult** PR: 118 mL × 1	6-8 hr
polyethylene glycol (Colyte, GoLYTELY, NuLYTELY, MiraLAX) (C)	Emollient laxative	**Adult only** PO: 4 L solution, usually ending before procedure; patient should fast at least 4 hr before drinking solution MiraLAX: 17 g once daily	1 hr
◆ psyllium (Metamucil, Fiberall, others) (B)	Bulk-forming laxative	**Pediatric 6-11 yr** PO: ½ rounded tsp in water or juice daily-tid **Pediatric 12 yr and older, and adult** PO: 1 rounded tsp in 8 oz water or juice daily-tid	12-24 hr

BM, Bowel movement; *PO*, oral; *PR*, by rectum.
*Docusate sodium is available in both capsule and liquid forms. Docusate calcium is available in capsule form only.
†Rectal route is sometimes used to reverse certain types of coma.

DOSAGES

Selected Laxatives—cont'd

Drug (Pregnancy Category)	Pharmacologic Class	Usual Dosage Range	Onset of Action
◆ senna (Senokot, others) (C)	Stimulant-irritant laxative	**Pediatric 2-5 yr‡** PO (liquid): 2.5 mL (max: ½ tsp bid) **Pediatric 6-11 yr‡** PO (tabs): 1 tab daily (max: 2 tabs bid) PO (liquid): 7.5-10 mL daily (max: 5 mL bid) **Pediatric 12 yr and older, and adult‡** PO (tabs): Start with 2 tabs daily (max: 4 tabs bid) PO (liquid): 15 mL daily (max: 30 mL bid)	6-24 hr

‡Many dosage forms; consult product labeling if in doubt. Most common dosage forms are 8.6-mg sennosides in tablet form and 8.8 mg/5 mL of sennosides in liquid form.

have shown a hypersensitivity reaction to it. It is available as a rectal solution and as both adult and pediatric suppositories.

◆ lactulose

Lactulose (Chronulac) is a synthetic derivative of the natural sugar lactose, which is not digested in the stomach or absorbed in the small bowel. Instead it passes unchanged into the large intestine, where it is metabolized. Colonic bacteria digest lactulose to produce lactic acid, formic acid, and acetic acid, which creates a hyperosmotic environment that draws water into the colon and produces a laxative effect. This drug-induced acidic environment also reduces blood ammonia levels by converting ammonia to ammonium. Ammonium is a water-soluble cation that is trapped in the intestines and cannot be reabsorbed into the systemic circulation. This effect has proved helpful in reducing serum ammonia levels in patients with hepatic encephalopathy. Lactulose use is contraindicated in patients on a low-galactose diet. It is available as a solution for either oral or rectal use.

polyethylene glycol 3350

PEG-3350 is most commonly given before diagnostic or surgical bowel procedures, because it is a very potent laxative that induces total cleansing of the bowel. The *3350* designation refers to the osmolality of the drug. It is usually available in a powdered dosage form that contains mixtures of electrolytes that also help stimulate bowel evacuation (e.g., Colyte, GoLYTELY, MoviPrep). The powder is usually reconstituted in a large volume of fluid (1 gal) that is then gradually drunk by the patient on the afternoon of the day before the procedure. Use of PEG is contraindicated in patients with GI obstruction, gastric retention, bowel perforation, toxic colitis, toxic megacolon, or ileus.

An oral solution of PEG-3350 and electrolytes is available for GI lavage. Diarrhea usually occurs within 30 to 60 minutes after ingestion; complete evacuation and cleansing of the bowel is accomplished within 4 hours. MiraLAX is a PEG-3350 product that is available OTC and can be used daily for constipation in much smaller amounts than those used for total bowel cleansing.

SALINE LAXATIVES

Saline laxatives consist of various magnesium or sodium salts. They increase osmotic pressure and draw water into the colon, producing a watery stool, usually within 3 to 6 hours of ingestion. The currently available saline laxatives are listed in Box 51-1. It should be noted that oral sodium phosphate–containing products used for bowel evacuation, such as Fleet Phospho-Soda, were taken off the market in 2008 because of concerns about acute phosphate nephropathy.

> ### BOX 51-1 Saline Laxatives
>
> **Magnesium Laxatives**
> **Sulfate**
> Epsom salts
> **Hydroxide**
> Milk of magnesia
> **Citrate**
> Citrate of magnesia
> **Sodium Laxatives**
> Fleet Enema

magnesium salts

The magnesium saline laxatives, magnesium citrate (Citroma), and magnesium hydroxide (Phillips Milk of Magnesia) are unpleasant-tasting OTC laxative preparations. They should be used with caution in patients with renal insufficiency, because they can be absorbed enough to cause hypermagnesemia. They are most commonly used to evacuate the bowel rapidly in preparation for endoscopic examination and to help remove unabsorbed poisons from the GI tract.

Use of magnesium salts is contraindicated in patients with renal disease, abdominal pain, nausea and vomiting, obstruction, acute surgical abdomen, or rectal bleeding. Magnesium hydroxide, more commonly referred to as *milk of magnesia,* is available in oral liquid and tablet form. It is also found in a variety of combination products, such as Haley's M-O (see mineral oil profile). Other magnesium products are listed in the discussion of saline laxatives earlier in the chapter. Note that magnesium *oxide* is used as a supplement, not as a laxative (see Chapter 53).

STIMULANT LAXATIVES

Stimulant laxatives induce intestinal peristalsis. In the past, several different stimulant laxatives were available; however, the U.S. Food and Drug Administration has required that all except bisacodyl (Dulcolax) and senna (Senokot) be removed from the market. Their site of action is the entire GI tract. The action of the stimulant laxatives is proportional to the dose. The stimulant class is the most likely of all laxative classes to cause dependence.

bisacodyl

Bisacodyl (Dulcolax) is the most commonly used stimulant laxative. It is available as an oral tablet and rectal suppository. It is used for constipation or for whole bowel evacuation prior to endoscopic examination. It is available OTC.

◆ **senna**

Senna (Senokot) is a commonly used OTC stimulant laxative. Senna is obtained from the dried leaves of the *Cassia acutifolia* plant. It may be used for relief of acute constipation or bowel preparation for surgery or examination. Because of its stimulating action on the GI tract, it may cause abdominal pain. It can produce complete bowel evacuation in 6 to 12 hours. Senna is available in a variety of dosages as tablets, syrup, and granules. One product, Senokot-S, includes both senna and the stool softener docusate sodium.

DRUGS FOR IRRITABLE BOWEL SYNDROME

Irritable bowel syndrome (IBS) is a condition of chronic intestinal discomfort characterized by cramps, diarrhea, and/or constipation. Patients usually cope with the symptoms by avoiding irritating foods and/or taking OTC laxatives and antidiarrheal drugs. Women are affected more often than men. Tegaserod (Zelnorm) is a serotonin (5-hydroxytryptamine 4) receptor agonist and is approved for treatment of IBS with constipation and chronic idiopathic constipation in women younger than 55 years of age for whom no alternative therapy exists. Tegaserod was approved in 2002 and taken off the market in 2007, then reintroduced under restricted availability in 2008. Tegaserod has been associated with serious adverse events including angina, heart attacks, and stroke. Patients must be registered with the manufacturer. It is pregnancy category B and is dosed at 6 mg twice a day for 4 to 6 weeks.

Lubiprostone (Amitiza) is a chloride channel activator that is indicated for the treatment of chronic idiopathic constipation and IBS with constipation in women 18 years and older. It is dosed at 24 mcg twice a day for idiopathic constipation and 8 mcg twice a day for IBS. The most common adverse effects are nausea, diarrhea, and abdominal pain. It is pregnancy category C drug. It is contraindicated in patients with known or suspected bowel obstruction.

NURSING PROCESS

Assessment

Before giving *antidiarrheal* preparations, the nurse should obtain a thorough history and perform an assessment of bowel patterns, general state of health, any recent illness, and any dietary changes. Abdominal assessment should include auscultation of bowel sounds in all four quadrants *after* inspection of the entire abdomen but *before* percussion and palpation. Performing auscultation and inspection before percussion prevents any possible stimulation of peristalsis or bowel sounds that would not occur otherwise. When the frequency of bowel sounds ranges from 6 to 32 per minute, it is important to describe exactly what is heard and the amount of activity in each of the four quadrants. Terms such as *high-pitched, low-pitched, gurgling,* or *tinkling* may be used to describe the character of the sounds, whereas activity may be described as *hypoactive* (less than 6 sounds per minute), *normoactive* (between 6 and 32 sounds per minute), or *hyperactive* (more than the normal range). The abdominal assessment should be performed for any

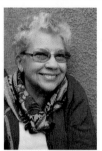
patient with GI complaints, including altered bowel status. The presence of tenderness, rigidity, changes in contour, bulges, and obvious peristaltic waves across the abdomen should be noted. Frequency, consistency, amount, color, and odor (if present) of stools should be assessed and documented. In addition, it is critical to patient safety and health to be sure that the possibility of *Clostridium difficile* infection or other infectious diarrhea is ruled out. Any contraindications, cautions, and drug interaction for all these drugs need to be assessed for and documented. Complaints of abdominal pain, bloody stools, confirmation of hypoactive to no bowel sounds, and/or fever should be reported to the prescriber immediately. With diphenoxylate there is an additional concern for use in patients with respiratory problems because of the risk for respiratory depression. Loperamide is not tolerated well in the elderly. Patients in this age group are also more susceptible to fluid and electrolyte depletion; thus, there is a need for close assessment of hydration status and age.

Laxative use requires further assessment in addition to the abdominal assessment and bowel pattern history described earlier. For example, questions should focus on changes in bowel patterns, long-term use of laxatives (because patients may become laxative dependent), and dietary and fluid intake. Vital signs (especially blood pressure), daily weight measurements, intake and output, and fluid and electrolyte levels should be assessed and the presence of any weakness noted because of the possibility of hypotension and volume or electrolyte depletion (with long-term laxative use). The type of laxative and the related mechanism of action dictate specific assessments because of differences in how strongly the patient reacts to the various laxative drugs. The bulk-forming laxatives are often used to treat chronic constipation and have few adverse effects, but a basic abdominal and bowel pattern assessment and related history taking are still needed. Contraindications, cautions, and drug interactions should be assessed for and documented. Docusate products must also be used cautiously in the elderly and require the same thorough assessment.

Magnesium-based laxatives act as osmotics, so assessment should include specific attention to baseline fluid and electrolyte levels to identify any deficits before these drugs are used. All of the previously mentioned assessment measures regarding abdominal examination and bowel patterns are appropriate for these drugs, but the patient should also be assessed for the presence of abdominal pain, the degree of peristalsis, and any history of recent abdominal surgery, nausea, vomiting, or weight loss. Serum magnesium, BUN, and creatinine levels should be evaluated if ordered. The elderly react more adversely to this class of laxatives, and their use in this patient group should be avoided. Patients who have diabetes or are on a low-sodium diet should be assessed carefully because of the drug-related elevation in blood glucose and serum sodium levels with the use of magnesium laxatives. Lactulose is an osmotic laxative and, in addition to collecting the previously mentioned assessment data, the nurse should document baseline mental status and ammonia levels.

Senna should be used with caution in the elderly because of possible dehydration and electrolyte loss. Patients taking a PEG-electrolyte solution, often used for GI cleansing or bowel preparation, should be assessed for the presence of ulcerative colitis, because the solution may be given differently and only in specific situations in these patients. The nurse should note whether other medications are to be given to the patient; if so, they should be given 1 hour before the polyethylene solution so that absorption of the other oral medication is not decreased.

Patients taking *drugs for IBS* need additional assessment of liver functioning as well as assessment for any underlying cardiac disease. The availability of tegaserod is restricted, and patients are to be registered with the manufacturer because of the severe adverse effects; thus a thorough history taking and assessment is crucial to patient safety. Lubiprostone is not to be used in patients with a known or suspected bowel obstruction.

Nursing Diagnoses

- Constipation related to improper diet and fluid intake
- Diarrhea related to GI irritation from food, bacteria or viruses, or pathology
- Fluid volume deficit related to excessive diarrhea and loss of fluids and electrolytes caused by frequent, loose stools
- Risk for injury related to the adverse effects of medication
- Noncompliance related to lack of knowledge about and/or experience with the medication regimen

Planning
Goals

- Patient regains normal bowel patterns.
- Patient remains free of fluid and electrolyte disturbances related to changes in bowel patterns and lack of proper management of bowel alterations.
- Patient is free from self-injury related to possible weakness and dizziness or the adverse effects of medications.
- Patient remains compliant with the regimen of medication and nonpharmacologic measures.

Outcome Criteria

- Patient reports the signs and symptoms of constipation or diarrhea to the prescriber if recommended measures and/or medications do not correct altered bowel patterns within a specified period of time.
- Patient reports the signs and symptoms of fluid and electrolyte loss, such as weakness, lethargy, decreased urinary output, and dizziness.
- Patient states measures to take to avoid adverse effects and injuries related to change in bowel patterns, changes in fluid and electrolyte status, and/or treatment, such as changing positions slowly, increasing intake of fluids, asking for assistance with ambulation as needed, and ambulating slowly.
- Patient states methods of administration that enhance effective and safe use of the recommended drugs, including following proper dosing, taking oral doses with water or fluids as appropriate, and reporting undesired adverse effects.
- Patient states nonpharmacologic measures to relieve constipation or diarrhea, such as forcing fluids, increasing intake of fiber or bulk for constipation, removing irritating foods from the diet, and increasing intake of bulk for diarrhea.

Implementation

Antidiarrheals should be taken exactly as prescribed, with strict adherence to the recommended dose, frequency, and duration of treatment. The nurse should encourage patients to be aware of their fluid intake and any dietary changes that would impact their health status or possibly exacerbate the symptoms already present. Patients should also be aware of the factors precipitating the diarrhea, and if symptoms persist, they should know to contact a prescriber immediately. Bowel pattern changes, weight, fluid volume status, intake and output, and mucous membrane status should be documented before, during, and after the initiation of treatment—whether for constipation or diarrhea. Bismuth subsalicylate should be taken as directed, and the patient should be aware that this medication will turn the stool black or gray. If tablets are used, they should be chewed thoroughly before swallowing with at least 6 oz of fluid. This medication is a salicylate and should not be taken with other salicylates to avoid risk of toxicity. Diphenoxylate hydrochloride may be given without regard to food intake but should be given with adequate fluid. Loperamide should be taken as ordered, and any specific directions should be followed (e.g., for the specific number of tablets recommended by the manufacturer after the first loose stool and the total number of tablets to be taken within a 24-hour time period). Maximum amounts should not be exceeded, and if diarrhea continues or other symptoms occur (e.g., fever, abdominal pain, bloody stools), the prescriber should be contacted immediately. See Patient Teaching Tips for more information.

Bulk-forming *laxatives* such as methylcellulose must be administered as specified by package insert or as ordered. Methylcellulose should be taken with at least 8 oz or 1 full glass of liquid after the powder form has been thoroughly stirred into it. The fluid must be taken immediately to avoid choking or swelling of the product in the throat or esophagus. The medication should not be taken in its dry form. See Patient Teaching Tips for more information.

Docusate is available in a variety of oral dosage forms (e.g., capsules, tablets, syrups, elixir), and all should be taken with at least 6 oz of water or other fluid. An additional 6 to 8 glasses of water a day should be drunk to help with stool softening. Milk or fruit juices may be used to help to disguise the taste, if needed. Bisacodyl, if ordered, should be taken on an empty stomach for faster action, and whole tablets should not be chewed or crushed. Milk, antacids, or juices should not be taken with the dose or within 1 hour of taking the medication. Rectal suppositories, if too soft, can be placed in a medicine cup with ice to harden them before insertion. Once the wrapper is removed, a water-soluble lubricant should be applied and the suppository inserted immediately into the rectum. A gloved hand or finger cot should be used for the insertion. The patient should attempt to keep the suppository in place by lying still on the left side for at least 15 to 30 minutes to allow the drug to dissolve. Lactulose may be taken with juice, milk, or water to increase palatability. It is important to note that the normal color of the oral solution is pale yellow. Rectal dosage forms are administered as a retention enema with dilution as ordered and should be retained for 30 to 60 minutes. For a retention enema, the tip of the apparatus should be well lubricated and inserted carefully with the nozzle pointed toward the umbilicus of the patient, who should be lying on the left side. Fluid should be released gradually, and administration should be discontinued if the patient experiences severe abdominal pain. If long-term use of the drug is indicated, electrolyte levels should be monitored.

Magnesium-based laxatives should be used only as ordered and in certain situations. Fluids should be forced and other instructions followed per the prescriber's order or the package instructions. Refrigeration may help increase the palatability of the oral solution. It is always important that this type of drug be taken exactly as prescribed for constipation, with consumption of plenty of fluids and careful attention to adverse effects. PEG-electrolyte solution should be mixed with water or flavored sports drink as directed and shaken well before drinking. Chilled solutions are tolerated better. Rapid drinking of each dose is recommended.

IBS drugs, such as tegaserod, should be given as ordered and usually on an empty stomach before meals. Lubiprostone should be given as prescribed and is usually ordered for twice-daily dosing. The patient should be monitored frequently by the prescriber and control (or lack of control) of symptoms of IBS should be assessed.

Evaluation

Therapeutic responses to any of these medications include an improvement in the GI-related signs and symptoms reported by the patient (e.g., decrease in diarrhea or constipation), return to normal bowel patterns with normal bowel sounds, and absence of abnormal findings on assessment of the abdomen and bowel patterns. Adverse effects for which to monitor patients vary according to drug. Goals and outcome criteria should also serve as a means to evaluate the nursing care plan related to each problem, whether it is constipation, diarrhea, or both.

PATIENT TEACHING TIPS

- Instructions should include information that antidiarrheals should be taken exactly as prescribed, giving close attention to indicated dosages with warnings of over-use!
- Antidiarrheal drugs should be taken with caution in performing tasks that require mental alertness or motor skills until it is clear how the drug actually affects the patient. With any of these drugs, any abdominal distention/firm/hard abdomen, abdominal pain, worsening (or no improvement) of symptoms, rectal bleeding, unrelieved constipation or diarrhea, fever, nausea, vomiting and other GI-related signs and symptoms, dizziness, muscle weakness, and muscle cramping should be reported immediately to the prescriber.
- The adverse effect of dry mouth may be helped by frequent mouth care, fluid intake, or use of sugarless gum or candy.
- Bismuth subsalicylate may turn the stool tarry black, so the patient should be warned of this and told to report any bloody stools to the prescriber. Other drugs containing salicylates should be avoided at this time. Always check for cautions and contraindications of this drug, especially for pediatric patients.

- Increasing the intake of fluids, preferably water, as well foods high in fiber and whole grain, green leafy vegetables, and fruits may help to minimize constipation. Exercise is also beneficial.
- Educate patient that what are normal bowel patterns for one person may not be normal for another.
- All antidiarrheals and laxatives must be kept out of the reach of children.
- For patients taking powder forms of methylcellulose, emphasize the need to have the powder thoroughly mixed with at least 6 oz of liquid which is stirred and drunk immediately to avoid esophageal or throat obstruction.
- Senna may turn the urine pink-red, red-violet, red-brown or yellowish brown. The patient should also be informed that other medications should not be taken within 1 hour of taking senna and that it often takes 6 to 12 hours for the laxative effect of the oral drug to occur.

POINTS TO REMEMBER

- Diarrhea is a leading cause of morbidity and mortality in under-developed countries.
- Drugs used to treat diarrhea include adsorbents, anticholinergics, opiates, and intestinal flora modifiers.
- Most acute diarrhea is self-limiting, subsiding in 3 days to 2 weeks.
- Fluid and electrolyte replacement is vital while a patient is experiencing diarrhea.

- Patients should be encouraged to check and recheck dosage instructions before taking medication and to note any drug-food and drug-drug interactions.
- Anticholinergics work by decreasing GI peristalsis through their parasympathetic blocking effects. Adverse effects include urinary retention, headache, confusion, dry skin, rash, and blurred vision.
- Adsorbents work by coating the walls of the GI tract. They remain in the intestine and bind the causative bacteria or toxin to

the adsorbent surface, so that it can be eliminated from the body through the stool. They may increase bleeding and cause constipation, dark stools, and black tongue.

- Intestinal flora modifiers are also used to manage diarrhea and consist of bacterial cultures of *Lactobacillus*. They reestablish normal intestinal flora destroyed by infection or antibiotics and suppress the growth of diarrhea-causing bacteria.
- Opiates are also used as antidiarrheals and help to decrease bowel motility and thus permit longer contact of intestinal contents with the absorptive surface of the bowel. Opiates also help to reduce the pain associated with rectal spasms.

- Laxatives, especially osmotic medications, may cause fluid and electrolyte loss.
- Patients must be made aware of the abuse potential of laxatives and the problems associated with their misuse as well as laxative dependency issues.
- Stool softeners and bulk-forming drugs are often preferred to other drug classes in the treatment of constipation because they are not as problematic with regard to fluid and electrolyte loss.

NCLEX EXAMINATION REVIEW QUESTIONS

1 A patient is being prepared for a colonoscopy. The nurse expects which laxative to be used as preparation for this procedure?
a Methylcellulose
b Docusate sodium
c PEG-3350
d Glycerin

2 The nurse is administering oral methylcellulose (Citrucel) and keeps in mind that a major potential concern with this drug is
a dehydration.
b tarry stools.
c renal calculi.
d esophageal obstruction.

3 A 45-year-old woman has been diagnosed with irritable bowel syndrome (IBS) and will be taking lubiprostone (Amitiza). The nurse assesses for conditions that may be contraindications to this drug, such as:
a Constipation
b Bowel obstruction
c Renal calculi
d Anemia

4 When the nurse teaches a patient about taking bisacodyl tablets, which instruction is correct?
a "Take this medication on an empty stomach."
b "Chew the tablet for quicker onset of action."

c "Take this medication with juice or milk."
d "Take this medication with an antacid if it upsets your stomach."

5 A patient has been receiving long-term antibiotic therapy as part of treatment for an infected leg wound. He tells the nurse that he has had "spells of diarrhea" for the last week. Which medication is most appropriate for him at this time?
a Bismuth subsalicylate
b *L. acidophilus*
c Diphenoxylate with atropine
d Codeine

6 A patient has been instructed to use an OTC form of the bulk-forming laxative methylcellulose (Citrucel) to prevent constipation. The nurse should advise the patient of potential adverse effects, including:
a Fluid and electrolyte disturbances
b Decreased absorption of vitamins
c Gas formation
d Darkened stools
e Discolored urine

1. c, 2. d, 3. b, 4. a, 5. b, 6. a, c.

CRITICAL THINKING ACTIVITIES: BEST ACTION

1 The nurse is explaining to a group of elderly patients the importance of seeking treatment for diarrhea. During the discussion with the group, a member asks, "If I have eaten something 'bad,' does it matter if I take something to stop the diarrhea?" What is the nurse's best response, considering the age of the group?

2 A woman calls the clinic because her 4-month-old daughter has had diarrhea for about 8 hours. What is the nurse's best response?

3 An 88-year-old patient is undergoing a bowel preparation for colonoscopy. What are the nurse's best actions regarding monitoring the patient during the bowel preparation?

For answers, see *http://evolve.elsevier.com/Lilley*.

CHAPTER 52

Antiemetic and Antinausea Drugs

OBJECTIVES

When you reach the end of this chapter, you should be able to do the following:

1 Discuss the pathophysiology of nausea and vomiting, including specific precipitating factors and/or diseases.
2 Identify the various antiemetic and antinausea drugs and their drug classification groupings.
3 Describe the mechanisms of action, indications for use, contraindications, cautions, and drug interactions of the various categories of antiemetic and antinausea drugs.
4 Develop a nursing care plan that includes all phases of the nursing process for patients taking antiemetic and antinausea drugs.

e-Learning Activities

http://evolve.elsevier.com/Lilley

NCLEX Review Questions • Animations • Nursing Care Plans • Audio Glossarys • Category Catchers • Medication Errors Checklists • IV Therapy Checklists • Calculators • Frequently Asked Questions • Content Updates • Supplemental Resources • Answers to Case Studies and Critical Thinking Activities

Drug Profiles

aprepitant, p. 816
dronabinol, p. 816
◆ meclizine, p. 814
◆ metoclopramide, p. 814
◆ ondansetron, p. 816

phosphorated carbohydrate
  solution, p. 816
◆ prochlorperazine, p. 814
promethazine, p. 814
scopolamine, p. 812

◆ *Key drug.*

Glossary

Antiemetic drugs Drugs given to relieve nausea and vomiting. (p. 810)
Chemoreceptor trigger zone (CTZ) The area of the brain that is involved in the sensation of nausea and the action of vomiting. (p. 810)
Emesis The forcible emptying or expulsion of gastric and, occasionally, intestinal contents through the mouth; also called *vomiting.* (p. 810)
Nausea Sensation often leading to the urge to vomit. (p. 810)
Vomiting center The area of the brain that is involved in stimulating the physiologic events that lead to nausea and vomiting. (p. 810)

• • •

Anatomy, Physiology, and Disease Overview

NAUSEA AND VOMITING

Nausea and vomiting are two gastrointestinal (GI) disorders that can be extremely unpleasant but also can lead to more serious complications if not treated promptly. **Nausea** is an unpleasant feeling

that often precedes vomiting. If it does not subside spontaneously or is not relieved by medication, it can lead to vomiting. Vomiting, which is also called **emesis,** is the forcible emptying or expulsion of gastric and, occasionally, intestinal contents through the mouth. A variety of stimuli can induce nausea and vomiting, including foul odors or tastes, unpleasant sights, irritation of the stomach or intestines, and certain drugs (ipecac or antineoplastic drugs).

The **vomiting center** is an area in the brain that is responsible for initiating the physiologic events that lead to nausea and vomiting. Neurotransmitter signals are sent to the vomiting center from the **chemoreceptor trigger zone (CTZ),** another area in the brain involved in the induction of nausea and vomiting. These signals alert those areas of the brain to the existence of nauseating substances (noxious stimuli) that need to be expelled from the body. Once the CTZ and vomiting center are stimulated, they initiate the events that trigger the vomiting reflex. The neurotransmitters involved in this process and their respective receptors are listed in Table 52-1. The various pathways and the areas of the body that send the signals to the vomiting center are illustrated in Figure 52-1. Two specific types of nausea and vomiting, chemotherapy-induced and postoperative, produce much more intense symptoms and are treated much more aggressively than general nausea and vomiting.

Pharmacology Overview

ANTIEMETIC DRUGS

Drugs used to relieve nausea and vomiting are called **antiemetic drugs.** The discovery of new drugs coupled with a better understanding of how the older drugs work has had a dramatic impact on the way in which nausea and vomiting are now treated. All antiemetic drugs work at some site in the vomiting pathways. There are six categories of such drugs with varying mechanisms of action. When drugs from different categories are combined, the antiemetic effectiveness is increased because more than one pathway becomes blocked. Some of the more commonly used antiemetics in the various categories are listed in Table 52-2. The sites at which antiemetics work in the vomiting pathway are shown in Figure 52-2.

Syrup of Ipecac

- Since November 2003 the American Academy of Pediatrics (AAP) has strongly advised *against* the use of syrup of ipecac as an emetic when children swallow a poisonous substance. In a statement published in the November 2003 issue of *Pediatrics,* the AAP recommended that syrup of ipecac no longer be used as a home treatment for poisoning. Syrup of ipecac is still not recommended for use at this time. See *http://www.aap.org/publiced/BR_Poison.htm* for more information.
- If a child has been exposed to a toxic substance, the caregiver should call the national poison control hotline at 800-222-1222. Calls are routed to the local poison control center.
- Steps to follow to prevent accidental poisoning, as identified by the AAP, include the following: (1) Keep potential poisons out of sight and out of reach. (2) Always check to make sure containers are securely closed and the cabinets where they are stored are securely shut and locked after poisonous substances are used. (3) Never transfer a substance from its original to an alternate container. (4) Safely dispose of all unused and unneeded medications. (5) *Never* refer to medicines as "candy."
- The AAP specifies that the following steps should be implemented for the treatment of poisoning in young children: (1) If the poison has been ingested, *first* call the national poison control hotline at 800-222-1222. (2) If the poison has touched the skin or eyes, run tap water over the skin or eyes for 15 to 20 minutes. (3) If the poison has been inhaled, remove the child from the hazardous environment. (4) In *all* cases of poisoning, *if the victim is conscious and alert, call the local poison control center. If the victim has collapsed or stopped breathing, call 911* for emergency transport to a hospital.

Modified from American Academy of Pediatrics: Poison treatment in the home, *Pediatrics* 112:1061-1064, 2003; Davis JL: Pediatricians advise calling poison control when child exposed to poison, November 2003, WebMD Medical News, available at *http://www.webmd.com.* Also visit *http://www.aap.org.*

Mechanism of Action and Drug Effects

Drugs used to prevent or treat nausea and vomiting have many different mechanisms of action. Most work by blocking one of the vomiting pathways, as shown in Figure 52-2. In doing so, they block the neurologic stimulus that induces vomiting. The mechanisms of action of the drugs in the six antiemetic drug categories are summarized in Table 52-3.

Anticholinergic drugs are discussed in Chapter 21 and have several uses. As antiemetics, they act by binding to and blocking acetylcholine (ACh) receptors in the vestibular nuclei, which are located deep within the brain. When ACh is prevented from binding to these receptors, nausea-inducing signals originating in this area cannot be transmitted to the chemotrigger receptor zone (CTZ). Anticholinergics also block receptors located in the reticular formation so that nausea-inducing signals originating in this area cannot be transmitted to the vomiting center. Anticholinergics also tend to dry GI secretions and reduce smooth muscle spasms, both of which effects are often helpful in reducing acute GI symptoms, including nausea and vomiting.

Antihistamines (histamine 1 [H_1] receptor blockers) act by inhibiting vestibular stimulation in a manner that is very similar to that of the anticholinergics. Although they bind primarily to H_1 receptors, they also have potent anticholinergic activity, in-

TABLE 52-1 Neurotransmitters Involved in Nausea and Vomiting

Neurotransmitter (Receptor)	Site in the Vomiting Pathway
Acetylcholine (ACh)	VC in brain; vestibular and labyrinthine pathways in inner ear
Dopamine (D_2)	GI tract and CTZ in brain
Histamine (H_1)	VC in brain; vestibular and labyrinthine pathways in inner ear
Prostaglandins	GI tract
Serotonin (5-HT_3)	GI tract; CTZ and VC in brain

CTZ, Chemoreceptor trigger zone; *ACh,* acetylcholine receptor; *D_2,* dopamine 2 receptor; *GI,* gastrointestinal; *H_1,* histamine 1 receptor; *5-HT_3,* 5-hydroxytryptamine 3 receptor; *VC,* vomiting center.

cluding antisecretory and antispasmodic effects. Thus the antihistamines prevent cholinergic stimulation in both the vestibular and reticular systems. Nausea and vomiting occur when these systems are stimulated. Note that these drugs are not to be confused with *histamine 2 [H_2] receptor blockers* used for gastric acid control (see Chapter 50).

Antidopaminergic drugs, although they are traditionally used for their antipsychotic effects (see Chapter 17), also prevent nausea and vomiting by blocking dopamine receptors in the CTZ. Many of the antidopaminergics also have anticholinergic actions similar to those of anticholinergic drugs. In addition, antidopaminergic drugs calm the central nervous system (CNS).

Prokinetic drugs, in particular metoclopramide, act as antiemetics by blocking dopamine receptors in the CTZ, which desensitizes the CTZ to impulses it receives from the GI tract. Their primary action, however, is to stimulate peristalsis in the GI tract. This enhances the emptying of stomach contents into the duodenum, as well as intestinal movements.

Serotonin blockers work by blocking serotonin receptors located in the GI tract, CTZ, and vomiting center. There are many subtypes of serotonin receptors, and they are located throughout the body (CNS, smooth muscles, platelets, and GI tract). The receptor subtype involved in the mediation of nausea and vomiting is the 5-hydroxytryptamine 3 (5-HT_3) receptor. These receptors are the site of action of the serotonin blockers such as ondansetron, granisetron, dolasetron, and palonosetron.

Tetrahydrocannabinol (THC), in a drug class by itself, is the major psychoactive substance in marijuana. Nonintoxicating doses in the form of the drug dronabinol are occasionally used as an antiemetic because of the drug's inhibitory effects on the reticular formation, thalamus, and cerebral cortex. These effects cause an alteration in mood and in the body's perception of its surroundings, which may be beneficial in relieving nausea and vomiting. Although this particular category of antiemetics is less commonly prescribed, there are occasionally patients who respond well to THC. Examples are patients being treated for cancer or acquired immunodeficiency syndrome (AIDS) who experience nausea and vomiting. In such patients, dronabinol may also stimulate the appetite, and nutritional wasting syndromes are common in both diseases. The drug also demonstrates some benefit in controlling symptoms of glaucoma. There is a large, but highly controversial, political movement with partici-

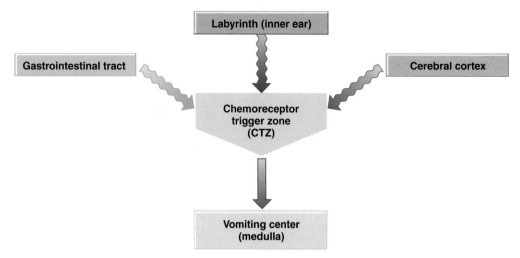

FIGURE 52-1 Various pathways and areas in the body sending signals to the vomiting center.

TABLE 52-2 Antiemetic Drugs: Common Drug Categories

Category	Antiemetic Drugs
Anticholinergics (acetylcholine blockers)	scopolamine
Antihistamines (H_1 receptor blockers)	dimenhydrinate, diphenhydramine, meclizine
Antidopaminergics	prochlorperazine, promethazine, droperidol
Prokinetics	metoclopramide
Serotonin blockers	dolasetron, granisetron, ondansetron, palonosetron
Tetrahydrocannabinoids	dronabinol

pation of many cancer, AIDS, and glaucoma patients in favor of legalization of the marijuana plant for these uses.

Indications

The therapeutic uses of the antiemetic drugs vary depending on the drug category. There are several indications for the drugs in each class. These are listed in Table 52-4.

Contraindications

The primary contraindication for all antiemetics is known drug allergy. Other contraindications for various specific drugs are mentioned in the drug profiles.

Adverse Effects

Most of the adverse effects of the antiemetics stem from their nonselective blockade of various receptors. Some of the more common adverse effects associated with the various categories of antinausea drugs are listed in Table 52-5.

Interactions

The drug interactions associated with the antiemetic drugs are also specific to the individual drug categories. Anticholinergics have additive drying effects when given with antihistamines and antidepressants. Increased CNS depressant effects are seen when antihistamine antiemetics are administered with barbiturates, opioids, hypnotics, tricyclic antidepressants, or alcohol. Increased CNS depression also occurs when alcohol or other CNS depressants are given together with antidopaminergic drugs. Combining metoclopramide with alcohol can result in additive CNS depression. Anticholinergics and analgesics can block the motility effects of metoclopramide. Serotonin blockers and THC have no significant drug interactions.

Dosages

For the recommended dosages of selected antiemetic drugs, see the Dosages table on p. 815.

Antiemetics are used to treat nausea and vomiting in a variety of clinical situations. The ultimate goals of antiemetic therapy are minimizing or preventing fluid and electrolyte disturbances and minimizing deterioration of the patient's nutritional status. Most of the antiemetics act by blocking receptors in the CNS, but some work directly in the GI tract. As previously mentioned, there are six major classes of antiemetic drugs. However, there are other drugs that may also be used to treat nausea and vomiting. These include corticosteroids such as dexamethasone (see Chapter 33) and anxiolytics such as lorazepam (see Chapter 17). When used in combination therapies, these latter drugs, as well as dronabinol, are very beneficial in preventing the nausea and vomiting caused by cancer chemotherapy. Lorazepam also helps to blunt the memory of the nausea and vomiting experience (especially with cancer chemotherapy). Chemotherapy-induced nausea and vomiting and postoperative nausea and vomiting can be especially difficult to treat. The serotonin blockers have proven to be very effective in preventing these types of nausea and vomiting.

ANTICHOLINERGIC
scopolamine

Scopolamine (Transderm-Scōp) is the primary anticholinergic drug used as an antiemetic. It has potent effects on the vestibular nuclei, which are located in the area of the brain that controls balance. Scopolamine works by blocking the binding of ACh to the

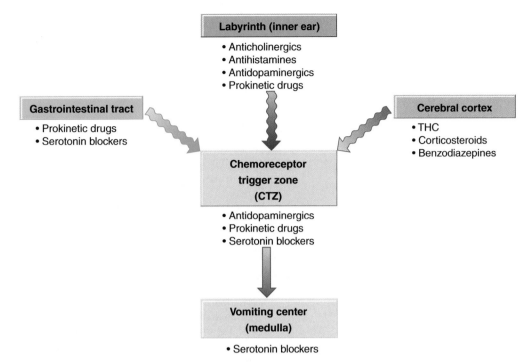

FIGURE 52-2   Sites of action of selected antinausea drugs. *THC,* Tetrahydrocannabinol.

TABLE 52-3 Antiemetic Drugs: Mechanisms of Action

Category	Mechanism of Action
Anticholinergics	Block ACh receptors in the vestibular nuclei and reticular formation
Antihistamines	Block H$_1$ receptors, thereby preventing ACh from binding to receptors in the vestibular nuclei
Antidopaminergics	Block dopamine in the CTZ and may also block ACh
Prokinetics	Block dopamine in the CTZ or stimulate ACh receptors in the GI tract
Serotonin blockers	Block serotonin receptors in the GI tract, CTZ, and VC
Tetrahydrocannabinoids	Have inhibitory effects on the reticular formation, thalamus, and cerebral cortex

ACh, Acetylcholine; *CTZ,* chemoreceptor trigger zone; *GI,* gastrointestinal; *VC,* vomiting center.

TABLE 52-4 Antiemetic Drugs: Indications

Category	Indications/Uses
Anticholinergics	Motion sickness, secretion reduction before surgery, nausea and vomiting
Antihistamines	Motion sickness, nonproductive cough, sedation, rhinitis, allergy symptoms, nausea and vomiting
Antidopaminergics	Psychotic disorders (mania, schizophrenia, anxiety), intractable hiccups, nausea and vomiting
Prokinetics	Delayed gastric emptying, gastroesophageal reflux, nausea and vomiting
Serotonin blockers	Nausea and vomiting associated with cancer chemotherapy, postoperative nausea and vomiting
Tetrahydrocannabinoids	Nausea and vomiting associated with cancer chemotherapy, anorexia associated with weight loss in patients with AIDS and cancer

AIDS, Acquired immunodeficiency syndrome.

cholinergic receptors in this region and thereby correcting an imbalance between the two neurotransmitters ACh and norepinephrine. These effects make scopolamine one of the most commonly used drugs for the treatment and prevention of the nausea and vomiting associated with motion sickness. Scopolamine is also used to treat postoperative nausea and vomiting. Use of the drug is contraindicated in patients with glaucoma. Scopolamine is available in oral, injectable, transdermal, and even ocular forms (see Chapter 57). The most commonly used formulation for nausea is the 72-hour transdermal patch, which releases a total of 1 mg of the drug.

PHARMACOKINETICS

Route	Onset of Action	Peak Plasma Concentration	Elimination Half-life	Duration of Action
Transdermal	1-2 hr	6-8 hr	9.5 hr	72 hr

ANTIHISTAMINES

Antihistamine antiemetics are some of the most commonly used and safest antiemetics. Some of the popular antihistamines are meclizine (Antivert), dimenhydrinate (Dramamine), and diphen-

TABLE 52-5 Antinausea Drugs: Adverse Effects

Body System	Adverse Effects
Anticholinergics	
Central nervous	Dizziness, drowsiness, disorientation
Cardiovascular	Tachycardia
Ears, eyes, nose, throat	Blurred vision, dilated pupils, dry mouth
Genitourinary	Difficult urination, constipation
Integumentary	Rash, erythema
Antihistamines	
Central nervous	Dizziness, drowsiness, confusion
Ears, eyes, nose, throat	Blurred vision, dilated pupils, dry mouth
Genitourinary	Urinary retention
Antidopaminergics	
Cardiovascular	Orthostatic hypotension, electrocardiographic changes, tachycardia
Central nervous	Extrapyramidal symptoms, pseudoparkinsonism, akathisia, dystonia, tardive dyskinesia, headache
Ears, eyes, nose, throat	Blurred vision, dry eyes
Genitourinary	Urinary retention
Gastrointestinal	Dry mouth, nausea and vomiting, anorexia, constipation
Prokinetics	
Cardiovascular	Hypotension, supraventricular tachycardia
Central nervous	Sedation, fatigue, restlessness, headache, dystonia
Gastrointestinal	Dry mouth, nausea and vomiting, diarrhea
Serotonin Blockers	
Central nervous	Headache
Gastrointestinal	Diarrhea, transient increase in AST and ALT levels
Other	Rash, bronchospasm
Tetrahydrocannabinoids	
Central nervous	Drowsiness, dizziness, anxiety, confusion, euphoria
Ears, eyes, nose, throat	Visual disturbances
Gastrointestinal	Dry mouth

ALT, Alanine aminotransferase; *AST,* aspartate aminotransferase.

hydramine (Benadryl), the latter of which is discussed in Chapter 36. Many of the antihistamines are available over the counter.

◆ meclizine

Meclizine (Antivert) is commonly used to treat the dizziness, vertigo, and nausea and vomiting associated with motion sickness. Contraindications include shock and lactation. It is available for oral use only.

PHARMACOKINETICS

Route	Onset of Action	Peak Plasma Concentration	Elimination Half-life	Duration of Action
PO	1 hr	Variable	6 hr	8-24 hr

ANTIDOPAMINERGICS

Prochlorperazine (Compazine), promethazine (Phenergan), and droperidol (Inapsine) are the most commonly used antiemetics in the antidopaminergic class. These drugs have antidopaminergic as well as antihistaminergic and anticholinergic properties. Droperidol was one of the most commonly used drugs to treat and prevent postop-

erative nausea and vomiting for several decades until the U.S. Food and Drug Administration (FDA) called for a black box warning and required continuous electrocardiographic monitoring with its use. These restrictions were in response to concerns over QTC widening and possible ventricular dysrhythmias. Some institutions still use droperidol, whereas others have banned its use.

◆ prochlorperazine

Prochlorperazine (Compazine), especially in the injectable form, is used frequently in the hospital setting. The drug is contraindicated in patients with hypersensitivity to phenothiazines, those in a coma, and those who have seizures, encephalopathy, or bone marrow depression. It is available for both injection and oral use.

PHARMACOKINETICS

Route	Onset of Action	Peak Plasma Concentration	Elimination Half-life	Duration of Action
IM	30-40 min	2-4 hr	6-8 hr	3-4 hr

promethazine

Promethazine (Phenergan) is commonly used in hospitalized patients as an antiemetic. The preferred route is oral or intramuscular. The intravenous route is not the preferred route but is commonly used. However, extreme care must be taken to avoid accidental intraarterial injection. When promethazine is inadvertently given intraarterially instead of intravenously, severe tissue damage, often requiring amputation, can occur. Promethazine should be diluted in at least 10 mL of fluid (the more dilute the better) and given in a running intravenous line at the port furthest from the patient's vein or through a large-bore vein (not hand or wrist vein). It should be discontinued immediately if burning or pain occurs with administration. Promethazine is contraindicated in children younger than 2 years of age. Sedation is the most common adverse effect and actually may be beneficial. The drug is also available as a rectal suppository. It should not be given subcutaneously.

PHARMACOKINETICS

Route	Onset of Action	Peak Plasma Concentration	Elimination Half-life	Duration of Action
IM	20 min	4.4 hr	9-16 hr	2-6 hr

PROKINETIC

Prokinetic drugs promote the movement of substances through the GI tract and increase GI motility. The only prokinetic drug that is also used to prevent nausea and vomiting is metoclopramide.

◆ metoclopramide

Metoclopramide (Reglan) is available only by prescription because it can cause some severe adverse effects if not used correctly. Metoclopramide is used for the treatment of delayed gastric emptying and gastroesophageal reflux and also as an antiemetic. Its use is contraindicated in patients with seizure disorder, pheochromocytoma, breast cancer, or GI obstruction and also in patients with a hypersensitivity to it or to procaine or procainamide. Metoclopramide is available in both oral and parenteral formulations. Extrapyramidal adverse effects can occur with its use, especially in young adults. In 2009, the FDA posted a public health advisory regarding the potential of developing tardive dyskinesia with long-term use of metoclopramide.

PHARMACOKINETICS

Route	Onset of Action	Peak Plasma Concentration	Elimination Half-life	Duration of Action
PO	20-60 min	1-2.5 hr	2.5-5 hr	3-4 hr

Dosages

Selected Antiemetic and Antinausea Drugs

Drug (Pregnancy Category)	Pharmacologic Class	Usual Dosage Range	Indications/Uses
Anticholinergics			
scopolamine (Transderm-Scōp) (C)	Anticholinergic, belladonna alkaloid	Apply 1 patch to hairless area behind ear every 3 days (starting at least 4 hr before travel)	Motion sickness prophylaxis
Antihistamines			
◆ meclizine (Antivert, Bonine) (B)	Anticholinergic, antihistamine	**Adult** PO: 25-50 mg 1 hr before travel and repeated daily during travel	Motion sickness prophylaxis
		PO: 25-100 mg/day, divided 1-4 times daily	Treatment of vertigo
Antidopaminergics			
◆ prochlorperazine (Compazine) (C)	Phenothiazine	**Pediatric** PO/PR: Less than 9 kg: 0.4 mg/kg/24 hr 9-13 kg: 2.5 mg q12-24h 13.1-17 kg: 2.5 mg q8-12h 17.1-37 kg: 2.5 mg q8h or 5 mg q12h IM: 0.13 mg/kg/dose **Adult** PO: 5-10 mg 3-4 times daily IM: 5-10 mg q3-4h (max 40 mg/day) PR: 25 mg twice daily IV: 5-10 mg q6h	Antiemetic
promethazine (Phenergan) C	Phenothiazine	**Pediatric older than 2 yr** 0.25-1 mg/kg/dose 4-6 times daily **Adult** 12.5-25 mg q4-6h	Antiemetic
Prokinetics			
◆ metoclopramide (Reglan) (B)	Dopamine antagonist	**Adult** IV: 1-2 mg/kg (30 min before chemotherapy; repeat q2h × 2 doses, then q3h × 3 doses)	Chemotherapy antiemetic
		IM: 10-20 mg × 1 dose near end of surgery	Prevention of postoperative nausea and vomiting
Serotonin Blockers			
◆ ondansetron (Zofran) (B)	Antiserotonergic	**Pediatric 4-11 yr*** PO: 4 mg 3 times daily, 30 min before chemotherapy, repeated 4 and 8 hr after first dose **Pediatric 6 mo-18 yr** IV: 0.15 mg/kg over 15 min, given 30 min before chemotherapy, repeated 4 and 8 hr after first dose **Adult** PO: 8 mg tid **Adult** IV: 24-32 mg once daily	Chemotherapy antiemetic
		Pediatric: 1 mo-12 yr Less than 40 kg: 0.1 mg/kg single dose More than 40 kg: 4 mg as single dose **Adult** 4 mg as single dose 30 min before surgery ends	Prevention and treatment of postoperative nausea
Tetrahydrocannabinoids			
dronabinol (Marinol) (C)	Marijuana-derived antiemetic	**Adult** PO: Initially, 5 mg/m^2 1-3 hr before chemotherapy, then q2-4h after chemotherapy up to 6 times daily for 3 days; this dose may, if needed, be increased in 2.5-mg/m^2 increments to a max dose of 15 mg/m^2	Chemotherapy antiemetic
		PO: 2.5-5 mg twice daily before lunch and before or after dinner, or 2.5 mg as single prn or bedtime dose for patients intolerant of 5-mg doses	Appetite stimulation in HIV/AIDS and cancer patients

AIDS, Acquired immunodeficiency syndrome; *HIV*, human immunodeficiency virus (infection); *IM*, intramuscular; *IV*, intravenous; *PO*, oral; *PR*, rectal.
*There are optional dosage regimens for chemotherapy-induced nausea and vomiting; the reader is referred to a drug information handbook.

SEROTONIN BLOCKERS

The serotonin blockers are also called *5-HT₃ receptor blockers* because they block the 5-HT$_3$ receptors in the GI tract, the CTZ, and the vomiting center. (The chemical name for serotonin is 5-hydroxytryptamine, or 5-HT.) Drugs in this class have very specific actions, and as a result they have very few adverse effects. No significant drug interactions are known to occur. These drugs are indicated for the prevention of nausea and vomiting associated with cancer chemotherapy and also for the prevention of postoperative or radiation-induced nausea and vomiting. Currently there are four drugs in this category: dolasetron (Anzemet), granisetron (Kytril), ondansetron (Zofran), and palonosetron (Aloxi). This class of drugs revolutionized the treatment of nausea and vomiting, especially in cancer patients and post-operative patients. When used to prevent postoperative nausea and vomiting, a dose is usually given approximately 30 minutes before the end of the surgical procedure. When used to prevent or treat nausea and vomiting associated with cancer treatment, the drug should be given in the first 24 to 48 hours of chemotherapy. All drugs in this class are pregnancy category B.

◆ ondansetron

Ondansetron (Zofran) is the prototypical drug in this class. Approved in 1992, it represented a major breakthrough in treating chemotherapy-induced nausea and vomiting and, later, postoperative nausea and vomiting. It is also used for the treatment of hyperemesis gravidarum (nausea and vomiting associated with pregnancy). Its only listed contraindication is drug allergy. It is available in both oral and injectable forms and as orally disintegrating tablets. Doses up to 8 mg can be given by intravenous push over 2 to 5 minutes. Ondansetron was the first of the class to become available as a generic formulation, which significantly increased its use.

PHARMACOKINETICS

Route	Onset of Action	Peak Plasma Concentration	Elimination Half-life	Duration of Action
IV	15-30 min	1-1.5 hr	3.5-5 hr	6-12 hr

TETRAHYDROCANNABINOID
dronabinol

Dronabinol (Marinol) is the only commercially available tetrahydrocannabinoid. It is a synthetic derivative of THC, the major active substance in marijuana. Dronabinol was approved by the FDA in 1985 for the treatment of nausea and vomiting associated with cancer chemotherapy. It is generally used as a second-line drug after treatment with other antiemetics has failed. It is also used to stimulate appetite and weight gain in patients with AIDS and chemotherapy patients. Its only listed contraindication is drug allergy. It is available for oral use only.

PHARMACOKINETICS

Route	Onset of Action	Peak Plasma Concentration	Elimination Half-life	Duration of Action
PO	30-60 min	1-3 hr	19-36 hr	4-6 hr

MISCELLANEOUS ANTINAUSEA DRUGS
phosphorated carbohydrate solution

Phosphorated carbohydrate solution (Emetrol) is a mint-flavored, pleasant-tasting oral solution used to relieve nausea. It works by direct local action on the walls of the GI tract, where it reduces cramping caused by excessive smooth muscle contraction. It can be used to control milder cases of nausea and vomiting resulting from causes such as stomach or intestinal "flu" and excessive (or

unhealthy) eating or drinking. It does not have a pregnancy category rating, but one of its listed unlabeled (non–FDA-approved) uses is for treatment of morning sickness during pregnancy. It is probably not sufficient for treatment of more severe nausea symptoms such as those associated with cancer chemotherapy. Its only contraindication is drug allergy. It is available for oral use only.

aprepitant

Aprepitant (Emend) is the first in a new class of antiemetic drugs and was approved in 2003. It is an antagonist of substance P–neurokinin 1 receptors in the brain. In contrast to other antiemetics, this drug has little affinity for 5-HT$_3$ (serotonin) and dopamine receptors. However, studies do show that aprepitant augments the antiemetic actions of both ondansetron and the corticosteroid dexamethasone. This drug is specifically indicated for the prevention of nausea and vomiting associated with *highly emetogenic* cancer chemotherapy regimens, including high-dose cisplatin. Common adverse effects include dizziness, headache, insomnia, and GI discomforts, but these are generally no more common than with other standard antiemetic regimens. Aprepitant may induce the metabolism of warfarin, and the prothrombin time/international normalized ratio should be checked before each cycle of aprepitant. The drug may reduce the effectiveness of oral contraceptives. Because it is a major inhibitor of the cytochrome P-450 enzyme system, caution should be used in giving it together with drugs that are primarily metabolized by cytochrome P-450 enzyme 3A4, including azole antifungals, clarithromycin, diltiazem, nicardipine, protease inhibitors, and verapamil. It may increase the bioavailability of steroids, including dexamethasone and methylprednisolone, and dosages of these drugs may need to be adjusted by 25% to 50%. Pregnancy category B.

NURSING PROCESS

Assessment

Before any antinausea or antiemetic drug is administered, a complete nursing history should be obtained and a thorough physical assessment completed, with attention to the following: history of the symptoms of nausea and vomiting; medical history and current medical status; medication history and drugs currently taken, including over-the-counter drugs, herbals, prescription drugs, and social drugs (e.g., cigarettes, alcohol); and any alternative therapies used. Any factors precipitating nausea or vomiting should be identified; weight loss should be noted; baseline vital signs should be measured; intake and output should be assessed; the skin and mucous membranes should be examined, with turgor and color noted; and capillary refill (which should be less than 5 seconds) should also be noted. If laboratory tests are ordered (e.g., serum sodium, potassium, and chloride levels; hemoglobin level and hematocrit; red and white blood cell counts; and urinalysis), the findings should be assessed and documented to establish baseline levels. The patient should be assessed for any contraindications or cautions to the use of these drugs and for drug interactions (previously discussed), as well as for any allergies. The *anticholinergic drug* scopolamine should be given only after careful assessment of the patient's health history and medication history. One very important concern to reemphasize with scopolamine, which is com-

HERBAL THERAPIES AND DIETARY SUPPLEMENTS

Ginger (Zingiber officinale)

■ *Overview*
Found naturally in the Asian tropics; now cultivated in other continents, including part of the United States; plant parts utilized are the rhizome and root; active ingredients include *gingerols* and *gingerdione*

■ *Common Uses*
Used as an antioxidant; also used for relief of such varied symptoms as sore throat, migraine headache, and nausea and vomiting (including that induced by cancer chemotherapy, morning sickness, and motion sickness); many other varied uses

■ *Adverse Effects*
Skin reactions, anorexia, nausea, vomiting

■ *Potential Drug Interactions*
Can increase absorption of all oral medications; may theoretically increase bleeding risk with anticoagulants (e.g., warfarin [Coumadin]) or antiplatelet drugs (e.g., clopidogrel [Plavix])

■ *Contraindications*
Contraindicated in cases of known product allergy; may worsen cholelithiasis (gallstones); anecdotal evidence of abortifacient properties—some clinicians recommend not using during pregnancy

CASE STUDY

Nausea and Chemotherapy

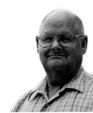
© Brocreative

Mr. S., a 68-year-old retired bus driver, has begun outpatient chemotherapy after a recent diagnosis of lung cancer. He has recovered well from a right lung lobectomy, the incisions are well healed, and he is now physically and emotionally ready for a 3-month regimen of chemotherapy. The premedication orders call for a variety of drugs, including granisetron (Kytril). He has a prescription for oral ondansetron (Zofran) for use at home.

1. What is the mechanism of action of granisetron that makes it effective in the management of chemotherapy-induced nausea and vomiting?
2. What important patient teaching points should you emphasize to Mr. S. about the ondansetron?
3. After 2 weeks of therapy, the oncologist discontinues the ondansetron because Mr. S. complains that it does nothing to help the nausea and vomiting. Mr. S. receives a prescription for dronabinol but expresses concern, exclaiming, "There's marijuana in that pill!" What would you explain to Mr. S.?

For answers, see *http://evolve.elsevier.com/Lilley*.

monly administered in patch form to prevent motion sickness, is the contraindication to its use in patients with narrow-angle glaucoma. If the patient has a history of this disorder, then other antiemetic or antinausea drugs should be used. The same concern regarding use in patients with narrow-angle glaucoma applies to *antihistamines* (e.g., meclizine); in addition, antihistamines should be used cautiously in pediatric patients, who may have severe paradoxical reactions, and in the elderly, who often develop agitation, mental confusion, hypotension, and even psychotic-type reactions in response to these drugs. Other medications should be considered for patients if these reactions occur.

Antidopaminergic drugs, such as promethazine, should be used only after cautious assessment for signs and symptoms of dehydration and electrolyte imbalance by evaluation of skin turgor and examination of the tongue for the presence of longitudinal furrows. Contraindications, cautions, and drug interactions for these drugs have been discussed earlier. Double-checking of the name and mechanism of action is also important (e.g., prochlorperazine may be confused with promethazine).

Prokinetic drugs (e.g., metoclopramide) are often reserved for the treatment of nausea and vomiting associated with antineoplastic drug therapy or radiation therapy and for the treatment of GI motility disturbances. The action of these drugs is decreased when they are taken with anticholinergics or opiates, and because this occurs commonly it is worthy of emphasis. Age is important to assess because of the increased risk of tardive dyskinesia in the young and the elderly. Remember the FDA public health advisory regarding untoward reactions with long-term use (see the Pharmacology section).

The *serotonin blocker* granisetron should be given only after assessment of baseline vital signs and age (its safety in those younger than 2 years of age has not been established). Ondansetron use requires assessment for the signs and symptoms of de-

hydration and electrolyte disturbances, with evaluation of skin turgor and examination for dry mucous membranes or longitudinal furrows in the tongue. Serum levels of bilirubin, aspartate aminotransferase, and alanine aminotransferase should also be assessed before initiation of therapy, especially in patients with liver dysfunction.

The *tetrahydrocannabinoid* dronabinol and its contraindications, cautions, and drug interactions have been discussed previously. Patients taking this drug should be assessed for signs and symptoms of dehydration with attention to low urine output, dry mucous membranes, poor skin turgor, and overall lethargy before this medication is given. A thorough assessment of hydration status is important because treatment of volume and electrolyte imbalances may be required in addition to treatment with antinausea or antiemetic drugs. In addition, motor and cognitive abilities should be assessed and a neurologic head-to-toe examination performed before and during drug therapy.

Nursing Diagnoses
- Risk for injury related to the adverse effects of antiemetic medications (e.g., sedation and dizziness)
- Risk for falls related to weakness and dizziness from vomiting and from the adverse effects of antiemetic medications
- Risk for deficient fluid volume related to nausea and vomiting and limited oral intake
- Impaired physical mobility related to weakness from fluid and electrolyte disturbances secondary to vomiting

Planning
Goals
- Patient remains free of injury and falls from weakness and dizziness secondary to nausea, vomiting, and/or the adverse effects of medication therapy.

- Patient manages the adverse effects of medications or identifies when to seek medical care.
- Patient regains normal fluid volume status and hydration status.
- Patient regains normal levels of activity without risk of falls and injury.

Outcome Criteria

- Patient states measures to implement to prevent injury, such as obtaining assistance while ill, rising slowly, changing positions slowly, taking medications as ordered, and initiating fluid intake once nausea and/or vomiting subside.
- Patient states adverse effects of drug therapy such as sedation, confusion, lethargy, hypotension, and CNS depression.
- Patient states measures to implement to prevent further fluid volume deficits, such as consumption of oral fluids (e.g., clear liquids) or chilled gelatin along with medications.
- Patient increases activity by 10 to 15 minutes per day with cautious rising and walking.

Implementation

Undiluted forms of diphenhydramine should be cautiously administered intravenously at the recommended rate of 25 mg/min as ordered. Intramuscular forms should be administered into large muscles (e.g., ventral gluteal), and sites should be rotated if repeated injections are necessary. Promethazine may be given orally without regard to meals, and suppository forms are available, if needed. Suppository dosage forms should remain in their foil covering until use and, once the wrap is removed, should be moistened with water or water-soluble lubricating gel before being inserted well into the rectum. Patients should be placed on the left side for suppository insertion and should remain there for several minutes and hold in the suppository for as long as possible to increase its absorption. Vital signs should be measured frequently, and the patient should be monitored for extrapyramidal symptoms throughout therapy, whether at home or in the hospital. The patient should be encouraged to avoid other CNS depressants and alcohol and to limit caffeine when this drug is used, as well as to avoid driving and other activities that require mental alertness or motor coordination.

Patients taking meclizine should have their blood pressure checked frequently, especially if they are elderly. Sedation raises a concern for patient safety, with the need for cautious movement at all times. Dry mouth produced by any of these medications may be alleviated by using sugarless gum or hard candy. Metoclopramide given orally should be administered 30 minutes before meals and at bedtime. Intravenous dosage forms should be given over the recommended time period. In addition, solutions for parenteral dosing should be kept for only 48 hours and protected from light. Metoclopramide should not be given in combination with any other medications, such as phenothiazines, that would lead to exacerbation of extrapyrami-

dal reactions. Extrapyramidal reactions should be reported immediately to the prescriber. The development of tardive dyskinesia, an involuntary neurologic movement, has been associated with the long-term use of metoclopramide. The FDA issued a public health advisory about this in 2009. Monitor for and educate patients about this potential problem.

The scopolamine transdermal patch should be applied behind the ear as directed. The area behind the ear should be cleansed and dried before the patch is applied. If the patch becomes dislodged, the residual drug should be washed off and a fresh patch put in place. The patient should be warned not to engage in tasks requiring mental clarity or motor skill while taking the medication. Granisetron may be given intravenously or orally. Intravenous doses should be infused over the recommended time period and diluted as appropriate. A transient taste disorder may occur, especially if the drug is taken with antineoplastic medications, but will pass with continued therapy. The patient should be encouraged to use relaxation techniques and imagery as complementary therapies. Ondansetron may be given orally, intramuscularly, or intravenously. Intramuscular doses should be injected into a large muscle mass. Intravenous push is usually given over 2 to 5 minutes and infusions over 15 minutes as ordered and as per manufacturer guidelines. Oral forms are well tolerated regardless of the relation of dosing to meals. The patient should be encouraged to avoid alcohol and other CNS depressants during this therapy and to avoid any activities requiring mental alertness or motor skill. Dronabinol, granisetron, and ondansetron are usually indicated before chemotherapy. Dronabinol should be administered 1 to 3 hours before antineoplastic therapy and may be taken at home before the scheduled treatment appointment. Relief of nausea and vomiting should occur within approximately 15 minutes of oral drug administration. Aprepitant is often used in combination with other medications to prevent nausea and vomiting associated with chemotherapy and is given, as ordered, for postoperative nausea and vomiting. The prescriber's orders may indicate other drugs to be administered as well as the timing of the dosage. Oral dosage forms should be given as ordered.

Evaluation

The therapeutic effects of antiemetic and antinausea drugs include a decrease in or elimination of nausea and vomiting, and avoidance or elimination of complications such as fluid and electrolyte imbalances and weight loss. The patient should be monitored for adverse effects such as GI upset, drowsiness, lethargy, weakness, extrapyramidal reactions, and orthostatic hypotension during the therapy. Laboratory testing (e.g., electrolyte levels, blood urea nitrogen level, urinalysis with specific gravity) may be ordered for evaluation purposes. Defined goals and outcomes may also be used to evaluate therapeutic effectiveness.

PATIENT TEACHING TIPS

- Use of antiemetic or antinausea drugs should carry a warning about drowsiness and caution while performing any hazardous tasks or driving (while taking these drugs). The patient should also be cautioned about taking antiemetic or antinausea drugs with alcohol and other CNS depressants because of the possible toxicity and exacerbation of CNS depression.
- Educate about the possible adverse effects of ondansetron, including headache, which may be relieved by taking a simple analgesic (e.g., acetaminophen).

- A patient taking dronabinol should be reminded to change positions slowly to prevent syncope or dizziness resulting from the hypotensive effects of the drug. The patient should also avoid taking any other CNS depressants with this antiemetic and should be cautious when engaging in activities that require mental alertness.
- The application sites for transdermal scopolamine patches should be rotated, and the patches should be applied to nonirritated areas behind the ear; the hands should be washed thoroughly before and after application.

POINTS TO REMEMBER

- Antiemetics help to control vomiting, or emesis, and are also useful in relieving or preventing nausea. Antiemetics are used to prevent motion sickness, reduce secretions before surgery, treat delayed gastric emptying, and prevent postoperative nausea and vomiting. Most of these drugs can cause drowsiness.
- Anticholinergics work by blocking ACh receptors in the vestibular nuclei and reticular formation. This blockade prevents areas in the brain from being activated by nauseous stimuli.
- Antihistamines work by blocking H_1 receptors, which has the same effect as the anticholinergics. Antidopaminergic antiemetics block dopamine receptors in the CTZ and may also block ACh receptors. Prokinetic drugs also block dopamine receptors in the CTZ.
- The serotonin-blocking drugs (granisetron and ondansetron) may be highly effective antiemetics. They are most commonly used for the prevention of chemotherapy-induced nausea and vomiting.

- Antiemetics are often given 30 to 60 minutes before a chemotherapy drug is administered (time may vary depending on the specific drug) and may also be given during the chemotherapeutic treatment.
- Dronabinol therapy is used to prevent chemotherapy-induced nausea and vomiting and is associated with postural hypotension.
- Patients taking antiemetic or antinausea drugs should be cautioned that drowsiness and hypotension may occur, so they should avoid driving and using heavy machinery while taking these medications.

NCLEX EXAMINATION REVIEW QUESTIONS

1 The nurse is providing patient teaching regarding scopolamine transdermal patches (Transderm-Scōp) to a patient who is planning an ocean cruise. Which instruction is most appropriate?
   a "Apply the patch the day before traveling."
   b "Apply the patch at least 4 hours before traveling."
   c "The patch should be applied to the shoulder area."
   d "The patch should be applied to the temple just above the ear."
2 A middle-aged woman is experiencing severe vertigo due to Ménière's disease. The nurse expects this patient to receive which drug, which is considered the most appropriate drug treatment for vertigo?
   a meclizine (Antivert)
   b prochlorperazine (Compazine)
   c metoclopramide (Reglan)
   d dronabinol (Marinol)
3 A 33-year-old patient is in the outpatient cancer center for his first round of chemotherapy. The nurse knows that which schedule is the most appropriate timing for the intravenous antiemetic drug?
   a Four hours before the chemotherapy begins
   b Thirty minutes before the chemotherapy begins
   c At the same time as the chemotherapy drugs
   d At the first sign of nausea
4 When reviewing the various types of antinausea medications, the nurse recognizes that prokinetic drugs are also used for
   a motion sickness.
   b vertigo.

   c delayed gastric emptying.
   d GI obstruction.
5 A patient who has been receiving chemotherapy tells the nurse that he has been searching the Internet for antinausea remedies and that he found a reference to a product called Emetrol (phosphorated carbohydrate solution). He wants to know if this drug would help him. Which would be the nurse's best answer?
   a "This may be a good remedy for you. Let's talk to your physician."
   b "This drug is used only after other drugs have not worked."
   c "This drug is used only to treat severe nausea and vomiting caused by chemotherapy."
   d "This drug may not help the more severe nausea symptoms associated with chemotherapy."
6 The nurse is preparing to administer dronabinol (Marinol) to a patient. Which statements about dronabinol therapy are true? (Select all that apply.)
   a It is approved for nausea and vomiting related to cancer chemotherapy.
   b It is approved for use with hyperemesis gravidarum (nausea and vomiting associated with pregnancy).
   c It is approved to help stimulate the appetite in patients with nutritional wasting due to cancer or AIDS.
   d It may cause extrapyramidal symptoms.
   e It may cause drowsiness or euphoria.

CRITICAL THINKING ACTIVITIES: BEST ACTION

1 A patient who has received chemotherapy with a highly emetogenic drug has orders for both ondansetron (Zofran) and prochlorperazine (Compazine). Which drug would be the best choice for the nurse to administer for the patient's nausea and vomiting, and how should it be administered? Explain your answer.

2 The nurse is administering antiemetic drugs to a patient who has been vomiting. What is the priority for assessment at this time? Explain.

3 The nurse has just given an 83-year-old patient a dose of an antinausea drug. Considering this patient's age, what is the nurse's best action regarding evaluation of the drug's effects?

For answers, see *http://evolve.elsevier.com/Lilley.*

CHAPTER 53

Vitamins and Minerals

OBJECTIVES

When you reach the end of this chapter, you should be able to do the following:

1 Discuss the importance of the various vitamins and minerals to the normal functioning of the human body.
2 Briefly describe the various acute and chronic disease states and conditions that may lead to various imbalances in vitamin and mineral levels.
3 Discuss the pathologies that result from vitamin and mineral imbalances.
4 Describe the treatment of these vitamin and mineral imbalances.
5 Identify mechanisms of action, indications, cautions, contraindications, drug interactions, dosages, recommended daily allowances, and routes of administration of each of the vitamins and minerals.
6 Develop a nursing care plan related to the use of vitamins and minerals that includes all phases of the nursing process.

e-Learning Activities

Drug Profiles

♦ *Key drug.*

Glossary

Beriberi A disease of the peripheral nerves caused by a dietary deficiency or an inability to assimilate thiamine (vitamin B₁). Symptoms are fatigue, diarrhea, appetite and weight loss, and disturbed nerve function, causing paralysis and wasting of limbs, edema, and heart failure. (p. 829)
Coenzyme A nonprotein substance that combines with a protein molecule to form an active enzyme. (p. 821)
Enzymes Specialized proteins that catalyze biochemical reactions in organic matter. (p. 821)
Fat-soluble vitamins Vitamins that can be dissolved (i.e., is soluble) in fat. (p. 822)
Minerals Inorganic substances that are ingested and attach to enzymes or other organic molecules. (p. 827)
Pellagra A disease resulting from a deficiency of niacin or a metabolic defect that interferes with the conversion of tryptophan to niacin (vitamin B₃). (p. 829)
Rhodopsin The purple pigment in the rods of the retina, formed by a protein, opsin, and a derivative of retinol (vitamin A). (p. 823)

Rickets A condition caused by a deficiency of vitamin D. (p. 826)
Scurvy A condition resulting from a deficiency of ascorbic acid (vitamin C). (p. 833)
Tocopherols Biologically active chemicals that make up vitamin E compounds. (p. 827)
Vitamins Organic compounds essential in small quantities for normal physiologic and metabolic functioning of the body. (p. 821)
Water-soluble vitamins Vitamins that can be dissolved (i.e., is soluble) in water. (p. 822)

• • •

Physiology and Disease Overview

For the body to grow and maintain itself, it needs the essential building blocks provided by carbohydrates, fats, and proteins. Vitamins and minerals are needed to efficiently utilize these nutrients. **Vitamins** are organic molecules needed in small quantities for normal metabolism and other biochemical functions, such as growth or repair of tissue. Equally important are **minerals,** inorganic elements or salts found naturally in the earth. **Enzymes** are proteins secreted by cells; they act as catalysts to induce chemical changes in other substances. A **coenzyme** is a substance that enhances or is necessary for the action of enzymes. Many enzymes are useless without the appropriate vitamins and/or minerals that chemically bind with them and cause them to function properly. Both vitamins and minerals act primarily as coenzymes, binding to enzymes (or other organic molecules) to activate anabolic (tissue-building) processes in the body. For example, coenzyme A is an important carrier molecule associated with the *citric acid cycle,* one of the body's major energy-producing metabolic reactions. However, it requires pantothenic acid (vitamin B₅) to complete its function in the citric acid cycle.

Vitamins and minerals are essential in our lives, whether or not we are conscientious in our food choices. Under most circumstances, daily requirements of vitamins and minerals are met by ingestion of fluids and balanced meals. Ingesting food helps us maintain adequate stores of essential vitamins and minerals and serves to preserve intestinal mass and structure, provide chemicals for hormones and enzymes, and prevent harmful overgrowth of bacteria.

Various illnesses can occur that can cause acute or chronic deficiencies of vitamins, minerals, electrolytes, and fluids. These conditions require replacement or supplementation of these nutrients. Common examples include extensive burn injuries and acquired immunodeficiency syndrome (AIDS). Excessive loss of vitamins and minerals may also be the result of poor dietary intake, an inability to swallow after cancer chemotherapy or radiation, or mental disorders such as anorexia nervosa. Poor dietary absorption can also be caused by various gastrointestinal malabsorption syndromes. In addition, drug and alcohol abuse are frequently associated with inadequate nutritional intake that warrants vitamin and mineral supplementation. Deficiencies in dietary protein, fat, and carbohydrates are also common. These nutrients are discussed in Chapter 54. Because of some of their distinct properties and functions in the body related to blood formation, iron and the vitamin folic acid (vitamin B_9) are discussed separately in Chapter 55.

Pharmacology Overview

VITAMINS

The human body requires vitamins in specific minimum amounts on a daily basis, and these can be obtained from both plant and animal food sources. In some cases, the body synthesizes some of its own vitamin supply. Supplemental amounts of vitamin B complex and vitamin K are synthesized by normal bacterial flora in the gastrointestinal tract. Vitamin D can be synthesized by the skin when the skin is exposed to sunlight.

An inadequate diet will cause various nutrition-related vitamin deficiencies. In 1941 the Food and Nutrition Board of the National Academy of Sciences published its first list of *recommended daily allowances (RDAs)* of essential nutrients. A newer published standard is the list of dietary reference intakes (DRIs). Whereas the RDAs represented *minimum* nutrient requirements, the DRIs are designed to represent *optimal* nutrient amounts for good health. Laws in the United States require that detailed nutritional information be listed on any packaged food product. The *percentage daily values* are the values that appear on the mandatory labels of commercial food products and indicate what per-

centage of the DRI for a specific nutrient is met by a single serving of the food product. Information regarding DRIs is available from the following sources:

1. Federal Food and Nutrition Information Center: *http://www.nal.usda.gov/fnic*
2. Institute of Medicine: Dietary Reference Intakes (DRIs): recommended intakes for individuals available at *http://www.iom.edu/?id521381*

Vitamins are classified as either fat or water soluble. **Water-soluble vitamins** can be dissolved in water and are easily excreted in the urine. **Fat-soluble vitamins** are dissolvable in fat and tend to be stored longer in the liver and fatty tissues. Because water-soluble vitamins (B-complex group and vitamin C) cannot be stored in the body in large amounts, daily intake is required to prevent the development of deficiencies. Conversely, fat-soluble vitamins (vitamins A, D, E, and K) do not need to be taken daily because substantial amounts are stored in the liver and fatty tissues. Deficiencies of these vitamins occur only after prolonged deprivation from an adequate supply or from disorders that prevent their absorption. Table 53-1 lists the fat-soluble and water-soluble vitamins.

One controversial topic related to vitamins is that of nutrient "megadosing," as a strategy both for health promotion and maintenance and for treatment of various illnesses. Some cancer patients elect to use supplemental megadosing of specific nutrients in hopes of strengthening their body's response to more conventional cancer treatments. The American Dietetic Association defines megadosing as "doses of a nutrient that are 10 or more times the recommended amount." A related term was coined in 1968 by the Nobel Prize–winning chemist Linus Pauling. He defined *orthomolecular medicine* to be "the preventive or therapeutic use of high-dose vitamins to treat disease." Probably the best-known claim of Dr. Pauling was that megadoses of vitamin C (at more than 100 times the U.S. RDA) could prevent or cure the common cold and cancer. Many studies since have not substantiated this claim. However, there are some situations in which nutrient megadosing is known to be helpful, including the following:

- When concurrent long-term drug therapy depletes vitamin stores or otherwise interferes with the function of a vitamin. A common clinical example is the use of vitamin B_6 (pyridoxine) supplementation in patients receiving the drug isoniazid for treatment of tuberculosis (see Chapter 41).
- In gastrointestinal malabsorption syndromes such as those seen in patients with severe colitis and cystic fibrosis (all

---

TABLE 53-1 Fat- and Water-Soluble Vitamins

Fat Soluble		Water Soluble	
Designation	Name	Designation	Name
vitamin A	retinol	vitamin B_1	thiamine
vitamin D	D_3, cholecalciferol; D_2, ergocalciferol, dihydrotachysterol	vitamin B_2	riboflavin
vitamin E	tocopherols	vitamin B_3	niacin
vitamin K	K_1, phytonadione	vitamin B_5	pantothenic acid
	K_2, menaquinone	vitamin B_6	pyridoxine
		vitamin B_9	folic acid
		vitamin B_{12}	cyanocobalamin
		biotin	
		vitamin C	ascorbic acid

major nutrient classes, including protein, fat, carbohydrates, vitamins, and minerals).

- For the treatment of pernicious anemia, which results from cyanocobalamin (vitamin B$_{12}$) deficiency. The gastrointestinal tract uses a fairly complex mechanism to drive cyanocobalamin absorption. Specifically, a glycoprotein known as *intrinsic factor* is secreted by the parietal cells of the gastric glands (see Chapter 50). Intrinsic factor facilitates absorption of cyanocobalamin in the intestine. When this process is compromised (e.g., by disease), administration of megadoses of cyanocobalamin can bypass this absorption mechanism by allowing a small amount of the vitamin to diffuse on its own through the intestinal mucosa.
- When the vitamin acts as a drug when megadosed. The most common example is niacin (vitamin B$_3$, also called *nicotinic acid*). At dosages of up to 20 mg daily, it functions as a vitamin, but at dosages 50 to 100 times higher, it reduces blood levels of both triglycerides and low-density lipoprotein cholesterol (see Chapter 29).

In contrast with the aforementioned examples, there are some situations in which nutrient megadosing is known to be harmful. For example, any excess of one or more nutrients can result in deficiencies of other nutrients due to their chemical competition for sites of absorption in the intestinal mucosa. This is more likely to be the case with megadosing of minerals, such as calcium, copper, iron, and zinc, and is less likely to result from vitamin megadosing. Vitamin megadosing can lead to toxic accumulations known as *hypervitaminosis,* especially with the fat-soluble vitamins A, D, and K. Vitamin E appears safer, however, even at doses 10 to 20 times the recommended DRI. Hypervitaminosis is much less likely to occur with the water-soluble vitamins (B complex and C) because they are readily excreted through the urinary system. Nevertheless, it is known that megadosing with vitamin B$_6$ (pyridoxine) at 50 to 100 times the DRI can cause nerve damage.

Persons with an illness may be the least able to tolerate nutrient megadosing, although megadosing regimens are often prescribed for them. For example, megadosing may be more of a strain for a gastrointestinal tract that is already weakened by illness. Megadosing can even interfere with chemotherapy drugs as well as radiation treatments, because these therapies work to destroy cancer cells through oxidation processes. Nutritional supplementation with antioxidants may impede such treatment mechanisms. Patients should be advised to share with their health care providers any unusual nutritional regimens that they plan to try, especially if they have a serious illness.

FAT-SOLUBLE VITAMINS

Fat-soluble vitamins are not readily excreted in the urine and are stored in the body. Thus, daily ingestion of these vitamins is not necessary to maintain good health and, in fact, is more likely to result in hypervitaminosis.

The fat-soluble vitamins are A, D, E, and K. As a group they share the following characteristics:
- They are present in both plant and animal foods.
- They are stored primarily in the liver.
- They exhibit slow metabolism or breakdown.
- They are excreted via the feces.
- They can reach toxic levels *(hypervitaminosis)* if excessive amounts are consumed.

VITAMIN A

Vitamin A (retinol) is derived from animal fats such as those found in dairy products, eggs, meat, liver, and fish liver oils. Vitamin A is also derived from carotenes, which are found in plants (e.g., green and yellow vegetables, yellow fruits). Therefore, vitamin A is an exogenous substance for humans because it must be obtained from either plant or animal foods. There are more than 600 naturally occurring carotenoid compounds in plant-based foods. Of these, 40 to 50 occur commonly in the human diet. Beta carotene is the most prevalent of these, followed by alpha carotene and cryptoxanthin. These are known as *provitamin A carotenoids,* because they are all metabolized to various forms of vitamin A in the body. Table 53-2 lists the food sources of several nutrients.

Mechanism of Action and Drug Effects

Vitamin A is essential for night vision and for normal vision, because it is part of one of the major retinal pigments called **rhodopsin.** Beta carotene is metabolized in the body to retinal (retinaldehyde), and some of this retinal is reduced to the alcohol compound known as *retinol.* The remainder of the retinal may be oxidized to the carboxylic acid compound retinoic acid. Unlike retinal, retinoic acid has no direct role in vision, but it is essential for normal cell growth and differentiation and for the development of the physical shapes of the body's many parts—a process known as *morphogenesis.* It is also involved in the growth and development of bones and teeth and in other body processes, including reproduction, maintenance of the integrity of mucosal and epithelial surfaces, and cholesterol and steroid synthesis.

Indications

Supplements of vitamin A may be used to satisfy normal body requirements or an increased demand, such as in infants and pregnant and nursing women. A normal diet should provide adequate amounts of vitamin A, but in cases of excessive need or inadequate dietary intake, vitamin A supplementation is indicated. Symptoms of vitamin A deficiency include night blindness, xerophthalmia, keratomalacia (softening of the cornea), hyperkeratosis of both the stratum corneum (outermost layer) of the skin and the sclera (outermost layer of eyeball), retarded infant growth, generalized weakness, and increased susceptibility of mucous membranes to infection. Vitamin A–related compounds, such as isotretinoin, are also used to treat various skin conditions, including acne, psoriasis, and *keratosis follicularis.*

Contraindications

Contraindications to vitamin A supplementation include known allergy to the individual vitamin product; known current state of hypervitaminosis; and excessive supplementation beyond recommended guidelines, especially during pregnancy or in oral malabsorption syndromes.

Adverse Effects

There are very few acute adverse effects associated with normal vitamin A ingestion. Only after long-term excessive ingestion of vitamin A do symptoms appear. Adverse effects are usually noticed in bones, mucous membranes, the liver, and the skin. Table 53-3 lists some of the symptoms of long-term excessive ingestion of vitamin A.

TABLE 53-2 Food Sources for Selected Nutrients

Vitamins/Minerals	Food Sources
vitamin A	Liver; fish; dairy products; egg yolks; dark green, leafy, yellow-orange vegetables and fruits
vitamin D	Dairy products, fortified cereals and fortified orange juice, liver, fish liver oils, saltwater fish, butter, eggs
vitamin E	Fish, egg yolks, meats, vegetable oils, nuts, fruits, wheat germ, grains, fortified cereals
vitamin K	Cheese, spinach, broccoli, brussels sprouts, kale, cabbage, turnip greens, soybean oils
vitamin B_1 (thiamine)	Yeast, liver, enriched whole-grain products, beans
vitamin B_2 (riboflavin)	Meats, liver, dairy products, eggs, legumes, nuts, enriched whole-grain products, green leafy vegetables, yeast
vitamin B_3 (niacin)	Liver, turkey, tuna, peanuts, beans, yeast, enriched whole-grain breads and cereals, wheat germ
vitamin B_6 (pyridoxine)	Organ meats, meats, poultry, fish, eggs, peanuts, whole grain products, vegetables, nuts, wheat germ, bananas, fortified cereals
vitamin B_{12} (cyanocobalamin)	Liver, kidney, shellfish, poultry, fish, eggs, milk, blue cheese, fortified cereals
vitamin C (ascorbic acid)	Broccoli, green peppers, spinach, Brussels sprouts, citrus fruits, tomatoes, potatoes, strawberries, cabbage, liver
calcium	Dairy products, fortified cereals and calcium-fortified orange juice, sardines, salmon
magnesium	Meats, seafood, milk, cheese, yogurt, green leafy vegetables, bran cereal, nuts
phosphorus	Milk, yogurt, cheese, peas, meat, fish, eggs
zinc	Red meats, liver, oysters, certain seafood, milk products, eggs, beans, nuts, whole grains, fortified cereals

Adapted from USDA Dietary Guidelines 2005. Available at *http://www.health.gov/DIETARYGUIDELINES/dga2005/document/html/AppendixB.htm.*

TABLE 53-3 Vitamin A: Adverse Effects

Body System	Adverse Effects
Central nervous	Headache, increased intracranial pressure, lethargy, malaise
Gastrointestinal	Nausea, vomiting, anorexia, abdominal pain, jaundice
Integumentary	Dry skin, pruritus, increased pigmentation, night sweats
Metabolic	Hypomenorrhea, hypercalcemia
Musculoskeletal	Arthralgia, retarded growth

Toxicity and Management of Overdose

The major toxic effects of vitamin A result from ingestion of excessive amounts, which occurs most commonly in children. A few hours after administration of an excess dose of vitamin A (over 25,000 units/kg), irritability, drowsiness, vertigo, delirium, coma, vomiting, and/or diarrhea may occur. In infants, excessive amounts of vitamin A can cause an increase in cranial pressure, resulting in symptoms such as bulging fontanelles, headache, papilledema, exophthalmos (bulging eyeballs), and visual disturbances. Papilledema is the presence of edematous fluid, often including blood, in the optic disc. This is the portion of the eye in the back of the retina, where nerve fibers converge to form the optic nerve. Over several weeks, a generalized peeling of the skin and erythema (skin reddening) may occur. These symptoms seem to disappear a few days after discontinuation of the drug, which is the only treatment necessary in situations of overdose.

Interactions

Vitamin A is absorbed less when used together with lubricant laxatives and cholestyramine. In addition, the concurrent use of isotretinoin and vitamin A supplementation can result in additive effects and possibly toxicity.

Dosages

For the recommended dosages of vitamin A, see the Dosages table on p. 825.

see the Dosages table on p. 825.

DRUG PROFILE

There are three forms of vitamin A: retinol, retinyl palmitate, and retinyl acetate. Medications containing vitamin A may require a prescription, but many over-the-counter (OTC) products, such as vitamin A–containing multivitamins, are also available. All vitamin A products are classified as pregnancy category A.

vitamin A

Vitamin A (Aquasol A), also known as *retinol, retinyl palmitate,* and *retinyl acetate,* is available in a variety of oral forms as well as an injectable form. Doses for vitamin A are expressed as *retinol activity equivalents (RAEs).* One RAE is approximately equal to the following:

- 1 mcg of retinol (either dietary or supplemental)
- 2 mcg of supplemental beta carotene
- 12 mcg of dietary beta carotene
- 24 mcg of dietary carotenoids

PHARMACOKINETICS

Route	Onset of Action	Peak Plasma Concentration	Elimination Half-life	Duration of Action
PO	42 days	4 hr	50-100 days	Unknown

VITAMIN D

Vitamin D, also called the *sunshine vitamin,* is responsible for the proper utilization of calcium and phosphorus in the body. The two most important members of the vitamin D family are vitamin D_2 (ergocalciferol) and vitamin D_3 (cholecalciferol). They have different sites of origin but similar functions in the body. Ergocalciferol (vitamin D_2) is plant derived and is therefore obtained through dietary sources. The natural form of vitamin D produced in the skin by ultraviolet irradiation (sun) is chemically known as

DOSAGES

Selected Vitamins

Drug	Pharmacologic Class	Usual Dosage Range	Indications/Uses
Vitamin D–Active Compounds			
calcifediol (hydroxy vitamin D$_3$) (Calderol)	Fat soluble	**Adult and pediatric 2-10 yr** PO: 50 mcg once daily **Infants** PO: 5-7 mcg/kg/day	Hypocalcemia in hemodialysis patients; hepatic osteodystrophy
calcitriol (dihydroxyvitamin D$_3$) (Rocaltrol, Calcijex)	Fat soluble	**Adult and pediatric 6 yr and older** PO/IV: 0.5-2 mcg/day **Pediatric 1-5 yr** PO/IV: 0.25-0.75 mcg/day	Hypoparathyroidism; hypocalcemia in patients receiving regular hemodialysis
dihydrotachysterol (DHT, Hytakerol)	Fat soluble (a form of vitamin D)	**Adult and pediatric 12 yr and older** PO: 0.8-2.4 mg/day × several days, followed by 0.2-1 mg/day **Pediatric younger than 12 yr** PO: 1-5 mg/day × 4 days, then 0.1-0.5 mg/day	Hypoparathyroidism
ergocalciferol (vitamin D$_2$) (Drisdol, Calciferol)	Fat soluble	**Adult*** PO/IM: 10,000-60,000 units/day **Pediatric*** 3000-5000 units/day	Rickets, hypoparathyroidism, renal failure
Vitamin B–Active Compounds			
vitamin B$_1$ (thiamine) (Thiamilate)	Water-soluble, B-complex group	**Adult** 1-2 mg/day **Infant/child** PO/IM/IV: 0.3-1.5 mg/day	Nutritional supplementation; alcohol-induced deficiency Nutritional supplementation; nutritional deficiency
vitamin B$_2$ (riboflavin) (Lactoflavin)	Water-soluble, B-complex group	**Adult** PO: 5-30 mg/day **Pediatric** 2.5-10 mg/day	Deficiency
vitamin B$_3$ (niacin, nicotinic acid) (Nicotinex)	Water-soluble, B-complex group	**Adult** PO: 1-6 g/day **Pediatric** PO: 50-100 mg 3 times daily	Hyperlipidemia; deficiency (pellagra)
Vitamin B$_6$ (pyridoxine) (Aminoxin, Vitelle)	Water-soluble, B-complex group	**Adult** PO/IV: 10-20 mg/day × 3 wk **Pediatric** PO/IV: 5-25 mg/day × 3 wk, then use a pediatric multivitamin product **Adult** PO/IV: 100-200 mg/day **Pediatric** 10-50 mg/day	Deficiency Drug-induced neuritis (e.g., isoniazid for tuberculosis)
vitamin B$_{12}$ (cyanocobalamin) (Nascobal)	Water-soluble, B-complex group	**Adult and pediatric** IM/subcut: 100 mcg/mo **Adult and pediatric** PO: 50-100 mcg/day **Adult only** Intranasal gel: 500 mcg/wk	Deficiency; anemia
Vitamins A, C, E, and K			
vitamin A (Aquasol A, others)	Fat soluble	**Adult and pediatric older than 8 yr** PO: Up to 500,000 units/day × 3 days, then 10,000-50,000 units/day for up to 2 mo **Pediatric 1-8 yr** PO: 5000-10,000 units/kg/day until recovery	Deficiency
vitamin C (ascorbic acid) (Vita-C, Dull-C, others)	Water soluble	**Adult and pediatric** PO/IV/IM/subcut: 100-250 mg 1-2 times daily × 2 wk	Deficiency (scurvy)

IM, Intramuscular; *IV,* intravenous; *PO,* oral; *subcut,* subcutaneous.
*Dosages should be individualized. Higher doses may be required based on response to therapy.

Continued

DOSAGES—cont'd

Selected Vitamins—cont'd

Drug	Pharmacologic Class	Usual Dosage Range	Indications/Uses
Vitamins A, C, E, and K—cont'd			
vitamin E (d-alpha tocopherol) (Aquavit E, Dry E 400, others)	Fat soluble	**Adult and pediatric older than 14 yr†** PO: 22.5 units/day **Pediatric 0-14 yr†** 4.5-16.5 units/day	Nutritional supplementation
vitamin K (phytonadione) (Mephyton, AquaMEPHYTON)	Fat soluble	**Adult** PO: 2.5-10 mg/day IM/IV: 1-10 mg single dose	Deficiency; warfarin-induced hypoprothrombinemia
		Infant and pediatric PO: 2.5-5 mg/day IM/IV: 1-2 mg single dose	Deficiency; hemorrhagic disease of newborn infant

†Dosage should be individualized by prescriber based on severity of deficiency.

7-dehydrocholesterol. It is more commonly referred to as *chole-calciferol* (vitamin D$_3$). This endogenous synthesis of vitamin D$_3$ usually produces sufficient amounts to meet daily requirements. Vitamin D is obtained through both endogenous synthesis and consumption of vitamin D$_2$–containing foods such as fish oils, salmon, sardines, and herring; fortified milk, bread, and cereals; and animal livers, tuna fish, eggs, and butter.

Mechanism of Action and Drug Effects

The basic function of vitamin D is to regulate the absorption and subsequent utilization of calcium and phosphorus. It is also necessary for the normal calcification of bone. Vitamin D in coordination with parathyroid hormone and calcitonin regulates serum calcium levels by increasing calcium absorption from the small intestine and extracting calcium from the bone when needed. Ergocalciferol and cholecalciferol are inactive and require transformation into active metabolites for biologic activity. Both vitamin D$_2$ and vitamin D$_3$ are biotransformed in the liver by the actions of parathyroid hormone. The resulting compound, calcifediol, is then transported to the kidney, where it is converted to calcitriol, which is believed to be the most physiologically active vitamin D analogue. Calcitriol promotes the intestinal absorption of calcium and phosphorus and the deposition of calcium and phosphorus into the structure of teeth and bones.

The drug effects of vitamin D are very similar to those of vitamin A and essentially all vitamin and mineral compounds. It is used as a supplement to satisfy normal daily requirements or an increased demand, as in infants and pregnant and nursing women.

Indications

Vitamin D can be used either to supplement dietary intake or to treat a deficiency of vitamin D. In the case of supplementation, it is given as a prophylactic measure to prevent deficiency-related problems. Vitamin D may also be used to treat and correct the result of a long-term deficiency that leads to such conditions as infantile rickets, tetany (involuntary sustained muscular contractions), and osteomalacia (softening of the bones). **Rickets** is specifically a vitamin D deficiency state. Symptoms include soft, pliable bones, which causes deformities such as bowlegs and knock knees; nodular enlargement on the ends and sides of the bones; muscle pain; enlarged skull; chest deformities; spinal

TABLE 53-4 Vitamin D: Adverse Effects

Body System	Adverse Effects
Cardiovascular	Hypertension, dysrhythmias
Central nervous	Fatigue, weakness, drowsiness, headache
Gastrointestinal	Nausea, vomiting, anorexia, cramps, metallic taste, dry mouth, constipation
Genitourinary	Polyuria, albuminuria, increased blood urea nitrogen level
Musculoskeletal	Decreased bone growth, bone and muscle pain

curvature; enlargement of the liver and spleen; profuse sweating; and general tenderness of the body when touched. Vitamin D can also help promote the absorption of phosphorus and calcium. For this reason, its use is important in preventing osteoporosis. Because of the role of vitamin D in the regulation of calcium and phosphorus, it may be used to correct deficiencies of these two elements. Other uses include dietary supplementation and treatment of osteodystrophy, hypocalcemia, hypoparathyroidism, pseudohypoparathyroidism, and hypophosphatemia.

Contraindications

Contraindications to vitamin D products include known allergy to the product, hypercalcemia, renal dysfunction, and hyperphosphatemia.

Adverse Effects

As with vitamin A, very few acute adverse effects are associated with normal vitamin D ingestion. Only after long-term excessive ingestion of vitamin D do symptoms appear. Such effects are usually noticed in the gastrointestinal tract or the central nervous system (CNS) and are listed in Table 53-4.

Toxicity and Management of Overdose

The major toxic effects from ingesting excessive amounts of vitamin D occur most commonly in children. Discontinuation of vitamin D and reduced calcium intake reverse the toxic state. The amount of vitamin D considered to be toxic varies considerably among individuals but is generally thought to be 1.25 to 2.5 mg of ergocalciferol daily in adults and 25 mcg daily in infants and children.

The toxic effects of vitamin D are those associated with hypertension, such as weakness, fatigue, headache, anorexia, dry mouth, metallic taste, nausea, vomiting, abdominal cramps, ataxia, and bone pain. If not recognized and treated, these symptoms can progress to impairment of renal function and osteoporosis.

Interactions

Reduced absorption of vitamin D occurs with the concurrent use of lubricant laxatives and cholestyramine. Patients taking digitalis preparations can develop cardiac dysrhythmias as a result of excessive vitamin D intake.

Dosages

For the recommended dosages of vitamin D, see the Dosages table on p. 825.

DRUG PROFILES

There are four forms of vitamin D: calcifediol, calcitriol, dihydrotachysterol, and ergocalciferol. Vitamin D is available in OTC medications, such as multivitamin products, or by prescription. Although various pharmaceutical manufacturers may list their individual vitamin D products as pregnancy category C, these products are generally considered to be category A or B as long as the patient is not dosed at higher levels than recommended.

calcifediol

Calcifediol (Calderol) is the 25-hydroxylated form of cholecalciferol (vitamin D_3). It is a vitamin D analogue used primarily for the management of hypocalcemia in patients with chronic renal failure who are undergoing hemodialysis. Calcifediol is also used for signs of hyperparathyroid disease. It is available only for oral use.

calcitriol

Calcitriol (Rocaltrol) is the 1,25-dihydroxylated form of cholecalciferol (vitamin D_3). It is a vitamin D analogue used for the management of hypocalcemia in patients with chronic renal failure who are undergoing hemodialysis. It is also used in the treatment of hypoparathyroidism and pseudohypoparathyroidism, vitamin D–dependent rickets, hypophosphatemia, and hypocalcemia in premature infants. It is available in both oral and injectable forms.

PHARMACOKINETICS

Route	Onset of Action	Peak Plasma Concentration	Elimination Half-life	Duration of Action
PO	Less than 3 hr	3-6 hr	3-6 hr	3-5 days

dihydrotachysterol

Dihydrotachysterol (Hytakerol) is a vitamin D analogue that is administered orally once daily for the treatment of any of the previously mentioned conditions. Intramuscular use is indicated for patients with gastrointestinal, liver, or biliary disease associated with malabsorption of vitamin D analogues. It is available orally and parenterally.

ergocalciferol

Ergocalciferol (Drisdol) is vitamin D_2. It is indicated for use in patients with gastrointestinal, liver, or biliary disease associated with malabsorption of vitamin D analogues. It is available orally and parenterally.

PHARMACOKINETICS

Route	Onset of Action	Peak Plasma Concentration	Elimination Half-life	Duration of Action
PO	30 days	Unknown	19 days	Months to years

VITAMIN E

Four biologically active chemicals called **tocopherols** (alpha, beta, gamma, and delta) make up the vitamin E compounds. Alpha tocopherol is the most biologically active natural form of vitamin E and can come from plant and animal sources.

Mechanism of Action and Drug Effects

Although vitamin E is a powerful biologic antioxidant and an essential component of the diet, its exact nutritional function has not been fully demonstrated. The only recognized significant deficiency syndrome for vitamin E occurs in premature infants. In this situation, vitamin E deficiency may result in irritability, edema, thrombosis, and hemolytic anemia.

The drug effects of vitamin E are not as well defined as those of the other fat-soluble vitamins. It is believed to protect polyunsaturated fatty acids, a component of cellular membranes. It has also been shown to hinder the deterioration of substances such as vitamin A and ascorbic acid (vitamin C), two substances that are highly oxygen sensitive and readily oxidized; thus it acts as an antioxidant.

Indications

Vitamin E is most commonly used as a dietary supplement to augment current daily intake or to treat a deficiency. Premature infants are those at greatest risk for complications from vitamin E deficiency. Vitamin E has received much attention as an antioxidant. Preventing the oxidation of various substances prevents the formation of toxic chemicals within the body, some of which are believed to cause cancer. There is a popular but unproved theory that vitamin E has beneficial effects for patients with cancer, heart disease, premenstrual syndrome, and sexual dysfunction. However, the American Heart Association no longer recommends the use of high-dose vitamin E to prevent heart disease. In fact, recent studies have shown no benefit and possible harm.

Contraindications

Contraindications for vitamin E include known allergy to a specific vitamin E product. There are currently no approved injectable forms of this vitamin.

Adverse Effects

Very few acute adverse effects are associated with normal vitamin E ingestion, because it is relatively nontoxic. Adverse effects are usually noticed in the gastrointestinal tract or CNS and are listed in Table 53-5.

Dosages

For the recommended dosages of vitamin E, see the Dosages table on p. 825.

TABLE 53-5 Vitamin E: Adverse Effects

Body System	Adverse Effects
Central nervous	Fatigue, headache, blurred vision
Gastrointestinal	Nausea, diarrhea, flatulence
Genitourinary	Increased blood urea nitrogen level
Musculoskeletal	Weakness

Vitamin E is available as an OTC medication. As noted, it has four forms: alpha, beta, gamma, and delta tocopherol. It is available in many multivitamin preparations and is also available by prescription. Vitamin E products are usually contraindicated only in cases of known drug allergy.

vitamin E

Vitamin E (Aquasol E) activity is generally expressed in U.S. Pharmacopeia (USP) or international units. It is available for oral and topical use.

VITAMIN K

Vitamin K is the last of the four fat-soluble vitamins (A, D, E, and K). There are three types of vitamin K: phytonadione (vitamin K_1), menaquinone (vitamin K_2), and menadione (vitamin K_3). The body does not store large amounts of vitamin K; however, vitamin K_2 is synthesized by the intestinal flora, which provides an endogenous supply.

Vitamin K is essential for the synthesis of blood coagulation factors, which takes place in the liver. Vitamin K–dependent blood coagulation factors are factors II, VII, IX, and X. Other names for these clotting factors are as follows: factor II (prothrombin); factor VII (proconvertin); factor IX (Christmas factor); and factor X (Stuart-Prower factor)

Mechanism of Action and Drug Effects

Vitamin K activity is essential for effective blood clotting because, as noted earlier, it facilitates the hepatic biosynthesis of factors II, VII, IX and X. Vitamin K deficiency results in coagulation disorders caused by hypoprothrombinemia. Coagulation defects affecting these clotting factors can be corrected with administration of vitamin K. Vitamin K deficiency is rare because intestinal flora are normally able to synthesize sufficient amounts. If a deficiency develops, it can be corrected with vitamin K supplementation.

Indications

Vitamin K is indicated for dietary supplementation and for treatment of deficiency states. Although rare, deficiency states can develop with inadequate dietary intake or inhibition of the intestinal flora resulting from the administration of broad-spectrum antibiotics. Deficiency states can also be seen in newborns because of malabsorption attributable to inadequate amounts of bile or selected drugs. For this reason, infants born in hospitals are often given a prophylactic intramuscular dose of vitamin K on arrival to the nursery. Vitamin K deficiency can also result from the administration and pharmacologic action of the oral anticoagulant warfarin (see Chapter 28). Warfarin works to thin the blood by inhibiting vitamin K–dependent clotting factors II, VII, IX, and X in the liver. Administration of vitamin K overrides the mechanism by which the anticoagulant inhibits production of vitamin K–dependent clotting factors. Thus vitamin K can be used to reverse the effects of warfarin. It is important to note that when vitamin K is used in this manner, the patient becomes unresponsive to warfarin for approximately 1 week after vitamin K administration.

Contraindications

The only usual contraindication to treatment with vitamin K is known drug allergy.

TABLE 53-6 Vitamin K: Adverse Effects

Body System	Adverse Effects
Central nervous	Headache, brain damage (large doses)
Gastrointestinal	Nausea, decreased liver enzyme levels
Hematologic	Hemolytic anemia, hemoglobinuria, hyperbilirubinemia
Integumentary	Rash, urticaria

Adverse Effects

Vitamin K is relatively nontoxic and thus causes very few adverse effects. Severe reactions limited to hypersensitivity or anaphylaxis have occurred rarely during or immediately after intravenous administration. Adverse effects are usually related to injection-site reactions and hypersensitivity. See Table 53-6 for a list of such major effects by body system.

Toxicity and Management of Overdose

Toxicity is primarily limited to use in the newborn. Hemolysis of red blood cells (RBCs) can occur, especially in infants with low levels of glucose-6-phosphate dehydrogenase. In severe cases, replacement with blood products may be indicated.

Dosages

For the recommended dosages of vitamin K, see the Dosages table on p. 825.

The most commonly used form of vitamin K is phytonadione (vitamin K_1). Both phytonadione and menadione (vitamin K_3) are available by prescription only in oral and parenteral forms. Menadione is classified as a pregnancy category X drug, whereas phytonadione is a category C drug. They are both contraindicated in patients who have shown a hypersensitivity reaction to them. Their use is also contraindicated in patients who are in the last few weeks of pregnancy and in patients with severe hepatic disease.

vitamin K_1

Vitamin K_1 (phytonadione) (Aqua-Mephyton) is available in both oral and injectable forms. Because of its potential to cause anaphylaxis (due to the formulation), for intravenous use it is usually diluted and given over 30 to 60 minutes. Vitamin K should be given subcutaneously and not intramuscularly when used to reverse warfarin effects.

PHARMACOKINETICS

Route	Onset of Action	Peak Plasma Concentration	Elimination Half-life	Duration of Action
PO	6-12 hr	24-48 hr	1.2 hr	24 hr
IV	1-2 hr	12-14 hr	1.2 hr	24 hr

WATER-SOLUBLE VITAMINS

The water-soluble vitamins include the vitamin B complex and vitamin C (ascorbic acid). They are present in a variety of plant and animal food sources. The vitamin B complex is a group of 10 vitamins that are often found together in food, although they are chemically dissimilar and have different metabolic functions.

BOX 53-1 Water-Soluble Vitamins: Alternate Names

Designation	Alternate Name
vitamin B complex	
vitamin B_1	thiamine
vitamin B_2	riboflavin
vitamin B_3	niacin
vitamin B_5	pantothenic acid
vitamin B_6	pyridoxine
vitamin B_9	folic acid
vitamin B_{12}	cyanocobalamin
vitamin C	ascorbic acid

Because the B vitamins were originally isolated from the same sources, they were grouped together as B-complex vitamins. Vitamin C (ascorbic acid), the other principal water-soluble vitamin, is concentrated in citrus fruits and is not classified as part of the B complex. The numeric subscripts associated with various B vitamins reflect the order in which they were discovered. In clinical practice, some B vitamins are more often referred to by their common name, whereas others are more often referred to by their numeric designation. For example, "vitamin B_{12}" is used more often in clinical practice than the corresponding common name "cyanocobalamin." However, "folic acid" is rarely referred to as "vitamin B_9." The most commonly used B-complex vitamins, as well as vitamin C, are listed in Box 53-1. Folic acid (vitamin B_9) has a special role in hematopoiesis and therefore is described further in Chapter 55.

Water-soluble vitamins are a chemically diverse group sharing only the characteristic of being dissolvable in water. Like fat-soluble vitamins, they act primarily as coenzymes or oxidation-reduction agents in important metabolic pathways. Unlike fat-soluble vitamins, water-soluble vitamins are not stored in the body in appreciable amounts. Their water-soluble properties promote urinary excretion and reduce their half-life in the body. Therefore, dietary intake must be adequate and regular or else deficiency states will develop. The body excretes what it does not need, which makes toxic reactions to water-soluble vitamins very rare.

VITAMIN B_1

A deficiency of vitamin B_1 (thiamine) results in the classic disease **beriberi** or Wernicke's encephalopathy (cerebral beriberi). Common findings in beriberi include brain lesions, polyneuropathy of peripheral nerves, serous effusions (abnormal collections of fluids in body tissues), and cardiac anatomic changes. Vitamin deficiency can result from poor diet, extended fever, hyperthyroidism, liver disease, alcoholism, malabsorption, and pregnancy and breast-feeding.

Mechanism of Action and Drug Effects

Vitamin B_1 (thiamine) is an essential precursor for the formation of *thiamine pyrophosphate*. When thiamine combines with *adenosine triphosphate (ATP)*, the result is *thiamine pyrophosphate coenzyme*. This is required for the *citric acid cycle (Krebs cycle)*, a major part of carbohydrate metabolism, as well as several other metabolic pathways. In addition, thiamine plays a key role in the integrity of the peripheral nervous system, cardiovascular system, and gastrointestinal tract.

Indications

The essential role of thiamine in many metabolic pathways makes it useful in treating a variety of metabolic disorders. These include subacute necrotizing encephalomyelopathy, maple syrup urine disease, and lactic acidosis associated with pyruvate carboxylase enzyme deficiency and hyper-beta-alaninemia. Some of the deficiency states treated by thiamine are beriberi, Wernicke's encephalopathy, peripheral neuritis associated with **pellagra** (niacin deficiency), and neuritis of pregnancy. Thiamine is used as a dietary supplement to prevent or treat deficiency in cases of malabsorption such as that induced by alcoholism, cirrhosis, or gastrointestinal disease. Other situations in which thiamine may have therapeutic value are the management of poor appetite, ulcerative colitis, chronic diarrhea, and cerebellar syndrome or ataxia (impaired muscular coordination). It is also used as an oral insect repellent.

Contraindications

The only usual contraindication to any of the B-complex vitamins is known allergy to a specific vitamin product.

Adverse Effects

Adverse effects are rare but include hypersensitivity reactions, nausea, restlessness, pulmonary edema, pruritus, urticaria, weakness, sweating, angioedema, cyanosis, and cardiovascular collapse. Administration by intramuscular injection can produce local tenderness, and intravenous injections can produce anaphylaxis.

Interactions

Thiamine is incompatible with alkaline- and sulfite-containing solutions.

Dosages

For the recommended dosages of vitamin B_1, see the Dosages table on p. 825.

DRUG PROFILE

thiamine

Thiamine is contraindicated only in individuals with a history of a hypersensitivity reaction. Thiamine is available for both oral use and injection. Pregnancy category A.

PHARMACOKINETICS

Route	Onset of Action	Peak Plasma Concentration	Elimination Half-life	Duration of Action
PO	Unknown	1-2 hr	1.2 hr	24 hr

VITAMIN B_2

A deficiency of vitamin B_2 (riboflavin) results in cutaneous, oral, and corneal changes that include cheilosis (chapped or fissured lips), seborrheic dermatitis, and keratitis.

Mechanism of Action and Drug Effects

Riboflavin serves several important functions in the body. Riboflavin is converted into two coenzymes (flavin mononucleotide and flavin adenine dinucleotide) that are essential for tissue respiration. Riboflavin also plays an important part in carbohydrate catabolism. Another B vitamin, vitamin B_6 (pyridoxine), requires riboflavin for activation. Riboflavin is also needed to convert tryptophan into niacin and to maintain erythrocyte integrity. Deficiency is rare and does not usually occur in healthy people.

Indications

Riboflavin is primarily used as a dietary supplement and for treatment of deficiency states. Patients who may experience riboflavin deficiency include those with longstanding infections, liver disease, alcoholism, or malignancy, and those taking probenecid. Riboflavin supplementation may also be beneficial in the treatment of microcytic anemia; acne; migraine headache; congenital methemoglobinemia (presence in the blood of an abnormal, nonfunctional hemoglobin pigment); muscle cramps; and Gopalan's syndrome, a symptom of suspected riboflavin (and possibly pantothenic acid [vitamin B_5]) deficiency that involves a sensation of tingling in the extremities (for this reason, it is also called *burning feet syndrome*).

Contraindications

The only usual contraindication to riboflavin is known allergy to a given vitamin product.

Adverse Effects

Riboflavin is a very safe and effective vitamin; to date, no adverse effects or toxic effects have been reported. In large dosages, riboflavin will discolor urine to a yellow-orange.

Dosages

For the commonly recommended dosages of riboflavin, see the Dosages table on p. 825.

DRUG PROFILE

riboflavin

Riboflavin (vitamin B_2) is needed for normal respiratory functions. It is a safe, nontoxic water-soluble vitamin with almost no adverse effects. It is available only for oral use. Pregnancy category A.

PHARMACOKINETICS

Route	Onset of Action	Peak Plasma Concentration	Elimination Half-life	Duration of Action
PO	Unknown	Unknown	66-84 min	24 hr

VITAMIN B_3

The body is able to produce a small amount of vitamin B_3 (niacin) from dietary tryptophan, an essential amino acid occurring in dietary proteins and some commercially available nutritional supplements. A dietary deficiency of niacin (vitamin B_3) will produce the classic symptoms known as *pellagra*. Symptoms of pellagra include various psychotic disorders; neurasthenic syndrome; crusting, erythema, and desquamation of the skin; scaly dermatitis; inflammation of the oral, vaginal, and urethral mucosa, including glossitis (inflamed tongue); and diarrhea or bloody diarrhea.

Mechanism of Action and Drug Effects

The metabolic actions of niacin (vitamin B_3) are not due to niacin in the ingested form but rather to its metabolic product, *nicotinamide*. Nicotinamide is required for numerous metabolic reactions, including those involved in carbohydrate, protein, purine, and lipid metabolism, as well as tissue respiration (Figure 53-1). A key example involves two compounds, *nicotinamide adenosine dinucleotide (NAD)* and *nicotinamide adenosine dinucleotide phosphate (NADP)*, both of which are necessary for the carbohydrate pathway known as *glycogenolysis* (the breakdown of stored glycogen into usable glucose). The parent compound, niacin itself, also has a pharmacologic role as an *antilipemic* drug (see Chapter 29). The doses of niacin required for its antilipemic effect are substantially higher than those required for the nutritional and metabolic effects.

Indications

Niacin is indicated for the prevention and treatment of pellagra, a condition caused by a deficiency of vitamin B_3 that is most commonly the result of malabsorption, and also for management of certain types of hyperlipidemia (see Chapter 29). It also has a beneficial effect in peripheral vascular disease.

Contraindications

Niacin, unlike certain other B-complex vitamins, has additional contraindications besides drug allergy. These include liver disease, severe hypotension, arterial hemorrhage, and active peptic ulcer disease.

Adverse Effects

The most frequent adverse effects associated with the use of niacin are flushing, pruritus, and gastrointestinal distress. These usually subside with continued use and are most frequently seen

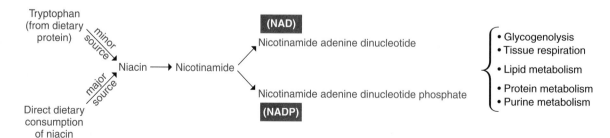

FIGURE 53-1 Niacin, once in the body, is converted to nicotinamide adenosine dinucleotide (NAD) and nicotinamide adenosine dinucleotide (NADP), which are coenzymes needed for many metabolic processes.

TABLE 53-7 Niacin (Vitamin B₃): Adverse Effects

Body System	Adverse Effects
Cardiovascular	Postural hypotension, dysrhythmias, atrial fibrillation
Central nervous	Headache, dizziness, anxiety, sensation of warmth
Gastrointestinal	Nausea, vomiting, diarrhea, peptic ulcer
Genitourinary	Hyperuricemia
Hepatic	Abnormal liver function test results, hepatitis
Integumentary	Flushing, dry skin, rash, pruritus, keratosis
Metabolic	Decreased glucose tolerance

when larger doses of niacin are used in the treatment of hyperlipidemia. Table 53-7 lists adverse effects by body system.

Dosages

For the commonly recommended dosages of niacin, see the Dosages table on p. 825.

DRUG PROFILE

niacin

Niacin is used to treat pellagra, hyperlipidemias, and peripheral vascular disease. Its use should be monitored closely in patients who have a history of coronary artery disease, gallbladder disease, jaundice, liver disease, or arterial bleeding. It is available only for oral use. Pregnancy category A.

PHARMACOKINETICS

Route	Onset of Action	Peak Plasma Concentration	Elimination Half-life	Duration of Action
PO	30-60 min	45 min	45 min	Variable

VITAMIN B₆

Vitamin B₆ (pyridoxine) is composed of three compounds: pyridoxine, pyridoxal, and pyridoxamine. Deficiency of vitamin B₆ can lead to a type of anemia known as *sideroblastic anemia*, neurologic disturbances, seborrheic dermatitis, cheilosis, and xanthurenic aciduria (formation of xanthine crystals or "stones" in urine). It may also result in convulsions, especially in neonates and infants; hypochromic microcytic anemia; and glossitis (inflamed tongue) and stomatitis (inflamed oral mucosa). Pyridoxine deficiency also affects the peripheral nerves, skin, mucous membranes. Inadequate intake or poor absorption of pyridoxine causes the development of these conditions. Vitamin B₆ deficiency may occur as a result of uremia, alcoholism, cirrhosis, hyperthyroidism, malabsorption syndromes, and heart failure. It may also be induced by various drugs, such as isoniazid, cycloserine, ethionamide, hydralazine, penicillamine, and pyrazinamide.

Mechanism of Action and Drug Effects

Pyridoxine, pyridoxal, and pyridoxamine are all converted in erythrocytes to the active coenzyme forms of vitamin B₆, *pyridoxal phosphate* and *pyridoxamine phosphate*. These compounds are necessary for many metabolic functions, such as protein, carbohydrate, and lipid utilization in the body. They also play an

TABLE 53-8 Pyridoxine (Vitamin B₆): Adverse Effects

Body System	Adverse Effects
Central nervous	Paresthesias, flushing, warmth, headache, lethargy
Integumentary	Pain at injection site

important part in the conversion of the amino acid tryptophan to niacin (vitamin B₃) and the neurotransmitter *serotonin*. They are also essential in the synthesis of gamma-aminobutyric acid, an inhibitory neurotransmitter in the CNS. They are important in the synthesis of heme and the maintenance of the hematopoietic system. In addition, these substances are necessary for the integrity of the peripheral nerves, skin, and mucous membranes.

Indications

Pyridoxine is used to prevent and treat vitamin B₆ deficiency. This includes deficiency that can result from therapy with certain medications, including isoniazid (for tuberculosis), hydralazine (for hypertension), and oral contraceptives. Although deficiency of vitamin B₆ is rare, it can occur in conditions of inadequate intake or poor absorption of pyridoxine. Seizures that are unresponsive to usual therapy, morning sickness during pregnancy, and various metabolic disorders may respond to pyridoxine therapy.

Contraindications

The only usual contraindication to pyridoxine use is drug allergy.

Adverse Effects

Adverse effects with pyridoxine use are rare and usually do not occur at normal dosages; high dosages and long-term use may produce the adverse effects listed in Table 53-8. Toxic effects are a result of very large dosages sustained for several months. Neurotoxicity is the most likely result, but this will subside upon discontinuation of the pyridoxine.

Interactions

Pyridoxine will reduce the activity of levodopa; therefore, vitamin formulations containing B₆ should be avoided in patients taking levodopa alone. However, the overwhelming majority of patients with Parkinson's disease take a combination of levodopa and carbidopa, and this interaction does not occur with combination therapy.

Dosages

For the commonly recommended dosages of vitamin B₆, see the Dosages table on p. 825.

DRUG PROFILE

pyridoxine

Pyridoxine is a water-soluble B-complex vitamin composed of three components: pyridoxine, pyridoxal, and pyridoxamine. It has several vital roles in the body but is primarily responsible for the integrity of peripheral nerves, skin, mucous membranes, and the hematopoietic system. It is available only for oral use. Pregnancy category A.

PHARMACOKINETICS

Route	Onset of Action	Peak Plasma Concentration	Elimination Half-life	Duration of Action
PO	Unknown	30-60 min	15-20 days	Unknown

VITAMIN B₁₂

Vitamin B_{12} (cyanocobalamin) is a water-soluble B-complex vitamin that contains cobalt (hence, its name; and *cyano-* means "blue"). It is synthesized by microorganisms and is present in the body as two different coenzymes: adenosylcobalamin and methylcobalamin. Cyanocobalamin is a required coenzyme for many metabolic pathways, including fat and carbohydrate metabolism and protein synthesis. It is also required for growth, cell replication, hematopoiesis, and nucleoprotein and myelin synthesis (Figure 53-2).

Vitamin B_{12} deficiency results in gastrointestinal lesions, neurologic changes that can result in degenerative CNS lesions, and megaloblastic anemia. The major cause of cyanocobalamin deficiency is malabsorption. Other possible but less likely causes are poor diet, chronic alcoholism, and chronic hemorrhage.

Mechanism of Action and Drug Effects

Humans must have an exogenous source of cyanocobalamin, because it is required for nucleoprotein and myelin synthesis, cell reproduction, normal growth, and the maintenance of normal erythropoiesis. The cells that have the greatest requirement for vitamin B_{12} are those that divide rapidly, such as epithelial cells, bone marrow, and myeloid cells.

Reduced sulfhydryl (–5H) groups are required to metabolize fats and carbohydrates and to synthesize protein. Cyanocobalamin is involved in maintaining sulfhydryl groups in the reduced form. Cyanocobalamin deficiency can lead to neurologic damage that begins with an inability to produce myelin and is followed by gradual degeneration of the axon and nerve head.

Cyanocobalamin activity is identical to the activity of the anti–pernicious anemia factor present in liver extract called *extrinsic factor* or *Castle factor.* The oral absorption of cyanocobalamin (extrinsic factor) requires the presence of *intrinsic factor,* which is a glycoprotein secreted by gastric parietal cells. A complex is formed between the two factors, which is then absorbed by the intestines. This is depicted in Figure 53-3.

Indications

Cyanocobalamin is used to treat deficiency states that develop because of an insufficient intake of the vitamin. It is also included in multivitamin formulations that are used as dietary supplements. Deficiency states are most often the result of malabsorption or poor dietary intake, including consumption of a strict vegetarian diet, because the primary source of cyanocobalamin is foods of animal origin.

The most common manifestation of untreated cyanocobalamin deficiency is pernicious anemia. The use of vitamin B_{12} to treat pernicious anemia and other megaloblastic anemias results in the rapid conversion of a megaloblastic bone marrow to a normoblastic bone marrow. The preferred route of administration of vitamin B_{12} in treating megaloblastic anemias is deep intramuscular injection. If not treated, deficiency states can lead to megaloblastic anemia and irreversible neurologic damage. Cyanocobalamin is also useful in the treatment of pernicious anemia caused by an endogenous lack of intrinsic factor.

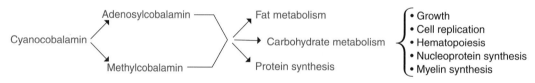

FIGURE 53-2   Cyanocobalamin is a required coenzyme for many body processes.

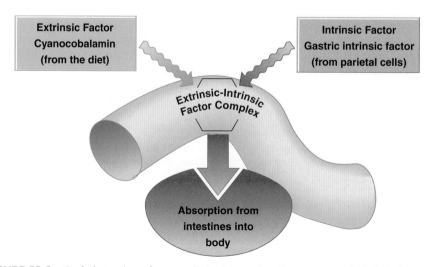

FIGURE 53-3   Oral absorption of cyanocobalamin requires the presence of intrinsic factor, which is secreted by gastric parietal cells.

TABLE 53-9 Cyanocobalamin (Vitamin B$_{12}$): Adverse Effects

Body System	Adverse Effects
Cardiovascular	Heart failure, peripheral, vascular thrombosis, pulmonary edema
Central nervous	Flushing, optic nerve atrophy
Gastrointestinal	Diarrhea
Integumentary	Itching, rash, pain at injection site
Metabolic	Hypokalemia

Contraindications

The only usual contraindication to cyanocobalamin (vitamin B$_{12}$) is known drug product allergy. This may include sensitivity to the chemical element cobalt, which is part of the structure of cyanocobalamin. Another contraindication is hereditary optic nerve atrophy (Leber's disease).

Adverse Effects

Vitamin B$_{12}$ is nontoxic, and large doses must be ingested to produce adverse effects, which include itching, transitory diarrhea, and fever. Other adverse effects are listed by body system in Table 53-9.

Interactions

Concurrent use with anticonvulsants, aminoglycoside antibiotics, or long-acting potassium preparations decreases the oral absorption of vitamin B$_{12}$. In addition, it has been suggested that chloramphenicol antagonizes the hematologic response of vitamin B$_{12}$.

Dosages

For the commonly recommended dosages of vitamin B$_{12}$, see the Dosages table on p. 825.

DRUG PROFILE

cyanocobalamin

Cyanocobalamin is a water-soluble B-complex vitamin required for maintenance of body fat and carbohydrate metabolism and protein synthesis. It is also needed for growth, cell replication, blood cell production, and the integrity of normal nerve function. Cyanocobalamin (vitamin B$_{12}$) is available both as OTC preparations and by prescription. Most of the OTC cyanocobalamin-containing products are oral multivitamin preparations, whereas many of the cyanocobalamin-only products contain large doses for parenteral injection and are available by prescription only. Another available dosage form is an intranasal gel. Pregnancy category A.

PHARMACOKINETICS

Route	Onset of Action	Peak Plasma Concentration	Elimination Half-life	Duration of Action
PO	Unknown	8-12 hr	6 days	Unknown

VITAMIN C

Vitamin C (ascorbic acid) can be used in many therapeutic situations. Prolonged ascorbic acid deficiency results in the nutritional disease **scurvy,** which is characterized by weakness, edema, gingivitis and bleeding gums, loss of teeth, anemia, subcutaneous hemorrhage, bone lesions, delayed healing of soft tissues and bones, and hardening of leg muscles. Scurvy has been recognized for several centuries, especially among sailors. In 1795, the British navy ordered the consumption of limes to prevent the disease.

Mechanism of Action and Drug Effects

Vitamin C is reversibly oxidized to dehydroascorbic acid and acts in oxidation-reduction reactions. It is required for several important metabolic activities, including collagen synthesis and the maintenance of connective tissue; tissue repair; maintenance of bone, teeth, and capillaries; and folic acid metabolism (specifically, the conversion of folic acid into its active metabolite). It is also essential for erythropoiesis. Vitamin C enhances the absorption of iron and is required for the synthesis of lipids, proteins, and steroids. It has also been shown to aid in cellular respiration and resistance to infections.

Indications

Vitamin C is used to treat diseases associated with vitamin C deficiency and as a dietary supplement. It is most beneficial in patients who have larger daily requirements because of pregnancy, lactation, hyperthyroidism, fever, stress, infection, trauma, burns, smoking, exposure to cold temperatures, and the use of certain drugs (e.g., estrogens, oral contraceptives, barbiturates, tetracyclines, and salicylates). Because vitamin C is an acid, it can also be used as a urinary acidifier. The benefits of other uses of vitamin C are less well documented. For example, taking vitamin C to prevent or treat the common cold is common practice. However, most large controlled studies have shown that ascorbic acid has little or no value as a prophylactic for the common cold.

Contraindications

The only usual contraindication for vitamin C use is known allergy to a specific vitamin product.

Adverse Effects

Vitamin C is usually nontoxic unless excessive dosages are consumed. Megadoses can produce nausea, vomiting, headache, and abdominal cramps and will acidify the urine, which can result in the formation of cystine, oxalate, and urate renal stones. Furthermore, individuals who discontinue taking excessive daily doses of ascorbic acid can experience scurvylike symptoms.

Interactions

Ascorbic acid has the potential to interact with many classes of drugs. However, clinical experience concerning many interactions is inconclusive. Coadministration with acid-labile drugs such as penicillin G or erythromycin should be avoided. Large doses of vitamin C can acidify the urine and may enhance the excretion of basic drugs and delay the excretion of acidic drugs.

Dosages

For the commonly recommended dosages of vitamin C, see the Dosages table on p. 825.

ascorbic acid

Ascorbic acid is a water-soluble vitamin required for the prevention and treatment of scurvy. It is also required for erythropoiesis and the synthesis of lipids, protein, and steroids. It is available both in OTC preparations such as multivitamin products and by prescription. Ascorbic acid is available in many oral dosage forms as well as an injectable form. Pregnancy category A.

MINERALS

Minerals are essential nutrients that are classified as inorganic compounds. They act as building blocks for many body structures and thus are necessary for a variety of physiologic functions. They are also needed for intracellular and extracellular body fluid electrolytes. Iron is essential for the production of hemoglobin, which is required for transport of oxygen throughout the body (see Chapter 55). Minerals are necessary for muscle contraction and nerve transmission, and are required components of essential enzymes.

Mineral compounds are composed of various metallic and nonmetallic elements that are chemically combined with ionic bonds. When these compounds are dissolved in water, they separate (dissociate) into positively charged metallic cations and electrolytes or negatively charged nonmetallic anions (Figure 53-4). Ingestion of minerals provides essential elements necessary for vital bodily functions. Elements that are required in larger amounts are called *macrominerals;* those required in smaller amounts are called *microminerals* or *trace elements.* Table 53-10 classifies these nutrient elements as either macrominerals or microminerals and as metal or nonmetal.

CALCIUM

Calcium is the most abundant mineral element in the human body, accounting for approximately 2% of the total body weight. The highest concentration of calcium is in bones and teeth. The efficient absorption of calcium requires adequate amounts of vitamin D.

Calcium deficiency results in hypocalcemia and can affect many bodily functions. Causes of calcium deficiency include inadequate calcium intake and/or insufficient vitamin D to facilitate absorption; hypoparathyroidism; and malabsorption syndrome, especially in older people. Calcium deficiency–

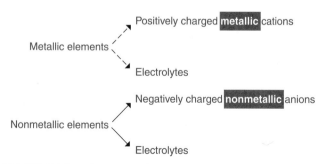

FIGURE 53-4 When mineral compounds are dissolved in water, they separate into positively charged metallic cations or negatively charged nonmetallic anions.

TABLE 53-10 Mineral Elements

Element	Symbol	Type	Ionic/Electrolyte Form
Macrominerals			
Calcium*	Ca	Metal	Ca^{2+} calcium cation
Chlorine	Cl	Nonmetal	Cl^- chloride anion
Magnesium*	Mg	Metal	Mg^{2+} magnesium cation
Phosphorous*	P	Nonmetal	PO_4^{3-} phosphate anion
Potassium	K	Metal	K^+ potassium cation
Sodium	Na	Metal	Na^+ sodium cation
Sulfur	S	Nonmetal	SO_4^{2-} sulfate anion
Microminerals			
Chromium	Cr	Metal	Cr^{3+} chromium cation
Cobalt	Co	Metal	Co^{2+} cobalt cation
Copper	Cu	Metal	Cu^{2+} copper cation
Fluorine	F	Nonmetal	F^+ fluoride anion
Iodine*	I	Nonmetal	I^+ iodide anion
Iron*	Fe	Metal	Fe^{2+} ferrous cation
Manganese	Mn	Metal	Mn^{2+} manganese cation
Molybdenum	Mo	Metal	Mo^{6+} molybdenum cation
Selenium*	Se	Metal	Se^{2-} selenium cation
Zinc*	Zn	Metal	Zn^{2+} zinc cation

*Mineral elements that have a current recommended daily allowance (RDA).

related disorders include infantile rickets, adult osteomalacia, muscle cramps, osteoporosis (especially in postmenopausal females), hypoparathyroidism, and renal dysfunction. Table 53-11 lists the possible causes of calcium deficiency and the resulting disorders.

Mechanism of Action and Drug Effects

Calcium participates in a variety of essential physiologic functions and is a building block for body structures. Specifically, calcium is involved in the proper development and maintenance of teeth and skeletal bones. It is an important catalyst in many of the coagulation pathways in the blood. Calcium acts as a cofactor in clotting reactions involving the intrinsic and extrinsic pathways of thromboplastin. It is also a cofactor in the conversion of prothrombin to thrombin by thromboplastin and the conversion of fibrinogen to fibrin. Calcium is essential for the normal maintenance and function of the nervous, muscular, and skeletal systems and for cell membrane and capillary permeability. It is an important catalyst in many enzymatic reactions, including transmission of nerve impulses; contraction of cardiac, smooth, and skeletal muscles; renal function; respiration; and, as noted earlier, blood coagulation. Calcium also plays a regulatory role in the release and storage of neurotransmitters and hormones, in white blood cell (WBC) and hormone activity, in the uptake and binding of amino acids, and in intestinal absorption of cyanocobalamin (vitamin B_{12}) and gastrin secretion.

Indications

Calcium salts are used for the treatment or prevention of calcium depletion in patients for whom dietary measures are inadequate. Calcium requirements are also high for growing children and for women who are pregnant or breast-feeding. Many

TABLE 53-11 Calcium Deficiency: Causes and Disorders

Cause	Disorder
Inadequate intake	Infantile rickets
Insufficient vitamin D	Adult osteomalacia
Hypoparathyroidism	Muscle cramps
Malabsorption syndrome	Osteoporosis

conditions may be associated with calcium deficiency, including the following:

- Achlorhydria
- Alkalosis
- Chronic diarrhea
- Hyperphosphatemia
- Hypoparathyroidism
- Menopause
- Pancreatitis
- Pregnancy and lactation
- Premenstrual syndrome
- Renal failure
- Sprue
- Steatorrhea
- Vitamin D deficiency

Calcium is also used to treat various manifestations of established deficiency states, including adult osteomalacia, hypoparathyroidism, infantile rickets or tetany, muscle cramps, osteoporosis, and renal insufficiency. In addition, calcium is used as a dietary supplement for women during pregnancy and lactation.

More than 12 different selected calcium salts are available for treatment or nutritional supplementation. Each calcium salt contains a different amount of elemental calcium per gram of calcium salt. Table 53-12 lists the available salts and their associated calcium content.

Contraindications

Contraindications for administration of exogenous calcium include hypercalcemia, ventricular fibrillation of the heart, and known allergy to a specific calcium drug product.

Adverse Effects

Although adverse effects and toxicity are rare, hypercalcemia can occur. Symptoms include anorexia, nausea, vomiting, and constipation. In addition, when calcium salts are administered by intramuscular or subcutaneous injection, mild to severe local reactions, including burning, necrosis and sloughing of tissue, cellulitis, and soft tissue calcification, may occur. Venous irritation may occur with intravenous administration. Other adverse effects associated with both oral and parenteral use of calcium salts are listed in Table 53-13.

Toxicity and Management of Overdose

Long-term excessive calcium intake can result in severe hypercalcemia, which can cause cardiac irregularities, delirium, and coma. Management of acute hypercalcemia may require hemodialysis, whereas milder cases will respond to discontinuation of calcium intake.

TABLE 53-12 Calcium Salts: Calcium Content

Calcium Salt	Elemental Calcium Content (per gram)
Phosphate tribasic	400 mg (20 mEq)
Carbonate	400 mg (20 mEq)
Phosphate dibasic anhydrous	290 mg (14.5 mEq)
Chloride	270 mg (13.5 mEq)
Acetate	253 mg (12.7 mEq)
Phosphate dibasic dihydrate	230 mg (11.5 mEq)
Citrate	211 mg (10.6 mEq)
Glycerophosphate	191 mg (9.6 mEq)
Lactate	130 mg (6.5 mEq)
Gluconate	90 mg (4.5 mEq)
Gluceptate	82 mg (4.1 mEq)
Glubionate	64 mg (3.2 mEq)

TABLE 53-13 Calcium Salts: Adverse Effects

Body System	Adverse Effects
Cardiovascular	Hemorrhage, rebound hypertension
Gastrointestinal	Constipation, nausea, vomiting, flatulence
Genitourinary	Renal dysfunction, renal stones, renal failure
Metabolic	Hypercalcemia, metabolic alkalosis

Interactions

Calcium salts will chelate (bind with) tetracyclines and quinolones to produce an insoluble complex. If hypercalcemia is present in patients taking digitalis preparations, serious cardiac dysrhythmias can occur.

Dosages

For the recommended dosages of calcium and other selected minerals, see the Dosages table on p. 836.

DRUG PROFILE

calcium

Calcium salts are primarily used in the treatment or prevention of calcium depletion in patients in whom dietary measures are inadequate. Many calcium salts are available, all with a different content of elemental calcium per gram of salt. Calcium is available in both oral and parenteral forms. Numerous calcium preparations are available that have different names and provide different doses. Manufacturer instructions should be consulted for recommended dosages. The pharmacokinetics of calcium are highly variable and depend on individual patient physiology and the characteristics of the specific drug product used. Medication errors and confusion are common with calcium products, because the amount of the salt is not the same as the amount of elemental calcium. For example, calcium carbonate 1250 mg is equal to 500 mg of elemental calcium. Depending on the institution, the drug may be profiled as 1250 mg, but the tablet is labeled as 500 mg. Additional confusion occurs with the injectable forms, calcium chloride and calcium gluconate. Calcium chloride provides about three times as much elemental calcium as does calcium gluconate, but they are both ordered as 1 g or 1 ampule. Calcium chloride can cause severe problems if it infiltrates from the intra-

DOSAGES

Selected Minerals

Drug	Pharmacologic Class	Usual Dosage Range	Indications/Uses
calcium carbonate (Tums, others)	Mineral salt	PO: 500 mg 2-4 times daily	Calcium supplementation, hypocalcemia, osteoporosis, renal insufficiency, rickets
magnesium oxide (Max-Ox 400, others)	Mineral salt	PO: 400 mg 1-2 times daily	Magnesium supplementation, hypomagnesemia

PO, Oral.

PREVENTING MEDICATION ERRORS

All Calcium Forms Are Not the Same!

When calcium is given, it is essential to use the correct form. Calcium chloride has many uses, including treatment of cardiac arrest and hypocalcemic tetany. Both calcium carbonate (Os-Cal, Tums, Caltrate) and calcium citrate (Citracal) are used as antacids and are also used to treat or prevent calcium deficiency and to treat hyperphosphatemia. However, calcium acetate (PhosLo) is *not* used for calcium replacement. It is used only to control hyperphosphatemia in patients with end-stage renal disease. Be cautious when giving calcium—the different forms are not interchangeable.

---

venous line. For that reason, it is recommended that it be diluted or given through a central line if it is given by intravenous push. Adding to the confusion is calcium acetate (PhosLo), which is used not for calcium replacement but to bind phosphate in renal patients. Nurses should contact the hospital pharmacist with any questions. Calcium products are pregnancy category C.

MAGNESIUM

Magnesium is one of the principal cations present in the intracellular fluid. It is an essential part of many enzyme systems associated with energy metabolism. Magnesium deficiency (hypomagnesemia) is usually caused by (1) malabsorption, especially in the presence of high calcium intake; (2) alcoholism; (3) long-term intravenous feeding; (4) diuretic use; and (5) metabolic disorders, including hyperthyroidism and diabetic ketoacidosis. Symptoms associated with hypomagnesemia include cardiovascular disturbances, neuromuscular impairment, and mental disturbances. Dietary intake from vegetables and other foods will usually prevent magnesium deficiency. However, magnesium is required in greater amounts in individuals with diets high in protein-rich foods, calcium, and phosphorus.

Mechanism of Action and Drug Effects

The precise mechanism for the effects of magnesium has not been fully determined. Magnesium is a known cofactor for many enzyme systems. It is required for muscle contraction and nerve function. Magnesium produces an anticonvulsant effect by inhibiting neuromuscular transmission in selected convulsive states.

Indications

Magnesium is used for treatment of magnesium deficiency and as a nutritional supplement in total parenteral nutrition and multivitamin preparations. It is used as an anticonvulsant in magnesium deficiency–induced seizure states; to manage complications of pregnancy, including preeclampsia and eclampsia; as a tocolytic drug for inhibition of uterine contractions in premature labor; for treatment of pediatric acute nephropathy; for management of various cardiac dysrhythmias; and for short-term treatment of constipation.

Contraindications

Contraindications to magnesium administration include known drug product allergy, heart block, renal failure, adrenal gland failure (Addison's disease), and hepatitis.

Adverse Effects

Adverse effects of magnesium are due to hypermagnesemia, which results in tendon reflex loss, difficult bowel movements, CNS depression, respiratory distress and heart block, and hypothermia.

Toxicity and Management of Overdose

Toxic effects are extensions of symptoms caused by hypermagnesemia, a major cause of which is the long-term use of magnesium products (especially antacids in patients with renal dysfunction). Severe hypermagnesemia is treated with intravenous calcium and possibly the diuretic furosemide.

Interactions

The use of magnesium with neuromuscular blocking drugs and CNS depressants produces additive effects.

DRUG PROFILE

magnesium

Magnesium is a mineral that has a variety of dosage forms and uses. It is an essential part of many enzyme systems. When it is absent or diminished in the body, cardiovascular, neuromuscular, and mental disturbances can occur. Magnesium sulfate is the most common form of magnesium used as a mineral replacement. It is available in both oral and injectable forms. Pregnancy category B.

PHOSPHORUS

Phosphorus is widely distributed in foods, and thus a dietary deficiency is rare. Deficiency states are primarily due to malabsorption, extensive diarrhea or vomiting, hyperthyroidism, hepatic disease, and long-term use of aluminum or calcium antacids.

Mechanism of Action and Drug Effects

Phosphorus in the form of the phosphate group and/or anion (PO_4^3) is a required precursor for the synthesis of essential body chemicals and an important building block for body structures. Phosphorus is required as a structural unit for the synthesis of nucleic acid and the adenosine phosphate compounds (adenosine monophosphate [AMP], adenosine diphosphate [ADP], and adenosine triphosphate [ATP]) responsible for cellular energy transfer. It is also necessary for the development and maintenance of the skeletal system and teeth. The skeletal bones contain up to 85% of the phosphorus content of the body. In addition, phosphorus is required for the proper utilization of many B-complex vitamins, and it is an essential component of physiologic buffering systems.

Indications

Phosphorus is used for treatment of deficiency states and as a dietary supplement in many multivitamin formulations.

Contraindications

Contraindications to phosphorous or phosphate administration include hyperphosphatemia and hypocalcemia.

Adverse Effects

Adverse effects are usually associated with the use of phosphorus replacement products. These effects include diarrhea, nausea, vomiting, and other gastrointestinal disturbances. Other adverse effects include confusion, weakness, and breathing difficulties.

Toxicity and Management of Overdose

Toxic reactions to phosphorus are extremely rare and usually occur only after ingestion of the pure element.

Interactions

Antacids can reduce the oral absorption of phosphorus.

■ DRUG PROFILE

phosphorus
Phosphorus is a mineral that is essential to our well-being. It is needed to make energy in the form of ADP and ATP for all bodily processes. Phosphorus is present in a large number of drug formulations and appears as a phosphate salt (PO_4). Phosphorus should be used with caution in patients with renal impairment. It is available in both oral and parenteral formulations.

ZINC

The metallic element zinc is often taken orally in the form of the sulfate salt as a mineral supplement. Normally a dietary trace element, zinc plays a crucial role in the enzymatic metabolic reactions involving both proteins and carbohydrates. This makes it especially important for normal tissue growth and repair. It therefore also has a major role in wound healing.

NURSING PROCESS

Assessment

Before administering *vitamins*, the nurse should assess the patient for nutritional disorders by reviewing the results of various laboratory tests, such as hemoglobin level, hematocrit, WBC and RBC counts, and serum albumin and total protein levels. The patient's dietary intake, dietary patterns, menu planning, grocery shopping/food practices and habits, and cultural influences should be assessed before any supplemental therapy is given. For vitamin A deficiencies, a baseline assessment of the patient's vision, including night vision, and examination of the skin and mucous membranes should be completed and documented. Serum *vitamin A* levels of less than 20 mcg/dL (in adults) indicate a deficiency. Contraindications, cautions, and drug interactions should be noted and have been previously discussed, (as for the other vitamins covered in this chapter).

For patients who are deficient in *vitamin D*, a baseline assessment of skeletal formation with attention to any deformities should be performed. Serum calcium levels should also be measured as ordered. During the assessment phase for vitamin D, it is important to remember that patients with a serum calcium level of less than 7.5 mg/dL may have deficient vitamin D levels. In addition, determination of baseline inorganic phosphorus and serum citrate levels may be helpful. Before *vitamin E* is administered, patients should be assessed for hypoprothrombinemia, because this condition may occur secondary to vitamin E deficiency. Any baseline bleeding or hematologic problems need to be documented and a thorough skin assessment performed with attention to skin integrity, presence of any edema, muscle weakness, easy bruising, and/or bleeding.

The last of the fat-soluble vitamins, *vitamin K*, is associated with clotting function; therefore, prior to its use, the patient's prothrombin time, international normalized ratio, and platelet counts should be documented. The skin should be assessed for bruises, petechiae, and erythema, and the gums should be examined for gingival bleeding. Urine and stool should also be assessed for the presence of blood before the use of this drug. Vital signs should be measured with attention to blood pressure and pulse rate. If intravenous dosage forms are used, it is important to assess baseline skin color, temperature, and vital signs because of the associated risk for facial flushing, chest pain, weak pulse rate, profuse diaphoresis, and hypotension with possible progression to shock and cardiac arrest. It is also important to remember that the fat-soluble vitamins are all stored in the body tissue when excessive quantities are consumed and may become toxic if taken in large dosages, so baseline values of vitamins A, D, E, and K should always be known before any ordered or recommended therapy is begun.

Vitamin B₁ (thiamine) hypersensitivity may cause skin rash and wheezing; therefore, the presence of any allergic reactions to vitamin B compounds needs to be documented. Because it is rare for a deficiency of only one B-complex vitamin to occur, deficiencies of all the B vitamins must be ruled out before treatment begins. Baseline assessments of vital signs and mental status should be performed, and urinary thiamine levels may also be ordered (in adults urinary thiamine levels of less than 27 mcg/dL indicate deficiency). *Vitamin C* is usually well tolerated; however, the patient

CASE STUDY

Vitamin Supplements

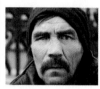

© Wrangler

S.C., aged 49, was found unconscious in a vacant house and was brought to the emergency department. He had an elevated blood alcohol level and eventually manifested delirium tremens. Now, a week later, he is in stable condition on a medical-surgical unit. He is weak and malnourished, and cannot remember how he got to the hospital. The nurse is reviewing his medication list and notes that several vitamin supplements are ordered.

1. Based on his history, what vitamin deficiencies are possible?
2. Which vitamin supplement is especially used to treat complications associated with alcoholism? Explain.
3. S.C. is receiving large doses of several vitamins, and the nurse is concerned about vitamin toxicities. Which type of vitamin, water-soluble or fat-soluble, carries the risk of toxicities? Explain.
4. Because of S.C.'s long-term malnourished state, the physician is concerned about the condition of his bones and starts S.C. on phosphorus and calcium supplementation, along with vitamin D. Explain the rationale behind the addition of vitamin D.

For answers, see *http://evolve.elsevier.com/Lilley*.

---

should be assessed for any history of nutritional deficits or problems with dietary intake, and any allergies should be noted.

With *macrominerals* (e.g., calcium, magnesium), a baseline assessment should include attention to contraindications, cautions, and drug interactions, as well as nutritional status and results of nutrition-related laboratory studies (e.g., hemoglobin level, hematocrit, RBC and WBC counts, levels of these macrominerals). Before calcium and magnesium are administered, the patient's serum levels should be obtained and recorded. Calcium interacts with many medications, as described previously, so a review to identify any potential for such interactions is important. If there is a history of cardiac disease, a baseline electrocardiogram (ECG) recording may be ordered prior to calcium therapy; if decreased QT wave and T wave inversion are observed, calcium may be discontinued or given in reduced dosages as ordered. Magnesium is also associated with several drug interactions, and a review for these potential interactions should be carried out before drug therapy is initiated. Because magnesium may be given for a desired systemic effect, the patient's renal status should be assessed. It is also important to assess the prescriber's order for completeness and reason for use, so that it is fully understood why the drug is being given (e.g., replacement, antacid, or laxative purposes). In addition, an order for the use of calcium, magnesium and/or zinc within total parenteral nutritional infusions should be thoroughly assessed.

Nursing Diagnoses

- Disturbed sensory perception (visual) related to night blindness from vitamin A deficiency
- Acute pain related to bone or skeletal deformities resulting from vitamin D deficiency
- Impaired physical mobility related to poorly developed muscles from vitamin D and/or vitamin E deficiency and from fatigue related to poor nutrition and vitamin B deficiency

- Diarrhea related to vitamin E adverse effects
- Risk for injury (e.g., bruising, bleeding) related to deficient levels of vitamin K and potential for bleeding disorders
- Acute pain in joints related to disease from vitamin C deficiency
- Impaired tissue integrity related to vitamin C deficiency and subsequent decreased healing

Planning

Goals

- Patient maintains sensory, perceptual, and skin/mucosal membrane integrity during therapy.
- Patient experiences minimal complaints and/or adverse effects related to vitamin and mineral therapy.
- Patient regains or maintains normal bowel elimination patterns during therapy.
- Patient reports improved comfort levels during drug therapy.
- Patient reports improved mental processes with therapy.
- Patient regains and maintains levels of activity considered normal for age, weight, and height.

Outcome Criteria

- Patient openly verbalizes fears and anxieties about possible visual, perceptual, and bodily changes due to vitamin and mineral deficiencies with positive reports of compliance to prescribed therapies.
- Patient states measures to minimize injury and maximize intactness of skin and mucous membranes, such as performing frequent mouth care, keeping skin clean and dry and applying moisturizers as needed, and drinking at least 6 to 8 glasses of water per day.
- Patient states measures to help prevent falls and injury on a daily basis (e.g., minimizing obstacles in the home; removing excess furniture or small, loose rugs; adding night lights).
- Patient uses dietary measures (e.g., increased consumption of bulk, fiber), hydration, and progressive exercise to assist in regaining normal bowel patterns.
- Patient increases stamina and energy to enhance tolerance for performing activities of daily living and/or progressive exercise, as tolerated.

Implementation

Before administering *vitamin A*, the nurse should document the patient's dietary intake for the preceding 24 hours. Any signs and symptoms of hypervitaminosis or hypercarotenemia (excess vitamin A; see previous discussion) should be documented. *Vitamin D* should be given with concurrent evaluations of renal function and serum calcium levels. The nurse should assess growth measurements in children, and all patients should be informed of signs and symptoms to report to their prescribers, such as constipation, anorexia, nausea, vomiting, metallic taste, and dry mouth. *Vitamin B_1* (thiamine) therapy should be given as ordered. Niacin should be administered with milk or food to decrease gastrointestinal upset. If pyridoxine is ordered to be given intravenously, the proper infusion rate and dilutional solutions need to be verified. Cyanocobalamin should be administered orally with meals to increase its absorption. Ascorbic acid should be given orally, and oral effervescent forms should be dissolved in at least 6 oz of water or juice. If *vitamin C* is given intravenously, the proper infusion rate and dilutional solutions should be checked. If it is administered for acidification of urine, the nurse should assess urinary pH frequently.

Various oral *calcium* products are available (see pharmacology discussion), and because of the differences in the amount of elemental calcium they provide (e.g., calcium carbonate 1250 mg is equal to only 500 mg of elemental calcium) medication errors may occur and confusion may arise about the various dosages available OTC. Injectable dosage forms of calcium may also be confusing, and so the order should be carefully followed and the medication checked, per policy and standards (see previous discussion in the pharmacology section and the Preventing Medication Errors box on p. 836). Because of problems with venous irritation, intravenous calcium should be given via an intravenous infusion pump and with proper dilution. Giving intravenous calcium too rapidly may precipitate cardiac irregularities or cardiac arrest; therefore it must be administered slowly, as ordered, and within the manufacturer guidelines (e.g., usually less than 1 mL/min). Patients should be kept recumbent for 15 minutes after the infusion to prevent further problems. Should extravasation of the intravenous calcium solution occur, the nurse should discontinue the infusion immediately but leave the intravenous catheter in place. The prescriber may then order an injection of 1% procaine and/or other antidotes or fluids to reduce vasospasm at the site and dilute the irritating effects of calcium on surrounding tissue. However, all facility policies and procedural guidelines and/or manufacturer insert information should be followed as deemed appropriate. In addition, documentation should include the appearance of the intravenous site (e.g., erythema, swelling, and any drainage). If oral dosage forms of calcium are used, they should be given 1 to 3 hours after meals.

Magnesium should be administered according to manufacturer guidelines and as ordered. Intravenous magnesium sulfate should always be given very cautiously; an infusion pump should be used, and manufacturer guidelines for dosage and dilutional concentration should be followed. During intravenous magnesium infusion, the patient's ECG and vital signs should be monitored, and patellar or knee-jerk reflexes should be rated. Impaired reflexes are used as an indication of drug-related CNS depressant effects. CNS depression may quickly lead to respiratory and/or cardiac depression; thus frequent monitoring is required. Documentation should be complete, and each set of vital sign measurements and ratings of reflexes should be recorded. Should there be a decrease in the strength of reflexes and/or a decrease in respirations to less than 12 breaths/min, the prescriber should be contacted immediately, the infusion stopped, and the patient monitored closely. Other signs that require immediate attention are confusion, irregular heart rhythm, cramping, unusual fatigue, lightheadedness, and dizziness. Calcium gluconate should be readily accessible for use as an antidote to magnesium toxicity. Oral dosage forms of magnesium should be administered as ordered and in the exact dosage prescribed. For other pointers related to the use of vitamins, minerals, and trace elements, see Patient Teaching Tips.

Evaluation

Evaluation should always include reviewing whether goals and outcome criteria have been met as well as monitoring for therapeutic responses and adverse effects of each vitamin or mineral. Therapeutic responses to *vitamin A* therapy include restoration of normal vision and intact skin, whereas adverse effects include lethargy, night blindness, skin and corneal changes, and, in infancy, failure to thrive. Therapeutic responses to *vitamin D* include improved bone growth and formation and an intact skeleton with decreased or no pain compared with baseline musculoskeletal deformity, weakness, and discomfort. Adverse effects include constipation, anorexia, metallic taste, and dry mouth. Therapeutic responses to *vitamin E* include improved muscle strength, improved skin integrity, and alpha tocopherol levels within normal limits; adverse effects include blurred vision, headache, fatigue, nausea, diarrhea, and weakness. Therapeutic responses to *vitamin K* include return to normal clotting; adverse effects are described in the pharmacology section of the chapter (as for all other vitamins and minerals covered in this chapter). Therapeutic response to *vitamin B_1* (thiamine) includes improved mental status and less confusion. Therapeutic responses to riboflavin, niacin, pyridoxine, and cyanocobalamin include improved skin integrity, normal vision, improved mental status, and normal RBC count, hemoglobin level, and hematocrit. Adverse effects from vitamin B are rare (see the Pharmacology section). Therapeutic responses to *vitamin C* include improvements in capillary intactness, integrity of the skin and mucous membranes, healing, energy level, and mental state. An adverse reaction associated with vitamin C is precipitate formation in the urine with possible stone development. Therapeutic responses to *macrominerals* include resolution of the deficient state and any associated signs and symptoms, which depend on the specific element or mineral.

PATIENT TEACHING TIPS

- Educate about the best dietary sources of both water- and fat-soluble vitamins (vitamins A, B, C, D, E, and K), as well as about the best sources of elements and minerals. See Table 53-2 for the nutrient content of various food items.
- Any patient taking vitamins, minerals, or elements should be closely monitored for therapeutic and adverse effects. The patient should be encouraged to monitor his or her own progress in how well the patient feels and to note any improvement in the related condition or health status. Intake of fluids should be encouraged with all vitamin and mineral therapy.
- Signs and symptoms of any related adverse effects should be shared with the patient, such as the adverse effects of diarrhea, blurred vision, dizziness, and flulike symptoms with vitamin E therapy.

- Patients who have had a gastrectomy or ileal resection and those with pernicious anemia should be informed of the necessity for vitamin B_{12} injections.
- Patients taking up to 600 mg/day of vitamin C should be told that there may be a slight increase in daily urination and that diarrhea is associated with intake of more than 1 g/day of vitamin C.
- Patients taking macrominerals (see Table 53-10) must take the medication as prescribed and with adequate amounts of fluids.
- The patient should be educated about calcium therapy and about food items and drugs that will chelate or bind with calcium. For example, calcium binds with tetracycline antibiotics and decreases or negates the effect of the antibiotic.

POINTS TO REMEMBER

- OTC use of vitamins and minerals may lead to serious problems and adverse effects; therefore, a prescriber should be consulted before supplements are taken.
- Nurses must incorporate the nutritional status of patients into the nursing care plan to provide comprehensive care during vitamin or mineral therapy.
- The nurse's participation in health promotion and wellness includes providing information about dietary needs and the body's need for vitamins and minerals.

- Patient education related to vitamin and mineral replacement must focus on dietary sources of the specific nutrient, drug and food interactions, and adverse effects. Patients must be instructed about when it is necessary to contact the prescriber.
- Vitamins and minerals can be dangerous to the patient if given without concern or caution for the patient's overall condition and underlying disease processes.
- It should never be assumed that because the drug is a vitamin or a mineral it does not have adverse reactions or toxicity. Most vitamins and minerals can become toxic at high levels.

NCLEX EXAMINATION REVIEW QUESTIONS

1 When giving calcium intravenously, the nurse needs to administer it slowly, keeping in mind that rapid intravenous administration of calcium may cause which problem?
  a Ototoxicity
  b Renal damage
  c Tetany
  d Cardiac dysrhythmias

2 The nurse will assess which laboratory test results before administration of vitamin K?
  a Prothrombin time and international normalized ratio
  b Red and white blood cell counts
  c Phosphorous and calcium levels
  d Total protein and albumin levels

3 A patient has sustained severe intestinal damage due to a gastrointestinal infection. The nurse will need to assess for signs of a deficiency of which vitamin?
  a Vitamin A (retinol)
  b Vitamin B_{12} (cyanocobalamin)
  c Vitamin B_6 (pyridoxine)
  d Vitamin E (tocopherols)

4 The nurse is providing wound care for a patient with a stage IV pressure ulcer and expects that the patient will receive which vitamin to assist in wound healing?
  a Vitamin K
  b Vitamin B_1

  c Vitamin C
  d Vitamin D

5 While caring for a newly admitted patient who has a long history of alcoholism, the nurse anticipates that part of the patient's medication regimen will include which vitamin?
  a Vitamin B_1 (thiamine)
  b Vitamin B_6 (pyridoxine)
  c Vitamin C (ascorbic acid)
  d Vitamin A (retinol)

6 When administering vitamin and mineral supplements, the nurse implements appropriate interventions, including: (Select all that apply.)
  a Not administering oral calcium tablets with oral tetracyclines
  b Administering intravenous calcium via a rapid intravenous push infusion
  c Monitoring the heart rhythm (ECG) of a patient receiving an intravenous magnesium infusion
  d Giving oral niacin with milk or food to decrease gastrointestinal upset
  e Monitoring for the formation of renal stones in patients taking large doses of vitamin C

1. d, 2. a, 3. b, 4. c, 5. a, 6. a, c, d, e.

CRITICAL THINKING ACTIVITIES: BEST ACTION

1 The nurse is about to administer calcium supplemental therapy to a patient with a history of cardiac disease. What is the most important assessment that is needed before the nurse gives the drug?

2 A patient with a stage III pressure ulcer is receiving daily doses of vitamin C and zinc. A new nurse asks the medication nurse, "Why is this patient receiving these two particular supplements?" What would be the nurse's best answer?

3 A patient receiving a magnesium infusion has developed tendon reflex loss, CNS depression, and some respiratory distress. The nurse monitoring this patient expects that these problems are a result of what condition, and the nurse prepares for what best actions?

For answers, see *http://evolve.elsevier.com/Lilley.*

CHAPTER 54

Nutritional Supplements

OBJECTIVES

When you reach the end of this chapter, you should be able to do the following:

1 Describe the various pathophysiologic processes and/or disease states that may lead to nutritional deficiencies and require nutritional supplemental support.

2 Discuss the various enteral and parenteral nutritional supplements used to treat the various deficiencies, including specific ingredients.

3 Describe the nurse's role in the process of initiating and maintaining continuous or intermittent enteral feedings, total parenteral nutrition, and other forms of nutritional supplementation.

4 Compare the various enteral feeding tubes, including specific uses, and detail the special needs of patients requiring this nutritional support.

5 Discuss the mechanisms of action, cautions, contraindications, routes of administration, drug interactions, adverse effects, and complications associated with enteral and parenteral nutritional supplementation.

6 Develop a nursing care plan that includes all phases of the nursing process for patients receiving enteral and parenteral supplemental feedings.

7 Discuss the various laboratory values related to nutritional deficits or altered nutritional status and their impact on monitoring the therapeutic effects of the therapy.

---

e-Learning Activities

http://evolve.elsevier.com/Lilley

NCLEX Review Questions • Animations • Nursing Care Plans • Audio Glossary • Category Catchers • Medication Errors Checklists • IV Therapy Checklists • Calculators • Frequently Asked Questions • Content Updates • Supplemental Resources • Answers to Case Studies and Critical Thinking Activities

Drug Profiles

amino acids, p. 846
carbohydrate formulation, p. 844
carbohydrates, p. 846

fat formulation, p. 844
lipid emulsions, p. 846
protein formulation, p. 844

◆ *Key drug.*

Glossary

Anabolism Constructive metabolism characterized by the conversion of simple substances into the more complex compounds of living matter. (p. 842)

Casein The principal protein of milk and the basis for curd and cheese. (p. 844)

Catabolism A complex metabolic process in which energy is liberated for use in work, energy storage, or heat production by the destruction of complex substances by living cells to form simple compounds. (p. 845)

Dumping syndrome A complex bodily reaction to the rapid entry of concentrated nutrients into the jejunum of the small intestine. The patient may experience nausea, weakness, sweating, palpitations,

syncope, sensations of warmth, and diarrhea. Most commonly occurs with eating following partial gastrectomy or with enteral feedings that are administered too rapidly into the stomach or jejunum via a feeding tube. (p. 843)

Enteral nutrition The provision of food or nutrients via the gastrointestinal tract, either naturally by eating or through a feeding tube in patients unable to eat. (p. 842)

Essential amino acids Those amino acids that cannot be manufactured by the body. (p. 846)

Essential fatty acid deficiency A condition that develops if fatty acids that the body cannot produce are not present in dietary or nutritional supplements. (p. 846)

Hyperalimentation An older term for parenteral nutrition; its use is now discouraged because it may be misinterpreted to mean overfeeding. (p. 844)

Malnutrition Any disorder of undernutrition. (p. 842)

Multivitamin infusion (MVI) A concentrated solution that contains several water- and fat-soluble vitamins and is used as part of an intravenous (parenteral) nutrition source. (p. 846)

Nonessential amino acids Those amino acids that the body can produce without extracting them from dietary intake. (p. 846)

Nutrients Substances that provide nourishment and affect the nutritive and metabolic processes of the body. (p. 842)

Nutritional supplements Oral, enteral, or intravenous nutritional preparations used to provide optimal nutrients to meet the body's nutritional needs. (p. 842)

Nutritional support The provision of nutrients orally, enterally, or parenterally for therapeutic reasons. (p. 842)

Parenteral nutrition The administration of nutrients by a route other than through the alimentary canal, such as intravenously. (p. 842)

Semiessential amino acids Those amino acids that can be produced by the body but not in sufficient amounts in infants and children. (p. 846)

Total parenteral nutrition (TPN) The intravenous administration of the total nutrient requirements of the patient with gastrointestinal dysfunction, accomplished via peripheral or central venous catheter. (p. 844)

Whey The thin serum of milk remaining after the casein and fat have been removed. It contains proteins, lactose, water-soluble vitamins, and minerals. (p. 844)

● ● ●

Anatomy, Physiology, and Disease Overview

Nutrients are dietary products that undergo chemical changes when ingested (and metabolized) and cause tissue to be enhanced and energy to be liberated. Nutrients are required for cell growth and division; enzyme activity; protein, carbohydrate, and fat synthesis; muscle contraction; secretion of hormones (e.g., vasopressin, gastrin); wound repair; immune competence; gut integrity; and numerous other essential cellular functions. Providing for these nutritional needs is known as **nutritional support.** Adequate nutritional support is needed to prevent the breakdown of tissue proteins for use as an energy supply to sustain essential organ systems, which is what occurs during starvation. Malnutrition can decrease organ size and impair the function of organ systems (e.g., cardiac, respiratory, gastrointestinal, hepatic, renal). Nutritional supplements are a means of providing adequate nutritional support to meet the body's nutritional needs.

Malnutrition is a condition in which the body's essential need for nutrients is not met by nutrient intake. The purpose of nutritional support is the successful prevention, recognition, and management of malnutrition. **Nutritional supplements** are dietary products used to provide nutritional support. Nutritional supplement products can be administered to patients in a variety of ways. They vary in the amount and chemical complexity of the carbohydrates, proteins, fats, electrolytes, vitamins, and minerals that compose them, as well as in their osmolality. These nutrients may be given in a digested form, a partially digested form, or an undigested form. Nutritional supplements can also be tailored for specific disease states.

Patients' nutrient requirements vary according to age, gender, size or weight, physical activity, preexisting medical conditions, nutritional status, and current medical or surgical treatment. Nutritional supplements are classified according to the method of administration as either enteral or parenteral. **Enteral nutrition** is the provision of food or nutrients via the gastrointestinal tract. Nutritional supplements may also be administered parenterally. **Parenteral nutrition** is the intravenous administration of nutrients. Its purpose is to promote **anabolism** (tissue building), nitrogen balance, and maintenance or improvement of body weight. It is used when the oral or enteral feeding routes cannot or should not be used (e.g., in postoperative patients or patients who are cachectic from advanced cancer or acquired immunodeficiency syndrome [AIDS]). The selection of either enteral nutrition or parenteral nutrition and the specific nutritional composition of the product used depend on the specific patient and the clinical situation. Enteral nutrition should be used when the patient has a functioning gastrointestinal tract.

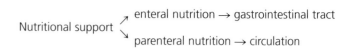

Pharmacology Overview

ENTERAL NUTRITION

Enteral nutrition is the provision of food or nutrients through the gastrointestinal tract. The most common and least invasive route of administration is oral consumption. A feeding tube is used in the other five enteral routes (Figure 54-1). The six routes of enteral nutrition delivery are listed in Table 54-1.

Patients who may benefit from feeding tube delivery of nutritional supplements include those with abnormal esophageal or stomach peristalsis, altered anatomy secondary to surgery, depressed consciousness, or impaired digestive capacity. The enteral route is considered to be the superior route of administration

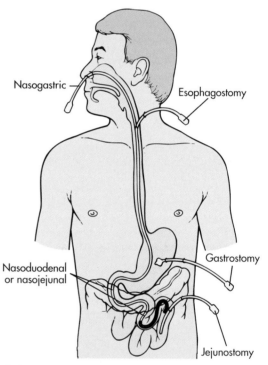

FIGURE 54-1 Tube feeding routes. (From Lewis SM et al: *Medical-surgical nursing: assessment and management of clinical problems,* ed 7, St Louis, 2007, Mosby.)

TABLE 54-1 Routes of Enteral Nutrition Delivery

Route	Description
Gastrostomy	Feeding tube surgically inserted directly into the stomach
Jejunostomy	Feeding tube surgically inserted into the jejunum
Nasoduodenal	Feeding tube placed from the nose to the duodenum
Nasojejunal	Feeding tube placed from the nose to the jejunum
Nasogastric	Feeding tube placed from the nose to the stomach
Oral	Nutritional supplements delivered by mouth

BOX 54-1 Enteral Formulations

Elemental Formulations

Peptamen
Vital HN
Vivonex Plus
Vivonex TEN

Contents: dipeptides, tripeptides, or crystalline amino acids; glucose oligosaccharides; and vegetable oil or medium-chain triglycerides (MCTs)

Comments: minimal digestion; minimal residue

Indications: malabsorption, partial bowel obstruction, irritable bowel disease, radiation enteritis, bowel fistula, short bowel syndrome

Polymeric Formulations

Complete
Ensure
Ensure Plus
Isocal
Osmolite
Portagen
Jevity
Sustacal

Contents: complex nutrients (proteins, carbohydrates, and fat)

Indications: preferred over elemental formulations for patients with fully functional gastrointestinal tracts and few specialized nutrient requirements

Modular Formulations

Carbohydrate
Moducal
Polycose

Contents: single-nutrient formulas (protein, carbohydrate, or fat)

Fat
MCT Oil
Microlipid

Indications: can be added to a monomeric or polymeric formulation to provide a more individualized nutrient formulation

Protein
Casec
ProMod
Propac
Stresstein

Altered Amino Acid Formulations

Amin-Aid
Hepatic-Aid
Travasorb Renal
Traum-Aid HBC

Contents: varying amounts of specific amino acids

Indications: for use in patients with diseases associated with altered metabolic capacities

Formulation for Impaired Glucose Tolerance

Glucerna

Contents: protein, carbohydrate, fat, sodium, potassium

Indications: for use in patients with impaired glucose tolerance (e.g., diabetic patients)

Box 54-2 Enteral Nutritional Supplements: Indications

Complete Nutritional Formulations (i.e., for General Nutritional Deficiencies)
- Inability to consume or digest normal foods
- Accelerated catabolic status
- Undernourishment because of disease

Incomplete Nutritional Formulations (i.e., for Specific Nutritional Deficiencies)
- Genetic metabolic enzyme deficiency
- Hepatic or renal impairment

Infant Nutritional Formulations
- Sole nutritional intake for premature and full-term infants
- Supplemental nutritional intake for older infants receiving solid foods
- Supplemental nutritional intake for breast-fed infants

Indications

Enteral nutrition can be used to supplement an oral diet that is currently insufficient for a patient's nutrient needs or used alone to meet all of the patient's nutrient needs. Box 54-2 lists the main types of enteral nutritional supplements and their indications.

Contraindications

The usual contraindication to nutritional supplements of any kind is known allergy to a specific product or genetic disease that renders a patient unable to metabolize certain types of nutrients.

Adverse Effects

The most common adverse effect of nutritional supplements is gastrointestinal intolerance, manifesting as diarrhea. Infant nutritional formulations are most commonly associated with allergies and digestive intolerance. The other nutritional supplements are most commonly associated with osmotic diarrhea. Rapid feeding or bolus doses can result in **dumping syndrome,** which produces intestinal disturbances. In addition, tube feeding places the patient at significant risk for aspiration pneumonia. This is especially true in patients in whom mental status, gag reflexes, and general mobility are compromised.

Interactions

Various nutrients can interact with drugs to produce significant food-drug interactions. With some exceptions, food usually delays the absorption of drugs when administered simultaneously. High gastric acid content or prolonged emptying time can result in decreased effects of certain antibiotics (cephalosporins, erythromycin, and penicillins). An increased absorption rate resulting in increased therapeutic effects can be seen when corticosteroids or vitamins A and D are given with nutritional supplements. The antibiotic effects of tetracyclines and quinolones are decreased when they are given with nutritional supplements as a result of chemical inactivation. These drugs should be given at least 2 hours before or after tube feedings. Tube feedings can also reduce the absorption of phenytoin, which may result in seizures. It is recommended that tube feedings be held for at least 2 hours before and after the administration of phenytoin. This can be problematic, because the

of nutritional supplements and should therefore be used whenever possible.

Approximately 100 different enteral supplement formulations are available. The enteral supplements have been divided into groups according to the basic characteristics of the individual formulations. The enteral formulation groups are elemental, polymeric, modular, altered amino acid, and impaired glucose tolerance. These are described in Box 54-1.

Mechanism of Action and Drug Effects

The enteral formula groups provide the basic building blocks for anabolism. Different combinations and amounts of these nutrients are used based on the individual patient's anabolic needs. Enteral nutrition supplies complete dietary needs through the gastrointestinal tract by the normal oral route or by feeding tube.

patient may not receive adequate nutrition due to withholding of feedings. This issue is somewhat controversial, and some suggest that the interaction is more theoretical than actual. Thus, some institutions have decided to ignore this possible interaction and just to monitor phenytoin levels and patient status, rather than holding the tube feedings, whereas others continue to hold the tube feedings. Often the patient requires intravenous phenytoin when continuous tube feedings are necessary.

Dosages

Because nutrient requirements vary greatly, dosages are individualized according to patient needs.

DRUG PROFILES

Enteral nutrition can be provided by a variety of supplements. Individual patient characteristics determine the appropriate enteral supplement. The four most commonly used enteral formulations are elemental, polymeric, modular, and altered amino acid.

ELEMENTAL FORMULATIONS
Elemental formulations are enteral supplements that contain dipeptides, tripeptides, or crystalline amino acids. Minimal digestion is required with elemental formulations. These supplements are indicated for patients with pancreatitis, partial bowel obstruction, irritable bowel disease, radiation enteritis, bowel fistulas, and short bowel syndrome. They are contraindicated in patients who have had hypersensitivity reactions to them. Elemental formulation supplements are available without a prescription and have no pregnancy category.

POLYMERIC FORMULATIONS
Polymeric formulations are enteral supplements that contain complex nutrients derived from proteins, carbohydrates, and fat. The polymeric formulations are some of the most commonly used enteral formulations because they most closely resemble normal dietary intake. They are preferred over elemental formulations in patients who have fully functional gastrointestinal tracts and have no specialized nutrient needs. Polymeric formulations are also less hyperosmolar than elemental formulations and therefore cause fewer gastrointestinal problems. They are contraindicated in patients who have had hypersensitivity reactions to them. They are available without a prescription and have no pregnancy category.

The most commonly used enteral supplement in the polymeric formulation category of enteral nutrition products is Ensure. It is lactose free and is also available in a higher-calorie formula called Ensure Plus. Other polymeric formulations are listed in Box 54-1. These drugs contain complex nutrients such as **casein** and soy protein for protein, corn syrup and maltodextrins for carbohydrates, and vegetable oil or milk fat for fat. They are available in liquid formulations only.

MODULAR FORMULATIONS
carbohydrate formulation
Moducal and Polycose are examples of commonly used enteral supplements in the carbohydrate modular formulation category. Both are carbohydrate supplements that supply carbohydrates only. They are intended to be used in addition to monomeric or polymeric formulations to provide a more individual specialized nutrient mix. They are available in liquid formulations only. These products are obtainable without a prescription, have no pregnancy category, and are contraindicated only in patients who have had hypersensitivity reactions to them.

fat formulation
Microlipid and MCT Oil are the formulations available in the fat category. Microlipid is a fat supplement supplying only fats. It is a concentrated source of calories and contains 4.5 kcal/mL. These drugs are given to help individualize nutrient formulations. They may be used in patients with malabsorption and other gastrointestinal disorders and in patients with pancreatitis. They are available in liquid formulations only. These products are obtainable without a prescription, have no pregnancy category, and are contraindicated only in patients who have had hypersensitivity reactions to them.

protein formulation
Casec, ProMod, and Propac are examples of protein modular formulations. They are used to increase patients' protein intake and provide additional proteins. They are derived from a variety of sources such as **whey**, casein, egg whites, and amino acids. All of the available products are dried powders that must be reconstituted with water. They may sometimes be reconstituted by placing them in enteral feedings that are already in liquid form. They are indicated for patients with increased protein needs. They are contraindicated in patients who have had hypersensitivity reactions to them. Protein formulation supplements are available without a prescription and have no pregnancy category.

ALTERED AMINO ACID FORMULATIONS
Amin-Aid is one of the many amino acid formulation nutritional supplements available. Many of the nutritional supplements in this category are also listed as modular formulations because they can be used as both single-nutrient formulas and as nutritional formulations for patients with genetic errors of metabolism. Specialized amino acid formulations are used most commonly in patients who have metabolic disorders such as phenylketonuria, homocystinuria, and maple syrup urine disease. They are also used to supply nutritional support to patients with illnesses such as renal impairment, eclampsia, heart failure, or liver failure.

PARENTERAL NUTRITION

Parenteral nutritional supplementation (intravenous administration) is the preferred method for patients who are unable to tolerate and/or maintain adequate enteral or oral intake. Instead of administration of partially digested nutrients into the gastrointestinal tract (as in enteral nutrition), vitamins, minerals, amino acids, dextrose, and lipids are administered intravenously directly into the circulatory system. This effectively bypasses the entire gastrointestinal system, which eliminates the need for absorption, metabolism, and excretion. Parenteral nutrition is also called **total parenteral nutrition (TPN)** or **hyperalimentation.**

TPN can supply all of the calories, carbohydrates, amino acids, fats, trace elements, vitamins, and minerals needed for growth, weight gain, wound healing, convalescence, immunocompetence, and other health-sustaining functions.

TPN can be administered through either a peripheral vein or a central vein. Each route of delivery of TPN has specific requirements and limitations. It is generally accepted that TPN should be considered only when oral or enteral support is impossible or when the gastrointestinal absorptive or functional capacity is not sufficient to meet the nutritional needs of the patient. Some of the factors that must be considered in deciding whether to use peripheral or central TPN for a given patient are listed in Table 54-2.

TABLE 54-2 Peripheral and Central Parenteral Nutrition: Characteristics

Characteristic	Peripheral	Central
Goal of nutritional therapy (total vs. supplemental)	Supplemental (total if moderate to low needs)	Total
Length of therapy	Short (fewer than 14 days)	Long (14 days or longer)
Osmolarity	Hyperosmolar (600-900 mOsm/L)	Hyperosmolar (600-900 mOsm/L)
Fluid tolerance	Must be high	Can be fluid restricted
Dextrose	Less than 12.5%	10%-35%
Amino acids	Less than 3%	More than 3%-7%
Fats	10%-20%	10%-20%
Calories per day	Less than 2000 kcal/day	Over 2000 kcal/day

PERIPHERAL TOTAL PARENTERAL NUTRITION

Peripheral TPN (PPN) is one route of administration of TPN. A peripheral vein is used to deliver nutrients to the patient's circulatory system. PPN is usually a temporary method of administration. The long-term administration of nutritional supplements via a peripheral vein may lead to phlebitis. There are a variety of indications for PPN. It should be considered a temporary measure to provide adequate nutrients in patients who have mild deficits or who are restricted from oral intake and have slightly elevated metabolic rates.

PPN is most valuable in patients who do not have large nutritional needs, can tolerate moderately large fluid loads, and need nutritional supplements only temporarily. PPN may be used alone or in combination with oral nutritional supplements to provide the necessary fat, carbohydrate, and protein needed by the patient to maintain health.

Mechanism of Action and Drug Effects

PPN provides the basic nutrient building blocks for anabolism. Different combinations and amounts of these nutrients are used based on the individual patient's anabolic needs.

Indications

PPN is used to administer nutrients to patients who need more nutrients than their current oral intake can supply or to provide complete daily nutrition. It is meant only as a temporary means (less than 2 weeks) of delivering TPN.

Circumstances under which patients may benefit from the delivery of PPN are as follows:
- The patient must undergo a procedure that restricts oral feedings.
- The patient has anorexia caused by radiation or cancer chemotherapy.
- The patient has a gastrointestinal illness that prevents oral food ingestion.
- The patient has just undergone surgery of any type.
- The patient's nutritional deficits are minimal, but oral nutrition will not be started for longer than 5 days

Contraindications

As mentioned previously for the enteral nutritional products, the only usual contraindication to nutritional supplementation of any kind is known drug allergy to a specific product or a genetic disease that renders a patient unable to assimilate certain types of nutrients.

TABLE 54-3 Amino Acids: Recommended Daily Dosage Guidelines

Healthy		Malnourished or Trauma/Burn
Adult	Infant/Child	Adult
0.9 g/kg	1.5-3 g/kg	Up to 2 g/kg

Adverse Effects

The most devastating adverse effect of PPN is phlebitis, which is vein irritation or inflammation of a vein. If phlebitis is severe enough and is not treated appropriately, it can lead to the loss of a limb. However, this is rare. Another potential adverse effect is fluid overload. PPN is limited to solutions with a lower dextrose concentration, generally less than 10%, to avoid sclerosing of the vein. Thus, large volumes are needed to meet a patient's daily nutritional requirements. Some patients, such as those with renal or heart failure, cannot tolerate large fluid volumes. In these patients, fluid restrictions may make it impossible to provide adequate calories through PPN.

Dosages

Dosage requirements vary from patient to patient. Age, gender, weight, and numerous other factors must be considered for proper administration of TPN. Guidelines for amino acids appear in Table 54-3.

DRUG PROFILES

The individual components of peripheral and central TPN are the same. The difference lies in the concentrations and amounts of the components delivered per volume of nutritional supplement. The basic components of peripheral or central TPN are amino acids, carbohydrates, lipids, trace elements, vitamins, fluids, and electrolytes. Most of the electrolyte components are discussed in Chapter 27.

AMINO ACIDS

Amino acids have many roles in the maintenance of normal nutritional status. The primary role is protein synthesis, or anabolism. Provision of adequate amino acids in nutritional supplements reduces the breakdown of proteins (**catabolism**) and also helps to promote normal growth and wound healing.

Amino acids are commonly classified as essential or nonessential according to whether they can or cannot be produced by the body. **Nonessential amino acids** are those that the body pro-

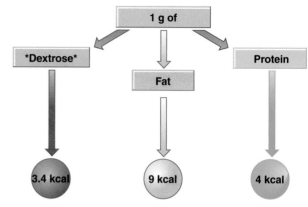

FIGURE 54-2   One gram of dextrose, fat, or protein will provide varying amounts of energy as calories.

duces and therefore need not be present in dietary intake. The body is able to manufacture, from nutritional nitrogen sources, all but eight of the available amino acids. **Essential amino acids** are those amino acids that cannot be produced by the body. Therefore, they must be included in daily dietary intake. Amino acids are used as building blocks for the protein that is needed for normal growth and development. Two amino acids, histidine and arginine, are not manufactured by the body in large enough quantities during rapid growth periods such as infancy or childhood. Thus, they are referred to as **semiessential amino acids.** Box 54-3 lists the amino acids according to their categories.

amino acids

Amino acid crystalline solutions (Aminosyn 3%, 5%, and 10%, and FreAmine III 8.5% and 10%) can be used in either peripheral or central TPN. Amino acids are a source of both protein and calories. They provide 4 kcal/g. The two currently available brands of amino acid solutions differ only in their respective concentrations. The dosage of these solutions varies depending on the patient's weight and requirements. These drugs have no restrictions regarding pregnancy and have no contraindications to use.

CARBOHYDRATES
carbohydrates

In nutritional support, carbohydrates are usually supplied to patients through dextrose. Dextrose is normally the greatest source of calories and provides 3.4 kcal/g. However, protein (amino acids) and lipids are also used as calorie sources (Figure 54-2). The concentration of dextrose in TPN is an important consideration. In PPN, dextrose concentrations are kept below 10% to decrease the possibility of phlebitis. In central TPN, dextrose concentrations can range from 10% to 50%, but they are commonly 25% to 35%. Because dextrose is a sugar, supplemental insulin may be given simultaneously in nutritional supplements. Use of a balanced nutritional supplement that contains dextrose and lipids as caloric sources decreases the need for large amounts of insulin.

FAT

The average North American diet contains 40% fat. This means that of the total calories supplied, 40% to 50% of the calories are obtained through fat grams. The ideal diet contains no more than 30% fat. Intravenous fat emulsions serve two functions: they supply essential fatty acids, and they are a source of energy or calories. As with the amino acids, certain fatty acids are essential because the body cannot produce them. Linoleic acid cannot be synthesized by the body. It is needed to produce linolenic and arachidonic acid. If these fatty acids are not present in dietary or nutritional supplements, an **essential fatty acid deficiency** may develop. Clinical signs of essential fatty acid deficiency are hair loss, scaly dermatitis, growth retardation, reduced wound healing, decreased platelet levels, and fatty liver (Figure 54-3).

lipid emulsions

The currently marketed lipid emulsions, Intralipid and Liposyn, are available as 10%, 20%, or 30% emulsions. They differ in fat origin. Liposyn is made from safflower oil, and Intralipid is made from soybean oil.

Lipid emulsions should normally be adjusted to deliver 20% to 30% of the total daily calories and should not exceed 60% of daily caloric intake. Fat emulsions are most beneficial when combined with dextrose solutions. The use of fat to meet caloric needs prevents potentially harmful conditions—such as hyperglycemia, hyperinsulinemia, and hyperosmolarity—that can occur when a patient's entire caloric needs are being met solely by dextrose.

TRACE ELEMENTS

Trace elements are available in individual solutions and in many different combinations. The following are considered trace elements:
- Chromium
- Copper
- Iodine
- Manganese
- Molybdenum
- Selenium
- Zinc

Specific dosages and frequencies depend on the individual patient's requirements. Vitamins and other minerals may also be added accordingly. A common multivitamin combination is **multivitamin infusion (MVI).**

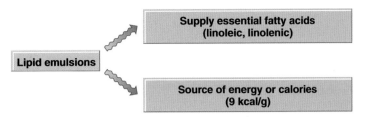

FIGURE 54-3   Lipid emulsions supply essential fatty acids and energy.

CENTRAL TOTAL PARENTERAL NUTRITION

In central TPN, a large central vein is used to deliver nutrients directly into the patient's circulation. Usually, the subclavian or internal jugular vein is used. Central TPN is generally indicated for patients who require nutritional supplements for a prolonged period, usually longer than 7 to 10 days. It can also be used in the home care setting. There are a variety of indications for central TPN. The disadvantages of central TPN are the risks associated with venous catheter insertion and the use and maintenance of the central vein. There is a greater potential for infection, more serious catheter-induced trauma and related events, metabolic alterations, and other technical or mechanical problems than with peripheral parenteral nutrition (PPN).

Mechanism of Action and Drug Effects

Central TPN is used to supply nutrients to patients who cannot ingest nutrients by mouth and cannot meet required daily nutritional needs by the enteral or peripheral parenteral routes. Like PPN, central TPN supplies the basic building blocks for anabolism. It provides the necessary fat, carbohydrate, and protein that the patient needs to maintain health.

Indications

TPN delivers total dietary nutrients to patients who require nutritional supplementation. Patients who may benefit from the delivery of TPN include the following:
- Patients who have large nutritional requirements (metabolic stress or hypermetabolism)
- Patients who need nutritional support for prolonged periods (longer than 7 to 10 days)
- Patients who are unable to tolerate large fluid loads

Contraindications

TPN is contraindicated in patients with allergy to any of its components. Rarely, a patient who is allergic to eggs may have cross-sensitivity to lipid formulations. TPN should be used only when the gastrointestinal tract cannot or should not be used (e.g., in postoperative patients or those who are otherwise unable to eat or digest and absorb nutrients).

Adverse Effects

The most common adverse effects of central TPN are those associated with the use of the central vein for delivery of the TPN. The risks associated with insertion of the infusion line, as well as the use and maintenance of the central vein for administration of TPN, can create some complications. As noted earlier, there is a greater potential for infection, serious catheter-induced trauma and related events, and other technical or mechanical problems than with PPN. Larger and more concentrated volumes of nutritional supplements are being delivered with central TPN, and therefore there is a greater chance for metabolic complications such as hyperglycemia.

Dosages

Administration is individualized according to patient needs.

> **DRUG PROFILE**
>
> The same formulations used in PPN are used in central TPN. Often the concentrations of fluids administered through the central vein are much higher than those used in nutritional formulations administered peripherally. Other than these minor differences, the nutritional supplements used are identical.

NURSING PROCESS

Assessment

The nurse should conduct a thorough nutritional assessment with attention to dietary history, weekly and daily food intake, weight, and height before initiation of any of these nutritional supplements. A nursing history should be completed and a thorough survey of all systems performed, including questions about any unusual symptoms, possible nutritional concerns, nausea, vomiting, loss of appetite, and weight gain or loss. Other questions should focus on past and present medical and health history; history of any difficulties with nutrition, gastrointestinal absorption, or food intolerance; stressors; and a complete medication profile, including a listing of all prescription drugs, over-the-counter drugs, herbals, and supplements. Consultation with a registered dietitian is crucial to identify the nutrients that are missing in a particular patient's diet. Total body metabolic rate, body mass index, muscle mass, and other variables linked to nutritional status should be assessed and are data that a nutritional consult may provide. Laboratory findings that may be assessed include some of the following: total protein level, albumin level, blood urea nitrogen level, red blood cell (RBC) count, white blood cell (WBC) count, vitamin B_{12} level, hemoglobin level, and hematocrit. Other laboratory studies may include cholesterol level, electrolyte levels, total lymphocyte count, serum transferrin level, iron level, urine creatinine clearance, lipid profile, and urinalysis. All of these objective and subjective data will help the prescriber, nutritionist/dietitian, and other members of the health care team to select the appropriate nutritional supplements for the patient.

Before administering an *enteral nutrition* supplement that is an elemental formulation, the nurse must also determine if the

Total Parenteral Nutrition

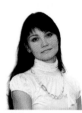

Mrs. C., a 28-year-old florist, has been unable to eat due to severe vomiting related to her pregnancy. She is at 13 weeks' gestation and has been admitted to the hospital because of dehydration and inability to eat due to her severe nausea and vomiting. The decision has been made to give her total parenteral nutrition (TPN) for at least a week. After a week of therapy, her obstetrician will then decide whether to continue or stop the infusion,

© Andry Starostin

based on her response. She will be receiving the TPN infusion via a peripheral intravenous catheter with infusion bags that will be changed every 24 hours.

1. Mrs. C. is anxious about this infusion and asks the nurse, "Why is that bag so large? What is in the bag?" How should the nurse answer these questions?
2. The nurse explains to Mrs. C. that her blood glucose levels will need to be monitored while she is receiving the TPN. Mrs. C. begins to cry, saying, "This morning sickness is bad enough, but now I have diabetes too? How can that be?" How should the nurse respond?
3. The nurse will monitor for what potential complication that can occur with peripherally administered TPN?
4. Before beginning the infusion, the nurse checks the ingredients of the TPN bag. The nurse notices that one of the contents is listed as 20% dextrose. What action should the nurse take at this time?

For answers, see *http://evolve.elsevier.com/Lilley*.

patient has a history of allergic reaction to any of the contents of the solution. Contraindications, cautions, and drug interactions must also be assessed for and documented. Of most concern is assessing the patient's cardiac and renal status and ensuring that the ingredients and the amount of solution are not too taxing on these systems. In addition, because these solutions are given orally, either by mouth or via tube feedings (see Chapter 10), it is most important to assess ability to swallow, gag reflex, and bowel sounds, and to note any nausea or vomiting. The nurse must also remember that protein-based formulations are to be avoided in patients with allergies to egg whites and whey.

Parenteral nutrition requires assessment of allergies to any of the ordered components of the intravenous solution as well as attention to age and metabolic needs. There are usually multiple combinations of products available; thus, the patient must be assessed carefully for allergies to essential proteins, amino acids, carbohydrates, trace elements, minerals, vitamins, lipids, high concentrations of dextrose, and fluids. It is important for the nurse to assess his or her own knowledge base about parenteral nutrition and the need for infusions through a central line, peripherally inserted central line, or peripherally inserted midline catheter. Some of the complications of parenteral nutrition include pneumothorax, infection, air emboli or emboli related to protein or lipid aggregation (associated with central catheter intravenous lines), septicemia related to the nutrient-rich solutions and invasive intravenous route of administration, and metabolic imbalances due to the solution ingredients and vomiting (seen with lipid administration in the parenteral nutrition). There must also

be a complete baseline assessment and thorough continuous monitoring of the following: (1) central line site, including patency, intactness, and appearance, (2) WBC and RBC counts as well as other laboratory values and parameters (listed earlier), (3) vital signs, (4) serum glucose levels, and (5) cardiac rhythm with electrocardiogram readings (as prescribed).

Nursing Diagnoses

- Diarrhea related to a decreased tolerance to enteral feedings and their ingredients
- Nutrition, less than body requirements, related to inability to take in sufficient oral nutrients
- Ineffective airway clearance related to possible aspiration of enteral feedings
- Deficient fluid volume related to altered nutritional status
- Risk for infection (sepsis) related to parenteral infusions and use of central venous access line
- Noncompliance related to lack of information about therapeutic regimen with enteral or parenteral supplementation

Planning

Goals

- Patient remains free of complications associated with enteral feedings and parenteral supplements.
- Patient regains near-normal or normal bowel patterns.
- Patient remains free of injury and infection during enteral or parenteral nutritional supplementation.
- Patient regains normal fluid volume status.
- Patient regains normal nutritional status through adequate dietary intake.
- Patient remains compliant with the treatment regimen and makes return visits to the prescriber as needed.

Outcome Criteria

- Patient identifies measures to decrease diarrhea while receiving enteral feedings, such as use of prescribed drugs to decrease motility and/or use of over-the-counter drugs or herbal products as ordered.
- Patient (or caregiver) demonstrates adequate technique for enteral tube feedings to decrease risk for aspiration, with emphasis on elevating the head of the bed and checking tube placement and residuals before feeding is initiated.
- Patient states measures to minimize risk for infection at total parenteral nutrition site (peripheral or central), such checking the site frequently for redness, swelling, drainage, or abnormal warmth, and reporting these to the prescriber or home health care nurse immediately.
- Patient begins to show proportional weight gain, adequate fluid volume status with improved skin turgor, and improved urinary output to at least 30 mL/hr, and laboratory values return to normal.
- Patient states symptoms to report to the prescriber, such as increased lethargy, fever, and shortness of breath.

Implementation

A prescriber's order must be complete and dated before enteral or parenteral (peripheral or central) nutrition supplementation is begun. In general, monitoring the status of the patient during and after *enteral feedings* is crucial to safe and prudent nursing care.

Tube feeding solutions are sometimes tinted with blue food coloring to help in detecting aspiration, but this should not replace checking for tube placement and for residuals. Gastric residual volumes should be measured and documented before each feeding as well as before each medication is administered. The tube feeding is usually stopped first, and stomach contents are aspirated using a syringe connected to the particular tube to detect any residual. If the volume aspirated is more than the volume delivered over the previous 2 hours (of continuous feeding), the nurse should return the aspirate, hold the feeding, and contact the prescriber while keeping the head of the patient's bed elevated. For intermittent bolus feedings, if the residual amount is more than 50% of the volume previously infused, the nurse should return the aspirate, withhold the feeding, and contact the prescriber. A reduction in the tube feeding volume will probably then be ordered. Hospital/facility policy or protocol should always be checked before use of enteral feedings, with checking and managing of residuals.

Newer tubes for nasogastric and other enteral feeding have smaller diameters and are thinner (5 French to 10 French) and more pliable for better patient tolerance. However, the smaller-diameter tubes make checking for gastric aspiration more difficult. The process of medication administration through a nasogastric tube is reviewed in Chapter 10 with step-by-step guidelines.

To prevent clogging of the feeding tube, it is often helpful to flush the tube with 30 mL of cranberry juice or other designated solution (per institutional policy) followed by 10 mL of water. The juice may help break up the formula residue and unclog certain types of feeding tubes, and the water helps to keep the tube clean and free of residue. Percutaneous enteral gastrostomy (PEG) tubes are also commonly used in many situations but do require surgical insertion by a gastroenterologist (often done under moderate sedation). Their care includes performing dressing changes during the initial period and then checking for residuals. Placement is not checked, but if it appears that the tube has come out of the opening and is longer than previously noted, the infusion should be stopped and the prescriber contacted.

Prescriber-ordered enteral feeding infusion rates and concentrations should be followed carefully. Usually the initial rate is 50 mL/hr at one-half strength, but this may be increased per patient tolerance to a rate ordered by the physician or appropriate health care provider. Although more rapid feeding increases the risk for hyperglycemia, dumping syndrome, and diarrhea, the nurse should continue to increase the patient's intake, because the total volume and number of calories to achieve recommended daily allowances is very important. Tube feeding formulas should always be at room temperature and should never be administered cold or warmed. If all the necessary steps to decrease or prevent diarrhea have been taken and have failed, antidiarrheal medications may be needed. Lactose-free solutions are available and should be used for patients who are lactose intolerant. Patients who have lactose intolerance may experience cramping, diarrhea, abdominal bloating, and flatulence with the ingestion of milk-based enteral feedings.

Parenteral nutrition infusions should be assessed every hour or per the facility's policies and procedures. The state of the entire infusion system and equipment as well as the condition of the patient should be documented, and it is the standard of care to examine the patient first and then check the insertion site, tubing,

infusion pump, and solution. To prevent infection, parenteral nutrition tubing is changed every time a new bag is added to the infusion. It is also recommended that tubing changes occur daily with the beginning of each new infusion. A 1.2-micron filter is used to trap bacteria, including *Pseudomonas* species. The patient's temperature should be recorded every 4 hours during the infusion, and any increase in temperature over 100° F (37.8° C) should be reported to the prescriber immediately. The patient should also be checked frequently for signs and symptoms of hyperglycemia, such as polydipsia (excessive thirst), polyuria (excessive urination), polyphagia (excessive hunger), headache, dehydration, nausea, vomiting, and weakness. These infusion rates should never be accelerated to increase plasma volume, because the rapid increase in the amount of dextrose solution may precipitate hyperglycemia and other related complications. Insulin replacement may be needed with the increase in dextrose; therefore, measurement of serum glucose levels by glucometer is important so that hyperglycemia may be immediately recognized and treated.

Hypoglycemia is manifested by cold, clammy skin; dizziness; tachycardia; and tingling of the extremities. Hypoglycemia associated with parenteral nutrition may be prevented by gradual reduction of the intravenous feeding rate to allow the pancreas time to adapt to the changing blood glucose levels. If parenteral nutrition is discontinued abruptly, rebound hypoglycemia may occur. This can be prevented by providing infusions of 5% to 10% glucose in situations in which parenteral nutrition must be discontinued immediately. Fluid overload may also occur with parenteral nutrition, manifested by weak pulse, hypertension, tachycardia, confusion, decreased urine output, and pitting edema. This may be prevented by maintaining infusion rates as ordered. If signs of fluid overload occur, the nurse should slow the infusion rate, measure vital signs, contact the prescriber, and remain with the patient until the patient's condition has stabilized. Auscultation of breath and heart sounds should always be a part of patient assessment, especially if additional therapies are administered that may precipitate fluid overload. Measurement of intake and output is usually indicated when parenteral nutrition is administered (and with enteral supplementation as well). See Patient Teaching Tips for further pointers on the use of nutritional supplements.

Evaluation

Therapeutic responses to nutritional supplementation include improved well-being, energy, strength, and performance of activities of daily living; an increase in weight; and laboratory test results that reflect an improved nutritional status. Specific laboratory values may include some of the following: albumin level, total protein level, hematocrit, hemoglobin level, RBC and WBC counts, BUN level, electrolyte levels, blood glucose and insulin levels, and iron values. Evaluation for adverse effects (see the Pharmacology section) associated with all enteral and/or parenteral nutrition infusions should be ongoing during and after therapy, and nutritional reevaluation should be carried out periodically so that the patient's nutritional needs are met. This may require frequent prescriber appointments or monitoring by a home health care nurse. The nurse should always refer to goals and outcome criteria to evaluate the effectiveness of therapy.

PATIENT TEACHING TIPS

- Because patients are often discharged with the need for various types of tube feedings, the patient and family or caregiver should receive education, instructions, and demonstrations about the daily care of the tube, preparation of tube feedings, and related procedures, which should be presented in a way that reflects the learning needs of the patient and those involved in the patient's care.
- The patient, family, and/or caregiver should be instructed about the need for correct placement of the tube, which should be checked before each tube feeding if a nasogastric tube is used. Incorrect placement of a nasogastric tube would be manifested by coughing, choking, difficulty in speaking, cyanosis, and subsequent respiratory distress. The head of the bed should remain elevated during infusions, and this positioning is more critical with nasogastric tube feedings than with gastrostomy tube feedings.
- Contact names and phone numbers for the prescriber, home health nurse, and other resources should be made available for use by the patient, family, and/or caregiver should any problems or concerns arise related to the feeding. A fever, difficulty breathing, sounds of lung congestion, high residual amounts, resistance to the flow of the feeding solution, and resistance in checking for residual are all causes for concern, and appropriate interventions should be implemented, including seeking emergency medical care if all else fails.
- Patients who are homebound and are receiving parenteral nutrition will need individualized education as well as support from home health care or related health care services. Practice is critical to acquisition of skill by the patient, family, and/or caregiver and should be an integral part of patient education. All procedures for storage, cleansing and care of the site, dressing changes, irrigation of the catheter, pump function and care, and changing of the bag, filters, and tubing should also be explained and demonstrated, with a return demonstration by the patient, before the patient is discharged. The patient should be told that parenteral nutrition will require home health care services by a registered nurse to help prevent the complications of infection at the site, sepsis, fever, and pneumonia.
- Educate about the need to check serum glucose levels at home as ordered by the prescriber if parenteral nutrition or other infused solutions high in dextrose are administered. The operation of a glucometer should be explained and specific steps for its use included in a demonstration to the patient, family, and/or caregiver. In addition, instructions in self-administration of insulin, based on sliding-scale coverage, may need to be included and reinforced.
- Signs and symptoms of potential complications of parenteral nutrition, including fever, cough, chest pains, dyspnea, and chills, (all of which are indicative of adverse reactions to lipid infusions) should be reported to the prescriber immediately. Restlessness, nervousness, fainting, and tachycardia are associated with hypoglycemia and should be reported; polyuria, polydipsia, polyphagia, nausea, vomiting, dehydration, headache, and/or weakness may indicate hyperglycemia and should also be reported.

POINTS TO REMEMBER

- A thorough nutritional assessment and possible consultation with a registered dietitian or nutritionist are essential for adequate intervention for the malnourished patient.
- Various enteral feeding formulations with different nutritional content are available, including some that are lactose free.
- Enteral feedings may result in complications such as hyperglycemia, dumping syndrome, and aspiration of the nutritional supplement.
- Parenteral nutrition supplementation (intravenously administered) is total parenteral nutrition (TPN) or hyperalimentation. PN or TPN may be administered through a central vein or through a peripheral vein (PPN).
- TPN is administered through a central venous catheter because of the hyperosmolarity of the substances used and the need for dilution provided by a larger-diameter vein to prevent damage to the vein. Parenteral nutrition given through a peripherally inserted central catheter (PPN) line is another option but uses a solution with a lower concentration of dextrose and other ingredients.
- Parenteral feedings may result in air embolism, fever, infection, fluid volume overload, hyperglycemia, or hypoglycemia. If they are discontinued abruptly, rebound hypoglycemia may result.
- Cautious and skillful nursing care may prevent or decrease the occurrence of complications associated with enteral or parenteral nutritional supplementation.

NCLEX EXAMINATION REVIEW QUESTIONS

1 The nurse is assessing an enteral feeding that is infusing via a nasogastric feeding tube. This tube is
a surgically inserted into the stomach.
b inserted through the nose into the jejunum.
c surgically inserted directly into the jejunum.
d inserted through the nose into the stomach.

2 When administering TPN, the nurse is aware that one purpose of intravenous fat (lipid) emulsions is to provide which nutrient?
a Calories
b Amino acids
c Minerals
d Immunoglobulins

3 The nurse is monitoring a patient who is receiving a TPN infusion and notes that the patient has cold clammy skin, shows tachycardia, and is complaining of feeling dizzy. The nurse should immediately
a stop the TPN infusion.
b check the patient's blood glucose level.
c order a stat (immediate) electrocardiogram.
d obtain an order for blood cultures.

4 A patient has new orders for administration of peripheral parenteral nutrition (PPN). The nurse knows that PPN is most appropriate in which situation?

a Therapy is expected to last longer than 2 weeks.
b Therapy is expected to last fewer than 14 days.
c A dextrose concentration of 20% is needed.
d Nutritional needs are 3000 kcal/day.

5 During the night shift, a patient's TPN infusion runs out, the pharmacy is closed, and a new TPN bag will not be available for about 6 hours. The nurse's most appropriate action at this time would be to
a hang a bottle of lipid solution.
b hang a bag of normal saline.
c hang a bag of 10% dextrose.
d call the prescriber for stat TPN orders.

6 The nurse is assessing a patient who is receiving an enteral tube feeding. Which of the following are possible adverse effects associated with enteral feedings? (Select all that apply.)
a Hyperglycemia
b Air embolism
c Aspiration
d Diarrhea
e Infection

CRITICAL THINKING ACTIVITIES: BEST ACTION

1 A patient who is receiving enteral nutrition through a percutaneous enteral gastrostomy tube is experiencing severe diarrhea. What is the nurse's best action?

2 A patient has been receiving TPN with a 25% glucose content, and the nurse has just discovered that the central intravenous access line is clogged. What is of the most immediate concern, and what is the nurse's best action at this time? Explain your answer.

3 At the beginning of the morning shift, the nurse is reviewing the medication orders of a patient who is receiving the impaired glucose tolerance formulation Glucerna through a nasogastric feeding tube. The patient has a history of seizures, and a dose of phenytoin is due later in the morning. What is the nurse's best action?

For answers, see *http://evolve.elsevier.com/Lilley.*

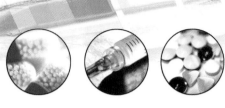

Miscellaneous Therapeutics: Hematologic, Dermatologic, Ophthalmic, and Otic Drugs

TIME MANAGEMENT

As you plan your study time for Part 10, it should be very clear that Chapter 57 will take significantly more time to complete than the other chapters. Do not let the length of the chapter overwhelm you. Apply the principles of time management to this chapter and you will succeed. The most important aspect of time management to apply to this chapter is the use of clear goal statements and action plan steps to help you achieve the goals.

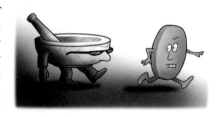

Goal Statements

Remember the criteria for goal statements. First, they must be realistic; the statements must be things you know you can accomplish. Second, they must be specific to the task. "I will study the chapter" is not a very specific goal. Specify what you expect to accomplish. "I will master the 33 terms in the chapter glossary" is a more specific goal statement. Third, there must be a time limit. How long will you spend in achieving this goal? Set a time limit for completion of each activity specifying the quantity of time to be spent in that learning activity. Finally, goal statements must be measurable. In the example about studying the glossary, including the number of terms contained in Chapter 57 helps clarify the goal.

Action Planning

The second segment of time management is the use of action planning. An action plan is a series of smaller, specific activities that you will accomplish to meet your goal statements. Your goal is to master the 33 terms. What will you do to meet that goal?

Action Steps Example

1. I will spend 1 hour from 3:00 to 4:00 PM on Monday making vocabulary drill cards for the terms found in the glossary in Chapter 57.
2. I will spend 15 minutes in rehearsal and review of these cards every day until the exam on this chapter is over.
3. Each time I cannot define and explain a term, I will put an X on the card to identify it as a term needing more review.
4. I will spend 1 hour the night before the exam doing a comprehensive review of the terms in Chapter 57, with special emphasis on those cards that have one or more X marks.

Action steps help ensure that you are spending your study time actively focusing on what you need to learn.

PURR

Prepare Example

Chapter 57, Objective 3 reads, "Discuss the mechanisms of action, indications, dosage forms with application techniques, adverse effects, cautions, contraindications, and drug interactions of the various ophthalmic drugs."

Question 1: What does *ophthalmic* mean? (literal question [LQ])

Question 2: What are ophthalmic drugs? (LQ)

Question 3: What is the mechanism of action of ophthalmic drugs? (LQ)

Question 4: Is there more than one mechanism of action? (LQ)

Question 5: If there is more than one mechanism of action, how are the mechanisms similar and how are they different? (interpretive question)

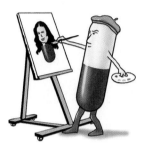

These questions are only suggestions for generated questions based on the chapter objectives. Many more questions can be asked about Objective 3. These questions are an essential part of the study process. Questions help make you an active reader and an active learner. The more questions you generate, the easier it will be to understand the chapter.

Outline Example

1. *Looking through the chapter, decide how much material is appropriate.* The section that begins with Antiglaucoma Drugs is probably too much material. Based on the chapter headings, this section could be broken down into six blocks of material. Block 1 would cover the material under the heading Cholinergic Drugs. Block 2 would be the material under the heading Sympathomimetics. The next four blocks would be Beta-Adrenergic Blockers, Carbonic Anhydrase Inhibitors, Osmotic Diuretics, and Prostaglandin Agonists.

2. *Apply the Prepare step to each block.* Beginning with "Cholinergic Drugs," generate some questions to guide your reading. Remember that it is important to ask both questions that will focus on literal information and questions that will help you interpret, evaluate, and analyze when you read.

3. *Read the material.* As soon as you have completed the self-questioning on the first block of material, read the material in the chapter. It is important that the reading be done immediately. Read for understanding, and as you read remember the questions you generated. This approach will help your concentration and comprehension.

4. *Take a short break.* Once you have completed the reading of this section of the chapter, give your mind a chance to reflect

and consolidate the learning. Limit the time you allow for a break and use the time for something pleasurable. Give yourself 5 or 10 minutes to read the newspaper, get a snack, or just take a short walk.

5. *Rehearse.* Before going on to the next section of the chapter it is important to spend a few minutes in rehearsal. Using the questions from step 2, go back over the material you read and try to respond to those questions. When you find yourself unable to answer a question, put a mark in the text beside the heading that caused the difficulty and move on. The mark will serve as a reminder for future review. At this point, the objective is not complete mastery of the material. The objective is to see what you have learned, so that you can move smoothly into the next section. Breaking a chapter into blocks is useful, but it is imperative that the links between sections be made as you study.

6. *Review.* After you have completed two or three major sections of the chapter, it is time to review. Start at the beginning of the chapter. Ask your questions. Try to answer them. If you cannot formulate a clear answer, then some rereading is necessary.

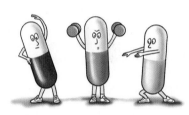

Also, pay attention to the marks made during the rehearsal step. Those marks indicate areas that you have already identified as needing review. When rereading, remember that the object is to read only as much of the material as needed to be able to respond to self-generated questions. There simply is not enough time to read the entire chapter a second or third time.

REPEAT THE STEPS

Prepare, read for understanding, take a short break, and then rehearse the material you've just read. It may seem that this process takes an excessive amount of time and involves a lot of repetition, but in the long run this process will produce better learning. The time spent in Prepare, Understand, and Rehearse will reduce the time needed to review. Frequent review as you move through the chapter will make the final review at exam time proceed more quickly and enable you to achieve mastery of the material.

CHAPTER **55**

Anemia Drugs

OBJECTIVES

When you reach the end of this chapter, you should be able to do the following:

1 Discuss the importance of iron, vitamin B_{12}, and folic acid in the formation of blood cells.

2 Describe the various types of anemia-related drug treatments.

3 Discuss the mechanisms of action, cautions, contraindications, drug interactions, uses, dosages, and special administration techniques of the various drugs used to treat anemia, as well as measures to enhance the effectiveness and decrease the adverse effects of these drugs.

4 Develop a nursing care plan that includes all phases of the nursing process for patients taking drugs used to treat anemia.

---

e-Learning Activities

http://evolve.elsevier.com/Lilley

NCLEX Review Questions • Animations • Nursing Care Plans • Audio Glossary • Category Catchers • Medication Errors Checklists • IV Therapy Checklists • Calculators • Frequently Asked Questions • Content Updates • Supplemental Resources • Answers to Case Studies and Critical Thinking Activities

Drug Profiles

ferric gluconate, p. 859
ferrous fumarate, p. 858
◆ ferrous sulfate, p. 858

◆ folic acid, p. 859
iron dextran, p. 858
iron sucrose, p. 859

◆ *Key drug.*

Glossary

Erythrocytes Another name for red blood cells (RBCs). (p. 854)

Erythropoiesis The process of erythrocyte production. (p. 854)

Globin The protein part of the *hemoglobin* molecule (see later); the four different structural globin chains most often found in adults are the $alpha_1$, $alpha_2$, $beta_1$, and $beta_2$ chains. (p. 855)

Hematopoiesis The normal formation and development of all blood cell types in the bone marrow. (p. 854)

Heme Part of the *hemoglobin* molecule; a nonprotein, iron-containing pigment. (p. 855)

Hemoglobin A complex protein-iron compound in the blood that carries oxygen to the cells from the lungs and carbon dioxide away from the cells to the lungs. (p. 855)

Hemolytic anemias Anemias resulting from excessive destruction of erythrocytes. (p. 856)

Hypochromic Pertaining to less than normal color. The term usually describes an RBC with decreased hemoglobin content and helps further characterize anemias associated with reduced synthesis of hemoglobin. (p. 855)

Microcytic Pertaining to or characterized by smaller than normal cells. (p. 855)

Pernicious anemia A type of megaloblastic anemia usually seen in older adults and caused by impaired intestinal absorption of vitamin B_{12} (cyanocobalamin) due to lack of availability of intrinsic factor. (p. 856)

Reticulocytes An immature erythrocyte characterized by a meshlike pattern of threads and particles at the former site of the nucleus. (p. 854)

Spherocytes Small, globular, completely hemoglobinated erythrocytes without the usual central concavity or pallor. (p. 856)

• • •

Anatomy, Physiology, and Disease Overview

ERYTHROPOIESIS

The formation of new blood cells is one of the primary functions of bones. This process is known as **hematopoiesis,** and it includes the production of **erythrocytes** (red blood cells, or RBCs), as well as *leukocytes* (white blood cells) and *thrombocytes* (platelets). This process takes place in the *myeloid* tissue or bone marrow. This specialized tissue is located primarily in the ends, or *epiphyses*, of certain long bones and also in the flat bones of the skull, pelvis, sternum, and ribs.

Erythropoiesis, the process of erythrocyte formation, is the focus of this chapter. This involves the maturation of a nucleated RBC precursor into a hemoglobin-filled, nucleus-free erythrocyte. This process is driven by the hormone *erythropoietin*, produced by the kidneys. Erythropoietin is also produced commercially and is used to treat anemia in certain specific circumstances. It is discussed in Chapter 49.

When RBCs are manufactured in the bone marrow by myeloid tissue, they are released into the circulation as immature RBCs called **reticulocytes.** Once in the circulation, reticulocytes undergo a 24- to 36-hour maturation process to become mature, fully functional RBCs. After this, they have a life span of about 120 days.

It is important to know the structural components of the RBC to understand how anemia develops. More than one third of an RBC is composed of hemoglobin. **Hemoglobin** (abbreviated *Hgb*) is composed of two parts: heme and globin. **Heme** is a red pigment. Each heme group contains one atom of iron. **Globin** is a protein chain. The four different structural globin chains most often found in adults are the alpha$_1$, alpha$_2$, beta$_1$, and beta$_2$ chains. Together, four heme groups, each linked to one protein chain of globin, make up one hemoglobin molecule (Figure 55-1).

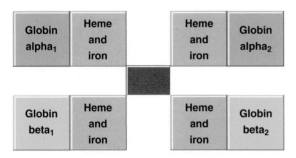

FIGURE 55-1 Schematic structure of a hemoglobin molecule.

TYPES OF ANEMIA

Anemias are classified into four main types based on the underlying causes (Figure 55-2). Anemias can be caused by maturation defects or they can be secondary to excessive RBC destruction. Two types of maturation defects lead to anemias, categorized by the location of the defect within the cell: *cytoplasmic* maturation defects occur in the cell cytoplasm, and *nuclear* maturation defects occur in the cell nucleus. Factors responsible for excessive RBC destruction can be either intrinsic or extrinsic.

Figure 55-3 summarizes the types of anemias arising from cytoplasmic maturation defects. Major examples include iron-deficiency anemia and genetic disorders such as *thalassemia,* which result in defective globin synthesis. The RBCs appear **hypochromic** (lighter red than normal) and **microcytic** (smaller than normal) on blood smear. Cytoplasmic maturation anemias occur as a result of reduced or abnormal hemoglobin synthesis. Because hemoglobin is synthesized from both iron and globin, a deficiency in either one can lead to a hemoglobin deficiency. Some common causes of iron-deficiency anemia are blood loss, surgery, childbirth, gastrointestinal bleeding, and hemorrhoids.

Figure 55-4 summarizes the types of anemias arising from nuclear maturation defects. These occur because of defects in deoxyribonucleic acid (DNA) or protein synthesis. Both DNA

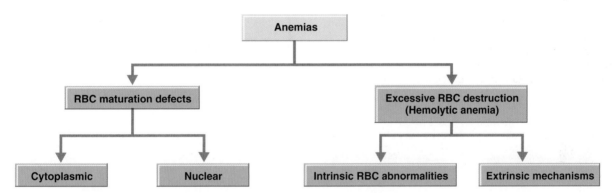

FIGURE 55-2 Underlying causes of anemia are red blood cell (RBC) maturation defects and factors secondary to excessive RBC destruction.

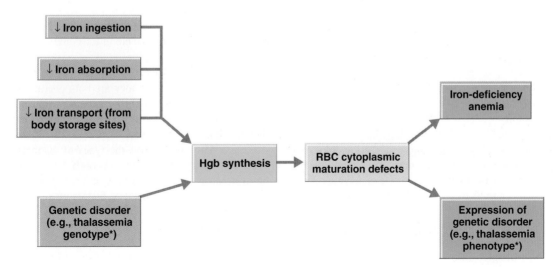

FIGURE 55-3 Schematic showing common causes and results of red blood cell (RBC) cytoplasmic maturation defects. ↓, Decreased.

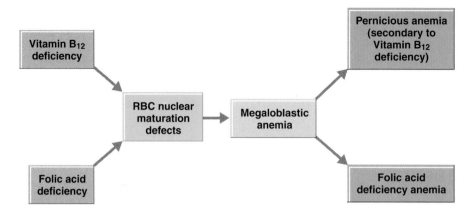

FIGURE 55-4   Schematic showing common causes and results of red blood cell (RBC) nuclear maturation defects.

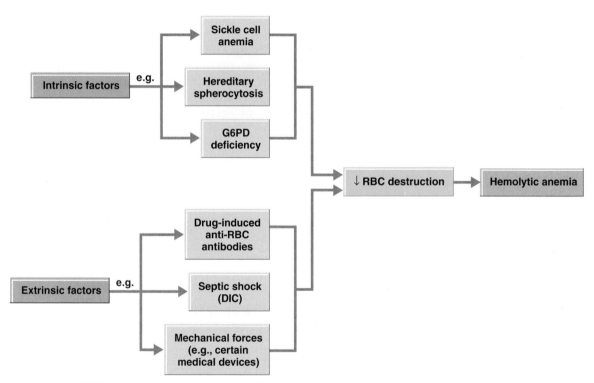

FIGURE 55-5   Increased red blood cell (RBC) destruction occurs as a result of intrinsic and extrinsic factors. ↓, Decreased; *DIC,* disseminated intravascular coagulation; *G6PD,* glucose-6-phosphate dehydrogenase.

and protein synthesis require vitamin B$_{12}$ and folic acid to be present in normal amounts for their proper production. If either of these two vitamins is absent or deficient, anemias secondary to nuclear maturation defects may develop. In such anemias, RBCs actually appear to be *normochromic* (normal in color) but are commonly *macrocytic* (larger than normal) on blood smear. One example is **pernicious anemia.** This type of anemia results from deficiency of vitamin B$_{12}$, which is used in the formation of new RBCs. The usual underlying cause is the failure of the stomach lining to produce intrinsic factor. *Intrinsic factor* is a gastric glycoprotein that allows vitamin B$_{12}$ to be absorbed in the intestine (see Chapter 53). Another example is the anemia caused by folic acid deficiency. Both pernicious anemia and folic acid deficiency anemia are also known as types of *mega-*

loblastic anemia, because they are both characterized by large, immature RBCs. Megaloblastic anemias are usually related to poor dietary intake and are most commonly seen in infancy, childhood, and pregnancy.

Figure 55-5 summarizes the types of anemias arising from excessive RBC destruction, or **hemolytic anemias.** These can occur because of abnormalities within the RBCs themselves *(intrinsic factors)* or as a result of factors outside of (*extrinsic* to) the RBCs. In both cases the erythrocytes appear on blood smear as **spherocytes,** which look fragmented. RBC abnormalities caused by intrinsic factors are usually the result of a genetic defect. Examples include *sickle cell anemia, hereditary spherocytosis,* and *glucose-6-phosphate dehydrogenase deficiency.* Examples of extrinsic mechanisms for excessive RBC destruction include drug-induced *antibodies* that target and destroy RBCs, septic shock that produces *disseminated intravascular coagulation,* and mechanical forces such as those created by *intraaortic balloon pumps* and *ventricular assist devices,* commonly used in cardiac intensive care units.

Pharmacology Overview

IRON

Iron is a mineral essential for the proper function of all biologic systems in the body. It is stored in many sites throughout the body (liver, spleen, and bone marrow). Deficiency of this mineral is also the principal nutritional deficiency resulting in anemia. Individuals who require the highest amount of iron are women (especially pregnant women) and children, and they are the groups most likely to develop iron-deficiency anemia. For women, this is partly due to ongoing menstrual blood losses. Most vitamin supplements for men contain little or no iron, because men are much less likely to develop iron-deficiency anemia. Nonetheless, dietary iron is usually sufficient for both men and women in developed countries.

Dietary sources of iron include meats and certain vegetables and grains (see *http://evolve.elsevier.com/Lilley* for specific examples). These forms of iron must be broken down by gastric juices before the iron can be absorbed. Other foods such as orange juice, veal, fish, and ascorbic acid may help with iron absorption. Conversely, eggs, corn, beans, and many cereal products containing chemicals known as *phytates* may impair iron absorption. However, it should be noted that both beans and eggs are themselves common dietary sources of iron. Oral iron preparations are available as ferrous salts. See Table 55-1 for a list of the currently available oral iron salts and their respective iron content. When a patient cannot tolerate oral iron, intravenous iron may be administered. There are three injectable iron products available: iron dextran (INFeD), iron sucrose (Venofer), and ferric gluconate (Ferrlecit).

Mechanism of Action and Drug Effects

Iron is an oxygen carrier in both hemoglobin and *myoglobin* (oxygen-carrying molecule in muscle tissue) and thus is critical for tissue respiration. Iron is also a required component of a number of enzyme systems in the body and is necessary for energy transfer in the *cytochrome oxidase* and *xanthine oxidase* enzyme systems. Administration of iron corrects iron-deficiency symptoms such as anemia, dysphagia, dystrophy of the nails and skin, and fissuring of the angles of the lips, and also maintains the bodily functions described earlier.

Indications

Supplemental iron contained in multivitamins plus iron or iron supplements alone are indicated for the prevention or treatment of iron-deficiency anemia. In all cases, an underlying cause should be identified. After identification of the cause, treatment should be aimed at attempting to correct the cause (e.g., chronic blood loss, such as from an ulcer) rather than simply alleviating the symptoms. Iron supplementation is also used in erythropoietin therapy (see Chapter 49), because it is essential for the production of RBCs.

TABLE 55-1 Ferrous Salts: Iron Content

Ferrous Salt	Iron Content
Ferrous fumarate	33% iron or 330 mg/g
Ferric gluconate	12% iron or 120 mg/g
Ferrous sulfate	20% iron or 200 mg/g
Ferrous sulfate (desiccated or dried)	30% iron or 300 mg/g

TABLE 55-2 Iron Preparations: Adverse Effects

Body System	Adverse Effects
Gastrointestinal	Nausea, constipation, epigastric pain, black and tarry stools, vomiting, diarrhea
Integumentary	Temporarily discolored tooth enamel and eyes, pain on injection

Contraindications

Contraindications to the use of iron products include known drug allergy, *hemochromatosis* (iron overload), hemolytic anemia, and any other anemia not associated with iron deficiency.

Adverse Effects

The most common adverse effects associated with iron preparations are nausea, vomiting, diarrhea, constipation, stomach cramps, and stomach pain. Excess iron intake can lead to accumulation and iron toxicity. See Table 55-2 for a more complete listing of the undesirable effects associated with iron preparations.

Toxicity and Management of Overdose

Iron overdose is the most common cause of pediatric poisoning deaths reported to U.S. poison control centers. Many iron supplements are enteric coated and resemble candy. Toxicity from iron ingestion results from a combination of the corrosive effects on the gastrointestinal mucosa and the metabolic and hemodynamic effects caused by the presence of excessive elemental iron.

Treatment is based on symptomatic and supportive measures, including suction and maintenance of the airway, correction of acidosis, and control of shock and dehydration with intravenous fluids or blood, oxygen, and vasopressors. Abdominal radiographs may be helpful, because iron preparations are radiopaque and may be visualized on x-ray film. Serum iron concentrations may be helpful in establishing the amount ingested. A serum iron concentration of more than 300 mcg/dL places the patient at serious risk for toxicity. The stomach should be emptied immediately by gastric lavage. Because many of the iron products are extended-release formulations that release the contents in the intestines rather than the stomach, whole-gut lavage is generally believed to be superior and more effective. This should be followed by a saline cathartic or possible surgical removal of ingested iron tablets. In patients with severe symptoms of iron intoxication, such as coma, shock, or seizures, chelation therapy with deferoxamine should be initiated.

DOSAGES

Selected Iron Preparations and Folic Acid

Drug (Pregnancy Category)	Pharmacologic Class	Usual Dosage Range	Indications/Uses
ferric gluconate (Ferrlecit) (B)	Parenteral iron salt	**Pediatric* older than 6 yr** 1.5 mg/kg/dose for 8 doses **Adult** 125 mg/dose for 8 doses	Iron deficiency associated with hemodialysis
ferrous fumarate (Feostat) (A)	Oral iron salt	**Pediatric*** 4-6 mg kg/day 3 mg/kg/day 1-2 mg/kg/day **Adult*** 100-200 mg given 1-3 times daily	Severe iron deficiency anemia Mild to moderate iron deficiency anemia Prophylaxis
◆ ferrous sulfate (A)	Oral iron salt	**Pediatric*** 4-6 mg/kg/day in 3 divided doses **Adult*** 300 mg 2 times daily, up to 300 mg 4 times daily	Iron deficiency
◆ folic acid (A)	Water-soluble B-complex vitamin	**Pediatric†** PO/IV/IM/subcut: 0.1-0.4 mg/day **Adult†** PO/IV/IM/subcut: Up to 1 mg/day	Folate deficiency; tropical sprue; nutritional supplementation; pregnancy-related supplementation
iron dextran (INFeD, Dexferrum) (C)	Parenteral iron salt	**Pediatric†** IM/IV: 5-10 kg: 25 mg/day (0.5 mL/day); greater than 10 kg: 50 mg/day (1 mL/day) **Adult†** IM/IV: 100 mg/day (2 mL/day)	Iron deficiency when oral iron therapy is unsatisfactory
iron sucrose (Venofer) (B)	Parenteral iron salt	IV: 100 mg 1-3 times weekly to a cumulative dose of 1000 mg; may give up to 500 mg as single dose on days 1 and 14	Iron deficiency in patients with chronic renal failure

IM, Intramuscular; *IV,* intravenous; *PO,* oral; *subcut,* subcutaneous.
*Doses are expressed in terms of elemental iron, not the salt itself.
†Expressed in milligrams of elemental iron. Dosages are calculated for each patient's weight according to manufacturer's label. Doses are approximate.

Interactions

The absorption of iron can be enhanced when it is given with ascorbic acid and decreased when it is given with antacids. Iron preparations can decrease the absorption of thyroid drugs, tetracyclines, and quinolone antibiotics.

Dosages

For the recommended dosages of iron preparations, see the Dosages table above.

DRUG PROFILES

Iron preparations are available by prescription and as over-the-counter (OTC) medications. They are contraindicated in patients with ulcerative colitis and regional enteritis, conditions of excessive body iron stores (e.g., *hemosiderosis, hemochromatosis*), peptic ulcer disease, hemolytic anemia, cirrhosis, gastritis, and esophagitis. Goals of therapy include maintenance of normal hemoglobin and hematocrit levels, and energy level.

ferrous fumarate

The ferrous fumarate iron salts (Femiron) contain the largest amount of iron per gram of salt consumed. Ferrous sulfate and ferric gluconate are two other forms of iron that are commonly used. Ferrous fumarate is 33% elemental iron; therefore, a 325-

mg tablet of ferrous fumarate provides 107 mg of elemental iron. Ferrous fumarate is available only for oral use.

PHARMACOKINETICS

Route	Onset of Action	Peak Plasma Concentration	Elimination Half-life	Duration of Action
PO	3-10 days	Unknown	6 hr	Variable

◆ ferrous sulfate

Ferrous sulfate is the most frequently used form of oral iron. Ferrous sulfate ($FeSO_4$) is dosed as 300 mg twice a day for most adult patients. Confusion arises with ferrous sulfate, because the dose is 300 mg, but many commercially available products are 324 mg. The two doses are used interchangeably. To add to the confusion, each 324-mg tablet contains 65 mg of elemental iron. It should be noted that pediatric dosing is based on elemental iron.

PHARMACOKINETICS

Route	Onset of Action	Peak Plasma Concentration	Elimination Half-life	Duration of Action
PO	1 wk	2 hr	6 hr	Variable

iron dextran

Iron dextran (INFeD, Dexferrum) is a colloidal solution of iron (as ferric hydroxide) and dextran. It is intended for intravenous or intramuscular use for treatment of iron deficiency. Anaphylactic reactions to iron dextran, including major orthostatic hypotension and fatal anaphylaxis, have been reported in 0.2% to 0.3% of patients. Because of this, a test dose of 25 mg of iron dextran should be administered by the chosen route before injection of the full dose. Although anaphylactic reactions usually occur within a few moments after the test dose, it is recommended that a period of at least 1 hour elapse before the remaining portion of the initial dose is given. Because of the potential of iron dextran to cause anaphylaxis, its use has been replaced by use of the newer products, ferric gluconate and iron sucrose. Iron dextran is available only for injection.

PHARMACOKINETICS

Route	Onset of Action	Peak Plasma Concentration	Elimination Half-life	Duration of Action
IM	Unknown	24-48 hr	5-20 hr	3 wk

ferric gluconate
Ferric gluconate (Ferrlecit) is an injectable iron product that is indicated for repletion of total body iron content in patients with iron-deficiency anemia who are undergoing hemodialysis. The risk of anaphylaxis is much less than with iron dextran, and a test dose is not required. Doses higher than 125 mg are associated with increased adverse events, including abdominal pain, dyspnea, cramps, and itching.

PHARMACOKINETICS

Route	Onset of Action	Peak Plasma Concentration	Elimination Half-life	Duration of Action
IV	End of infusion	7 min	1 hr	4 days

iron sucrose
Iron sucrose (Venofer) is another injectable iron product indicated for the treatment of iron-deficiency anemia in patients with chronic renal disease. It is also used for patients without kidney disease. Its risk of precipitating anaphylaxis is much less than that of iron dextran, and a test dose is not required. Hypotension is the most common adverse effect and appears to be related to infusion rate. Large doses of iron sucrose should be infused over 2.5 to 3.5 hours. Low-weight elderly patients appear to be at greatest risk of hypotension.

PHARMACOKINETICS

Route	Onset of Action	Peak Plasma Concentration	Elimination Half-life	Duration of Action
IV	End of infusion	Unknown	6 hr	Unknown

FOLIC ACID

Folic acid is a water-soluble B-complex vitamin. It is also referred to as *folate,* the name of its anionic form. The human body requires oral intake of folic acid. Dietary sources of folic acid include dried beans, peas, oranges, and green vegetables. Several conditions can lead to folic acid deficiency. However, because folic acid is absorbed in the upper duodenum, malabsorption syndromes are the most common cause of deficiency.

Mechanism of Action and Drug Effects

Folic acid is converted in the body to *tetrahydrofolic acid,* which is used for erythropoiesis and for synthesis of nucleic acids (DNA and ribonucleic acid [RNA]). Dietary ingestion of folate is required for the production of DNA and RNA. It is also essential for normal erythropoiesis. Folic acid is not active in the ingested form. It must first be converted to tetrahydrofolic acid, which is a cofactor for reactions in the biosynthesis of nucleic acids.

Indications

Folic acid is primarily used to prevent and treat folic acid deficiency. Anemias caused by folic acid deficiency can be treated by exogenous supplementation of folic acid. There is also much evidence to support the use of folic acid in the prevention of neural tube defects such as spina bifida, anencephaly, and encephalocele. It is recommended that administration begin at least 1 month before pregnancy and continue through early pregnancy to reduce the risk for fetal neural tube defects. Folic acid is also indicated for the treatment of tropical sprue, a malabsorption syndrome.

Contraindications

Contraindications to the use of folic acid include known allergy to a specific drug product and any anemia not related to folic acid deficiency (e.g., pernicious anemia). It should be emphasized that folic acid should not be used to treat anemias until the underlying cause and type of anemia have been determined. For example, administering folic acid to a patient with pernicious anemia may correct the hematologic changes of anemia while deceptively masking other symptoms of pernicious anemia.

Adverse Effects

Adverse effects associated with folic acid use are rare. Allergic reaction or yellow discoloration of urine may occur.

Interactions

Oral contraceptives (see Chapter 34), corticosteroids (see Chapter 33), sulfonamides (see Chapter 38), and dihydrofolate reductase inhibitors (including the antineoplastic drug methotrexate [see Chapter 47] and the antibiotic trimethoprim [see Chapter 38]) can all cause signs of folic acid deficiency. Folic acid can also lower the serum levels of phenytoin, which can possibly lead to breakthrough seizures.

Dosages

For recommended dosages of folic acid, see the Dosages table on p. 858.

DRUG PROFILE

◆ folic acid
Folic acid is a water-soluble B-complex vitamin that is used primarily in the treatment and prevention of folic acid deficiency and anemias caused by folic acid deficiency. Folic acid is available as an OTC medication in multivitamin preparations and by prescription as a single drug. It is contraindicated in patients with anemias other than megaloblastic or macrocytic anemia. These conditions representing contraindications include vitamin B_{12} deficiency anemia and uncorrected pernicious anemia. Folic acid is available for both oral and injectable use.

PHARMACOKINETICS

Route	Onset of Action	Peak Plasma Concentration	Elimination Half-life	Duration of Action
PO	Unknown	60-90 min	Unknown	Unknown

OTHER ANEMIA DRUGS

Other drugs that may be used in the prevention and treatment of anemia are cyanocobalamin (vitamin B_{12}) and erythropoietin (Epogen, Procrit). Cyanocobalamin is discussed in detail in Chapter 53, and erythropoietin is discussed in Chapter 49. Cyanocobalamin is used to treat pernicious anemia and other megaloblastic anemias. It can be given orally or intranasally to treat vitamin B_{12} deficiency but is usually given by deep intramuscular injection to treat pernicious anemia. Once remission of the anemia is seen, cyanocobalamin can be dosed once a month.

PHARMACOKINETIC BRIDGE
to Nursing Practice

Iron preparations provide a perfect example of how pharmacokinetic properties can impact drug dosing and efficacy. Oral iron is available in a variety of salt forms, such as ferrous fumarate, ferrous sulfate, and ferric gluconate. Although very similar in mechanism of action, the specific salt form is associated with different pharmacokinetics and offers varying amounts of elemental iron. The ferrous fumarate iron salts contain some of the largest amount of iron per gram of salt consumed. For example, each 100 mg of ferrous fumarate provides 33 mg of elemental iron, whereas each 100 mg of ferrous gluconate contains 11.6 mg of elemental iron. Ferrous sulfate, yet another iron salt, provides 20 mg elemental iron in each 100 mg. Ferrous fumarate has an onset of action of 4 days and peaks 7 to 10 days with durations of up to 4 months, as does ferrous gluconate and ferrous sulfate. Therefore, even though the pharmacokinetics of the different oral iron salts are similar, the amount of elemental iron varies significantly per 100 mg. Because of these varying amounts of elemental iron, the iron salts should never be exchanged for one another and should be given with caution to avoid medication errors. Other similar pharmacokinetic properties of oral iron products, such as absorption and excretion, must be understood because unabsorbed iron—though harmless—turns the stool black and may possibly mask melena (blood in the stools). It is recommended to take oral iron with juice (orange juice is preferred) or water but not with milk or antacids because they decrease drug absorption.

NURSING PROCESS

Assessment

Before any drug is given to treat an anemia, it is important to assess the patient's past and present medical history; to compile a medication profile, including all prescription, OTC, and herbal medications the patient is taking; and to assess for drug allergies. The patient should also be assessed to identify contraindications, cautions, and drug interactions prior to beginning treatment with any of these medications. Some of the laboratory studies that may be ordered before, during, and after therapy include RBC count, hemoglobin level, hematocrit, reticulocyte count, bilirubin level, and baseline levels of folate and/or B-complex vitamins. A nutritional assessment should also be performed with a focus on the amount of iron in the patient's diet. A 24-hour recall of all food intake with serving sizes may prove to be beneficial. A nutritional and dietary consult may also be ordered. In addition, asking questions about the patient's energy levels, ability to carry

---

LIFE SPAN CONSIDERATIONS: The Elderly Patient

Iron Products

- Instructions on how to take oral forms of iron are crucial to safe administration, and all types of teaching strategies should be implemented to reinforce all verbal and/or written instructions. Make sure education is individualized and geared to patients with alterations in sensory perception. Patients should be cautioned not to make changes in their medication regimen, such as doubling doses or discontinuing a drug, without a prescriber's order.
- Elderly patients and their spouses and/or caregivers should be instructed regarding which food sources are high in iron and how to include these foods in their menu planning. Patients should be told to steam vegetables and not to overcook them through excessive boiling. Avoiding overcooking or boiling of vegetables is important to preserve the content of vitamins and minerals, including iron.
- Remind older patients that gastrointestinal upset may occur with many drugs, including vitamins and iron. Iron products should be taken with food or a snack to help decrease this upset.
- Always educate elderly patients, as well as their spouses, other family members or significant others, and/or caregivers, about appropriate community resources (e.g., Meals on Wheels, senior citizen community centers, public recreation centers). A list of these community resources is often made available through a city web page, social services department, and other outlets.

out the activities of daily living, overall immunity to illnesses, and state of health may also provide invaluable information.

Nursing Diagnoses

- Activity intolerance related to fatigue and lethargy associated with anemias
- Risk for injury related to adverse effects of iron products
- Deficient knowledge related to limited exposure to the use of the medication
- Imbalanced nutrition, less than body requirements, related to the disease process

Planning
Goals

- Patient regains his or her normal level of activity, as ordered.
- Patient remains free of symptoms related to adverse effects of blood-forming drugs (e.g., iron products).
- Patient discusses the rationale for use, adverse effects, and patient education guidelines related to the use of blood-forming drugs.
- Patient attains normal nutritional status through the use of pharmacologic and non-pharmacologic measures.

Outcome Criteria

- Patient is able to tolerate gradual increase in activity as ordered (e.g., performing activities of daily living, walking 10 minutes a day with increases as tolerated) while taking a blood-forming drug.
- Patient implements measures to minimize the occurrence of adverse effects of blood-forming drugs, such as taking the drugs with food.

- Patient takes medication exactly as prescribed to enhance its efficacy.
- Patient reports symptoms associated with worsening of the disease process or adverse reactions to medications, such as abdominal distention, cramping, nausea, and vomiting.
- Patient keeps a daily journal of dietary intake to share with the health care provider every week.
- Patient uses examples of a balanced diet for daily menu planning.

Implementation

Oral liquid dosage forms of iron products should be diluted per manufacturer instructions and sipped through a plastic straw to avoid discoloration of tooth enamel. Other oral forms of iron should always be given with plenty of fluids such as juice but not with antacids or milk, and preferably not with meals, because these decrease absorption of the drug. However, most individuals find that they do need to take oral iron products with meals or food because of the commonly encountered adverse effect of gastrointestinal upset, even though altered absorption occurs. If antacids or milk products are used, they should be taken at least 1 to 2 hours before or after the oral dosage of iron. Iron products are generally packaged in a light-resistant, airtight container. Patients should be cautioned to remain in an upright or sitting position for up to 30 minutes after taking oral dosage forms of iron, ferrous products, and related drugs to help minimize esophageal irritation or corrosion. Patients should also be warned that the use of any iron product will turn the stools from brown to a black, tarry color. See Patient Teaching Tips for more information.

If a patient cannot tolerate oral iron, intravenous iron (e.g., iron dextran, iron sucrose, or ferric gluconate) may be prescribed. A test dose of iron may be ordered, with the remaining dose given an hour later if no adverse reaction occurs. Intramuscularly administered iron should be given deep in a large muscle mass using the Z-track method (see Chapter 10). Intravenous iron dextran should be given after the intravenous line is flushed with 10 mL of normal saline and should be administered with the recommended amount of diluent and at the recommended drip rate. Epinephrine and resuscitative equipment should always be available in case of anaphylactic reaction (to iron or any drug that has an increased risk of causing anaphylaxis). In addition, it may

be necessary for the patient to remain recumbent for 30 minutes after the intravenous injection to prevent drug-induced orthostatic hypotension. The patient should move slowly and purposefully during this time.

Evaluation

Evaluation of therapeutic responses to blood-forming drugs should focus on ensuring that goals and outcome criteria have been met as well as monitoring for therapeutic and adverse effects. Therapeutic responses to iron products include improved nutritional status, increased weight, increased activity tolerance and well-being, and absence of fatigue. Adverse effects include nausea, constipation, epigastric pain, black and tarry stools, and vomiting. Signs of toxicity include nausea, diarrhea, hematemesis, pallor, cyanosis, shock, and coma.

CASE STUDY

Iron Supplements

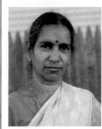
© Arvind Balarman

Mrs. E. is recovering from surgery and is in the office for a 1-month follow-up visit. She has been complaining of feeling "very tired" and having no energy, and blames it on the surgery. The physician orders some laboratory work and calls Mrs. E. a week later to tell her that she has iron-deficiency anemia. Her hemoglobin level is 10.2 g/dL and her hematocrit is 35%; her stool test result was negative for occult blood. She is given a prescription for ferrous sulfate, 300 mg, twice a day.

1. During the teaching session, what adverse effects should the nurse tell Mrs. E. to expect?
2. Mrs. E. complains about having a "sensitive stomach." What should she be taught about taking this drug?
3. When she takes the prescription to a local pharmacy, the label on the medication she receives reads "Ferrous sulfate (generic) 324 mg." Mrs. E. asks the pharmacist, "Is this dose correct?" Did a medication error occur?
4. How will Mrs. E.'s response to therapy be monitored?

For answers, see *http://evolve.elsevier.com/Lilley.*

PATIENT TEACHING TIPS

- The patient should be told to take iron products cautiously and to be aware of the potential for poisoning if these drugs are taken in greater than the recommended amounts. Oral iron products should be taken without alteration of the original dosage form, for example, no crushing. Oral dosages of iron should be taken with at least 4 to 6 oz of water or other fluid to help minimize gastrointestinal upset and increase absorption.
- Oral dosage forms of iron are not interchangeable, and prescription forms of these products may be very different from one another. Each product contains different forms of the iron salt

and also comes in different dose amounts. (One exception is that the 300-mg and 324-mg dosage forms of ferrous sulfate are used interchangeably.)
- The patient should be instructed to remain upright for up to 30 minutes after taking an iron product to prevent esophageal irritation or corrosion. The patient should also be reminded that iron products may turn the stools a black, tarry color.
- A diet high in iron should be encouraged including foods such as meat; dark green, leafy vegetables; dried beans; dried fruits; and eggs.

- Iron and folic acid are very important in the treatment of many disorders and diseases (e.g., malignancies) to achieve RBC and hemoglobin formation that is as adequate as possible and to help prevent nutritional deficits that can affect all body systems, especially the immune system.

- Blood-forming drugs are often used in the treatment of pernicious anemia, malabsorption syndromes, hemolytic anemias, hemorrhage, and renal and liver diseases.
- Iron products should be taken exactly as ordered. Parenteral dosage forms may cause anaphylaxis and orthostatic hypotension.

NCLEX EXAMINATION REVIEW QUESTIONS

1 When administering oral iron tablets, the nurse should keep in mind that the most appropriate substance, other than water, to give with these tablets is
   a pudding.
   b an antacid.
   c milk.
   d orange juice.
2 The nurse is teaching a patient about oral iron supplements. Which statement is correct?
   a "You need to take this medication on an empty stomach or else it won't be absorbed."
   b "It is better absorbed on an empty stomach, but if that causes your stomach to be upset, you can take it with food."
   c "Take this medication with a sip of water, then lie down to avoid problems with low blood pressure."
   d "If you have trouble swallowing the tablet, you may crush it."
3 The nurse is administering an intravenous dose of iron dextran. For which potential adverse effect is it most important for the nurse to monitor at this time?
   a Anaphylaxis
   b Gastrointestinal distress
   c Black, tarry stools
   d Bradycardia

4 The nurse is assessing a patient who is to receive folic acid supplements. It is important to rule out which condition before giving the folic acid?
   a Malabsorption syndromes
   b Pernicious anemia
   c Tropical sprue
   d Pregnancy
5 A patient who is taking oral iron supplements calls the office, quite upset about having "very black, shiny stools." What should be the nurse's response?
   a "You may be bleeding, and you should come to the office immediately."
   b "Are you taking this medication on an empty stomach?"
   c "This is an unusual reaction, and you should stop the tablets immediately."
   d "It is normal for oral iron products to change the stools to a black and tarry color."
6 When iron sucrose is administered, which nursing interventions are correct? (Select all that apply.)
   a Administer a test dose before giving the full dose
   b Give via deep intramuscular injection into a large muscle mass using the Z-track method
   c Administer large doses over 2.5 to 3.5 hours, intravenously
   d Monitor the patient for hypertension
   e Monitor for hypotension, especially in elderly or low-weight patients

For answers: 1. d, 2. b, 3. a, 4. b, 5. d, 6. c, e.

CRITICAL THINKING ACTIVITIES: BEST ACTION

1 The nurse is administering an intravenous dose of iron dextran. A test dose has just been given. What important action should the nurse take next? Explain.
2 J.J., a 27-year-old female, has decided that she wants to start a family. She asks the nurse, "Are there any vitamins I need to take now to make sure I'm healthy?" What is the nurse's best answer?

3 D.V. has a new prescription for an oral iron tablet. He asks the nurse, "What do I need to know about taking this pill?" What is the nurse's best answer?

For answers, see *http://evolve.elsevier.com/Lilley.*

CHAPTER 56

Dermatologic Drugs

OBJECTIVES

When you reach the end of this chapter, you should be able to do the following:

1 Discuss the normal anatomy, physiology, and functions of the skin.

2 Describe the different disorders, infections, and other conditions commonly affecting the skin.

3 Identify the various dermatologic drugs used to treat these disorders, infections, and other conditions and describe the various classifications of these drugs.

4 Discuss the mechanisms of action, indications, contraindications, cautions, other drug interactions, application techniques, and adverse effects of the various topical dermatologic drugs.

5 Develop a nursing care plan that includes all phases of the nursing process for patients using topical dermatologic drugs.

e-Learning Activities

http://evolve.elsevier.com/Lilley

NCLEX Review Questions • Animations • Nursing Care Plans • Audio Glossary • Category Catchers • Medication Errors Checklists • IV Therapy Checklists • Calculators • Frequently Asked Questions • Content Updates • Supplemental Resources • Answers to Case Studies and Critical Thinking Activities

Drug Profiles

anthralin, p. 870
♦ bacitracin, p. 865
♦ benzoyl peroxide, p. 866
calcipotriene, p. 870
clindamycin, p. 867
♦ clotrimazole, p. 868
fluorouracil, p. 871
imiquimod, p. 872
♦ isotretinoin, p. 867
♦ lindane, p. 871

miconazole, p. 868
minoxidil, p. 871
mupirocin, p. 866
neomycin and polymyxin B, p. 865
♦ pimecrolimus, p. 872
♦ silver sulfadiazine, p. 866
tar-containing products, p. 870
tazarotene, p. 870
tretinoin, p. 867

♦ *Key drug.*

Glossary

Acne vulgaris A chronic inflammatory disease of the *pilosebaceous* glands of the skin, involving lesions such as *papules* and *pustules* ("pimples"); referred to in this chapter as *acne*. (p. 866)

Actinic keratosis A slowly developing, localized thickening of the outer layers of the skin resulting from long-term, prolonged exposure to the sun. Also called *solar keratosis*. (p. 871)

Atopic dermatitis A chronic skin inflammation seen in patients with hereditary susceptibility to *pruritus*. (p. 865)

Basal cell carcinoma The most common form of skin cancer; it arises from epidermal cells known as *basal cells* and is rarely metastatic. (p. 865)

Carbuncles Necrotizing infections of skin and subcutaneous tissue caused by multiple furuncles (boils). They are usually caused by the bacterium *Staphylococcus aureus*. (p. 865)

Cellulitis An acute, diffuse, spreading infection involving the skin, subcutaneous tissue, and sometimes muscle as well. It is usually caused by infection of a wound with *Streptococcus* or *Staphylococcus* species. (p. 865)

Dermatitis Any inflammation of the skin. (p. 865)

Dermatophytes Any of common groups of fungi that infect skin, hair, and nails. These fungi are most commonly from the genera *Microsporum, Epidermophyton,* and *Trichophyton.* (p. 867)

Dermatosis The general term for any abnormal skin condition. (p. 865)

Dermis The layer of the skin just below the epidermis, consisting of papillary and reticular layers and containing blood and lymphatic vessels, nerves and nerve endings, glands, and hair follicles. (p. 864)

Eczema A pruritic, papulovesicular dermatitis occurring as a reaction to many endogenous and exogenous agents, and characterized by erythema, edema, and an inflammatory infiltrate of the dermis accompanied by oozing, crusting, and scaling. (p. 865)

Epidermis The superficial, avascular layers of the skin, made up of an outer dead, cornified portion and a deeper living, cellular portion. (p. 864)

Folliculitis Inflammation of a follicle, usually a hair follicle. A follicle is defined as any sac or pouchlike cavity. (p. 865)

Furuncles Painful skin nodules caused by *Staphylococcus* organisms that enter the skin through the hair follicles. Also called a *boil*. (p. 865)

Impetigo A pus-generating, contagious superficial skin infection, usually caused by staphylococci or streptococci. It generally occurs on the face and is most commonly seen in children. (p. 865)

Papules Small, circumscribed, superficial, solid elevations of the skin that are usually pink and less than 0.5 to 1 cm in diameter. (p. 865)

Pediculosis An infestation with lice of the family Pediculidae. (p. 870)

Pruritus An unpleasant cutaneous sensation that provokes the desire to rub or scratch the skin to obtain relief. (p. 868)

Psoriasis A common, chronic squamous cell dermatosis with polygenic (multigene) inheritance and a fluctuating pattern of recurrence and remission. (p. 865)

Pustules Visible collections of pus within or beneath the epidermis. (p. 865)

Scabies A contagious disease caused by *Sarcoptes scabiei,* the itch mite, characterized by intense itching of the skin and injury to the skin (excoriation) resulting from scratching. (p. 871)

Tinea A fungal skin disease caused by a dermatophyte and characterized by itching, scaling, and, sometimes, painful lesions. *Tinea* is a general term for an infection with any of various dermatophytes that occur at several sites. Also called *ringworm*. (p. 867)

Topical antimicrobials Substances applied to any surface that either kill microorganisms or inhibit their growth or replication. (p. 865)

Vesicles Small sacs containing liquid; also called *cysts*. (p. 865)

• • •

Anatomy, Physiology, and Disease Overview

The skin is the largest organ of the body. It covers the body and serves several functions. It acts as a protective barrier for the internal organs. Without skin, harmful external agents such as microorganisms and chemicals would gain access to and damage or destroy many of our delicate internal organs. Part of this protection includes the skin's ability to maintain a surface pH of 4.5 to 5.5. This weakly acidic environment discourages the growth of microorganisms that thrive at a more alkaline pH of 6 to 7.5. The skin also has the ability to sense changes in temperature (heat or cold), pressure, or pain—information that is then transmitted along nerve endings. The temperature of the environment changes continually; despite this, the body maintains an almost constant internal temperature due in large part to the skin, which plays a major role in the regulation of body temperature. Heat loss and conservation are regulated in coordination with the blood vessels that supply blood to the skin and by means of perspiration. The skin is also able to excrete fluid and electrolytes through sweat glands. In addition, it stores fat, synthesizes vitamin D, and provides a site for drug absorption.

The skin is made up of two layers: the **dermis** and the **epidermis** (Figure 56-1). The outer skin layer, or epidermis, is itself composed of four layers. From the outermost to innermost, these are the stratum corneum, stratum lucidum, stratum granulosum, and stratum germinativum. The respective functions of these layers are described in Table 56-1.

None of these layers has a direct blood supply of its own. Instead, nourishment is provided through diffusion from the dermis below. The dermis lies between the epidermis and subcutaneous fat and differs from the epidermis in many ways. It is approximately 40 times thicker than the epidermis. Traversing the dermis is a rich supply of blood vessels, nerves, lymphatic tissue, elastic tissue, and connective tissue, which provide extra support and nourishment to the skin. Also contained in the dermis are the exocrine glands—the eccrine, apocrine, and sebaceous glands—and the hair follicles. The functions of the various types of exocrine glands are explained in Table 56-2.

Below the dermis is a layer of loose connective tissue called the *hypodermis*. It helps make the skin flexible. It is also here that the subcutaneous fat tissue is located, which provides thermal insulation and cushioning or padding. It is also the source of nutrition for the skin.

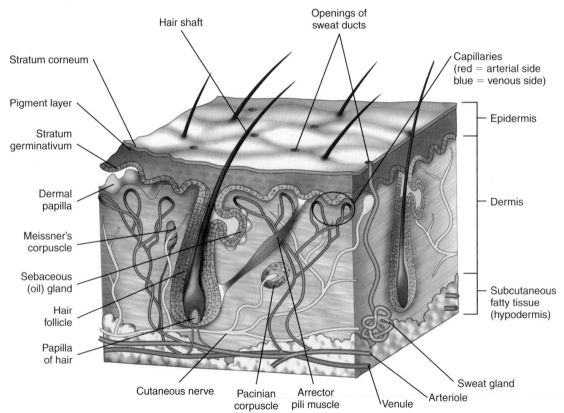

FIGURE 56-1 Microscopic view of the skin. The epidermis, shown in longitudinal section, is raised at one corner to reveal the ridges in the dermis. (Modified from Thibodeau GA, Patton KT: *Anatomy and physiology*, ed 5, St Louis, 2003, Mosby.)

TABLE 56-1 Epidermal Layers

Layer	Description
Stratum corneum ("horny layer," so named because keratin is the same protein that makes up the horns of animals)	Outermost layer consisting of dead skin cells that are made of a converted water-repellant protein known as *keratin;* it is the protective layer for the entire body. After it is desquamated or shed, it is replaced by new cells from below.
Stratum lucidum ("clear layer")	Layer where keratin is formed; it is translucent and contains flat cells.
Stratum granulosum ("granular layer")	Cells die in this layer; granulated cells are located here, which gives this layer the appearance for which it is named.
Stratum germinativum ("germinative layer")	New skin cells are made in this layer; it contains melanocytes, which produce melanin, the skin color pigment.

TABLE 56-2 Exocrine Glands of the Skin

Gland	Function
Sebaceous	Large lipid-containing cells that produce oil or film that covers the epidermis, protects and lubricates the skin, and is water repellent and antiseptic
Eccrine	Sweat glands that are located throughout the skin surface; help regulate body temperature and prevent skin dryness
Apocrine	Mainly in axilla, genital organs, and breast areas; emit an odor; believed to be scent or sex glands

Reactions or disorders of the skin are common and numerous. A **dermatosis** is any abnormal skin condition. Dermatoses include a variety of types of **dermatitis** (skin inflammation). Among these are conditions such as **atopic dermatitis, eczema,** and **psoriasis.** In addition, there are also a variety of skin cancers, including **basal cell carcinoma,** squamous cell carcinoma, and melanoma.

Pharmacology Overview

Drugs that are administered directly to a skin site are called *topical dermatologic drugs.* These drugs are available in a variety of formulations that are suitable for specific indications. Each formulation has certain characteristics that make it beneficial for certain uses. The formulations, their characteristics, and examples are provided in Table 56-3. Note that the focus of this chapter is topically administered medications. Because so many topical drugs are available, the scope of this chapter is limited to some of the more commonly used medications. Systemically administered drugs are also used to treat several skin disorders (see Part 7) and are cross-referenced throughout this chapter.

There are many therapeutic categories of dermatologic drugs. Some of the most common ones are the following:

- Antibacterial drugs
- Antifungal drugs
- Antiinflammatory drugs
- Antineoplastics
- Antipruritic drugs (for itching)
- Antiviral drugs
- Burn drugs
- Débriding drugs (promote wound healing)
- Emollients (skin softeners)
- Keratolytics (cause softening and peeling of the stratum corneum)
- Local anesthetics
- Sunscreens
- Topical vasodilators

ANTIMICROBIALS

Topical antimicrobials are antibacterial, antifungal, and antiviral drugs that, as the name implies, are applied topically. Although topical antimicrobials have many of the same properties as the systemic forms, there are differences in terms of their toxicities and adverse effects.

GENERAL ANTIBACTERIAL DRUGS

Common skin disorders caused by various bacteria are **folliculitis, impetigo, furuncles, carbuncles, papules, pustules, vesicles,** and **cellulitis.** The bacteria responsible are most commonly *Streptococcus pyogenes* and *Staphylococcus aureus.* Dermatologic antibacterial drugs are used to treat or prevent these skin infections. The most commonly used drugs are bacitracin, polymyxin, and neomycin. Unfortunately, due to the high incidence of infection with methicillin-resistant *S. aureus* (MRSA), mupirocin is now also commonly used.

DRUG PROFILES

◆ bacitracin

Bacitracin is a polypeptide antibiotic that is applied topically for the treatment or prevention of local skin infections caused by susceptible aerobic and anaerobic gram-positive organisms such as staphylococci, streptococci, anaerobic cocci, corynebacteria, and clostridia. It works by inhibiting bacterial cell wall synthesis, which leads to cell death. It can be either bactericidal or bacteriostatic, depending on the causative organism. Its antimicrobial spectrum is broadened in several available combination drug products. Most of these also contain neomycin and/or polymyxin B (see later).

Adverse reactions are usually minimal; however, reactions ranging from skin rash to allergic anaphylactoid reactions have occurred. If itching, burning, inflammation, or other signs of sensitivity occur, bacitracin should be discontinued. This drug is available in ointment form and is usually applied to the affected area one to three times daily. It is also available in systemic and ophthalmic (see Chapter 57) formulations.

neomycin and polymyxin B

Neomycin and polymyxin B are two additional broad-spectrum antibiotics that are available as the popular nonprescription product known as Neosporin. Neosporin cream is a combination of these two drugs alone, whereas Neosporin ointment also contains bacitracin. Several brand name and generic combinations of these three topical antibiotics are available, and all are commonly used as topical antiseptics for minor skin wounds. Although neomycin/polymyxin B is still a very popular over-the-counter (OTC) product,

TABLE 56-3 Dermatologic Formulations: Characteristics and Examples

Formulation	Characteristics	Examples
Aerosol foam	Can cover large area; useful for drug delivery into a body cavity (e.g., vagina, rectum) or hair areas	ProctoFoam, Epifoam, contraceptive foams
Aerosol spray	Spreads thin liquid or powder film; covers large areas; useful when skin is tender to touch (e.g., burns)	Solarcaine, Desenex, Kenalog
Bar	Similar to a bar of soap; useful as a wash with water	PanOxyl (benzoyl peroxide)
Cleanser	Nongreasy; used as an astringent (oil remover) and/or wash with water	ZoDerm
Cream	Contains water and can be removed with water; not greasy or occlusive; usually white semisolid; good for moist areas	hydrocortisone cream (Cortaid), Benadryl cream
Gel/jelly	Contains water and possibly alcohol; easily removed and good lubricator; usually clear, semisolid substance; useful when lubricant properties are desirable	K-Y jelly, Saligel, Surgilube
Lotion	Contains water, alcohol, and solvents; may be a suspension, emulsion, or solution; good for large or hairy areas	Calamine lotion, Lubriderm lotion, Kwell lotion
Oil	Contains very little if any water; occlusive, liquid; not removable with water	Lubriderm bath oil
Ointment	Contains no water; not removable with water; occlusive, greasy, and semisolid; desirable for dry lesions because of occlusiveness	Vaseline (petrolatum), zinc oxide ointment, A & D ointment
Paste	Similar properties to those of ointments; contains more powder than ointments; excellent protectant properties	zinc oxide paste (Balmex)
Pledget (pad)	Moistened pad that is applied to or wiped over affected area	EryPads (erythromycin)
Powder	Slight lubricating properties; may be shaken on affected area; promotes drying of area where applied	Tinactin powder, Desenex powder
Shampoo	Soapy liquid for washing hair and/or skin	Nizoral (ketoconazole)
Solution	Nongreasy liquid; dries quickly	erythromycin topical solution (Eryderm)
Stick	Spreads thin chalky or viscous liquid film; often better for smaller areas	Benadryl Itch Relief
Tape	Most occlusive formulation; consistent topical drug delivery; useful when small, straight areas require drug application	Cordran tape

there is evidence that use of the drug can increase the likelihood of future allergic reactions of the skin.

mupirocin

Mupirocin (Bactroban) is an antibacterial product available only by prescription. It is used on the skin for treatment of staphylococcal and streptococcal impetigo. It is used topically and intranasally to treat nasal colonization with *MRSA*. The drug is applied topically three times daily and intranasally twice daily. Adverse reactions are usually limited to local burning, itching, or minor pain.

◆ silver sulfadiazine

Silver sulfadiazine (Silvadene) has been proven both effective and safe in the prevention and treatment of infections in burns. One of the major concerns for burn victims is infection at the burn site. However, because increased systemic absorption of a drug can occur in compromised skin areas such as burns, topical burn drugs must not be too potent or toxic to avoid causing dangerous systemic effects. This is especially true when larger burned areas must be treated, because the drug may be applied over a large surface area of skin and therefore may be absorbed in greater quantities. On the other hand, the blood supply to burned areas is often drastically reduced, so that systemically administered antibiotics either cannot reach the site or do so only in quantities too low to be effective. Therefore, the only way of applying these drugs to ensure that they reach the burn site is to do so topically.

Silver sulfadiazine is a synthetic antimicrobial drug produced when silver nitrate reacts with the chemical sulfadiazine. It appears to act on the cell membrane and cell wall of susceptible bacteria and is used as an adjunct in the prevention and treatment of infection in second- and third-degree burns. The adverse effects of silver sulfadiazine are similar to those of other topical drugs and include pain,

burning, and itching. This medication should not be used in patients who are allergic to sulfonamide drugs. It is available only as a 1% cream and should be applied topically to cleansed and débrided burned areas once or twice daily using a sterile-gloved hand.

ANTIACNE DRUGS

Acne vulgaris is the most common skin infection. Its precise cause is unknown and somewhat controversial. Likely causative factors include heredity, stress, drug reactions, hormones, and bacterial infections. Common bacterial causes include Staphylococcus species (spp.) and *Propionibacterium acnes*. Some of the most commonly used antiacne drugs are benzoyl peroxide, clindamycin, erythromycin, tetracycline, isotretinoin, and the vitamin A acid known as *retinoic acid*. Many other drugs are also used in the treatment and prevention of acne, including systemic formulations of the antibiotics minocycline, doxycycline, and tetracycline (see Chapter 38). Some practitioners also prescribe oral contraceptives (see Chapter 34) for female acne patients, because in some controlled studies estrogen has been shown to have beneficial effects against acne, especially hormone-driven acne.

DRUG PROFILES

◆ benzoyl peroxide

The microorganism that most commonly causes acne, *P. acnes*, is an anaerobic bacterium; that is, it needs an environment that is poor in oxygen to grow. Benzoyl peroxide is effective in combating such infection because it slowly and continuously liberates active oxygen in the skin, resulting in antibacterial, antiseptic, drying, and keratolytic actions. These actions create an environment that is unfavorable for the continued growth of the *P. acnes* bacteria, and they soon die. Drugs such as benzoyl peroxide that soften scales and loosen the outer horny layer of the skin are referred to as *keratolytics.*

Benzoyl peroxide generally produces signs of improvement within 4 to 6 weeks. Adverse effects tend to be related to dose (including overuse) and include peeling skin, red skin, or a sensation of warmth. Blistering or swelling of the skin is generally considered an allergic reaction to the product and is an indication to stop treatment. Overuse of this drug and also of tretinoin is common in teenaged patients who are attempting to cure their acne quickly. The result can be painful, reddened skin, which usually resolves on return to use of these medications as prescribed.

Benzoyl peroxide is available in multiple topical dosage forms, including a cleansing bar, liquid, lotion, mask, cream, gel, and cleanser. It is also available in various combination drug products. It is usually applied topically one to four times daily, depending on the dosage form and prescriber's instructions. Pregnancy category C.

clindamycin

Clindamycin (Cleocin T) is a topical form of the systemic antibiotic described in Chapter 39. It is most commonly prescribed for acne. Adverse reactions are usually limited to minor, local skin reactions, including burning, itching, dryness, oiliness, and peeling. The drug is available in gel, lotion, suspension, and foam. It is usually applied once or twice daily. Pregnancy category B.

◆ isotretinoin

Isotretinoin (Accutane) is an oral product indicated for the treatment of severe recalcitrant cystic acne. Isotretinoin inhibits sebaceous gland activity and has antikeratinizing (anti–skin hardening) and antiinflammatory effects. Isotretinoin is one of relatively few medications that are classified as pregnancy category X drugs. This means that it is a proven human *teratogen,* or a chemical that is known to induce birth defects. It is imperative that female patients of childbearing age be counseled and agree not to become pregnant during use of the drug. For these reasons, in 2005, the U.S. Food and Drug Administration (FDA) approved more stringent guidelines regarding the prescription and use of this medication. It is now officially required that at least two contraceptive methods be used by sexually active women during therapy with isotretinoin and for 1 month after completion of therapy. A risk management program of unprecedented size and scope has been designed and approved by the FDA especially for this drug. It is known as *iPLEDGE* and was fully implemented as of March 1, 2006. As a result, federal law now requires that any health care provider who prescribes this drug be a registered and active member of this program, and patients must also be qualified and registered. Further information is available at the iPLEDGE call center at 866-495-0654 or online at *http://www.ipledgeprogram.com.* In addition, there have been case reports of suicide and suicide attempts in patients receiving this medication. Patients should be educated to report any signs of depression immediately to their prescribers. Follow-up treatment may be needed, and simply stopping the drug may be insufficient. Despite these rather strong concerns, this drug does prove to be very helpful in treating severe acne cases. Isotretinoin is available only for oral use.

tretinoin

Tretinoin (retinoic acid, vitamin A acid) (Renova, Retin-A) is a derivative of vitamin A that is used to treat acne and ameliorate the dermatologic changes (e.g., fine wrinkling, mottled hyperpigmentation, roughness) associated with photodamage (sun damage). The drug appears to act as an irritant to the skin, in particular to the follicular epithelium. Specifically, it stimulates the turnover of epidermal cells, which results in skin peeling. While this is occurring, the free fatty acid levels of the skin are reduced, and horny cells of the outer epidermis cannot then adhere to one another. Without fatty acids and horny cells, acne and its comedo, or pimple, cannot exist.

Topically administered tretinoin has been shown to enhance the repair of skin damaged by ultraviolet (UV) radiation, or sunlight. It does this by increasing the formation of fibroblasts and collagen, both of which are needed to rebuild skin. The drug also may reduce collagen degradation by inhibiting the enzyme collagenase that breaks down collagen.

Tretinoin's main adverse effects are local inflammatory reactions, which are reversible when therapy is discontinued. Some of the most common adverse effects are excessively red and edematous blisters, crusted skin, and temporary alterations in skin pigmentation. Tretinoin is available in many topical formulations, including creams, gels, and a liquid. Because of its potential to cause severe irritation and peeling, it may initially be applied once every 2 or 3 days, and treatment often starts with a lower-strength product.

Retin-A Micro has been approved for the treatment of acne vulgaris. This particular acne product contains tretinoin formulated inside a synthetic polymer called a *Microsponge system.* This system is made of round microscopic particles of synthetic polymer. These microspheres act as reservoirs for tretinoin, allowing the skin to absorb small amounts of the drug over time. Retin-A Micro is currently available only in gel form. All topical forms of tretinoin are rated pregnancy category C. They are not to be confused with the oral capsule form of tretinoin that is used to treat leukemia and is rated pregnancy category D. Another antiacne retinoid is adapalene, a topical solution.

ANTIFUNGAL DRUGS

A few fungi produce keratolytic enzymes, which allows them to live on the skin. Topical fungal infections are primarily caused by *Candida* spp. (candidiasis), **dermatophytes,** and *Malassezia furfur* (tinea versicolor). These fungi are found in moist, warm environments, especially in dark areas such as the feet or groin.

Candidal infections are most commonly caused by *Candida albicans,* a yeastlike opportunistic fungus present in the normal flora of the mouth, vagina, and intestinal tract. Two significant factors that commonly predispose a person to a candidal infection are broad-spectrum antibiotic therapy, which promotes an overgrowth of nonsusceptible organism in the natural body flora, and immunodeficiency disorders such as those that occur in patients with cancer or acquired immunodeficiency syndrome (AIDS) and those undergoing organ transplantation. Because these infections favor warm, moist areas of the skin and mucous membranes, they most commonly occur orally (e.g., thrush in infants), vaginally, and cutaneously in sites such as beneath the breasts and in diapered areas. They may also cause nail infections.

Dermatophytes are a group of three closely related genera consisting of *Epidermophyton* spp., *Microsporum* spp., and *Trichophyton* spp. that use the keratin found on the skin to feed their growth. They produce superficial mycotic (fungal) infections of keratinized tissue (hair, skin, and nails). Infections caused by dermatophytes are called **tinea,** or *ringworm,* infections. The name *ringworm* comes from the fact that the infection sometimes assumes a circular pattern at the site of infection.

TABLE 56-4 Topical Antifungal Drugs

Drug	Trade Name	Dosage Form	Indications	Legal Status
butenafine	Mentax, Lotrimin Ultra	1% cream	Tinea pedis	Rx
butoconazole	Femstat 3	2% vaginal cream	Candidiasis	OTC
ciclopirox olamine	Loprox	0.77% cream and lotion, 8% solution (for nails)	Candidiasis, dermatophytoses, tinea versicolor	Rx
clotrimazole	Gyne-Lotrimin 3	2% vaginal cream, 100- and 200-mg vaginal tabs	Candidiasis	OTC
	Lotrimin	2% cream, 1% lotion and solution	Candidiasis, tinea versicolor	Rx
	Lotrimin AF	1% cream, lotion, and solution	Dermatophytoses	OTC
	Mycelex	1% cream and solution	Dermatophytoses	Rx
	Mycelex	10-mg troches	Oropharyngeal candidiasis	Rx
	Mycelex-7	1% vaginal cream, 100-mg vaginal tabs	Candidiasis	OTC
ketoconazole	Nizoral	2% cream and shampoo	Candidiasis, dermatophytoses, tinea versicolor	Rx
miconazole	Micatin	2% cream, powder, and spray	Dermatophytoses	OTC
	Monistat-Derm	2% cream	Candidiasis, dermatophytoses, tinea versicolor	Rx
nystatin	Nilstat, Mycostatin	Cream, ointment, powder	Candidiasis	Rx
terbinafine	Lamisil	1% cream and spray	Dermatophytoses	OTC
tolnaftate	Tinactin	1% cream, solution, gel, powder, and spray	Dermatophytoses	OTC
undecylenic acid	Cruex, Desenex	Powder, cream, solution, soap	Dermatophytoses	OTC

OTC, Available over the counter without prescription; *Rx,* currently available by prescription only.

Tinea infections are further identified by the body location where they occur: tinea pedis (foot), tinea cruris (groin), tinea corporis (body), and tinea capitis (scalp). Tinea infections of the foot are also known as *athlete's foot* and those of the groin as *jock itch.*

Fungi usually invade the stratum corneum, which is the dead layer of desquamated (shed) cells. Inflammation occurs when the fungi invade this layer; sensitivity (e.g., itching) occurs when they penetrate the epidermis and dermis.

Many of the fungi that cause topical infections are very difficult to eradicate. The organisms are very slow growing, and antifungal therapy may be required for periods ranging from several weeks to as long as 1 year. However, many topical antifungal drugs are available for the treatment of both dermatophytic infections and those caused by yeast and yeastlike fungi. Some of these drugs, their dosage forms, and their uses are listed in Table 56-4. Systemically administered antifungal drugs are sometimes used to treat skin conditions as well. These drugs were discussed in Chapter 42.

The most commonly reported adverse effects of topical antifungals are local irritation, **pruritus,** a burning sensation, and scaling. Ciclopirox and clotrimazole are classified as pregnancy category B drugs, and econazole, ketoconazole, and miconazole are classified as pregnancy category C drugs. Hypersensitivity is the one contraindication to the use of any of these drugs.

DRUG PROFILES

♦ clotrimazole

Clotrimazole (Lotrimin, Mycelex-G) is available both OTC and by prescription. It is available as a lozenge for the treatment of oropharyngeal candidiasis, commonly known as *thrush.* It is also available as a cream, lotion, or solution for the treatment of dermatophytoses (e.g., athlete's foot), superficial mycoses, and cutaneous candidiasis. Similar topical preparations are available for intravaginal administration in the treatment of vulvovaginal candidiasis, commonly called

a *yeast infection,* and vaginal trichomoniasis. Clotrimazole is available in many topical formulations: a powder; a 10-mg oral topical lozenge; a 1% cream, lotion, and solution; 1% and 2% vaginal creams; and 100- and 500-mg vaginal tablets. Different dosages and dosage forms are used for the treatment of different fungal infections. Pregnancy category B.

miconazole

Miconazole (Monistat) is a topical antifungal drug that is available in several OTC and prescription products. It inhibits the growth of several fungi, including dermatophytes and yeast, as well as gram-positive bacteria, and is commonly used to treat dermatophytoses, superficial mycoses, cutaneous candidiasis, and vulvovaginal candidiasis. It is present in many OTC remedies for athlete's foot, jock itch, and yeast infections.

For the treatment of athlete's foot, jock itch, ringworm, and other susceptible fungal infections, miconazole should be applied sparingly to the cleansed, dry, infected area twice daily in the morning and evening. For the treatment of yeast infections, one 200-mg suppository should be inserted in the vagina once daily at bedtime for 3 consecutive days or 100 mg (one suppository or 5 g of the 2% cream) should be administered intravaginally once daily at bedtime for 7 days. The most common adverse effects of topically administered miconazole are vulvovaginal burning and itching, pelvic cramps and rash, urticaria, stinging, and contact dermatitis. It is available in a variety of topical formulations: as a 2% aerosol spray and powder, a 2% powder, a 2% cream, a 2% vaginal cream, and a 100- and 200-mg vaginal suppository. It is also now available as a 1200-mg vaginal suppository for one-time dosing. Pregnancy category C.

ANTIVIRAL DRUGS

Topical antivirals are now used less frequently than before, because systemic antiviral drug therapy has generally been shown to be superior for controlling such viral skin conditions. Nevertheless, two antiviral ointments are described here. As is the case with systemic drug therapy, these products are best used early in a viral skin lesion outbreak. Topical antivirals are more likely to be used for acute outbreaks, whereas systemic drugs are used for acute outbreaks as well as ongoing prophylaxis against outbreaks. As noted in Chapter 40, viral infections are very difficult to treat because they live in the body's own healthy cells and use their cell mechanisms to reproduce. The same holds true for topical viral infections. Infections caused by herpes simplex virus types 1 and 2 and human papillomavirus (which causes anogenital warts) are particularly serious and are becoming more common.

The only topical antiviral drugs currently available to treat such viral infections are acyclovir (Zovirax) and penciclovir (Denavir). They work by comparable mechanisms as described for similar antiviral drugs in Chapter 40. Acyclovir and penciclovir are available as topical ointments (5% and 1%, respectively). Acyclovir is applied every 3 hours, or six times daily, for 1 week. Penciclovir is applied every 2 hours while awake for 4 days. A finger cot or rubber glove should be worn for the application of the ointment to prevent the spread of infection. The most common adverse effects are stinging, itching, and rash. Acyclovir is classified as a pregnancy category C drug and penciclovir as a pregnancy category B drug.

ANESTHETIC, ANTIPRURITIC, AND ANTIPSORIATIC DRUGS

TOPICAL ANESTHETICS

Topical anesthetic drugs are drugs that are used to numb the skin. They accomplish this by inhibiting the conduction of nerve impulses from sensory nerves, thereby reducing or eliminating the pain or pruritus associated with insect bites, sunburn, and allergic reactions to plants such as poison ivy, as well as many other uncomfortable skin disorders. They are also used to numb the skin before a painful injection (e.g., insertion of an intravenous line in a pediatric patient). Topical anesthetics are available as ointments, creams, sprays, liquids, and jellies, and are discussed in Chapter 12. A lidocaine/prilocaine combination drug (EMLA) and lidocaine alone (Ela-max) are topical anesthetic drugs that are used frequently, especially in pediatric patients. EMLA should be applied 1 hour before the procedure, whereas Ela-max is effective within 30 minutes.

TOPICAL ANTIPRURITICS AND ANTIINFLAMMATORIES

Topical antipruritic (antiitching) drugs contain antihistamines or corticosteroids. Many exert a combined anesthetic and antipruritic action when applied topically. The antihistamines and their therapeutic effects are covered in Chapter 36. New recommendations for the use of topical antihistamines state that these drugs should not be used to treat the following conditions because of systemic absorption and subsequent toxicity: chickenpox, widespread poison ivy lesions, and other lesions involving large body surface areas.

The most commonly used topical antiinflammatory drugs are the corticosteroids (see Chapter 33). They are generally indicated for the relief of inflammatory and pruritic dermatoses. When topically administered corticosteroids are used, many of the undesirable systemic adverse effects associated with the use of the sys-

TABLE 56-5	Commonly Used Topical Corticosteroids (in Order of Decreasing Potency)
Range of Potency*	**Corticosteroid**
1. Higher potency	betamethasone dipropionate (cream and ointment), clobetasol propionate, halobetasol propionate, diflorasone diacetate
2. Moderate potency	amcinonide, betamethasone dipropionate (cream), betamethasone benzoate, betamethasone valerate (0.1% cream, ointment, and lotion), desoximetasone (0.05% cream), desoximetasone, fluocinolone, halcinonide, fluocinolone (cream and ointment), flurandrenolide, mometasone, triamcinolone acetonide (0.5% cream and ointment)
3. Lower potency	alclometasone, desonide, fluocinolone (0.01% solution), triamcinolone (0.1% cream, lotion), hydrocortisone, dexamethasone

*Skin penetration and thus potency is enhanced by the vehicle (dosage form) containing the steroid. In decreasing order of effectiveness are ointments, gels, creams, and lotions.

temically administered corticosteroids are avoided. The beneficial drug effects of topically administered corticosteroids are their antiinflammatory, antipruritic, and vasoconstrictive actions.

The many different available dosage forms of the various corticosteroids vary in their relative potency, and this often guides their selection for treating various conditions. For instance, corticosteroids that are fluorinated (which increases the potency) are used for the treatment of dermatologic disorders such as psoriasis. The vehicle in which the corticosteroid is contained also may alter its vasoconstrictor properties and therapeutic efficacy. Ointments are generally the most penetrating, followed next by gels, creams, and lotions. Propylene glycol also enhances the penetration of the corticosteroid and its vasoconstrictor effects. Most corticosteroids are available in many topical formulations, which provide a variety of options. The currently available topical corticosteroids, along with their respective potencies, are listed in Table 56-5.

Adverse effects of these drugs include skin reactions such as acne eruptions, allergic contact dermatitis, burning sensations, dryness, itching, skin fragility, hypopigmentation, purpura, hirsutism (usually facial), folliculitis, round and swollen face, and alopecia (usually of the scalp). Another adverse effect is the opportunistic overgrowth of bacteria, fungi, or viruses as a result of the immunosuppressive effects of this class of drugs. *Tachyphylaxis* (weakening of drug effect over time) may also occur with these drugs, especially with long-term use or overuse. They should generally be applied no more than twice daily as a thin layer over the affected area. The usual adult dosage of these drugs is one or two applications daily, as directed. Less potent topical corticosteroids are used in children, but the same schedule is followed. Corticosteroids are classified as pregnancy category C drugs and are contraindicated in patients with hypersensitivity to them. Because many of these products are available orally as well as topically, the potential exists for both to be administered simultaneously. This is not recommended and is potentially harmful. The combined use of topical and oral preparations of the same drug can lead to toxicity.

ANTIPSORIATIC DRUGS

Psoriasis is a common skin condition in which areas of the skin become thick, reddened, and covered with silvery scales. Psoriasis is actually a result of a disordered immune system, although it is generally referred to as a skin condition. It is believed to involve *polygenic* (multigene) inheritance. Psoriasis has fluctuating patterns of recurrence and remission. Flare-ups can be triggered by changes in climate, infection, stress, excessive alcohol intake, or dry skin. Although there are many subtypes, the most classic one is known as *plaque psoriasis* and typically manifests as large, dry, erythematous scaling patches of the skin that are often white or silver on top. Commonly affected skin areas include nails, scalp, genitals, and lower back. Treatment usually begins with a topical corticosteroid for mild to moderate cases. When this therapy is not successful, topical antipsoriatic drugs are used. In addition to these topical drugs, there are also newer systemically administered antipsoriatic drugs. A thorough discussion of these drugs is beyond the scope of this chapter on topical medications, but those given by systemic injection include etanercept (Enbrel) and alefacept (Amevive). Another drug, efalizumab (Raptiva), was pulled from the U.S. market in 2009. Etanercept is discussed in more detail in Chapter 49 on biologic response modifiers. In addition, the antineoplastic drug methotrexate (see Chapter 47) is also used for its antipsoriatic properties.

■ DRUG PROFILES

tazarotene

Tazarotene is a receptor-selective retinoid. It is thought to normalize epidermal differentiation, reducing the influx of inflammatory cells into the skin. Synthetic retinoids are vitamin A analogues and are thought to play a role in skin cell differentiation and proliferation. Tazarotene is available in gel form and is approved for the treatment of stable plaque psoriasis and mild to moderately severe facial acne. Like isotretinoin, tazarotene is a pregnancy category X drug, and a negative pregnancy test 2 weeks before starting therapy is required for female patients.

tar-containing products

Drug products containing coal tar derivatives were among the first medications used to treat psoriasis and are still used today for this purpose. Tar derivatives are known to have antiseptic, antibacterial, and *antiseborrheic* properties, and they work to soften and loosen scaly or crusty areas of the skin. *Seborrhea* is excessive secretion of *sebum*, a normal skin secretion containing fat and epithelial cell debris. Tar-containing products are available in a variety of shampoo forms (for scalp psoriasis), as well as solution, oil, ointment, cream, lotion, gel, and even soap forms for bathing. These products typically contain 1% to 10% coal tar. Adverse reactions usually include minor skin burning, photosensitivity, and other irritations. These products may be applied from one to four times daily or once or twice weekly as prescribed.

anthralin

Anthralin (Anthra-Derm) is a unique drug that is believed to work by inhibition of deoxyribonucleic acid (DNA) synthesis and mitosis within the epidermis to the development of reduce psoriatic lesions. It is available in ointment and cream form and is usually applied once daily. Adverse reactions are generally limited to minor skin irritation. Pregnancy category C.

calcipotriene

Calcipotriene (Dovonex) is a synthetic vitamin D_3 analogue that works by binding to vitamin D_3 receptors in skin cells known as *keratinocytes,* the abnormal growth of which contributes to psoriatic lesions. Calcipotriene helps to regulate the growth and reproduction of keratinocytes. The most common adverse reaction is minor skin irritation. However, more serious reactions can occur in some cases, including worsening of psoriasis, dermatitis, skin atrophy, and folliculitis. Calcipotriene is usually applied twice daily. Pregnancy category C. Taclonex is a combination product containing calcipotriene and betamethasone, a topical steroid.

MISCELLANEOUS DERMATOLOGIC DRUGS

There are many other topically applied drugs. Those discussed in this section are the topical ectoparasiticides (scabicides and pediculicides), hair growth drugs, sunscreens, antineoplastics, and immunomodulating drugs. Many of these drugs are available both OTC and by prescription. Aloe vera herbal preparations (see the Herbal Therapies and Dietary Supplements box) are also available OTC.

■ DRUG PROFILES

ECTOPARASITICIDAL DRUGS

Ectoparasites are insects that live on the outer surface of the body, and the drugs that are used to kill them are called *ectoparasiticidal drugs.* Lice are transmitted from person to person by close contact with infested individuals, clothing, combs, or towels. A parasitic infestation on the skin with lice is called **pediculosis,** and such infestations go by one of three different names, depending on the location of the infestation:

- Pediculosis pubis—pubic louse or "crabs," infestation by *Phthirus pubis*
- Pediculosis corporis—body louse, infestation by *Pediculus humanus corporis*
- Pediculosis capitis—head louse, infestation by *Pediculus humanus capitis*

Common findings in infested persons include itching; eggs of the lice attached to hair shafts (called *nits*); lice on the skin or clothes; and, in the case of pubic lice, sky blue macules (discolored skin patches) on the inner thighs or lower abdomen. Pediculoses are treated with a class of drugs called *pediculicides*. A second common parasitic skin infection known as **scabies** is that caused by the itch mite *Sarcoptes scabiei*. Scabies is transmitted from person to person by close contact, such as by sleeping next to an infested person. The scabies mite causes irritation and itching by boring into the horny layers of skin located in cracks and folds. Itching seems to occur most commonly in the evening. The drugs used to treat these infestations are called *scabicides*.

Treatment of these parasitic infestations should begin with identification of the source of infestation to prevent reinfestation. Next, the clothing and personal articles of the infested person should be decontaminated. This is best accomplished by washing them in hot, soapy water or by dry-cleaning them. All close contacts of the person should also be treated to prevent reinfestation.

In addition to lindane, profiled here, malathion (Ovide) and crotamiton (Eurax) are also ectoparasiticidal drugs.

◆ lindane

Lindane (Kwell) is a chlorinated hydrocarbon originally developed as an agricultural insecticide. It is both a scabicide and a pediculicide because it is effective in treating both scabies and pediculosis. It is available in two topical formulations: a 1% lotion and a 1% shampoo.

For the treatment of pubic or body lice, the cream or lotion is applied in a sufficient quantity to cover the skin and hair of the infested and surrounding areas. It is left on for 12 hours and then thoroughly washed off. A second application is seldom needed. Head lice can be treated with lindane shampoo, which should be worked into the hair and left on for 4 minutes. The hair should then be rinsed and dried, after which the nits (eggs) should be combed from the hair shafts. The treatment for scabies is similar. It involves the application of lindane over the entire body, from the neck down. It is left on for 8 to 12 hours and then washed off. A similar second application 1 week later is often recommended. The OTC products are applied in similar fashion, although details may vary among individual products. Adverse effects of lindane are an eczematous skin rash and, rarely, central nervous system toxicity. The latter is more common in young children and in cases of overuse. For many years, lindane was the most widely used pediculicide, but it has been superseded to some degree by permethrin. This is because of case reports of neurotoxicity, including dizziness, seizures, and deaths, caused by lindane. Most of the adverse events occurred due to product misuse (e.g., ingestion) or overuse. Children are at higher risk of neurotoxicity because their skin surface area is larger in relation to body weight. Lindane is still recommended as second-line therapy for lice and scabies after failure of one of the OTC preparations. However, the FDA has recommended that it be sold in smaller containers (1 to 2 oz) with definitive patient instructions on proper use.

HAIR GROWTH DRUGS
minoxidil

Minoxidil (Rogaine) is a vasodilating drug that is administered systemically to control hypertension (see Chapter 25). Topically it has the same vasodilating effect, but when used in this way it is applied to the scalp to stimulate hair growth. The vasodilation it causes is one possible explanation for how it promotes hair growth. It may also act at the level of the hair follicle, possibly stimulating hair follicle growth directly.

Minoxidil can be used by both men and women who experience baldness or hair thinning. Treatment involves administering the drug to the affected areas (those with balding and anticipated balding) twice daily, usually morning and evening. It generally takes 4 months before results are seen. Systemic absorption of topically applied minoxidil may occur with possible adverse effects, including tachycardia, fluid retention, and weight gain. Local effects may include skin irritation, and the drug should not be applied to skin that is already irritated, nor should it be used concurrently with other topical medications applied to the same site. Pregnancy category C. Note that the beneficial effects of this drug can be reduced by heat, including the use of a blow dryer. The systemically administered drug finasteride (Proscar, 5 mg) is used to treat benign prostatic hyperplasia, as discussed in Chapter 35. A lower-strength version known as Propecia (1 mg) is also used to treat male pattern alopecia.

SUNSCREENS

Sunscreens are topical products used to protect the skin from damage caused by the UV radiation of sunlight. There are currently nearly 160 specific sunscreen products on the market. None requires a prescription for use. Each is composed of typically three to five various chemical ingredients that work together to provide UV protection and, usually, a moisturizing effect as well. Common examples of these ingredients are titanium dioxide, octyl methoxycinnamate, homosalate, and parabens. Sunscreens are given a *sun protection factor* (SPF) rating. This is a number ranging from 2 to 50 (and even higher in some newer products) in order of increasing potency of UV protection. Most sunscreens come in lotion, cream, or gel form. A smaller number of lip balms are also available.

ANTINEOPLASTIC DRUGS

Skin cancer is the most common form of cancer. There are two types of nonmelanoma skin cancer: basal cell carcinoma and squamous cell carcinoma. Basal cell carcinoma is the most common and is rarely fatal, but it can be highly disfiguring. Squamous cell carcinoma, on the other hand, can be fatal, with 2500 deaths reported annually. The most aggressive skin cancer, melanoma, accounts for only 3% of all skin cancers but is responsible for 75% of deaths associated with skin cancer. The most common cause of skin cancer is exposure to the sun and tanning beds. Early detection and prevention (with the use of sunscreen) are of the utmost importance.

fluorouracil

Various premalignant skin lesions and basal cell carcinomas may be treated with the topically applied antineoplastic drug fluorouracil (Efudex). As noted in Chapter 47, this drug is an antimetabolite that acts by interfering with key cellular metabolic reactions, destroying rapidly growing cells, such as premalignant and malignant cells. It is also used topically in the treatment of *solar* or **actinic keratosis** and superficial basal cell carcinomas of the skin—often in addition to local surgical excision. More aggressive skin cancers, *squamous cell carcinoma* and *malignant melanoma*, are not treated with fluorouracil but are usually treated with more aggressive surgery, radiation therapy, and/or systemic chemotherapy (see Chapters 47 and 48).

The adverse effects associated with the topical use of this antineoplastic are generally limited to local inflammatory reactions such as dermatitis, stomatitis, and photosensitivity. More serious affects include swelling, scaling, pain, pruritus,

TABLE 56-6 Selected Wound Care Products

Product Name	Advantages	Disadvantages	Contraindications
acetic acid (vinegar)	Low cost	Cytotoxic	Allergy
sodium hypochlorite (Dakin's bleach solution)	Aids débridement; reduces microbial count	Partly toxic and irritating to healing tissue	Clean, noninfected wounds
cadexomer iodine (Iodosorb, others)	Slow release; safe for viable cells; absorbs exudates; promotes wound healing	Partly toxic to fibroblast cells; stains tissue	Iodine allergy
collagenase (Santyl)	Good for patients taking anticoagulants or in whom surgery is contraindicated; selectively removes necrotic tissue; does not harm normal tissue; OK for infected wounds	Requires prescriber's order; not for use with other common wound products such as silver sulfadiazine (Silvadene) or Dakin's solution; expensive	Clean, well-granulating wound; product allergy
Biafine topical emulsion	Can be used for "tunneling" wounds as well as full-thickness wounds and radiation dermatitis	Must not be applied within 4 hr of radiation therapy	Bleeding wounds, skin rashes related to food or drug allergies

burning, soreness, tenderness, suppuration, scarring, and hyperpigmentation.

Fluorouracil is available in both cream and solution form. It can be applied with a nonmetallic applicator, clean fingertips, or gloved fingers. If the fingers are used, they should be washed thoroughly immediately after application. Either a 1% or 2% fluorouracil solution should be used for the treatment of multiple actinic keratoses of the head and neck. The solution should be applied twice daily to the lesions. Superficial basal cell carcinoma may be treated with 5% fluorouracil, administered twice daily for at least 2 to 6 weeks. Another topical drug also used for the treatment of actinic keratoses and basal cell carcinomas is the immunomodulator imiquimod, discussed below.

IMMUNOMODULATORS
◆ pimecrolimus
Pimecrolimus (Elidel) is available in a cream form for use in treating atopic dermatitis. Atopic dermatitis is caused by a hereditary susceptibility to pruritus and is often associated with allergic rhinitis, hay fever, and asthma. This drug works through a mechanism similar to that of the anti–transplant-rejection drug tacrolimus (Prograf), which was discussed in Chapter 45. A topical form of tacrolimus (Protopic) is also used and has similar actions and indications. Adverse reactions to both drugs are usually limited to minor skin irritations.

imiquimod
Imiquimod (Aldara) is an immunomodulating drug that has demonstrated efficacy in treating actinic keratosis, superficial basal cell carcinoma, and anogenital warts. Its exact mechanism of action is unknown, but it is believed somehow to enhance the body's immune response to these conditions. It is applied two to five times per week, as prescribed, depending on the condition being treated. Adverse reactions include mild skin reactions such as burning, induration (hardness), irritation, pain, and bleeding, which can occur both locally (at the site of medication administration) and at skin areas remote from the site of administration. More severe adverse skin reactions include edema, erosion or ulceration, scaling, scabbing, exudation, and vesicle formation. Systemic reactions, likely related to systemic immunomodulating effects, include cough, upper respiratory tract infection, musculoskeletal reactions (e.g., back pain), and lymphadenopathy. This drug is available only in cream form.

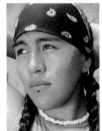
WOUND CARE DRUGS

Although superficial skin wounds usually require minimal interventions, deeper skin wounds often require more definitive care for optimal healing. Such care includes addressing the systemic issues (e.g., body nutritional status) that are critical to tissue repair. Vitamin C (ascorbic acid) and zinc have been shown to improve wound healing when they are given orally. Topical wound care medications are key to one of the fundamental steps of wound care, referred to in the literature as *preparation of the wound bed*. Wound

TABLE 56-7 Skin Preparation Drugs

Drug	Effective Against	Adverse Effects
isopropyl alcohol	Bacteria, fungi, virus	Excessive dryness of skin
chlorhexidine (Hibiclens)	Bacteria, fungi	Central nervous system toxicity in neonates and burn patients
povidone-iodine (Betadine)	Bacteria, fungi, virus	Staining of skin, irritation and pain at wound sites
benzalkonium chloride (Zephiran)	Bacteria, fungi	Chemical burns if left in contact with skin for too long

débridement is removal of nonviable tissue and elimination of bacteria by suitable cleansing. It should be noted that up until 2009, drugs containing papain or papain/urea were commonly used as topical débriding drugs. However, the FDA no longer allows these drugs to be manufactured, because they never received FDA approval. Table 56-6 provides information regarding selected currently available wound care medications.

SKIN PREPARATION DRUGS

The skin should be disinfected before any invasive procedure. Isopropyl alcohol (70%) is most commonly used to prepare the skin before minor procedures such as drawing blood or giving injections. Isopropyl alcohol has been shown to lower the bacterial count for 20 to 40 minutes after application. Other drugs that are used to prepare the skin include povidone-iodine (Betadine), chlorhexidine (Hibiclens), and benzalkonium chloride (Zephiran). Benzalkonium chloride is a surface-active drug that works by denaturing the microorganism or essentially destroying its protein. Chlorhexidine acts by disrupting bacterial membranes and inhibiting cell wall synthesis. It is used primarily as a surgical scrub or hand-washing agent by health care professionals. Povidone-iodine is an antiseptic that kills bacteria, fungi, and viruses. It is used for the prevention or treatment of topical infections associated with surgery, burns, and minor cuts and scrapes, and for relief of minor vaginal infections. It is the most widely used antiseptic, but patients should be screened for iodine or shellfish allergies before using it. It is available in many different dosage forms. See Table 56-7 for more information on selected skin preparation drugs.

NURSING PROCESS

Assessment

Before any dermatologic preparation is administered, the patient should be assessed for any allergies (including allergies to all drug ingredients, such as benzoyl or peroxide), contraindications, cautions, and drug interactions, and the findings should be documented (see previous discussion in the pharmacology section). Topical antibacterials are associated with a wide range of reactions because of the generalized sensitivity of patients to antibiotics, even when in a different dosage form; therefore, if a patient is allergic to a systemic antibacterial, he or she will also be allergic to topical dosage forms. The nurse should also assess the results of any culture and sensitivity testing that was ordered before giving the antibacterial to ensure appropriate identification of effective drugs. Before administering any type of topical medication (e.g., antimicrobial, corticosteroid, antiacne drug), the nurse should always consider the concentration of the medication, length of exposure to the skin, condition of the skin, size of the area affected, and hydration of the skin. All of these factors have a significant influence on the action of the medication.

The skin or affected area must be inspected thoroughly under an adequate light source and the area palpated with a gloved hand. In dark-skinned patients, an erythematous area may not be visible but may be palpated as an area of warmth. Should there be any possibility of systemic absorption of topical drugs—for example, tretinoin—results of liver function studies should be assessed prior to drug therapy. For various antibacterial drugs, the possibility of systemic absorption warrants assessment of baseline renal and hepatic functioning. Baseline hearing levels should also be assessed for drugs that are known to be ototoxic (e.g., silver sulfadiazine). Physical assessment of the skin should be accompanied by assessment of surrounding structures, including lymph nodes. The patient's overall health status and hygiene practices should also be assessed, including whether the patient has experienced any trauma and whether there is any history of immunosuppression. The nurse should also remember that the skin of the very young and the elderly is more fragile and permeable to certain topical dermatologic preparations. These characteristics also lead to a higher risk for systemic absorption from the skin. It is also important to note other possible situations that may result in a drug effect that is less than therapeutic, such as the use of topical drugs over an area that is full of pus or debris. The use of herbal products, such as topical aloe vera, also requires thorough assessment and notation of any allergies, contraindications, cautions, and drug interactions (see the Herbal Therapies and Dietary Supplements box on p. 870).

Nursing Diagnoses

- Impaired skin integrity related to specific diseases, reactions, conditions, or breaks in the skin barrier
- Acute pain related to the skin condition or the adverse effects of the topical drug
- Deficient knowledge related to lack of experience with and exposure to use of topical drugs
- Ineffective therapeutic regimen management related to lack of information about the importance of adhering to the drug regimen and maintaining frequent dosing

Planning

Goals

- Patient's skin remains intact and healed in appearance, and integrity is maintained.
- Patient remains compliant with drug therapy and uses the appropriate drug application technique.
- Patient remains free of injury to the skin while receiving therapy.
- Patient experiences minimal or no complications of therapy.

Outcome Criteria

- Patient's skin improves daily as stated by the patient, with less redness, drainage, discomfort, itching, and/or rash.
- Patient reports increased comfort and minimal pain and itching at the site of the skin disorder.

- Patient demonstrates how to apply medication in keeping with the prescriber's orders, with specific attention to the requirements for emollient, lotion, solution, spray, cream, and ointment dosage forms.
- Patient states the rationale for treatment, adverse effects of the specific dermatologic preparation, and symptoms associated with the dermatologic therapy that should be reported to the prescriber.
- Patient remains compliant with the medication therapy with resulting improvement in the condition of the skin or affected area within 2 to 4 weeks of treatment.

Implementation

Generally speaking, before any topical medication is applied, the affected area should be cleansed of any debris, drainage, and/or residual medication, with care taken to follow any specific directions such as removing water- or alcohol-based topical preparations with soap and water. Standard Precautions should be used at all times (see Box 10-1). All dosage forms of medication should be stored as recommended. Gloves should be worn, not only to prevent contamination from secretions but also to prevent absorption of the medication through the skin. Application of the topical drug using a finger cot, tongue depressor, or cotton-tipped applicator is recommended. Lotions and solutions should be shaken or mixed thoroughly before use and applied evenly (see earlier for more information and refer to Chapter 10). The hands should be washed not only *before* but also *after* application of the medication. Any dressings should be applied as ordered, with special attention to directions concerning occlusive, wet, or wet-to-dry dressing changes. It is important to note, however, that most topical dermatologic drugs do not require use of a dressing once the medication is applied. The medication order may also say to avoid any type of dressing or coverage of the area. When medications are used for wound care, there is usually a step-by-step protocol for application of a cleansing agent, possible débridement drug, and rinsing solution, and final application of an antibacterial, antifungal, burn, antiseptic, or other solution that may have been ordered. Patient education regarding wound care and/or use of topical dermatologic drugs should be comprehensive. If home health care is needed after discharge, arrangements should be in place before the patient returns home. Information about the site of drug application, including drainage (color and amount), swelling, temperature, odor, color, and pain or other sensations, as well as the type of treatment rendered and the response, should be documented with each treatment or application and a comparative before-and-after assessment noted.

The manufacturer's guidelines regarding the use of any of the dermatologic preparations should always be followed, because each medication has a different type of base solution. Specific application procedures may be required for different dosage forms. It is also important to follow any instructions or orders regarding other treatments to the affected area, such as the use of an occlusive or wet dressing (see earlier). Medicated areas may also need to be protected from exposure to air or sunlight. Strict adherence to the proper method of application and dosage of any dermatologic preparation is important to its effectiveness, and doubling up of a missed dose is not recommended. After the patient or nurse has completed the medication administration process, all contaminated dressings, gloves, or equipment should be disposed of properly. Safety and comfort should be maintained at all times. See *http://evolve.elsevier. com/Lilley* for more information about the classifications of topical dermatologic drugs and associated nursing implications. Further pointers for patient education are presented in Patient Teaching Tips. Also see Table 56-6 for information about specific drugs for wound care and their advantages and disadvantages.

Evaluation

Evaluation should always begin with monitoring to ensure that goals and outcome criteria are being met. Therapeutic responses to the various dermatologic preparations include improved condition of the skin and healing of lesions or wounds; a decrease in the size of lesions with eventual resolution; and a decrease in swelling, redness, weeping, itching, and burning of the area. The prescriber should be notified if a therapeutic response is not observed within an appropriate time (anywhere from 48 hours to 72 hours or longer, depending on the drug, disorder or skin problem, acute or chronic nature of the condition, etc.) or if signs and symptoms worsen or new ones appear. Adverse effects for which to evaluate include increased severity of symptoms—for example, increased redness, swelling, pain, and drainage; fever; or any other unusual problems at the affected area. Adverse effects may range from slight irritation of the site where the topical drug has been applied to an allergic reaction to toxic systemic effects.

PATIENT TEACHING TIPS

- Patient instructions should include keeping the skin clean and dry and maintaining adequate general hygiene, cleanliness, adequate hydration, and proper nutrition during drug therapy. The patient should understand how to prepare the skin for application of the medication and how to follow instructions as provided.
- If indicated or ordered, dressings should be applied to the area after the medication has been applied. Proper disposal of contaminated dressings or equipment should be encouraged. The need for thorough hand washing before and after application of medication should be emphasized and demonstrated to all those involved in the care of the patient. The importance of compliance with the drug regimen should also be emphasized.
- The patient should be instructed to notify the prescriber if any unusual or adverse reactions occur or if the original condition worsens or fails to improve within a designated period.
- All female patients of childbearing age should be counseled regarding the birth defect hazards associated with exposure to certain dermatologic drugs. All sexually active women must use contraception during treatment with any teratogenic medication and for at least 1 month after discontinuation of the drug.
- The patient should be educated regarding ways to prevent exposure to the sun through the use of sunscreen and protective clothing, and avoidance of overexposure. Tanning beds create risk for skin cancer as well, and the patient should be instructed to use them in moderation and to apply sunscreen beforehand. All skin moles or lesions should be monitored for any unusual changes in color, size, texture, and/or shape.

POINTS TO REMEMBER

- Dermatologic drugs are used to treat topical infections.
- Common skin disorders caused by bacteria are folliculitis, impetigo, furuncles, carbuncles, and cellulitis.
- The bacterium most commonly responsible for acne is *P. acnes.*
- The fungi that are responsible for causing topical fungal infections are *Candida,* dermatophytes, and *M. furfur.*
- The most common topical fungal infections are *Candida* infections, for example, yeast infections.
- One of the most common topical viral infections is infection with herpes simplex virus types 1 and 2.
- Topical anesthetics are used therapeutically to numb the skin. Indications for topical anesthetics include insect bites, sunburn, poison ivy, and prevention of pain from injections.

- Corticosteroids are some of the most widely used topical drugs and are indicated for relief of topical inflammatory and pruritic disorders.
- Beneficial effects of corticosteroids include antiinflammatory, antipruritic, and vasoconstrictor actions.
- Adverse and toxic reactions to dermatologic drugs can and do occur; therefore, these drugs should be administered cautiously, and the prescriber's orders and manufacturer's guidelines should be followed. This is critical to ensure safe and effective treatment.
- Patient education about the medication, its administration, and its effectiveness are important to ensure compliance with the treatment regimen.

NCLEX EXAMINATION REVIEW QUESTIONS

1 The nurse is assessing the skin of a teenaged patient who has been using a benzoyl peroxide product for 2 weeks as part of treatment for acne. Which assessment findings indicate that the patient is having an allergic reaction and will need to stop treatment?
  a Reddened skin over the treatment area
  b Blistering skin over the treatment area
  c Peeling skin over the treatment area
  d Sensation of warmth when the product is applied
2 When considering the variety of OTC topical corticosteroid products, the nurse is aware that which type of preparation is generally most effective?
  a Gel
  b Lotion
  c Spray
  d Ointment
3 The nurse is monitoring for an allergic reaction to topical bacitracin, which would be evident by presence of
  a petechia.
  b thickened skin.
  c itching and burning.
  d purulent drainage.
4 When the nurse is teaching a patient about the mechanism of action of tretinoin, which statement by the nurse is correct?
  a "This medication acts by killing the bacteria that cause acne."
  b "This medication actually causes skin peeling."

  c "This medication acts by protecting your skin from UV sunlight."
  d "This medication has antiinflammatory actions."
5 When the nurse is providing wound care with Dakin's solution for a patient who has a stage III pressure ulcer, the patient exclaims, "I smell bleach! Why are you putting bleach on me?" The nurse's best explanation is:
  a "This is a very dilute solution and acts to reduce the bacteria in the wound so that it can heal."
  b "This solution is used instead of medication to promote wound healing."
  c "This solution is used to dissolve the dead tissue in your wound."
  d "Don't worry, we would never use bleach on a patient!"
6 The nurse is performing wound care on a burned area using silver sulfadiazine cream in a patient with an arm wound. Which actions by the nurse are correct? (Select all that apply.)
  a Applying the cream over the previous layer to avoid disturbing the wound bed
  b Gently cleansing the wound to remove the previous layer of cream and wound debris
  c Using clean gloves to apply the ointment
  d Using sterile gloves to apply the ointment
  e Always covering the wound with a dressing after applying the cream
  f Washing hands before and after the procedure

1. b, 2. d, 3. c, 4. b, 5. a, 6. b, d, f.

CRITICAL THINKING ACTIVITIES: BEST ACTION

1 A 22-year-old woman with severe acne is receiving counseling before taking isotretinoin (Accutane). She has read the online iPLEDGE information (see *http://www.iPLEDGEprogram.com*) and is shocked to see that two negative pregnancy test results are required before therapy is started and that a pregnancy test must be performed monthly during therapy. What is the nurse's best answer to her concerns?
2 A hospitalized patient has been transferred to a regular medical-surgical unit after spending 3 days in the intensive care unit as part of treatment for severe pneumonia. The nurse comes in to give medications and explains that one of the medications,

mupirocin (Bactroban), has been ordered to be given twice a day, intranasally. As the nurse prepares to apply the ointment, the patient asks, "What happened? Do I have an infection inside my nose on top of everything else?" What is the nurse's best answer?
3 The preoperative nurse is about to perform skin preparation with a povidone-iodine (Betadine) preparation kit before a minor surgical procedure. What is the most important thing for the nurse to assess before the nurse performs this preparation?

For answers, see http://evolve.elsevier.com/Lilley.

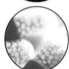

CHAPTER 57

Ophthalmic Drugs

OBJECTIVES

When you reach the end of this chapter, you should be able to do the following:

1 Discuss the anatomy and physiology of the structures of the eye and the impact of glaucoma and other disorders and disease processes on these structures.

2 List the various classifications of ophthalmic drugs, with examples of specific drugs in each class.

3 Discuss the mechanisms of action, indications, dosage forms with application techniques, adverse effects, cautions, contraindications, and drug interactions of the various ophthalmic drugs.

4 Develop a nursing care plan that includes all phases of the nursing process for patients receiving ophthalmic drugs.

e-Learning Activities

http://evolve.elsevier.com/Lilley

NCLEX Review Questions • Animations • Nursing Care Plans • Audio Glossary • Category Catchers • Medication Errors Checklists • IV Therapy Checklists • Calculators • Frequently Asked Questions • Content Updates • Supplemental Resources • Answers to Case Studies and Critical Thinking Activities

Drug Profiles

acetylcholine, p. 883
apraclonidine, p. 884
◆ artificial tears, p. 895
◆ atropine sulfate, p. 894
◆ bacitracin, p. 891
◆ betaxolol, p. 886
◆ ciprofloxacin, p. 891
cromolyn, p. 894
cyclopentolate, p. 894
dapiprazole, p. 894
◆ dexamethasone, p. 893
◆ dipivefrin, p. 885
◆ dorzolamide, p. 887
◆ echothiophate p. 883
◆ erythromycin, p. 891

fluorescein, p. 894
flurbiprofen, p. 893
◆ gentamicin, p. 890
glycerin, p. 888
ketorolac, p. 893
◆ latanoprost, p. 889
mannitol, p. 888
natamycin, p. 891
olopatadine, p. 894
◆ pilocarpine, p. 883
◆ sulfacetamide, p. 891
tetracaine, p. 894
tetrahydrozoline, p. 895
◆ timolol, p. 886
trifluridine p. 891

◆ *Key drug.*

Glossary

Accommodation The adjustment of the *lens* of the eye for variations in distance. (p. 879)

Angle-closure glaucoma Glaucoma that occurs as a result of a narrowed anatomic angle between the lens and cornea. Also called *closed-angle glaucoma, narrow-angle glaucoma, congestive glaucoma,* and *pupillary closure glaucoma.* (p. 880)

Anterior chamber The bubblelike portion of the front of the eye between the *iris* and the *cornea.* (p. 879)

Aqueous humor The clear, watery fluid circulating in the *anterior* and *posterior chambers* of the eye. (p. 878)

Bactericidal Referring to any substance that kills bacteria. (p. 891)

Bacteriostatic Referring to any substance that stops the growth and reproduction of bacteria. (p. 891)

Canal of Schlemm A tiny circular vein at the angle of the anterior chamber of the eye through which the aqueous humor is drained and ultimately funneled into the bloodstream. Also called *Schlemm canal.* (p. 879)

Cataract An abnormal progressive condition of the *lens* of the eye, characterized by loss of transparency with resultant blurred vision. (p. 879)

Ciliary muscle The circular muscle between the *anterior* and *posterior* chambers of the eye behind the *iris.* It is connected to the suspensory ligaments that modulate the curvature of the *lens.* (p. 879)

Cones Photoreceptive (light-receiving) cells in the retina of the eye that enable a person to perceive colors and play a large role in central (straight-ahead) vision. (p. 879)

Cornea The convex, transparent anterior part of the eye. (p. 878)

Cycloplegia Paralysis of the *ciliary muscles,* which prevents the *accommodation* of the *lens* for variations in distance. (p. 879)

Cycloplegics Drugs that paralyze the ciliary muscles of the eye. (p. 879)

Dilator muscle A muscle that constricts the *iris* of the eye but dilates the pupil. Also called *dilator pupillae.* (p. 879)

Glaucoma An abnormal condition of elevated pressure within an eye because of obstruction of the outflow of *aqueous humor.* (p. 880)

Intraocular pressure The pressure of the fluids of the eye against the tunics (retina, choroid, and sclera). (p. 879)

Iris The round, muscular portion of the eye that gives the eye its color and serves as an aperture controlling the amount of light passing through the *pupil.* (p. 878)

Lacrimal ducts Small tubes that drain *tears* from the *lacrimal glands* into the nasal cavity. (p. 878)

Lacrimal glands Glands located at the medial corners of the eyelids that produce *tears.* (p. 878)

Lens The transparent, crystalline, curved structure of the eye that is located directly behind the *iris* and the *pupil* and is attached to the ciliary body by ligaments. (p. 879)

Lysozyme An enzyme with antiseptic actions that destroys some foreign organisms. It is normally present in tears, saliva, sweat, and breast milk. (p. 878)

Miotics Drugs that constrict the pupil. (p. 879)

Mydriatics Drugs that dilate the pupil. (p. 879)

Open-angle glaucoma A type of glaucoma that is often bilateral, develops slowly, is genetically determined, and does not involve a narrowing of the angle between the *iris* and the *cornea.* (Also called

876

chronic glaucoma, wide-angle glaucoma, and *simple glaucoma.*) (p. 880)

Optic nerve A major nerve that connects the posterior end of each eye to the brain, to which it transmits visual signals. (p. 879)

Posterior chamber The part of the eye behind the *iris* but in front of the *vitreous body.* It includes the *lens* and its suspensory ligaments, as well as *aqueous humor.* (p. 880)

Pupil A circular opening in the *iris* of the eye, located slightly to the nasal side of the center of the iris. The pupil lies behind the *anterior chamber* of the eye and the *cornea* and in front of the *lens.* (p. 878)

Retina The innermost layer of the eye, containing both *rods* and *cones* that receive visual stimuli and transmit them to the *optic nerve.* (p. 879)

Rods The tiny cylindrical photoreceptor elements arranged perpendicularly to the surface of the retina. Rods are especially sensitive to low-intensity light and are responsible for black and white and peripheral ("off-to-the-side") vision. (p. 879)

Sphincter pupillae A muscle that expands the *iris* while constricting or narrowing the diameter of the *pupil.* (p. 879)

Tears Watery saline or alkaline fluid secreted by the *lacrimal glands* to moisten the conjunctiva (see Figure 57-1). (p. 878)

Uvea The fibrous tunic beneath the sclera that includes the *iris,* the ciliary body, and the choroid of the eye (see Figure 57-1). Also called *tunica vasculosa bulbi* or *uveal tract.* (p. 878)

Vitreous body A transparent, semigelatinous substance contained in a thin membrane filling the cavity behind the *lens.* Also called the *corpus vitreum.* (p. 879)

Vitreous humor The fluid component of the vitreous body. (p. 879)

• • •

Anatomy and Physiology Overview

The eye is the organ responsible for the sense of sight. Figure 57-1 illustrates the structures of the eye, all of which are needed for accurate eyesight. Each eyeball is nearly spherical and approximately 1 inch in diameter. Each eye is recessed into a small frontal skull cavity known as an *orbit.* The exposed anterior (front) portion of the eye is covered by three layers: the protective external layer (*cornea* and *sclera*), a vascular middle layer known as the *uvea* (includes the *choroid, iris,* and *ciliary body*), and the internal layer, known as the *retina.* All of these layers are protected by the *eyelid,* which serves as an external protective tissue.

Each eye is held in place and moved by six muscles that are controlled by cranial nerves. These muscles include the *rectus* and *oblique* muscles. There are four types of rectus muscles: *inferior, superior, medial,* and *lateral.* There are two types of oblique muscles: *inferior* and *superior.* These muscles are shown in Figure 57-2. (The medial rectus muscle is hidden from view in this figure but is directly across from the lateral rectus muscle.) The *levator palpebrae superioris* muscle opens the eyelid (see later). This muscle rests on top of the superior rectus muscle. There are several other important structures that are either part of or adjacent to the eye. The structures and the purpose of each are as follows:

• *Eyebrow:* Rows of short hair above (superior to) the upper eyelids. The eyebrow protects the eye from direct light, falling dust or other small particles, and perspiration coming from the forehead.

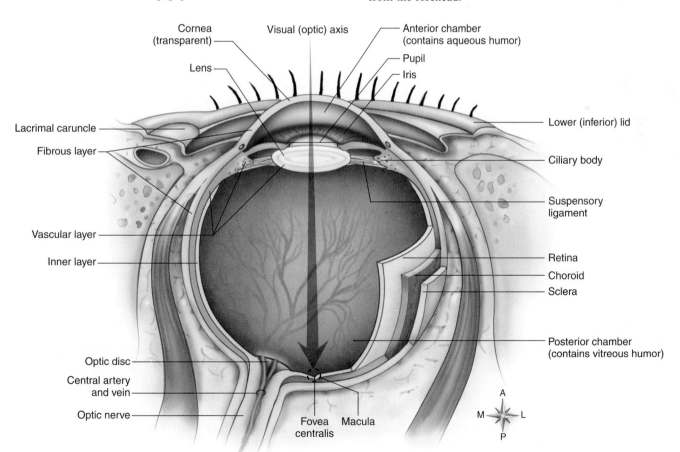

FIGURE 57-1   Horizontal section through the left eyeball, looking from the top down. (Modified from Patton KT, Thibodeau GA: *Anatomy and physiology,* ed 7, St Louis, 2010, Mosby.)

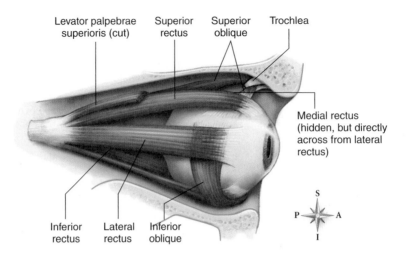

Levator palpebrae superioris (cut)   Superior rectus   Superior oblique   Trochlea

Medial rectus (hidden, but directly across from lateral rectus)

Inferior rectus   Lateral rectus   Inferior oblique

S
P — A
I

FIGURE 57-2   Extrinsic muscles of the right eye, lateral view. (Modified from Patton KT, Thibodeau GA: *Anatomy and physiology,* ed 7, St Louis, 2010, Mosby.)

- *Eyelid:* The layer of muscle and skin lined interiorly by the *conjunctiva.* The conjunctiva also covers the outer anterior surface of the eye, which includes the cornea.

   The eyelid is moveable and can open or close. It protects the eye when closed and allows vision when open. The eyelid is raised by contraction of the *levator palpebrae superioris* muscle and is lowered by relaxation of this muscle (see Figure 57-2).
- *Cornea:* The *convex* (outward-projecting; opposite of *concave*), transparent, anterior portion of the eye. It can be thought of as a window that sits in front of the *lens* and allows the passage of light.
- *Eyelashes:* Two or three rows of hairs that are located on the edge *(margin)* of the eyelids. They help prevent small particles from falling into the eye when it is open.
- *Palpebral fissure:* The space between the upper and lower eyelids when the eyelids are open but relaxed.
- *Sclera:* A tough, white coat of fibrous tissue that surrounds the entire eyeball except for the cornea. It helps maintain the shape of the eye. Commonly called the *white* of the eye, the sclera is nonvascular and allows light to pass through it to the lens.
- *Choroid:* One of the middle-layer structures of the eyeball that contains the blood vessels which supply the eye; it also absorbs light.
- *Ciliary body:* The structure that supports the *ciliary muscles* which control the curvature of the lens via attached *suspensory ligaments.*
- *Conjunctiva:* The mucous membrane that lines the eyelids and also covers the exposed anterior surface of the eyeball.
- *Iris:* The colored *(pigmented)* muscular apparatus behind the cornea.
- *Pupil:* The variable-sized opening in the center of the iris that allows light to enter into the eyeball when the eyelids are open. Its diameter changes with contraction and relaxation of the muscular fibers of the iris as the eye responds to changes in light, emotional states, and other types of stimulation. The pupil is the rear portion of the window of the eye through

which light passes to the lens and the retina (the cornea is the front part of this window).
- *Medial canthus:* The site of union of the upper and lower eyelids near the nose.
- *Lacrimal caruncle:* A small, red, rounded elevation covered by modified skin at the medial angle of the eye; the site of the *lacrimal glands* (see later).
- *Lateral canthus:* The site of union of the upper and lower eyelids away from the nose.

LACRIMAL GLANDS

The eye is kept moist and healthy by an intricate network of connected canals, ducts, and sacs that work together. The **lacrimal glands** produce tears that bathe and cleanse the exposed anterior portion of the eye. **Tears** are composed of an isotonic, aqueous solution that contains an enzyme called **lysozyme,** which acts as an antibacterial to help prevent eye infections. Tears drain into the nasal cavity through the **lacrimal ducts.**

LAYERS OF THE EYE

Overall, the eye can be conceived as having three separate anatomic layers. The fibrous *outer layer* of the eye has two parts that are continuous with each other: the *sclera* and the **cornea.** The sclera is a tough, fibrous layer that protects and maintains the shape of the eye. The cornea is a nonvascular transparent portion of the outer layer that allows light to enter the eye. It is located at the very front of the eye and is continuous with the sclera. It is pain sensitive (a protective function) and obtains nutrition from the **aqueous humor,** the clear watery fluid that circulates in the anterior and posterior chambers of the eye.

   The vascular *middle layer* of the eye is composed of the **iris** (to the anterior), ciliary body, and choroid (to the posterior). These three structures are collectively called the **uvea.** The iris gives color to the eye and has an adjustable opening in the center called the **pupil.** The main function of the iris is to regulate the

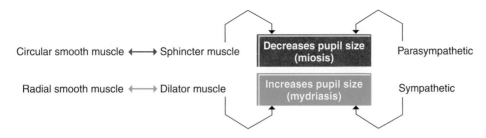

FIGURE 57-3 Different nervous systems control pupil size.

amount of light that enters the eye by causing the size of the pupil to vary. Pupil size is controlled by two smooth muscles. The **sphincter pupillae** muscle is controlled by the parasympathetic nervous system and constricts the diameter of the pupil (called *miosis*) (Figure 57-3). A sphincter is any circular band of muscle fibers that constricts a passage or closes a natural opening in the body (e.g., pyloric sphincter). Impulses from the parasympathetic nervous system operate this muscle. In contrast, the pupil is opened (called *mydriasis*) by a radial smooth muscle called the **dilator muscle.** It is composed of radiating fibers, like spokes of a wheel, that converge from the circumference of the iris toward its center. Sympathetic nervous system impulses control this muscle (see Figure 57-3).

The anterior portions of both the retina and choroid merge to become the *ciliary body,* which produces aqueous humor. This is the clear, watery fluid that circulates in both the *anterior* and *posterior chambers,* and it should not be confused with *tears* (described earlier). Aqueous humor also contributes, along with **vitreous humor** (see later), to the **intraocular pressure** of the eye. This is the internal pressure of all fluids against the *tunics* (retina, choroid, sclera) of the eye. Obviously, given the already small space of the eye, any change in the volume of aqueous humor present can lead to increased or reduced intraocular pressure. Normally, the aqueous humor is removed from the **anterior chamber** via the **canal of Schlemm** at a rate that balances out its production by the ciliary body. The ciliary body also provides a support for the suspensory ligaments to which the lens (see later) is attached. The choroid is a thin, dark layer that lines most of the internal side of the sclera. The function of the choroid is to absorb light and prevent its reflection out of the eye. The choroid is also the major location of the network of blood vessels that supply the eye.

The **lens** is the transparent crystalline structure of the eye, located directly behind the iris and the pupil. It has a *biconvex* (oval-spherical) shape and is held in place by *suspensory ligaments* that are attached to the **ciliary muscle.** Contraction of the ciliary muscle modifies the tension of the suspensory ligaments, which changes the shape of the lens. This function is important for visual accommodation as well as the focusing of light (and visual images) onto the retina. The ciliary muscle is controlled by the parasympathetic nervous system through the oculomotor cranial nerve (cranial nerve III). Accordingly, the lens divides the interior of the eyeball into posterior (rear) and anterior (forward) chambers. The larger chamber behind the lens is filled with a jellylike fluid called the **vitreous body.** The

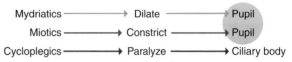

FIGURE 57-4 Drug classes and their effects on pupil size.

lens is normally transparent to allow light to pass through easily. It is composed of uniform layers of protein fibers that are encased by a clear connective tissue capsule. A loss of lens transparency results in a visual condition called a **cataract.** A cataract is a gray-white opacity that can be seen within the lens. If cataracts are untreated, sight may eventually be completely lost. At the onset of a cataract, vision is blurred and may be further worsened by the glare of bright lights. *Diplopia* or double vision may also develop.

Before light rays reach the retina, they are focused into a sharp image by the lens of the eye. The elasticity of the lens enables it to change its shape and focusing power. This process is called **accommodation** and is facilitated by the ciliary body. Paralysis of accommodation is called **cycloplegia. Mydriatics** are drugs that dilate the pupil (e.g., apraclonidine). Drugs that constrict the pupil are called **miotics** (e.g., acetylcholine, pilocarpine). Drugs that paralyze the ciliary body are called **cycloplegics,** but they also have mydriatic properties (e.g., atropine, cyclopentolate) (Figure 57-4). All of these medications are used to facilitate visualization of the inner eye during ophthalmic examinations.

The third and *inner layer* of the eye is a thin delicate layer known as the **retina.** It contains light-sensitive *photoreceptors* called **rods** and **cones.** The basic function of the retina is to receive the light image formed by the lens and to convert it via the rods and cones into the neural signals that support vision. Both types of photoreceptors are located near the surface of the retina. Rods produce black and white vision, including shades of gray, and are especially sensitive in low light; cones are responsible for color vision (Figure 57-5). In addition, rods are more active in providing peripheral (to-the-side) vision, whereas cones are more active in central (straight-ahead) vision. In the posterior central part of the retina, the nerve fibers of retinal cells join to form the **optic nerve.** The function of this nerve is to connect the retina with the visual center of the brain, located within the occipital lobe that extends above and behind the cerebellum. It is this portion of the brain that interprets incoming visual stimuli.

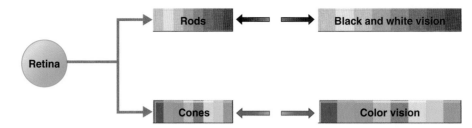

FIGURE 57-5   Function of rods and cones in relation to color vision.

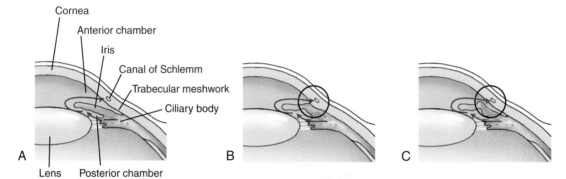

FIGURE 57-6   Main structures of the eye and an enlargement of the canal of Schlemm showing the flow of aqueous humor. **A,** Flow in a normal eye. **B,** In angle-closure glaucoma, the closure of the anterior angle due to contact between the iris and the trabecular meshwork prevents aqueous humor from exiting through the canal of Schlemm, which leads to increased intraocular pressure. **C,** In open-angle glaucoma, the anterior angle remains open, but the canal of Schlemm is obstructed by tissue abnormalities. (Modified from McKenry LM, Tessier E, Hogan MA: *Mosby's pharmacology in nursing,* ed 22, St Louis, 2006, Mosby.)

Pharmacology Overview

Medications used to treat disorders of the eye can be divided into several major drug groups: antiglaucoma drugs, antimicrobials, antiinflammatory drugs, topical anesthetics, diagnostic drugs, antiallergic drugs, and lubricants and moisturizers. There are also a variety of combination drug products that include two or more medications from different subclasses. These products are not discussed further in this chapter because of space limitations due to the large number of other drug classes and products that are described in detail. However, the reader can assume the same therapeutic indications and drug effects for these combination products as for the single-ingredient drug products corresponding to their individual components. The focus of this chapter is on commonly used therapeutic medications. A multitude of various products are also available for use in the care of contact lenses, including contact lens–cleaning enzymes, irrigating solutions, and eye washes. Again, because of space limitations, these products are not discussed further in this chapter. Their use is fairly straightforward, and they carry limited risk. More exotic surgical drugs are also beyond the scope of this chapter. The reader is advised to refer to the manufacturer's packaging information for details about any unfamiliar product encountered in clinical practice.

ANTIGLAUCOMA DRUGS

The aqueous humor is a nourishing liquid that is produced by the ciliary body and flows from the **posterior chamber** (behind the iris) to the anterior chamber (in front of the iris). The aqueous humor is removed via the canal of Schlemm, which is located adjacent to the union of the sclera and cornea in the anterior chamber. When the normal flow and drainage of aqueous humor is inhibited, intraocular pressure can be raised to dangerous levels. This creates a serious ocular condition called **glaucoma.** The two major types of glaucoma for purposes of this chapter are **angle-closure glaucoma** and **open-angle glaucoma.** Figure 57-6 shows the pathophysiology of each and provides an enlarged view of the involved eye structures. Table 57-1 lists additional characteristic features of each type. Glaucoma can be a *primary* illness (occurring on its own) or can be *secondary* to another eye condition or injury (e.g., posttraumatic glaucoma). Congenital glaucoma can also occur in infants. The visual and optic nerve changes typical of glaucoma can also occur in the absence of increased intraocular pressure (normotensive glaucoma). There are a few other more exotic forms of glaucoma (e.g., pigmentary glaucoma, pseudoexfoliative glaucoma) that are also beyond the scope of this chapter.

In summary, glaucoma is an eye disorder usually associated with excessive intraocular pressure caused by abnormally elevated levels of aqueous humor. This occurs when the aqueous humor is not drained through the canal of Schlemm as quickly as it is formed by the ciliary body. The accumulated aqueous humor creates a backward pressure that pushes the vitreous humor against the retina. Continued pressure on the retina destroys its neurons, which leads to impaired vision and eventual blindness (Figure 57-7). Unfortunately, glaucoma is often without early symptoms, and therefore many people are not diagnosed until some permanent sight loss has occurred.

TABLE 57-1 Glaucoma: Types and Characteristics

	Angle-Closure Glaucoma	Open-Angle Glaucoma
Synonyms	Closed-angle glaucoma, narrow-angle glaucoma, congestive glaucoma, pupillary closure glaucoma	Chronic glaucoma, wide-angle glaucoma, simple glaucoma
Chronicity	Acute (can cause rapid vision loss)	Chronic
Relative incidence	Less common	More common
Nature of angle	Narrow	Larger
Most common age of onset and race	Older than 30 yr, white	30 yr or older, African American
Major symptoms	Blurred vision, severe headaches, eye pain	Blurred vision, occasional headaches
Treatment	Topical or systemic drugs, surgery	Topical or systemic drugs, surgery

TABLE 57-2 Antiglaucoma Drugs: Effects on Aqueous Humor

Drug Class	Increased Drainage	Decreased Production	Color-Coded Eyedropper
Miotics			
Direct-acting cholinergics	+++	0	Green
Indirect-acting cholinergics (cholinesterase inhibitors)	+++	0	Green
Mydriatics			
Sympathomimetics	++	+++	Purple
Others			
Beta-blockers	+	+++	Yellow, blue
Carbonic anhydrase inhibitors	0	+++	Orange
Osmotic diuretics	+++	0	
Prostaglandin agonists	+++	0	Clear, teal

0, No effect; +, minor effect; ++, moderate effect; +++, pronounced effect.

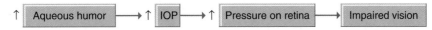

FIGURE 57-7 How increased aqueous humor can result in impaired vision. *IOP,* Intraocular pressure.

Effective treatment of glaucoma involves reducing intraocular pressure by either increasing the drainage of aqueous humor or decreasing its production. Some drugs may do both. Effective drug therapy can delay and possibly even prevent the development of glaucoma. Glaucoma eyedrops are color coded according to medication class to aid the patient in identification, and they are listed in Table 57-2. Drug classes used to reduce intraocular pressure include the following:

- Direct-acting cholinergics (also called *miotics* and *parasympathomimetic drugs*)
- Indirect-acting cholinergics (also called *miotics, cholinesterase inhibitors,* and *parasympathomimetic drugs*)
- Adrenergics (also called *mydriatics* and *sympathomimetic drugs*)
- Antiadrenergics (beta-blockers; also called *sympatholytic drugs*)
- Carbonic anhydrase inhibitors
- Osmotic diuretics
- Prostaglandin agonists

See Table 57-2 for a comparison of the effects of these drugs on aqueous humor flow.

CHOLINERGIC DRUGS

There are two categories of ocular parasympathetic drugs, more concisely referred to as *cholinergic* drugs: direct acting and indirect acting. Directing-acting cholinergics include acetylcholine, carbachol, and pilocarpine. Indirect-acting drugs, which are also called *cholinesterase inhibitors,* include echothiophate, currently the only available drug in this class. Because one primary drug effect of these drugs is pupillary constriction, or *miosis* (see later), they are also commonly called *miotics.*

Mechanism of Action and Drug Effects

As discussed in Chapters 20 and 21, *acetylcholine* is the endogenous neurochemical mediator of nerve impulses in the *parasympathetic nervous system.* It stimulates parasympathetic or *cholinergic* receptors located in the brain and throughout the body along parasympathetic nerve branches. This results in several effects on the eye: miosis (pupillary constriction), vasodilation of blood vessels in and around the eye, contraction of ciliary muscles, drainage of aqueous humor, and reduced intraocular pressure. Ciliary muscle contraction promotes aqueous humor drainage by widening the space where the drainage occurs. Miosis promotes aqueous humor drainage by causing the iris to stretch, which also serves to widen this space. The action of acetylcholine is normally short lived. It is rapidly hydrolyzed to *choline* and *acetic acid* by two *cholinesterase* enzymes known as *acetylcholinesterase* and *pseudocholinesterase* (Figure 57-8).

Both direct- and indirect-acting miotics have effects similar to those of acetylcholine, but their actions are more prolonged (Figure 57-9). The direct-acting miotics are able to directly stimulate ocular cholinergic receptors and actually mimic acetylcholine. Indirect-acting miotics work by binding to and inactivating the cholinesterases (*acetylcholinesterase* and *pseudocholinesterase*), the enzymes that break down acetylcholine by *hydrolysis,* as noted earlier. As a result, acetylcholine accumulates and acts longer at the cholinergic receptor sites. This leads to drug effects that include miosis, ciliary muscle contraction, enhanced aqueous humor drainage, and reduced intraocular pressure by an average of 20% to 30% (Figure 57-10). Drug-induced miotic effects may be less pronounced in individuals with dark eyes (e.g., brown or hazel) than in those with lighter eyes (e.g., blue). This is because the pigment of the iris also absorbs the drug (which reduces its therapeutic effects), and dark eyes have more pigment.

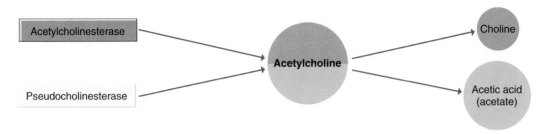

FIGURE 57-8   Metabolism of acetylcholine by endogenous enzymes.

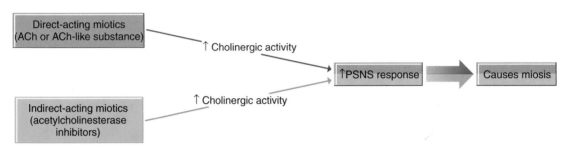

FIGURE 57-9   Cholinergic response of miosis to parasympathomimetic drugs. *ACh,* Acetylcholine; *PSNS,* parasympathetic nervous system.

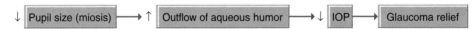

FIGURE 57-10   Therapeutic effects of direct- and indirect-acting miotics on glaucoma. *IOP,* Intraocular pressure.

Indications

The direct- and indirect-acting miotics are used for treatment of open-angle glaucoma, angle-closure glaucoma, and convergent strabismus (a condition in which one eye points toward the other, or "cross-eye") and in ocular surgery. They are also used to reverse the effect of mydriatic (pupil-dilating) drugs after ophthalmic examination. Specific indications may vary for different drugs, as shown in Table 57-3.

Contraindications

Contraindications to the use of miotics include known drug allergy and any serious active eye disorder in which induction of miosis might be harmful. An ophthalmologist will usually make this judgment.

Adverse Effects

Most of the adverse effects associated with the use of cholinergic and anticholinesterase drugs (miotics) are local and limited to the eye. This is an advantage of ocular drug administration. Adverse effects are more likely with indirect-acting miotics because they have longer-lasting effects (it takes time for the ocular tissues to synthesize new cholinesterase enzymes). Effects include blurred vision, drug-induced *myopia* (nearsightedness), and accommodative spasms. Such effects are secondary to contraction of the ciliary muscle, which results in spasm (paralysis) of visual accommodation by the lens. Miotic drugs also cause vasodilation of blood vessels supplying the conjunctiva, iris, and ciliary body. This results in increased permeability of the blood-aqueous barrier, which may lead to vascular

TABLE 57-3 Miotics: Indications

Drug	Indications
acetylcholine	Need for complete and rapid miosis after cataract lens extraction, iridectomy
carbachol	Open-angle glaucoma
echothiophate	Accommodative esotropia, obstructive aqueous humor outflow, open- and angle-closure glaucoma after iridectomy
pilocarpine	Open-angle glaucoma, secondary glaucoma after iridectomy, reversal of cycloplegia

congestion and ocular inflammation. The *blood-aqueous barrier* is the anatomic barrier that normally prevents exchange of fluids between eye chambers and the bloodstream, comparable to the blood-brain barrier mentioned in Chapter 2. Other undesirable effects include temporary stinging upon drug instillation, reduced nighttime or low-light vision, conjunctivitis, *lacrimation* (tearing), twitching of the eyelids *(blepharospasm),* and eye or brow pain. Prolonged use can result in iris cysts, lens opacities, and, rarely, retinal detachment.

Systemic effects are uncommon but are more likely to occur with cholinesterase inhibitors (indirect-acting miotics). When they do occur, they are due to generalized cholinergic stimulation. Sufficient drug must be absorbed into the general circulation for systemic effects to appear. Possible systemic effects are listed in Table 57-4.

TABLE 57-4 Miotics: Adverse Effects

Body System	Adverse Effects
Cardiovascular	Hypotension, bradycardia, tachycardia
Central nervous	Headache
Genitourinary	Urinary incontinence
Gastrointestinal	Salivation, nausea, vomiting, cramps, diarrhea
Respiratory	Bronchoconstriction, including asthma attacks
Dermatologic	Sweating

Toxicity and Management of Overdose

Occasionally, toxicity may develop after the use of topically applied miotic drugs. Toxic effects are an extension of the drugs' systemic effects and are more common with prolonged use of high doses. The most severe and prolonged effects are seen with long-acting anticholinesterases. Excessive parasympathetic nervous system effects are treated with intravenous or intramuscular atropine. Epinephrine may be used for bronchoconstriction or bradycardia.

Interactions

Drug interactions are unlikely because of primarily local actions of these drugs. When miotic drugs are given with topical adrenergics, antiadrenergics (e.g., beta-blockers), or carbonic anhydrase inhibitors, additive lowering effects on intraocular pressure can be seen. Systemic cholinergic drugs can theoretically have additive cholinergic effects when given with miotics. Indirect-acting miotics (cholinesterase inhibitors) may also potentiate the effects of the neuromuscular blocker succinylcholine (see Chapter 12), possibly even leading to cardiorespiratory arrest.

Dosages

For recommended dosages of selected miotic drugs, see the Dosages table below.

DRUG PROFILES

Direct-acting ocular cholinergics include acetylcholine (Miochol-E), carbachol (Carboptic), and pilocarpine (Pilocar). Indirect-acting drugs, which are also called *cholinesterase inhibitors,* include echothiophate (Phospholine Iodide). These drugs are used for management of glaucoma, as adjuncts for ocular surgery, and for treatment of various other ophthalmic conditions.

DIRECT-ACTING MIOTICS
acetylcholine

Acetylcholine (Miochol-E) is a direct-acting parasympathomimetic drug that is used to produce miosis during ophthalmic surgery. It is a pharmaceutical form of the naturally occurring neurotransmitter in the body. It has very quick onset and may begin to work almost immediately. It is administered directly into the anterior chamber of the eye before and after securing one or more sutures.

PHARMACOKINETICS

Route	Onset of Action	Peak Plasma Concentration	Elimination Half-life	Duration of Action
Ocular	Instant	Instant	3 min	10 min

◆ pilocarpine

Pilocarpine (Pilocar) is a direct-acting parasympathomimetic drug that is used as a miotic in the treatment of glaucoma. Pilocarpine is available in many different strengths as an ocular gel and solution. One special formulation is the pilocarpine ocular insert system (Ocusert Pilo-20), which is applied once weekly by the patient.

PHARMACOKINETICS (IMMEDIATE-RELEASE FORMULATION)

Route	Onset of Action	Peak Plasma Concentration	Elimination Half-life	Duration of Action
Ocular	10-30 min	75 min	Unknown	4-8 hr

INDIRECT-ACTING MIOTIC
◆ echothiophate

Echothiophate (Phospholine Iodide) is an indirect-acting parasympathomimetic that has an organophosphate structure and acts by phosphorylating cholinesterase enzymes. This effect is normally irreversible until new enzymes are synthesized by the body, which may take days or even weeks. For these reasons, this drug is considered to be long acting.

PHARMACOKINETICS

Route	Onset of Action	Peak Plasma Concentration	Elimination Half-life	Duration of Action
Ocular	10-30 min	24 hr	Long	7-28 days

SYMPATHOMIMETICS

Sympathomimetic drugs are used for the treatment of glaucoma and ocular hypertension. These drugs include the alpha receptor agonists brimonidine (Alphagan P) and apraclonidine (Iopidine), as well as the alpha and beta receptor agonists epinephryl (Epinal) and dipivefrin (Propine).

DOSAGES

Selected Miotics

Drug (Pregnancy Category)	Pharmacologic Class	Usual Dosage Range	Indications
acetylcholine (Miochol-E) (C)	Direct acting cholinergic	0.5 to 2 mL preoperatively	Need for surgical miosis
◆ echothiophate (Phospholine Iodide) (C)	Indirect acting cholinergic	1 drop 1-2 times daily	Early and advanced chronic open-angle glaucoma; glaucoma secondary to cataract surgery; accommodative esotropia
◆ pilocarpine (Pilocar, Isopto Carpine, Akarpine, Pilopine HS) (C)	Direct acting cholinergic	Solution: 1-2 drops 3-4 times daily Gel: 0.5 inch into lower conjunctival sac at bedtime (use any other eyedrops at least 5 min before gel)	Chronic open-angle and angle-closure glaucoma; acute angle-closure glaucoma; preoperative and postoperative intraocular hypertension; need for reversal of drug-induced mydriasis

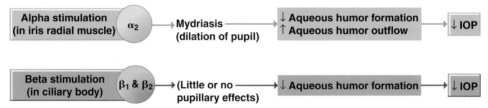

FIGURE 57-11   Mechanism of mydriasis.

FIGURE 57-12   Ocular effects of alpha (α) and beta (β) stimulation. *IOP,* Intraocular pressure.

Mechanism of Action and Drug Effects

Sympathomimetic drugs mimic the sympathetic neurotransmitters norepinephrine and epinephrine and stimulate the dilator muscle to contract by means of alpha and/or beta receptor interaction. This stimulation results in increased pupil size or *mydriasis* (Figure 57-11). Dilation is seen within minutes of instillation of the ophthalmic drops and lasts for several hours, during which time the intraocular pressure is reduced (Figure 57-12). The exact mechanism of action is unknown. However, alpha receptor stimulation is known to reduce intraocular pressure by enhancing aqueous humor outflow through the canal of Schlemm. Production of aqueous humor by the ciliary body may also be reduced as another drug effect. Both of these effects appear to be dose dependent.

Indications

Both epinephrine and dipivefrin may be used to reduce elevated intraocular pressure in the treatment of chronic open-angle glaucoma, either as initial therapy or as long-term therapy. Increases in intraocular pressure during ophthalmic surgery are usually mediated via increased catecholamine stimulation of the sympathetic nervous system. Apraclonidine stimulates primarily the alpha$_2$ receptors, which oppose these effects, and thus corrects the surgery-induced elevation in intraocular pressure. Brimonidine also has primarily alpha$_2$ activity but is used to lower intraocular pressure in patients with open-angle glaucoma or ocular hypertension.

Contraindications

Contraindications for the sympathomimetic ophthalmics include drug allergy and may include the presence of active, severe ophthalmic problems that, in the judgment of an ophthalmologist, might be aggravated by the effects of these drugs.

Adverse Effects

The adverse effects of the sympathomimetic mydriatics are primarily limited to ocular effects and include burning, eye pain, and lacrimation. Such effects are usually temporary and may subside as the patient grows accustomed to the medication. Other ocular effects may include conjunctival hyperemia, localized melanin deposits in the conjunctiva, and release of pigment granules from the iris. Although systemic effects associated with the use of sympathomimetic mydriatics are uncommon, they are

theoretically possible, especially with the use of larger doses or prolonged drug therapy. They include cardiovascular effects such as extrasystoles, tachycardia, and hypertension. Other effects that may be noticed are headache and faintness.

Toxicity and Management of Overdose

Rare toxic reactions are primarily the result of an extension of the therapeutic and adverse effects of these drugs. The most significant are cardiac dysrhythmias. Discontinuation of the drugs usually alleviates the toxic symptoms.

Interactions

With sufficient topical absorption, sympathomimetic mydriatics have the potential to react with other drugs. Cardiac dysrhythmias are potentiated when mydriatic drugs are given with halogenated anesthetics, cardiac glycosides, thyroid hormones, or tricyclic antidepressants.

Dosages

For recommended dosages of sympathomimetic drugs, see the Dosages table on p. 885.

DRUG PROFILES

Sympathomimetic ophthalmic drugs include dipivefrin (Propine), epinephryl (Epinal), apraclonidine (Iopidine), and brimonidine (Alphagan P). These drugs are used for management of glaucoma and ocular hypertension, and for ocular surgery.

apraclonidine

Apraclonidine (Iopidine) is structurally and pharmacologically related to the alpha$_2$ stimulant clonidine. It reduces intraocular pressure 23% to 39% by stimulating alpha$_2$ and beta$_2$ receptors. It also prevents ocular vasoconstriction, which reduces ocular blood pressure as well as aqueous humor formation. Apraclonidine is primarily used to inhibit perioperative intraocular pressure increases, rather than to treat glaucoma. Brimonidine (Alphagan P) is a similar drug but is used primarily for glaucoma.

PHARMACOKINETICS

Route	Onset of Action	Peak Plasma Concentration	Elimination Half-life	Duration of Action
Ocular	1 hr	3-5 hr	8 hr	12 hr

DOSAGES

Selected Ocular Sympathomimetics

Drug (Pregnancy Category)	Pharmacologic Class	Usual Dosage Range	Indications/Uses
apraclonidine (Iopidine) (C)	Direct acting	0.5% solution: 1-2 drops 3 times daily	Short-term adjunctive therapy for glaucoma not controlled by other drugs
◆ dipivefrin (Propine) (C)	Direct acting	1 drop q12h	Chronic open-angle glaucoma

◆ dipivefrin

Dipivefrin (Propine) is a synthetic sympathomimetic miotic drug. It is a prodrug of epinephrine. The prodrug has little or no pharmacologic activity until hydrolyzed in the eye to two chemically modified forms of epinephrine. These chemical alterations account for the main advantage of this drug over epinephrine: it has enhanced lipophilicity (fat solubility) and can better penetrate into the tissues of the anterior chamber of the eye. This quality also reduces the likelihood of any systemic adverse effects. Dipivefrin typically reduces mean intraocular pressure approximately 15% to 25%. On a weight basis, dipivefrin is 4 to 11 times as potent as epinephrine in reducing intraocular pressure and 5 to 12 times as potent as epinephrine in terms of its mydriatic effects. Epinephryl (Epinal) is a newer drug with similar properties and uses.

PHARMACOKINETICS

Route	Onset of Action	Peak Plasma Concentration	Elimination Half-life	Duration of Action
Ocular	30 min	1 hr	1-3 hr	12 hr

BETA-ADRENERGIC BLOCKERS

The antiglaucoma beta-adrenergic blockers that reduce intraocular pressure include the beta$_1$-selective drugs betaxolol and levobetaxolol. Recall from Chapter 19 that beta$_1$-selective beta-blockers are also called *cardioselective*. Nonselective ocular beta$_1$- and beta$_2$-blockers include carteolol, levobunolol, metipranolol, and timolol.

Mechanism of Action and Drug Effects

The ophthalmic beta-blockers reduce both elevated and normal intraocular pressure. They do this without affecting pupillary size, accommodation, or night vision. They appear to reduce intraocular pressure by reducing aqueous humor formation. In addition, timolol may produce a minimal increase in aqueous outflow.

Indications

Ophthalmic beta-blockers are used to reduce elevated intraocular pressure in various conditions, including chronic open-angle glaucoma and ocular hypertension. They may also be used alone or in combination with a topical miotic (e.g., echothiophate iodide, pilocarpine), topical dipivefrin, and/or systemic carbonic anhydrase inhibitors. When used in combination, these drugs may have an additive intraocular pressure-lowering effect. They may also be used to treat some forms of angle-closure glaucoma.

Contraindications

Contraindications for ophthalmic beta-blockers include known drug allergy and any ocular condition for which beta-receptor blockade might be harmful.

Adverse Effects

The adverse effects of antiglaucoma beta-blockers are primarily limited to ocular effects and limited systemic effects. The most common ocular effects are transient burning and discomfort. Other effects include blurred vision, pain, photophobia, lacrimation, blepharitis, keratitis (inflammation of the cornea), and decreased corneal sensitivity. Because these drugs are administered topically, few, if any, systemic effects are expected. Theoretical systemic effects include bradycardia, bronchospasm, headache, and dizziness as described for systemic beta-blockers in Chapter 19. However, ocular beta-blockers have not been shown to affect glucose metabolism.

Toxicity and Management of Overdose

Toxic reactions to beta-blockers are rare and primarily involve the cardiovascular system. Symptoms include bradycardia, cardiac failure, hypotension, and bronchospasms. Treatment involves discontinuation of the drug and supportive care (e.g., administration of adrenergic and anticholinergic drugs).

Interactions

Drug interactions with systemic drugs are unlikely due to the primarily localized nature of ophthalmically administered drugs. Theoretically, ophthalmic beta-blockers can have additive therapeutic and/or adverse effects when given with systemically administered beta-blockers or other cardiovascular drugs (e.g., calcium channel blockers), up to and including cardiorespiratory arrest.

Dosages

For recommended dosages of beta-adrenergic blockers, see the Dosages table on p. 886.

DRUG PROFILES

The currently available ophthalmic beta-blocking drugs are betaxolol (Betoptic), carteolol (Ocupress), levobunolol (Betagan), levobetaxolol (Betaxon), metipranolol (OptiPranolol), and timolol (Timoptic). These drugs are used to treat glaucoma and ocular hypertension.

DOSAGES

Selected Ocular Beta-Blockers

Drug (Pregnancy Category)	Pharmacologic Class	Usual Dosage Range	Indications
◆ betaxolol (Betoptic, Betoptic S) (C)	Direct acting	1-2 drops twice daily	Chronic open-angle glaucoma; ocular hypertension
◆ timolol (Betimol, Timoptic, Timoptic-XE) (C)	Direct acting	Solution: 1 drop twice daily Gel-forming solution: 1 drop daily	Open-angle glaucoma; ocular hypertension

◆ betaxolol

Betaxolol (Betoptic) is a beta$_1$-selective beta-blocker. It is structurally related to the systemic beta receptor blocker metoprolol that is used primarily to treat cardiovascular disorders. Betaxolol is one of the most potent and selective beta-blocking drugs. Its ability to decrease aqueous humor formation and consequently intraocular pressure has made it an excellent drug for the treatment of ocular disorders such as open-angle glaucoma and ocular hypertension.

PHARMACOKINETICS

Route	Onset of Action	Peak Plasma Concentration	Elimination Half-life	Duration of Action
Ocular	0.5-1 hr	2 hr	Unknown	More than 12 hr

◆ timolol

Timolol (Timoptic) may differ slightly from the other ophthalmic beta-blockers in that it may increase the outflow of aqueous humor as well as decrease its formation. The drug acts at both beta$_1$ and beta$_2$ receptors and is indicated for the treatment of open-angle glaucoma and ocular hypertension. It is available in various liquid forms, both with and without preservatives. Preservative-free products were developed because of patient allergies to benzalkonium chloride, a commonly used preservative. Timolol is also available in a gel-forming solution (with preservatives). The gel-forming products are longer acting and allow for once-daily dosing, a convenience over the twice-daily dosing that many patients require of the other timolol formulations.

PHARMACOKINETICS

Route	Onset of Action	Peak Plasma Concentration	Elimination Half-life	Duration of Action
Ocular	15-30 min	1-2 hr	Unknown	12-24 hr

CARBONIC ANHYDRASE INHIBITORS

Ophthalmic carbonic anhydrase inhibitors include brinzolamide and dorzolamide. Both drugs are also sulfonamides and are therefore chemically related to the sulfonamide antibiotics (see Chapter 38). These two drugs are available only in topical ophthalmic form. Systemic carbonic anhydrase inhibitors for oral use are described in Chapter 26 on diuretics and are sometimes also used as adjunct drug therapy for glaucoma.

Mechanism of Action and Drug Effects

These drugs work by inhibiting the enzyme *carbonic anhydrase*, which exists throughout the body and is involved in acid-base balance. In the eye, however, the inhibition of this enzyme results in

TABLE 57-5 Carbonic Anhydrase Inhibitors: Adverse Effects

Body System	Adverse Effects
Central nervous	Drowsiness, confusion, paresthesias, seizures
Eyes, ears, nose, throat	Transient myopia, tinnitus
Gastrointestinal	Anorexia, vomiting, diarrhea, liver failure
Genitourinary	Polyuria, hematuria
Integumentary	Urticaria, rarely photosensitivity, severe skin reactions (e.g., Stevens-Johnson syndrome)
Hematologic	Blood dyscrasias
Metabolic	Acidotic states and electrolyte imbalance with long-term therapy

decreased intraocular pressure by reduction of aqueous humor formation.

Indications

Ocular carbonic anhydrase inhibitors are used primarily for management of glaucoma, including both open-angle and angle-closure glaucoma; they may also be used preoperatively to control intraocular pressure.

Contraindications

Contraindications include known drug allergy and any ocular condition for which their use might be harmful in the judgment of an ophthalmologist.

Adverse Effects

Systemic absorption of these drugs occurs, and although systemic adverse effects are unlikely, the same adverse effects listed for sulfonamide antibiotics in Chapter 38 can theoretically occur with these drugs. Patients with sulfa allergies may develop cross-sensitivities to the carbonic anhydrase inhibitors. Specific adverse effects are listed in Table 57-5.

Toxicity and Management of Overdose

Toxicity associated with the use of carbonic anhydrase inhibitors is rare. Their use may predispose the patient to possible acidotic states and electrolyte imbalances. These toxic reactions generally require only supportive care. This may include the repletion of electrolytes, especially potassium, and the administration of bicarbonate to correct any acidotic state.

DOSAGES

Ocular Carbonic Anhydrase Inhibitor

Drug (Pregnancy Category)	Pharmacologic Class	Usual Dosage Range	Indications
◆ dorzolamide (Trusopt) (C)	Carbonic anhydrase inhibitor	1 drop 3 times daily	Open-angle glaucoma; ocular hypertension

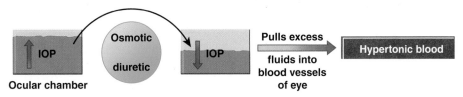

FIGURE 57-13 Mechanism and ocular effects of osmotic diuretics. *IOP,* Intraocular pressure.

Interactions

The systemic use of carbonic anhydrase inhibitors can result in several significant drug interactions, and the ocular carbonic anhydrase inhibitors have a theoretical (but less likely) potential for these interactions. These drugs can cause hypokalemia and increase the likelihood of digitalis toxicity. Hypokalemia is also more likely to occur when these drugs are coadministered with corticosteroids and diuretics. They increase renal excretion of lithium, which reduces its therapeutic effects, and also tend to increase the drug effects of basic drugs as a result of decreased renal excretion.

Dosages

For recommended dosages of the carbonic anhydrase inhibitor dorzolamide, see the Dosages table above.

DRUG PROFILE

There are currently two ocular carbonic anhydrase inhibitors: brinzolamide (Azopt) and dorzolamide (Trusopt).

◆ dorzolamide
Dorzolamide (Trusopt) is solely indicated for treatment of elevated intraocular pressure associated with either ocular hypertension or open-angle glaucoma. It is available only as an ophthalmic solution. The other drug in this class, brinzolamide, has comparable indications, dosages, and pharmacokinetics.

PHARMACOKINETICS

Route	Onset of Action	Peak Plasma Concentration	Elimination Half-life	Duration of Action
Ocular	Rapid	Variable	3-4 mo	Variable

OSMOTIC DIURETICS

Osmotic drugs may be administered either intravenously, orally, or topically to reduce intraocular pressure. The osmotic diuretics that are most commonly used for this purpose are glycerin and mannitol. Isosorbide and urea are two other less commonly used osmotic diuretics.

Mechanism of Action and Drug Effects

The osmotic diuretics reduce ocular hypertension by causing the blood to become hypertonic in relation to both intraocular and spinal fluids. This creates an osmotic gradient that draws water from the aqueous and vitreous humors into the bloodstream, which causes a reduction in the volume of intraocular fluid; the result is a decrease in intraocular pressure (Figure 57-13). Systemic (nonocular) effects of these drugs are discussed in Chapter 26.

Indications

Ocular uses for osmotic diuretics include treatment of acute glaucoma episodes and reduction of intraocular pressure before or after ocular surgery. Typically, glycerin is used first; if the treatment is unsuccessful, mannitol is tried. Isosorbide and urea are two other osmotic drugs that may also be used in similar situations. They are usually administered after glycerin or mannitol has failed. Isosorbide may be especially beneficial for diabetic patients because it is not metabolized into sugar calories, unlike glycerin, which can cause hyperglycemia.

Contraindications

Osmotic diuretics are contraindicated in patients with known drug allergy, pronounced anuria, acute pulmonary edema, cardiac decompensation, and severe dehydration, because they can worsen all of these conditions.

Adverse Effects

The most frequent reactions to osmotic diuretic drugs are nausea, vomiting, and headache. The most significant adverse effects are fluid and electrolyte imbalance. Other effects are possible irritation and thrombosis at the injection site. A variety of other potential adverse effects are listed in Table 57-6.

Interactions

Increased lithium excretion caused by both mannitol and urea are the only significant drug interactions that have been reported.

Toxicity and Management of Overdose

Toxic reactions are primarily a result of the hyperosmolarity of the blood. The most significant toxic reactions are hypovolemia (secondary to diuresis), cardiac dysrhythmias, and hyperosmo-

TABLE 57-6 Osmotic Diuretics: Adverse Effects

Body System	Adverse Effects
Cardiovascular	Edema, thrombophlebitis, hypotension, hypertension, tachycardia, angina-like chest pains, fever, chills
Central nervous	Dizziness, headache, convulsions, rebound increased intracranial pressure, confusion
Electrolytes	Fluid electrolyte imbalances, acidosis, dehydration
Eyes, ears, nose, throat	Loss of hearing, blurred vision, nasal congestion
Gastrointestinal	Nausea, vomiting, dry mouth, diarrhea
Genitourinary	Marked diuresis, urinary retention, thirst

lar nonketotic coma. Treatment involves discontinuation of the drug and management of presenting symptoms with fluids and electrolytes.

Dosages

For recommended dosages of osmotic drugs, see the Dosages table below.

DRUG PROFILES

Osmotic diuretics include mannitol (Osmitrol), glycerin (Osmoglyn), urea (Ureaphil), and isosorbide (Ismotic). These drugs are normally reserved for acute reduction of intraocular pressure during glaucoma crises and perioperative reduction of intraocular pressure in ophthalmic surgery.

glycerin
Glycerin (Osmoglyn) is an osmotic drug given orally to lower intraocular pressure or topically to reduce superficial corneal edema. Another common use is before iridectomy in individuals with acute narrow-angle glaucoma. It is also used preoperatively and/or postoperatively in procedures such as treatment of congenital glaucoma, repair of retinal detachment, cataract extraction, and keratoplasty (corneal transplant). It may also be used in management of some secondary glaucomas.

PHARMACOKINETICS

Route	Onset of Action	Peak Plasma Concentration	Elimination Half-life	Duration of Action
Ocular	10-30 min	1-1.5 hr	30-45 min	4-5 hr

mannitol
Mannitol (Osmitrol) is administered only by intravenous infusion to reduce elevated intraocular pressure when the pressure cannot be lowered by other methods. Mannitol has been shown to be effective in treating acute episodes of angle-closure, absolute, or secondary glaucoma and in lowering intraocular pressure before intraocular surgery. Mannitol does not penetrate the eye and may be used when irritation is present, unlike some of the other osmotic drugs, such as urea.

PHARMACOKINETICS

Route	Onset of Action	Peak Plasma Concentration	Elimination Half-life	Duration of Action
IV	30-60 min	1 hr	15-100 min	6-8 hr

PROSTAGLANDIN AGONISTS

Latanoprost (Xalatan) is the most popular of three drugs in this newer class of ophthalmic drugs used to treat glaucoma—the prostaglandin agonists. The other two drugs are travoprost (Travatan) and bimatoprost (Lumigan).

Mechanism of Action and Drug Effects

Prostaglandins reduce intraocular pressure primarily by increasing the outflow of aqueous fluid, not by reducing its production. They are believed to accomplish this by increasing the outflow of aqueous humor between the uvea and sclera as well as via the usual exit through the trabecular meshwork, a filterlike structure within the eye (see Figure 57-6). A single dose of prostaglandin agonist lowers intraocular pressure for 20 to 24 hours, which allows a single daily dosing regimen. The drug effects are primarily limited to these ocular effects.

Indications

Prostaglandin agonists are used in the treatment of glaucoma.

Contraindications

The only usual contraindication is known drug allergy.

Adverse Effects

Prostaglandin agonists are generally well tolerated. Adverse effects reported in clinical trials included foreign body sensation, punctate epithelial keratopathy (dotted appearance of the cornea), stinging, conjunctival hyperemia ("bloodshot" eyes), blurred vision, itching, and burning. Systemic effects occur in a small percentage of patients and include skin reactions, upper respiratory tract infections, and headache. There is one unique

DOSAGES

Osmotic Diuretics

Drug (Pregnancy Category)	Pharmacologic Class	Usual Dosage Range	Indications/Uses
glycerin (Ophthalgan) (C)	Organic alcohol	1-2 drops before eye exam as lubricant, more if needed during exam	Gonioscopy of edematous cornea
mannitol (Osmitrol) (C)	Organic alcohol	IV: 1.5-2 g/kg infused over at least 30 min; for preoperative use give 1-1.5 hr before surgery	Acute reduction of elevated intraocular pressure

IV, Intravenous.

DOSAGES

Ocular Prostaglandin Agonist

Drug (Pregnancy Category)	Pharmacologic Class	Usual Dosage Range	Indications
◆ latanoprost (Xalatan) (C)	Prostaglandin	1 drop every day in evening	Open-angle glaucoma and ocular hypertension in patients who are intolerant of or whose conditions is uncontrolled by other drugs

adverse effect associated with all prostaglandin agonists: in some people with hazel, green, or bluish brown eye color, eye color will turn permanently brown, even if the medication is discontinued. This adverse effect appears to be cosmetic only with no known ill effects on the eye.

Interactions

Concurrent administration of prostaglandin agonists with any other eyedrops containing the preservative thimerosal may result in precipitation. It is recommended that the two medications be administered at least 5 minutes apart.

Dosages

For recommended dosages of the prostaglandin agonist latanoprost, see the Dosages table above.

DRUG PROFILE

◆ latanoprost

About 3% to 10% of patients treated with latanoprost (Xalatan) have shown increased iris pigmentation after 3 to 4½ months of treatment. Latanoprost is a prodrug of a naturally occurring prostaglandin known as prostaglandin F_2-alpha. When this ester prodrug is administered, it is converted by hydrolysis (with water from ocular fluids) to the prostaglandin F_2-alpha, which in turn reduces intraocular pressure. Latanoprost is available only in eyedrop form.

PHARMACOKINETICS

Route	Onset of Action	Peak Plasma Concentration	Elimination Half-life	Duration of Action
Ocular	30-60 min	2 hr	17 min	24 hr

ANTIMICROBIAL DRUGS

Topical antimicrobials used to treat ocular infections include antibacterial, antifungal, and antiviral drugs. All require a prescription. Many of these drugs are also available for systemic administration for treatment of infections elsewhere in the body. A variety of infections can occur in the eye; many are self-limiting and rarely result in harm. However, some infections require the use of ocular antimicrobials to be eliminated. The most commonly used antimicrobials from the main antimicrobial drug classes are discussed in this chapter. Some common eye infections that may require antibiotic therapy are listed in Table 57-7. The choice of a particular ophthalmic antimicrobial drug should be based on the following:
- Clinical experience
- Sensitivity and characteristics of the organisms most likely to have caused the infection

TABLE 57-7 Common Ocular Infections

Infection	Description
Blepharitis	Inflammation of the eyelids.
Conjunctivitis	Inflammation of the conjunctiva (the mucous membrane lining the back of the eyelids and the front of the eye except the cornea). It may be bacterial or viral and is often associated with common colds. When caused by *Haemophilus* organisms, it is commonly called *pink eye*. It is highly contagious but usually self-limiting.
Hordeolum (sty)	Acute localized infection of the eyelash follicles and the glands of the anterior lid. It results in the formation of a small abscess or cyst.
Keratitis	Inflammation of the cornea caused by bacterial infection. Herpes simplex keratitis is caused by viral infection.
Uveitis	Infection of the uveal tract or the vascular layer of the eye, which includes the iris, ciliary body, and choroid.
Endophthalmitis	Inflammation of the inner eye structure caused by bacteria.

- Characteristics of the disease itself
- Sensitivity and response of the patient
- Laboratory results (cultures and sensitivity testing)

Mechanism of Action and Drug Effects

The drugs used to treat infections of the eye work in a variety of ways to destroy the invading organism. Their specific antimicrobial actions are similar to those described for systemically administered drugs. These are discussed in Chapters 38, 39, 40, and 42. The drug effects are focused on the microorganism invading the eye. Some antimicrobials destroy the causative organism, whereas others simply inhibit the organism's growth, allowing the body's immune system to fight the infection.

Indications

The indication for ocular antimicrobials is known or suspected infection with one or more specific microorganisms. Empirical treatment (without confirmation of the causative organism through culture and sensitivity testing) should be based on reasonable clinical evaluation of presenting signs and symptoms. Topical use of antimicrobials helps prevent the antimicrobial drug resistance that could arise from unnecessary systemic use. However, systemic antimicrobials may be administered to treat more severe ocular infections.

DOSAGES

Selected Ocular Antimicrobials

Drug (Pregnancy Category)	Pharmacologic Class	Usual Dosage Range	Indications
Antibacterial Drugs			
◆ bacitracin (AK-Tracin) (C)	Miscellaneous antibiotic	Solution: 1-2 drops q1-4h Ointment: 0.5-inch ribbon into lower conjunctival sac 3-4 times daily	
◆ ciprofloxacin (Ciloxan) (C)	Quinolone	Solution: 1-2 drops every 2 hr for 2 days, then 2 drops every 4 hr for 5 days Ointment: ½ inch tid for 2 days, then ½ inch daily for 5 days	Bacterial ocular infections
◆ erythromycin (Ilotycin) (C)	Macrolide	Ointment: ½ inch 2-6 times/day	
◆ gentamicin (Genoptic, others) (C)	Aminoglycoside	Solution: 1-2 drops every 2-4 hr Ointment: ½ inch 2-3 times/day	
◆ sulfacetamide (Bleph-10, others) (C)	Sulfonamide	Solution: 1-2 drops every 2-3 hr Ointment: Apply 1-4 times/day	
Antifungal Drug			
natamycin (Natacyn) (C)	Antifungal	1 drop into conjunctival sac q1-2h, then usually reduce after first 3-4 days to 6-8 drops/day; therapy usually continues for 14-21 days	Fungal ocular infections
Antiviral Drug			
trifluridine (Viroptic) (C)	Antiviral	Initially 1 drop q2h while awake (max 9 drops/day); may later decrease to 5 drops/day	Viral ocular infections: keratitis and keratoconjunctivitis due to HSV types 1 and 2

HSV, Herpes simplex virus.
Note: Dosages vary based on the type and severity of infection.

Contraindications

Contraindications to the use of antimicrobials include known drug allergy or other severe previous adverse drug reaction. Also, use of any drug class for the wrong type of infection (e.g., use of an antibacterial drug to treat a viral infection) may obviously worsen the infection and delay treatment. This situation should be avoided whenever possible, and the patient should be monitored for signs of progress or treatment failure.

Adverse Effects

The most common adverse effects of ocular antibiotics are local and transient inflammation, burning, stinging, urticaria, dermatitis, angioedema, and drug hypersensitivity. Other effects are listed in the profiles of the specific drugs. Topical application of antimicrobial drugs may also interfere with growth of the normal bacterial flora of the eye, which may encourage the growth of other, more harmful organisms.

Interactions

Systemic drug interactions are unlikely due to the primarily local effects of ocular antimicrobials. One possible interaction involves the concurrent use of corticosteroids (e.g., dexamethasone). Such drugs have immunosuppressive effects, which may impede the therapeutic effects of ocular antimicrobials, as is also the case with systemic antimicrobials.

Dosages

For recommended dosages of ocular antimicrobials, see the Dosages table above.

DRUG PROFILES

ANTIBACTERIAL DRUGS
AMINOGLYCOSIDES

Aminoglycosides (see Chapter 39) are potent antimicrobials that destroy bacteria by interfering with protein synthesis in bacterial cells by binding to ribosomal subunits, which eventually leads to bacteria death. Aminoglycosides used to treat ocular infections include gentamicin (Garamycin) and tobramycin (Tobrex). Adverse effects include swollen eyelids, mydriasis, and local erythema. Toxic reactions are rare because of poor topical absorption. Another possible toxic reaction is the overgrowth of nonsusceptible organisms, which can lead to eye infections that are resistant to treatment.

◆ gentamicin

Gentamicin (Garamycin) is effective against a wide variety of gram-negative and gram-positive organisms. It is particularly useful against *Pseudomonas, Proteus,* and *Klebsiella* organisms. Gram-positive organisms that are effectively destroyed by gentamicin include staphylococci and streptococci that have developed resistance to other antibiotics. Gentamicin is available as an ophthalmic ointment and a solution.

PHARMACOKINETICS

Route	Onset of Action	Peak Plasma Concentration	Elimination Half-life	Duration of Action
Ocular	Variable	Immediate	Unknown	6-12 hr

MACROLIDES

Macrolide antibiotics include erythromycin, azithromycin, and other drugs (see Chapter 38). Erythromycin is the most commonly used macrolide for ophthalmic use.

◆ erythromycin

Erythromycin (Ilotycin) is a macrolide antibiotic indicated for the treatment of various ophthalmic infections. It is available only as an ophthalmic ointment. In normal concentrations, it inhibits the growth of an organism but does not destroy it. Erythromycin relies on the body's defense mechanisms to destroy the bacteria; however, in high concentrations, it becomes **bactericidal.** It is indicated for the treatment of neonatal conjunctivitis caused by *Chlamydia trachomatis* and for the prevention of eye infections in newborns that may be caused by *Neisseria gonorrhoeae* or other susceptible organisms.

PHARMACOKINETICS

Route	Onset of Action	Peak Plasma Concentration	Elimination Half-life	Duration of Action
Ocular	Variable	Immediate	Unknown	Variable

POLYPEPTIDES

Bacitracin and polymyxin B are polypeptide antibiotics. These drugs are rarely used systemically because of their potent nephrotoxic effects. They are bactericidal antimicrobials that inhibit protein synthesis in susceptible organisms, which leads to cell death. They are most commonly used in the treatment of superficial infections caused by gram-positive bacteria.

◆ bacitracin

Bacitracin (AK-Tracin) is an ophthalmic antimicrobial drug used to treat various eye infections. It is available as a single-ingredient product and as a combination product with polymyxin or neomycin and polymyxin. These combinations were developed to make bacitracin a broader-spectrum antibiotic. Bacitracin is available in ointment form.

PHARMACOKINETICS

Route	Onset of Action	Peak Plasma Concentration	Elimination Half-life	Duration of Action
Ocular	Variable	Immediate	Unknown	Variable

QUINOLONES

Quinolone antibiotics are very effective broad-spectrum antibiotics. They are discussed in detail in Chapter 39. They are bactericidal, destroying a wide spectrum of organisms that are often very difficult to treat. Currently five ophthalmic quinolones are available: ciprofloxacin (Ciloxan), gatifloxacin (Zymar), moxifloxacin (Vigamox), levofloxacin (Quixin), and ofloxacin (Ocuflox).

Significant adverse effects include formation of corneal precipitates during treatment for bacterial keratitis. Other reactions include corneal staining and infiltrates. Toxic reactions are limited because of poor topical absorption. Those that occur are usually taste disorders and nausea. There are no significant drug interactions.

◆ ciprofloxacin

Ciprofloxacin (Ciloxan) is a synthetic quinolone antibiotic. It is available in ointment and solution form. Ciprofloxacin is indicated for the treatment of bacterial keratitis and conjunctivitis caused by susceptible gram-positive and gram-negative bacteria. One notable adverse reaction to ophthalmic ciprofloxacin has been the appearance on the corneal surface of a white, crystalline precipitate occurring within any corneal lesions for which the patient was being treated. This has occurred in approximately 17% of patients, and within 1 to 7 days of starting therapy. However, in all cases to date the condition has been self-limiting, has not required drug discontinuation, and has not adversely affected clinical outcome.

PHARMACOKINETICS

Route	Onset of Action	Peak Plasma Concentration	Elimination Half-life	Duration of Action
Ocular	Variable	Immediate	1-2 hr	Variable

SULFONAMIDES

Sulfonamides are synthetic **bacteriostatic** antibiotics that work by blocking the synthesis of folic acid in susceptible bacteria. Sulfacetamide sodium (Bleph-10) and sulfisoxazole (Gantrisin) are used to treat conjunctivitis and other ocular infections caused by susceptible bacteria.

The adverse effects are primarily limited to local reactions and include local irritation and stinging. Sulfonamide use can result in the overgrowth of nonsusceptible organisms. No significant topical toxic effects have been reported with the use of ophthalmic sulfonamides.

◆ sulfacetamide

Sulfacetamide (Bleph-10) is the most commonly used ophthalmic sulfonamide antibacterial drug. It is available in solution and ointment form.

PHARMACOKINETICS

Route	Onset of Action	Peak Plasma Concentration	Elimination Half-life	Duration of Action
Ocular	Variable	Immediate	Unknown	Variable

ANTIFUNGAL DRUG
natamycin

Natamycin (Natacyn) is a polyene antifungal drug and therefore is related to two other antifungal drugs, amphotericin B and nystatin (see Chapter 42). It destroys fungi in the eye by binding to sterols in the fungal cell membrane, which disrupts the protective capabilities of the cell and results in cell death. Natamycin is used topically in the treatment of blepharitis, conjunctivitis, and keratitis caused by susceptible fungi (*Candida* and *Aspergillus* species). It is available only in suspension form.

PHARMACOKINETICS

Route	Onset of Action	Peak Plasma Concentration	Elimination Half-life	Duration of Action
Ocular	Variable	Immediate	Unknown	Variable

ANTIVIRAL DRUGS

Three antiviral ophthalmic drugs are currently available: fomivirsen (Vitravene), ganciclovir (Vitrasert), and trifluridine (Viroptic). Fomivirsen and ganciclovir are used to treat cytomegalovirus infections; they are implanted in the eye by an ophthalmologist and are beyond the scope of this chapter.

trifluridine

Trifluridine (Viroptic, 1% ophthalmic drops) is a pyrimidine nucleoside. This medication inhibits viral replication because its metabolites block the synthesis of viral deoxyribonucleic acid (DNA) by inhibiting viral DNA polymerase, an enzyme needed for DNA synthesis. This ophthalmic drug is used against ocular infections (keratitis and keratoconjunctivitis) caused by types 1 and 2 of the herpes simplex virus. Significant adverse effects include secondary glaucoma, corneal punctate defects, uveitis, and stromal edema (edema in the tough, fibrous, transparent portion of the cornea known as the *stroma*). The drugs exhibit no appreciable topical absorption, and no significant drug interactions have been reported.

ANTIINFLAMMATORY DRUGS

Many of the same antiinflammatory drug classes that are used systemically may also be used ophthalmically to treat various ocular inflammatory disorders and surgery-related pain and in-

---

BOX 57-1 Ophthalmic Antiinflammatory Drugs

Nonsteroidal Antiinflammatories
- bromfenac (Xibrom)
- diclofenac (Voltaren)
- flurbiprofen (Ocufen)
- ketorolac (Acular)

Corticosteroids
- dexamethasone (Decadron, others)
- fluocinonide (Retisert)
- fluorometholone (Fluor-Op, others)
- loteprednol (Lotemax, others)
- medrysone (HMS)
- prednisolone (Pred Forte, others)
- rimexolone (Vexol)

---

flammation. These drugs include both nonsteroidal antiinflammatory drugs (NSAIDs) and corticosteroids and are listed in Box 57-1.

Mechanism of Action and Drug Effects

Corticosteroids and NSAIDs, as discussed in Chapters 33 and 44, respectively, both act to reduce inflammatory responses that arise from the body's metabolic pathway (series of biochemical reactions) for the naturally occurring biochemical arachidonic acid. Each of these two drug classes acts at different enzymatic sites in this complex metabolic pathway, as illustrated in Figure 57-14.

When tissues are damaged, the membranes of affected cells release phospholipids in response to the damage. These phospholipids are then broken down by several different enzymes within the arachidonic acid metabolic pathway. Phospholipase is one of the first enzymes involved, and it is the enzyme that is inhibited by corticosteroids. A second enzyme, cyclooxygenase, occurs farther down the pathway and is the site of action of the NSAIDs. Both drug actions reduce the production of various inflammatory mediators, such as leukotrienes, prostaglandins, and thromboxanes. This in turn reduces pain, erythema, and other inflammatory processes.

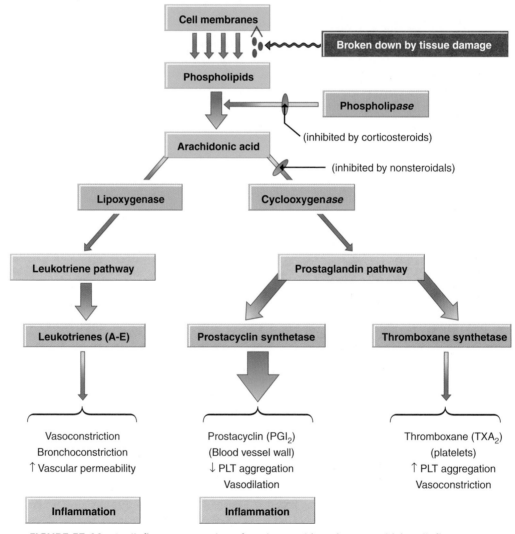

FIGURE 57-14 Antiinflammatory action of corticosteroids and nonsteroidal antiinflammatory drugs (NSAIDs). *PGI₂*, Prostaglandin I₂; *PLT*, platelet; *TXA₂*, thromboxane A₂.

Indications

Corticosteroids and NSAIDs are applied topically for the symptomatic relief of many ophthalmic inflammatory conditions. They may be used to treat corneal, conjunctival, and scleral injuries from chemical, radiation, or thermal burns or from penetration of foreign bodies. They are used during the acute phase of the injury process to prevent fibrosis and scarring, which result in visual impairment. The immunosuppressant effect is more notable with corticosteroids than with NSAIDs. Consequently, NSAIDs are considered less toxic and are often preferred as initial topical therapy for such injuries. NSAIDs are also used in the symptomatic treatment of seasonal allergic conjunctivitis.

Corticosteroids and NSAIDs are used prophylactically before ocular surgery to prevent or reduce the intraoperative miosis that may occur secondary to surgery-induced trauma. They are also used prophylactically after ocular surgery, such as cataract extraction, glaucoma surgery, and corneal transplantation, to prevent inflammation and scarring.

Contraindications

These drugs are contraindicated in cases of known drug allergy. In addition, they should not be used for minor abrasions or wounds because they may suppress the ability of the eye to resist bacterial, viral, or fungal infections. This is especially true of corticosteroids, which, as noted earlier, have stronger immunosuppressant effects.

Adverse Effects

The most common adverse effect of corticosteroids is transient burning or stinging on application. The extended use of corticosteroids may result in cataracts, increased intraocular pressure, and optic nerve damage.

DRUG PROFILES

Corticosteroids and NSAIDs that are used to treat ophthalmic inflammatory disorders are listed in Box 57-1. These ophthalmic formulations share many of the same characteristics as their systemic drug counterparts. However, the ophthalmic derivatives have limited systemic absorption. Therefore, most therapeutic and toxic effects are restricted to the eye.

CORTICOSTEROID
◆ dexamethasone

Dexamethasone (Decadron) is a synthetic corticosteroid that is available in many systemic and ophthalmic formulations. It is used to treat inflammation of the eye, eyelids, conjunctiva, and cornea, and it may also be used in the treatment of uveitis, iridocyclitis, allergic conditions, and burns and in the removal of foreign bodies. Dexamethasone is available in ointment, suspension, and solution form.

PHARMACOKINETICS

Route	Onset of Action	Peak Plasma Concentration	Elimination Half-life	Duration of Action
Ocular	Variable	Immediate	Unknown	Variable

NONSTEROIDAL ANTIINFLAMMATORY DRUGS
flurbiprofen

Flurbiprofen (Ocufen) is an NSAID that is used to treat inflammatory ophthalmic conditions, such as postoperative inflammation after a cataract extraction. It is also used to inhibit intraoperative miosis that may be induced by operative trauma and tissue injury. It is available in solution form.

PHARMACOKINETICS

Route	Onset of Action	Peak Plasma Concentration	Elimination Half-life	Duration of Action
Ocular	30 min	90 min	Unknown	3 hr

ketorolac

Ketorolac (Acular) is an NSAID that is available in both oral and injectable formulations for systemic use. The ophthalmic formulation is used to reduce certain manifestations of ocular inflammation caused by trauma, such as ocular surgery, and inflammation secondary to external agents, such as allergens and bacteria. Ketorolac is contraindicated in patients who have exhibited hypersensitivity to it. It is available in solution form. It is important to know that this drug may delay eye wound healing and lead to corneal epithelial breakdown; therefore, constant monitoring of the eye should continue through the duration of therapy.

PHARMACOKINETICS

Route	Onset of Action	Peak Plasma Concentration	Elimination Half-life	Duration of Action
Ocular	Rapid	Immediate	Unknown	4-6 hr

TOPICAL ANESTHETICS

Topical anesthetic ophthalmic drugs are local anesthetics that are used to alleviate eye pain. The two currently available topical anesthetics used for ophthalmic purposes are proparacaine and tetracaine.

Mechanism of Action and Drug Effects

As described in Chapter 12, local anesthetics stabilize the membranes of nerves, which results in a decrease in the movement of ions into and out of the nerve endings. When nerves are stabilized in this way, they cannot transmit signals about painful stimuli to the brain. Usually, the application of topical anesthetic drugs to the eye results in local anesthesia in less than 30 seconds.

Indications

Ophthalmic topical anesthetic drugs are used to produce ocular anesthesia for short corneal and conjunctival procedures. They prevent pain during surgical procedures and certain painful ophthalmic examinations.

Contraindications

Contraindications to local ophthalmic anesthetics include known drug allergy. These medications are recommended only for short-term use and are not recommended for self-administration.

Adverse Effects

Adverse effects are rare with ophthalmic anesthetic drugs and are limited to local effects such as stinging, burning, redness, and lacrimation. These drugs also have mydriatic and cycloplegic effects because they dilate the pupil and paralyze the ciliary muscle, which prevents accommodation of vision. Systemic toxicity is rare but can theoretically lead to central nervous system (CNS) stimulation and/or CNS or cardiovascular depression.

Medications for Eye Trauma

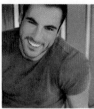

Jason, a construction worker, is being seen in the emergency department because of a possible eye injury. He was working without eye protection, and a gust of wind sprayed metal shavings into his face. The physician has instilled fluorescein sodium and has noted areas in the eyeball with green halos around them.

© CURAphotography

1. What is the purpose of the fluorescein sodium, and what is indicated by the green halos?
2. Jason is sent to an ophthalmologist for further treatment. What eye medication do you expect will be used for the next procedure?
3. After the procedure, Jason receives a prescription for dexamethasone ocular ointment, to be administered three times a day. What specific patient teaching information should be shared with Jason?

For answers, see *http://evolve.elsevier.com/Lilley*.

Interactions

Because of limited systemic absorption and short duration of action, ophthalmic anesthetic drugs have no significant drug interactions.

DRUG PROFILE

Topical ophthalmic anesthetic drugs are a small class of the many available ophthalmic drugs. There are currently only two drugs available for this purpose: proparacaine (Alcaine) and tetracaine (generic only). They are very similar in their indications and dosing regimens.

tetracaine

Tetracaine is a local anesthetic of the ester type (see Chapter 12). It is applied as an eyedrop to numb the eye for various ophthalmic procedures. Tetracaine begins to work in about 25 seconds and lasts for about 15 to 20 minutes. Additional drops are applied as needed. It is currently available only in solution form.

PHARMACOKINETICS

Route	Onset of Action	Peak Plasma Concentration	Elimination Half-life	Duration of Action
Ocular	Less than 30 sec	1-5 min	Short	15-20 min

DIAGNOSTIC DRUGS

DRUG PROFILES

CYCLOPLEGIC MYDRIATICS
◆ atropine sulfate

Atropine sulfate (Isopto Atropine) solution and ointment are used as mydriatic and cycloplegic drugs. The drug dilates the pupil (mydriasis) and paralyze the ciliary muscle (cycloplegic refraction), which prevents accommodation. Such drug action may be needed either to assist in eye examination or to treat uveal tract inflammatory states that benefit from pupillary dilation. The usual dosage for uveitis (inflammation of the choroid, iris, or ciliary body) in children and adults is 1 to 2 drops of the solution, or 0.3 to 0.5 cm of ointment, 2 to 3 times daily. The dosage for eye examina-

tion is 1 drop of solution, ideally 1 hour before the procedure.

cyclopentolate

Cyclopentolate solution (Cyclogyl) is used primarily as a diagnostic mydriatic and cycloplegic drug. Unlike atropine, it is not normally used to treat uveitis. The usual adult dose is 1 to 2 drops (0.5%, 1%, or 2%). This is repeated in 5 to 10 minutes if needed. The dose for children is the same as that for adults. The drug effects usually subside within 24 hours. Other cycloplegic mydriatics are scopolamine (Isopto Hyoscine), homatropine (Isopto Homatropine), and tropicamide (Mydriacyl). All three are topical ophthalmic solutions with indications similar to those of atropine and cyclopentolate, except that tropicamide, like cyclopentolate, is generally used for diagnostic purposes only and not for treatment of inflammatory states.

MYDRIASIS-REVERSAL DRUG
dapiprazole

Dapiprazole (Rev-Eyes) is the only currently available alpha-adrenergic ophthalmic blocking drug. It is used to reverse the effects of mydriatic drugs and restore normal pupillary function. Its use is contraindicated only in cases of known drug allergy or circumstances in which pupillary constriction is undesirable, such as in acute iritis. The recommended dosage is 2 drops in the affected eye following ophthalmologic examination. This dose is repeated once after 5 minutes.

OPHTHALMIC DYE
fluorescein

Fluorescein (AK-Fluor) is an ophthalmic diagnostic dye used to identify corneal defects and to locate foreign objects in the eye. It is also used in fitting hard contact lenses. After the instillation of fluorescein, various defects are highlighted in either bright green or yellow-orange, and foreign objects have a green halo around them. Fluorescein is available for use as an ophthalmic injection, solution, and diagnostic applicator strips. Dose determination and drug administration are usually carried out by an ophthalmologist.

ANTIALLERGIC DRUGS

DRUG PROFILES

ANTIHISTAMINES
olopatadine

Olopatadine (Patanol) is a popular ocular antihistamine used to treat symptoms of allergic conjunctivitis (hay fever), which can be seasonal or nonseasonal. It works by competing at the receptor sites for histamine, an inflammatory mediator produced by mast cells. Histamine normally produces ocular symptoms such as itching and tearing. Other ocular antihistamines include azelastine (Optivar), emedastine (Emadine), ketotifen (Zaditor), and epinastine (Elestat). These drugs have mechanisms of action, therapeutic and adverse effects, and drug interactions similar to those of the systemic antihistamines described in Chapter 36, although systemic effects are less likely with ophthalmic administration. Dosages for olopatadine can be found in the Dosages table on p. 895.

MAST CELL STABILIZERS
cromolyn

Cromolyn sodium (Crolom) is an antiallergic drug that inhibits the release of inflammation-producing mediators from sensitized inflammatory cells called *mast cells*. It is used in the treatment of

DOSAGES

Ocular Antiallergics

Drug (Pregnancy Category)	Pharmacologic Class	Usual Dosage Range	Indications
cromolyn (Crolom) (C)	Mast cell stabilizer	1-2 drops in each eye 4-6 times daily	Vernal (springtime) conjunctivitis and/or keratitis (corneal inflammation)
olopatadine (Patanol 0.1%) (C)	Antihistamine	1-2 drops in each affected eye 2 times per day at an interval of 6-8 hours	Allergic conjunctivitis
olopatadine (Patanol 0.2%) (C)	Antihistamine	1 drop in each affected eye once a day	Allergic conjunctivitis

vernal keratoconjunctivitis (springtime inflammation of the cornea and conjunctiva). Other mast cell stabilizers with similar effects are pemirolast (Alamast), nedocromil (Alocril), and lodoxamide (Alomide). Dosages for cromolyn can be found in the Dosages table on p. 895.

DECONGESTANTS
tetrahydrozoline
Tetrahydrozoline is an ocular decongestant. It works by promoting vasoconstriction of blood vessels in and around the eye. This reduces the edema associated with allergic and inflammatory processes. It is specifically indicated to control redness, burning, and other minor irritations. Other ocular decongestants include phenylephrine (Neo-Synephrine), oxymetazoline (Visine LR), and naphazoline (Clear Eyes). Dosages for tetrahydrozoline can be found in the Dosages table on p. 895.

LUBRICANTS AND MOISTURIZERS
◆ artificial tears
An array of products are available over the counter to provide lubrication or moisture for the eyes. This is often helpful to patients with dry or otherwise irritated eyes. Artificial tears are isotonic and contain buffers to adjust pH. In addition, they contain preservatives for microbial control and may contain viscosity agents for extension of ocular activity. Selected over-the-counter brand names include Moisture Drops, Murine, Nu-Tears, Akwa Tears, and Tears Plus. Many similar products are available on the market both as solutions (eyedrops) and as lubrication ointments. They are often dosed to patient comfort as needed. Restasis is an ophthalmic form of the immunosuppressant drug cyclosporine (see Chapter 45). It is also used to promote tear production in the condition technically known as *keratoconjunctivitis sicca* (dry eyes). It can be used together with artificial tears, if the drugs are given 15 minutes apart.

NURSING PROCESS

Assessment

Before administering any ophthalmic drug per the prescriber's orders, a baseline assessment of the eye and its structures should be completed and normal and abnormal findings documented. Any redness, swelling, pain, excessive tearing, eye drainage or discharge, decrease in visual acuity, or other unusual symptoms should be documented. The patient should also be assessed for hypersensitivity to medications and for any drug- or disorder-related contraindications, cautions, and drug interactions. A visual acuity test (e.g., Snellen chart test) should be performed, if indicated, and the findings noted before, during, and after drug treatment, when appropriate. Any loss of or change in vision or loss of peripheral vision in either or both eyes should be noted. A nursing history should focus on past or present systemic disease processes and exposure to any chemicals that could be topical irritants to the eye, skin, or mucous membranes, including past or present occupational and environmental exposures. All known sensitivities to drugs, chemicals, or other product ingredients should be documented as well. The systemic effects associated with ophthalmic dosage forms are usually minimal if drugs are given as prescribed and directed; however, systemic absorption may occur, with possible adverse effects, if poor application technique is used (see Implementation later and Chapter 10). Should the drug gain access to the circulation, adverse effects should be anticipated.

Nursing Diagnoses

- Risk for infection related to eye disease, condition, or irritation due to a lack of information about various eye problems and lack of motivation to follow directions
- Risk for injury to self (eye) related to improper use of medication and improper instillation procedures
- Acute pain related to the eye disorder, infection, and/or inflammatory eye condition
- Deficient knowledge related to lack of information about the eye disorder and associated medication therapy

Planning
Goals

- Patient remains free of signs and symptoms of infection or irritation of the eye.
- Patient remains compliant with the therapy regimen.
- Patient remains free from self-injury related to adverse effects of therapy.
- Patient is without eye pain related to the eye disorder.

Outcome Criteria

- Patient states the signs and symptoms of infection of the eye, such as eye pain, drainage, redness, and decreased activity, and reports them immediately to the prescriber.
- Patient states ways to become more compliant with the therapy regimen by taking medications as prescribed, including

following proper timing and installation technique; and using other nondrug therapy aids, such as application of warm or cool compresses as recommended.

- Patient minimizes self-injury related to the adverse effects of therapy by creating a safe environment at home, including reducing clutter and moving out any unused rugs or furniture; putting in more lighting, especially night lights; and using assistive devices as needed, if vision is altered.
- Patient minimizes eye pain related to the eye disorder by applying compresses or using nonaspirin analgesics as ordered.

Implementation

It is important to administer only clear products (e.g., drops, ointments, solutions) to the eye. All solutions should be shaken and the contents mixed thoroughly. Solutions with any particulate matter should not be used. One of the most important standards to follow during instillation of drops or ointment is to avoid touching the eye with the tip of the dropper or container to prevent contamination of the product. Any excess medication must be removed promptly, and pressure should be applied to the inner canthus for 1 minute (or other specified period). Application of pressure to the inner canthus after instillation of medication is needed to prevent or decrease systemic absorption and subsequent systemic adverse effects. Ointments and any other ophthalmic topical drug dosage form should always be applied to the conjunctival sac and never directly onto the eye itself (cornea). To facilitate the instillation of ophthalmic medication, the patient should tilt the head back and look up at the ceiling. Several ophthalmic drugs with different actions are often ordered, and each drug must be given exactly as prescribed and within the specified time period. This is particularly important when surgical procedures are being performed on the eye, because several drugs with different actions may be ordered and must be given at specific times (as ordered). Ointments may cause a temporary blurring of vision because of the film that bathes the eye. This film will decrease once the drug is absorbed, and vision should become clearer. The nurse should refer to an authoritative drug source for specific instructions and guidelines regarding application technique, length of time to apply pressure to the inner canthus, and any other special directions. See Chapter 10 for administration technique for ophthalmic drugs.

Directions for the use of *antiviral ophthalmic preparations* should be followed closely. *Topical anesthetics* should be administered, as ordered, for use in removal of a foreign body or treatment of eye injury. Repeated and continuous use should be avoided because of the risk for delayed wound healing, corneal perforation, permanent corneal opacification, and vision loss. When there is an abrasion or other injury to the eye and appropriate medications are ordered, patching of the affected eye is recommended. This helps prevent further injury resulting from loss of the blink reflex due to overuse of topical anesthetic. Additional patient instructions should include any appropriate information about any change in eye color. For example, *latanoprost* actually changes the eye color permanently from hazel, green, or bluish brown to brown. Although this color change occurs, no known injury to the eye is associated with this color change.

Ophthalmic *ketorolac* should be given as ordered. *Artificial tear solutions* are often used in long-term care and are available over the counter. Once therapy has been initiated, the prescriber may order periodic intraocular pressure measurements and visual field and funduscopic examinations. The importance of follow-up visits for such monitoring should be shared with the patient (see Patient Teaching Tips).

Evaluation

Therapeutic responses to *miotics* include decreased aqueous humor of the eye with resultant decreased intraocular pressure and decreased signs, symptoms, and long-term effects associated with glaucoma. Possible adverse effects are included in Table 57-4. *Beta-adrenergic blockers* are therapeutic if there is a resultant decrease in intraocular pressure. Possible adverse effects for which to evaluate include weakness, eye irritation, rash, bradycardia, hypotension, and dysrhythmias. Therapeutic responses to *antibiotic, antifungal, and antiviral ophthalmic drugs* include elimination of the infection or condition and resolution of symptoms, and prevention of complications. Therapeutic responses to *ophthalmic anesthetics* include prevention/relief of pain associated with the injury. Adverse effects may include CNS excitation (e.g., dizziness, tremors, restlessness, nervousness) if the drug is systemically absorbed. *Antiinflammatory ophthalmic solutions* should result in a decrease in allergic reactions with a decrease in itching, tearing, redness, and eye discharge. Potential complications of these solutions include swelling of the conjunctiva (chemosis). Further monitoring should include reevaluation of goals and outcome criteria.

PATIENT TEACHING TIPS

- When a parasympathomimetic drug—or any other class of ophthalmic drug—is to be used, the patient should be educated about the correct administration technique. A demonstration with return demonstrations by the patient should be used as a teaching strategy.
- The patient should be reminded that solutions with eye droppers as well as solutions in containers for direct application should be kept sterile by avoiding touching the tip of the eye dropper or container to the surface of the eye.
- Indirect parasympathomimetics (cholinergics) should be given to the patient only after the patient demonstrates adequate knowledge of the medication and the technique for administration. The patient should be educated about adverse effects associated with these cholinergic drugs, such as blurred vision, bronchospasm, nausea, vomiting, bradycardia, hypotension, and sweating.
- With any ophthalmic drug, the following should be reported to the prescriber: severe stinging, burning, itching, and redness of the eye, excessive tearing or excessive dryness of the eye, puffiness of the eye/eyelids, discharge from the eye, fever, eye pain, and/or loss or change of vision.
- Sympatholytic drugs should be instilled as ordered. Once these drugs (and many other drugs used in the eye) are instilled, the patient should be instructed to apply pressure to the inner canthus with a tissue or 2 × 2 inch gauze pad for 1 full minute or as directed. Application of pressure to the inner canthus helps to minimize absorption and decrease risk of systemic adverse effects. Blurred vision, difficulty breathing, wheezing, sweating, flushing, and loss of sight should be reported to the prescriber.
- Photosensitivity is an expected adverse effect of mydriatics; therefore, when these drugs are administered, the patient should be encouraged to wear sunglasses to help minimize eye discomfort and/or headaches while in sunlight.
- With topical anesthetics, the patient should not rub or touch the eye while it is numb, because eye damage may result. The patient should also wear a patch to protect the eye because of loss of the blink reflex.
- Ophthalmic medications should be used as prescribed and never overused. Products whose expiration dates have passed should be discarded appropriately. Medications should not be stopped without consulting the prescriber first because of the possibility of adverse reactions.
- Contact lenses should not be worn while ophthalmic drugs are being instilled and for the duration of therapy, because the lenses may lead to further irritation.
- Ophthalmic ketorolac, an antiinflammatory drug, may delay eye wound healing and lead to corneal epithelial breakdown, so if these problems are present or suspected, they should be reported.

POINTS TO REMEMBER

- Glaucoma is a disorder of the eye caused by inhibition of the normal flow and drainage of aqueous humor, and its treatment helps to reduce intraocular pressure either by increasing the drainage of aqueous humor or decreasing its production.
- Drugs that increase aqueous humor drainage are direct parasympathomimetics, indirect parasympathomimetics, sympathomimetics, and beta-blockers.
- A large proportion of the inflammatory diseases of the eye are caused by viruses, and many ocular antimicrobials are available to treat bacterial, viral, and fungal infections of the eye.
- Common ocular infections include conjunctivitis, hordeolum (sty), keratitis, uveitis, and endophthalmitis.
- Antiinflammatory ophthalmic drugs include corticosteroids and are used to inhibit inflammatory responses to mechanical forces, chemicals, and immunologic reactions.
- Topical anesthetics are used to prevent pain to the eye and are beneficial during surgery, ophthalmic examinations, and removal of foreign bodies.
- All ophthalmic preparations must be administered exactly as ordered and into the conjunctival sac. Safe and accurate application or instillation technique must be used and contact of the dropper or tube to the eye avoided to prevent contamination of the drug.
- Patients should report any increase in symptoms, such as eye pain or drainage and fever, to the prescriber immediately.

NCLEX EXAMINATION REVIEW QUESTIONS

1 The ophthalmologist has given a patient a dose of ocular atropine drops. Which statement by the nurse accurately explains to the patient the reason for these drops?

   a "These drops will cause the surface of your eye to become numb, so that the doctor can do the examination."

   b "These drops are used to check for any possible foreign bodies or corneal defects that may be in your eye."

   c "These drops cause your pupils to constrict, which makes the eye examination easier."

   d "These drops cause your pupils to dilate, which makes the eye examination easier."

2 When assessing a patient who is receiving a direct-acting sympathomimetic eyedrop as part of treatment for glaucoma, the nurse notes that the drug affects the pupil in which way?

   a It causes mydriasis, or pupil dilation.

   b It causes miosis, or pupil constriction.

   c It changes the color of the pupil.

   d It causes no change in pupil size.

3 During patient teaching regarding self-administration of ophthalmic drops, which statement by the nurse is correct?

   a "Hold the eyedrops over the cornea and squeeze out the drop."

   b "Apply pressure to the lacrimal duct area for 5 minutes after administration."

   c "Be sure to place the drop in the conjunctival sac of the lower eyelid."

   d "Squeeze your eyelid closed tightly after placing the drop into your eye."

4 When the nurse is providing teaching about eye medications for glaucoma, the nurse tells the patient that miotics help glaucoma by which mechanism of action?

   a Decreasing intracranial pressure

   b Decreasing intraocular pressure

   c Increasing tear production

   d Causing pupillary dilation

5 During an assessment of a glaucoma patient who may be receiving a carbonic anhydrase inhibitor as part of treatment, the nurse recognizes that which condition would be considered a problem?

   a Allergy to sulfa drugs

   b Allergy to penicillins

   c Diabetes mellitus

   d Hypertension

6 A patient has undergone an eye procedure during which ophthalmic mydriatics and anesthetic drops were used. The nurse gives which instructions to the patient before the patient is discharged? (Select all that apply.)

   a "Do not rub or touch the numb eye."

   b "You may reinsert your contact lenses before you leave."

   c "Be sure to wear sunglasses when you go outside."

   d "Your pupils will appear very tiny until the medication wears off."

   e "Report any increase in eye pain or drainage to the ophthalmologist immediately."

1. d, 2. b, 3. c, 4. b, 5. a, 6. a, c, e.

CRITICAL THINKING ACTIVITIES: BEST ACTION

1 A patient has a prescription for latanoprost (Xalatan). What is the most important piece of information that the nurse should tell the patient *before* the patient starts taking this medication?

2 A patient with type 2 diabetes mellitus has a new prescription for an ophthalmic beta-blocker for treatment of glaucoma. Two days later, the patient calls the office and tells the nurse, "I looked this drug up on the Internet, and it says that this type of drug can mess up my blood sugar levels. I don't want to take the drops if that happens." What is the nurse's best response to the patient?

3 The nurse is assessing the eyes of a patient who had ocular surgery a week earlier. The patient has been receiving ketorolac (Acular) ophthalmic solution. What is the most important thing the nurse must keep in mind when assessing the eyes of this patient?

For answers, see *http://evolve.elsevier.com/Lilley.*

Otic Drugs

e-Learning Activities

http://evolve.elsevier.com/Lilley
NCLEX Review Questions • Animations • Nursing Care Plans • Audio Glossary • Category Catchers • Medication Errors Checklists • IV Therapy Checklists • Calculators • Frequently Asked Questions • Content Updates • Supplemental Resources • Answers to Case Studies and Critical Thinking Activities

Drug Profiles

◆ carbamide peroxide, p. 901
Cortic (hydrocortisone/pramoxine/chloroxylenol), Acetasol HC (hydrocortisone/acetic acid), p. 901

Cortisporin Otic (hydrocortisone/neomycin/polymyxin B), Ciprodex (ciprofloxacin), Cipro HC Otic (ciprofloxacin/hydrocortisone), Floxin Otic (ofloxacin), p. 901

◆ *Key drug.*

Glossary

Cerumen A yellowish or brownish waxy excretion produced by modified sweat glands in the external ear canal. Also called *earwax.* (p. 901)

Otitis externa Inflammation or infection of the external auditory canal. (p. 899)

Otitis media Inflammation or infection of the middle ear. (p. 899)

• • •

Anatomy, Physiology, and Disease Overview

The ear is made up of four parts: the external, outer, middle, and inner ears. The external ear is composed of the *pinna* (outer projecting part of the ear) and the *external auditory meatus* or opening of the ear canal. Synonyms for the pinna are *auricle* and *ala.*

The term *outer ear* refers primarily to the *external auditory canal.* This is the space between the external auditory meatus and the *tympanic membrane* (eardrum). The middle ear is composed of the *tympanic cavity,* which is the space that begins with the tympanic membrane and ends with the *oval window.* Included in the middle ear are three bony structures of the *mastoid* bone—the *malleus* ("hammer"), *incus* ("anvil"), *and stapes* ("stirrup")—as well as the *auditory* or *eustachian tube.* The inner ear includes the *cochlea* and *semicircular canals.* The ear and its associated structures are illustrated in Figure 58-1.

Disorders of the ear can be categorized according to the portion of the ear affected. External ear (pinna) disorders are generally the result of physical trauma to the ear and consist of lacerations or scrapes to the skin and localized infection of the hair follicles, which often causes the development of a boil. These disorders also tend to be self-limiting and heal with time. Other examples of external ear disorders are contact dermatitis, seborrhea, and psoriasis, as evidenced by itching, local redness, inflammation, weeping, or drainage. These conditions usually respond to the same topical medications used for any other local skin disorders, as discussed in Chapter 56. However, symptoms such as drainage, pain, and dizziness are sometimes also the first signs of a more serious underlying condition (e.g., head trauma, meningitis) and warrant prompt medical evaluation. Medications for disorders affecting the outer (ear canal) and middle ear are the focus of this chapter. Diseases of the inner ear involve highly specialized medical practices that are beyond the scope of this book.

The most common disorders affecting the outer and middle ear are bacterial and fungal infections, inflammation, and earwax accumulation. Such disorders are often self-limiting, and treatments are usually successful. If problems persist or are left untreated, however, more serious problems such as hearing loss may result. Infections affecting the ear canal are known as **otitis externa,** whereas those affecting the middle ear are known as **otitis media.** Otitis media is a common disease of infancy and early childhood. It is often preceded by an upper respiratory tract

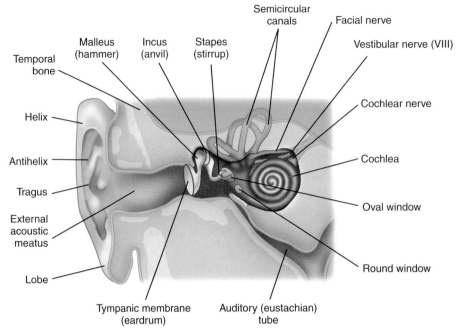

FIGURE 58-1   Structure of the ear.

infection. It may also occur in adults, but it is then generally associated with trauma to the tympanic membrane. Foreign objects and infection or inflammation associated with water sports are the usual sources of such trauma. In adults, the condition is also more likely to manifest as otitis externa, involving the ear canal and/or external tympanic membrane. Common symptoms of both otitis media and otitis externa are pain, fever, malaise, pressure, a sensation of fullness in the ears, and impaired hearing. If the condition is left untreated, tinnitus (ringing in the ears), nausea, vertigo, mastoiditis, and even temporary or permanent hearing deficits may occur.

Pharmacology Overview

TREATMENT OF EAR DISORDERS

Some of the minor ailments that affect the outer or middle ear can be treated with over-the-counter medications, but persistent, painful conditions generally require prescription medications. Drugs used to treat ear conditions are known as *otic drugs,* and most are applied topically to the ear canal. Because of this they generally are involved in no drug interactions. Adverse effects are uncommon and usually do not extend beyond localized irritation, and otic drugs are normally contraindicated only in cases of known drug allergy. Pertinent classes of otic drugs include the following:

- Antibacterials (antibiotics)
- Antifungals
- Antiinflammatory drugs
- Local analgesics
- Local anesthetics
- Steroids
- Wax emulsifiers

TABLE 58-1 Common Antibacterial Otic Products

Steroid Component	Antibiotic Component	Trade Name
hydrocortisone (1%)	5 mg of neomycin and 10,000 units of polymyxin B per 10-mL bottle	Cortisporin Otic, others
hydrocortisone (1%)	ciprofloxacin 2 mg/mL	Cipro HT Otic
dexamethasone (0.1%)	ciprofloxacin 3 mg/mL	Ciprodex
None	ofloxacin 3 mg/mL	Floxin Otic

More serious cases of ear disorders may require treatment with systemic drugs such as antimicrobial drugs, analgesics, antiinflammatory drugs, and antihistamines. These medications are discussed in detail in previous chapters dealing with the respective drug classes.

ANTIBACTERIAL AND ANTIFUNGAL OTIC DRUGS

Antibacterial and antifungal otic drugs are often combined with steroids to take advantage of the antiinflammatory, antipruritic, and antiallergic effects of the latter drugs. These drugs are used to treat outer and middle ear infections. Because they all work and are dosed very similarly, four products are profiled together here. Systemic antibiotics are also commonly prescribed for these conditions (e.g., amoxicillin; see Chapter 38), either alone or in addition to the otic drugs described in the following sections. Tables 58-1 and 58-2 list several commonly used products and their component amounts.

TABLE 58-2 Common Antifungal Otic Products

Ingredients	Trade Name
hydrocortisone, 1%; pramoxine, 1%; chloroxylenol, 0.1%; propylene glycol diacetate, 3%; benzalkonium chloride (amount not specified)	Cortic
hydrocortisone, 1%; acetic acid, 2%; propylene glycol diacetate, 3%; sodium acetate, 0.015%; benzethonium chloride, 0.02%	Acetasol HC

DRUG PROFILES

ANTIBACTERIAL PRODUCTS
Cortisporin Otic, Ciprodex, Cipro HC Otic, Floxin Otic
Cortisporin (and other brands) is a three-drug combination that includes hydrocortisone and two antimicrobials, neomycin (an *aminoglycoside;* see Chapter 39) and polymyxin B. Hydrocortisone is the steroid most commonly used in otic drugs, although there is one preparation (Ciprodex) that contain ciprofloxacin (a *fluoroquinolone;* see Chapter 39) and dexamethasone. In either case, the purpose of the steroid component is to reduce the inflammation and itching associated with ear infections. Ciprofloxacin is also available in combination with hydrocortisone (Cipro HC Otic). Ofloxacin (Floxin Otic) is another fluoroquinolone available only as a single-drug product. All of these products are used for the treatment of bacterial otitis externa or otitis media caused by susceptible bacteria such as *Staphylococcus aureus, Escherichia coli, Klebsiella* species, and others. Their usual dosage is 4 drops three to four times daily, except for ofloxacin, which is dosed at 5 to 10 drops twice daily (5-drop dose for children under 12 years). With some otic drugs, it is recommended to saturate a retrievable cotton or tissue *wick* and let this wick soak inside the ear canal, as a means of dosing the drug. The wick can be periodically remoistened with additional drug or removed and further eardrops inserted directly into the ear canal. The nurse should follow the specific instructions on the drug package or the method recommended by the prescriber or pharmacist.

ANTIFUNGAL PRODUCTS
Cortic, Acetasol HC
Although fungal infections of the ear are uncommon, otic drugs are available for their treatment. These drugs may also have antibacterial and even antiviral properties. Two commonly used preparations are Cortic and Acetasol HC. Cortic is composed of hydrocortisone (a steroid), pramoxine (a local anesthetic), chloroxylenol (an antiseptic antifungal), propylene glycol diacetate (an emulsifying drug), and benzalkonium chloride (an antiseptic preservative). Acetasol HC consists of hydrocortisone, acetic acid (an antifungal), propylene glycol diacetate, sodium acetate (a preservative), and benzethonium chloride (an antiseptic preservative). The local anesthetic components help ease both the pain and itching common in ear infections.

EARWAX EMULSIFIERS
An additional common ear problem is the accumulation and eventual *impaction* (hardening) of earwax, or **cerumen,** which can also contribute to or complicate the infectious and inflammatory conditions described earlier. Products that soften and help to eliminate earwax are referred to as *earwax emulsifiers*. Wax, or cerumen, is a natural product of the ear and is produced by modified sweat glands in the ear canal. However, it can occasionally build up and become impacted, which results in pain and

CASE STUDY

Ear Medications

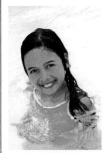

© Juriah Mosin

Trixie is 8 years old and loves to swim in the neighborhood pool. Lately she has had a feeling of fullness in her left ear, and today she tells her mother that her ear is hurting and itching and that she feels "awful." Her mother takes her temperature and finds that it is 101° F (38.3° C). She calls the pediatrician's office for an appointment, and Trixie is seen the next morning. After examining Trixie, the pediatrician says that Trixie has otitis media in the left ear and some earwax buildup in both ears. The pediatrician removes some of the earwax manually, writes prescriptions for oral antibiotics for Trixie, and gives instructions to use an earwax emulsifier. The nurse meets with them to review the instructions.

1. Trixie's mother asks, "Why is the antibiotic a pill? It seems to me that if she has an ear infection, she should take eardrops!" What is the nurse's best response?
2. Trixie's mother has another question: "What will happen if this ear infection does not get better?"
3. Trixie complains that her ear "really hurts and itches." What can be given to her for this problem? How will it be given?

For answers, see *http://evolve.elsevier.com/Lilley.*

partial temporary deafness. From chemistry, a nonpolar substance is one that is not water soluble. Such a substance is said to be *emulsified* when it is chemically and/or physically converted to a more water-soluble form. *Earwax emulsifiers* loosen impacted cerumen, which allows it to be flushed out of the ear canal through irrigation (with water).

DRUG PROFILE

◆ carbamide peroxide
Carbamide peroxide (Debrox) is a commonly used earwax emulsifier. It is combined with other components (e.g., glycerin, a lubricant) that help soften and lubricate cerumen prior to irrigation. Carbamide peroxide slowly releases hydrogen peroxide and oxygen when exposed to moisture. This release of oxygen imparts a weak antibacterial action to this otic drug. In addition, the *effervescence* (foaming) resulting from the release of oxygen has the mechanical effect of emulsifying impacted cerumen to release it from the walls of the ear canal. Earwax emulsifiers should not be used without prescription when ear drainage, tympanic membrane rupture, or significant pain or other irritation is present. After allowing the drug to dissolve the earwax, one can remove it by gentle flushing the ear canal with warm water from a bulb syringe. Some earwax removal products include such a syringe in the package.

NURSING PROCESS

Assessment
Before administering any of the otic preparations, baseline hearing or auditory status should be assessed, as deemed appropriate, and the findings documented. The patient's symptoms, past and

present medical history, and use of prescription drugs, over-the-counter drugs, and herbals should also be documented. Any drug or food allergies should also be recorded. A basic understanding of the anatomy of the ear, especially anatomic variations in patients of different age groups, is needed to ensure proper application technique. Contraindications, cautions, and drug interactions for the otic drugs, chemicals, and/or solutions have been discussed previously in the pharmacology section, and the patient should always be assessed for these and the findings documented. In addition, if the patient has a perforated eardrum, this is usually a contraindication to the use of otic drugs.

Nursing Diagnoses

- Impaired verbal communication related to possible hearing impairment stemming from damage induced by long-term ear disorders or infections
- Risk for injury related to symptoms of the ear disorder and possible vestibular dysfunction
- Risk for infection related to inadequate treatment
- Disturbed sensory perception related to complications from untreated or undertreated ear infections or disorders
- Deficient knowledge related to lack of experience with otic drugs and their method of administration
- Noncompliance related to a lack of motivation for frequent instillation of eardrops as ordered

Planning

Goals

- Patient regains normal patterns of hearing and communicating.
- Patient is free of discomfort and symptoms related to the ear disorder.
- Patient remains free of or experiences minimal signs and symptoms of ear infection with the course of treatment.
- Patient is free of adverse reactions or adverse effects.
- Patient is free of complications associated with medication therapy.
- Patient adheres to the recommended drug therapy regimen as ordered.

Outcome Criteria

- Patient openly verbalizes feelings related to ear problems and therapy, such as a decrease in or loss of hearing related to ear infections or disorders, or to therapy.

- Patient reports immediately to the prescriber any increased hearing loss; increased symptoms of ear pain, redness, and swelling of the ear canal; or fever.
- Patient states measures to take to increase the effectiveness of the medication regimen, such as accurately applying or instilling the medication and then remaining supine or sitting with the affected ear upward for a short period.
- Patient demonstrates accurate medication administration technique as appropriate for age group and in keeping with specific directions.

Implementation

Eardrops should be instilled only after the ear has been thoroughly cleansed, all cerumen (earwax) has been removed (by irrigation if necessary, or as ordered), and the dropper has been cleansed as recommended. Eardrops, solutions, and ointments should be at room temperature before instillation. Administration of solutions that are too cold may cause a vestibular type of reaction with vomiting and dizziness. If the solution has been refrigerated, it should be allowed to warm to room temperature. Higher temperatures may affect the potency of these solutions; therefore, administration at room temperature is recommended. Generally speaking, eardrops should be administered according to the above guidelines and as ordered. Adults should be given eardrops while the pinna is held up and back, whereas in children younger than 3 years of age the pinna should be held down and back. Time should be allowed for adequate coverage of the ear by the medication. Gentle massage to the tragus area of the ear may also help to increase coverage of the medication after the solution is given. See Patient Teaching Tips and also Chapter 10 for further information on eardrop instillation.

Evaluation

The therapeutic effects of otic drugs, as with all drugs, should be gauged by evaluating whether goals and objectives have been met. Therapeutic effects should include less pain, redness, and swelling in the ear; a reduction in fever and white blood cell counts; and negative culture results if the previous culture has yielded positive findings. The ear canal should be monitored for the occurrence of rash and/or any signs of local irritation, such as redness and heat at the site. The patient should be evaluated for adverse effects with each application or instillation, and any unusual appearance of the outer ear and ear canal should be reported immediately to the prescriber and documented.

PATIENT TEACHING TIPS

- Thorough instructions should be given to the patient about the proper use of eardrops or instillation of any medication into the ear. The patient should be warned that dizziness may occur after application of the medication; therefore, the patient should remain supine during instillation and for a few minutes thereafter.
- Medication to be applied to the ear should be at room temperature. This may be achieved by running warm water over the medication bottle, but care must be taken to prevent water from getting into the container, damaging the label so that the directions are unreadable, or making the solution too warm to use. The patient should take care not to heat the medication—for

example, a microwave oven should not be used for warming—because eardrops that are overheated may lose potency. If the pharmacy indicates that the drug should be kept in a refrigerator, the drug should be taken out of the refrigerator up to 1 hour before it is to be instilled so that it may warm up to room temperature. Most medications for the ear are stored at room temperature.

- The patient should lie on the side opposite to that of the affected ear for about 5 minutes after instillation of the drug. If the patient prefers, a small cotton ball may be inserted gently into the ear canal to keep the drug in place, but it should not be forced into the ear or jammed down into the ear canal.

POINTS TO REMEMBER

- Otic drugs may include the following ingredients, either by themselves or mixed together (depending on the prescriber's order): steroids, antibacterials, antifungals, antiinflammatories, and wax-emulsifying compounds. Many of the antiinfective drugs are combined with steroids (in solution) to take advantage of the additional antiinflammatory, antipruritic, and antiallergic drug effects of the steroids.
- Some ear infections require additional drug therapy with systemic dosage forms of corticosteroids, antibiotics, antifungals, and antiinflammatory drugs, so the patient may need to be reminded of oral and other dosage forms.
- Some disorders of the ear are self-limiting to a degree, but appropriate treatment is important to prevent complications to the

ear and/or systemic complications. If left untreated, ear infections or disorders may lead to a decrease in or loss of hearing.

- Wax, or cerumen, is a natural product of the ear and is normally produced by modified sweat glands in the auditory canal; emulsifying otic drugs (such as carbamide peroxide) loosen and help remove this wax.
- Single drugs and combination drug products are used to treat many ear conditions, and the nurse must know the indications for and specific information about these drugs to ensure their safe use.

NCLEX EXAMINATION REVIEW QUESTIONS

1 While teaching a patient about treatment of otitis media, the nurse should mention that untreated otitis media may lead to
  a mastoiditis.
  b throat infections.
  c fungal ear infection.
  d decreased cerumen production.
2 During a teaching session about eardrops, the patient tells the nurse, "I know why an antibiotic is in this medicine, but why do I need to take a steroid?" The nurse's best answer would be which statement?
  a "The steroid will help to soften the cerumen."
  b "The steroid reduces itching and inflammation."
  c "The steroid also has antifungal effects."
  d "This medication helps to anesthetize the area to decrease pain."
3 The nurse is preparing to administer eardrops. Which technique for administering eardrops is correct?
  a Warm the solution to 106° F (41° C) before using.
  b Position the patient so that the unaffected ear is accessible.
  c Massage the tragus before administering the eardrops.
  d Gently insert a cotton ball into the outer ear canal after the drops are given.

4 The nurse is discussing treatment of earwax buildup with a patient. Which statement about earwax emulsifiers is true?
  a These drugs are useful for treatment of ear infections.
  b These drugs loosen impacted cerumen so that it may be removed by irrigation.
  c These drugs are used to rinse out excessive earwax.
  d These drugs enhance the secretion of earwax.
5 During an examination, the nurse notes that a patient has a perforated tympanic membrane. There is an order for eardrops. Which action by the nurse is most appropriate?
  a Give the medication as ordered.
  b Check the patient's hearing, then give the drops.
  c Hold the medication and check with the prescriber.
  d Administer the drops with a cotton wick.
6 The nurse is preparing to administer carbamide peroxide (Debrox) to an adult patient with impacted cerumen. Which actions by the nurse are correct? (Select all that apply.)
  a Have the patient lie on his side with the affected ear up.
  b Chill the medication before administering it.
  c Pull the pinna of the ear down and back.
  d Pull the pinna of the ear up and back.
  e Vigorously irrigate the ear with warm water to remove the softened earwax.

CRITICAL THINKING ACTIVITIES: BEST ACTION

1 A nurse is explaining about wax emulsifiers to a patient who has decreased hearing because of impacted cerumen. The patient asks, "How can this help me? What will this medication do for me?" What is the nurse's best answer?

2 When discussing eardrop administration with a patient, the patient says, "I'll keep these in the refrigerator so that they'll be cold when I give them to myself." What is the nurse's best response?

3 The nurse is observing while the mother of an infant administers eardrops for the first time. The mother says, "When I give the drops, I will pull the ear up and back like this, give the drops, then massage the ear lobe." What is the best action of the nurse at this time?

For answers, see *http://evolve.elsevier.com/Lilley.*

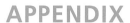

Pharmaceutical Abbreviations

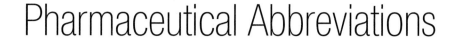

Abbreviation	Translation
Drug Dosage	
cc*	Cubic centimeter (equivalent to 1 mL)
g or gm	Gram
gr	Grain
gtt	Drop
IU*	International unit
L	Liter
lb	Pound
℔ or min	Minim
mEq	Milliequivalent
min	Minute
ml or mL	Milliliter
no	Number
os	Quantity sufficient, as much as needed
ss	One half
oz	Ounce
tbsp	Tablespoon
tsp	Teaspoon
u or U*	Unit
μg or mcg*	Microgram
Drug Route	
AD	Right ear
AS	Left ear
AU	Both ears
ID	Intradermal
IM	Intramuscular
IV	Intravenous
NG	Nasogastric
OD	Right eye
OS	Left eye
OU	Both eyes
PO	By mouth
SC, SQ, subcut	Subcutaneous
SL	Sublingual

Abbreviation	Translation
Drug Administration	
aa	Of each
ac	Before meals
ad lib	As desired, freely
bid	Twice a day
h or hr	Hour
hs	Hour of sleep, at bedtime
noct	Night
NPO	Nothing by mouth
pc	After meals
prn	When needed
qd*	Every day, once a day
qh	Every hour
qid	Four times a day
qod*	Every other day
Rx	Prescribe, take
stat	Immediately
tid	Three times a day

*Note: As part of its 2004 National Patient Safety Goals, and affirmed in 2005, the Joint Commission announced that all accredited organizations must discontinue using the following abbreviations, acronyms, and symbols: U, IU, qd, qod, MS, MSO_4, and $MgSO_4$. Also to be discontinued are trailing zeros and lack of leading zeros. In other words, a zero should never appear by itself *after* a decimal point (1 mg instead of 1.0 mg), and a zero should always be used *before* a decimal point (0.1 mg instead of .1 mg). In addition, abbreviations for drug names should not be used because they can be misinterpreted. Other items are being considered for future inclusion on the official "do not use" list, such as the @ sign (write out the word at) and the symbols > and < (write out as *greater than* and *less than*). The abbreviations "cc" and "μg" should also be avoided and are being considered for inclusion on future lists. For more information, please see *http://www.jointcommission.org/PatientSafety/DoNotUseList*.

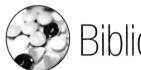

Bibliography

General

American Heart Association/American Stroke Association: *Heart disease and stroke statistics—2006 update* (At-a-Glance Version), Dallas, Tex, 2006, The Associations, available at *http://www.americanheart.org/downloadable/heart/1140534985281Statsupdate06book.pdf.*

Black JM: *Medical-surgical nursing: clinical management for positive outcomes*, ed 7, St Louis, 2004, Saunders.

Brunton L et al: *Goodman and Gilman's the pharmacological basis of therapeutics*, ed 11, New York, 2006, McGraw-Hill.

Burkhart PV, Rayens MK, Bowman RK: An evaluation of children's metered-dose inhaler technique for asthma medications, *Nurs Clin North Am* 40(1):167-182, 2005.

Christensen BL, Kockrow EO: *Adult health nursing*, ed 5, St Louis, 2006, Mosby.

Clayton BD: *Basic pharmacology for nurses*, ed 14, St Louis, 2006, Mosby.

Crouch MA: Chronic heart failure: developments and perspectives, *Consult Pharm* 20(9):751-765, 2005.

D'Arcy Y: What you need to know about fentanyl patches, *Nursing* 36(8):73, 2005.

Deglin JH, Vallerand AH: *Med notes: nurse's pocket pharmacology guide*, Philadelphia, 2004, FA Davis.

Dorland's illustrated medical dictionary, ed 31, Philadelphia, 2007, Saunders.

Drug facts and comparisons, St Louis, 2008, Wolters-Kluwer.

Emsam (selegiline transdermal system) [prescribing information], Morgantown, WVa, 2008, Somerset Pharmaceuticals, available at *http://www.emsam.com.*

Ferri FF: *Ferri's 2008 clinical advisor*, Philadelphia, 2008, Mosby.

Goldman L et al: *Cecil textbook of medicine*, ed 23, Philadelphia, 2007, Saunders.

Hausman KA: *Clinical companion for medical-surgical nursing: critical thinking for collaborative care*, ed 5, St Louis, 2006, Saunders.

Joint Commission: National patient safety goals, 2008, available at *http://www.jointcommission.org/PatientSafety/NationalPatientSafetyGoals/08_hap_npsgs.htm.*

Kee JL: *Pharmacology: a nursing process approach*, ed 5, St Louis, 2006, Saunders.

Kryger MH et al: *Principles and practices of sleep medicine*, ed 4, Philadelphia, 2005, Saunders.

Lacy CF et al, editors: *Drug information handbook*, ed 17, Hudson, Ohio, 2008, Lexi-Comp.

Maurer FA, Smith CA: *Community/public health nursing practice: health for families and populations*, ed 5, St Louis, 2009, Saunders.

McEvoy GK et al: *AHFS drug information 2005*, Bethesda, Md, 2005, American Society of Health-System Pharmacists.

McKenry LM, Tessier E, Hogan M: *Mosby's pharmacology in nursing*, ed 22, St Louis, 2006, Mosby.

Munoz C, Hilgenberg C: Ethnopharmacology, *Am J Nurs* 105(8):40-49, 2005.

Nathan DM et al: Management of hyperglycemia in type 2 diabetes: a consensus algorithm for the initiation and adjustment of therapy (update), *Diabetes Care* 31:173-175, 2008.

Perry AG, Potter PA: *Clinical nursing skills and techniques*, ed 6, St Louis, 2006, Mosby.

Potter PA: *Basic nursing: essentials for practice*, ed 6, St Louis, 2006, Mosby.

Rosso R et al: Calcium channel blockers and beta-blockers versus beta-blockers alone for preventing exercise-induced arrhythmias in catecholaminergic polymorphic ventricular tachycardia, *Heart Rhythm* 4(9):1140-1154, 2007.

Saag K et al: American College of Rheumatology 2008 recommendations for the use of nonbiologic and biologic disease-modifying antirheumatic drugs in rheumatoid arthritis, *Arthritis Rheum* 59(6):762-784, 2008.

Springhouse: Nursing 2010 drug handbook with Web toolkit, ed 13, Philadelphia, 2009, Lippincott Williams.

Sweetman SC et al: *Martindale: the complete drug reference*, ed 34, London, 2005, Pharmaceutical Press.

UpToDate online, version 16.2 [database online], 2008, available at *http://www.uptodate.com.*

US Food and Drug Administration: Sales of supplements containing ephedrine alkaloids (Ephedra) prohibited, April 12, 2004, available at *http://www.fda.gov/oc/initiatives/ephedra/february2004.*

Weir R et al: Heart failure in older patients, *Br J Cardiol* 13(4):257-266, 2006.

Woods A, Moshang J: Triple threat: diabetes, hypertension, and heart disease, *Nurs Manage* 36(11):27-33, 2005.

Chapter 1

Bulechek S: *Nursing interventions classification (NIC)*, ed 5, St Louis, 2008, Mosby.

Fesler-Birch DM: Critical thinking and patient outcomes: a review, *Nurs Outlook* 53(2):59-65, 2005.

Michalopoulos A, Michalopoulos H: Management's possible benefits from teamwork and the nursing process, *Nurse Leader* 4(3):52-55, 2006.

Moorhead SL, Johnson M, Mass ML, Swanson E: *Nursing outcomes classification (NOC)*, ed 4, St Louis, 2008, Mosby.

Mosby's pocket dictionary of medicine, nursing and health professions, ed 6, St Louis, 2010, Mosby.

NANDA International: *NANDA-I nursing diagnoses: definitions and classification 2009-2011*, Kaukauna, Wisc, 2008, NANDA International.

O'Connell D, Reifsteck SW: Disclosing unexpected outcomes and medical error, *J Med Pract Manage* 19(6):317-323, 2004.

Smetzer J: Take ten giant steps to medication safety, *Nursing* 31(11):49-53, 2001.

Chapter 3

Brager R, Sloand E: The spectrum of polypharmacy, *Nurse Pract* 30(6):44-50, 2005.

Chang CM et al: Use of the Beers criteria to predict adverse drug reaction among first-visit elderly outpatients, *Pharmacotherapy* 25(6):831-838, 2005. Available at *http://medscape.com/viewpublication/132_index.*

DiPiro JT et al: *Pharmacotherapy: a pathophysiologic approach*, ed 6, New York, 2005, McGraw-Hill.

Gallagher N, Petal AH: Inappropriate prescribing in the elderly, *J Clin Pharm Ther* 32(2):113-121, 2007.

Harrison JP, Ford D, Wilson K: The impact of hospice programs on U.S. hospitals, *Nurs Econ* 23(2):78-90, 2005.

Institute for Safe Medication Practices: Tablet splitting: do it only when you "half" to, and then do it safely, *ISMP Medication Safety Alert! Acute Care*, May 18, 2006. Available at *http://www.ismp.org/newsletters/acutecare/articles/20060518.asp*.

Mitchell SL et al: Terminal care for persons with advanced dementia in the nursing home and home care settings, *J Palliat Care Med* 7(6):808-816, 2004.

Molony S: Beers criteria for potentially inappropriate medication use in the elderly, 2004, 16(6): 547-548, available at *http://www.medscape.com/viewpublication/786_index*.

National Hospice and Palliative Care Organization: *NHPCO's facts and figures: hospice care in America*, Alexandria, Va, October 2008, National Hospice and Palliative Care Organization.

Osterberg L, Blaschke T: Adherence to medication, *NEJM* 353(5):487-497, 2005.

Shepler S et al: Keep your older patients out of medication trouble: learn why aging puts your patient at greater risk for adverse drug reactions and what you can do to protect her, *Nursing* 36(9):44-47, 2006.

Skidmore-Roth L: *Mosby's nursing drug reference*, ed 21, St Louis, 2008, Mosby.

Sutton PD: Births, marriages, divorces and deaths: provisional data for September 2007, *National Vital Statistics Reports*, 56(18), Hyattsville, Md, 2008, National Center for Health Statistics

Wick JY: The Beers criteria: red flags for elders, *Pharmacy Times*, p 56, June 2006. Available at *http://www.pharmacytimes.com/issues/articles/2006-06_3593.asp*.

Wooten J, Glass J: Polypharmacy: keeping the elderly safe, *RN* 68(8):44-50, 2005.

Chapter 4

Adams M: FDA under scrutiny as criticisms mount, March 26, 2005, available at *http://www.newstarget.com/005991.html*.

Lobiondo-Wood G: *Nursing research: methods and critical appraisal for evidence-based practice*, ed 6, St Louis, 2005, Mosby.

US Census Bureau: US Census Bureau news: an older and more diverse nation by midcentury, August 2008, *http://www.census.gov/Press-Release/www/releases/archives/population/012496.html*.

US Department of Defense, Tricare military health plan: Medicare Part D, September 2007, available at *http://www.tricare.mil/mybenefit/ProfileFilter.do*.

US Department of Health and Human Services, Centers for Medicare and Medicaid Services: Overview of Medicare Part D, available at *http://www.cms.hhs.gov/MMAUpdate/01_Overview.asp*.

US Department of Health and Human Services, Office of Civil Rights: Summary of the HIPAA privacy rule, May 2003, available at *http://www.hhs.gov/OCR/privacysummary.pdf*.

US Food and Drug Administration: Dietary supplements, July 2005, available at *http://www.cfsan.fda.gov/~dms/supplmnt.html*.

US Food and Drug Administration: FDA issues public health advisory on Vioxx as its manufacturer voluntarily withdraws the product, September 30, 2004, available at *http://www.fda.gov/bbs/topics/news/2004/NEW01122.html*.

US Food and Drug Administration: FDA issues safety alert on Avandia, May 21, 2007, available at *http://www.fda.gov/bbs/topics/NEWS/2007/NEW01636.html*.

US Food and Drug Administration: Timeline: chronology of drug regulation in the United States, available at *http://www.fda.gov/cder/about/history/time1.htm*.

US Food and Drug Administration, Office of Regulatory Affairs: Compliance policy guidelines, sec 420.200, compendium revisions and deletions (CPG 7132.02), available at *http://www.fda.gov/ora/compliance_ref/cpg/cpgdrg/cpg420-200.html*.

Chapter 5

Gates BJ et al: AmpliChip for cytochrome P-450 genotyping: the epoch of personalized prescriptions, *Hosp Pharm* 41:442-445, 2006.

Gene testing, gene therapy, pharmacogenomics, Human Genome Project Information website, June 11, 2003, available at *http://www.ornl.gov/TechResources/Human_Genome/home.html*.

Greco KE: Nursing in the genomic era: nurturing our genetic nature, *Medsurg Nurs* 12(5):307-312, 2003.

Kenna GA et al: Pharmacotherapy, pharmacogenomics, and the future of alcohol dependence treatment, part 2, *Am J Health Syst Pharm* 61:2380-2388, 2004.

Kreiner T, Buck KT: Moving toward whole-genome analysis: a technology perspective, *Am J Health Syst Pharm* 62:296-305, 2005.

Lea DH: Genetic and genomic healthcare: ethical issues of importance to nurses, *Online J Issues Nurs* 13(1):6, 2008.

Lea DH: Look back to move forward: how genetics changes daily practice, *Nurs Manage* 34(11):19-25, 2003.

Lea DH: Tailoring drug therapy with pharmacogenetics, *Nursing* 35(4):22-23, 2005.

Nicol MJ: The variation of response to pharmacotherapy: pharmacogenetics—a new perspective to "the right drug for the right person," *Medsurg Nurs* 12(4):242-249, 2003.

Nussbaum RL, McInnes RR, Willard HE: *Thompson and Thompson genetics in medicine*, ed 6, Philadelphia, 2004, Saunders.

Paice JA: Pharmacokinetics, pharmacodynamics, and pharmacogenomics of opioids, *Pain Manag Nurs* 8(3):82-85, 2007.

Pauli EK: Pharmacogenomics: going down the rabbit hole, *Formulary* 30(11):667-669, 2005.

Prows C: Genetics Summer Institute course, 2002.2004, available at *http://gepn.cchmc.org*.

Prows CA, Prows DR: Medication selection by genotype, *Am J Nurs* 104(5):60-70, 2004.

Teagarden JR: Pharmacogenomics and its potential uses in managed care pharmacy, *Hosp Pharm* 41:477-481, 2006.

Turnpenny P, Ellard S: *Emery's elements of medical genetics*, ed 12, London, 2005, Churchill Livingstone.

US Food and Drug Administration: FDA news: FDA clears first of kind genetic lab test, December 23, 2004, available at *http://www.fda.gov/bbs/topics/news/2004/new01149.html*.

Wooten JM: Drug watch 2006: new frontiers, *RN* 69(3):36-41, 2006.

Workman ML: Genetic concepts for medical-surgical nursing. In Ignatavicius DD, Workman ML, editors: *Medical-surgical nursing: critical thinking for collaborative care*, ed 6, St Louis, 2009, Saunders.

Chapter 6

American Medical Association: Physicians with disruptive behavior, January 2005, available at *http://www.ama-assn.org/ama/pub/category/8533.html*.

Barnsteiner JH: Medication reconciliation, *Am J Nurs* 105(3 suppl):31-36, 2005.

Clarin OA: Strategies to overcome barriers to effective nurse practitioner and physician collaboration, *J Nurse Pract*, 3(8):538-548, 2007, available at *http://www.medscape.com/viewarticle/568013*.

Cohen H: Protecting patients from harm: reduce the risks of high-alert drugs, *Nursing*, 37(9):49-55, 2007.

Cohen M: Medication errors: reconciling medications, safeguarding transitions, *Nursing* 34(7):14-16, 2005.

Dennison RD: Creating an organizational culture for medication safety, *Nurs Clin North Am* 40(1):1-23, 2005.

Feldman J: Magnet nursing and the healthcare team: a physician's view, 2007, available at *http://www.medscape.com/viewarticle/562949*.

Hughes RE, Edgerton EA: First, do no harm: reducing pediatric medication errors: children are especially at risk for medication errors, *Am J Nurs* 105(5):79-89, 2005.

Hughes RG, Ortiz E: Medication errors: why they happen and how they can be prevented, *Am J Nurs* 105(3 suppl):14-24, 2005.

Institute for Healthcare Improvement: Five million lives campaign, 2006.2008, available at *http://www.ihi.org//IHI/Programs/Campaign.*

Institute for Safe Medication Practices: High-reliability organizations (HROs): what they know that we don't (part I), July 14, 2005, available at *http://www.ismp.org/MSAarticles/20050714.htm.*

Institute for Safe Medication Practices: High-reliability organizations (HROs): what they know that we don't (part II), July 28, 2005, available at *http://www.ismp.org/MSAarticles/20050728.htm.*

Institute for Safe Medication Practices: ISMP's list of error-prone abbreviations, symbols, and dose designations, 2006, available at *http://www.ismp.org/Tools/errorproneabbreviations.pdf.*

Institute for Safe Medication Practices: ISMP's list of high-alert medications, 2007, available at *http://www.ismp.org/Tools/highalertmedications.pdf.*

Institute for Safe Medication Practices: Medication safety alert (regarding student nurse errors), *ISMP Safety Alert! Acute Care,* 12(21):1-3, 2007, available at *http://www.ismp.org/Newsletters/acutecare/articles/20071018.asp.*

Intravenous Nurses Society: Medication safety (symposium summary), *J Infus Nurs* 28:42-47, 2005.

The Joint Commission Speak Up, available at *www.jointcommission.org/generalpublic/speak+upabout_speakup.htm.*

Lafleur KJ: Tackling med errors with technology, *RN* 67(5):29-34, 2004.

Lazoritz S, Carlson PJ: Don't tolerate disruptive physician behavior, *Am Nurse Today* 3(3), 2008, available at *http://www.americannursetoday.com/article.aspx?id=4882&fid=4860#.*

Lindeke LL, Sieckert AM: Nurse-physician workplace collaboration, *Online J Issues Nurs* 10(1), 2005.

Manno MS, Hayes DD: Best-practice interventions: how medication reconciliation saves lives, *Nursing* 36(3):63-64, 2006.

Metules TJ, Bauer J: Part 1: JCAHO's patient safety goals: a practical guide, *RN* 69(12):21-27, 2006.

Metules TJ, Bauer J: Part 2: JCAHO's patient safety goals: a practical guide, *RN* 70(1):39-43, 2007.

O'Connell D et al: Disclosing unanticipated outcomes and medical errors, *J Clin Outcomes Manage* 10(1):25-29, 2003.

O'Reilly MA: Change and change again: nurse leaders in the new millennium: highlights of the National Association of Neonatal Nurses' 23rd annual conference, January 2008, available at *http://www.medscape.com/viewarticle/568013.*

Richardson WC et al: *To err is human: building a safer health system,* Washington DC, 1999, National Academies Press.

Rosenstein AH: Nurse-physician relationships: impact on nurse satisfaction and retention, *Am J Nurs* 102(6):26-34, 2002.

Rosenstein AH, O'Daniel M: Disruptive behavior and clinical outcomes: perceptions of nurses and physicians, *Am J Nurs* 105(1):54-65, 2005.

Smith DS, Haig K: Reduction of adverse drug events and medication errors in a community hospital setting, *Nurs Clin North Am* 40(1):25-32, 2005.

Spencer DC et al: Effect of a computerized prescriber-order-entry system on reported medication errors, *Am J Health Syst Pharm* 62(4):416-419, 2005.

Stetina P, Groves M, Pafford L: Managing medication errors—a qualitative study, *Medsurg Nurs* 14(3):174-178, 2005.

Tuohy N, Paparella S: Look-alike and sound-alike drugs: errors waiting to happen, *J Emerg Nurs* 31(6):569-571, 2005.

Wager N et al: The effects on ambulatory blood pressure of working under favourably and unfavourably perceived supervisors, *Occup Environ Med* 60:468-474, 2003.

Chapter 7

Aiken L et al: Educational levels of hospital nurses and surgical patient mortality, *JAMA* 290(12):1617-1623, 2003.

American Nurses Association: *Nursing: scope and standards of practice,* Silver Spring, Md, 2004, The Association.

Billings DM: *Teaching in nursing: a guide for faculty,* ed 2, St Louis, 2004, Saunders.

Broome B: Culture 101, *Urol Nurs* 26(6):486-489, 2006.

Canobbio MM: *Mosby's handbook of patient teaching,* ed 3, St Louis, 2006, Mosby.

Chang M, Kelly AE: Patient education: addressing cultural diversity and health literacy issues, *Urol Nurs* 27(5):411-417, 2007.

Cutilli CC: Do your patients understand? Determining your patient's health literacy skills, *Orthop Nurs* 24(5):372-377, 2005.

Joint Commission on Accreditation of Healthcare Organizations: *Accreditation manual for hospitals,* Oakbrook, Ill, 2006, The Commission.

Leininger MM: *Culture care diversity and universality: a worldwide nursing theory,* ed 2, Boston, 2006, Jones & Bartlett.

Nies MA: *Community/public health nursing: promoting the health of populations,* ed 4, St Louis, 2006, Saunders.

Rankin SH, Stallings KD, London F: *Patient education in health and illness,* ed 5, Philadelphia, 2005, Lippincott Williams & Wilkins.

Redman BK: *The practice of patient education,* ed 9, St Louis, 2001, Mosby.

US Department of Commerce: An older and more diverse nation by midcentury [press release], August 14, 2008, available at *http://www.census.gov/Press-Release/www/releases/archives/population/012496.html.*

Chapter 8

Aschenbrenner DS: The conversion of a prescription drug to OTC status, *Am J Nurs* 107(3):54-57, 2007.

Berardi RR et al: *Handbook of nonprescription drugs,* ed 14, Washington, DC, 2004, American Pharmacists Association.

Bressler R: Herb-drug interactions: interactions between ginseng and prescription medications, *Geriatrics* 60(7):16-17, 2005.

Bressler R: Herb-drug interactions: St. John's wort and prescription medications, *Geriatrics* 60(7):21-23, 2005.

D'Arcy Y: Safety first: what you need to know about NSAIDs, *Nursing made incredibly easy!* 5(2):13-15, 2007.

Hoblyn J: Herbal supplements in older adults, *Geriatrics* 60(2):18-23, 2005.

Huang SM et al: Drug interactions with herbal products and grapefruit juice, *Clin Pharmacol Ther* 75(1):1-12, 2004.

Hulisz D: Top herbal products: efficacy and safety concerns [continuing medical education module], MedscapeCME website, 2007, available at *http:www.cme.medscape.com/viewprogram/8494.*

Hussar DA: Introduction to over-the-counter drugs, Merck Manual of Medical Information—Second Home Edition [online], April 2007, available at *http://www.merck.com/mmhe/print/sec02/ch018/ch018b.html.*

Ignatavicius DD, Workman ML: *Medical-surgical nursing: critical thinking for collaborative care,* ed 5, St Louis, 2006, Saunders.

Institute for Safe Medication Practices: A call to action: protecting U.S. citizens from inappropriate medication use, available at *http://www.ismp.org/pressroom/viewpoints/CommunityPharmacy.pdf.*

Institute for Safe Medication Practices, Medicine cabinet, available at *http://www.ismp.org/pressroom/viewpoints/CommunityPharmacy.pdf.*

Lam A, Bradley G: Use of self-prescribed non-prescription mediations and dietary supplements in assisted living facility residents, *J Am Pharm Assoc* 46:574-581, 2006.

Mennick F: Infant deaths with cold medications, *Am J Nurs* 107(3):22, 2007.

Miller L, editor: *Chain pharmacy industry profile*, ed 9, Alexandria, Va, 2006, National Association of Chain Drug Stores Foundation, p 8.

Miller S: Drug watch '06: vitamins and minerals, *RN* 69(10):37-43, 2006.

Millions suffer from addiction to OTC nasal sprays, Medical News Today website, July 13, 2005, available at *http://www.medicalnewstoday. com/articles/27323.php.*

National Center for Complementary and Alternative Medicine website, available at *http://nccam.nih.gov.*

Sand-Jecklin K, Hoggatt B, Badzek L: Know the benefits and risks of using common herbal therapies, *Holist Nurs Pract* 18(4):192-198, 2004.

Soeken K: Selected CAM therapies for arthritis-related pain: the evidence from systematic reviews, *Clin J Pain* 20(1):13-18, 2004.

Tall J, Raja S: Dietary constituents as novel therapies for pain, *Clin J Pain* 20(1):19-26, 2004.

US Food and Drug Administration: Consumer update: OTC cough and cold products: not for infants and children under 2 years of age, January 17, 2008, available at *http://www.fda.gov/consumer/updates/ coughcold011708.html.*

US Food and Drug Administration: Evidence on the safety and effectiveness of ephedra: implications for regulation, February 23, 2003, available at *http://www.fda.gov/bbs/topics/NEWS/ephedra/whitepaper.html.*

US Food and Drug Administration: FDA facts sheet: dietary supplement current good manufacturing practices (CGMPs) and interim final rule (IFR) facts, June 22, 2007, available at *http://www.cfsan.fda.gov/ ~dms/dscgmps6.html.*

US Food and Drug Administration: FDA news: FDA releases recommendations regarding use of over-the-counter cough and cold products, January 17, 2008, available at *http://www.fda.gov/bbs/topics/ NEWS/2008/NEW01778.html.*

US Food and Drug Administration: Kava-containing dietary supplements may be associated with severe liver injury, March 25, 2002, available at *http://www.cfsan.fda.gov/~dms/addskava.html.*

US Food and Drug Administration: The new over-the-counter medicine label: take a look, March 7, 2006, available at *http://www.fda.gov/ cder/consumerinfo/OTClabel.htm.*

US Food and Drug Administration: Overview of dietary supplements, August 17, 2005, available at *http://www.cfsan.fda.gov/~dms/ ds-oview.html#what.*

US Food and Drug Administration: Public health advisory: nonprescription cough and cold medicine use in children, January 17, 2008, available at *http://www.fda.gov/cder/drug/advisory/cough_cold_2008.htm.*

US Food and Drug Administration, Office of Nonprescription Products: What we do, May 2003, available at *http://www.fda.gov/cder/Offices/ OTC/whatwedo.htm.*

Chapter 9

Bauer J: Smokers get another option to help them kick the habit, *RN* 69(7):58, 2006.

Campral (acamprosate calcium) delayed-release tablets [prescribing information], St Louis, August 2005, Forest Pharmaceuticals, available at *http://www.campral.com.*

Carpenter-Palumbo KM: New York Office of Alcoholism and Substance Abuse Services (OASAS), Albany, NY, 2005, available at *http://www. oasas.state.ny.us/index.cfm?level=communications#.*

Copello AG, Templeton L, Velleman R: Family interventions for drug and alcohol misuse: is there a best practice? *Curr Opin Psychiatry* 12(3):271-276, 2006.

Ewing JA: Detecting alcoholism: the CAGE questionnaire, *JAMA* 252:1905-1907, 1984.

Flammer M: Chantix (varenicline) package insert [safety] update, January 17, 2008, available at *http://www.chantix.com.*

Greenberg M: *Occupational, industrial, and environmental toxicology*, ed 2, Philadelphia, 2003, Mosby.

Hamid H, El-Mallakh R, Vandeveir K: Substance abuse: medical and slang terminology, *South Med J* 98(3):350-362, 2005.

Quitting can be different this time, Chantix website, 2009, available at *http://www.chantix.com.*

Stoll D, King LE Jr: Disulfiram-alcohol skin reaction to beer-containing shampoo, *JAMA* 244(18):2045, 1980.

Substance Abuse and Mental Health Services Administration: Legal but lethal: the danger of abusing over-the-counter drugs, available at *http://www.family/samhsa.gov/get/otcdrugs.asp.*

Substance Abuse and Mental Health Services Administration, Office of Applied Studies: National Survey on Drug Use and Health: misuse of over-the-counter cough and cold medications among persons aged 12 to 25, January 10, 2008, available at *http://www.oas.samhsa. gov/2k8/cough/cough.htm.*

Substance Abuse and Mental Health Services Administration, Office of Applied Studies: Substance Abuse and Mental Health Data Archive (SAMHDA), July 2008, available at *http://oas.samhsa.gov/ SAMHDA.htm.*

US Department of Justice: Intelligence brief: huffing: the abuse of inhalants, November 2001, available at *http://www.usdoj.gov/ndic/pub07/ 708/708p.pdf.*

US Food and Drug Administration: Early communication about an ongoing safety review: varenicline (marketed as Chantix), November 20, 2007, available at *http://www.fda.gov/cder/drug/early_comm/ varenicline.htm.*

US Food and Drug Administration: FDA approves novel medication for smoking cessation, May 11, 2006, available at *http://www.fda.gov/ bbs/topics/NEWS/2006/NEW01370.html.*

US Food and Drug Administration: FDA issues early communication for Chantix, November 20, 2007, available at *http://www.fda.gov/bbs/ topics/NEWS/2007/NEW01749.html.*

US Food and Drug Administration: FDA talk paper: FDA approves new drug for treatment of alcoholism, July 29, 2004, available at *http:// www.fda.gov/bbs/topics/answers/2004/ANS01302.html.*

US Food and Drug Administration, Center for Drug Evaluation and Research: Legal requirements for the sale and purchase of drug products containing pseudoephedrine, ephedrine, and phenylpropanolamine, May 8, 2006, available at *http://www.fda.gov/cder/news/ methamphetamine.htm.*

US Food and Drug Administration, Center for Drug Evaluation and Research: OxyContin: questions and answers, July 2001, available at *http://www.fda.gov/cder/drug/infopage/oxycontin/oxycontin-qa.htm.*

Chapter 10

Bower MLM: Is your patient's metered-dose inhaler technique up to snuff? *Nursing* 35(8):50-51, 2005.

Carter-Templeton H, McCoy T: Are we on the same page? A comparison of intramuscular injection explanations in nursing fundamental texts, *Medsurg Nurs* 17(4):237-240, 2008.

Hadaway LC: IV rounds: delivering multiple medications via backpriming, *Nursing* 34(3):24-26, 2004.

Hockenberry MJ et al: *Wong's nursing care of infants and children*, ed 8, St Louis, 2007, Mosby.

Ignatavicius DD: Asking the right questions about medication safety, *Nursing* 30(9):51-54, 2000.

Institute for Safe Medication Practices: Hazard alert! Asphyxiation possible with syringe tip caps, *ISMP Medication Safety Alert!* August 2001. Available at *http://www.ismp.org/hazardalerts/Hypodermic. asp.*

Institute for Safe Medication Practices: How fast is too fast for IV push medication? *ISMP Medication Safety Alert!* May 15, 2003. Available at *http://www.ismp.org/Newsletters/acutecare/articles/ 20030515.asp?ptr=y.*

Jacobs B: Using an infusion pump safely, *Nursing* 36(10):24, 2006.

Karch A: Not so fast! IV push drugs can be dangerous when given too rapidly, *Am J Nurs* 103(8):71, 2003.

Lee M, Phillips J: FDA safety page—transdermal patches: high risk for error? *Drug Topics*, pp 54-55, April 1, 2002.

Love GH: Clinical do's and don'ts: administering an intradermal injection, *Nursing* 36(6):20, 2006.

McConnell E: Clinical do's and don'ts: applying nitroglycerin ointment, *Nursing* 31(6):17, 2001.

McErlane K: Keeping track of the patch: transdermal delivery in obese patients, *Am J Nurs* 105(6):36-37, 2005.

Miller D, Miller H: To crush or not to crush? *Nursing* 30(2):50-52, 2000.

Moshang J: Making a point about insulin pens, *Nursing* 35(2):46-47, 2005.

National Drug Data File Plus: intravenous module, First Data Bank website, September 9, 2008, available at *http://www.firstdatabank.com/products/nddf/clinical/intravenous.aspx*.

Nicoll LH, Hesby A: Intramuscular injection: an integrative research review and guideline for evidence-based practice, *Appl Nurs Res* 16(2):149-162, 2002.

Padula CA et al: Enteral feedings: what the evidence says, *Am J Nurs* 104(7):62-70, 2004.

Pruitt W: Teaching your patient to use a peak flowmeter, *Nursing* 35(3):54-55, 2005.

Pullen R: Clinical do's and don'ts: administering medication by the Z-track method, *Nursing* 35(7):24, 2005.

Pullen R: Clinical do's and don'ts: administering an orally disintegrating tablet, *Nursing* 38(1):18, 2008.

Pullen R: Clinical do's and don'ts: managing IV patient-controlled analgesia, *Nursing* 33(7):24, 2003.

Reising DL, Neal RS: Enteral tube flushing, *Am J Nurs* 105(3):58-63, 2005.

Rushing J: Clinical do's and don'ts: administering eyedrops, *Nursing* 37(5):18, 2007.

Schulmeister L: Transdermal drug patches: medicine with muscle, *Nursing* 35(1):48-52, 2005.

Stein HG: Glass ampules and filter needles: an example of implementing the sixth "r" in medication administration, *Medsurg Nurs* 15(5):290-294, 2006.

Uko-Ekpenyong G: Improving medication adherence with orally disintegrating tablets, *Nursing* 36(9):20-21, 2006.

Chapter 11

Abboud L: Actiq's use and abuse raise concern, *Wall Street Journal*, May 17, 2004.

Acetadote (acetylcysteine) injection [prescribing information], Nashville, Tenn, February 2006, Cumberland Pharmaceuticals, available at *http://www.acetadote.net*

American Pain Society: Definitions related to the use of opioids for the treatment of pain, 2008, available at *http://www.ampainsoc.org/advocacy/opioids2.htm*.

American Society for Pain Management Nursing: ASPMN position statement: pain management in patients with addictive disease, September 2002, available at *http://www.aspmn.org/Organization/documents/addictions_9pt.pdf*.

Cohen MR: Acetylcysteine routes: mistakes in the mist? *Nursing* 35(6):12, 2005.

Cohen MR: Epidural injection: long-acting concerns, *Nursing* 35(6):12, 2005.

D'Arcy Y: Conquering pain: have you tried these new techniques? *Nursing* 35(3):36-41, 2005.

D'Arcy Y: New pain management options: delivery systems and techniques, *Nursing* 37(2):26-27, 2007.

D'Arcy Y: Which analgesic is right for my patient? *Nursing* 36(7):50-55, 2006.

DepoDur [prescribing information], San Diego, Calif, February 2007, Pacira Pharmaceuticals, available at *http://www.depodur.com*.

Drug news: FDA advisory: more deaths linked to methadone, *Nursing* 37(2)31, 2007.

Drug news: new non-narcotic eases chronic pain, *Nursing* 35(6): 2005.

Drug update: a longer-lasting option for chronic pain patients (Ultram ER), *RN* 69(8):58, 2006.

Drug round-up: announcement on hazards of alcohol with opiates such as Avinza, *RN* 68(12):32hf3, 2005.

Duragesic (fentanyl) transdermal system [prescribing information], Titusville, NJ, April 2007, Ortho-McNeil-Janssen Pharmaceuticals, available at *http://www.duragesic.com*.

Grace PJ: The clinical use of placebos: is it ethical? Not when it involves deceiving patients, *Am J Nurs* 106(2):58-61, 2006.

Keller DL: Pain relievers, *RN* 69(4):22-27, 2006.

Kim HS et al: Strategies of pain assessment used by nurses on surgical units, *Pain Manag Nurs* 6(1):3-9,2005.

Kolcaba K: *Comfort theory and practice: a vision for holistic health care research*, Portland, Ore, 2003, Springer Publishing.

Lidoderm (lidocaine patch 5%) [prescribing information], Chadds Ford, Pa, April 2006, Endo Pharmaceuticals, available at *http://www.lidoderm.com/prescrib.aspx*.

Lillefjell M, Kroskstad S, Espnes GA: Prediction of function in daily life following multidisciplinary rehabilitation for individuals with chronic musculoskeletal pain: a prospective study, *BMC Musculoskelet Disord*, 2007, available at *http://www.medscapenursing.com/viewarticle/563476*.

McCaffery M, Arnstein P: The debate over placebos in pain management, *Am J Nurs* 106(2):62-65, 2006.

Nanna B et al: An evidence-based algorithm for the treatment of neuropathic pain, *MedGenMed* 9(2):36, 2007.

National Cancer Institute: Basic principles of cancer pain management, November 2005, available at *http://www.nci.nih.gov/cancertopics/pdq/supportivecare/pain/Patient/page4*.

Natural Standard: Feverfew, 2007, available at *http://www.naturalstandard.com*.

Olson J: *Clinical pharmacology made ridiculously simple*, Miami, Fla, 2003, MedMaster.

Opana and Opana ER: information for health care professionals, 2006-2007, available at *http://www.opana.com*.

Pasero C, McCaffery M: Authorized and unauthorized use of PCA pumps: clarifying the use of patient-controlled analgesia, in light of recent alerts. *AJN* 105(7):30-32, 2005

Plaisance L, Logan C: Nursing students' knowledge and attitudes regarding pain, *Pain Manag Nurs* 7(4):167-175, 2006.

Portenoy RK: Chronic pain, Merck Manuals Online Medical Library, February 2007, available at *http://www.merck.com/mmpe/print/sec16/ch209/ch209b.html*.

Portenoy RK: Pain: introduction, Merck Manuals Online Medical Library, February 2007, available at *http://www.merck.com/mmpe/print/sec16/ch209/ch209a.html*.

Prialt (ziconotide intrathecal infusion) [prescribing information], South San Francisco, Calif, April 2007, Elan Pharmaceuticals, available at *http://www.prialt.com*.

Raffanello TW: To do no harm: strategies for preventing prescription drug abuse, DEA Congressional testimony, February 9, 2004, available at *http://www.usdoj.gov/dea/pubs/cngrtest/ct020904.htm*.

Roman M, Cabaj T: Epidural analgesia, *Medsurg Nurs* 14(4):257-259, 2005.

Schulmeister L: Stuck on you: transdermal drug patches, *Nursing Made Incredibly Easy!* March/April:17, 2007.

Snow M: Shutting down shingles, *Nursing* 36(4):18-19, 2006.

US Food and Drug Administration: FDA approves Actiq for marketing, November 5, 1998, available at *http://www.fda.gov/bbs/topics/ ANSWERS/ANS00921.html*.

US Food and Drug Administration: FDA news: FDA issues second safety warning on fentanyl skin patch, December 21, 2007, available at *http://www.fda/gov/bbs/topics/NEWS/2007/NEW01762.html*.

US Food and Drug Administration: Proper use of fentanyl patches, March-April 2006, available at *http://www.fda.gov/fdac/features/ 2006/206_fentanyl.html*.

World Health Organization: Pain ladder for cancer pain, 2008, available at *http://www.who.int/cancer/palliative/painladder/en/print.html*.

Chapter 12

American Association of Nurse Anesthetists: Conscious sedation: what patients should expect, available at *http://www.aana.com/uploadedFiles/ For_Patients/sedation_brochure03.pdf*.

Brenman EK, editor: Pain management: spinal headaches, 2007, available at *http://www.webmd.com*.

Carter-Templeton H: Malignant hyperthermia, *Nursing* 35(6):88, 2005.

Drain CB: *Perianesthesia nursing: a critical care approach*, ed 4, St Louis, 2003, Saunders.

Dripps RD et al: *Introduction to anesthesia: the principles of safe practice*, ed 7, Philadelphia, 1988, Saunders.

Halliday AB: Shades of sedation: learning about moderate sedation and analgesia, *Nursing* 36(4):36-41, 2006.

Koda-Kimble M et al: *Applied therapeutics: the clinical use of drugs*, ed 8, Baltimore, 2005, Lippincott Williams & Wilkins.

Litman DO, Rosenberg H: Malignant hyperthermia, *JAMA* 293(23):2918-2924, 2005.

Miller R et al: *Miller's anesthesia*, ed 6, Philadelphia, 2005, Churchill Livingstone.

Pasero C, McCaffery M: Ketamine: low doses may provide some relief for painful conditions, *Am J Nurs* 105(4):60-64, 2005.

Schwartz A: Learning the essentials of epidural anesthesia, *Nursing* 36(1):44-49, 2006.

Chapter 13

Lunesta (eszopiclone) tablets [prescribing information], Marlborough, Mass, April 2007, Sepracor Pharmaceuticals, available at *http://www. lunesta.com*.

Monthly Prescribing Reference 24(1), January 2008, available at *http:// www.PrescribingReference.com*.

Roberts I: Barbiturates for acute traumatic brain injury, *Cochrane Database Syst Rev* Issue 2:CD000033, 1999 [last assessed as up to date March 1, 2006].

Rozerem (ramelteon) tablets [prescribing information], Deerfield, Ill, 2006, Takeda Pharmaceuticals, available at *http://www.rozerem.com*.

Scheid CD et al: Treatment options for insomnia, *Am Fam Physician* 76(4):517-526, 2007.

Tariq SH et al: Pharmacotherapy for insomnia, *Clin Geriatr Med* 24:93-105, 2008.

Watanabe N, Churchill R, Furukawa TA: Combination of psychotherapy and benzodiazepines versus either therapy alone for panic disorder: a systematic review, *BMC Psychiatry* 7:18-20, 2007. Available at *http:// www.medscape.com*.

Chapter 14

Apnea of prematurity, Merck Manuals Online Medical Library, November 2005, available at *http://www.merck.com/mmpe/print/sec19/ch277/ ch277c.html*.

Aschenbrenner DS: ADHD drug withdrawn: risk of liver failure outweighs favorable effects, *Am J Nurs* 106(2):29-30, 2006.

Attention-deficit/hyperactivity disorder, Merck Manuals Online Medical Library, November 2005, available at *http://www.merck.com/mmpe/ print/sec19/ch299/ch299b.html*.

Centers for Disease Control and Prevention: Body mass index, December 2004, available at *http://www.cdc.gov/nccdphp/dnpa/bmi/index.htm*.

Centers for Disease Control and Prevention: Body mass index formula for adults, July 2005, available at *http://www.cdc.gov/nccdphp/dnpa/ bmi/bmi-adult-formula.htm*.

Centers for Disease Control and Prevention: Overweight and obesity, September 2005, available at *http://www.cdc.gov/nccdphp/dnpa/obesity*.

Centers for Disease Control and Prevention: Overweight and obesity: defining overweight and obesity, September 2005, available at *http:// www.cdc.gov/nccdphp/dnpa/obesity/defining.htm*.

Centers for Disease Control and Prevention, National Center for Health Statistics: Obesity still a major problem, new data show, October 2004, available at *http://www.cdc.gov/nchs/pressroom/04facts/obesity.htm*.

Centers for Disease Control and Prevention, National Center for Health Statistics: Prevalence of overweight and obesity among adults: United States, 1999.2002, December 2004, available at *http://www.cdc.gov/ nchs/products/pubs/pubd/hestats/obese/obse99.htm*.

Cohen AL et al: Stimulant medications and attention deficit-hyperactivity disorder, *N Engl J Med*, 354(21):2294-2295, 2006.

Jones HR: *Netter's neurology*, Teterboro, NJ, 2005, Icon Learning Systems.

Metabolic syndrome, Merck Manuals Online Medical Library, November 2005, available at *http://www.merck.com/mmpe/print/sec01/ch006/ ch006b.html*.

Migraine, Merck Manuals Online Medical Library, November 2005, available at *http://www.merck.com/mmpe/print/sec16/ch216/ch216d.html*.

Moss SB et al: Attention deficit/hyperactivity disorder in adults, *Prim Care* 34:445-473, 2007.

Narcolepsy, Merck Manuals Online Medical Library, November 2005, available at *http://www.merck.com/mmpe/print/sec16/ch215/ch215d.html*.

National Institutes of Health: Statistics related to overweight and obesity, October 2004, available at *http://win.niddk.nih.gov/statistics/index.htm*.

Nishino S: Narcolepsy, *Sleep Med Clin* 1:47-61, 2006.

Nissen S: ADHD drugs and cardiovascular risk, *NEJM* 354(14):1445-1448, 2006

Obesity, Merck Manuals Online Medical Library, November 2005, available at *http://www.merck.com/mmpe/print/sec01/ch006/ch006a.html*.

Orzano JA, Scott JG: Diagnosis and treatment of obesity in adults: an applied evidence-based review, *J Am Board Fam Pract* 17(5):359-369, 2004. Available at *http://www.medscape.com/viewarticle/489073_print*.

SayNo, a "eDrugRehab" website available at *http://www.sayno.com/ stimlant.html*.

Schardt D: Caffeine: the inside scoop, *Nutrition Action Health Letter, Center for the Science in the Public Interest*, March 2008, 1-6, available at *http://cspinet.org/nah/02_08/caffeine.pdf*.

US Department of Health and Human Services: FDA approves orlistat for obesity, 2001, available at *http://www.fda.gov/bbs/topics*.

US Food and Drug Administration: FDA announces rule prohibiting sale of dietary supplements containing ephedrine alkaloids effective April 12, April 12, 2004, available at *http://www.fda.gov/bbs/topics/ NEWS/2004/NEW01050.html*.

US Food and Drug Administration: FDA issues public health advisory on Strattera (atomoxetine) for attention deficit disorder, available at *http://www.fda.gov/bbs/topics/news/2005/new01237.html*.

US Food and Drug Administration: FDA issues regulation prohibiting sale of dietary supplements containing ephedrine alkaloids and reiterates its advice that consumers stop using these products, February 6, 2004, available at *http://www.fda.gov/bbs/topics/NEWS/2004/NEW01050.html*.

US Food and Drug Administration: FDA news: FDA approves orlistat for over-the-counter use, February 2007, available at *http://www.fda.gov/ bbs/topics/NEWS/2007/NEW01557.html*.

US Food and Drug Administration: Public health advisory: suicidal thinking in children and adolescents being treated with Strattera (atomoxetine), August 2005, available at *http://www.fda.gov/cder/drug/ advisory/atomoxetine.htm*.

US Food and Drug Administration: Talk paper: FDA approves Xyrem for cataplexy attacks in patients with narcolepsy, July 17, 2002, available at *http://www.fda.gov/bbs/topics/ANSWERS/2002/ANS01157.html.*

WebMD website, 2009, available at *http://www.webmd.com/add-adhd/default.htm.*

Chapter 15

Bergey GK: Initial treatment of epilepsy: special issues in treating the elderly, *Neurology* 63(10 suppl 4):S40-S48, 2004.

Brodie MJ, Kwan P: Epilepsy in elderly people, *BMJ* 331:1317-1322, 2005.

Chen JWY, Wasterlain CG: Status epilepticus: pathophysiology and management in adults, *Lancet Neurol* 5:246-256, 2006.

Drugs news: fibromyalgia: anticonvulsant offers pain relief, *Nursing* 37(2):31, 2007.

Drug news: seizure control: easy to use gel approved for home use, *Nursing* 36(2):30, 2006.

Duncan JS et al: Adult epilepsy, *Lancet* 367:1087-1100, 2006.

Gabitril [prescribing information], Frazer, Penn, Cephalon Inc., 2008, available at *http://www.gabitril.com.*

Gold Standard: Pregabalin, Clinical Pharmacology [database online], September 2007, available at *http://www.clinicalpharmacology.com.*

Hussar DA: New drugs '06: part II: pregabalin, *Nursing* 36(8):56-57, 2006.

International League Against Epilepsy: Seizure types, 2008, available at *http://www.ilae-epilepsy.org/Visitors/Centre/ctf/seizure_types.cfm.*

Keppra [prescribing information], S.A. Belgium, UCB, 2007, available at *http://www.keppra.com.*

Lamictal [prescribing information], Research Triangle Park, NC, Glaxo-SmithKlein, 2008, available at *http://www.lamictal.com.*

Living with epilepsy: day-to-day, Keppra website, available at *http://www.keppra.com/pc/living_with_epilepsy/day-to-day_activities2.asp.*

Living with epilepsy: epilepsy and seniors: age-old question, Keppra website, 2009, available at *http://www.keppra.com/pc/living_with_epilespy/seniors.asp.*

Lyrica [prescribing information], NewYork, NY, Pfizer, 2008, available at *http://www.lyrica.com.*

Neurontin [prescribing information], New York, NY, Pfizer, 2007, available at *http://www.neurontin.com.*

Seizure disorders, Merck Manuals Online Medical Library, November 2005, available at *http://www.merck.com/mmpe/print/sec16/ch214/ch214a.html.*

Springhouse nurse's drug guide 2005, Philadelphia, 2005, Lippincott Williams & Wilkins.

Sullivan MG: Drug information: drug updates story: coverage policies shouldn't influence anticonvulsant prescribing, says American Academy of Neurology, Mosby's Nursing Consult [database online], April 16, 2007, available at *http://www.nursingconsult.com/das/news/body/2/drug/674810905/185058/1.html.*

Szocke CE et al: Update on pharmacogenetics in epilepsy: a brief review, *Lancet Neurol* 5:189-196, 2006.

Tebb Z, Tobias JD: New anticonvulsants—new adverse effects, *South Med J* 99:375-379, 2006.

Tocco S: Evidence-based nursing monographs: epilepsy, December 26, 2007, Mosby's Nursing Consult [database online], available at *http://www.nursingconsult.com/das/news/body/2/ebnm/674810902/190851/1.html.*

Trileptal [prescribing information], Basel, Switzerland, Novartis Pharmaceuticals, 2008, available at *http://www.trileptal.com.*

Types of seizures, Epilepsy Canada website, 2005, available at *http://www.epilepsy.ca/eng/content/types.html.*

US Food and Drug Administration: Consumer update: serious health risks with antiepileptic drugs, February 5, 2008, available at *http://www.fda.gov/consumer/updates/antiepileptic020508.html.*

US Food and Drug Administration: FDA news: FDA alerts health care providers to risk of suicidal thoughts and behavior with antiepileptic medications, January 31, 2008, available at *http://www.fda.gov/bbs/topics/NEWS/2008/NEW01786.html.*

US Food and Drug Administration: Information for healthcare professionals: suicidality and antiepileptic drugs, January 31, 2008, available at *http://www.fda.gov/cder/drug/InfoSheets/HCP/antiepilepticsHCP.htm.*

US Food and Drug Administration: News alert: FDA requires warnings about risk of suicidal thoughts and behavior for antiepileptic medications, available at *http://www.fda.gov/bbs/topics/NEWS/2008/NEW01927.html.*

US Food and Drug Administration: Suicidal behavior and ideation and antiepileptic drugs, February 1, 2008, available at *http://www.fda.gov/cder/drug/infopage/antiepileptics/default.htm.*

US Food and Drug Administration: Tiagabine hydrochloride (marketed as Gabitril) information: seizures in patients without epilepsy, February 18, 2005, available at *http://www.fda.gov/cder/drug/infopage/tiagabine/default.htm.*

Vigevano F: Levetiracetam in pediatrics, *J Child Neurol* 20(2):87-93, 2005.

Waknine Y: FDA approvals: Keppra and Soliris, available at *http://www.medscape.com/viewarticle/2008.*

Wilby J et al: Clinical effectiveness, tolerability and cost-effectiveness of newer drugs for epilepsy in adults: a systematic review and economic evaluation, *Health Technol Assess* 9(15):1-157, iii-iv, 2005.

Zoler ML: Drug information: drug updates story: bioequivalence of epilepsy drugs questioned, Mosby's Nursing Consult [database online], December 20, 2007, available at *http://www.nursingconsult.com/das/news/body/2/drug/674810905/190966/1.html.*

Zonegran [prescribing information]. Woodclif Lake, NJ, Eisai Pharmaceuticals, 2008, available at *www.zonegran.com.*

Chapter 16

American Academy of Neurology: An algorithm (decision tree) for the management of Parkinson's disease: treatment guidelines, MD Consult [database online], 2001, available at *http://www.mdconsult.com/das/article/body/87782159-2.*

Apokyn (apomorphine hydrochloride injection) [prescribing information], Morristown, NJ, 2007, Vernalis Pharmaceuticals, available at *http://www.apokyn.com.*

Azilect (rasagiline tablets) [prescribing information], Kansas City, Mo, 2007, Teva Neuroscience, available at *http://www.azilect.com.*

Bonuccelli U: Role of dopamine agonists in Parkinson's disease: an update, *Expert Rev Neurother* 7(10):1391-1399, 2007.

Bradley WG et al: *Neurology in clinical practice*, Philadelphia, 2004, Butterworth-Heinemann.

Chen JJ, Ly A: Resagiline: a second-generation monoamine oxidase type-B inhibitor for the treatment of Parkinson's disease, *American Journal of Health-System Pharmacy*, 2006, available at *http://www.medscape.com/viewarticle/532116.*

Edwards KR: Conference report: highlights of the 8th International Conference on Alzheimer's and Parkinson's Disease, 2007, available at *http://www.medscape.com.*

Eidelberg D, Pourfar M: Parkinson's disease, Merck Manuals Online Medical Library, available at *http://www.merck.com/mmpe.*

Gasser T: Update on the genetics of Parkinson's disease, *Mov Disord* 22(17 suppl):S343-S350, 2007.

Hauser RA: Long-term care of Parkinson's disease: strategies for managing "wearing off" symptom re-emergence and dyskinesias, *Geriatrics* 61(9):14-20, 2006.

Juri CC: Levodopa for Parkinson's disease: what have we learned? *Rev Med Chil* 134(7):893-901, 2006.

Linton AD: *Introduction to medical-surgical nursing*, ed 4, St Louis, 2007, Saunders.

National Institutes of Health, National Institute of Neurological Disorders and Stroke: NINDS Parkinson's disease information page, April 2008, available at *http://www.ninds.nih.gov/disorders/parkinsons_disease/parkinsons_disease.htm*.

Neupro recall information, March 2008, available at *http://www.neupro.com*.

Nyholm D: Pharmacokinetic optimisation in the treatment of Parkinson's disease: an update. *Clin Pharmacokinet* 45(2):109-136, 2006.

Pahwa R: *Practice parameter: treatment of Parkinson disease with motor fluctuations and dyskinesia (an evidence-based review): report of the Quality Standards Subcommittee of the American Academy of Neurology*, St Paul, Minn, February 2006, American Academy of Neurology.

Parkinson's disease, MedlinePlus website, 2009, available at *http://www.nlm.nih.gov/medlineplus/parkinsonsdisease.html*.

Parkinson's disease: the basics, WebMD website, June 2005, available at *http://www.webmd.com/parkinsons-disease/parkinsons-overview*.

Scatena R: An update on pharmacological approaches to neurodegenerative diseases, *Expert Opin Investig Drugs* 16(1):59-72, 2007.

Singh C: Pesticides and metals induced Parkinson's disease: involvement of free radicals and oxidative stress, *Mol Biol* 53(5):19-28, 2007.

Suchowersky O: *Practice parameter: neuroprotective strategies and alternative therapies for Parkinson disease (an evidence-based review): report of the Quality Standards Subcommittee of the American Academy of Neurology*, St Paul, Minn, January 2006, American Academy of Neurology.

Thomure A: Helping your patient manage Parkinson's disease, *Nursing* 36(8):20-21, 2006.

US Food and Drug Administration: Consumer health information: Neupro patch for Parkinson's approved, May 2007, available at *http://www.fda.gov/consumer/updates/neupro051407.html*.

US Food and Drug Administration: FDA news: FDA approves new treatment for Parkinson's disease, May 2006, available at *http://www.fda.gov/bbs/topics/NEWS/2006/NEW01373.html*.

US Food and Drug Administration: FDA talk paper: FDA approves expanded use of brain implant for Parkinson's disease, January 2002, available at *http://www.fda.gov/bbs/topics/ANSWERS/2002/ANS01130.html*.

US Food and Drug Administration: FDA talk paper: new warnings for Parkinson's drug, Tasmar, November 16, 1998, available at *http://www.fda/gov/bbs/topiccs/ANSWERS/ANS00924.html*.

van Eimeren T: An update on functional neuroimaging of parkinsonism and dystonia, *Curr Opin Neurol* 19(4):412-419, 2006.

van Hilten JJ: Bromocriptine/levodopa combined versus levodopa alone for early Parkinson's disease, *Cochrane Database Syst Rev* Issue 4:CD003634, January 2007.

van Hilten JJ: Bromocriptine versus levodopa in early Parkinson's disease, *Cochrane Database Syst Rev* Issue 4:CD002258, January 2007.

Vivancos-Matellano F: Ropinirole in the treatment of Parkinson's disease: an update, *Rev Neurol* 42(9):542-548, 2006.

Chapter 17

Anxiety disorders, Merck Manuals Online Medical Library, November 2005, available at *http://www.merck.com/mmpe/print/sec19/ch300/ch300b.html*.

Aschenbrenner DS: Additional precaution concerning antidepressants: further risk to liver function is noted, *Am J Nurs* 106(2):29, 2006.

Buchanan RW et al: Olanzapine treatment of residual positive and negative symptoms, *Am J Psychiatry* 162(1):124-129, 2005.

Calabrese JR: A randomized, double-blind, placebo-controlled trial of quetiapine in the treatment of bipolar I or II depression, *Am J Psychiatry* 162(7):1351-1360, 2005.

Capriotti T: Nursing pharmacology: update on depression and antidepressant medications, *Medsurg Nurs* 15(4):241-246, 2006.

Catalano G et al: Acute akathisia associated with quetiapine use, *Psychosomatics* 46(4):291-301, 2005.

Depressive disorders, Merck Manuals Online Medical Library, November 2005, available at *http://www.merck.com/mmpe/print/sec19/ch300/ch300d.html*.

Diagnostic and statistical manual of mental disorders, ed 4, text revision (DSM-IV-TR), Washington, DC, 2000, American Psychiatric Association.

Drew BL: What should I do when I suspect that a patient is suicidal? Available at *http://www.medscape.com/viewarticles/572760*.

Drug news: antidepressants and triptans: beware of serotonin syndrome, *Nursing* 3(10):32, 2006.

Drug news: schizophrenia: older drug performs as well as newcomers, *Nursing* 35(12):30, 2007.

Duckworth K: Bipolar disorder, National Alliance on Mental Illness website, October 2006, available at *http://www.nami.org*.

Duckworth K: Major depression, National Alliance on Mental Illness website, September 2006, available at *http://www.nami.org*.

Duckworth K: Schizophrenia, National Alliance on Mental Illness website, February 2007, available at *http://www.nami.org*.

Edlinger M: Trends in the pharmacological treatment of patients with schizophrenia over a 12 year observation period, *Schizophr Res* 77(1):25-34, 2005.

Factsheet: anxiety disorders: what you need to know, Mental Health America website, November 2007, available at *http://www.mentalhealthamerica.net/go/information/gen-info/anxiety-disorders*.

Factsheet: bipolar disorder: what you need to know, Mental Health America website, January 2007, available at *http://www.nmha.org*.

Factsheet: depression: what you need to know, Mental Health America website, January 2008, available at *http://www.nmha.org*.

Factsheet: post-traumatic stress disorder, Mental Health America website, available at *http://www.nmha.org*.

Gijsman HJ et al: Antidepressants for bipolar depression: a systematic review of randomized, controlled trials, *Am J Psychiatry* 161(9):1537-1547, 2004.

Gorman J: Post-traumatic stress disorder, National Alliance on Mental Illness website, May 2003, available at *http://www.nami.org*.

Grunze H: Reevaluating therapies for bipolar depression, *J Clin Psychiatry* 66(suppl 5):17-25, 2005.

Hamrin V, Scahill L: Selective serotonin reuptake inhibitors for children and adolescents with major depression: current controversies and recommendations, *Issues Ment Health Nurs* 26(4):433-450, 2005.

Hunt N: *Your questions answered: bipolar disorder*, London, 2005, Elsevier Limited.

Institute for Safe Medication Practices: ISMP's list of confused drug names, 2008, available at *http://www.ismp.org*.

Institute for Safe Medication Practices: ISMP's list of high-alert medications, 2008, available at *http://www.ismp.org*.

Invega (paliperidone) extended-release tablets [prescribing information], Titusville, NJ, 2008, Ortho-McNeil-Janssen Pharmaceuticals, available at *http://www.invega.com/invega/hcp.html*.

Kessler RC et al: Prevalence, severity, and comorbidity of twelve-month DSM-IV disorders in the National Comorbidity Survey Replication (NCS-R), *Arch Gen Psychiatry* 62(6):617-627, 2005.

Moore DP, Jefferson JW: *Handbook of medical psychiatry*, ed 2, Philadelphia, 2004, Mosby.

Muzina DJ: Bipolar spectrum disorder: differential diagnosis and treatment, *Prim Care* 34:521-550, 2007.

National Institute of Mental Health: Anxiety disorders factsheet, available at *http://www.nimh.nih.gov/health/topics/anxiety-disorders/index.shtml*.

National Institute of Mental Health: Bipolar disorder factsheet, available at *http://www.nimh.nih.gov/health/publications/bipolar-disorder/introduction.shtml*.

National Institute of Mental Health: Generalized anxiety disorder factsheet, April 2008, available at *http://www.nimh.nih.gov/health/publications/anxiety-disorders/generalized-anxiety-disorder-gad.shtml*.

National Institute of Mental Health: What are the different forms of depression (fact sheet), available at *http://www.nimh.nih.gov/health/publications/depression/what-is-a-depressive-disorder.shtml*.

National Institute of Mental Health: What is schizophrenia? (fact sheet), April 2008, available at *http://www.nimh.nih.gov/health/publications/schizophrenia/what-is-schizophrenia.shtml*.

Nelson JC et al: Are there differences in the symptoms that respond to a selective serotonin or norepinephrine reuptake inhibitor? *Biol Psychiatry* 57(12):1535-1542, 2005.

Phelan KM et al: Lithium interaction with the cyclo-oxygenase 2 inhibitors rofecoxib and celecoxib and other nonsteroidal anti-inflammatory drugs, *J Clin Psychiatry* 64:1328-1334, 2003.

Rapkin JA: Journal scan: focus on PMDD and SSRIs, 2007, available at *http://www.medscape.com/viewarticle/561265*.

Razadyne [prescribing information], Tuitville, NJ Ortho-McNeil-Janssen Pharmaceuticals, 2007, available at *http://www.razadyne.com*.

Risperdal Consta [prescribing information], Tuitsville, NJ, 2008, Ortho-McNeil-Janssen Pharmaceuticals, available at *http://www.risperdalconsta.com*.

Schizophrenia, Merck Manuals Online Medical Library, November 2005, available at *http://www.merck.com/mmpe/print/sec15/ch202/ch202e.html*.

Shastry BS: Genetic diversity and new therapeutic concepts, *J Hum Genet* 50:321-328, 2005.

Shastry BS: Role of SNP/haplotype in gene discovery and drug development: an overview, *Drug Dev Res* 62:143-150, 2004.

Silva de Lima M et al: Quality of life in schizophrenia: a multicenter, randomized, naturalistic, controlled trial comparing olanzapine to first-generation antipsychotics, *J Clin Psychiatry* 66(7):831-838, 2005.

Simpson GM et al: Randomized, controlled, double-blind multicenter comparison of the efficacy and tolerability of ziprasidone and olanzapine in acutely ill inpatients with schizophrenia or schizoaffective disorder, *Am J Psychiatry* 161(10):1837-1847, 2004.

Simpson GM et al: Six-month, blinded, multicenter continuation study of ziprasidone versus olanzapine in schizophrenia, *Am J Psychiatry* 162(8):1535-1538, 2005.

Stoner SC, Dubisar B: Drug watch '06: psychotropics, *RN* 69(7):31-38, 2006.

Talbott JA: *Yearbook of psychiatry and applied mental health 2005*, Philadelphia, 2005, Mosby.

Texas Department of State Health Services: Algorithm for mania/hypomania, available at *http://www.dshs.state.tx.us/mhprograms/timabd1algo.pdf*.

Texas Department of State Health Services: Algorithm for the treatment of depression in bipolar disorder, available at *http://www.dshs.state.tx.us/mhprograms/timabd2algo.pdf*.

US Food and Drug Administration: Antidepressant drugs that have healthcare professional and patient information sheets, June 2005, available at *http://www.fda.gov/cder/drug/antidepressants/antidepressantList.htm*.

US Food and Drug Administration: Atypical antipsychotic drugs information, April 2005, available at *http://www.fda.gov/cder/drug/infopage/antipsychotics/default.htm*.

US Food and Drug Administration: Class suicidality labeling language for antidepressants, January 2005, available at *http://www.fda.gov/cder/drug/antidepressants/PI_template.pdf*.

US Food and Drug Administration: FDA issues public health advisory for antipsychotic drugs used for treatment of behavioral disorders in elderly patients, April 2005, available at *http://www.fda.gov/bbs/topics/ANSWERS/2005/ANS01350.html*.

US Food and Drug Administration: FDA public health advisory: deaths with antipsychotics in elderly patients with behavioral disturbances, April 2005, available at *http://www.fda.gov/cder/drug/advisory/antipsychotics.htm*.

US Food and Drug Administration: FDA public health advisory: suicidality in adults being treated with antidepressant medications, June 2005, available at *http://www.fda.gov/cder/drug/advisory/SSRI200507.htm*.

US Food and Drug Administration: FDA talk paper: FDA reviews data for antidepressant use in adults, July 2005, available at *http://www.fda.gov/bbs/topics/ANSWERS/2005/ANS01362.html*.

US Food and Drug Administration: List of drugs receiving a boxed warning, other product labeling changes, and a medication guide pertaining to pediatric suicidality, January 2005, available at *http://www.fda.gov/cder/drug/antidepressants/MDD_alldruglist.pdf*.

US Food and Drug Administration: Medication guide (for parents) about using antidepressants in children and teenagers, January 2005, available at *http://www.fda.gov/cder/drug/antidepressants/MG_template.pdf*.

US Food and Drug Administration: 2004 Safety alert: Risperdal (risperidone), available at *http://www.fda.gov/medwatch/SAFETY/2004/risperdal.htm*.

Vieta E: The package of care for patients with bipolar depression, *J Clin Psychiatry* 66(suppl 5):34-39, 2005.

Ward KS: New developments in antidepressant therapy, *Nurs Clin North Am* 40(1):95-105, 2005.

Yatham LN et al: Atypical antipsychotics in bipolar depression: potential mechanisms of action, *J Clin Psychiatry*, 66(suppl 5):40-48, 2005.

Zheng CJ et al: Drug ADME associated protein data base as a resource for facilitating pharmacogenomics research, *Drug Dev Res* 62:134-142, 2004.

Chapter 18

Colbert K, Greene MH: Nesiritide (Natrecor): a new treatment for acute decompensated congestive heart failure, *Crit Care Nurs* 26(1):40-43, 2003.

Sauls JM, Rone T: Emerging trends in the management of heart failure: beta blocker therapy. *Nurs Clin North Am* 40(1):135-148, 2005.

Chapter 19

Flomax Oral, 2009, available at *http://www.healthcentral.com/incontinence/find-drug-1039-150.htmlat*.

Sauls JL, Rone T: Emerging trends in the management of heart failure: beta blocker therapy, *Nurs Clin North Am* 40(1):135-148, 2005.

Chapter 20

Azpiroz F, Malagelada JR: Current concepts and considerations and post vagotomy gastroparesis: effect of metoclopramide and bethanechol, *Gastroenterology* 134(1):82-85, January 2008, available at *http://www.medscape.com*.

Eckert GP, Muller WE, Wood WG: Cholesterol-lowering drugs and Alzheimer's disease, *Future Lipidol* 2(4):423-432, 2007.

Jeffery S: Exercise may improve cognition in adults with memory impairment, *JAMA* 300:1027-1037, 2008.

Johns Hopkins health alert: do Alzheimer's disease medications really work?, 2008, available at *http://www.johnshopkinshealthalerts.com/alerts/memory/JohnsHopkinsHealthAlertsMemory_1749-1.html*.

Ortho-McNeil Pharmaceutical: Dear healthcare professional [letter], March 31, 2005, available at *http://www.WebMD.com;* more information available at *http://www.ortho-mcneilneurologics.com*.

Razadyne [prescribing information], Tuitville, NJOrtho-McNeil Neurologics, Ortho-McNeil-Janssen Pharmaceuticals, 2007, available at *http://www.razadyne.com*.

Chapter 21

Drug news: oxybutynin: skin patch calms busy bladders, *Nursing* 30, 2007.

Hussar DA: New drugs: 2007; part 1, *Nursing* 37(2):51-58, 2007.

Monthly Prescribing Reference 24(4), April 2008, available at *http://www.prescribingreference.com*.

Physicians' desk reference, ed 60, Montvale, NJ, 2006, Medical Economics.

Sand-Jecklin K: Know the benefits and risks of using common herbal therapies, *Holistic Nurs Pract* 18(4):192-198, 2004.

Wolf ZR: Pursuing safe medication use and the promise of technology, *Medsurg Nurs* 16(2):92-99, 2007.

Chapter 22

Adams K et al: Executive summary: HFSA 2006 Comprehensive Heart Failure Practice Guideline, *J Card Failure* 12(1):10-38, 2006.

FDA warning letter: nesiritide, Scios, Inc., available at *http://www.pharmcast.com/WarningLetters/Yr2007/Nov2007/Scios1107.htm*.

Hunt SA: American College of Cardiology/American Heart Association 2005 Guideline update for the diagnosis and management of chronic heart failure in adults, *Circulation* 112:e154-e235, September 2005.

Koda-Kimble MA et al: *Applied therapeutics: the clinical use of drugs*, ed 8, Philadelphia, 2005, Lippincott Williams & Wilkins.

Shaddy RE, Webb G: Applying heart failure guidelines to adult congenital heart disease patients, *Expert Rev Cardiovasc Ther* 6(2):165-174, 2008.

Swan BA, Conway-Phillips R, Griffin K: Demonstrating the value of the RN in ambulatory care, *Nurs Econ* 24(6):315-322, 2006.

Wright J: Drug watch '06: cardiovascular meds, *RN* 69(5):33-39, 2006.

Yancy CW: Evidence-based medical therapy and device therapy for heart failure: points of emphasis in the new 2005 AHA/ACC guidelines [continuing medical education/continuing education module], MedscapeCME website, January 2006, available at *http://www.medscapenursing.com; http://www.medscape.com/viewprogram/4916*.

Chapter 23

2005 American Heart Association guidelines for cardiopulmonary resuscitation and emergency cardiovascular care, *Circulation* 112(24 suppl):IV1-203, 2005.

Brodsky MA et al: A history of heart failure predicts arrhythmia treatment efficacy: data from the Antiarrhythmics versus Implantable Defibrillators (AVID) study, *Am Heart J* 152(4):724-730, 2006.

Goldstein RN, Stambler BS: New antiarrhythmic drugs for prevention of atrial fibrillation, *Prog Cardiovasc Dis* 48(3):193-208, 2005.

Hanna IR et al: Approaching cardiac arrhythmias in the elderly patient, *MedGenMed* 7(4):24, 2005.

Kannankeril PJ: Drug induced long QT and torsades de pointes: recent advances, *Curr Opin Cardiol* 22(1):39-43, 2007.

Kannankeril PJ: Understanding drug induced torsades de pointes, *Expert Opin Drug Saf* 7(3):231-239, 2008.

Pharmacologic treatment of arrhythmias. UpToDate website, 2008. available at *http:/www.uptodate.com*.

Springhouse nursing 2009 student drug handbook,, Philadelphia, 2009, Lippincott Williams & Wilkins.

Tikosyn [prescribing information], New York, NY, Pfizer, 2006, available at *http://www.Tikosyn.com*.

Chapter 24

Abrams J: Clinical practice: chronic stable angina, *N Engl J Med* 352:2524-2533, 2005.

Anderson S et al: Dosage of beta-adrenergic blockers after myocardial infarction, *Am J Health Syst Pharm* 60:2471-2474, 2003.

Boden WE et al: Optimal medical therapy with or without PCI for stable coronary disease, *N Engl J Med* 356:1503-1516, 2007.

Brogden NK, Dunn S: Advances in the treatment of chronic stable angina [continuing education module], US Pharmacist website, February 1, 2008, available at *http://www.uspharmacist.com*.

2007 Chronic angina focused update of the American College of Cardiology/American Heart Association guidelines for the management of patients with chronic stable angina, available at *http://www.americanheart.org*.

Henderson RA et al: Seven-year outcome in the RITA-2 trial: coronary angioplasty versus medical therapy, *J Am Coll Cardiol* 42(7):1161-1170, 2003.

ISMP Medication Safety Alert!, *NurseAdvise-ERR* 3(6), 2005, available at *http://www.ismp.org/Newsletters/nursing/Issues/NurseAdviseERR200506.pdf*.

Itsik Ben-Dor, Battler A: Treatment of stable angina, *Heart* 93:868-874, 2007.

Mahler DA, Fierro-Carrion G, Mejia-Alfaro R, Ward J, Baird JC: Responsiveness of continuous ratings of dyspnea during exercise in patients with COPD, *Medicine & Science in Sports and Exercise*, 37(4):529-535, 2005.

Oparil S, Weber MA: *Hypertension: companion to Brenner & Rector's the kidney*, ed 2, Philadelphia, 2005, Saunders.

Trujillo TC, Nolan PE: Ischemic heart disease: anginal. In Koda-Kimble MA et al, editors: *Applied therapeutics: the clinical use of drugs*, ed 9, Philadelphia, 2007, Lippincott Williams & Wilkins.

Webb AJ, Patel N, Loukogeorgakis S, et al: Acute blood pressure lowering, vasoprotective, and antiplatelet properties of dietary nitrate via bioconversion to nitrite, *Hypertension* 51:543-547, 2008.

Wood S: New AHA statement sets lower BP targets for high-risk and established CAD patients, June 2007, available at *http://www.medscape.com/viewarticle/55870*.

Zimetbaum R: Inpatient or outpatient initiation of antiarrhythmic medications for atrial fibrillation, February 8, 2006, available at *http://www.americanheart.org/downloadable/heart/1023122768115zimetbaum_inpatient_vs_outpatient.pdf*.

Chapter 25

Agency for Healthcare Research and Quality, National Guideline Clearinghouse: Essential hypertension: managing adult patients in primary care, September 2005, available at *http://www.guideline.gov*.

Agency for Healthcare Research and Quality, National Guideline Clearinghouse: Medical management of adults with essential hypertension, September 2005, available at *http://www.guideline.gov*.

American Heart Association guidelines for treating resistant hypertension, available at *http://www.americanheart.org*.

The Antihypertensive and Lipid Lowering Treatment to Prevent Heart Attack Trial website, *http://www.allhat.org*.

Bystolic [prescribing information], St. Louis, Mo, Forest Pharmaceutics 2009, available at *http://www.bystolic.com*.

Dressler RL: Antihypertensive agents for the prevention of diabetic nephropathy, *Am Fam Physician* 74(1):77-79, 2006.

Flack JM, Sica DA: Therapeutic considerations in the African-American patient with hypertension: considerations with calcium channel blocker therapy, J Clin Hypertens (Greenwich) 7(4 suppl 1):9-14, 2005.

Inspra [prescribing information], New York, NY, Pfizer, 2007, available at *http://www.pfizer.com/products/rx/rx_product_inspra.jsp*.

JNC 7 Express: The seventh report of the Joint National Committee on Detection, Evaluation, and Treatment of High Blood Pressure (JNC-7), Bethesda, Md, 2003, National Institutes of Health.

Monthly Prescribing Reference 21(10), 2005, available at *http://www.presribingref.com*.

New guidelines for hypertension treatment, newsletter no. 1518, May 2008, available at *http://www.ASHP.org*.

Remodulin [prescribing information], Research Triangle Park, NC, United Therapeutics, 2008, available at *http://www.remodulin.com*.

The seventh report of the Joint National Committee on Detection, Evaluation and Treatment of High Blood Pressure (JNC-7), available at *http://www.nhlbi.nih.gov/guidelines/hypertension*.

Tekturna prescribing information, East Hanover, NJ, Novartis, 2008, available at *http://www.tekturna.com*.

Tracleer [prescribing information], San Francisco, Calif, Actelion Pharmaceuticals, 2009, available at *http://www.tracleer.com*.

Chapter 26

Bauer J: Blood pressure cuffs, *RN* 65(8), 2002, available at *http://www.rnweb.com*.

Brookes L: Prehypertension, the elderly, dementia, and sleep—how to treat the blood pressure? *Medscape Cardiol* 10(1), 2006.

Coleman WL, Garfield C, Committee on Psychosocial Aspects of Child and Family Health: Fathers and pediatricians: enhancing men's role in the care and development of their children, *Pediatrics* 113:1406-1411, 2004.

Imazio M et al: Management of heart failure in elderly people, *Int J Clin Pract* 62(2):270-280, 2008.

Johnson K et al: Sulfonamide cross-reactivity: fact or fiction, *Ann Pharmacother* 39(2):290-301, 2005.

Klabunder RE: Cardiovascular pharmacology concepts, available at *http://www.cvpharmacology.com*.

Monthly Prescribing Reference, 24(6), June 2008, available at *http://www.prescribingreference.com*.

Opie LH, Gersh BJ: *Drugs for the heart*, ed 6, Philadelphia, 2005, Saunders.

Ponka D: Approach to managing patients with sulfa allergy, *Can Fam Physician* 52:1434-1438, 2006.

Chapter 27

Fulcher EM: *Introduction to intravenous therapy for health professionals*, Philadelphia, 2007, Saunders.

Gahart BL: *Intravenous medications: a handbook for nurses and health professionals*, ed 24, St Louis, 2007, Mosby.

Rosenthal K: Intravenous fluids: the whys and wherefores, *Nursing* 36(7):26-27, 2006.

Chapter 28

Aronow WS: Treatment of peripheral arterial disease in the elderly person, *Ann Long Term Care* 13(9):34-37, 2005.

Bhatt DL et al for the CHARISMA investigators: Clopidogrel and aspirin versus aspirin alone for the prevention of atherothrombotic events, *N Engl J Med* 354:1706-1717, 2006.

The eighth ACCP Conference of Antithrombotic and Thrombolytic Therapy: evidence-based guidelines, *Chest* 133(6 suppl):141s-159s, 2008.

Fugate S et al: Impaired warfarin response secondary to high-dose vitamin K1 for rapid anticoagulation reversal: case series and literature review, *Pharmacotherapy* 24(9):1213-1220, 2004.

Greenblat D: Cranberry juice and warfarin: is there an interaction? *Anticoag Forum* 10(spring):1-4, 2006.

Howard P et al: An update on the diagnosis, complications, and treatment of heparin-induced thrombocytopenia, *Hosp Pharmacy* 39:408-417, 2004.

Important information to know when you are taking Coumadin and vitamin K, Bethesda, Md, December 2003, National Institutes of Health, Warren Grant Magnuson Clinical Center. Available at *http://ods.od.nih.gov/factsheets/cc/coumadin1.pdf*.

Kerr JL et al: Role of clopidogrel in unstable angina and non-ST-segment elevation in myocardial infarction: from literature and guidelines to practice, *Pharmacotherapy* 24(8):1037-1049, 2004.

2009 National Patient Safety Goals, available at *http://www.jointcommission.org/PatientSafety/NationalPatientSafetyGoals*

Warfarin (marketed as Coumadin), August 16, 2007, available at *http://www.fda.gov/Safety/MedWatch/SafetyInformation/SafetyAlertsforHumanMedicalProducts/ucm152972.htm*.

Wittkowsky A et al: Effect of age on international normalized ratio at the time of major bleeding episodes in patients treated with warfarin, *Pharmacotherapy* 24(5):600-605, 2004.

Chapter 29

Briel M et al: Effects of statins on stroke prevention in patients with and without coronary heart disease, *Evidence Based Nursing* 8:86, 2005.

Brown BG, Taylor AJ: Does ENHANCE diminish confidence in lowering LDL or in ezetimibe? *N Engl J Med* 358:1504-1507, 2008.

Cleveland Clinic Heart Center: Update on cholesterol guidelines: more intensive treatment options for higher risk patients, report endorsed by National Heart, Lung, and Blood Institute, American College of Cardiology, and American Heart Association, July 13, 2004, available at *http://www.clevelandclinic.org/heartcenter/pub/news/archive/2004/NCEPLDL7_13print.htm*.

Expert Panel on Detection, Evaluation, and Treatment of High Blood Cholesterol in Adults (Adult Treatment Panel III), available at *http://www.guideline.gov*.

Gandhi GY et al: Patient important outcomes in registered diabetes trials, *JAMA* 229:2543-2549, 2008.

Kastelein JTP, Akdin F, Stroes EJG: Simvastatin with or without ezetimibe in hypercholesterolemia, *N Engl J Med* 358:1431-1443, 2008.

Kinlay S: Vascular form and function: two mechanisms for cardiovascular prevention, *Eur Heart J* 29:1711-1713, 2008.

Ky B, Rader DJ: The effects of statin therapy on plasma markers of inflammation in patients without vascular disease, *Clin Cardiol* 28:67-70, 2005.

Mikhailidis DP et al: The use of ezetimibe in achieving low density lipoprotein lowering goals in clinical practice: position statement of a United Kingdom consensus panel, *Curr Med Res Opin* 21(6):959-969, 2005.

Natural Standard: Red yeast rice, available at *http://www.naturalstandard.com*.

Steinmetz KL, Schonder KS: Colesevelam: potential uses for the newest bile resin, *Cardiovasc Drug Rev* 23(1):15-30, 2005.

Talbert RL: Role of the National Cholesterol Education Program Adult Treatment Panel III guidelines in managing dyslipidemia, *Am J Health Syst Pharm* 60(2):S3-S8, 2003.

US Food and Drug Administration: FDA public health advisory on Crestor (rosuvastatin), March 2, 2005, available at *http://www.fda/gov/cder/drug/advisory/crestor_3_2005.htm*.

Chapter 30

Gavoli C et al: Effect of growth hormone deficiency and recombinant hGH replacement on the hypothalamic-pituitary-adrenal axis in children with idiopathic isolation GH deficiency, *Clin Endocrinol* 68(2):247-251, 2008.

Physiological homeostasis, available at *http://www.biology-online.org/4/1_physiological_homeostasis.htm*.

Russell JA et al: Vasopressin versus norepinephrine infusion in patients with septic shock, *N Engl J Med* 358(9):877-887, 2008.

Sandostatin (octreotide) [prescribing information], Basel, Switzerland, Novartis, 2007, available at *http://www.sandostatin.com*.

Thomson ABR et al: Dumping syndrome, eMedicine website, 2008, available at *http://www.emedicine.com/med/topic589.htm*.

Zhang XP et al: Protective effects of baicalin and octreotide on multiple organ injury in severe acute pancreatitis, *Dig Dis Sci* 53(2):581-591, 2008.

Chapter 31

Monthly Prescribing Reference, 10(2), September 2006, available at *http://www.uic.edu/classes/pcol*.

Nazario B: Thyroid Q&A [WebMD live events transcript], available at *http://www.webmd.com/content/chat_transcripts/1/103872.htm*.

Chapter 32

ACCORD Study Group: Effects of intensive glucose lowering in type 2 diabetes, *N Engl J Med* 358:2545-2569, 2008.

American Diabetes Association: Drug therapy for high cholesterol, available at *http://www.diabetes.org/diabetes-cholesterol/drug-therapy.jsp*.

American Diabetes Association: People with diabetes should use aspirin to lower heart-attack risk, available at *http://www.diabetes.org/diabetes-research/summaries/persell-asprin.jsp*.

American Diabetes Association: Standards of medical care in diabetes—2008, *Diabetes Care* 31(suppl 1):S12-S54, 2008.

Bickston TH: *Medical-surgical nursing recall*, Philadelphia, 2004, Lippincott Williams & Wilkins.

Bolen S et al: Systematic review: comparative effectiveness and safety of oral medications for type 2 diabetes mellitus, *Ann Intern Med* 147:386-399, 2007.

Davis T, Edelman SV: Insulin therapy in type 2 diabetes, *Med Clin North Am* 88(4):865-895, 2004.

Diabetes Control and Complications Research Trial Group: The effect of intensive treatment of diabetes on the development and progression of long-term complications of insulin-dependent diabetes mellitus, *N Engl J Med* 329:977-986, 1993.

Dow NE: Tight insulin control: making it work, *RN* 68(7):45-52, 2005.

Edmisson KW: Multidimensional pharmacologic strategies for diabetes, *Nurs Clin North Am* 40(1):107-117, 2005.

Haas L: Management of diabetes mellitus medications in the nursing home, *Drugs Aging* 22(3):209-218, 2005.

Hirsch IR: Treatment of patients with severe insulin deficiency: what we have learned over the past 2 years, *Am J Med* 116(3A):17-22, 2004.

Hirsch I, Braithwate S: Sliding scale insulin therapy: an ineffective option of inpatient glycemic control, *Resid Staff Physician* 53(2):8, 2007.

Lebovitz HE: Oral antidiabetic agents: 2004, *Med Clin North Am* 88(4):847-863, ix-x, 2004.

Lien LF, Bethel MA, Feinglos MN: In-hospital management of type 2 diabetes mellitus, *Med Clin North Am* 88(4):1085-1105, xii, 2004.

National Institute of Diabetes and Digestive and Kidney Diseases: Diabetes control and complications trial (DCCT) and follow-up study, available at *http://diabetes.niddk.nih.gov/dm/pubs/control*.

National Institute of Diabetes and Digestive and Kidney Diseases: National diabetes statistics, 2007, available at *http://diabetes.niddk.nih.gov/dm/pubs/statistics/index.htm*.

Nissen SE, Wolski K: Effect of rosiglitazone on the risk of myocardial infarction and death from cardiovascular causes, *N Engl J Med* 356:2457-2471, 2007.

Ohkubo Y et al: Intensive insulin therapy prevents the progression of diabetic microvascular complications in Japanese patients with non-insulin-dependent diabetes mellitus: a randomized prospective 6-year study, *Diabetes Res Clin Pract* 28:103-106, 1995.

Riddle MC: Glycemic management of type 2 diabetes: an emerging strategy with oral agents, insulins, and combinations, *Endocrinol Metab Clin North Am* 34:77-98, 2005.

Riddle MC: Making the transition from oral to insulin therapy, *Am J Med* 118(suppl 5A):14S-20S, 2005.

Stoneking K: Initiating basal insulin therapy in patients with type 2 diabetes mellitus, *Am J Health Syst Pharm* 62(5):510-518, 2005.

Turner RC et al: Intensive blood glucose control with sulphonylureas of insulin compared with conventional treatment and risk of complications in patients with type 2 diabetes (UKPDS 33), *Lancet* 352:837-853, 1998.

US Food and Drug Administration: FDA approves new drug to treat type 1 and type 2 diabetes, 2005, available at *http://www.fda.gov/bbs/topics/ANSWERS/2005/ANS01345.html*.

Chapter 33

Goroll AH, Mulley AG, Mulley AG Jr: *Primary care medicine: office evaluation and management of the adult patient*, Philadelphia, 2006, Lippincott Williams & Wilkins.

Royal College of Surgeons of Edinburgh, Surgical Knowledge and Skills website, available at *http://www.edu.rcseng.ac*.

Chapter 34

Bolland MJ et al: Vascular events in healthy older women receiving calcium supplementation: randomized controlled trial, *BMJ* 336:262-265, 2008.

Estrogen and progestogen use in postmenopausal women: July 2008 position statement of the North American Menopause Society, *Menopause* 15(4):584-603, 2008.

FDA MedWatch: Bisphosphonates: a possible cause of severe and sometimes incapacitating bone, joint and/or muscle pain, available at *http://www.fda.gov/medwatch/safety/2008/safety08.htm#bisphophonates*.

Heiss G et al for the WHI investigators: Health risks and benefits 3 years after stopping randomized treatment with estrogen and progestin, *JAMA* 299:1036-1045, 2008.

Hodis H: Assessing benefits and risks of hormone therapy in 2008: new evidence, especially with regard to the heart, *Cleve Clin J Med* 75(suppl 4):S3-S11, 2008.

National Cancer Institute: Women's Health Initiative study, available at *http://www.cancer.gov*.

National Heart, Lung, and Blood Institute: Calcium and vitamin D supplements offer modest bone improvements, no benefits for colorectal cancer, February 2006, available at *http://www.nhlbi.nih.gov/new/press/06-02-15.htm*.

National Heart, Lung, and Blood Institute: NHLBI advisory for physicians on the WHI trial of conjugated equine estrogens versus placebo, March 2006, available at *http://www.nhlbi.nih.gov/whi/e-a_advisory.htm*.

National Institutes of Health: NIH News: NIH asks participants in Women's Health Initiative estrogen-alone study to stop study pills, begin follow-up phase, March 2, 2004, available at *http://www.nhlbi.nih.gov/new/press/04-03-02.htm*.

National Osteoporosis Foundation website, available at *http://www.nof.org*.

NuvaRing [prescribing information], Kenilworth, NJ, Schering-Plough 2008, available at *http://www.nuvaring.com*.

Parsons LC: Osteoporosis: incidence, prevention, and treatment of the silent killer, *Nurs Clin North Am* 40(1):119-133, 2005.

Piascik P: Recent advances in oral and transdermal contraception, *US Pharm*, September 2008, available at *http://www.medscape.com/viewarticle/582386*.

US Food and Drug Administration: Estrogen and estrogen with progestin therapies, February 2006, available at *http://www.fda.gov/cder/drug/infopage/estrogens_progestins/default.htm*.

US Food and Drug Administration: FDA public health advisory: sepsis and medical abortion, November 2005, available at *http://www.fda.gov/cder/drug/advisory/mifeprex.htm*.

US Food and Drug Administration: Mifeprex (mifepristone) information, March 2006, available at *http://www.fda.gov/cder/drug/advisory/mifeprex200603.htm*.

Women's Health Initiative, National Heart, Lung, and Blood Institute, available at *http://www.nhlbi.nih.gov/whi*.

Chapter 35

Avodart [prescribing information], Research Triangle Park, NC, GlaxoSmithKlein, 2008, available at *http://www.avodart.com*.

Benign prostatic hypertrophy drugs available in U.S., *Health Med Week* 83, 2003.

Blanchard N, Abu-Baker A: The treatment of benign prostatic hypertrophy [continuing education module], US Pharmacist website, August 1, 2008, available at *http://www.uspharmacist.com*.

Gaines K: Tadalafil (Cialis) and vardenafil (Levitra): recently approved drugs for erectile dysfunction, *Urol Nurs* 24(1), 2004.

Levitra [prescribing information], Research Triangle Park, NC, Glaxo-SmithKlein, 2008, available at *http://www.levitra.com*.

Viagra [prescribing information], New York, NY, Pfizer, 2008, available at *http://www.viagra.com*.

Chapter 36

Barclay L: Evidence limited to recommend antihistamines for nonspecific cough in children, available at *http://www.medscape.com/viewarticle/573321_print*.

Baren J: Dextromethorphan abuse is on the rise nationwide, Journal Watch Emergency Medicine website, January 5, 2007, available at *http://emergency-medicine.jwatch.org/cgi/content/citation/2007/105/5*.

Clarinex (desloratadine) [professional product information and package insert], Kenilworth, NJ, Schering Corporation, available at *http://www.clarinex.com*.

Hitti M: Cough, cold drugs not for kids under 4, available at *http://www.medscape.com/viewarticle/581715*.

Jellin J et al: *Natural medicines comprehensive database*, ed 6, Stockton, Calif, 2004, Therapeutic Research Faculty.

Skidmore-Roth L: *Mosby's handbook of herbs and natural supplements*, ed 2, St Louis, 2004, Mosby.

US Food and Drug Administration: FDA public health advisory, nonprescription cough and cold medicine use in children, August 2007, available at *http://www.fda.gov/medwatch*.

Chapter 37

Asthma and Allergy Foundation of America: HFA inhalers, patient information, available at *http://www.aafa.org*.

Donohue JF: Asthma medications: black box warnings—where do we go from here? Available at *http://www.medscape.com/viewarticle/555291*.

National Asthma Education and Prevention Program, available at *http://www.nhlbi.nih.gov/about/naepp*.

National Heart, Lung, and Blood Institute: NAEPP Expert Panel Report guidelines for the diagnosis and management of asthma, executive summary, 2007, available at *http://www.nhlbi.nih.gov/guidelines/asthma/execsumm.pdf*.

Tamesis GP, Covar RA: Long-term effects of asthma medications in children, *Curr Opin Allergy Clin Immunol*, July 2008, available at *http://www.medscape.com/viewarticle/577778*.

Tezky T, Holquist C: FDA safety page: misadministration of capsules for inhalation, April 4, 2005, available at *http://www.drugtopics.com/drugtopics/article/articleDetail.jsp?id=153758*.

US Food and Drug Administration: FDA talk paper: FDA publishes final rule on chlorofluorocarbons in metered dose inhalers, available at *http://www.fda.gov/cder/mdi/default.htm*.

US Food and Drug Administration, Edelman NH, and American Lung Association: FDA talk paper: statement of support on the FDA's recommendation to ban CFC inhalers, January 2006, available at *http://www.lungusa.org*.

Xolair [product information], available at *http://www.xolair.com*.

Chapter 38

Clarithromycin (Biaxin) [prescribing information], Abbott Park, Ill, Abbott Labs, 2008, available at *http://www.biaxinxl.com*.

Doribax [prescribing information], New York, NY, Pfizer, 2009, available at *http://www.doribax.com*.

Fowler SB: Community-acquired pneumonia: follow the guidelines to better outcomes, *Am Nurse Today* 3(9):26-31, 2008.

Hussar DA: New drugs '08, *Nursing* 38(7):41-48, 2008.

Ketek [prescribing information], Bridgewater, NJ, Sanofi-Aventis, 2007, available at *http://www.ketek.com*.

Shain C, Baure J: Drug watch '06 antibiotics, *RN* 69(9):41-48, 2006.

Tygacil [prescribing information], Madison, NJ, Wyeth, 2008, available at *http://www.tygacil.com*.

Wold GH: *Basic geriatric nursing*, ed 3, St Louis, 2004, Mosby.

Zhanel GG et al: Carbapenems, *Drugs* 67:1027-1032, 2007.

Chapter 39

Centers for Disease Control and Prevention: Environmental management of staph and MRSA in community settings, July 2008, available at *http://www.cdc.gov/ncidod/dhqp/ar_mrsa_Enviro_Manage.html*.

Centers for Disease Control and Prevention: Strategies for clinical management of MRSA in the community, available at *http://www.cdc.gov*.

Daum R: Skin and soft tissue infections caused by methicillin-resistant *Staphylococcus aureus*, N Engl J Med 357:380-390, 2007.

Gaynes R, Edwards J, the National Nosocomial Infections Surveillance System: Overview of nosocomial infections caused by gram-negative bacilli, *Clin Infect Dis* 41:848-854, 2005.

Gorwitz RJ et al, participants in the CDC Convened Experts' Meeting on Management of MRSA in the Community: Strategies for clinical management of MRSA in the community. Summary of an experts' meeting convened by the Centers for Disease Control and Prevention, March 2006, available at *http://www.cdc.gov/ncidod/dhqp/pdf/ar/CAMRSA_ExpMtgStrategies.pdf*.

Handwashing technique overview, available at *http://www.webmd.com/cold-and-flu/tc/hand-washing-topic-overview*.

Harbarth S, Emonet S: Navigating the World Wide Web in search of resources on antimicrobial resistance, *Clin Infect Dis* 43:72-78, 2006.

Jernigan JA et al: Methicillin-resistant *Staphylococcus aureus* as community pathogen (conference summary), *Emerg Infect Dis* 12(11), 2006. Available at *http://www.cdc.gov/ncidod/EID/vol12no11/06-0911.htm*.

Pop-Vicas A, D'Agata E: The rising influx of multidrug-resistant gram-negative bacilli into a tertiary care hospital, *Clin Infect Dis* 40:1792-1798, 2005.

Sheff B: Multidrug-resistant microorganisms, *Nursing* 33(11):59-63, 2003.

Society for Healthcare Epidemiology of America and Infectious Diseases Society of America Joint Committee on the Prevention of Antimicrobial Resistance: Guidelines for the prevention of antimicrobial resistance in hospitals, *Infect Control Hosp Epidemiol* 18(4):275-329, 2007.

Chapter 40

Centers for Disease Control and Prevention: Antiviral agents for seasonal influenza: information for health professionals, available at *http://www.cdc.gov/flu/professionals/antivirals*.

Centers for Disease Control and Prevention: Avian influenza: current situation, April 2006, available at *http://www.cdc.gov/flu/avian/outbreaks/current.htm*.

Centers for Disease Control and Prevention: Avian influenza infection in humans, March 2006, available at *http://www.cdc.gov/flu/avian/gen-info/avian-flu-humans.htm*.

Centers for Disease Control and Prevention: HIV statistics, available at *http://www.cdc.gov/hiv/topics/surveillance/basic.htm#hivest*.

Centers for Disease Control and Prevention: Key facts about avian influenza (bird flu) and avian influenza A (H5N1) virus, February 2006, available at *http://www.cdc.gov/flu/avian/gen-info/facts.htm*.

Centers for Disease Control and Prevention: West Nile Virus: treatment information and guidance for clinicians, available at *http://www.cdc.gov/ncidod/dvbid/westnile/clinicians/treatment.htm*.

De Clercq E: Antivirals: current state of the art, *Future Virol* 3(4):393-405, 2008.

DePestel DD et al: Magnitude and duration of elevated gastric pH in patients infected with human immunodeficiency virus after administration of chewable, dispersible, buffered didanosine tablets, *Pharmacotherapy* 24(11):1539-1545, 2004.

Deutsch KF: Hepatitis C: the silent epidemic, *Clin Advisor* 6(5):10-18, 2003.

Ellis JM et al: Fosamprenavir: a novel protease inhibitor and prodrug of amprenavir, *Formulary* 39:151-160, 2004.

Havliv D: HIV integrase inhibitors—out of the pipeline and into the clinic, *NEJM* 359(4):416-418, 2008.

Moscona A: The role of antivirals in prevention of avian influenza: an expert interview with Anne Moscona, MD, 2007, Medscape Infectious Diseases, available at *http://www.medscape.com/viewarticle/551914.*

Musial BL et al: Atazanavir: a new protease inhibitor to treat HIV infection, *Am J Health Syst Pharm* 61:1365-1374, 2004.

National Institute of Allergy and Infectious Diseases: Course of HIV infection, available at *http://www.niaid.nih.gov/publications/hivaids/9.htm.*

National Institute of Allergy and Infectious Diseases: HIV infection and AIDS: an overview, available at *http://www.niaid.nih.gov/factsheets/hivinf.htm.*

San Francisco AIDS Foundation: Stages of HIV, available at *http://www.sfaf.org/aids101/hiv_disease.html.*

US Department of Health and Human Services: AIDSinfo website, available at *http://www.aidsinfo.nih.gov.*

US Food and Drug Administration: FDA approved drugs for AIDS, 2008, available at *http://www.fda.gov/oashi/aids/virals.html.*

Chapter 41

American Thoracic Society: International standards for tuberculosis treatment, 2006, available at *http://www.thoracic.org/sections/about-ats/assemblies/mtpi/resources/istc-report.pdf.*

American Thoracic Society: Tuberculosis: patients' rights and responsibilities, 2006, available at *http://www.thoracic.org/sections/about-ats/assemblies/mtpi/resources/istc-charter.pdf.*

Barclay L: Options for screening and treatment of tuberculosis reviewed, 2008, available at *http://www.medscape.com/viewarticle/579389.*

Centers for Disease Control and Prevention: Emergence of *Mycobacterium tuberculosis* with extensive resistance to second-line drugs—worldwide, 2000.2004, March 2006, available at *http://www.cdc.gov/mmwr/preview/mmwrhtml/mm5511a2.htm.*

Centers for Disease Control and Prevention: Extensively drug-resistant tuberculosis: an overview, available at *http://www.cdc.gov/tb/xdrtb/overview.htm.*

Centers for Disease Control and Prevention: Trends in tuberculosis—United States, 2006, March 2007, available at *http://www.cdc.gov/mmwr/preview/mmwrhtml/mm5511a3.htm.*

Centers for Disease Control and Prevention: Tuberculosis control activities after Hurricane Katrina—New Orleans, Louisiana, 2005, March 2006, available at *http://www.cdc.gov/mmwr/preview/mmwrhtml/mm5512a2.htm.*

Centers for Disease Control and Prevention: World TB Day, March 2006, available at *http://www.cdc.gov/mmwr/preview/mmwrhtml/mm5511a1.htm.*

Mitnick CD, Appleton SC, Shin SS: Epidemiology and treatment of multidrug resistant tuberculosis, *Semin Respir Crit Care Med* 29(5):499-524, 2008. Available at *http://www.medscape.com/viewarticle/581866.*

Wright A, Matteo Zignol M: Anti-tuberculosis drug resistance in the world: fourth global report: the World Health Organization/International Union Against Tuberculosis and Lung Disease (WHO/UNION) Global Project on Anti-Tuberculosis Drug Resistance Surveillance, 2002-2007, available at *http://www.who.int/tb/publications/2008.*

Chapter 42

Antifungal drugs, *Treat Guidel Med Lett* 3(30):7-14, 2005.

Brown J: Zygomycosis: an emerging fungal infection, *Am J Health Syst Pharm* 62(24):2593-2596, 2005.

Dodds Ashley E et al: Pharmacology of systemic antifungal agents, *Clin Infect Dis* 43(suppl 1): S28-S39, 2006.

Pappas PG et al: Combating invasive fungal infections: reports from the 45th Annual Interscience Conference on Antimicrobial Agents and Chemotherapy, *Contagion* 3(3, suppl 1):101s-109s 2006.

van Till JW et al: Single-drug therapy or selective decontamination of the digestive tract as antifungal prophylaxis in critically ill patients: a systematic review, *Critical Care* 1(6):126-132 2007.

Chapter 43

Centers for Disease Control and Prevention: Amebiasis fact sheet, September 2008, available at *http://www.cdc.gov/ncidod/dpd/parasites/amebiasis/factsht_amebiasis.htm.*

Centers for Disease Control and Prevention: General approach to uncomplicated malaria, available at *http://www.cdc.gov/malaria/diagnosis_treatment/clinicians2.htm.*

Centers for Disease Control and Prevention: Giardiasis fact sheet, 2008, available at *http://www.cdc.gov/ncidod/dpd/parasites/giardiasis/factsht_giardiasis.htm.*

Centers for Disease Control and Prevention: Information for health care providers: prescription drugs for malaria, February 2006, available at *http://www.cdc.gov/travel/malariadrugs2.htm.*

Centers for Disease Control and Prevention: Parasitic roundworm diseases, February 2005, available at *http://www.niaid.nih.gov/factsheets/roundwor.htm.*

Centers for Disease Control and Prevention: Traveler's health: destinations, August 2008, available at *http://www.cdc.gov/travel/destinat.htm.*

Centers for Disease Control and Prevention: Traveler's health: destinations: Mexico and Central America, January 2006, available at *http://www.cdc.gov/travel/camerica.htm.*

Centers for Disease Control and Prevention: Treatment of malaria (guidelines for clinicians), 2008, available at *http://www.cdc.gov/malaria/pdf/clinicalguidance.pdf.*

National Institute of Allergy and Infectious Diseases, available at *http://www.niaid.nih.gov/factsheets/ictdr.htm.*

Nogid B, Nogid A: A microscopic look at parasitic infections, *Pharm Times*, pp 34-37, February 2006.

Swiss Pharmaceutical Society: *Index nominum international drug directory*, Stuttgart, Germany, 2004, MedPharm GmbH Scientific Publishers.

Timbury MC et al: *Notes on medical microbiology*, Edinburgh, 2002, Churchill Livingstone.

Chapter 44

Durrance SA: Older adults and NSAIDs: avoiding adverse reactions, *Geriatr Nurs* 24(6):348-352, 2003. Available at *http://www.medscape.com/viewarticle/466796.*

Simon LS et al: Cardiovascular safety of celecoxib: a meta-analysis of 41 clinical studies in 44,300 patients [paper presented at American College of Rheumatology annual meeting, November 2005], *Arthritis Rheumatism* 52(9):S406, 2005 (abstract 1049).

Solomon S et al: Cardiovascular risk associated with celecoxib in a clinical trial for colorectal adenoma prevention, *N Engl J Med* 352(11):1071-1080, 2005.

Treatment of acute gout, version 16.3, October 1, 2008, available at *http://UptoDate.com.*

US Food and Drug Administration: NSAID black box warning template, January 2006, available at *http://www.fda.gov/medwatch/SAFETY/2006/Jan_PI/AdultNSAIDRxTemplate.pdf.*

Zanni GR: Gout: treatment considerations for the practicing pharmacist, *Pharmacy Times*, pp 76-77, January 2006.

Chapter 45

Hijnen DJ et al: Cyclosporin: a treatment is associated with increased serum immunoglobulin E levels in a subgroup of topic dermatitis patients, *Dermatitis* 18(3):163-165, 2007.

Ingelfinger J, Schwartz R: Immunosuppression—the promise of specificity, *N Engl J Med* 353:836-839, 2005.

Meldrum M: Immunosuppressant pharmacology 2, available at *http://www.ufpdnotes.com/PCol_II_pdf/Immunosuppressant2.pdf*.

Plevey S: Immunosuppressants: continue or stop?, available at *http://www.medscape.com/viewarticle/567868*.

Rex D: Effects of immunosuppressants on antibodies to infliximab, available at *http://gastroenterology.jwatch.org/cgi/content/citation/2007/1019/4*.

Vincenti F et al: Costimulation blockade with belatacept in renal transplantation, *N Engl J Med* 353:770-781, 2005.

Chapter 46

Adult smokers need pneumococcal vaccine, available at *http://www.WebMD.com*.

Centers for Disease Control and Prevention: Anthrax case definition, February 2006, available at *http://www.bt.cdc.gov/agent/anthrax/anthrax-hcp-factsheet.asp*.

Centers for Disease Control and Prevention: Bioterrorism case definitions, 2006, available at *http://www.bt.cdc.gov/bioterrorism/casedef.asp*.

Centers for Disease Control and Prevention: Botulism case definition, December 2005, available at *http://www.bt.cdc.gov/agent/botulism/casedef.asp*.

Centers for Disease Control and Prevention: Brucellosis case definition, March 2005, available at *http://www.bt.cdc.gov/agent/brucellosis/casedef.asp*.

Centers for Disease Control and Prevention: CDC statement regarding autism-related advertisement in *USA Today*, April 2006, available at *http://www.cdc.gov/od/oc/media/pressrel/s060406.htm*.

Centers for Disease Control and Prevention: Chemical terrorism, April 2006, available at *http://www.cdc.gov/nceh/dls/chemical_terrorism.htm*.

Centers for Disease Control and Prevention: Chemical terrorism: laboratory response, February 2006, available at *http://www.cdc.gov/nceh/dls/laboratory_response.htm*.

Centers for Disease Control and Prevention: Chemical terrorism: rapid toxic screen, December 2005, available at *http://www.cdc.gov/nceh/dls/rapid_toxic_screen.htm*.

Centers for Disease Control and Prevention, Child and adolescent immunization schedule, 2008, available at *http://www.cdc.gov/vaccines/recs/schedules/child-schedule.htm*.

Centers for Disease Control and Prevention: Control of influenza, 2008, available at *http://www.cdc.gov*.

Centers for Disease Control and Prevention: Guide to vaccinations contraindications, available at *http://www.cdc.gov/vaccines/recs/vac-admin/contraindications.htm*.

Centers for Disease Control and Prevention: Herpes zoster vaccine Q&A, available at *http://www.cdc.gov/vaccines/vpd-vac/shingles/vac-faqs.htm*.

Centers for Disease Control and Prevention: Mercury and vaccines (thimerosal), available at *http://www.cdc.gov/vaccinesafety/concerns/thimerosal.htm*.

Centers for Disease Control and Prevention: Mumps factsheet, 2006, available at *http://www.cdc.gov/nip/diseases/mumps/vac-chart.htm*.

Centers for Disease Control and Prevention: Plague case definition, March 2005, available at *http://www.bt.cdc.gov/agent/plague/casedef.asp*.

Centers for Disease Control and Prevention: Recommended adult immunization schedule by vaccine and age group, United States, 2005-2006, available at *http://www.cdc.gov/nip/recs/adult-schedule.pdf*.

Centers for Disease Control and Prevention: Smallpox case definition, February 2006, available at *http://www.bt.cdc.gov/agent/smallpox/diagnosis/casedefinition.asp*.

Important information about Gardasil, Gardasil website, available at *http://www.gardisil.com*.

Shingles vaccine, available at *http://www.webmd.com/skin-problems-and-treatments/shingles/news/20060526/fda-approves-shingles-vaccine*.

US Department of Health and Human Services: Vaccine adverse event reporting system, available at *http://vaers.hhs.gov*.

US Department of Health and Human Services, Health Resources and Services Administration: National Childhood Vaccine Injury Act vaccine injury table, available at *http://www.hrsa.gov/vaccinecompensation/table.htm*.

US Department of Justice: National Vaccine Injury Compensation Program fact sheet, available at *http://www.usdoj.gov/civil/torts/const/vicp/about.htm*.

US Department of Justice: National Vaccine Injury Compensation Program website, available at *http://www.usdoj.gov/civil/torts/const/vicp/index.htm*.

US Food and Drug Administration: Drug preparedness and response to bioterrorism, February 2006, available at *http://www.fda.gov/cder/drugprepare*.

Chapters 47 and 48

American Society of Clinical Oncology, available at *http://www.asco.org*.

Kaplow R: Innovations in antineoplastic therapy, *Nurs Clin North Am* 40(1):77-94, 2005.

National Cancer Institute, available at *http://www.nci.hih.gov*.

Chapter 49

Morrow T: Natalizumab: FDA is concerned—should managed care be too? *Formulary* 41:184-189, 2006.

Pell LJ et al: Epoetin alfa protocol and multidisciplinary blood-conservation program for critically ill patients, *Am J Health Syst Pharm* 62(4): 400-405, 2005.

Rheumatoid arthritis, MedlinePlus website, available at *http://www.nlm.nih.gov/medlineplus/rheumatoidarthritis.html*.

US Food and Drug Administration: FDA approves resumed marketing of Tysabri under a special distribution program, available at *http://www.fda.gov/bbs/topics/NEWS/2006/NEW01380.html*.

US Food and Drug Administration: Public health advisory: recombinant erythropoietic agents, available at *http://www.fda.gov/Cder/drug/advisory/RHE.htm*.

Chapter 50

Acid reflux drugs may up fractures, WebMD website, 2008, available at *http://www.webmd.com*.

American Society of Health-System Pharmacists: Guidelines for stress ulcer prophylaxis, available at *http://www.ASHP.org*.

Chey WD et al: American College of Gastroenterologists guideline on management of *H. Pylori* infection, *Am J Gastroenterol* 102:1808-1825, 2007.

Spirt MJ, Stanley S: Update of stress ulcer prophylaxis in critically ill patients, *Crit Care Nurse* 26(1):18-27, 2006.

Weinstein WM, Hawkey CJ, Bosh J: *Clinical gastroenterology and hepatology*, ed 1, 2005, Mosby.

Chapter 51

Amitiza [prescribing information], Deerfield, Ill, Takeda Pharmaceuticals, 2009, available at *http://www.amitiza.com*.

US Food and Drug Administration: FDA announces discontinued marketing of GI drug, Zelnorm, for safety reasons, March 2007, available at *http://www.fda.gov*.

US Food and Drug Administration: FDA approves Relistor for opioid-induced constipation, April 24, 2008, available at *http://www.fda.gov/NewsEvents/Newsroom/PressAnnouncements/2008/ucm116885.htm*.

US Food and Drug Administration: FDA requires new safety measures for oral sodium phosphate products to reduce risk of acute kidney injury, available at *http://www.fda.gov/NewsEvents/Newsroom/PressAnnouncements/2008/ucm116988.htm*.

Chapter 52

American Society of Health-System Pharmacists: Guidelines on the prevention of chemotherapy induced nausea and vomiting, available at *http://www.ashp.org.*

Hesketh PJ: Chemotherapy induced nausea and vomiting, *N Engl J Med* 258(23):2482-2494, 2008.

Oncology Nursing Society website, available at *http://www.ons.org.*

Post operative nausea and vomiting: an overview, available at *http://www.anesthesiologyinfo.com/articles/04252004.php.*

US Food and Drug Administration: Labeling changes to droperidol, available at *http://www.fda.gov/cder/foi/appletter/2001/16796s39ltr.pdf.*

Chapter 53

American Heart Association: ACC/AHA release revised guidelines for the management of unstable angina (UA) and non-ST-elevation myocardial infarction (NSTEMI), August 2007, available at *http://www.americanheart.org/presenter.jhtml?identifier=3049500.*

Insel P, Turner RE, Ross D: *Discovering nutrition*, Boston, 2003, Jones & Bartlett.

National Institutes of Health, Office of Dietary Supplements website, available at *http://ods.od.nih.gov.*

Wilbert C: Kids who take vitamins may not need them, 2009, available at *http://www.medscape.com/viewarticle/587773.*

Chapter 54

Fitzgerald MA: What do I need to know about drug interactions with enteral feedings?, 2005, available at *http://www.medscape.com/viewarticle/498270.*

Hamidon BB et al: A prospective comparison of percutaneous endoscopic gastrostomy and nasogastric tube feeding in patients with acute dysphagic stroke, *Med J Malaysia* 61(1):59-66, 2006.

Lewis SM, Heitkemper MM, Dirksen SR: *Medical-surgical nursing: assessment and management of clinical problems*, ed 6, St Louis, 2004, Mosby.

Seifert CF et al, the Institute for Healthy Aging at Texas Tech University Health Sciences Center: Consensus recommendations for administering medications through an enteral feeding tube, 2004, available at *http://www.ttuhsc.edu/Centers/Aging/seifert.htm.*

Suzuki Y et al: Covering the percutaneous endoscopic gastrostomy (PEG) tube prevents peristomal infection, *World J Surg* 30(8):1450-1458, 2006.

Chapter 55

Lebwohl MG et al: *Treatment of skin disease: comprehensive therapeutic strategies*, ed 2, 2006, Mosby.

Chapter 56

American Osteopathic College of Dermatology: Psoriasis, available at *http://www.aocd.org/skin/dermatologic_diseases/psoriasis.html.*

Beitz JM: Wound débridement: therapeutic options and care considerations, *Nurs Clin N Am* 40(2):233-249, 2005.

Biafine topical emulsion, available at *http://www.biafine.com.*

Doughty D: Dressings and more: guidelines for topical wound management, *Nurs Clin N Am* 40(2):217-231, 2005.

Lebwohl MG et al: *Treatment of skin disease: comprehensive therapeutic strategies*, ed 2, St Louis, 2006, Mosby.

Questions and answers about FDA's enforcement action regarding unapproved topical drug products containing papain, available at *http://www.fda.gov/Drugs/GuidanceComplianceRegulatoryInformation/EnforcementActivitiesbyFDA/SelectedEnforcementActionsonUnapprovedDrugs/ucm119646.htm.*

Skin Cancer Foundation: Skin cancer facts, 2008, available at *http://www.skincancer.org/Skin-Cancer/2008-Skin-Cancer-Facts.html.*

Smith R: Wound care product selection [continuing education module], US Pharmacist website, April 2005, available at *http://www.uspharmacist.com/index.asp?page=ce/2716/default.htm.*

US Food and Drug Administration: FDA talk paper: FDA issues health advisory regarding labeling changes for lindane products, March 2003, available at *http://www.fda.gov/bbs/topics/ANSWERS/2003/ANS01205.html.*

US Food and Drug Administration: iPLEDGE update, March 2006, available at *http://www.fda.gov/cder/drug/infopage/accutane/iPLEDGEupdate200603.htm.*

US Food and Drug Administration: Isotretinoin (marketed as Accutane) capsule information, March 2006, available at *http://www.fda.gov/cder/drug/infopage/accutane/default.htm.*

Chapter 57

American Academy of Ophthalmology: *Preferred practice pattern: comprehensive adult medical eye evaluation*, San Francisco, 2005, The Academy. Available at *http://www.aao.org/education.*

Bielory L et al: Treating the ocular component of allergic rhinoconjunctivitis and related eye disorders, *Medscape Gen Med* 9(3):35, 2007.

Goldberg DE et al: HIV associated retinopathy in the HAART era, *Retina* 25:633-641, 2005.

Miller J et al: Endophthalmitis caused by bacillus species, *Am J Ophthalmol* 145:883-884, 2008.

Ophthalmic azithromycin (AzaSite), *Med Lett Drugs Ther* 50:11, 2008.

Chapter 58

Roland PS et al: A comparison of ciprofloxacin/dexamethasone with neomycin/polymyxin for otitis externa pain, *Adv Ther* 24:671-675, 2007.

Rosenfeld RM et al: Clinical practice guideline: acute otitis externa, *Otolaryngol Head Neck Surg* 134:s4-s23, 2006.

Rovers MM et al: Predictors of pain/fever at 3 to 7 days for children with acute otitis media not treated initially with antibiotics: a meta-analysis of individual patient data, *Pediatrics* 119(3):579-585, 2007.

Spiro DM et al: Wait and see prescription for treatment of acute otitis media: a randomized controlled trial, *JAMA* 296:1235-1241, 2006.

Williams ME: Examining the ears, nose and oral cavity in the older patient [continuing medical education/continuing education module], MedscapeCME website, available at *http://cme.medscape.com/viewprogram/7064_pnt.*

Index

A

Abacavir (Ziagen), 638
Abatacept (Orencia), drug profile, 776
Abbreviations, usage, 72*b*
Abdomen, subcutaneous injections, 127*f*
Absolute refractory period, 350
Absorption
  pharmokinetic term, 26
  substance penetration, 798
Abstinence syndrome, 161
Abused substances, 98*b*
Acarbose (Precose), 499
  drug profile, 500
  pharmacokinetics, 500*t*
Accelerated Drug Review Regulations, 52*t*
Accommodation, 876
  process, 879
Accredited hospitals, The Joint Commission
    requirements, 56
ACE inhibitors, 336
  availability, 336
Acellular pertussis vaccine, drug profile,
    709-713
Acetaldehyde syndrome, 103*t*
Acetaminophen, 166
  action mechanism, 165
  pharmacokinetics, 166*t*
  suppository dosage forms, 171
  tolerance, 165
Acetaminophen (Tylenol), 32
Acetasol HC, drug profile, 901
Acetazolamide (Diamox)
  drug profile, 406
  effectiveness, 405
  pharmacokinetics, 406*t*
  usage, 405
Acetic acid
  derivatives, drug profiles, 685
  hydrolysis, 881
Acetylcholine (ACh), 312
  binding, 186
  blockade, anticholinergic drugs (usage),
      253
  breakdown, hydrolysis (usage), 881
  bronchial tree receptor, 569
  concentrations, increase, 314
  definition, 312
  endogenous neurochemical mediator, 881
  excitatory neurotransmitter, 244-245
  metabolism, endogenous enzymes (usage),
      882*f*
  neurotransmitter, 312
  receptor, 786
    binding, 313-314
Acetylcholine (Miochol-E)
  drug profile, 883
  pharmacokinetics, 883*t*
Acetylcholinesterase, 312, 881
  action, inhibition, 312-313
  definition, 312
  inactivation, 881
Acetylsalicylic acid (ASA) (aspirin)
  drug profile, 684
  marketing, 679
  pharmacokinetics, 684*t*
Acid, hypersecretion, 785

Acid-controlling drugs, 792-793
  administration, 793
  anatomy/physiology/disease, overview, 784-787
  assessment, 793
  drug profiles, 792-793*b*
  evaluation, 795
  implementation, 794-795
  nursing diagnoses, 793-794
  nursing process, 793-795
  outcome criteria, 794
  pharmacology, overview, 787-793
  planning, 794
    goals, 794
Acid-related pathophysiology, 784-787
Acne vulgaris, 863
  infection, 866
Acquired brain disorder, 227
Acquired disease, 61
  definition, 61
  disease development, 62
Acquired immunodeficiency syndrome (AIDS),
    623, 725
  acquisition, 100
  AIDS-associated cancer, 626-627
  AIDS-related complex (ARC), 633
  defining conditions, 634
  drugs
    dosages, list, 638*t*
    FDA approval (web site), 626
  function, 624
  immunosuppressive disease, 646
  indicator diseases, 634*b*
  infection, overview, 631-634
  U.S. cases, recognition, 631
  virus, impact, 635
Actinic keratosis, 863
  treatment, 871
    effectiveness, demonstration, 872
Action
  duration, 17
    definition, 17
    time length, 27
  mechanism, 28-29
  onset, 17
    definition, 17
    time requirement, 27
Action potential, 347
  aspects, 350*f*
  change, 349
  comparison, 351*t*
  creation, 349
  definition, 347
  duration, 347
    definition, 347
    phase interval, 350
  phases, 349
    waveforms, 348*f*
  waveform, 349*f*
Activated clotting factors, 433
Active childhood varicella (chickenpox), 627
Active immunization, 704, 706-707
  artificial/natural process, 705-706
  passive immunization, contrast, 706*t*
Active immunizing drugs, 704
  availability, 707
  drug profiles, 709-715

Active immunizing drugs (Continued)
  information, 717-718
  vaccines/toxoids, 708
Active questioning, 287
Active transport, 36
  definition, 36
  energy expenditure, 36-37
Active tubular reabsorption, 26
Active tubular secretion, 26
Acute diabetic complications, 491-492
Acute diarrhea, 797
Acute muscle spasms, 203
Acute pain, 151
  chronic pain, contrast, 155*t*
  definition, 151
  suddenness, 153
Acute salicylate intoxication
  signs/symptoms, 682*t*
  treatment, 682*t*
Acute salicylate toxicity, signs/symptoms, 682
Acute therapy, 29
  drug treatment, 29
Acyclovir (Zovirax)
  drug profile, 629
  pharmacokinetics, 629*t*
Adalimumab (Humira), drug profile, 771
Addict, label, 157
Addiction, 97, 151
  definition, 97, 151
  treatment strategies, 98
Addison disease, 509
  adrenocortical hormones, undersecretion/
      hyposecretion, 510
Additive effects, 16
  definition, 16
  drug combinations, 31
Adenine (A), 63
Adenosine (Adenocard)
  drug profile, 363
  pharmacokinetics, 363*t*
Adenosine deaminase (ADA) deficiency, gene
    therapy, 64*f*, 731
Adenosine diphosphate (ADP), 837
Adenosine monophosphate (AMP), 837
Adenosine triphosphate (ATP), 786, 837
  molecules, pump, 348-349
  niacin, combination, 829
Adenoviruses, 64
Adjunct anesthetics (adjuncts), 178
  definition, 178
  drugs, 179
Adjunctive anesthetic drugs, 180*t*
Adjuvant, 761
Adjuvant analgesic drugs, 151
  addition, 152
  definition, 151
Adjuvant drugs, usage, 157-158
Administration route, 20
  nursing considerations, 22*t*
Adolescence, medication administration (age-
    related considerations), 40*b*
Adolescents
  huffing practices, 109
  life span considerations, 40
  OTC drug abuse, 109
  substance abuse, case study, 107*b*

Page numbers followed by *b, t,* or *f* indicate boxes, tables, or figures, respectively. Entries in blue indicate disorders. Boldface entries indicate generic drug names.

Special Features

Note: Case Studies, Patient Teaching Tips, Points to Remember, NCLEX Examination Review Questions, and Critical Thinking Activities are provided for each chapter.